HEALTH ALERTS

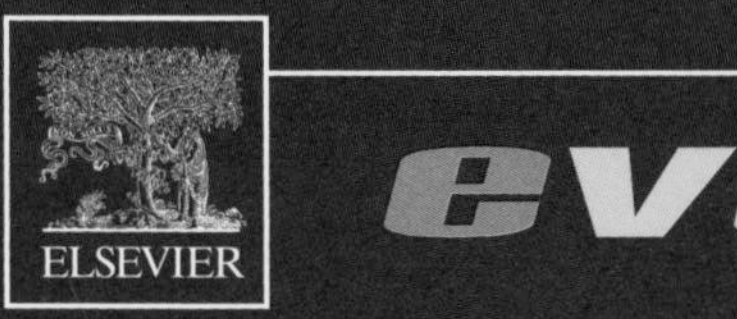

To access your Student and Instructor Resources, visit:

http://evolve.elsevier.com/Huether

Evolve® Student Learning Resources for ***Huether and McCance: Understanding Pathophysiology,* Fourth Edition** offer the following features:

Student Resources (NOTE: Instructors also have access to Student material.)

- **Answers to Quick Checks**
  Short answers are provided for the questions in Quick Check boxes interspersed throughout each chapter of the textbook.
- **Algorithm Completion**
  Algorithm completion exercises for every chapter focus on the path of progression in cellular mechansims, body system functions, and diseases.
- **Key Terms Matching**
  Match key terms to definitions and descriptions.
- **Critical Thinking**
  Critical thinking questions with suggested answers for each chapter.
- **WebLinks**
  Link to hundreds of websites carefully chosen to supplement the content of the textbook. The WebLinks are regularly updated, with new ones added as they develop.

Understanding Pathophysiology

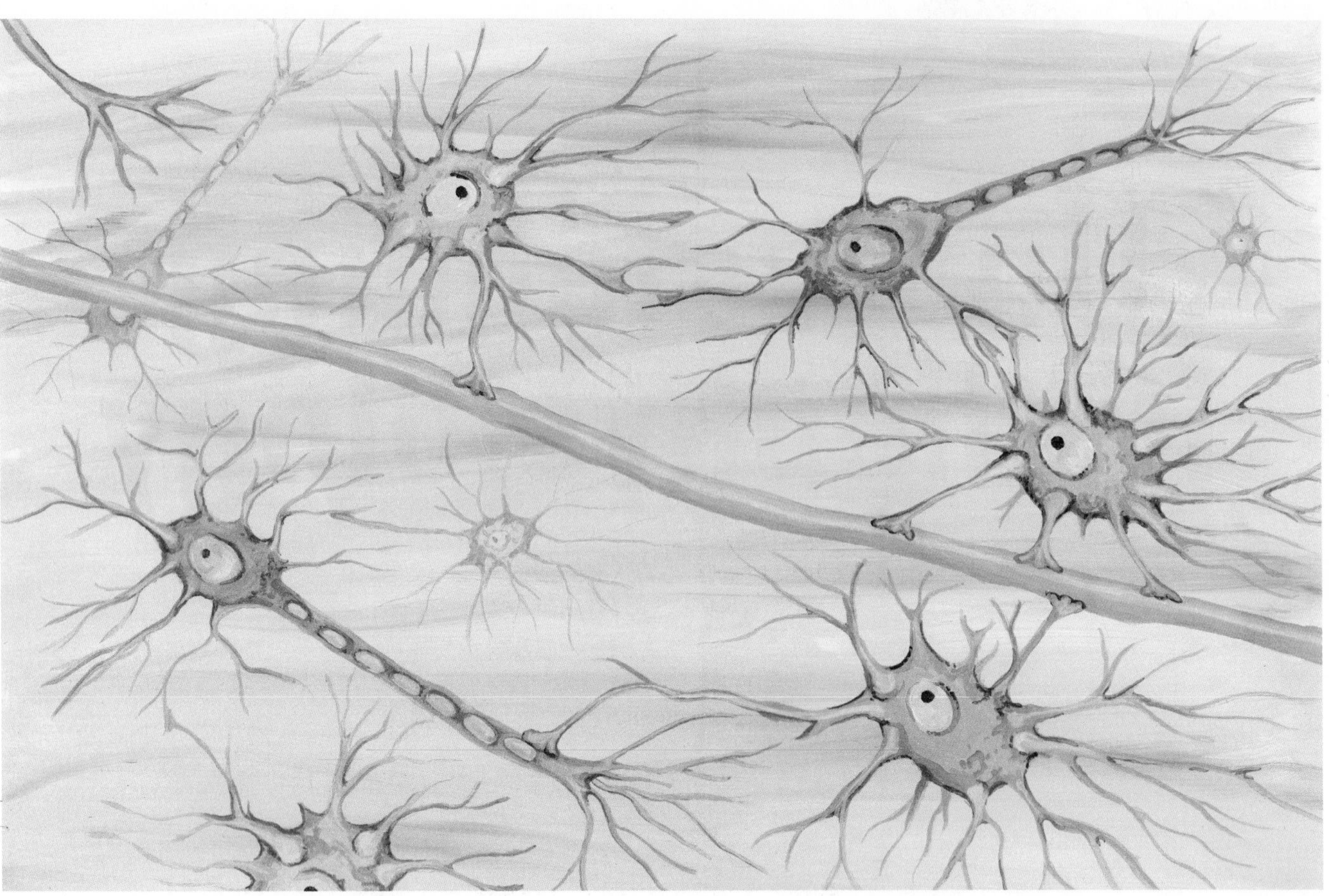

ABOUT THE COVER

The illustration on the cover is a painting by graphic designer Anne Wolfer created especially for this edition of the textbook. The painting represents astrocytes connected to neurons and a blood vessel. Much of the current research into brain communication focuses on astrocytes, the star-shaped glia that hold neurons in place. Historically, investigators focused on cells that generated action potentials, which astrocytes do not do. Consequently, the important role of these cells has not been studied until recently. Astrocytes communicate with neurons and modify signals sent and received and thus they are vital for chemical (rather than electrical) communication with neighboring neurons and information transmittal at the synapse. Astrocytes generate chemical signals called gliotransmitters, which are small molecules that travel to nearby cells and deliver messages. Knowledge of astrocyte function helps support our understanding of communication patterns in such diseases as Alzheimer, AIDS, and brain cancer.

Understanding Pathophysiology

Sue E. Huether, RN, PhD
Professor Emeritus
College of Nursing
University of Utah
Salt Lake City, Utah

Kathryn L. McCance, RN, PhD
Professor
College of Nursing
University of Utah
Salt Lake City, Utah

SECTION EDITORS

Valentina L. Brashers, MD
Professor Nursing and Attending Physician in Internal Medicine
University of Virginia Health System
Charlottesville, Virginia

Neal S. Rote, PhD
Academic Vice-Chair and Director of Research
Department of Obstetrics and Gynecology
University Hospitals of Cleveland;
Professor of Reproductive Biology and Pathology
Case School of Medicine
Case Western Reserve University
Cleveland, Ohio

Fourth Edition
with 900 illustrations

MOSBY

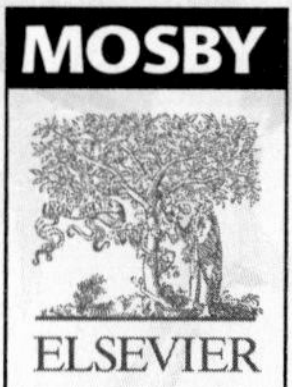

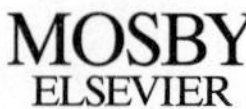

11830 Westline Industrial Drive
St. Louis, Missouri 63146

UNDERSTANDING PATHOPHYSIOLOGY, FOURTH EDITION ISBN: 978-0-3230-4990-0

Notice

Knowledge and best practice in this field are constantly changing. As new research and experience broaden our knowledge, changes in practice, treatment and drug therapy may become necessary or appropriate. Readers are advised to check the most current information provided (i) on procedures featured or (ii) by the manufacturer of each product to be administered, to verify the recommended dose or formula, the method and duration of administration, and contraindications. It is the responsibility of the practitioner, relying on their own experience and knowledge of the patient, to make diagnoses, to determine dosages and the best treatment for each individual patient, and to take all appropriate safety precautions. To the fullest extent of the law, neither the Publisher nor the Authors assumes any liability for any injury and/or damage to persons or property arising out of or related to any use of the material contained in this book.

The Publisher

Previous editions copyrighted 2004, 2000, 1996
ISBN: 9780323049900

Library of Congress Cataloging-in-Publication Data
Library of Congress Control Number: 2007935686

Managing Editor: Brian Dennison
Developmental Editor: Betsy Stream
Publishing Services Manager: Jeffrey Patterson
Editorial Assistant: Tina Kaemmerer
Project Manager: Jeanne Genz
Book Designer: Kimberly E. Denando

Printed in China
Last digit is the print number: 9 8 7 6 5 4 3 2

CONTRIBUTORS

Phillip Barnette, MD
Assistant Professor
Pediatric Hematology/Oncology
University of Utah School of Medicine
Salt Lake City, Utah

Barbara J. Boss, RN, PhD, CFNP, CANP
Professor of Nursing
University of Mississippi Medical Center
Jackson, Mississippi

Kristen Lee Carroll, MD
Associate Professor
Department of Orthopaedics
University of Utah
Salt Lake City, Utah

Christy L. Crowther, RN, MS, CRNP
Adult Nurse Practitioner
Anne Arundel Orthopaedic Surgeons
Annapolis, Maryland

Curtis B. DeFriez, MD
Professor, Health Sciences
Weber State University
Ogden, Utah

Angela Deneris, PhD, CNM, FACNM
Associate Professor, Clinical
Nurse-Midwifery and Women's Health Nurse Practitioners Programs
University of Utah College of Nursing
Salt Lake City, Utah

Beth A. Forshee, PhD
Assistant Professor of Physiology
Lake Erie College of Osteopathic Medicine
Erie, Pennsylvania

Deborah K. Froh, MD
Associate Professor of Pediatrics
University of Virginia
Charlottesville, Virginia

Mikel Gray, PhD, FNP, PNP, CUNP, CCCN, FAANP, FAAN
Nurse Practitioner and Professor
Department of Urology and School of Nursing
University of Virginia
Charlottesville, Virginia

Todd Cameron Grey, MD
Chief Medical Examiner, State of Utah;
Associate Clinical Professor of Pathology
University of Utah School of Medicine
Salt Lake City, Utah

Robert E. Jones, MD, FACP, FACE
Adjunct Associate Professor of Medicine
University of Utah School of Medicine
Salt Lake City, Utah

Lynn B. Jorde, PhD
H.A. and Edna Benning Presidential Professor
Department of Human Genetics
University of Utah School of Medicine
Salt Lake City, Utah

Nancy E. Kline, PhD, RN, CPNP, FAAN
Director, Research and Evidence-Based Practice
Department of Nursing
Memorial Sloan-Kettering Cancer Center
New York, New York

Nancy L. McDaniel, MD, FAAP, FACC
Associate Professor of Pediatrics
Medical Director of UVA Children's Hospital
Vice Chair Department of Pediatrics
Charlottesville, Virginia

Katherine Morgan, MSN, WHNP, ANP
Associate Clinical Professor
University of Utah College of Nursing
Salt Lake City, Utah

Richard A. Sugerman, PhD
Professor of Anatomy
Assistant Vice President for Academic Program Development
Western University of Health Sciences
College of Osteopathic Medicine of the Pacific
Pomona, California

David M. Virshup, MD
Professor and Director
Program in Cancer and Stem Cell Biology
Duke-NUS Graduate Medical School
Singapore

Robin R. Wilkerson, RN, PhD
Professor
School of Nursing
University of Mississippi
Jackson, Mississippi

REVIEWERS

Cathy Abell, RN, MSN
Assistant Professor
Department of Nursing,
Western Kentucky University
Bowling Green, Kentucky

Patricia McCallig Bates, RN, BSN, CURN
Urological Nurse
Portland, Oregon

Beth Anne Batturs, RN, MSN
Director of Nursing
Anne Arundel Community College
Arnold, Maryland

Julia A. Eggert, PhD, APRN-BC GNP, AOCN
Associate Professor
School of Nursing
Clemson University
Clemson, South Carolina

Kelly Fisher, PhD, RN
Assistant Professor of Nursing
University of Massachusetts Lowell
Haverhill, Massachusetts

Dorothy Fraser, MSN, FNP
Director Fresno Teaching Center
University of California–Davis
Davis, California

Susan K. Frazier, PhD, RN
Associate Professor
College of Nursing
University of Kentucky
Lexington, Kentucky

Laurel Halloran, PhD, BSN, MSN, APRN
Professor
Department of Nursing
Western Connecticut State University
Danbury, Connecticut

Lisa Anne Bemis Hardy, RN, BSN
Emergency Department
Huntsville Hospital
Huntsville, Alabama

Nancy Smith Haugen, PhD, MN, BSN, AS, RN
Professor
Nursing Department Chair
Florida Hospital College of Health Sciences
Orlando, Florida

Misty Kirby-Nolan, MSN, CNP
Regional Anesthesia Pain Management
Northwestern Memorial Hospital
Chicago, Illinois

Sarah M. Magnuson-Whyte, MN, RN
Director of Nursing
Pierce College
Puyallup, Washington

Lora McGuire, RN, MS
Professor of Nursing
Joliet Junior College
Joliet, Illinois

Sandra A. Mitchell, CRNP, MScN, AOCN
Predoctoral Fellow, National Institutes of Health
Nurse Practitioner National Cancer Institute
Bethesda, Maryland
Doctoral Candidate, University of Utah, College of Nursing,
Distance Education PhD in Cancer Research
Salt Lake City, Utah

Phyllis D. Morgan, PhD, APRN, BC
Assistant Professor
Department of Nursing
Fayetteville State University
Fayetteville, North Carolina

Nancy L. Oldenburg, RN, MS, CPNP
Assistant Professor
School of Nursing
Northern Illinois University
DeKalb, Illinois

Kevin N. Sheth, MD
Neuro-Critical Care & Stroke Fellow
Department of Neurology
Massachusetts General Hospital
Boston, Massachusetts

Bernadette White, RN, MSN, APRNc
Assistant Professor
School of Nursing
Creighton University
Omaha, Nebraska

PREFACE

This edition, like the previous one, has been rigorously updated and revised, with many sections completely rewritten to reflect recent findings. The pace of current progress in areas such as immunity, inflammation, cancer, genetics, and cardiovascular disease is astounding. And although some of this progress already has been translated into clinical practice, many challenges remain on just *how* to use this new information to help improve diagnostic and disease management practices. Nonetheless, we believe students should be exposed to these emerging understandings as they unfold and be encouraged to follow these developments throughout their professional lives.

A major goal of this edition of *Understanding Pathophysiology* was to make it even more understandable. Toward that end we have edited the book to improve clarity by defining more of the terms used, by explaining some concepts more fully, by simplifying the more difficult content, and by revising and adding more color illustrations and photos. For example, the chapters on inflammation and immunity were rewritten entirely for simplification. We believe we have met our challenge without deleting any key information.

Although the primary focus of the text is pathophysiology, we continue to include discussions of the following interconnected topics to highlight their importance for clinical practice:

- A life span approach that includes special sections on aging and separate chapters on children
- Epidemiology and incidence rates showing dramatic, worldwide differences that reflect the importance of environmental and lifestyle factors on disease initiation and progression
- Clinical manifestations and summaries of treatment
- Gender differences that affect epidemiology and pathophysiology
- Molecular biology—mechanisms of normal cell function and how their alteration leads to disease
- Health promotion/risk reduction

ORGANIZATION OF THE BOOK

The book is organized into two parts: Part One, Basic Concepts of Pathophysiology and Part Two, Body Systems and Diseases.

Part One: Basic Concepts of Pathophysiology

Part One introduces basic principles and processes. The concepts include descriptions of cellular communication; genes and genetic disease; forms of cell injury; fluid and electrolytes and acid and base balance; immunity and inflammation; mechanisms of infection; stress, coping, and illness; and tumor biology. Knowledge of these processes is essential to gaining a contemporary understanding of the pathophysiology of common diseases.

Significant revisions to Part One include new or updated information on the following topics:

- Cellular communication and the extracellular matrix (Chapter 1)
- Oxidative stress, agents of cell injury, cell death, and aging (Chapter 3)
- Mechanisms of human defense—characteristics of innate and adaptive immunity, antigen recognition and response, induction of the immune response, clonal diversity and selection (Chapter 6)
- Mechanisms of hypersensitivity, autoimmunity, and immune deficiency (Chapter 7)
- The effects of stress and the role of cortisol and immunity (Chapter 8)
- The significance of infection, inflammation, immunity, genetics, and the microenvironment to cancer (Chapter 9)
- Cancer epidemiology, manifestations, and treatment of cancer (Chapter 10)

Part Two: Body Systems and Diseases

Part Two presents the pathophysiology of the most common alterations according to body system. To guarantee readability and comprehension we have used a logical sequence and uniform approach in presenting the content of the units and chapters. Each unit focuses on a specific organ system and contains chapters related to anatomy and physiology, the pathophysiology of the most common diseases, and common alterations in children. The anatomy and physiology content is presented as a review to enhance the learner's understanding of the structural and functional changes inherent in pathophysiology. A brief summary of normal aging effects is included at the end of these review chapters. The general organization of each disease/disorder discussion includes an introductory paragraph on relevant risk factors and epidemiology, then related pathophysiology, clinical manifestations, and a brief review of treatment.

Significant revisions to Part Two include new or updated information on the following topics:

- Neurotransmitters (Chapter 12)
- Clinical pain syndromes and classification of sleep disorders (Chapter 13)
- Pathogenesis of degenerative brain diseases and diffuse brain injury (Chapters 14 and 15)
- Mechanisms of hormone receptors and insulin action (Chapter 17)
- Obesity, insulin resistance, and inflammatory cytokines; complications of diabetes and autoimmune mechanisms of thyroid disease (Chapter 18)

- Platelet function and coagulation; alterations of leukocyte function, and myeloid tumors (Chapters 19 and 20)
- Mechanisms of cardiac workload, cardiac angiogenesis and growth factors, and myocardial hypoxia (Chapter 22)
- Mechanisms of aneurysm formation, atherosclerosis, hypertension, coronary artery disease, heart failure, and shock (Chapter 23)
- Pediatric valvular disorders, heart failure, and classification of hypertension (Chapter 24)
- Mechanisms of dyspnea, asthma, and pulmonary hypertension (Chapter 26)
- Inflammation in cystic fibrosis; bronchopulmonary dysplasia (Chapter 27)
- Nephrons and the regulation of blood pressure and fluid and electrolyte balance (Chapter 28)
- Urinary tract obstruction, neurogenic bladder, overactive bladder syndrome, and systemic manifestation of chronic renal failure (Chapter 29)
- Grading of vesicoureteral reflux; pediatric glomerular disorders (Chapter 30)
- Prostate cancer; breast diseases, and mechanisms of breast cancer (Chapter 32)
- Gastroesophageal reflux disease, cytokines, and obesity (Chapter 34)
- Gluten sensitive enteropathy, intestinal malrotation, and rotavirus (Chapter 35)
- Bone remodeling, osteoporosis, rheumatoid arthritis, and osteoarthritis (Chapter 37)
- Itch receptors, bee stings, immune mechanisms of skin disease, and Lyme disease (Chapter 39)

FEATURES TO PROMOTE LEARNING

A number of features are incorporated into this text that guide and support learning and understanding, including:

- NEW! A *Glossary* of more than 850 terms related to pathophysiology
- NEW! Marginal *CD icons* point to more than 40 animations on the Companion CD
- *Chapter Outlines* including page numbers for easy reference
- *Quick Check* questions strategically placed throughout each chapter to help readers confirm their understanding of the material; answers are included on the textbook's Evolve website
- *Health Alerts* with concise discussions of the latest research
- *Risk Factors* boxes for selected diseases
- End-of-chapter *Did You Understand?* summaries that condense the major concepts of each chapter into an easy-to-review list format
- *Key Terms* set in boldface in text and listed, with page numbers, at the end of each chapter
- Special headings for *Aging* and *Pediatrics* content that highlight discussions of life span alterations

ART PROGRAM

The art program, which is crucial for explaining pathophysiology, was given the same careful attention as the text and comprises more than 900 images. This edition includes more than 200 new full-color drawings and photographs. Hundreds of high-quality photographs show clinical manifestations, pathologic specimens, and clinical imaging techniques. Numerous micrographs show normal and abnormal cellular structure. These visual presentations were carefully chosen to help the learner more easily understand and appreciate even the most complex concepts of physiology and pathophysiology.

TEACHING/LEARNING PACKAGE

For Students

A **Companion CD** comes with every new copy of the book and includes review questions and answers and numerous animations to help students master pathophysiology. CD icons in the margins of the text direct readers to animations on related content.

The free **Student Learning Resources** on Evolve include answers to the Quick Check questions in the book, algorithm completion exercises, key term/definition matching exercises, critical thinking questions with answers, and WebLinks. Go to http://evolve.elsevier.com/Huether.

The **Study Guide and Workbook** includes learning objectives, *Memory Check!* anatomy and physiology reviews, concise summaries of key chapter concepts, a practice examination for each chapter, and case studies with critical-thinking questions. Answers to the practice examinations and a discussion of each case study can be found in the back of the Study Guide.

For Instructors

The **Instructor's Electronic Resource CD** is available free to instructors with qualified adoptions of the textbook and includes: an *Instructor's Manual* with learning objectives, difficult concepts discussions, and critical thinking exercises with answers; a *Test Bank* of approximately 1,400 items (available as text files or in ExamView computerized testing software); a *PowerPoint Presentation* of more than 2,000 lecture slides; an *Image Collection* of approximately 800 key figures from the text; and *Audience Response Questions* for use with i-clicker and other systems.

All of these teaching resources are also available to instructors at the book's **Evolve site,** along with access to the WebLinks and other student learning resources. Plus the *Evolve Learning System* provides a comprehensive suite of course communication and organization tools that allow you to upload your class calendar and syllabus, post scores and announcements, and more. Go to http://evolve.elsevier.com/Huether.

The newest and most exciting part of the package is **Pathophysiology Online,** a complete set of online modules that provide thoroughly developed lessons on the most important and difficult topics in pathophysiology supplemented with illustrations, animations, interactive activities, interactive algorithms, self-assessment reviews, and exams. Instructors can use it to enhance traditional classroom lecture courses or for distance and online-only courses. Students can use it as a self-guided study tool.

Acknowledgments

Although we can never really thank our contributors adequately, we would like to try by expressing our enormous gratitude for their generous contributions of time, knowledge, and talent. Without their expertise, we would not have a textbook.

For this edition Tina Brashers, MD, and Neal Rote, PhD, joined our team as Section Editors. Both have worked with us for years as contributing authors. Tina is an exceptional teacher, has received numerous awards for her work with nursing and medical students and faculty, and brings innovation and clarity to the subject of pathophysiology. Her work on Pathophysiology Online continues to be intensive and creative and a significant learning enhancement for students. Her own *Clinical Applications of Pathophysiology* book brings pathophysiology to the real world of clinical practice and assists students to advance their skill in critical thinking and decision making. Thank you, Tina, for your writing, guidance of authors, review of manuscript, and great sense of humor. Neal has passion, precision, and expertise in immunity and human defenses. His experience in teaching and research contributes to the clarity with which he presents this complex content. Neal spent enormous amounts of time rethinking and drawing several new figures. Thank you, Neal, for your persistence in promoting understanding and your continuing support.

The reviewers for this edition were outstanding and made many helpful recommendations—thank you all. Special thanks to Lisa Hardy and Susan Frazier for your meticulous reviews of the page proofs.

Once again we are deeply indebted to Sue Meeks. Sue orchestrates the various stages of manuscript preparation and single-handedly word processes the entire revision of the manuscript. She continues to amaze us with her sincere level of enthusiasm for attending to detail, and the extraordinary effort she devotes to organizing, preparing, and accomplishing the task. Thank you, Sue.

Brian Dennison, our Managing Editor, is world-class. Brian's organizational skill, penchant for detail, patience, and overall perspective are exceptional. Notable for this edition has been Brian's goal of simplification and length management. We especially appreciate Brian's keen eye and discerning guidance regarding the artwork. Thank you, Brian. We also thank Executive Publisher Darlene Como, who was responsible for overseeing the entire project. As always, Darlene's gift for seeing the big picture is a steady source of guidance and perspective. Thank you, Darlene. A person very significant to the publication of our textbooks is Executive Vice President Sally Schrefer. Her years of unwavering support and enthusiasm have been essential—thanks again, Sally.

Jeanne Genz, the Project Manager for this edition, was an early bird with alerting e-mails sent to us by 5:30 AM. Always courteous, Jeanne was focused and exacting. It was a pleasure to work with you, Jeanne—thank you. The Book Designer for this edition was Kim Denando and we appreciate the beautiful color scheme and style that she provided. Thank you, Kim.

Betsy Stream, our Development Editor, and Tina Kaemmerer, Editorial Assistant, were diligent in keeping the details of revision on track. Betsy processed all the chapters and reviewed page proofs. Tina routed materials to authors, contributors, and reviewers, obtained the permissions, and coordinated the companion CD and Study Guide. Thank you, Betsy and Tina, for a job well done.

We thank the Department of Dermatology at the University of Utah School of Medicine, which provided numerous photos of skin lesions. Thanks also to Arthur R. Brothman, PhD, of the University of Utah School of Medicine, for the *N-myc* gene amplification slides used to illustrate the discussion of neuroblastoma and John Hoffman, MD, for the PET scan figure of cancer metastases. Patty Bassman from Graphic World created numerous new illustrations with great accuracy and detail. Thank you, Patty.

Thank you to our many colleagues and friends at the University of Utah College of Nursing, School of Medicine, Eccles Medical Library, and College of Pharmacy. In particular, we would like to thank Lyn Pearse for handling details related to submission of the manuscript. A special thanks to Margaret Clayton and Blaine Winters for their very organized and thorough approach in preparing the instructor's manual. A big thanks to Beth Forshee for her excellent revisions to the glossary, review questions, test bank, quick check answers, and other resources on the student website. Beth and Tina Brashers also updated the interactive online lessons and activities for Pathophysiology Online. Thanks to Celeste Davis for revising the lecture slides. And thanks as always to Clayton Parkinson for revising the Study Guide.

The challenging task of creating the textbook's cover art was accomplished by graphic designer Anne Wolfer. Her remarkable eye for color and gifted sense for visually defining a concept helped her create this spectacular cover. Thank you, Anne.

Special thanks to colleagues and students, particularly nursing, medical, and pharmacy students for your letters, e-mail messages, and phone calls. It's because of you, the future clinicians, that we are so motivated to put our best efforts into this work.

Sincerely and with great affection we thank our families, especially Mae, John, Anne, Ray, Mark, Eric, Greg, Sue, Kallie, Rosie, Margot, and Sarah. Always supportive, you make the work possible!

Sue E. Huether
Kathryn L. McCance

CONTENTS

UNIT 3 CELLULAR PROLIFERATION: CANCER

PART TWO **Body Systems and Disease**

UNIT 4 THE NEUROLOGIC SYSTEM

INTRODUCTION TO PATHOPHYSIOLOGY

Pathophysiology is the study of the underlying changes in body physiology that result from disease or injury. The science of pathophysiology seeks to provide an understanding of the mechanisms of disease and how and why alterations in body structure and function lead to the signs and symptoms of disease. Understanding pathophysiology guides health care professionals in the planning, selection, and evaluation of therapies and treatments.

Knowledge of human anatomy and physiology and the interrelationship among the various cells and organ systems of the body is an essential foundation for the study of pathophysiology. Review of this subject matter enhances comprehension of pathophysiologic events and processes. Understanding pathophysiology also entails the use of principles, concepts, and basic knowledge from other fields of study including pathology, genetics, immunology, and epidemiology. A number of terms are used to focus the discussion of pathophysiology; they may be used interchangeably at times but that does not necessarily indicate that they have the same meaning. Those terms are reviewed here for the purpose of clarification.

Pathology is the investigation of structural alterations in cells, tissues, and organs, which can help identify the cause of a particular disease. Pathology differs from **pathogenesis,** which is the pattern of tissue changes associated with the *development* of disease. **Etiology** refers to the study of the *cause* of disease. Diseases may be caused by infection, heredity, alterations in immunity, malignancy, malnutrition, degeneration, or trauma. Diseases that have no identifiable cause are termed **idiopathic.** Diseases that occur as a result of medical treatment are termed **iatrogenic.** For example, some antibiotics can injure the kidney and cause renal failure. Diseases that are acquired as a consequence of being in a hospital environment are called **nosocomial.** An infection that develops as a result of a person's immune system being depressed after receiving cancer treatment during a hospital stay is defined as a nosocomial infection.

Diagnosis is the naming or identification of a disease. A **prognosis** is the expected outcome of a disease. **Acute disease** is the sudden appearance of signs and symptoms that last only a short time. **Chronic disease** develops more slowly and the signs and symptoms last for a long time, perhaps for a lifetime. Chronic diseases may have a pattern of remission and exacerbation. **Remissions** are periods when symptoms disappear or diminish significantly. **Exacerbations** are periods when the symptoms become worse or more severe. A **complication** is the onset of a disease in a person who is already coping with another existing disease. For example, a person who has had surgery to remove a diseased appendix may develop the complication of a wound infection or pneumonia. **Sequelae** are unwanted outcomes of having a disease or are the result of trauma, such as paralysis resulting from a stroke or severe scarring resulting from a burn.

Clinical manifestations are the signs and symptoms or *evidence* of disease. **Signs** are objective alterations that can be observed or measured by another person, measures of bodily functions such as pulse rate, blood pressure, body temperature, or white blood cell count. Some signs are **local** such as redness or swelling and other signs are **systemic** such as fever. **Symptoms** are subjective experiences reported by the person with disease, such as pain, nausea, or shortness of breath. The **prodromal period** of a disease is the time during which a person experiences vague symptoms such as fatigue or loss of appetite before the onset of specific signs and symptoms. The term **insidious symptoms** refers to vague or nonspecific feelings and an awareness that there is a change within the body. Some diseases have a **latent period,** a time during which no symptoms are readily apparent in the affected person, but the disease is nevertheless present in the body; an example is the incubation phase of an infection or the early growth phase of a tumor. A **syndrome** is a group of symptoms that occur together and may be caused by several interrelated problems or a specific disease. Severe acute respiratory syndrome (SARS), for example, presents with a set of symptoms that include headache, fever, body aches, an overall feeling of discomfort, and sometimes dry cough and difficulty breathing. A **disorder** is an abnormality of function; this term also can refer to an illness or a particular problem such as a bleeding disorder.

Epidemiology is the study of tracking patterns or disease occurrence and transmission among populations and by geographic areas. **Incidence** of a disease is the number of new cases occurring in a specific period. **Prevalence** of a disease is the number of existing cases within a population during a specific period.

Risk factors, also known as **predisposing factors,** increase the probability that disease will occur, but these factors are not the *cause* of disease. Risk factors include heredity, age, gender, race, environment, and lifestyle. A **precipitating factor** is a condition or event that *does* cause a pathologic event or disorder. For example, asthma is precipitated by exposure to an allergen, or angina (pain) is precipitated by exertion.

Pathophysiology is an exciting field of study that is ever changing as discoveries are made. Understanding pathophysiology empowers health care professionals with the knowledge of how and why disease develops and informs their decision making to ensure optimal health care outcomes.

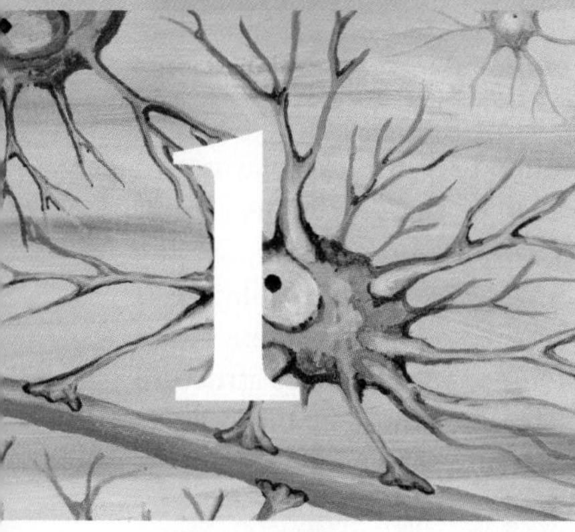

1 CELLULAR BIOLOGY

Kathryn L. McCance

CHAPTER OUTLINE

ELECTRONIC RESOURCES

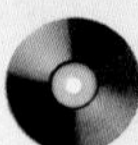

Companion CD
- Review Questions and Answers
- Animations

evolve Website
http://evolve.elsevier.com/Huether/
- Quick Check Answers
- Key Terms Exercises
- Critical Thinking Questions with Answers
- Algorithm Completion Exercises
- WebLinks

All body functions depend on the integrity of cells. Therefore an understanding of cellular biology is increasingly necessary to comprehend disease processes. An overwhelming amount of information reveals how cells behave as a multicellular "social" organism. At the heart of it all is cellular communication (cellular "crosstalk")—how messages originate and are transmitted, received, interpreted, and used by the cell. Streamlined conversation between, among, and within cells maintains cellular function. Cells must demonstrate a "chemical fondness" for other cells to maintain the integrity of the entire organism. When they no longer tolerate this fondness, the conversation breaks down, and cells either adapt (sometimes altering function) or become vulnerable to isolation, injury, or disease.

PROKARYOTES AND EUKARYOTES

Living cells generally are divided into eukaryotes and prokaryotes. The cells of higher animals and plants are eukaryotes, as are the single-celled organisms, fungi, protozoa, and most algae. Prokaryotes include cyanobacteria (blue-green algae), bacteria, and rickettsiae. Prokaryotes traditionally were studied as core subjects of molecular biology. Today, emphasis is on the eukaryotic cell; much of its structure and function have no counterpart in bacterial cells.

Eukaryotes (*eu* = good; *karyon* = nucleus) are larger and have more extensive intracellular anatomy and organization than prokaryotes. Eukaryotic cells have a characteristic set of membrane-bound intracellular compartments, called *organelles,* that includes a well-defined nucleus. The **prokaryotes** contain no organelles, and their nuclear material is not encased by a nuclear membrane. Prokaryotic cells are characterized by lack of a distinct nucleus.

Besides having structural differences, prokaryotic and eukaryotic cells differ in chemical composition and biochemical activity. The *nuclei* of prokaryotic cells carry genetic information in a single circular chromosome, and they lack a class of proteins called *histones,* which in eukaryotic cells bind with deoxyribonucleic acid (DNA) and are involved in the supercoiling of DNA. Eukaryotic cells have several or many chromosomes. Protein production, or synthesis, in the two classes of cells also differs because of major structural differences in ribonucleic acid

(RNA) protein complexes. Other distinctions include differences in mechanisms of transport across the outer cellular membrane and in enzyme content.

CELLULAR FUNCTIONS

Cells become specialized through the process of **differentiation,** or maturation, so that some cells eventually perform one kind of function and other cells perform other functions. Cells with a highly developed function, such as movement, often lack some other property, such as hormone production, which is more highly developed in other cells.

The eight chief cellular functions are as follows:

1. *Movement.* Muscle cells can generate forces that produce motion. Muscles that are attached to bones produce limb movements, whereas those that enclose hollow tubes or cavities move or empty contents when they contract, for example, the colon.
2. *Conductivity.* Conduction as a response to a stimulus is manifested by a wave of excitation, an electrical potential that passes along the surface of the cell to reach its other parts. Conductivity is the chief function of nerve cells.
3. *Metabolic absorption.* All cells can take in and use nutrients and other substances from their surroundings.
4. *Secretion.* Certain cells, such as mucous gland cells, can synthesize new substances from substances they absorb and then secrete the new substances to serve as needed elsewhere.
5. *Excretion.* All cells can rid themselves of waste products resulting from the metabolic breakdown of nutrients. Membrane-bound sacs (lysosomes) within cells contain enzymes that break down, or digest, large molecules, turning them into waste products that are released from the cell.
6. *Respiration.* Cells absorb oxygen, which is used to transform nutrients into energy in the form of adenosine triphosphate (ATP). Cellular respiration, or oxidation, occurs in organelles called mitochondria.
7. *Reproduction.* Tissue growth occurs as cells enlarge and reproduce themselves. Even without growth, tissue maintenance requires that new cells be produced to replace cells that are lost normally through cellular death. Not all cells are capable of continuous division, and some cells, such as nerve cells, cannot reproduce.
8. *Communication.* Communication is vital for cells to survive as a society of cells. Appropriate communication allows the maintenance of a dynamic steady state.

STRUCTURE AND FUNCTION OF CELLULAR COMPONENTS

Figure 1-1 shows a "typical" eukaryotic cell. It consists of three components: an outer membrane called the **plasma membrane,** or **plasmalemma;** a fluid "filling" called **cytoplasm;** and the "organs" of the cell—the membrane-bound intracellular **organelles,** among them the nucleus.

Nucleus

The **nucleus,** which is surrounded by the cytoplasm and generally is located in the center of the cell, is the largest membrane-bound organelle. Two membranes compose the **nuclear envelope** (Figure 1-2, *A*). The outer membrane is continuous with membranes of the endoplasmic reticulum. The nucleus contains the **nucleolus,** a small dense structure composed largely of ribonucleic acid, most of the cellular DNA, and the DNA-binding proteins, the histones, that regulate its activity. The DNA "chain" in eukaryotic cells is so long that it is easily broken. Therefore the histones that bind to DNA cause DNA to fold into chromosomes (Figure 1-2, *C*), which decreases the risk of breakage and is essential for cell division in eukaryotes.

The primary functions of the nucleus are cell division and control of genetic information. Other functions include the replication and repair of DNA and the transcription of the information stored in DNA. Genetic information is transcribed into RNA, which can be processed into messenger, transport, and ribosomal RNA and introduced into the cytoplasm, where it directs cellular activities. Most of the processing of RNA occurs in the nucleolus. (The role of DNA and RNA in protein synthesis is discussed in Chapter 2.)

Cytoplasmic Organelles

Cytoplasm is an aqueous solution (cytosol) that fills the **cytoplasmic matrix**—the space between the nuclear envelope and the plasma membrane. The cytosol represents about half the volume of a eukaryotic cell. It contains thousands of enzymes involved in intermediate metabolism and is crowded with ribosomes making proteins. Newly synthesized proteins remain in the cytosol if they lack a signal for transport to a cell organelle.[1] The organelles suspended in the cytoplasm are enclosed in biologic membranes, so they can simultaneously carry out functions requiring different biochemical environments. Many of these functions are directed by coded messages carried from the nucleus by RNA. They include synthesis of proteins and hormones and their transport out of the cell, isolation and elimination of waste products from the cell, metabolic processes, breakdown and disposal of cellular debris and foreign proteins (antigens), and maintenance of cellular structure and motility. The cytosol is a storage unit for fat, carbohydrates, and secretory vesicles. Table 1-1 lists the principal cytoplasmic organelles.

✓ QUICK CHECK 1-1

1. Why is the process of differentiation essential to specialization? Give an example.
2. Describe at least two cellular functions.

Plasma Membranes

Whether they surround the cell or enclose an intracellular organelle, membranes are exceedingly important to normal physiologic function because they control the composition of

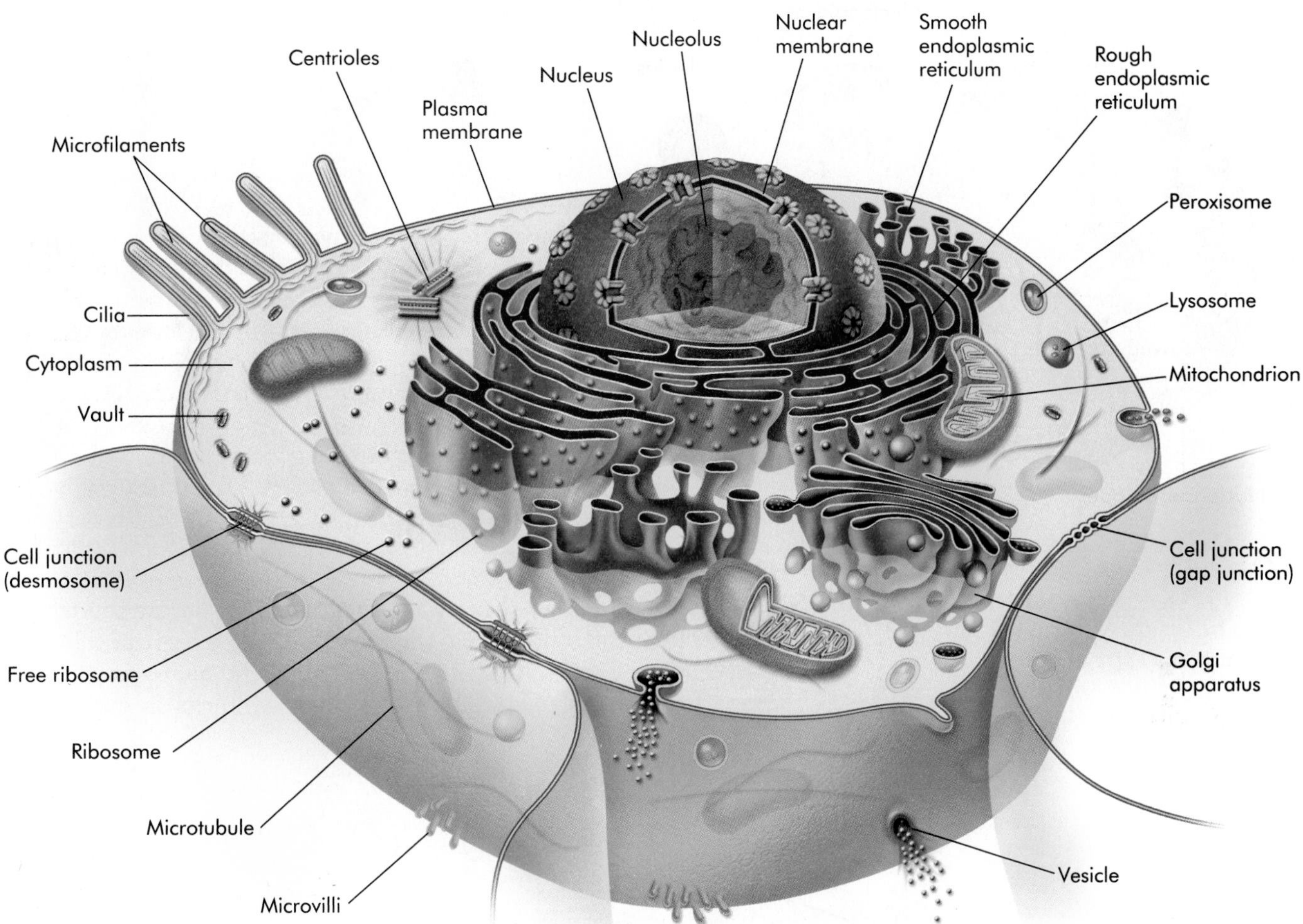

Figure 1-1 ■ **Typical Components of a Eukaryotic Cell.**

the space, or compartment, they enclose. Membranes can include or exclude various molecules, and by controlling the movement of substances from one compartment to another, membranes exert a powerful influence on metabolic pathways. The plasma membrane also has an important role in cell-to-cell recognition. Other functions of the plasma membrane include cellular mobility and the maintenance of cellular shape (Table 1-2).

Membrane composition

The outer surface of the plasma membrane is not smooth but dimpled with cavelike indentations known as **caveolae** ("tiny caves"). Caveolae serve as a storage site for many receptors and provide a route for transport into the cell. (See p. 20.)

The major chemical components of all membranes are lipids and proteins, but the percentage of each varies among different membranes. Intracellular membranes have a higher percentage of proteins than plasma membranes have, presumably because most enzymatic activity occurs within organelles. Carbohydrates are associated mainly with plasma membranes, where they combine chemically with lipids, forming glycolipids, and with proteins, forming glycoproteins.

Lipids

The basic component of the plasma membrane is a bilayer of lipid molecules—phospholipids, glycolipids, and cholesterol. Lipids are responsible for the structural integrity of the membrane. Each lipid molecule is said to be polar, or **amphipathic,** which means that one part is hydrophobic (uncharged, or "water hating") and another part is hydrophilic (charged, or "water loving") (Figure 1-3).

The membrane spontaneously organizes itself into two layers because of these two incompatible solubilities. The hydrophobic region (hydrophobic tail) of each lipid molecule is protected from water, whereas the hydrophilic region (hydrophilic head) is immersed in it. The bilayer serves as a barrier to the diffusion of water and hydrophilic substances, while allowing lipid-soluble molecules, such as oxygen (O_2) and carbon dioxide (CO_2), to diffuse through it readily.

Proteins

Proteins can be classified as integral or peripheral membrane proteins. **Integral membrane proteins** are embedded in the lipid bilayer linked to either *phosphatidylinositol,* a minor phospholipid, or a fatty acid chain. The integral proteins can be removed from the membrane only by

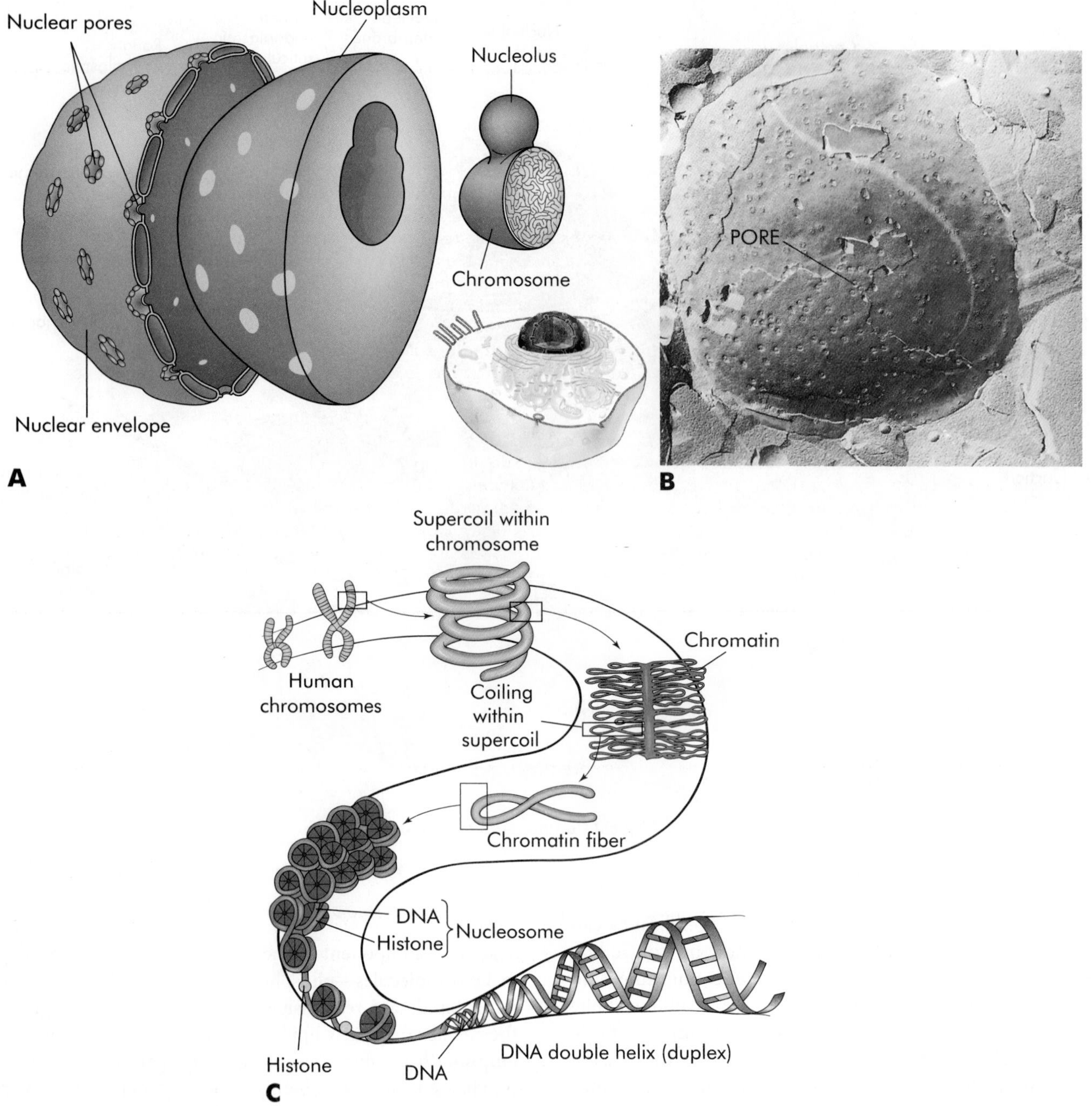

Figure 1-2 ■ **The Nucleus.** The nucleus is composed of a double membrane, called a *nuclear envelope,* that encloses the fluid-filled interior, called *nucleoplasm.* The chromosomes are suspended in the nucleoplasm (here shown much larger than real size to show the tightly packed DNA strands). Swelling at one or more points of the chromosome, shown in **A,** occurs at a nucleolus where genes are being copied into RNA. The nuclear envelope is studded with pores. **B,** The pores are visible as dimples in this freeze etch of a nuclear envelope. **C,** Histone-folding DNA in chromosomes. (**B** from Raven PH, Johnson GB: *Biology,* St Louis, 1992, Mosby.)

detergents that solubilize (dissolve) the lipid. **Peripheral membrane proteins** are not embedded in the bilayer but reside at one surface or the other, bound to an integral protein.

Proteins exist in densely folded molecular configurations rather than straight chains, so most hydrophilic units are at the surface of the molecule and most hydrophobic units are inside. Although membrane structure is determined by the lipid bilayer, membrane functions are determined largely by proteins. Proteins act as (1) recognition and binding units (receptors) for substances moving into and out of the cell; (2) pores or transport channels for various electrically charged particles, called *ions* or *electrolytes,* and specific carriers for amino acids and monosaccharides; (3) specific enzymes that drive active pumps to promote concentration of certain ions, particularly potassium (K^+), within the cell while keeping concentrations of other ions, for example, sodium (Na^+), below concentrations found in the extracellular environment; (4) cell surface markers, such as **glycoproteins** (proteins attached to carbohydrates) that identify a cell to its neighbor; (5) **cell adhesion molecules (CAMs),** or proteins that allow cells to hook

TABLE 1-1

Principal Cytoplasmic Organelles

Organelle	Characteristics and Description
Ribosomes	RNA-protein complexes synthesized in the nucleolus and secreted into the cytoplasm. Provide sites for cellular protein synthesis.
Endoplasmic reticulum	A network of tubular channels (cisternae) that extend throughout the outer nuclear membrane. Specializes in the synthesis and transport of protein and lipid components of most organelles.
Golgi complex	A network of smooth membranes and vesicles located near the nucleus. Is responsible for processing and packaging proteins onto secretory vesicles that break away from the complex and migrate to various intracellular and extracellular destinations, including the plasma membrane. The best-known vesicles are those that have coats largely made of the protein *clathrin.*
Lysosomes	Saclike structures that originate from the Golgi complex and contain enzymes for digesting most cellular substances down to their basic form, such as amino acids, fatty acids, and sugars. Cellular injury leads to release of lysosomal enzymes that cause cellular self-destruction.
Peroxisomes	Similar to lysosomes but contain several oxidative enzymes (e.g., catalase, urate oxidase) that produce hydrogen peroxide; reactions detoxify various wastes.
Mitochondria	Contain the metabolic machinery needed for cellular energy metabolism. Enzymes of respiratory chain (electron-transport chain), found in inner membrane of mitochondria, generate most of cell's ATP (oxidative phosphorylation). Has a role in osmotic regulation, pH control, calcium homeostasis, and cell signaling.
Cytoskeleton	"Bone and muscle" of the cell. Composed of a network of protein filaments, including microtubules and actin filaments (microfilaments); forms cell extensions (microvilli, cilia, flagella).
Caveolae	Tiny indentations (caves) that can capture extracellular material and shuttle it inside the cell or across the cell.
Vaults	Newly identified cytoplasmic ribonucleoproteins shaped like octagonal barrels. They are thought to act as "trucks," shuttling molecules from the nucleus to elsewhere in the cell.

TABLE 1-2

Plasma Membrane Functions

Cellular Mechanism	Membrane Functions
Structure	Usually thicker than the membranes of intracellular organelles
	Containment of cellular organelles
	Maintenance of relationship with cytoskeleton, endoplasmic reticulum, and other organelles
	Maintenance of fluid and electrolyte balance
	Outer surfaces of plasma membranes in many cells are not smooth but are dimpled with cave-like indentations called *caveolae;* they are also studded with cilia or even smaller cylindrical projections called *microvilli;* both are capable of movement
Protection	Barrier to toxic molecules and macromolecules (proteins, nucleic acids, polysaccharides)
	Barrier to foreign organisms and cells
Activation of cell	Hormones (regulation of cellular activity)
	Mitogens (cellular division; see Chapter 2)
	Antigens (antibody synthesis; see Chapter 6)
	Growth factors (proliferation and differentiation; see Chapter 9)
Storage	Storage site for many receptors
	Transport
	Diffusion and exchange diffusion
	Endocytosis (pinocytosis, phagocytosis)
	Exocytosis (secretion)
	Active transport
Cell-to-cell interaction	Communication and attachment at junctional complexes
	Symbiotic nutritive relationships
	Release of enzymes and antibodies to extracellular environment
	Relationships with extracellular matrix

Modified from King DW, Fenoglio CM, Lefkowitch JH: *General pathology: principles and dynamics,* Philadelphia, 1983, Lea & Febiger.

together and form attachments of the cytoskeleton for maintaining cellular shape; and (6) catalysts of chemical reactions, for example, conversion of lactose to glucose (Figure 1-4).

The interaction of plasma membrane proteins with lipids is complex. The role of proteins in the onset and progression of disease is important because of their enzymatic, transport, and recognition-receptor functions in cellular physiology.

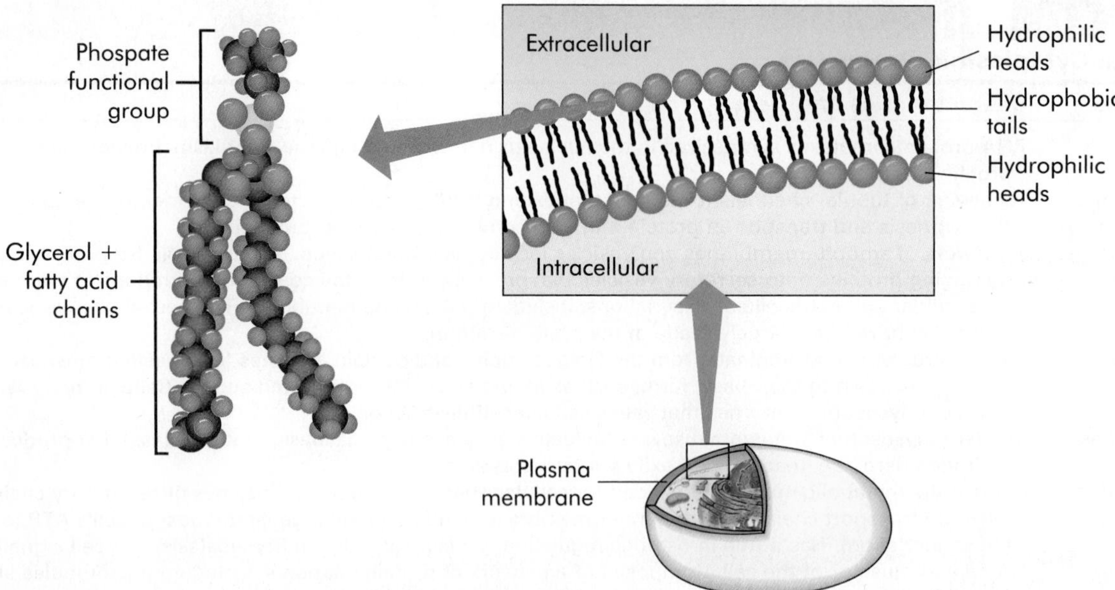

Figure 1-3 ■ **Amphipathic Molecule.** In cellular membranes, amphipathic phospholipid molecules are organized in a bimolecular layer. The hydrophilic regions of the molecules are located at the membrane surfaces, and the hydrophobic regions are oriented toward the center of the membrane.

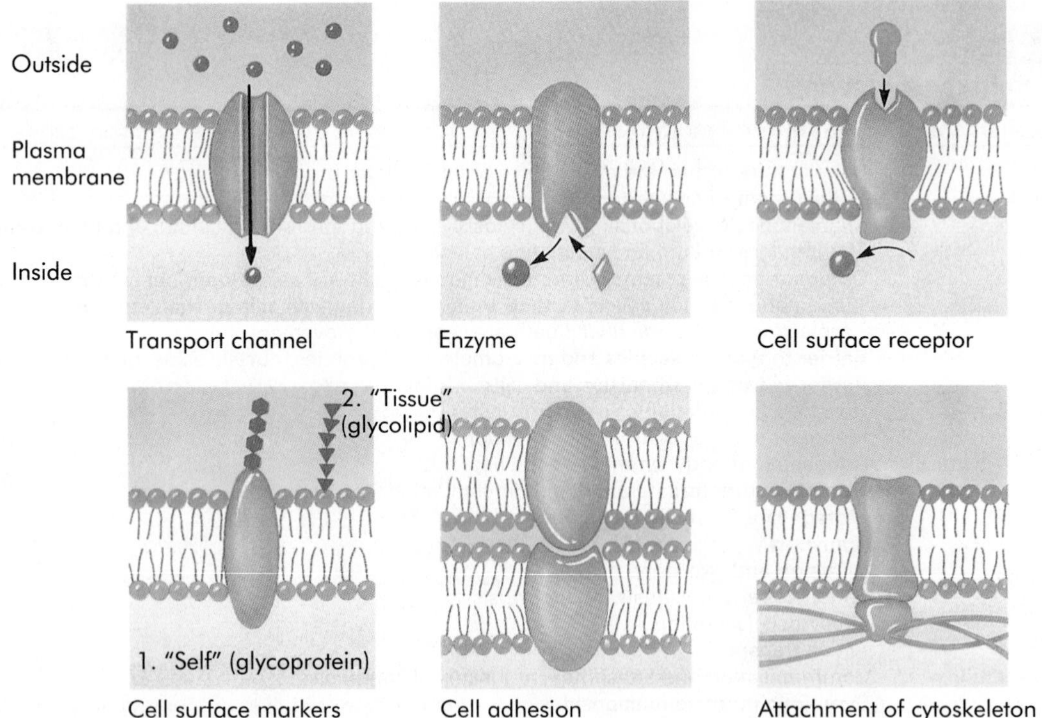

Figure 1-4 ■ **Functions of Plasma Membrane Proteins.** The plasma membrane proteins illustrated here show a variety of functions performed by the different types of plasma membranes. (From Raven PH, Johnson GB: *Understanding biology,* ed 3, Dubuque, Iowa, 1995, Brown.)

Carbohydrates

The carbohydrate contained within the plasma membrane is generally in the form of glycoprotein. Intercellular recognition, required for tissue formation, is an important function of membrane glycoproteins.

Fluid mosaic model

In the 1960s, G.L. Nicholson and S.J. Singer proposed the popular **fluid mosaic model** for biologic membranes (Figure 1-5). The model, which is continually being modified, presents integral proteins as pieces of a mosaic that float

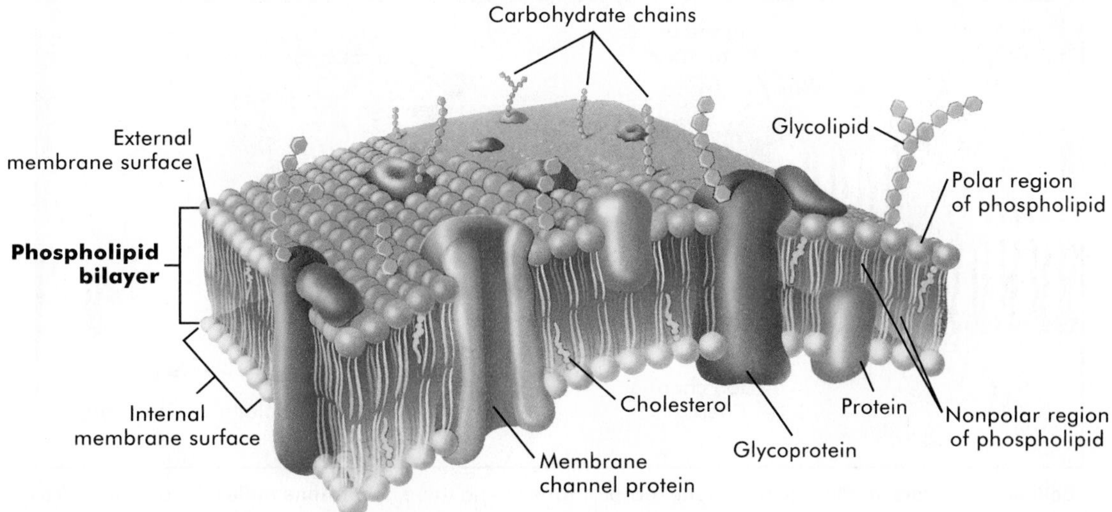

Figure 1-5 ■ **Fluid Mosaic Model.** Schematic, three-dimensional view of the fluid mosaic model of membrane structure. The lipid bilayer provides the basic structure and serves as a relatively impermeable barrier to most water-soluble molecules. (Modified from Thibodeau GA, Patton KT: *Anatomy & physiology,* ed 6, St Louis, 2007, Mosby.)

singly or as aggregates in the fluid lipid bilayer. The protein molecules (1) transport other molecules into and out of the cell; (2) facilitate (catalyze) membrane reactions; (3) receive messages, thus acting as receptors for extracellular and intracellular signals; and (4) create structural linkages between the external and internal cellular environments.

The fluid mosaic model accounts for the flexibility of cellular membranes, their self-sealing properties, and their impermeability to many substances. The degree of a membrane's fluidity depends on temperature. At lower temperatures the lipids are in a gel crystalline state, and at higher temperatures they become highly fluid. These properties are critical for cellular growth, division, and receptor function. Because *some* proteins are free to move within the plasma membranes (like floating icebergs), certain foreign proteins (antigens) may become buried in the bilayer, emerging at the surface only after injury and then attracting antibodies (proteins produced by the immune system), which attack host cells. Antigens and antibodies, which are integral to the immune response, are discussed in Chapter 6. The burial and reemergence of antigens may cause autoimmune disease, described in Chapter 7.

In the fluid mosaic model, cellular membranes are dynamic. Lipids and proteins can move laterally on the membrane, and ions and other molecules move through it. Cells, however, can immobilize specific membrane proteins in a region of the membrane. Confinement may be needed for certain functions to occur. The fluid mosaic model describes the membrane as existing in a state of change and modulation, which allows the cell to protect itself actively against injurious agents. Hormones, bacteria, viruses, drugs, antibodies, chemicals that transmit nerve impulses (neurotransmitters), and other substances attach to the plasma membrane by means of receptor molecules on its outer layer. The number of receptors present may vary at different times, and the cell can modulate the effects of injurious agents by altering receptor number and pattern.[2] This aspect of the fluid mosaic model has drastically modified previously held concepts concerning the onset of disease.

The concentration of cholesterol in the plasma membrane affects membrane fluidity. Increased concentration means less fluidity on the membrane's hydrophilic outer surface and more fluidity at its hydrophobic core. Cholesterol content changes are factors in some diseases. In cirrhosis of the liver, for example, the cholesterol content of the red blood cell's plasma membrane increases, causing a decrease in membrane fluidity that seriously affects the cell's ability to transport oxygen.

Cellular Receptors

Cellular receptors are protein molecules on the plasma membrane, in the cytoplasm, or in the nucleus that can recognize and bind with specific smaller molecules called **ligands.** Hormones, for example, are ligands. Recognition and binding depend on the chemical configuration of the receptor and its smaller ligand, which must fit together somewhat like pieces of a jigsaw puzzle (see Chapter 17).

Plasma membrane receptors protrude from or are exposed at the external surface of the membrane and often are attached to integral proteins (Figure 1-6). Some of these recognition units have all the mobile properties related to membrane fluidity. The ligands that bind with membrane receptors include hormones, neurotransmitters, antigens, complement components, lipoproteins, infectious agents, drugs, and metabolites. Many new discoveries concerning the specific interactions of cellular receptors with their respective ligands have provided a basis for understanding disease.

Although the chemical nature of ligands and their receptors differs, receptors are classified based on their location and function. Cellular type determines overall cellular function, but plasma membrane receptors determine which

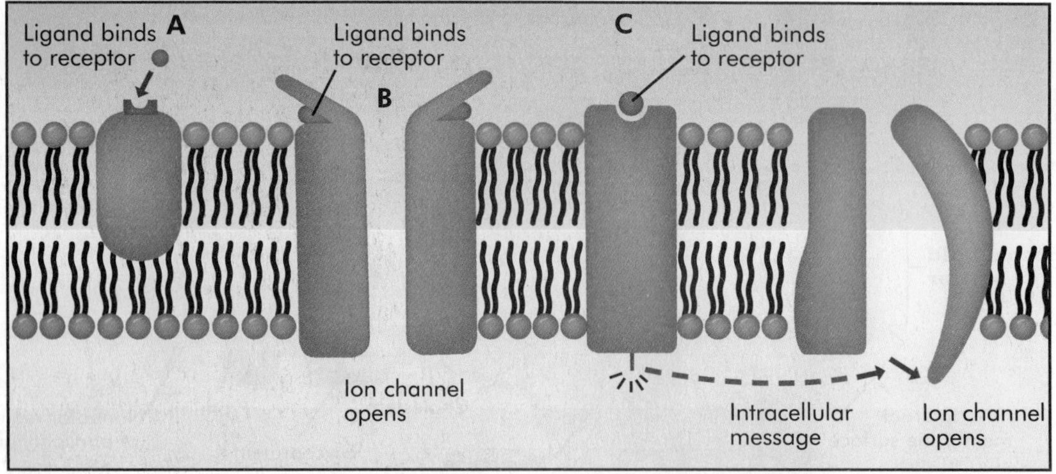

Figure 1-6 ■ **Cellular Receptors. A,** Plasma membrane receptor for a ligand (here, a hormone molecule) on the surface of an integral protein. A neurotransmitter can exert its effect on a postsynaptic cell by means of two fundamentally different types of receptor proteins: **B,** channel-linked receptors, and **C,** non–channel-linked receptors. Channel-linked receptors are also known as *ligand-gated channels.*

ligands a cell will bind with and how the cell will respond to the binding. Specific processes also control intracellular mechanisms.

Receptors for different drugs are found on the plasma membrane, in the cytoplasm, and in the nucleus. Membrane receptors have been found for certain anesthetics, opiates, endorphins, enkephalins, antibiotics, cancer chemotherapeutic agents, digitalis, and other drugs. Membrane receptors for endorphins, which are opiate-like peptides isolated from the pituitary gland, are found in large quantities in pain pathways of the nervous system (see Chapters 12 and 13). With binding, the endorphins (or drugs such as morphine) change the cell's permeability to ions, increase the concentration of molecules that regulate intracellular protein synthesis, and initiate molecular events that modulate pain perception.

Receptors for infectious microorganisms, or antigen receptors, bind bacteria, viruses, and parasites. Antigen receptors on white blood cells (lymphocytes, monocytes, macrophages, granulocytes) recognize and bind with antigenic microorganisms and activate the immune and inflammatory responses (see Chapters 5 and 6).

CELL-TO-CELL ADHESIONS

Cells are small and squishy, *not* like bricks. They are enclosed by only a flimsy membrane, yet the cell depends on the integrity of this membrane for its survival. How can cells be formed together strongly, with their membranes intact, to form a muscle that can lift this textbook? Plasma membranes not only serve as the outer boundaries of all cells but also allow groups of cells to be held together robustly, in **cell-to-cell adhesions,** to form tissues and organs. Once arranged, cells are held together by three different means: (1) cell adhesion molecules in the cell's plasma membrane (see p. 4), (2) the extracellular matrix, and (3) specialized cell junctions.

Adhesion receptors can either directly activate or modulate many of the signals initiated by circulating growth factors.[3] Adhesion receptors and their cytoskeleton partners can regulate the trafficking of signaling molecules between the cytoplasm and nucleus.[3] In addition, deficiencies of certain adhesion molecules can increase predispositions to pathologic alterations.

Extracellular Matrix

Cells can be bound together by attachment to one another or through the extracellular matrix (also including the **basement membrane**), which the cells secrete around themselves. The **extracellular matrix** is an intricate meshwork of fibrous proteins embedded in a watery, gel-like substance composed of complex carbohydrates (Figure 1-7). The matrix is like glue; however, it provides a pathway for diffusion of nutrients, wastes, and other water-soluble traffic between the blood and tissue cells. Interwoven within the matrix are three groups of **macromolecules**: (1) fibrous structural proteins, including collagen and elastin; (2) adhesive glycoproteins, such as fibronectin; and (3) proteoglycans and hyaluronic acid.

1. **Collagen** forms cable-like fibers or sheets that provide tensile strength or resistance to longitudinal stress. Collagen breakdown, such as occurs in osteoarthritis, destroys the fibrils that give cartilage its tensile strength.
2. **Elastin** is a rubber-like protein fiber most abundant in tissues that must be capable of stretching and recoiling, such as those found in the lungs.
3. **Fibronectin** promotes cell adhesion and cell anchorage. Reduced amounts have been found in certain types of cancerous cells; this allows cancer cells to travel or metastasize to other parts of the body.

All of these macromolecules occur in intercellular junctions and cell surfaces and may assemble into two different components: interstitial matrix and basement membrane (BM) (see Figure 1-7).

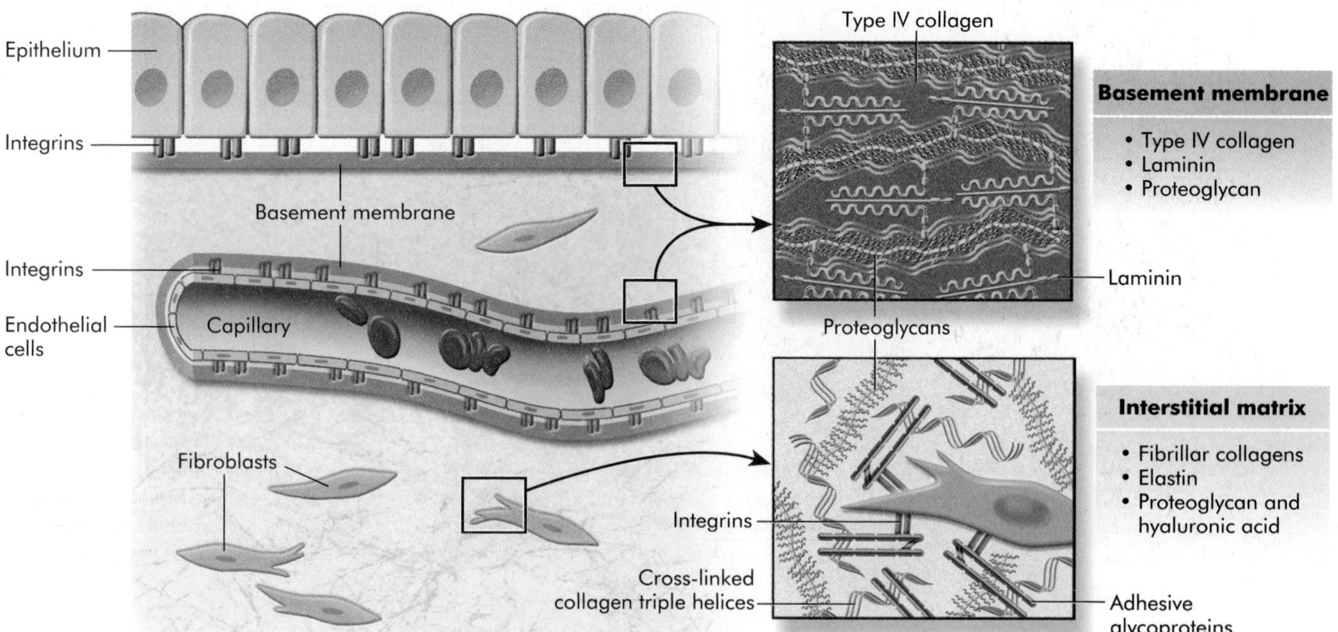

Figure 1-7 ■ **Extracellular Matrix.** Tissues are not just cells but also extracellular space. The extracellular space is an intricate network of macromolecules called the *extracellular matrix (ECM).* The macromolecules that constitute the ECM are secreted locally (by mostly fibroblasts) and assembled into a meshwork in close association with the surface of the cell that produced them. Two main classes of macromolecules include proteoglycans, which are bound to polysaccharide chains called *glycosaminoglycans,* and fibrous proteins (e.g., collagen, elastin, fibronectin, and laminin), which have structural and adhesive properties. Together the proteogylcan molecules form a gel-like ground substance in which the fibrous proteins are embedded. The gel permits rapid diffusion of nutrients, metabolites, and hormones between the blood and the tissue cells. Matrix proteins modulate cell-matrix interactions including normal tissue remodeling (which can become abnormal, for example, with chronic inflammation). Disruptions of this balance results in serious diseases such as arthritis, tumor growth, and others. (Modified from Kumar V, Abbas A, Fausto N: *Robbins and Cotran pathologic basis of disease,* ed 7, Philadelphia, 2005, Saunders.)

The extracellular matrix is secreted by **fibroblasts** ("fiber formers"), local cells that are present in the matrix. The matrix and the cells within it are known collectively as **connective tissue,** because they connect cells together to form tissue and organs. Human connective tissues are enormously varied. They can be hard and dense, like bone; flexible, like tendons or the dermis of the skin; resilient and shock absorbing, like cartilage; or soft and transparent, like the jelly that fills the eye. In all these examples, the majority of the tissue is composed of extracellular matrix, and the cells that produce the matrix are scattered within it like raisins in a pudding (see Figure 1-7).

The matrix is not just a passive scaffolding for cellular attachment; it also helps regulate the function of the cells with which it interacts. The matrix helps regulate such important functions as cell growth and differentiation.

Specialized Cell Junctions

Cells in direct physical contact with neighboring cells are often linked together at specialized plasma membrane regions called **cell junctions.** Cell junctions have two main functions: (1) to hold cells together and (2) to permit small molecules to pass from cell to cell, allowing coordination of the activities of cells that form tissues.

The three main types of cell junctions are (1) desmosomes (macula adherens), (2) tight junctions (zonula occludens), and (3) gap junctions, or adhering junctions (Figure 1-8). Together they form the **junctional complex. Desmosomes** hold cells together by forming either continuous bands or belts of epithelial sheets or button-like points of contact. Desmosomes also act as a system of braces to maintain structural stability. **Tight junctions** are barriers to diffusion, prevent the movement of substances through transport proteins in the plasma membrane, and prevent the leakage of small molecules between the plasma membranes of adjacent cells. **Gap junctions** are clusters of communicating tunnels or connexons that allow small ions and molecules to pass directly from the inside of one cell to the inside of another. **Connexons** are joining proteins that extend outward from each of the adjacent plasma membranes. Cells connected by gap junctions are considered ionically (electrically) and metabolically coupled. Gap junctions coordinate the activities of adjacent cells. They are important, for example, for synchronizing contractions of heart muscle cells through ionic coupling and for permitting action potentials to spread rapidly from cell to cell in neural tissues. Why gap junctions occur in tissues that are not electrically active is unknown. Although most gap junctions are associated with junctional complexes, they sometimes exist as independent structures.

The junctional complex is a highly permeable part of the plasma membrane. Its permeability is controlled by a process called **gating,** which depends on concentrations of

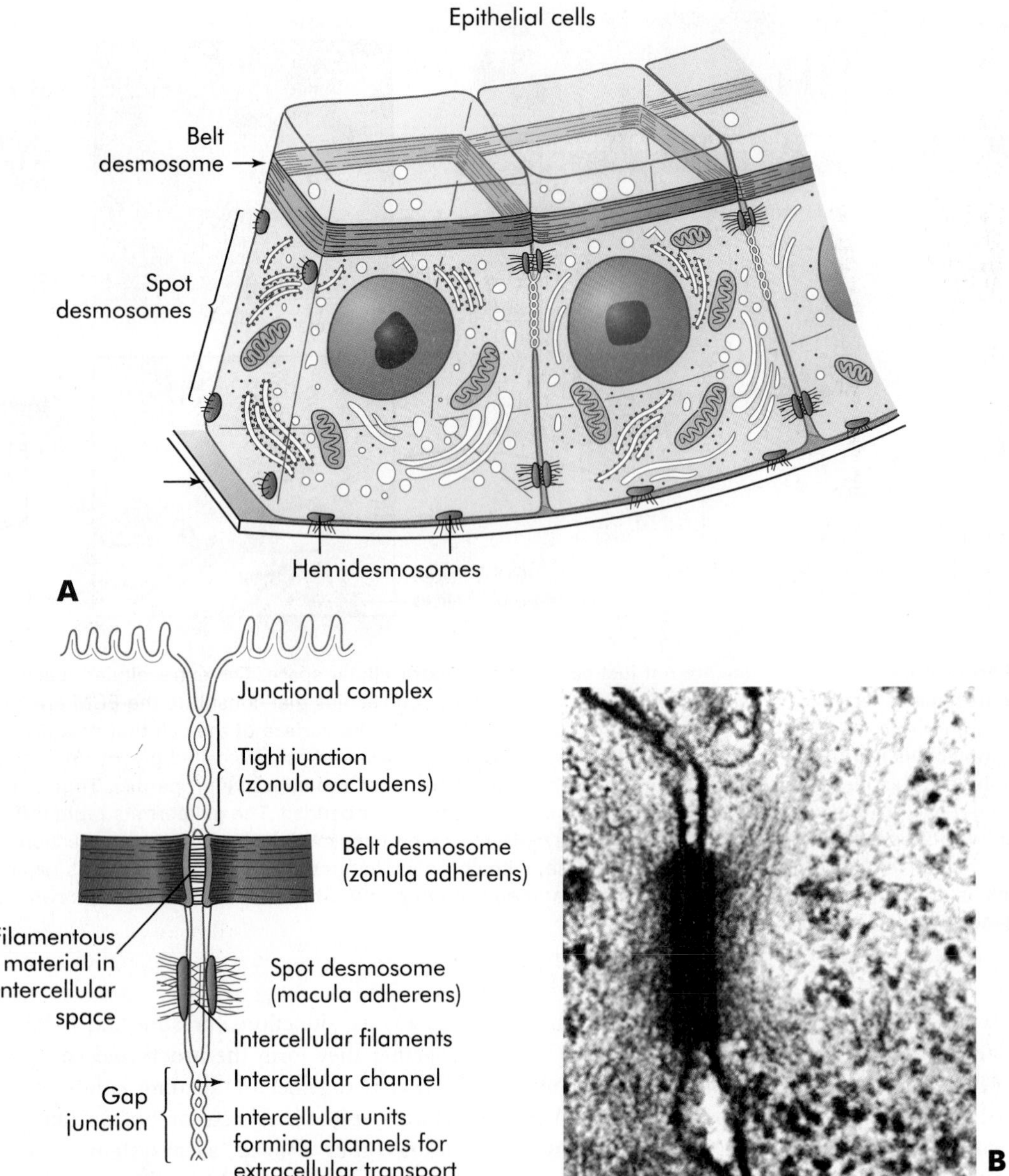

Figure 1-8 ■ **Junctional Complex. A,** Schematic drawing of a belt desmosome between epithelial cells. This junction, also called the *zonula adherens,* encircles each of the interacting cells. The spot desmosomes and hemidesmosomes, like the belt desmosomes, are adhering junctions. This tight junction is an impermeable junction that holds cells together but seals them in such a way that molecules cannot leak between them. The gap junction, as a communicating junction, mediates the passage of small molecules from one interacting cell to the other. **B,** Electron micrograph of desmosomes. (From Raven PH, Johnson GB: *Biology,* St Louis, 1992, Mosby.)

calcium ions in the cytoplasm. Increased cytoplasmic calcium causes decreased permeability at the junctional complex. Gating enables uninjured cells to seal themselves off from injured neighbors. Calcium is released from injured cells.

CELLULAR COMMUNICATION AND SIGNAL TRANSDUCTION

Cells need to communicate with each other to maintain a stable internal environment, or **homeostasis;** to regulate their growth and division; to oversee their development and organization into tissues; and to coordinate their functions. Cells communicate in three ways: (1) they form protein channels (gap junctions) that directly coordinate the activities of adjacent cells; (2) they display plasma membrane–bound signaling molecules (receptors) that affect the cell itself and other cells in direct physical contact; and (3) they secrete chemicals that signal to cells some distance away (Figure 1-9). Alterations in cellular communication affect disease onset and progression. In fact, if a cell cannot perform gap junctional intercellular communication, normal growth control and cell differentiation is compromised, thereby favoring cancerous tumor development

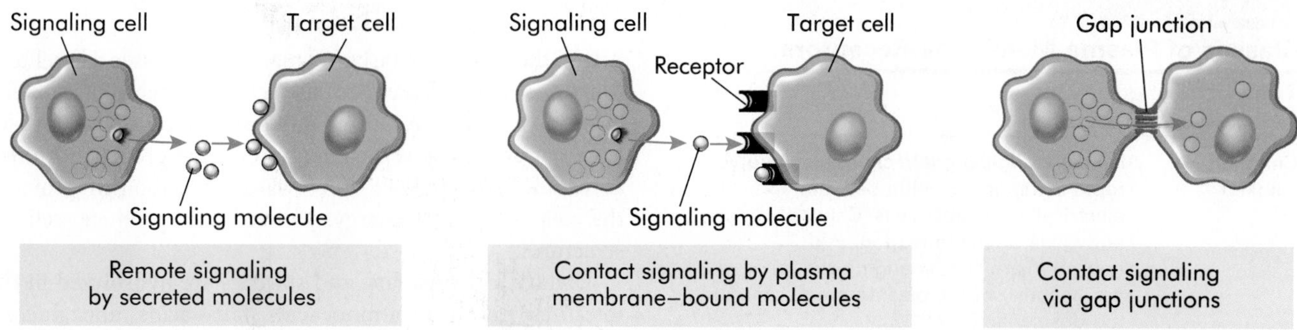

Figure 1-9 ■ **Cellular Communication.** Three primary ways in which cells communicate with one another.

(see Chapter 9). (Communication through gap junctions was discussed earlier, and contact signaling by plasma membrane–bound molecules is discussed on this page and on p. 12.) Secreted chemical signals involve communication locally and at a distance. Primary modes of chemical signaling are hormonal, neurohormonal, paracrine, and autocrine (Figure 1-10).

Hormonal signaling involves specialized endocrine cells that secrete hormone chemicals released by one set of cells that travel through the tissue through the bloodstream to produce a response in other sets of cells (see Chapter 17). In **neurohormonal signaling,** hormones are released into the blood by neurosecretory neurons. Like endocrine cells, neurosecretory neurons release blood-borne chemical messengers, whereas ordinary neurons secrete short-range neurotransmitters into a small discrete space (i.e., synapse). In **paracrine signaling,** cells secrete local chemical mediators that are quickly taken up, destroyed, or immobilized. The mediators act only on nearby cells. In **autocrine signaling,** signaling molecules may act back on the cells of origin (i.e., autostimulation). Autocrine circuits function as a component of normal growth-regulatory mechanisms in many adult tissue types. Neurons communicate directly with the cells they innervate by releasing chemicals or **neurotransmitters** at specialized junctions called **chemical synapses;** the neurotransmitter diffuses across the synaptic cleft and acts on the postsynaptic target cell (see Figure 1-10). Many of these same signaling molecules are receptors used in hormonal, neurohormonal, paracrine, and autocrine signaling. Important differences lie in the speed and selectivity with which the signals are delivered to their targets.[1]

Plasma membrane receptors belong to one of three classes that are defined by the signaling (transduction) mechanism used. Table 1-3 summarizes these receptors. Cells respond to external stimuli by activating a variety of **signal transduction pathways,** communication pathways, or signaling cascades (Figure 1-11, *C*). Signals are passed between cells when a particular type of molecule is produced by one cell—the **signaling cell**—and received by another—the **target cell**—by means of a **receptor protein** that recognizes and responds specifically to the signal

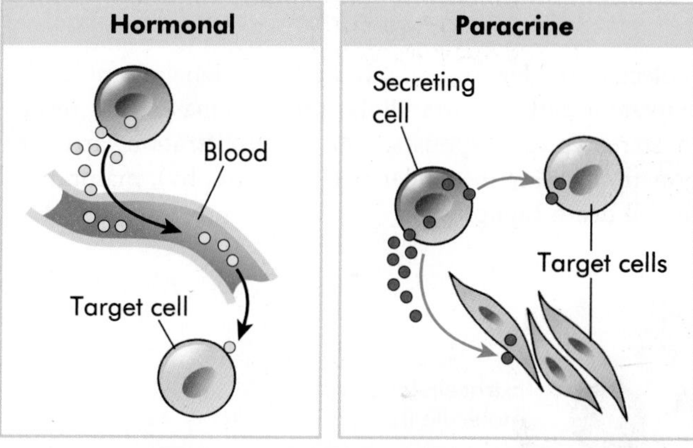

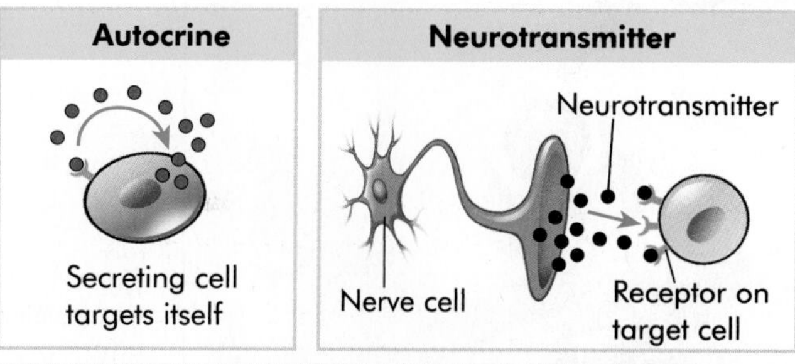

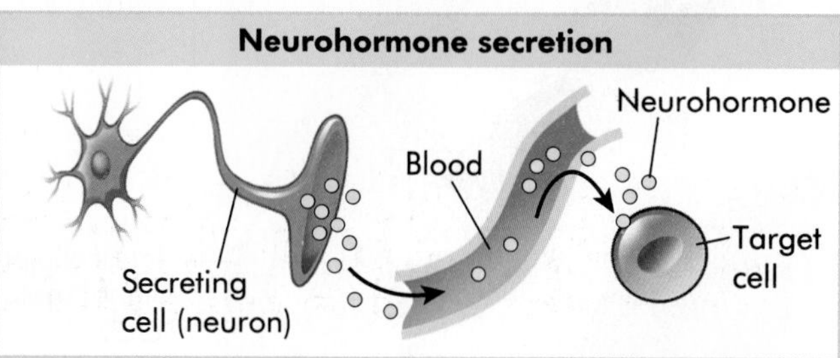

Figure 1-10 ■ **Primary Modes of Chemical Signaling.** Five forms of signaling mediated by secreted molecules. Hormones, paracrines, autocrines, neurotransmitters, and neurohormones are all intracellular messengers that accomplish communication between cells. Not all neurotransmitters act in the strictly synaptic mode shown; some act in a paracrine mode as local chemical mediators that influence multiple target cells in the area.

TABLE 1-3

Classes of Plasma Membrane Receptors

Type of Receptor	Description
Channel linked	Also called *ligand-gated* channels; involve rapid synaptic signaling between electrically excitable cells. Channels open and close briefly in response to neurotransmitters, changing the ion permeability of the plasma membrane of the postsynaptic cell.
Catalytic	Once activated by ligands, function directly as enzymes.
G-protein linked	Indirectly activate or inactivate plasma membrane enzyme or ion channel; interaction mediated by *GTP-binding regulatory protein (G-protein).* May also interact with inositol phospholipids, which are significant in cell signaling, and molecules involved in the *inositol-phospholipid transduction pathway.*

molecule (see Figure 1-11). In turn, the signaling molecules activate a path of intracellular protein kinases that results in stereotypical responses, such as proliferation, arrest of growth, increase in cellular size (hypertrophy), maturation, or cell death (apoptosis).

CELLULAR METABOLISM

All of the chemical tasks of maintaining essential cellular functions are referred to as **cellular metabolism.** The energy-using process of metabolism is called **anabolism** (*ana* = upward), and the energy-releasing process is known as **catabolism** (*kata* = downward). Metabolism provides the cell with the energy it needs to produce cellular structures.

Dietary proteins, fats, and starches are hydrolyzed in the intestinal tract into amino acids, fatty acids, and glucose. These constituents are then absorbed, circulated, and taken up by the cell, where they may be used for various vital cellular processes, including the production of ATP. The process by which ATP is produced is one example of a series of reactions called a **metabolic pathway.** A metabolic pathway involves several steps whose end products are not always detectable. A key feature of cellular metabolism is the directing of biochemical reactions by protein catalysts or enzymes. Each enzyme has a high affinity for a **substrate,** a specific substance converted to a product of the reaction.

Role of Adenosine Triphosphate

For a cell to function, it must be able to extract and use the chemical energy in organic molecules. When 1 mole of glucose metabolically breaks down in the presence of oxygen into carbon dioxide and water, 686 kilocalories (kcal) of

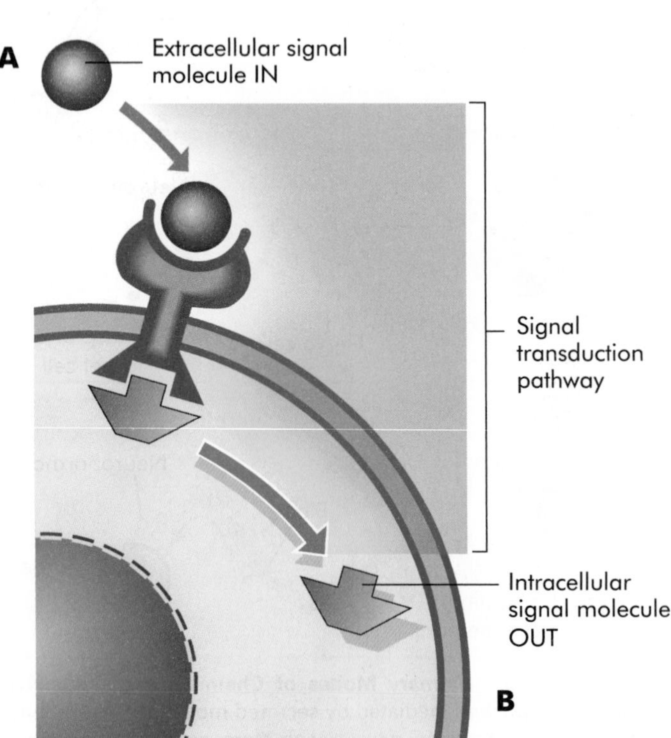

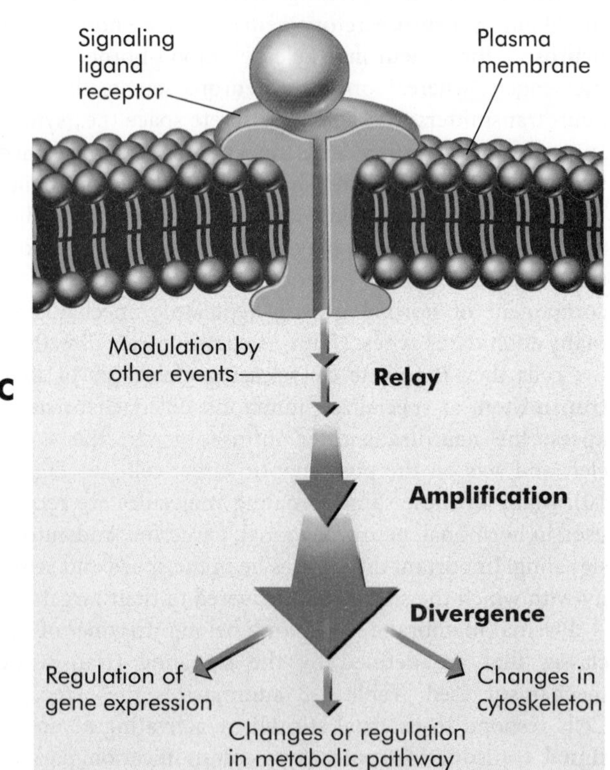

Figure 1-11 ■ **Schematic of a Signal Transduction Pathway.** Like a telephone receiver that converts an electrical signal into a sound signal, a cell converts an extracellular signal, **A,** into an intracellular signal, **B. C,** An extracellular chemical messenger (ligand) bonds to a receptor protein located on the plasma membrane where it is transduced into an intracellular signal. This process initiates a signaling cascade that relays the signal into the cell interior, amplifying and distributing it en route. Steps in the cascade can be modulated by other events in the cell.

chemical energy are released. The chemical energy lost by one molecule is transferred to the chemical structure of another molecule by an energy-carrying or transferring molecule, such as ATP. The energy stored in ATP can be used in various energy-requiring reactions and in the process is generally converted to adenosine diphosphate (ADP) and inorganic phosphate (Pi). The energy available as a result of this reaction is about 7 kcal/mol of ATP. The cell uses ATP for muscle contraction and active transport of molecules across cellular membranes. ATP not only stores energy but also *transfers* it from one molecule to another. Energy stored by carbohydrate, lipid, and protein is catabolized and transferred to ATP.

Food and Production of Cellular Energy

Catabolism of the proteins, lipids, and polysaccharides found in food can be divided into the following three phases (Figure 1-12):

Phase 1: **Digestion.** Large molecules are broken down into smaller subunits: proteins into amino acids, polysaccharides into simple sugars, and fats into fatty acids and glycerol. These processes occur outside the cell and are activated by secreted enzymes.

Phase 2: **Glycolysis** and **oxidation.** The most important part of phase 2 is glycolysis, the splitting of glucose. Glycolysis produces two molecules of ATP per glucose molecule through oxidation, or the removal and transfer of a pair of electrons. The total process is called *oxidative cellular metabolism* and involves nine biochemical reactions (Figure 1-13).

Phase 3: **Citric acid cycle (Krebs cycle, tricarboxylic acid cycle).** Most of the ATP is generated during this final phase. It begins with the citric acid cycle and ends with oxidative phosphorylation. About two thirds of the total oxidation of carbon compounds in most cells is accomplished during this phase. The major end products are carbon dioxide (CO_2) and two dinucleotides, reduced

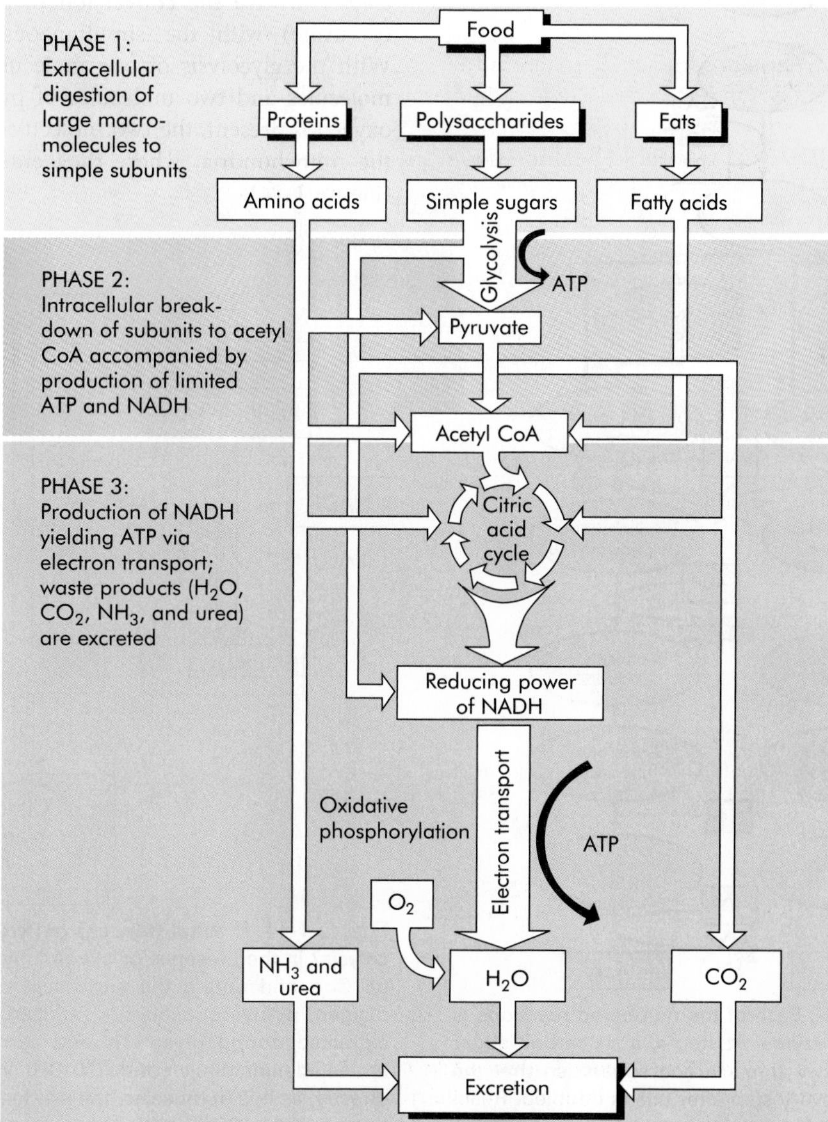

Figure 1-12 ■ **Three Phases of Catabolism: From Breakdown of Food to Elimination of Waste Products.** These reactions produce adenosine triphosphate (ATP), which is used to power other processes in the cell.

nicotinamide adenine dinucleotide (NADH), and the reduced form of flavin adenine dinucleotide ($FADH_2$), which transfer their electrons into the electron-transport chain.

Oxidative Phosphorylation

Oxidative phosphorylation occurs in the mitochondria and is the mechanism by which the energy produced from carbohydrates, fats, and proteins is transferred to ATP. During the catabolism of foods, many reactions involve the removal of electrons from various intermediates. These reactions generally require a coenzyme (a nonprotein carrier molecule), such as nicotinamide adenine dinucleotide (NAD), to transfer the electrons and thus are called **transfer reactions.**

Molecules of NAD and flavin adenine nucleotide (FAD) transfer electrons they have gained from the oxidation of substrates to molecular oxygen, O_2. The electrons from reduced NAD and FAD, NADH and $FADH_2$, are transferred to the **electron-transport chain** on the inner surfaces of the mitochondria with the release of hydrogen ions. Some carrier molecules are brightly colored, iron-containing proteins known as cytochromes that accept a pair of electrons. These electrons eventually combine with molecular oxygen.

If oxygen is not available to the electron-transport chain, ATP will not be formed by the mitochondria. Instead, an anaerobic (without oxygen) metabolic pathway synthesizes ATP. This process, called **substrate phosphorylation** or **anaerobic glycolysis,** is linked to the breakdown (glycolysis) of carbohydrate (see Figure 1-13). Because glycolysis occurs in the cytoplasm of the cell, it provides energy for cells that lack mitochondria. The reactions in anaerobic glycolysis involve the conversion of glucose to pyruvic acid (pyruvate) with the simultaneous production of ATP. With the glycolysis of one molecule of glucose, two ATP molecules and two molecules of pyruvate are liberated. If oxygen is present, the two molecules of pyruvate move into the mitochondria, where they enter the citric acid cycle (Figure 1-14).

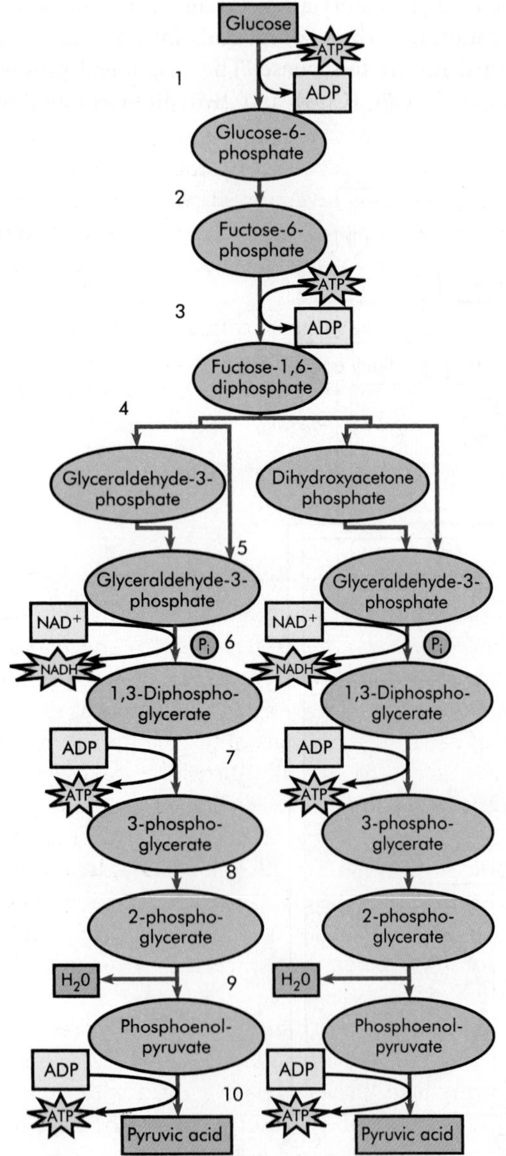

Figure 1-13 ■ **Glycolysis.** Each of the numbered reactions is catalyzed by a different enzyme. At step *4,* a six-carbon sugar is broken down to give two three-carbon sugars, so that the number of molecules at every step after this is doubled. Reactions *5* and *6* are responsible for the net synthesis of adenosine triphosphate (ATP) and reduced nicotinamide adenine dinucleotide (NADH) molecules.

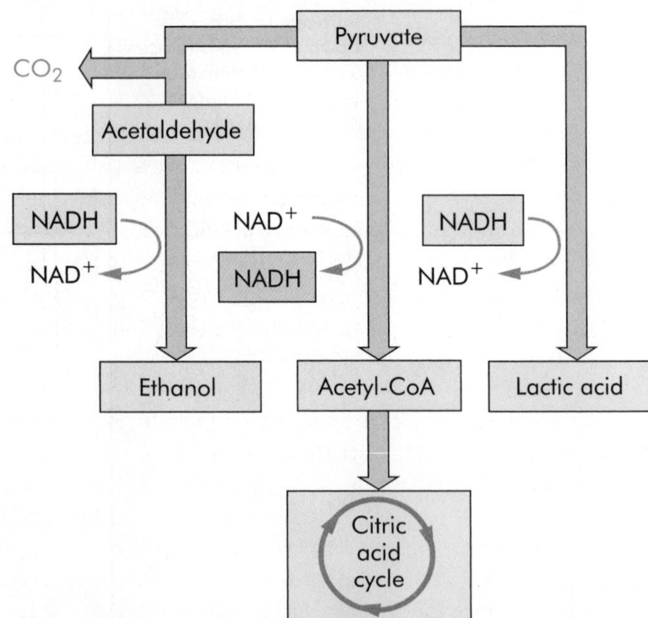

Figure 1-14 ■ **What Happens to Pyruvate, the Product of Glycolysis?** In the presence of oxygen, pyruvate is oxidized to acetyl CoA and enters the citric acid cycle. In the absence of oxygen, pyruvate instead is reduced, accepting the electrons extracted during glycolysis and carried by reduced nicotinamide adenine dinucleotide (NADH). When pyruvate is reduced directly, as it is in muscles, the product is lactic acid. When carbon dioxide (CO_2) is first removed from pyruvate and the remainder is reduced, as it is in yeasts, the resulting product is ethanol.

If oxygen is absent, pyruvate is converted to lactic acid which is released into the extracellular fluid. The conversion of pyruvic acid to lactic acid is reversible; therefore, once oxygen is restored, lactic acid is quickly converted back to either pyruvic acid or glucose. The anaerobic generation of ATP from glucose through glycolysis is not as efficient as the aerobic generation process. Adding an oxygen-requiring stage to the catabolic process (phase 3; see Figure 1-12) provides cells with a much more powerful method for extracting energy from food molecules.

MEMBRANE TRANSPORT: CELLULAR INTAKE AND OUTPUT

Cells continually take in nutrients, fluids, and chemical messengers from the extracellular environment and expel metabolites, or the products of metabolism, and end products of lysosomal digestion. The mechanisms involved depend on the characteristics of the substance to be transported. In **passive transport,** water and small, electrically uncharged molecules move easily through pores in the plasma membrane's lipid bilayer. This process occurs naturally through any semipermeable barrier. It is driven by osmosis, hydrostatic pressure, and diffusion, all of which depend on the laws of physics and do not require life. The process does not require any energy expenditure by the cell.

Other molecules are too large to pass through pores or are ligands bound to receptors on the cell's plasma membrane. Some of these molecules are moved into and out of the cell by **active transport,** which requires life, biologic activity, and the cell's expenditure of metabolic energy. Unlike passive transport, active transport occurs across only living membranes that (1) use energy generated by cellular metabolism and (2) have receptors that can recognize and bind with the substance to be transported. Large molecules (macromolecules), along with fluids, are transported by endocytosis (taking in) and exocytosis (expelling). Water and electrically charged molecules are transported by protein channels embedded in the plasma membrane. Ligands enter the cell by means of receptor-mediated endocytosis.

Movement of Water and Solutes

Cellular membranes are semipermeable and generally allow passage of water and small particles of dissolved substances called **solutes,** depending on their size, solubility, electrical properties, and concentration on either side of the membrane. Small, lipid-soluble particles, such as oxygen, carbon dioxide, and urea, readily pass through the lipid bilayers of the plasma membrane. Larger, water-soluble particles may pass through pores in the membranes. Although large protein molecules, such as albumin and globulin, pass through membranes by endocytosis, they exert an osmotic effect on the movement of water (see p. 16).

Body fluids are composed of **electrolytes,** which are electrically charged and dissociate into constituent **ions** when placed in solution, and nonelectrolytes, such as glucose, urea, and creatinine, which do not dissociate. Electrolytes account for approximately 95% of the solute molecules in body water. Electrolytes exhibit **polarity** by orienting themselves toward the positive or negative pole. Ions with a positive charge are known as **cations** and migrate toward the negative pole, or cathode, if an electrical current is passed through the electrolyte solution. **Anions** carry a negative charge and migrate toward the positive pole, or anode, in the presence of electrical current. Anions and cations are located in both the intracellular fluid (ICF) and extracellular fluid (ECF) compartments, although their concentration depends on their location. (Fluid and electrolyte balance between body compartments is discussed in Chapter 4.) For example, sodium (Na^+) is the predominant extracellular cation, and potassium (K^+) is the principal intracellular cation. The difference in ICF and ECF concentrations of these ions is important to the transmission of electrical impulses across the plasma membranes of nerve and muscle cells.

Electrolytes are measured in milliequivalents per liter (mEq/L) or milligrams per deciliter (mg/dl). The term *milliequivalent* indicates the chemical-combining activity of an ion, which depends on the electrical charge, or **valence,** of its ions. In abbreviations, valence is indicated by the number of plus or minus signs. One milliequivalent of any cation can combine chemically with 1 mEq of any anion: one monovalent anion will combine with one monovalent cation. Divalent ions combine more strongly than monovalent ions. To maintain electrochemical balance, one divalent ion will combine with two monovalent ions (e.g., $Ca^{++} + 2Cl^- = CaCl_2$).

Passive transport: diffusion, filtration, and osmosis

Diffusion

Diffusion is the movement of a solute molecule from an area of greater solute concentration to an area of lesser solute concentration. This difference in concentration is known as a **concentration gradient.** Although particles in a solution move randomly in any direction, if the concentration of particles in one part of the solution is greater than in another part, the particles distribute themselves evenly throughout the solution. According to the same principle, if the concentration of particles is greater on one side of a *permeable membrane* than on the other side, the particles diffuse spontaneously from the area of greater concentration to the area of lesser concentration until equilibrium is reached. The higher the concentration on one side, the greater the diffusion rate.

The diffusion rate is influenced by differences of electrical potential across the membrane (see p. 22). Because the pores in the lipid bilayer are often lined with Ca^{++}, other cations (e.g., Na^+ and K^+) diffuse slowly because they are repelled by positive charges in the pores.

The rate of diffusion of a substance depends also on its size (diffusion coefficient) and its lipid solubility (Figure 1-15). Usually, the smaller the molecule and the more soluble it is in oil, the more hydrophobic or nonpolar it is and the more rapidly it will diffuse across the bilayer. Oxygen, carbon dioxide, and steroid hormones are all nonpolar

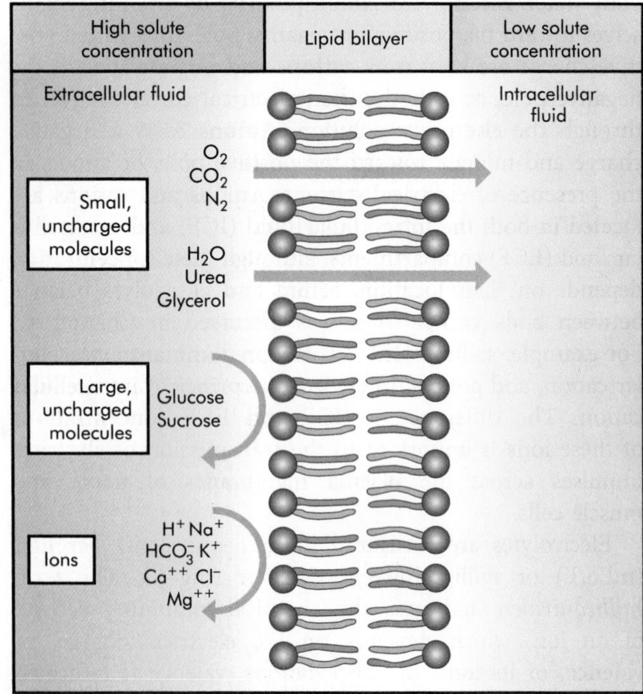

Figure 1-15 ■ Passive Diffusion of Solute Molecules Across the Plasma Membrane. Oxygen (O_2), nitrogen (N_2), water (H_2O), urea, glycerol, and carbon dioxide (CO_2) can diffuse readily down the concentration gradient. Macromolecules are too large to diffuse through pores in the plasma membrane. Ions may be repelled if the pores contain substances with identical charges. If the pores are lined with cations, for example, other cations will have difficulty diffusing because the positive charges will repel one another. Diffusion can still occur, but it occurs more slowly. (From Thibodeau GA, Patton KT: *Anatomy & physiology,* ed 6, St Louis, 2007, Mosby.)

molecules. Water-soluble substances, such as sugars and inorganic ions, diffuse very slowly, whereas uncharged lipophilic ("lipid-loving") molecules, such as fatty acids and steroids, diffuse rapidly. Ions and other polar molecules generally diffuse across cellular membranes more slowly than lipid-soluble substances.

Water readily diffuses through biologic membranes because water molecules are small and uncharged. The dipolar structure of water allows it to cross rapidly the regions of the bilayer containing the lipid head groups. Their groups constitute the two outer regions of the lipid bilayer.

Filtration: hydrostatic pressure

Filtration is the movement of water and solutes through a membrane because of a greater pushing pressure (force) on one side of the membrane than on the other side. **Hydrostatic pressure** is the mechanical force of water pushing against cellular membranes. In the vascular system, hydrostatic pressure is the blood pressure generated in vessels when the heart contracts. Blood reaching the capillary bed has a hydrostatic pressure of 25 to 30 mm Hg, which is sufficient force to push water across the thin capillary membranes into the interstitial space. Hydrostatic pressure is partially balanced by osmotic pressure, whereby water moving *out* of the capillaries is partially balanced by osmotic forces that tend to *pull* water into the capillaries. Water that is not osmotically attracted back into the capillaries moves into the lymph system (see the discussion of Starling's forces in Chapter 4).

Osmosis

Osmosis is the movement of water "down" a concentration gradient—that is, across a semipermeable membrane from a region of higher water concentration to one of lower concentration. For osmosis to occur, (1) the membrane must be more permeable to water than to solutes and (2) the concentration of solutes must be greater so that water moves more easily. Osmosis is directly related to both hydrostatic pressure and solute concentration but *not* to particle size or weight. For example, particles of the plasma protein albumin are small but are more concentrated in body fluids than the larger and heavier particles of globulin. Therefore, albumin exerts a greater osmotic force than does globulin.

Osmolality controls the distribution and movement of water between body compartments. The terms *osmolality* and *osmolarity* often are used interchangeably in reference to osmotic activity, but they define different measurements. **Osmolality** measures the number of milliosmoles per kilogram of water, or the concentration of molecules per *weight* of water. **Osmolarity** measures the number of milliosmoles per liter of solution, or the concentration of molecules per *volume* of solution.

In solutions that contain only dissociable substances, such as sodium and chloride, the difference between the two measurements is negligible. In considering all the different solutes in plasma (e.g., proteins, glucose, lipids), however, the difference between osmolality and osmolarity becomes more significant. Less of plasma's weight is water, and the overall concentration of particles is therefore greater. The osmolality will be greater than the osmolarity because of the smaller proportion of water. Osmolality is thus preferred in human clinical assessment.

The normal osmolality of body fluids is 280 to 294 mOsm/kg (milliosmoles per kilogram). The osmolality of intracellular and extracellular fluid tends to equalize and so provides a measure of body fluid concentration and thus the body's hydration status. Hydration is affected also by hydrostatic pressure, because the movement of water by osmosis can be opposed by an equal amount of hydrostatic pressure. The amount of hydrostatic pressure required to oppose the osmotic movement of water is called the **osmotic pressure** of the solution. Factors that determine osmotic pressure are the type and thickness of the plasma membrane, the size of the molecules, the concentration of molecules or the concentration gradient, and the solubility of molecules within the membrane.

Effective osmolality is sustained osmotic activity and depends on the concentration of solutes remaining on one side of a permeable membrane. If the solutes penetrate the membrane and equilibrate with the solution on the other side of the membrane, the osmotic effect will be diminished or lost.

Plasma proteins influence osmolality because they have a negative charge. The principle involved is known as

Gibbs-Donnan equilibrium; it occurs when fluid in one compartment contains small, diffusible ions, such as Na^+ and chloride (Cl^-), together with large, nondiffusible, charged particles, such as plasma proteins. Because the body tends to maintain an electrical equilibrium, the nondiffusible protein molecules cause asymmetry in the distribution of small ions. Anions such as Cl^- are thus driven out of the cell or plasma, and cations such as Na^+ are attracted. The protein-containing compartment maintains a state of electroneutrality, but the osmolality is higher. The overall osmotic effect of colloids, such as plasma proteins, is called the **oncotic pressure,** or **colloid osmotic pressure.**

Tonicity describes the effective osmolality of a solution. (The terms *osmolality* and *tonicity* may be used interchangeably.) Solutions have relative degrees of tonicity. An **isotonic solution** (or isosmotic solution) has the same osmolality or concentration of particles (285 mOsm) as the ICF or ECF. A **hypotonic solution** has a lower concentration and is thus more dilute than body fluids. A **hypertonic solution** has a concentration of more than 285 to 294 mOsm/kg. The concept of tonicity is important when correcting water and solute imbalances by administering different types of replacement solutions (see Chapter 4).

QUICK CHECK 1-2

1. Glycolysis results in the production of what?
2. Describe the difference between diffusion and osmosis.
3. Why do water and small, electrically charged molecules move easily through pores in the plasma membrane?

Mediated and active transport

Mediated transport

Mediated transport (passive and active) involves integral or transmembrane proteins with receptors that are highly specific for the substance being transported. Inorganic anions and cations (e.g., Na^+, K^+, Ca^{++}, Cl^-, HCO_3^-) and charged and uncharged organic compounds require specific transport systems to facilitate movement through different cellular membranes. Mediated transport is much faster than simple diffusion.

A **transport protein** *(carrier protein)* is a transmembrane or integral protein that binds with and transfers a specific solute molecule across the lipid bilayer. Each transport protein, or **transporter,** has receptors for a specific solute. When the transporter is saturated—that is, when all receptor sites are occupied by solute molecules—the rate of transport is maximal. Solute binding can be blocked by **competitive inhibitors** that compete for the same receptor site and may or may not be transported by the transport protein. Noncompetitive inhibitors bind elsewhere but can alter the structure of the transporter.

The polypeptide chain of the transport protein crosses the lipid bilayer multiple times. This chain forms a continuous pathway enabling solutes to pass across the membrane without directly contacting the hydrophobic interior of the lipid bilayer (Figure 1-16).[1]

Another mechanism of mediated transport is the channel protein. The protein transporter creates a water-filled pore or channel across the bilayer through which specific ions can diffuse. These channels are sometimes called *ion channels* or *K^+ leak channels* (Figure 1-17). The channel is controlled by a gate mechanism that determines which receptor-bound solutes can move into it. Binding stimulates conformational changes in the protein transporter that move the solute through the channel short distances until it reaches the other side of the membrane. Ion channels

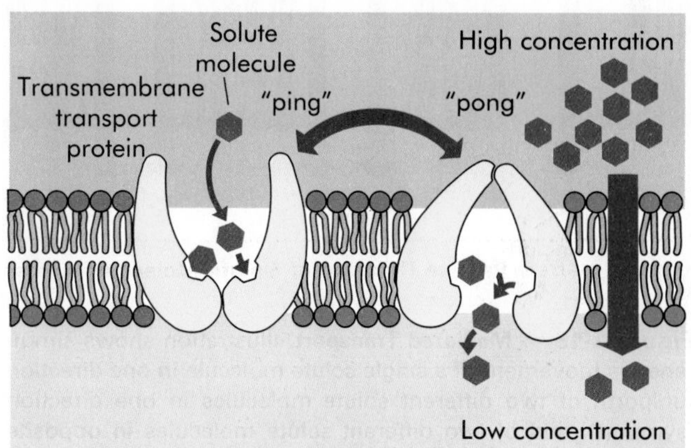

Figure 1-16 ■ Conformational-change Model of Mediated Transport (Facilitated Diffusion). The transporter protein has two states, "ping" and "pong." In the ping state, sites for molecules of a specific solute are exposed on the outside of the bilayer. In the pong state, the sites are exposed to the inner side of the bilayer.

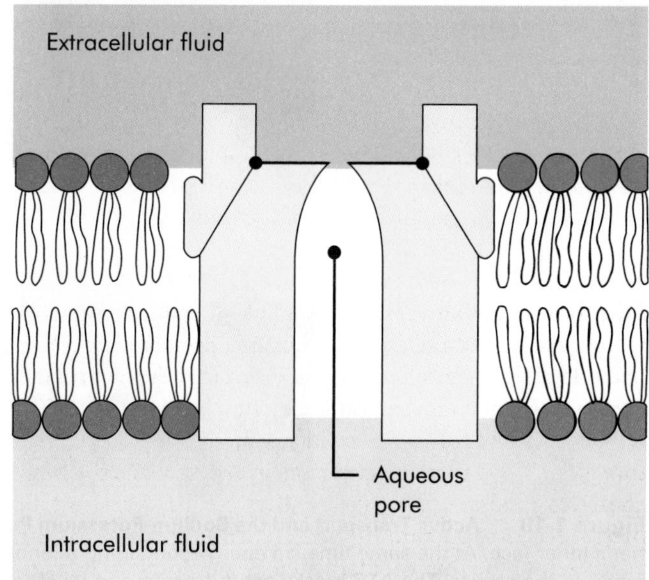

Figure 1-17 ■ Channel Mode of Mediated Transport (Facilitated Diffusion). A channel protein forms a water-filled pore across the bilayer through which specific ions can diffuse.

are responsible for the electrical excitability of nerve and muscle cells and play a critical role in the membrane potential.

Mediated transport systems can move solute molecules singly or two at a time. Two molecules can be moved simultaneously in one direction (a process called **symport**) or in opposite directions (called **antiport**), or a single molecule can be moved in one direction (called **uniport**) (Figure 1-18).

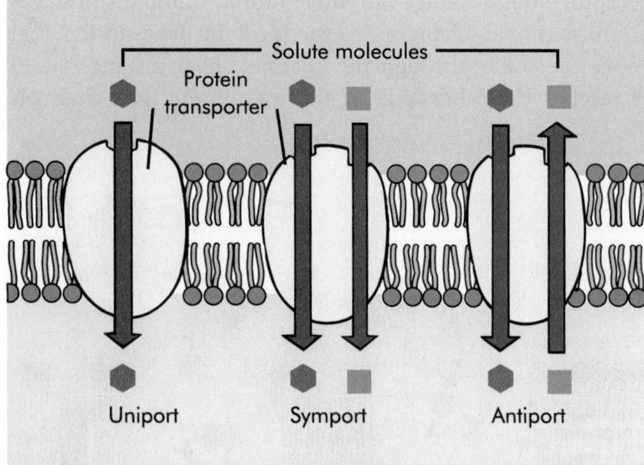

Figure 1-18 ■ **Mediated Transport.** Illustration shows simultaneous movement of a single solute molecule in one direction (uniport), of two different solute molecules in one direction (symport), and of two different solute molecules in opposite directions (antiport).

In **passive mediated transport,** or **facilitated diffusion,** the protein transporter moves solute molecules through cellular membranes without expending metabolic energy. The direction of movement is the same as in simple diffusion—down the concentration gradient. A well-known passive transport system is that for glucose in erythrocytes (red blood cells). Glucose is transported by a uniport mechanism and demonstrates saturation kinetics—that is, the transport system is saturated when all the glucose-specific receptors on the membrane are occupied and operating at their maximal capacity.

In **active mediated transport,** or active transport, the protein transporter moves molecules against, or up, the concentration gradient. Unlike passive mediated transport, active mediated transport requires the expenditure of energy. Many, but not all, active mediated transport systems, or pumps, have ATP as their primary energy source. Some use the electrochemical gradient of Na^+ across the membrane (Figure 1-19). Energy in the form of ATP, however, is required for activation of the Na^+ gradient.

A "carrier" mechanism in the plasma membrane mediates the transport of ions and nutrients. The best-known pump is the $Na^+ + K^+$–dependent ATPase pump. It continuously regulates the cells' volume by controlling leaks through pores or protein channels and maintaining the ionic concentration gradients needed for cellular excitation and membrane conductivity (see p. 22). The maintenance of intracellular K^+ concentrations is required also for enzyme activity, including enzymes involved in protein synthesis.

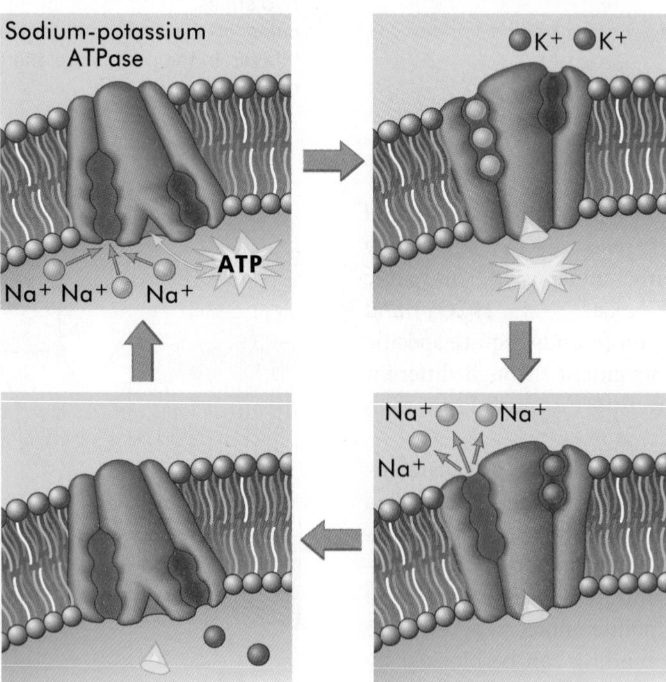

Figure 1-19 ■ **Active Transport and the Sodium-Potassium Pump.** Three sodium (Na^+) ions bind to sodium-binding sites on the carrier's inner face. At the same time, an energy-containing adenosine triphosphate (ATP) molecule produced by the cell's mitochondria binds to the carrier. The ATP breaks apart, transferring its stored energy to the carrier. The carrier then changes shape, releases the three Na^+ ions to the outside of the cell, and attracts two potassium (K^+) ions to its potassium-binding sites. The carrier then returns to its original shape, releasing the two K^+ ions and the remnant of the ATP molecule to the inside of the cell. The carrier is now ready for another pumping cycle. (From Thibodeau GA, Patton KT: *Anatomy & physiology,* ed 6, St Louis, 2007, Mosby.)

Active transport of Na^+ and K^+

The active transport system for Na^+ and K^+ is found in virtually all mammalian cells. The Na^+, K^+ antiport system (i.e., Na^+ moving out of and K^+ moving into the cell) uses the direct energy of ATP to move these cations. The transporter protein is ATPase, which requires Na^+, K^+, and magnesium (Mg^{++}) ions. The concentration of ATPase in plasma membranes is directly related to Na^+, K^+ transport activity. Approximately 60% to 70% of the ATP synthesized by cells, especially muscle and nerve cells, is used to maintain the Na^+, K^+ transport system. Excitable tissues have a high concentration of Na^+, K^+ ATPase, as do other tissues that transport significant amounts of Na^+. For every ATP molecule hydrolyzed, three molecules of Na^+ are transported out of the cell, whereas only two molecules of K^+ move into the cell. The process leads to an electrical potential and is called *electrogenic*, with the inside of the cell more negative than the outside. Although the exact mechanism for this transport is uncertain, it is possible that ATPase induces the transporter protein to undergo several conformational changes, causing Na^+ and K^+ to move short distances (see Figure 1-19). The conformational change lowers the affinity for Na^+ and K^+ to the ATPase transporter, resulting in the release of the cations after transport.

Table 1-4 summarizes the major mechanisms of transport through pores and protein transporters in the plasma membranes. Many disease states are caused or manifested by loss of these membrane transport systems.

Transport by Vesicle Formation

Endocytosis and exocytosis

The active transport mechanisms by which the cells move large proteins, polynucleotides, or polysaccharides (macromolecules) across the plasma membrane are very different from those that mediate small solute and ion transport. Transport of macromolecules involves the sequential formation and fusion of membrane-bound vesicles.

In **endocytosis,** a section of the plasma membrane enfolds substances from outside the cell, invaginates (folds inward), and separates from the plasma membrane, forming a vesicle that moves into the cell (Figure 1-20, *A*). Two types of endocytosis are designated based on the size of the vesicle formed. **Pinocytosis** (cell drinking) involves the ingestion of fluids and solute molecules through formation of small

TABLE 1-4

Major Transport Systems in Mammalian Cells

Substance Transported	Mechanism of Transport	Tissues
SUGARS		
Glucose	Passive: protein channel	Most tissues
Fructose	Active: symport with Na^+ Passive	Small intestines and renal tubular cells Intestines and liver
AMINO ACIDS		
Amino acid specific transporters	Coupled channels	Intestines, kidney, and liver
All amino acids except proline	Active: symport with Na^+	Liver
Specific amino acids	Active: group translocation Passive	Small intestine
OTHER ORGANIC MOLECULES		
Cholic acid, deoxycholic acid, and taurocholic acid	Active: symport with Na^+	Intestines
Organic anions (e.g., malate, α-ketoglutarate, glutamate)	Antiport with counter-organic anion	Mitochondria of liver cells
ATP-ADP	Antiport transport of nucleotides; can be active	Mitochondria of liver cells
INORGANIC IONS		
Na^+	Passive	Distal renal tubular cells
Na^+/H^+	Active antiport, proton pump	Proximal renal tubular cells and small intestines
Na^+/K^+	Active: ATP driven, protein channel	Plasma membrane of most cells
Ca^{++}	Active: ATP driven, antiport with Na^+	All cells, antiporter in red cells
H^+/K^+	Active	Parietal cells of gastric cells secreting H^+
Cl^-/HCO_3^- (perhaps other anions)	Mediated: antiport (anion transporter–band 3 protein)	Erythrocytes and many other cells
WATER	Osmosis passive	All tissues

Data from Alberts B et al: *Molecular biology of the cell,* ed 4, New York, 2001, Garland; Devlin TM, editor: *Textbook of biochemistry: with clinical correlations,* ed 3, New York, 1992, Wiley; Raven PH, Johnson GB: *Understanding biology,* ed 3, Dubuque, Iowa, 1995, Brown.

Note: The known transport systems are listed here; others have been proposed. Most transport systems have been studied in only a few tissues, and their sites of activity may be more limited than indicated.

ATP, Adenosine triphosphate; *ADP,* adenosine diphosphate.

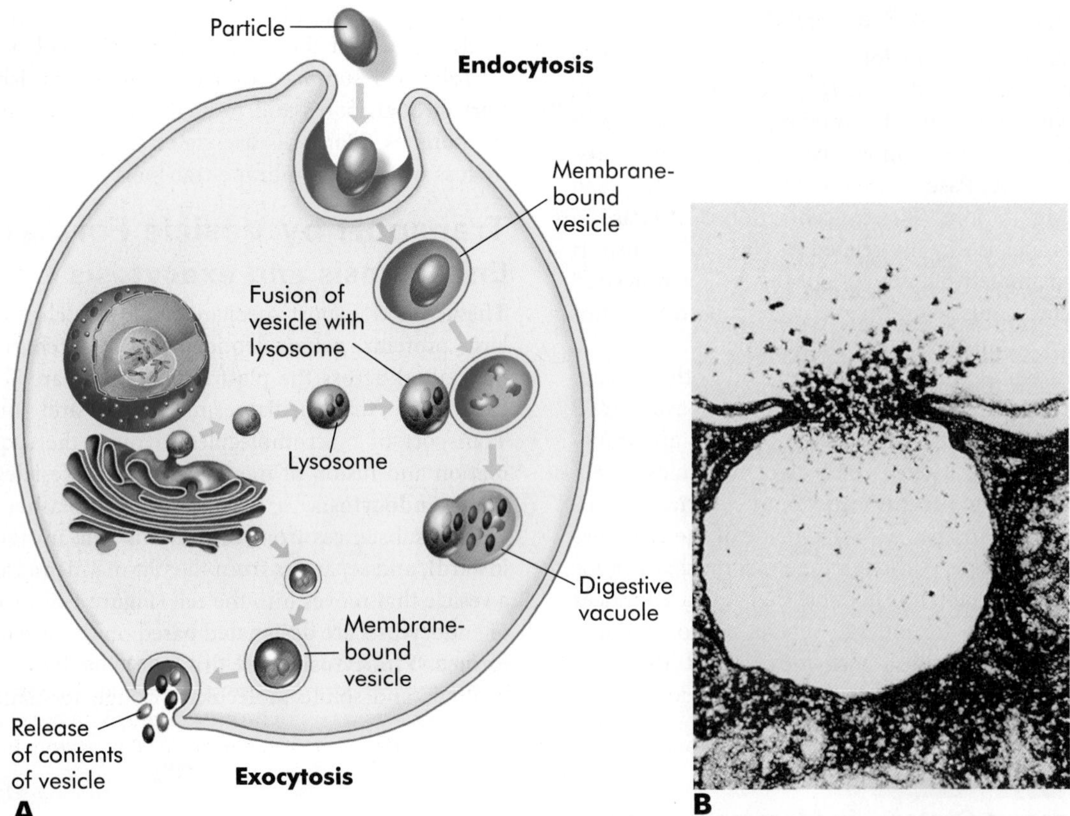

Figure 1-20 ■ **Endocytosis and Exocytosis. A,** Endocytosis and fusion with lysosome and exocytosis. **B,** Electron micrograph of exocytosis. (**B** from Raven PH, Johnson GB: *Biology,* ed 5, New York, 1999, McGraw-Hill.)

vesicles, and **phagocytosis** (cell eating) involves the ingestion of large particles, such as bacteria, through formation of large vesicles (vacuoles).

Because most cells continually ingest fluid and solutes by pinocytosis, the terms *pinocytosis* and *endocytosis* often are used interchangeably. In pinocytosis, the vesicle containing fluids, solutes, or both fuses with a lysosome, and lysosomal enzymes digest them for use by the cell. In phagocytosis, the large molecular substances are engulfed by the plasma membrane and enter the cell so that they can be isolated and destroyed by lysosomal enzymes (see Chapter 5). Substances that are not degraded by lysosomes are isolated in residual bodies and released by exocytosis. Both pinocytosis and phagocytosis require metabolic energy and often involve binding of the substance with plasma membrane receptors before membrane invagination and fusion with lysosomes in the cell.

In eukaryotic cells, secretion of macromolecules almost always occurs by exocytosis (see Figure 1-20). **Exocytosis** has two main functions: (1) replacement of portions of the plasma membrane that have been removed by endocytosis and (2) release of molecules synthesized by the cells into the extracellular matrix.

Receptor-mediated endocytosis

Ligand binding to *some* plasma membrane receptors leads to clustering, aggregation, and immobilization of the receptors in specialized areas of the membrane called **coated pits** (Figure 1-21). The pits, which are coated with bristle-like structures (clathrin), deepen and enfold (invaginate), internalizing ligand-receptor complexes and forming a coated vesicle. The clathrin coat or bristles may be responsible for trapping membrane receptors in coated pits. This internalization process, called **receptor-mediated endocytosis (ligand internalization),** is rapid and enables the cell to ingest large amounts of specific ligands without ingesting large volumes of extracellular fluid. The cellular uptake of cholesterol, for example, depends on receptor-mediated endocytosis.

Caveolae

The outer surface of the plasma membrane is dimpled with tiny flask-shaped pits (cavelike) called *caveolae.* Caveolae are also called **microdomains.** Caveolae are cholesterol-rich domains where protein caveolin are involved in several processes, including clathrin-independent endocytosis, the regulation and transport of cellular cholesterol, and cell communication.[4] Many proteins, including a variety of receptors, cluster in these tiny chambers. Cellular uptake through the opening and closing of caveolae is called **potocytosis.** Potocytosis is thought to be an uptake mechanism for a variety of small molecules, including the B vitamin, folic acid. Potocytosis is in contrast to receptor-mediated endocytosis that also transports molecules into the cell

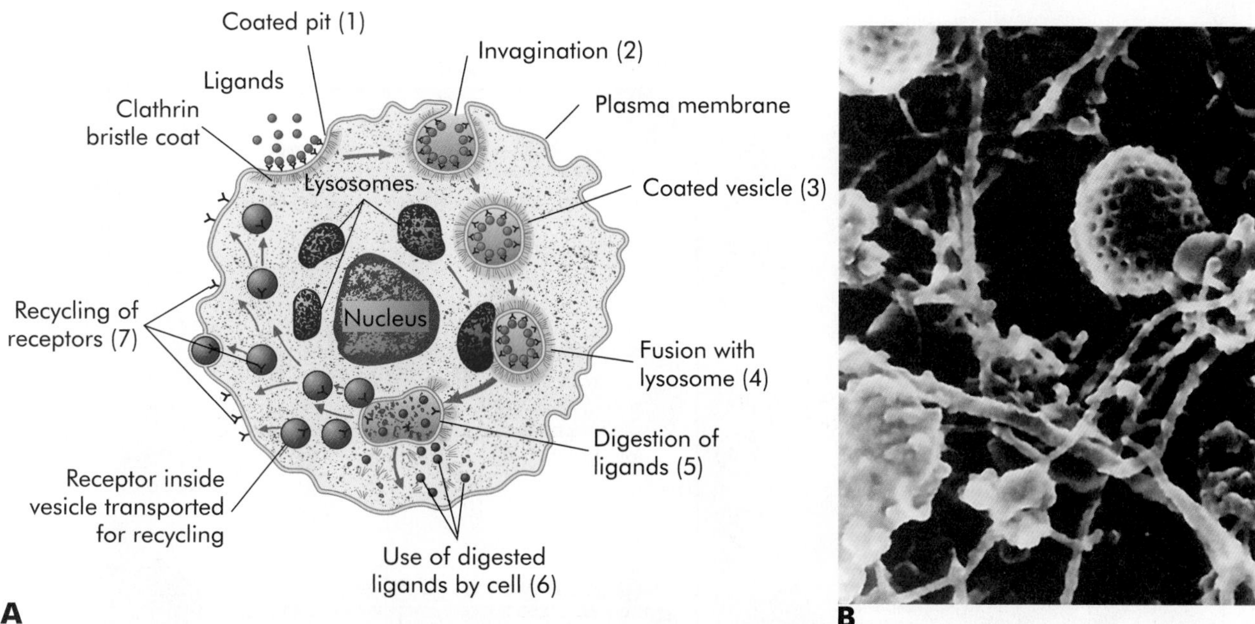

Figure 1-21 ■ **Ligand Internalization by Means of Receptor-Mediated Endocytosis. A,** The ligand attaches to its surface receptor (through the bristle coat or clathrin coat) and, through receptor-mediated endocytosis, enters the cell. The ingested material fuses with a lysosome and is processed by hydrolytic lysosomal enzymes. Processed molecules can then be transferred to other cellular components. **B,** Electron micrograph of a coated pit showing different sizes of filaments of the cytoskeleton (× 82,000). (**B** from Erlandsen SL, Magney JE: *Color atlas of histology,* St Louis, 1992, Mosby.)

but with the formation of a vesicle. In potocytosis, the caveolae are thought to remain attached to the plasma membrane.

Caveolae are not only uptake vehicles but also important sites for signal transduction, a tedious process in which extracellular chemical messages or *signals* are communicated to the cell's interior for execution (see p. 10). For example, strong evidence now exists that plasma membrane estrogen receptors localize in caveolae, and crosstalk with estradiol facilitates several intracellular biologic actions.[5]

Movement of Electrical Impulses: Membrane Potentials

All body cells are electrically polarized, with the inside of the cell more negatively charged than the outside. The difference in electrical charge, or voltage, is known as the **resting membrane potential** and is about −70 to −85 millivolts. The difference in voltage across the plasma membrane results from the differences in ionic composition of ICF and ECF. Sodium ions are more concentrated in the ECF, and potassium ions are in greater concentration in the ICF. The concentration difference is maintained by the active transport of Na^+ and K^+ (the sodium-potassium pump), which transports sodium outward and potassium inward (Figure 1-22). Because the resting plasma membrane is more permeable to K^+ than to Na^+, K^+ diffuses easily from the ICF to the ECF. Because both sodium and potassium are cations, the net result is an excess of anions inside the cell, resulting in the resting membrane potential.

Nerve and muscle cells are excitable and can change their resting membrane potential in response to electrochemical stimuli. Changes in resting membrane potential convey messages from cell to cell. When a nerve or muscle cell receives a stimulus that exceeds the membrane threshold value, a rapid change occurs in the resting membrane potential, known as the **action potential.** The action potential carries signals along the nerve or muscle cell and conveys information from one cell to another. (Nerve impulses are described in Chapter 12.) When a resting cell is stimulated through voltage-regulated channels, the cell membranes become more permeable to sodium, so a net movement of sodium into the cell occurs and the membrane potential decreases, or moves forward, from a negative value (in millivolts) to zero. This decrease is known as **depolarization.** The depolarized cell is more positively charged, and its polarity is neutralized.

To generate an action potential and the resulting depolarization, the **threshold potential** must be reached. Generally this occurs when the cell has depolarized by 15 to 20 millivolts. When the threshold is reached, the cell will continue to depolarize with no further stimulation. The sodium gates open, and sodium rushes into the cell, causing the membrane potential to reduce to zero and then become positive (depolarization). The rapid reversal in polarity results in the action potential.

During **repolarization,** the negative polarity of the resting membrane potential is reestablished. As the voltage-gated sodium channels begin to close, voltage-gated potassium

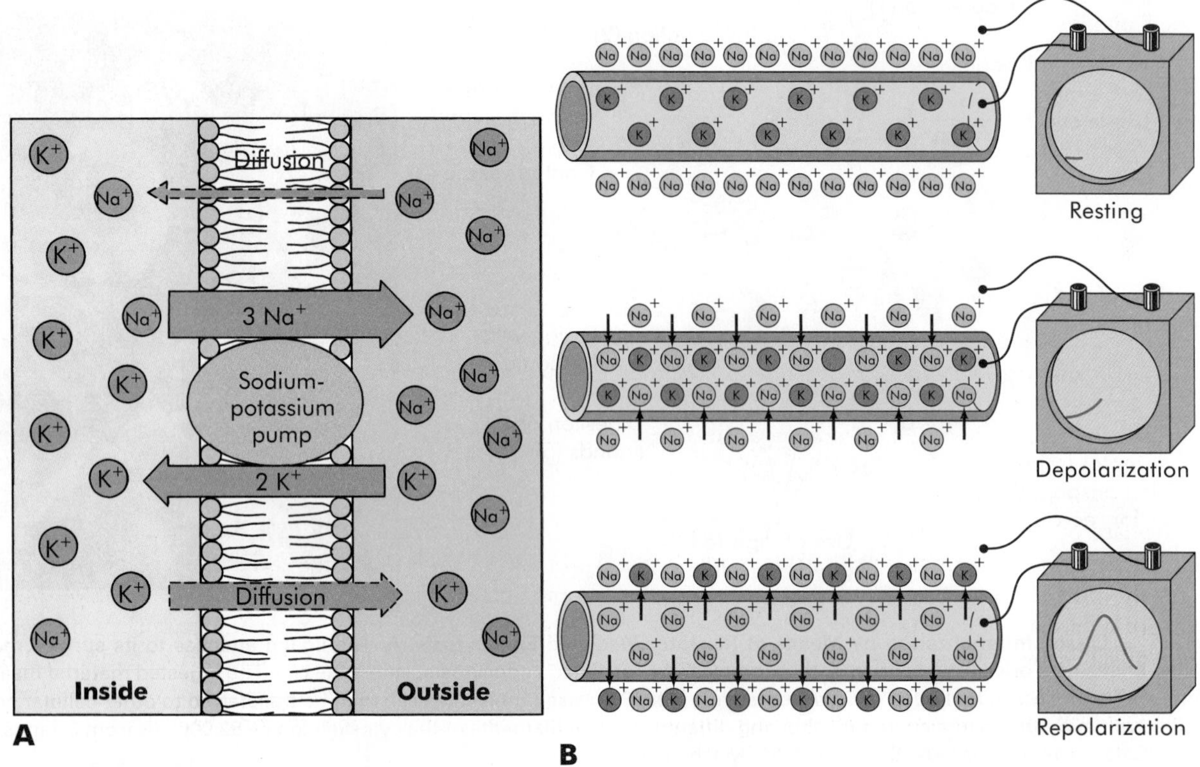

Figure 1-22 ■ **Sodium-Potassium Pump and Propagation of an Action Potential. A,** Concentration difference of sodium (Na^+) and potassium (K^+) intracellularly and extracellularly. The direction of active transport by the sodium-potassium pump is also shown. **B,** The top diagram represents the polarized state of a neuronal membrane when at rest. The lower diagrams represent changes in sodium and potassium membrane permeabilities with depolarization and repolarization. (From Thibodeau GA, Patton KT: *Anatomy & physiology,* ed 6, St Louis, 2007, Mosby.)

channels open. Membrane permeability to sodium decreases, and potassium permeability increases, so potassium ions leave the cell. The sodium gates close, and with the loss of potassium, the membrane potential becomes more negative. The Na^+, K^+ pump then returns the membrane to the resting potential by pumping potassium back into the cell and sodium out of the cell.

During most of the action potential, the plasma membrane cannot respond to an additional stimulus. This time is known as the **absolute refractory period** and is related to changes in permeability to sodium. During the latter phase of the action potential, when permeability to potassium increases, a stronger-than-normal stimulus can evoke an action potential known as the **relative refractory period.**

When the membrane potential is more negative than normal, the cell is in a **hyperpolarized** (less excitable) state. A stronger-than-normal stimulus is then required to reach the threshold potential and generate an action potential. When the membrane potential is more positive than normal, the cell is in a **hypopolarized** (more excitable than normal) state and a weaker-than-normal stimulus is required to reach the threshold potential. Changes in the intracellular and extracellular concentration of ions or a change in membrane permeability can cause these alterations in membrane excitability.

QUICK CHECK 1-3

1. Identify examples of molecules transported in one direction (symport) and opposite directions (antiport).
2. If oxygen is no longer available to make ATP, what happens to the transport of Na^+?
3. Why are caveolae important to the cell?

CELLULAR REPRODUCTION: THE CELL CYCLE

Cells of the human body are subject to wear and tear, and most do not last for the lifetime of the individual. In most tissues, new cells are created as fast as old cells die. Cellular reproduction is therefore necessary for the maintenance of life. Reproduction of gametes (sperm and egg cells) occurs through a process called *meiosis,* described in Chapter 2. The reproduction, or division, of other body cells (somatic cells) involves two sequential phases: **mitosis,** or nuclear division, and **cytokinesis,** or cytoplasmic division. Before a cell can divide, however, it must double its mass and duplicate all its contents. Separation for division occurs during the growth phase, called **interphase.** The alternation between mitosis and interphase in all tissues with cellular turnover is known as the **cell cycle.**

The four designated phases of the cell cycle (Figure 1-23) are (1) the **S phase** (S = synthesis), in which DNA is synthesized in the cell nucleus; (2) the **G_2 phase** (G = gap), in which RNA and protein synthesis occurs, namely, the period between the completion of DNA synthesis and the next phase (M); (3) the **M phase** (M = mitosis), which includes both nuclear and cytoplasmic division; and (4) the **G_1 phase,** which is the period between the M phase and the start of DNA synthesis.

Phases of Mitosis and Cytokinesis

Interphase (the G_1, S, and G_2 phases) is the longest phase of the cell cycle. During interphase, the chromatin consists of very long, slender rods jumbled together in the nucleus. Late in interphase, strands of **chromatin** (the substance that gives the nucleus its granular appearance) begin to coil, causing shortening and thickening.

The M phase of the cell cycle, mitosis and cytokinesis, begins with **prophase,** the first appearance of chromosomes. As the phase proceeds, each chromosome is seen as two identical halves called **chromatids,** which lie together and are attached by a spindle site called a **centromere.** (The two chromatids of each chromosome, which are genetically identical, are sometimes called sister chromatids.) The nuclear membrane, which surrounds the nucleus, disappears. **Spindle fibers** are microtubules formed in the cytoplasm. They radiate from two centrioles located at opposite poles of the cell and pull the chromosomes to opposite sides of the cell, beginning **metaphase.** Next, the centromeres become aligned in the middle of the spindle, which is called the **equatorial plate** (or **metaphase plate**) of the cell. In this stage, chromosomes are easiest to observe microscopically because they are highly condensed and arranged in a relatively organized fashion.

Anaphase begins when the centromeres split and the sister chromatids are pulled apart. The spindle fibers shorten, causing the sister chromatids to be pulled, centromere first, toward opposite sides of the cell. When the sister chromatids are separated, each is considered to be a chromosome. Thus, the cell has 92 chromosomes during this stage. By the end of anaphase, there are 46 chromosomes lying at each side of the cell. Barring mitotic errors, each of the two groups of 46 chromosomes is identical to the original 46 chromosomes present at the start of the cell cycle.

During **telophase,** the final stage, a new nuclear membrane is formed around each group of 46 chromosomes, the spindle fibers disappear, and the chromosomes begin to uncoil. Cytokinesis causes the cytoplasm to divide into roughly equal parts during this phase. At the end of telophase, two identical diploid cells, called **daughter cells,** have been formed from the original cell.

Rates of Cellular Division

Although the complete cell cycle lasts 12 to 24 hours, generally about 1 hour is required for the four stages of mitosis

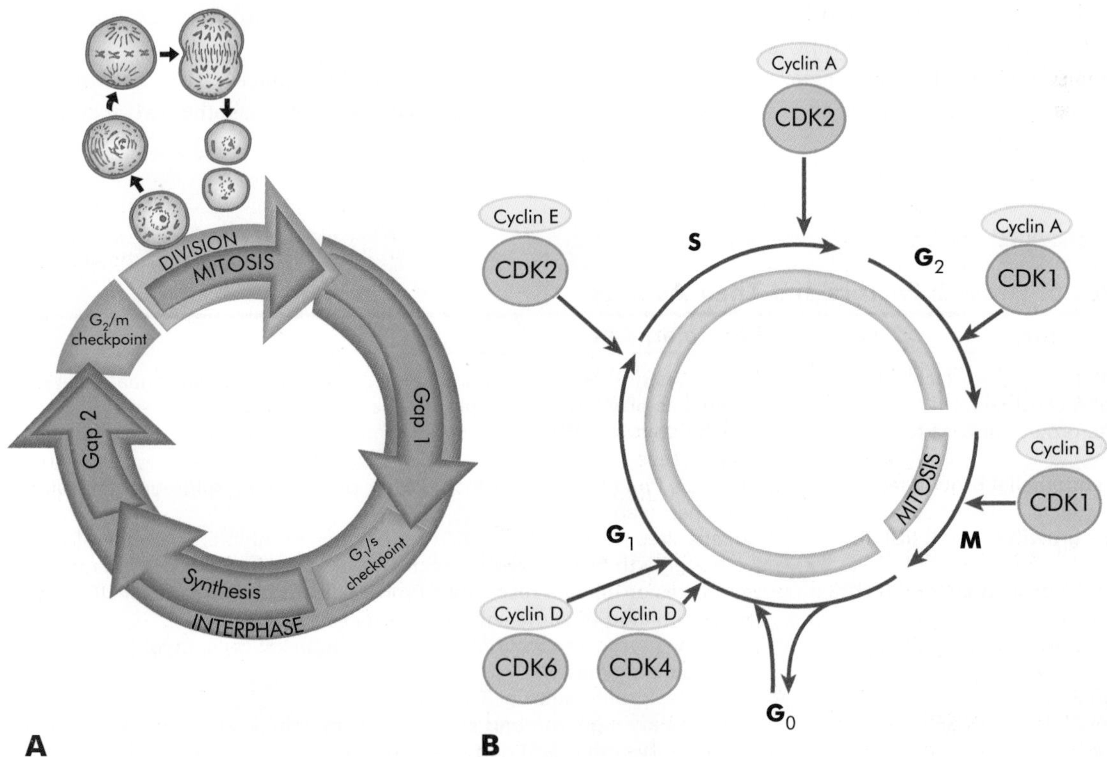

Figure 1-23 ■ **Interphase and the Phases of Mitosis. A,** The G_1/S checkpoint is to "check" for cell size, nutrients, growth factors, and DNA damage. The G_0 is the resting state. The G_2/M checkpoint checks for cell size and DNA replication. **B,** The orderly progression through the phases of the cell cycle is regulated by *cyclins* (so called because levels rise and fall) and *cyclin-dependent protein kinases* (CdKs) and their inhibitors. When cyclins are complexed with CdKs, it triggers cell cycle events.

and cytokinesis. All types of cells undergo mitosis during formation of the embryo, but many adult cells, such as nerve cells, lens cells of the eye, and muscle cells, lose their ability to replicate and divide. The cells of other tissues, particularly epithelial cells (e.g., of the intestine, lung, skin), divide continuously and rapidly, completing the entire cell cycle in less than 10 hours.

The difference between cells that divide slowly and cells that divide rapidly is the length of time spent in the G_1 phase of the cell cycle. Once the S phase begins, however, progression through mitosis takes a relatively constant amount of time.

The mechanisms that control cell division depend on genes and protein growth factors. Protein growth factors govern the proliferation of different cell types. Individual cells are members of a complex cellular society in which survival of the entire organism is key—not survival or proliferation of just the individual cells. When a need arises for new cells, as in repair of injured cells, previously nondividing cells must be triggered rapidly to reenter the cell cycle. With continual wear and tear, the cell birth rate and the cell death rate must be kept in balance.

Growth Factors

Growth factors, also called **cytokines,** are peptides (protein fractions) that transmit signals within and between cells. They have a major role in the regulation of tissue growth and development (Table 1-5). Having nutrients is not enough for a cell to proliferate; it must also receive stimulatory chemical signals (growth factors) from other cells, usually its neighbors or the surrounding supporting tissue called **stroma** (Figure 1-24). These signals act to overcome intracellular braking mechanisms that tend to restrain cell growth and block progress through the cell cycle (see Figure 1-24).

An example of a brake that regulates cell proliferation is the **retinoblastoma (Rb) protein,** first identified through studies of a rare childhood eye tumor called *retinoblastoma,* in which the Rb protein is missing or defective (see p. 25). The Rb protein is abundant in the nucleus of all vertebrate cells. It binds to gene regulatory proteins, preventing them from stimulating the transcription of genes required for cell proliferation (see Figure 1-24). Extracellular signals, such as growth factors, activate intracellular signaling pathways that inactivate the Rb protein, leading to cell proliferation.

Different types of cells require different growth factors; for example, **platelet-derived growth factor (PDGF)** stimulates the production of connective tissue cells. Table 1-5 summarizes the most significant growth factors. Evidence shows that some growth factors also regulate other cell processes, such as cellular differentiation. In addition to growth factors that stimulate cellular processes, there are factors that inhibit these processes; these factors are not well understood. Cells that are starved of growth factors come to a halt after mitosis and enter the **arrested (resting) (G0)** state of the cell cycle (see p. 28 for cell cycle).[1]

TISSUES

Cells of one or more types are organized into tissues, and different types of tissues compose organs. Finally, organs are integrated to perform complex functions as tracts or systems.

All cells are in contact with a network of extracellular macromolecules known as the **extracellular matrix** (see

TABLE 1-5

Examples of Growth Factors and Their Actions

Growth Factor	Physiologic Actions
Platelet-derived growth factor (PDGF)	Stimulates proliferation of connective tissue cells and neuroglial cells
Epidermal growth factor (EGF)	Stimulates proliferation of epidermal cells and other cell types
Insulin-like growth factor I (IGF-I)	Collaborates with PDGF and EGF; stimulates proliferation of fat cells and connective tissue cells
Vascular endothelial growth factor	Mediates functions of endothelial cells; proliferation, migration, invasion, survival, and permeability
Insulin-like growth factor II (IGF-II)	Collaborates with PDGF and EGF; stimulates or inhibits response of most cells to other growth factors; regulates differentiation of some cell types (e.g., cartilage)
Transforming growth factor β (TGBβ; multiple subtypes)	Stimulates or inhibits response of most cells to other growth factors; regulates differentiation of some cell types (e.g., cartilage)
Fibroblast growth factor (FGF; multiple subtypes)	Stimulates proliferation of fibroblasts, endothelial cells, myoblasts, and other multiple subtypes
Interleukin-2 (IL-2)	Stimulates proliferation of T lymphocytes
Nerve growth factor (NGF)	Promotes axon growth and survival of sympathetic and some sensory and central nervous system (CNS) neurons
Hemopoietic cell growth factors (IL-3, GM-CSF, G-CSF, erythropoietin)	Promote proliferation of blood cells

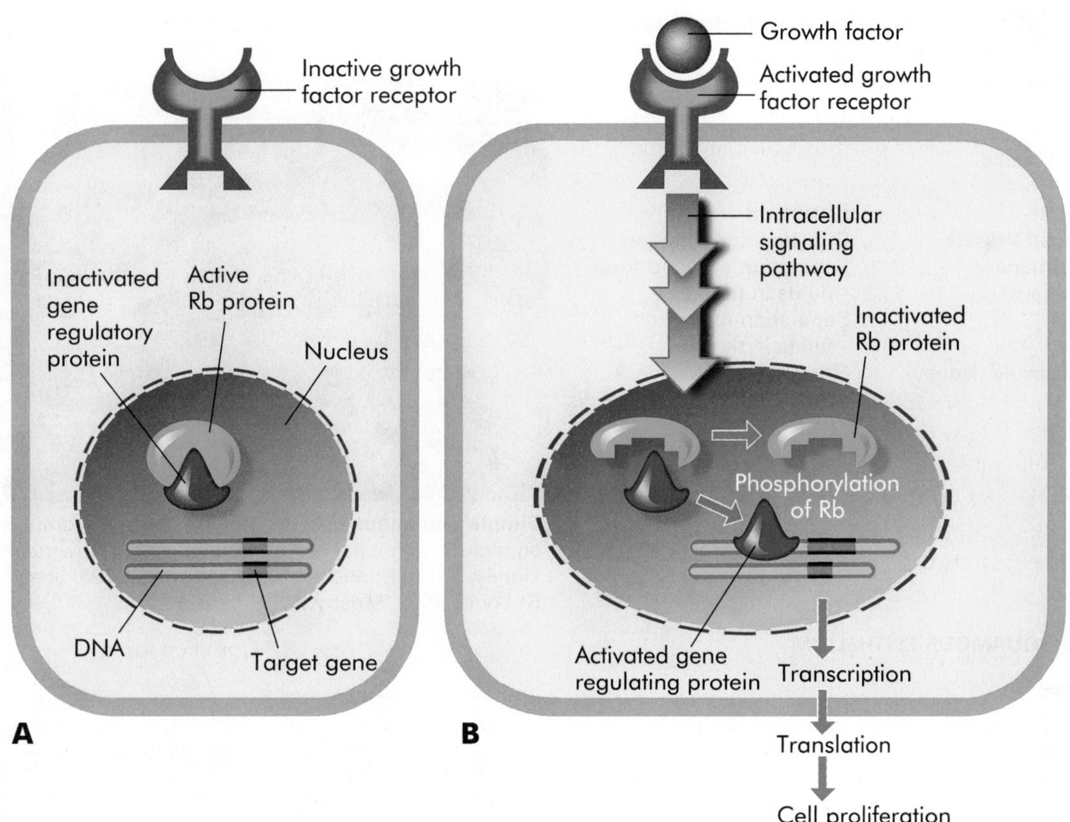

Figure 1-24 ■ **How Growth Factors Stimulate Cell Proliferation. A,** Resting cell. With the absence of growth factors, the retinoblastoma (Rb) protein is not phosphorylated; thus, it holds the gene regulatory proteins in an inactive state. The gene regulatory proteins are required to stimulate the transcription of genes needed for cell proliferation. **B,** Proliferating cell. Growth factors bind to the cell surface receptors and activate intracellular signaling pathways leading to activation of intracellular proteins. These intracellular proteins phosphorylate and thereby inactivate the Rb protein. The gene regulatory proteins are now free to activate the transcription of genes, leading to cell proliferation.

p. 8). This matrix not only holds cells and tissues together but also provides an organized latticework within which cells can migrate and interact with one another.

Tissue Formation

The process by which differentiated cells create tissues and organs is called **pattern formation.**[6] To form tissues, cells must exhibit intercellular recognition and communication, adhesion, and memory. Specialized cells sense their environment through signals, such as growth factors, from other cells. This type of communication ensures that new cells are produced only when and where they are required. Different cell types have different adhesion molecules in their plasma membranes, sticking selectively to other cells of the same type. They can also adhere to extracellular matrix components. Cells have memory because of specialized patterns of gene expression evoked by signals that acted during embryonic development. Memory allows cells to autonomously preserve their distinctive character and pass it on to their progeny.[1]

Types of Tissues

The four basic types of tissues are nerve, epithelial, connective, and muscle. The structure and function of these four types underlie the structure and function of each organ system. Neural tissue is composed of highly specialized cells called *neurons,* which receive and transmit electrical impulses rapidly across junctions called *synapses* (see Figure 12-1). Different types of neurons have special characteristics that depend on their distribution and function within the nervous system. Epithelial, connective, and muscle tissues are summarized in Boxes 1-1 to 1-3.

✔ QUICK CHECK 1-4

1. Why is cell cycle communication so important?
2. Discuss the five types of intracellular communication.
3. Why is cell-to-cell adhesion so important?
4. Why is the extracellular matrix important for tissue cells?

BOX 1-1 Characteristics of Epithelial Tissues

SIMPLE SQUAMOUS EPITHELIUM

Structure
Single layer of cells

Location	Function
Lining of blood vessels	Diffusion and filtration
Lining of pulmonary alveoli (air sacs)	Separation of blood from fluids in tissues Separation of air from fluids in tissues
Bowman's capsule (kidney)	Filtration of substances from blood, forming urine

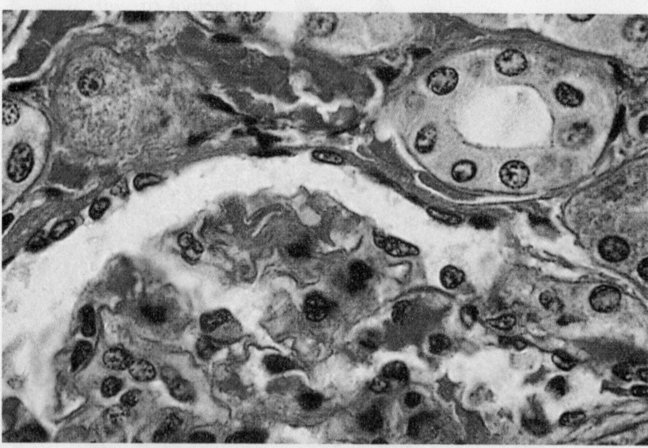

Simple Squamous Epithelial Cell. Photomicrograph of simple squamous epithelial cell in parietal wall of Bowman's capsule in kidney. (From Erlandsen SL, Magney JE: *Color atlas of histology,* St Louis, 1992, Mosby.)

STRATIFIED SQUAMOUS EPITHELIUM

Structure
Two or more layers, depending on location, with cells closest to basement membrane tending to be cuboidal

Location	Function
Epidermis of skin	Protection and secretion
Linings of mouth, pharynx, esophagus, anus	

Cornified layer
Basement membrane
Basal cells
Dermis

Cornified Stratified Squamous Epithelium. Diagram of stratified squamous epithelium of the skin. (Copyright Ed Reschke. Used with permission.)

TRANSITIONAL EPITHELIUM

Structure
Vary in shape from cuboidal to squamous depending on whether basal cells of the bladder are columnar or are composed of many layers; when the bladder is full and stretched, the cells flatten and stretch like squamous cells

Location	Function
Linings of urinary bladder and other hollow structures	Stretching that permits expansion of hollow organs

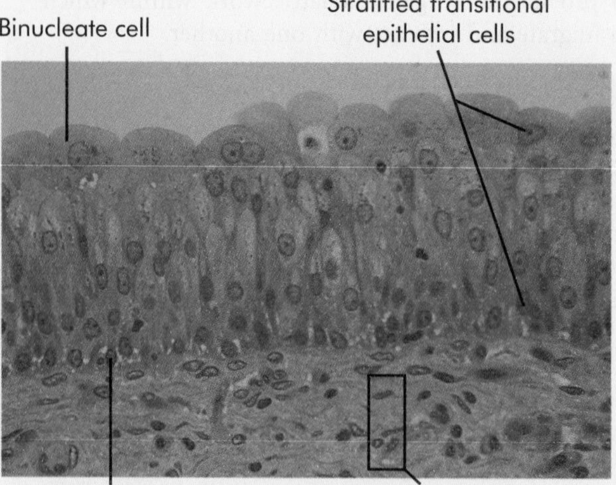

Stratified Squamous Transitional Epithelium. Photomicrograph of stratified squamous transitional epithelium of the urinary bladder. (Copyright Ed Reschke. Used with permission.)

(Continued)

BOX 1-1 Characteristics of Epithelial Tissues—Cont'd

SIMPLE CUBOIDAL EPITHELIUM

Structure
Simple cuboidal cells; rarely stratified (layered)

Location	Function
Glands (e.g., thyroid, sweat, salivary) Parts of kidney tubule and outer covering of the ovary	Secretion

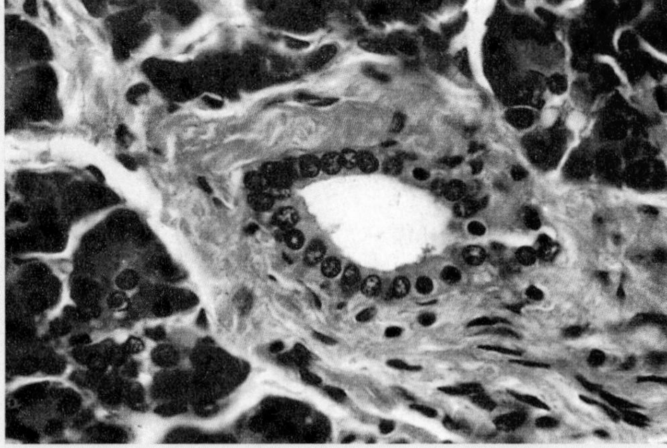

Simple Cuboidal Epithelium. Photomicrograph of simple cuboidal epithelium of the pancreatic duct. (From Erlandsen SL, Magney JE: *Color atlas of histology,* St Louis, 1992, Mosby.)

SIMPLE COLUMNAR EPITHELIUM

Structure
Large amounts of cytoplasm and cellular organelles

Location	Function
Lining of digestive tube Ducts of many glands	Secretion and absorption from stomach to anus

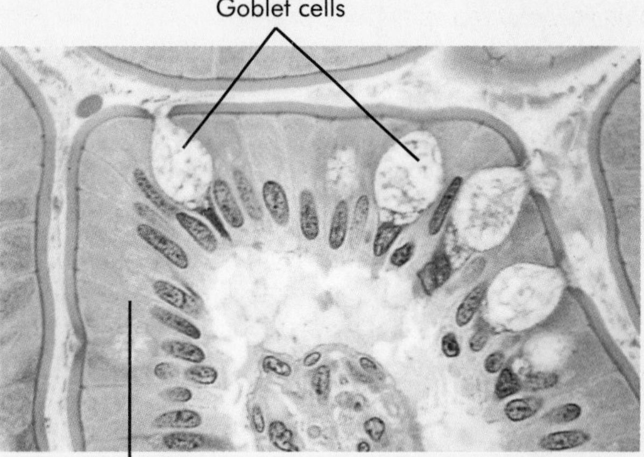

Simple Columnar Epithelium. Photomicrograph of simple columnar epithelium. (Copyright Ed Reschke. Used with permission.)

CILIATED SIMPLE COLUMNAR EPITHELIUM

Structure
Same as simple columnar epithelium but ciliated

Location	Function
Linings of bronchi of the lungs, nasal cavity, and oviducts	Secretion, absorption, and propulsion of fluids and particles

STRATIFIED COLUMNAR EPITHELIUM

Structure
Small and rounded basement membrane (columnar cells do not touch basement membrane)

Location	Function
Linings of epiglottis, part of pharynx, anus, and male urethra	Protection

PSEUDOSTRATIFIED CILIATED COLUMNAR EPITHELIUM

Structure
All cells in contact with basement membrane
Nuclei found at different levels within the cell, giving stratified appearance
Free surface often ciliated

Location	Function
Linings of large ducts of some glands (parotid, salivary), male urethra, respiratory passages, and eustachian tubes of ears	Transport of substances

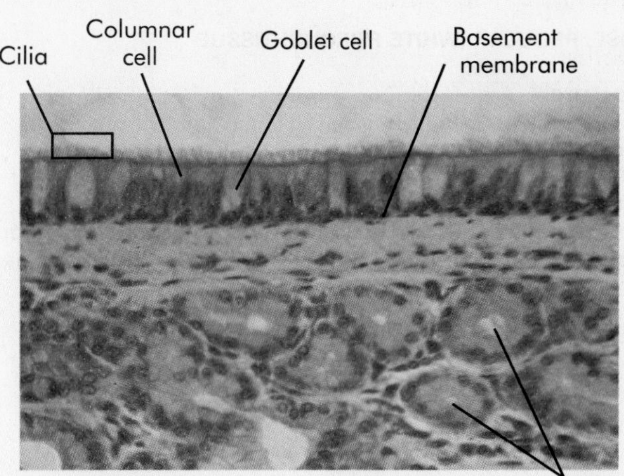

Pseudostratified Ciliated Columnar Epithelium. Photomicrograph of pseudostratified ciliated columnar epithelium of the trachea. (Copyright Robert L. Calentine. Used with permission.)

BOX 1-2 Connective Tissues

LOOSE OR AREOLAR TISSUE

Structure

Unorganized; spaces between fibers
Most fibers collagenous, some elastic and reticular
Includes many types of cells (fibroblasts and macrophages most common) and large amount of intercellular fluid

Location and Function

Attaches skin to underlying tissue, holds organs in place by filling the spaces between them, supports blood vessels
Intercellular fluid transports nutrients and waste products
Fluid accumulation causes swelling (edema)

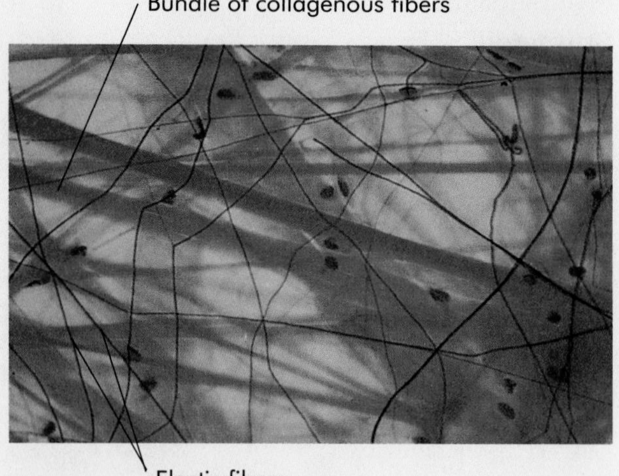

Loose Areolar Connective Tissue. (Copyright Ed Reschke. Used with permission.)

DENSE, IRREGULAR TISSUE

Structure

Dense, compact, and areolar tissue, with fewer cells and more, closely woven collagenous fibers than in loose tissue

Location and Function

Dermis layer of the skin; acts as protective barrier

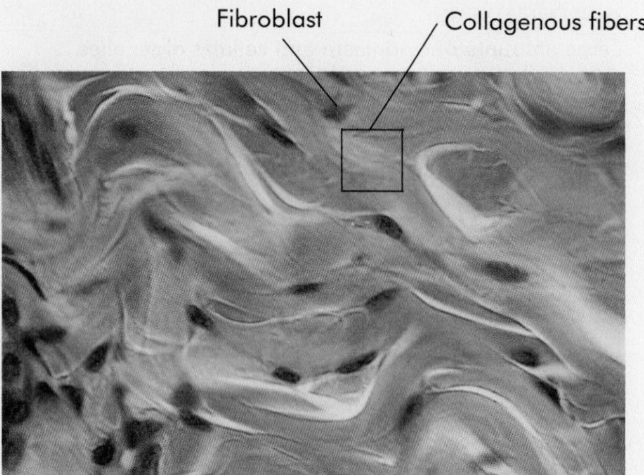

Dense, Irregular Connective Tissue. (Copyright Ed Reschke. Used with permission.)

DENSE, REGULAR (WHITE FIBROUS) TISSUE

Structure

Collagenous fibers and some elastic fibers, tightly packed into parallel bundles, with only fibroblast cells

Location and Function

Forms strong tendons of muscle, ligaments of joints, some fibrous membranes, and fascia that surrounds the organs and muscles

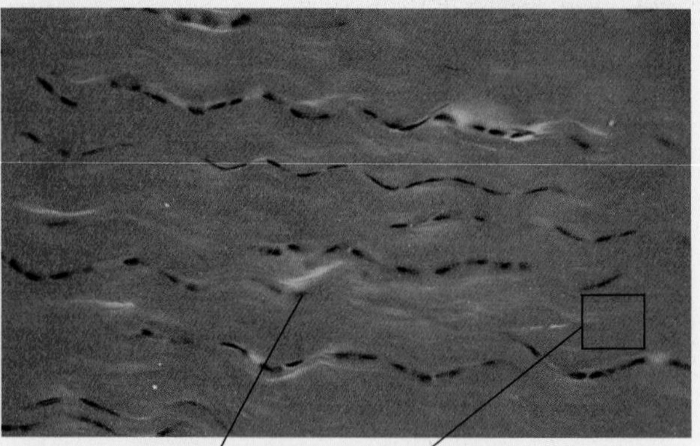

Dense, Regular (White Fibrous) Connective Tissue. (Copyright Phototake. Used with permission).

(Continued)

BOX 1-2 Connective Tissues—Cont'd

ELASTIC TISSUE

Structure

Elastic fibers, some collagenous fibers, fibroblasts

Location and Function

Lends strength and elasticity to walls of arteries, trachea, vocal chords, and other structures

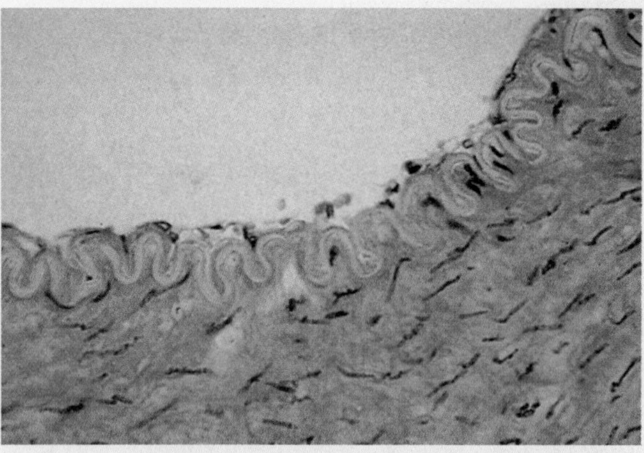

Elastic Connective Tissue. (From Erlandsen SL, Magney JE: *Color atlas of histology,* St Louis, 1992, Mosby.)

ADIPOSE TISSUE

Structure

Fat cells dispersed in loose tissues; each cell containing a large droplet of fat flattens nucleus and forces cytoplasm into a ring around cell's periphery

Location and Function

Stores fat, which provides padding and protection

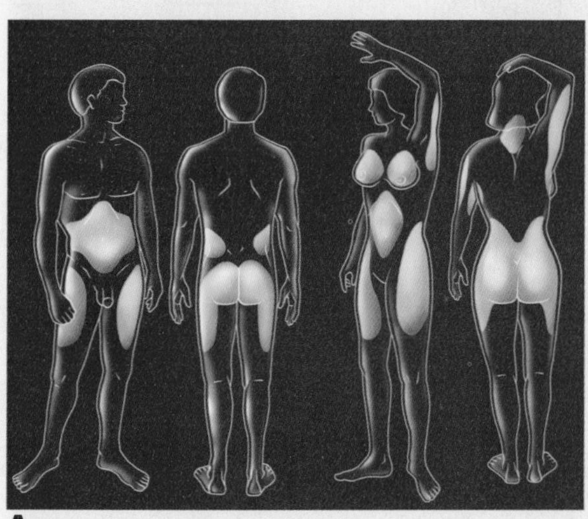

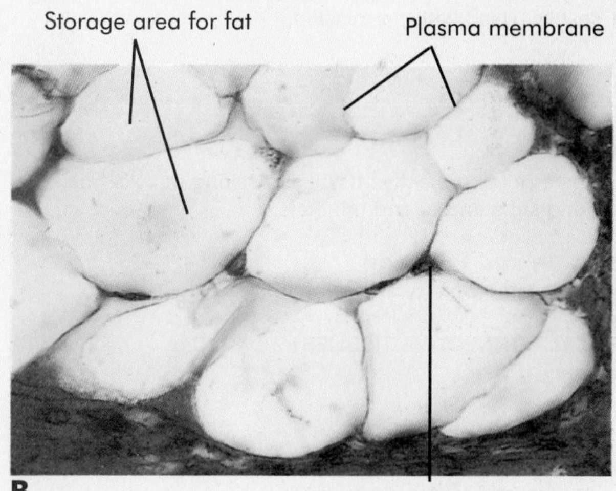

Adipose Tissue. A, Fat storage areas—distribution of fat in male and female bodies. **B,** Photomicrograph of adipose tissue. (**A** from Thibodeau GA, Patton KT: *Anatomy & physiology,* ed 6, St Louis, 2007, Mosby; **B** Copyright Ed Reschke. Used with permission.)

(Continued)

BOX 1-2 Connective Tissues—Cont'd

CARTILAGE (HYALINE, ELASTIC, FIBROUS)

Structure
Collagenous fibers embedded in a firm matrix (chondrin); no blood supply

Location and Function
Gives form, support, and flexibility to joints, trachea, nose, ear, vertebral disks, embryonic skeleton, and many internal structures

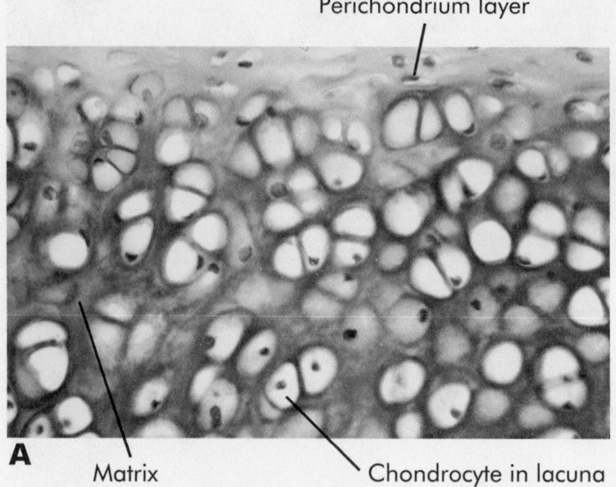

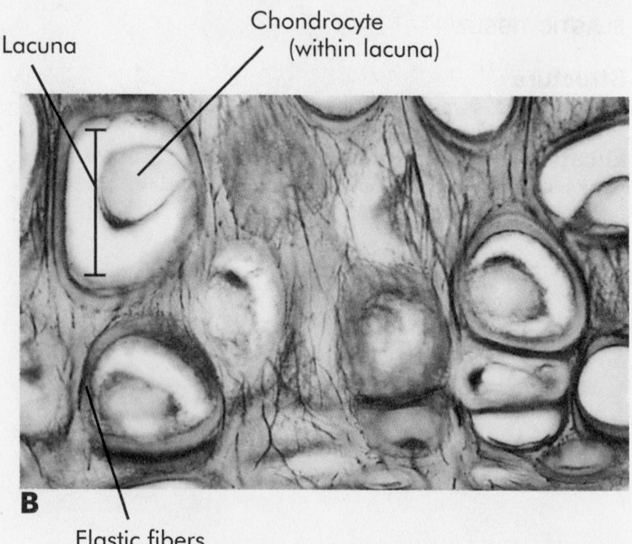

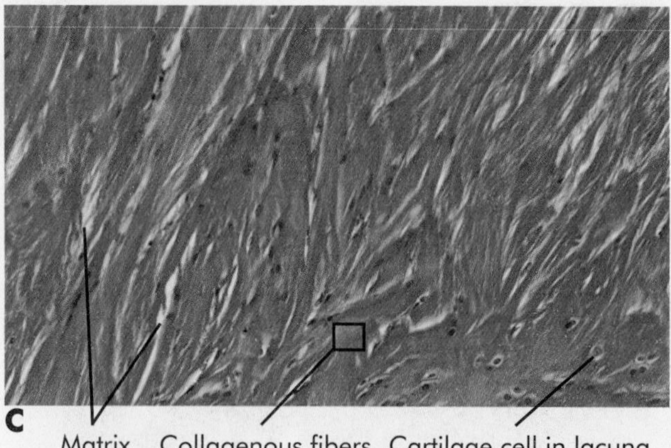

Cartilage. A, Hyaline cartilage. **B,** Elastic cartilage. **C,** Fibrous cartilage. (**A** and **C** copyright Robert L. Calentine; **B** copyright Ed Reshke. Used with permission.)

BONE

Structure
Bone is a rigid connective tissue consisting of cells, fibers, ground substances, and minerals.

Location and Function
Lends skeleton rigidity and strength

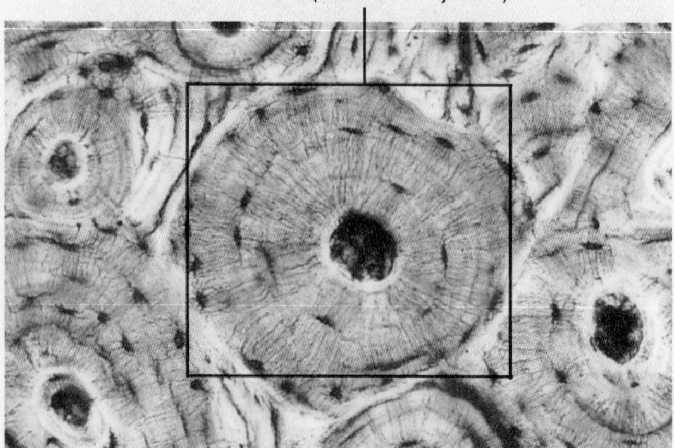

Bone. (Copyright Phototake. Used with permission.)

SPECIAL CONNECTIVE TISSUES
Plasma

Structure
Fluid

Location and Function
Serves as matrix for blood cells

Macrophages in tissue, reticuloendothelial, or macrophage system

Structure
Scattered macrophages (phagocytes) called Kupffer's cells (in liver), alveolar macrophages (in lungs), microglia (in central nervous system)

Location and Function
Facilitate inflammatory response and carry out phagocytosis in loose connective, lymphatic, digestive, medullary (bone marrow), splenic, adrenal, and pituitary tissues

BOX 1-3 Muscle Tissues

SKELETAL (STRIATED) MUSCLE

Structure Characteristics of Cells

Long, cylindrical cells that extend throughout length of muscles
Striated myofibrils (proteins)
Many nuclei on periphery

Location

Attached to bones directly or by tendons

Function

Voluntary movement of skeleton; maintenance of posture

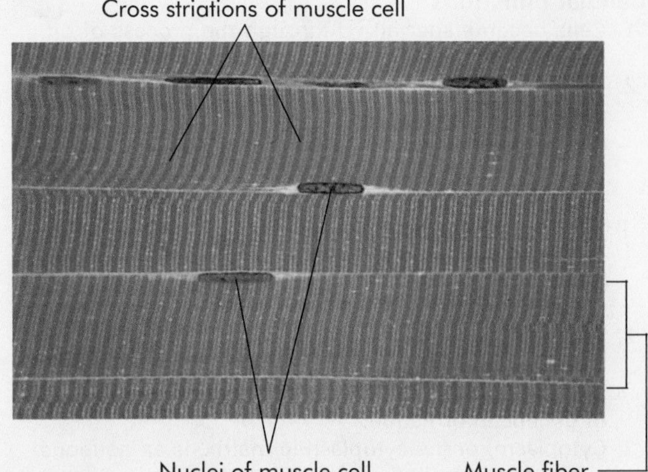

Skeletal (Striated) Muscle. (From Thibodeau GA, Patton KT: *Anatomy & physiology*, ed 6, St Louis, 2007, Mosby.

CARDIAC MUSCLE

Structure Characteristics of Cells

Branching networks throughout muscle tissue
Striated myofibrils

Location

Cells attached end-to-end at intercalated disks; tissue forms walls of heart (myocardium)

Function

Involuntary pumping action of heart

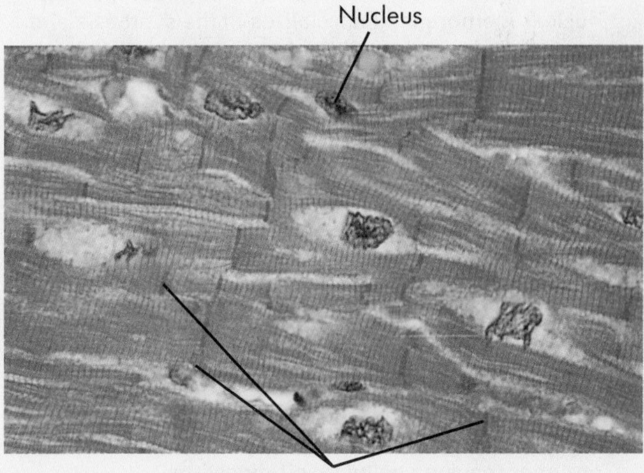

Cardiac Muscle. (Copyright Ed Reschke. Used with permission.)

SMOOTH (VISCERAL) MUSCLE

Structure Characteristics of Cells

Long spindles that taper to a point
Absence of striated myofibrils

Location

Walls of hollow internal structures, such as digestive tract and blood vessels (viscera)

Function

Voluntary and involuntary contractions that move substances through hollow structures

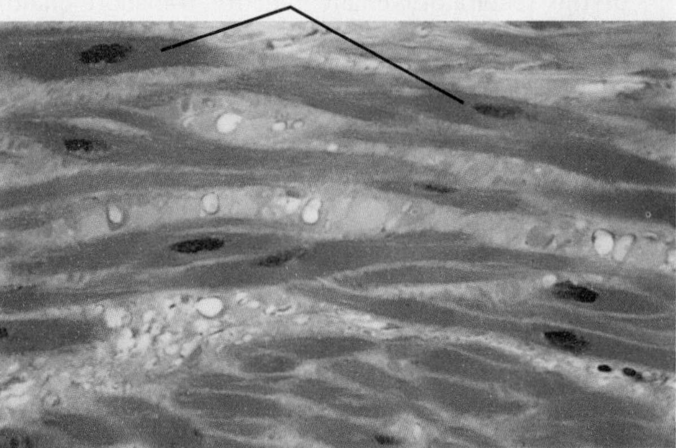

Smooth (Visceral) Muscle. (Copyright Phototake. Used with permission.)

Did You Understand?

Cellular Functions

1. Cells become specialized through the process of differentiation or maturation.
2. The eight specialized cellular functions are movement, conductivity, metabolic absorption, secretion, excretion, respiration, reproduction, and communication.

Structure and Function of Cellular Components

1. The eukaryotic cell consists of three general components: the plasma membrane, the cytoplasm, and the intracellular organelles.
2. The nucleus is the largest membrane-bound organelle and is found usually in the cell's center. The chief functions of the nucleus are cell division and control of genetic information.
3. Cytoplasm, or the cytoplasmic matrix, is an aqueous solution (cytosol) that fills the space between the nucleus and the plasma membrane.
4. The organelles are suspended in the cytoplasm and are enclosed in biologic membranes.
5. The endoplasmic reticulum is a network of tubular channels (cisternae) that extend throughout the outer nuclear membrane. It specializes in the synthesis and transport of protein and lipid components of most of the organelles.
6. The Golgi complex is a network of smooth membranes and vesicles located near the nucleus. The Golgi complex is responsible for processing and packaging proteins into secretory vesicles that break away from the Golgi complex and migrate to a variety of intracellular and extracellular destinations, including the plasma membrane.
7. Lysosomes are saclike structures that originate from the Golgi complex and contain digestive enzymes. These enzymes are responsible for digesting most cellular substances down to their basic form, such as amino acids, fatty acids, and sugars.
8. Cellular injury leads to a release of the lysosomal enzymes, causing cellular self-digestion.
9. Peroxisomes are similar to lysosomes but contain several enzymes that either produce or use hydrogen peroxide.
10. Mitochondria contain the metabolic machinery necessary for cellular energy metabolism. The enzymes of the respiratory chain (electron-transport chain), found in the inner membrane of the mitochondria, generate most of the cell's ATP.
11. The cytoskeleton is the "bone and muscle" of the cell. The internal skeleton is composed of a network of protein filaments, including microtubules and actin filaments (microfilaments).
12. The plasma membrane encloses the cell and, by controlling the movement of substances across it, exerts a powerful influence on metabolic pathways.
13. Protein receptors (recognition units) on the plasma membrane enable the cell to interact with other cells and with extracellular substances.
14. The plasma membrane is a bilayer of lipids (phospholipids, glycolipids) and cholesterol, which gives the membrane its structural integrity.
15. Membrane functions are determined largely by proteins. These functions include recognition by protein receptors and transport of substances into and out of the cell.
16. The fluid mosaic model accounts for the fluidity of the lipid bilayer and the flexibility, self-sealing properties, and selective impermeability of the plasma membrane.
17. Cellular receptors are protein molecules on the plasma membrane, in the cytoplasm, or in the nucleus that are capable of recognizing and binding smaller molecules, called *ligands.*
18. The dynamic nature of the fluid plasma membrane enables it to vary the number of receptors on its surface. The cell is therefore capable of "hiding" from injurious agents by altering receptor number and pattern.
19. The ligand-receptor complex initiates a series of protein interactions, causing adenylate cyclase to catalyze the transformation of cellular ATP to messenger molecules that stimulate specific responses within the cell.

Cell-to-Cell Adhesions

1. Cell-to-cell adhesions are formed on plasma membranes, thereby allowing the formation of tissues and organs. Cells are held together by three different means: (a) the extracellular membrane, (b) cell adhesion molecules in the cell's plasma membrane, and (c) specialized cell junctions.
2. The extracellular matrix includes three groups of macromolecules: (1) fibrous structural proteins (collagen and elastin), (2) adhesive glycoproteins, and (3) proteoglycans and hyaluronic acid. The matrix helps regulate cell growth, movement, and differentiation.
3. The three major types of cell junctions are desmosomes, tight junctions, and gap junctions.

Cellular Communication and Signal Transduction

1. Cells communicate in three ways: (a) they form protein channels (gap junctions); (b) they display receptors that affect intracellular processes or other cells in direct physical contact; and (c) they secrete signals for long-distance communication.
2. Primary modes of chemical signaling include hormonal, neurohormonal, neurotransmitters, paracrine, and autocrine.
3. Signal transduction involves signals or instructions from extracellular chemical messengers that are conveyed to the cell's interior for execution.

Cellular Metabolism

1. The chemical tasks of maintaining essential cellular functions are referred to as *cellular metabolism.* Anabolism is the energy-using process of metabolism, whereas catabolism is the energy-releasing process.
2. Adenosine triphosphate (ATP) functions as an energy-transferring molecule. Energy is stored by molecules of carbohydrate, lipid, and protein, which, when catabolized, transfer energy to ATP.
3. Oxidative phosphorylation occurs in the mitochondria and is the mechanism by which the energy produced from carbohydrates, fats, and proteins is transferred to ATP.

Did You Understand?—Cont'd

Membrane Transport: Cellular Intake and Output

1. Water and small, electrically uncharged molecules move through pores in the plasma membrane's lipid bilayer in the process called *passive transport.*
2. Passive transport does not require the expenditure of energy; rather, it is driven by the physical effects of osmosis, hydrostatic pressure, and diffusion.
3. Larger molecules and molecular complexes (e.g., ligand-receptor complexes) are moved into the cell by active transport, which requires the cell to expend energy (by means of ATP).
4. The largest molecules (macromolecules) and fluids are transported by the processes of endocytosis (ingestion) and exocytosis (expulsion).
5. Two types of solutes exist in body fluids: electrolytes and nonelectrolytes. Electrolytes are electrically charged and dissociate into constituent ions when placed in solution. Nonelectrolytes do not dissociate when placed in solution.
6. Diffusion is the passive movement of a solute from an area of higher solute concentration to an area of lower solute concentration.
7. Filtration is the measurement of water and solutes through a membrane because of a greater pushing pressure.
8. Hydrostatic pressure is the mechanical force of water pushing against cellular membranes.
9. Osmosis is the movement of water across a semipermeable membrane from a region of lower solute concentration to a region of higher solute concentration.
10. The amount of hydrostatic pressure required to oppose the osmotic movement of water is called the *osmotic pressure of the solution.*
11. The overall osmotic effect of colloids, such as plasma proteins, is called the *oncotic pressure or colloid osmotic pressure.*
12. Mediated transport can be passive or active. Mediated transport includes the movement of two molecules simultaneously in one direction (symport) or in opposite directions (antiport) or the movement of a single molecule in one direction (uniport).
13. Passive mediated transport is also called *facilitated diffusion.* It does not require the expenditure of metabolic energy.
14. Active mediated transport requires metabolic energy (ATP) to move molecules against the concentration gradient.
15. Active transport occurs also by endocytosis, or vesicle formation, in which the substance to be transported is engulfed by a segment of the plasma membrane, forming a vesicle that moves into the cell.
16. Pinocytosis is a type of endocytosis in which fluids and solute molecules are ingested through formation of small vesicles.
17. Phagocytosis is a type of endocytosis in which large particles, such as bacteria, are ingested through formation of large vesicles, called *vacuoles.*
18. In receptor-mediated endocytosis, the plasma membrane receptors are clustered, along with bristle-like structures, in specialized areas called *coated pits.*
19. Endocytosis occurs when coated pits invaginate, internalizing ligand-receptor complexes in coated vesicles.
20. Inside the cell, lysosomal enzymes process and digest material ingested by endocytosis.
21. Caveolae are cavelike pits, and uptake through their opening and closing is called *potocytosis.*
22. All body cells are electrically polarized, with the inside of the cell more negatively charged than the outside. The difference in voltage across the plasma membrane is the resting membrane potential.
23. When an excitable (nerve or muscle) cell receives an electrochemical stimulus, cations enter the cell, causing a rapid change in the resting membrane potential known as the *action potential.* The action potential "moves" along the cell's plasma membrane and is transmitted to an adjacent cell. This is how electrochemical signals convey information from cell to cell.

Cellular Reproduction: The Cell Cycle

1. Cellular reproduction in body tissues involves mitosis (nuclear division) and cytokinesis (cytoplasmic division).
2. Only mature cells are capable of division. Maturation occurs during a stage of cellular life called *interphase (growth phase).*
3. The cell cycle is the reproductive process that begins after interphase in all tissues with cellular turnover. There are four phases of the cell cycle: (1) the S phase, during which DNA synthesis takes place in the cell nucleus; (2) the G_2 phase, the period between the completion of DNA synthesis and the next phase (M); (3) the M phase, which involves both nuclear (mitotic) and cytoplasmic (cytokinetic) division; and (4) the G_1 phase (growth phase), after which the cycle begins again.
4. The M phase (mitosis) involves four stages: prophase, metaphase, anaphase, and telophase.
5. The mechanisms that control cell division depend on "social control genes" and protein growth factors.

Tissues

1. Cells of one or more types are organized into tissues, and different types of tissues compose organs. Organs are organized to function as tracts or systems.
2. Three key factors that maintain the cellular organization of tissues are (a) recognition and cell communication, (b) selective cell-to-cell adhesion, and (c) memory.
3. Tissue cells are linked at cell junctions, which are specialized regions on their plasma membranes called *desmosomes, tight junctions,* and *gap junctions.* Cell junctions attach adjacent cells and allow small molecules to pass between them.
4. The four basic types of tissues are epithelial, muscle, nerve, and connective tissues.
5. Neural tissue is composed of highly specialized cells called neurons that receive and transmit electrical impulses rapidly across junctions called *synapses.*

(Continued)

Did You Understand?—Cont'd

6. Epithelial tissue covers most internal and external surfaces of the body. The functions of epithelial tissue include protection, absorption, secretion, and excretion.
7. Connective tissue binds various tissues and organs together, supporting them in their locations and serving as storage sites for excess nutrients.
8. Muscle tissue is composed of long, thin, highly contractile cells or fibers called *myocytes*. Muscle tissue that is attached to bones enables voluntary movement. Muscle tissue in internal organs enables involuntary movement, such as the heartbeat.

Key Terms

Absolute refractory period, 22
Action potential, 21
Active mediated transport, 18
Active transport, 15
Amphipathic, 3
Anabolism, 12
Anaphase, 23
Anion, 15
Antiport, 18
Arrested (resting) (G_0) state, 24
Autocrine signaling, 11
Basement membrane, 8
Catabolism, 12
Cation, 15
Caveolae, 3, 20
Cell adhesion molecule (CAM), 4
Cell cycle, 22
Cell junction, 9
Cell-to-cell adhesions, 8
Cellular metabolism, 12
Cellular receptor, 7
Centromere, 23
Chemical synapses, 11
Chromatid, 23
Chromatin, 23
Citric acid cycle (Krebs cycle tricarboxylic acid cycle), 13
Coated pit, 20
Collagen, 8
Competitive inhibitor, 17
Concentration gradient, 15
Connective tissue, 9
Connexon, 9
Cytokinesis, 22
Cytoplasm, 2
Cytoplasmic matrix, 2
Daughter cell, 23
Depolarization, 21
Desmosome, 9
Differentiation, 2
Diffusion, 15
Digestion, 13
Effective osmolality, 16
Elastin, 8
Electrolyte, 15
Electron-transport chain, 14
Endocytosis, 19
Equatorial plate (metaphase plate), 23
Eukaryote, 1
Exocytosis, 20
Extracellular matrix, 8, 24
Fibroblast, 9
Fibronectin, 8
Filtration, 16
Fluid mosaic model, 6
G_1 phase, 23
G_2 phase, 23
Gap junction, 9
Gating, 9
Glycolysis, 13
Glycoprotein, 4
Growth factor (cytokines), 24
Homeostasis, 10
Hormonal signaling, 11
Hydrostatic pressure, 16
Hyperpolarized, 22
Hypertonic solution, 17
Hypopolarized, 22
Hypotonic solution, 17
Integral membrane protein, 3
Interphase, 22
Ion, 15
Isotonic solution, 17
Junctional complex, 9
Ligand, 7
M phase, 23
Macromolecule, 8
Mediated transport, 17
Metabolic pathway, 12
Metaphase, 23
Microdomains, 20
Mitosis, 22
Neurohormonal signaling, 11
Neurotransmitter, 11
Nuclear envelope, 2
Nucleolus, 2
Nucleus, 2
Oncotic pressure (colloid osmotic pressure), 17
Organelle, 2
Osmolality, 16
Osmolarity, 16
Osmosis, 16
Osmotic pressure, 16
Oxidation, 13
Oxidative phosphorylation, 14
Paracrine signaling, 11
Passive mediated transport (facilitated diffusion), 18
Passive transport, 15
Pattern formation, 25
Peripheral membrane protein, 4
Phagocytosis, 20
Pinocytosis, 19
Plasma membrane (plasmalemma), 2
Plasma membrane receptor, 7
Platelet-derived growth factor (PDGF), 24
Polarity, 15
Potocytosis, 20
Prokaryote, 1
Prophase, 23
Receptor protein, 11
Receptor-mediated endocytosis (ligand internalization), 20
Relative refractory period, 22
Repolarization, 21
Resting membrane potential, 21
Retinoblastoma (Rb) protein, 24
S phase, 23
Signal transduction pathway, 11
Signal transduction, 11
Signaling cell, 11
Solute, 15
Spindle fiber, 23
Stroma, 24
Substrate, 12
Substrate phosphorylation (anaerobic glycolysis), 14
Symport, 18
Target cell, 11
Telophase, 23
Threshold potential, 21
Tight junction, 9
Tonicity, 17
Transfer reaction, 14
Transport protein (transporter), 17
Uniport, 18
Valence, 15

References

1. Alberts B et al: *Molecular biology of the cell*, ed 4, New York, 2002, Garland.
2. Catt KJ et al: Hormonal regulation of peptide receptors and target cell responses, *Nature* 280(5718):109–116, 1979.
3. Aplin AE: Cell adhesion molecule regulation of nucleocytoplasmic trafficking, *FEBS LeH* 534(1–3):11–4 review, 2003.
4. Quest AF, Leyton L, Parraga M: Caveolins, caveolae, and lipid rafts in cellular transport, signaling, and disease, *Biochem Cell Biol* 82(1):129–144, 2004.
5. Kiss AL et al: Oestrogen-mediated tyrosine phosphorylation of caveolin-1 and its effect on the oestrogen receptor localization: an in vivo study, *Mol Cell Endocrinol* 245(1-2):128–137, 2005.
6. Jorde LB et al: *Medical genetics*, ed 3, updated, St Louis, 2006, Mosby.

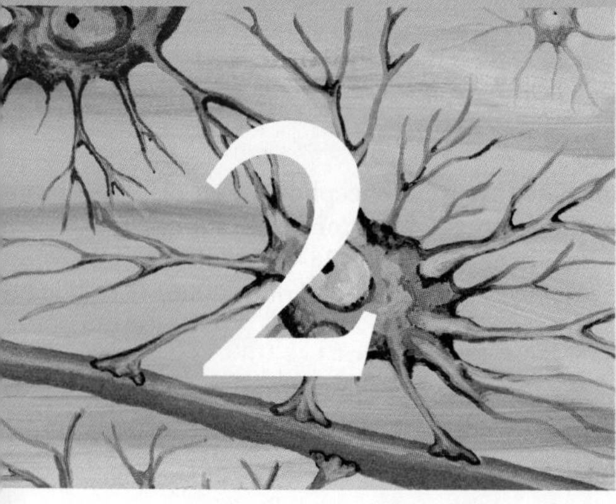

2 GENES AND GENETIC DISEASES

Lynn B. Jorde

CHAPTER OUTLINE

ELECTRONIC RESOURCES

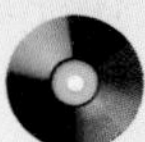

Companion CD
- Review Questions and Answers
- Animations

evolve Website
http://evolve.elsevier.com/Huether/
- Quick Check Answers
- Key Terms Exercises
- Critical Thinking Questions with Answers
- Algorithm Completion Exercises
- WebLinks

In the nineteenth century, microscopic studies of cells led scientists to suspect that the nucleus of the cell contained the important mechanisms of inheritance. Scientists found that chromatin, the substance that gives the nucleus a granular appearance, is observable in nondividing cells. Just before the cell divides, the chromatin condenses to form discrete, dark-staining organelles, which are called **chromosomes.** (Cell division is discussed in Chapter 1.) With the rediscovery of Mendel's important breeding experiments at the turn of the twentieth century, it soon became apparent that the chromosomes contained **genes,** the basic units of inheritance.

The primary constituent of chromatin is **deoxyribonucleic acid (DNA).** Genes are composed of sequences of DNA. By serving as the blueprints of proteins in the body, genes ultimately influence all aspects of body structure and function. Structural genes dictate the makeup of proteins. Estimates suggest that there are approximately 20,000 to 25,000 structural genes. An error in one of these genes often leads to a recognizable genetic disease.

To date, more than 16,000 genetic conditions have been identified and cataloged. As infectious diseases continue to come under increasingly effective control, the proportion of beds in pediatric hospitals occupied by children with genetic diseases has risen. In addition, many common diseases that primarily affect adults, such as hypertension, coronary heart disease, diabetes, and cancer, are now known to have important genetic components.

Great progress is being made in the diagnosis of genetic diseases and in the understanding of genetic mechanisms underlying them. With the huge strides being made in molecular genetics, "gene therapy"—the insertion of normal genes to correct genetic disease—has begun.

DNA, RNA, AND PROTEINS: HEREDITY AT THE MOLECULAR LEVEL

Definitions

Composition and structure of DNA

Genes are composed of DNA, which has three basic components: the pentose sugar molecule, deoxyribose; a phosphate molecule; and four types of nitrogenous bases. Two of the bases, **cytosine** and **thymine,** are single carbon-nitrogen rings called **pyrimidines.** The other two bases, **adenine** and **guanine,** are double carbon-nitrogen rings called **purines.** The four bases are commonly represented by their first letters: A, C, T, and G.

Watson and Crick demonstrated how these molecules are physically assembled together as DNA, proposing the **double-helix model,** in which DNA appears like a twisted ladder with chemical bonds as its rungs (Figure 2-1). The two sides of the ladder are made up of the sugar and phosphate molecules, held together by strong phosphodiester

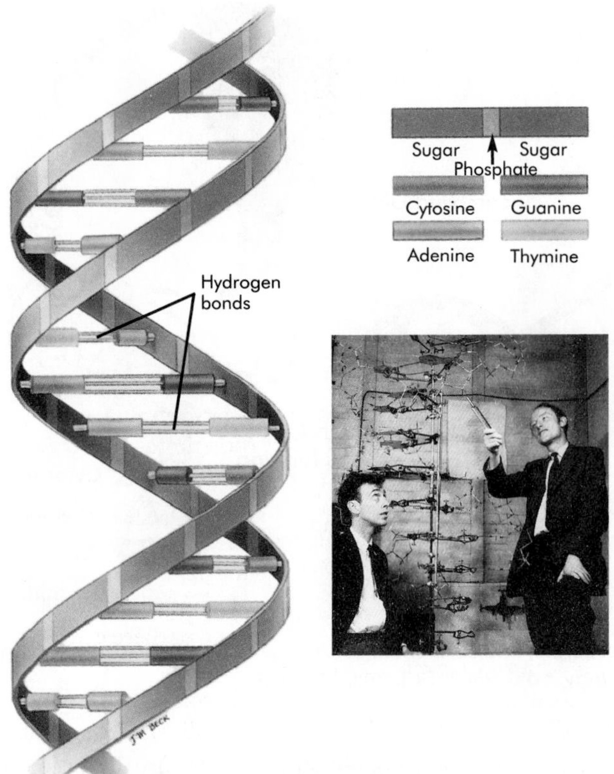

Figure 2-1 ■ **Watson-Crick Model of the DNA Molecule.** The DNA structure illustrated here is based on that published by James Watson *(photograph, left)* and Francis Crick *(photograph, right)* in 1953. Note that each side of the DNA molecule consists of alternating sugar and phosphate groups. Each sugar group is united to the sugar group opposite it by a pair of nitrogenous bases (adenine-thymine or cytosine-guanine). The sequence of these pairs constitutes a genetic code that determines the structure and function of a cell. (From Thibodeau GA, Patton KT: *Anatomy & physiology,* ed 6, St Louis, 2007, Mosby.)

bonds. Projecting from each side of the ladder, at regular intervals, are the nitrogenous bases. The base projecting from one side is bound to the base projecting from the other by a weak hydrogen bond. Therefore, the nitrogenous bases form the rungs of the ladder; adenine pairs with thymine, and guanine pairs with cytosine. Each DNA subunit—consisting of one deoxyribose molecule, one phosphate group, and one base—is called a **nucleotide.**

DNA as the genetic code

DNA directs the synthesis of all the body's proteins. Proteins are composed of one or more **polypeptides** (intermediate protein compounds), which are in turn composed of sequences of **amino acids.** The body contains 20 different types of amino acids, which are specified by the four nitrogenous bases. To specify (code for) 20 different amino acids with only four bases, different combinations of bases, occurring in groups of three, are used. These triplets of bases are known as **codons**. Each codon specifies a single amino acid in a corresponding protein. Because there are 64 ($4 \times 4 \times 4$) possible codons but only 20 amino acids, there are many cases in which several codons correspond to the same amino acid.

The genetic code is universal: *all* living organisms use precisely the same DNA codes to specify proteins except for mitochondria, the cytoplasmic organelles in which cellular respiration takes place (see Chapter 1)—they have their own extranuclear DNA. Several codons of mitochondrial DNA encode different amino acids than do the same nuclear DNA codons.

Replication of DNA

DNA replication consists of breaking the weak hydrogen bonds between the bases, leaving a single strand with each base unpaired. The consistent pairing of adenine with thymine and of guanine with cytosine, known as **complementary base pairing,** is the key to accurate replication. The unpaired base attracts a free nucleotide only if the nucleotide has the proper complementary base. When replication is complete, a new double-stranded molecule identical to the original is formed (Figure 2-2). The single strand is said to be a **template,** or molecule on which a complementary molecule is built, and is the basis for synthesizing the new double strand.

Several different proteins are involved in DNA replication. The most important of these proteins is an enzyme known as **DNA polymerase.** This enzyme travels along the single DNA strand, adding the correct nucleotides to the free end of the new strand and checking to make sure that its base is actually complementary to the template base. This mechanism of DNA proofreading substantially enhances the accuracy of DNA replication.

Mutation

A **mutation** is any inherited alteration of genetic material. Mutations may cause disease or be subtle, silent substitutions that do not change amino acids. One type of mutation is the **base pair substitution,** in which one base pair replaces another.

The **frameshift mutation** involves the insertion or deletion of one or more base pairs of the DNA molecule. As Figure 2-3 shows, these mutations can change the entire "reading frame" of the DNA sequence if the deletion or insertion is not a multiple of three base pairs (the number of base pairs in a codon). Frameshift mutations can thus greatly alter the amino acid sequence.

Agents known as **mutagens** increase the frequency of mutations. Examples include radiation and chemicals such as nitrogen mustard, vinyl chloride, alkylating agents, formaldehyde, and sodium nitrite.

Mutations are rare events. The rate of **spontaneous mutations** (those occurring in the absence of exposure to known mutagens) in humans is about 10^{-4} to 10^{-7} per gene per generation. This rate varies from one gene to another. Some chromosome regions have particularly high mutation rates and are known as **mutational hot spots.**

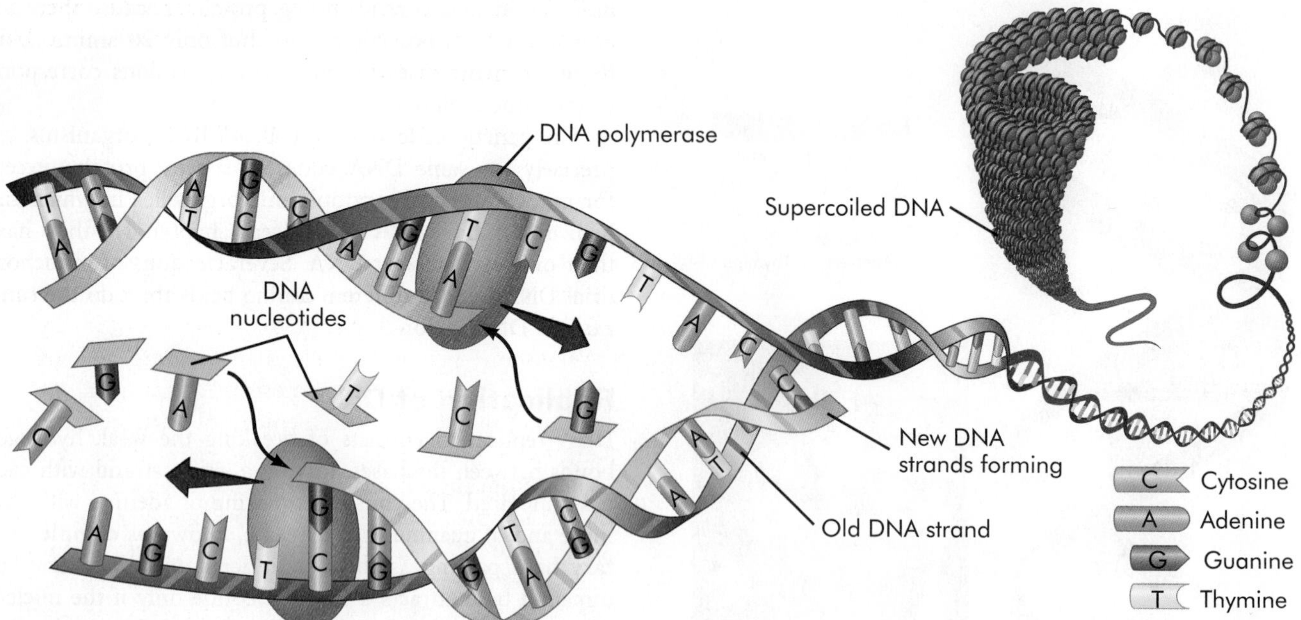

Figure 2-2 ■ **Replication of DNA.** The two chains of the double helix separate, and each chain serves as the template for a new complementary chain. (From Thibodeau GA, Patton KT: *Anatomy & physiology,* ed 6, 2007, St Louis, Mosby.)

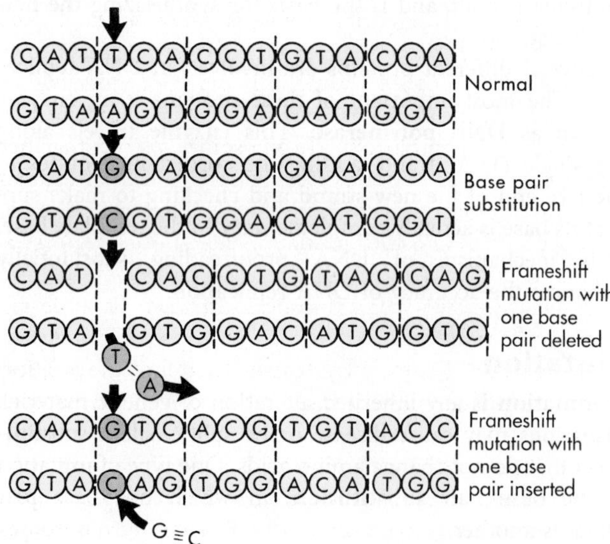

Figure 2-3 ■ **Different Kinds of Mutations.** *C,* Cytosine; *A,* adenine; *T,* thymine; *G,* guanine.

From Genes to Proteins

DNA is formed and replicated in the cell nucleus, but protein synthesis takes place in the cytoplasm. The DNA code is transported from nucleus to cytoplasm, and subsequent protein is formed through two basic processes: transcription and translation. These processes are mediated by **ribonucleic acid (RNA),** which is chemically similar to DNA except that the sugar molecule is ribose rather than deoxyribose, and uracil rather than thymine is one of the four bases. The other bases of RNA, as in DNA, are adenine, cytosine, and guanine. Uracil is structurally similar to thymine, so it also can pair with adenine. Whereas DNA usually occurs as a double strand, RNA usually occurs as a single strand.

Transcription

In **transcription,** RNA is synthesized from a DNA template, forming **messenger RNA (mRNA). RNA polymerase** binds to a **promoter site,** a sequence of DNA that specifies the beginning of a gene. RNA polymerase then separates a portion of the DNA, exposing unattached DNA bases. One DNA strand then provides the template for the sequence of mRNA nucleotides.

The sequence of bases in the mRNA is thus complementary to the template strand, and except for the presence of uracil instead of thymine, the mRNA sequence is identical to the other DNA strand. Transcription continues until a **termination sequence** is reached. Then the RNA polymerase detaches from the DNA, and the transcribed mRNA is freed to move out of the nucleus and into the cytoplasm (Figures 2-4 and 2-5).

Gene splicing

When the mRNA is first transcribed from the DNA template, it reflects exactly the base sequence of the DNA and is called **heterogeneous nuclear RNA (hnRNA).** In eukaryotes, many RNA sequences are removed by nuclear enzymes, and the remaining sequences are spliced together to form the functional mRNA that migrates to the cytoplasm. The excised sequences are called **introns,** and the sequences that are left to code for proteins are called **exons.**

Translation

In **translation,** RNA directs the synthesis of a polypeptide (see Figure 2-5), interacting with **transfer RNA (tRNA),** a cloverleaf-shaped strand of about 80 nucleotides. The

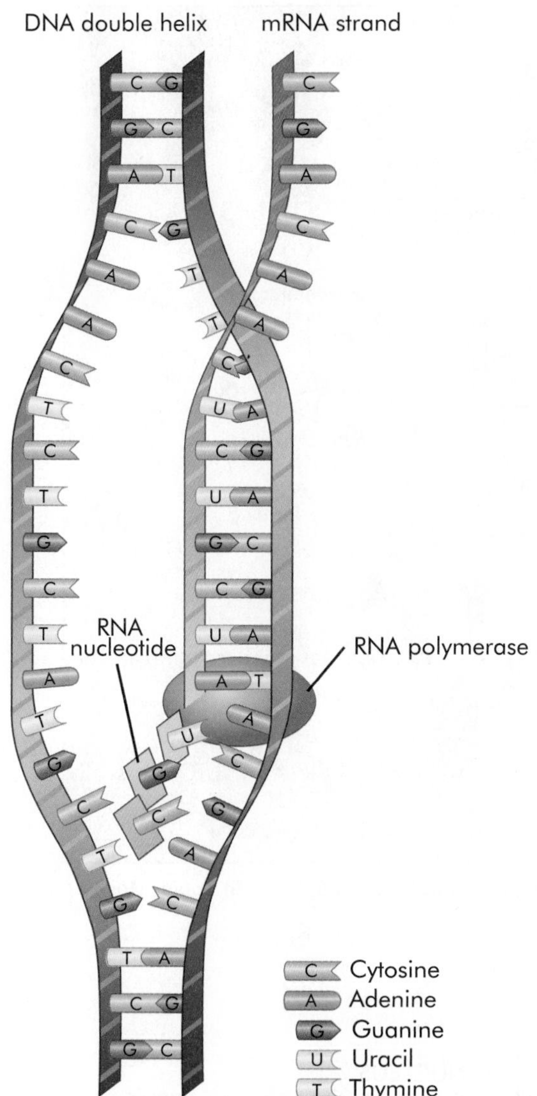

Figure 2-4 ■ **General Scheme of Ribonucleic Acid (RNA) Transcription. (See text for explanation.)** (From Thibodeau GA, Patton KT: *Anatomy & physiology,* ed 6, 2007, St Louis, Mosby.)

tRNA molecule has a site where an amino acid attaches. The three-nucleotide sequence at the opposite side of the cloverleaf is called the **anticodon.** It undergoes complementary base pairing with an appropriate codon in the mRNA, which specifies the sequence of amino acids through tRNA.

The site of actual protein synthesis is in the **ribosome,** which consists of roughly equal parts of protein and **ribosomal RNA (rRNA).** During translation, the ribosome first binds to an initiation site on the mRNA sequence and then binds to its surface, so that base pairing can occur between tRNA and mRNA. The ribosome then moves along the mRNA sequence, processing each codon and translating an amino acid by way of the interaction of mRNA and tRNA.

The ribosome provides an enzyme that catalyzes the formation of covalent peptide bonds between the adjacent amino acids, resulting in a growing polypeptide. When the ribosome arrives at a termination signal on the mRNA sequence, translation and polypeptide formation cease; the mRNA, ribosome, and polypeptide separate from one another; and the polypeptide is released into the cytoplasm to perform its required function.

CHROMOSOMES

Human cells can be categorized into **gametes** (sperm and egg cells) and **somatic cells,** which include all cells other than gametes. Each somatic cell nucleus has 46 chromosomes in 23 pairs (Figure 2-6). These are **diploid cells,** and the individual's father and mother each donate one chromosome per pair. New somatic cells are formed through **mitosis** and **cytokinesis.** Gametes are **haploid cells:** they have only one member of each chromosome pair, for a total of 23 chromosomes. Haploid cells are formed from diploid cells by **meiosis** (Figure 2-7).

In 22 of the 23 chromosome pairs, the two members of each pair are virtually identical in microscopic appearance: thus, they are **homologous.** These 22 chromosome pairs are homologous in both males and females and are termed **autosomes.** The remaining pair of chromosomes, the sex chromosomes, consists of two homologous X chromosomes in females and a nonhomologous pair, X and Y, in males.

Figure 2-8, *A,* illustrates a **metaphase spread,** which is a photograph of the chromosomes as they appear in the nucleus of a somatic cell during metaphase. (Chromosomes are easiest to visualize during this stage of mitosis.) In Figure 2-8, *B,* the chromosomes are arranged according to size, with the homologous chromosomes paired together (this is now typically done by a computer). The 22 autosomes are numbered according to length, with chromosome number 1 the longest and chromosome 22 the shortest. A **karyotype** is an ordered display of chromosomes. Some natural variation in relative chromosome length can be expected from person to person, so it is not always possible to distinguish each chromosome by its length. Therefore, the position of the centromere also is used to classify chromosomes (Figure 2-9).

The chromosomes in Figure 2-8 were stained with Giemsa stain, resulting in distinctive **chromosome bands.** These form various patterns in the different chromosomes so that each chromosome can be distinguished easily. Using banding techniques, researchers can number chromosomes and study individual variations. Missing or duplicated portions of chromosomes, which often result in serious diseases, also are readily identified. More recently, techniques have been devised that permit each chromosome to be visualized with a different color.

Chromosome Aberrations and Associated Diseases

Chromosome abnormalities are the leading known cause of mental retardation and miscarriage. Estimates indicate that a major chromosome aberration occurs in at least 1 in 12 conceptions. Most of these fetuses do not survive to term; about 50% of all recovered first-trimester spontaneous abortuses have major chromosome aberrations.[1] The number of live births affected by these abnormalities is,

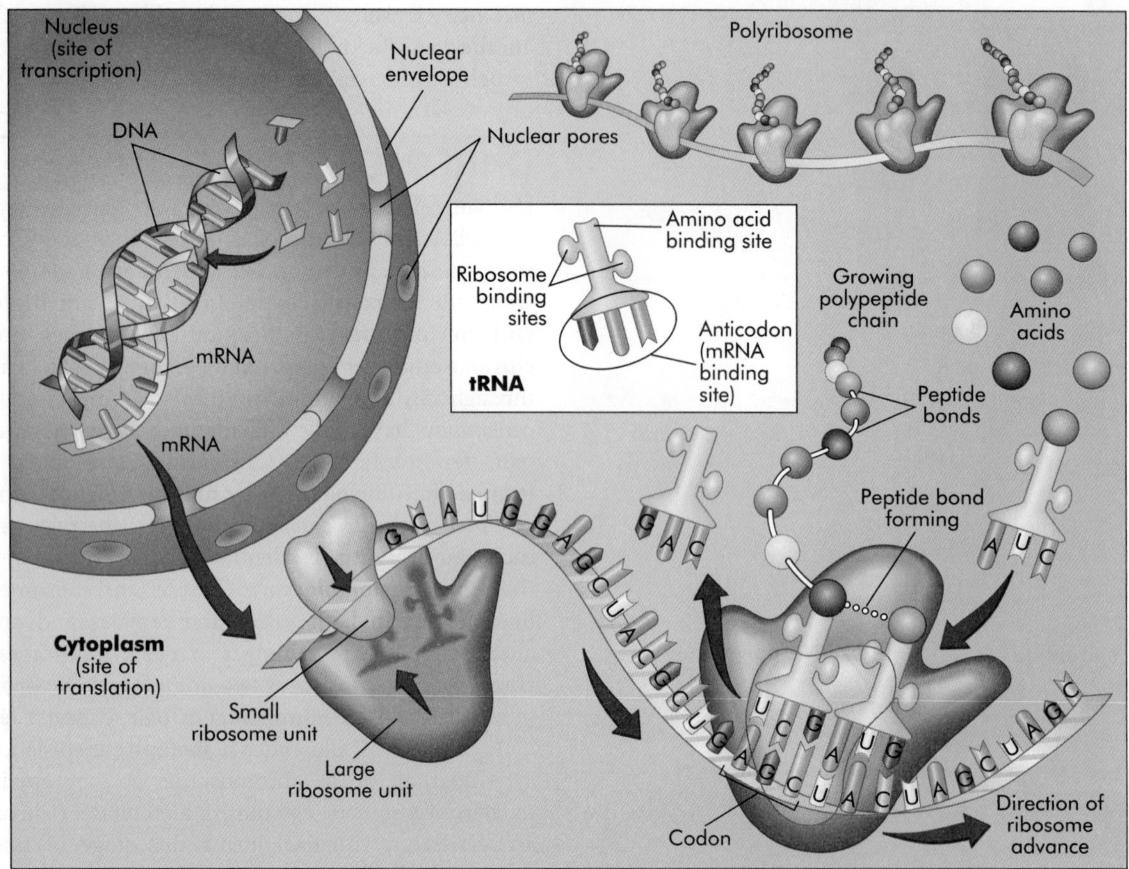

Figure 2-5 ■ **Protein Synthesis.** (From Thibodeau GA, Patton KT: *Anatomy & physiology,* ed 6, 2007, St Louis, Mosby.)

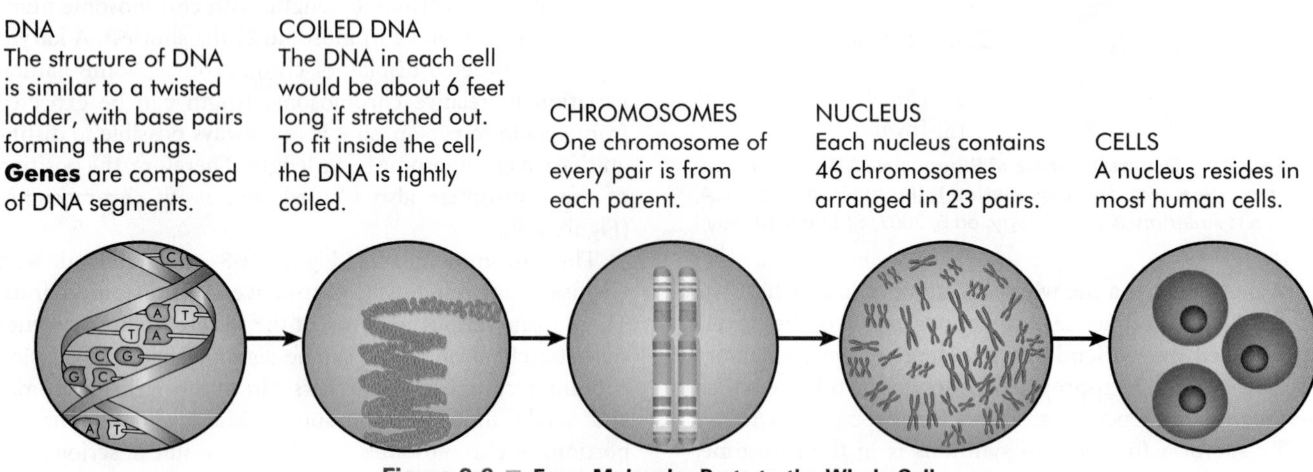

DNA
The structure of DNA is similar to a twisted ladder, with base pairs forming the rungs. **Genes** are composed of DNA segments.
COILED DNA
The DNA in each cell would be about 6 feet long if stretched out. To fit inside the cell, the DNA is tightly coiled.
CHROMOSOMES
One chromosome of every pair is from each parent.
NUCLEUS
Each nucleus contains 46 chromosomes arranged in 23 pairs.
CELLS
A nucleus resides in most human cells.

Figure 2-6 ■ **From Molecular Parts to the Whole Cell.**

however, significant; about 1 in 150 has a major diagnosable chromosome abnormality.[1]

Polyploidy

Cells with a multiple of the normal number of chromosomes are **euploid cells** (Greek *eu* = good or true). Because normal gametes are haploid and most normal somatic cells are diploid, they are both euploid forms. When a euploid cell has more than the diploid number of chromosomes, it is said to be a **polyploid cell.** Several types of body tissues, including some liver, bronchial, and epithelial tissues, are normally polyploid. A zygote that has three copies of each chromosome, rather than the usual two, has a form of polyploidy called **triploidy. Tetraploidy**, a condition in which euploid cells have 92 chromosomes, has been observed also. Both of these conditions are incompatible with postnatal survival. Nearly all triploid fetuses are spontaneously aborted or stillborn. The prevalence of triploidy among live births is approximately 1:10,000. Tetraploidy has been found primarily in early

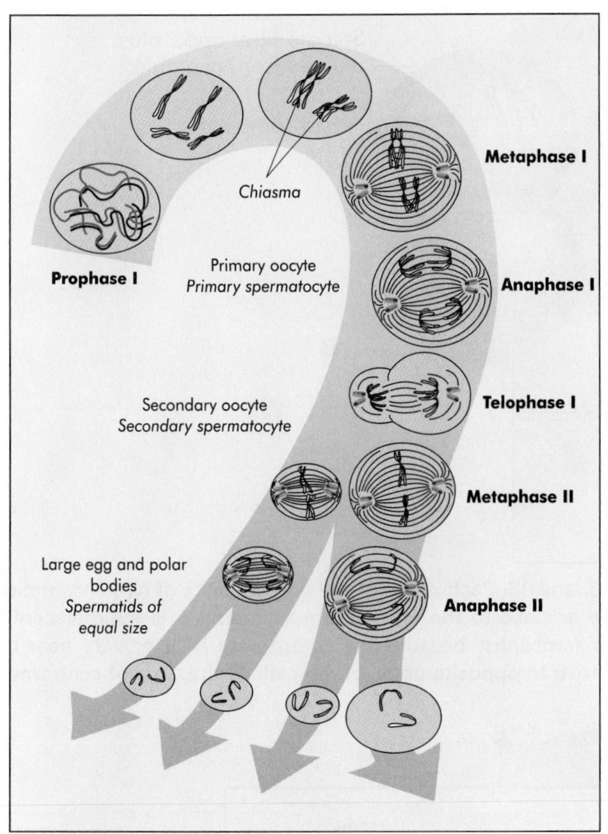

Figure 2-7 ■ **Phases of Meiosis.** (From Jorde LB et al, *Medical genetics,* ed 3, updated, St Louis, 2006, Mosby.)

abortuses, although occasionally, affected infants have been born alive. Like triploid infants, however, they do not survive. Triploidy and tetraploidy are relatively common conditions, accounting for approximately 10% of all known miscarriages.[2]

Aneuploidy

A cell that does not contain a multiple of 23 chromosomes is an **aneuploid cell.** A cell containing three copies of one chromosome is said to be trisomic (a condition termed **trisomy**) and is aneuploid. Monosomy, the presence of only one copy of a given chromosome in a diploid cell, is the other common form of aneuploidy. Among the autosomes, monosomy of any chromosome is lethal, but newborns with trisomy of some chromosomes can survive. This difference illustrates an important principle: *in general, loss of chromosome material has more serious consequences than duplication of chromosome material.*

Aneuploidy of the sex chromosomes is less serious than that of the autosomes. Very little genetic material–only about 40 genes–is located on the Y chromosome. For the X chromosome, inactivation of extra chromosomes (see p. 52) largely diminishes their effect. A zygote bearing *no* X chromosome, however, will not survive.

Aneuploidy is usually the result of **nondisjunction,** an error in which homologous chromosomes or sister chromatids fail to separate normally during meiosis or mitosis (Figure 2-10). Nondisjunction during either stage

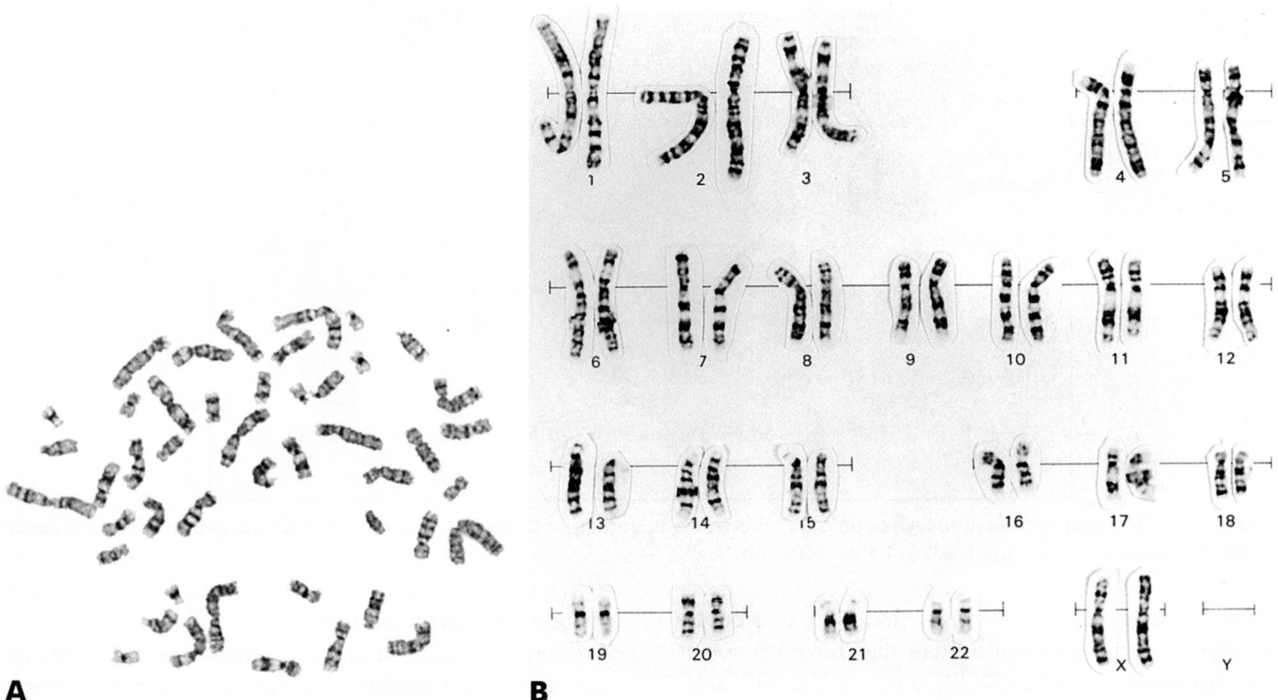

Figure 2-8 ■ **Karyotype of Chromosomes. A,** G-banded metaphase of a normal cell showing the bands of all normal chromosomes. **B,** G-banded karyotype of a normal female cell showing the banding patterns of the various chromosomes. Identical patterns characterize homologous chromosomes. The chromosomes are arranged from largest to smallest in size. (From Damjanov I, Linder J: *Anderson's pathology,* ed 10, vol 1, St Louis, 1996, Mosby.)

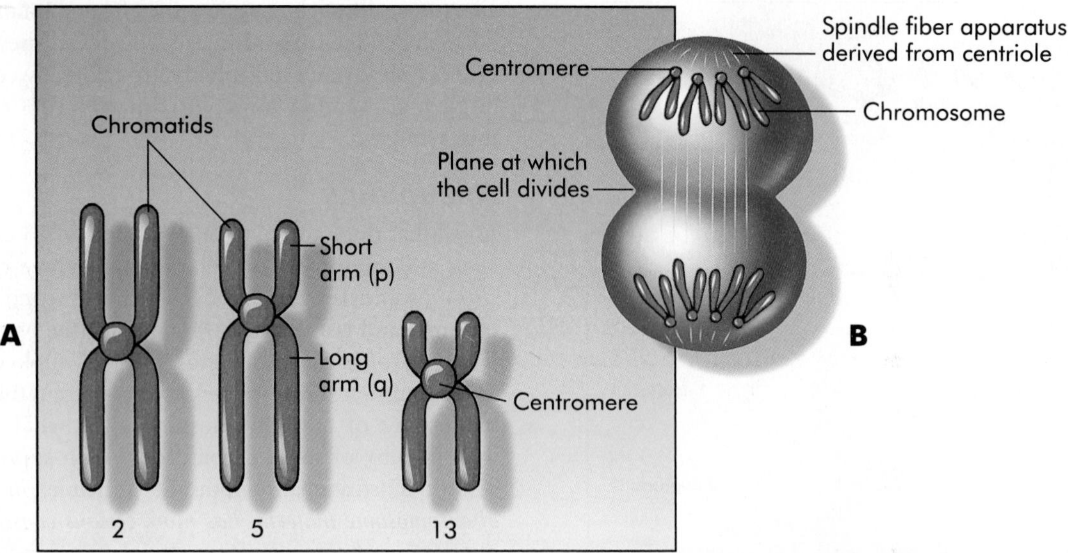

Figure 2-9 ■ **Structure of Chromosomes.** **A,** Human chromosomes 2, 5, and 13. Each is replicated and consists of two chromatids. Chromosome 2 is a metacentric chromosome because the centromere is close to the middle; chromosome 5 is submetacentric because the centromere is set off from the middle; chromosome 13 is acrocentric because the centromere is at or very near the end. **B,** During mitosis, the centromere divides and the chromosomes move to opposite poles of the cell. At the time of centromere division, the chromatids are designated as chromosomes.

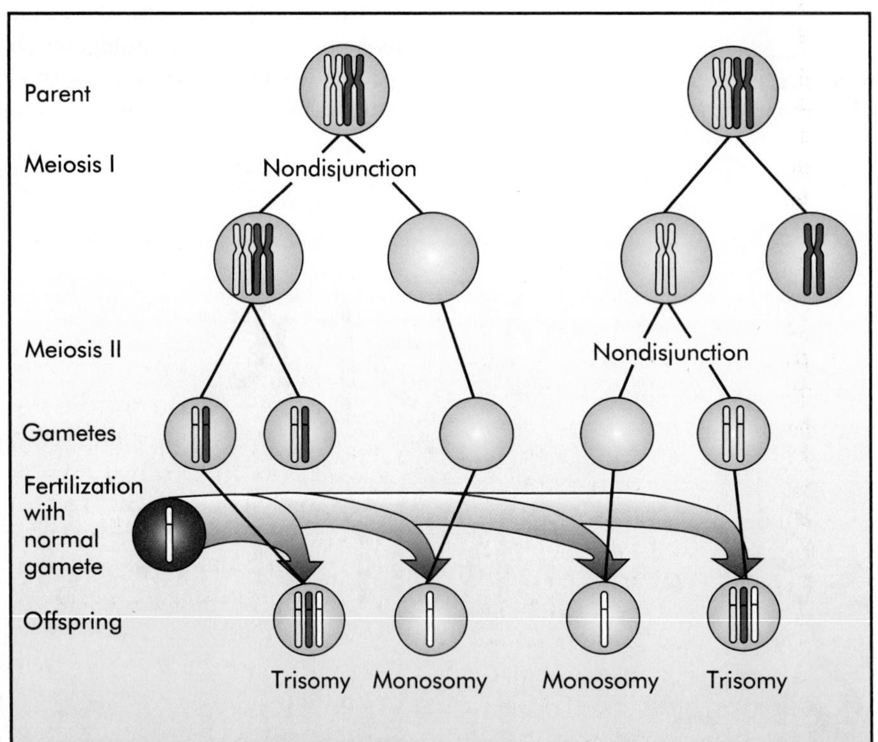

Figure 2-10 ■ **Nondisjunction.** Causes aneuploidy when chromosomes or sister chromatids fail to divide properly. (From Jorde LB et al: *Medical genetics,* ed 3, updated, St Louis, 2006, Mosby.)

of meiosis produces some gametes that have two copies of a given chromosome and others that have no copies of the chromosome. When such gametes unite with normal haploid gametes, the resulting zygote is monosomic or trisomic for that chromosome. Occasionally, a cell can be monosomic or trisomic for more than one chromosome.

Autosomal aneuploidy

Trisomy can occur for any chromosome, but the only forms seen with an appreciable frequency in live births are trisomies of the thirteenth, eighteenth, or twenty-first chromosomes. Fetuses with most other chromosomal trisomies do not survive to term. Trisomy 16, for example, is the most common trisomy among abortuses, but it is not seen in live births.[3]

Partial trisomy, in which only an extra portion of a chromosome is present in each cell, can occur also. The consequences of partial trisomies are not as severe as those of complete trisomies. Trisomies may occur in only some cells of the body. Individuals thus affected are said to be **chromosomal mosaics**, meaning that the body has two or more different cell lines, each of which has a different karyotype. Mosaics are often formed by early mitotic nondisjunction occurring in one embryo cell but not in others.

The best-known example of aneuploidy in an autosome is trisomy of the twenty-first chromosome, which causes **Down syndrome** (named after J. Langdon Down, who first described the disease in 1866). Down syndrome is seen in approximately 1 in 800 to 1 in 1000 live births[4]; its principal features are shown and outlined in Figure 2-11 and Table 2-1.

The risk of having a child with Down syndrome increases greatly with maternal age. As Figure 2-12 demonstrates, women younger than 30 years have a risk ranging from about 1 in 1000 births to 1 in 2000 births. The risk begins to rise substantially after 35 years of age, and it reaches 3% to 5% for women older than 45 years. This dramatic increase in risk may be caused by the age of maternal egg cells, which are held in an arrested state of prophase I from the time they are formed in the female embryo until they are shed in ovulation. Thus, an egg cell formed by a 45-year-old woman is itself 45 years old. This long suspended state may allow defects to accumulate in the cellular proteins responsible for meiosis, leading to nondisjunction. The risk of Down syndrome, as well as other trisomies, does not increase with paternal age.[4]

Sex chromosome aneuploidy

The incidence of sex chromosome aneuploidies is fairly high. Among live births, about 1 in 500 males and 1 in 900 females has a form of sex chromosome aneuploidy.[5] Because these conditions are generally less severe than autosomal aneuploidies, all forms except complete absence of any X chromosome material allow at least some individuals to survive.

One of the most common sex chromosome aneuploidies, affecting about 1 in 1000 newborn females, is trisomy X. Instead of two X chromosomes, these females have three X chromosomes in each cell. Most of them have no overt physical abnormalities, although sterility, menstrual irregularity, or mental retardation is sometimes seen. Some females have four X chromosomes, and they are more often mentally retarded. Those with five or more X chromosomes generally have more severe mental retardation and various physical defects.

A condition that leads to somewhat more serious problems is the presence of a single X chromosome and no homologous X or Y chromosome, so that the individual has a total of 45 chromosomes. The karyotype is usually designated 45,X, and it causes a set of symptoms known as **Turner syndrome** (Figure 2-13; see Table 2-1).

Individuals with at least two X chromosomes and one Y chromosome in each cell (47,XXY karyotype) have a disorder known as **Klinefelter syndrome** (Figure 2-14; see Table 2-1).

Abnormalities of chromosome structure

In addition to the loss or gain of whole chromosomes, parts of chromosomes can be lost or duplicated as gametes are formed, and the arrangement of genes on chromosomes can be altered. Unlike aneuploidy and polyploidy, these changes sometimes do not have serious consequences for an individual's health. Some of them can even go entirely unnoticed, especially when very small pieces of chromosomes are involved. Nevertheless, abnormalities of chromosome structure can also produce serious disease in individuals or their offspring.

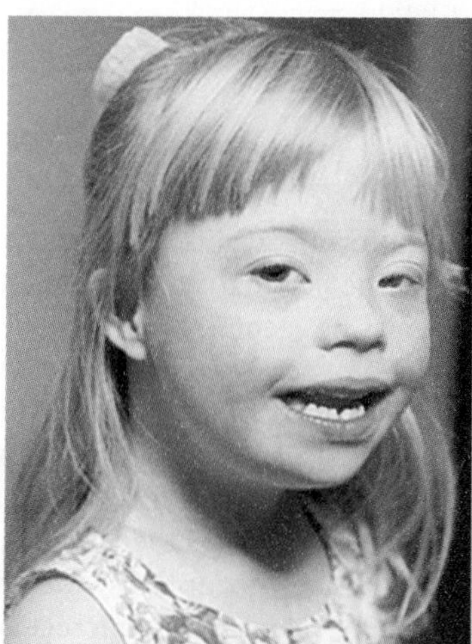

Figure 2-11 ■ **Child with Down Syndrome.** (Courtesy Drs. A. Olney and M. MacDonald, University of Nebraska Medical Center, Omaha.)

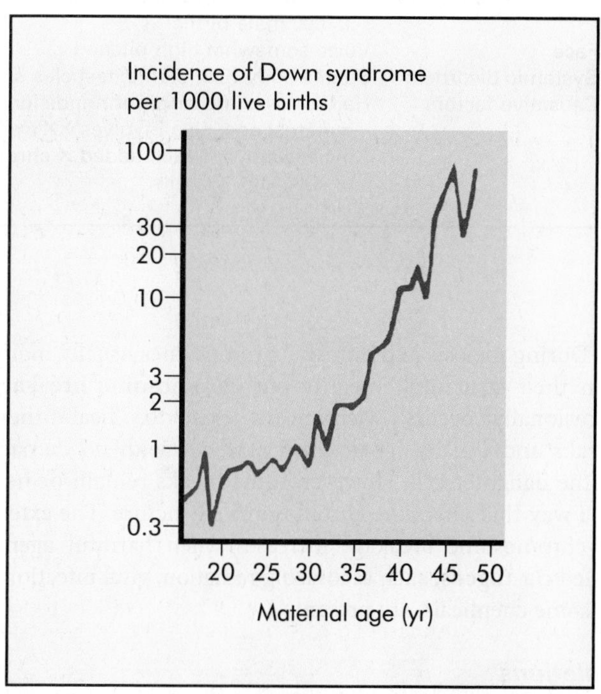

Figure 2-12 ■ **Down Syndrome Increases with Maternal Age.** Rate is per 1000 live births related to maternal age.

TABLE 2-1

Characteristics of Various Chromosome Disorders

Disease/Disorder	Features
DOWN SYNDROME	
Trisomy of chromosome 21	
IQ	Usually ranges from 20 to 70 (mental retardation)
Male/female findings	Virtually all males are sterile; some females can reproduce
Face	Distinctive: low nasal bridge, epicanthal folds, protruding tongue, low-set ears
Musculoskeletal system	Poor muscle tone (hypotonia), short stature
Systemic disorders	Congenital heart disease (one third to one half of cases), reduced ability to fight respiratory infections, increased susceptibility to leukemia—overall reduced survival rate; by age 40 years usually develop symptoms similar to those of Alzheimer disease
Mortality	About three fourths of fetuses with Down syndrome abort spontaneously or are stillborn; 20% of infants die before age 10 years; those who live beyond 10 years have life expectancy of about 60 years
Causative factors	97% caused by nondisjunction during formation of one of parent's gametes or during early embryonic development; 3% result from translocations; in 95% of cases, nondisjunction occurs when mother's egg cell is formed; remainder involve paternal nondisjunction; 1% are mosaics—these have a large number of normal cells, and the effects of the trisomic cells are attenuated and symptoms are generally less severe
TURNER SYNDROME	
(45,X) Monosomy of the X chromosome	
IQ	Not considered retarded, although some impairment of spatial and mathematical reasoning ability is found
Male/female findings	Found only in females
Musculoskeletal system	Short stature common, characteristic webbing of the neck, widely spaced nipples, reduced carrying angle at the elbow
Systemic disorders	Coarctation (narrowing) of the aorta, edema of the feet in newborns, usually sterile and have gonadal streaks rather than ovaries; streaks are sometimes susceptible to cancer
Mortality	About 15% to 20% of spontaneous abortions with chromosome abnormalities have this karyotype, most common single-chromosome aberration; highly lethal during gestation, only about 0.5% of these conceptions survive to term
Causative factors	Three fourths inherit X chromosome from mother, thus caused by meiotic error in the father; frequency low compared with other sex chromosome aneuploidies (1:5000 newborn females); half have simple monosomy of X chromosome; remainder have more complex abnormalities; combinations of 45X cells with XX or XY cells common
KLINEFELTER SYNDROME	
(47,XXY)	
IQ	Moderate degree of mental impairment may be present
Male/female findings	Have a male appearance but usually sterile; half develop female-like breasts (gynecomastia); occurs in 1:1000 male births
Face	Voice somewhat high pitched
Systemic disorders	Sparse body hair, sterile, testicles small
Causative factors	Half of cases the result of nondisjunction of X chromosomes in mother, frequency rises with increasing maternal age; also involves XXY and XXXY karyotypes with degree of physical and mental impairment increasing with each added X chromosome; mosaicism fairly common with most prevalent combination of XXY and XY cells

During meiosis and mitosis, chromosomes usually maintain their structural integrity but **chromosome breakage** occasionally occurs. Mechanisms exist to "heal" these breaks and usually repair them perfectly with no damage to the daughter cell. However, some breaks remain or heal in a way that alters the chromosome's structure. The extent of chromosome breakage increases when harmful agents called **clastogens,** such as ionizing radiation, viral infections, or some chemicals, are present.

Deletions

Broken chromosomes and lost DNA cause **deletions** (Figure 2-15). Usually, a gamete with a deletion unites with a normal gamete to form a zygote. The zygote thus has one chromosome with the normal complement of genes and one with some missing genes. Because many genes can be lost in a deletion, serious consequences result even though one normal chromosome is present. The most often cited example of a disease caused by a chromosomal deletion is the **cri du chat syndrome.** The term literally means "cry of the cat" and describes the characteristic cry of the affected child. Other symptoms include low birth weight, severe mental retardation, microcephaly (smaller than normal head size), and heart defects. The disease is caused by a deletion of part of the short arm of chromosome 5.

Duplications

A deficiency of genetic material is more harmful than an excess, so **duplications** usually have less serious consequences than deletions. For example, a deletion of a region of chromosome 5 causes cri du chat syndrome, but a duplication of the same region causes mental retardation but less serious physical defects.

Inversions

An **inversion** occurs when two breaks take place on a chromosome, followed by the reinsertion of the missing fragment at its original site but in inverted order. Therefore a chromosome symbolized as ABCDEFG might become ABEDCFG after an inversion.

Unlike deletions and duplications, no loss or gain of genetic material occurs, so inversions are "balanced" alterations of chromosome structure, and they often have no apparent physical effect. Some genes are influenced by neighboring genes, however, and this **position effect,** a change in a gene's expression caused by its position, sometimes results in physical defects in these persons. Inversions can cause serious problems in the offspring of individuals carrying the inversion because the inversion can lead to duplications and deletions in the chromosomes transmitted to the offspring.

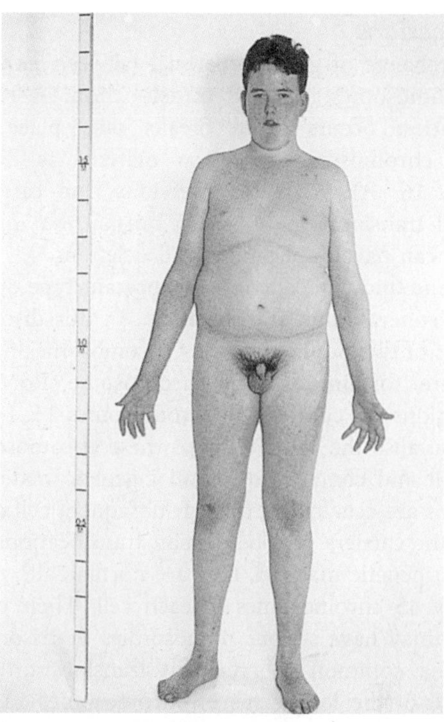

Figure 2-14 ■ **Klinefelter Syndrome.** This young man exhibits many characteristics of Klinefelter syndrome: small testes, some development of the breasts, sparse body hair, and long limbs. This syndrome results from the presence of two or more X chromosomes with one Y chromosome (genotypes XXY or XXXY, for example). (From Thibodeau GA, Patton KT: *Anatomy & physiology,* ed 6, 2007, St Louis, Mosby.)

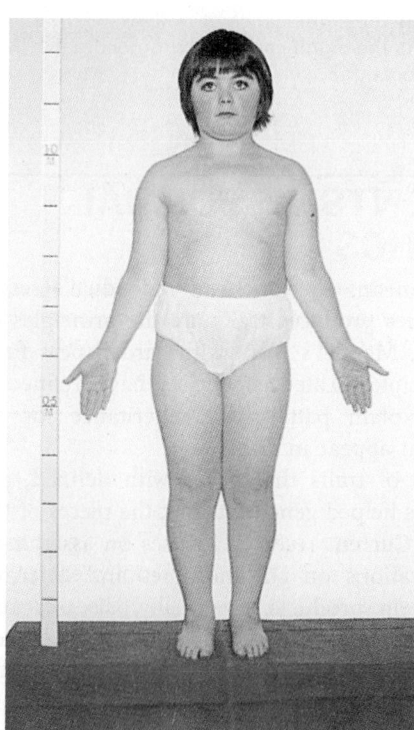

Figure 2-13 ■ **Turner Syndrome.** A sex chromosome is missing, and the person's chromosomes are 45,X. Characteristic signs are short stature, female genitalia, webbed neck, shield-like chest with underdeveloped breasts and widely spaced nipples, and imperfectly developed ovaries. (From Thibodeau GA, Patton KT: *Anatomy & physiology,* ed 6, 2007, St Louis, Mosby.)

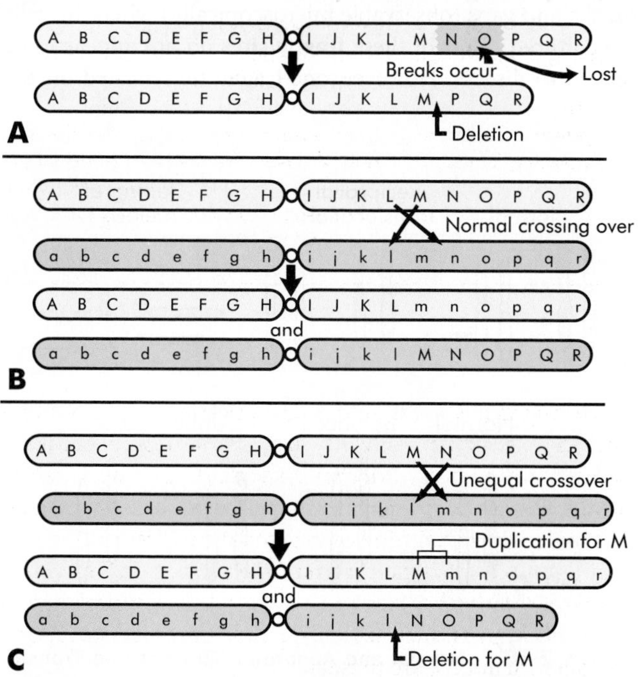

Figure 2-15 ■ **Abnormalities of Chromosome Structure.** **A,** Deletion occurs when a chromosome segment is lost. **B,** Normal crossing over. **C,** The generation of duplication and deletion through unequal crossing over.

Translocations

The interchange of genetic material between nonhomologous chromosomes is called **translocation.** A **reciprocal translocation** occurs when breaks take place in two different chromosomes and the material is exchanged (Figure 2-16, *A*). As with inversions, the carrier of a reciprocal translocation is usually normal, but his or her offspring can have duplications and deletions.

A second and clinically more important type of translocation is **robertsonian translocation.** In this disorder, the long arms of two nonhomologous chromosomes fuse at the centromere, forming a single chromosome. Robertsonian translocations are confined to chromosomes 13, 14, 15, 21, and 22 because the short arms of these chromosomes are very small and contain no essential genetic material. The short arms are usually lost during subsequent cell divisions. Because the carriers of robertsonian translocations lose no important genetic material, they are normal, although they have only 45 chromosomes in each cell. Their offspring, however, may have serious monosomies or trisomies. For example, a common robertsonian translocation involves the fusion of the long arms of chromosomes 21 and 14. An offspring who inherits a gamete carrying the fused chromosome can receive an extra copy of the long arm of chromosome 21 and develop Down syndrome. Robertsonian translocations are responsible for approximately 3% to 5% of Down syndrome cases. Parents who carry a robertsonian translocation involving chromosome 21 have an increased risk for producing multiple offspring with Down syndrome.

Fragile sites

A number of areas on chromosomes develop distinctive breaks and gaps (observable microscopically) when the cells are cultured. Most of these **fragile sites** do not appear to be related to disease. However, one fragile site, located on the long arm of the X chromosome, is associated with *fragile X syndrome.* The most important feature of this syndrome is mental retardation. With a relatively high population prevalence (affecting approximately 1 in 4000 males and 1 in 8000 females), the fragile X syndrome is the second most common genetic cause of mental retardation (after Down syndrome).

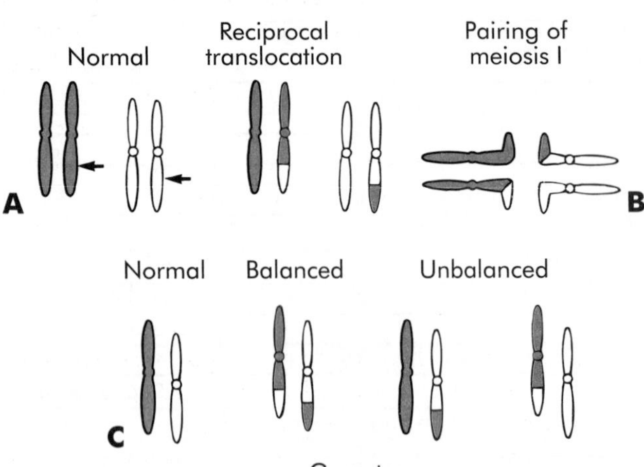

Figure 2-16 ■ Normal and Abnormal Chromosome Translocation. A, Normal chromosomes and reciprocal translocation. **B,** Pairing at meiosis. **C,** Consequences of translocation in gametes; unbalanced gametes result in zygotes that are partially trisomic and partially monosomic and consequently develop abnormally.

In fragile X syndrome, females who inherit the mutation do not necessarily express the disease condition but they can pass it on to descendants who do express it. Ordinarily, a male who inherits a disease gene on the X chromosome expresses the condition, because he has only one X chromosome. An uncommon feature of this disease is that about one third of carrier females are affected, although less severely than males. Unaffected transmitting males have been shown to have more than about 50 repeated DNA sequences near the beginning of the fragile X gene. These "repeats" consist of CGG sequences duplicated again and again. Affected males have 230 or more.[6] Increased numbers of these repeated sequences in successive generations can lead to expression of the fragile X syndrome. More than a dozen other genetic diseases, including Huntington disease and myotonic dystrophy, also are caused by this mechanism.[7]

QUICK CHECK 2-1

1. What is the major composition of DNA?
2. Define the terms *mutation, autosomes,* and *sex chromosomes.*
3. What is the significance of mRNA?
4. What is the significance of chromosomal translocation?

ELEMENTS OF FORMAL GENETICS

The mechanisms by which an individual's set of paired chromosomes produces traits are the principles of genetic inheritance. Mendel's work with garden peas first defined these principles. Later geneticists have refined Mendel's work to explain patterns of inheritance for traits and diseases that appear in families.

Analysis of traits that occur with defined, predictable patterns has helped geneticists link the pieces of the human gene map. Current research focuses on assigning genes to specific locations on chromosomes and determining the genes' protein products. Eventually, diseases and defects caused by single genes can be traced and therapies to prevent and treat such diseases can be developed.

Traits caused by single genes are called mendelian traits (after Gregor Mendel). Each gene occupies a position along a chromosome known as a **locus.** The genes at a particular locus can take different forms (i.e., they can be composed of different nucleotide sequences) called **alleles.** A locus that has two or more alleles that each occur with an appreciable frequency in a population is said to be **polymorphic** (or a **polymorphism**).

Because humans are diploid organisms, each chromosome is represented twice, with one member of the chromosome pair contributed by the father and one by the mother. At a given locus, an individual has one allele whose origin is paternal and one whose origin is maternal. When the two alleles are identical, the individual is **homozygous** at that locus. When the alleles are not identical, the individual is **heterozygous** at that locus.

Phenotype and Genotype

The composition of genes at a given locus is known as the **genotype.** The outward appearance of an individual, which is the result of both genotype and environment, is the **phenotype.** For example, an infant who is born with an inability to metabolize the amino acid phenylalanine has the single-gene disorder known as phenylketonuria (PKU) and thus has the PKU genotype. If the condition is left untreated, abnormal metabolites of phenylalanine will begin to accumulate in the infant's brain and irreversible mental retardation will occur. Mental retardation is thus one aspect of the PKU phenotype. By imposing dietary restrictions to exclude food that contains phenylalanine, however, retardation can be prevented. Although the child still has the PKU genotype, a modification of the environment (in this case, the child's diet) produces an outwardly normal phenotype.

Dominance and Recessiveness

In many loci, the effects of one allele mask those of another when the two are found together in a **heterozygote.** The allele whose effects are observable is said to be **dominant.** The allele whose effects are hidden is said to be **recessive** (from the Latin root for "hiding"). Traditionally, for loci having two alleles, the dominant allele is denoted by an uppercase letter and the recessive allele is denoted by a lowercase letter. When one allele is dominant over another, the heterozygote genotype Aa has the same phenotype as the dominant homozygote AA. For the recessive allele to be expressed, it must exist in the **homozygote** form, *aa.* When the heterozygote is distinguishable from both homozygotes, the locus is said to exhibit **codominance.**

A **carrier** is an individual who has a disease gene but is phenotypically normal. Many genes for a recessive disease occur in heterozygotes who carry one copy of the gene but do not express the disease. When recessive genes are lethal in the homozygous state, they are eliminated from the population when they occur in homozygotes. By "hiding" in carriers, however, recessive genes for diseases are passed on to the next generation.

TRANSMISSION OF GENETIC DISEASES

The pattern in which a genetic disease is inherited through generations is termed the **mode of inheritance.** Knowing the mode of inheritance can reveal much about the disease gene itself, and members of families with the disease can be given reliable genetic counseling.

Gregor Mendel systematically studied modes of inheritance and formulated two basic laws of inheritance. His **principle of segregation** states that homologous genes separate from one another during reproduction and that each reproductive cell carries only one homologous gene. Mendel's second law, the **principle of independent assortment,** states that the hereditary transmission of one gene does not affect the transmission of another. Mendel discovered these laws in the mid-nineteenth century by performing breeding experiments with garden peas, even though he had no knowledge of chromosomes. Early twentieth-century geneticists found that chromosomal behavior essentially corresponds to Mendel's laws, which now form the basis for the **chromosome theory of inheritance.**

The known single-gene diseases can be classified into four major modes of inheritance: autosomal dominant, autosomal recessive, X-linked dominant, and X-linked recessive. The first two types involve genes known to occur on the 22 pairs of autosomes. The last two types occur on the X chromosome; very few disease genes occur on the Y chromosome.

The **pedigree** chart summarizes family relationships and shows which members of a family are affected by a genetic disease (Figure 2-17). Generally, the pedigree begins with one individual in the family, the **proband,** also termed the **propositus** (male) or **proposita** (female). This individual is usually the first person in the family diagnosed or seen in a clinic.

Autosomal Dominant Inheritance

Characteristics of pedigrees

Diseases caused by autosomal dominant genes are rare, with the most common occurring in fewer than 1 in 500 individuals. Therefore, it is uncommon for two individuals that are both affected by the same autosomal dominant disease to produce offspring together. Figure 2-18, *A,* illustrates this unusual pattern. Affected offspring are usually produced by the union of a normal parent with an affected heterozygous parent. The Punnett square in Figure 2-18, *B,* illustrates this mating. The affected parent can pass either a disease gene or a normal gene to the next generation. On average, half the children will be heterozygous and will express the disease, and half will be normal.

The pedigree in Figure 2-19 shows the transmission of an autosomal dominant gene. Several important characteristics of this pedigree support the conclusion that the trait is caused by an autosomal dominant gene:

1. The two sexes exhibit the trait in approximately equal proportions, and males and females are equally likely to transmit the trait to their offspring.
2. No generations are skipped. If an individual has the trait, one parent must also have it. If neither parent has the trait, none of the children have it (with the exception of new mutations, as discussed later).
3. Affected heterozygous individuals transmit the trait to approximately half their children, and because gamete transmission is subject to chance fluctuations, all or

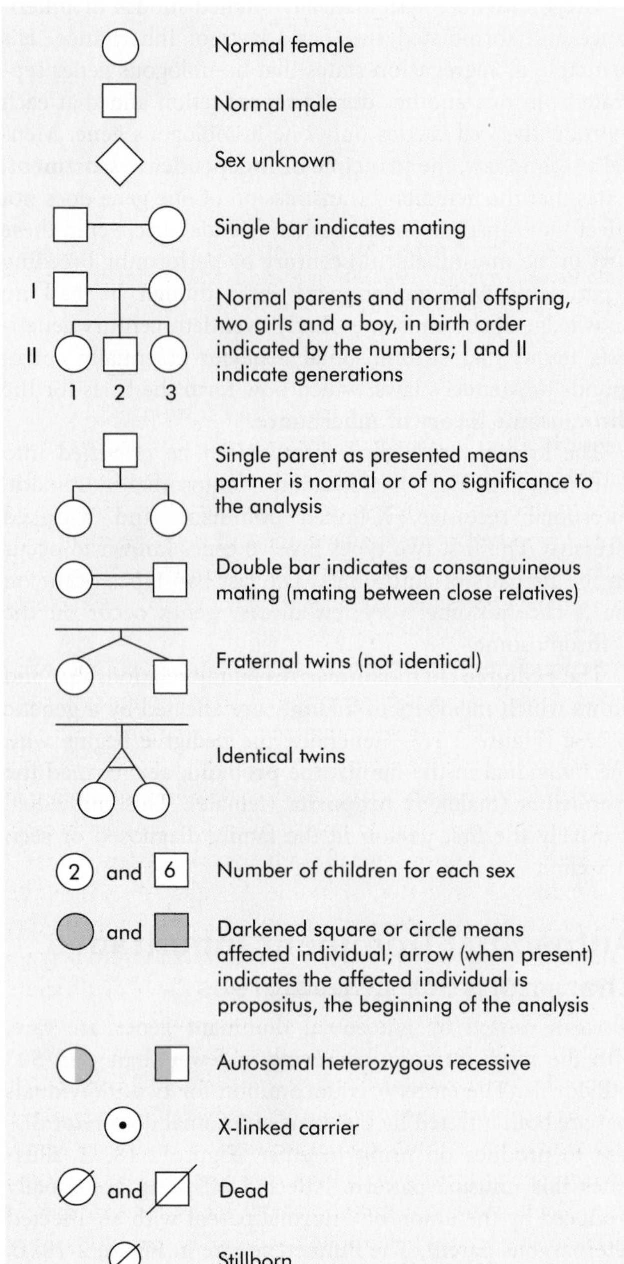

Figure 2-17 ■ **Symbols Commonly Used in Pedigrees.** (From Jorde LB et al: *Medical genetics,* ed 3, updated, St Louis, 2006, Mosby.)

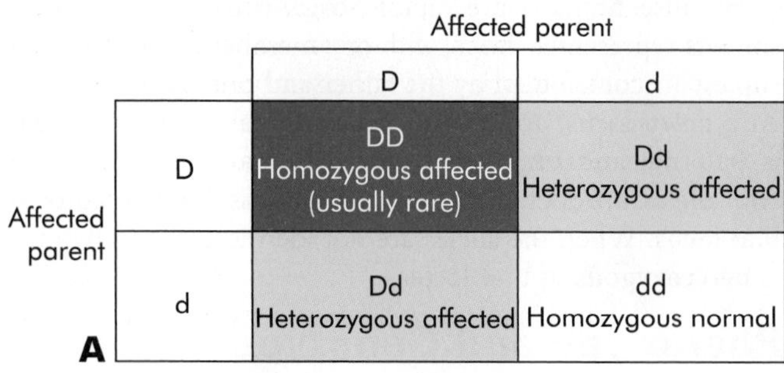

B

		Normal parent	
		d	d
Affected parent	D	Dd Heterozygous affected	Dd Heterozygous affected
	d	dd Homozygous normal	dd Homozygous normal

Figure 2-18 ■ **Punnett square and autosomal dominant traits. A,** Punnett square for the mating of two individuals with an autosomal dominant gene. Here both parents are affected by the trait. **B,** Punnett square for the mating of a normal individual with a carrier for an autosomal dominant gene.

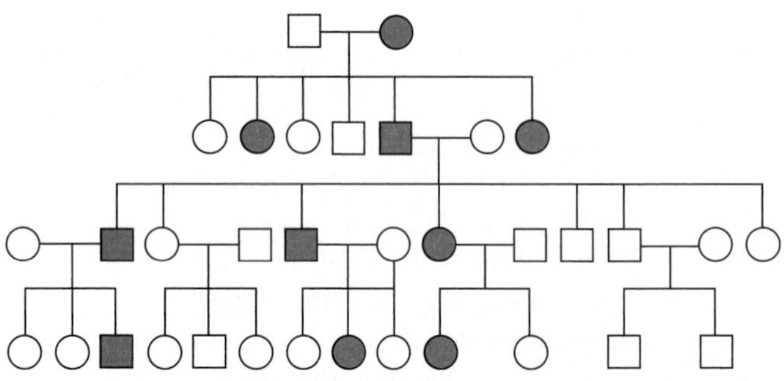

Figure 2-19 ■ **Pedigree for Achondroplasia.** Pedigree showing the transmission of an autosomal dominant disease.

none of the children of an affected parent may have the trait. When large numbers of matings of this type are studied, however, the proportion of affected children closely approaches one half.

Recurrence risks

Parents at risk for producing children with a genetic disease nearly always ask the question, "What is the *chance* that our child will have this disease?" When one child has already been born with a genetic disease, the parents can be given a **recurrence risk,** which is the probability that subsequent children will also have the disease. When one parent is affected by an autosomal dominant disease (and is a heterozygote) and the other is unaffected, the recurrence risk for each child is one half.

An important principle is that each birth is an independent event, much like a coin toss. Thus, even though parents may have already had a child with the disease, their recurrence risk remains one half. Even if they have had several children, all affected (or all unaffected) by the disease, the law of independence dictates that the probability that their next child will have the disease is still one half. Parents' misunderstanding of this principle is a common problem encountered in genetic counseling.

If a child is born with an autosomal dominant disease and there is no history of the disease in the family, the child is probably the product of a new mutation. The gene transmitted by one of the parents has thus undergone a mutation from a normal to a disease-causing allele. The genes at this locus in most of the parent's other germ cells are still normal. In this situation the recurrence risk for the parent's subsequent offspring is not greater than that of the general population. The offspring of the affected child, however, will have a recurrence risk of one half. Because these diseases often reduce the potential for reproduction, many autosomal dominant diseases result from new mutations.

Occasionally, two or more offspring have symptoms of an autosomal dominant disease when there is no family history of the disease. Because mutation is a rare event, it is unlikely that this disease would be a result of multiple mutations in the same family. The mechanism most likely responsible is termed **germline mosaicism.** During the embryonic development of one of the parents, a mutation occurred that affected all or part of the germline but few or none of the somatic cells of the embryo. Thus, the parent carries the mutation in his or her germline but does not actually express the disease. As a result, the unaffected parent can transmit the mutation to multiple offspring. This phenomenon, although relatively rare, can have significant effects on recurrence risks.[8]

Delayed age of onset

One of the best-known autosomal dominant diseases is Huntington disease, a neurologic disorder whose main features are progressive dementia and increasingly uncontrollable limb movements (chorea; discussed further in Chapter 15). A key feature of this disease is its **delayed age of onset:** symptoms usually are not seen until 40 years of age or later. Thus, those who develop the disease often have had children before they are aware that they have the gene. If the disease were present at birth, nearly all affected persons would die before reaching reproductive age and the occurrence of the gene in the population would be much lower. An individual whose parent has the disease has a 50% chance of developing it during middle age. He or she is thus confronted with a torturous question: Should I have children, knowing that there is a 50:50 chance that I may have this disease gene and will pass it to half of my children? A DNA test is now used to determine whether an individual has inherited the mutation that causes Huntington disease.

Penetrance and expressivity

The **penetrance** of a trait is the percentage of individuals with a specific genotype who also exhibit the expected phenotype. Incomplete penetrance means that individuals who have the gene for a disease may not exhibit the disease phenotype at all, even though the gene and the associated disease may be transmitted to the next generation. A pedigree illustrating the transmission of an autosomal dominant gene with incomplete penetrance is given in Figure 2-20. Retinoblastoma, the most common malignant eye tumor affecting children, typically exhibits incomplete penetrance. About 10% of the individuals who are **obligate carriers** of the gene (i.e., those who have an affected parent and affected children and therefore must themselves carry the gene) do not have the disease. The penetrance of the gene is then said to be 90%.

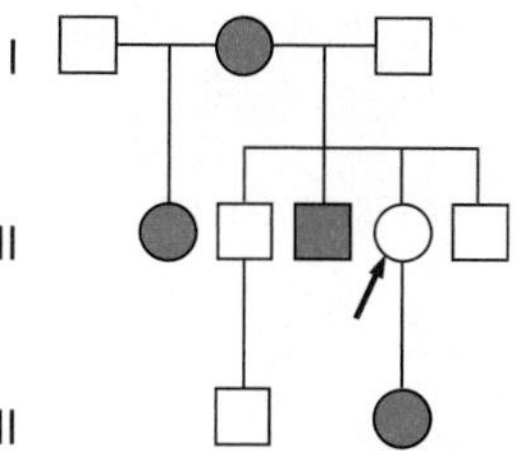

Figure 2-20 ■ Pedigree for Retinoblastoma Showing Incomplete Penetrance. Female with marked arrow in line II must be heterozygous, but she does not express the trait.

The gene responsible for retinoblastoma has been mapped to the long arm of chromosome 13, and its DNA sequence has been studied extensively. This gene is known as a **tumor-suppressor gene:** the normal function of its protein product is to regulate the cell cycle so that cells do not divide uncontrollably. When the protein is altered, its tumor-suppressing capacity is lost and a tumor can form[9] (see Chapters 9 and 15).

Expressivity is the extent of variation in phenotype associated with a particular genotype. If the expressivity of a disease is variable, penetrance may be complete but the severity of the disease can vary greatly. A good example of variable expressivity in an autosomal dominant disease is neurofibromatosis type 1, or von Recklinghausen disease. The gene that causes neurofibromatosis has been mapped to the long arm of chromosome 17, and studies of its DNA sequence indicate that, like the retinoblastoma gene, it is a tumor-suppressor gene.[10] The expression of this gene varies from a few harmless caf-au-lait (light brown) spots on the skin to numerous neurofibromas, scoliosis, seizures, gliomas, neuromas, malignant peripheral nerve sheath tumors, hypertension, and learning disorders (Figure 2-21).

Several factors cause variable expressivity. Genes at other loci sometimes modify the expression of a disease gene. Environmental factors can influence expression of a disease gene. Finally, different mutations at a locus can cause variation in severity. For example, a mutation that alters only one amino acid of the factor VIII gene usually produces a mild form of hemophilia A, whereas a "stop" codon (premature termination of translation) usually produces a more severe form of this clotting disorder.

Epigenetics and genomic imprinting

Although this chapter focuses on DNA sequence variation and its consequence for disease, there is increasing evidence that the same DNA sequence can produce dramatically different phenotypes depending on chemical modifications that alter the *expression* of genes (these modifications are collectively termed **epigenetic**). An important example of such a modification is **DNA methylation**, the attachment of a methyl group to a cytosine base that is followed by a guanine base in the DNA sequence (Figure 2-22). These sequences, which are common near many genes, are termed **CpG islands**. When the CpG islands located near a gene become heavily methylated, the gene is less likely to be

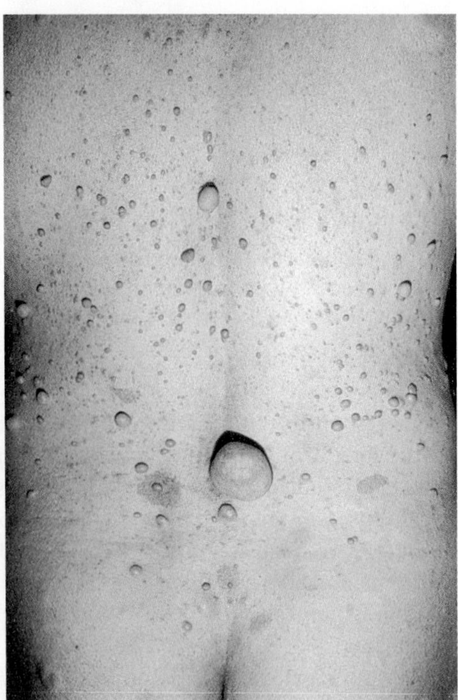

Figure 2-21 ■ **Neurofibromatosis.** Tumors. The most common is sessile or pedunculated. Early tumors are soft, dome-shaped papules or nodules that have a distinctive violaceous hue. Most are benign. (From Habif et al: *Skin disease: diagnosis and treatment,* ed 2, St Louis, 2005, Mosby.)

transcribed into mRNA. In other words, the gene becomes transcriptionally inactive. One study showed that identical (monozygotic) twins accumulate different methylation patterns in the DNA sequences of their somatic cells as they age, causing increasing numbers of phenotypic differences.[11] Intriguingly, twins with more differences in their lifestyles (e.g., smoking versus nonsmoking) accumulated larger numbers of differences in their methylation patterns. The twins, despite having identical DNA sequences, become more and more different as a result of epigenetic changes, which in turn affect the expression of genes.

Epigenetic alteration of gene activity can have important disease consequences. For example, a major cause of one form of inherited colon cancer (termed hereditary nonpolyposis colorectal cancer [HNPCC]) is the methylation of a gene whose protein product repairs damaged DNA. When this gene becomes inactive, damaged DNA accumulates eventually resulting in colon tumors. Epigenetic changes are also discussed in Chapter 9. Approximately 100 human genes are thought to be methylated differently, depending on which parent transmits the gene. This epigenetic modification, characterized by methylation and other changes, is termed **genomic imprinting.** For each of these genes, one of the parents *imprints* the gene (inactivates it) when it is transmitted to the offspring. An example is the insulin-like growth factor 2 gene (IGF2) on chromosome 11, which is transmitted by both parents, but the copy inherited from the mother is normally methylated and inactivated (imprinted). Thus, only one copy of IGF2 is active in normal individuals. However, the maternal imprint is occasionally lost resulting in two active copies of IGF2. This causes excess fetal growth and a condition known as *Beckwith-Weidemann syndrome.*

A second example of genomic imprinting is a deletion of part of the long arm of chromosome 15 (15q11-q13), which, when inherited from the father, causes the offspring to manifest a disease known as *Prader-Willi syndrome* (short stature, obesity, hypogonadism). When the same deletion is inherited from the mother, the offspring develop *Angelman syndrome* (mental retardation, seizures, ataxic gait). The two different phenotypes reflect the fact that different genes are normally active in the maternally and paternally transmitted copies of this region of chromosome 15.

Autosomal Recessive Inheritance

Characteristics of pedigrees

Like autosomal dominant diseases, diseases caused by autosomal recessive genes are rare in populations, although there can be numerous carriers. The most common lethal recessive disease in white children, cystic fibrosis, occurs in about 1 in 2500 births. Approximately 1 in 25 whites carries one copy of the gene for cystic fibrosis (see Chapter 27). Carriers are phenotypically normal. Some autosomal recessive diseases are characterized by delayed age of onset, incomplete penetrance, and variable expressivity.

Figure 2-23 shows a pedigree for cystic fibrosis. The cystic fibrosis gene, which has been mapped to the long arm of chromosome 7, encodes a chloride ion channel in some epithelial cells. Defective transport of chloride ions leads to a salt imbalance that results in secretions of abnormally thick, dehydrated mucus. Some digestive organs, particularly the pancreas, become obstructed, causing malnutrition, and the lungs become clogged with mucus, making them highly susceptible to bacterial infections. Death from lung disease or heart failure occurs before 30 years of age in about one half of persons with cystic fibrosis.

The important criteria for discerning autosomal recessive inheritance include the following:

1. Males and females are affected in equal proportions.
2. Consanguinity (marriage between related individuals) is sometimes present, especially for rare recessive diseases.
3. The disease may be seen in siblings of affected individuals but usually not in their parents.
4. On average, one fourth of the offspring of carrier parents will be affected.

Recurrence risks

In most cases of recessive disease, both of the parents of affected individuals are heterozygous carriers. On average, one fourth of their offspring will be normal homozygotes, one half will be phenotypically normal carrier heterozygotes, and one fourth will be homozygotes with the disease (Figure 2-24). Thus, the recurrence risk for the offspring of carrier parents is 25%. However, in any given family, there are chance fluctuations.

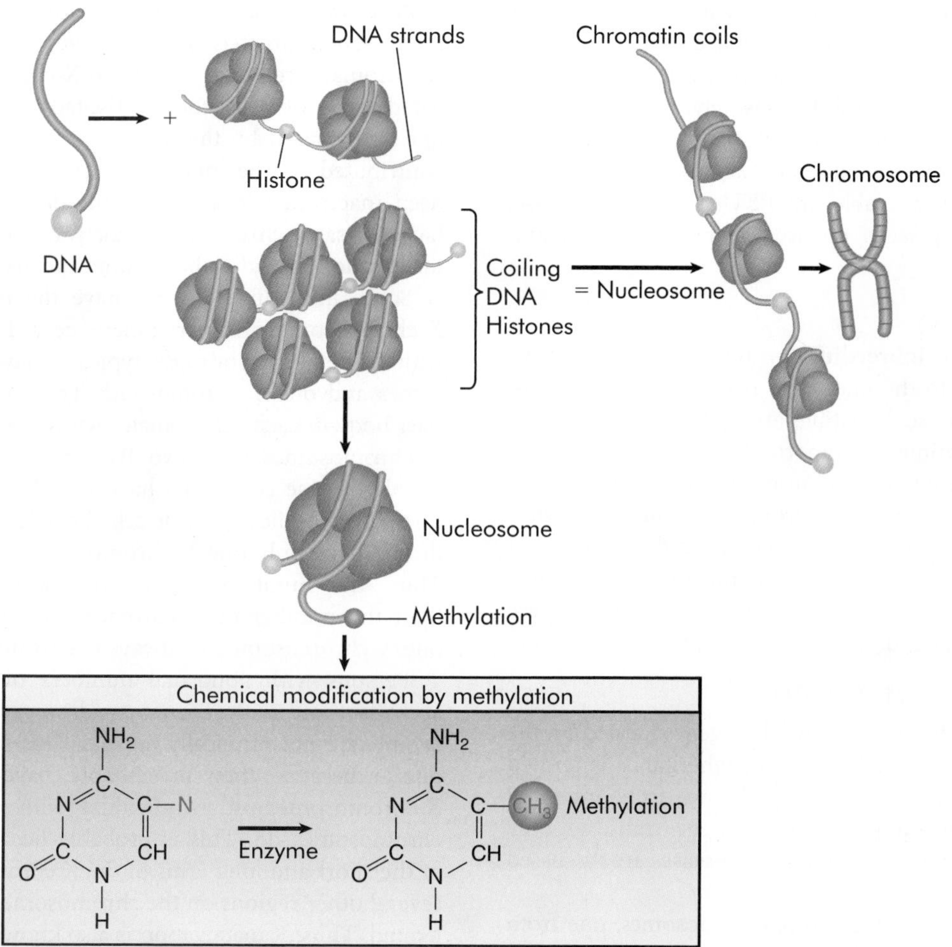

Figure 2-22 ■ **Epigenetic Modifications.** Because DNA is a long molecule, it needs packaging to fit in the tiny nucleus. Packaging involves *coiling* of the DNA in a "left-handed" spiral around spools, made of four pairs of proteins individually known as histones and collectively as the histone octamer. The entire spool is called a nucleosome (also see Figure 1-2). Nucleosomes are organized into chromatin, the repeating building blocks of a chromosome. Histone modifications are correlated with methylation, are reversible, and occur at multiple sites. Methylation occurs at the 5 position of cytosine and provides a "footprint" or signature as a unique epigenetic alteration (red). When genes are expressed, chromatin is open or active; however, when chromatin is condensed because of methylation and histone modification, genes are inactivated.

If two parents have a recessive disease, they each must be homozygous for the disease. Therefore, all their children also must be affected. This distinguishes recessive from dominant inheritance because two parents both affected by a dominant gene are nearly always both heterozygotes and thus one fourth of their children will be unaffected.

Because carrier parents usually are unaware that they both carry the same recessive gene, they often produce an affected child before knowing of their condition. **Carrier detection tests** can identify heterozygotes by measuring

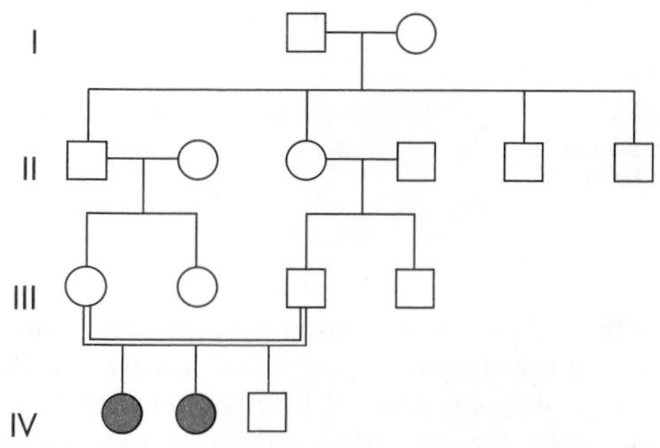

I
II
III
IV

Figure 2-23 ■ **Pedigree for Cystic Fibrosis.** The double bar denotes a consanguineous mating. Because cystic fibrosis is relatively common in European populations, most cases do not involve consanguinity.

	D	d
D	DD Homozygous normal	Dd Heterozygous carrier
d	Dd Heterozygous carrier	dd Homozygous affected

Figure 2-24 ■ **Punnett Square for the Mating of Heterozygous Carriers Typical of Most Cases of Recessive Disease.**

the reduced amount of a critical enzyme. This enzyme is totally lacking in a homozygous recessive individual, but a carrier, although phenotypically normal, will typically have half the normal enzyme level. Increasingly, carriers are now detected by direct examination of their DNA to reveal a mutation. Some recessive diseases for which carrier detection tests are now available are PKU, sickle cell disease, cystic fibrosis, Tay-Sachs disease, hemochromatosis, and galactosemia.

Consanguinity

Consanguinity and **inbreeding** are related concepts. **Consanguinity** refers to the mating of two related individuals, and the offspring of such matings are said to be *inbred.* Consanguinity is sometimes an important characteristic of pedigrees for recessive diseases because relatives share a certain proportion of genes received from a common ancestor. The proportion of shared genes depends on the closeness of their biologic relationship. Consanguineous matings produce a significant increase in recessive disorders and are seen most often in pedigrees for rare recessive disorders.

X-Linked Inheritance

Some genetic conditions are caused by genes located on the sex chromosomes, and that mode of inheritance is termed **sex linked.** Only a few diseases are known to be inherited as X-linked dominant or Y chromosome traits, so only the more common X-linked recessive diseases are discussed here.

Because females receive two X chromosomes, one from the father and one from the mother, they can be homozygous for a disease allele at a given locus, homozygous for the normal allele at the locus, or heterozygous. Males, having only one X chromosome, are **hemizygous** for genes on this chromosome. If a male inherits a recessive disease gene on the X chromosome, he will be affected by the disease because the Y chromosome does not carry a normal allele to counteract the effects of the disease gene. Because a single copy of an X-linked recessive gene will cause disease in a male, whereas two copies are required for disease expression in females, more males are affected by X-linked recessive diseases than are females.

X inactivation

In the late 1950s, Mary Lyon proposed that one X chromosome in the somatic cells of females is permanently inactivated, a process termed **X inactivation.**[12,13] This proposal, the Lyon hypothesis, explains why most gene products coded by the X chromosome are present in equal amounts in males and females, even though males have only one X chromosome and females have two X chromosomes. This phenomenon is called **dosage compensation.** The inactivated X chromosomes are observable in many interphase cells as highly condensed intranuclear chromatin bodies, termed **Barr bodies** (after Barr and Bertram, who discovered them in the late 1940s). Normal females have one Barr body in each somatic cell, whereas normal males have no Barr bodies.

Inactivation occurs very early in embryonic development—approximately 7 to 14 days after fertilization. In each somatic cell, one of the two X chromosomes is inactivated. In some cells, the inactivated X chromosome is the one contributed by the father; in other cells it is the one contributed by the mother. Once the X chromosome has been inactivated in a cell, all the descendants of that cell have the same chromosome inactivated (Figure 2-25). Thus inactivation is said to be random but *fixed.*

Some individuals do not have the normal number of X chromosomes in their somatic cells. For example, males with Klinefelter syndrome typically have two X chromosomes and one Y chromosome. These males do have one Barr body in each cell. Females whose cell nuclei have three X chromosomes have two Barr bodies in each cell, and females whose cell nuclei have four X chromosomes have three Barr bodies in each cell. Females with Turner syndrome have only one X chromosome and no Barr bodies. Thus, the number of Barr bodies is always one less than the number of X chromosomes in the cell. All but one X chromosome are always inactivated.

Persons with abnormal numbers of X chromosomes, such as those with Turner syndrome or Klinefelter syndrome, are not physically normal. This situation presents a puzzle because they presumably have only one active X chromosome, just as individuals with normal numbers of chromosomes do. This is probably because the distal tips of the short and long arms of the X chromosome, as well as several other regions on the chromosome arm, are not inactivated. Thus, X inactivation is also known to be *incomplete.*

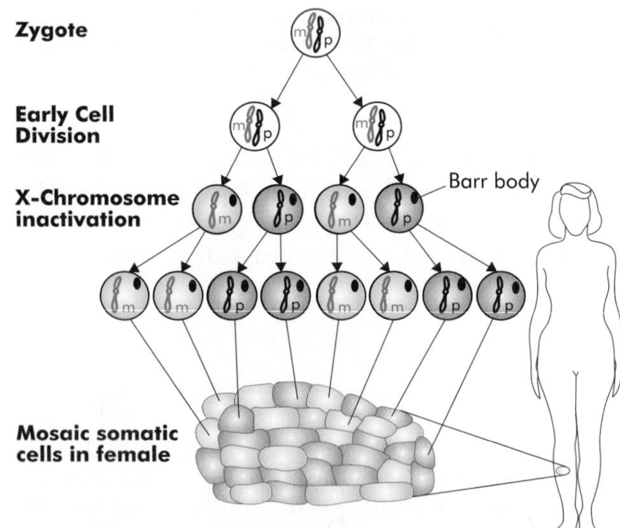

Figure 2-25 ■ **The X Inactivation Process.** The maternal (m) and paternal (p) X chromosomes are both active in the zygote and in early embryonic cells. X inactivation then takes place, resulting in cells having either an active paternal X or an active maternal X. Females are thus X chromosome mosaics, as shown in the tissue sample at the bottom of the page. (From Jorde LB et al: *Medical genetics,* ed 3, updated, St Louis, 2006, Mosby.)

Methylation of X chromosome DNA, a process in which DNA is inactivated when cytosine bases are enzymatically converted to 5-methylcytosine, appears to be involved in X inactivation. Inactive X chromosomes can be at least partially reactivated in vitro by administering 5-azacytidine, a demethylating agent.

Sex determination

The process of sexual differentiation, in which the embryonic gonads become either testes or ovaries, begins during the sixth week of gestation. A key principle of sex determination in the human is that one copy of the Y chromosome is sufficient to initiate the process of gonadal differentiation that produces a male fetus. The number of X chromosomes does not alter this process. For example, an individual with two X chromosomes and one Y chromosome in each cell is still phenotypically a male. Thus, the Y chromosome must contain a gene that begins the process of male gonadal development.

This gene, termed *SRY* (for "sex-determining region on the Y"), has been located on the short arm of the Y chromosome.[14] The *SRY* gene lies just outside the **pseudoautosomal** region (Figure 2-26), which pairs with the distal tip of the short arm of the X chromosome during meiosis and exchanges genetic material with it (crossover), just as autosomes do. The DNA sequences of these regions on the X and Y chromosomes are highly similar. The rest of the X and Y chromosomes, however, do not exchange material and are not similar in DNA sequence.

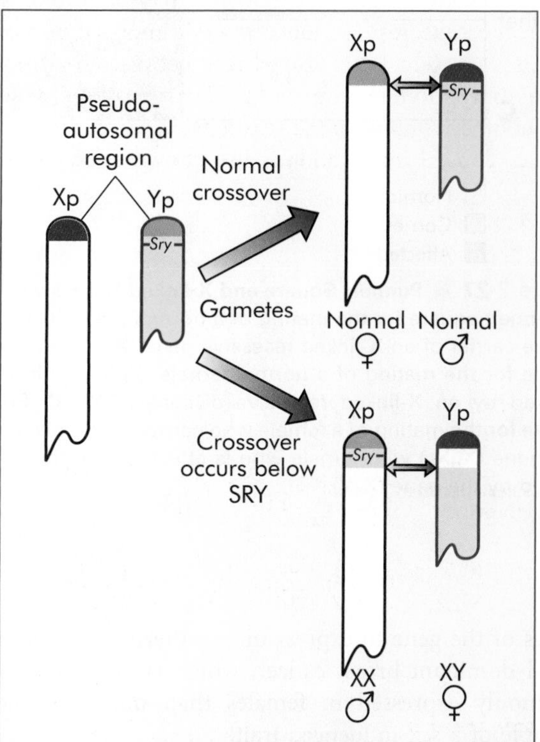

Figure 2-26 ■ **Distal Short Arms of the X and Y Chromosomes Exchange Material During Meiosis in the Male.** The region of the Y chromosome in which this crossover occurs is called the *pseudoautosomal region.* The *SRY* gene, which triggers the process leading to male gonadal differentiation, is located just outside the pseudoautosomal region. Occasionally, the crossover occurs on the centrometric side of the *SRY* gene, causing it to lie on an X chromosome instead of a Y chromosome. An offspring receiving this X chromosome will be an XX male, and an offspring receiving the Y chromosome will be an XY female.

Other genes that contribute to male differentiation are located on other chromosomes. Thus, *SRY* triggers the action of genes on other chromosomes. This concept is supported by the fact that the *SRY* protein product is similar to other proteins known to regulate gene expression.

Occasionally, the crossover between X and Y occurs closer to the centromere than it should, placing the *SRY* gene on the X chromosome after crossover. This variation can result in offspring with an apparently normal XX karyotype but a male phenotype. Such XX males are seen in about 1 in 20,000 live births and resemble males with Klinefelter syndrome. Conversely, it is possible to inherit a Y chromosome that has lost the *SRY* gene (the result of either a crossover error or a deletion of the gene). This situation produces an XY female. Such females have gonadal streaks rather than ovaries and have poorly developed secondary sex characteristics.

✔ QUICK CHECK 2-2

1. Why is the influence of environment significant to phenotype?
2. Discuss the differences between a dominant and recessive allele.
3. Why are the concepts of variable expressivity, incomplete penetrance, and delayed age of onset so important in relation to genetic diseases?
4. What is the recurrence risk for autosomal dominant inheritance and recessive inheritance?

Characteristics of pedigrees

X-linked pedigrees show distinctive modes of inheritance. The most striking characteristic is that females seldom are affected. To express an X-linked recessive trait, a female must be homozygous: either both her parents are affected, or her father is affected and her mother is a carrier. Such matings are rare.

The following are important principles of X-linked recessive inheritance:

1. The trait is seen much more often in males than in females.
2. Because a father can give a son only a Y chromosome, the trait is never transmitted from father to son.
3. The gene can be transmitted through a series of carrier females, causing the appearance of one or more "skipped generations."
4. The gene is passed from an affected father to all his daughters, who, as phenotypically normal carriers, transmit it to approximately half their sons, who are affected.

The most common and severe of all X-linked recessive disorders is Duchenne muscular dystrophy (DMD), which affects approximately 1 in 3500 males. As its name suggests, this disorder is characterized by progressive muscle degeneration. Affected individuals usually are unable to walk by age 10 or 12 years. The disease affects the heart and respiratory muscles, and death caused by respiratory or cardiac failure usually occurs before 20 years of age. Identification of the disease gene (on the short arm of the X chromosome) has greatly increased our understanding of the disorder.[15] The DMD gene is the largest gene ever found in the human, spanning more than 2 million DNA bases. It encodes a previously undiscovered muscle protein, termed **dystrophin.** Extensive study of dystrophin indicates that it plays an essential role in maintaining the structural integrity of muscle cells: it may also help to regulate the activity of membrane proteins. When dystrophin is absent, as in DMD, the cell cannot survive, and muscle deterioration ensues. Most cases of DMD are caused by frameshift deletions of portions of the DMD gene and thus involve alterations of all the amino acids encoded by the DNA following the deletion.

Recurrence risks

The most common mating type involving X-linked recessive genes is the combination of a carrier female and a normal male (Figure 2-27, *A*). On average, the carrier mother will transmit the disease gene to half her sons (who are affected) and half her daughters (who are carriers).

The other common mating type is an affected father and a normal mother (Figure 2-27, *B*). In this situation, all the sons must be normal because the father can transmit only his Y chromosome to them. Because all the daughters must receive the father's X chromosome, they will all be heterozygous carriers. Because the sons *must* receive the Y chromosome and the daughters *must* receive the X chromosome with the disease gene, these are precise outcomes and not probabilities. None of the children will be affected.

The final mating pattern, less common than the other two, involves an affected father and a carrier mother (Figure 2-27, *C*). With this pattern, on average, half the daughters will be heterozygous carriers, and half will be homozygous for the disease gene and thus affected. Half the sons will be normal, and half will be affected. Some X-linked recessive diseases, such as DMD, are fatal or incapacitating before the affected individual reaches reproductive age, and therefore affected fathers are rare or nonexistent.

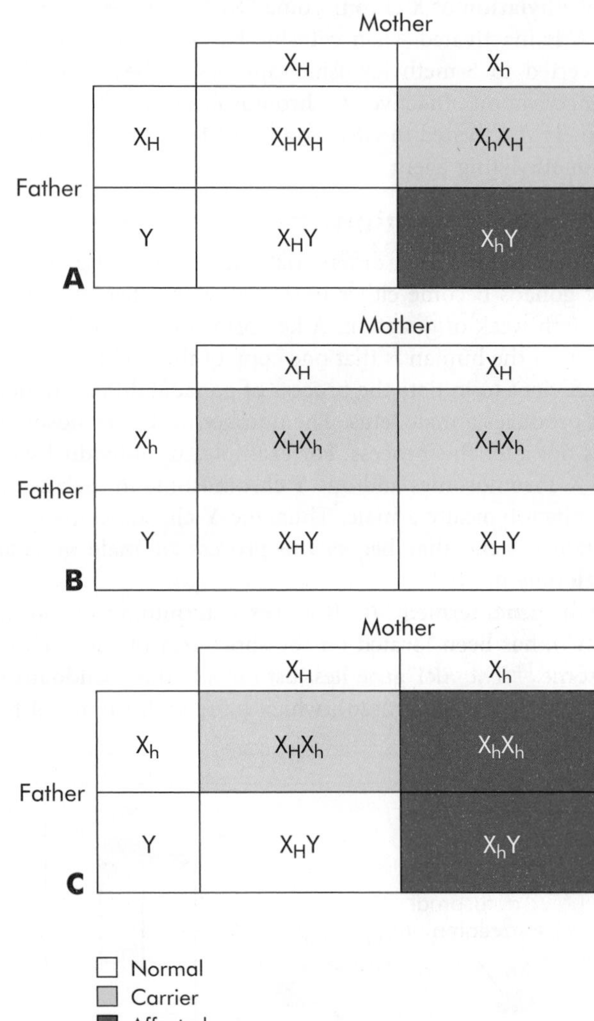

Figure 2-27 ■ Punnett Square and X-linked Recessive Traits. A, Punnett square for the mating of a normal male (X_HY) and a female carrier of an X-linked recessive gene (X_HX_h). **B,** Punnett square for the mating of a normal female (X_HX_H) with a male affected by an X-linked recessive disease (X_hY). **C,** Punnett square for the mating of a female who carries an X-linked recessive gene (X_HX_h) with a male who is affected with the disease caused by the gene (X_hY).

Sex-limited and sex-influenced traits

A **sex-limited trait** can occur in only one sex, often because of anatomic differences. Inherited uterine and testicular defects are two obvious examples. A **sex-influenced trait** occurs much more often in one sex than the other. For example, male-pattern baldness occurs in both males and females but is much more common in males. In males it is inherited as an autosomal dominant trait, whereas in females it is inherited as an autosomal recessive trait. Because of their hormonal constitution, females need two copies of the gene to express male-pattern baldness. Autosomal dominant breast cancer, which is now much more commonly expressed in females than males, is another example of a sex-influenced trait.

Evaluation of Pedigrees

With complications such as incomplete penetrance, variable expressivity, delayed age of onset, and sex-influenced traits, it is not always possible simply to look at a disease pedigree and determine the mode of inheritance. A sophisticated statistical methodologic approach has evolved to deal with such complications. Incorporated into computer programs, these statistical techniques assess the probability of observing a certain pedigree if a particular mode of inheritance (e.g., autosomal dominant with incomplete penetrance) is in effect.

LINKAGE ANALYSIS AND GENE MAPPING

Locating genes on specific regions of chromosomes is one of the most important endeavors in human genetics. The location and identification of a gene can tell much about the function of the gene, its interaction with other genes, and the likelihood that certain individuals will develop a genetic disease.

Classical Pedigree Analysis

Mendel's second law, the principle of independent assortment, states that an individual's genes will be transmitted to the next generation independently of one another. This law is only partly true, however, because genes located close together on the same chromosome do tend to be transmitted together to the offspring. Thus Mendel's principle of independent assortment holds true for most pairs of genes but not those that occupy the same region of a chromosome. Such loci demonstrate **linkage** and are said to be linked.

During the first meiotic stage, the arms of homologous chromosome pairs intertwine and sometimes exchange portions of their DNA (Figure 2-28) in a process known as **crossing over** (or **crossover**). During crossover, new combinations of alleles can be formed. For example, two loci on a chromosome have alleles A and a and alleles B and b. Alleles A and B are located together on one member of a chromosome pair, and alleles a and b are located on the other member. The genotype of this individual is denoted as AB/ab.

As Figure 2-28, *A*, shows, the allele pairs AB and ab would be transmitted together when no crossover occurs. However, when crossover occurs (Figure 2-28, *B*), all four possible pairs of alleles can be transmitted to the offspring: AB, aB, Ab, and ab. The process of forming such new arrangements of alleles is called **recombination.** Crossover does not necessarily lead to recombination, however, because double crossover between two loci can result in no actual recombination of the alleles at the loci (Figure 2-28, *C*).

Once a close linkage has been established between a disease locus and a "marker" locus (a DNA sequence that varies among individuals) and once the alleles of the two loci that are inherited together within a family have been determined, reliable predictions can be made as to whether a member of a family will develop the disease. This ability is especially important for diseases with delayed age of onset. Linkage has been established between several DNA polymorphisms and each of the two genes for autosomal dominant breast cancer (about 5% of breast cancer cases are caused by these autosomal dominant genes). Determining this kind of linkage means that it is possible for offspring of an individual with autosomal dominant breast cancer to know whether they also carry the gene and thus could pass it on to their own children. Other diseases for which linked markers have been found include adult polycystic kidney disease, familial Alzheimer disease, Huntington disease, and neurofibromatosis, type 1. In addition, specific mutations that cause these diseases have been identified, enabling direct detection of disease-causing mutations.

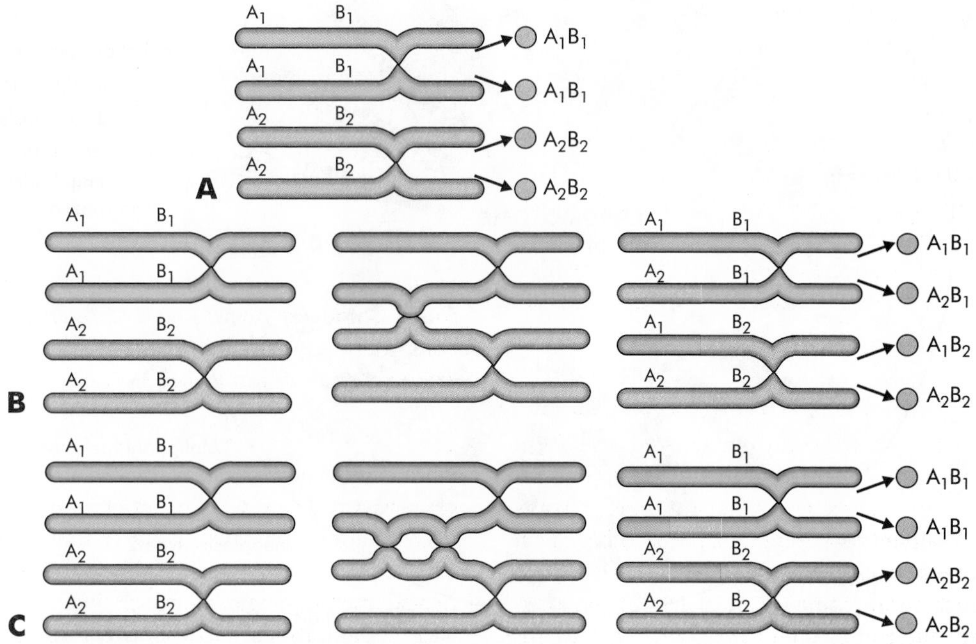

Figure 2-28 ■ **Genetic Results of Crossing Over. A,** No crossing over. **B,** Crossing over with recombination. **C,** Double crossing over, resulting in no recombination.

For some genetic diseases, prophylactic treatment is available if the condition can be diagnosed in time. An example of this is hemochromatosis, a recessive genetic disease in which excess iron is absorbed, causing degeneration of the heart, liver, brain, and other vital organs. The gene for hemochromatosis is closely linked to the human leukocyte antigen (HLA) (see Chapter 5) complex on chromosome 6. Individuals at risk for developing the disease can be determined by testing for a mutation in the hemochromatosis gene, and preventive therapy (periodic phlebotomy) can be initiated to deplete iron stores and ensure a normal life span.

Complete Human Gene Map: Prospects and Benefits

Rapid progress is being made in assigning genes to their chromosomal locations. A number of important genetic diseases have been located on specific areas of individual chromosomes: these include Huntington disease, retinoblastoma, DMD, hemophilia A, cystic fibrosis, PKU, neurofibromatosis, and several forms of familial Alzheimer disease (Figure 2-29).[1,16] Table 2-2 contains a partial list of mapped diseases. The development of thousands of new DNA markers is especially helpful in this effort. Mapping a disease gene is an important step toward isolating and **cloning** the gene (clones are identical copies of genes). Once a gene is cloned, its DNA sequence can be studied to determine the nature and function of the protein encoded by the gene. Cloning the genes that cause diseases such as cystic fibrosis and DMD has contributed immensely to our understanding of the pathophysiology of these disorders. In addition, the ability to clone a gene opens up the possibility of gene therapy for the disorder.

HEALTH ALERT
Gene Therapy

More than 6000 individuals are enrolled in more than 900 protocols. Most of these protocols involve the genetic alteration of cells to combat various types of cancer. Other protocols involve the treatment of inherited diseases, such as cystic fibrosis and familial hypercholesterolemia.

Data from Cavazzana-Calvo M, Thrasuer A, Mavilio F: The future of gene therapy, *Nat* 427:779–781, 2004.

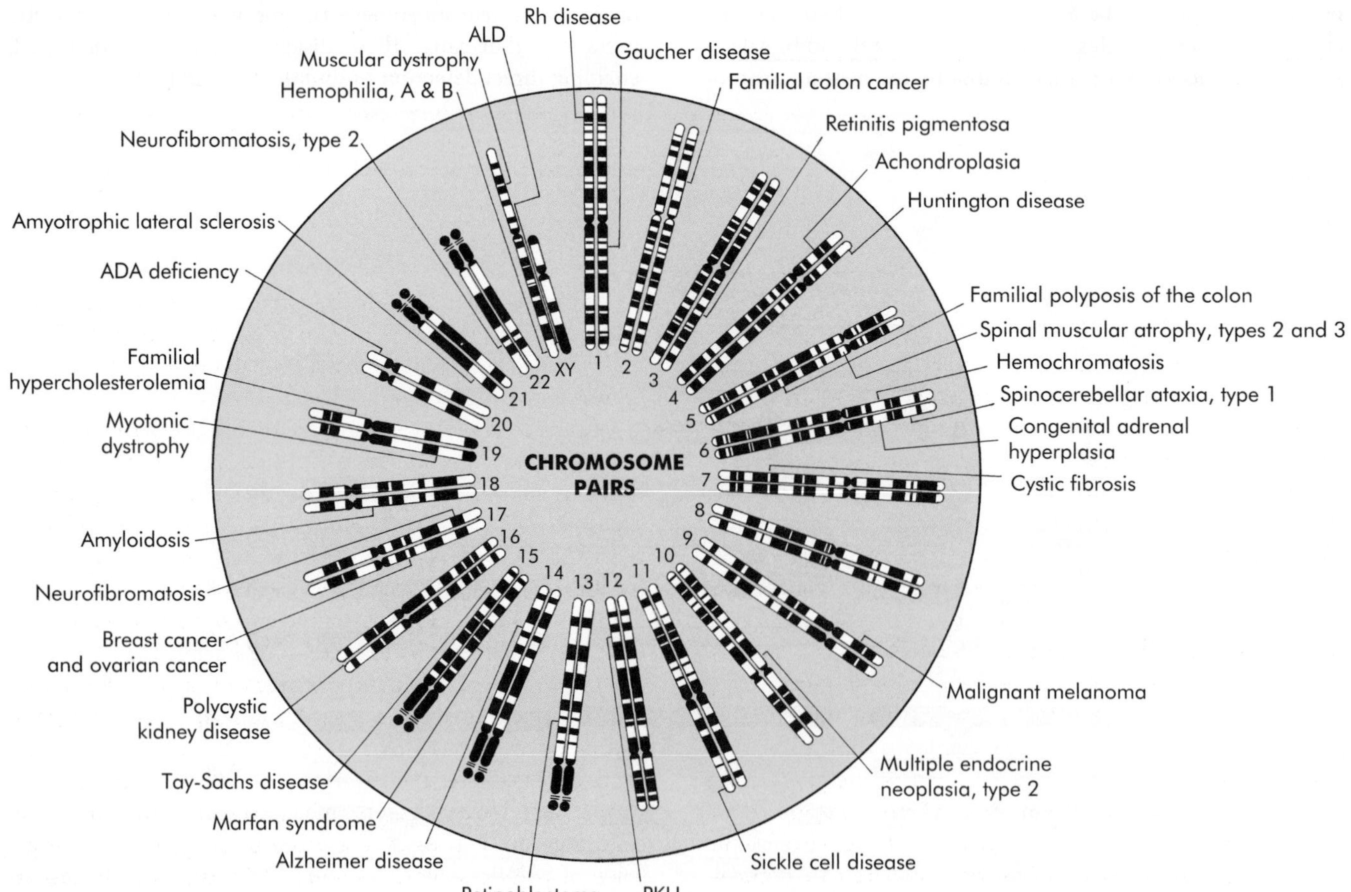

Figure 2-29 ■ **Example of Diseases: A Gene Map.** *PKU,* phenylketonuria; *ALD,* adrenoleukodystrophy; *ADA,* adenosine deaminase.

TABLE 2-2

Some Important Genetic Diseases That Have Been Mapped to Specific Chromosome Locations and Cloned

Disease	Chromosome Location
Huntington disease	4p16
Cystic fibrosis	7q31
Hemophilia A	Xq28
Marfan syndrome	15q15-21
Sickle cell anemia	11p15
α-Thalassemia	11p15
β-Thalassemia	16pter-p12
Familial breast cancer	
BRCA1	17q21
BRCA2	13q
Fragile X syndrome	Xq27
Phenylketonuria	12q21-qter
Duchenne muscular dystrophy	Xp21
Becker muscular dystrophy*	Xp21
Retinoblastoma	13q14
Hemochromatosis	6p21
Familial hypercholesterolemia	19p13 (LDL receptor defect)
Polycystic kidney disease	16p,4
α1-Antitrypsin deficiency	14q31-32
Familial Alzheimer disease†	21q11-q21, 14, 19, 1
Tay-Sachs disease	15q22-q25
Neurofibromatosis, type 1	17q11 19p13 (classical)
Neurofibromatosis, type 2	22q11-13 17q11 (bilateral acoustic form)
Familial polyposis coli	5q21-22

*Becker muscular dystrophy is an allelic form of Duchenne muscular dystrophy.
†Familial Alzheimer disease is a complex, heterogenous disease. The single genes now located for this disease are associated with only some of the known causes.

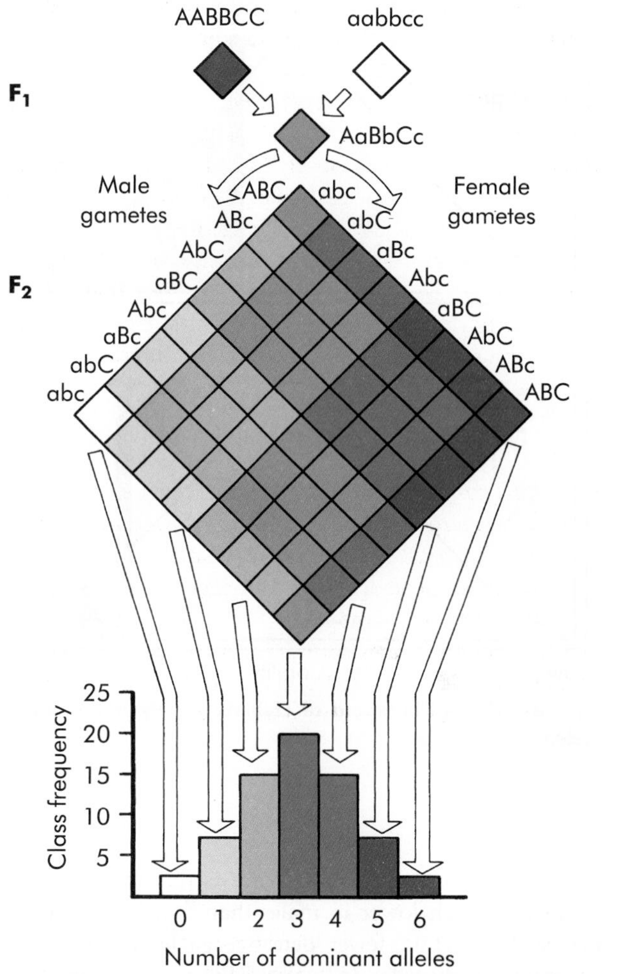

Figure 2-30 ■ **Multifactorial Inheritance.** Analysis of mode of inheritance for grain color in wheat. The trait is controlled by three independently assorted gene loci.

MULTIFACTORIAL INHERITANCE

Not all traits are produced by single genes; some traits result from several genes acting together. These are called **polygenic traits.** When environmental factors influence the expression of the trait (as is usually the case), the term **multifactorial inheritance** is used. Many multifactorial and polygenic traits tend to follow a normal distribution in populations (the familiar bell-shaped curve). Figure 2-30 shows how three loci acting together can cause grain color in wheat to vary in a gradual way from white to red, exemplifying multifactorial inheritance. If both the alleles at each of the three loci are white alleles, the color is pure white. If most alleles are white but a few are red, the color is somewhat darker; if all are red, the color is dark red.

Other examples of multifactorial traits include height and IQ. Although both height and IQ are determined in part by genes, they are influenced also by environment. For example, the average height of many human populations has increased by 5 to 10 cm in the past 100 years because of improvements in nutrition and health care. Also, IQ scores can be improved by exposing individuals (especially children) to enriched learning environments. Thus, both genes and environment contribute to variation in these traits.

A number of diseases do not follow the bell-shaped distribution. Instead they appear to be either present in or absent from an individual. Yet they do not follow the patterns expected of single-gene diseases. Many of these are probably polygenic or multifactorial, but a certain **threshold of liability** must be crossed before the disease is expressed. Below the threshold the individual appears normal; above it, the individual is affected by the disease (Figure 2-31).

One of the best-known examples of such a threshold trait is pyloric stenosis, a disorder characterized by a narrowing or obstruction of the pylorus, the area between the stomach and intestine. Chronic vomiting, constipation, weight loss, and electrolyte imbalance can result from the condition, but it is easily corrected by surgery. The prevalence of pyloric stenosis is about 3 in 1000 live births in whites. This disorder is much more common in males than females, affecting 1 in 200 males and 1 in 1000 females. The

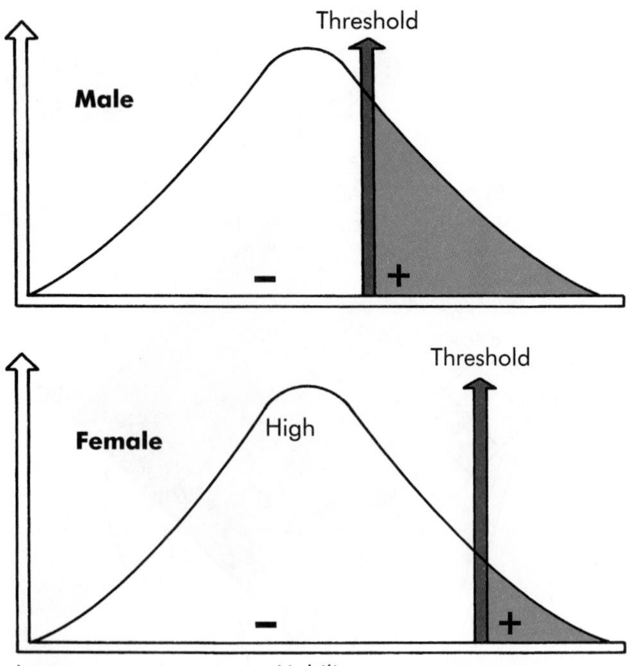

Figure 2-31 ■ **Threshold of Liability for Pyloric Stenosis in Males and Females.**

apparent reason for this difference is that the threshold of liability is much lower in males than females, as shown in Figure 2-30. Thus, fewer defective alleles are required to generate the disorder in males. This situation also means that the offspring of affected females are more likely to have pyloric stenosis because affected females necessarily carry more disease-causing alleles than do most affected males.

A number of other common diseases are thought to correspond to a threshold model. They include cleft lip and cleft palate, neural tube defects (anencephaly, spina bifida), clubfoot (talipes), and some forms of congenital heart disease.

Although recurrence risks can be given with confidence for single-gene diseases (e.g., 50% for autosomal dominants, 25% for autosomal recessives), it is considerably more difficult to do so for multifactorial diseases. The number of genes contributing to the disease is not known, the precise allelic constitution of the parents is not known, and the extent of environmental effects can vary from one population to another. For most multifactorial diseases, **empirical risks** (i.e., those based on direct observation) have been derived. To determine empirical risks, a large sample of families in which one child has developed the disease is examined. Then the siblings of each child are surveyed to calculate what percentage of them also develop the disease.

Another difficulty is distinguishing polygenic or multifactorial diseases from single-gene diseases that have incomplete penetrance or variable expressivity (Box 2-1). Large data sets and good epidemiologic data often are necessary to make the distinction. Box 2-1 lists criteria that are commonly used to define multifactorial diseases.

The genetics of common disorders such as hypertension, heart disease, and diabetes is complex and often confusing. Nevertheless, the public health impact of these diseases, together with the evidence for hereditary factors in their etiology, demands that genetic studies be pursued. Specific genes contributing to susceptibility for each of these diseases have been discovered, and the next decade will undoubtedly witness substantial advancements in our understanding of these disorders.

QUICK CHECK 2-3

1. Define linkage analysis; cite an example.
2. Why is "threshold of liability" an important consideration in multifactorial inheritance?
3. Discuss the concept of multifactorial inheritance, and include two examples.

BOX 2-1 Criteria Used to Define Multifactorial Diseases

1. The recurrence risk becomes higher if more than one family member is affected. For example, the recurrence risk for neural tube defects in a British family increases to 10% if two siblings have been born with the disease. By contrast, the recurrence risk for single-gene diseases remains the same regardless of the number of siblings affected.
2. If the expression of the disease is more severe, the recurrence risk is higher. This is consistent with the liability model; a more severe expression indicates that the individual is at the extreme end of the liability distribution. Relatives of the affected individual are thus at a higher risk for inheriting disease genes. Cleft lip or cleft palate is a condition in which this has been shown to be true.
3. Relatives of probands of the less commonly affected are more likely to develop the disease. As with pyloric stenosis, this occurs because an affected individual of the less susceptible sex is usually at a more extreme position on the liability distribution.
4. Generally, if the population frequency of the disease is f, the risk for offspring and siblings of probands is approximately $\sqrt{f}$. This does not usually hold true for single-gene traits.
5. The recurrence risk for the disease decreases rapidly in more remotely related relatives. Although the recurrence risk for single-gene diseases decreases by 50% with each degree of relationship (e.g., an autosomal dominant disease has a 50% recurrence risk for siblings, 25% for uncle-nephew relationship, 12.5% for first cousins), the risk for multifactorial inheritance decreases much more quickly.

Did You Understand?

DNA, RNA, and Proteins: Heredity at the Molecular Level

1. Genes, the basic units of inheritance, are composed of deoxyribonucleic acid (DNA) and are located on chromosomes.
2. DNA is composed of deoxyribose, a phosphate molecule, and four types of nitrogenous bases. The physical structure of DNA is a double helix.
3. The DNA bases code for amino acids, which in turn make up proteins. The amino acids are specified by triplet codons of nitrogenous bases.
4. DNA replication is based on complementary base pairing, in which a single strand of DNA serves as the template for attracting bases that form a new strand of DNA.
5. DNA polymerase is the primary enzyme involved in replication. It adds bases to the new DNA strand and performs "proofreading" functions.
6. A mutation is an inherited alteration of genetic material (i.e., DNA).
7. Substances that cause mutations are called *mutagens.*
8. The mutation rate in humans varies from locus to locus and ranges from 10^{-4} to 10^{-7} per gene per generation.
9. Transcription and translation, the two basic processes in which proteins are specified by DNA, both involve ribonucleic acid (RNA). RNA is chemically similar to DNA, but it is single-stranded, has a ribose sugar molecule, and has uracil rather than thymine as one of its four nitrogenous bases.
10. Transcription is the process by which DNA specifies a sequence of messenger RNA (mRNA).
11. Much of the RNA sequence is spliced from the mRNA before the mRNA leaves the nucleus. The excised sequences are called *introns,* and those that remain to code for proteins are called *exons.*
12. Translation is the process by which RNA directs the synthesis of polypeptides. This process takes place in the ribosomes, which consist of proteins and ribosomal RNA (rRNA).
13. During translation, mRNA interacts with transfer RNA (tRNA), a molecule that has an attachment site for a specific amino acid.

Chromosomes

1. Human cells consist of diploid somatic cells (body cells) and haploid gametes (sperm and egg cells).
2. Humans have 23 pairs of chromosomes. Twenty-two of these pairs are autosomes. The remaining pair consists of the sex chromosomes. Females have two homologous X chromosomes as their sex chromosomes; males have an X and a Y chromosome.
3. A karyotype is an ordered display of chromosomes arranged according to length and the location of the centromere.
4. Various types of stains can be used to make chromosome bands more visible.
5. About 1 in 150 live births has a major diagnosable chromosome abnormality. Chromosome abnormalities are the leading known cause of mental retardation and miscarriage.
6. Polyploidy is a condition in which a euploid cell has some multiple of the normal number of chromosomes. Humans have been observed to have triploidy (three copies of each chromosome) and tetraploidy (four copies of each chromosome); both conditions are lethal.
7. Somatic cells that do not have a multiple of 23 chromosomes are aneuploid. Aneuploidy is usually the result of nondisjunction.
8. Trisomy is a type of aneuploidy in which one chromosome is present in three copies in somatic cells. A partial trisomy is one in which only part of a chromosome is present in three copies.
9. Monosomy is a type of aneuploidy in which one chromosome is present in only one copy in somatic cells.
10. In general, monosomies cause more severe physical defects than do trisomies, illustrating the principle that the loss of chromosome material has more severe consequences than the duplication of chromosome material.
11. Down syndrome, a trisomy of chromosome 21, is the best-known disease caused by a chromosome aberration. It affects 1 in 800 live births and is much more likely to occur in the offspring of women older than 35 years.
12. Most aneuploidies of the sex chromosomes have less severe consequences than those of the autosomes.
13. The most commonly observed sex chromosome aneuploidies are the 47,XXX karyotype, 45,X karyotype (Turner syndrome), 47,XXY karyotype (Klinefelter syndrome), and 47,XYY karyotype.
14. Abnormalities of chromosome structure include deletions, duplications, inversions, and translocations.

Elements of Formal Genetics

1. Mendelian traits are caused by single genes, each of which occupies a position, or locus, on a chromosome.
2. Alleles are different forms of genes located at the same locus on a chromosome.
3. At any given locus in a somatic cell, an individual has two genes, one from each parent. An individual may be homozygous or heterozygous for a locus.
4. An individual's genotype is his or her genetic makeup, and the phenotype reflects the interaction of genotype and environment.
5. In a heterozygote, a dominant gene's effects mask those of a recessive gene. The recessive gene is expressed only when it is present in two copies.

Transmission of Genetic Diseases

1. Genetic diseases caused by single genes usually follow autosomal dominant, autosomal recessive, or X-linked recessive modes of inheritance.
2. Pedigree charts are important tools in the analysis of modes of inheritance.
3. Recurrence risks specify the probability that future offspring will inherit a genetic disease. For single-gene diseases, recurrence risks remain the same for each offspring, regardless of the number of affected or unaffected offspring.

(Continued)

Did You Understand?—Cont'd

4. The recurrence risk for autosomal dominant diseases is usually 50%.
5. Germline mosaicism can alter recurrence risks for genetic diseases because unaffected parents can produce multiple affected offspring. This situation occurs because the germline of one parent is affected by a mutation but the parent's somatic cells are unaffected.
6. Skipped generations are not seen in classical autosomal dominant pedigrees.
7. Males and females are equally likely to exhibit autosomal dominant diseases and to pass them on to their offspring.
8. Many genetic diseases have a delayed age of onset.
9. A gene that is not always expressed phenotypically is said to have incomplete penetrance.
10. Variable expressivity is a characteristic of many genetic diseases.
11. Genomic imprinting, which is associated with methylation, results in differing expression of a disease gene, depending on which parent transmitted the gene.
12. Epigenetics involves changes, such as the methylation of DNA bases, that do not alter the DNA sequence but can alter the expression of genes.
13. Most commonly, parents of children with autosomal recessive diseases are both heterozygous carriers of the disease gene.
14. The recurrence risk for autosomal recessive diseases is 25%.
15. Males and females are equally likely to be affected by autosomal recessive diseases.
16. Consanguinity is sometimes present in families with autosomal recessive diseases, and it becomes more prevalent with rarer recessive diseases.
17. Carrier detection tests for an increasing number of autosomal recessive diseases are available.
18. The frequency of genetic diseases approximately doubles in the offspring of first-cousin matings.
19. In each normal female somatic cell, one of the two X chromosomes is inactivated early in embryogenesis.
20. X inactivation is random, fixed, and incomplete (i.e., only part of the chromosome is actually inactivated). It may involve methylation.
21. Gender is determined embryonically by the presence of the *SRY* gene on the Y chromosome. Embryos that have a Y chromosome (and thus the *SRY* gene) become males, whereas those lacking the Y chromosome become females. When the Y chromosome lacks the *SRY* gene, an XY female can be produced. Similarly, an X chromosome that contains the SRY gene can produce an XX male.
22. X-linked genes are those that are located on the X chromosome. Nearly all known X-linked diseases are caused by X-linked recessive genes.
23. Males are hemizygous for genes on the X chromosome.
24. X-linked recessive diseases are seen much more often in males than in females because males need only one copy of the gene to express the disease.
25. Fathers cannot pass X-linked genes to their sons.
26. Skipped generations often are seen in X-linked recessive disease pedigrees because the gene can be transmitted through carrier females.
27. Recurrence risks for X-linked recessive diseases depend on the carrier and affected status of the mother and father.
28. A sex-limited trait is one that occurs only in one sex (gender).
29. A sex-influenced trait is one that occurs more often in one sex than in the other.

Linkage Analysis and Gene Mapping

1. During meiosis I, crossover occurs and can cause recombinations of alleles located on the same chromosome.
2. The frequency of recombinations can be used to infer the map distance between loci on the same chromosome.
3. A marker locus, when closely linked to a disease-gene locus, can be used to predict whether an individual will develop a genetic disease.
4. A more complete gene map will facilitate marker studies, gene cloning, studies of gene function and interaction, and gene therapy.

Multifactorial Inheritance

1. Traits that result from the combined effects of several loci are polygenic. When environmental factors also influence the trait, it is multifactorial.
2. Many multifactorial traits have a threshold of liability. Once the threshold of liability has been crossed, the disease may be expressed.
3. Empiric risks, based on direct observation of large numbers of families, are used to estimate recurrence risks for multifactorial diseases.
4. Recurrence risks for multifactorial diseases become higher if more than one family member is affected or if the expression of the disease in the proband is more severe.
5. Recurrence risks for multifactorial diseases decrease rapidly for more remote relatives.

Key Terms

Adenine, 36
Allele, 46
Amino acid, 37
Aneuploid cell, 41
Anticodon, 39
Autosome, 39
Barr body, 52
Base pair substitution, 37
Carrier detection test, 51
Carrier, 47
Chromosomal mosaic, 43
Chromosome band, 39
Chromosome breakage, 45
Chromosome theory of inheritance, 47
Chromosome, 36
Clastogen, 45
Cloning, 56
Codominance, 47
Codon, 37
Complementary base pairing, 37
Consanguinity, 52
CpG islands, 49
Cri du chat syndrome, 45
Crossing over (crossover), 55
Cytokinesis, 39
Cytosine, 36
Delayed age of onset, 49
Deletion, 45
Deoxyribonucleic acid (DNA), 36
Diploid cell, 39
DNA methylation, 50
DNA polymerase, 37
Dominant, 47
Dosage compensation, 52
Double-helix model, 36
Down syndrome, 43
Duplication, 45
Dystrophin, 54
Empirical risk, 58
Epigenetic, 49
Euploid cell, 40
Exon, 38
Expressivity, 49
Fragile site, 46
Frameshift mutation, 37
Gamete, 39
Gene, 36
Genomic imprinting, 50
Genotype, 47
Germline mosaicism, 49
Guanine, 36
Haploid cell, 39
Hemizygous, 52
Heterogeneous nuclear RNA (hnRNA), 38
Heterozygote, 47
Heterozygous, 47
Homologous, 39
Homozygote, 47
Homozygous, 47
Inbreeding, 52
Intron, 38
Inversion, 45
Karyotype, 39
Klinefelter syndrome, 43
Linkage, 55
Locus, 46
Meiosis, 39
Messenger RNA (mRNA), 38
Metaphase spread, 39
Methylation, 53
Mitosis, 39
Mode of inheritance, 47
Multifactorial inheritance, 57
Mutagen, 37
Mutation, 37
Mutational hot spot, 37
Nondisjunction, 41
Nucleotide, 37
Obligate carrier, 49
Partial trisomy, 43
Pedigree, 47
Penetrance, 49
Phenotype, 47
Polygenic trait, 57
Polymorphic (polymorphism), 46
Polypeptide, 37
Polyploid cell, 40
Position effect, 45
Principle of independent assortment, 47
Principle of segregation, 47
Proband (propositus/proposita), 47
Promoter site, 38
Pseudoautosomal, 53
Purine, 36
Pyrimidine, 36
Recessive, 47
Reciprocal translocation, 46
Recombination, 55
Recurrence risk, 48
Ribonucleic acid (RNA), 38
Ribosomal RNA (rRNA), 39
Ribosome, 39
RNA polymerase, 38
Robertsonian translocation, 46
Sex-influenced trait, 54
Sex-limited trait, 54
Sex linked (inheritance), 52
Somatic cell, 39
Spontaneous mutation, 37
Template, 37
Termination sequence, 38
Tetraploidy, 40
Threshold of liability, 57
Thymine, 36
Transcription, 38
Transfer RNA (tRNA), 38
Translation, 38
Translocation, 46
Triploidy, 40
Trisomy, 41
Tumor-suppressor gene, 49
Turner syndrome, 43
X inactivation, 52

References

1. Jorde LB et al: *Medical genetics*, ed 3, updated, St Louis, 2006, Mosby.
2. Hassold TJ: Chromosome abnormalities in human reproductive wastage, *Trends Genet* 2:105–110, 1986.
3. Hassold T, Hunt PA: To err (meiotically) is human: the genesis of human aneuploidy, *Nat Rev Genet* 2(4):280–291, 2001.
4. Roizen NJ, Patterson D: Down's syndrome, *Lancet* 361 (9365):1281–1289, 2003.
5. Allanson JE, Graham GE: Sex chromosome abnormalities, In Rimoin DL et al, editors: *Emery and Rimoin's principles and practice of medical genetics*, ed 4, London, 2002, Churchill Livingstone.
6. Terracciano A, Chiurazzi P, Neri G: Fragile X syndrome, *Am J Med Genet C Semin Med Genet* 137(1):32–37, 2005.
7. Gatchel JR, Zoghbi HY: Diseases of unstable repeat expansion: mechanisms and common principles, *Nat Rev Genet* 6 (10):743–755, 2005.
8. Zlotogora J: Germ line mosaicism, *Hum Genet* 102(4): 381–386, 1998.
9. Vogelstein G, Kinzler KW, editors: *The genetic basis of human cancer*, ed 2, New York, 2002, McGraw-Hill.
10. Arun D, Gutmann DH: Recent advances in neurofibromatosis type 1, *Curr Opin Neurol* 17(2):101–105, 2004.
11. Fraga MF et al: Epigenetic differences arise during the lifetime of monozygotic twins, *Proc Natl Acad Sci USA* 102: 10604–10609, 2005.
12. Lyon MF: X-chromosome inactivation, *Curr Biol* 9(7): R235–R237, 1999.
13. Brown CJ, Greally JM: A stain upon the silence: genes escaping X inactivation, *Trends Genet* 19(8):432–438, 2003.
14. Fleming A, Vilain E: The endless quest for sex determination genes, *Clin Genet* 67(1):15–25, 2005.
15. Emery AEH: Duchenne and other X-linked muscular dystrophies, In Rimoin DL et al, editors: *Emery and Rimoin's principles and practice of medical genetics*, ed 4, London, 2002, Churchill Livingstone.
16. Collins FS, Morgan M, Patrinos A: The Human Genome Project: lessons from large-scale biology, *Science* 300(5617): 286–290, 2003.

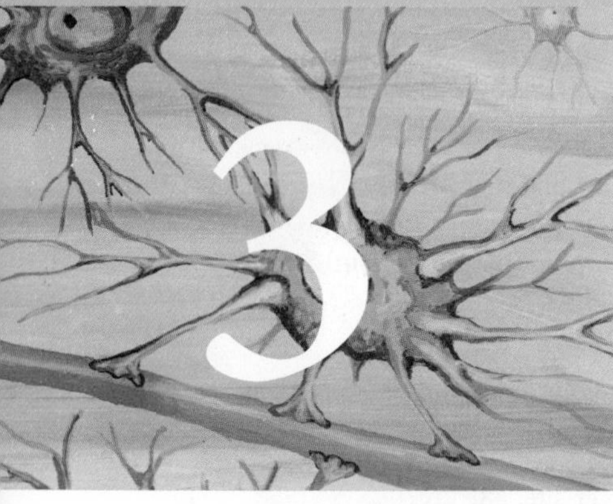

3 ALTERED CELLULAR AND TISSUE BIOLOGY

Kathryn L. McCance ▪ Todd Cameron Grey

CHAPTER OUTLINE

ELECTRONIC RESOURCES

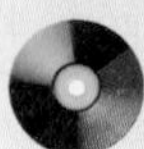

Companion CD
- Review Questions and Answers
- Animations

evolve Website
http://evolve.elsevier.com/Huether/
- Quick Check Answers
- Key Terms Exercises
- Critical Thinking Questions with Answers
- Algorithm Completion Exercises
- WebLinks

Knowledge of the structural and functional reactions of cells and tissues to injurious agents, including genetic defects, is key for the understanding of disease processes. Altered cellular and tissue biology can result from adaptation, injury, neoplasia, aging, or death. (Neoplasia is discussed in Chapters 9 to 11.) Adaptation occurs in response to both normal, or physiologic, conditions and adverse, or pathologic, conditions. For example, the uterus adapts to pregnancy—a normal physiologic state—by enlarging. Enlargement occurs because of an increase in the size and number of uterine cells. In an adverse condition such as high blood pressure, myocardial cells are stimulated to enlarge by the increased work of pumping. Like most of the body's adaptive mechanisms, however, cellular adaptations to adverse conditions are usually only temporarily successful. Severe or long-term stressors overwhelm adaptive processes, and cellular injury or death ensues.

Injury may be reversible (sublethal) or irreversible (lethal) and is classified broadly as chemical, hypoxic (lack of sufficient oxygen), free radical, intentional, unintentional, immunologic, infection, and inflammatory. Cellular injuries from various causes have different clinical and pathophysiologic manifestations. Cellular death is confirmed by structural changes seen when cells are stained and examined under a microscope.

Cellular aging causes structural and functional changes that eventually may lead to cellular death or a decreased capacity to recover from injury. Mechanisms explaining how and why cells age are not known, and distinguishing between pathologic changes and physiologic changes that occur with aging is often difficult. Aging clearly causes alterations in cellular structure and function, yet senescence is both inevitable and normal.

CELLULAR ADAPTATION

Cells adapt to their environment to escape and protect themselves from injury. An adapted cell is neither normal nor injured—its condition lies somewhere between these two states. Cellular adaptations, however, are a common and central part of many disease states. In the early stages of a successful adaptive response, cells may have enhanced function; thus, it is hard to know whether the response is pathologic or an extreme adaptation to an excessive functional demand. The most significant adaptive changes in cells include atrophy (decrease in cell size), hypertrophy (increase in cell size), hyperplasia (increase in cell number), and metaplasia (reversible replacement of one mature cell type by another less mature cell type). Dysplasia (deranged cellular growth) is not considered a true cellular adaptation but rather an atypical hyperplasia. These changes are shown in Figure 3-1.

Atrophy

Atrophy is a decrease or shrinkage in cellular size. If atrophy occurs in a sufficient number of an organ's cells, the entire organ shrinks or becomes atrophic. Atrophy can affect any organ, but it is most common in skeletal muscle, the heart, secondary sex organs, and the brain. Atrophy can be classified as *physiologic* or *pathologic*. **Physiologic atrophy** occurs with early development. For example, the thymus gland undergoes physiologic atrophy during childhood. **Pathologic atrophy** occurs as a result of decreases in workload, pressure, use, blood supply, nutrition, hormonal stimulation, and nervous stimulation. Individuals immobilized in bed for a prolonged time exhibit a type of skeletal muscle atrophy called **disuse atrophy.** Aging causes brain cells to become atrophic and endocrine-dependent organs, such as the gonads, to shrink as hormonal stimulation decreases. Whether atrophy is caused by normal physiologic conditions or by pathologic conditions, atrophic cells exhibit the same basic changes.

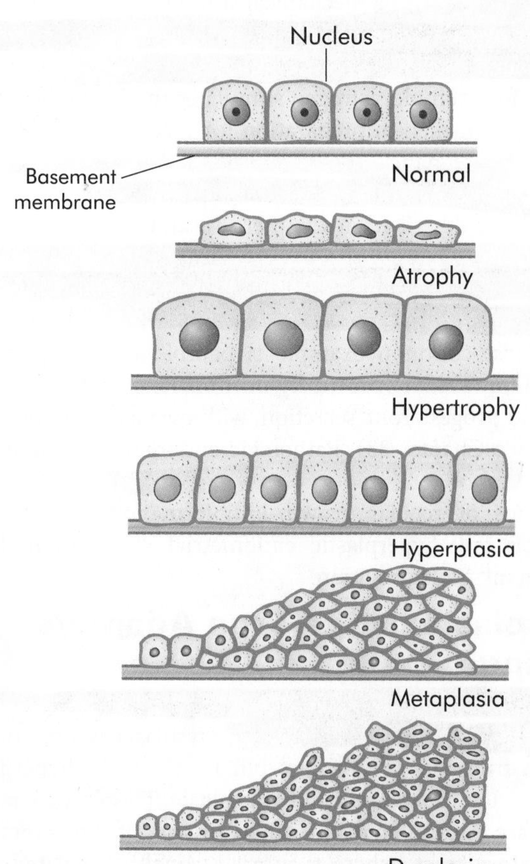

Figure 3-1 ■ **Adaptive and Dysplastic Alterations in Simple Cuboidal Epithelial Cells.**

The atrophic muscle cell contains less endoplasmic reticulum and fewer mitochondria and myofilaments (part of the muscle fiber that controls contraction) than does the normal cell. In muscular atrophy caused by nerve loss, oxygen consumption and amino acid uptake are immediately reduced. The biochemical changes of atrophy are just beginning to be understood. The mechanisms probably include decreased protein synthesis, increased protein catabolism, or both.[1]

Protein catabolism involves **proteosomes,** a large protein catabolic complex in the cytoplasm, and **ubiquitin-proteosome pathway,** where proteins are degraded first to ubiquitin (another small protein) and then degraded in the cytoplasm (see Figure 3-8). Protein ubiquitination and proteolysis play a central role in controlling protein turnover. Deregulation of this pathway often leads to abnormal cell growth and is associated with cancer and other diseases. This pathway is responsible for the rapid breakdown of proteins in hypercatabolic states, including cancer cachexia.

Atrophy resulting from chronic malnutrition is often accompanied by more **autophagic vacuoles,** which are membrane-bound vesicles within the cell that contain cellular debris and hydrolytic enzymes. The level of hydrolytic enzymes rises rapidly in atrophy. The enzymes are isolated in autophagic vacuoles to prevent uncontrolled cellular destruction. Thus, the vacuoles form as needed to protect uninjured organelles from the injured organelles and are eventually taken up and destroyed by lysosomes. Certain contents of the autophagic vacuole may resist destruction by lysosomal enzymes and persist in membrane-bound residual bodies. An example of this is granules that contain **lipofuscin,** the yellow-brown age pigment. Lipofuscin accumulates primarily in liver cells, myocardial cells, and atrophic cells.

Hypertrophy

Hypertrophy is an increase in the size of cells and consequently in the size of the affected organ (Figure 3-2). The cells of the heart and kidneys are particularly prone to enlargement. The increased cellular size is associated with an increased accumulation of protein in the cellular components (plasma membrane, endoplasmic reticulum, myofilaments, mitochondria) and *not* with an increase in cellular fluid. Hypertrophy can be *physiologic* or *pathologic* and is caused by specific hormone stimulation or by increased

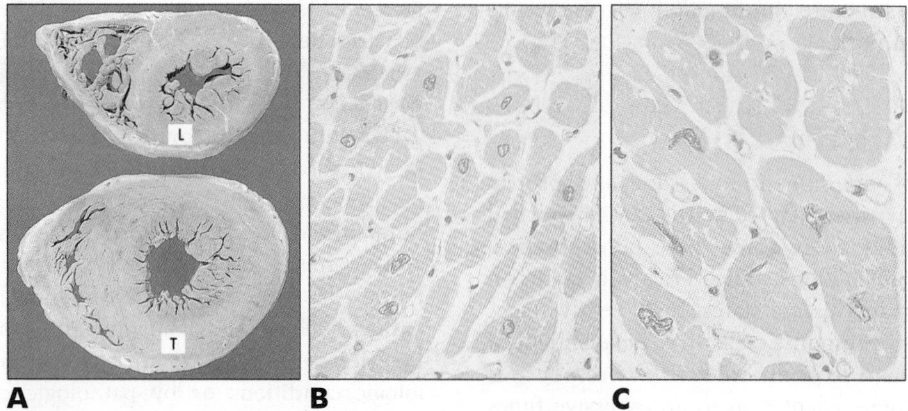

Figure 3-2 ■ **Hypertrophy of Cardiac Muscle in Response to Valve Disease. A**, Transverse slices of a normal heart and a heart with hypertrophy of the left ventricle (*L*, normal thickness of left ventricular wall; *T*, thickened wall from heart in which severe narrowing of aortic valve caused resistance to systolic ventricular emptying). **B**, Histology of cardiac muscle from the normal heart. **C**, Histology of cardiac muscle from a hypertrophied heart. (From Stevens A, Lowe J: *Pathology: illustrated review in color*, ed 2, Edinburgh, 2000, Mosby.)

functional demand. The triggers for hypertrophy include two types of signals: (1) mechanical signals, such as stretch, and (2) trophic signals, such as growth factors, hormones, and vasoactive agents. For example, in skeletal muscles, physiologic hypertrophy occurs in response to heavy work. Muscular hypertrophy tends to diminish if the excessive workload diminishes. When a diseased kidney is removed, the remaining kidney adapts to the increased workload with an increase in both the size and the number of cells. The major contributing factor to this renal enlargement is hypertrophy. Another example of normal or physiologic hypertrophy is the increased growth of the uterus and mammary glands in response to pregnancy. A pathologic example is pathophysiologic hypertrophy in the heart secondary to hypertension or problem valves.

Hyperplasia

Hyperplasia is an increase in the number of cells resulting from an increased rate of cellular division. Hyperplasia, as a response to injury, occurs when the injury has been severe and prolonged enough to have caused cell death. Loss of epithelial cells and cells of the liver and kidney triggers deoxyribonucleic acid (DNA) synthesis and mitotic division. Increased cell growth is a multistep process involving the production of growth factors, which stimulate the remaining cells to synthesize new cell components and, ultimately, to divide. Hyperplasia and hypertrophy often occur together, and both take place if the cells can synthesize DNA; however, in *nondividing cells* (e.g., myocardial fibers) only hypertrophy occurs.

Two types of normal, or physiologic, hyperplasia are (1) compensatory and (2) hormonal. **Compensatory hyperplasia** is an adaptive mechanism that enables certain organs to regenerate. For example, removal of part of the liver leads to hyperplasia of the remaining liver cells (hepatocytes) to compensate for the loss. Even with removal of 70% of the liver, regeneration is complete in about 2 weeks. **Hepatocyte growth factor (HGF)** is an important mediator in vitro of liver regeneration.[2]

Some cells—such as nerve, skeletal muscle, and myocardial cells and the lens cells of the eye—do not regenerate. Additional skeletal muscle cells, however, can be made by the fusion of myoblasts.[3] Significant compensatory hyperplasia occurs in epidermal and intestinal epithelia, hepatocytes, bone marrow cells, and fibroblasts, and some hyperplasia is noted in bone, cartilage, and smooth muscle cells. Another example of compensatory hyperplasia is the callus, or thickening, of the skin as a result of hyperplasia of epidermal cells in response to a mechanical stimulus.

Hormonal hyperplasia occurs chiefly in estrogen-dependent organs, such as the uterus and breast. After ovulation, for example, estrogen stimulates the endometrium to grow and thicken in preparation for receiving the fertilized ovum. If pregnancy occurs, hormonal hyperplasia, as well as hypertrophy, enables the uterus to enlarge. (Hormone function is described in Chapters 18 and 32.)

Pathologic hyperplasia is the abnormal proliferation of normal cells, usually in response to excessive hormonal stimulation or growth factors on target cells (Figure 3-3). The most common example is pathologic hyperplasia of the endometrium (caused by an imbalance between estrogen and progesterone secretion, with oversecretion of estrogen) (see Chapter 33). Pathologic endometrial hyperplasia, which causes excessive menstrual bleeding, is under the influence of regular growth-inhibition controls. If these controls fail, hyperplastic endometrial cells can undergo malignant transformation.

Dysplasia: Not a True Adaptive Change

Dysplasia refers to abnormal changes in the size, shape, and organization of mature cells. Dysplasia is not considered a true adaptive process but is related to hyperplasia and is often called **atypical hyperplasia.** Dysplastic changes often are encountered in epithelial tissue of the cervix and respiratory tract, where they are strongly associated with common neoplastic growths and often are found adjacent to cancerous cells. Data indicate that atypical hyperplasia

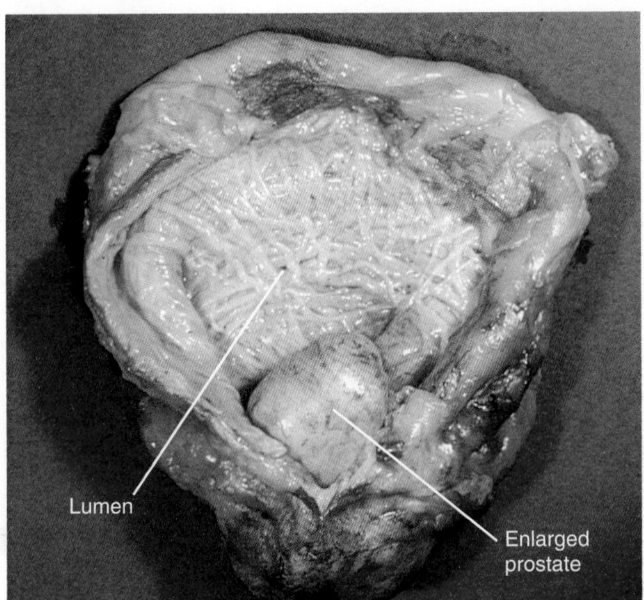

Figure 3-3 ■ Hyperplasia of the Prostate with Secondary Thickening of the Obstructed Urinary Bladder. The enlarged prostate is seen protruding into the lumen of the bladder, which appears trabeculated. These "trabeculae" result from hypertrophy and hyperplasia of smooth muscle cells that occurs in response to increased intravesical pressure caused by urinary obstruction. (From Damjanov I: *Pathology for the health professions,* ed 3, St Louis, 2006, Saunders.)

appears to be involved in breast cancer development.[4-6] Dysplasia is often classified as mild, moderate, or severe; however, because this classification scheme is somewhat subjective, it has prompted some to recommend the use of either "low grade" or "high grade" instead. If the inciting stimulus is removed, dysplastic changes often are reversible.

Metaplasia

Metaplasia is the reversible replacement of one mature cell type by another, sometimes less differentiated, cell type. It is thought to develop from a reprogramming of stem cells that exist on most epithelia or of undifferentiated (embryonic) mesenchymal cells present in connective tissue. These precursor cells mature along a new pathway because of signals generated by cytokines and growth factors in the cell's environment. The best example of metaplasia is replacement of normal columnar ciliated epithelial cells of the bronchial (airway) lining by stratified squamous epithelial cells (Figure 3-4). The newly formed cells do not secrete mucus or have cilia, causing loss of a vital protective mechanism. Bronchial metaplasia can be reversed if the inducing stimulus, usually cigarette smoking, is removed. With prolonged exposure to the inducing stimulus, however, dysplasia and cancerous transformation can occur.

CELLULAR INJURY

Most diseases begin with cell injury. Cellular injury occurs if the cell is unable to maintain homeostasis—a normal or adaptive steady state—in the face of injurious stimuli. Injured cells may recover **(reversible injury)** or die **(irreversible injury).** Injurious stimuli include chemical agents, lack of sufficient oxygen (hypoxia), free radicals, infectious agents, physical and mechanical factors, immunologic reactions, genetic factors, and nutritional imbalances. Types of injuries and their responses are summarized in Table 3-1 and Figure 3-5.

The extent of cellular injury depends on the type, state (including level of cell differentiation and increased susceptibility to fully differentiated cells), and adaptive processes of the cell, as well as the type, severity, and duration of the injurious stimulus. Two individuals exposed to an identical stimulus may incur varying degrees of cellular injury. Modifying factors, such as nutritional status, can profoundly influence the extent of injury. The precise "point of no return" that leads to cellular death is a biochemical puzzle, and the exact mechanisms responsible for the transition from reversible to irreversible cellular damage are currently being debated.

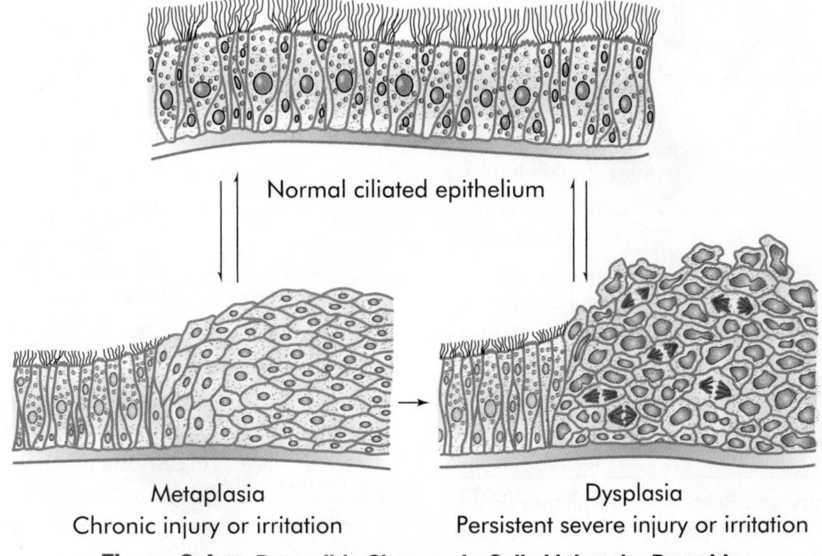

Figure 3-4 ■ Reversible Changes in Cells Lining the Bronchi.

TABLE 3-1

Types of Progressive Cell Injury and Responses

Type	Responses
Adaptation	Atrophy, hypertrophy, hyperplasia, metaplasia
Active cell injury	Immediate response of "entire" cell
Reversible	Loss of ATP, cellular swelling, detachment of ribosomes, autophagy of lysosomes
Irreversible	"Point of no return" structurally when severe vacuolization of the mitochondria occurs and Ca^{++} moves into the cell
Necrosis	Common type of cell death with severe cell swelling and breakdown of organelles
Apoptosis, or programmed cell death	Cellular self-destruction for elimination of unwanted cell populations
Chronic cell injury (subcellular alterations)	Persistent stimuli response may involve only specific organelles or cytoskeleton (e.g., phagocytosis of bacteria)
Accumulations or infiltrations	Water, pigments, lipids, glycogen, proteins
Pathologic calcification	Dystrophic and metastatic calcification

ATP, Adenosine triphosphate; *Ca^{++}*, calcium.

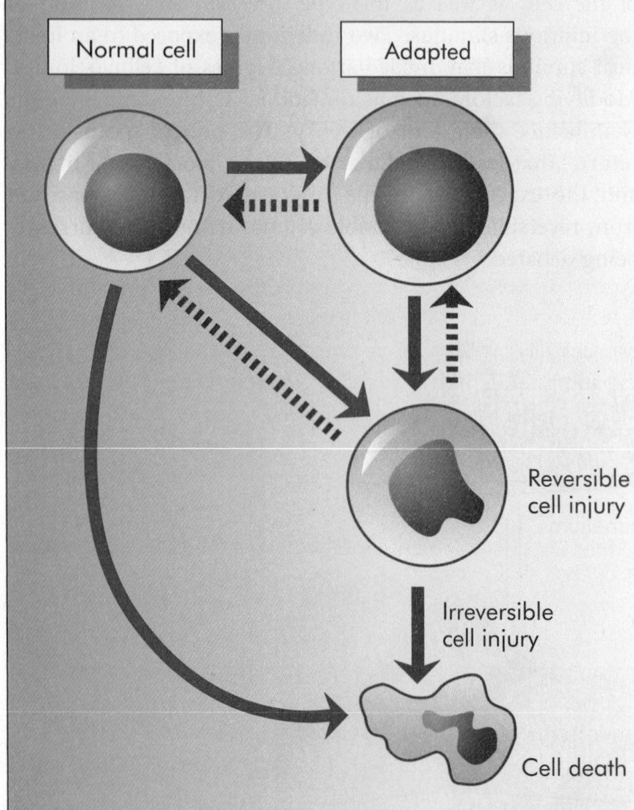

Figure 3-5 ■ **Cellular Injury and Responses.** Depiction of the relationship among normal, adapted (hypertrophied), and reversibly injured cells and cell death of myocardial cells.

General Mechanisms of Cell Injury

Four common biochemical themes are important to understanding cell injury and cell death regardless of the injuring agent. These include ATP depletion, oxygen and oxygen-derived free radicals, calcium alterations, and defects in membrane permeability (Table 3-2). The common forms of cell injury are (1) hypoxic injury, (2) free radicals and reactive oxygen species injury, and (3) chemical injury.

Hypoxic Injury

Hypoxia, or lack of sufficient oxygen, is the single most common cause of cellular injury (Figure 3-6). Hypoxia can result from a decreased amount of oxygen in the air, loss of hemoglobin or hemoglobin function, decreased production of red blood cells, diseases of the respiratory and cardiovascular systems, and poisoning of the oxidative enzymes (cytochromes) within the cells. The most common cause of hypoxia is **ischemia** (reduced blood supply).

Ischemic injury often is caused by the gradual narrowing of arteries (arteriosclerosis) and complete blockage by blood clots (thrombosis). Progressive hypoxia caused by gradual arterial obstruction is better tolerated than the sudden acute **anoxia** (total lack of oxygen) caused by a sudden obstruction, as with an embolus (a blood clot or other plug in the circulation). An acute obstruction in a coronary artery can cause myocardial cell death (infarction) within minutes if the blood supply is not restored, whereas the gradual

TABLE 3-2

Common Themes in Cell Injury and Cell Death

Theme	Comments
ATP depletion	Loss of mitochondrial ATP and decreased ATP synthesis; results include cellular swelling, decreased protein synthesis, decreased membrane transport, and lipogenesis, all changes that contribute to loss of integrity of plasma membrane
Oxygen and oxygen-derived free radicals	Lack of oxygen is key in progression of cell injury in ischemia (reduced blood supply); activated oxygen species (free radicals, O_2^-, H_2O_2, $OH\cdot$) cause destruction of cell membranes and cell structure
Intracellular calcium and loss of calcium steady state	Normally intracellular cytosolic calcium concentrations are very low; ischemia and certain chemicals cause an increase in cytosolic Ca^{++} concentrations; sustained levels of Ca^{++} continue to increase with damage to plasma membrane; Ca^{++} causes intracellular damage by activating a number of enzymes
Defects in membrane permeability	Early loss of selective membrane permeability found in all forms of cell injury

ATP, Adenosine triphosphate; *Ca^{++}*, calcium.

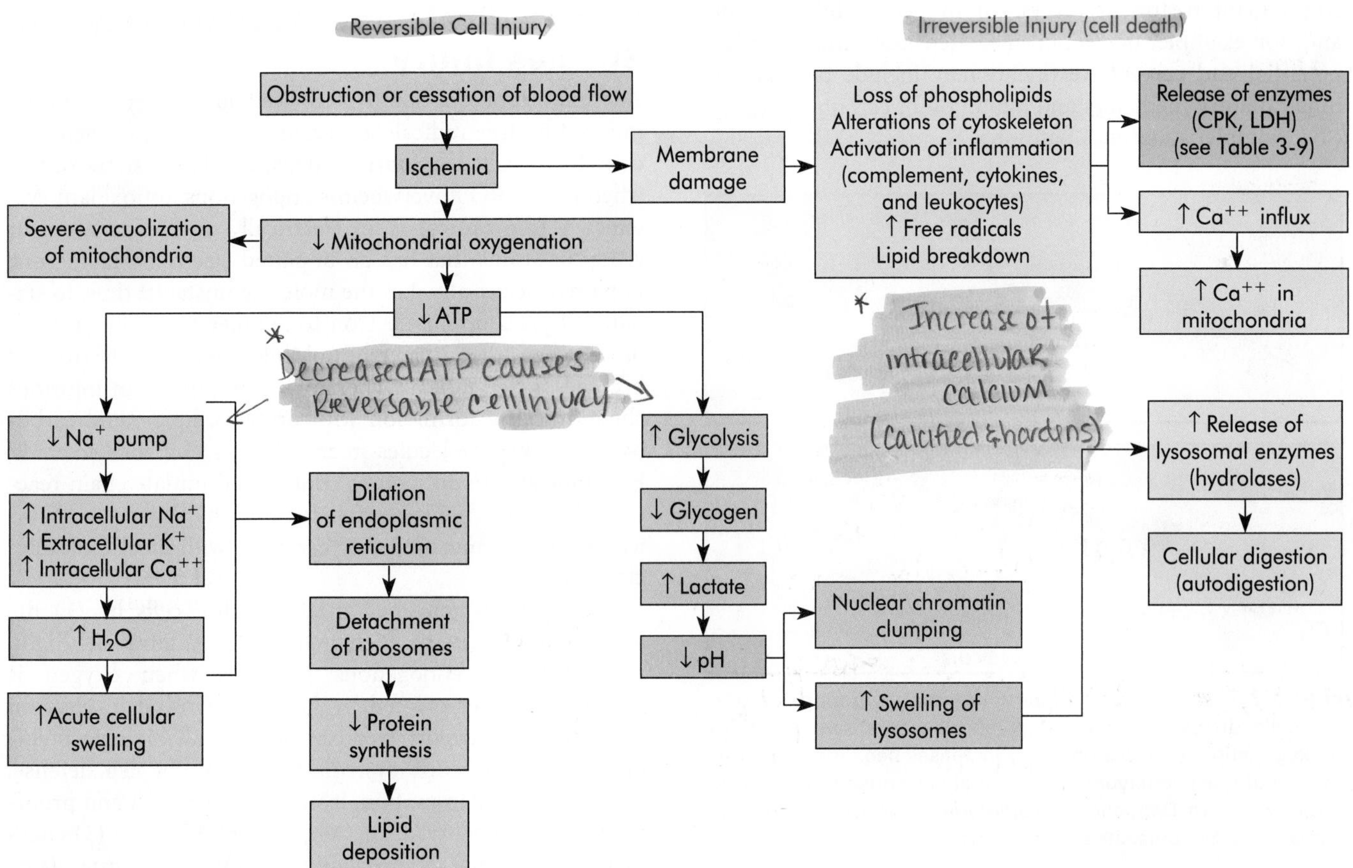

Figure 3-6 ■ **Hypoxic Injury Induced by Ischemia.** Purple boxes involve reversible cell injury, light blue boxes involve irreversible cell death, and green boxes are clinical manifestations.

onset of ischemia usually results in myocardial adaptation. Myocardial infarction and stroke, which are common causes of death in the United States, generally result from atherosclerosis (a type of arteriosclerosis) and consequent ischemic injury. (Vascular obstruction is discussed in Chapter 23.)

Cellular responses to hypoxic injury caused by ischemia have been demonstrated in studies of the heart muscle. Within 1 minute after blood supply to the myocardium is interrupted, the heart becomes pale and has difficulty contracting normally. Within 3 to 5 minutes, the ischemic portion of the myocardium ceases to contract because of a rapid decrease in mitochondrial phosphorylation, causing insufficient adenosine triphosphate (ATP) production. Lack of ATP leads to increased anaerobic metabolism, which generates ATP from glycogen when there is insufficient oxygen. When glycogen stores are depleted, even anaerobic metabolism ceases.

A reduction in ATP levels causes the plasma membrane's sodium-potassium (Na^+-K^+) pump and sodium-calcium exchange to fail, which leads to an intracellular accumulation of sodium and calcium and diffusion of potassium out of the cell. Sodium and water then can enter the cell freely, and cellular swelling, as well as early dilation of the endoplasmic reticulum, results. Dilation causes the ribosomes to detach from the rough endoplasmic reticulum, reducing protein synthesis. With continued hypoxia, the entire cell becomes markedly swollen, with increased concentrations of sodium, water, and chloride and decreased concentrations of potassium. These disruptions are reversible if oxygen is restored. If oxygen is not restored, however, **vacuolation** (formation of vacuoles) occurs within the cytoplasm and swelling of lysosomes and marked mitochondrial swelling result from damage to the outer membrane. Continued hypoxic injury with accumulation of calcium subsequently activates multiple enzyme systems resulting in membrane damage, cytoskeleton disruption, activation of inflammation, DNA degradation, and eventual cell death (see Figure 3-23). Structurally, with plasma membrane damage, extracellular calcium readily moves into the cell and intracellular calcium stores are released. Intracellular calcium activates enzymes that can further damage membrane proteins, ATP, and nucleic acids. The substrates necessary to reconstitute ATP are lost and calcium accumulates in the mitochondria. Irreversible damage is characterized by two events: (1) lack of ATP generation because of mitochondrial damage and (2) major disturbances and damage in membrane function.

Restoration of oxygen, however, can cause additional injury called **reperfusion injury** (Figure 3-7). Reperfusion injury results from the generation of highly reactive oxygen intermediates, sometimes called *oxidative stress,* including hydroxyl radical (OH^-), superoxide (O_2^-), and hydrogen peroxide (H_2O_2). These radicals can all cause further membrane damage and mitochondrial calcium overload. Neutrophils are especially affected with reperfusion injury, including neutrophil adhesion to the endothelium.

Antioxidant treatment reverses both neutrophil adhesion and, for example, neutrophil-mediated heart injury. Other potential and current treatments may include blockage of inflammatory mediators and inhibition of certain cell death (for example, apoptotic) pathways.

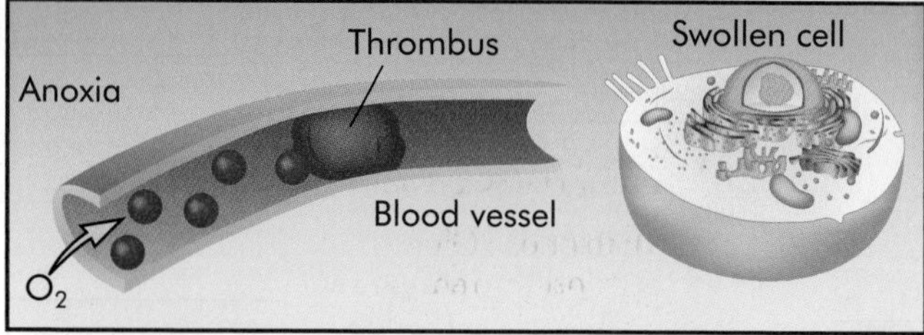

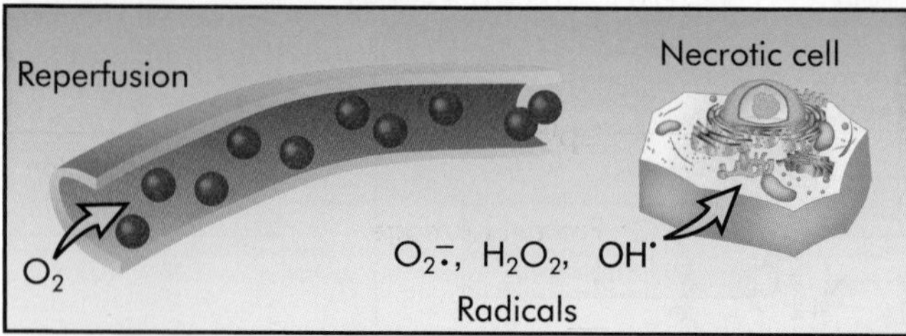

Figure 3-7 ■ **Reperfusion Injury.** Without oxygen, or anoxia, the cells display hypoxic injury and become swollen. With reoxygenation, reperfusion injury increases because of the formation of reactive oxygen radicals that can cause cell necrosis. (Redrawn from Damjanov I: *Pathology for the health professions*, ed 3, St Louis, 2006, Saunders.)

HEALTH ALERT
Natural Antioxidants

Nutrient antioxidants—vitamin C, vitamin E, and β-carotene, a precursor to vitamin A—work by inactivating free radicals. Especially important is the prevention of oxidative damage to mitochondrial DNA. Vitamin C, found in citrus fruits, broccoli, and potatoes, is probably the most notable of the antioxidant nutrients. A water-soluble vitamin, it is the first line of defense, scavenging free radicals before they enter cell membranes. Vitamin C promotes wound healing, growth, and tissue repair. It also enhances the effect of vitamin E. It is known to lower the risk of cataracts and heart disease. Vitamin E, which is fat soluble and available in unprocessed oils, wheat germ, hazelnuts, almonds, egg yolk, and butter, does much of its protective antioxidant work within the lipid-rich cell membrane. It is an anticoagulant and important in the formation of blood cells. It also helps to utilize vitamin K, and it reduces the risk of cataracts. β-Carotene, found in carrots, dark green and yellow-orange vegetables and fruits, leafy vegetables, sweet potatoes, tomatoes, spinach, squash, and broccoli, is converted to vitamin A in the small intestine and *may* be associated with reduced risk of cancer, cataracts, and heart disease.

✔ QUICK CHECK 3-1

1. When does a cell become irreversibly injured?
2. Why are oxidative free radicals damaging to cells?
3. How do cells become markedly swollen with hypoxic injury?

Free Radicals and Reactive Oxygen Species Injury

An important mechanism of cellular injury is injury induced by free radicals, especially by reactive oxygen species (ROS) called **oxidative stress.** Oxidative stress occurs when excess ROS overwhelms endogenous antioxidant systems. A **free radical** is an electrically uncharged atom or group of atoms that has an unpaired electron. Having one unpaired electron makes the molecule unstable; thus, to stabilize, it gives up an electron to another molecule or steals one. When the attacked molecule loses its electron, it becomes a free radical. Therefore, it is capable of injurious chemical bond formation with proteins, lipids, and carbohydrates—key molecules in membranes and nucleic acids. Free radicals are difficult to control and initiate chain reactions. They are *highly* reactive because they have low chemical specificity, meaning they can react with most molecules close by.

Free radicals may be initiated within cells by (1) the absorption of extreme energy sources (e.g., ultraviolet light, radiation), (2) endogenous reactions when oxygen is reduced to water created by systems involved in electron and oxygen transport (redox reactions; all biologic membranes contain redox systems important for cell defense, for example, inflammation, iron uptake, growth, and proliferation and signal transduction) (Figure 3-8), and (3) enzymatic metabolism of exogenous chemicals or drugs (e.g., CCl_3, a product of carbon tetrachloride [CCl_4]). Table 3-3 describes the most significant free radicals.

During normal metabolism, the mitochondria are the greatest source and target of ROS. These ROS contribute to mitochondria dysfunction and are related to many human diseases and aging. Usually ROS are reduced by intracellular antioxidant enzymes, including superoxide dismutase (SOD), glutathione peroxidase, and catalase, as well as antioxidant molecules such as glutathione and vitamin E (alpha-tocopherol). In pathologic conditions, however, the large numbers of ROS overwhelm the balance by antioxidants. This inefficiency of antioxidants is even more serious in mitochondria because mitochondria in most cells lack catalase.[7] Consequently, the excessive production of hydrogen peroxide and eventually hydroxyl radical (OH) in mitochondria will damage lipid, proteins, and **mitochondrial DNA (mDNA),** which then causes cells to die of necrosis or apoptosis.[7–10] Mitochondrial oxidative stress has been implicated in heart disease, Alzheimer disease, Parkinson disease, prion diseases, and amyotropic lateral sclerosis (ALS), as well as aging itself.[11–14] Currently, investigators are trying to identify the polypeptides (i.e., proteomes) directly involved in diseases associated with mitochondrial dysfunction.

Free radicals cause several damaging effects by (1) **lipid peroxidation,** which is the destruction of polyunsaturated lipids (the same process by which fats become rancid) leading to membrane damage and increased permeability; (2) attacking critical proteins that affect ion pumps and transport mechanisms; (3) fragmenting DNA, causing

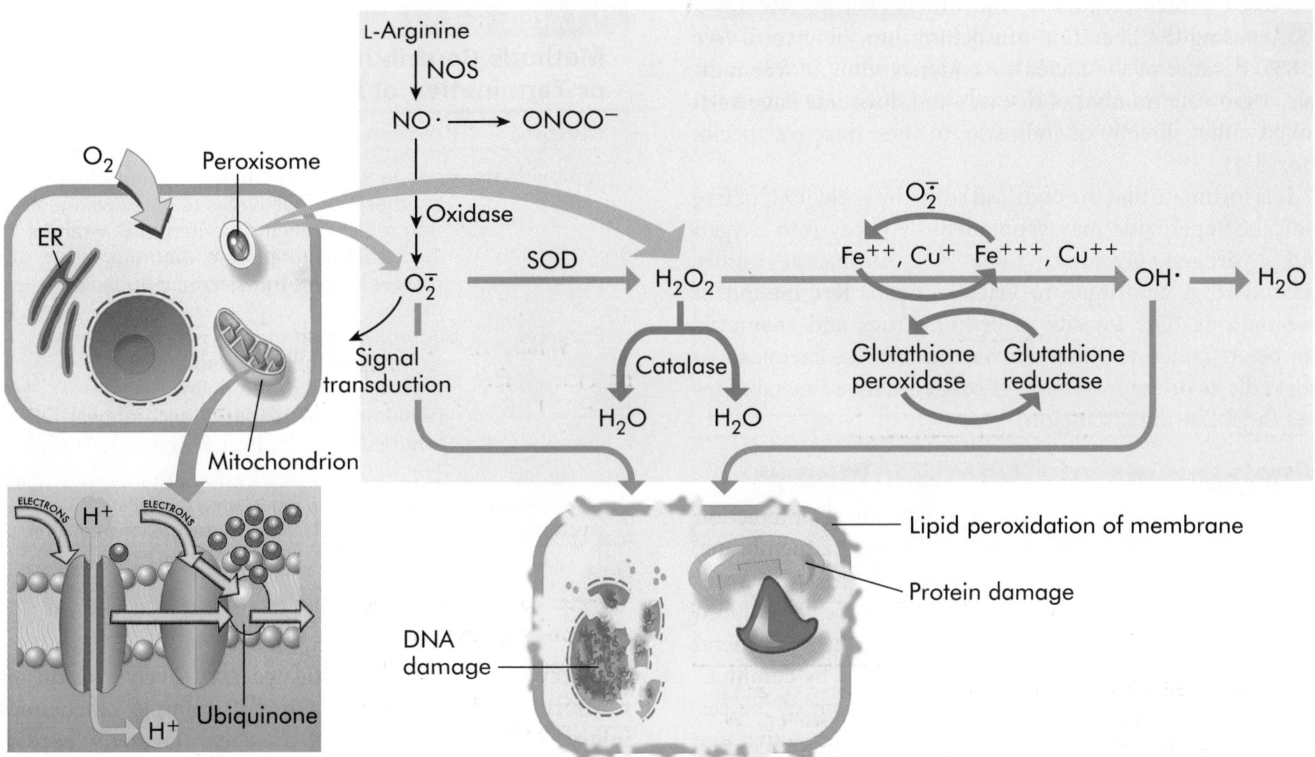

Figure 3-8 ■ **Generation of Reactive Oxygen Species and Antioxidant Mechanisms in Biologic Systems.** Mitochondria have four sites of entry for electrons coming into the electron transport system: one for reduced nicotinamide adenine dinucleotide (NADH) and three for the reduced form of flavin adenine dinucleotide ($FADH_2$). These pathways meet at the small, lipophilic molecule, ubiquinone (coenzyme Q), at the beginning of the common electron transport pathway. Ubiquinone transfers electrons in the inner membrane, ultimately enabling their interaction with oxygen (O_2) and hydrogen (H_2) to yield water (H_2O). In so doing, the transport allows free energy change and the synthesis of one mole of adenosine triphosphate (ATP). With the transport of electrons, free radicals are generated within the mitochondria. Reactive oxygen species (O_2^-, H_2O_2, OH·, and nitric oxide [NO]) act as physiologic modulators of some mitochondrial functions but may also cause cell damage. O_2 is converted to superoxide (O_2^-) by oxidative enzymes in the mitochondria, endoplasmic reticulum (ER), plasma membrane, peroxisomes, and cytosol. O_2 is converted to H_2O_2 by superoxide dismutase (SOD) and further to OH· by the Cu/Fe Fenton reaction. Superoxide catalyzes the reduction of Fe^{++} to Fe^{+++}, thus increasing OH· formation by the Fenton reaction. H_2O_2 is also derived from oxidases in peroxisomes. The three reactive oxygen species (H_2O_2, OH·, and O_2^-), cause free radical damage to lipids (peroxidation of the membrane), proteins (ion pump damage), and DNA (impaired protein synthesis). The major antioxidant enzymes include SOD, catalase, and glutathione peroxidase. (Data from Drge W: *Physiol Rev* 82:47–95, 2002; Buetler TM, Krauskopf A, Ruegg UT: *News Physiol Sci* 19:120–123, 2004.)

TABLE 3-3

Biologically Relevant Free Radicals

Free Radical	Comments
Reactive oxygen species (ROS) Superoxide O_2^- $O_2 \xrightarrow{\text{Oxidase}} O_2^-$	Generated either (1) directly during autoxidation in mitochondria or (2) enzymatically by enzymes in the cytoplasm, such as xanthine oxidase or cytochrome P-450; once produced, it can be inactivated spontaneously or more rapidly by the enzyme superoxide dismutase (SOD): $O_2^- + O_2^- + -H_2^- \xrightarrow{\text{SOD}} H_2O_2 + O_2$
Hydrogen peroxide (H_2O_2) $O_2^- + O_2^- + -H_2^- \xrightarrow{\text{SOD}} H_2O_2 + O_2$ Or oxidases present in peroxisomes O_2 peroxisome $O_2^- \xrightarrow{\text{SOD}} H_2O_2$	Generated by the enzyme SOD or directly by oxidases in intracellular peroxisomes (Note: SOD is considered an antioxidant because it converts superoxide to H_2O_2; catalase [another antioxidant] can then decompose H_2O_2 to $O_2 + H_2O$.)
Hydroxyl radicals (OH^-) $H_2O \rightarrow H\cdot + OH\cdot$ Or $Fe^{++} + H_2O_2 \rightarrow Fe^{++} + OH\cdot + OH^-$ Or $H_2O_2 + O_2^- \rightarrow OH\cdot + OH^- + O_2$	Generated by the hydrolysis of water caused by ionizing radiation or by interaction with metals—especially iron (Fe) and copper (Cu); iron is important in toxic oxygen injury because it is required for maximal oxidative cell damage
Nitric oxide (NO) $NO\cdot + O_2^- \rightarrow ONOO^- + H^+$	NO by itself is an important mediator that can act as a free radical; it can be converted to another radical—peroxynitrite anion ($ONOO^-$), as well as NO_2 and CO_3^-

Data from Cotran RS, Kumar V, Collins T: *Robbins' pathologic basis of disease*, ed 6, Philadelphia, 1999, Saunders.

decreased protein synthesis; and (4) damaging mitochondria, causing the liberation of calcium into the cytosol (see p. 85). Because of the increased understanding of free radicals, a growing number of diseases and disorders have been linked either directly or indirectly to these reactive species (Box 3-1).

It is fortunate that the body can sometimes rid itself of free radicals. Superoxide may spontaneously decay into oxygen and hydrogen peroxide. Table 3-4 summarizes other methods that contribute to inactivation or termination of free radicals. The toxicity of certain drugs and chemicals can be attributed to either conversion of these chemicals to free radicals or the formation of oxygen-derived metabolites (see the following discussion).

Mechanisms of Chemical Injury

Chemical injury begins with a biochemical interaction between a toxic substance and the cell's plasma membrane, which is ultimately damaged, leading to increased permeability. Not all the mechanisms causing chemically induced membrane destruction are known; however, the two general mechanisms include (1) direct toxicity caused by combination of a chemical with a molecular component of the cell membrane or organelles and (2) formation of reactive free radicals and lipid peroxidation.

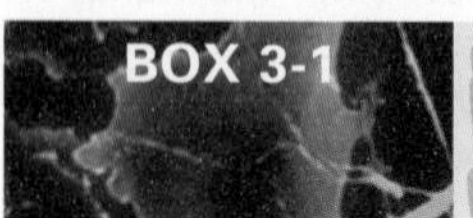

BOX 3-1 Diseases and Disorders Linked to Oxygen-Derived Free Radicals

- Deterioration noted in aging
- Atherosclerosis
  - Ischemic brain injury
  - Alzheimer disease
  - Neurotoxins
- Cancer
- Cardiac myopathy
- Chronic granulomatous disease
- Diabetes mellitus
- Eye disorders
  - Macular degeneration
  - Cataracts
- Inflammatory disorders
- Iron overload
- Lung disorders
  - Asbestosis
  - Oxygen toxicity
  - Emphysema
- Nutritional deficiencies
- Radiation injury
- Reperfusion injury
- Rheumatoid arthritis
- Skin disorders
- Toxic states
  - Xenobiotics (CCl_4, paraquat, cigarette smoke, etc.)
  - Metal irons (Ni, Cu, Fe, etc.)

Adapted from Knight JA: Review: free radicals, antioxidants, and the immune system, *Ann Clin Lab Sci* 30(2):145, 2000.

TABLE 3-4 Methods Contributing to Inactivation or Termination of Free Radicals

Method	Process
Antioxidants	Endogenous or exogenous; either blocks synthesis or inactivates (e.g., scavenges) free radicals; includes vitamin E, vitamin C, cysteine, glutathione, albumin, ceruloplasmin, transferrin, γ-lipoacid, others
Enzymes	Superoxide dismutase,* which converts superoxide to H_2O_2; catalase* (in peroxisomes) decomposes H_2O_2; glutathione peroxidase* decomposes OH· and H_2O_2

*These enzymes are important in modulating the cellular destructive effects of free radicals, also released in inflammation.

Because it has been investigated extensively, carbon tetrachloride (CCl_4) injury is a useful example of chemical injury. Carbon tetrachloride, an agent formerly used in dry cleaning, is converted by an enzyme system in the smooth endoplasmic reticulum of liver cells into $CCl_3^{\cdot}$ (chloromethyl), a highly toxic free radical. The newly formed $CCl_3^{\cdot}$, rapidly destroys the endoplasmic reticulum of the liver cell by lipid peroxidation, breaking down the reticulum's lipid component.

The lipid molecules accumulate within the cytoplasm, starting within cisternae of the endoplasmic reticulum (Figure 3-9). Fatty liver develops because CCl_4 poisoning blocks the synthesis of **lipid-acceptor proteins (apoproteins)** that normally bind with triglycerides to form lipoproteins, which are then transported out of the cell. Blockage of triglyceride (lipoprotein) secretion begins 10 to 15 minutes after CCl_4 exposure. Fat droplets that accumulate in cisternae of the endoplasmic reticulum combine to form larger droplets and fill vacuoles that, in turn, fill the entire cytoplasm. Approximately 10 to 12 hours later, the liver appears grossly enlarged and pale because of the accumulation of fat. Fatty change is reversible if the abnormality responsible for the change is removed. At this point, the cellular changes are the same as in hypoxic injury (see p. 66).

Chemical agents

Many chemical agents cause cellular injury. Highly toxic substances are known as **poisons.** Minute amounts of some, such as arsenic and cyanide, can rapidly destroy enough cells to cause death of the individual. Chronic exposure to air pollutants, insecticides, and herbicides can cause cellular injury. Carbon monoxide, carbon tetrachloride, and social drugs, such as alcohol, can significantly alter cellular function and injure cellular structures. Recreational, over-the-counter, and prescribed drugs also may cause cellular injury, sometimes leading to death. Accidental or suicidal

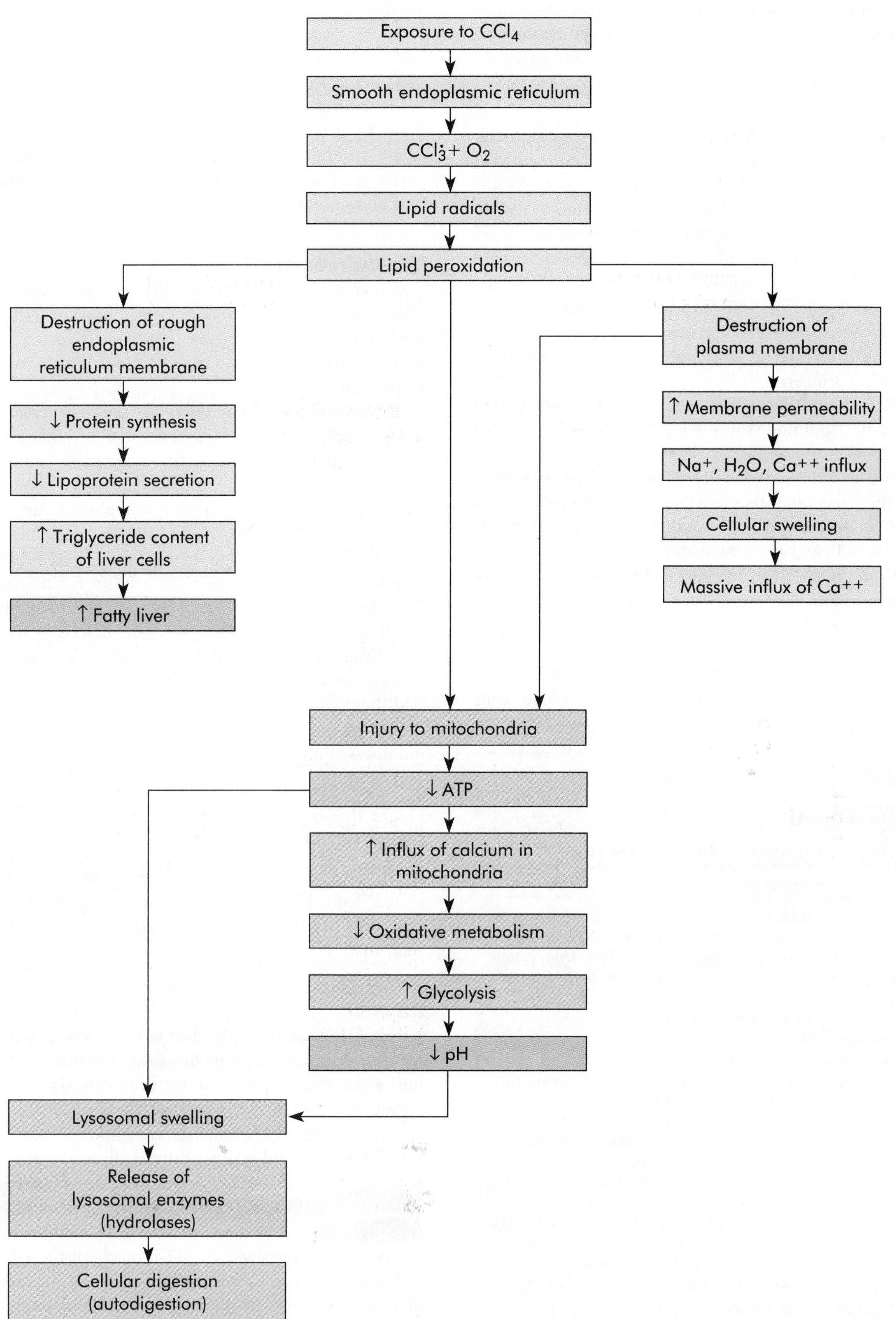

Figure 3-9 ■ Chemical Injury of Liver Cells Induced by Carbon Tetrachloride (CCl_4) Poisoning. Light blue boxes are mechanisms unique to chemical injury, purple boxes involve hypoxic injury, and green boxes are clinical manifestations.

poisonings by chemical agents cause numerous deaths. The injurious effects of some agents—lead, carbon monoxide, ethyl alcohol, mercury—are common cellular injuries.

Lead

Lead is a heavy metal that persists in the environment. Despite efforts to reduce exposure through government regulation, lead toxicity is still a primary hazard for children.[15] Compared to adults, children absorb lead more readily through the intestines. If nutrition is compromised, especially if dietary intake of iron, calcium, zinc, and vitamin D is insufficient, lead's toxic effects are enhanced.[16,17] Particularly worrisome is lead exposure during pregnancy because the developing fetal nervous system is especially vulnerable and can result in learning disorders, hyperactivity, and attention problems.[15]

Lead-based paint has a sweet taste and is often ingested by children. Common sources of lead are included in Table 3-5.

The organ systems primarily affected by lead ingestion include the nervous system, the hematopoietic system (tissues that produce blood cells), and the kidneys. Lead affects many different biologic activities, many of which may be related to the function of calcium.[15] Alterations in calcium may play a role in the interference with neurotransmitters, which may cause hyperactive behavior and proliferation of capillaries of the white matter and arteries.[15] Lead inhibits several enzymes involved in hemoglobin synthesis and causes anemia as a result of lysis of red blood cells (hemolysis). Other manifestations of brain involvement include convulsions and delirium and, with peripheral nerve involvement, wrist, finger, and sometimes foot paralysis. Renal lesions can cause tubular dysfunction resulting in glycosuria (glucose in the urine), aminoaciduria (amino acids in the urine), and hyperphosphaturia (excess phosphate in the urine). Gastrointestinal symptoms are less severe and include nausea, loss of appetite, weight loss, and abdominal cramping.

TABLE 3-5

Common Sources of Lead Exposure

Exposure	Source
Environmental	Lead paint, soil, or dust near roadways or lead-painted homes, plastic window blinds, plumbing materials (from pipes or solder), pottery glazes and ceramic ware, lead-core candle wicks, leaded gasoline, water (pipes)
Occupational	Lead mining and refining, plumbing and pipe fitting, auto repair, glass manufacturing, battery manufacturing and recycling, printing shop, construction work, plastic manufacturing, gas station attendant, firing-range attendant
Hobbies	Glazed pottery making, target shooting at firing ranges, lead soldering, preparing fishing sinkers, stained-glass making, painting, car or boat repair
Other	Gasoline sniffing, costume jewelry, cosmetics, contaminated herbal products

Data from Sanborn MD et al: Identifying and managing adverse environmental health effects, 3, lead exposure, *CMAJ* 166(10):1287–1292, 2002.

Carbon monoxide

Gaseous substances can be classified according to their ability to asphyxiate (interrupt respiration) or irritate. Toxic asphyxiants, such as carbon monoxide, hydrogen cyanide, and hydrogen sulfide, directly interfere with cellular respiration.

Carbon monoxide (CO) is an odorless, colorless, and undetectable gas unless it is mixed with a visible or odorous pollutant. It is produced by the incomplete combustion of fuels such as gasoline. Although CO is a chemical agent, the ultimate injury it produces is a hypoxic injury—namely, oxygen deprivation. Normally, oxygen molecules are carried to tissues bound to hemoglobin in red blood cells (see Chapter 26). Because CO's affinity for hemoglobin is 300 times greater than that of oxygen, it quickly binds with the hemoglobin, preventing oxygen molecules from doing so. Minute amounts of CO can produce a significant percentage of **carboxyhemoglobin** (carbon monoxide bound with hemoglobin).

Symptoms related to CO poisoning include headache, giddiness, tinnitus (ringing in the ears), nausea, weakness, and vomiting. At risk for carbon monoxide exposure are those who (1) breathe air polluted by gasoline engines or defective furnaces; (2) work in occupations such as coal mining, fire fighting, welding, or engine repair; and (3) smoke cigarettes, cigars, or pipes. The fetus is especially at risk from the effects of carbon monoxide because fetal carboxyhemoglobin levels are likely to be 10% to 15% more than maternal levels.

Ethanol

Alcohol **(ethanol)** is the primary choice among mood-altering drugs available in the United States. Because alcohol is not only a psychoactive drug but also a food, it is considered part of the basic food supply in many societies. A large intake of alcohol has enormous effects on nutritional status. Liver and nutritional disorders are the most serious consequences of alcohol abuse. Major nutritional deficiencies include magnesium, vitamin B_6, thiamine, and phosphorus. How ethanol affects folate metabolism is currently under investigation. The mechanisms of ethanol-induced liver injury have emerged through the clarification of a newly proposed pathway for ethanol oxidation, the microsomal P-450 oxidase pathway (see the discussion that follows).

The major effects of acute alcoholism involve the CNS. After alcohol is ingested, it is absorbed, unaltered, in the stomach and small intestine. Fatty foods and milk slow absorption. Alcohol then is distributed to all tissues and fluids of the body in direct proportion to the blood concentration.

Most of the alcohol in the blood is metabolized in the liver through one major and two accessory pathways. The major pathway involves hepatic alcohol dehydrogenase (ADH), an enzyme of the cytosol that catalyzes the conversion of ethanol to acetaldehyde (Figure 3-10).

The microsomal ethanol oxidizing system (MEOS) depends on cytochrome P-450, an enzyme needed for cellular oxidation. Activation of MEOS requires a high ethanol concentration and thus is thought to be important in the accelerated ethanol metabolism (i.e., tolerance) noted in persons with chronic alcoholism.

Individuals differ in their capability to metabolize alcohol. Genetic differences in metabolism of liver alcohol, including aldehyde dehydrogenases, have been identified.[18] These genetic polymorphisms may account for ethnic and gender differences in ethanol metabolism. Persons with chronic alcoholism develop tolerance because of production of enzymes, leading to an increased rate of metabolism (e.g., P-450).

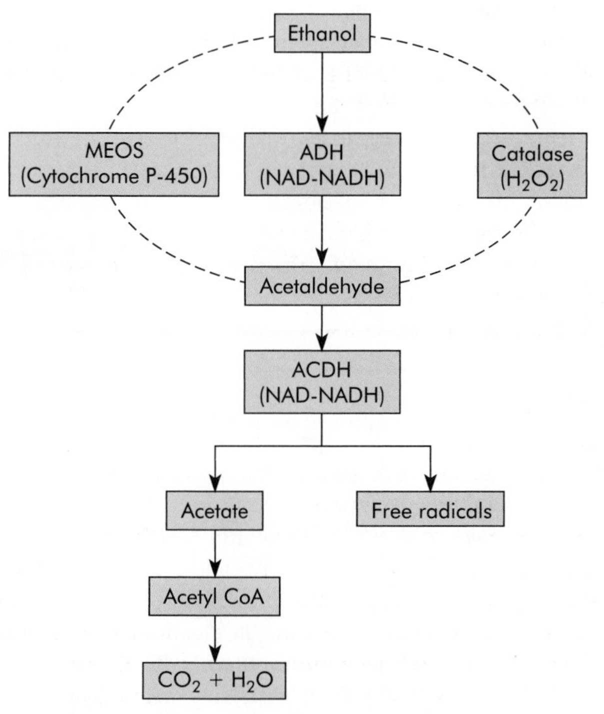

Figure 3-10 ■ **Major Pathway of Metabolism of Alcohol in the Liver through ADH.**

Since 1997, studies have consistently validated the so-called *J-* or *U-shaped* inverse association between alcohol and cardiovascular disease. Consistent epidemiologic studies show that people who daily consume light-to-moderate (*not* excessive) amounts of alcohol reduce their risk of coronary heart disease (CHD) as compared to nondrinkers. The suggested mechanisms for cardioprotection include increased levels of high-density lipoprotein cholesterol (HDL-c), decreased levels of low-density lipoprotein cholesterol (LDL-C), prevention of clot formation, reduction in platelet aggregation, and lowering of plasma apolipoprotein (a) levels.[19] Limited data suggest that the level for optimal benefit may be slightly lower for women; therefore, the American Heart Association recommends no more than two drinks per day for men and one drink per day for women.

Acute alcoholism affects mainly the CNS but may induce reversible hepatic and gastric changes.[20–23] The hepatic changes, initiated by acetaldehyde, include inflammation, deposition of fat, enlargement of the liver, interruption of microtubular transport of proteins and their secretion, increase in intracellular water, depression of fatty acid oxidation in the mitochondria, increased membrane rigidity, increased reactive oxygen species, and acute liver cell necrosis (see Chapter 34). In the CNS, alcohol is, itself, a depressant, initially affecting subcortical structures (probably the brain stem reticular formation).[20–22] Consequently, motor and intellectual activity becomes disoriented. At higher blood levels, medullary centers become depressed, affecting respiration. Much investigation is under way concerning the relationship of alcohol and snoring and obstructive sleep apnea (cessation of breathing).[24,25]

Chronic alcoholism causes structural alterations in practically all organs and tissues in the body because most tissues contain enzymes capable of ethanol oxidation or nonoxidative metabolism. The most significant activity, however, occurs in the liver and to a lesser extent in the stomach.[26] The following alterations occur in the liver: fatty liver, alcoholic hepatitis, and cirrhosis. Acute gastritis is a direct toxic effect and chronic use can lead to acute and chronic pancreatitis. Cellular damage is increased by reactive oxygen species (ROS) and oxidative stress (see p. 68). Activation of proinflammatory cytokines from neutrophils and lymphocytes mediate liver damage.[26] Oxidative stress is associated with cell membrane phospholipid depletion, which alters the fluidity and function of cell membranes as well as intercellular transport. Chronic alcoholism is related to several disorders, including increased tendency to hypertension and regressive changes in skeletal muscle (see Chapter 35).

Ethanol is implicated in the onset of a variety of immune defects, including effects on the production of cytokines involved in inflammatory responses (tumor necrosis factor, interleukin-1, interleukin-6).[20,22] The deleterious effects of prenatal alcohol exposure can cause mental retardation and neurobehavioral disorders, as well as fetal alcohol syndrome. **Fetal alcohol syndrome** includes growth retardation, facial anomalies, cognitive impairment, and ocular malformations (Figure 3-11). The specific mechanisms of injury are unknown.

Whatever the cause, persons with chronic alcoholism have a significantly shortened life span related mainly to damage to the liver, stomach, brain, and heart. Alcohol is a well-known cause of hepatic injury, terminating in cirrhosis (Figure 3-12) (see Chapter 34), yet moderate amounts of alcohol may decrease the incidence of coronary heart disease.

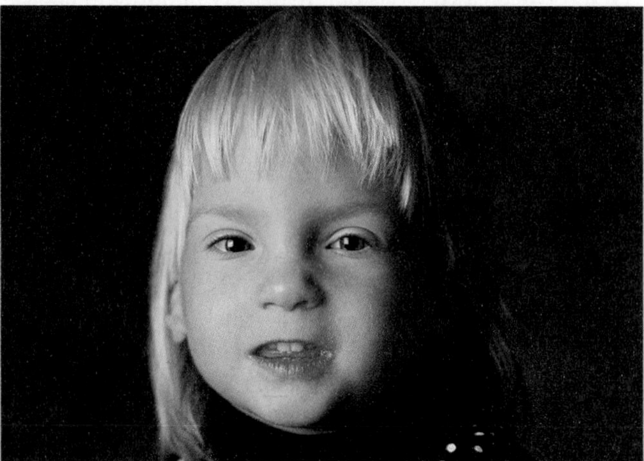

Figure 3-11 ■ **Fetal Alcohol Syndrome.** When alcohol enters the fetal blood, the potential result can cause tragic congenital abnormalities, such as microcephaly ("small head"), low birth weight, and cardiovascular defects, as well as developmental disabilities, such as physical and mental retardation, and even death. Note the small head, thinned upper lip, small eye openings (palpebral fissures), epicanthal folds, and receded upper jaw (retrognathia) typical of fetal alcohol syndrome. (From Fortinash KM, Holoday Worret PA: *Psychiatric mental health nursing,* ed 3, St Louis, 2004, Mosby.)

Mercury

Mercury has been used medically and commercially for centuries. Today people are exposed to mercury from three major sources: fish consumption, dental amalgams, and vaccines. Table 3-6 summarizes these sources and their health effects.

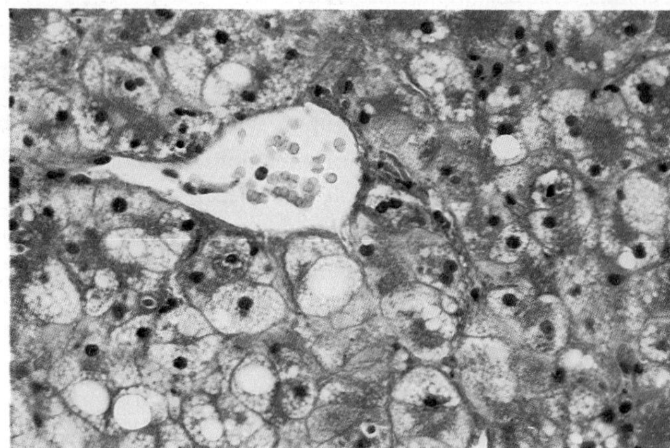

Figure 3-12 ■ **Alcoholic Hepatitis.** Chicken-wire fibrosis extending between hepatocytes (Mallory trichrome stain.) (From Damjanov I, Linder J, editors: *Anderson's pathology,* ed 10, St Louis, 1996, Mosby.)

TABLE 3-6

Major Sources of Mercury Exposure and Health Effects

Source	Comments
Dental amalgams	Amalgams consist of 50% mercury combined with other metals
	Controversial whether amalgams can release mercury vapors into the mouth and when fillings are removed cause transient elevations
	Health concerns from claims that mercury vapor can cause or worsen degenerative diseases (e.g., Alzheimer disease); however, several epidemiologic studies have failed to provide evidence
	A difficult problem is that mercury can inhibit biochemical process *in vitro* without the same effects *in vivo*
Fish consumption	Consumption of fish and sea mammals is major source of exposure to methyl mercury
	Faroe Islands study showed methyl mercury exposure from whale consumption
	U.S. study showed methyl mercury levels slightly higher than EPA guideline
	FDA recommends pregnant women, nursing mothers, and young children avoid eating fish with a high mercury content (>1 parts per million [ppm]), such as shark, swordfish, tile fish, king mackerel, and whale meat
Vaccines	Thimerosal, a preservative in many multidose vials of vaccines, contains ethyl mercury
	Single-dose vials do not require preservatives
	Several vaccines containing thimerosal were given to infants until 1999
	With the exception of some flu vaccines, removal of thimerosal is currently being completed in the United States
	It is presumed that the mercury children receive in vaccines containing thimerosal is excreted with no accumulation during the 2-month periods between vaccinations

Data from Center for Disease Control, 2004; available at www.cdc.gov/nip/vacsafeconcerns/thimerosal/flags-thimerosal.htm#4; ClarksonTW, Magos L, Myers GI: The toxicology of mercury—current exposures and clinical manifestations, *N Engl J Med* 349(18):1731–1737, 2003.

Social or street drugs

The social or "recreational" use of psychoactive drugs is widespread around the world. Most popular and dangerous are the drugs methamphetamine (METH), marijuana, cocaine, and heroin. Although the prevalence of cocaine use in the general population decreased in 1986, morbidity and mortality related to cocaine increased sharply in the 1990s. "Illicit use of drugs" is a prevalent risk behavior among adolescents. Table 3-7 summarizes the effects of these drugs.

QUICK CHECK 3-2

1. Discuss the possible mechanisms of cell injury related to chronic alcoholism.
2. What are some of the systemic effects of METH, cocaine, marijuana, and heroin use?

TABLE 3-7

Social or Street Drugs and Their Effects

Type of Drug	Description and Effects
Marijuana	*Active substance:* delta 9-tetrahydrocannabinol (THC), found in resin of the cannabis sativa plant With smoking (e.g., "joints"), about 50% is absorbed through the lungs; when ingested only 10% is absorbed; with heavy use the following adverse effects have been reported: alterations of sensory perceptions, cognitive and psychomotor impairment (e.g., inability to judge time, speed, distance); smoking 3 or 4/day is similar to smoking 20 cigarettes/day in regard to frequency of chronic bronchitis and may contribute to lung cancer; data from animal studies only indicate reproductive changes include reduced fertility, decreased sperm motility, and decreased circulatory testosterone; fetal abnormalities include low birth weight and increased frequency of childhood leukemia; increased frequency of infectious illness is thought to be the result of depressed cell-mediated and humoral immunity
Methamphetamine (Meth)	An amine derivation of amphetamine ($C_{10}H_{15}N$) used as crystalline hydrochloride CNS stimulant; in large doses causes irritability, aggressive (violent) behavior, anxiety, excitement, auditory hallucinations, and paranoia (delusions and psychosis); mood changes are common and the abuser can swiftly change from friendly to hostile; paranoiac swings can result in suspiciousness, hyperactive behavior, and dramatic mood swings Appeals to abusers because body's metabolism is increased and produces euphoria, alertness, and perception of increased energy Stages: *Low intensity:* user is not psychologically addicted and uses methamphetamine by swallowing or snorting *Binge* and *high intensity:* user has psychologic addiction and smokes or injects to achieve a faster, stronger high *Tweaking:* most dangerous stage, user is continually under the influence, not sleeping for 3 to 15 days, extremely irritated, and paranoid
Cocaine and crack	Extracted from the leaves of the cocoa plant and sold as a water-soluble powder (cocaine hydrochloride) liberally diluted with talcum powder or other white powders; extraction of pure alkaloid from cocaine hydrochloride is "free-base" called *crack* because it "cracks" when heated Crack is more potent than cocaine; cocaine is widely used as an anesthetic, usually in procedures involving the oral cavity; it is a potent CNS stimulant, blocking reuptake of neurotransmitters norepinephrine, dopamine, and serotonin; also increases synthesis of norepinephrine and dopamine; dopamine induces a sense of euphoria, and norepinephrine causes adrenergic potentiation, including hypertension, tachycardia, and vasoconstriction; cocaine can therefore cause severe coronary artery narrowing and ischemia; not clear is why cocaine increases thrombus formation; other cardiovascular effects include dysrhythmias, sudden death, dilated cardiomyopathy, rupture of descending aorta (i.e., secondary to hypertension); effects on the fetus include premature labor, retarded fetal development, stillbirth, hyperirritability
Heroin	An opiate closely related to morphine, methadone, and codeine Highly addictive, and withdrawal causes intense fear ("I'll die without it"); sold "cut" with similar-looking white powder; dissolved in water it is often highly contaminated; feeling of tranquility and sedation lasts only a few hours and thus encourages repeated intravenous or subcutaneous injections; acts on the receptors enkephalins, endorphins, and dynorphins, which are widely distributed throughout the body with high affinity to the CNS; effects can include infectious complications, especially *Staphylococcus aureus,* granulomas of the lung, septic embolism, and pulmonary edema—in addition, viral infections from casual exchange of needles and HIV; sudden death is related to overdosage secondary to respiratory depression, decreased cardiac output, and severe pulmonary edema

Data from Cotran RS, Kumar V, Colllins T: *Robbins pathologic basis of disease,* ed 7, Philadelphia, 2005, Elsevier/Saunders; Nahas G, Sutin K, Bennett WM: Review of marijuana and medicine, *N Engl J Med* 343(7):514, 2000.

CNS, Central nervous system; *HIV,* human immunodeficiency virus.

Unintentional and Intentional Injuries

Unintentional and intentional injuries are an important health problem in the United States. In 2002, there were 161,269 deaths, an injury death rate of 55.67/100,000.[27] Death is significantly more common for men than women; the overall rate for men is 81.77/100,000 versus 31.60/100,000 for women. Significant racial differences are noted in the death rate, with whites at 55.01/100,000, blacks at 65.65/100,000, and other racial groups at a combined rate of 35.58/100,000. There also is a bimodal age distribution for injury-related deaths, with peaks in the young adult and elderly groups. Unintentional injury is the leading cause of death for people between the ages of 1 and 34 years; intentional injury (suicide, homicide) ranks at between the second and fourth leading cause of death in this age group. The 1999 report published by the Institute of Medicine (IOM) indicated that between 44,000 and 98,000 unnecessary deaths per year occurred in hospitals alone as a result of errors by medical professionals. Speculation has been considerable that these statistics are either overestimated or underestimated. Despite disagreements over the reported statistics, an accurate account is a tremendous challenge (Kopec et al, 2006).[27a] Statistics on nonfatal injuries are harder to document accurately, but they are known to be a significant cause of morbidity and disability and to cost society billions of dollars annually. The more common terms used to describe and classify unintentional and intentional injuries and brief descriptions of important features of these injuries are discussed here.

Blunt-force injuries

Injuries by **blunt force** are caused by the application of mechanical energy to the body resulting in the tearing, shearing, or crushing of tissues. They are the most common type of injuries seen in most health care settings. Blunt-force injury may be caused by blows (where a moving object strikes the body), impacts (where the moving body strikes a fixed object), or a combination of both. Motor vehicle accidents and falls are the most common causes, accounting for 45,579 and 17,116 deaths, respectively, in 2002.

Contusion

A contusion (bruise) is bleeding into the skin or underlying tissues as a consequence of a blow that squeezes or crushes the soft tissues and ruptures blood vessels without breaking the skin. It may take several hours after injury before any change in skin color is seen. A bruise will be red-purple initially, eventually becoming blue-black, and then gradually changing to yellow-brown or green before fully disappearing (see Figure 3-22). These color changes reflect the progression of tissue damage and healing that develops in the area of underlying injury. The length of time depends on factors such as the extent and location of the injury and the degree of vascularization in the area. Small contusions may resolve in a matter of days, whereas larger ones can take weeks to completely heal. Bruising of soft tissues may sometimes be confined to deeper structures; thus, no injury is visible externally. Blood in deeper structures may dissect along fascial planes, so discoloration of the skin may be seen in areas not directly injured by the initiating blow or impact, such as bruising of the thigh in a hip or pelvis fracture or "black eyes" in orbital plate fractures. Contusions also may be seen in internal organs in cases of severe injury.

A collection of blood in soft tissues or an enclosed space also may be referred to as a **hematoma.** A **subdural hematoma** is a collection of blood between the inner surface of the dura mater and the surface of the brain, resulting in the shearing of small veins that bridge the subdural space. Subdural hematoma can result from blows, falls, or sudden acceleration/deceleration of the head, as occurs in shaken baby syndrome. An **epidural hematoma** is a collection of blood between the inner surface of the skull and the dura. It is caused by a torn artery and is almost always associated with a skull fracture.

Contusions of the brain may result from (1) a blow or (2) a fall or impact. In blows, when a moving object strikes the stationary head, a cerebral contusion grouped in the portions of the brain underlying the area of scalp and skull injury is known as a *coup* pattern of injury. In falls or impacts, when the moving head strikes a fixed object, a cerebral contusion seen in the area of the brain opposite the external injury is known as a *contrecoup* pattern of injury. Contrecoup injury results when the head accelerates and the brain lags behind and presses into the areas of the skull directly opposite the direction of motion. When the head suddenly stops, the areas of the brain pressing into the skull are injured. For example, a person who falls directly backward, striking the occiput (back of the head), will have cerebral contusions of the frontal and temporal tips (these injuries are discussed further in Chapter 15).

Abrasion

An abrasion (scrape) results from removal of the superficial layers of the skin that was caused by friction between the skin and the injuring object. Abrasions vary in size and severity from fine, thin scratches to large areas of denudation (road rash). In cases where force is applied in a tangential, nonperpendicular direction to the skin surface, tags of tissue may be heaped up at the trailing or downstream edge of the abrasion. An abrasion will have a pale, moist, yellow-brown appearance at first. The color darkens to brown or even black as the injury dries. The injury may ooze fluid for 1 or 2 days until it is completely covered by a crust, or scab, which eventually flakes off of the underlying regenerated skin.

Abrasions and contusions may have a patterned appearance that mirrors the shape and features of an injuring object (Figure 3-13). Patterning of injuries can be of crucial importance in cases of automobile accidents, assaults, or homicides; they document the connection between the victim's injuries and a suspect vehicle or weapon. Bite marks

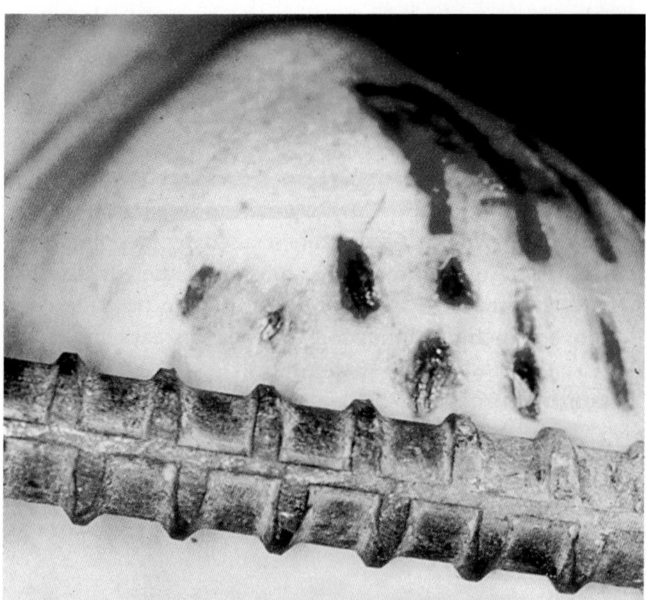

Figure 3-13 ■ **Patterned Abrasion Caused by a Piece of Rebar.** Note the tissue tags at the inferior margins indicating a downward direction to the blow that caused this injury.

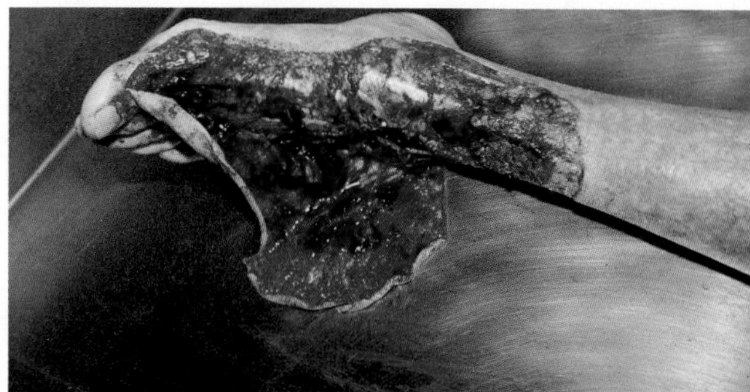

Figure 3-14 ■ **Avulsed Laceration in Motor Vehicle Accident Victim.** The victim was the driver, and this injury most likely was caused by the brake pedal.

(usually a combination of abrasion and contusion) are another example of a patterned injury that can demonstrate a link between an assailant and a victim.

Laceration

A **laceration** is a tear or rip resulting when the tensile strength of the skin or tissue is exceeded. Unlike an incision, where the tissue is cleanly divided by a sharp edge, a laceration is much more jagged and irregular, and the edges are abraded. The depths of a laceration are irregular, and there are often tissue "bridges" of small vessels or nerves that have been stretched but not broken, crossing from one side of the wound to the other. If the injuring force is applied perpendicularly to the skin, there will be crushing of the surrounding tissue with associated abrasion and contusion. If force is applied tangentially, there will also be undermining of the wound, with tissues at the trailing edge of the wound lifted away from the underlying structures creating a pocket in the direction opposite from where the blow came. An extreme example is an **avulsion** (Figure 3-14), in which a wide area of tissue may be pulled away creating a large flap. Usually, the shallower the angle of incidence of the blow, the more extensive the undermining.

Lacerations of internal organs are common in blunt-impact injuries. Lacerations of the liver, spleen, kidneys, and bowel may occur in cases of blows to the abdomen, often with no visible injury to the abdominal wall seen externally. The thoracic aorta may be lacerated in sudden deceleration accidents. This results because the arch of the aorta is freely mobile, whereas the descending portion is attached to the spinal column. Rapid deceleration causes horizontal shearing with either partial or complete transection just below the take-off of the left subclavian artery. Severe blows or impacts to the chest also may cause rupturing of the heart with lacerations of the atria or ventricles.

Fractures

Blunt-force blows or impacts also can cause bone to break or shatter. See Chapter 37 for an in-depth discussion of fractures.

Sharp-force injuries

Cutting and piercing injuries accounted for 2762 deaths in 2002. As with all injuries, men have a higher rate (1.44/100,000) than women (0.49/100,000). There also are differences among races, with rates in whites at 0.73/100,000, blacks at 2.33/100,000, and other racial groups at 0.96/100,000.

Incised wounds

An **incised wound** is a cut that is *longer* than it is *deep*. The wound may be straight or jagged, depending on the object used and how the injury occurred, with sharp, distinct edges without abrasion. Because the wound is caused by a sharp edge, the tissues are cleanly divided and there is no tissue bridging or undermining. Incised wounds may be thin and narrow or more elliptic and gaping in appearance because of varying lines of tension in the skin, location, and orientation. They tend to produce significant external bleeding with minimal internal hemorrhage. These wounds are often seen in sharp-force injury suicides. In most cases, in addition to a deep, lethal cut, there will be multiple superficial incisions grouped in the same area; these are known as hesitation marks (Figure 3-15).

Stab wounds

A **stab wound** is a penetrating sharp-force injury that is *deeper* than it is *long*. Because a sharp instrument is used, the depths of the wound are clean and distinct with no underlying or associated crushing injury. The edges usually are clean but may be abraded if the object is inserted deeply with enough force so that a wider, blunter portion of the instrument (e.g., hilt of a knife) impacts the skin. Figure 3-16 illustrates this type of wound.

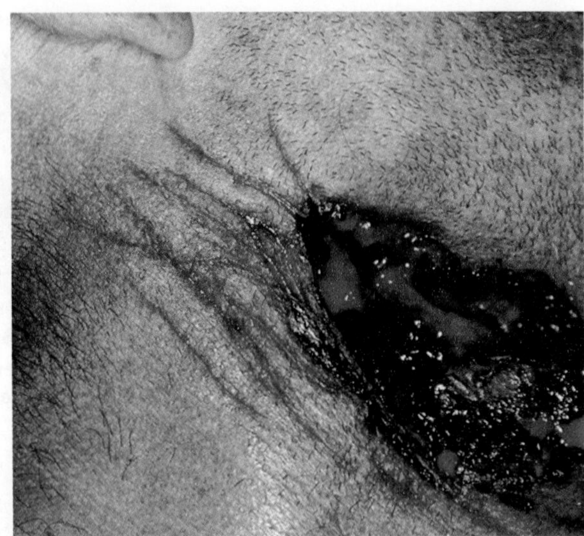

Figure 3-15 ■ **Self-inflicted Incised Wound of the Neck with Multiple Hesitation Marks.**

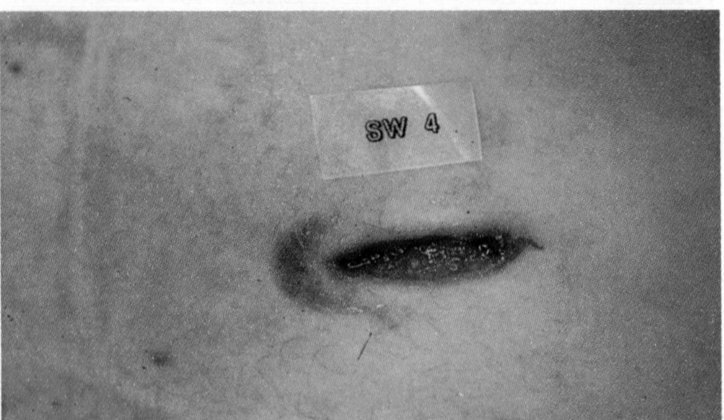

Figure 3-16 ■ **Stab Wound with Associated Hilt Mark.** Note the sharp margin away from the hilt mark with the blunt margin toward it. This wound was caused by a single-edge knife.

A number of features of the blade used to inflict injury may be determined by careful examination of the stab wound. If a *single-edge* blade is used, one margin of the wound will be sharp and the other blunt; if a *double-edge* blade causes the wound, both margins will have a sharp appearance. Stab wounds produced by a *serrated-edge* blade are often indistinguishable from those made by a *smooth-edge* blade. If there was any hesitation or scraping of the skin edges by the blade, an interrupted pattern of abrasion may be seen but is uncommon. Once the edges are in opposition, the thickness of the blade may be estimated from the width of the wound. Depth of the wound may not correlate with the length of the blade because the blade may not be inserted fully, or, as a consequence of compression of tissues from a forceful thrust, the wound may be deeper than the length of the blade.

Depending on size and location of the stab wound, the amount of external bleeding may be surprisingly small. After an initial spurt, even if a major vessel or the heart is struck, the wound track may be almost completely closed by tissue pressure, allowing only a trickle of visible blood despite copious internal bleeding.

Puncture wounds

Instruments or objects with sharp points but without sharp edges may produce penetrating **puncture wounds.** A classic example is a wound of the foot caused by stepping on a nail. These injuries often have abrasion of the edges of the wound, are prone to infection, and also can be quite deep despite a sometimes innocuous external appearance.

Chopping wounds

Heavy, edged instruments (axes, hatchets, propeller blades) produce injuries—**chopping wounds**—with a combination of sharp- and blunt-force characteristics. In addition to cutting, associated crushing of the wound edges and underlying tissues is usually present.

Gunshot wounds

Injuries caused by gunfire accounted for more than 30,242 deaths in the United States in 2002. Of these, 17,108 were suicides, 11,829 were homicides, 762 were accidents, and 243 were classified as undetermined. Men are much more likely to die from gunshot injury than women. The male death rate in 2002 was 18.60/100,000, and it was only 2.82/100,000 for women. Black men between the ages of 15 and 24 years have the greatest gunfire injury death rate: 86.95/100,000. To put this statistic into perspective, if this was the rate for the United States as a whole, there would be more than 250,000 gunshot wound deaths per year.

Gunshot wounds may be either penetrating (bullet retained in the body) or perforating (bullet exits). In some cases the bullet may fragment, so pieces of the missile are retained even though there is an exit wound. The most important factors determining the appearance of a gunshot injury are whether it is an entrance or an exit wound and the range of fire.

Entrance wounds

Although all **entrance wounds** share some common features, the overall appearance is most affected by the range of fire.

Contact range entrance wounds occur when the gun is held so the muzzle rests on or presses into the skin surface, causing a distinctive type of wound. In addition to the hole made by the bullet, there is searing of the edges of the wound from the flame, hot gases exiting the barrel, and soot or smoke deposited on the edges of and in the depths of the wound. In hard contact wounds, where the barrel is firmly pressed into the skin, there may be minimal soot and searing on the outside of the wound but deep penetration of smoke, burning gunpowder fragments, and hot gases into the depths of the injury. In hard contact wounds of the head, where there is only a thin layer of skin and muscle overlying bone, the large amount of gas and explosive energy sent into the wound may cause severe tearing and disruption of the tissues, giving the wound a large, gaping, and jagged appearance—a phenomenon known as **blow back.** In areas of the body with thicker layers of soft tissue, the blow back may not cause tearing but will forcefully drive the skin back onto the end of the barrel, producing a patterned abrasion that mirrors the features of the weapon, known as a **muzzle imprint** (Figure 3-17).

Intermediate (distance) range entrance wounds are surrounded by gunpowder tattooing or stippling (Figure 3-18). **Tattooing** results from fragments of burning or unburned pieces of gunpowder exiting the barrel and striking the skin surface with enough force to be driven into the epidermis or superficial dermis. **Stippling** results when fragments of powder strike with enough force to abrade the skin but not actually penetrate the surface. This phenomenon can be seen when the muzzle-to-target range of most handguns is less than 48 inches. Beyond this distance, pieces of gunpowder disperse and slow down so much that tattooing or stippling cannot occur. The closer the muzzle is to the skin, the tighter the distribution and greater the density of powder fragments is around the actual entrance hole. Soot also may be deposited.

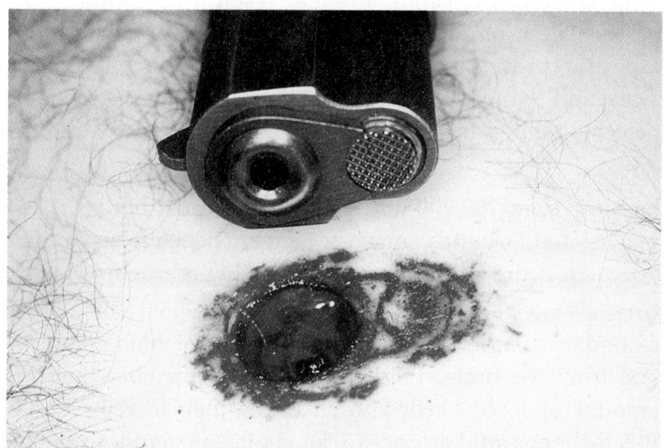

Figure 3-17 ■ Contact Range Gunshot Wound of the Chest with a Muzzle Abrasion.

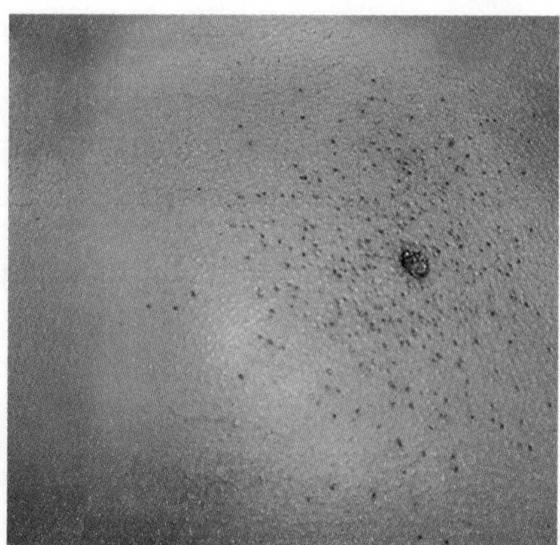

Figure 3-18 ■ Intermediate Range Gunshot Wound with Stippling and Tattooing.

An **indeterminate range entrance wound** occurs when flame, soot, or gunpowder does not reach the skin surface and the only thing striking the body is the bullet. The term *indeterminate* is used rather than *distant* because it does not imply that one can actually determine the range of fire from the appearance of the wound. For example, if an individual is shot through multiple layers of clothing, the entrance wound may have no soot, searing, or stippling even though the actual range of fire is only a matter of inches; the wound looks the same as if the shot came from a range of 6 meters (20 feet) or more. Indeterminate wounds are characterized by a hole surrounded by a rim of abrasion. The size of the hole can vary according to a number of factors. It is important to remember that one cannot say what caliber of weapon inflicted the wound based solely on the size of the entrance wound. The collar of abrasion results from the fact that the bullet first causes stretching and scraping of the skin before it actually perforates. If the bullet strikes perpendicular to the skin, the margin of abrasion collar is concentrically distributed about the defect; if it strikes at an angle, the collar is eccentric, with the wider margin pointing in the direction from which the bullet came (Figure 3-19). If the bullet has struck an intermediary target before hitting the skin, it can be turning and tumbling, producing an irregular abrasion collar.

Exit wounds

Exit wounds have the same general appearance no matter what the range of fire. Their shape can vary from round to slitlike to completely irregular. As with entrance wounds, the size does not correlate well with the caliber of the projectile making the wound. The most important factors affecting exit wounds are the speed of the projectile and the degree of deformation. A smaller, highly deformed bullet exiting at high speed can produce a large, irregular wound, whereas a larger, intact, slower-moving bullet may make only a small hole. Size *cannot* be used to determine if the hole is an exit or entrance wound. In most cases, the margins of an exit wound do *not* have an abrasion collar. An exit wound has clean edges that often can be reapproximated to cover the defect. The exception is when something is pressing against the skin surface at the exit

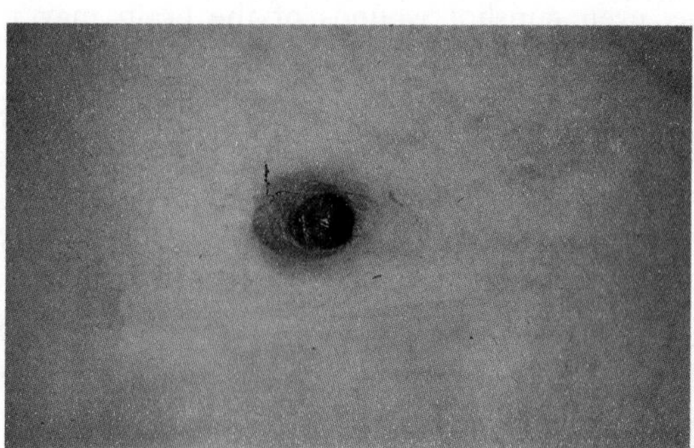

Figure 3-19 ■ Indeterminate Range Entrance Wound with Eccentric Collar of Abrasion Resulting from the Bullet Striking the Skin at an Angle.

site, such as tight clothing or the back of a chair. In that situation, the bullet pushes the skin against the supporting surface, causing rubbing and scraping around the exit defect as it comes out; this is known as a **shored exit wound.**

It is important to remember that because the skin is so elastic and deformable, it is one of the toughest structures for a bullet to go through. It is not uncommon for a bullet to pass entirely through the body and be stopped just beneath the skin. Often no visible injury of the overlying skin is present; however, careful palpation of the area may allow one to locate the bullet.

Wounding potential of firearms

The amount of damage done by a bullet is a function of a number of variables. For the most part, the damage caused is a result of the amount of energy transferred to the tissues impacted. The energy a bullet has is determined by the following formula:

$$KE = \frac{1}{2} MV^2$$

where KE is kinetic energy, M is the mass, and V is the speed.

Clearly, increasing the speed of a bullet has a much greater effect on its potential to cause damage than increasing its size. As the bullet passes through tissue and slows down, its energy is dissipated into the surrounding structures. This energy transfer causes tissue destruction in a zone that can be much larger than the actual size of the bullet; the zone of destruction may be several inches in diameter with very high-powered bullets. This transfer of energy in head wounds may lead to orbital plate fractures and palpebral ecchymosis (black eyes) or blood draining from the ears even though the path of the bullet did not come near the base of the skull. The amount of damage caused may be exacerbated by the generation of secondary missiles of bone fragments when portions of the skeleton are struck. Some bullets are designed to expand or fragment when they strike an object, thereby increasing the cross-sectional area of the projectile, increasing drag, and enhancing the transfer of energy into the tissues. "Hollow-point" ammunition is an example of this kind of bullet.

Obviously, the lethality of a gunshot injury depends on what structures are damaged. Depending on the extent of damage, even gunshot wounds of the brain may not be lethal; however, they are usually immediately incapacitating and lead to significant long-term disability. It is important to remember that a victim with a "lethal" injury (wound of the heart or aorta) may not be immediately incapacitated and may engage in varying degrees of physical activity after being injured. Just because the victim is active or even combative when first evaluated does not mean the individual may not have experienced a potentially lethal injury.

Asphyxial injuries

Asphyxial injuries are caused by a failure of cells to receive or utilize oxygen. Deprivation of oxygen may be partial *(hypoxia)* or total *(anoxia)*. Asphyxial injuries can be grouped into four general categories: suffocation, strangulation, chemical, and drowning.

Suffocation

Suffocation, or oxygen failing to reach the blood, can result from a lack of oxygen in the environment (entrapment in an enclosed space or filling of the environment with a suffocating gas) or blockage of the external airways. Classic examples of these types of asphyxial injuries are a child who is trapped in an abandoned refrigerator or a person who commits suicide by putting a plastic bag over his or her head. A reduction in the ambient oxygen level to 16% (normal is 21%) is immediately dangerous. If the level is below 5%, death can ensue within a matter of minutes. The diagnosis of these types of asphyxial injuries depends on knowing the history of what happened because there will be no specific physical findings.

Diagnosis and treatment in **choking asphyxiation** (obstruction of the internal airways) depend on locating and removing the obstructing material. Injury or disease also may cause swelling of the soft tissues of the airway leading to partial or complete obstruction and subsequent asphyxiation. Suffocation also may result from compression of the chest or abdomen (mechanical or compressional asphyxia) preventing normal respiratory movements. Usual signs and symptoms include florid facial congestion and petechiae (pinpoint hemorrhages) of the eyes and face.

Strangulation

Strangulation is caused by compression and closure of the blood vessels and air passages resulting from external pressure on the neck. This causes cerebral hypoxia or anoxia secondary to the alteration or cessation of blood flow to and from the brain. It is important to remember that the amount of force needed to close the jugular veins (2 kg [4.5 lb]) or carotid arteries (5 kg [11 lb]) is significantly less than that required to crush the trachea (15 kg [33 lb]). It is the alteration of cerebral blood flow in most types of strangulation that causes injury or death—not the lack of airflow. With complete blockage of the carotid arteries, unconsciousness can occur within 10 to 15 seconds.

A noose is placed around the neck, and the weight of the body is used to cause constriction of the noose and compression of the neck in **hanging strangulations.** The body does not need to be completely suspended to produce severe injury or death. Depending on the type of ligature used, there usually is a distinct mark on the neck, an inverted V with the base of the V pointing toward the point of suspension. Internal injuries of the neck are actually quite rare in hangings, and only in judicial hangings, where the body is weighted and dropped, will significant soft tissue or cervical spinal trauma be seen. Petechiae of the eyes or face may be seen, but they are rare.

In **ligature strangulation,** the mark on the neck is horizontal without the inverted V pattern seen in hangings. Petechiae may be more common because intermittent opening and closure of the blood vessels may occur as a result of the victim's struggles. Internal injuries of the neck are rare.

Variable amounts of external trauma on the neck are found with contusions and abrasions in **manual strangulation** caused either by the assailant or by the victim clawing at his or her own neck in an attempt to remove the assailant's hands. Internal damage can be quite severe, with bruising of deep structures and even fractures of the hyoid bone and tracheal and cricoid cartilages. Petechiae are common.

Chemical asphyxiants

Chemical asphyxiants either prevent the delivery of oxygen to the tissues or block its utilization. Carbon monoxide is the most common chemical asphyxiant (see p. 72). **Cyanide** acts as an asphyxiant by combining with the ferric iron atom in cytochrome oxidase, thereby blocking the intracellular utilization of oxygen. A victim of cyanide poisoning will have the same cherry-red appearance as a carbon monoxide intoxication victim because cyanide blocks the utilization of circulating oxyhemoglobin. An odor of bitter almonds also may be detected. (The ability to smell cyanide is a genetic trait that is absent in a significant portion of the general population.) **Hydrogen sulfide** (sewer gas) is a chemical asphyxiant in which victims of hydrogen cyanide poisoning may have brown-tinged blood in addition to the nonspecific signs of asphyxiation.

Drowning

Drowning is an alteration of oxygen delivery to tissues resulting from the breathing in of fluid, usually water. In 2002, there were 4146 drowning deaths in the United States. Although research in the 1940s and 1950s indicated that changes in blood electrolyte levels and volume as a result of absorption of fluid from the lungs may be an important factor in some drownings, the major mechanism of injury is hypoxemia (low blood oxygen levels). Even in freshwater drownings, where large amounts of water can pass through the alveolar-capillary interface, there is no evidence that increases in blood volume cause significant electrolyte disturbances or hemolysis, or that the amount of fluid loading is beyond the compensatory capabilities of the kidneys and heart. Airway obstruction is the more important pathologic abnormality, underscored by the fact that in as many as 15% of drownings little or no water enters the lungs because of vagal nerve-mediated laryngospasms. This phenomenon is called **dry-lung drowning.**

No matter what mechanism is involved, cerebral hypoxia will lead to unconsciousness in a matter of minutes. Whether this progresses to death depends on a number of factors, including the age and the health of the individual. One of the most important factors is the temperature of the water. Irreversible injury will develop much more rapidly in warm water than it will in cold water. Submersion times of up to 1 hour with subsequent survival have been reported in children who were submerged in very cold water. Complete submersion is not necessary for a person to drown. An incapacitated or helpless individual (epileptic, alcoholic, infant) may drown in water that is only a few inches deep.

It is important to remember that no specific or diagnostic findings *prove* that a person recovered from the water is actually a drowning victim. In cases where water has entered the lung, there may be large amounts of foam coming out of the nose and mouth, although this also can be seen in certain types of drug overdoses. A body recovered from water with signs of prolonged immersion could just as easily be a victim of some other type of injury that has been put in the water to obscure the actual cause of death. When working with a living victim recovered from water, it is essential to keep in mind that an underlying condition may have led to the person's becoming incapacitated and submerged—a condition that also may need to be treated or corrected while correcting hypoxemia and dealing with its sequelae.

✓ QUICK CHECK 3-3

1. Correlate the changes in color of a contusion to its mechanism of injury.
2. Why is it important to understand "patterning of injuries"?
3. Distinguish between a laceration, an abrasion, and a contusion.
4. What is the major mechanism of injury with drowning?

Infectious Injury

The pathogenicity (virulence) of microorganisms lies in their ability to survive and proliferate in the human body, where they injure cells and tissues. The disease-producing potential of a microorganism depends on its ability to (1) invade and destroy cells, (2) produce toxins, and (3) produce damaging hypersensitivity reactions. (See Chapter 7 for a description of infection and infectious organisms.)

Immunologic and Inflammatory Injury

Cellular membranes are injured by direct contact with cellular and chemical components of the immune and inflammatory responses, such as phagocytic cells (lymphocytes, macrophages) and substances such as histamine, antibodies, lymphokines, complement, and proteases (see Chapter 5). Complement is responsible for many of the membrane alterations that occur during immunologic injury.

Membrane alterations are associated with a rapid leakage of potassium (K^+) out of the cell and a rapid influx of water. Antibodies can interfere with membrane function by binding to and occupying receptor molecules on the plasma membrane. Antibodies also can block or destroy cellular junctions, interfering with intercellular communication. Other mechanisms of cellular injury are genetic factors, nutritional imbalances, and physical agents. These are summarized in Table 3-8.

TABLE 3-8
Mechanisms of Cellular Injury

Mechanism	Characteristics	Examples
GENETIC FACTORS	Alter cell's nucleus and the plasma membrane's structure, shape, receptors, or transport mechanisms	Sickle cell anemia, Huntington disease, muscular dystrophy, abetalipoproteinemia, familial hypercholesterolemia
NUTRITIONAL IMBALANCES	Pathophysiologic cellular effects develop when nutrients are not consumed in diet and transported to the body's cells *or* when excessive amounts of nutrients are consumed and transported	Protein deficiency, protein-calorie malnutrition, glucose deficiency, lipid deficiency (hypolipidemia), hyperlipidemia (increased lipoproteins in the blood causing deposits of fat in the heart, liver, and muscle), vitamin deficiencies
PHYSICAL AGENTS		
Temperature extremes	Hypothermic injury results from chilling or freezing of cells, creating high intracellular sodium concentrations; abrupt drops in temperature lead to vasoconstriction and increased viscosity of blood, causing ischemic injury, infarction, and necrosis; reactive oxygen species (ROS) is gaining importance	Frostbite
	Hyperthermic injury is caused by excessive heat and varies in severity according to the nature, intensity, and extent of the heat	Burns, burn blisters, heat cramps, heat exhaustion, heat stroke
Atmospheric pressure	Tissue injury caused by compressive waves of air or fluid impinging on the body, followed by a sudden wave of decreased pressure; changes may collapse the thorax, rupture internal solid organs, and cause widespread hemorrhage: carbon dioxide and nitrogen that are normally dissolved in blood come out of solution and form small bubbles (gas emboli), causing hypoxic injury and pain	Blast injury (air or immersion), decompression sickness (caisson disease or "the bends"); recently reported in a few individuals with subdural hematomas after riding high-speed roller coasters
Ionizing radiation	Refers to any form of radiation that can remove orbital electrons from atoms; source is usually the environment, and damage is mainly to the DNA molecule, thus causing chromosomal aberrations; also induces growth factors and extracellular matrix remodeling; uncertainty exists regarding effects of low levels of radiation	X-rays, γ-rays, and α- and β-particles cause skin redness, skin damage, chromosomal damage, cancer
Illumination	Fluorescent lighting and halogen lamps create harmful stresses; ultraviolet light has been linked to skin cancer	Eyestrain, obscured vision, cataracts, headaches, melanoma
Mechanical stresses	Injury is caused by physical impact or irritation; they may be overt or cumulative	Faulty occupational biomechanics, leading to overexertion disorders
Noise	Can be caused by acute loud noise or the cumulative effects of various intensities, frequencies, and duration of noise; considered a public health threat	Hearing impairment or loss; tinnitus, temporary threshold shift (TTS), or loss can occur as a complication of critical illness, from mechanical trauma, ototoxic medications, infections, vascular disorders, and noise

MANIFESTATIONS OF CELLULAR INJURY

Cellular accumulations, also known as **infiltrations,** occur not only when injury is sublethal and sustained in injured cells but also in normal cells. Common accumulations consist of substances that are normally present, such as fluids and electrolytes, triglycerides (lipids), glycogen, calcium, uric acid, proteins, melanin, and bilirubin. Abnormal accumulations of these substances can occur in the cytoplasm (often in the lysosomes) or in the nucleus if (1) the normal, endogenous substance is produced in excess or at an increased rate; (2) an endogenous substance (normal or abnormal) is not effectively catabolized, usually because of lack of a vital lysosomal enzyme; or (3) harmful exogenous materials, such as heavy metals, mineral dusts, or microorganisms, accumulate because of inhalation, ingestion, or infection.

In all storage diseases, the cells attempt to digest, or catabolize, the "stored" substances. As a result, excessive amounts of metabolites (products of catabolism) accumulate in the cells and are expelled into the extracellular matrix, where they are taken up by phagocytic cells called *macrophages* (see Chapter 5). Some of these scavenger cells circulate throughout the body, whereas others remain fixed in certain tissues, such as the liver or spleen. As more and more macrophages and other phagocytes migrate to tissues that are producing excessive metabolites, the affected tissues begin to swell. This is the mechanism that causes enlargement of the liver (hepatomegaly) or the spleen (splenomegaly) as a clinical manifestation of many storage diseases.

Water

Cellular swelling, the most common degenerative change, is caused by the shift of extracellular water into the cells. In hypoxic injury, movement of fluid and ions into the cell is associated with acute failure of metabolism and loss of ATP production. Normally, the pump that transports sodium ions out of the cell is maintained by the presence of ATP and ATPase, the active-transport enzyme. In metabolic failure caused by hypoxia, reduced ATP and ATPase permit sodium to accumulate in the cell while potassium diffuses outward. The increased intracellular sodium increases osmotic pressure, drawing more water into the cell. The cisternae of the endoplasmic reticulum become distended, rupture, and coalesce to form large vacuoles that isolate the water from the cytoplasm, a process called *vacuolation.* Progressive vacuolation results in **oncosis** (a new term replacing *hydropic degeneration*) or **vacuolar degeneration** or swelling (degeneration by water) (Figure 3-20). If cellular swelling affects all the cells in an organ, the organ increases in weight and becomes distended and pale.

Oncosis (*ónkosis,* means swelling) as a term has gained attention. It is a form of cell death where the mechanism is failure of the sodium/potassium (Na^+/K^+) pumps of the plasma membrane. It is caused, typically, by ischemia and possibly by toxic agents that interfere with ATP generation.[28] It evolves within 24 hours to cell death. It is usually accompanied by nuclear dissolution.[29-31]

Cellular swelling is reversible and is considered sublethal. It is, in fact, an early manifestation of almost all types of cellular injury, including severe or lethal cell injury. It is also associated with high fever, hypokalemia (abnormally low concentrations of potassium in the blood; see Chapter 4), and certain infections.

Lipids and Carbohydrates

Certain metabolic disorders result in the abnormal intracellular accumulation of carbohydrates and lipids. These substances may accumulate throughout the body but are found primarily in the spleen, liver, and CNS. Accumulations in cells of the CNS can cause neurologic dysfunction and severe mental retardation. Lipids accumulate in Tay-Sachs disease, Niemann-Pick disease, and Gaucher disease, whereas in the diseases known as mucopolysaccharidoses, carbohydrates are in excess. The mucopolysaccharidoses are progressive disorders that usually involve multiple organs, including liver, spleen, heart, and blood vessels. The accumulated mucopolysaccharides are found in reticuloendothelial cells, endothelial cells, intimal smooth muscle cells, and fibroblasts throughout the body. These carbohydrate accumulations can cause clouding of the cornea, joint stiffness, and mental retardation.

Although lipids sometimes accumulate in heart and kidney cells, the most common site of intracellular lipid accumulation, or **fatty change,** is liver cells. Because hepatic

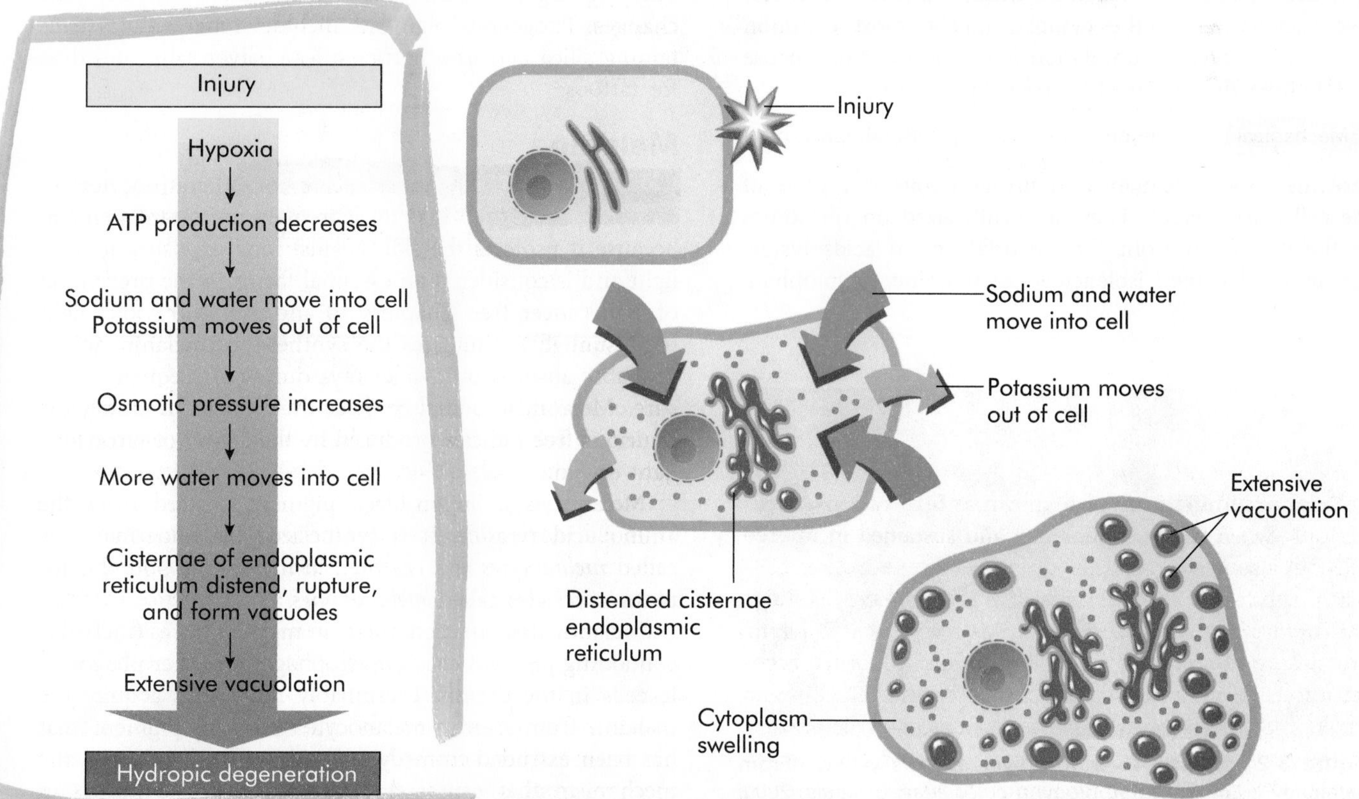

Figure 3-20 ■ **The Process of Oncosis (formerly referred to as "Hydropic Degeneration").** *ATP,* Adenosine triphosphate.

metabolism and secretion of lipids are crucial to proper body function, imbalances and deficiencies in these processes lead to major pathologic changes. Lipid accumulation in liver cells causes fatty liver, or fatty change (Figure 3-21). As lipids fill the cells, vacuolation pushes the nucleus and other organelles aside. Grossly, the liver looks yellowish and greasy.

Lipid accumulation in liver cells occurs after cellular injury sets one or more of the following mechanisms in motion:

1. Increased movement of free fatty acids into the liver (starvation, for example, increases breakdown of triglycerides in adipose tissue, releasing fatty acids that subsequently enter liver cells)
2. Failure of the metabolic process that converts fatty acids to phospholipids, resulting in the preferential conversion of the fatty acids to triglycerides
3. Increased synthesis of triglycerides from fatty acids (increases in an enzyme, α-glycerophosphatase, can accelerate triglyceride synthesis)
4. Decreased synthesis of apoproteins (lipid-acceptor proteins)
5. Failure of lipids to bind with apoproteins and form lipoproteins
6. Failure of mechanisms that transport lipoproteins out of the cell

Glycogen

Intracellular accumulations of glycogen are seen in genetic disorders called *glycogen storage diseas*es and in disorders of glucose and glycogen metabolism. As with water and lipid accumulation, glycogen accumulation results in excessive vacuolation of the cytoplasm. The most common cause of glycogen accumulation is the disorder of glucose metabolism, diabetes mellitus (see Chapter 18).

Proteins

Proteins provide cellular structure and constitute most of the cell's dry weight. They are synthesized on ribosomes in the cytoplasm from the essential amino acids lysine, threonine, leucine, isoleucine, methionine, tryptophan, valine, phenylalanine, and histidine. Protein accumulation probably damages cells in two ways. First, metabolites, produced when the cell attempts to digest some proteins, are enzymes that, when released from lysosomes, can damage cellular organelles. Second, excessive amounts of protein in the cytoplasm push against cellular organelles, disrupting organelle function and intracellular communication.

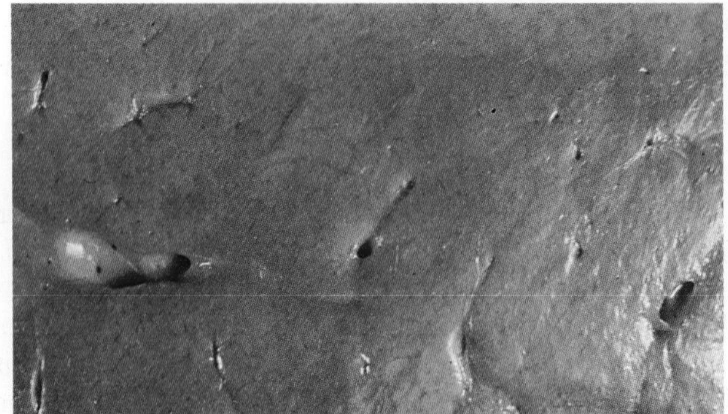

Figure 3-21 ■ **Fatty Liver.** The liver appears yellow. (From Damjanov I, Linder J: *Pathology: a color atlas,* St Louis, 2000, Mosby.)

Protein excess accumulates primarily in the epithelial cells of the renal convoluted tubule and in the antibody-forming plasma cells (B lymphocytes) of the immune system. Several types of renal disorders cause excessive excretion of protein molecules in the urine (proteinuria). Normally, little or no protein is present in the urine, and its presence in significant amounts indicates cellular injury and altered cellular function. Protein accumulations in the cytoplasm of renal tubular cells do not cause direct cellular dysfunction, but they do signify a pathologic process.

Accumulations of protein in B lymphocytes can occur during active synthesis of antibodies during the immune response. The excess aggregates of protein are called *Russell bodies* (see Chapter 5). Russell bodies have been identified in multiple myeloma (plasma cell tumor) (see Chapters 20).

Pigments

Pigment accumulations may be normal or abnormal, endogenous (produced within the body) or exogenous (produced outside the body). Endogenous pigments are derived, for example, from amino acids (e.g., tyrosine, tryptophan). They include melanin and the blood proteins—porphyrins, hemoglobin, and hemosiderin. Lipid-rich pigments, such as lipofuscin (the aging pigment), give a yellow-brown color to cells undergoing slow, regressive, and often atrophic changes. Exogenous pigments include mineral dusts containing silica and iron particles, lead, silver salts, and dyes for tattoos.

Melanin

Melanin accumulates in epithelial cells (keratinocytes) of the skin and retina. It is an extremely important pigment because it protects the skin against long exposure to sunlight and is considered an essential factor in the prevention of skin cancer (see Chapters 10 and 39). Ultraviolet light (e.g., sunlight) stimulates the synthesis of melanin, which probably absorbs ultraviolet rays during subsequent exposure. Melanin also may protect the skin by trapping the injurious free radicals produced by the action of ultraviolet light on skin.

Melanin is a brown-black pigment derived from the amino acid *tyrosine.* It is synthesized by epidermal cells called *melanocytes* and is stored in membrane-bound cytoplasmic vesicles called *melanosomes.*

Melanin also can accumulate in melanophores (melanin-containing pigment cells), macrophages, or other phagocytic cells in the dermis. Presumably these cells acquire the melanin from nearby melanocytes or from pigment that has been extruded from dying epidermal cells. This is the mechanism that causes freckles. Melanin also occurs in the benign form of pigmented moles called *nevi* (see

Chapter 39). Malignant melanoma is a cancerous skin tumor that contains melanin.

A decrease in melanin production occurs in the inherited disorder of melanin metabolism called *albinism.* Albinism is often diffuse, involving all the skin, the eyes, and the hair. Albinism is also related to phenylalanine metabolism. In classic types, the person with albinism is unable to convert tyrosine to DOPA (3,4-dihydroxyphenylalanine), an intermediate in melanin biosynthesis. Melanin-producing cells are present in normal numbers, but they are unable to make melanin. Individuals with albinism are very sensitive to sunlight and quickly become sunburned. They are also at high risk for skin cancer.

Hemoproteins

Hemoproteins are among the most essential of the normal endogenous pigments. They include hemoglobin and the oxidative enzymes, the **cytochromes.** Central to an understanding of disorders involving these pigments is knowledge of iron uptake, metabolism, excretion, and storage (see Chapter 19). Hemoprotein accumulations in cells are caused by excessive storage of iron, which is transferred to the cells from the bloodstream. Iron enters the blood from three primary sources: (1) tissue stores, (2) the intestinal mucosa, and (3) macrophages that remove and destroy dead or defective red blood cells. The amount of iron in blood plasma depends also on the metabolism of the major iron-transport protein, *transferrin.*

Iron is stored in tissue cells in two forms: as ferritin and, when increased levels of iron are present, as hemosiderin. **Hemosiderin** is a yellow-brown pigment derived from hemoglobin. With pathologic states, excesses of iron cause hemosiderin to accumulate within cells, often in areas of bruising and hemorrhage and in the lungs and spleen after congestion caused by heart failure. With local hemorrhage, the skin first appears red-blue and then lysis of the escaped red blood cells occurs, causing the hemoglobin to be transformed to hemosiderin. The color changes noted in bruising reflect this transformation (Figure 3-22).

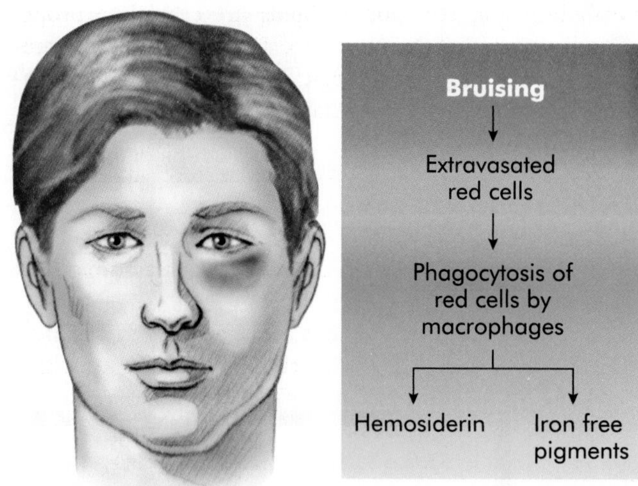

Figure 3-22 ■ **Hemosiderin Accumulation Is Noted as the Color Changes in a "Black Eye."**

Hemosiderosis is a condition in which excess iron is stored as hemosiderin in the cells of many organs and tissues. This condition is common in individuals who have received repeated blood transfusions or prolonged parenteral administration of iron. Hemosiderosis is associated also with increased absorption of dietary iron, conditions in which iron storage and transport are impaired, and hemolytic anemia. Excessive alcohol (wine) ingestion also can lead to hemosiderosis. Normally, absorption of excessive dietary iron is prevented by an iron-absorption process in the intestines. Failure of this process can lead to total body iron accumulations in the range of 60 to 80 g, compared with normal iron stores of 4.5 to 5 g. Excessive accumulations of iron, such as occur in hemochromatosis (a genetic disorder of iron metabolism and the most severe example of iron overload), are associated with liver and pancreatic cell damage.

It is debatable whether iron accumulation itself causes cellular injury or whether injury is the result of the basic defect that leads to iron storage. The finding that the extent of liver injury (cirrhosis) is related to the extent of iron accumulation suggests that excessive iron accumulation does injure cells.[32,33]

Bilirubin is a normal, yellow-to-green pigment of bile derived from the porphyrin structure of hemoglobin. Excess bilirubin within cells and tissues causes jaundice (icterus), or yellowing of the skin. Jaundice occurs when the bilirubin level exceeds 1.5 to 2 mg/dl of plasma, compared with the normal values of 0.4 to 1 mg/dl. Hyperbilirubinemia occurs with (1) destruction of red blood cells (erythrocytes), such as in hemolytic jaundice; (2) diseases affecting the metabolism and excretion of bilirubin in the liver; and (3) diseases that cause obstruction of the common bile duct, such as gallstones or pancreatic tumors. Certain drugs (specifically chlorpromazine and other phenothiazine derivatives), estrogenic hormones, and halothane, an anesthetic, can cause the obstruction of normal bile flow through the liver.

Because unconjugated bilirubin is lipid soluble, it can injure the lipid components of the plasma membrane. Albumin, a plasma protein, provides significant protection by binding unconjugated bilirubin in plasma. Unconjugated bilirubin causes two cellular effects: uncoupling of oxidative phosphorylation and a loss of cellular proteins. These two effects could cause structural injury to the various membranes of the cell.

Calcium

Calcium salts accumulate in both injured and dead tissues (Figure 3-23). An important mechanism of cellular calcification is the influx of extracellular calcium in injured mitochondria (see p. 65). Another mechanism that causes calcium accumulation in alveoli (gas-exchange airways of the lungs), gastric epithelium, and renal tubules is the excretion of acid at these sites, leading to the local production of hydroxyl ions. Hydroxyl ions result in precipitation of calcium hydroxide ($Ca[OH]^2$) and hydroxyapatite

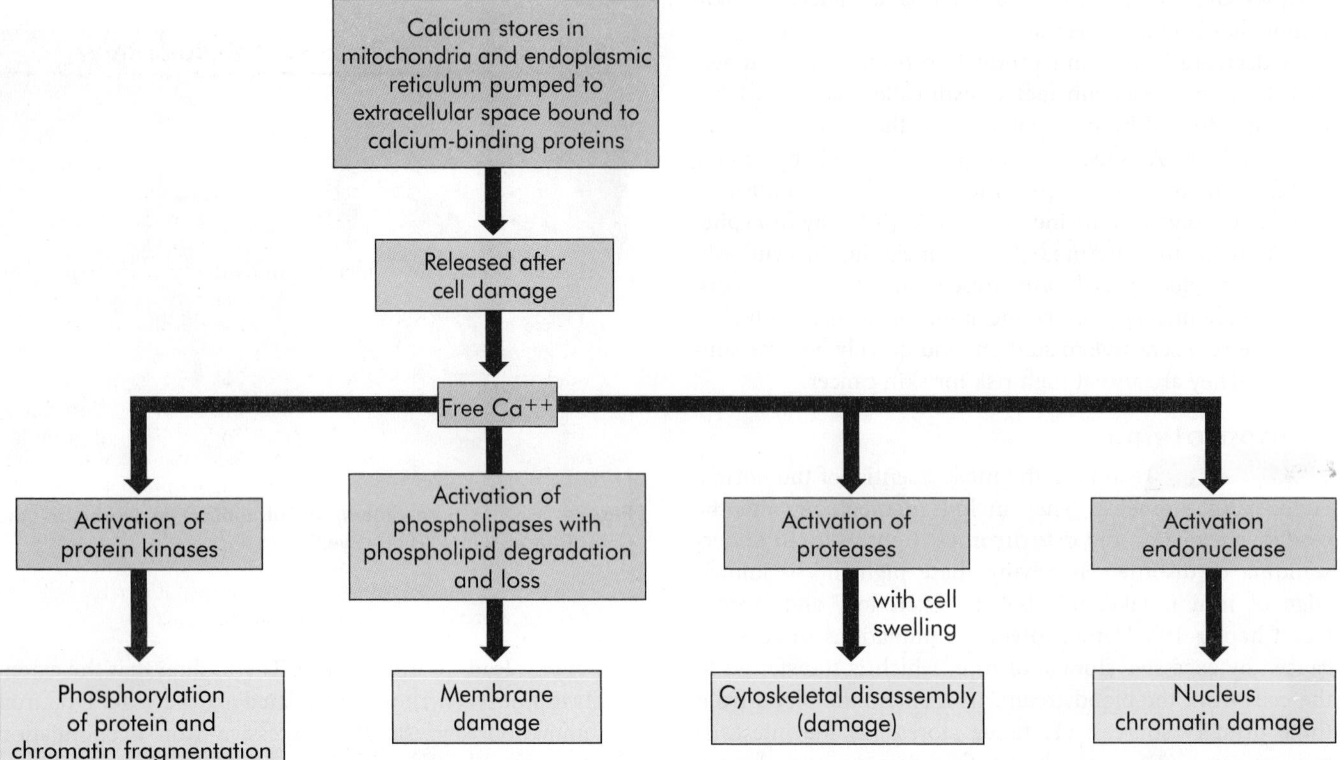

Figure 3-23 ■ **Free Cytosolic Calcium: A Destructive Agent.** Normally, calcium is removed from the cytosol by adenosine triphosphate (ATP)-dependent calcium pumps. In normal cells, calcium is bound to buffering proteins, such as calbindin or paralbumin, and is contained in the endoplasmic reticulum and the mitochondria. If there is abnormal permeability of calcium-ion channels, direct damage to membranes, or depletion of ATP (i.e., hypoxic injury), calcium increases in the cytosol. If the free calcium cannot be buffered or pumped out of cells, uncontrolled enzyme activation takes place, causing further damage. Uncontrolled entry of calcium into the cytosol is an important final common pathway in many causes of cell death.

($3Ca^3[PO^4]^2Ca[OH]^2$), a mixed salt. Damage occurs when calcium salts clump and harden, interfering with normal cellular structure and function.

Pathologic calcification can be dystrophic or metastatic. **Dystrophic calcification** occurs in dying and dead tissues, chronic tuberculosis of the lungs and lymph nodes, advanced atherosclerosis (narrowing as a result of plaque accumulation), and heart valve injury (Figure 3-24). Calcification of the heart valves interferes with their opening and closing, causing heart murmurs (see Chapter 23). Calcification of the coronary arteries predisposes them to severe narrowing and thrombosis, which can lead to myocardial infarction. Another site of dystrophic calcification is the center of tumors. Over time, the center is deprived of its oxygen supply, dies, and becomes calcified. The calcium salts appear as gritty, clumped granules that can become hard as stone. When several layers clump together, they resemble grains of sand and are called **psammoma bodies.**

Metastatic calcification consists of mineral deposits that occur in undamaged normal tissues as the result of hypercalcemia (excess calcium in the blood; see Chapter 4). Conditions that cause hypercalcemia include hyperparathyroidism, toxic levels of vitamin D, hyperthyroidism, idiopathic hypercalcemia of infancy, Addison disease (adrenocortical insufficiency), systemic sarcoidosis, milk-alkali syndrome, and the increased bone demineralization that results from bone tumors, leukemia, and disseminated cancers. Hypercalcemia also may occur in advanced renal failure with phosphate retention, resulting in hyperparathyroidism.

Urate

In humans, uric acid (**urate**) is the major end product of purine catabolism in the absence of urate oxidase. Serum urate concentration is, in general, stable: approximately 5 mg/dl in postpubertal males and 4.1 mg/dl in postpubertal females. Disturbances in maintaining serum urate levels result in hyperuricemia and the deposition of sodium urate crystals in the tissues, leading to painful disorders collectively called *gout.* These disorders include acute arthritis, chronic gouty arthritis, tophi (firm, nodular, subcutaneous deposits of urate crystals surrounded by fibrosis), and nephritis (inflammation of the nephron). Chronic hyperuricemia results in the deposition of urate in tissues, cell injury, and inflammation. Because urate crystals are not degraded by lysosomal enzymes, they persist in dead cells.

Systemic Manifestations

Systemic manifestations of cellular injury include a general sense of fatigue and malaise, a loss of well-being, and altered appetite. Fever is often present because of biochemicals produced during the inflammatory response. Table 3-9

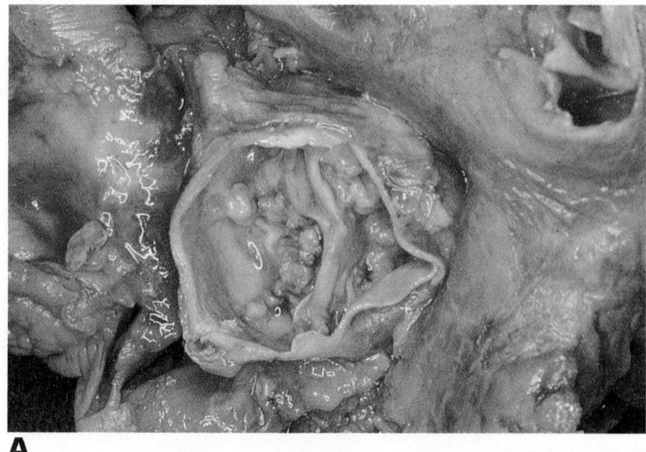

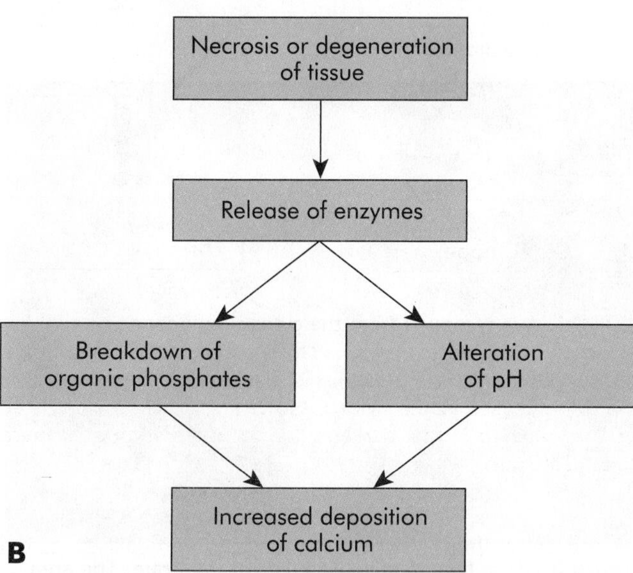

Figure 3-24 ■ **Aortic Valve Calcification. A,** This calcified aortic valve is an example of dystrophic calcification. **B,** This algorithm shows the dystrophic mechanism of calcification. (**A** from Damjanov I: *Pathology for the health professions,* ed 3, St Louis, 2006, Saunders.)

TABLE 3-9
Systemic Manifestations of Cellular Injury

Manifestation	Cause
Fever	Release of endogenous pyrogens (interleukin-1, tumor necrosis factor-α, prostaglandins) from bacteria or macrophages; acute inflammatory response
Increased heart rate	Increase in oxidative metabolic processes resulting from fever
Increase in leukocytes (leukocytosis)	Increase in total number of white blood cells because of infection; normal is 5000–9000/mm^3 (increase is directly related to the severity of the infection)
Pain	Various mechanisms, such as release of bradykinins, obstruction, pressure
Presence of cellular enzymes	Release of enzymes from cells of tissue* in extracellular fluid
Lactate dehydrogenase (LDH) (LDH isoenzymes)	Release from red blood cells, liver, kidney, skeletal muscle
Creatine kinase (CK) (CK isoenzymes)	Release from skeletal muscle, brain, heart
Aspartate aminotransferase (AST/SGOT)	Release from heart, liver, skeletal muscle, kidney, pancreas
Alanine aminotransferase (ALT/SGPT)	Release from liver, kidney, heart
Alkaline phosphatase (ALP)	Release from liver, bone
Amylase	Release from pancreas
Aldolase	Release from skeletal muscle, heart

*The rapidity of enzyme transfer is a function of the weight of the enzyme and the concentration gradient across the cellular membrane. The specific metabolic and excretory rates of the enzymes determine how long levels of enzymes remain elevated.

summarizes the most significant systemic manifestations of cellular injury.

CELLULAR DEATH

Necrosis

Cellular death eventually leads to cellular dissolution, or **necrosis.** Necrosis is the sum of cellular changes after local cell death and the process of cellular self-digestion known as autodigestion, or **autolysis** (Figure 3-25). Cells die long before any necrotic changes are noted by light microscopy.[30] The structural signs that indicate irreversible injury and progression to necrosis are dense clumping and progressive disruption of genetic material and disruption of the plasma and organelle membranes. In later stages of necrosis, most organelles are disrupted, and **karyolysis** (nuclear dissolution and lysis of chromatin from the action of hydrolytic enzymes) is under way. In some cells, the nucleus shrinks and becomes a small, dense mass of genetic material **(pyknosis).** The pyknotic nucleus eventually dissolves (by karyolysis) as a result of the action of hydrolytic lysosomal enzymes on DNA. **Karyorrhexis** means fragmentation of the nucleus into smaller particles or "nuclear dust."

Different types of necroses tend to occur in different organs or tissues and sometimes can indicate the mechanism or cause of cellular injury. The four major types of necroses are coagulative, liquefactive, caseous, and fatty. Another type, gangrenous necrosis, is *not* a distinctive type of cell death but refers instead to larger areas of tissue death. These necroses are summarized as follows:

1. **Coagulative necrosis.** Occurs primarily in the kidneys, heart, and adrenal glands; commonly results from hypoxia caused by severe ischemia or hypoxia caused by chemical injury, especially ingestion of mercuric chloride. Coagulation is caused by protein denaturation, which causes the protein albumin to change from a

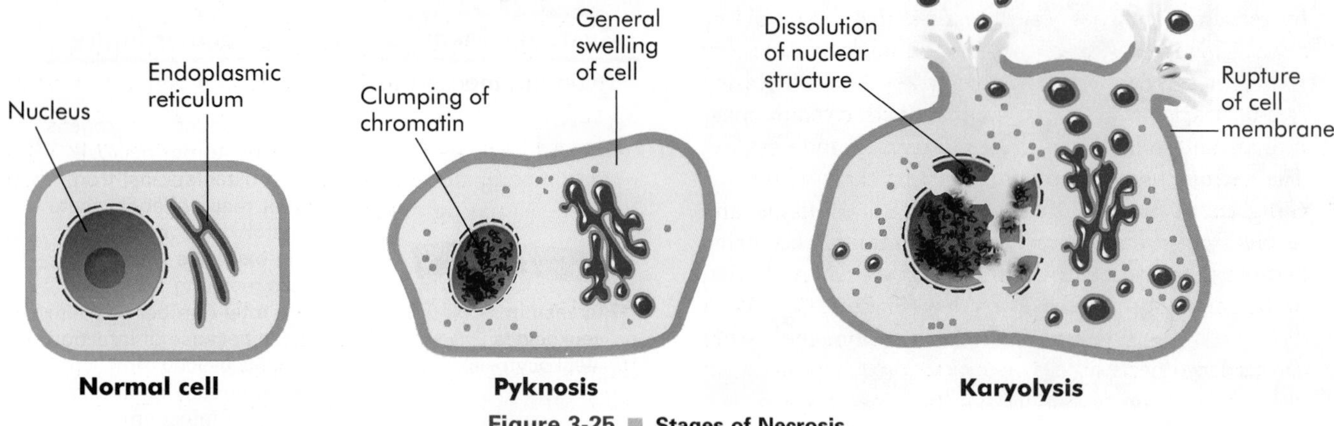

Figure 3-25 ■ **Stages of Necrosis.**

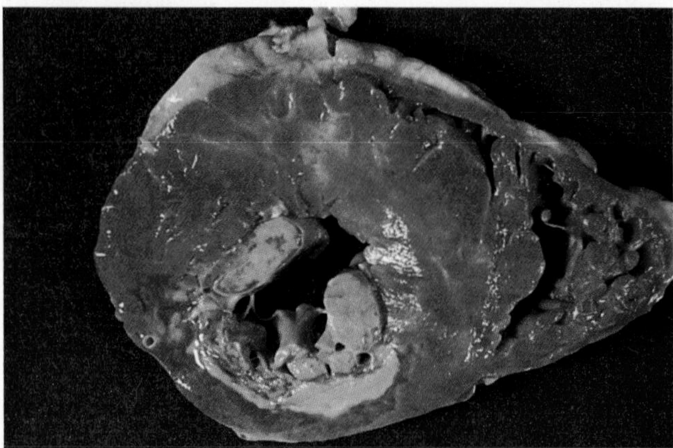

Figure 3-26 ■ **Coagulative Necrosis of Myocardium of Posterior Wall of Left Ventricle of Heart.** A large, anemic (white) infarct is readily apparent; note also the necrosis of papillary muscle. (From Damjanov I, Linder J, editors: *Anderson's pathology*, ed 10, St Louis, 1996, Mosby.)

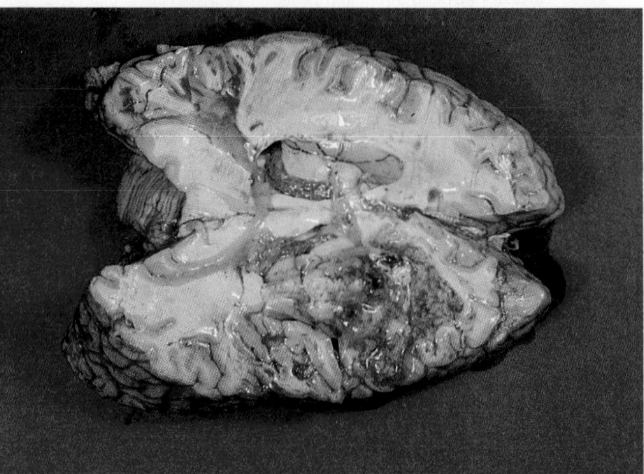

Figure 3-27 ■ **Liquefactive Necrosis of the Brain.** The area of infarction is softened as a result of liquefaction necrosis. (From Damjanov I: *Pathology for the health professions*, ed 3, St Louis, 2006, Saunders.)

gelatinous, transparent state to a firm, opaque state (Figure 3-26).

2. **Liquefactive necrosis.** Commonly results from ischemic injury to neurons and glial cells in the brain (Figure 3-27). Dead brain tissue is readily affected by liquefactive necrosis because brain cells are rich in the digestive hydrolytic enzymes and lipids and the brain contains little connective tissue. Cells are digested by their own hydrolases, so the tissue becomes soft, liquefies, and is walled off from healthy tissue, forming cysts. This can be caused by bacterial infection, especially staphylococci, streptococci, and *Escherichia coli.*
3. **Caseous necrosis.** Usually results from tuberculous pulmonary infection, especially by *Mycobacterium tuberculosis* (Figure 3-28). It is a combination of coagulative and liquefactive necroses. The dead cells disintegrate, but the debris is not completely digested by the hydrolases. Tissues resemble clumped cheese in that they are soft and granular. A granulomatous inflammatory wall encloses areas of caseous necrosis.

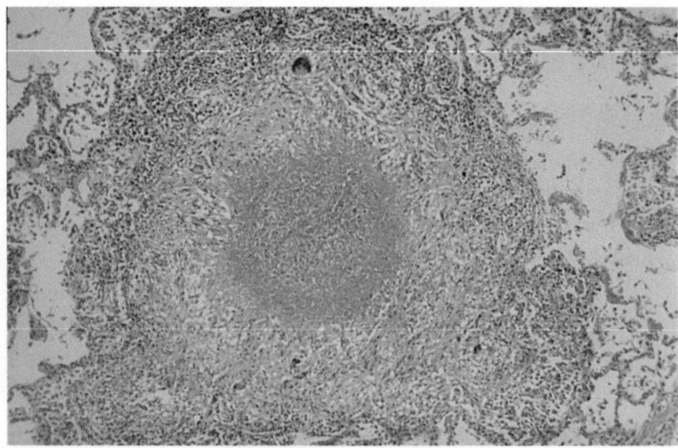

Figure 3-28 ■ **Granuloma with Central Caseous Necrosis Typical of Pulmonary Tuberculosis.** (From Damjanov I, Linder J, editors: *Anderson's pathology,* ed 10, St Louis, 1996, Mosby.)

4. **Fat necrosis.** Fat necrosis is cellular dissolution caused by powerful enzymes, called *lipases*, that occur in the breast, pancreas, and other abdominal structures (Figure 3-29). Lipases break down triglycerides, releasing free fatty acids, which then combine with calcium, magnesium, and sodium ions, creating soaps (saponification). The necrotic tissue appears opaque and chalk-white.
5. **Gangrenous necrosis.** Refers to death of tissue and results from severe hypoxic injury, commonly occurring because of arteriosclerosis, or blockage, of major arteries, particularly those in the lower leg (Figure 3-30). With hypoxia and subsequent bacterial invasion, the tissues can undergo necrosis. *Dry gangrene* is usually the result of coagulative necrosis. The skin becomes very dry and shrinks, resulting in wrinkles, and its color changes to dark brown or black. *Wet gangrene* develops when neutrophils invade the site, causing liquefactive necrosis. This usually occurs in internal organs, causing the site to become cold, swollen, and black. A foul odor is present, and if systemic symptoms become severe, death can ensue.
6. **Gas gangrene.** A special type of gangrene caused by infection of injured *tissue* by one of many species of *Clostridium*. These anaerobic bacteria produce hydrolytic enzymes and toxins that destroy connective tissue and cellular membranes and cause bubbles of gas to form in muscle cells. This can be fatal if enzymes lyse the membranes of red blood cells, destroying their oxygen-carrying capacity. Death is caused by shock.

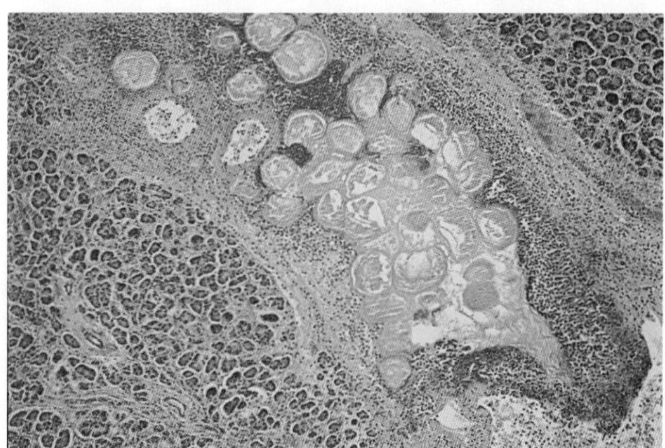

Figure 3-29 ■ Fat Necrosis of Pancreas. Interlobular adipocytes are necrotic; acute inflammatory cells surround these. (From Damjanov I, Linder J, editors: *Anderson's pathology,* ed 10, St Louis, 1996, Mosby.)

Apoptosis

Apoptosis ("dropping off") is an important, distinct type of cell death that differs from necrosis in several ways (Figure 3-31). Apoptosis is an active process of cellular self-destruction called programmed cell death—that is, cells need to die otherwise endless proliferation would lead to gigantic bodies. Every day the average adult may create 10 billion new cells—and kill off the same number.[34] A specific set of enzymes and genes are activated to cause apoptosis. These genes are sometimes called *suicide cells* because their activation by the nucleus inactivates so-called life-sustaining genes and promotes pathways leading to killer genes.

Apoptosis affects scattered, single cells; however, there are examples of it occurring in widespread areas. The process of apoptosis is nuclear and cytoplasmic shrinkage of a cell followed by fragmentation into membrane-bound fragments and subsequent phagocytosis by neutrophils and neighboring healthy cells. As a controlled process in normal development, apoptosis determines the size, patterning, and function of many tissues.[35,36] Apoptosis occurs throughout the life span—embryonic to old age. It can be activated by exogenous factors, for example, a long-lasting viral infection, or endogenously by the absence of certain growth factors. Accordingly, apoptosis can be classified as *physiologic* or *pathologic*.

Physiologic apoptosis is important in the development of body tissue. For example, it is responsible for local deletion of cells during tissue turnover and normal embryonic development. It has been shown to occur in endocrine-dependent tissues undergoing normal atrophic change. **Pathologic apoptosis** is the result of intracellular events

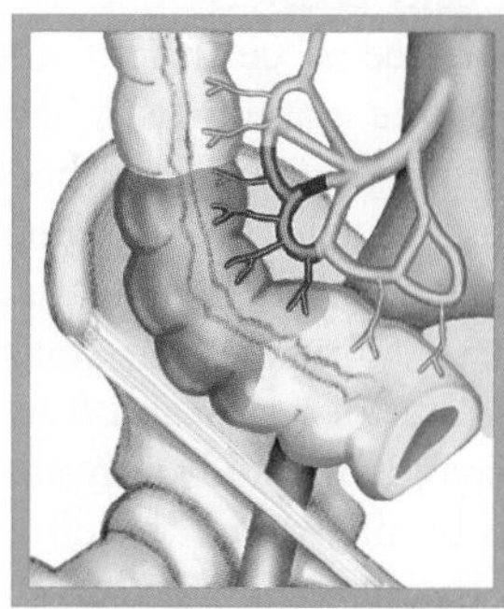

Thrombosis or embolism

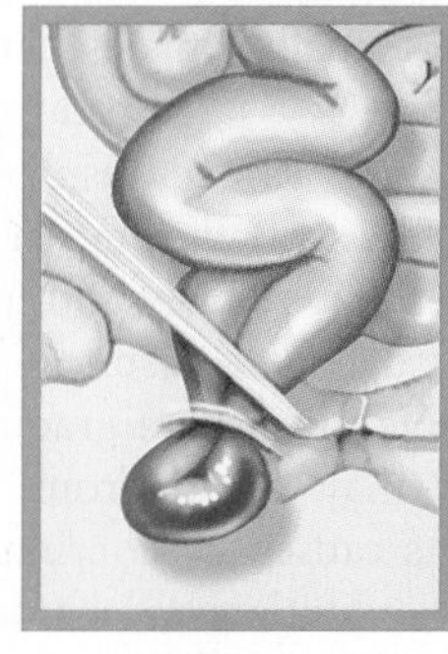

Strangulated hernia

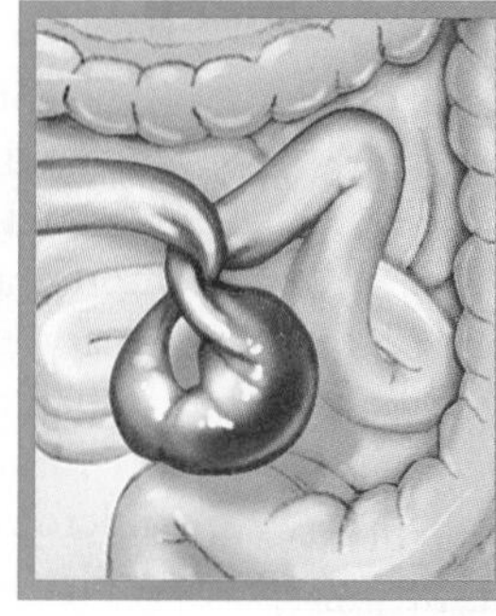

Volvulus

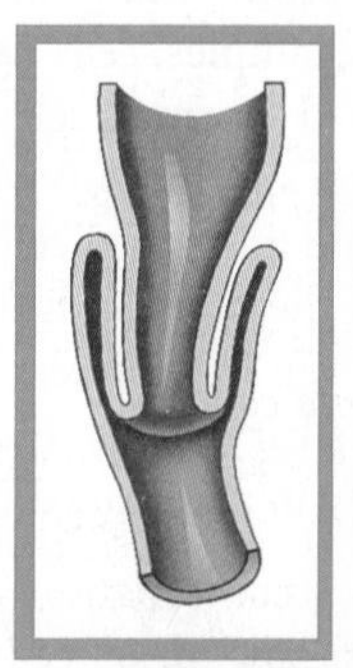

Intussusception

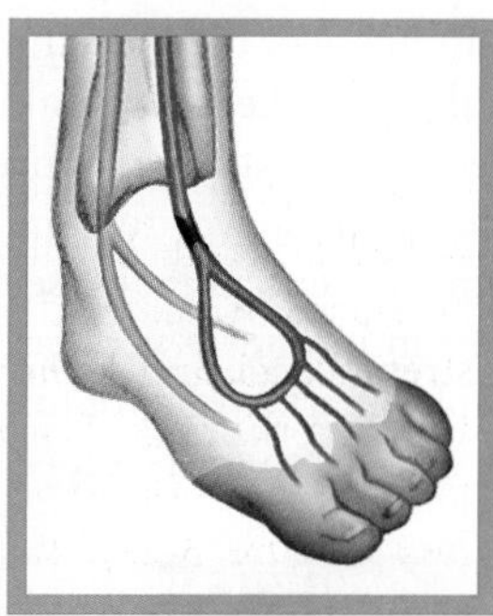

Gangrene

Figure 3-30 ■ Gangrene, a Complication of Necrosis. In certain circumstances, necrotic tissue will be invaded by putrefactive organisms that are both saccharolytic and proteolytic. Foul-smelling gases are produced, and the tissue becomes green or black as a result of breakdown of hemoglobin. Obstruction of the blood supply to the bowel almost inevitably is followed by gangrene.

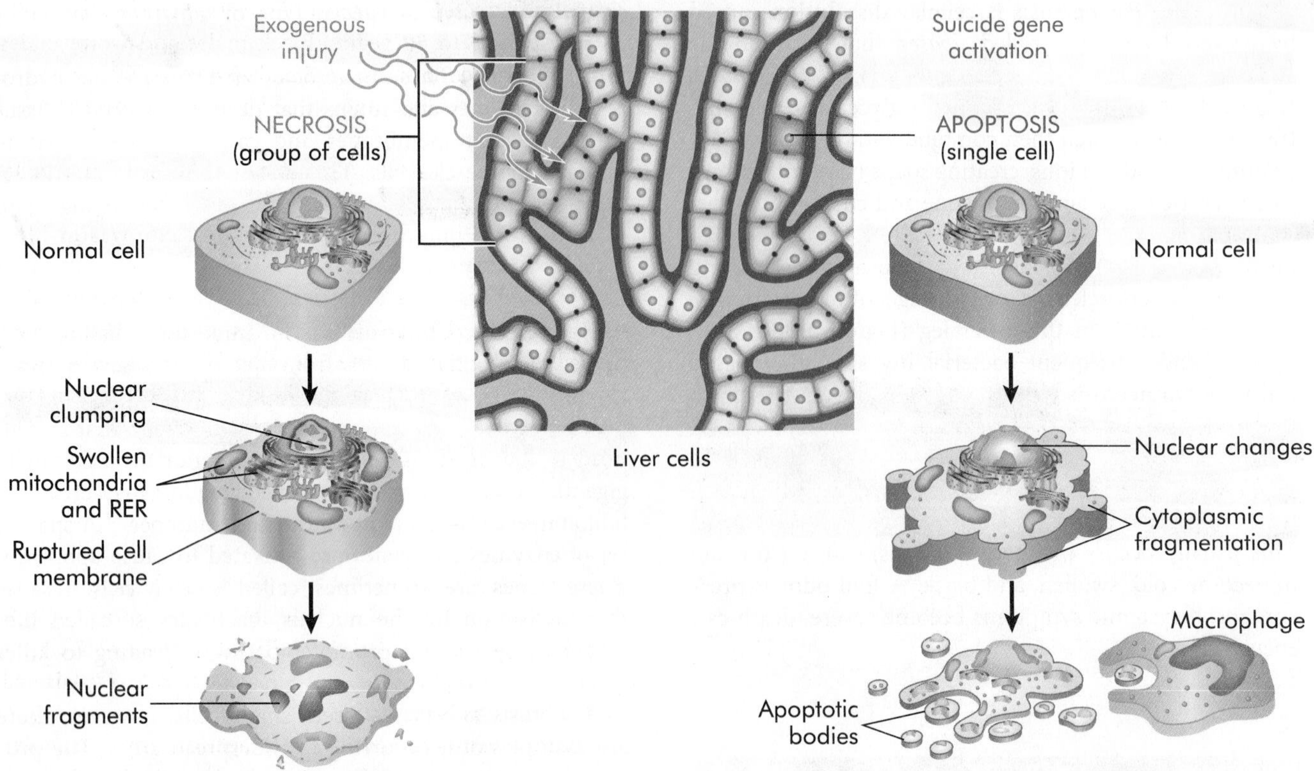

Figure 3-31 ■ **Necrosis and Apoptosis in Liver Cells.** Necrosis is caused by exogenous injury whereby cells are swollen and have nuclear changes in ruptured cell membrane. Apoptosis is single cell death. It is genetically programmed (suicide genes) and depends on energy. Apoptotic bodies contain part of the nucleus and cytoplasmic organelles, which are ultimately taken up by macrophages or adjacent cells. *RER,* Rough endoplasmic reticulum. (Redrawn from Damjanov I: *Pathology for the health professions,* ed 3, St Louis, 2006, Saunders.)

or adverse exogenous stimuli. For example, deficiencies of specific enzymes can lead to diseases where cells have undergone apoptosis. Liver cells infected with viral hepatitis C, for example, can undergo apoptosis. Apoptosis in hemopoietic cells has been linked to the production of free radicals[37] and can spontaneously occur in some malignant tumors and cells treated with ionizing radiation and chemotherapy. *Absence of apoptosis* can cause pathologic change. A mutation in a gene (*bcl-2,* for example) that promotes apoptosis may only give the signal to proliferate and not die. Thus, lymphocytes may accumulate, enlarging lymph nodes and eventually proliferating into the blood.

In many of the preceding examples, cells deprived of survival signals die by programmed (normal) cell death. It seems reasonable that dependence on specific survival signals provides a simple way to eliminate misplaced cells, regulate cell numbers, and, perhaps, select the fittest cells.[38–40] Apoptosis can run its course very fast, even in minutes. Thus, the best cellular marker of apoptosis is karyohexis (fragmentation of the nucleus to dust), especially in an isolated cell.[30]

QUICK CHECK 3-4

1. Why is an increase in intracellular calcium injurious?
2. Compare and contrast necrosis and apoptosis.
3. Why is apoptosis significant?

AGING & Altered Cellular and Tissue Biology

Aging usually is defined as a normal physiologic process that is both universal and inevitable. The basic mechanisms of aging depend on the irreversible and universal processes at the cellular and molecular level. To understand aging requires the separation of irreversible processes from potentially reversible mechanisms (i.e., those that result from disease or age-related debilities).

Aging traditionally has not been considered a disease because it is "normal"; disease is usually considered "abnormal." Conceptually, this distinction seems clear until the concept of injury is introduced; some pathologists have defined disease as the result of injury. Aging has been defined as the time-dependent loss of structure and function that proceeds slowly and in such small increments that it appears to be the result of the accumulation of small, imperceptible injuries—a gradual result of "wear and tear."

Injuries may result from unavoidable and universal microinsults caused by continuous bombardment by ultraviolet light, countless mechanical insults, and reactions to metabolites (Figure 3-32).[41] In this context, the distinction between aging and disease is unclear. For example, some degree of atrophy of the brain is considered normal in old age until it proceeds far enough to cause clinically significant

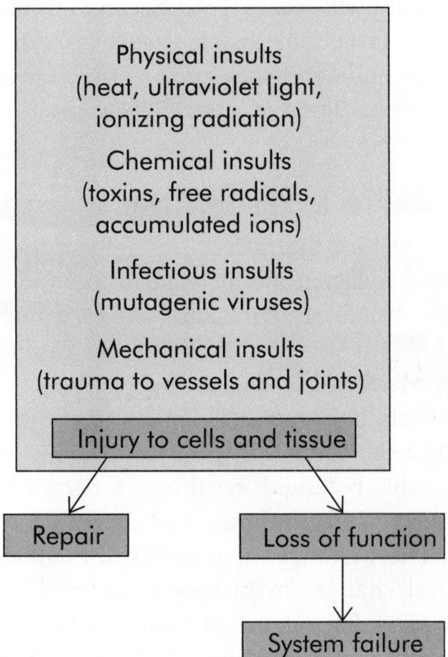

Figure 3-32 **Microinsults.** (Redrawn from Johnson HA, editor: *Is aging physiological or pathological? Relations between normal aging and a disease,* New York, 1985, Raven.)

disability and is called a *disease.* Likewise, most human beings have atherosclerosis, and the plaques progress with age, but at what point in this progression is atherosclerosis considered abnormal? These conceptual distinctions have given rise to two general categories of theories of aging. The first category proposes that aging is the result of the accumulation of random injuries and events. The second category proposes that aging is the result of a genetically controlled developmental program, or built-in self-destructive processes.

Normal Life Span

The **maximal life span** of humans is between 80 and 100 years and does not vary significantly among populations. However, in primitive societies few individuals reach the maximal life span; most die in infancy or the early years. In societies with improved sanitation, housing, nutrition, and health care, many persons do attain the maximal life span. Although the maximal life span has not changed significantly over time, the average life span, or life expectancy, has increased. Recently, the death rate for people 65 years of age and older has declined significantly, largely as a result of decreased cardiovascular disease.

Life Expectancy and Gender Differences

Life expectancy is a summary measure of mortality—the average number of years of life expected if current death rates were constant. As of 2004, life expectancy at birth for the total population reached a record high of 77.9 years. The **gender gap** between male and female life expectancy was 5.2 years, down from 5.4 years in 2002. The difference between male and female life expectancy at birth has been decreasing since a peak of 7.8 years in 1979. Life expectancy for males increased to a record 75 years. Female life expectancy increased to 80 years.. Black males and white males both reached record highs (69.2 and 75.4 years, respectively), as well as black females and white females (76 and 80 years, respectively).

In the United States, Hawaii had the lowest mortality with an age-adjusted death rate of 650.1 deaths per 100,000 population; the highest mortality rate was in Mississippi with 1015.2 deaths per 100,000.[42] Japan still ranks first for life expectancy (males, 82.8 years; females, 87.7 years) and the United States ranks twelfth. Longer life expectancies in many other developing countries suggest the possibility of increasing the life expectancy in the United States.[42]

Theories and Mechanisms of Aging

Relatively little indisputable knowledge exists on the subject of aging. Table 3-10 presents the historical development of aging research. Many theories have focused on a single mechanism—the so-called magic bullet approach to arrest aging. It is doubtful that a single theory will explain all the mechanisms of aging.

Evidence exists both for and against any particular theory of aging. However, three major mechanisms of aging have retained their appeal or have been extensively tested (1) cellular changes produced by genetic and envi-

TABLE 3-10
Theories of Aging

Theory	Year	Proponent
Waste product theory	1923	Carrell & Ebeling
Wear-and-tear theory	1924	Pearl
Rate of living theory*	1928	Pearl
Endocrine theory	1947	Korenchevsky & Jones
Free-radical theory†	1955	Harman
Collagen theory‡	1957	Verzar
Metabolic theory*	1957; 1961	Carlson et al; Johnson et al
Somatic mutation theory	1959	Sziliard
Error-catastrophe theory	1963; 1970	Orgel
Cross-linking theory‡	1968	Bjorksten
Programmed senescence theory	1969	Hayflick
Immunologic theory	1969	Walform
Evolution theory	1977	Kirkwood
Mitochondrial theory	1980	Miguel & Fleming

Data from Schneider EL: Theories of aging: a perspective. In Warner HR et al, editors: *Modern biological theories of aging,* New York, 1987, Raven Press; Melov S: Mitochondrial oxidative stress: physiologic consequences and potential for a role in aging, *Ann NY Acad Sci* 908:219–225, 2000; Biesalsk HK: Free radical theory of aging, *Curr Opin Clin Nutr Metab Care* 5(1):5–10, 2002.
*May represent the same theory.
†Current emphasis on mitochondrial oxidative stress and genetic variability for antioxidant protection.
‡May represent the same theory.

ronmental-lifestyle factors; (2) changes in cellular regulatory, or control, mechanisms, especially in cells of the neuroendocrine, immune, and central nervous systems; and (3) degenerative extracellular and vascular alterations.[43–46]

Genetic and environmental lifestyle factors

Cellular aging results from wear and tear that causes functional changes and eventual cellular death. Cells may become damaged during replication as a result of factors within the cell, such as DNA and protein mechanisms, or factors outside the cell, such as ionizing radiation. Cells may already be programmed at birth or injured during life so as to cause errors in mitotic division and in the replication of genetic material, eventually leading to either cellular atrophy or death. Atrophy is common in the thymus, testis, ovary, uterus, and breast of aged individuals, although these organs age differently.

One genetic mechanism of aging is programmed aging. Regardless of damaging environmental factors, some investigators think that each normal cell may have a finite life span during which it can replicate. A classic experiment done by Hayflick demonstrated that fibroblasts are limited to a finite number of generations (40 to 60 doublings).[47] Proponents believe that an intrinsic program within the human genome progressively slows or shuts down certain physiologic mechanisms, including mitosis.

The **somatic mutation hypothesis** proposes that aging is the result of DNA damage, inefficiency of repair, and loss of integrity of DNA synthesis. Most experimental evidence thus far does not support the hypothesis that aging is the result of somatic mutation.

The **catastrophic** or **error-prone theory,** initially proposed by Orgel in 1963, stated that the presence of errors in those enzymes involved in transcription and translation, and thus their own synthesis, leads to an increase in errors and eventually to the death of the cell. Most of the evidence, however, argues against this theory as originally formulated. The accumulation of altered proteins in aging may result from an increased production or a decreased ability of aged cells to degrade their cellular proteins or both.

Alterations of cellular control mechanisms

The overall effects of aging may be caused by changes in certain cell populations that exert regulatory or control functions, such as cells of the CNS, neuroendocrine system, and immune system. The **neuroendocrine theory** of aging purports that a genetic program for aging is encoded in the brain and is controlled and relayed to peripheral tissues through hormonal and neural agents. Possible mechanisms include (1) increased hormonal degradation, (2) decreased rate of hormonal synthesis and secretion; and (3) decreased target-organ sensitivity related to the number of cellular receptors for hormonal ligands, ligand-receptor binding, or ligand internalization.

Proponents of immune theories of aging believe that the immune system is implicated in aging because (1) immune function declines with age; (2) the decline in immune function is related to certain diseases, such as cancer, and to many other secondary effects; and (3) the number of autoantibodies (antibodies that attack body tissues) increases with age.

Degenerative extracellular changes

Extracellular factors that affect the aging process include the binding of collagen; the increase in free radicals' effects on cells; the structural alterations of fascia, tendons, ligaments, bones, and joints; and peripheral vascular disease, particularly arteriosclerosis (see Chapter 23).

Aging affects the extracellular matrix with increased cross-linking (e.g., aging collagen becomes more insoluble, chemically stable but rigid, resulting in decreased cell permeability), decreased synthesis, and increased degradation of collagen. These changes, together with the disappearance of elastin and changes in proteoglycans and plasma proteins, cause disorders of the ground substance that result in dehydration and wrinkling of the skin (see Chapter 39). Other age-related defects in the extracellular matrix include skeletal muscle alterations (e.g., atrophy, decreased tone, loss of contractility), cataracts, diverticula, hernias, and rupture of intervertebral disks.

Free radicals of oxygen that result from oxidative cellular metabolism, *oxidative stress* (e.g., respiratory chain, phagocytosis, prostaglandin synthesis), damage tissues during the aging process. The oxygen radicals produced include superoxide radical, hydroxyl radical, and hydrogen peroxide (see p. 68). These oxygen products are extremely reactive and can damage nucleic acids, destroy polysaccharides, oxidize proteins, peroxidize unsaturated fatty acids, and kill and lyse cells. Oxidant effects on target cells can give rise to malignant transformation, presumably through DNA damage. That progressive and cumulative damage from oxygen radicals may lead to harmful alterations in cellular function is consistent with those alterations of aging. This hypothesis is founded on the wear-and-tear theory of aging, which states that damages accumulate with time, decreasing the organism's ability to maintain a steady state. Because these oxygen-reactive species not only can permanently damage cells but also may lead to cell death, there is new support for their role in the aging process. Current emphasis is on oxidative damage to the DNA in mitochondria (mDNA). It is well established that mitochondrial deficits accumulate with age in rodent tissues.[48] Furthermore, levels of oxidative damage to mDNA are several times higher than those of nuclear DNA. Superoxide radicals produced during mitochondrial respiration react with nitric oxide inside mitochondria to produce damaging **peroxynitrite.**[49]

Of much interest is the relationship between aging and the disappearance or alteration of extracellular substances important for vessel integrity. With aging, lipid, calcium, and plasma proteins are deposited in the walls of vessels. These depositions cause serious basement membrane thickening and alterations in smooth muscle functioning, resulting in arteriosclerosis (a progressive disease that causes such problems as stroke, myocardial infarction, renal disease, and peripheral vascular disease).

Cellular Aging

Cellular changes characteristic of aging include atrophy, decreased function, and loss of cells, possibly caused by apoptosis. Loss of cellular function from any of these causes initiates the compensatory mechanisms of hypertrophy and hyperplasia of remaining cells, which can lead to metaplasia, dysplasia, and neoplasia. All of these changes can alter receptor placement and function, nutrient pathways, secretion of cellular products, and neuroendocrine control mechanisms. In the aged cell, DNA, RNA, cellular proteins, and membranes are most susceptible to injurious stimuli. DNA is particularly vulnerable to such injuries as breaks, deletions, and additions. Lack of DNA repair increases the cell's susceptibility to mutations that may be lethal or may promote the development of neoplasia (see Chapter 9).

Tissue and Systemic Aging

It is probably safe to say that every physiologic process functions less efficiently with increasing age. The most characteristic tissue change with age is a progressive stiffness or rigidity that affects many systems, including the arterial, pulmonary, and musculoskeletal systems. A consequence of blood vessel and organ stiffness is a progressive increase in peripheral resistance to blood flow. The movement of intracellular and extracellular substances also decreases with age, as does the diffusion capacity of the lung. Blood flow through organs also decreases.

Aging occurs in part because of declines in the function of tissue stem cells. Normal tissue function requires that the rate of cell loss be matched by the rate of cell renewal. Aging is increased by changes that either accelerates cellular loss or slows tissue repair.[50]

Changes in the endocrine and immune systems include thymus atrophy. Although this occurs at puberty, causing a decreased immune response to T-dependent antigens (foreign proteins), increased autoantibodies and immune complexes (antibodies that are bound to antigens) and an overall decrease in the immunologic tolerance for the host's own cells further diminish the effectiveness of the immune system later in life. In women, the reproductive system loses ova, and in men, spermatogenesis decreases. Responsiveness to hormones decreases in the breast and endometrium.

The stomach experiences decreases in the rate of emptying and secretion of hormones and hydrochloric acid. Muscular atrophy diminishes mobility by decreasing motor tone and contractility. **Sarcopenia,** loss of muscle mass and strength, can occur into old age. The skin of the aged individual is affected by atrophy and wrinkling of the epidermis and alterations in underlying dermis, fat, and muscle.

Total body changes include a decrease in height; a reduction in circumference of the neck, thighs, and arms; widening of the pelvis; and lengthening of the nose and ears. Several of these changes are the result of tissue atrophy and of decreased bone mass caused by osteoporosis and osteoarthritis. Although growth hormone function, reflected in diminished levels of insulin-like growth factor-1, is a current hypothesis for explaining decreased bone and lean body mass, recent research has found advancing age rather than declining levels of these hormones as a major determinant.[51]

Body composition changes with age. With middle age, there is an increase in body weight (men gain until 50 years of age and women until 70 years) and fat mass, followed by a decrease in stature, weight, **fat-free mass** (FFM; includes all minerals, proteins, and water plus all other constituents except lipids), and body cell mass at older ages. As fat increases, total body water decreases. Increased body fat and centralized fat distribution (abdominal) are associated with non-insulin-dependent diabetes and heart disease. Total body potassium also decreases because of decreased cellular mass. An increased sodium/potassium ratio suggests that the decreased cellular mass is accompanied by an increased extracellular fluid compartment.

Although some of these alterations are probably inherent in aging, others represent consequences of the process. Advanced age increases susceptibility to disease, and death occurs after an injury or insult because of diminished cellular, tissue, and organic function.

Frailty

Frailty is imprecisely defined as a wasting syndrome of aging, leaving a person vulnerable to falls, functional decline, disease, and death. Age-related changes in the musculoskeletal system are thought to be important determinants of frailty.[52] Criteria to define frailty often include mobility, balance, muscle strength, motor activity, cognition, nutritional status, endurance, falls, fractures, and bone density.[52] Endocrine-immune dysregulation occurs in aging including declining hormones (for example, estrogens, testosterone, IGF-1), and increasing proinflammatory cytokines (for example, IL-6 and C-reactive protein [CRP]). The joint effects of low levels of IGF-1 and increased levels of interleukin-6 are related to high risk for progressive disability and death in older women.[53] These alterations may be significant for the development of frailty.

Elevated levels of other catabolic cytokines including tumor necrosis factor-alpha (TNF-α), as well as IL-6, have been linked to sarcopenia.[54] Declines in ovarian function also may lead to increased proinflammatory cytokines (such as IL-1, IL-6, and TNF-α).[55,56] Because the effects of dehydroepiandrosterone (DHEA) and testosterone can be mediated by their metabolism to estrogen, androgen deficiency could increase proinflammatory cytokines.[52] Thus, an important mechanism of frailty may be endocrine-immune dysregulation and future studies are needed to evaluate the specific mechanisms to various biologic markers of frailty.

SOMATIC DEATH

Somatic death is death of the entire person. Unlike the changes that follow cellular death in a live body, **postmortem change** is diffuse and does not involve components of the inflammatory response. Within minutes after death, postmortem changes appear, eliminating any difficulty in determining that death has occurred. The most notable manifestations are complete cessation of respiration and circulation. The surface of the skin usually becomes pale and yellowish; however, the lifelike color of the cheeks and lips may persist after death that is caused by carbon monoxide poisoning, drowning, or chloroform poisoning.[57]

Body temperature falls gradually immediately after death and then more rapidly (approximately 1.0° to 1.5° F/hr) until, after 24 hours, body temperature equals that of the environment.[58] After death caused by certain infective diseases, body temperature may continue to rise for a short time. Postmortem reduction of body temperature is called **algor mortis.**

Blood pressure within the retinal vessels decreases, causing muscle tension to decrease and the pupils to dilate. The face, nose, and chin become sharp or peaked-looking as blood and fluids drain away.[57] Gravity causes blood to settle in the most dependent, or lowest, tissues, which develop a purple discoloration called **livor mortis.** Incisions made at this time usually fail to cause bleeding. The skin loses its elasticity and transparency.

Within 6 hours after death, acidic compounds accumulate within the muscles because of the breakdown of carbohydrate and depletion of ATP. This interferes with ATP-dependent detachment of myosin from actin (contractile proteins), and muscle stiffening, or **rigor mortis,** sets in. The smaller muscles are usually affected first, particularly the muscles of the jaw. Within 12 to 14 hours, rigor mortis usually affects the entire body.

Signs of putrefaction are generally obvious about 24 to 48 hours after death. Rigor mortis gradually diminishes, and the body becomes flaccid at 36 to 62 hours. Putrefactive changes vary depending on the temperature of the environment. The most visible is greenish discoloration of the skin, particularly on the abdomen. The discoloration is thought to be related to the diffusion of hemolyzed blood into the tissues and the production of sulfhemoglobin.[46] Slippage or loosening of the skin from underlying tissues occurs at the same time. After this, swelling or bloating of the body and liquefactive changes occur, sometimes causing opening of the body cavities. At a microscopic level, putrefactive changes are associated with the release of enzymes and lytic dissolution called **postmortem autolysis.**

QUICK CHECK 3-5

1. Why are microinsults important to aging?
2. What are the body composition changes that occur with aging?
3. Define frailty and possible endocrine-immune involvement.

Did You Understand?

Cellular Adaptation

1. Cellular adaptation is an alteration that enables the cell to maintain a steady state despite adverse conditions.
2. Atrophy is a decrease in cellular size caused by aging, disuse, or lack of blood supply, hormonal stimulation, or neural stimulation. The amounts of endoplasmic reticulum, mitochondria, and microfilaments decrease.
3. Hypertrophy is an increase in the size of cells caused by increased work demands or hormonal stimulation. The amounts of protein in the plasma membrane, endoplasmic reticulum, microfilaments, and mitochondria increase.
4. Hyperplasia is an increase in the number of cells caused by an increased rate of cellular division. Normal hyperplasia is stimulated by hormones or the need to replace lost tissues.
5. Dysplasia, or atypical hyperplasia, is an abnormal change in the size, shape, and organization of mature tissue cells.
6. Metaplasia is the reversible replacement of one mature cell type by another less mature cell type.

Cellular Injury

1. Cellular injury occurs if the cell is unable to maintain homeostasis. Injured cells may recover (reversible injury) or die (irreversible injury). Injury is caused by lack of oxygen (hypoxia), free radicals, caustic or toxic chemicals, infectious agents, inflammatory and immune responses, genetic factors, insufficient nutrients, or physical trauma from many causes.
2. Four biochemical themes are important to cell injury: (a) ATP depletion, (b) oxygen and oxygen-derived free radicals, (c) intracellular calcium and loss of calcium steady state, and (d) defects in membrane permeability.
3. The sequence of events leading to cell death is commonly decreased ATP production, failure of active-transport mechanisms (the sodium-potassium pump), cellular swelling, detachment of ribosomes from the endoplasmic reticulum, cessation of protein synthesis, mitochondrial swelling as a result of calcium accumulation, vacuolation, leakage of digestive enzymes from lysosomes, autodigestion of intracellular structures, lysis of the plasma membrane, and death.
4. The initial insult in hypoxic injury is usually ischemia (the cessation of blood flow into vessels that supply the cell with oxygen and nutrients).
5. Free radicals cause cellular injury because they have an unpaired electron that makes the molecule unstable. To stabilize itself, the molecule gives up an electron to another molecule or steals one. Therefore it forms injurious chemical bonds with proteins, lipids, and carbohydrates—key molecules in membranes and nucleic acids.

Did You Understand?—Cont'd

6. The damaging effects of free radicals, especially activated oxygen species (O_2^-, OH·, H_2O_2), include (a) lipid peroxidation, (b) alteration of ion pumps and transport mechanisms, (c) fragmentation of DNA, and (d) damage to mitochondria-releasing calcium into the cytosol.
7. Restoration of oxygen, however, can cause additional injury called *reperfusion injury.*
8. The initial insult in chemical injury is damage or destruction of the plasma membrane. Examples of chemical agents that cause cellular injury are carbon tetrachloride, lead, carbon monoxide, and ethyl alcohol.
9. Unintentional and intentional injuries are an important health problem in the United States. Death as a result of these injuries is more common for men than women and higher among blacks than whites and other racial groups.
10. Injuries by blunt force are the result of the application of mechanical energy to the body, resulting in tearing, shearing, or crushing of tissues. The most common types of blunt-force injuries include motor vehicle accidents and falls.
11. A contusion is bleeding into the skin or underlying tissues as a consequence of a blow. A collection of blood in soft tissues or an enclosed space may be referred to as a hematoma.
12. An abrasion (scrape) results from removal of the superficial layers of the skin caused by friction between the skin and injuring object. Abrasions and contusions may have a patterned appearance that mirrors the shape and features of the injuring object.
13. A laceration is a tear or rip resulting when the tensile strength of the skin or tissue is exceeded.
14. An incised wound is a cut that is longer than it is deep. A stab wound is a penetrating sharp-force injury that is deeper than it is long.
15. Gunshot wounds may be either penetrating (bullet retained in the body) or perforating (bullet exits). The most important factors determining the appearance of a gunshot injury are whether it is an entrance or an exit wound and the range of fire.
16. Asphyxial injuries are caused by a failure of cells to receive or utilize oxygen. These injuries can be grouped into four general categories: suffocation, strangulation, chemical, and drowning.
17. Activation of inflammation and immunity, which occurs after cellular injury or infection, involves powerful biochemicals and proteins capable of damaging normal (uninjured and uninfected) cells.
18. Genetic disorders injure cells by altering the nucleus and the plasma membrane's structure, shape, receptors, or transport mechanisms.
19. Deprivation of essential nutrients (proteins, carbohydrates, lipids, vitamins) can cause cellular injury by altering cellular structure and function, particularly of transport mechanisms, chromosomes, the nucleus, and DNA.
20. Injurious physical agents include temperature extremes, changes in atmospheric pressure, ionizing radiation, illumination, mechanical stresses (e.g., repetitive body movements), and noise.

Manifestations of Cellular Injury

1. Cellular manifestations of cellular injury include accumulations of water, lipids, carbohydrates, glycogen, proteins, pigments, hemosiderin, bilirubin, calcium, and urate.
2. Accumulations harm cells by "crowding" the organelles and by causing excessive (and sometimes harmful) metabolites to be produced during their catabolism. The metabolites are released into the cytoplasm or expelled into the extracellular matrix.
3. Cellular swelling, the accumulation of excessive water in the cell, is caused by the failure of transport mechanisms and is a sign of many types of cellular injury. Oncosis is a type of cellular death resulting from cellular swelling.
4. Accumulations of organic substances—lipids, carbohydrates, glycogen, proteins, pigments—are caused by disorders in which (a) cellular uptake of the substance exceeds the cell's capacity to catabolize (digest) or use it or (b) cellular anabolism (synthesis) of the substance exceeds the cell's capacity to use or secrete it.
5. Dystrophic calcification (accumulation of calcium salts) is always a sign of pathologic change because it occurs only in injured or dead cells. Metastatic calcification, however, can occur in uninjured cells in individuals with hypercalcemia.
6. Disturbances in urate metabolism can result in hyperuricemia and deposition of sodium urate crystals in tissue—leading to a painful disorder called *gout.*
7. Systemic manifestations of cellular injury include fever, leukocytosis, increased heart rate, pain, and serum elevations of enzymes in the plasma.

Cellular Death

1. Cellular death is manifested as cellular dissolution, or necrosis. Necrosis is the sum of the changes after local cell death and includes the process of autolysis, or cellular self-destruction.
2. There are four major types of necroses: coagulative, liquefactive, caseous, and fat necroses. Different types of necroses occur in different tissues.
3. Structural signs that indicate irreversible injury and progression to necrosis are the dense clumping and disruption of genetic material and the disruption of the plasma and organelle membranes.
4. Apoptosis, a distinct type of sublethal injury, is a process of selective cellular self-destruction that occurs in both normal and pathologic tissue changes.
5. Gangrenous necrosis, or gangrene, is tissue necrosis caused by hypoxia and the subsequent bacterial invasion.

AGING & Altered Cellular and Tissue Biology

1. It is difficult to determine the physiologic (normal) from the pathologic changes of aging.
2. Humans have an inherent maximal life span (80 to 100 years) that is dictated by currently unknown intrinsic mechanisms.
3. Although the maximal life span has not changed significantly over time, the average life span, or life expectancy, has increased. Life expectancy for men is about 75 years, and for women it is 80 years.

(Continued)

Did You Understand?—Cont'd

4. The physiologic mechanisms of aging apparently are associated with (a) cellular changes produced by genetic and environmental-lifestyle factors, (b) changes in cellular regulatory or control mechanisms, and (c) degenerative extracellular and vascular alterations.
5. Frailty is imprecisely defined as a wasting syndrome of aging leaving a person vulnerable to falls, functional decline, disease, and death.

Somatic Death

1. Somatic death is death of the entire organism. Postmortem change is diffuse and does not involve the inflammatory response.
2. Manifestations of somatic death include cessation of respiration and circulation, gradual lowering of body temperature, pupil dilation, loss of elasticity and transparency in the skin, muscle stiffening (rigor mortis), and skin discoloration (livor mortis). Signs of putrefaction are obvious about 24 to 48 hours after death.

Key Terms

References

1. Kornitzer D, Chiechanover A: Modes of regulation of ubiquitin mediated protein degradation, *J Cell Physiol* 183(1):1–11, 2000.
2. Mohammed FF et al: Metalloproteinase inhibitor TIMP-1 affects hepatocyte cell cycle via HGF activation in murine liver regeneration, *Hepatology* 41(4):857–867, 2005.
3. Pisconti A et al: Follistatin induction by nitric oxide through cyclic GMP: a tightly regulated signaling pathway that controls myoblast fusion, *J Cell Biol* 172(2):233–244, 2006.
4. Allred DC, Moshin SK, Fugua SA: Histological and biological evolution of human premalignant breast disease, *Endocr Relat Cancer* 8(1):47–61, 2001.

References—Cont'd

5. Dabbs DJ et al: Molecular alterations in columnar cell lesions of the breast, *Mod Pathol* 19(3):344–349, 2006.
6. Renshaw AA et al: Atypical ductal hyperplasia in breast core needle: correlation of size of the lesion, complete removal of the lesion, and the incidence of carcinoma in follow-up biopsies, *Am J Clin Pathol* 116(1):92–96, 2001.
7. Bai J, Cederbaum AI: Mitochondrial catalase and oxidative injury, *Biol Signals Recept* 10(3–4):189–199, 2001.
8. Lee HC, Wei YH: Mitochondrial biogenesis and mitochondrial DNA maintenance of mammalian cells under oxidative stress, *Int J Biochem Cell Biol* 37(4):822–834, 2005.
9. Lopez MF, Melov S: Applied proteomics: mitochondrial proteins and effect on function, *Circ Res* 90(4):380–389, 2002.
10. Melov S: Therapeutics against mitochondrial oxidative stress in animal models of aging, *Ann N Y Acad Sci* 959:330–340, 2002.
11. Golden TR, Melov S: Mitochondrial DNA mutations, oxidative stress, and aging, *Mech Ageing Dev* 122(14):1577–1589, 2001.
12. Kelso GF et al: Selective targeting of a redox-active ubiquinone to mitochondria with cells: antioxidant and antiapoptotic properties, *J Biol Chem* 276(7):4588–4596, 2001.
13. Lee HC, Wei YH: Mitochondrial alterations, cellular response to oxidative stress and defective degradation of proteins in aging, *Biogerontology* 2(4):231–244, 2001.
14. Lenaz G et al: Role of mitochondria in oxidative stress and aging, *Ann N Y Acad Sci* 959:199–213, 2002.
15. Costa LG et al: Developmental neuropathy of environmental agents, *Annu Rev Pharmacol Toxicol* 44:87–110, 2004.
16. Marshall L et al: Identifying and managing adverse environmental health effects. 1. Taking an exposure history, *CMAJ* 166(8):1049–1055, 2002.
17. Weir E: Identifying and managing adverse environmental health effects: a new series, *Can Med Assoc J* 166 (8):1041–1043, 2002.
18. Hines LM et al: Alcoholism: the dissection for endophenotypes, *Dialogues Clin Neurosci* 7(2):153–163, 2005.
19. Agarwal DP: Cardioprotective effects of light-moderate consumption of alcohol: a review of putative mechanisms, *Alcohol Alcohol* 37(5):409–415, 2002.
20. Molina PE et al: Mechanisms of alcohol-induced tissue injury, *Alcohol Clin Exp Res* 27(3):563–575, 2003.
21. Cotran RS, Kumar V, Collins T: *Robbins' pathologic basis of disease*, ed 6, Philadelphia, 1999, Saunders.
22. Jaeschke H et al: Mechanisms of hepatotoxicity, *Toxicol Sci* 65(2):166–176, 2002.
23. Kurose I et al: CD18/ICAM-1-dependent nitric oxide production of Kupffer cells as a cause of mitochondrial dysfunction in hepatoma cells: influence of chronic alcohol feeding, *Free Radic Biol Med* 22(1–2):229–239, 1997.
24. Traviss KA et al: Lifestyle-related weight gain in obese men with newly diagnosed obstructive sleep apnea, *J Am Diet Assoc* 102(5):703–706, 2002.
25. Young T, Peppard PE, Gottlieb DJ: Epidemiology of obstructive sleep apnea: a population health perspective, *Am J Respir Crit Care Med* 165(9):1217–1239, 2002.
26. Leiber CS: Metabolism of alcohol, *Clin Liver Dis* 9(1):1–35, 2005.
27. Centers for Disease Control and Prevention, National Center for Injury Prevention and Control Injury statistics website, http://webapp.cdc.gov/sasweb/ncipc/mortrate10.html Washington, DC, 2006, CDC.
27a. Kopec D et al: The state of the art in the reduction of medical errors, *Stud Health Technol Inform* 121:126–137, 2006.
28. Levin ST: Apoptosis, necrosis or oncosis: what is your diagnosis? A report from the Cell Death Nomenclature Committee of the Society of Toxicologic Pathologists, *Toxicol Sci* 41(2):155–156, 1998.
29. Kern JC, Kehrer JP: Acrolein-induced cell death: a caspase-influenced decision between apoptosis and oncosis/necrosis, *Chem Biol Interact* 139(1):79–95, 2002.
30. Majno G, Joris I: Apoptosis, oncosis, and necrosis: an overview of cell death, *Am J Pathol* 146(1):3–15, 1995.
31. Mills EM et al: Regulation of cellular oncosis by uncoupling protein 2, *J Biol Chem* 2002.
32. Eaton JW, Qian M: Molecular bases of cellular iron toxicity (1,2), *Free Radic Biol Med* 32(9):833–840, 2002.
33. Philpott CC: Molecular aspects of iron absorption: insights into the role of HFE in hemochromatosis, *Hepatology* 35 (5):993–1001, 2002.
34. Raloff J: Coming to terms with death: accurate descriptions of a cell's demise may offer clues to diseases and treatments, *Sci News* 159:378–380, 2001.
35. D'Mello SR: Molecular regulation of neuronal apoptosis, *Curr Top Dev Biol* 39:187–213, 1998.
36. Zakeri Z, Lockshin RA: Cell death during development, *J Immunol Methods* 265(1–2):3–20, 2002.
37. Garland JM, Sondergaard KL, Jolly J: Redox regulation of apoptosis in interleukin-3-dependent haemopoietic cells, *Br J Haematol* 99(4):756–765, 1997.
38. al-Rubeai M: Apoptosis and cell culture technology, *Adv Biochem Eng Biotechnol* 59:225–249, 1998.
39. Raff MC: Social controls on cell survival and cell death, *Nature* 356(6368):397–401, 1992.
40. Chow SC, Kass CE, Orrenius S: Purines and their roles in apoptosis, *Neuropharmacology* 36(9):1149–1156, 1997.
41. In: Johnson HA, editor: *Is aging physiological or pathological? In relations between normal aging and disease* New York, 1985, Raven.
42. National Center for Health Statistics: Health, United States, *NVSR* 53(15):.
43. Chang E et al: Aging and survival of the cutaneous microvasculature, *J Invest Dermatol* 118(5):752–758, 2002.
44. Fossel M: Cell senescence in human aging and disease, *Ann N Y Acad Sci* 959:14–23, 2002.
45. Shringarpure R, Davies KJ: Protein turnover by the proteasome in aging and disease, *Free Radic Biol Med* 32 (11):1084–1089, 2002.
46. Riley MW: Foreword: the gender paradox, In: MG Ory MG and HR Warner HR, editors. *Gender, health, and longevity: multidisciplinary perspectives*, New York, 1990, Springer.
47. Hayflick L: The limited in vitro lifetime of human diploid cell strains, *Exp Cell Res* 37:614, 1965.
48. Melov S: Mitochondrial oxidative stress: physiologic consequences and potential for a role in aging, *Ann N Y Acad Sci* 908:219–225, 2000.
49. Czarnecka AM, Golik P, Bartnik E: Mitochondrial DNA mutations in human neoplasia, *J Appl Genet* 47(1):67–78, 2006.
50. Sharpless NE, DePinho RA: Telomeres, stem cells, senescence, and cancer, *J Clin Invest* 113:160–168, 2004.
51. O'Connor KG et al: Serum levels of insulin-like growth factor-I are related to age and not to body composition in healthy women and men, *J Gerontol A Biol Sci Med Sci* 53 (3):M176–M182, 1998.
52. Joseph C et al: Role of endocrine-immune dysregulation in osteoporosis, sarcopenia, frailty, and fracture risk, *Molec Aspects Med* 26(3):181–201, 2005.
53. Capopola AR et al: Insulin-like growth factor I ad interleukin-6 contribute synergistically to disability and mortality in older women, *J Clin Endocrinol Metab* 88:2019–2025, 2003.
54. Roubenoff R et al: Cytokines, insulin-like growth factor 1, sarcopenia, and mortality in very old community-dwelling men and women: the Framingham Heart Study, *Am J Med* 1156:429–435, 2003.

References—Cont'd

55. Lambert KC et al: Estrogen receptor-alpha deficiency promotes increased TNF-alpha secretion and bacterial killing by murine macrophages in response to microbial stimuli in vitro, *J Leukoc Biol* 75(6):1166–1172, 2004.
56. Yang SX, Kuchel GA: Estrogen, cerebrovascular system and dementia, In: RH Paul RH, RA Cohen RA, and BR Ott BR, editors. *Vascular dementia: cerebrovascular mechanisms and clinical management*, Totowa, NJ, 2004, Humana Press.
57. Shennan T: *Postmortems and morbid anatomy*, ed 3, Baltimore, 1935, William Wood.
58. Minckler J, Anstall HB, Minckler TM: *Pathobiology: an introduction*, St Louis, 1971, Mosby.

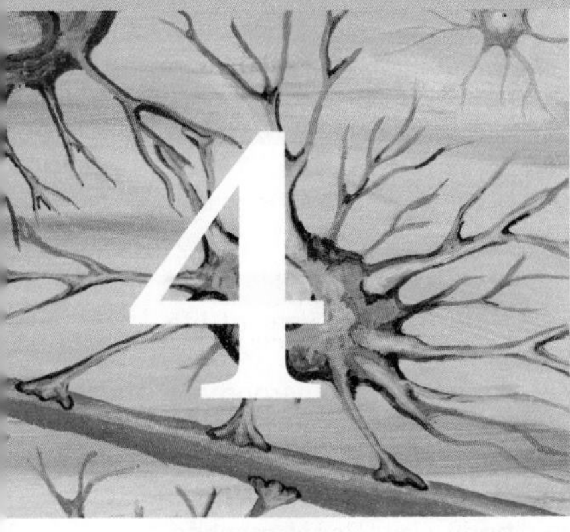

4 FLUIDS AND ELECTROLYTES, ACIDS AND BASES

Sue E. Huether

CHAPTER OUTLINE

ELECTRONIC RESOURCES

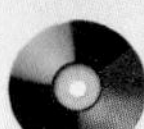

Companion CD
- Review Questions and Answers
- Animations

evolve Website
http://evolve.elsevier.com/Huether/
- Quick Check Answers
- Key Terms Exercises
- Critical Thinking Questions with Answers
- Algorithm Completion Exercises
- WebLinks

The cells of the body live in a fluid environment with an electrolyte and acid-base concentration maintained within a narrow range. Changes in electrolyte concentration affect the electrical activity of nerve and muscle cells and cause shifts of fluid from one compartment to another. Alterations in acid-base balance disrupt cellular functions. Fluid fluctuations also affect blood volume and cellular function. Disturbances in these functions are common and can be life threatening. Understanding how alterations occur and how the body compensates or corrects the disturbance is important for understanding many pathophysiologic conditions.

DISTRIBUTION OF BODY FLUIDS

The sum of fluids within all body compartments constitutes **total body water (TBW)**—about 60% of body weight (Table 4-1). The volume of TBW is usually expressed as a percentage of body weight in kilograms. One liter of water weighs 2.2 lb (1 kg). The rest of the body weight is made up of fat and fat-free solids, particularly bone.

Body fluids are distributed among functional compartments, or spaces, and provide a transport medium for cellular and tissue function. **Intracellular fluid (ICF)** comprises all the fluid within cells, about two thirds of TBW. **Extracellular fluid (ECF)** is all the fluid outside the cells (about one third of TBW) and is divided into smaller compartments. The two main ECF compartments are the **interstitial fluid** (the space between cells and outside the blood vessels) and the **intravascular fluid** (blood plasma) (Table 4-2). The total volume of body water for a 70-kg person is about 42 liters. Other ECF compartments include lymph and transcellular fluids, such as synovial, intestinal, and cerebrospinal fluid; sweat; urine; and pleural, peritoneal, pericardial, and intraocular fluids.

Although the amount of fluid within the various compartments is relatively constant, solutes (i.e., salts) and water are exchanged between compartments to maintain their unique compositions. The percentage of TBW varies with the amount of body fat and age. Because fat is water repelling (hydrophobic), very little water is contained in adipose (fat) cells. Individuals with more body fat have proportionately less TBW and tend to be more susceptible to dehydration.

Maturation and the Distribution of Body Fluids

The distribution and the amount of TBW change with age (see the *Pediatric* and *Aging* boxes), and although daily fluid intake may fluctuate widely, the body regulates water volume within a relatively narrow range. The primary sources of body water are drinking, ingestion of water in food, and water derived from oxidative metabolism. Normally, the largest amounts of water are lost through renal excretion, with lesser amounts lost through the stool and through vaporization from the skin and lungs (insensible water loss) (Table 4-3).

TABLE 4-1

Total Body Water (%) in Relation to Body Weight

Body Build	Adult Male	Adult Female	Infant
Normal	60	50	70
Lean	70	60	80
Obese	50	42	60

Note: Total body water is a percentage of body weight.

TABLE 4-2

Distribution of Body Water

Fluid Compartment	Percentage of Body Weight	Volume (L)
Intracellular fluid (ICF)	40	28
Extracellular fluid (ECF)	20	14
Interstitial	(15)	(11)
Intravascular	(5)	(3)
Total body water (TBW)	60	42

TABLE 4-3

Normal Water Gains and Losses (70-kg Man)

Daily Intake (ml)		Daily Output (ml)	
Drinking	1400–1800	Urine	1400–1800
Water in food	700–1000	Stool	100
Water of oxidation	300–400	Skin	300–500
		Lungs	600–800
Total	2400–3200	Total	2400–3200

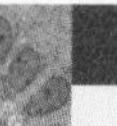

PEDIATRICS & Distribution of Body Fluids

Newborn Infants

At birth, TBW represents about 75% to 80% of body weight and decreases to about 67% during the first year of life. Physiologic loss of body water amounting to 5% of body weight occurs as an infant adjusts to a new environment. Infants are particularly susceptible to significant changes in TBW because of a high metabolic rate and greater body surface area. Consequently, they have a greater fluid intake and output in relation to their body size. Renal mechanisms of fluid and electrolyte conservation may not be mature enough to counter abnormal losses related to vomiting or diarrhea, thereby allowing dehydration to occur. Symptoms of dehydration include thirst, decreased urine output, decreased body weight, decreased skin elasticity, sunken fontanels, absent tears, dry mucous membranes, increased heart rate, and irritability.

Children and Adolescents

TBW slowly decreases to 60% to 65% of body weight. At adolescence, the percentage of TBW approaches adult levels and differences according to gender appear. Males have a greater percentage of body water because of increased muscle mass, and females have more body fat because of the influence of estrogen and thus less water.

AGING & Distribution of Body Fluids

The further decline in the percentage of TBW in the elderly is in part the result of a decreased free fat mass and decreased muscle, as well as reduced ability to regulate sodium and water balance. Kidneys are less efficient in producing concentrated urine, and sodium-conserving responses are sluggish. Thirst perception also may decline and loss of cognitive function can influence access to beverages. Healthy older adults can adequately maintain their hydration status. When disease is present, a decrease in TBW and dehydration can become life threatening.

Data from Bossingham MJ, Carnell NS, Campbell WW: Water balance, hydration status, and fat-free mass hydration in younger and older adults, *Am J Clin Nutr* 81(6):1342–1350, 2005; Luckey AE, Parsa CJ: Fluid and electrolytes in the aged, *Arch Surg* 138 (10):1055–1060, 2003.

Water Movement Between Plasma and Interstitial Fluid

The distribution of water and the movement of nutrients and waste products between the capillary and interstitial spaces occur as a result of changes in hydrostatic pressure (pushes water) and osmotic (oncotic) pressure (pulls water) at the arterial and venous ends of the capillary. Because water, sodium, and glucose readily move across the capillary membrane, plasma proteins (particularly albumin) maintain effective osmolality by generating plasma oncotic pressure.

As plasma flows from the arterial to the venous end of the capillary, four forces determine if fluid moves out of the capillary and into the interstitial space (filtration) or if fluid moves back into the capillary from the interstitial space (reabsorption):

1. **Capillary hydrostatic pressure (blood pressure)** facilitates the outward movement of water from the capillary to the interstitial space.
2. **Capillary oncotic pressure** osmotically attracts water from the interstitial space back into the capillary.
3. **Interstitial hydrostatic pressure** facilitates the inward movement of water from the interstitial space into the capillary.
4. **Interstitial oncotic pressure** osmotically attracts water from the capillary into the interstitial space.

The movement of fluid back and forth across the capillary wall is called **net filtration** and is best described as **Starling's forces:**

Net filtration =
(Forces favoring filtration) − (Forces opposing filtration)

Forces favoring filtration =
Capillary hydrostatic pressure and interstitial oncotic pressure

Forces opposing filtration =
Capillary oncotic pressure and interstitial hydrostatic pressure

At the arterial end of the capillary, hydrostatic pressure exceeds capillary oncotic pressure and fluid moves into the interstitial space (filtration). At the venous end of the capillary, capillary oncotic pressure exceeds capillary hydrostatic pressure and fluids are attracted back into the circulation (reabsorption). Interstitial hydrostatic pressure promotes the movement of about 10% of the interstitial fluid along with small amounts of protein into the lymphatics, which then returns to the circulation. Because albumin does not normally cross the capillary membrane, interstitial oncotic pressure is normally minimal. Figure 4-1 illustrates net filtration.

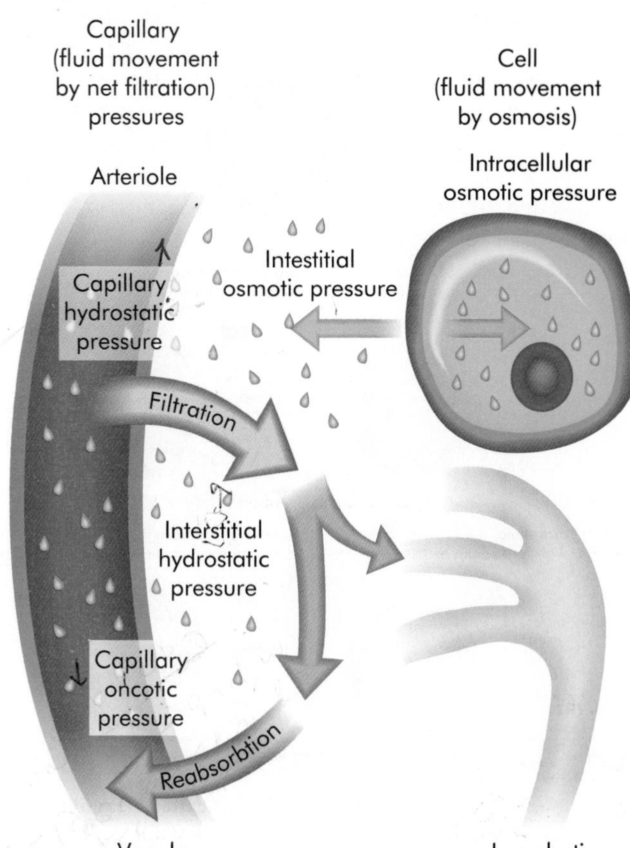

Figure 4-1 ■ Fluid Movement Between Plasma and Interstitial Space. The movement of fluid between the vascular, interstitial spaces, and the lymphatics is the result of net filtration of fluid across the semipermeable capillary membrane. *Capillary hydrostatic pressure* is the primary force for fluid movement out of the arteriolar end of the capillary and into the interstitial space. At the venous end, *capillary oncotic pressure* (from plasma proteins) attracts water back into the vascular space. *Interstitial hydrostatic pressure* promotes the movement of fluid and proteins in to the lymphatics. *Osmotic pressure* accounts for the movement of fluid between the interstitial space and the intracellular space. Normally intracellular and extracellular fluid osmotic pressures are equal (280 to 294 mOsm) and water is equally distributed between the interstitial and intracellular compartments.

Water Movement Between ICF and ECF

Water moves between ICF and ECF compartments primarily as a function of osmotic forces (see Chapter 1, for definitions). Sodium is responsible for the ECF osmotic balance, and potassium maintains the ICF osmotic balance. The osmotic force of ICF proteins and other nondiffusible substances is balanced by the active transport of ions out of the cell. Water crosses cell membranes freely, so the osmolality of TBW is normally at equilibrium. Normally the ICF is not subject to rapid changes in osmolality, but when ECF osmolality changes, water moves from one compartment to another until osmotic equilibrium is reestablished. Examples of the maintenance of osmotic equilibrium are illustrated in Figure 4-2.

ALTERATIONS IN WATER MOVEMENT

Edema

Edema is the excessive accumulation of fluid within the interstitial spaces. The forces favoring fluid movement from the capillaries or lymphatic channels into the tissues are increased capillary hydrostatic pressure, lowered plasma oncotic pressure, increased capillary membrane permeability, and lymphatic channel obstruction[1] (Figure 4-3).

PATHOPHYSIOLOGY Hydrostatic pressure increases as a result of venous obstruction or salt and water retention. Venous obstruction causes hydrostatic pressure to increase behind the obstruction pushing fluid from the capillaries into the interstitial spaces. Thrombophlebitis (inflammation of veins), hepatic obstruction, tight clothing around the extremities, and prolonged standing are common causes of venous obstruction. Congestive heart failure and renal failure are associated with salt and water retention,

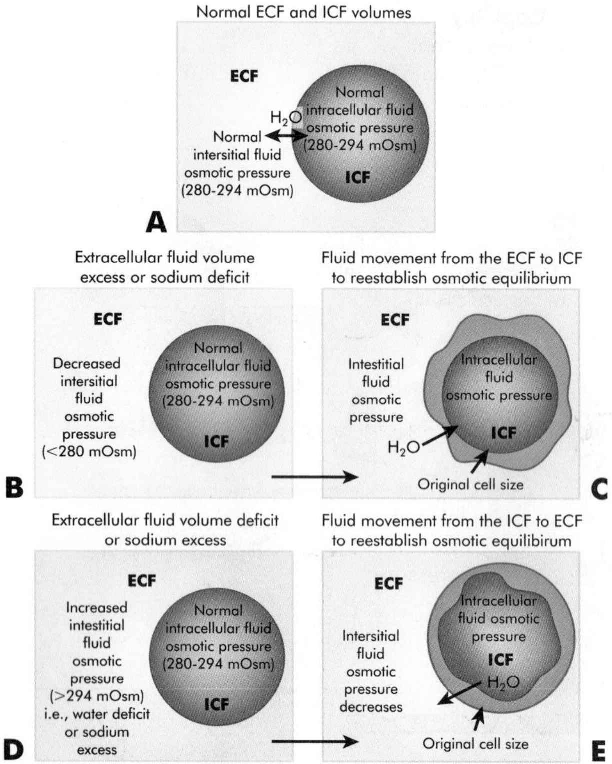

Figure 4-2 ■ Examples of Changes in Osmotic Equilibrium Between ECF and ICF. A, Normal ECF and ICF volumes. Intracellular and extracellular fluid osmotic pressures are equal and water is equally distributed between the compartments. **B,** Extracellular fluid volume excess or sodium deficit. ECF volume excess or sodium deficit decreases the ECF osmotic pressure and water is attracted to the ICF space (see *C*). **C,** Fluid movement from the ECF to ICF to reestablish osmotic equilibrium. The intracellular osmotic pressure attracts water from the ECF causing an increase in ICF water volume with a balancing of osmotic forces between the ECF and ICF. The consequence is an increase in ICF volume and cell swelling. **D,** Extracellular fluid volume deficit or sodium excess. ECF volume deficit increases the ECF osmotic pressure and intracellular water is attracted to the ECF space (see *E*). **E,** Fluid movement from the ICF to the ECF to reestablish osmotic equilibrium. Water from the intracellular space has moved to the extracellular space until the osmotic forces are equal. The consequence is a decrease in ICF water volume and cell size. *ICF,* Intracellular fluid; *ECF,* extracellular fluid.

which cause plasma volume overload, increased capillary hydrostatic pressure, and edema.

Lost or diminished plasma albumin production (liver disease or protein malnutrition) contributes to decreased plasma oncotic pressure. Plasma proteins are lost in glomerular diseases of the kidney, serous drainage from open wounds, hemorrhage, burns, and cirrhosis of the liver. The decreased oncotic attraction of fluid within the capillary causes filtered capillary fluid to remain in the interstitial space, resulting in edema.

Capillaries become more permeable with inflammation and immune responses, especially with trauma such as burns or crushing injuries, neoplastic disease, and allergic reactions. Proteins escape from the vascular space and produce edema through decreased capillary oncotic pressure and interstitial fluid protein accumulation.

The lymphatic system normally absorbs interstitial fluid and a small amount of proteins. When lymphatic channels are blocked or surgically removed, proteins and fluid accumulate in the interstitial space causing **lymphedema.**[2] For example, lymphedema of the arm or leg occurs after surgical removal of axillary and femoral lymph nodes for treatment of carcinoma. Inflammation or tumors may cause lymphatic obstruction, leading to edema of the involved tissues.

CLINICAL MANIFESTATIONS Edema may be localized or generalized. *Localized edema* is usually limited to a site of trauma, as in a sprained finger. Another kind of localized edema occurs within particular organ systems and includes cerebral edema, pulmonary edema, pleural effusion (fluid accumulation in the pleural space), pericardial effusion (fluid accumulation within the membrane around the heart), and ascites (accumulation of fluid in the peritoneal space). *Generalized edema* is manifested by a more uniform distribution of fluid in interstitial spaces. Dependent edema, in which fluid accumulates in gravity-dependent areas of the body, might signal more generalized edema. Dependent edema appears in the feet and legs when standing and in the sacral area and buttocks when supine (face up). It can be identified by pressing on tissues overlying bony prominences. A pit left in the skin indicates edema (hence the term *pitting edema*).

Edema usually is associated with weight gain, swelling and puffiness, tight-fitting clothes and shoes, limited movement of affected joints, and symptoms associated with the underlying pathologic condition. Fluid accumulations increase the distance required for nutrients and waste products to move between capillaries and tissues. Blood flow may be impaired also. Therefore, wounds heal more slowly, and with prolonged edema, the risks of infection and pressure sores over bony prominences increase. Edema of specific organs, such as the brain, lung, or larynx, can be life threatening.

As edematous fluid accumulates, it is trapped in a "third space" (i.e., the interstitial space, pleural space, pericardial space) and is unavailable for metabolic processes. Dehydration can develop as a result of this sequestering. Such sequestration occurs with severe burns, where large amounts of vascular fluid are lost to the interstitial spaces, reducing plasma volume and causing shock (see Chapter 23).

✓ QUICK CHECK 4-1

1. How does an increase in capillary hydrostatic pressure cause edema?
2. How does a decrease in capillary oncotic pressure cause edema?

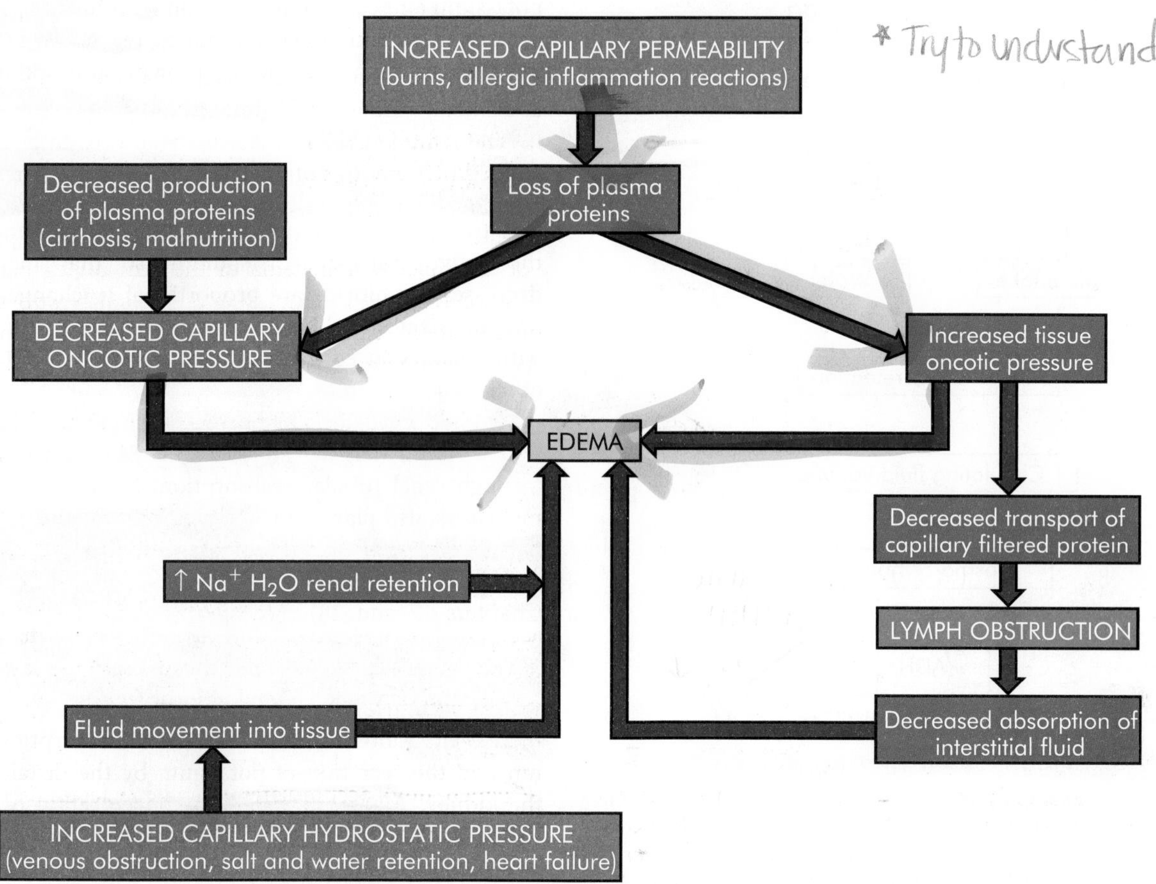

Figure 4-3 ■ **Mechanisms of Edema Formation.** *Na^+*, sodium; *H_2O*, water.

SODIUM, CHLORIDE, AND WATER BALANCE

The kidneys and hormones have a central role in maintaining sodium and water balance. Because water follows the osmotic gradients established by changes in salt concentration, sodium and water balance are intimately related. Water balance is regulated primarily by antidiuretic hormone (ADH; also known as *vasopressin*); sodium is regulated by renal effects of aldosterone (see p. 104).

Water Balance

Water balance is regulated by the secretion of ADH. ADH is secreted when plasma osmolality increases or circulating blood volume decreases and blood pressure drops. Increased plasma osmolality occurs with water deficit or sodium excess in relation to water (see Figure 4-2, *D*). The increased osmolality stimulates hypothalamic **osmoreceptors**. In addition to causing thirst, these osmoreceptors signal the posterior pituitary gland to release ADH. Thirst stimulates water drinking and ADH increases the permeability of renal tubular cells to water. Water is then reabsorbed into the plasma from the distal tubules and collecting ducts of the kidney (see Chapter 28). Urine concentration increases, and the reabsorbed water decreases plasma osmolality, returning it toward normal (see Figure 4-2, *E*).

With fluid loss (dehydration) from vomiting, diarrhea, or excessive sweating, a decrease in blood volume and blood pressure often occurs. **Volume-sensitive receptors** and **baroreceptors** (nerve endings that are sensitive to changes in volume and pressure) also stimulate the release of ADH from the pituitary gland. The volume receptors are located in the right and left atria and thoracic vessels; baroreceptors are found in the aorta, pulmonary arteries, and carotid sinus. ADH secretion also occurs when atrial pressure drops, as occurs with decreased blood volume. The reabsorption of water mediated by ADH then promotes the restoration of plasma volume and blood pressure (Figure 4-4).

Sodium and Chloride Balance

Sodium (Na^+) accounts for 90% of the ECF cations (positively charged ions). (The distribution of electrolytes in body compartments is summarized in Table 4-4.) Along

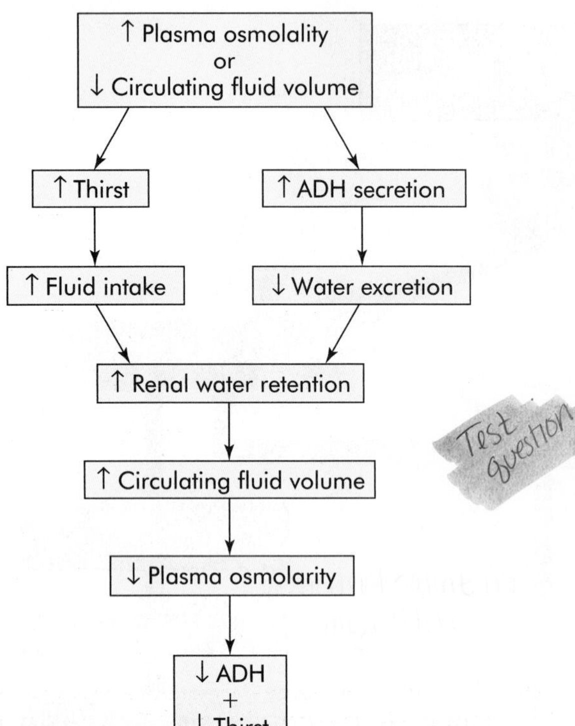

Figure 4-4 ■ **The Antidiuretic Hormone (ADH) System.**

TABLE 4-4

Representative Distribution of Electrolytes in Body Compartments

Electrolytes	ECF (mEq/L)	ICF (mEq/L)
CATIONS		
Sodium	142	12
Potassium	4.2	150
Calcium^{++}	5	0
Magnesium^{++}	2	24
Totals	153	186
ANIONS		
Bicarbonate	24	12
Chloride	103	4
Phosphate	2	100
Proteins	16	65
Other anions	8	6
Totals	153	186

ECF, Extracellular fluid; *ICF,* intracellular fluid.

with its constituent anions (negatively charged ions) chloride and bicarbonate, sodium regulates extracellular osmotic forces and therefore regulates water balance. Sodium is important in other functions, including working with potassium and calcium to maintain neuromuscular irritability for conduction of nerve impulses, regulation of acid-base balance (through sodium bicarbonate and sodium phosphate), participation in cellular chemical reactions, and membrane transport.

Chloride (Cl^-) is the major anion in the ECF and provides electroneutrality, particularly in relation to sodium. The transport of chloride is generally passive and follows the active transport of sodium, so that increases or decreases in chloride are proportional to changes in sodium. The concentration of chloride tends to vary inversely with changes in concentration of bicarbonate (HCO_3^-), the other major anion.

The kidney maintains normal serum sodium concentration within a narrow range (136 to 145 mEq/L) primarily through renal tubular reabsorption. Neural and hormonal mediators also play a role. Hormonal regulation of sodium balance is mediated by **aldosterone,** a mineralocorticoid synthesized and secreted from the adrenal cortex (see Chapters 17 and 28). Aldosterone secretion is influenced by both circulating blood volume and plasma concentrations of sodium and potassium (aldosterone is secreted when sodium levels are depressed or potassium levels are increased). Aldosterone increases the reabsorption of sodium and the secretion of potassium by the distal tubule of the kidney. As a result, sodium concentration of the ECF is enhanced, and potassium is excreted with the urine.

When circulating blood volume and blood pressure are reduced, **renin,** an enzyme secreted by the juxtaglomerular cells of the kidney, is released. Renin stimulates the formation of **angiotensin I,** an inactive polypeptide. Angiotensin-converting enzyme (ACE) in pulmonary vessels converts angiotensin I to angiotensin II, which stimulates the secretion of aldosterone and also causes vasoconstriction. The aldosterone then promotes sodium and water reabsorption, increasing blood volume (Figure 4-5). Vasoconstriction elevates the systemic blood pressure and restores renal perfusion (blood flow). This restoration inhibits the further release of renin. This complete mechanism is known as the **renin-angiotensin-aldosterone system** (see Chapter 28).

Natriuretic hormones (peptides) promote urinary excretion of sodium and water and decreases blood pressure. Atrial natriuretic hormone is produced by the atrial muscle of the heart and functions in renal elimination of sodium to control sodium and water balance. Natriuretic hormone is sometimes called the "third factor" in sodium regulation, after increased glomerular filtration rate and aldosterone.[3] Its effect is apparent when there is prolonged aldosterone elevation from chronic retention of fluid or excessive secretion from an adrenal tumor. The sodium-retaining action of aldosterone is overcome by the action of natriuretic hormone, and salt is excreted, followed by a water diuresis (Figure 4-6). Natriuretic hormones can also decrease concentrations of plasma renin-aldosterone and reduce blood pressure.[4]

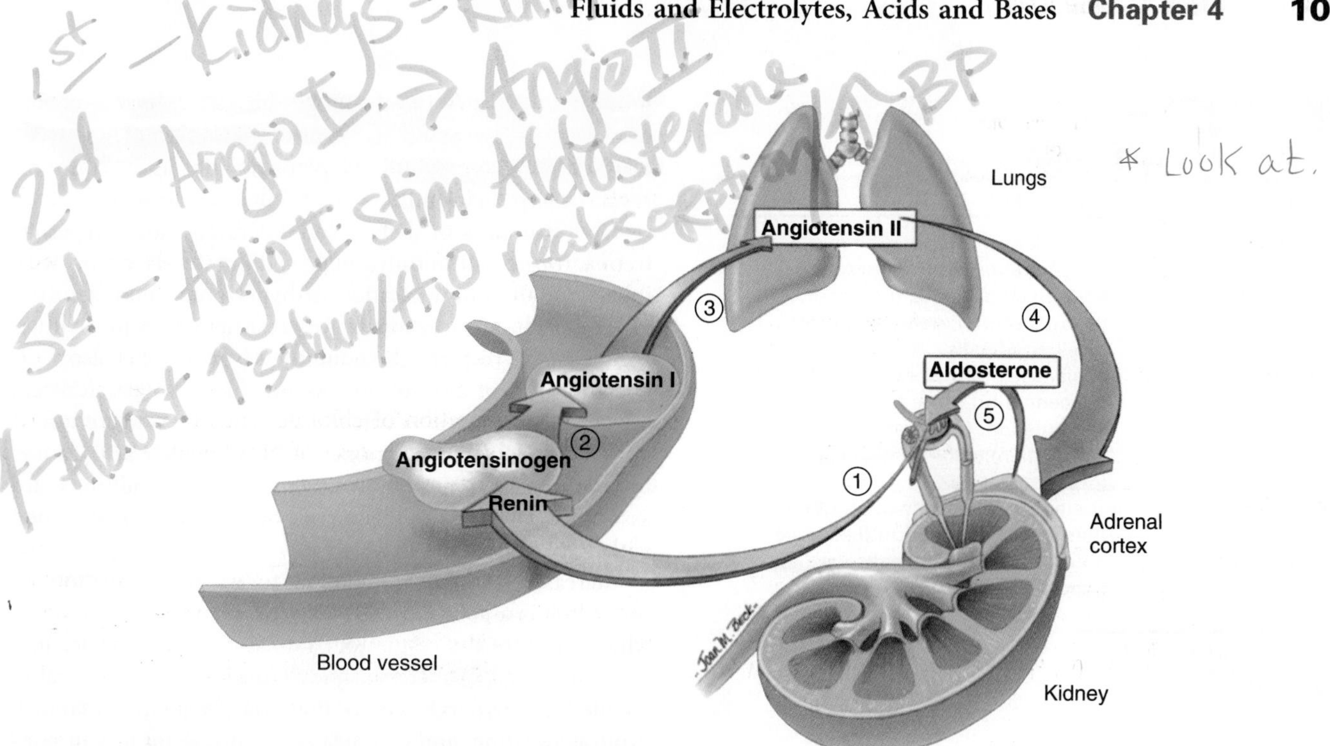

Figure 4-5 ■ **The Renin-Angiotensin-Aldosterone System. (1)** Renal juxtaglomerular cells sense decrease in blood pressure and release renin; **(2)** Renin activates angiotensinogen to angiotensin I; **(3)** Angiotensin I is converted to angiotensin II via angiotensin-converting enzyme (ACE) in the lung; **(4)** Angiotensin II promotes vasoconstriction and stimulates aldosterone secretion from the adrenal cortex resulting in renal sodium and water retention and an increase in blood pressure. (From Thibodeau GA, Patton KT: *Anatomy & physiology,* ed 6, St Louis, 2007, Mosby.)

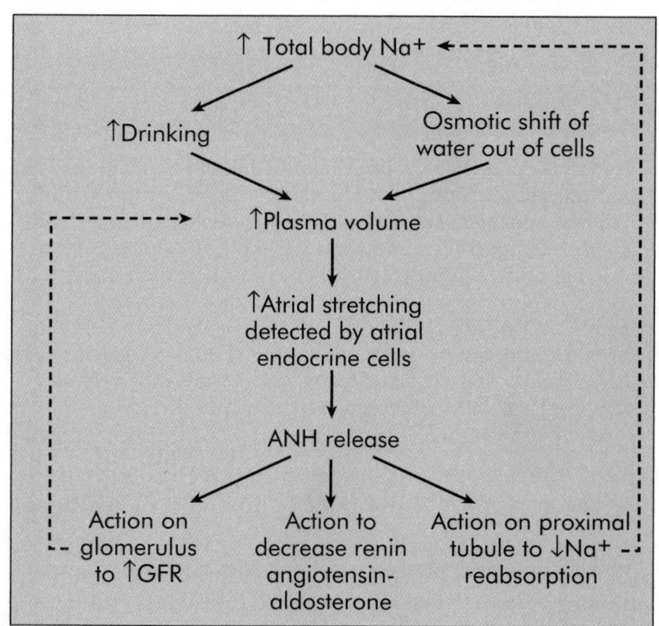

Figure 4-6 ■ **The Atrial Natriuretic Hormone (ANH) System.** *Na^+,* sodium; *GFR,* glomerular filtration rate. (From Thibodeau GA, Patton KT: *Anatomy & physiology,* ed 5, St Louis, 2003, Mosby.)

✓ QUICK CHECK 4-2

1. What forces promote net filtration?
2. What hormones regulate salt and water balance?

ALTERATIONS IN SODIUM, CHLORIDE, AND WATER BALANCE

Alterations in sodium and water balance are closely related.[5] Water imbalances may develop with gains or losses of salt. Likewise, sodium imbalances occur with alterations in body water volume. Generally, these alterations can be classified as changes in tonicity—the change in the concentration of solutes with relation to water (see Chapter 1). Alterations can therefore be classified as isotonic, hypertonic, or hypotonic (Table 4-5).

Isotonic Alterations

Isotonic alterations occur when TBW changes are accompanied by proportional changes in electrolytes (osmolality remains within normal range [280 mOsm to 294 mOsm]). For example, if an individual loses pure plasma or ECF, fluid volume is depleted but the concentration and type of electrolytes and the osmolality remain in the normal range. Excessive amounts of isotonic body fluids can result from excessive administration of intravenous normal saline or oversecretion of aldosterone with renal retention of both sodium and water. Losses of isotonic body fluids include hemorrhage, severe wound drainage, and excessive diaphoresis (sweating).

Isotonic fluid loss (isotonic dehydration) causes contraction of the ECF volume with weight loss, dryness of skin and mucous membranes, decreased urine output, and

TABLE 4-5
Water and Solute Imbalances

Tonicity	Mechanism
Isotonic (isoosmolar) imbalance	Gain or loss of ECF resulting in a concentration equivalent to a 0.9% sodium chloride (salt) solution (normal saline); no shrinking or swelling of cells
Hypertonic (hyperosmolar) imbalance	Imbalances that result in an ECF concentration more than 0.9% salt solution, (i.e., water loss or solute gain); cells shrink in a hypertonic fluid
Hypotonic (hypoosmolar) imbalance	Imbalance that results in an ECF less than 0.9% salt solution (i.e., water gain or solute loss); cells swell in a hypotonic fluid

ECF, Extracellular fluid.

symptoms of hypovolemia. Indicators of hypovolemia include a rapid heart rate, flattened neck veins, and normal or decreased blood pressure. In severe states, hypovolemic shock can occur (see Chapter 23).

Isotonic fluid excesses are most commonly the result of excessive administration of intravenous fluids, hypersecretion of aldosterone, or the effects of drugs such as cortisone (which causes renal reabsorption of sodium and water). As plasma volume expands, hypervolemia develops with weight gain. The diluting effect of excess plasma volume leads to decreased hematocrit and decreased plasma protein concentration. The neck veins may distend, and the blood pressure increases. Increased capillary hydrostatic pressure leads to edema formation. Ultimately, pulmonary edema and heart failure may develop.

Hypertonic Alterations

Hypertonic fluid alterations develop when the osmolality of the ECF is elevated above normal (greater than 294 mOsm). The most common causes are increased concentration of ECF sodium (hypernatremia) or deficit of ECF water. In both instances, ECF hypertonicity attracts water from the intracellular space, causing ICF dehydration (see Figure 4-2, *D-E*). A primary increase in ECF sodium causes an osmotic attraction of water and symptoms of hypervolemia. In contrast, a hypertonic state caused primarily by water loss leads to hypovolemia (Table 4-6).

Hypernatremia

PATHOPHYSIOLOGY **Hypernatremia** occurs when serum sodium levels exceed 147 mEq/L. Increased serum sodium may be caused by an acute gain in sodium or a net loss of water.[6] Because sodium is largely in the ECF, sodium gains cause intracellular dehydration. The movement of water to the ECF may cause hypervolemia, or with an accompanying water loss, both ICF and ECF dehydration may occur. Hyperosmolality is a common result of hypernatremia.

High amounts of dietary sodium rarely cause hypernatremia. More commonly, high sodium levels occur with inappropriate administration of hypertonic saline solution (e.g., as sodium bicarbonate for treatment of acidosis during cardiac arrest). High sodium levels can occur also with oversecretion of aldosterone, as in primary hyperaldosteronism or Cushing syndrome caused by excess secretion of adrenocorticotropic hormone (ACTH), which also causes increased secretion of aldosterone. These conditions are associated with hypervolemia as some water is reabsorbed with sodium.

Increased sodium in relation to water deprivation or water loss is associated with fever or respiratory infections, which increase the respiratory rate and enhance water loss from the lungs. Diabetes insipidus (decreased ADH), diabetes mellitus (hyperglycemia), polyuria (frequent urination), profuse sweating, and diarrhea also cause water loss in relation to sodium. Infants with severe diarrhea are particularly vulnerable. Insufficient water intake can cause hypernatremia, particularly in individuals who are comatose, confused, or immobilized; these conditions are also associated with hypovolemia.

HEALTH ALERT
Breastfeeding and Hypernatremia

Hypernatremic dehydration (serum sodium >150 mEq/L) is an uncommon but serious complication of breastfed infants. At risk are babies older than 48 hours who have lost greater than 10% of body weight and have not regained original birthweight by day 10. The most common presenting symptom is nonhemolytic jaundice. Nonmetabolic symptoms include apnea or bradycardia or both. Higher breast milk sodium levels also are found. Babies with significant weight loss require increased efforts and maternal support to establish successful breastfeeding.

Data from Moritz ML et al: Breastfeeding-associated hypernatremia: are we missing the diagnosis? *Pediatrics* 116(3): e343-e347, 2005; Tarcan A et al: Weight loss and hypernatremia in breast-fed babies: frequency in neonates with non-hemolytic jaundice, *J Paediatr Child Health* 41(9–10):484–487, 2005; Shroff R et al: Life-threatening hypernatraemic dehydration in breastfed babies, *Arch Dis Child* 91(12):1025–6, 2006.

CLINICAL MANIFESTATIONS Water is redistributed to the extracellular space, and intracellular dehydration ensues. Thirst, fever, dry mucous membranes, and restlessness are associated with hypernatremia as a result of water loss. Central nervous system symptoms include muscle twitching and hyperreflexia (hyperactive reflexes). Convulsions are the most serious symptoms.

TABLE 4-6

Causes and Consequences of Hypertonic Imbalances

Causative Factor	Mechanism	Extracellular Fluid Effects	Intracellular Effects
Increased sodium (hypernatremia)	Excessive intake	Hypervolemia	Intracellular dehydration
	Intravenous hypertonic sodium	Weight gain	Thirst
	Saline-induced abortions	Bounding pulse	Fever
	Selected infant formulas	Increased blood pressure	Decreased urine output
	Decreased sodium loss	Edema	Shrinkage of brain cells
	Hyperaldosteronism	Venous distention	Confusion
	Cushing syndrome	Neuromuscular symptoms	Coma
	Renal failure	Muscle weakness	Cerebral hemorrhage
	Congestive heart failure	Seizures	
Water deficit	Water deprivation	Hypovolemia	Intracellular dehydration
	Confusion or coma	Weight loss	See above
	Inability to communicate	Weak pulses	
	Loss of thirst	Postural hypotension	
	Inability to swallow	Tachycardia	
	Water loss		
	Watery diarrhea		
	Diabetes insipidus (↓ ADH)		
	Excessive diuresis		
	Excessive diaphoresis		
Other factors	Hyperglycemia	Initial dilutional hyponatremia	Intracellular dehydration
		Polyuria	See above
		Polydipsia	
		Weight loss	
		Hypovolemia	
		Late hypernatremia	

Water Deficit

PATHOPHYSIOLOGY **Dehydration** describes water deficit but also is commonly used to indicate both sodium loss and water loss (isotonic or isoosmolar dehydration).[7] Pure **water deficits** (hyperosmolar or hypertonic dehydration) are rare because most people have access to water. Individuals who are comatose or paralyzed continue to have insensible water losses through the skin and lungs with a minimal obligatory formation of urine. Hyperventilation caused by fever also may precipitate water deficit. The most common cause of water loss is increased renal clearance of free water as a result of impaired tubular function or inability to concentrate the urine, as with diabetes insipidus (decreased ADH) (see Chapter 18).

CLINICAL MANIFESTATIONS Marked water deficit is manifested by symptoms of dehydration: thirst, dry skin and mucous membranes, elevated temperature, weight loss, and concentrated urine (with the exception of diabetes insipidus). Skin turgor may be normal or decreased. Symptoms of hypovolemia include tachycardia, weak pulses, and postural hypotension (a decrease in blood pressure with movement from lying or sitting to standing) (see Table 4-6).

Hyperchloremia

Hyperchloremia occurs clinically when there is too much sodium or too little bicarbonate. More than normal amounts of chloride can be expected with hypernatremia or metabolic acidosis (see p. 115). Ingestion of excessive chloride infrequently accompanies the use of an ammonium chloride diuretic. No specific symptoms are associated with chloride excess.

Hypotonic Alterations

Hypotonic fluid imbalances occur when the osmolality of the ECF is less than normal (i.e., less than 280 mOsm) (see Figure 4-2, *B-C*). The most common causes are sodium deficit (hyponatremia) or water excess. Either leads to *intracellular overhydration* (cellular edema) and cell swelling. When there is a sodium deficit, the osmotic pressure of the ECF decreases and water moves into the cell, where the osmotic pressure is greater. The plasma volume then decreases, leading to symptoms of hypovolemia. With a water excess, increases in both the ICF and ECF volume occur, causing symptoms of hypervolemia and water intoxication with cerebral and pulmonary edema (Table 4-7).

Hyponatremia

PATHOPHYSIOLOGY **Hyponatremia** develops when the serum sodium concentration falls below 135 mEq/L. Sodium deficits usually cause hypoosmolality with movement of water into cells. Among the clinical syndromes causing hyponatremia are sodium loss, inadequate sodium

TABLE 4-7
Causes and Consequences of Hypotonic Imbalances

Causative Factor	Mechanism	Extracellular Fluid Effects	Intracellular Fluid Effects
Decreased sodium (hyponatremia)	Inadequate intake of Na^+ Hypoaldosteronism Increased loss of Na^+ Diuresis Profuse sweating Gastrointestinal losses	Extracellular volume contraction and hypovolemia (but may not occur if there is water excess)	Increased intracellular water; edema Brain cell swelling, irritability, depression, confusion Systemic cellular edema, including weakness, anorexia, nausea, and diarrhea
Water excess	Sodium dilution Excessive administration of hypotonic intravenous solutions Drinking water to replace isotonic fluid losses Tap water enemas Psychogenic polydipsia Renal water retention Increased antidiuretic hormone	Extracellular volume expands with hypervolemia (but may not occur if fluid is trapped in intracellular space)	Edema (see above)
Other factors	Isotonic dehydration treated with intravenous D_5W; glucose in D_5W solution is metabolized to water, contributing to hyponatremia Nephrotic syndrome Cirrhosis Cardiac failure	Hypervolemia or hypovolemia	Edema (see above)

intake, or dilution of the body's sodium level by water excess.[8]

Pure sodium deficits usually are caused by extrarenal losses, such as vomiting, diarrhea, gastrointestinal suctioning, and burns, or renal losses from use of diuretics. **Inadequate intake** of dietary sodium is rare but possible in individuals on low-sodium diets, particularly when diuretics are taken. **Dilutional hyponatremias** occur when the proportion of TBW to total body sodium is excessive. Replacement of fluid loss with intravenous 5% dextrose in water also can cause a dilutional hyponatremia once the glucose is metabolized to carbon dioxide and water, leaving a hypotonic solution with a diluting effect. Excessive sweating may stimulate thirst and intake of large amounts of water, which dilute sodium. Hyponatremia also may be hypoosmolar or hypertonic. During acute oliguric renal failure, severe congestive heart failure, or cirrhosis, renal excretion of water is impaired. Both TBW and sodium levels are increased, but TBW exceeds the increase in sodium, producing a **hypoosmolar hyponatremia. Hypertonic hyponatremia** develops with hyperlipidemia, hyperproteinemia, and hyperglycemia. Increases in plasma lipids and proteins displace water volume and decrease sodium concentration. Hyperglycemia increases ECF osmolality and attracts water from the ICF compartment. The osmotic fluid shift to the ECF in turn dilutes the concentration of sodium and other electrolytes.

CLINICAL MANIFESTATIONS Deficits of sodium alter the cell's ability to depolarize and repolarize normally (see Chapter 1). Behavioral and neurologic changes characteristic of hyponatremia include lethargy, confusion, apprehension, depressed reflexes, seizures, and coma. Pure sodium losses may be accompanied by loss of ECF, causing an isotonic **hypovolemia** with symptoms of hypotension, tachycardia, and decreased urine output. Weight gain, edema, ascites, and jugular vein distention are characteristic of dilutional hyponatremias. Water restriction is a common treatment.

Water excess

PATHOPHYSIOLOGY When the body is functioning normally, it is almost impossible to produce an excess of TBW. Some individuals with psychogenic disorders develop water intoxication from **compulsive water drinking.** Acute renal failure, severe congestive heart failure, and cirrhosis can precipitate water excess during intravenous infusion of 5% dextrose in water. **Decreased urine formation** from renal disease or decreased renal blood flow contributes to water excess. The overall effect is dilution of the ECF, with water moving to the intracellular space by osmosis. Water excess produces a hypotonic or hypoosmolar water imbalance and is usually accompanied by hyponatremia.

The **syndrome of inappropriate secretion of ADH (SIADH)** occurs when factors other than hyperosmolality or hypovolemia stimulate the secretion of ADH.[5,9] Several clinical conditions that result in SIADH are fear, pain, acute infection, brain trauma, surgery, and drugs such as analgesics and anesthetics. The most common cause is bronchogenic cancer because the cancer cells produce ADH. SIADH is not caused by excess water intake but by decreased renal excretion of water. Therefore, SIADH increases the risk of water excess if intravenous fluids are being administered. Serum sodium and osmolality are reduced. The kidney continues to excrete sodium, and urine-specific gravity elevates, but urine volume decreases. Treatment includes water restriction medications and treatment of the underlying cause of the disorder.[9]

CLINICAL MANIFESTATIONS The symptoms of water excess are related to the rate at which water loading has occurred. Acute excesses cause confusion and convulsions. Weakness, nausea, muscle twitching, headache, and weight gain are common symptoms of long-term water accumulation.

Hypochloremia

Loss of chloride, **hypochloremia,** is usually the result of hyponatremia or elevated bicarbonate concentration, as in metabolic alkalosis (see p. 116). Hypochloremia develops with vomiting and loss of hydrochloric acid (metabolic alkalosis). Sodium deficit related to restricted intake or use of diuretics is accompanied by chloride deficiency. Cystic fibrosis, for example, also is characterized by hypochloremia (see Chapter 27).

✓ QUICK CHECK 4-3

1. What causes isotonic imbalance?
2. Give two examples of hypertonic alterations, and explain the mechanisms of action for each.
3. What is a hypotonic imbalance? Give two examples.

ALTERATIONS IN POTASSIUM AND OTHER ELECTROLYTES

Potassium

Potassium (K^+) is the major intracellular electrolyte and is essential for normal cellular functions. Total body potassium content is about 4000 mEq, with most of it (98%) located in the cells. The ICF concentration of potassium is 150 to 160 mEq/L; the ECF concentration is 3.5 to 5.0 mEq/L. The difference in concentration is maintained by a sodium-potassium adenosine triphosphatase active transport system (Na^+, K^+ ATPase pump) (see Chapter 1).

As the predominant ICF ion, potassium exerts a major influence in regulating ICF osmolality and fluid balance and for intracellular electrical neutrality in relation to hydrogen (H^+) and sodium. Potassium is required for glycogen and glucose deposition in liver and skeletal muscle cells. It also maintains the resting membrane potential, as reflected in transmission and conduction of nerve impulses, maintenance of normal cardiac rhythms, and skeletal and smooth muscle contraction.

Dietary potassium moves rapidly into cells after dietary ingestion. However, the distribution of potassium between intracellular and extracellular fluids is influenced by several factors. Insulin, aldosterone, epinephrine, and alkalosis facilitate the shift of potassium into cells. Insulin deficiency, aldosterone deficiency, acidosis, cell lysis, and strenuous exercise facilitate the shift of potassium out of cells. Glucagon blocks entry of potassium into cells, and glucocorticoids promote potassium excretion. Potassium also will move out of cells along with water when there is increased ECF osmolarity.

Although potassium is found in most body fluids, the kidney is the most efficient regulator of potassium balance. Potassium is freely filtered by the renal glomerulus, and 90% is reabsorbed by the proximal tubule and loop of Henle. In the distal tubules, principal cells secrete potassium and intercalated cells reabsorb potassium. These cells determine the amount of potassium excreted from the body.

The potassium concentration in the distal tubular cell is determined primarily by the plasma concentration in the peritubular capillaries. When plasma potassium concentration increases from increased dietary intake or shifts of potassium from the ICF to the ECF occur, potassium is secreted into the urine by the distal tubules. Decreased plasma potassium results in decreased distal tubular secretion, although approximately 5 to 15 mEq per day will continue to be lost. Changes in the rate of filtrate (urine) flow through the distal tubule also influence the concentration gradient for potassium secretion. When the flow rate is high, as with the use of diuretics, potassium concentration in the distal tubular urine is lower, leading to the secretion of potassium into the urine.[10]

Changes in pH and thus in hydrogen ion concentration also affect potassium balance. During acute acidosis, hydrogen ions accumulate in the ICF and potassium shifts out of the cell to the ECF to maintain a balance of cations across the cell membrane. This occurs in part because of a decrease in sodium-potassium ATPase pump activity. Decreased ICF potassium results in decreased secretion of potassium by the distal tubular cells, contributing to hyperkalemia. In acute alkalosis, intracellular fluid levels of hydrogen diminish and potassium shifts into the cell and the distal tubular cells increase their secretion of potassium further contributing to hypokalemia.

Besides conserving sodium, aldosterone also regulates potassium. When plasma potassium concentration increases, aldosterone is released, stimulating the release of potassium into the urine by the distal renal tubules. Aldosterone also increases the secretion of potassium from the sweat glands.

Insulin helps regulate plasma potassium levels by stimulating the sodium potassium ATPase pump, thus promoting the movement of potassium into liver and muscle cells, particularly after eating. Insulin can also be used to treat hyperkalemia. Dangerously low levels of plasma potassium can result when insulin is given while potassium levels are depressed. Potassium balance is especially significant in the treatment of conditions requiring insulin administration, such as insulin-dependent diabetes mellitus.

Potassium tolerance is the ability of the body to adapt to increased levels of potassium intake over time. A sudden increase in potassium may be fatal, but if the intake of potassium is slowly increased by amounts of more than 120 mEq per day, the kidney can increase the urinary excretion of potassium and maintain potassium balance.

Hypokalemia

PATHOPHYSIOLOGY Potassium deficiency, or **hypokalemia,** develops when the serum potassium concentration falls below 3.5 mEq/L. Because cellular and total body stores of potassium are difficult to measure, changes in potassium balance are described, although not always accurately, by the plasma concentration. Generally, lowered serum potassium indicates loss of total body potassium. With potassium loss from the ECF, the concentration gradient change favors movement of potassium from the cell to the ECF. The ICF/ECF concentration ratio is maintained, but total body potassium is depleted.

ECF hypokalemia can develop without losses of total body potassium. For example, potassium shifts into the cell during respiratory or metabolic alkalosis or after administration of insulin. In alkalosis, potassium shifts into the cell in exchange for hydrogen to maintain plasma acid-base balance. Insulin also promotes cellular uptake of potassium and may cause an ECF potassium deficit.

Potassium shifts from the ICF to the ECF in conditions such as diabetic ketoacidosis, in which the increased hydrogen ion concentration in the ECF causes H^+ to shift into the cell in exchange for potassium. A normal level of potassium is maintained in the plasma, but potassium continues to be lost in the urine, causing a deficit in total body potassium. Severe, even fatal, hypokalemia may occur if insulin is administered without also providing potassium supplements. Thus, total body potassium depletion becomes evident when insulin treatment and rehydration therapy are initiated. Potassium replacement is instituted cautiously to prevent hyperkalemia.

Factors contributing to the development of hypokalemia include reduced intake of potassium, increased entry of potassium into cells, and increased losses of body potassium. Dietary deficiency of potassium is a rare cause but may occur in elderly individuals with both low protein intake and inadequate intake of fruits and vegetables and in individuals with alcoholism or anorexia nervosa. Generally, reduced potassium intake becomes a problem when combined with other causes of potassium depletion.

Shifts of potassium from the extracellular to intracellular space cause apparent deficits in total body potassium. Alkalosis, particularly respiratory alkalosis, is the most common clinical problem. Extracellular fluid potassium exchanges with ICF hydrogen in an attempt to correct alkalosis by decreasing the pH of the ECF.

Losses of potassium from body stores are usually caused by gastrointestinal and renal disorders. Diarrhea, intestinal drainage tubes or fistulae, and laxative abuse also result in hypokalemia. Normally, only 5 to 10 mEq of potassium and 100 to 150 ml of water are excreted in the stool each day. With diarrhea, fluid and electrolyte losses can be voluminous, with several liters of fluid and 100 to 200 mEq of potassium lost per day. Vomiting or continuous nasogastric suctioning often is associated with potassium depletion, partly because of the potassium lost from the gastric fluid but principally because of renal compensation for volume depletion and the metabolic alkalosis (elevated bicarbonate levels) that occurs from sodium, chloride, and hydrogen ion losses. The loss of fluid and sodium stimulates the secretion of aldosterone, which in turn causes renal losses of potassium. During alkalosis, the elevated flow of bicarbonate at the distal tubule also contributes to renal excretion of potassium because the increased tubular lumen electronegativity attracts potassium.

Renal potassium losses occur with increased secretion of potassium by the distal tubule. Use of potassium-wasting diuretics, excessive aldosterone secretion, increased distal tubular flow rate, and low plasma magnesium concentration all may contribute to urinary losses of potassium. Many diuretics inhibit the reabsorption of sodium chloride, causing the diuretic effect. The distal tubular flow rate then increases, promoting potassium excretion. If sodium loss is severe, the compensating aldosterone secretion may further deplete potassium stores. Primary hyperaldosteronism with excessive secretion of aldosterone from an adrenal adenoma (tumor) also causes potassium wasting. Many kidney diseases reduce one's ability to conserve sodium. The disordered sodium reabsorption produces a diuretic effect, and the increased distal tubule flow rate favors the secretion of potassium. Magnesium deficits stimulate renin release and hyperaldosteronism, causing hypokalemia. Several antibiotics are known to cause hypokalemia by increasing the rate of potassium excretion.

CLINICAL MANIFESTATIONS Mild losses of potassium are usually asymptomatic. Neuromuscular and cardiac effects of hypokalemia produce the most common symptoms with severe loss of potassium. Neuromuscular excitability decreases, causing skeletal muscle weakness, smooth muscle atony, and cardiac dysrhythmias.[11]

Symptoms occur in relation to the rate of potassium depletion. Because the body can accommodate slow losses of potassium, the decrease in ECF concentration may allow potassium to shift from the intracellular space, restoring the potassium concentration gradient toward normal, with less severe neuromuscular changes. With acute and severe losses of potassium, changes in neuromuscular excitability are more profound. Skeletal muscle weakness occurs initially in the larger muscles of the legs and arms and ultimately affects the diaphragm and depresses ventilation. Paralysis and respiratory arrest can occur. Loss of smooth muscle tone is manifested by constipation, intestinal distention, anorexia, nausea, vomiting, and paralytic ileus (paralysis of the intestinal muscles).

The cardiac effects of hypokalemia are related also to changes in membrane excitability. Because potassium contributes to the repolarization phase of the action potential, hypokalemia delays ventricular repolarization. Various dysrhythmias may occur, including sinus bradycardia, atrioventricular block, and paroxysmal atrial tachycardia. The characteristic changes in the electrocardiogram (ECG) reflect delayed repolarization. For instance, the amplitude of the T wave decreases, the amplitude of the U wave increases, and the ST segment is depressed (Figure 4-7). In severe states of hypokalemia, P waves peak and the QRS complex is prolonged. Hypokalemia also increases the risk of digitalis toxicity.

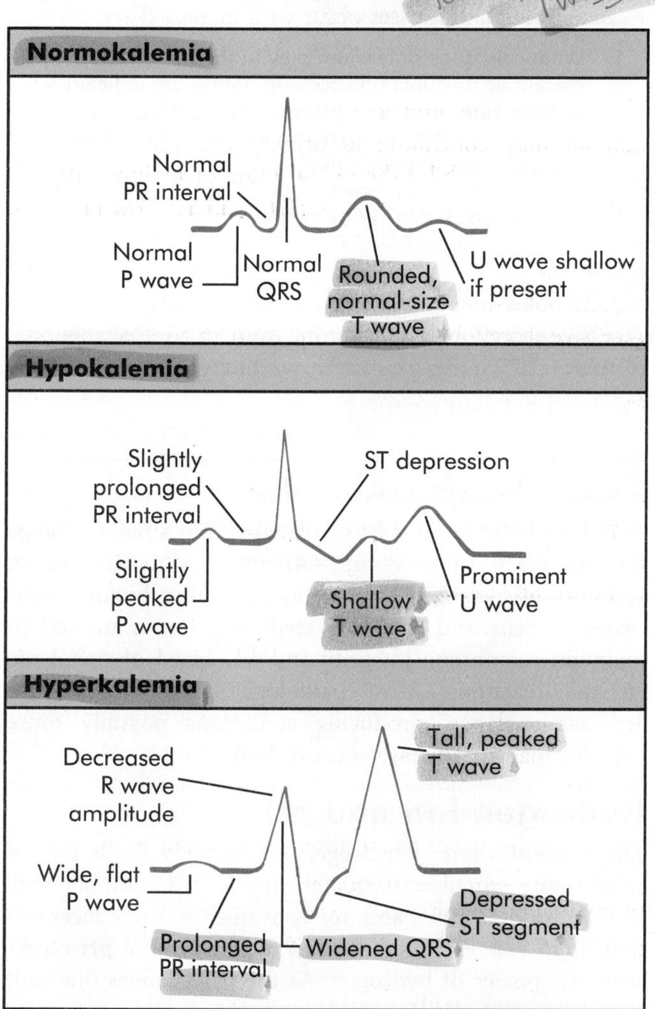

Figure 4-7 ■ **Electrocardiogram Changes with Potassium Imbalance.**

A wide range of metabolic dysfunctions may result from potassium deficiency (Table 4-8). Carbohydrate metabolism is affected because hypokalemia depresses insulin secretion and alters hepatic and skeletal muscle glycogen synthesis. Renal function is impaired, with a decreased ability to concentrate urine. Polyuria (increased urine) and polydipsia (increased thirst) are associated with decreased responsiveness to ADH. Long-term potassium deficits lasting more than 1 month may damage renal tissue, with interstitial fibrosis and tubular atrophy.

Hyperkalemia

PATHOPHYSIOLOGY Elevation of ECF potassium above 5.5 mEq/L constitutes **hyperkalemia.**[12] Because of efficient renal excretion, increases in total body potassium are relatively rare. Acute increases in serum potassium are handled quickly through increased cellular uptake and renal excretion of body potassium excesses. Excretion is partially mediated by the secretion of aldosterone, because it facilitates excretion of potassium in the urine.

Potassium excesses may be caused by increased intake, a shift of potassium from cells to the ECF, or decreased renal excretion. If renal function is normal, slow, long-term increases in potassium intake are usually well tolerated through potassium adaptation, although short-term potassium loading can exceed renal excretion rates. Use of stored whole blood and intravenous boluses of potassium penicillin G or replacement potassium can precipitate hyperkalemia, particularly with impaired renal function. Dietary excesses of potassium are uncommon, but accidental ingestion of potassium salt substitutes can cause toxicity.

Potassium moves from the ICF to the ECF with cell trauma or a change in cell membrane permeability, acidosis, insulin deficiency, or cell hypoxia. Burns, massive crushing injuries, and extensive surgeries can cause loss of potassium to the ECF as a result of cell trauma. If renal function is sustained, potassium is excreted. As cell repair begins, hypokalemia develops without an adequate replacement of potassium.

In acidosis, hydrogen ions shift into the cells in exchange for ICF potassium and sodium; hyperkalemia and acidosis therefore often occur together. Because insulin promotes cellular entry of potassium, insulin deficits, which occur with such conditions as diabetic ketoacidosis, are accompanied by hyperkalemia. Hypoxia can lead to hyperkalemia by diminishing the efficiency of cell membrane active transport, resulting in the potassium escaping to the ECF. Digitalis overdose may cause hyperkalemia by inhibiting the Na^+, K^+ ATPase pump, which maintains increased intracellular potassium and extracellular sodium (see Chapter 1).

Decreased renal excretion of potassium commonly is associated with hyperkalemia. Renal failure that results in oliguria (urine output of 30 ml/hr or less) is accompanied by elevations of serum potassium. The severity of hyperkalemia is related to the amount of potassium intake, the

TABLE 4-8

Clinical Manifestations of Potassium Alterations

Organ System	Hypokalemia	Hyperkalemia
Cardiovascular	Dysrhythmias Electrocardiogram changes Cardiac arrest Weak irregular pulse Postural hypotension	Dysrhythmias Bradycardia Heart block Cardiac arrest
Nervous	Lethargy Fatigue Confusion Paresthesias	Anxiety Tingling Numbness
Gastrointestinal	Nausea and vomiting Decreased motility Distention Decreased bowel sounds Ileus	Nausea and vomiting Diarrhea Colicky pain
Kidney	Water loss Thirst Inability to concentrate urine Kidney damage	Oliguria Kidney damage
Skeletal and smooth muscle	Weakness Flaccid paralysis Respiratory arrest Constipation Bladder dysfunction	Early: hyperactive muscles Late: weakness and flaccid paralysis

degree of acidosis, and the rate of cell damage. Decreases in the secretion or renal effects of aldosterone also can cause decreases in the urinary excretion of potassium. For example, Addison disease (a disease of the adrenal gland) results in decreased production and secretion of aldosterone and thus contributes to hyperkalemia. Potassium-sparing diuretics (e.g., spironolactone), which inhibit sodium reabsorption and potassium and hydrogen secretion by the distal tubule, also may contribute to hyperkalemia.

CLINICAL MANIFESTATIONS Symptoms of hyperkalemia vary with the severity of hyperkalemia. During mild attacks, increased neuromuscular irritability may be manifested as restlessness, intestinal cramping, and diarrhea. Severe hyperkalemia causes muscle weakness, loss of muscle tone, and paralysis. Hyperkalemia causes decreased cardiac conduction and more rapid repolarization of heart muscle. In mild states of hyperkalemia, the more rapid repolarization is reflected in the ECG as narrow and taller T waves with a shortened QT interval. Severe hyperkalemia depresses the ST segment, prolongs the PR interval, and widens the QRS complex due to decreased conduction velocity (see Figure 4-7). Bradydysrhythmias are common in hyperkalemia, with alterations in cardiac conduction causing ventricular fibrillation or cardiac arrest.

As with hypokalemia, changes in the ratio of intracellular to extracellular potassium concentration contribute to the symptoms of hyperkalemia (see Table 4-8). The neuromuscular effects of hyperkalemia are related to the increase in rate of repolarization and the presence of other contributing factors, such as acidosis and calcium balance. Long-term increases in ECF potassium concentration result in shifts of potassium into the cell, because the tendency is to maintain a normal ratio of ICF to ECF potassium concentrations. Acute elevations of extracellular potassium affect neuromuscular irritability as this ratio is disrupted. Increases in extracellular fluid calcium concentration can override the neuromuscular effects of hyperkalemia because calcium is also a cation.

QUICK CHECK 4-4

1. What role does potassium play in the body? What metabolic dysfunctions occur in potassium deficiency? In potassium excess?
2. How can you not have a deficit in total body potassium and still have hypokalemia?
3. What is the most prominent ECG change associated with hyperkalemia? With hypokalemia?

Other Electrolytes

The specifics of balance for the other body electrolytes—calcium (Ca^{++}), phosphate (P^{+}), and magnesium (Mg^{++})—are summarized in Table 4-9.

ACID-BASE BALANCE

Acid-base balance must be regulated within a narrow range for the body to function normally. Slight changes in amounts of hydrogen can significantly alter biologic processes in cells and tissues.[13] Hydrogen ion is needed to maintain membrane integrity and the speed of metabolic enzyme reactions. Most pathologic conditions disturb acid-base balance, producing conditions possibly more harmful than the disease process itself.

Hydrogen Ion and pH

The concentration of hydrogen ion in body fluids is very small—approximately 0.0000001 mg/L. This number may be expressed as 10^{-7}, and, for convenience, the concentration of 10^{-7} is indicated as pH 7.0. The symbol *pH* represents the power of hydrogen. As the pH changes one unit (e.g., 7.0 to 6.0), the $[H^+]$ ($[H^+]$ = hydrogen ion concentration) changes tenfold. The greater the $[H^+]$, the more acidic the solution and the lower the pH. The lower the $[H^+]$, the

TABLE 4-9

Alterations in Other Body Electrolytes

Parameter	Calcium	Phosphate	Magnesium
Normal values	Serum: 8.8-10.5 mg/dl (total), 4.5-5.6 mg/dl (ionized); 99% in bone as hydroxyapatite; remainder in plasma and body cells with 50% bound to plasma proteins; 40% free or ionized; ionized form most important physiologically	Serum: 2.5-5.0 mg/dl, but may be as high as 6.0-7.0 mg/dl in infants and young children; mainly in bone with some in ICF and ECF; exists as phospholipids, phosphate esters, and inorganic phosphate (ionized form)	Serum: 1.8-3.0 mEq/L; 40%-60% stored in muscle and bone, one third bound to plasma proteins
Function	Needed for fundamental metabolic processes; major cation for structure of bone and teeth; enzymatic cofactor for blood clotting; required for hormone secretion and the function of cell receptors; directly related to plasma membrane stability and permeability, as well as transmission of nerve impulses and contraction of muscles	Intracellular and extracellular anion buffer in regulation of acid-base balance; provides energy for muscle contraction (as ATP)	A cofactor in intracellular enzymatic reactions and causes neuromuscular excitability; often interacts with calcium and potassium in reactions at cellular level and has an important role in smooth muscle contraction and relaxation
Excess	Hypercalcemia (serum concentrations >10-12 mg/dl)	Hyperphosphatemia (serum concentrations >4.7 mg/dl)	Hypermagnesemia (serum concentrations >3.0 mEq/L)
Causes	Hyperparathyroidism; bone metastases with calcium resorption from breast, prostate, renal, and cervical cancer; sarcoidosis; excess vitamin D; many tumors that produce PTH	Acute or chronic renal failure with significant loss of glomerular filtration; treatment of metastatic tumors with chemotherapy that releases large amounts of phosphate into serum; long-term use of laxatives or enemas containing phosphates; hypoparathyroidism	Usually renal failure; also excessive intake of magnesium-containing antacids, adrenal insufficiency
Effects	Many nonspecific; fatigue, weakness, lethargy, anorexia, nausea, constipation; impaired renal function, kidney stones; dysrhythmias, bradycardia, cardiac arrest; bone pain, osteoporosis	Symptoms primarily related to low serum calcium levels (caused by high phosphate levels) similar to the results of hypocalcemia; when prolonged, calcification of soft tissues in lungs, kidneys, joints	Skeletal smooth muscle contraction; excess nerve function; loss of deep tendon reflexes; nausea and vomiting; muscle weakness; hypotension; bradycardia; respiratory distress
Deficit	Hypocalcemia (serum calcium concentration <8.5 mg/dl)	Hypophosphatemia (serum phosphate concentration <2.0 mg/dl)	Hypomagnesemia (serum magnesium concentration <1.5 mEq/L)
Causes	Related to inadequate intestinal absorption, deposition of ionized calcium into bone or soft tissue, blood administration, or decreases in PTH and vitamin D; nutritional deficiencies occur with inadequate sources of dairy products or green leafy vegetables	Most commonly by intestinal malabsorption related to vitamin D deficiency, use of magnesium- and aluminum-containing antacids, long-term alcohol abuse, and malabsorption syndromes; respiratory alkalosis; increased renal excretion of phosphate associated with hyperparathyroidism	Malnutrition, malabsorption syndromes, alcoholism, renal tubular dysfunction, loop diuretics
Effects	Increased neuromuscular excitability; tingling, muscle spasm (particularly in hands, feet, and facial muscles), intestinal cramping, hyperactive bowel sounds; severe cases show convulsions and tetany; prolonged QT interval, cardiac arrest	Conditions related to reduced capacity for oxygen transport by red blood cells and disturbed energy metabolism; leukocyte and platelet dysfunction; deranged nerve and muscle function; in severe cases, irritability, confusion, numbness, coma, convulsions; possibly respiratory failure (because of muscle weakness), cardiomyopathies, bone resorption (leading to rickets or osteomalacia)	Behavioral changes, irritability, increased reflexes, muscle cramps, ataxia, nystagmus, tetany, convulsions, tachycardia, hypotension

ATP, Adenosine triphosphate; *PTH*, parathyroid hormone.

more basic the solution and the higher the pH. In biologic fluids, a pH of less than 7.4 is defined as acidic and a pH greater than 7.4 is defined as basic or alkaline (Table 4-10).

Body acids are formed as end products of the metabolism of protein, carbohydrates, and fats. This must be balanced by the amount of basic substances in the body to maintain normal pH. The lungs, kidneys, and bones are the major organs involved in regulating acid-base balance. The systems work together to regulate short- and long-term changes in acid-base status.

Body acids exist in two forms: **volatile** (can be eliminated as CO_2 gas) and **nonvolatile** (can be eliminated by the kidney). The volatile acid is carbonic acid (H_2CO_3), a weak acid (does not release its hydrogen easily). In the presence of the enzyme carbonic anhydrase, it readily dissociates into carbon dioxide (CO_2) and water (H_2O). The carbon dioxide is then eliminated by pulmonary ventilation.

Sulfuric, phosphoric, and other organic acids are nonvolatile strong acids (readily give up their hydrogen). Nonvolatile acids are secreted into the urine by the renal tubules in amounts of about 60–100 mEq of hydrogen per day or about 1 mEq per kilogram of body weight.

Buffer Systems

Buffering occurs in response to changes in acid-base status. **Buffers** can absorb excessive hydrogen (H^+) (acid) or hydroxyl ion (OH^-) (base) and prevent a significant change in pH. The buffer systems are located in both the ICF and ECF compartments, and they function at different rates (Table 4-11). The most important plasma buffer systems are carbonic acid-bicarbonate and the protein hemoglobin (Figure 4-8). Phosphate and protein are the most important intracellular buffers.

Carbonic acid–bicarbonate buffering

The carbonic acid–bicarbonate buffer pair *operates in both the lung and the kidney* and is a major extracellular buffer. The lungs can decrease the amount of carbonic acid by blowing off carbon dioxide and leaving water. The kidneys can reabsorb bicarbonate or regenerate new bicarbonate from carbon dioxide and water. The relationship between bicarbonate and carbonic acid is usually expressed as a ratio. Normal bicarbonate level is about 24 mEq/L, and normal carbonic acid level is about 1.2 mEq/L (when the arterial CO_2 partial pressure [$PaCO_2$] is 40 mm Hg), producing a 20:1 ratio and the normal pH of 7.4. These two systems are very effective together because the lungs can adjust acid concentration rapidly and bicarbonate is easily reabsorbed or regenerated by the kidneys.

Renal and respiratory adjustments to changes in pH are known as **compensation**. The respiratory system compensates for changes in pH by increasing or decreasing carbon dioxide by changing ventilation. The renal system compen-

TABLE 4-10
pH of Body Fluids

Body Fluid	pH	Factors Affecting pH
Gastric juices	1.0–3.0	Hydrochloric acid production
Urine	5.0–6.0	H^+ ion excretion from waste products
Arterial blood	7.38–7.42	pH is slightly higher because there is less carbonic acid (H_2CO_3)
Venous blood	7.37	pH is slightly lower because there is more carbonic acid
Cerebrospinal fluid	7.32	Decreased bicarbonate and higher carbon dioxide content decreases pH
Pancreatic fluid	7.8–8.0	Contains bicarbonate produced by exocrine cells

TABLE 4-11
Buffer Systems

Buffer Pairs	Buffer System	Reaction	Rate
HCO_3^-/H_2CO_3	Bicarbonate	$H^+ + HCO_3^- \rightleftharpoons H_2O + CO_2$	Instantaneous
Hb^-/HHb	Hemoglobin	$HHb \rightleftharpoons H^+ + Hb^-$	Instantaneous
$HPO_4^=/H_2PO_4^-$	Phosphate	$H_2PO_4^- + H^+ + HPO_4^=$	Instantaneous
Pr^-/HPr	Plasma proteins	$HPr \rightleftharpoons H^+ + Pr^-$	Instantaneous

Organs	Mechanism	Rate
Lungs	Regulates retention or elimination of CO_2 and therefore H_2CO_3 concentration	Minutes–hours
Ionic shifts	Exchange of intracellular potassium and sodium for hydrogen	2–4 hours
Kidneys	Bicarbonate reabsorption and regeneration, ammonia formation, phosphate buffering	Hours–days
Bone	Exchanges of calcium and phosphate and release of carbonate	Hours–days

HCO_3^-, Bicarbonate; *H_2CO_3*, carbonic acid; *Hb*, hemoglobin; *HHb*, hydrogenated hemoglobin; *$H_2PO_4^=$*, dibasic phosphate; *$H_2PO_4^-$*, monobasic phosphate; *Pr^-*, protein; *HPr*, hydrogenated protein; *CO_2*, carbon dioxide.

sates by producing more acidic or more alkaline urine. **Correction** occurs when the values for both components of the buffer pair (carbonic acid and bicarbonate) return to normal levels.

Protein buffering

Both intracellular and extracellular proteins have negative charges and can serve as buffers for hydrogen, but because most proteins are inside cells, they are primarily an intracellular buffer system. Hemoglobin (Hb) is an excellent intracellular buffer because it can bind with hydrogen (H^+) (forming HHb) and carbon dioxide (forming $HHbCO_2$). Hemoglobin bound to hydrogen becomes a weak acid. Hemoglobin not saturated with oxygen (venous blood) is a better buffer than hemoglobin saturated with oxygen (arterial blood). The pH control mechanism is illustrated in Figure 4-8.

Renal buffering

The distal tubule of the kidney regulates acid-base balance by secreting hydrogen into the urine and reabsorbing bicarbonate. Dibasic phosphate ($HPO_4^=$) and ammonia (NH_3) are two important renal buffers. The renal buffering of hydrogen ions requires the use of carbon dioxide (CO_2) and water (H_2O) to form H_2CO_3. The enzyme carbonic anhydrase catalyzes the reaction. The hydrogen is then secreted from the tubular cell and buffered in the lumen by phosphate and ammonia (i.e., forms $H_2PO_3^-$ and NH_4^+). The remaining bicarbonate is reabsorbed. The end effect is the addition of new bicarbonate to the plasma, which contributes to the alkalinity of the plasma because the hydrogen ion is excreted from the body.

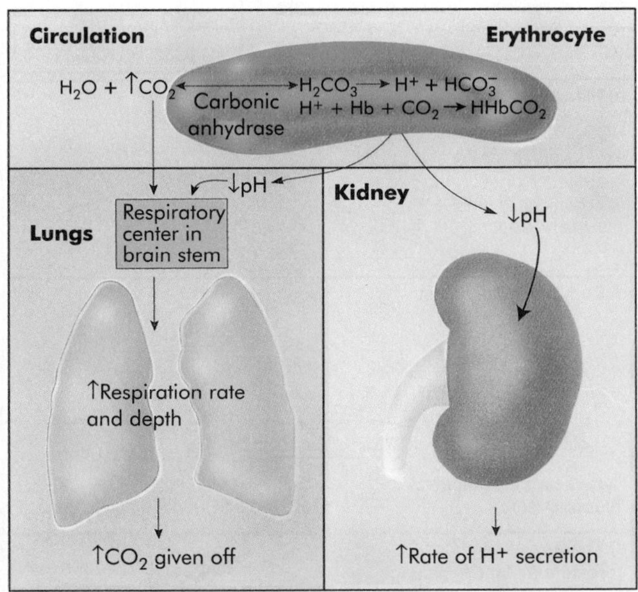

Figure 4-8 ■ **Integration of pH Control Mechanisms.** Elevated carbon dioxide (CO_2) levels result in increased formation of carbonic acid (H_2CO_3) in red blood cells. The resulting increase in hydrogen ions (H^+), coupled with elevated CO_2 levels, results in $HHbCO_2$ and an increase in respiratory rate and secretion of H^+ by the kidneys, thus helping to regulate the pH of body fluids. (From Thibodeau GA, Patton KT: *Anatomy & physiology,* ed 6, St Louis, 2007, Mosby.)

Acid-Base Imbalances

Pathophysiologic changes in the concentration of hydrogen ion in the blood lead to acid-base imbalances.[14] In **acidemia** the pH of arterial blood is less than 7.4. A systemic increase in hydrogen ion concentration is termed **acidosis.** In **alkalemia,** the pH of arterial blood is greater than 7.4. A systemic decrease in hydrogen ion concentration is termed **alkalosis.** These changes may be caused by metabolic or respiratory processes. Figure 4-9 summarizes the relationship among pH, the partial pressure of carbon dioxide, and bicarbonate during different primary acid-base states.

Metabolic acidosis

In **metabolic acidosis,** noncarbonic acids increase or bicarbonate is lost from extracellular fluid (Table 4-12). This can occur either quickly (e.g., in lactic acidosis caused by poor oxygenation) or over an extended period of time (e.g., in renal failure or diabetic ketoacidosis).[15]

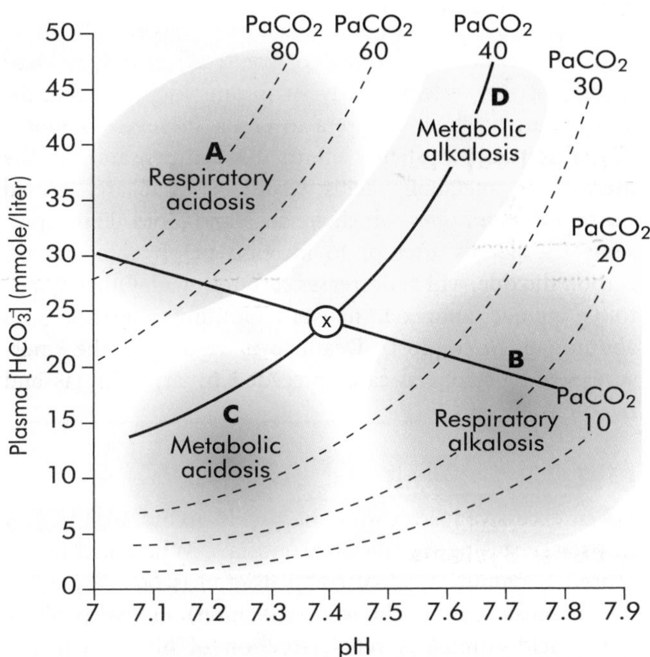

Figure 4-9 ■ **Davenport Diagram: Classic Working Diagram for Studying Primary Uncompensated Acid-Base Imbalance.** The point ⊗ represents a normal pH value (7.4) and normal values for partial pressure of carbon dioxide ($PaCO_2$ = 40 mm Hg) and bicarbonate (HCO_3^- = 24 mEq/L). Note that as the $PaCO_2$ increases toward 60 mm Hg *(A)*, the pH decreases (respiratory acidosis), and that as it decreases toward 20 mm Hg *(B)*, the pH increases (respiratory alkalosis). Metabolic acidosis develops as the concentration of HCO_3^- decreases *(C)*, and metabolic alkalosis develops as the concentration of HCO_3^- increases *(D)*.

TABLE 4-12
Causes of Metabolic Acidosis

Increased Noncarbonic Acids (Elevated Anion Gap)	Bicarbonate Loss (Normal Anion Gap)
Increased H^+ load	Diarrhea
Ketoacidosis (e.g., diabetes mellitus, starvation)	Ureterosigmoidoscopy
Lactic acidosis (e.g., shock, hypoxemia)	
Ingestion (e.g., ammonium chloride, ethylene glycol, methanol, salicylates, paraldehyde)	
Decreased H^+ excretion	
Proximal renal tubule acidosis	Renal HCO_3^- loss
Distal renal tubule acidosis	Decreased renal H^+secretion

Anion gap refers to anions not usually measured in laboratory reports (e.g., sulfate, phosphate, and lactate). The anions usually measured are chloride (Cl^-) and bicarbonate (HCO_3^-). When the sum of the measured anions is subtracted from the sum of usually measured cations (e.g., sodium and potassium), there is a "gap" of approximately 10 to 12 mEq/L; this is the anion gap. An elevated anion gap provides clues to the cause of the acidosis.
H^+, Hydrogen.

The buffering systems normally compensate for excess acid and maintain arterial pH within normal range. When acidosis is severe, buffers become depleted, cannot compensate, and the ratio of bicarbonate to carbonic acid decreases to less than 20:1 (Figure 4-10). The specific type of acidosis can be determined by examining the anion gap (Box 4-1).

Metabolic acidosis is manifested by changes in the function of the neurologic, respiratory, gastrointestinal, and cardiovascular systems. Early symptoms include headache and lethargy, which progress to coma in severe acidosis. The respiratory system's efforts to compensate for the increase in metabolic acids result in what are termed *Kussmaul respirations,* which are deep and rapid. This represents the body's attempt to increase pH by blowing off carbon dioxide, which decreases carbonic acid. Other symptoms include anorexia, nausea, vomiting, diarrhea, and abdominal discomfort. Death can result in the most severe and prolonged cases preceded by arrhythmias and hypotension.

Metabolic alkalosis

When excessive loss of metabolic acids occurs, bicarbonate increases, causing **metabolic alkalosis.**[16] When acid loss is caused by vomiting, renal compensation is not very effective because loss of chloride (an anion) in hydrochloric (HCl) acid stimulates renal retention of bicarbonate (an anion). Hyperaldosteronism also can lead to alkalosis as a result of sodium bicarbonate retention and loss of hydrogen and potassium. Diuretics may produce a mild alkalosis because they promote greater excretion of sodium, potassium, and chloride than of bicarbonate (Figure 4-11).

Some common signs and symptoms of metabolic alkalosis are weakness; muscle cramps; hyperactive reflexes; tetany; shallow, slow respirations; confusion; convulsions; and atrial tachycardia. The manifestations vary with the cause and severity of the alkalosis. The symptoms of hyperactive reflexes and tetany occur because alkalosis increases binding of Ca^{++} to plasma proteins thus decreasing ionized calcium. The decreased ionized calcium causes excitable cells to become hypopolarized, initiating an action potential more easily and causing muscle contraction.

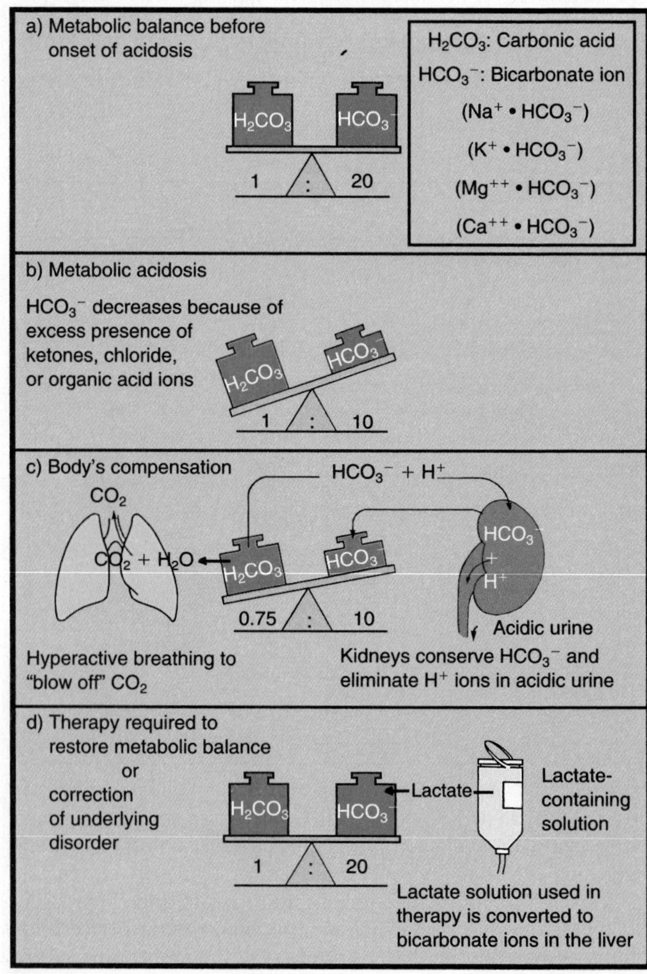

Figure 4-10 ■ **Metabolic Acidosis.** (From Thibodeau GA, Patton KT: *Anatomy & physiology,* ed 6, St Louis, 2007, Mosby.)

BOX 4-1 Anion Gap

The evaluation of the anion gap can be useful for distinguishing different types of metabolic acidosis. Normally, the concentrations of cations and anions in the plasma are equivalent. Some anions, such as protein, sulfates, phosphates, and organic acids, however, are not measured in the common laboratory evaluations of the blood. Therefore the normal anion gap represents the difference between the sum of sodium (Na^+) and potassium (K^+) and the sum of bicarbonate (HCO_3^-) and chloride (Cl^-), or about 10 to 12 mEq.

In metabolic acidosis a normal anion gap is characteristic of conditions related to bicarbonate loss with retention of chloride to maintain an ionic balance. This is called *hyperchloremic metabolic acidosis.* An elevated anion gap is characteristic of acidosis associated with accumulation of anions other than chloride (e.g., lactate, ketoacids [i.e., acetoacetate and beta butyrate]) (see Table 4-12).

Respiratory acidosis

A decrease in alveolar ventilation in relation to the metabolic production of carbon dioxide produces **respiratory acidosis** by an increase in carbonic acid.[17] The arterial carbon dioxide tension (or pressure) ($PaCO_2$) is >45 mm Hg. This occurs with depression of ventilation, resulting in an excess of carbon dioxide (hypercapnia) in the blood. Respiratory acidosis can be acute or chronic. Common causes include depression of the respiratory center (i.e., from drugs or head injury), respiratory muscle paralysis, disorders of the chest wall (kyphoscoliosis or broken ribs), and disorders of the lung parenchyma (pneumonia, pulmonary edema, emphysema, asthma, bronchitis). Renal compensation occurs by elimination of hydrogen and retention of bicarbonate (Figure 4-12).

The signs and symptoms seen often include headache, blurred vision, breathlessness, restlessness, and apprehension followed by lethargy, disorientation, muscle twitching, tremors, convulsions, and coma. Respiratory rate is rapid at first and gradually becomes depressed as the respiratory center adapts to increasing levels of carbon dioxide. The skin may be warm and flushed as the elevated carbon dioxide causes vasodilation.

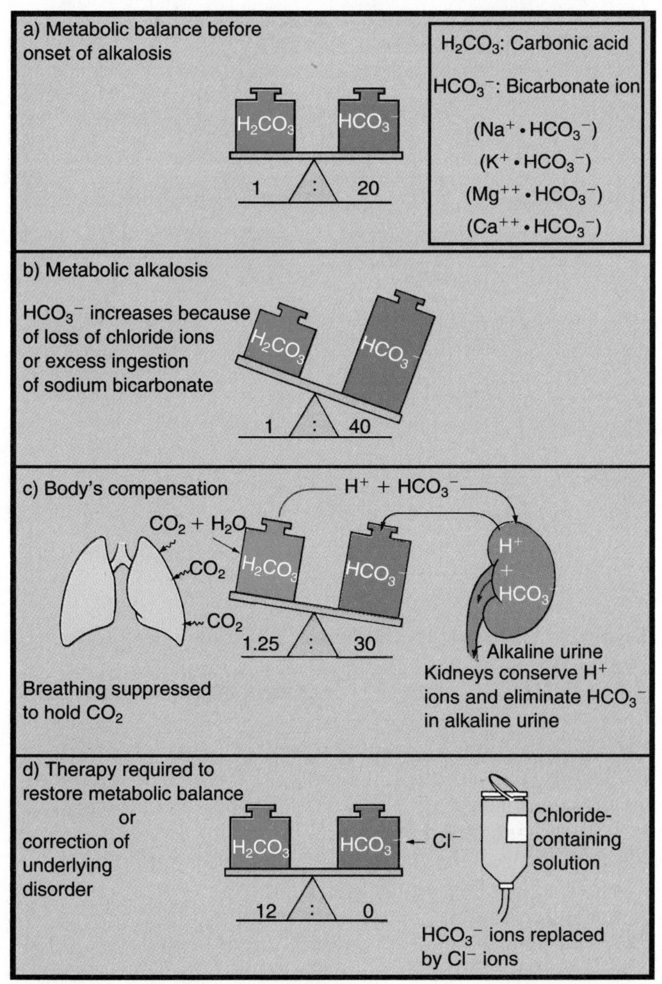

Figure 4-11 ■ **Metabolic Alkalosis.** (From Thibodeau GA, Patton KT: *Anatomy & physiology,* ed 6, St Louis, 2007, Mosby.)

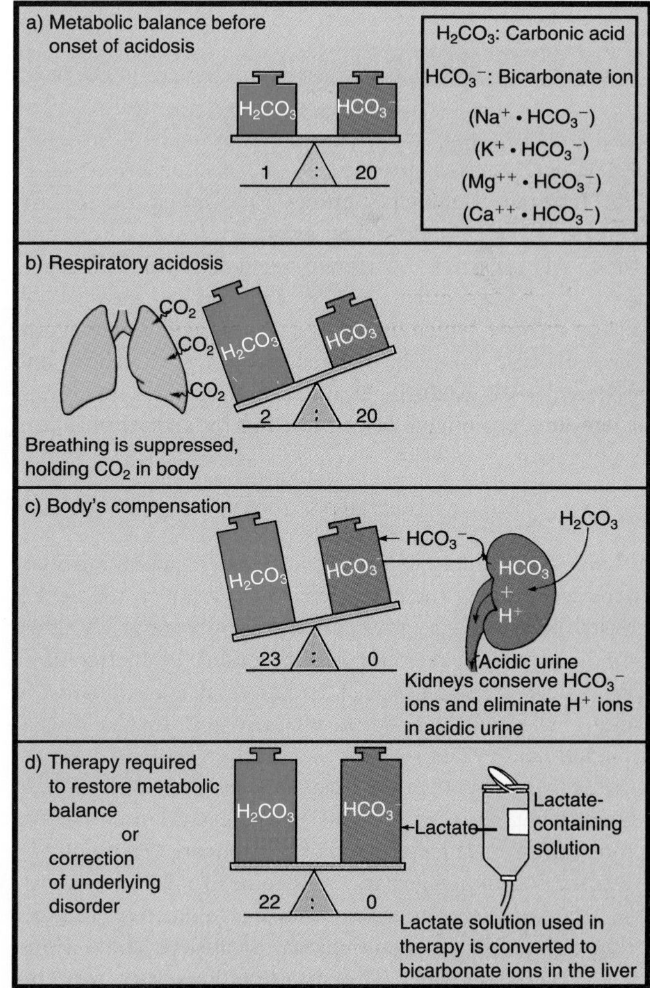

Figure 4-12 ■ **Respiratory Acidosis.** (From Thibodeau GA, Patton KT: *Anatomy & physiology,* ed 6, St Louis, 2007, Mosby.)

Respiratory alkalosis

Respiratory alkalosis occurs when there is alveolar hyperventilation and excessive reduction in plasma carbon dioxide levels (hypocapnia).[18] The $PaCO_2$ is <35 mm Hg. Respiratory alkalosis can be chronic or acute. Hypoxemia (caused by pulmonary disease, congestive heart failure, or high altitudes), hypermetabolic states (fever, anemia, thyrotoxicosis), early salicylate intoxication, hysteria, cirrhosis, and gram-negative sepsis stimulate hyperventilation. Improper use of mechanical ventilators also can cause iatrogenic (treatment-related) respiratory alkalosis, and secondary alkalosis may develop as a result of hyperventilation stimulated by metabolic or respiratory acidosis. The kidneys compensate by decreasing hydrogen excretion and bicarbonate reabsorption (Figure 4-13).

The central and peripheral nervous systems are stimulated by respiratory alkalosis, causing dizziness, confusion, tingling of extremities (paresthesias), convulsions, and coma. Cerebral vasoconstriction reduces cerebral blood flow. Carpopedal spasm (spasm of muscles in the fingers and toes), tetany, and other symptoms of hypocalcemia (see Table 4-9) are similar to those of metabolic alkalosis. Deep, rapid respirations are primary symptoms that cause respiratory alkalosis.

QUICK CHECK 4-5

1. Metabolic acid-base disturbances are caused by alterations in what two chemicals?
2. How do alterations in carbon dioxide influence acid-base states?

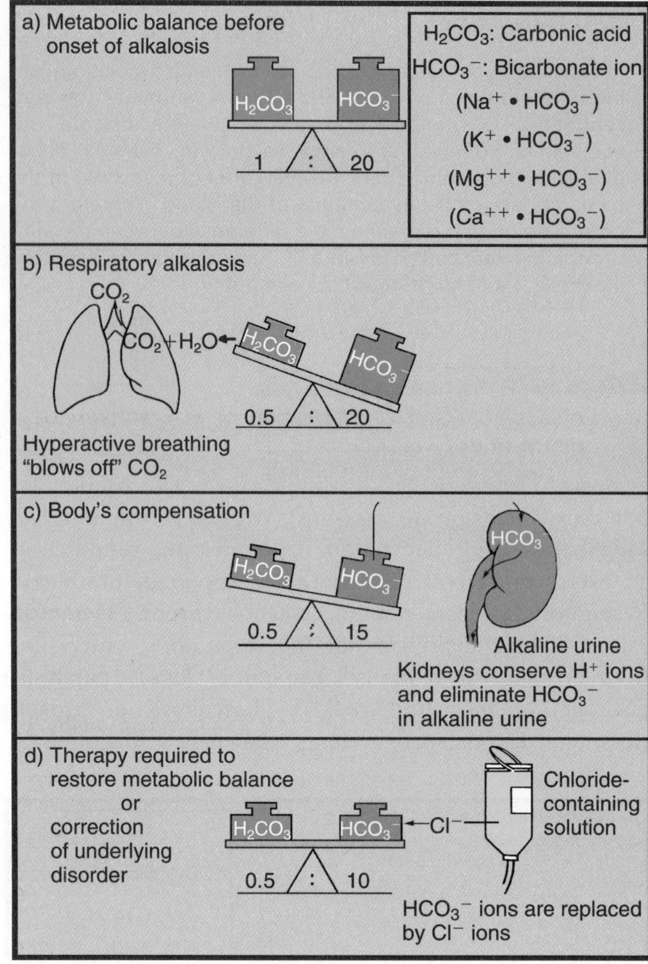

Figure 4-13 ■ **Respiratory Alkalosis.** (From Thibodeau GA, Patton KT: *Anatomy & physiology,* ed 6, St Louis, 2007, Mosby.)

Did You Understand?

Distribution of Body Fluids

1. Body fluids are distributed among functional compartments and are classified as intracellular fluid (ICF) and extracellular fluid (ECF).
2. The sum of all fluids is the total body water (TBW), which varies with age and amount of body fat.
3. Water moves between the ICF and ECF compartments principally by osmosis.
4. Water moves between the plasma and interstitial fluid by osmosis (pulling of water) and hydrostatic pressure (pushing of water), which occur across the capillary membrane.
5. Movement across the capillary wall is called *net filtration* and is described according to Starling's law (the balance between hydrostatic and osmotic forces).

Alterations in Water Movement

1. Edema is a problem of fluid distribution that results in accumulation of fluid within the interstitial spaces.
2. The pathophysiologic process that leads to edema is related to an increase in forces favoring fluid filtration from the capillaries or lymphatic channels into the tissues.
3. Edema is caused by arterial dilation, venous or lymphatic obstruction, increased vascular volume, or increased capillary permeability.
4. Edema may be localized or generalized and usually is associated with weight gain, swelling and puffiness, tighter-fitting clothes and shoes, and limited movement of the affected area.

Sodium, Chloride, and Water Balance

1. Sodium and water balance are intimately related; chloride levels are generally proportional to change in sodium levels.
2. Water balance is regulated by the sensation of thirst and by antidiuretic hormone (ADH), which is secreted in response to by an increase in plasma osmolality or a decrease in circulating blood volume.
3. Sodium balance is regulated by aldosterone, which increases reabsorption of sodium from the urine into the blood by the distal tubule of the kidney.
4. Renin and angiotensin are enzymes that promote secretion of aldosterone and thus regulate sodium and water balance.

Did You Understand?—Cont'd

5. Atrial natriuretic hormone also is involved in decreasing tubular reabsorption and promoting urinary excretion of sodium.

Alterations in Sodium, Chloride, and Water Balance

1. Alterations in water balance may be classified as isotonic, hypertonic, or hypotonic.
2. Isotonic alterations occur when changes in TBW are accompanied by proportional changes in electrolytes.
3. Hypertonic alterations develop when the osmolality of the ECF is elevated above normal, usually because of an increased concentration of ECF sodium or a deficit of ECF water.
4. Hypernatremia (sodium levels more than 147 mEq/L) may be caused by an acute increase in sodium or a loss of water.
5. Water deficit, or hypertonic dehydration, is rare but can be caused by lack of access to water, pure water losses, hyperventilation, arid climates, and increased renal elimination of water.
6. Hyperchloremia is caused by an excess of sodium or a deficit of bicarbonate.
7. Hypotonic alterations occur when the osmolality of the ECF is less than normal.
8. Hyponatremia (serum sodium concentration less than 135 mEq/L) usually causes movement of water into cells.
9. Hyponatremia may be caused by sodium loss, inadequate sodium intake, or dilution of the body's sodium level with excess water.
10. Water excess is rare but can be caused by compulsive water drinking, decreased urine formation, or the syndrome of inappropriate secretion of ADH (SIADH).
11. Hypochloremia usually is the result of hyponatremia or elevated bicarbonate concentrations.

Alterations in Potassium and Other Electrolytes

1. Potassium is the predominant ICF ion; it regulates ICF osmolality, maintains the resting membrane potential, and is required for deposition of glycogen in liver and skeletal muscle cells.
2. Potassium balance is regulated by the kidney, by aldosterone and insulin secretion, and by changes in pH.
3. The mechanism of potassium tolerance or adaptation allows the body to accommodate slowly to increased levels of potassium intake.
4. Hypokalemia (serum potassium concentration less than 3.5 mEq/L) indicates loss of total body potassium, although ECF hypokalemia can develop without losses of total body potassium, and plasma potassium levels may be normal or elevated when total body potassium is depleted.
5. Hypokalemia may be caused by reduced potassium intake, a shift from ECF to ICF potassium, increased aldosterone, and increased renal excretion.
6. Hyperkalemia (potassium levels that are more than 5.5 mEq/L) may be caused by increased potassium intake, a shift from ICF to ECF potassium, or decreased renal excretion.
7. Calcium is a necessary ion in the structure of bones and teeth, in blood clotting, in hormone secretion and the function of cell receptors, and in membrane stability.
8. Phosphate acts as a buffer in acid-base regulation and provides energy for muscle contraction.
9. Calcium and phosphate concentrations are rigidly controlled by parathyroid hormone (PTH), vitamin D, and calcitonin.
10. Hypocalcemia (serum calcium concentration less than 8.5 mg/dl) is related to inadequate intestinal absorption, deposition of calcium into bone or soft tissue, blood administration, or decreased PTH and vitamin D levels.
11. Hypercalcemia (serum calcium concentration more than 12 mg/dl) can be caused by a number of diseases, including hyperparathyroidism, bone metastases, sarcoidosis, and excess vitamin D.
12. Hypophosphatemia is usually caused by intestinal malabsorption and increased renal excretion of phosphate.
13. Hyperphosphatemia develops with acute or chronic renal failure when there is significant loss of glomerular filtration.
14. Magnesium is a major intracellular cation and is regulated principally by PTH.
15. Magnesium functions in enzymatic reactions and often interacts with calcium at the cellular level.
16. Hypomagnesemia (serum magnesium concentrations less than 1.5 mEq/L) may be caused by malabsorption syndromes.
17. Hypermagnesemia (serum magnesium concentrations more than 2.5 mEq/L) is rare and usually is caused by renal failure.

Acid-Base Balance

1. Hydrogen ions, which maintain membrane integrity and the speed of enzymatic reactions, must be concentrated within a narrow range if the body is to function normally.
2. Hydrogen ion concentration [H^+] is expressed as pH, which represents the negative logarithm (i.e., 10^{-7}) of hydrogen ions in solution (i.e., .0000001).
3. Different body fluids have different pH values.
4. The renal and respiratory systems, together with the body's buffer systems, are the principal regulators of acid-base balance.
5. Buffers are substances that can absorb excessive acid or base without a significant change in pH.
6. Buffers exist as acid-base pairs; the principal plasma buffers are carbonic acid–bicarbonate, protein (hemoglobin), and phosphate.
7. The lungs and kidneys act to compensate for changes in pH by increasing or decreasing ventilation and by producing more acidic or more alkaline urine.
8. Correction is a process different from compensation; correction occurs when the values for both components of the buffer pair return to normal.
9. Acid-base imbalances are caused by changes in the concentration of hydrogen in the blood; an increase causes acidosis, and a decrease causes alkalosis.

(Continued)

Did You Understand?—Cont'd

10. An abnormal increase or decrease in bicarbonate concentration causes metabolic alkalosis or metabolic acidosis; changes in the rate of alveolar ventilation and removal of carbon dioxide produce respiratory acidosis or respiratory alkalosis.
11. Metabolic acidosis is caused by an increase in noncarbonic acids or loss of bicarbonate from the extracellular fluid.
12. Metabolic alkalosis occurs with an increase in bicarbonate usually caused by loss of metabolic acids from conditions such as vomiting or gastrointestinal suctioning or from excessive bicarbonate intake, hyperaldosteronism, and diuretic therapy, which increase plasma bicarbonate.
13. Respiratory acidosis occurs with a decrease in alveolar ventilation, which in turn causes hypercapnia (an increase in carbon dioxide) and increases in carbonic acid concentration.
14. Respiratory alkalosis occurs with alveolar hyperventilation and excessive reduction of carbon dioxide, or hypocapnia with decreases in carbonic acid.

Key Terms

References

1. O'Brien JC, Chennubhotla SA, Chennubhotla RV: Treatment of edema, *Am Fam Physician* 17(11):2111–2117, 2005.
2. Linnitt N: Lymphoedema: recognition, assessment and management, *Br J Community Nurs* 10(3):S20–S26, 2005.
3. Suzuki T, Yamazaki T, Yazaki Y: The role of natriuretic peptides in the cardiovascular system, *Cardiovasc Res* 51 (3):489–494, 2001.
4. Cea LB: Natriuretic peptide family: new aspects, *Curr Med Chem Cardiovasc Hematol Agents* 3(2):87–87, 2005.
5. Lin M, Liu SJ, Lim IT: Disorders of water balance, *Emerg Med Clin North Am* 23(3):749–770, 2005ix.
6. Offenstadt G, Das V: Hyponatremia, hypernatremia: a physiological approach, *Minerva Anestesiol* 72(6):353–356, 2006.
7. Lee CAB, Barrett CA, Ignatavicius D: *Fluids and electrolytes: a practical approach,* ed 4, Philadelphia, 1996, FA Davis.
8. Yeates KE, Singer M, Morton AR: Salt and water: a simple approach to hyponatremia, *CMAJ* 170(3):365–369, 2004.
9. Siragy HM: Hyponatremia, fluid-electrolyte disorders and the syndrome of inappropriate antidirectic hormone secretion: diagnosis and treatment options, *Endocr Prac* (4):446–457, 2006.
10. Guyton AC, Hall JE: *Textbook of medical physiology,* Philadelphia, 2006, Saunders p. 370, 2006.
11. Schaefer TJ, Wolford RW: Disorders of potassium, *Emerg Med Clin North Am* 23(3):723–747, 2005.
12. Evans KJ, Greenberg A: Hyperkalemia: a review, *J Intensive Care Med* 20(5):272–290, 2005.
13. Simpson H: Interpretation of arterial blood gases: a clinical guide for nurses, *Br J Nurs* 13(9):522–528, 2004.
14. Herd AM: An approach to complex acid-base problems: keeping it simple, *Can Fam Physician* 51:226–232, 2005.
15. Casaletto JJ: Differential diagnosis of metabolic acidosis, *Emerg Med Clin North Am* 23(3):771–787, 2005.
16. Khanna A, Kurtzman NA: Metabolic alkalosis, *J Nephrol* 19 (Suppl 9):S86–96, 2006.
17. Epstein SK, Singh N: Respiratory acidosis, *Respir Care* 46 (4):366–383, 2001.
18. Foster GT, Vaziri ND, Sassoon CS: Respiratory alkalosis, *Respir Care* 46(4):384–391, 2001.

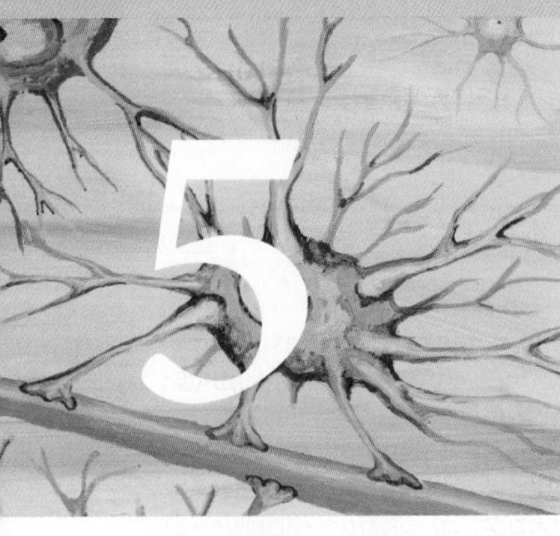

5 INNATE DEFENSES: INFLAMMATION

Neal S. Rote

CHAPTER OUTLINE

ELECTRONIC RESOURCES

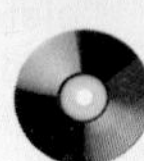

Companion CD
- Review Questions and Answers
- Animations

evolve Website
http://evolve.elsevier.com/Huether/
- Quick Check Answers
- Key Terms Exercises
- Critical Thinking Questions with Answers
- Algorithm Completion Exercises
- WebLinks

The human body is continually exposed to a large variety of conditions that result in damage, such as sunlight, pollutants, agents that can cause physical trauma, and infectious agents (viruses, bacteria, fungi, parasites). Damage can also arise from within, such as cancers. The damage may be at the level of a single cell, which can be easily repaired, or may be at the level of multiple cells or tissues or organs, which can result in disease and potentially the death of the individual.

To protect us from these conditions, the body has developed a highly sophisticated, multilevel system of interactive defense mechanisms. These mechanisms include highly effective physical (e.g., skin, mucous membranes) and chemical (e.g., enzymes in perspiration and tears) barriers that minimize the damaging effects of environmental agents. These barriers are supplemented by rapidly activated biochemical and cellular responses (inflammation) that limit damage and initiate repair and inducible responses (immune response) that increase the body's long-term protective capacity against specific and highly dangerous infectious agents.

HUMAN DEFENSE MECHANISMS

The human body has developed several means of protecting itself from injury and infection. **Innate resistance,** also known as natural or native immunity, includes natural barriers (physical, mechanical, and biochemical) and inflammation (Table 5-1). A variety of innate barriers form the first line of defense at the body's surfaces and are in place at birth to prevent damage by substances in the environment and thwart infection by pathogenic microorganisms.[1]

TABLE 5-1

Overview of Human Defenses

	INNATE IMMUNITY		
Characteristics	**Barriers**	**Inflammatory Response**	**Adaptive (Acquired) Immunity**
Level of defense	First line of defense against infection and tissue injury	Second line of defense; occurs as a response to tissue injury or infection	Third line of defense; becomes active when innate immune system signals the cells of adaptive immunity
Timing of defense	Constant	Immediate response	Delay between exposure to antigen and maximum response
Specificity	Broadly specific	Broadly specific	Very specific
Cells	Epithelial cells forming anatomic barriers (i.e., skin and mucous membranes)	Mast cells, granulocytes (neutrophils, eosinophils, basophils), monocytes/ macrophages, NK cells, platelets, endothelial cells	T lymphocytes, B lymphocytes, macrophages, dendritic cells
Memory	No memory	No memory	Specific immunologic memory by T and B lymphocytes
Protein factors	Toxins from epithelial cells, lysozyme, bacterial toxins	Complement, clotting factors, kinins	Antibodies, complement
Cytokines and chemokines	Few	Many	Many

If the surface barriers are breached, the second line of defense, the **inflammatory response,** is activated to protect the body from further injury, prevent infection of the injured tissue, and promote healing. The inflammatory response is a rapid activation of biochemical and cellular mechanisms that are relatively nonspecific, with similar responses being initiated against a wide variety of causes of tissue damage. The third line of defense, **adaptive immunity** (also known as acquired or specific immunity), is induced in a relatively slower and more specific process. The immune response targets particular invading microorganisms for the purpose of eradicating them. Adaptive immunity also involves "memory," which results in a more rapid response during future exposure to the same microorganism.

FIRST LINE OF DEFENSE: PHYSICAL, MECHANICAL, AND BIOCHEMICAL BARRIERS

Physical and Mechanical Barriers

The physical barriers that cover the external parts of the human body offer considerable protection from damage and invasion by pathogens. These barriers are composed of tightly associated epithelial cells of the skin and of the membranes lining the gastrointestinal, genitourinary, and respiratory tracts. When pathogens attempt to penetrate this physical barrier, they may be removed by mechanical means—sloughed off with dead skin cells as they are routinely replaced, expelled by coughing or sneezing, vomited from the stomach, or flushed from the urinary tract by urine. Epithelial cells of the upper respiratory tract also produce mucus and have hairlike cilia that trap and move pathogens upward to be expelled by coughing or sneezing. Additionally, the low temperature on the body's surface generally inhibits microorganisms, most of which routinely require temperatures near 37° C for efficient growth.

Biochemical Barriers

Epithelial surfaces also secrete substances meant to trap or destroy pathogens. Mucus, perspiration (or sweat), saliva, tears, and earwax are all examples of biochemical secretions that can trap potential invaders and contain substances that will kill microorganisms. Perspiration, tears, and saliva contain an enzyme (lysozyme) that attacks the cell walls of gram-positive bacteria. Sebaceous glands in the skin also secrete fatty acids and lactic acid that kill bacteria and fungi. These glandular secretions create an acidic (pH 3 to 5) and inhospitable environment for most bacteria. Epithelial cells secrete small molecular weight proteins, generically termed **antimicrobial peptides,** that are toxic to certain bacteria, fungi, and viruses.

A spectrum of nonpathogenic bacteria, which is collectively called the **normal bacterial flora,** resides on the body's surfaces. The normal flora contributes to our innate protection against pathogenic microorganisms. Colonization of the lower gut begins quickly after birth, and the number and concentration of microorganisms increases progressively during the first year of life. Many of these microorganisms help digest fatty acids, large polysaccharides, and other dietary substances; produce vitamin K; and assist in the absorption of various ions, such as calcium, iron, and magnesium. They also produce chemicals (ammonia, phenols, indols, and other toxic chemicals) that inhibit colonization by pathogenic microorganisms.

Prolonged antibiotic treatment can alter the normal intestinal flora, decreasing its protective activity, and lead to an overgrowth of pathogenic microorganisms, such as the yeast *Candida albicans* or the bacteria *Clostridium difficile.*

The bacterium *Lactobacillus* is a major constituent of the normal vaginal flora in healthy women. This microorganism produces chemicals (hydrogen peroxide, lactic acid, and other molecules) that help prevent infections of the vagina and urinary tract by other bacteria and yeast. Diminished colonization with lactobacilli (e.g., as a result of prolonged antibiotic treatment) increases the risk for urologic or vaginal infections, such as vaginosis.

SECOND LINE OF DEFENSE: INFLAMMATION

Virtually any injury to vascularized (having a blood supply) tissues will activate inflammation. The classic symptoms of inflammation include redness, heat, swelling, pain, and loss of function. Characteristic microscopic changes also occur within seconds (Figure 5-1). These include the following:

1. Vasodilation (increased size of the blood vessels), which causes slower blood velocity and increases blood flow to the injured site
2. Increased vascular permeability (the blood vessels become porous) and leakage of fluid out of the vessel, causing swelling (edema) at the site of injury; as plasma moves outward, blood in the microcirculation becomes more viscous and flows more slowly, and the increased blood flow and increasing concentration of red cells at the site of inflammation cause locally increased warmth and redness
3. White blood cell adherence to the inner walls of vessels and their migration through enlarged junctions between the endothelial cells lining the vessels into the surrounding tissue

Each of the characteristic changes associated with inflammation is the direct result of the activation and interactions of a host of chemicals and cellular components found in the blood and tissues (Figure 5-2). The vascular changes deliver leukocytes, plasma proteins, and other biochemical mediators to the site of injury, where they act in

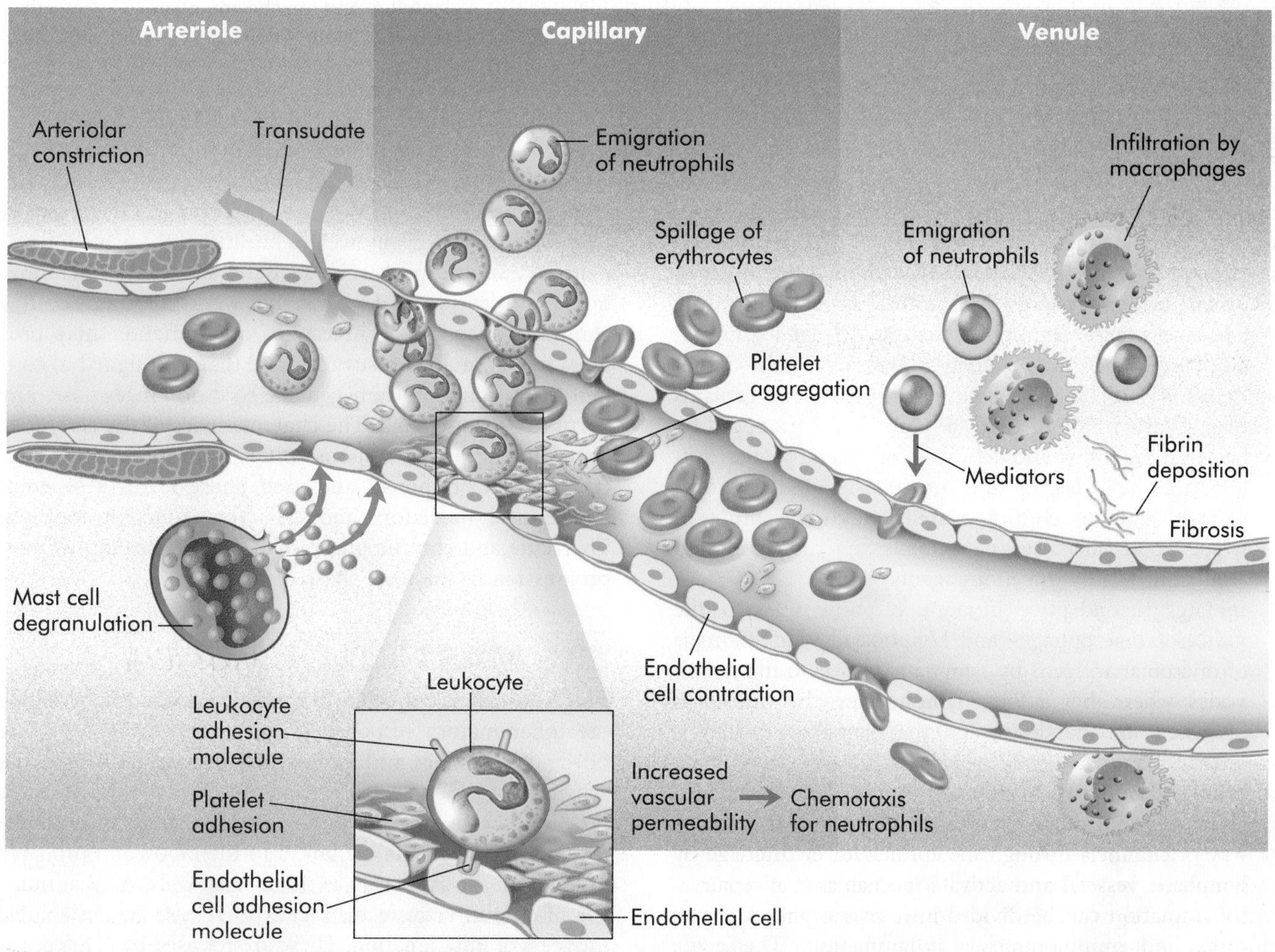

Figure 5-1 ■ **The Sequence of Events in the Process of Inflammation.** See the text for details.

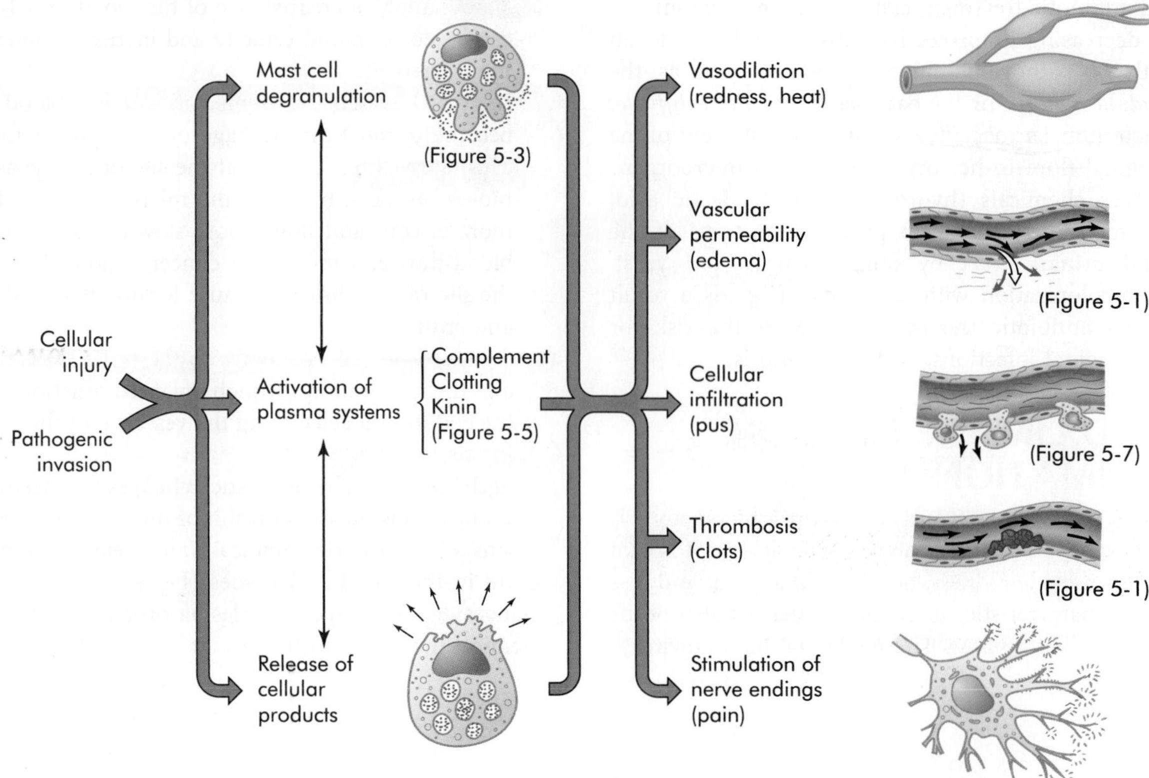

Figure 5-2 ■ **Acute Inflammatory Response.** Inflammation is usually initiated by cellular injury and may be complicated by infection. Mast cell degranulation, the activation of three plasma systems, and the release of subcellular components from the damaged cells occur as a consequence. These systems are interdependent, so that induction of one (e.g., mast cell degranulation) can result in the induction of the other two. The result is the development of the characteristic microscopic and clinical hallmarks of inflammation. The figure numbers refer to additional figures in which more detailed information may be found on that portion of the response.

concert. There are several benefits of inflammation. They include the following:

1. Limits and controls tissue damage through the influx of plasma protein systems (e.g., clotting system) and white blood cells (e.g., eosinophils) that prevent the inflammatory response from spreading to areas of healthy tissue
2. Prevents infection by contaminating microorganisms through the influx of fluid to dilute toxins produced by bacteria, the influx and activation of plasma protein systems that help destroy and contain bacteria (e.g., complement system, clotting system), and the influx of white blood cells (e.g., neutrophils, macrophages) that "eat" and destroy infectious agents
3. Initiates the adaptive immune response through the influx of macrophages and lymphocytes and drainage of microbial antigens by lymphatic vessels to the lymph nodes, where they activate lymphocytes (this process is discussed in Chapter 6, and the lymphatic system is described in Chapter 22)
4. Initiates healing through removal of bacterial products, dead cells, and other products of inflammation (e.g., by way of channels through the epithelium or drainage by lymphatic vessels) and activate mechanisms of repair

Inflammation can be divided into several phases: acute, chronic, and granulomatosus inflammation. The acute inflammatory response is self-limiting—that is, it continues only until the threat to the host is eliminated. This usually takes 8 to 10 days from onset to healing. If the acute inflammatory response proves inadequate, a chronic inflammation may develop and persist for weeks or months. If a continued response is necessary, inflammation may progress to a granulomatosus response that is designed to contain the infection or damaged site so it no longer poses any harm to the individual. The characteristics of the early (i.e., acute) inflammatory response differ from those of the later (i.e., chronic) response, and each phase involves different biochemical mediators and cells that function together. The acute and chronic phases may lead to healing without progression to the next phase.

THE MAST CELL * starts it all

The mast cell is probably the most important activator of the inflammatory response (Figure 5-3).[2] **Mast cells** are filled with granules and located in the loose connective tissues close to blood vessels near the body's outer surfaces (i.e., in the skin and lining the gastrointestinal and respiratory tracts). Basophils are found in the blood and probably function in the same way as tissue mast cells. A great number of stimuli activate mast cells to release potent soluble inducers of inflammation. These are released by (1) **degranulation** (the release of the contents of mast cell granules) and

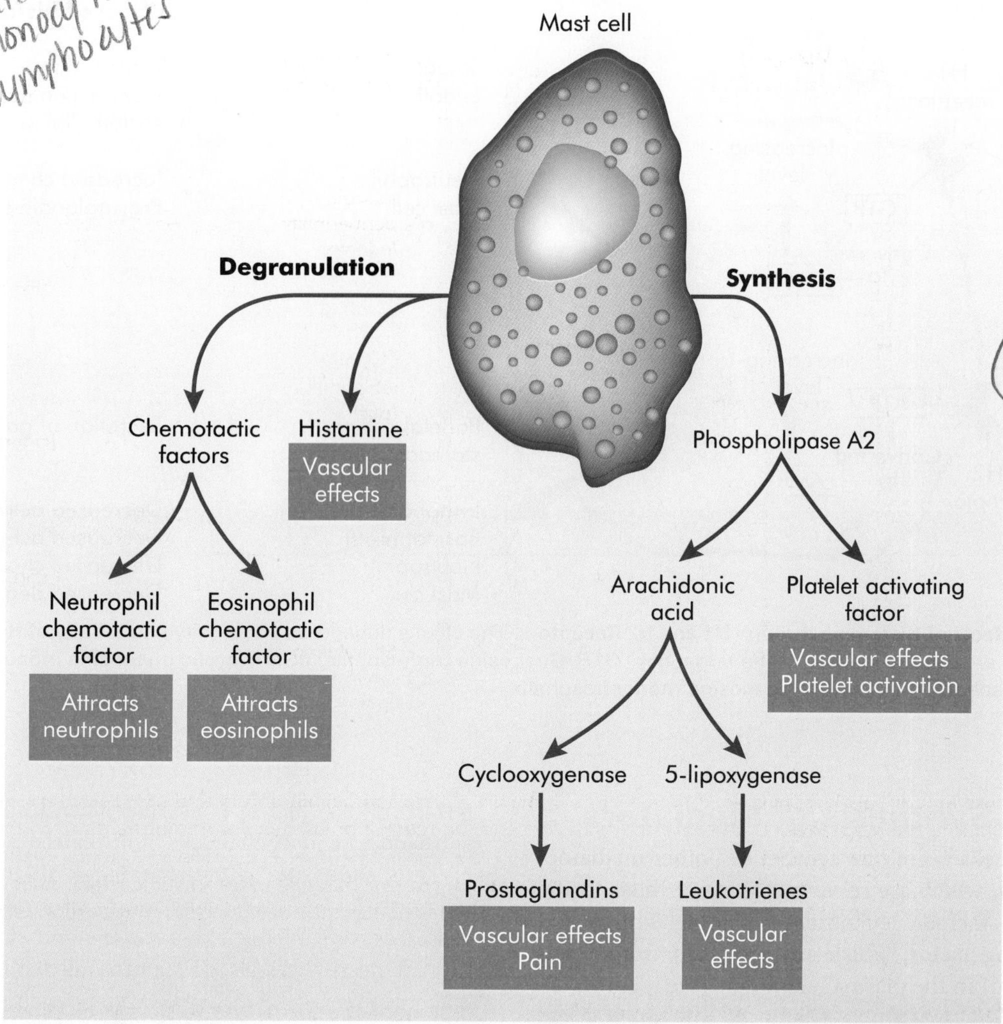

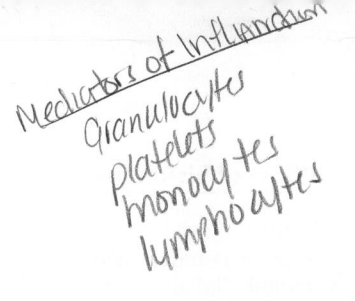

Figure 5-3 **Degranulation (left) and Synthesis (right) of Biologic Mediators by Mast Cells during Inflammation.** Mast cells are filled with darkly staining granules that contain a large number of biologically active substances. Among these are histamine, which is a major initiator of vascular changes, and a variety of chemotactic factors. These substances are released immediately after stimulation of mast cells. Other substances are synthesized in response to mast cell stimulation. These include lipid-based molecules that originate from plasma membrane phospholipids as a result of the action of phospholipase A2. These include platelet-activating factor and a variety of prostaglandins and leukotrienes.

(2) *synthesis* (the new production and release of mediators in response to a stimulus).

Mast Cell Degranulation

In response to a stimulus, biologically active molecules are released from the mast cell granules within seconds and exert their effects immediately. These molecules include histamine and chemotactic factors.

Histamine is a small weight molecule with potent effects on many other cells, particularly those that control the circulation. Histamine, along with serotonin (found in many cells, but not human mast cells), is called a vasoactive amine. These molecules cause temporary, rapid constriction of smooth muscle and dilation of the postcapillary venules, which results in increased blood flow into the microcirculation. Histamine also causes increased vascular permeability resulting from retraction of endothelial cells lining the capillaries (see Figures 5-1 and 5-7) and increased adherence of leukocytes to the endothelium. Histamine affects cells by binding to histamine H1 and H2 receptors on the target cell surface (Figure 5-4). Antihistamines are drugs that block the binding of histamine to its receptors, resulting in decreased inflammation.

Mast cell granules also contain **chemotactic factors.** Chemotactic factors diffuse from a site of inflammation forming a gradient and causing the directional movement (**chemotaxis**) of cells toward the inflammation (see Figure 5-7). The mast cell contains two specific chemotactic factors: **neutrophil chemotactic factor** and **eosinophil chemotactic factor of anaphylaxis (ECF-A).** Neutrophils are the predominant cell needed to kill bacteria in the early stages of inflammation. Eosinophils help regulate the inflammatory response. Both cells are discussed in more detail later in this chapter.

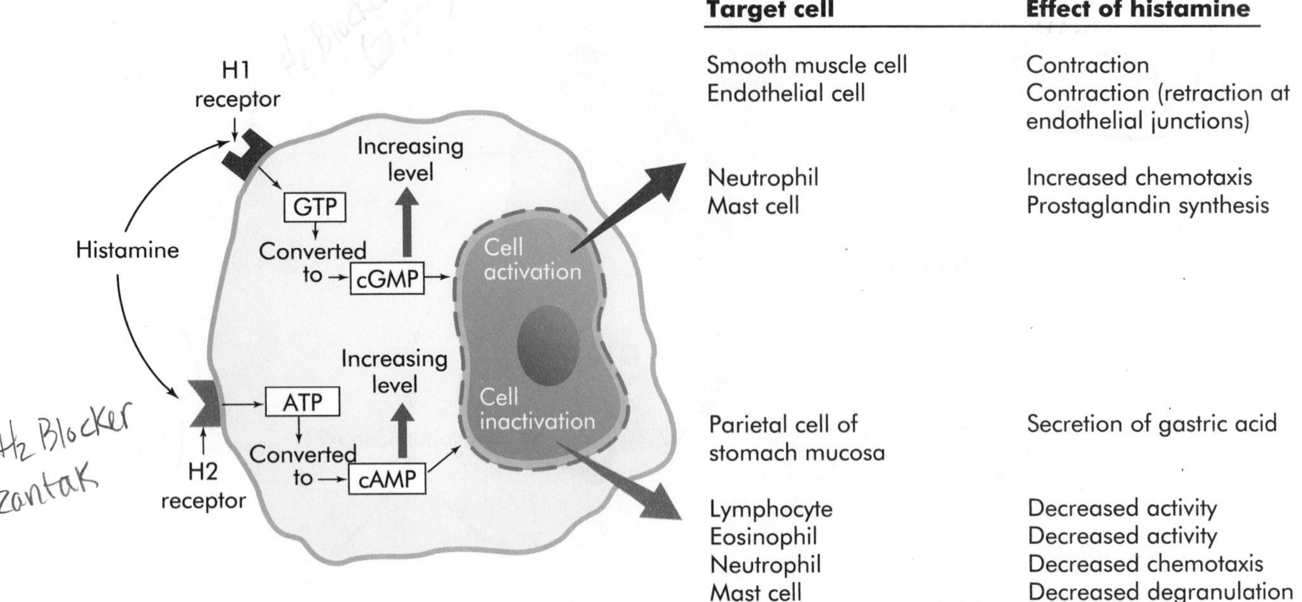

H1
receptor
Increasing
level
GTP
Histamine
Converted
to
cGMP
Cell
activation
Increasing
level
ATP
Cell
inactivation
Converted
to
cAMP
H2
receptor
Target cell
Effect of histamine
Smooth muscle cell
Contraction
Endothelial cell
Contraction (retraction at endothelial junctions)
Neutrophil
Increased chemotaxis
Mast cell
Prostaglandin synthesis
Parietal cell of stomach mucosa
Secretion of gastric acid
Lymphocyte
Decreased activity
Eosinophil
Decreased activity
Neutrophil
Decreased chemotaxis
Mast cell
Decreased degranulation

Figure 5-4 ■ **Effects of Histamine through H1 and H2 Receptors.** The effects depend on (1) density and affinity of H1 or H2 receptors on the target cell and (2) the identity of the target cell. *GTP,* Guanosine triphosphate; *cGMP,* cyclic guanosine monophosphate; *ATP,* adenosine triphosphate; *cAMP,* cyclic adenosine monophosphate.

Mast Cell Synthesis of Mediators

Activated mast cells begin new synthesis of other mediators of inflammation, which are released later than those in the granules. These include leukotrienes, prostaglandins, and platelet-activating factor, which are produced from lipids (arachidonic acid) in the plasma membrane (see Figure 5-4). **Leukotrienes (slow-reacting substances of anaphylaxis [SRS-A])** are sulfur-containing lipids that produce histamine-like effects: smooth muscle contraction and increased vascular permeability. Leukotrienes appear to be important in the later stages of the inflammatory response because they stimulate slower and more prolonged responses than do histamines.

Prostaglandins cause increased vascular permeability, neutrophil chemotaxis, and pain by direct effects on nerves. They are long-chain, unsaturated fatty acids produced by the action of the enzyme cyclooxygenase on arachidonic acid from membrane phospholipids and are classified into groups (E, D, A, F, and B) according to their structure. Prostaglandins E_1 and E_2 cause increased vascular permeability and smooth muscle contraction. Aspirin and some other nonsteroidal anti-inflammatory drugs (NSAIDs) block the synthesis of prostaglandins of the E series and other arachidonic acid derivatives, thereby inhibiting inflammation.

Platelet-activating factor (PAF) is produced by removal of a fatty acid from the plasma membrane phospholipid by phospholipase A2. Although mast cells are a major source of PAF, this molecule also can be produced during inflammation by neutrophils, monocytes, endothelial cells, and platelets. The biologic activity of PAF is virtually identical to that of leukotrienes, namely causing endothelial cell retraction to increase vascular permeability, leukocyte adhesion to endothelial cells, and platelet activation.

Thus, at a site of tissue damage all the hallmarks of inflammation are caused by mast cell products. Histamine causes dilation of the blood vessels and slows the circulation in nearby vessels. Histamine also causes endothelial cells to change their shapes and open intercellular junctions, which allows fluid to leak from the blood into the surrounding tissues. Increased blood flow and vasodilation result in increased redness and warmth, and increased vascular permeability results in local swelling from increased fluid in the tissues. Lipid-derived mediators are released later and continue the inflammatory process through histamine-like effects and cause pain.

QUICK CHECK 5-1

1. How are the five classic superficial symptoms of inflammation related to the process of inflammation?
2. What two phagocytic cell types are involved in the acute inflammatory response? What is the role of each?
3. What products do the mast cells release during inflammation, and what are their effects?
4. How do leukotrienes and prostaglandins function in inflammation?

PLASMA PROTEIN SYSTEMS

Three key **plasma protein systems** are essential to an effective inflammatory response. These are the complement system, the clotting system, and the kinin system (Figure 5-5). Although each system has a unique role in inflammation,

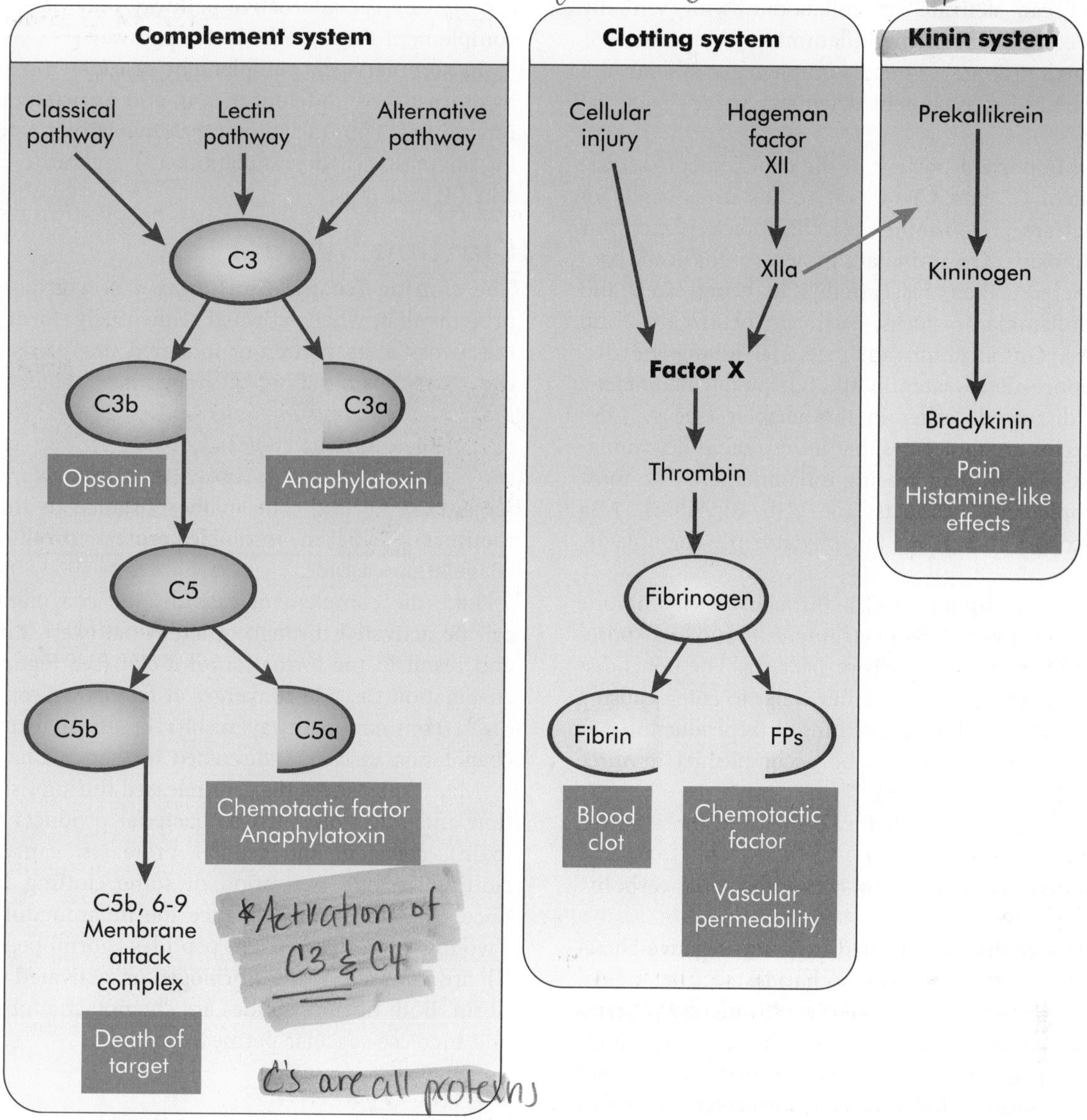

Figure 5-5 ■ **Plasma Protein Systems in Inflammation: Complement, Clotting, and Kinin Systems.** See the text for more detailed information. In this scheme some systems are activated by multiple pathways that come together (at C3 for the complement system and factor X for the clotting system). Some of the components of the pathways are activated by being split into two active components (C3 and C5 of the complement system and fibrinogen of the clotting system). The larger of the components usually activates the next component of the pathway (as do C3b and C5b of the complement system). Hageman factor participated in both the clotting and kinin pathways (i.e., activated factor XII [XIIa] helps activate factor X and prekallikrein). Many of the components of each pathway have potent biologic activities (in red colored boxes). Many other components of each pathway are not shown in this drawing but play very important roles in activation of the pathway. *FP,* Fibrinopeptides.

they have many similarities. Each system consists of multiple proteins in the blood. To prevent activation in unnecessary situations, each protein is normally in an inactive form. Several of the proteins are enzymes that circulate in inactive forms as proenzymes. Each system contains a few proteins that can be activated by products of tissue damage or infection. Activation of the first component results in sequential activation of other components of the system, leading to a biologic function that helps protect the individual. This sequential activation is referred to as a cascade. Thus, we refer to the complement cascade, the clotting cascade, or the kinin cascade. In some cases, activation of a protein may require that it be enzymatically cut into two pieces of different size. Usually the larger fragment continues the cascade by activating the next component. The smaller fragment frequently has potent biologic activities to promote inflammation.

Complement System

The **complement system** consists of a large number of proteins (sometimes called complement components) that together constitute about 10% of the total circulating serum protein.[3] The complement system is extremely important because activated components can destroy pathogens directly and can activate or collaborate with virtually every other component of the inflammatory response. For these reasons, proteins of the complement system are among the body's most potent defenders against bacterial infection.

The most important portion of the complement cascade is activation of C3 and C5, which results in a variety of subunits that are (1) opsonins, (2) chemotactic factors, or (3) anaphylatoxins. **Opsonins** are molecules that coat bacteria and increase their susceptibility to being eaten and killed by inflammatory cells, such as neutrophils and macrophages. Opsonization and bacterial killing are discussed in more detail later in this chapter. Chemotactic factors are discussed earlier in this chapter (see p. 125). **Anaphylatoxins** are molecules that induce rapid degranulation of mast cells, thus increasing inflammation. The most potent complement products are C3b (opsonin), C3a (anaphylatoxin), and C5a (anaphylatoxin, chemotactic factor).

Complement components C5b through C9 (membrane attack complex, or MAC) form a complex that creates pores in the outer membranes of cells or bacteria. The pores disrupt the cell's membrane and permit water to enter, causing the cell to burst or at least preventing its reproduction.

Complement activation can be accomplished in three different ways (see Figure 5-5):

1. **Classical pathway:** activated by proteins of the acquired immune system (antibodies)
2. **Lectin pathway:** activated by certain bacterial carbohydrates
3. **Alternative pathway:** activated by gram-negative bacterial and fungal cell wall polysaccharides

The classical pathway is primarily activated by proteins of the acquired immune system, antibodies.[4] Antibody must first bind to their targets, called antigens. Antigens can be proteins or carbohydrates from bacteria or other infectious agents. Antigens and antibodies are discussed in more detail in Chapter 6. Antibody activates the first component of complement, C1, which through other complement components leads to activation of C3 and C5. Thus, the acquired immune response (Chapter 6) can use the complement system to kill bacteria and activate inflammation.

The alternative pathway is activated by several substances found on the surface of infectious organisms (e.g., lipopolysaccharides [endotoxin] on the bacterial surface or yeast cell wall carbohydrates [zymosan]).[5] This pathway uses unique proteins (factor B, factor D, and properdin) to form a complex that activates C3. C3 activation leads to C5 activation and convergence with the classical pathway. Thus, the complement system can be directly activated by certain infectious organisms without antibody being present.

The lectin pathway is similar to the classic pathway but is independent of antibody. It is activated by a plasma protein called mannose-binding lectin (MBL). MBL is similar to C1 and binds to bacterial polysaccharides containing the carbohydrate mannose. Thus, infectious agents that do not activate the alternative pathway may be susceptible to complement through the lectin pathway.

In summary, the complement cascades can be activated by at least three different means, and its products have four functions: (1) opsonization, (2) anaphylatoxic activity resulting in mast cell degranulation, (3) leukocyte chemotaxis, and (4) cell lysis.

Clotting System

The **clotting (coagulation) system** is a group of plasma proteins that, when activated sequentially, form a fibrinous meshwork at an injured or inflamed site.[6] This (1) forms a clot that stops bleeding, (2) traps infectious organisms and prevents their spread to adjacent tissues, (3) keeps microorganisms and foreign bodies at the site of greatest inflammatory cell activity, and (4) provides a framework for future repair and healing. The main substance in this fibrinous mesh is fibrin, an insoluble protein produced by the coagulation cascade.

Like the complement cascade, the coagulation cascade can be activated through different pathways that converge and result in the formation of a clot (see Figure 5-5). The coagulation cascade converges at factor X. From that point on, a common pathway results in fibrin formation. The coagulation cascade is discussed further in Chapter 19.

Many substances that are released during tissue destruction and infection, such as bacterial products (e.g., endotoxin), collagen, and cellular proteases, can activate the clotting system. Activation of some clotting factors produces fragments that enhance the inflammatory response. Two low-molecular-weight peptides (fibrinopeptides A and B) are released when fibrinogen is activated to produce fibrin. Both fibrinopeptides are chemotactic for neutrophils and increase vascular permeability.

Kinin System

The third plasma protein system, the **kinin system,** interacts closely with the coagulation system (see Figure 5-5). Both the clotting and kinin systems are activated through activated factor XII (factor XIIa). Another name for factor XIIa is prekallikrein activator because it enzymatically activates the first component of the kinin system, prekallikrein. The final product of the kinin system is a small-molecular-weight molecule, **bradykinin,** which is produced from a larger precursor molecule, kininogen. At low doses, bradykinin causes dilation of blood vessels, acts with prostaglandins to induce pain, causes smooth muscle cell contraction, and increases vascular permeability (see Figures 5-2 and 5-7). Bradykinin induces smooth muscle contraction more slowly than histamine and may be more important during the later phases of inflammation.

Control and Interaction of Plasma Protein Systems

The three plasma protein systems described previously are highly interactive so that activation of one results in secondary activation of the other two. It is beneficial to the individual to activate all three systems, but it would be detrimental if the systems continued producing potent proinflammatory molecules indefinitely. Therefore, the systems are tightly regulated to control and localize inflammation to the appropriate sites. For instance, during clot formation the enzyme **plasmin** is produced from plasminogen. Plasmin limits clot formation by degrading fibrin and fibrinogen and also can activate the complement cascade through components C1, C3, and C5.

Inflammation is tightly regulated at many other levels. Products of these pathways are rapidly modified or destroyed within seconds by enzymes from the plasma. For instance, the anaphylatoxic activities of C3a and C5a are inactivated by the plasma enzyme **carboxypeptidase.** Another inhibitor, **C1 esterase inhibitor (C1 inh)** binds to C1 to inhibit further activation of the classical complement pathway. It also binds to elements of the kinin and clotting systems to prevent or limit their activation. Hereditary angioneurotic edema is an autosomal dominant disease characterized by a deficiency of this inhibitor. In individuals with this disease, emotional stress and other stimuli often cause recurrent edema in the gastrointestinal tract, respiratory tract, and skin, with swelling around the larynx sometimes causing death. The mechanism appears to be episodic, uncontrolled activation of plasmin, resulting in Hageman factor (XII) activation, bradykinin production, and C1 activation.

CELLULAR COMPONENTS OF INFLAMMATION

Several types of cells participate in the inflammatory response. The primary circulating white blood cells are granulocytes, so called because of the many enzyme-containing granules in their cytoplasm. These include neutrophils, eosinophils, and basophils. Other blood components include platelets, monocytes (precursors of macrophages that are found in the tissues), and various forms of lymphocytes. Lymphocyte-like natural killer cells (NK cells) are found both in the circulation and tissues.

Under normal conditions, these circulating cells move unimpeded with the flow of blood. Many of the biochemical mediators are produced by mast cells or from activation of plasma protein systems or are released from dying cells diffuse to the vessels and affect **endothelial cells** that line the vessels and cells in the circulation (see Figure 5-1). All the cells respond by producing new **adhesion molecules** on their surfaces. (Chapter 1 contains information on selectins and integrins.) The change in adhesion molecules on leukocytes, as well as platelets, increases their "stickiness" with the endothelial cells.[7] Thus, at a site of inflammation, white blood cells (particularly neutrophils) and platelets accumulate on the vessel wall.

Additionally, endothelial cells release **nitric oxide (NO),** which has at least two effects on inflammation. First, NO causes vasodilation by inducing relaxation of vascular smooth muscle, a response that is local and short lived. Secondly, NO may suppress mast cell release of inflammatory molecules and decrease platelet adhesion and aggregation.

Neutrophils

The **neutrophil,** or **polymorphonuclear neutrophil (PMN),** is a member of the granulocytic series of white blood cells and is named for the characteristic staining pattern of its granules as well as its multilobed nucleus.[8] Neutrophils are the predominant phagocytes in the early inflammatory site, arriving within 6 to 12 hours after the initial injury. Several inflammatory mediators (e.g., some bacterial proteins, complement fragments C3a and C5a, and mast cell neutrophil chemotactic factor) specifically and rapidly attract neutrophils from the circulation and activate them.

Because the neutrophil is a mature cell that is incapable of division and sensitive to acidic environments, it is short lived at the inflammatory site and becomes a component of the purulent exudate, or pus, which is removed from the body through the epithelium or via the lymphatic system. (The lymphatic system is described in Chapter 22.) The primary roles of the neutrophil are removal of debris and dead cells in sterile lesions, such as burns, and phagocytosis of bacteria in nonsterile lesions.

Monocytes and Macrophages

Monocytes (the immature form of this white blood cell in the blood) and **macrophages** (the mature cell in the tissues) have fewer and larger lysosomes in their cytoplasm than do granulocytes.[9] Monocytes are the largest normal blood cells and have a nucleus that is often indented or horseshoe shaped. Monocytes are produced in the bone marrow, enter the circulation, and migrate to the inflammatory site, where they develop into macrophages. Monocytes also appear to be the precursors of macrophages that are fixed in tissues (tissue macrophages), including Kupffer's cells in the liver, alveolar macrophages in the lungs, and microglia in the brain. Macrophages are generally larger and are more active as phagocytes than their monocytic precursors (Figure 5-6).

Macrophages enter the site after 24 hours or later, and they gradually replace the neutrophils. They migrate to the site after neutrophils because they move more sluggishly and because many of the chemotactic factors that attract them, such as macrophage chemotactic factor, must first be released by neutrophils. Macrophages are better suited than neutrophils to long-term defense against infectious agents because macrophages can survive and divide in the acidic inflammatory site.

Several bacteria are resistant to killing by granulocytes and can even survive inside macrophages. Microorganisms such as *Mycobacterium tuberculosis* (tuberculosis), *Mycobacterium leprae* (leprosy), *Salmonella typhi* (typhoid fever), *Brucella abortus* (brucellosis), and *Listeria monocytogenes* (listeriosis) can remain dormant or multiply inside the phagolysosomes of macrophages. The bactericidal activity of macrophages can increase markedly with the help of inflammatory **cytokines** produced by cells of the acquired immune system (subsets of T lymphocytes) or cells activated through Toll-like receptors (see p. 131). (Cytokines are a family of proteins that are secreted and activate other

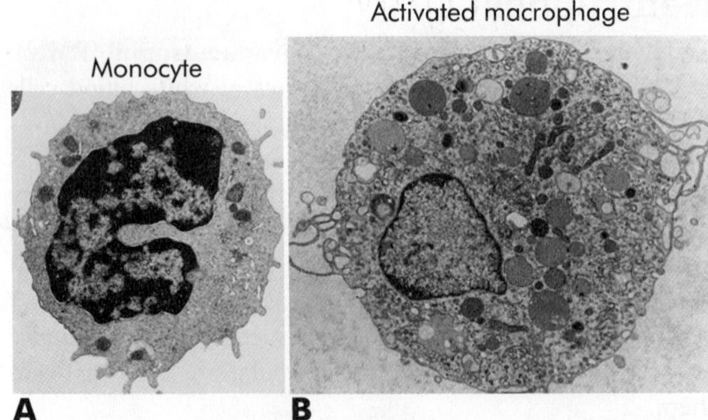

Figure 5-6 ■ Activation of a Macrophage by Cytokines. Some cytokines produced by lymphocytes can react with surface receptors on macrophages and greatly increase their ability to kill bacteria. **A,** Electron micrograph of a peripheral blood monocyte. **B,** Electron micrograph of an activated tissue macrophage showing increases in cytoplasmic volume, plasma membrane, and numbers of lysosomal granules. Additionally, activation includes increases in glucose metabolism, phagocytic activity, and bacterial killing. (**A,** From Abbas AK, Lichtman AH: *Cellular and molecular immunology,* ed 5, Philadelphia, 2003, Saunders; **B,** from Bloom W, Fawcett DW: *A textbook of histology,* ed 11, Philadelphia, 1986, Saunders.)

inflammatory cells. They are discussed in detail later in this chapter.) Macrophages have cell surface receptors for these cytokines and are further activated to become more effective killers of infectious microorganisms.

Eosinophils

Although **eosinophils** are only mildly phagocytic, they have two specific functions: (1) they serve as the body's primary defense against parasites, and (2) they help regulate vascular mediators released from mast cells.[10] Their role in resistance to parasites occurs in collaboration with specific antibodies produced by the acquired immune system and is discussed in Chapter 6.

The second function, regulation of mast cell-derived inflammatory mediators, is a critical function of eosinophils and helps limit inflammation. Mast cells produce eosinophil chemotactic factor-A (ECF-A), which attracts eosinophils to the site of inflammation. Eosinophil lysosomes contain several enzymes that degrade vasoactive molecules, thereby controlling the vascular effects of inflammation. These enzymes include histaminase, which mediates the degradation of histamine, and arylsulfatase B, which degrades some of the lipid-derived mediators produced by mast cells.

Natural Killer (NK) Cells

The main function of **natural killer (NK) cells** is to recognize and eliminate cells infected with viruses and abnormal host cells, specifically cancer cells. Along with Toll-like receptors, NK cells have additional inhibitory and activating receptors that allow them to recognize differences between infected or tumor cells and normal cells. If the NK cell binds to a target cell through activating receptors, it produces several cytokines and toxic molecules that can kill the target. (Mechanisms of cell-to-cell killing by NK cells are discussed further in Chapter 6.)

Platelets

Platelets are cytoplasmic fragments formed from megakaryocytes. They circulate in the bloodstream until vascular injury occurs. After injury, platelets are activated by many products of tissue destruction and inflammation, including collagen, thrombin, and platelet-activating factor. Activation results in (1) their interaction with components of the coagulation cascade to stop bleeding and (2) degranulation, releasing biochemical mediators such as serotonin, which has vascular effects similar to those of histamine. (Platelet function is described in detail in Chapter 19.)

Phagocytosis

Phagocytosis is the process by which a cell ingests and disposes of foreign material, including microorganisms (Figure 5-7). Cells that perform this process are called **phagocytes.** The two most important phagocytes are neutrophils and macrophages. Both cells are circulating in the blood and must first leave the circulation and migrate to the site of inflammation before initiating phagocytosis. The change of surface molecules described earlier increases the adhesion, or stickiness, between leukocytes and endothelial cells, causing the leukocytes to adhere more avidly to the walls of the capillaries and venules in a process called **margination,** or **pavementing.**[11] Adhesion molecules that are expressed later lead to **diapedesis,** or emigration of the cells through the endothelial junctions that have retracted in response to inflammatory mediators.

Once inside the tissue, leukocytes are attracted to the inflammatory site by chemotactic factors. The primary chemotactic factors include many bacterial products, neutrophil chemotactic factor from mast cells, complement fragments C3a and C5a, and products of the clotting and kinin systems.

At the inflammatory site, the process of phagocytosis involves five steps: (1) adherence of the phagocyte to its target, (2) engulfment (ingestion or endocytosis), (3) formation of a phagosome, (4) fusion of the phagosome with lysosomal granules within the phagocyte, and (5) destruction of the target (see Figure 5-7) (lysosomes are described in Chapter 1). Throughout the process, both the target and digestive enzymes are isolated within membrane-bound vesicles. Isolation protects the phagocyte itself from the harmful effects of the target microorganisms, as well as its own enzymes.

Most phagocytes can trap and engulf bacteria that have not been coated with an opsonin. Adherence occurs through groups of innate receptors, **pattern recognition receptors (PRRs),** that bind to unique molecular "patterns" on infectious agents or their products **(pathogen-associated molecular patterns [PAMPs])** or products of cellular

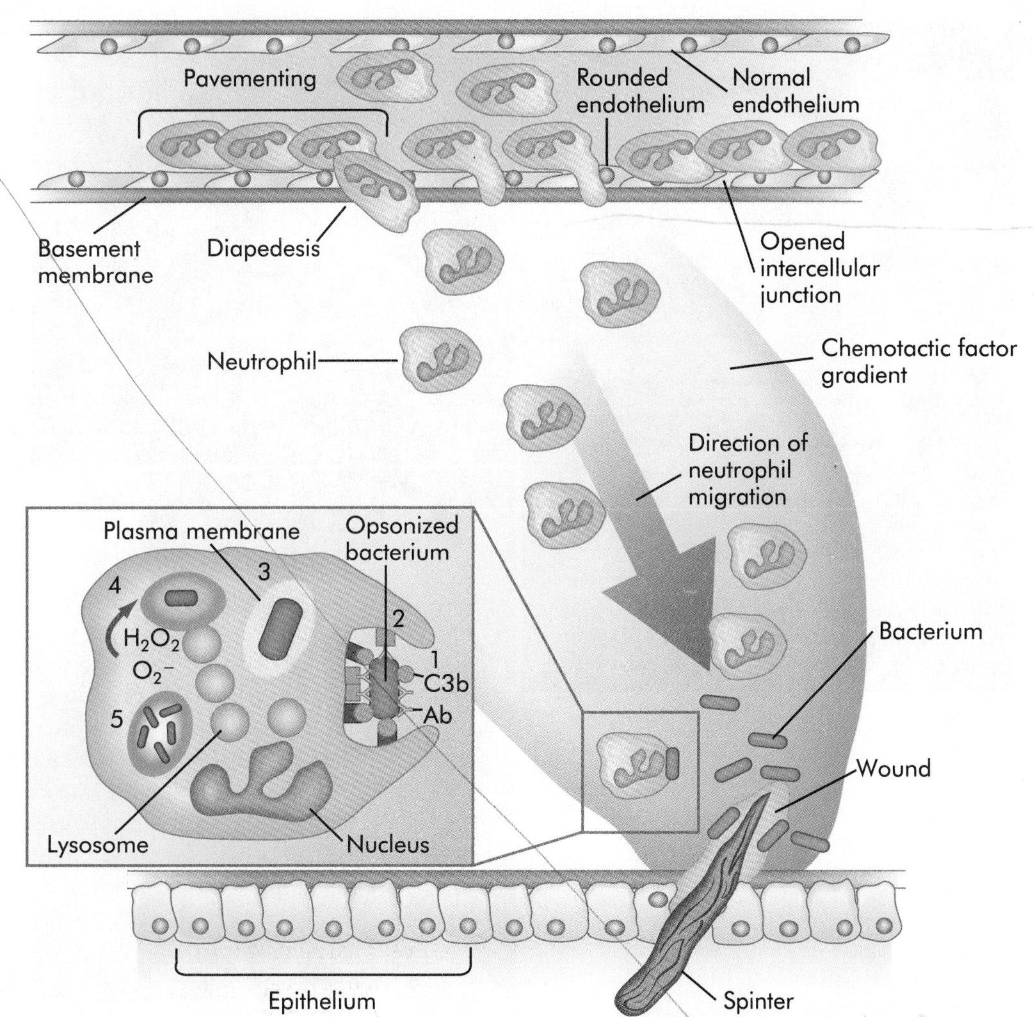

Figure 5-7 ■ **Process of Phagocytosis.** Phagocytosis is a multistep process that involves diffusion of chemotactic factors from a site of injury. Many additional factors affect the blood vessels and increase adhesion molecules on endothelial cells and neutrophils, resulting in adherence of the neutrophils to the vessel wall (pavementing), retraction of endothelial cells (vascular permeability), and movement of the neutrophils through the opened intercellular junctions (diapedesis) and into the tissue. The cells move up the gradient toward the highest concentration of chemotactic factors (chemotaxis). At the site of injury, neutrophils begin phagocytosis of contaminating bacteria. The actual process of phagocytosis involves several steps (see enlargement): **(1)** adherence to the bacteria, which is increased by opsonins such as antibody (Ab) and complement component C3b; **(2)** engulfment of the bacteria by extensions of the neutrophil's membrane (pseudopods); **(3)** formation of a phagosome containing the bacterium surrounded by the neutrophil's plasma membrane; **(4)** fusion of lysosomes with the vacuole to form a phagolysosome and the production of toxic oxygen molecules (H_2O_2, hydrogen peroxide; O_2^-, superoxide); and **(5)** killing and breakdown of the bacterium.

damage.[12] One set of PRRs consists of **Toll-like receptors (TLRs),** at least 10 of which have been described in humans.[13] They are expressed on the surface of phagocytes as well as many cells that have direct contact with potential pathogenic microorganisms. These include mucosal epithelial cells, mast cells, neutrophils, macrophages, and some subpopulations of lymphocytes. TLRs recognize a large variety of chemicals located on the microorganism's cell wall or surface (e.g., bacterial lipopolysaccharide [LPS], peptidoglycans, lipoproteins, yeast zymosan, and viral coat proteins) and on other surface structures (e.g., bacterial flagellin).

Phagocytosis using innate receptors is a relatively slow process. Opsonization greatly enhances adherence by acting as a glue to tighten the affinity of adherence between the phagocyte and the target cell. The most efficient opsonins are antibody and C3b produced by the complement system. Antibodies are made against antigens on the surface of bacteria and are highly specific to that particular microorganism. Certain bacterial and fungal polysaccharide coatings activate the alternative and lectin pathways of complement activation, which deposits C3b on the bacterial surface and increases phagocytosis. The surface of phagocytes contains a variety of specific receptors that will strongly bind to opsonins. These include **complement receptors** that bind to C3b and **Fc receptors** that bind to a site on antibody molecules (discussed in Chapter 6).

Engulfment (endocytosis) is carried out by small pseudopods that extend from the plasma membrane and surround the adherent microorganism (Figure 5-8 and see Figure 5-7)

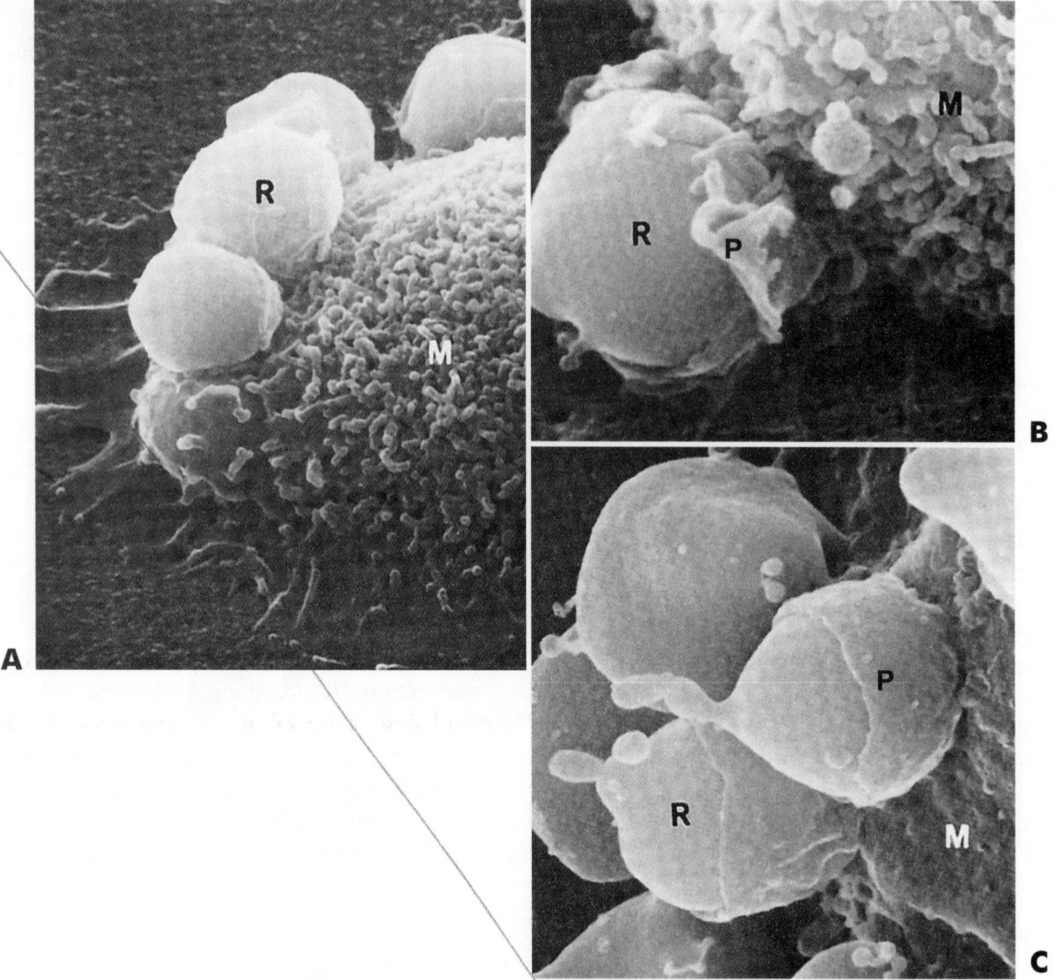

Figure 5-8 ■ **Steps in Phagocytosis.** This scanning electron micrograph shows the progressive steps in phagocytosis of red blood cells by a macrophage. **A,** The macrophage *(M)* attaches to the red blood cells *(R)*. **B,** An extension of the macrophage membrane (*P*; pseudopod) starts to enclose the red cell. **C,** The red blood cells are almost totally engulfed by the macrophage. (Modified from King DW, Fenoglio CM, Lefkowitch JH: *General pathology: principles and dynamics,* Philadelphia, 1983, Lea & Febiger.)

forming an intracellular phagocytic vacuole, or **phagosome.** After the formation of the phagosome, lysosomes converge, fuse with the phagosome, and discharge their contents, creating a **phagolysosome.** Destruction of the bacterium takes place within the phagolysosome and is accomplished by both oxygen-dependent and oxygen-independent mechanisms.[14]

Oxygen-dependent killing mechanisms result from the production of toxic oxygen species. Phagocytosis is accompanied by a burst of oxygen uptake by the phagocyte; this is termed the *respiratory burst* and results from a shift in much of the cell's glucose metabolism to the **hexose-monophosphate shunt,** which produces nicotinamide adenine dinucleotide phosphate (NADPH). A membrane-associated enzyme, NADPH oxidase uses NADPH to generate superoxide (O_2^-), hydrogen peroxide (H_2O_2), and other reactive oxygen species that can be highly damaging to bacteria. Hydrogen peroxide also can collaborate with the lysosomal enzyme myeloperoxidase and halide anions (Cl^- and Br^-) to form acids that kill bacteria and fungi.

Oxygen-independent mechanisms of microbial killing include (1) the acidic pH (3.5 to 4.0) of the phagolysosome, (2) cationic proteins that bind to and damage target cell membranes, (3) enzymatic attack of the microorganism's cell wall by lysozyme and other enzymes, and (4) inhibition of bacterial growth by lactoferrin binding of iron.

When a phagocyte dies at an inflammatory site, it frequently lyses (breaks open) and releases its cytoplasmic contents, including the lysosomal enzymes, into the tissue. They can digest the connective tissue matrix, causing much of the tissue destruction associated with inflammation. The destructive effects of many enzymes released by dying phagocytes are minimized by natural inhibitors found in the blood, such as **α1-antitrypsin,** a plasma protein produced by the liver. An inherited deficiency of α_1-antitrypsin often leads to chronic lung damage and emphysema as a result of inflammation. (The pulmonary effects of α_1-antitrypsin deficiency are described in Chapter 26.) Released lysosomal products also may contribute to inflammation by increasing vascular permeability, attracting additional monocytes, and activating the complement and kinin systems.

QUICK CHECK 5-2

1. What are the four major functions of the complement system?
2. How is the coagulation cascade activated? How is it related to the plasma kinin cascade?
3. What factors control the plasma protein systems?
4. What are the four steps in the process of phagocytosis?

CELLULAR PRODUCTS

For inflammation to occur, many different kinds of cells must cooperate. That cooperation is achieved by the secretion of a variety of proteins that affect other cells. These factors are referred to as cytokines or chemokines.[15] They can be either proinflammatory or anti-inflammatory in nature, depending on whether they tend to induce or inhibit the inflammatory response. These molecules usually diffuse over short distances, bind to the appropriate target cells, and affect the function of the target cell. Some effects occur over long distances, such as the systemic induction of fever by some cytokines (i.e., endogenous pyrogens) that are produced at an inflammatory site. Cytokine and chemokine effects on another cell are mediated through specific cell-surface receptors. The binding of cytokines or chemokines to a target cell often induces synthesis of additional cellular products.

Cytokines

The majority of important cytokines are classified as interleukins (ILs) or interferons (IFNs) (Figure 5-9). Other critical cytokines, however, are not classified as either. Many of these same cytokines are produced by cells of the acquired immune system in response to specific antigens and are discussed further in Chapter 6.

Interleukins

The **interleukins (IL)** are produced predominantly by macrophages and lymphocytes in response to their recognition of a pathogen or stimulation by other products of inflammation.

Interleukin-1 (IL-1) is a proinflammatory cytokine produced mainly by macrophages. IL-1 is an endogenous pyrogen (i.e., fever-causing cytokine) that reacts with receptors on cells of the hypothalamus and affects the body's thermostat resulting in fever. It also activates phagocytes and lymphocytes, thereby enhancing both the innate and acquired immunity, and acts as a growth factor for many cells. It has several effects on neutrophils, including induction of proliferation (resulting in an increase in the number of circulating neutrophils), chemotaxis, increased cellular respiration, and increased lysosomal enzyme activity.

Interleukin-6 (IL-6) is produced by macrophages, lymphocytes, fibroblasts, and other cells. It directly induces hepatocytes (liver cells) to produce many of the proteins

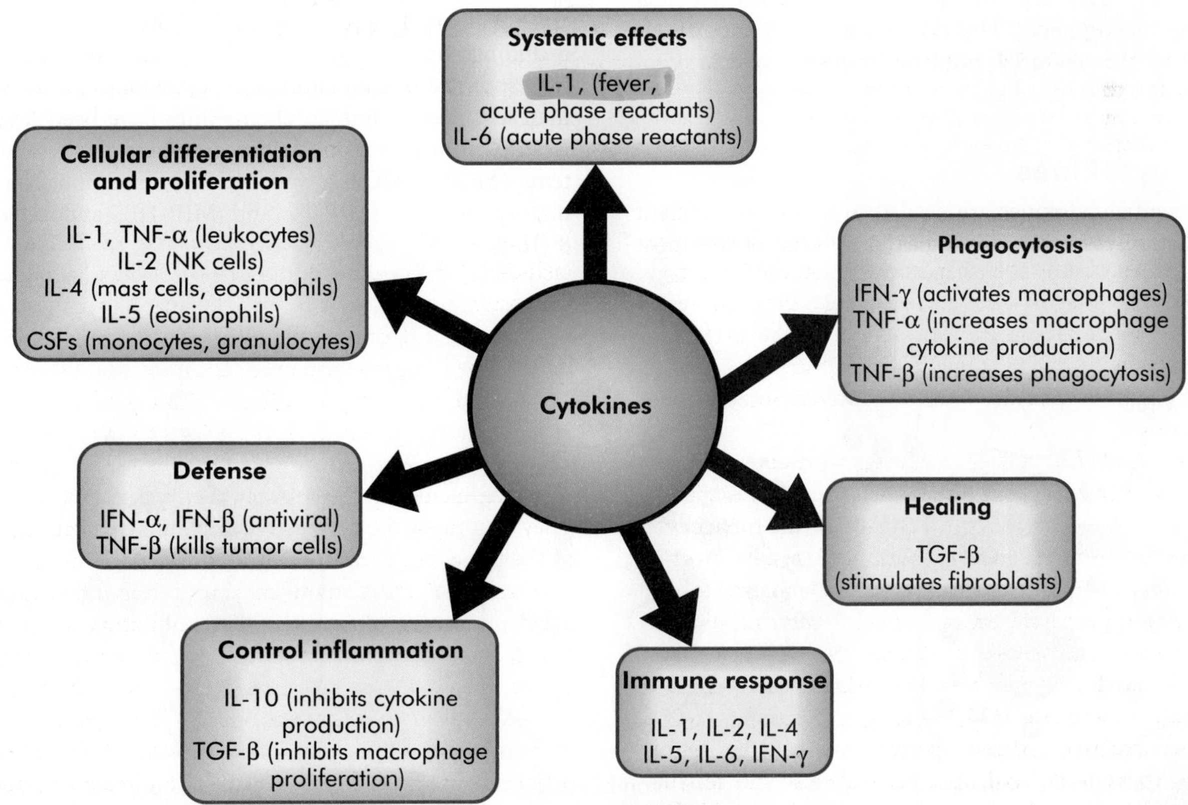

Figure 5-9 ■ **Selected Cytokines that Mediate Inflammation and the Acquired Immune Response.** See the text for a more detailed description. *IL,* Interleukin; *IFN,* interferon; *TNF,* tumor necrosis factor; *TGF,* transforming growth factor; *CSFs,* colony stimulating factors.

needed in inflammation (acute-phase reactants, discussed later in this chapter). IL-6 also stimulates growth and differentiation of precursors of blood cells in the bone marrow and the growth of fibroblasts.

Interleukin-10 (IL-10) is an example of an anti-inflammatory cytokine and is primarily produced by lymphocytes to down-regulate both the inflammatory and acquired immune responses. IL-10 suppresses the growth of lymphocytes and the production of proinflammatory cytokines by macrophages.

More than 30 interleukins have been identified. Their varied effects include the following:

1. Alteration of adhesion molecule expression on many types of cells
2. Induction of leukocyte chemotaxis
3. Induction of proliferation and maturation of leukocytes in the bone marrow
4. General enhancement or suppression of inflammation

Interferons

Interferons (INFs) are a family of cytokines that protect against viral infections. (Mechanisms of viral infection are described in Chapter 7.) Different types of cells produce different kinds of INFs; macrophages and other cells are the primary producers of both IFN-α and IFN-β, whereas lymphocytes release IFN-γ. IFN-α and IFN-β induce production of antiviral proteins, thereby conferring protection on uninfected cells (Figure 5-10). IFN-γ enhances the inflammatory response by increasing the microbiocidal activity of macrophages. This cytokine also facilitates development of the acquired immune response against viral antigens on infected cells.

Other cytokines

Other essential cytokines are needed to mount an efficient inflammatory response (see Figure 5-9). One of the most important is **tumor necrosis factor-alpha** (TNF-α). Macrophages secrete TNF-α in response to recognition of foreign materials by Toll-like receptors. Other cells, such as mast cells, are additional and crucial sources of this proinflammatory cytokine. TNF-α induces a multitude of proinflammatory effects, including enhancement of endothelial cell adhesion molecule expression, which results in increased adherence of neutrophils, and induction of chemokine production by both endothelial cells and macrophages. When secreted in large amounts, TNF-α has systemic effects that include the following:

1. Inducing fever by acting as an endogenous pyrogen
2. Causing increased synthesis of inflammation-related serum proteins by the liver
3. Causing muscle wasting (cachexia) and intravascular thrombosis in cases of severe infection and cancer

Very high levels of TNF-α can be lethal and are probably responsible for fatalities from shock caused by gram-negative bacterial infections.

Transforming growth factors are produced by many types of cells in response to inflammation, tumor growth, and cellular differentiation. Cytokines that are growth factors induce the cell division and differentiation of many cell types, such as hemopoietic blood cells. **Colony-stimulating factors** are cytokines that stimulate differentiation of blood cells (see Chapter 19.)

Chemokines

Chemokines are a family of low-molecular-weight (8 to 10 kDa) peptides that primarily induce leukocyte chemotaxis. Chemokines are synthesized by many cell types, including macrophages, fibroblasts, and endothelial cells, in response to proinflammatory cytokines. To date, more than 40 different human chemokines have been described. Examples include monocyte/macrophage chemotactic proteins (MCP-1, MCP-2, and MCP-3), macrophage inflammatory proteins (MIP-1α and MIP-1β), and interleukin 8 (IL-8).

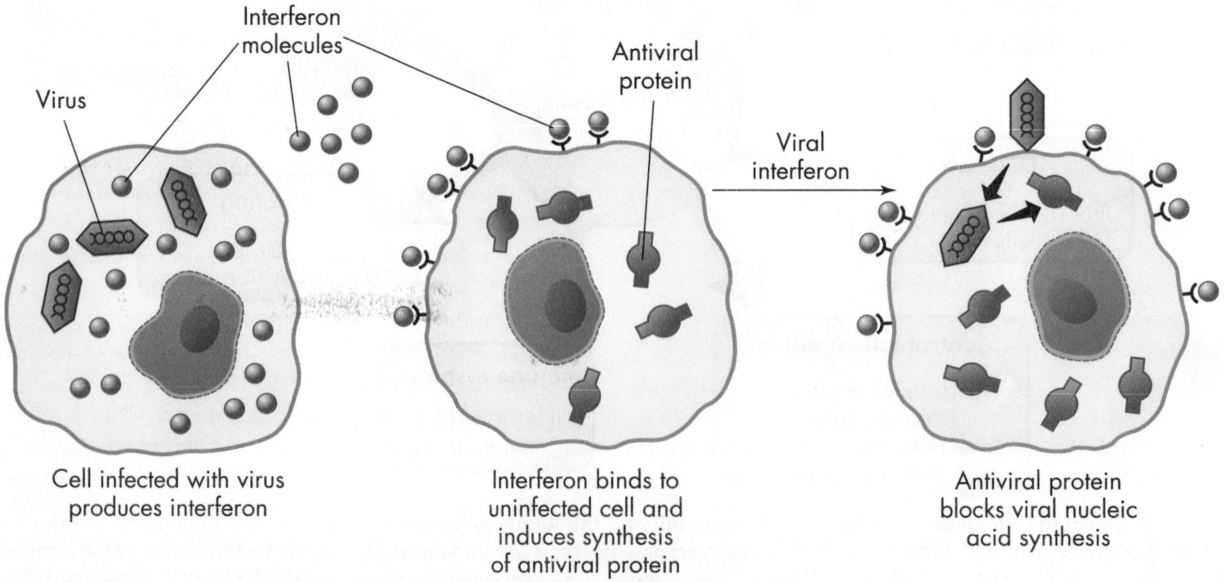
Interferon molecules
Virus
Antiviral protein
Viral interferon
Cell infected with virus produces interferon
Interferon binds to uninfected cell and induces synthesis of antiviral protein
Antiviral protein blocks viral nucleic acid synthesis

Figure 5-10 ■ **The Action of Interferon.**

QUICK CHECK 5-3

1. What are cytokines?
2. How do cytokines promote inflammation?

HEALTH ALERT

Fat Is "Inflammatory"

Obesity has increased dramatically in recent years and is a significant health problem in the United States. The many health-related problems linked to obesity appear to be secondary to a chronic systemic low-grade inflammatory response mediated by the adipose tissue itself. Proinflammatory molecules produced by adipose tissue include TNF-α. IL-6, and several other cytokines and chemokines. These lead to increases in circulating C-reactive protein (CRP) and other inflammatory mediators that place the individual at increased risk for cardiovascular disease and other complications.

Data from Fantuzzi G: Adipose tissue, adipokines, and inflammation, *J Allergy Clin Immunol* 115:911–909, 2005; and Schaffler A, Muller-Ladner U, Scholmerich J, Buchler C: Role of adipose tissue as an inflammatory organ in human diseases, *Endocr Rev* 27(5):449–467, 2006.

LOCAL MANIFESTATIONS OF ACUTE INFLAMMATION

The cells and plasma protein systems described previously interact to produce all the characteristics of inflammation, whether local or systemic, as well as determine the duration of inflammation, either acute or chronic. Local inflammation accompanies all types of cellular and tissue injury, whether infected or sterile, and is responsible for initiating healing.

All the local characteristics of acute inflammation (i.e., swelling, pain, heat, and redness) result from vascular changes and the subsequent leakage of circulating components into the tissue. *Heat* and *redness* are the result of vasodilation and increased blood flow through the injured site. *Swelling* (edema) occurs as exudate (fluid and cells) accumulates in the tissues. Swelling is usually accompanied by *pain* caused by pressure exerted by exudate accumulation, as well as the presence of soluble biochemical mediators such as prostaglandins and bradykinin.

Exudate varies in composition, depending on the stage of the inflammatory response and, to some extent, the injurious stimulus. In early or mild inflammation, the exudate is watery **(serous exudate)** with very few plasma proteins or leukocytes. An example of serous exudate is the fluid in a blister. In more severe or advanced inflammation, the exudate may be thick and clotted **(fibrinous exudate),** such as in the lungs of individuals with pneumonia. If a large number of leukocytes accumulate, as in persistent bacterial infections, the exudate consists of pus and is called a **purulent (suppurative) exudate.** Purulent exudate is characteristic of walled-off lesions (**cysts** or **abscesses**). If bleeding occurs, the exudate is filled with erythrocytes and is described as a **hemorrhagic exudate.**

SYSTEMIC MANIFESTATIONS OF ACUTE INFLAMMATION

The three primary systemic changes associated with the acute inflammatory response are fever, leukocytosis (a transient increase in circulating leukocytes), and increased levels in circulating plasma proteins.

Fever

Fever is partially induced by specific cytokines (e.g., IL-1, released from neutrophils and macrophages).[16] These are known as **endogenous pyrogens** to differentiate them from pathogen-produced **exogenous pyrogens. Pyrogens** act directly on the hypothalamus, the portion of the brain that controls the body's thermostat. (Mechanisms of temperature regulation are discussed in Chapter 13.)

A fever can be beneficial because some microorganisms (e.g., syphilis, gonococcal urethritis) are highly sensitive to small increases in body temperature. On the other hand, fever may have harmful side effects because it may enhance the host's susceptibility to the effects of endotoxins associated with gram-negative bacterial infections (bacterial toxins are described in Chapter 7).

Leukocytosis

Leukocytosis is an increase in the number of circulating white blood cells. During many infections, leukocytosis may be accompanied by a "left shift" in the ratio of immature to mature neutrophils, so that the more immature forms of neutrophils, such as band cells, metamyelocytes, and occasionally myelocytes, are present in relatively greater than normal proportions. (Chapter 19 discusses the development and maturation of blood cells.) Production of immature leukocytes increases primarily from proliferation and release of granulocyte and monocyte precursors in the bone marrow, which is stimulated by several products of inflammation.

Plasma Protein Synthesis

The synthesis of many plasma proteins, mostly products of the liver, is increased during inflammation. These proteins, which can be either pro-inflammatory or anti-inflammatory in nature, are referred to as **acute-phase reactants** (Table 5-2). Acute-phase reactants reach maximal circulating levels within 10 to 40 hours after the start of inflammation. IL-1 indirectly induces the synthesis of acute-phase reactants by increasing production of IL-6, which directly stimulates synthesis of acute-phase reactants by liver cells.

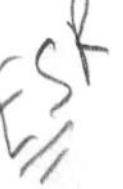

Common laboratory tests for inflammation measure levels of acute phase reactants. For example, an increase in blood levels of acute-phase reactants, primarily fibrinogen, is associated with an increased erythrocyte sedimentation rate. Although increased erythrocyte sedimentation is a

TABLE 5-2

Acute-Phase Reactants: Proteins That Are Increased or Decreased in the Blood During Inflammation

Function	Increased	Decreased
Coagulation components	Fibrinogen, prothrombin, factor VIII, plasminogen	None
Protease inhibitors	α_1-Antitrypsin, α_1-antichymotrypsin	Inter-α-antitrypsin
Transport proteins	Haptoglobin, hemopexin, ceruloplasmin, ferritin	Transferrin
Complement components	C1s, C2, C3, C4, C5, C9, factor B, C1 inhibitor	Properdin
Miscellaneous proteins	α_1-Acid glycoprotein, fibronectin, serum amyloid A (SAA), C-reactive protein (CRP)	Albumin, prealbumin, α_1-lipoprotein, β-lipoprotein

nonspecific reaction, it is considered a good indicator of an acute inflammatory response.

CHRONIC INFLAMMATION

Superficially, the difference between acute and chronic inflammation is duration; chronic inflammation lasts 2 weeks or longer, regardless of cause. Chronic inflammation is sometimes preceded by an unsuccessful acute inflammatory response (Figure 5-11). For example, if bacterial contamination or foreign objects (e.g., dirt, wood splinter, glass) persist in a wound, an acute response may be prolonged beyond 2 weeks. Pus formation, suppuration (purulent discharge), and incomplete wound healing may characterize this type of chronic inflammation.

Chronic inflammation can occur also as a distinct process without previous acute inflammation. Some microorganisms (e.g., mycobacteria that cause tuberculosis) have cell walls with a very high lipid and wax content, making them relatively insensitive to breakdown by phagocytes. Other microorganisms (e.g., those that cause leprosy, syphilis, and brucellosis) can survive within the macrophage and avoid removal by the acute inflammatory response. Other microorganisms produce toxins that damage tissue and

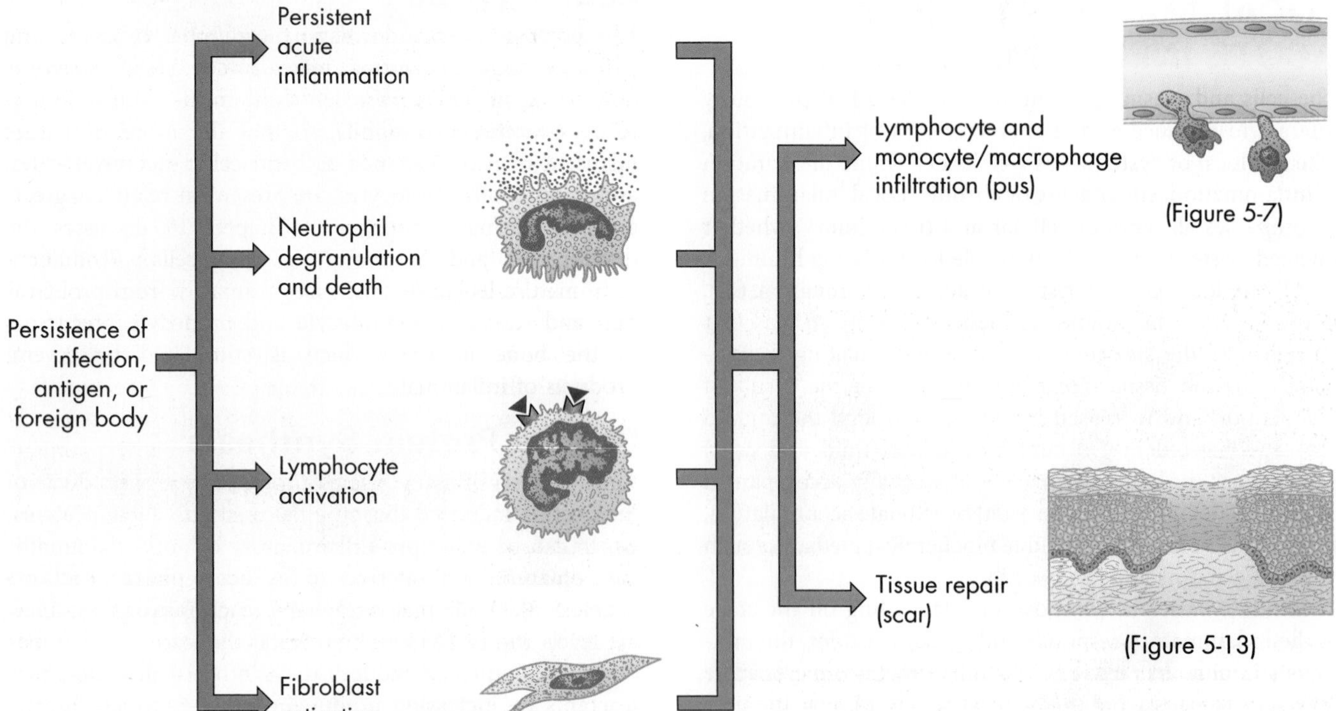

Figure 5-11 ■ **The Chronic Inflammatory Response.** Inflammation usually becomes chronic because of the persistence of an infection, an antigen, or a foreign body in the wound. Chronic inflammation is characterized by the persistence of many of the processes of acute inflammation. In addition, large amounts of neutrophil degranulation and death, the activation of lymphocytes, and the concurrent activation of fibroblasts result in the release of mediators that induce the infiltration of more lymphocytes and monocytes/macrophages and the beginning of wound healing and tissue repair. For more detailed information on each portion of the response, see the figures referred to in this illustration.

cause persistent inflammation even after the organism is killed. Finally, chemicals, particulate matter, or physical irritants (e.g., inhaled dusts, wood splinters, and suture material) can cause a prolonged inflammatory response.

Chronic inflammation is characterized by a dense infiltration of lymphocytes and macrophages. If macrophages are unable to protect the host from tissue damage, the body attempts to wall off and isolate the infected area, thus forming a **granuloma** (Figure 5-12). For example, infections caused by some bacteria (*Listeria* sp., *Brucella* sp.), fungi (histoplasmosis, coccidioidomycosis), and parasites (leishmaniasis, schistosomiasis, toxoplasmosis) can result in granuloma formation. The process of granuloma formation begins when some macrophages differentiate into large **epithelioid cells,** which are incapable of phagocytosing large bacteria but are capable of taking up debris and other small particles. Other macrophages fuse into multinucleated **giant cells,** which are active phagocytes that can engulf very large particles—larger than can be engulfed by a single macrophage. These two types of differentiated macrophages form the center of the granuloma, which is surrounded by a wall of lymphocytes. The granuloma itself is often encapsulated by fibrous deposits of collagen and may become cartilaginous or possibly calcified by deposits of calcium carbonate and calcium phosphate.

The classic granuloma associated with tuberculosis is characterized by a wall of epithelioid cells surrounding a center of dead and decaying tissue (caseous necrosis; see Chapter 3) and mycobacteria. Decay of cells within the granuloma results in the release of acids and the enzymatic contents of lysosomes from dead phagocytes. In this inhospitable environment, the cellular debris is broken down into its basic constituents, and a clear fluid remains (liquefaction necrosis; see Chapter 3). Eventually, this fluid diffuses out and leaves a hollow, thick-walled structure in the tissue that may remain for the life of the individual.

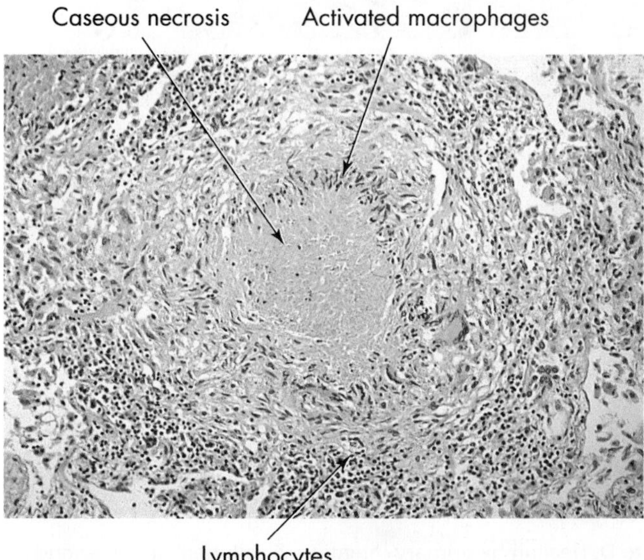

Figure 5-12 ■ **Tuberculous Granuloma.** Granulomas frequently form around areas of infection with the organism that causes tuberculosis. The granulomas consist of a central area of amorphous caseous (cheeselike) necrosis that is surrounded by a zone of activated macrophages, in which multinucleate macrophages (Langerhans giant cells) are present. There are outer layers of lymphocytes and fibroblasts. A wall of fibrin is laid down around the granulomas, and the contents eventually breakdown and liquefy. (From Stevens A, Lowe J: *Pathology,* ed 2, Edinburgh, 2000, Mosby.)

QUICK CHECK 5-4

1. Describe the basic steps in acute inflammation.
2. Describe how acute inflammation differs from chronic inflammation. What characteristics do they share?
3. List the types of exudate produced in inflammation.

RESOLUTION AND REPAIR

Tissue damage is followed by a period of healing that begins during acute inflammation and may last for as long as 2 years (Figure 5-13).[17] The most favorable outcome is a return to normal structure and function. The repaired tissues may be close to normal if damage is minor, no complications occur, and destroyed tissues are capable of **regeneration.** This restoration is called **resolution.** Resolution may not be possible if extensive damage is present, the tissue is not capable of regeneration, infection results in abscess or granuloma formation, or fibrin persists in the lesion. In those cases, repair takes place instead of resolution. **Repair** is the replacement of destroyed tissue with scar tissue. **Scar tissue** is composed primarily of collagen that fills in the lesion and restores strength but cannot carry out the physiologic functions of destroyed tissue. Both resolution and repair begin with phagocytic "cleaning up" **(débridement)** of the site of injury by removal of fibrin clots after dissolution by fibrinolytic enzymes and removal of microorganisms, erythrocytes, and dead tissue cells.

Healing involves processes that (1) fill in, (2) seal, and (3) shrink the wound. These characteristics of healing vary in importance and duration among different types of wounds. A clean incision, such as a paper cut or a sutured surgical wound, heals primarily through the process of collagen synthesis. Because this type of wound has minimal tissue loss and close apposition of the wound edges, very little sealing **(epithelialization)** and shrinkage **(contraction)** are required. Wounds that heal under conditions of minimal tissue loss are said to heal by **primary intention.**

Other wounds do not heal as easily. Healing of an open wound, such as a stage IV pressure ulcer (decubitus ulcer), requires a great deal of tissue replacement so that epithelialization, scar formation, and contraction take longer and healing occurs through **secondary intention** (see Figure 5-13). Healing by either primary or secondary intention may occur at different rates for different types of tissue injury.

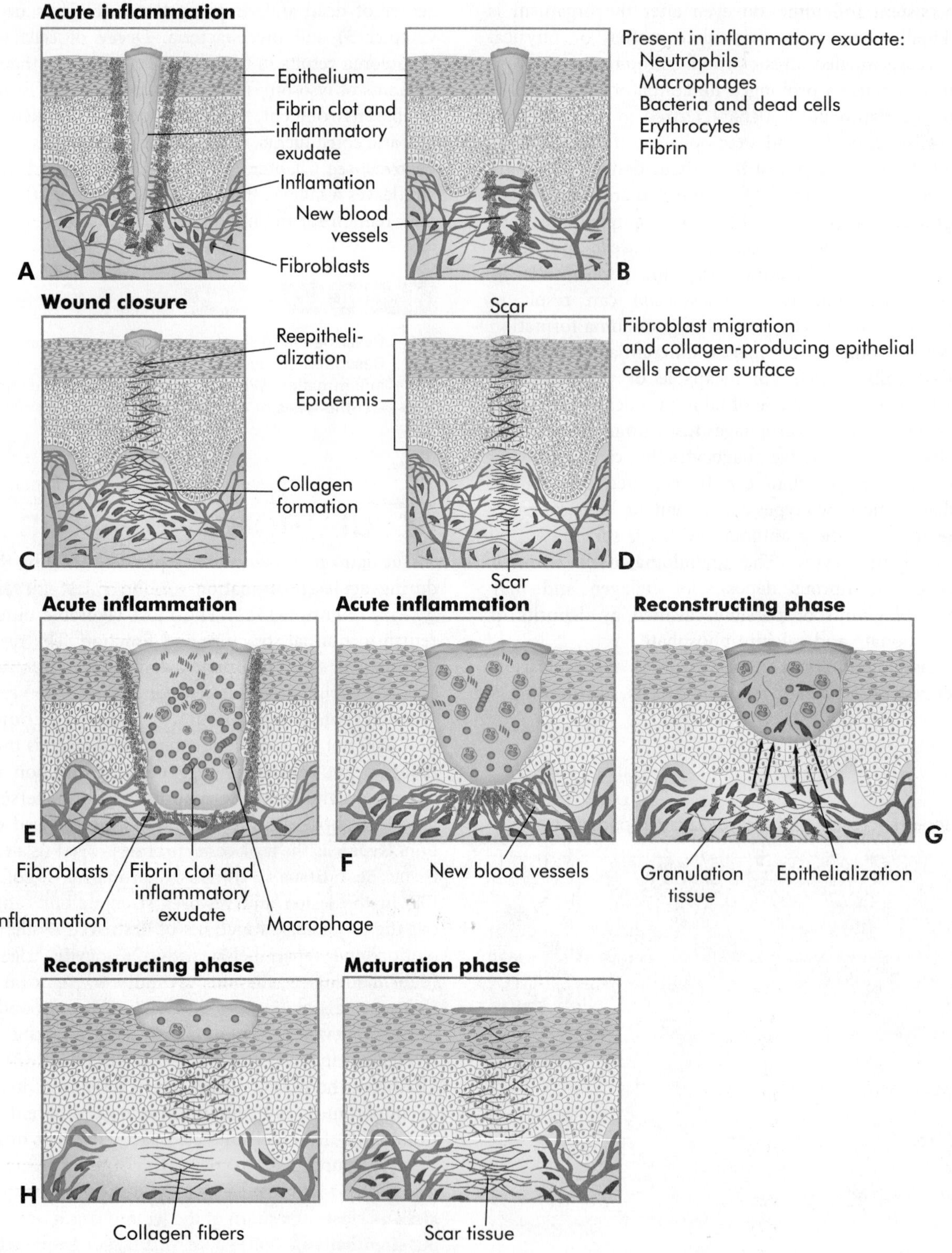

Figure 5-13 ■ **Wound Repair by Primary or Secondary Intention. A** to **D,** Healing by primary intention. **E** to **I,** Healing by secondary intention. Please see the text for more details.

Both resolution and repair occur in two overlapping phases. The **reconstructive phase** begins 3 to 4 days after the injury and continues for as long as 2 weeks. This phase is characterized by fibroblast (connective tissue cell) proliferation, followed by collagen synthesis by the fibroblasts, epithelialization, contraction of the wound, and cellular differentiation. The second phase, the **maturation phase,** begins several weeks after injury and is normally complete within 2 years. During this phase, there is continuation of cellular differentiation, scar formation, and scar remodeling.

Reconstructive Phase

Surgical and penetrating wounds are useful models of both normal and abnormal (dysfunctional) healing. Bleeding is initially sealed off by a blood clot containing a cross-linked mesh of fibrin and trapped platelets. Most surgical wounds are completely sealed within hours after closure. This sealing helps unite the wound edges and creates a physical barrier to bacterial invasion. The fibrin mesh acts as a scaffold for fibroblasts and collagen deposition that ultimately fills the wound.

For healing to proceed, the fibrin clot must be replaced by normal tissue (resolution) or scar tissue (repair).[18] Enzymatic digestion of the clot usually results from activation of the plasma fibrinolytic system (plasmin generation) or release of lysosomal enzymes from dead neutrophils. Macrophages invade the dissolving clot and clear away debris and dead cells. Macrophages secrete the following biochemical mediators, which promote healing:

1. **Transforming growth factor–beta (TGF-β)** stimulates fibroblasts entering the lesion to synthesize and secrete the collagen precursor procollagen
2. **Angiogenesis factors** such as vascular endothelial growth factor (VEGF) and fibroblast growth factor-2 (FGF-2) stimulate vascular endothelial cells to form capillary buds that grow into the lesion
3. **Matrix metalloproteinases (MMPs)** degrade and remodel extracellular matrix proteins (e.g., collagen and fibrin) at the site of injury

Granulation tissue grows into the wound from surrounding healthy connective tissue. Granulation tissue is filled with new capillaries (angiogenesis) derived from capillaries in the surrounding tissue, giving the granulation tissue a red, granular appearance. New lymphatic vessels also grow into the granulation tissue by a similar process.

During this process the healing wound must be protected. Epithelialization is the process by which epithelial cells grow into the wound from surrounding healthy tissue. Epithelial cells migrate under the clot or scab using MMPs to unravel collagen. Migrating epithelial cells contact similar cells from all sides of the wound and seal it, thereby halting migration and proliferation. The epithelial cells remain active, undergoing differentiation to give rise to the various epidermal layers (see Chapter 39). Epithelialization of a skin wound can be hastened if the wound is kept moist, preventing the fibrin clot from becoming a scab.

Fibroblasts are the most important cells during healing because they secrete collagen and other connective tissue proteins, which are deposited in débrided areas about 6 days after the fibroblasts have entered the lesion. **Collagen** is the most abundant protein in the body. It contains high concentrations of the amino acids glycine, proline, and lysine, many of which are enzymatically modified. Modification of proline and lysine requires several cofactors and is absolutely necessary for proper collagen polymerization and function. These include iron, ascorbic acid (vitamin C), and molecular oxygen (O_2); absence of any of these results in impaired wound healing. As healing progresses, collagen molecules are cross-linked by intermolecular covalent bonds to form collagen fibrils that are further cross-linked to form collagen fibers. The complete process takes several months.

Wound contraction is necessary for closure of all wounds, especially those that heal by secondary intention. Contraction is noticeable 6 to 12 days after injury. The granulation tissue contains **myofibroblasts**—specialized cells that are responsible for wound contraction. Myofibroblasts have features of both smooth muscle cells and fibroblasts. They appear microscopically similar to fibroblasts but differ in that their cytoplasm contains bundles of parallel fibers similar to those found in smooth muscle cells. Wound contraction occurs as extensions from the plasma membrane of myofibroblasts establish connections between neighboring cells, contract their fibers, and exert tension on the neighboring cells while anchoring themselves to the wound bed.

Maturation Phase

Collagen matrix assembly, tissue regeneration, and wound contraction continue into the maturation phase—a phase that can persist for years. Scar tissue is remodeled and capillaries disappear, leaving the scar avascular. Within 2 to 3 weeks after maturation has begun, the scar tissue has gained about two thirds of its eventual maximum strength.

Epidermal wounds that heal by secondary intention and unsutured internal lesions are not completely restored by healing. At best, repaired tissue regains 80% of its original tensile strength. Only epithelial, hepatic (liver), and bone marrow cells are capable of the complete mitotic regeneration of the normal tissue known as compensatory hyperplasia (hyperplasia is described in Chapter 3). In fibrous connective tissue such as joints and ligaments, normal healing results in replacement of the original tissue with new tissue that does not have exactly the same structure or function as that of the original. Some tissues heal without replacement of cells. For example, damage resulting from myocardial infarction heals with a scar composed of fibrous tissue rather than with cardiac muscle.

Dysfunctional Wound Healing

Dysfunctional healing may occur during any phase of the process and may involve insufficient repair, excessive repair, or infection. The cause of dysfunctional healing can be related to a predisposing disorder, such as diabetes mellitus; to an acquired condition, such as hypoxemia (insufficient oxygen in arterial blood); or to numerous drugs and nutrients. Wound repair delays healing by reactivating inflammatory processes.

Dysfunction during the inflammatory response

Healing is prolonged if bleeding is not stopped during acute inflammation. Large clots increase the amount of space that granulation tissue must fill and serve as mechanical barriers to oxygen diffusion. Excess blood cells resulting from hemorrhage must be cleared before repair and prolong the process. Accumulated blood is an excellent culture medium for bacteria and promotes infection, thereby prolonging inflammation by increasing exudation and pus formation.

Excessive fibrin deposition is detrimental to healing. Fibrin released in response to injury must eventually be reabsorbed to prevent organization into fibrous adhesions. Adhesions formed in the pleural, pericardial, or abdominal cavities can bind organs together by fibrous bands and distort or strangulate the affected organ.

Decreased blood volume also inhibits inflammation because of vessel constriction rather than the dilation required to deliver inflammatory cells to the site of injury. Anti-inflammatory steroids prevent macrophages from migrating to the site of injury and inhibit their release of collagenase and plasminogen activator; they also inhibit fibroblast migration into the wound during the reconstructive phase.

Optimal nutrition is important during all phases of healing because metabolic needs increase. The substances most needed are glucose, oxygen, and protein. Leukocytes need glucose to produce the adenosine triphosphate 5′(ATP) needed for chemotaxis, phagocytosis, and intercellular killing, therefore the wounds of persons with diabetes who receive insufficient insulin heal poorly. Persons with diabetes are at risk for ischemic wounds because they are likely to have both small-vessel diseases that impair the microcirculation and altered (glycosylated) hemoglobin, which has an increased affinity for oxygen and thus does not readily release oxygen in tissues. Oxygen-deprived (ischemic) tissue is susceptible to infection, which prolongs inflammation. Hypoproteinemia also prolongs inflammation because it impairs fibroblast proliferation.

Wound infection is treated in several ways. Most important is the removal or débridement of necrotic tissue and foreign bodies. Débridement is accomplished by surgery or use of absorbent dressings. Wound irrigation and antibiotic therapy also combat infection.

Dysfunction during the reconstructive phase

Impaired collagen synthesis

Most of the factors that interfere with the production of collagen in healing tissues are nutritional.[18] Scurvy, for example, is caused by lack of ascorbic acid—one of the cofactors required for collagen formation by fibroblasts. The results of scurvy are poorly formed connective tissue and greatly impaired healing.

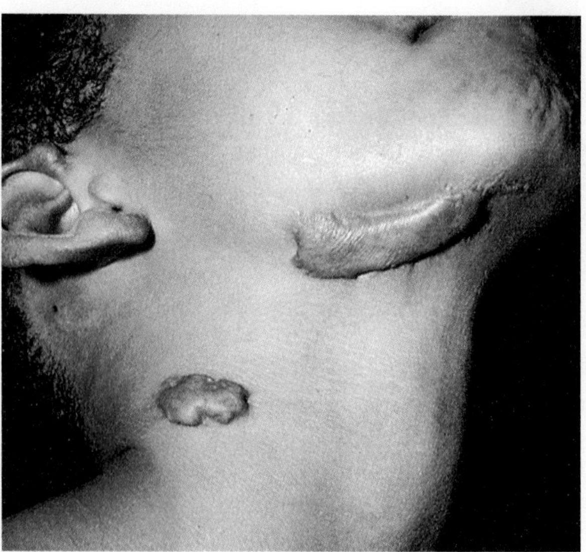

Figure 5-14 ■ Keloid (scar) Formation. Scar and keloid caused by excessive synthesis of collagen at a suture site. (From Damjanov I, Linder J: *Anderson's pathology,* ed 10, St Louis, 1996, Mosby.)

Protein and other nutrients are required for collagen synthesis. These include iron, oxygen, ketoglutarate, manganese, copper, and calcium. Usually such minute amounts of these substances are required as cofactors that deficiencies are not clinically significant.

Dysfunctional collagen synthesis also may involve excessive production of collagen, causing surface overhealing leading to a keloid or a hypertrophic scar (Figure 5-14). A **keloid** is a raised scar that extends beyond the original boundaries of the wound. It invades surrounding tissue and is likely to recur after surgical removal. A familial tendency to keloid formation has been observed, with a greater incidence in blacks than whites. A **hypertrophic scar** is raised but remains within the original boundaries of the wound. Hypertrophic scars tend to regress over time.

Impaired epithelialization

Epithelialization is suppressed by anti-inflammatory steroids, hypoxemia, ionizing radiation, and zinc deficiencies. Wound care technique may greatly influence epithelial cell migration. External wounds that are draining or healing by secondary intention often are débrided and protected with dressings. The ideal dressing absorbs some drainage without being incorporated into the clot or granulation tissue. Because epithelial cells must migrate across the wound during healing, dressings that débride healthy epithelial cells along with necrotic tissue prolong epithelialization.

Many solutions that traditionally have been used to clean or irrigate wounds are deleterious to the fragile new cells in the wound bed. Normal saline is the most innocuous solution that can be used to cleanse or irrigate a wound that is healing primarily by epithelialization. Solutions such as iodine and hydrogen peroxide are very drying and subsequently inhibit rather than promote epithelial cell migration.

Wound disruption

A potential complication of wounds that are sutured closed is **dehiscence,** in which the wound pulls apart at the suture line. Dehiscence generally occurs 5 to 12 days after suturing, when collagen synthesis is at its peak. Approximately half of dehiscence occurrences are associated with wound infection, but they also may be the result of sutures breaking because of excessive strain. Obesity increases the risk for dehiscence because adipose tissue is difficult to suture. Wound dehiscence usually is heralded by increased serous drainage from the wound and a feeling that "something gave way." Prompt surgical attention is required.

Impaired contraction

Wound contraction, although necessary for healing, may become pathologic when contraction is excessive, resulting in a deformity or **contracture.** Burns are especially susceptible to contracture development. Internal contraction deformities include duodenal strictures caused by dysfunctional healing of an ulcer and esophageal strictures caused by lye burns. Contracture may occur in cirrhosis of the liver. Scar tissue that becomes contracted constricts vascular flow and contributes to the development of portal hypertension and esophageal varices. Proper positioning and range-of-motion exercises and surgery are among the physical means used to overcome myofibroblast pull and prevent contractures.

QUICK CHECK 5-5

1. How does regeneration of tissue differ from repair of tissue?
2. What does it mean to heal by primary intention?
3. What is the role of fibroblasts in wound healing?
4. Describe various ways wound healing may be dysfunctional.

PEDIATRICS & Factors Affecting Mechanisms of Self-Defense in the Newborn Child

- Transiently depressed inflammatory function
- Neutrophils incapable of chemotaxis, lacking fluidity in plasma membrane
- Tendency for infections associated with chemotactic defects, for example, cutaneous abscesses caused by staphylococci and cutaneous candidiasis
- Diminished oxidative and bacterial responses in those stressed by in utero infection or respiratory insufficiency
- Partial deficiency in complement, especially components of alternative pathways (e.g., factor B)
- Tendency to develop severe overwhelming sepsis and meningitis when infected by bacteria against which no maternal antibodies are present

AGING & Factors Affecting Mechanisms of Self-Defense in the Elderly

- At risk for impaired wound healing—often associated with chronic illness, for example, diabetes mellitus or cardiovascular disease
- Taking required medications that may interfere with healing, for example, antiinflammatory steroids
- At risk for sustaining wounds because of impaired sensation or mobility and physiologic changes in skin
- Loss of subcutaneous fat, which diminishes layer of protection
- Thickened and less elastic collagen fibers, which contribute to less protection
- Atrophied epidermis, including underlying capillaries, which decreases perfusion and increases risk of hypoxia in wound bed

Data from Crighton MH, Puppione AA: Geriatric neutrophils: implications for older adults, *Sem Oncol Nurs* 22:3–9, 2006.

Did You Understand?

Human Defense Mechanisms

1. There are two types of human defense: innate resistance, which includes natural barriers and the inflammatory response, and the adaptive (acquired) immune system.

First Line of Defense: Physical, Mechanical, and Biochemical Barriers

1. Physical and mechanical barriers are the first lines of defense that prevent damage to the individual and prevent invasion by pathogens; these include the skin and mucous membranes.
2. Antibacterial peptides in mucous secretions, perspiration, saliva, tears, and other secretions provide a biochemical barrier against pathogenic microorganisms.
3. The normal bacterial flora provides protection by releasing chemicals that prevent colonization by pathogens.

Second Line of Defense: Inflammation

1. Inflammation is a rapid and nonspecific protective response to cellular injury from any cause. It can occur only in vascularized tissue.
2. The macroscopic hallmarks of inflammation are redness, swelling, heat, pain, and loss of function of the inflamed tissues.
3. The microscopic hallmark of inflammation is an accumulation of fluid and cells at the inflammatory site.

The Mast Cell

1. The most important activator of the inflammatory response is the mast cell, which initiates inflammation by releasing biochemical mediators (histamine, chemotactic factors) from preformed cytoplasmic granules and synthesizing other mediators (prostaglandins, leukotrienes) in response to a stimulus.

(Continued)

Did You Understand?—Cont'd

2. Histamine is the major vasoactive amine released from mast cells. It causes constriction of vascular smooth muscles, dilation of capillaries, and retraction of endothelial cells lining the capillaries, which increases vascular permeability.

Plasma Protein Systems

1. Inflammation is mediated by three key plasma protein systems: the complement system, the clotting system, and the kinin system. The components of all three systems are a series of inactive proteins that are activated sequentially.
2. The complement system can be activated by antigen-antibody reactions (through the classical pathway) or by other products, especially bacterial polysaccharides (through the lectin pathway or the alternative pathway), resulting in the production of biologically active fragments and target cell lysis.
3. The most biologically potent products of the complement system are C3b (opsonin), C3a (anaphylatoxin), and C5a (anaphylatoxin, chemotactic factor).
4. The clotting system stops bleeding, localizes microorganisms, and provides a meshwork for repair and healing.
5. Bradykinin is the most important product of the kinin system and causes vascular permeability, smooth muscle contraction, and pain.

Cellular Components of Inflammation

1. Many different types of cells are involved in the inflammatory process including neutrophils, monocytes and macrophages, eosinophils, natural killer (NK) cells, and platelets.
2. Phagocytic cells (neutrophils and macrophages) engulf and destroy microorganisms by enclosing them in phagocytic vacuoles (phagolysosomes), within which toxic products (especially metabolites of oxygen) and degradative lysosomal enzymes kill and digest the microorganisms.
3. Opsonins, such as antibody and complement component C3b, coat microorganisms and make them more susceptible to phagocytosis by binding them more tightly to the phagocyte.
4. The polymorphonuclear neutrophil (PMN), the predominant phagocytic cell in the early inflammatory response, exits the circulation by diapedesis through the retracted endothelial cell junctions and moves to the inflammatory site by chemotaxis.
5. The macrophage, the predominant phagocytic cell in the late inflammatory response, is highly phagocytic, responsive to cytokines, and promotes wound healing.
6. Eosinophils release products that control the inflammatory response and are the principal cell that kills parasitic organisms.
7. Natural killer cells recognize and eliminate cells infected with viruses, cancer cells, and other abnormal cells.
8. Platelets interact with proteins of the clotting system to stop bleeding and release a number of mediators that promote and control inflammation.
9. Phagocytosis is a multistep cellular process for the elimination of pathogens and foreign debris. The steps include recognition and attachment, engulfment, formation of a phagosome and phagolysosome, and destruction of pathogens or foreign debris.

Cellular Products

1. The cells involved in inflammation stimulate other cells by secreting cytokines, which include interleukins, interferons, and other molecules.
2. Interferons are produced by cells that are already infected by viruses. Once released from infected cells, interferons can stimulate neighboring healthy cells to produce substances that prevent viral infection.
3. Chemokines are synthesized by a number of different cells and induce leukocytes chemotaxis.

Local Manifestations of Acute Inflammation

1. Local manifestations of inflammation are the result of the vascular changes associated with the inflammatory process, including vasodilation and increased capillary permeability. The symptoms include redness, heat, swelling, and pain.
2. The functions of the vascular changes are to dilute toxin molecules produced by dying cells or contaminating microorganisms, carry plasma proteins and leukocytes to the injury site, carry debris away from the site, and initiate healing and repair.

Systemic Manifestations of Acute Inflammation

1. The principal systemic effects of inflammation are fever and increases in levels of circulating leukocytes and plasma proteins (acute phase reactants).

Chronic Inflammation

1. Chronic inflammation can be a continuation of acute inflammation that lasts 2 weeks or longer. It also can occur as a distinct process without much preceding acute inflammation.
2. Chronic inflammation is characterized by a dense infiltration of lymphocytes and macrophages. The body may wall off and isolate the infection to protect against tissue damage by formation of a granuloma.

Resolution and Repair

1. Resolution (regeneration) is the return of tissue to nearly normal structure and function. Repair is healing by scar tissue formation.
2. Damaged tissue proceeds to resolution (restoration of the original tissue structure and function) if little tissue has been lost or injured tissue is capable of regeneration. This is called healing by primary intention.
3. Tissues that sustained extensive damage or those incapable of regeneration heal by the process of repair resulting in the formation of a scar. This is called healing by secondary intention.
4. Resolution and repair occur in two separate phases, the reconstructive phase in which the wound begins to heal and the maturation phase in which the healed wound is remodeled.
5. Dysfunctional wound healing can occur as a result of abnormalities in either the inflammatory response or the reconstructive phase of resolution and repair.

IL-1 = proinflam. IL-10 = antiinflammatory cytokine
IL-6 = Proteins

Did You Understand?—Cont'd

PEDIATRICS & Factors Affecting Mechanisms of Self-Defense in the Newborn Child

1. Neonates often have transiently depressed inflammatory function, particularly neutrophil chemotaxis and alternative complement pathway activity.

AGING & Factors Affecting Mechanisms of Self-Defense in the Elderly

1. Elderly persons are at risk for impaired wound healing, usually because of chronic illnesses.

Key Terms

α_1-antitrypsin, 132
Abscess, 135
Acute-phase reactant, 135
Adaptive immunity, 122
Adhesion molecule, 129
Alternative pathway, 128
Anaphylatoxin, 128
Angiogenesis factor, 139
Antimicrobial peptide, 122
Bradykinin, 128
C1 esterase inhibitor (C1-Inh), 129
Carboxypeptidase, 129
Chemokine, 134
Chemotactic factor, 125
Chemotaxis, 125
Classical pathway, 128
Clotting (coagulation) system, 128
Collagen, 139
Colony-stimulating factor, 134
Complement receptor, 131
Complement system, 127
Contraction, 137
Contracture, 141
Cyst, 135
Cytokine, 129
Débridement, 137
Degranulation, 124
Dehiscence, 141
Diapedesis, 130
Endogenous pyrogen, 135
Endothelial cell, 129
Eosinophil chemotactic factor of anaphylaxis (ECF-A), 125
Eosinophil, 130
Epithelialization, 137
Epithelioid cell, 137
Exogenous pyrogens, 135
Exudate, 135
Fc receptor, 131
Fever, 135
Fibrinous exudate, 135
Fibroblast, 139
Giant cell, 137
Granulation tissue, 139
Granuloma, 137
Hemorrhagic exudate, 135
Hexose-monophosphate shunt, 132
Histamine, 125
Hypertrophic scar, 140
Inflammatory response, 122
Innate resistance, 121
Interferon (INF), 134
Interleukin (IL), 133
Interleukin-1 (IL-1), 133
Interleukin-6 (IL-6), 133
Interleukin-10 (IL-10), 134
Keloid, 140
Kinin system, 128
Lectin pathway, 128
Leukocytosis, 135
Leukotriene (slow-reacting substances of anaphylaxis [SRS-A]), 126
Macrophage, 129
Margination (pavementing), 130
Mast cell, 124
Matrix metalloproteinase (MMP), 139
Maturation phase, 139
Monocyte, 129
Myofibroblast, 139
Natural killer (NK) cell, 130
Neutrophil chemotactic factor, 125
Neutrophil, 129
Nitric oxide (NO), 129
Normal bacterial flora, 122
Opsonin, 128
Pathogen-associated molecular pattern (PAMP), 130
Pattern recognition receptor (PRR), 130
Phagocyte, 130
Phagocytosis, 130
Phagolysosome, 132
Phagosome, 132
Plasma protein system, 126
Plasmin, 129
Platelet, 130
Platelet-activating factor (PAF), 126
Polymorphonuclear neutrophil (PMN), 129
Primary intention, 137
Prostaglandin, 126
Purulent (suppurative) exudate, 135
Pyrogens, 135
Reconstructive phase, 139
Regeneration, 137
Repair, 137
Resolution, 137
Scar tissue, 137
Secondary intention, 137
Serous exudate, 135
Toll-like receptor (TLR), 131
Transforming growth factor, 134
Transforming growth factor-beta (TGF-β), 139
Tumor necrosis factor-alpha (TNF-α), 134
Wound contraction, 139

References

1. Tosi MF: Innate immune responses to infection, *J Allergy Clin Immunol* 116:241–249, 2005.
2. Vliagoftis H, Befus AD: Mast cells at mucosal frontiers, *Curr Mol Med* 5:573–589, 2005.
3. Goldfarb RD, Parrillo JE: Complement, *Crit Care Med* 33: S482–S484, 2005.
4. Lutz HU, Jelezarova E: Complement amplification revisited, *Mol Immunol* 43:2–12, 2006.
5. Thurman JM, Holers VM: The central role of the alternative complement pathway in human disease, *J Immunol* 176:1305–1310, 2006.
6. Aird WC: Coagulation, *Crit Care Med* 33:S485–S487, 2005.
7. Garrood T, Lee L, Pitzalis C: Molecular mechanisms of cell recruitment to inflammatory sites: general and tissue-specific pathways, *Rheumatol* 45:250–260, 2006.
8. Marshall JC: Neutrophils in the pathogenesis of sepsis, *Crit Care Med* 33:S502–S505, 2005.
9. Cavaillon J-M, Adib-Conquy M: Monocytes/macrophages and sepsis, *Crit Care Med* 33:S506–S509, 2005.
10. Rothenberg ME, Hogan SP: The eosinophil, *Annu Rev Immunol* 24:5.1–5.28, 2006.
11. Panés J, Perry M, Granger DN: Leukocyte-endothelial cell adhesion: avenues for therapeutic intervention, *Br J Pharmacol* 126:537–550, 1999.
12. Kawai T, Akira S: Pathogen recognition and toll-like receptors, *Cur Opin Immunol* 17:338–344, 2005.
13. Hawlisch H, Kohl J: Complement and toll-like receptors: key regulators of adaptive immune responses, *Mol Immunol* 43:13–21, 2006.

References—Cont'd

14. Segal AW: How neutrophils kill microbes, *Ann Rev Immunol* 23:197–223, 2005.
15. Steinke JW, Borish L: Cytokines and chemokines, *J Allergy Clin Immunol* 117:S441–S445, 2006.
16. Thompson HJ: Fever, a concept analysis, *J Adv Nurs* 51:484–492, 2005.
17. Broughton GB, Janis JE, Attinger CE: Wound healing: an overview, *Plast Reconstr Surg* 117(suppl):1e-S–32e-S, 2006.
18. Broughton GB, Janis JE, Attinger CE: The basic science of wound healing, *Plast Reconstr Surg* 117(suppl):12S–34S, 2006.

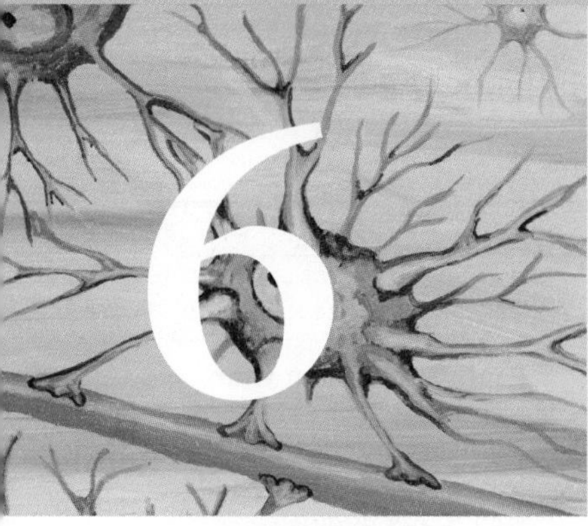

6 ADAPTIVE IMMUNITY

Neal S. Rote

CHAPTER OUTLINE

ELECTRONIC RESOURCES

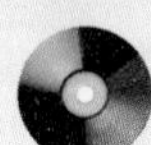

Companion CD
- Review Questions and Answers
- Animations

evolve Website
http://evolve.elsevier.com/Huether/
- Quick Check Answers
- Key Terms Exercises
- Critical Thinking Questions with Answers
- Algorithm Completion Exercises
- WebLinks

The third line of defense is adaptive (acquired) immunity, often called the immune response. It develops more slowly than the inflammatory response and is specific and has memory, so that it can confer permanent or long-term protection against specific microorganisms. Many components of innate resistance are necessary for the development of the adaptive immune response. Conversely, products of the adaptive immune response protect the individual by activating components of innate resistance. Thus, both systems are essential for complete protection against infectious disease.

GENERAL CHARACTERISTICS OF ADAPTIVE IMMUNITY

The immune system continually is challenged by a spectrum of substances that it recognizes as foreign, or "nonself." These substances are called antigens. Antigens are on infectious agents (e.g., viruses, bacteria, fungi, or parasites), on noninfectious substances from the environment (e.g., pollens, foods, or bee venoms), or on drugs, vaccines, transfusions, and transplanted tissues (Table 6-1).

The body's reaction to antigenic challenges is the immune response, which involves two types of **lymphocytes:** B lymphocytes (B cells) and T lymphocytes (T cells). The **B lymphocytes (B cells)** produce antibodies that enter the blood and react with the antigen, and the **T lymphocytes (T cells)** attack the antigen directly. Both cells are extremely specific, so that each individual B or T cell recognizes only one specific antigen.

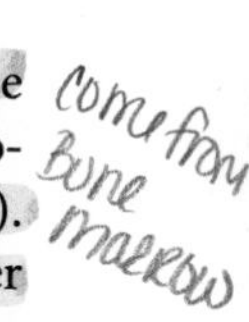

An immune response can be divided into two phases (Figure 6-1). Before birth, humans produce a large population of T cells and B cells that have the capacity to recognize almost any foreign antigen found in the environment. Each individual T or B cell, however, specifically recognizes only one particular antigen, but the sum of the population of lymphocytes may recognize millions of foreign antigens. This process is called the *generation of* ***clonal diversity*** and occurs in specialized (primary) lymphoid organs: the thymus for T cells and the bone marrow for B cells. Lymphocytes are released from these organs into the circulation as mature cells that have the capacity to react with antigen (immunocompetent). These cells migrate to other (secondary) lymphoid organs in the body in preparation for future exposure to antigen (Figure 6-2).

Antigen initiates the second phase of the immune response, **clonal selection**. This process involves a complex interaction among cells. To initiate an effective immune response, most antigens must be *processed,* in that they cannot react directly with cells of the immune system but must be shown or *presented* to the immune cells in a specific manner. This is the job of antigen-processing (antigen-presenting) cells (usually macrophages or similar cells), generally referred to as APCs (Figure 6-3). The interaction among APCs, subpopulations of T cells that facilitate immune responses **(helper T cells; Th cells),** and immunocompetent B or T cells results in differentiation of B cells

TABLE 6-1
Clinical Use of Antigen or Antibody

Antigen Source	USE OF ANTIGEN OR ANTIBODY			
	Protection: Combat Active Disease	Protection: Vaccination	Diagnosis	Therapy
Infectious agents	Neutralize or destroy pathogenic microorganisms (e.g., antibody response against viral infections)	Induce safe and protective immune response (e.g., recommended childhood vaccines)	Measure circulating antigen from infectious agent or antibody (e.g., diagnosis of hepatitis B infection)	Passive treatment with antibody to treat or prevent infection (e.g., administration of antibody against hepatitis A)
Cancers	Prevent tumor growth or spread (e.g., immune surveillance to prevent early cancers)	Prevent cancer growth or spread (e.g., vaccination with cancer antigens)	Measure circulating antigen (e.g., circulating PSA for diagnosis of prostate cancer)	Immunotherapy (e.g., treatment of cancer with antibodies against cancer antigens)
Environmental substances	Prevent entrance into body (e.g., secretory IgA limits systemic exposure to potential allergens)	No clear example	Measure circulating antigen or antibody (e.g., diagnosis of allergy by measuring circulating IgE)	Immunotherapy (e.g., substances administration of antigen for desensitization of individuals with severe allergies)
Self-antigens	Immune system tolerance to self-antigens, which may be altered by an infectious agent leading to autoimmune disease (see Chapter 7)	Some cases of vaccination alter tolerance to self-antigens leading to autoimmune disease	Measure circulating antibody against self-antigen for diagnosis of autoimmune disease (see Chapter 7)	Oral administration of self-antigens in order to diminish the production of autoimmune disease associated autoantibodies.

PSA, Prostate-specific antigen.

into active antibody-producing cells (plasma cells) and T cells into effector cells, such as cytotoxic T cells. Both lines also develop into memory cells that "remember" the antigen and respond even faster when that antigen enters the body again. Thus, the immune system possesses memory and specificity and is inducible, resulting in long-lasting protection against specific antigens.

Humoral and Cell-Mediated Immunity

The immune response has two arms: antibody and T cells, both of which protect against infection.[1] Antibody circulates in the blood and binds to antigens on infectious agents. This interaction can result in direct inactivation of the microorganism or activation of a variety of inflammatory mediators that will destroy the pathogen. Antibody is primarily responsible for protection against many bacteria and viruses. This arm of the immune response is termed **humoral immunity.**

T cells also undergo differentiation during an immune response and develop into several subpopulations of effector T cells that react directly with antigen on the surface of cells or infectious agents. Some develop into T cells that can stimulate the activities of other leukocytes through cell-to-cell contact or through the secretion of cytokines. Others develop into **cytotoxic T cells (Tc cells)** that attack and kill targets directly. Targets for Tc cells include cells infected by a variety of viruses, as well as cells that have become cancerous. This arm of the immune response is termed **cellular** or **cell-mediated immunity.**

The success of an acquired immune response depends on the functions of both the humoral and cellular responses, as well as the appropriate interactions between them. Additionally, both arms produce specialized subpopulations of **memory cells,** which are capable of "remembering" the antigen and responding more rapidly and efficiently if the associated pathogen invades again.

Active and Passive Immunity

Adaptive immunity can be either active or passive, depending on whether the antibodies or T cells are produced by the individual in response to antigen or are administered directly to the individual. **Active acquired immunity (active immunity)** is produced by an individual after either natural exposure to an antigen or after immunization, whereas **passive acquired immunity (passive immunity)** does not involve the host's immune response at all. Rather, passive immunity occurs when preformed antibodies or T cells are transferred from a donor to the recipient. This can occur naturally, as during pregnancy when maternal antibodies cross the placenta to the fetus, or artificially, as when antibodies are injected to fight against a specific disease. For instance, unvaccinated individuals who are exposed to particular infectious agents (e.g., hepatitis A virus, rabies virus) often will be given immune globulins, which are prepared from individuals who already have

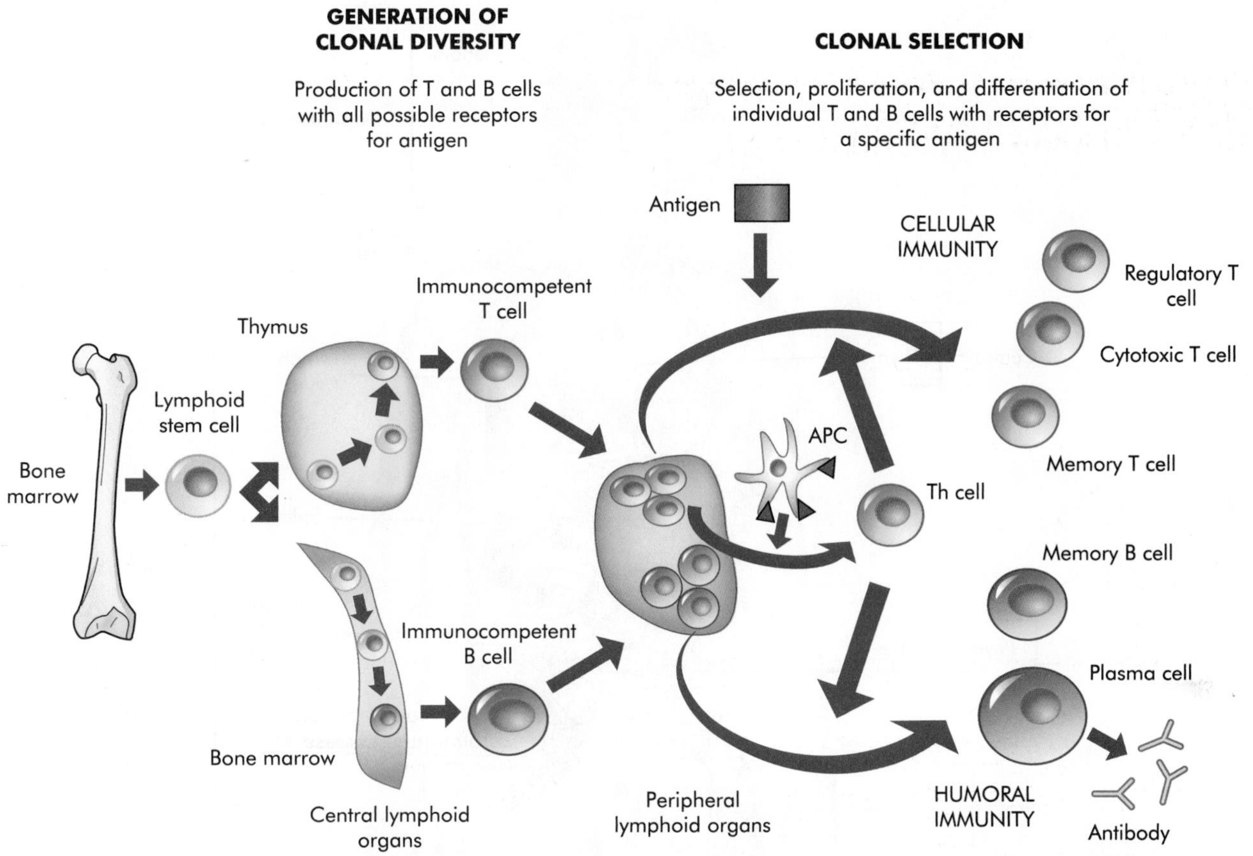

Figure 6-1 ■ **Overview of the Immune Response.** The immune response can be separated into two phases: the generation of clonal diversity and clonal selection. During the generation of clonal diversity, lymphoid stem cells from the bone marrow migrate to the central lymphoid organs (the thymus or regions of the bone marrow) where they undergo a series of cellular divisions and differentiation stages resulting in either immunocompetent T cells from the thymus or immunocompetent B cells from the bone marrow. These cells have never encountered foreign antigen. The immunocompetent cells enter the circulation and migrate to the secondary lymphoid organs (e.g., spleen and lymph nodes), where they take up residence in B and T cell–rich areas (more detail in Figure 6-14). The clonal selection phase is initiated by exposure to foreign antigen. The antigen is usually processed by antigen-presenting cells (APCs) for presentation to helper T cells (Th cells) (more detail in Figures 6-16 and 6-17). The intercellular cooperation among APCs, Th cells, and immunocompetent T and B cells results in a second stage of cellular proliferation and differentiation (more detail in Figures 6-19 and 6-20). Because antigen has "selected" those T and B cells with compatible antigen receptors, only a small population of T and B cells undergo this process at one time. The end result is an active cellular immunity or humoral immunity or both. Cellular immunity is mediated by a population of "effector" T cells that can kill targets (cytotoxic T cells) or regulate the immune response (regulatory T cells), as well as a population of memory T cells that can respond more quickly to a second challenge with the same antigen. Humoral immunity is mediated by a population of soluble proteins (antibodies) produced by plasma cells and by a population of memory B cells that can produce more antibody rapidly to a second challenge with the same antigen.

antibodies against that particular pathogen. Whereas active acquired immunity is long lived, passive immunity is only temporary because the donor's antibodies or T cells are eventually destroyed.

QUICK CHECK 6-1

1. Define acquired immunity.
2. Distinguish between innate and acquired immunity.
3. Distinguish between humoral and cell-mediated immunity.

ANTIGENS AND IMMUNOGENS

An **antigen** is a molecule that can *react with* antibodies or antigen receptors on B and T cells. Most, but not all, antigens are also **immunogens.** An antigen that is immunogenic will *induce* an immune response resulting in the production of antibodies or functional T cells. Although the terms *antigen* and *immunogen* commonly are used as synonyms, there are important differences between the two.

To be antigenic, part of a molecule's chemical structure must be recognized by and bound to an antibody or to specific receptors on a lymphocyte. The precise area of the molecule that is recognized is called its **antigenic determinant,** or **epitope.** The matching portion on the antibody or the lymphocyte receptor is sometimes referred to as the **antigen-binding site,** or **paratope.** The size of an antigenic determinant is relatively small, perhaps just a few amino acids or sugar residues (Figure 6-4). A large molecule (e.g., proteins, polysaccharides, nucleic acids) usually contains multiple and diverse antigenic determinants. Thus,

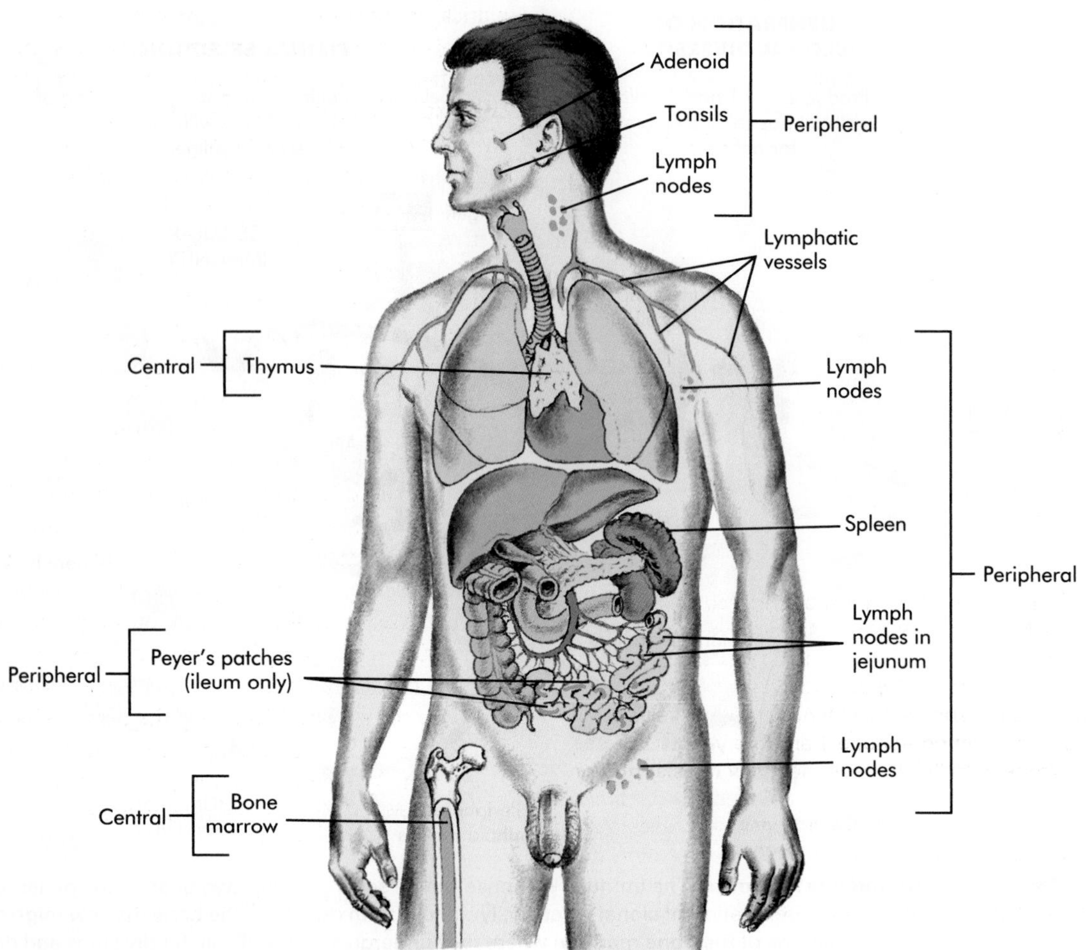

Figure 6-2 ■ **Lymphoid System.** Immature lymphocytes migrate through central (primary) lymphoid tissues: the bone marrow (central lymphoid tissue for B lymphocytes) and the thymus (central lymphoid tissue for T lymphocytes). Mature lymphocytes later reside in the T and B lymphocyte–rich areas of the peripheral (secondary) lymphoid tissues.

the immune response against the molecule may consist of a mixture of specific antibodies against several of these determinants.

Certain criteria influence the degree to which an antigen is immunogenic. These include (1) foreignness to the host, (2) adequate size, (3) adequate chemical complexity, and (4) being present in a sufficient quantity. These criteria are important for development of vaccines, which must be highly immunogenic to produce protective immune responses against pathogenic microorganisms.

Foremost among the criteria for immunogenicity is the antigen's foreignness. A **self-antigen** that fulfills all the criteria listed above *except* foreignness does not normally elicit an immune response. Thus, most individuals are *tolerant* to their own antigens. Some pathogens are successful because they develop the capacity to mimic self-antigens and avoid inducing an immune response. In Chapter 7 we will discuss specific diseases resulting from a breakdown of tolerance that leads to an individual's immune system attacking its own antigens (autoimmune diseases).

Molecular size also contributes to an antigen's immunogenicity. In general, large molecules (those bigger than 10,000 daltons), such as proteins, polysaccharides, and nucleic acids, are most immunogenic. Low-molecular-weight molecules such as amino acids, monosaccharides, fatty acids, and the purine and pyrimidine bases, tend to be unable to induce an immune response. Many molecules in this size range can function as **haptens:** antigens that are

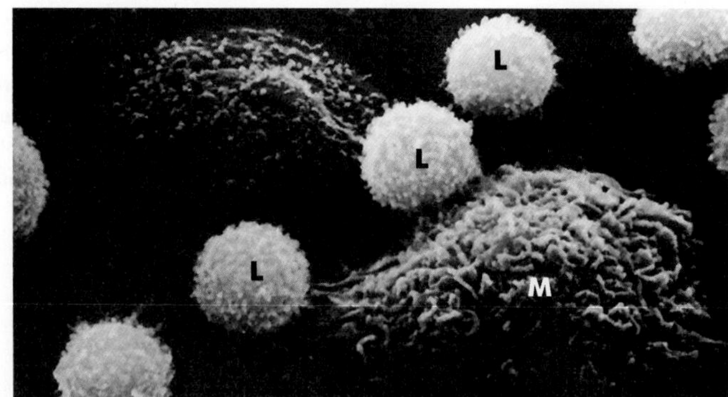

Figure 6-3 ■ **Scanning Electron Micrograph of Lymphocytes and Macrophages.** The lymphocytes are small and spherical; the macrophages are larger and more irregular in shape. (From Raven PH, Johnson GB: *Biology,* ed 5, New York, 1999, McGraw-Hill.)

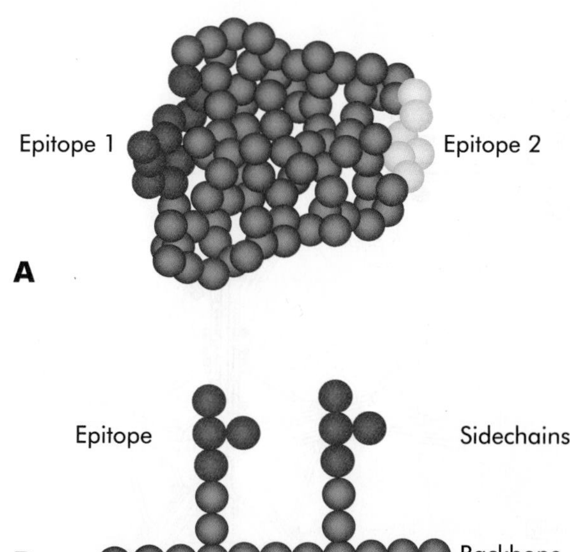

Figure 6-4 ■ **Antigenic Determinants (Epitopes).** Generic examples of epitopes on protein **(A)** and polysaccharide **(B)** molecules are shown. In **A,** an antigenic protein may have multiple different epitopes (epitopes 1 and 2) that react with different antibodies. Each sphere represents an amino acid with the red spheres representing epitope 1 and the yellow spheres representing epitope 2. Individual epitopes may consist of 8 or 9 amino acids. In **B,** a polysaccharide is constructed of a backbone with branched side chains. Each sphere represents an individual carbohydrate with the red spheres representing the carbohydrates that form the epitope. In this example, two identical epitopes are shown that would bind two identical antibodies.

too small to be immunogens by themselves but become immunogenic after combining with larger molecules that function as carriers for the hapten. For example, the antigens of poison ivy are haptens, but they initiate allergic responses in individuals after binding to large-molecular-weight proteins in the skin. Antigens that induce an allergic response are also called **allergens.**

Chemical complexity affects immunogenicity. The best immunogens contain a diversity of chemically different components. For instance, a large synthetic protein consisting only of the amino acid alanine would not be very immunogenic, despite its size and foreignness. Immunogenicity increases greatly after other amino acids, such as tyrosine, tryptophan, or phenylalanine, are inserted into the structure.

Finally, antigens that are present in extremely small or large quantities may be unable to elicit an immune response. In many cases, high or low extremes of antigen quantities may induce a state of tolerance rather than immunity.

Even if an antigen fulfills all these criteria, the quality and intensity of the immune response may still be affected by a variety of additional factors. For example, the route and vehicle of antigen entry or administration are critical to the immunogenicity of some antigens. This has important clinical implications. The most common routes for clinical administration of antigen are intravenous, intraperitoneal, subcutaneous, intranasal, and oral. Each route preferentially stimulates a different set of lymphocyte-containing (lymphoid) tissues and therefore results in the induction of different types of cell-mediated or humoral immune responses. For some vaccines, the route may affect the protectiveness of the immune response so that the individual is protected if immunized by one route, but may be less protected if administered through a different route (e.g., oral versus injected polio vaccines, discussed later in this chapter under Secretory Immune System). Immunogenicity of an antigen also may be altered by being delivered along with substances that stimulate the immune response; these substances are known as adjuvants. Finally, the genetic makeup of the individual can play a critical role in the immune system's ability to respond to many antigens. Some individuals appear to be unable to respond to immunization with a particular antigen, whereas they respond well to other antigens. For instance, a small percentage of the population may fail to produce a measurable immune response to a common vaccine, despite multiple injections. An individual's immune response can also be affected by the person's age, nutritional status, genetic background, and reproductive status, as well as exposure to traumatic injury, concurrent disease, or the use of immunosuppressive medications.

HUMORAL IMMUNE RESPONSE

Antibodies

An **antibody,** or immunoglobulin (Ig), is a serum glycoprotein produced by mature B cells **(plasma cells)** in response to a challenge by an antigen. The term *immunoglobulin* is used for all molecules that are known to have specificity for antigen, whereas the term *antibody* is generally used to denote one particular set of immunoglobulins known to have specificity for a particular antigen. There are five classes of immunoglobulins (IgG, IgA, IgM, IgE, and IgD), which are characterized by antigenic, structural, and functional differences (Figure 6-5). Within two of the immunoglobulin classes are several distinct subclasses including four subclasses of IgG and two subclasses of IgA.

Classes of immunoglobulins

IgG is the most abundant class of immunoglobulins, constituting 80% to 85% of the immunoglobulin in the blood and accounting for most of the protective activity against infections (Table 6-2). As a result of selective transport across the placenta, maternal IgG is the major class of antibody found in blood of the fetus and newborn. Four subclasses of IgG have been described: IgG1, IgG2, IgG3, and IgG4.

IgA has two subclasses, IgA1 and IgA2. IgA1 is found predominantly in the blood, whereas IgA2 is the predominant class found in body secretions (secretory IgA). Secretory IgA is a *dimer* of two IgA molecules held together through a J chain and secretory piece. The secretory piece is attached to IgA inside mucosal epithelial cells to protect

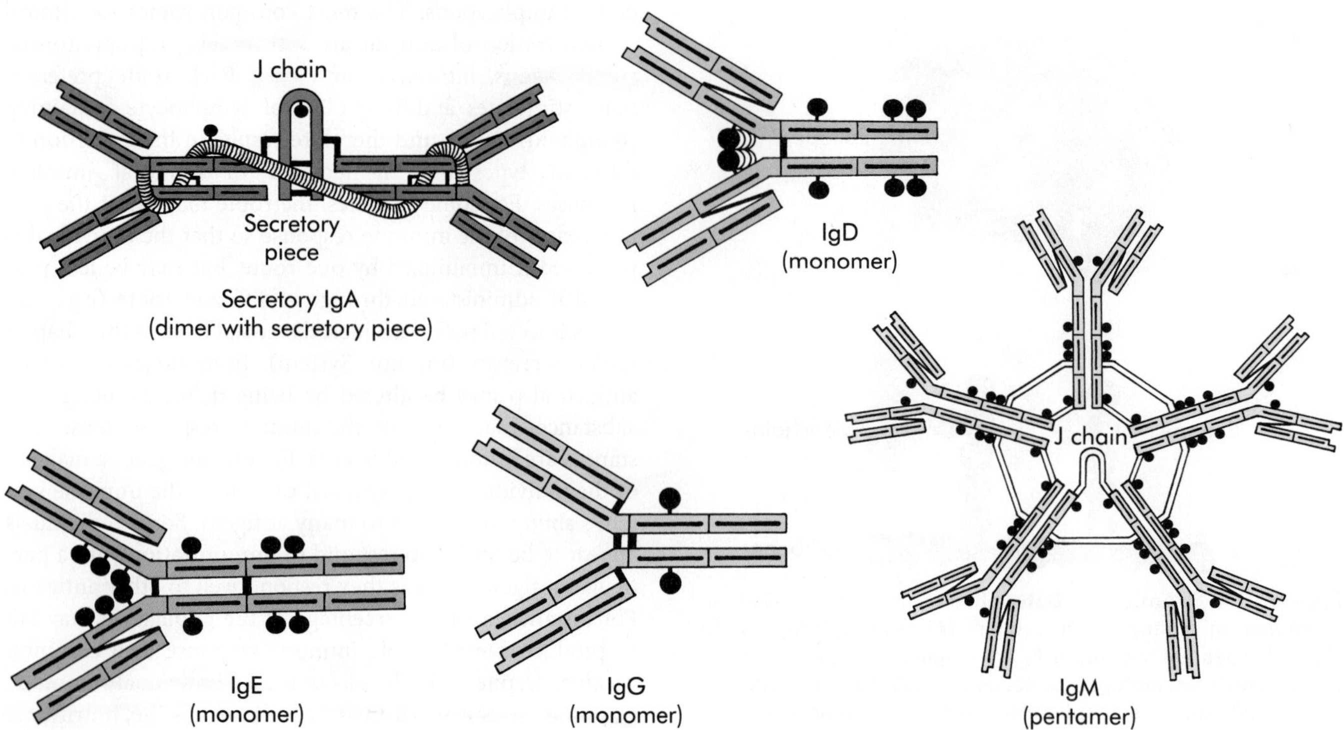

Figure 6-5 ■ **Structure of Different Immunoglobulins.** Secretory IgA, IgD, IgE, IgG, and IgM. The black circles attached to each molecule represent carbohydrate residues.

TABLE 6-2

Properties of Immunoglobulins

Class	Subclass	Adult Serum Levels (mg/dl)	Present in Secretions	Complement Activation	Opsonin	Agglutinin	Mast Cell Activation	Placental Transfer
IgG	IgG1	800–900	+	++	++	+	−	+++
	IgG2	280–300	+	+	−	+	−	+
	IgG3	90–100	+	+++	++	+	−	+++
	IgG4	50	−	−	−	+	+	++
IgM	IgM	120–150	+	++++	−	++++	−	−
IgA	IgA1	280–300	+	−	−	+	−	−
	IgA2	50	+	−	−	+	−	−
	sIgA	5	++++	−	−	+	−	−
IgD	IgD	3	−	−	−	−	−	−
IgE	IgE	0.03	+	−	−	−	+++	−

sIgA, Secretory immunoglobulin A; − indicates lack of activity; + to ++++ indicate relative activity or concentration.

these immunoglobulins against degradation by enzymes also found in secretions.

IgM is the largest of the immunoglobulins and usually exists as a pentamer that is stabilized by a J chain. It is the first antibody produced during the initial, or primary, response to antigen. IgM is synthesized early in neonatal life, and its synthesis may be increased as a response to infection *in utero*.

IgD is found in low concentrations in the blood. Its primary function is as an antigen receptor on the surface of early B cells.

IgE is normally at low concentrations in the circulation. It has very specialized functions as a mediator of many common allergic responses (see Chapter 7) and in the defense against parasitic infections.

Molecular structure

The parts of an antibody molecule were named based on studies using the enzyme papain to treat IgG. Three fragments resulted, two of which were identical. The two identical fragments retained the ability to bind antigen and were termed **antigen-binding fragments (Fab).** The third fragment crystallized and was termed the **crystalline fragment (Fc)** (Figure 6-6). The Fab portions contain the recognition sites (receptors) for antigenic determinants and confer the molecule's specificity toward a particular anti-

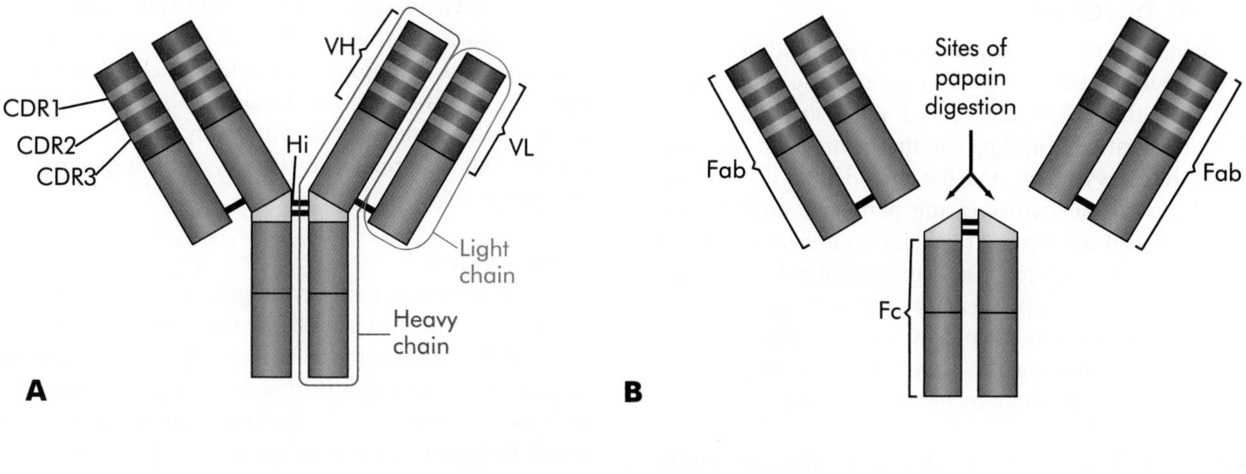

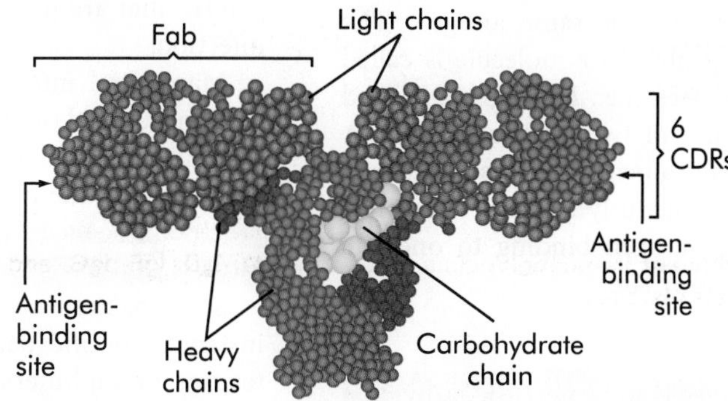

Figure 6-6 ■ **Molecular Structure of an Antibody. A,** The typical antibody molecule consists of four chains—two identical light (*L*) and two identical heavy (*H*)—held together by intrachain and interchain disulfide linkages. The primary interchain disulfides between heavy chains occur in the hinge region (*Hi*) and provide flexibility in some classes of antibody. Each heavy chain and light chain is divided into regions that have relatively constant amino acid sequences (*green* areas) and regions with a variable amino acid sequence (*VH, VL*). Within the VH and VL regions are three highly variable complementary-determining regions (CDR1, CDR2, CDR3). **B,** Fragmentation of IgG by limited digestion with the enzyme papain has identified three important portions of the molecule: an Fc and two identical Fab fragments. Both Fab fragments could bind antigen. **C,** In this molecular model of a typical antibody molecule, the light chains are represented by strands of red spheres (each represents an individual amino acid), and heavy chains are represented by strands of blue spheres. Note that the heavy chain contains sites where carbohydrates are bound. As the chains fold and interact, the six CDRs within a Fab region are placed in close proximity to form the antigen-binding site. (**C** from Thibodeau GA, Patton KT: *Anatomy & physiology,* ed 6, St Louis, 2007, Mosby.)

gen. The Fc portion is responsible for most of the biologic functions of antibodies.

Immunoglobulins consist of four polypeptide chains: two identical light (L) chains and two identical heavy (H) chains. The class of antibody is determined by which heavy chain is used: gamma (IgG), mu (IgM), alpha (IgA), epsilon (IgE), or delta (IgD). The light chains of an antibody molecule are of either the kappa (κ) or lambda (λ) type. The light and heavy chains are held together by noncovalent bonds and disulfide linkages. A set of disulfide linkages between the heavy chains occurs in the hinge region and, in some instances, lends a degree of flexibility at that site. An individual plasma cell produces only one H chain and one L chain at a time.

Each L and H chain is further subdivided into constant (C) and variable (V) regions. The constant regions have relatively stable amino acid sequences within a particular immunoglobulin class or subclass. Thus, the amino acid sequence of the constant region of one IgG1 should be almost identical with the sequence of the same region of another IgG1, even if they react with different antigens. Conversely, among different antibodies, the sequences of the variable regions are characterized by a large number of amino acid differences. Therefore, two IgG1 molecules against different antigens may have many differences in the amino acid sequence of their variable regions. The variable regions can be further subdivided because most of the region's viability in amino acid sequence is localized into three areas within the variable region. These three areas were once called *hypervariable regions* but are now called **complementary-determining regions (CDRs).** The four regions surrounding the CDRs have relatively stable amino acid sequences and are called framework regions (FRs).

Antigen binding

The variable regions of both the heavy (V_H) and light (V_L) chains fold and interact. The FRs control the accuracy of folding, and the CDRs are moved into close proximity, resulting in a antigen-binding site that is lined by the three CDRs of the heavy chain and the three CDRs of the light chain. The chemical nature of the particular amino acids in those sites and the shape of the site determine specificity toward a particular antigen. The antigen that will bind most strongly must have complementary chemistry and topography with the binding site formed by the antibody. The antigen fits into this binding site with the specificity of a key into a lock and is held there by noncovalent chemical interactions (Figure 6-7).

Because the heavy and light chains are identical within the same antibody molecule, the two binding sites are also identical and have specificity for the same antigen. The number of functional binding sites on a molecule is called its valence. Most antibody classes (i.e., IgG, IgE, IgD, and circulating IgA) have a valence of two, but secretory IgA has a valence of four. IgM, being a pentamer, has a theoretic valence of 10, but it can simultaneously use only about five binding sites because a large antigen binding to one site blocks antigen binding to another site.

Function of antibodies

The chief function of antibodies is to protect the individual from infection. The mechanism can be either direct or indirect (Figure 6-8). Directly, antibody can affect infectious agents or their toxic products by **neutralization** (inactivating or blocking the binding of antigen to receptors), **agglutination** (clumping insoluble particles that are in suspension), or **precipitation** (making a soluble antigen into an insoluble precipitate). Indirectly, antibodies activate components of innate resistance, including complement and phagocytes.

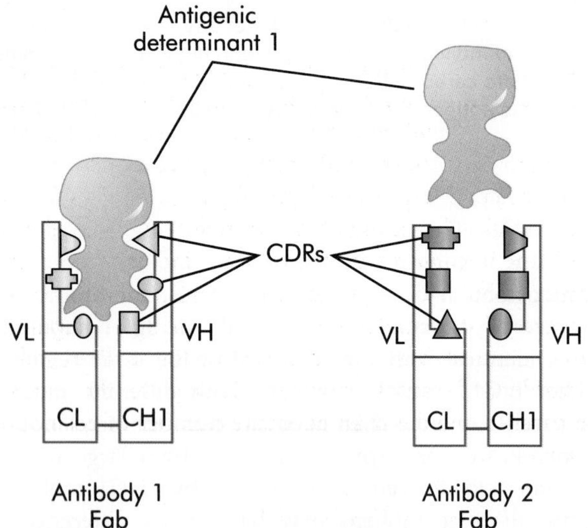

Figure 6-7 ■ **Antigen-Antibody Binding.** The specificity of an antibody binding with an antigen is determined by the shape and chemistry of the six complementary-determining regions (CDRs) in the combining site on the variable region of the antibody. This figure indicates two different antibodies (Fab portions of antibody 1 and antibody 2), which have different sets of CDRs and, therefore, different specificities. As indicated, the antigenic determinant that reacts well with antibody 1 is unable to react with antibody 2 because of differences in the antibody-combining site. *Fab,* Antigen-binding fragment.

Direct effects

To cause infection, many pathogens must attach to specific receptors on the host's cells. For instance, viruses that cause the common cold or the influenza virus must attach to specific receptors on respiratory epithelial cells. Some bacteria, such as *Neisseria gonorrhoeae* that causes gonorrhea, must attach to specific sites on urogenital epithelial cells. Antibodies may protect the host by covering sites on the microorganism that are needed for attachment, thereby preventing infection.

Many viral infections can be prevented by vaccination with inactivated or attenuated (weakened) viruses to induce neutralizing antibody production at the site of the virus' entrance into the body. A good indication of the degree of protection against viral infection is the level of antibodies found in the blood, which is called antibody **titer.**

Some bacteria secrete toxins that harm individuals. For instance, specific bacterial toxins cause the symptoms of tetanus or diphtheria. Most toxins bind to surface molecules on the host's cells and damage those cells. Protective antibodies can bind to the toxins, prevent their interaction with host cells, and neutralize their biologic effects. Detection of the presence of an antibody response against a specific toxin (antibodies referred to as *antitoxins*) can aid in the diagnosis of diseases. For example, laboratory tests that detect antistreptolysin O can be useful in diagnosing group A streptococcal infections. Antibodies that neutralize bacterial toxins can be induced to confer immunity against bacterial pathogens by means of immunization. To prevent harming the recipient of immunization, bacterial toxins are chemically inactivated so that they have lost most of their harmful properties but still retain their immunogenicity. These are referred to as *toxoids.* Examples of bacterial pathogens for which immunization with toxoids can provide immunologic protection include those that cause diphtheria and tetanus.

Indirect effects

Antibody is protective by interacting with or activating components of inflammation (Figure 6-9). The Fc portion is responsible for opsonic activity leading to enhanced phagocytosis and activation of the complement system that may lead to destruction of the pathogen or increased opsonic activity through deposition of C3b.

IgE

IgE is a special class of antibody that protects the individual from infection with large parasites. However, when IgE is produced against relatively innocuous environmental antigens, it is also the primary cause of common allergies

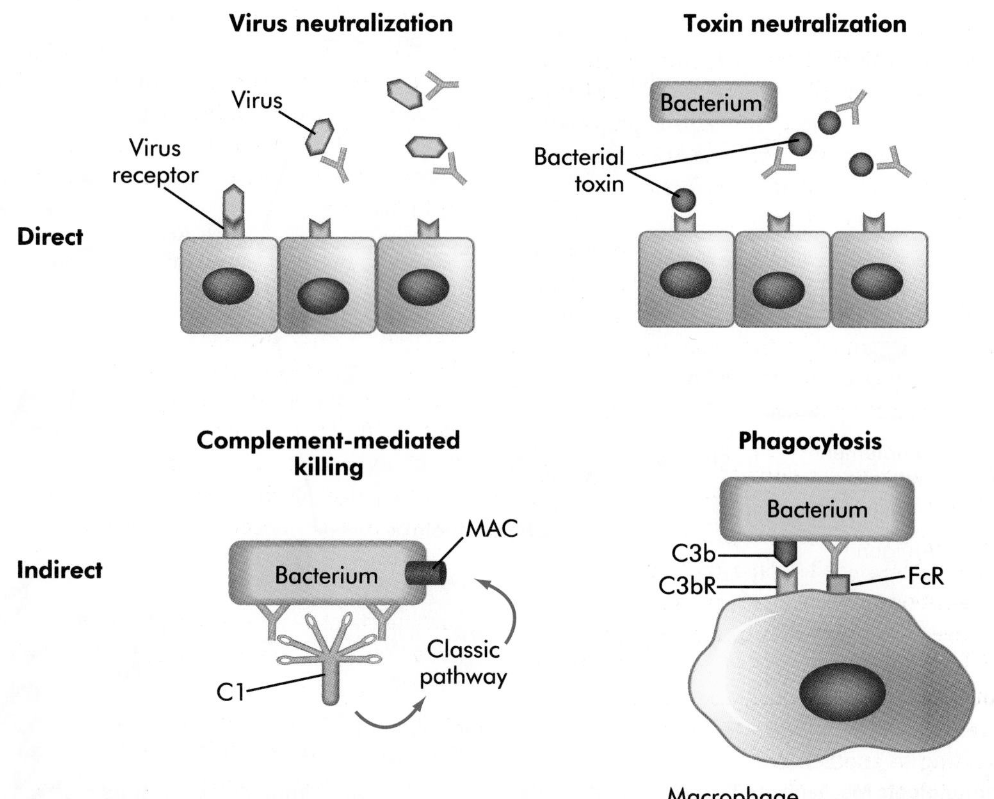

Figure 6-8 ■ **Direct and Indirect Functions of Antibody.** Activities of antibodies can be direct (through the action of antibody alone) or indirect (requiring activation of other components of inflammation, usually through the Fc region). Direct means they include neutralization of viruses or bacterial toxins before they bind to receptors on the surface of the host's cells. Indirect means they include activation of the classical complement pathway through C1 resulting in formation of the membrane-attack complex (MAC) or by increased phagocytosis of bacteria opsonized with antibody and complement components bound to appropriate surface receptors (FcR and C3bR) on the phagocyte.

(e.g., hay fever, dust allergies, bee stings). The role of IgE in allergies is discussed in Chapter 7.

Large multicellular parasites usually invade mucosal tissues (Figure 6-10). Many antigens from the parasites induce IgE, as well as other antibody classes. IgG, IgM, and IgA bind to the surface of parasites, activate complement, generate chemotactic factors for neutrophils and macrophages, and serve as opsonins for those phagocytic cells. This response, however, does not greatly damage parasites. The only inflammatory cell that can adequately damage a parasite is the eosinophil because of the special contents of its granules, particularly major basic protein. Thus, IgE is designed to specifically initiate an inflammatory reaction that preferentially attracts eosinophils to the site of parasitic infection.

Mast cells in the tissues have Fc receptors that specifically and with high affinity bind IgE. IgE against antigens of the parasite are rapidly bound to the mast cell surface. Soluble parasite antigens with multiple antigenic determinants diffuse to neighboring mast cells and simultaneously bind to multiple IgE molecules. This reaction initiates mast cell degranulation and secretion of eosinophil chemotactic factor of anaphylaxis (ECF-A). ECF-A is specifically chemotactic for eosinophils, resulting in eosinophil migration from the circulation into the tissues as well as an increase of surface receptors for IgG and complement component C3b. The eosinophil attaches to the surface of the parasite through these receptors and attempts phagocytosis. Because of the extremely large size of typical parasites, engulfment is unsuccessful. The eosinophilic granules move to the cell membrane in contact with the parasite and undergo normal degranulation, releasing major basic protein and other antimicrobial peptides onto the parasite's surface. Being highly cationic, major basic protein acts almost like sodium hydroxide and causes extensive damage to the parasite. The parasite will die if an adequate number of eosinophils are involved.

B cell antigen receptor

Another form of antibody serves as an antigen receptor on the B cell, the **B cell receptor (BCR).** Its role is to recognize antigen and communicate that information to the cell's nucleus. Therefore, the BCR complex consists of antibody bound to the cell surface and other molecules involved in intracellular signaling. BCRs on the surface of B cells that have not yet reacted with antigen are membrane-associated IgM and IgD immunoglobulins that have identical specificities. The IgM is a monomer rather than the pentamer

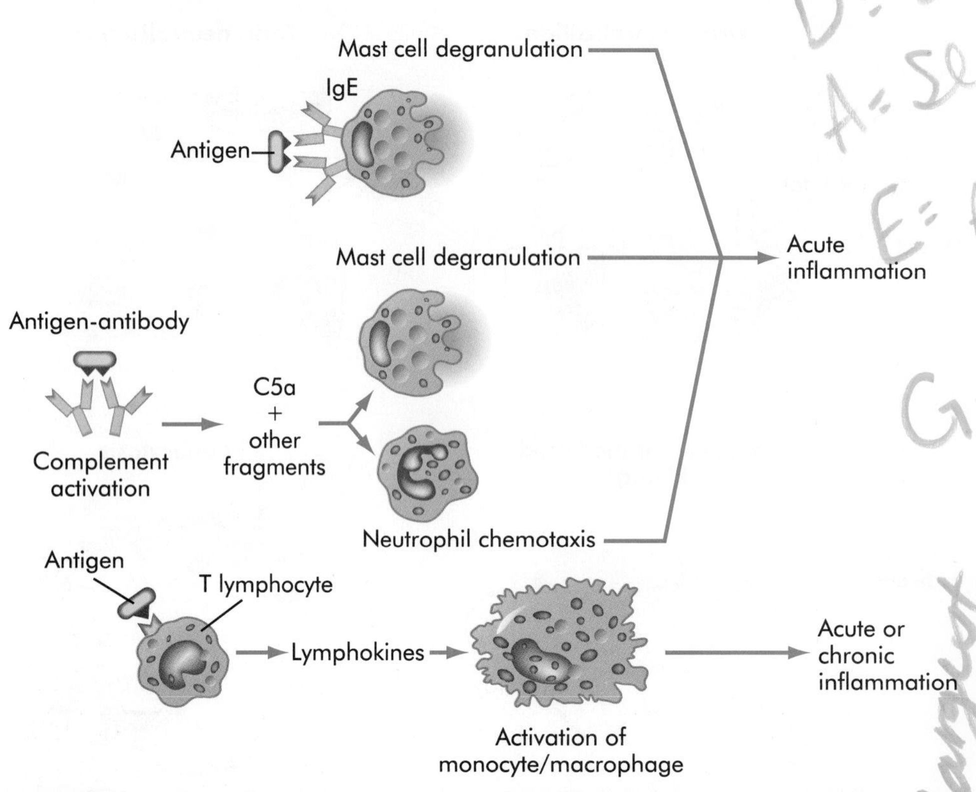

Figure 6-9 ■ **Immunologic Mechanisms That Activate the Inflammatory Response.** Immunologic factors may activate inflammation through three mechanisms: (1) IgE can bind to the surface of a mast cell and, after binding antigen, induce the cell's degranulation (see Figure 6-9); (2) antigen and antibody can activate the complement system, releasing anaphylatoxins and chemotactic factors, especially C5a that result in mast cell degranulation and neutrophil chemotaxis; and (3) antigen may also react with T lymphocytes, resulting in the production of lymphokines that may contribute to the development of either acute or chronic inflammation.

primarily found in the blood. After having reacted with antigen, the BCR on the developing plasma cell may change to other classes of antibody.

Secretory immune system

The entire body is protected by the **systemic immune system.** Another, partially independent, immune system protects the external surfaces of the body. This system is called the **secretory (mucosal) immune system** (Figure 6-11).[2] Antibodies in bodily secretions such as tears, sweat, saliva, mucus, and breast milk, provide local protection against infectious microorganisms. Pathogens can infect the body's surfaces and possibly penetrate to cause systemic disease. Alternatively, the microorganisms may reside in the membranes without causing disease and be a source of infection for other individuals. Thus, an individual may become a carrier for a particular infectious organism. For instance, in the 1950s two vaccines were developed to prevent a virus that entered through the gastrointestinal tract. The Sabin vaccine was administered orally as an attenuated (i.e., inactivated so as to render relatively harmless) live virus. This route caused a transient, limited infection and induced effective systemic and secretory immunity that prevented both the disease and the establishment of a carrier state. The Salk vaccine, on the other hand, consisted of killed viruses administered by injection in the skin. It induced adequate systemic protection but did not generally prevent an intestinal carrier state. Thus, recipients of the Salk vaccine were protected from disease but could still shed the virus and infect others.

IgA is the dominant **secretory immunoglobulin,** although IgM and IgG also are present in secretions. The primary role of IgA is to prevent the attachment and invasion of pathogens through mucosal membranes, such as those of the gastrointestinal, pulmonary, and genitourinary tracts. Antibodies in secretions are produced by plasma cells of the secretory (mucosal) immune system.

The B cells of the secretory immune system follow a different pattern of migration through the body than cells of the systemic immune system, residing in a different group of lymphoid tissues including the lacrimal and salivary glands and the lymphoid tissues of the breasts, bronchi, intestines, and genitourinary tract. The lymphoid tissues of secretory immune system are connected, thus many antigens that a mother has been exposed to in the gastrointestinal tract (e.g., polio virus) induce secretion of specific IgAs, IgMs, and IgGs into the breast milk. Antibodies in the milk may protect the nursing newborn against these infectious disease agents. Although colostral antibodies (i.e., found in colostrum of breast milk) provide the newborn with passive immunity against gastrointestinal infections, they do not provide systemic immunity because they do not cross the newborn's gut into the bloodstream after the first 24 hours of life. Maternal antibodies that pass across the placenta into the fetus before birth provide passive systemic immunity.

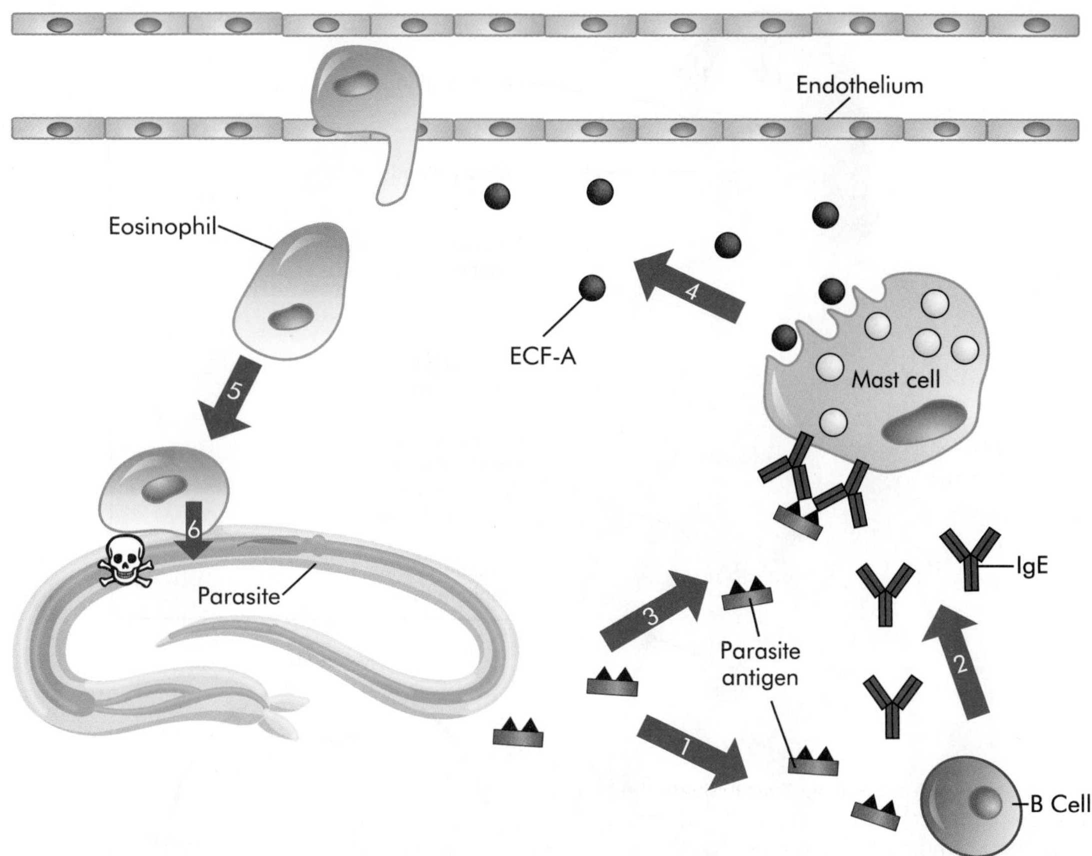

Figure 6-10 ■ **IgE-Mediated Destruction of a Parasite.** **(1)** Soluble antigens from a parasitic infection cause production of IgE antibody by B cells. **(2)** Secreted IgE binds to IgE-specific receptors on the mast cell. **(3)** Additional soluble parasite antigen cross-links the IgE on the mast cell surface, **(4)** leading to mast cell degranulation and release of many proinflammatory products, including eosinophil chemotactic factor of anaphylaxis (ECF-A). **(5)** ECF-A attracts eosinophils from the circulation. **(6)** The eosinophil attaches to the surface of the parasite and releases potent lysosomal enzymes that damage microorganisms.

Monoclonal antibodies

Most humoral immune responses are polyclonal—that is, a mixture of antibodies produced from multiple B lymphocytes. Most antigenic molecules have multiple antigenic determinants, each of which induces a different group of antibodies. Thus, a polyclonal response is a mixture of antibody classes, specificities, and function, some of which are more protective than others.

Monoclonal antibody is produced in the laboratory from one B cell that has been cloned, thus all the antibody is of the same class, specificity, and function. The advantages of monoclonal antibodies are that (1) a single antibody of known antigenic specificity is generated rather than a mixture of different antibodies; (2) monoclonal antibodies have a single, constant binding affinity; (3) monoclonal antibodies can be diluted to a constant titer (concentration in fluid) because the actual antibody concentration is known; and (4) the antibody can be easily purified. Thus, a highly concentrated antibody with optimal function has been used to develop extremely specific and sensitive laboratory tests (e.g., home and laboratory pregnancy tests) and therapies (e.g., several experimental therapies for cancer).

✔ QUICK CHECK 6-2

1. What is an antigen?
2. What are the major functions of antibody?
3. What is the difference between the secretory and systemic immune systems?

CELL-MEDIATED IMMUNE RESPONSE

There are several types of mature T cells, each with a different function. Memory cells induce the secondary immune response; **lymphokine-producing cells** secrete cytokines that activate other cells, such as macrophages; cytotoxic (Tc) cells attack antigens directly and destroy cells that bear foreign antigens; and regulatory cells, primarily helper T (Th) cells, control both cell-mediated and humoral immune responses. T cells are particularly important in protection against viruses, tumors, and pathogens that are resistant to killing by normal neutrophils and macrophages. They are also absolutely essential for the development of most humoral responses.

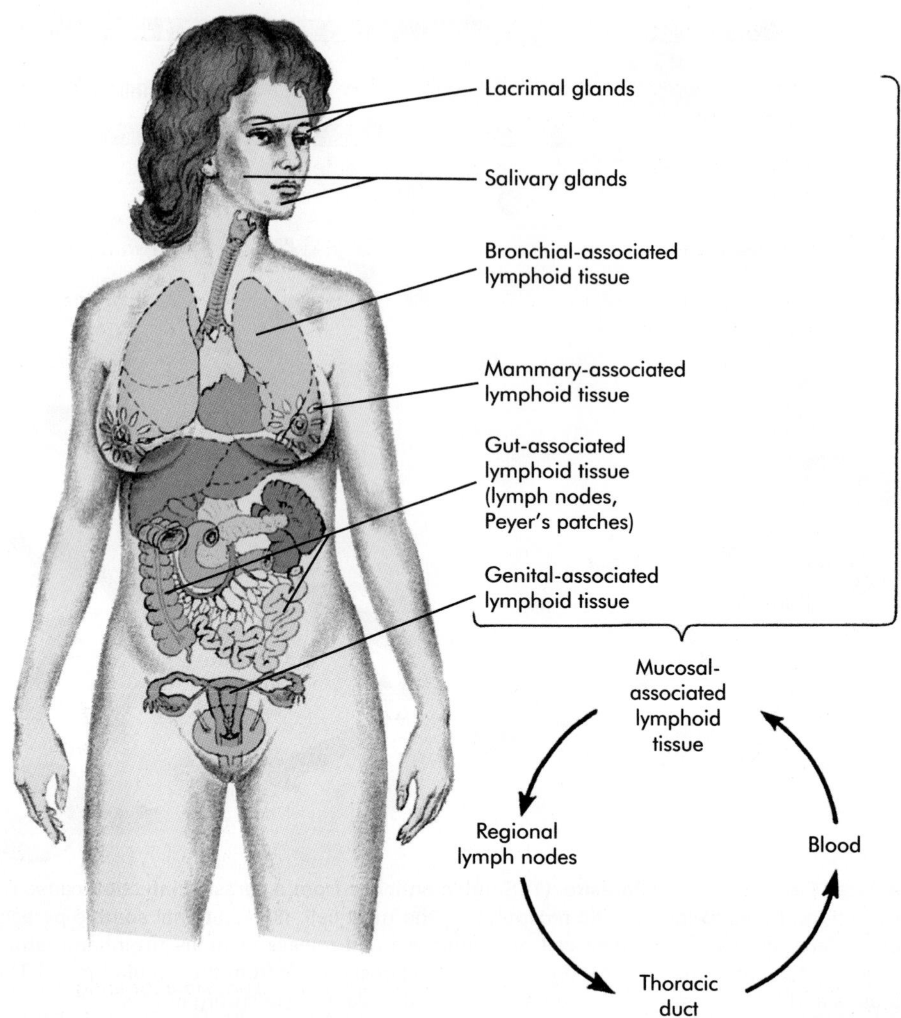

Figure 6-11 ■ **Secretory Immune System.** Lymphocytes from the mucosal-associated (secretory) lymphoid tissues circulate throughout the body in a pattern separate from other lymphocytes. For example, lymphocytes from the gut-associated lymphoid tissue circulate through the regional lymph nodes, the thoracic duct, and the blood and return to other mucosal-associated lymphoid tissues rather than to lymphoid tissue of the systemic immune system.

The process by which T cells recognize and destroy a target is highly complex and requires an understanding of three different concepts: the T cell receptor, antigen presentation, and CD molecules. Defects in any of these will lead to major defects in cell-mediated immunity and potentially the individual's death (Chapter 7).

T Cell Recognition of a Target Cell

T cell receptor complex

T lymphocytes use an antigen receptor that is similar to the B cell receptor. The **T cell receptor (TCR)** complex is composed of an antibody-like protein (TCR) and a group of accessory proteins that are involved in signaling to the nucleus. Although the components of the TCR resemble antibody, they are encoded by different genes. All of the TCRs on a single T cell are identical in structure and specificity.

Antigen presentation molecules

Unlike B cells, T cells do not react with soluble antigens. Protein antigen must be presented in a specific manner on the surface of the target cell; it must be held by molecules of the **major histocompatibility complex (MHC).** These molecules are discussed in more detail in Chapter 7.

MHC molecules are glycoproteins found on the surface of all human cells except red blood cells (Figure 6-12). They are divided into two general classes, class I and class II, based on their molecular structure, distribution among cell populations, and function in antigen presentation. MHC class I molecules are composed of a large alpha (α) chain along with a smaller chain called beta $(\beta)_2$ microglobulin. MHC class II molecules are composed of α and β chains that differ from the ones used for MHC class I.

The α and β transmembrane chains of the two MHC molecules are encoded from different genetic loci located

	Class I MHC	Class II MHC
Structure	Single transmembrane chain (α) complexed with β2-microglobulin	Two transmembrane chains (α and β)
Genes	3 different α chains: HLA-A, HLA-B, and HLA-C	3 different pairs of α and β chains: HLA-DR, HLA-DP, and HLA-DQ
Distribution	On all nucleated cells and platelets	On B cells, APCs, and some epithelial cells
Presentation	Presents "endogenous" antigens from intracellular proteins	Presents "exogenous" antigens from digested extracellular pathogens
Reacts with	CD8 on Tc cells	CD4 on Th cells

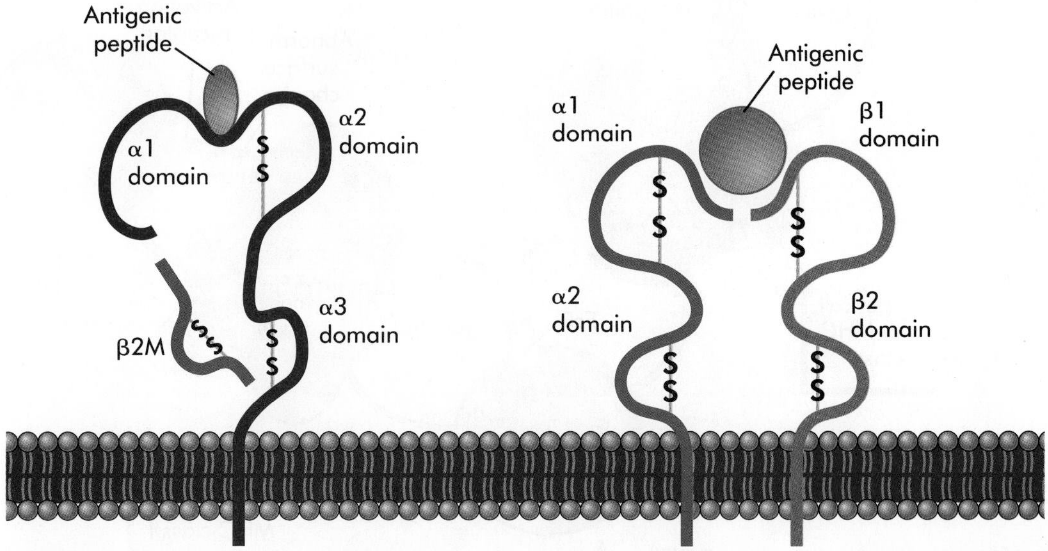

Figure 6-12 ■ **Antigen-Presenting Molecules.** Two sets of molecules are primarily responsible for antigen presentation: MHC class I and MHC class II. The MHC molecules are encoded from the major histocompatibility complex on chromosome 6. This complex also contains genes for several other molecules that participate in the innate or immune responses, including some complement proteins and cytokines, which are referred to as MHC class III molecules. This region contains information for the α chains of three principal class I molecules, called HLA-A, HLA-B, and HLA-C. These will be discussed in more detail in Chapter 7. Each of the MHC class I α chains complex with β2 microglobulin, which is encoded by a gene on chromosome 15. The MHC class I molecules present small peptide antigens (8 or 9 amino acids in length) in a pocket formed by the α1 and α2 domains of the α chain. The conformation of the molecule is stabilized by β2 microglobulin as well as by intrachain disulfide bonds (-S-S-). The α and β chains of class II molecules are also encoded in the MHC region. The principal class II molecules are HLA-DR, HLA-DP, and HLA-DQ. The MHC class II molecules present peptide antigens in a pocket formed by the α1 domain of the α chain and β1 domain of the β chain. Both MHC class I and II molecules are anchored to the plasma membrane by hydrophobic regions on the ends of the α and β chains.

as a large complex of genes on human chromosome 6 (β_2 microglobulin is found on a different chromosome). Most T cell functions (e.g., T cell–mediated cytotoxicity) require that fragments of antigen be presented by MHC class I molecules. Th cells require that antigen be presented by MHC class II molecules.

CD molecules

Cells express a large number of molecules on their surfaces, many of which are important in the immune response. Many of the molecules are part of a nomenclature that uses the prefix CD (cluster of differentiation) followed by a number (e.g., CD1 or CD2). The list of **CD molecules** is constantly increasing (currently in excess of 250). We will focus on a small number of highly important examples to illustrate the immensely complicated, but highly effective, interactions that take place to produce a protective immune response.

T Lymphocyte Function

Killing abnormal cells

Cytotoxic T lymphocytes

Cytotoxic T lymphocytes (Tc cells or CTLs) are responsible for the cell-mediated destruction of tumor cells or cells infected with viruses. The Tc cell must directly adhere to the target cell through antigen presented by MHC class I molecules and appropriate CD molecules (Figure 6-13). Tc cell–mediated killing is therefore *class I restricted.* Because of the cellular distribution of MHC class I

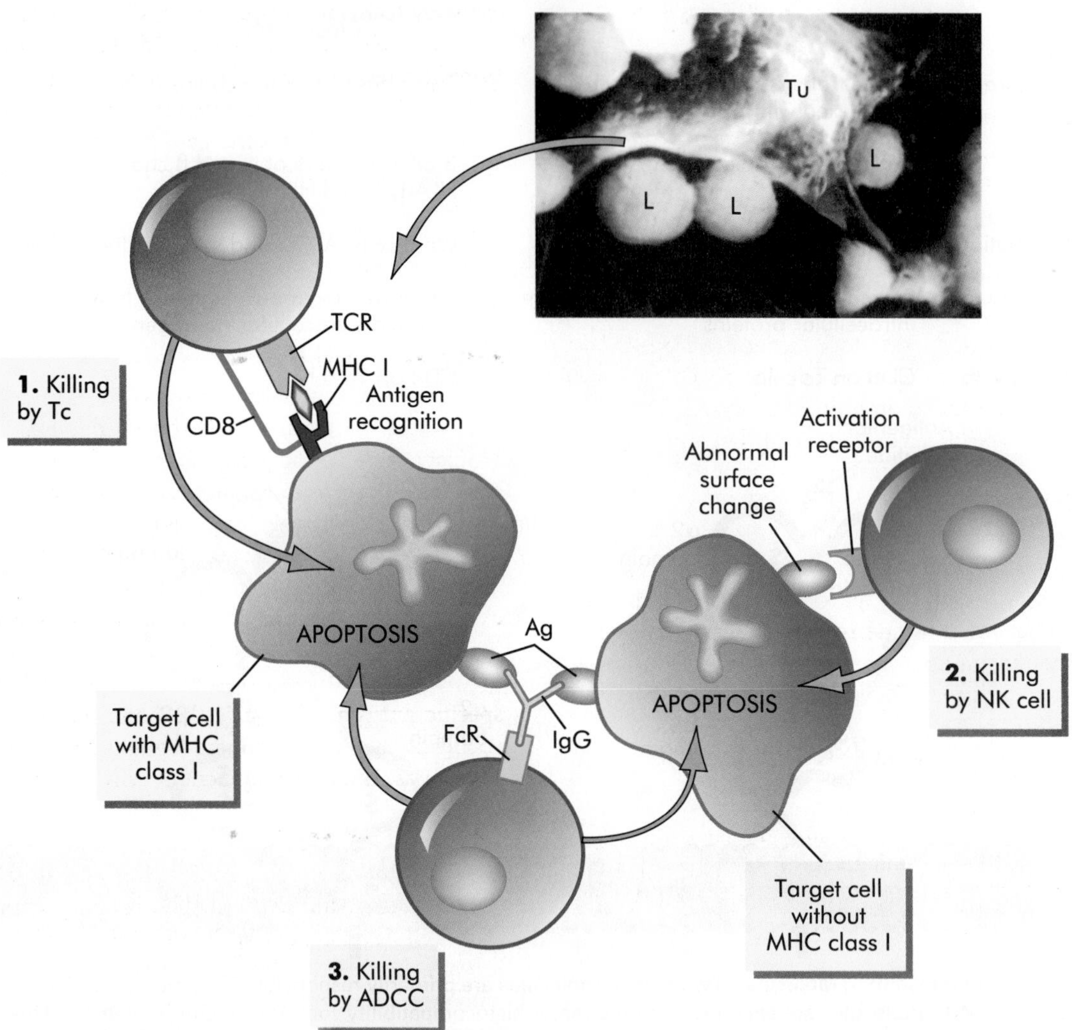

Figure 6-13 ■ **Cellular Killing Mechanisms.** Several cells have the capacity to kill abnormal (e.g., virally infected, cancerous) target cells. **(1)** Cytotoxic T (Tc) cells recognized endogenous antigen presented by MHC class I molecules. The Tc cell mobilizes multiple killing mechanisms that induce apoptosis of the target cell. **(2)** Natural killer (NK) cells identify and kill target cells through receptors that recognize abnormal surface changes. NK cells specifically kill targets that do not express surface MHC class I molecules. **(3)** Several cells, including macrophages and NK cells, can kill by antibody-dependent cellular cytotoxicity (ADCC). IgG antibodies bind to foreign antigen on the target cell, and cells involved in ADCC bind IgG through Fc receptors (FcR) and initiate killing. The insert is a scanning electron microscopic view of Tc cells (L) attacking a much larger tumor cell (Tu). (Insert from Thibodeau GA, Patton KT: *Anatomy & physiology,* ed 6, St Louis, 2007, Mosby).

molecules, Tc cells can recognize antigen on the surface of almost any type of cell that has been infected by a virus or has become cancerous. Most Tc cell killing also requires CD8 on the Tc cell that binds to MHC class I on the target. After attachment to a target cell, killing occurs by induction of apoptosis.

Other cells that kill abnormal cells

Various other cells kill targets in a fashion similar to Tc lymphocytes. Prominent among these cells are NK (natural killer) cells (see Chapter 5). NK cells are a special group of lymphoid cells that are similar to T cells but lack antigen-specific receptors.[3] Instead, they express Fc receptors for IgG and a variety of cell surface receptors that identify protein changes on the surface of cells infected with viruses or that have become cancerous. After attachment, the NK cell kills its target in a manner similar to that of Tc cells. NK cells also have receptors for MHC class I. However, these receptors are not CD8 and result in the NK cells being inactivated. Thus, NK cells primarily kill target cells that have suppressed the expression of MHC class I, as do some tumors.

NK cells, as well as some macrophages, can specifically kill targets through use of antibody. These cells express Fc receptors on their surface. If antigens on a pathogen or abnormal cell bind IgG, the NK cell can attach through Fc receptors and activate its normal killing mechanisms. This is referred to as **antibody-dependent cellular cytotoxicity (ADCC)** (see Figure 6-13).

T cells that activate macrophages

During chronic inflammation T cells produce cytokines that activate macrophages (see Chapter 5). The cytokines (particularly IFN-γ) stimulate the macrophage to become a more efficient phagocyte and increase production of proteolytic enzymes and other antimicrobial substances (see Figure 5-8).

Regulatory T lymphocytes

Regulatory T (Treg) cells are a group of T cells that control the immune response.[4] The most characterized is the T-helper (Th) cell, which is necessary for development of most humoral and cellular immune responses. The virus that causes AIDS specifically infects and destroys Th cells, thus leading to the onset of life-threatening infections. This cell will be discussed in more detail later in this chapter and in Chapter 7.

Other Treg cells suppress immune responses. This population, sometimes called T-suppressor cells, is a mixture of cells that affect the immune response in multiple ways. Some affect the recognition of antigen, and others suppress the proliferative steps that follow antigen recognition.

QUICK CHECK 6-3

1. What are the different types of T cells?
2. Define the primary and secondary immune responses.
3. What are antigen-presenting cells?
4. Why are cytokines important to the immune response?

GENERATION OF CLONAL DIVERSITY

The immune response occurs in two phases (Table 6-3). The **generation of clonal diversity** mostly occurs in the **primary (central) lymphoid organs** of the fetus and results in the development of **lymphoid stem cells** into B and T lymphocytes with the ability to react against almost any antigen that will be encountered throughout life. It is estimated that B and T cells can collectively recognize more than 10^8 different antigenic determinants. When the individual is exposed to an antigen, the process of clonal selection (discussed later in this chapter) begins, during which the particular antigen selects and induces further development of only a small group of B and T cells.

B Lymphocytes

In birds, an organ called the bursa of Fabricius is responsible for the maturation of B (bursal-derived) lymphocytes. Humans have no discrete bursa, but the bone marrow makes up the **human bursal equivalent** and serves as the primary lymphoid organ for B cell development (see Figure 6-1). Lymphocytes destined to become B cells circulate through the bursal equivalent, where they are exposed to hormones that, without the presence of antigen, induce proliferation and differentiation into B cells (see Figure 6-8). Each B cell, however, responds to only one specific antigen. They exit the bone marrow and take up residence in other lymphoid organs (secondary lymphoid organs) as immunocompetent B cells.

T Lymphocytes

The process of T cell proliferation and differentiation is similar to that for B cells.[5] The primary lymphoid organ for T cell development is the thymus. Lymphoid stem cells journey through the thymus, where, under the pressure and guidance of thymic hormones (thymosin, thymopoietin, thymostimulin, and several other hormones produced by the epithelium) and without the presence of antigen, they are driven to undergo cell division and simultaneously produce receptors (TCRs) against the diversity of antigens the

TABLE 6-3
Generation of Clonal Diversity vs. Clonal Selection

	Generation of Clonal Diversity	Clonal Selection
Purpose?	To produce large numbers of T and B lymphocytes with the maximum diversity of antigen receptors	Select, expand, and differentiate clones of T and B cells against a specific antigen
When does it occur?	Primarily in the fetus	Primarily after birth and throughout life
Where does it occur?	Central lymphoid organs: thymus for T cells, bone marrow for B cells	Peripheral lymphoid organs, including lymph nodes, spleen, and other lymphoid tissues
Is foreign antigen involved?	No	Yes, antigen determines which clones of cells will be selected
What hormones/ cytokines are involved?	Thymic hormones, IL-7, others	Many cytokines produced by Th cells and APCs
Final product?	Immunocompetent T and B cells that can react with antigen, but have not seen antigen, and migrate to the secondary lymphoid organs	Plasma cells that produce antibody, effector T cells that help (Th cells), kill targets (Tc cells), or regulate immune responses (Treg cells); memory B and T cells

Th cells, Helper T cells; *APCs,* antigen-presenting cells; *Tc cells,* cytotoxic T cells; *Treg cells,* regulatory T cells.

individual will encounter throughout life. They exit the thymus through the blood vessels and lymphatics as mature (immunocompetent) T cells with antigen-specific receptors on the cell surface and take up residence in secondary lymphoid organs.

INDUCTION OF THE IMMUNE RESPONSE

An immune response is triggered by antigen by a process called clonal selection. This generally occurs in lymphoid organs called the secondary (peripheral) lymphoid organs in which antigen selectively reacts with B or T cells (Figure 6-14). The secondary lymphoid organs include the spleen, lymph nodes, adenoids, tonsils, Peyer's patches (intestines), and the appendix (see Figure 6-2). Under the control of a variety of cytokines and complex cellular interactions, the selected B or T cells further proliferate and differentiate into plasma cells that produce antibody, T cells that can attack cellular targets, or B or T memory cells that will respond more quickly to a second exposure to the same antigen.

Primary and Secondary Immune Responses

The immune response to antigen has classically been divided into two phases—the primary and secondary responses—that are most easily demonstrated by measuring concentrations of circulating antibody over time (Figure 6-15). After a single initial exposure to most antigens, there is a latent period, or lag phase, during which B cell differentiation and proliferation occurs. After approximately 5 to 7 days, IgM antibody is detected in the circulation. The lag phase is the time necessary for the process of clonal selection. This is the **primary immune response,** characterized typically by initial IgM followed by IgG against the same antigen. The quantity of IgG may be about equal to or less than the amount of IgM. If no further exposure to the antigen occurs, the circulating antibody is catabolized (broken down) and measurable quantities fall. The individual's immune system, however, has been primed.

A second challenge by the same antigen results in the **secondary immune response,** which is characterized by the more rapid production of a larger amount of antibody

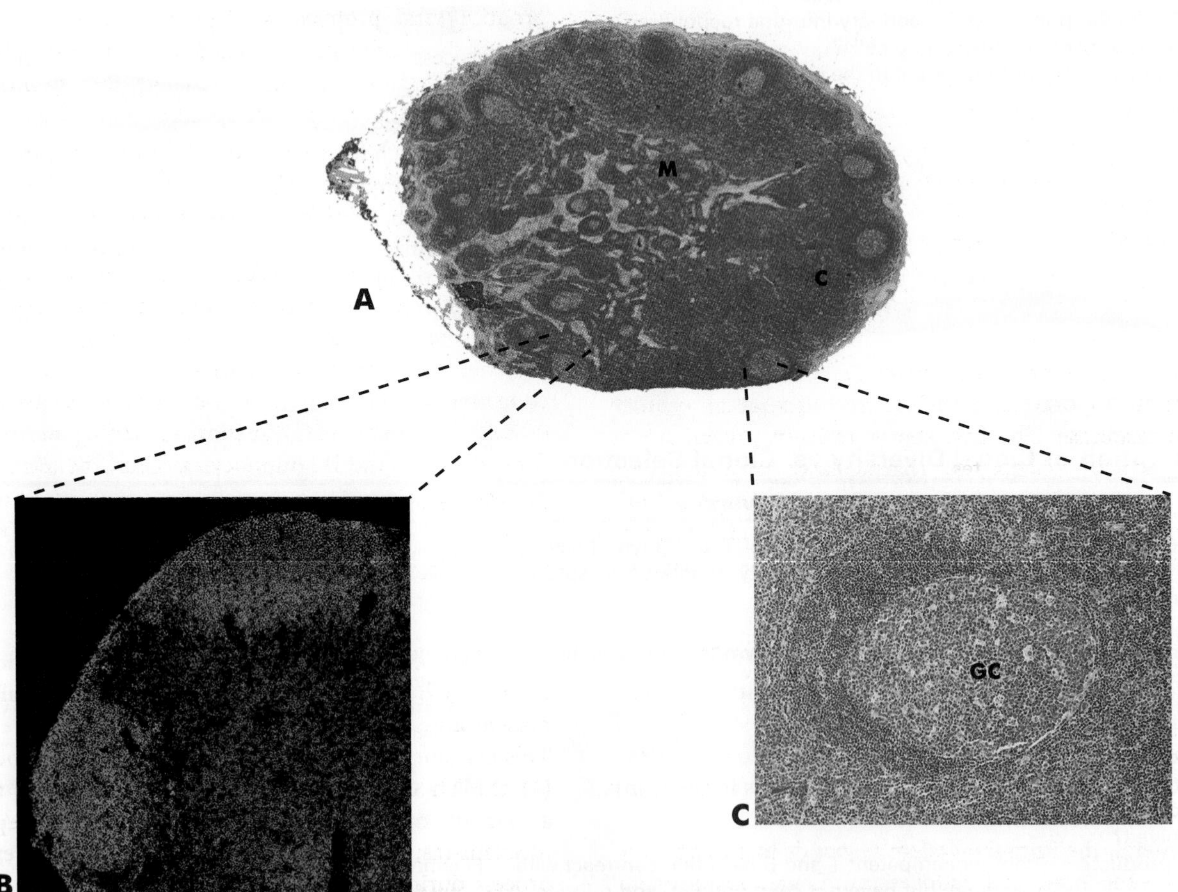

Figure 6-14 ■ Secondary Lymphoid Tissues: Sites of B Cell and T Cell Differentiation. A, A lymph node is organized into an outer cortex **(C)** and an inner medulla **(M)**. **B,** The lymph node contains areas that are rich in immunocompetent B cells (stained green) and T cells (stained red). **C,** In response to antigen, B cells undergo proliferation resulting in the formation of germinal centers (GC). (From Kumar V, Abbas A, Fausto N: *Robbins and Cotran pathologic basis of disease,* ed 7, Philadelphia, 2005, Saunders.)

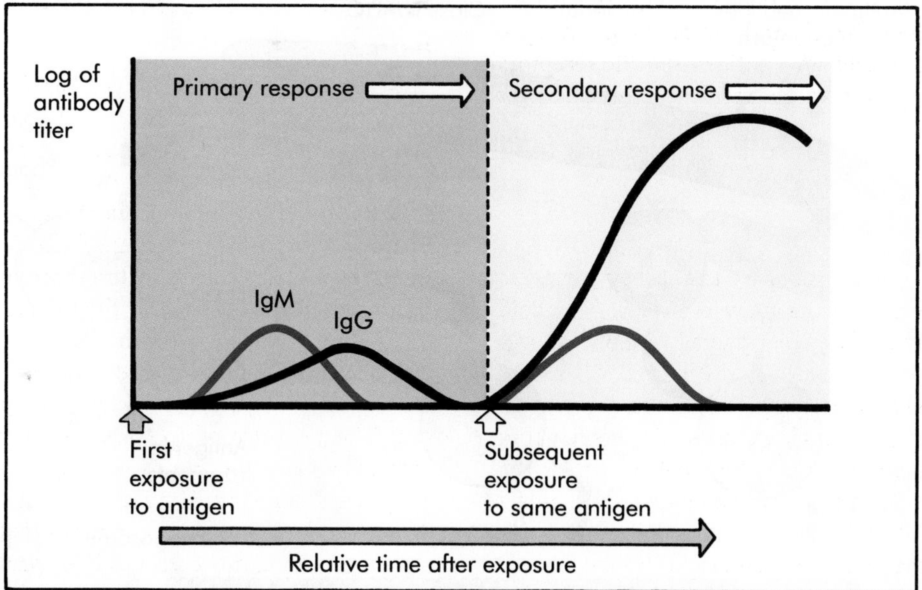

Figure 6-15 ■ **Primary and Secondary Immune Responses.** The initial administration of antigen induces a primary response during which IgM is initially produced, followed by IgG. Another administration of the antigen induces the secondary response in which IgM is transiently produced and larger amounts of IgG are produced over a longer period of time.

than the primary response. The rapidity of the secondary immune response is the result of memory cells that do not require further differentiation. IgM may be transiently produced in the secondary response, but IgG production is increased considerably, making it the predominant antibody class. If the antigenic challenge is in the form of a vaccine or occurs through natural infection, the level of protective IgG may remain elevated for decades.

Cellular Interactions in the Immune Response

In most cases, several steps involving cellular interactions must occur to produce a protective humoral or cellular immune response. The first step is **antigen presentation,** during which phagocytes (particularly macrophages) phagocytose, break up (process), and present antigenic fragments on the cell surface.[6] Antigen-presenting cells interact with Th cells to induce B cell to mature into plasma cells or T cells to mature into effector T cells.

Antigen processing and presentation

Antigens that enter the bloodstream or lymphatics encounter a variety of antigen presenting cells (APCs), including macrophages and macrophage-like cells in tissue (i.e., dendritic cells in the lymph nodes, Langerhans cells in the skin) (see Figures 6-1 and 6-2).

In general, the immune system responds to two types of antigens: exogenous and endogenous. Exogenous antigens originate from outside the body, such as infectious microorganisms. Endogenous antigens are synthesized within a cell. These include viral antigens because viruses infect cells and use the normal cellular protein-synthesizing machinery to produce viral proteins. Endogenous antigens also may include those uniquely produced by cancerous cells. When many cells undergo malignant change, they begin producing unique antigens that are specific to the cancer cell.

Exogenous and endogenous antigens are preferentially presented by different classes of MHC molecules: class I MHC molecules generally present endogenous antigens, and class II molecules prefer exogenous antigens (Figure 6-16). Because class I MHC molecules are expressed on all cells, except red blood cells, any change in that cell caused by viral infection or malignancy may result in foreign antigen being presented by MHC class I. Class II MHC molecules are co-expressed with MHC class I on a more limited number of cells that have APC function, including macrophages, dendritic cells, and B lymphocytes. Thus, the term **antigen processing** relates to the process by which exogenous and endogenous antigens are broken up and linked with the appropriate MHC molecules.

Helper T lymphocytes

Regardless of whether an antigen primarily induces a cellular or humoral immune response, APCs usually must present antigen to helper T cells (Th cells) (Figure 6-17).[7] This extremely important role involves three distinct steps: (1) the Th cell directly interacts with the APC through a variety of antigen-specific and antigen-independent mechanisms; (2) the Th cell undergoes a differentiation process during which a variety of cytokine genes are activated; and (3) depending on the pattern of cytokines expressed, the mature Th cell interacts with either immunocompetent B or T cells to cause their differentiation into either plasma cells or effector T cells.

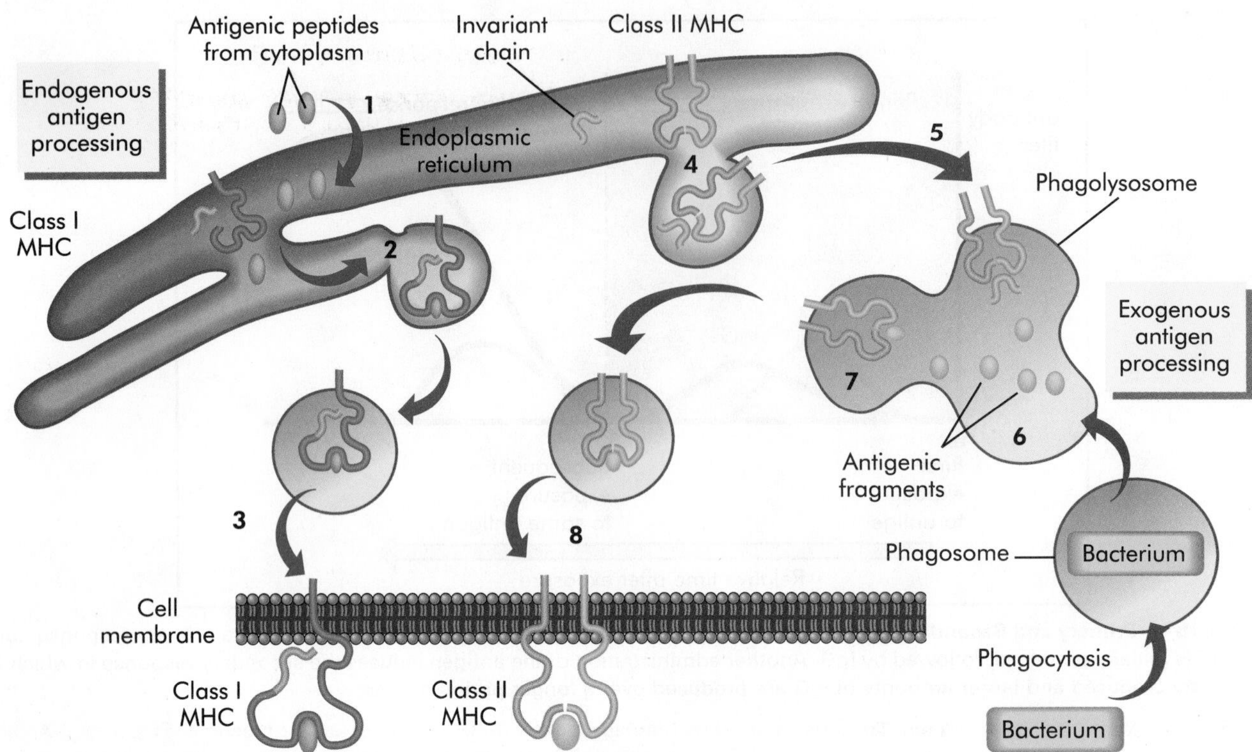

Figure 6-16 ■ **Antigen Processing.** Antigen processing and presentation are required for initiation of most immune responses. Foreign antigen may be either endogenous (cytoplasmic protein) or exogenous (e.g., bacterium). Endogenous antigenic peptides are transported into the endoplasmic reticulum **(1)** where the MHC molecules are being assembled. In the ER, antigenic peptides bind to the α chains of the MHC class I molecule **(2)**, and the complex is transported to the cell surface **(3)**. The α and β chains of the MHC class II molecules are also being assembled in the endoplasmic reticulum **(4)**, but the antigen-binding site is blocked by a small molecule (invariant chain) to prevent interactions with endogenous antigenic peptides. The MHC class II–invariant chain complex is transported to phagolysosomes **(5)** where exogenous antigenic fragments have been produced as a result of phagocytosis **(6)**. In the phagolysosomes, the invariant chain is digested and replaced by exogenous antigenic peptides **(7)**, after which the MHC class II–antigen complex is inserted into the cell membrane **(8)**.

When T cells develop in the thymus, two different populations are produced. T cells that are destined to become Th cells emerge from the thymus with a characteristic cell surface protein, called CD4. Cells destined to become Tc cells have a different cell surface protein, called CD8. The role of CD4 and CD8 is to help the interaction between T cells and APCs by reacting with antigen-presenting molecules. Thus, the T cell receptor and CD4 or CD8 both attach to the antigen presenting molecules on the surface of another cell. CD4 can only interact with MHC class II molecules, whereas CD8 reacts only with MHC class I molecules.

To mature into a functional helper cell, the Th cell must receive several signals, including the TCR binding to antigen and CD4 binding to MHC class II. Other signals between cell-surface adhesion molecules are important but will not be discussed here. If all the appropriate signaling pathways are activated, the cell will differentiate into a functional Th cell.

Additional signals are provided by cytokines. At this early stage of Th cell differentiation, IL-1 secreted by the APC provides this signal. The Th cell then produces IL-2, which is secreted and acts in an autocrine (self-stimulating) fashion to induce further maturation and proliferation of the Th cell. Without IL-2 production, the Th cell cannot efficiently mature into a functional helper cell.

At this point, Th cells undergo differentiation into either **Th1** or **Th2 cells** (see Figure 6-17). These subsets have different functions: Th1 cells appear to provide more help in developing cell-mediated immunity, whereas Th2 cells provide more help for developing humoral immunity. The two Th subsets differ considerably in the spectrum of cytokines produced by each. Additionally, each Th cell may suppress the other so that the immune response may favor either antibody formation, with suppression of a cell-mediated response, or the opposite. For example, antigens derived from viral or bacterial pathogens and those derived from cancer cells seem to induce a greater number of Th1 cells relative to Th2 cells, whereas antigens derived from multicellular parasites and allergens are hypothesized to result in production of more Th2 cells. Many antigens (e.g., tetanus vaccine), however, will produce excellent humoral and cell-mediated responses simultaneously.

Superantigens

Certain diseases are produced by a group of molecules called **superantigens (SAGs).**[8] SAGs bind to the variable

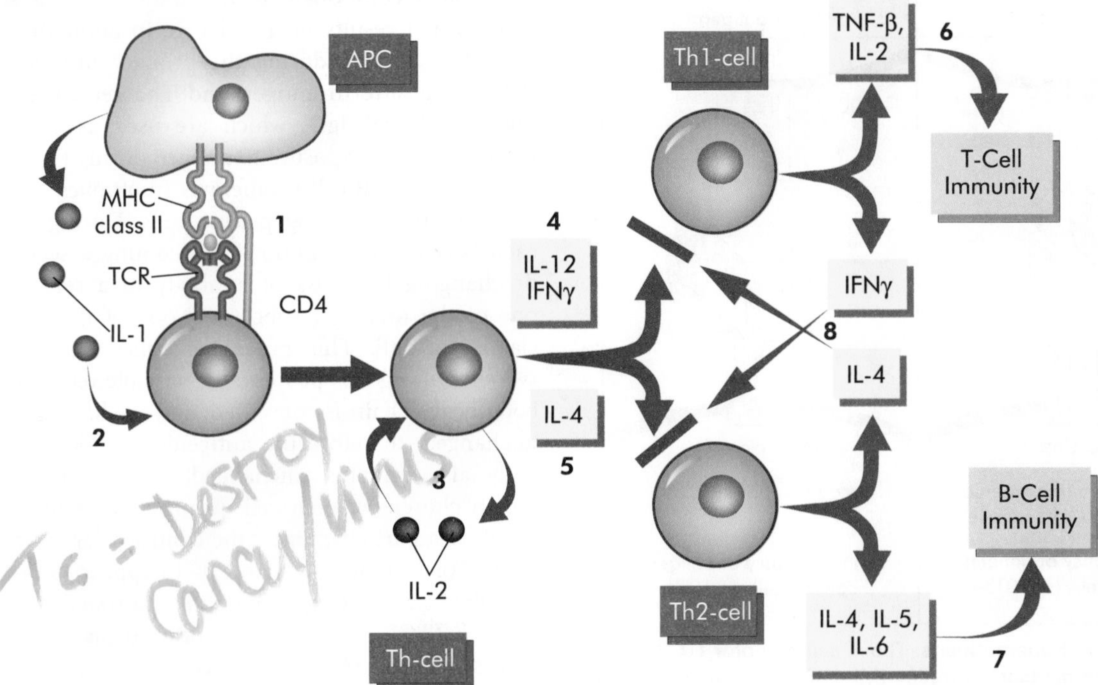

Figure 6-17 ■ Development of Th1 and Th2 Cells. Antigen presenting cells (APC) present antigen to a precursor Th cells. (1) An antigen signal is produced by the interaction of the T cell receptor (TCR) and CD4 with antigen presented by MHC class II molecules. (2) Cytokines (particularly IL-1) produced by the APC provide a second signal. (3) In response to these signals, the precursor Th cells begin producing the cytokine IL-2, which binds with the same cell to accelerate differentiation and proliferation. Commitment to a Th1 or Th2 phenotype results from the effects of other cytokines. (4) IL-12 and IFN-γ favor differentiation into the Th1 cell phenotype, whereas (5) IL-4 favors differentiation into the Th2 cell phenotype. (6) The Th1 cell produces cytokines that assist in the differentiation of cytotoxic T (Tc) cells (e.g., TNF-β, IL-2), whereas (7) the Th2 cell produces cytokines that favor B cell differentiation (e.g., IL-4, IL-5, IL-6). (8) Th1 and Th2 cells affect each other through the production of inhibitory cytokines: IFN-γ will inhibit development of Th2 cells, and IL-4 will inhibit the development of Th1 cells.

portion of the TCR outside of its normal antigen-specific binding site, as well as to MHC class II molecules outside of their antigen-presentation sites (Figure 6-18). Thus, SAGs are not digested and processed by an APC to be presented to an immune cell. This binding, which is independent of antigen-recognition, provides a signal for Th cell activation, proliferation, and cytokine production. The normal antigen-specific recognition between Th cells and APCs results in activation of a relatively few cells—only those cells with specific TCRs against that antigen. SAGs activate a large population of Th cells, regardless of antigen specificity, and induce excessive production of cytokines, including IL-2, IFN-γ, and TNF-α. The overproduction of inflammatory cytokines results in symptoms of a systemic inflammatory reaction, including fever, low blood pressure, and, potentially, fatal shock. Some examples of SAGs are the bacterial toxins produced by *Staphylococcus aureus* and *Streptococcus pyogenes* (SAGs that cause toxic shock syndrome and food poisoning).

T cell clonal selection: The cellular immune response

For T cells to mature, another set of cellular interactions is required (Figure 6-19).[9] Cytotoxic T cells (Tc) must react with antigen presented by MHC class I molecules on the surface of antigen-presenting cells or other target cells. The Tc cell binds antigen with a TCR identical with that found on Th cells. Tc cells express CD8, rather than CD4, which interacts with class I molecules and provides another differentiation signal. Additional adhesion molecules also must participate. A cytokine must also interact with the Tc cell to induce complete maturation and development of cytotoxic activity. IL-2 from the Th1 cell fulfills this role. Thus, the development of Tc cells is dependent on Th1 cell function.

B cell clonal selection: The humoral immune response

A sequence of cellular interactions is required to produce an effective antibody response (Figure 6-20).[10] The immunocompetent B cell is also an APC and expresses surface IgM and IgD B cell receptors (BCRs). Unlike the T cell receptor that can only "see" processed and presented antigen, the BCR can react with soluble antigen. Antigen binding to the BCR activates the B cell resulting in internalization of the antigen, antigen processing, and presentation of antigen fragments by MHC class II molecules. The antigen presented on the B cell surface is recognized by a Th2 cell through the TCR and CD4. The intercellular bridge created through antigen and other intercellular adhesion molecules induces the Th2 cell to secrete cytokines (particularly IL-4) that cause B cell proliferation and maturation into plasma cells.

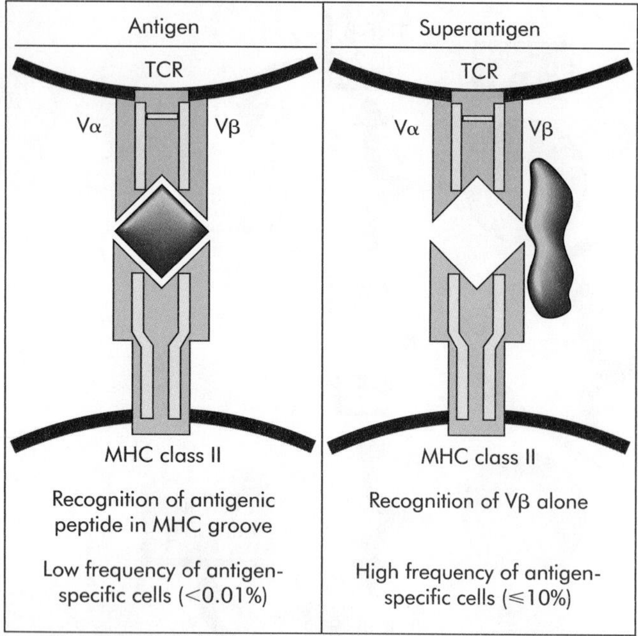

Figure 6-18 ■ **Superantigens.** The T cell receptor (TCR) and major histocompatibility complex (MHC) class II molecule are normally held together by processed antigen. Superantigens, such as some bacterial exotoxins, bind directly to the variable region of the TCR-β chain and the MHC class II molecule. Each superantigen activates sets of V-β chains independently of the antigen specificity of the TCR.

A major component of maturation is **class switch;** the process that results in the change in antibody production from IgM to IgG during the primary immune response. Before exposure to antigen and Th2 cells, the B cell produces IgM and IgD, which are used as cell membrane receptors. After exposure to antigen during the clonal selection process, a B cell proliferates (multiplies) and develops into antibody-secreting plasma cells. During that process, each B cell has the option of becoming a secretor of IgM or changing the class of antibody to a secreted form of one of the four IgG subclasses, one of the two IgA subclasses, or IgE. This process is called class- or isotype-switch. During this process, the variable region of the antibody heavy chain is conserved, and the light chain remains unchanged, therefore the antigenic specificity of the antibody also remains unchanged. The particular constant region chosen by each cell during class switch appears to be, at least partially, under the control of specific Th2 cytokines. For instance, IL-4 and IL-13 appear to preferentially stimulate switch to IgE secretion, and transforming growth factor-β (TGF-β) and IL-5 appear to play major roles in class switch to IgA secretion. Thus, during clonal selection, a B cell may produce a population of plasma cells that are capable of producing many different classes of antibody against the same antigen.

A few antigens can bypass the need for Th cells and can directly stimulate B cell maturation and proliferation. These

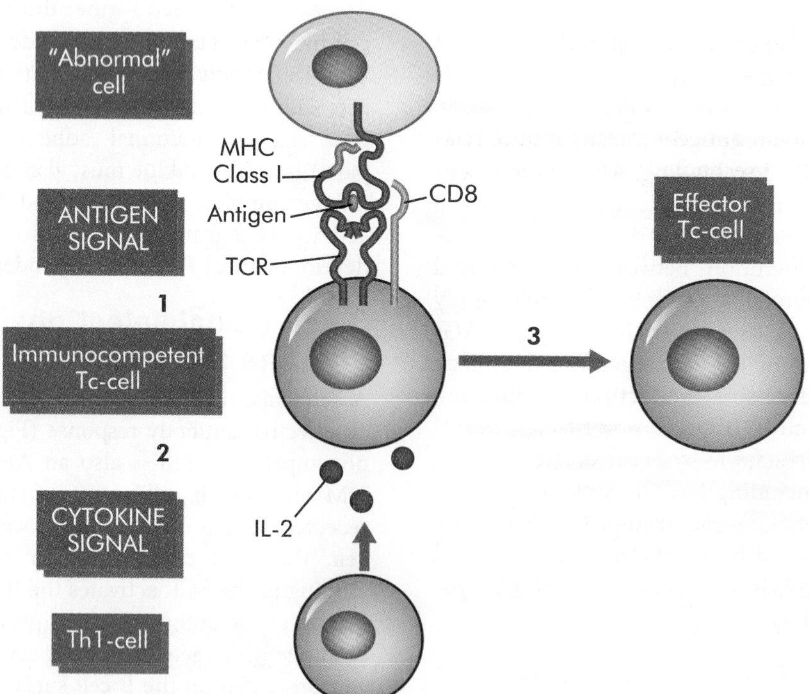

Figure 6-19 ■ **Tc-Cell Clonal Selection.** The immunocompetent Tc cell can react with antigen but cannot yet "kill" target cells. During clonal selection, this cell reacts with antigen presented by MHC class I molecules on the surface of a virally infected or cancerous "abnormal" cell. **(1)** The antigen–MHC class I complex is recognized simultaneously by the T cell receptor (TCR), which binds to antigen, and CD8, which binds to the MHC class I molecule. **(2)** A separate signal is provided by cytokines, particularly IL-2 from Th1 cells. **(3)** In response to these signals, the Tc cell develops into an "effector" Tc cell with the ability to kill abnormal cells.

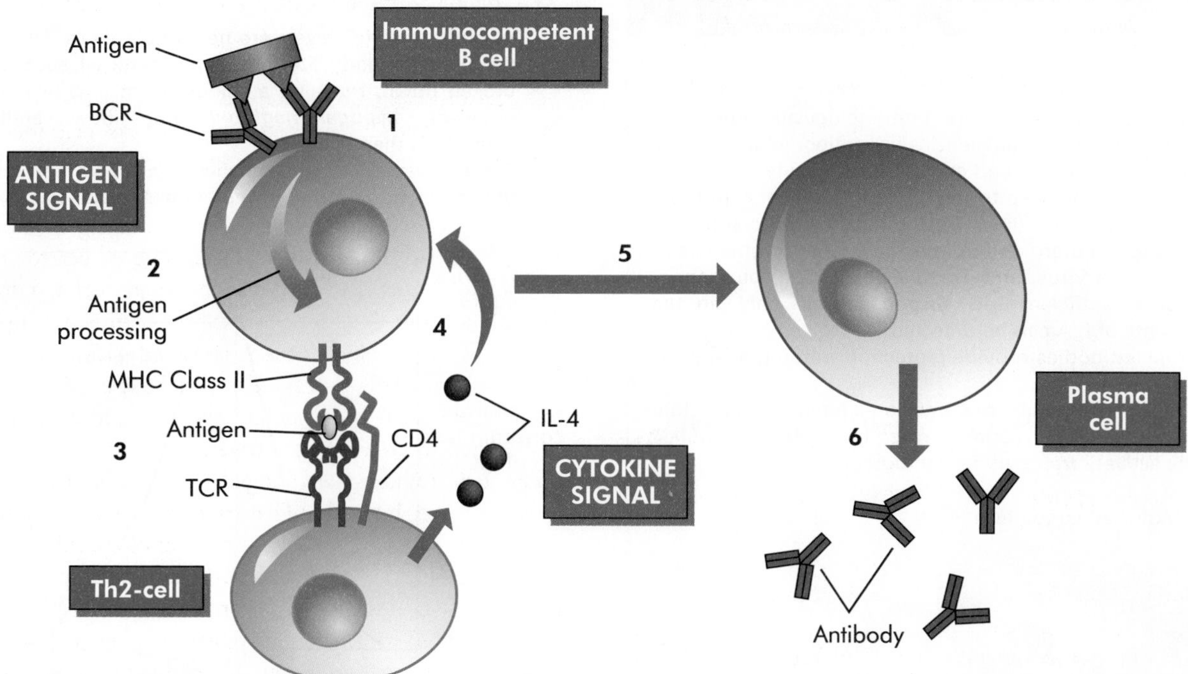

Figure 6-20 ■ **B Cell Clonal Selection.** Immunocompetent B cells undergo proliferation and differentiation into antibody-secreting plasma cells. Multiple signals are necessary **(1)**. The B cell itself can directly bind soluble antigen through the B cell receptor (BCR) and act as an antigen processing cell. Antigen is internalized, processed **(2)**, and presented **(3)** to the TCR on a Th2 cell by MHC class II molecules **(4)**. A cytokine signal is provided by the Th2 cell cytokines (e.g., IL-4) that react with the B cell **(5)**. The B cell differentiates into plasma cells that secrete antibody **(6)**.

are called *T cell-independent antigens* (Figure 6-21). They are mostly bacterial products that are large and are likely to have repeating identical antigenic determinants that bind and cross-link several B cell receptors. The accumulated intracellular signal is adequate to induce differentiation to a plasma cell but is not adequate to induce class switch. Therefore, T cell-independent antigens usually induce relatively pure IgM primary and secondary immune responses.

Memory cells

During the clonal selection process, both B cells and T cells differentiate into sets of long-lived memory cells.[11] The memory cells remain inactive until subsequent exposure to the same antigen. Upon reexposure, these memory cells do not require much further differentiation and will therefore rapidly become new plasma cells or effector T cells without the cellular interactions described previously.

✔ QUICK CHECK 6-4

1. What is meant by presentation of antigen?
2. Define class switch.
3. What is the function of memory cells?

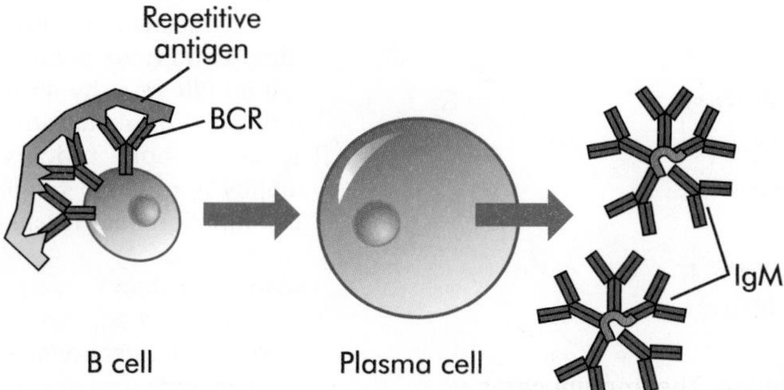

Figure 6-21 ■ **Activation of a B Cell by a T Cell-Independent Antigen.** Molecules containing repeating identical antigenic determinants may interact simultaneously with several receptors on the surface of the B cell and induce the proliferation and production of immunoglobulins. Because Th2 cells do not participate, class switch does not occur and the resultant antibody response is IgM.

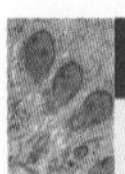

PEDIATRICS & Immune Function

Normal human infants are immunologically immature when born, with deficiencies in antibody production, phagocytic activity, and complement activity.

The fetus in the last trimester can produce a primary immune response (IgM; T cell independent) to antigenic challenge in utero and to infections (e.g., cytomegalovirus, rubella virus, and *Toxoplasma gondii*) but cannot produce sufficient IgG response, and only limited amounts of IgA can be detected.

Maternal antibodies provide protection within the fetal circulation.

Trophoblasts separate maternal and fetal blood so that immunoglobulins cannot cross; however, trophoblast cells actively *transport* immunoglobulins.

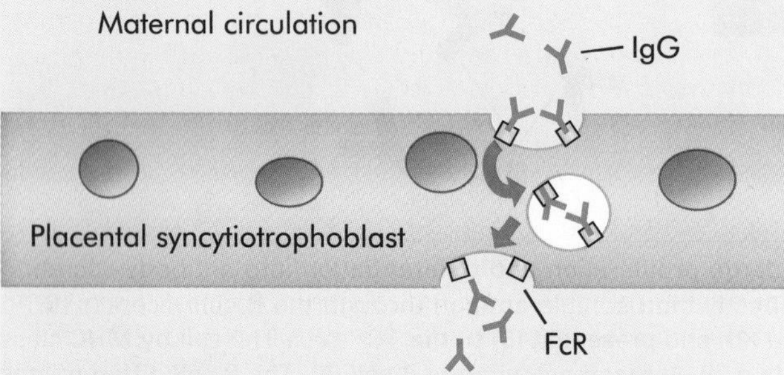

Transport of IgG Across the Syncytiotrophoblast. The human placenta is covered with a specialized multinucleate cell, the syncytiotrophoblast. Transport of maternal IgG across the syncytiotrophoblast and into the fetal circulation is an active process. Maternal IgG binds to Fc receptors on the surface of the syncytiotrophoblast and is internalized by the process of endocytosis. Receptors on the syncytiotrophoblast are specific for the Fc portion of IgG and do not bind other classes of immunoglobulins. Interaction of IgG with Fc receptors protects the antibody from lysosomal digestion during transport of the vacuole across the cell (i.e., transcytosis). On the fetal side of the syncytiotrophoblast, IgG is released by exocytosis (see Chapter 1).

At birth, total IgG levels are near adult levels.

After birth, antibody titers drop as maternal antibody is broken down, reaching a minimum at 5 to 6 months; transient *hypogammaglobulinemia* (low antibody levels) can then occur.

Recurrent respiratory tract infections are common during this transient period of immune insufficiency.

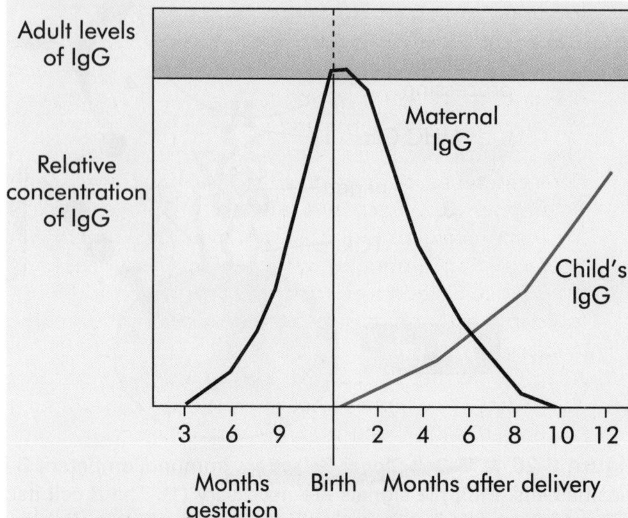

Antibody Levels in Umbilical Cord Blood and in Neonatal Circulation. Early in gestation, maternal IgG begins active transport across the placenta and enters the fetal circulation. At birth, the fetal circulation may contain nearly adult levels of IgG, which is almost exclusively from the maternal source. The fetal immune system has the capacity to produce IgM and small amounts of IgA before birth (not shown). After delivery, maternal IgG is rapidly destroyed and neonatal IgG production increases

AGING & Immune Function

Immune function decreases with age, with diminished T cell function and antibody responses to antigenic challenge; however, circulating autoantibodies and immune complexes increase.

Spontaneous monoclonal antibody production also increases without B cell malignancies (myeloma).

Thymus reaches maximum size at sexual maturity and then undergoes involution until it is a vestigial remnant by middle age; by 45 to 50 years of age, the thymus is only 15% of maximum size.

Thymic hormone production drops, as does the organ's ability to mediate T cell differentiation.

T cell function deteriorates, although the number of T cells does not drop.

Those older than 60 years have decreased delayed hypersensitivity responses, decreased T cell–mediated responses to infections, and decreased T cell activity.

Data from Min H: Effects of aging on early B- and T-cell development, *Immunol Rev* 205:1–17, 2005.

Did You Understand?

General Characteristics of the Immune Response

1. Adaptive immunity is a state of protection, primarily against infectious agents, that differs from inflammation by being slower to develop, being more specific, and having memory that makes it much longer lived.
2. Natural immunity is innate resistance, and acquired immunity is gained after birth.
3. The adaptive immune response is most often initiated by cells of the innate system. These cells process and present portions of invading pathogens (i.e., antigens) to lymphocytes in peripheral lymphoid tissue.
4. The adaptive immune response is mediated by two different types of lymphocytes—B lymphocytes and T lymphocytes. Each has distinct functions. B cells are responsible for humoral immunity that is mediated by circulating antibodies, whereas T cells are responsible for cell-mediated immunity, in which they kill targets directly or stimulate the activity of other leukocytes.
5. Adaptive immunity can be either active or passive depending on whether immune response components originated in the host or came from a donor.

Antigens and Immunogens

1. Antigens are molecules that react with components of the immune response, such as antibodies and receptors on B and T cells. Most antigens can induce an immune response, and thus the antigens are also immunogens.
2. The antigenic-determinant or epitope is the precise chemical structure with which an antibody or B cell/T cell receptor reacts.
3. Self-antigens are antigens on an individual's own cells. The individual's immune system does not normally recognize self-antigens as immunogenic, a condition known as tolerance.
4. Very small antigens may not normally be immunogenic (haptens) unless they are bound to a larger molecular weight molecule (carrier).

Humoral Immune Response

1. The humoral immune response is provided by molecules (antibodies) produced by B cells.
2. Antibodies are plasma glycoproteins that can be classified by chemical structure and biologic activity as IgG, IgM, IgA, IgE, or IgD.
3. The protective effects of antibodies may be direct or indirect.
4. Direct effects result from the binding of antibody directly to a harmful antigen or infectious agent. These include inhibition of processes that are necessary for infection, such as the reaction of an infectious agent with a particular cell in the body or neutralization of harmful bacterial toxins.
5. Indirect effects result from activation of inflammation by antibodies through the Fc portion of the molecule. These include opsonization to increase phagocytosis, killing the infectious agent through activation of complement, and widespread activation of inflammation through the production of biologically active complement components, such as C5a.
6. IgE is a special class of antibody that helps defend against parasitic infections.
7. Antibodies of the systemic immune system function internally, in the bloodstream and tissues. Antibodies of the secretory, or mucosal, immune system (primarily secretory IgA) function externally, in the secretions of mucous membranes.

Cell-Mediated Immune Response

1. T cells are responsible for the cell-mediated immune response.
2. There are several types of mature T cells: cytotoxic T cells (Tc), regulatory T cells including T helper (Th), and T suppression (Ts), and memory cells.
3. T cells have antigen specific receptors (T cell receptor or TCR) that must "see" antigen presented on cell surfaces by special antigen-presenting molecules of the major histocompatibility complex (MHC molecules).
4. Tc cells bind to and kill cellular targets such as cells infected with viruses or cancer cells.
5. The natural killer (NK) cell has some characteristics of the Tc cells and is important for killing target cells in which viral infection or malignancy has resulted in the loss of cellular MHC molecules.
6. Development of cell-mediated or humoral immune responses usually depends on populations of Th cells.

Generation of Clonal Diversity

1. The production of B and T lymphocytes with receptors against millions of antigens that will be possibly encountered in an individual's lifetime occurs in the fetus in the primary lymphoid organs: the thymus for T cells and portions of the bone marrow for B cells.
2. Immunocompetent T and B cells migrate from the primary lymphoid organs into the circulation and secondary lymphoid organs to await antigen.

Induction of the Immune Response

1. Induction of an immune response, or clonal selection, begins when antigen enters the individual's body.
2. The response to antigen can be divided into two phases: the primary and secondary responses. The primary response of humoral immunity is usually dominated by IgM, with lesser amounts of IgG. The secondary immune response has a more rapid production of a larger amount of antibody, predominantly IgG.
3. Most antigens must first interact with antigen-presenting cells (APCs), i.e., macrophages.
4. Antigen is processed in the APCs and presented on the cell surface by molecules of the MHC. The particular MHC molecule (class I or class II) that presents antigen determines which cell will respond to that antigen. Th cells require that the antigen be presented in a complex with MHC class II molecules. Tc cells require that antigen be presented by MHC class I molecules.
5. The T cell "sees" the presented antigen through the T cell receptor and accessory molecules: CD4 or CD8. CD4 is found on Th cells and reacts specifically with MHC class II. CD8 is found on Tc cells and reacts specifically with MHC class I.
6. A subgroup of Th cells (the Th2 cells) helps B cells respond to antigen and develop into antibody-secreting plasma cells.

(Continued)

Did You Understand?—Cont'd

7. A second subgroup of Th cells (the Th1 cells) helps Tc cells respond to antigen and develop into functional effector Tc cells.

PEDIATRICS & Immune Function

1. Mechanisms of self-defense are naturally somewhat deficient in the fetus, the neonate, and the elderly individual.
2. The T cell–independent immune response is adequate in the fetus and neonate, but the T cell–dependent immune response develops slowly during the first 6 months of life.
3. Maternal IgG antibodies are transported across the placenta into the fetal blood and protect the neonate for the first 6 months, after which they are replaced by the child's own antibodies.

AGING & Immune Function

1. T cell function and antibody production are somewhat deficient in elderly persons. Elderly individuals also tend to have increased levels of circulating autoantibodies (antibodies against self-antigens).

Key Terms

Active acquired immunity (active immunity), 146
Agglutination, 152
Allergen, 148
Antibody, 149
Antibody-dependent cellular cytotoxicity (ADCC), 158
Antigen presentation, 161
Antigen processing, 161
Antigen, 147
Antigen-binding fragment (Fab), 150
Antigen-binding site (paratope), 147
Antigenic determinant (epitope), 147
B lymphocyte (B cell), 145
B cell receptor (BCR), 153
CD molecule, 157
Cell-mediated immunity, 146
Cellular immunity, 146
Class switch, 164
Clonal selection, 145
Complementary-determining region (CDR), 151
Crystalline fragment (Fc), 150
Cytotoxic (Tc) cell, 146
Generation of clonal diversity, 159
Hapten, 148
Helper T (Th) cell, 145
Human bursal equivalent, 159
Humoral immunity, 146
Immunogen, 147
Lymphocyte, 145
Lymphoid stem cell, 159
Lymphokine-producing cell, 155
Major histocompatibility complex (MHC), 156
Memory cell, 146
Monoclonal antibody, 155
Neutralization, 152
Passive acquired immunity (passive immunity), 146
Plasma cell, 149
Precipitation, 152
Primary (central) lymphoid organ, 159
Primary immune response, 160
Regulatory T (Treg) cell, 159
Secondary immune response, 160
Secretory (mucosal) immune system, 154
Secretory immunoglobulin, 154
Self-antigen, 148
Superantigen (SAG), 162
Systemic immune system, 154
T lymphocyte (T cell), 145
T cell receptor (TCR), 156
Th1 cell, 162
Th2 cell, 162
Titer, 152

References

1. Chaplin DD: Overview of the human immune response, *J Allergy Clin Immunol* 117:S430–S435, 2006.
2. Brandtzaeg P, Johansen F-E: Mucosal B cells: phenotypic characteristics, transcriptional regulation, and homing properties, *Immunol Rev* 206:32–63, 2005.
3. Lanier LL: NK cell recognition, *Ann Rev Immunol* 23:225–274, 2005.
4. D'Ambrosio D: Regulatory T cells: how do they find their space in the immunological arena? *Semin Canc Biol* 16:91–97, 2006.
5. Ciofani M, Zúñiga-Pflücker JC: A survival guide to early T cell development, *Immunol Res* 34:117–132, 2006.
6. Trombetta ES, Mellman I: Cell biology of antigen processing in vitro and in vivo, *Ann Rev Immunol* 23:975–1028, 2005.
7. Jiang H, Chess L: Regulation of immune responses by T cells, *N Eng J Med* 354:1166–1176, 2006.
8. Silverman GJ, Goodyear CS: Confounding B cell defenses: lessons from a staphylococcal superantigen, *Nat Rev Immunol* 6:465–475, 2006.
9. Ochoa JB, Makarenkova V: T lymphocytes, *Crit Care Med* 33: S510–S5123, 2005.
10. MacConmara M, Lederer JA: B cells, *Crit Care Med* 33: S514–S516, 2005.
11. Kalia V et al: Differentiation of memory B and T cells, *Cur Opin Immunol* 18:255–264, 2006.

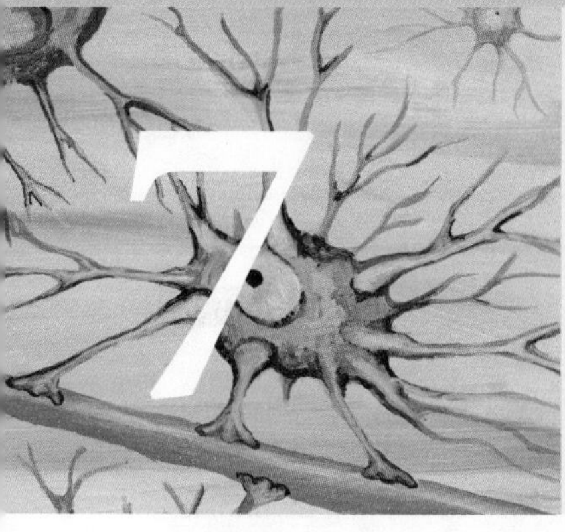

7 HYPERSENSITIVITIES, INFECTION, AND IMMUNE DEFICIENCIES

Neal S. Rote

CHAPTER OUTLINE

ELECTRONIC RESOURCES

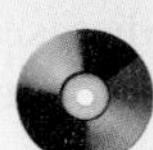

Companion CD
- Review Questions and Answers
- Animations

evolve Website
http://evolve.elsevier.com/Huether/
- Quick Check Answers
- Key Terms Exercises
- Critical Thinking Questions with Answers
- Algorithm Completion Exercises
- WebLinks

The immune system is a finely tuned network that protects the host against foreign antigens, particularly infectious agents. Sometimes this network breaks down, causing the immune system to react inappropriately. Inappropriate immune responses may be (1) exaggerated against environmental antigens (allergy); (2) misdirected against the host's own cells (autoimmunity); (3) directed against beneficial foreign tissues, such as transfusions or transplants (alloimmunity); or (4) insufficient to protect the host (immune deficiency). All of these can be serious or life threatening. Exaggerated immune responses (allergy) are the most common, but they are usually the least life threatening.

HYPERSENSITIVITY: ALLERGY, AUTOIMMUNITY, AND ALLOIMMUNITY

Allergy, autoimmunity, and alloimmunity are classified as *hypersensitivity reactions*. **Hypersensitivity** is an altered immunologic response to an antigen that results in disease or damage to the individual. Allergy, autoimmunity, and alloimmunity (also termed *isoimmunity*) can be most easily understood in relationship to the source of the antigen against which the hypersensitivity response is directed (Table 7-1). **Allergy** refers to a hypersensitivity to environmental antigens. These can include medicines, natural products (e.g., pollens, bee stings), infectious agents, and any other antigen that is not naturally found in the individual.

Autoimmunity is a disturbance in the immunologic tolerance of self-antigens. The immune system normally does not strongly recognize the individual's own antigens. Healthy individuals of all ages, but particularly the elderly, may produce low quantities of antibodies against their own antigens *(autoantibodies)* without developing overt autoimmune disease. Therefore, the presence of low quantities of autoantibodies does not necessarily indicate a disease state. Autoimmune diseases occur when the immune system reacts against self-antigens to such a degree that autoantibodies or autoreactive T cells damage the individual's tissues. Many clinical disorders are associated with autoimmunity and are generally referred to as **autoimmune diseases** (Table 7-2).

Alloimmune diseases occur when the immune system of one individual produces an immunologic reaction against tissues of another individual. Alloimmunity can be observed during immunologic reactions against transfusions, transplanted tissue, or the fetus during pregnancy.

The mechanism that initiates the onset of hypersensitivity, whether allergy, autoimmunity, or alloimmunity, is not completely understood. It is generally accepted that genetic, infectious, and possibly environmental factors contribute to hypersensitivity.

TABLE 7-1

Relative Incidence and Examples of Hypersensitivity Diseases*

	MECHANISM			
Target Antigen	Type I (IgE-Mediated)	Type II (Tissue Specific)	Type III (Immune Complex)	Type IV (Cell Mediated)
ALLERGY	++++	+	+	++
Environmental antigens	Hay fever	Hemolysis in drug allergies	Gluten (wheat) allergy	Poison ivy allergy
AUTOIMMUNITY	+	++	+++	++
Self-antigens	May contribute to some type III reactions	Autoimmune thrombocytopenia	Systemic lupus erythematosus	Hashimoto thyroiditis
ALLOIMMUNITY	+	++	+	++
Another person's antigens	May contribute to some type III reactions	Hemolytic disease of the newborn	Individuals who do not make their own IgA may have an anaphylactic response against IgA in human immune globulin	Graft rejection

*The frequency of each reaction is indicated in a range from rare (+) to very common (++++). An example of each reaction is given.

Mechanisms of Hypersensitivity

Diseases caused by hypersensitivity reactions can be characterized also by the particular immune mechanism that results in the disease (see Table 7-1). These mechanisms are apparent in most hypersensitivity reactions and have been divided into four distinct types: *type I* (IgE-mediated reactions), *type II* (tissue-specific reactions), *type III* (immune complex-mediated reactions), and *type IV* (cell-mediated reactions) (Table 7-3). This classification is artificial and seldom is a particular disease associated with only a single mechanism. The four mechanisms are interrelated, and in most hypersensitivity reactions several mechanisms can be at work simultaneously or sequentially.

As with all immune responses, hypersensitivity reactions require sensitization against a particular antigen that results in a primary immune response. Disease symptoms appear after an adequate secondary immune response occurs. Hypersensitivity reactions are immediate or delayed, depending on the time required to elicit clinical symptoms after reexposure to the antigen. Reactions that occur within minutes to a few hours after exposure to antigen are termed **immediate hypersensitivity reactions. Delayed hypersensitivity reactions** may take several hours to appear and are at maximum severity days after reexposure to the antigen.

The most rapid and severe immediate hypersensitivity reaction is **anaphylaxis.** Anaphylaxis occurs within minutes of reexposure to the antigen and can be either systemic (generalized) or cutaneous (localized). Symptoms of systemic anaphylaxis include itching, erythema, vomiting, abdominal cramps, diarrhea, and breathing difficulties. Severe anaphylactic reactions may include contraction of bronchial smooth muscle, edema of the throat, breathing difficulties, decreased blood pressure, shock, and death. An example of systemic anaphylaxis is an allergic reaction to bee stings. Cutaneous anaphylaxis results in local symptoms, such as pain, swelling, and redness, which occur at the site of exposure to an antigen (e.g., a painful local reaction to an injected vaccine or drug).

Type I: IgE-mediated hypersensitivity reactions

Type I reactions are mediated by antigen-specific IgE and the products of tissue mast cells (Figure 7-1).[1] Most common allergic reactions are type I reactions. In addition, most type I reactions occur against environmental antigens and are therefore allergic. Because of this strong association, many health care professionals use the term *allergy* to indicate only IgE-mediated reactions. However, IgE can contribute to some autoimmune and alloimmune diseases, and many common allergies (e.g., poison ivy) are not mediated by IgE.

IgE has a relatively short life span in the blood because it rapidly binds to Fc receptors on mast cells (see Figure 7-1). Unlike Fc receptors on phagocytes, which bind IgG that has reacted with antigen, the Fc receptors on mast cells specifically bind IgE that has not previously interacted with antigen. After a large amount of IgE has bound to the mast cells, an individual is considered sensitized. Further exposure of a sensitized individual to the allergen results in degranulation of the mast cell and the release of mast cell products (see Chapter 5).

Mechanisms of IgE-mediated hypersensitivity

The most potent mediator of IgE-mediated hypersensitivity is histamine, which affects several key target cells.[2] Acting through H1 receptors, histamine contracts bronchial smooth muscles (bronchial constriction), increases vascular permeability (edema), and causes vasodilation (increased blood flow) (see Chapter 5). The interaction of histamine

TABLE 7-2

Examples of Autoimmune Disorders

System Disease	Organ or Tissue	Probable Self-Antigen
ENDOCRINE SYSTEM		
Hyperthyroidism (Graves disease)	Thyroid gland	Receptors for thyroid-stimulating hormone on plasma membrane of thyroid cells
Hashimoto hypothyroidism	Thyroid gland	Thyroid cell surface antigens, thyroglobulin
Insulin-dependent diabetes	Pancreas	Islet cells, insulin, insulin receptors on pancreatic cells
Addison disease	Adrenal gland	Surface antigens on steroid-producing cells; microsomal antigens
Male infertility	Testis	Surface antigens on spermatozoa
SKIN		
Pemphigus vulgaris	Skin	Intercellular substances in stratified squamous epithelium
Bullous pemphigoid	Skin	Basement membrane
Vitiligo	Skin	Surface antigens on melanocytes (melanin-producing cells)
NEUROMUSCULAR TISSUE		
Polymyositis (dermatomyositis)	Muscle	Nuclear materials; myosin
Multiple sclerosis	Neural tissue	Surface antigens of nerve cells
Myasthenia gravis	Neuromuscular junction	Acetylcholine receptors; striations of skeletal and cardiac muscle
Rheumatic fever	Heart	Cardiac tissue antigens that cross reaction with group A streptococcal antigen
Cardiomyopathy	Heart	Cardiac muscle
GASTROINTESTINAL SYSTEM		
Ulcerative colitis	Colon	Mucosal cells
Pernicious anemia	Stomach	Surface antigens of parietal cells; intrinsic factor
Primary biliary cirrhosis	Liver	Cells of bile duct
Chronic active hepatitis	Liver	Surface antigens of hepatocytes, nuclei, microsomes, smooth muscle
EYE		
Sjögren syndrome	Lacrimal gland	Antigens of lacrimal gland, salivary gland, thyroid, and nuclei of cells
CONNECTIVE TISSUE		
Ankylosing spondylitis	Joints	Sacroiliac and spinal apophyseal joint
Rheumatoid arthritis	Joints	Collagen, IgG
Systemic lupus erythematosus	Multiple sites	Numerous antigens in nuclei, organelles, and extracellular matrix
Mixed connective tissue disease	Multiple sites	Ribonucleoprotein and numerous other nucleoproteins
Polyarteritis nodosa (necrotizing vasculitis)	Arterioles (small arteries)	Unknown
Antiphospholipid antibody syndrome	Platelets, endothelium, placenta	Membrane phospholipids, especially phosphatidylserine
RENAL SYSTEM		
Immune complex glomerulonephritis	Kidney	Numerous immune complexes
Goodpasture disease	Kidney	Glomerular basement membrane
HEMATOLOGIC SYSTEM		
Idiopathic neutropenia	Neutrophil	Surface antigens on polymorphonuclear neutrophils
Idiopathic lymphopenia	Lymphocytes	Surface antigens on lymphocytes
Autoimmune hemolytic anemia	Erythrocytes	Surface antigens on erythrocytes
Autoimmune thrombocytopenic purpura	Platelets	Surface antigens on platelets
RESPIRATORY SYSTEM		
Goodpasture disease	Lung	Septal membrane of alveolus

with H2 receptors results in increased gastric acid secretion. Some type I allergic responses can be controlled by blocking histamine receptors with antihistamines.

CLINICAL MANIFESTATIONS The clinical manifestations of type I reactions are attributable mostly to the biologic effects of histamine. The tissues most commonly affected by type I responses contain large numbers of mast cells and are sensitive to the effects of histamine released from them. These tissues are found in the gastrointestinal tract, the skin, and the respiratory tract (Figure 7-2 and Table 7-4).

TABLE 7-3
Immunologic Mechanisms of Tissue Destruction

Type	Name	Rate of Development	Class of Antibody Involved	Principal Effector Cells Involved	Participation of Complement	Examples of Disorders
I	IgE-mediated reaction	Immediate	IgE	Mast cells	No	Seasonal allergic rhinitis Asthma
II	Tissue-specific reaction	Immediate	IgG IgM	Macrophages in tissues	Frequently	Autoimmune thrombocytopenic purpura, Graves disease, autoimmune hemolytic anemia
III	Immune complex-mediated reaction	Immediate	IgG IgM	Neutrophils	Yes	Systemic lupus erythematosus
IV	Cell-mediated reaction	Delayed	None	Lymphocytes Macrophages	No	Contact sensitivity to poison ivy and metals (jewelry)

Gastrointestinal allergy is caused primarily by allergens that enter through the mouth—usually foods or medicines. Symptoms include vomiting, diarrhea, or abdominal pain. Foods most often implicated in gastrointestinal allergies are milk, chocolate, citrus fruits, eggs, wheat, nuts, peanut butter, and fish. When food is the allergen, the active immunogen may be an unidentifiable product of food breakdown by digestive enzymes. Sometimes the allergen is a drug, an additive, or a preservative in the food. For example, cows treated for mastitis with penicillin yield milk containing trace amounts of this antibiotic. Thus, hypersensitivity apparently caused by milk proteins may instead be the result of an allergy to penicillin.

Urticaria, or hives, is a dermal (skin) manifestation of allergic reactions (Figure 7-3). The underlying mechanism is the localized release of histamine and increased vascular permeability, resulting in limited areas of edema. Urticaria is characterized by white fluid-filled blisters (wheals) surrounded by areas of redness (flares). The **wheal and flare reaction** is usually accompanied by itching. Not all urticarial symptoms are caused by immunologic reactions. Some, termed *nonimmunologic urticaria,* result from exposure to cold temperatures, emotional stress, medications, systemic diseases, or malignancies (e.g., lymphomas).

Effects of allergens on the mucosa of the eyes, nose, and respiratory tract include conjunctivitis (inflammation of the membranes lining the eyelids) (see Figure 7-3), rhinitis (inflammation of the mucous membranes of the nose), and asthma (constriction of the bronchi). Symptoms are caused by vasodilation, hypersecretion of mucus, edema, and swelling of the respiratory mucosa. Because the mucous membranes lining the respiratory tract are continuous, they are all adversely affected. The degree to which each is affected determines the symptoms of the disease.

The central problem in allergic diseases of the lung is obstruction of the large and small airways (bronchi) of the lower respiratory tract by bronchospasm (constriction of smooth muscle in airway walls), edema, and thick secretions. This leads to ventilatory insufficiency, wheezing, and difficult or labored breathing (see Chapter 26).

Certain individuals are genetically predisposed to develop allergies and are called **atopic.** In families in which one parent has an allergy, allergies develop in about 40% of the offspring. If both parents have allergies, the incidence may be as high as 80%. Atopic individuals tend to produce higher quantities of IgE and to have more Fc receptors for IgE on their mast cells. The airways and the skin of atopic individuals have increased responsiveness to a wide variety of both specific and nonspecific stimuli.

EVALUATION AND TREATMENT Allergic reactions can be life threatening; therefore, it is essential that severely allergic individuals be made aware of the specific allergen against which they are sensitized and instructed to avoid contact with that material. Several tests are available to evaluate allergic individuals. These include food challenges, skin tests with allergens, and laboratory tests for total IgE and allergen-specific IgE.

Clinical **desensitization** to allergens can be achieved in some individuals. Minute quantities of the allergen to which the person is sensitive are injected in increasing doses over a prolonged period. This procedure may reduce the severity of the allergic reaction in the treated individual. However, this form of therapy is associated with a risk of systemic anaphylaxis, which can be severe and life threatening.

Type II: Tissue-specific hypersensitivity reactions

Type II hypersensitivities are generally reactions against a specific cell or tissue. Cells express a variety of antigens on their surfaces, some of which are called **tissue-specific antigens** because they are expressed on the plasma membranes of only certain cells. Platelets, for example, have groups of antigens that are found on no other cells of the body. The symptoms of many type II diseases are determined by which tissue or organ expresses the particular antigen. Environmental antigens (e.g., drugs or their

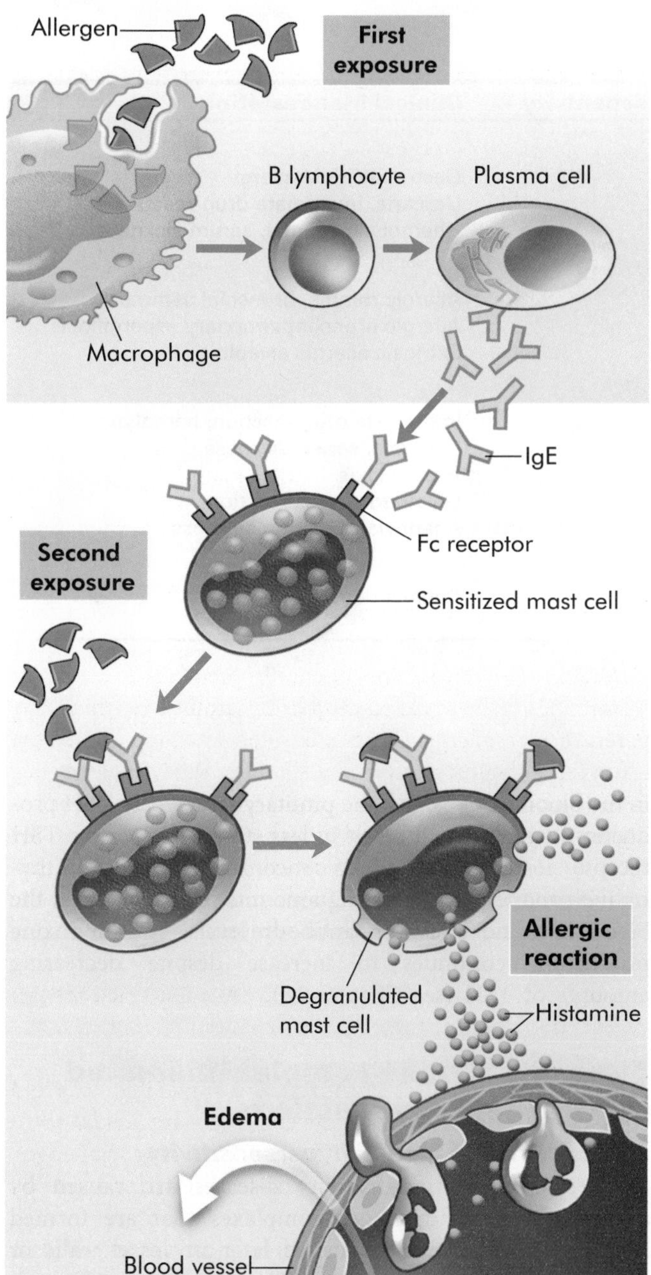

Figure 7-1 ■ **Mechanism of Type I, IgE-Mediated Reactions.** First exposure to an allergen stimulates B lymphocytes to mature into plasma cells that produce IgE. The IgE is adsorbed to the surface of the mast cell by binding with IgE-specific Fc receptors. When an adequate amount of IgE is bound the mast cell is "sensitized." During a second exposure, the allergen cross-links the surface-bound IgE and causes degranulation of the mast cell. The initial phase is characterized by vasodilation, vascular leakage, and smooth muscle spasm or glandular secretions, usually within 5 to 30 minutes after exposure to antigen. The late phase occurs 2 to 8 hours later without additional exposure to antigen and results from infiltration of tissues with inflammatory cells, including eosinophils, neutrophils, and basophils. (See Chapter 5 for more details on the role of mast cells in inflammation.)

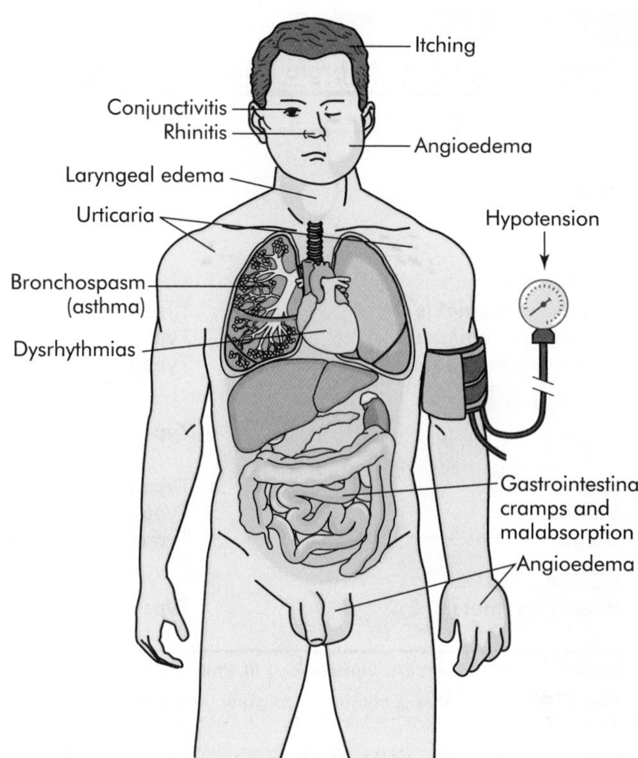

Figure 7-2 ■ **Type I Hypersensitivity Reactions.** Symptoms of type I allergic reactions are indicated.

metabolites) may bind to the plasma membranes of specific cells (especially erythrocytes and platelets) and function as targets of type II reactions.

The five general mechanisms by which type II hypersensitivity reactions can affect cells are shown in Figure 7-4. All of these mechanisms begin with antibody binding to tissue-specific antigens or antigens that have attached to particular tissues. First, *the cell may be destroyed by antibody and complement.* The antibody (IgM or IgG) reacts with an antigen on the surface of the cell, causing activation of the complement cascade through the classical pathway. Formation of the membrane attack complex (C5–9) damages the membrane and may result in lysis of the cell (see Figure 7-4, *A*). For example, erythrocytes are destroyed by complement-mediated lysis in individuals with autoimmune hemolytic anemia (see Chapters 20 and 21) or as a result of an alloimmune reaction to mismatched transfused blood cells.

Second, *antibody may cause cell destruction through phagocytosis by macrophages.* The antibody may additionally activate complement, resulting in the deposition of C3b on the cell surface. Receptors on the macrophage recognize and bind opsonins (e.g., antibody or C3b) and increase phagocytosis of the target cell (Figure 7-4, *B*; phagocytosis is illustrated in Chapter 5). For example, antibodies against platelet-specific antigens or against red blood cell antigens of the Rh system cause their removal by phagocytosis in the spleen.

The third mechanism involves *toxic products produced by neutrophils.* Soluble antigen such as medications, molecules

TABLE 7-4

Causes of Clinical Allergic Reactions

Typical Allergen	Mechanism of Hypersensitivity	Clinical Manifestation
INGESTANTS		
Foods	Type I	Gastrointestinal allergy
Drugs	Types I, II, III	Urticaria, immediate drug reaction, hemolytic anemia, serum sickness
INHALANTS		
Pollens, dust, molds	Type I	Allergic rhinitis, bronchial asthma
Aspergillus fumigatus	Types I, III	Allergic bronchopulmonary aspergillosis
Thermophilic actinomycetes*	Types III, IV	Extrinsic allergic alveolitis
INJECTANTS		
Drugs	Types, I, II, III	Immediate drug reaction, hemolytic anemia, serum sickness
Bee venom	Type I	Anaphylaxis
Vaccines	Type III	Localized Arthus reaction
Serum	Types I, III	Anaphylaxis, serum sickness
CONTACTANTS		
Poison ivy, metals	Type IV	Contact dermatitis

Modified from Bellanti JA: *Immunology III,* Philadelphia, 1985, Saunders.

*An order of fungi that is stimulated to grow by warmth.

released from infectious agents, or molecules released from an individual's own cells may enter the circulation. In some instances, the antigens are deposited on the surface of tissues, where they bind antibody (see Figure 7-4, *C*). The antibody may activate complement, resulting in the release of C3a and C5a, which are chemotactic for neutrophils, and deposition of complement component C3b. Neutrophils are attracted, bind to the tissues through receptors for the Fc portion of antibody (Fc receptor) or for C3b, and release their granules onto the healthy tissue. The components of neutrophil granules, as well as the toxic oxygen products produced by these cells, will damage the tissue.

The fourth mechanism is **antibody-dependent cell-mediated cytotoxicity (ADCC)** (see Figure 7-4, *D*). This mechanism involves natural killer (NK) cells. Antibody on the target cell is recognized by Fc receptors on the NK cells, which release toxic substances that destroy the target cell.

The fifth mechanism does not destroy the target cell but rather *causes the cell to malfunction.* The antibody is usually directed against antigenic determinants associated with specific cell-surface receptors (see Figure 7-4, *E*).[3] The antibody changes the function of the receptor by preventing interactions with their normal ligands, replacing the ligand and inappropriately stimulating the receptor, or destroying the receptor. For example, in the hyperthyroidism (excessive thyroid activity) of Graves disease, autoantibody binds to and activates receptors for thyroid-stimulating hormone (TSH) (a pituitary hormone that controls the production of the hormone thyroxine by the thyroid).[4] In this way, the antibody stimulates the thyroid cells to produce thyroxine. Under normal conditions, the increasing levels of thyroxine in the blood would signal the pituitary to decrease TSH production, which would result in less stimulation of the TSH receptor in the thyroid and a concomitant decrease in thyroxine production. Increasing amounts of thyroxine in the blood have no effect on antibody levels, and thyroxine production continues to increase despite decreasing amounts of TSH (see Chapter 18).

Type III: Immune complex–mediated hypersensitivity reactions

Mechanisms of type III hypersensitivity

Most type III hypersensitivity diseases are caused by antigen-antibody (immune) complexes that are formed in the circulation and deposited later in vessel walls or other tissues (Figure 7-5).[5] The primary difference between type II and type III mechanisms is that in type II hypersensitivity antibody binds to the antigen on the cell surface, whereas in type III the antibody binds to soluble antigen that was released into the blood or body fluids, and the complex is then deposited in the tissues. Type III reactions are not organ specific, and symptoms have little to do with the particular antigenic target of the antibody. The harmful effects of immune complex deposition are caused by complement activation, particularly through the generation of chemotactic factors for neutrophils. The neutrophils bind to antibody and C3b contained in the complexes and attempt to ingest the immune complexes. They are often unsuccessful because the complexes are bound to large areas of tissue. During the attempted phagocytosis, large quantities of lysosomal enzymes are released into the inflammatory site instead of into phagolysosomes. The attraction of neutrophils

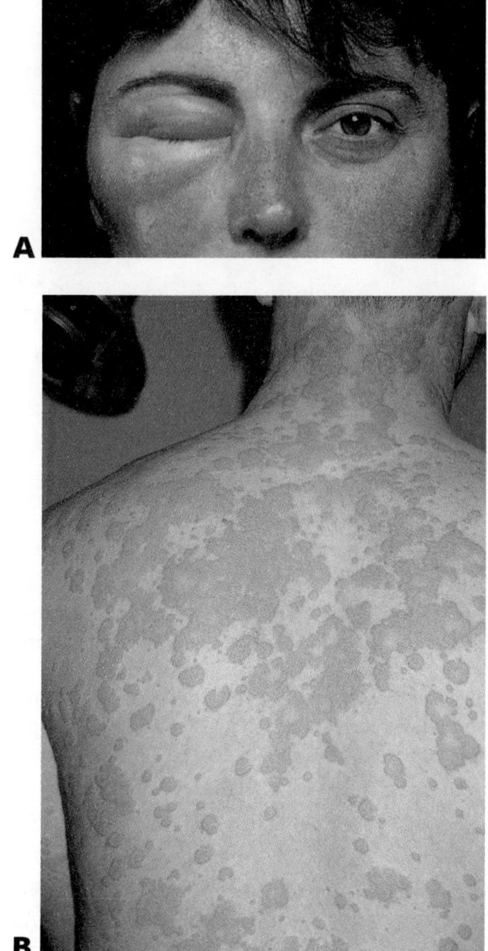

Figure 7-3 ■ **Type I Hypersensitivity Reactions.** Photographs show diffuse allergic-like **(A)** eye (angioedema) and **(B)** skin (allergic urticaria) reactions. The skin lesions have raised edges and develop within minutes or hours, with resolution occurring after about 12 hours. (From Male D et al: *Immunology,* ed 7, St Louis, 2006, Mosby.)

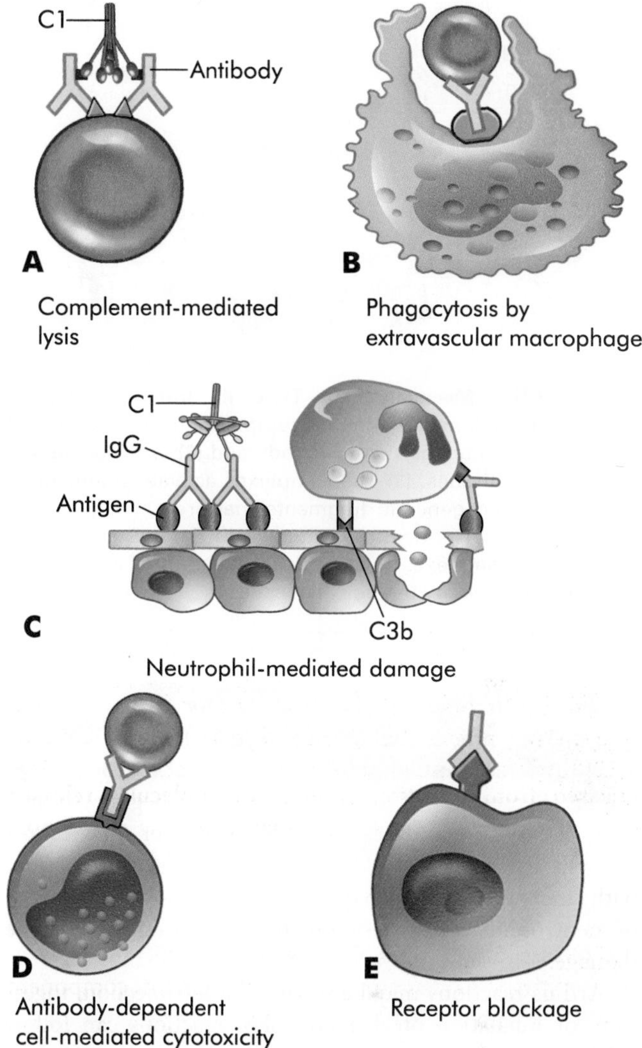

Figure 7-4 ■ **Mechanisms of Type II, Tissue-Specific Reactions.** Antibody binds to antigens on the cell surface and destroys or prevents the cell from functioning by **A,** complement-mediated lysis (an erythrocyte target is illustrated here); **B,** phagocytosis by macrophages in the tissue; **C,** neutrophil-mediated destruction; **D,** antibody-dependent cell-mediated cytotoxicity (ADCC); or **E,** modulation or blocking the normal function of receptors by antireceptor antibody. C1, Complement component C1; C3b, complement fragment produced from C3, which acts as an opsonin.

and the subsequent release of lysosomal enzymes cause most of the resulting tissue damage.

Immune complex disease

Two prototypic models of type III hypersensitivity help explain the variety of diseases in this category. Serum sickness is a model of systemic type III hypersensitivities, and the Arthus reaction is a model of localized or cutaneous reactions.

Serum sickness–type reactions are caused by the formation of immune complexes in the blood and their subsequent generalized deposition in target tissues. Typically affected tissues are the blood vessels, joints, and kidneys. Other symptoms include fever, enlarged lymph nodes, rash, and pain at sites of inflammation. Serum sickness was initially described as a complication of therapeutic administration of horse serum that contained antibody against tetanus toxin. Foreign serum generally is not administered to individuals today, although serum sickness reactions can be caused by the repeated intravenous administration of other antigens, such as drugs, and the characteristics of serum sickness are observed in systemic type III autoimmune diseases.

A form of serum sickness is **Raynaud phenomenon,** a condition caused by the temperature-dependent deposition of immune complexes in the capillary beds of the peripheral circulation. Certain immune complexes precipitate at temperatures below normal body temperature, particularly in the tips of the fingers, toes, and nose, and are called **cryoglobulins.** The precipitates block the circulation and cause localized pallor and numbness, followed by cyanosis (a bluish tinge resulting from oxygen deprivation) and eventually gangrene if the circulation is not restored.

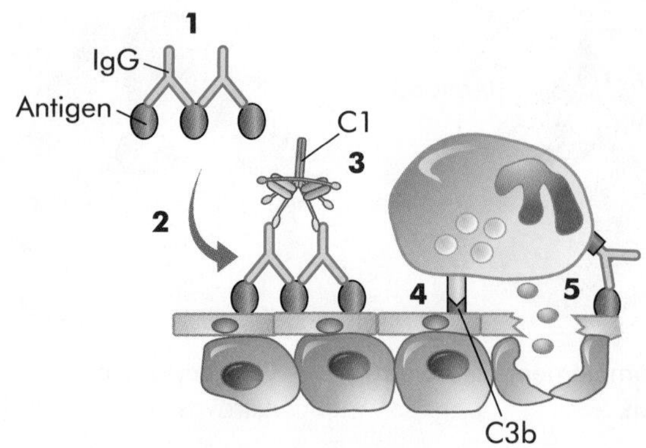

Figure 7-5 ■ Mechanism of Type III, Immune-Complex-Mediated Reactions. **(1)** Immune complexes form in the blood from circulating antigen and antibody and **(2)** are deposited in certain target tissues. **(3)** The complexes activate complement through C1 and generate fragments that are chemotactic for neutrophils. **(4)** The neutrophils attach to the IgG and C3b in the immune complexes and **(5)** release a variety of degradative enzymes that destroy the healthy tissues.

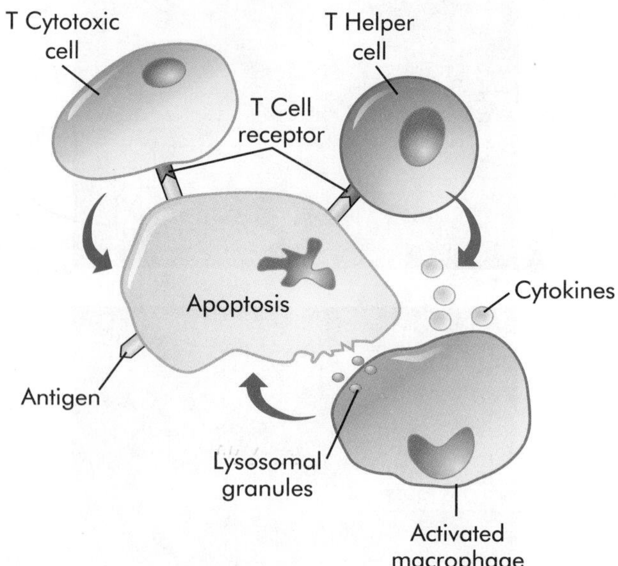

Figure 7-6 ■ Mechanism of Type IV Cell-Mediated Reactions. Antigens from target cells stimulate T cells to differentiate into T cytotoxic cells, which have direct cytotoxic activity, and T helper cells, which produce cytokines (especially interferon-γ) that activate macrophages. The macrophages can attach to targets and release enzymes and reactive oxygen species that induce apoptosis of the target.

An **Arthus reaction** is caused by repeated local exposure to an antigen that reacts with preformed antibody and forms immune complexes in the walls of the local blood vessels. Symptoms of an Arthus reaction begin within 1 hour of exposure and peak 6 to 12 hours later. The lesions are characterized by a typical inflammatory reaction, with increased vascular permeability, an accumulation of neutrophils, edema, hemorrhage, clotting, and tissue damage.

Arthus reactions may be observed after injection, ingestion, or inhalation of allergens. Skin reactions can follow subcutaneous or intradermal inoculation with drugs, fungal extracts, or antigens used in skin tests. Gastrointestinal reactions, such as gluten-sensitive enteropathy (celiac disease), follow ingestion of antigen, usually gluten from wheat products (see Chapter 35). Allergic alveolitis (farmer's lung, pigeon breeder's disease) is an Arthus-like acute hemorrhagic inflammation of the air sacs (alveoli) of the lungs resulting from inhalation of fungal antigens, usually particles from moldy hay or pigeon feces (see Chapter 26).

Type IV: Cell-mediated hypersensitivity reactions

Whereas types I, II, and III hypersensitivity reactions are mediated by antibody, type IV reactions are mediated by T lymphocytes and do not involve antibody (Figure 7-6). Type IV mechanisms occur through either cytotoxic T lymphocytes (Tc cells) or cytokine-producing Th1 cells.[6] Tc cells attack and destroy cellular targets directly. Th1 cells produce cytokines that recruit and activate phagocytic cells, especially macrophages. Destruction of the tissue is usually caused by direct killing by Tc cells or the release of soluble factors, such as lysosomal enzymes and toxic reactive oxygen species, from activated macrophages.

Clinical examples of type IV hypersensitivity reactions include graft rejection, the skin test for tuberculosis, and allergic reactions resulting from contact with such substances as poison ivy and metals. A type IV component also may be present in many autoimmune diseases. For example, T cells against type II collagen (a protein present in joint tissues) contribute to the destruction of joints in rheumatoid arthritis; T cells against a thyroid cell surface antigen contribute to the destruction of the thyroid in autoimmune thyroiditis (Hashimoto disease); and T cells against an antigen on the surface of pancreatic beta cells (the cell that normally produces insulin) are responsible for beta cell destruction in insulin-dependent (type 1) diabetes mellitus.

In 1891, Ehrlich was the first to thoroughly describe a type IV hypersensitivity reaction in the skin, leading to the development of a diagnostic skin test for tuberculosis. The reaction follows an intradermal injection of tuberculin antigen into a suitably sensitized individual and is called a **delayed hypersensitivity skin test** because of its slow onset—24 to 72 hours to reach maximum intensity. The reaction site is infiltrated with T lymphocytes and macrophages, resulting in a clear hard center **(induration)** and a reddish surrounding area **(erythema).**

Allergic type IV reactions are elicited by some environmental antigens that are haptens (Chapter 6) that become immunogenic after binding to larger (carrier) proteins in the individual. In allergic **contact dermatitis,** the carrier protein is in the skin. The best-known example is poison ivy (Figure 7-7). The antigen is a plant catechol, urushiol, which reacts with normal skin proteins and evokes a cell-mediated immune response. Skin reactions to industrial

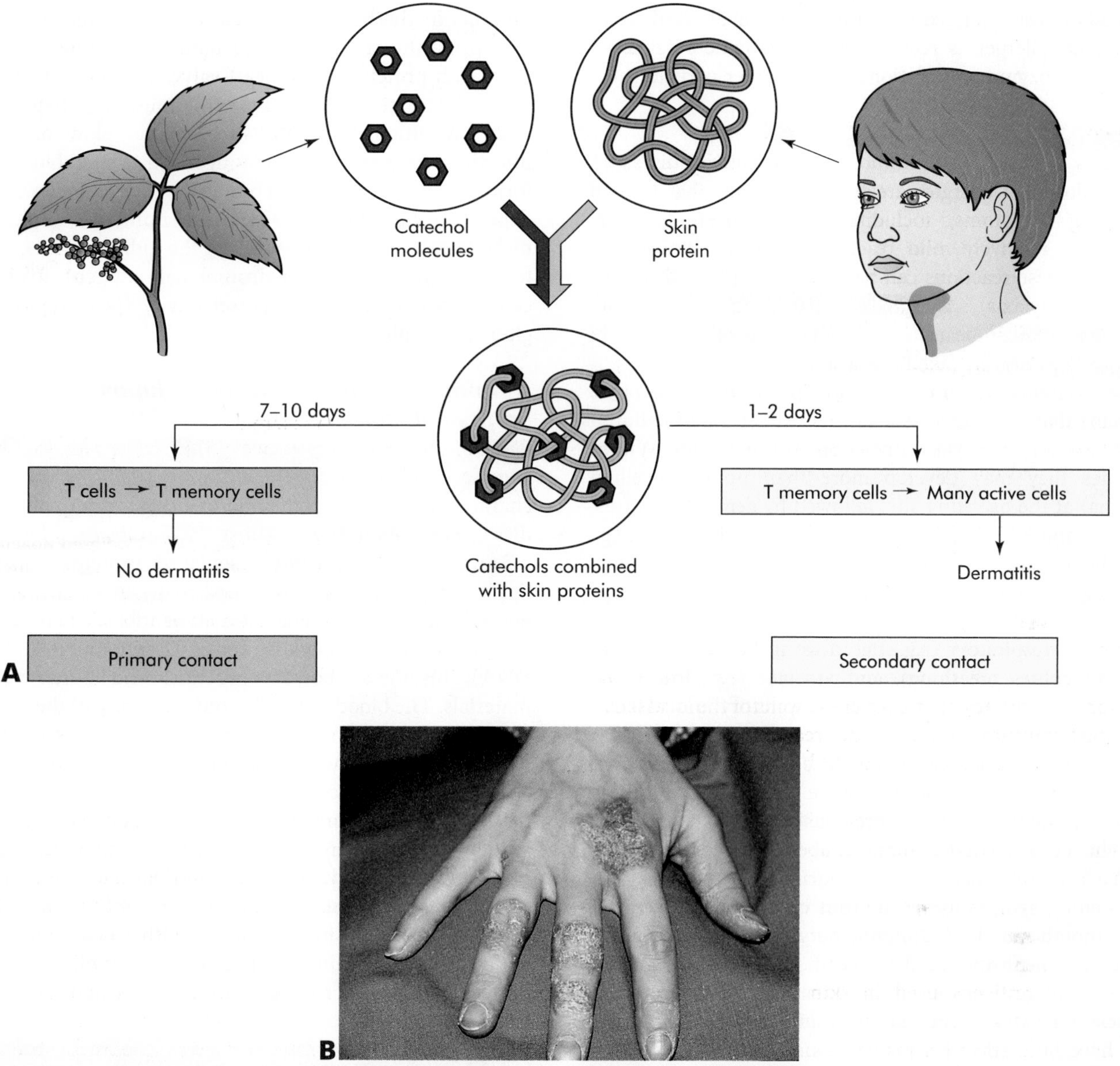

Figure 7-7 ■ Development of Allergic Contact Dermatitis. A, The development of allergy to poison ivy. The first (primary) contact with allergen sensitizes (produces reactive T cells) the individual but does not produce a rash (dermatitis). Secondary contact activates a type IV cell-mediated reaction that causes dermatitis. **B,** Contact dermatitis caused by a delayed hypersensitivity reaction leading to vesicles and scaling at the sites of contact. (From Damjanov I, Linder J: *Anderson's pathology,* ed 10, St Louis, 1996, Mosby.)

chemicals, cosmetics, detergents, clothing, food, metals, and topical medicines (such as penicillin) are elicited by the same mechanism. Contact dermatitis consists of lesions only at the site of contact with the allergen, such as a metal allergy to jewelry.

QUICK CHECK 7-1

1. Distinguish among the four types of hypersensitivity mechanisms.
2. What is the mechanism of anaphylaxis?
3. What are some clinical examples of type IV hypersensitivity?

Antigenic Targets of Hypersensitivity Reactions

Allergy

Allergens

Environmental antigens that cause allergic responses are called **allergens**. It is not known why some antigens are allergens and others are not. Typical allergens include pollens (e.g., ragweed), molds and fungi (e.g., *Penicillium notatum*), foods (e.g., milk, eggs, fish), animals (e.g., cat dander, dog dander), cigarette smoke, and components of house dust (e.g., fecal pellets of house mites). Often the allergen is contained within a particle that is too large to be phagocytosed or is surrounded by a protective nonallergenic coat. The actual allergen is released after enzymatic breakdown (e.g., by lysozyme in secretions) of the larger particle.

Allergic disease: bee sting allergy

Allergies are the most common hypersensitivity diseases.[7] The majority of allergies are type I reactions that lead to annoying symptoms, including runny noses, sneezing, and other relatively mild reactions. In some individuals, however, these reactions can be excessive and life threatening (anaphylaxis). Anaphylactic reactions have been described against peanuts and other nuts, shellfish, fish, milk, eggs, and some medications.

Bee venoms contain a mixture of enzymes and other proteins that may serve as allergens. About 1% of children may have an anaphylactic reaction to bee venom. Within minutes they may develop more than normal swelling (edema) at the bee sting site, followed by generalized hives, itching, and swelling in areas distal from the sting (e.g., eyes, lips), and other systemic symptoms including flushing, sweating, dizziness, and headache. The most severe symptoms may include gastrointestinal (e.g., stomach cramps, vomiting), respiratory (e.g., tightness in the throat, wheezing, difficulties breathing), and vascular (e.g., low blood pressure, shock) reactions. Severe respiratory and vascular reactions may lead to death.

For an individual with known bee sting hypersensitivity, lifestyle changes include avoidance of stinging or biting insects. If a child has had a previous anaphylactic reaction, the chance of having another is about 60%. Most individuals carry self-injectable epinephrine. The primary life-threatening symptoms result from contraction of respiratory smooth muscle. Autonomic nervous system mediators, such as epinephrine, bind to specific receptors on smooth muscle and reverse the effects of histamine and result in muscle relaxation. The administration of antihistamines will have little effect because histamine has already bound H1 receptors and initiated severe bronchial smooth muscle contraction. Long-term protection may be afforded by desensitization in most individuals.

Autoimmunity

It is fairly well established that autoimmune diseases can be familial. Affected family members may not all develop the same disease, but several members may have different disorders characterized by a variety of hypersensitivity reactions, including autoimmune and allergic.

Breakdown of tolerance

An individual is usually tolerant to his or her own antigens. **Tolerance** is a state of immunologic control so that the individual does not make a detrimental immune response against his or her own cells and tissues. Autoimmune disease results from a breakdown of this tolerance.

Although many theories exist concerning the initial cause of autoimmune diseases, only one example is known: acute rheumatic fever. In a small number of individuals with group A streptococcal sore throats, the M proteins in the bacterial capsule mimic (antigenic mimicry) normal heart antigens and induce antibodies that also react with proteins in the heart valve, damaging the valve.[8] Thus, rheumatic fever is a type II autoimmune hypersensitivity. Additionally, some streptococcal skin or throat infections release bacterial antigens into the blood that form circulating immune complexes. The complexes may deposit in the kidneys and initiate an immune complex glomerulonephritis (inflammation of the kidney). Thus, streptococcal antigens (an environmental antigen) may also cause a type III allergic hypersensitivity (poststreptococcal glomerulonephritis).

Autoimmune disease: systemic lupus erythematosus

Systemic lupus erythematosus (SLE) is the most common, complex, and serious of the autoimmune disorders. SLE is characterized by the production of a large variety of antibodies (autoantibodies) against self-antigens, including nucleic acids, erythrocytes, coagulation proteins, phospholipids, lymphocytes, platelets, and many other self-components.[9] The most characteristic autoantibodies are against nucleic acids (e.g., single-stranded DNA, double-stranded DNA), histones, ribonucleoproteins, and other nuclear materials. The blood normally contains many of these products of cellular turnover and breakdown. Excessive levels of autoantibodies react with the circulating antigen and form circulating immune complexes. The deposition of circulating DNA/anti-DNA complexes in the kidneys can cause severe kidney inflammation. Similar reactions can occur in the brain, heart, spleen, lung, gastrointestinal tract, peritoneum, and skin. Thus, some of the symptoms of SLE result from a type III hypersensitivity reaction. Other symptoms, such as destruction of red blood cells (anemia), lymphocytes (lymphopenia), and other cells, may be type II hypersensitivity reactions.

SLE, like most autoimmune diseases, occurs more often in women (approximately a 10:1 predominance of females), especially in the 20- to 40-year-old age group. Blacks are affected more often than whites (about an eightfold increased risk). A genetic predisposition for the disease has been implicated on the basis of increased incidence in twins and the existence of autoimmune disease in the families of individuals with SLE.

Clinical manifestations of SLE include arthralgias or arthritis (90% of individuals), vasculitis and rash (70% to 80% of individuals), renal disease (40% to 50% of individuals), hematologic abnormalities (50% of individuals, with anemia being the most common complication), and cardiovascular diseases (30% to 50% of individuals). As with most autoimmune diseases, SLE is characterized by frequent remissions and exacerbations. Because the signs and symptoms affect almost every body system and tend to come and go, SLE is extremely difficult to diagnose. This has led to the development of a list of 11 common clinical findings. The serial or simultaneous presence of at least four of them indicates that the individual has SLE. The findings are as follows:[10]

1. Facial rash confined to the cheeks (malar rash)
2. Discoid rash (raised patches, scaling)
3. Photosensitivity (skin rash developed as a result of exposure to sunlight)
4. Oral or nasopharyngeal ulcers
5. Nonerosive arthritis of at least two peripheral joints
6. Serositis (inflammation of membranes of lung [pleurisy] or heart [pericarditis])
7. Renal disorder (proteinuria of 0.5 g/day or cellular casts)
8. Neurologic disorders (seizures or psychosis)
9. Hematologic disorders (hemolytic anemia, leukopenia, lymphopenia, or thrombocytopenia)
10. Immunologic disorders (positive lupus erythematosus [LE] cell preparation, anti–double stranded DNA, anti-Smith [Sm] antigen, false-positive serologic test for syphilis, or antiphospholipid antibodies [anticardiolipin antibody or lupus anticoagulant])
11. Presence of antinuclear antibody (ANA)

HEALTH ALERT

Autoimmune Diseases Affect Women More Than Men

To explain why women are especially susceptible to autoimmune disorders, researchers are investigating whether the sex hormones estrogen and testosterone affect the immune system. Although inconclusive, there are several findings that support the idea that differences between gender are based on sex hormones. Disappointing, however, is that treating affected individuals with sex hormones have had inconclusive results. Other hormones may affect the progress of autoimmune diseases. In mice, the cells of males and females differ in how they process newly made proteins. These differences may also contribute to the increased susceptibility to autoimmune diseases in women.

From Christensen D: Vaccine verity: New studies weigh benefits and risks, *Sci News* 16:110-111, 2001; Cohen-Solal JF et al: Sex hormones and SLE: influencing the fate of autoreactive B cells, *Curr Top Microbiol Immunol* 305:67-88, 2006; Tomassini V, Pozzilli C: Sex hormones: a role in the control of multiple sclerosis? *Expert Opin Pharmacother* 7(7):857-868, 2006.

There is no cure for SLE or most other autoimmune diseases. The goals of treatment are to control symptoms and prevent further damage by suppressing the autoimmune response. Nonsteroidal antiinflammatory drugs, such as aspirin, ibuprofen, or naproxen, reduce inflammation and relieve pain. Corticosteroids are often prescribed for more serious active disease. Immunosuppressive drugs (e.g., methotrexate, azathioprine, or cyclophosphamide) are used to treat severe symptoms involving internal organs. Ultraviolet light can worsen symptoms (known as flares), and protection from sun exposure is helpful. Prolonged use of certain drugs can cause transient SLE-like symptoms, and the medication history is important for diagnostic evaluation. Improved outcomes may be available in the future with the continued advances in medical research and the use of stem cell treatments.[11]

Alloimmunity

Alloantigens

Genetic diversity is the norm in humans. Diversity is also observed among self-antigens, so that two individuals may have different antigens on their tissues and, therefore, be able to make an immune response against each other's tissues. Some self-antigens, such as the ABO blood group, have limited diversity with very few different antigens being expressed in the population, whereas others, such as the HLA system, have tremendous diversity.

Alloimmune disease: transfusion reactions

Red blood cells (erythrocytes) express several important surface antigens, known collectively as the **blood group antigens,** which can be targets of alloimmune reactions.[12] More than 80 different red cell antigens are grouped into several dozen blood group systems. The most important of these, because they provoke the strongest humoral alloimmune response, are the ABO and Rh systems.

ABO system. The **ABO blood group** consists of two major carbohydrate antigens, labeled A and B (Figure 7-8), that are expressed on virtually all cells. These are codominant so that both A and B can be simultaneously expressed, resulting in an individual having any one of four different blood types. The erythrocytes of persons with blood type A have the type A carbohydrate antigen (i.e., carry the A antigen), those with blood type B carry the B antigen, those with blood type AB carry both A and B antigens, and those of blood type O carry neither the A nor the B antigen. A person with type A blood also has circulating antibodies to the B carbohydrate antigen. If this person receives blood from a type AB or B individual, a severe transfusion reaction occurs, and the transfused erythrocytes are destroyed by agglutination or complement-mediated lysis. Similarly, a type B individual (whose blood contains anti-A antibodies) cannot receive blood from a type A or AB donor. Type O individuals, who have neither antigen but have both anti-A and anti-B antibodies, cannot accept blood from any of the other three types. These naturally occurring antibodies, called **isohemagglutinins,** are IgM immunoglobulins and are induced early in life by similar antigens expressed on naturally occurring bacteria in the intestinal tract.

Because individuals with type O blood lack both types of antigens, they are considered **universal donors,** meaning that anyone can accept their red blood cells. Similarly, type AB individuals are considered **universal recipients** because they lack both anti-A and anti-B antibodies and can be transfused with any ABO blood type. Agglutination and lysis cause harmful transfusion reactions that can be prevented only by complete and careful ABO matching between donor and recipient.

Rh system. The **Rh blood group** is a group of antigens expressed only on red blood cells. This is most diverse group of red cell antigens, consisting of at least 45 separate antigens, although only one is considered very important. The most important is the D antigen. Individuals who express the D antigen on their red cells are Rh-positive, whereas

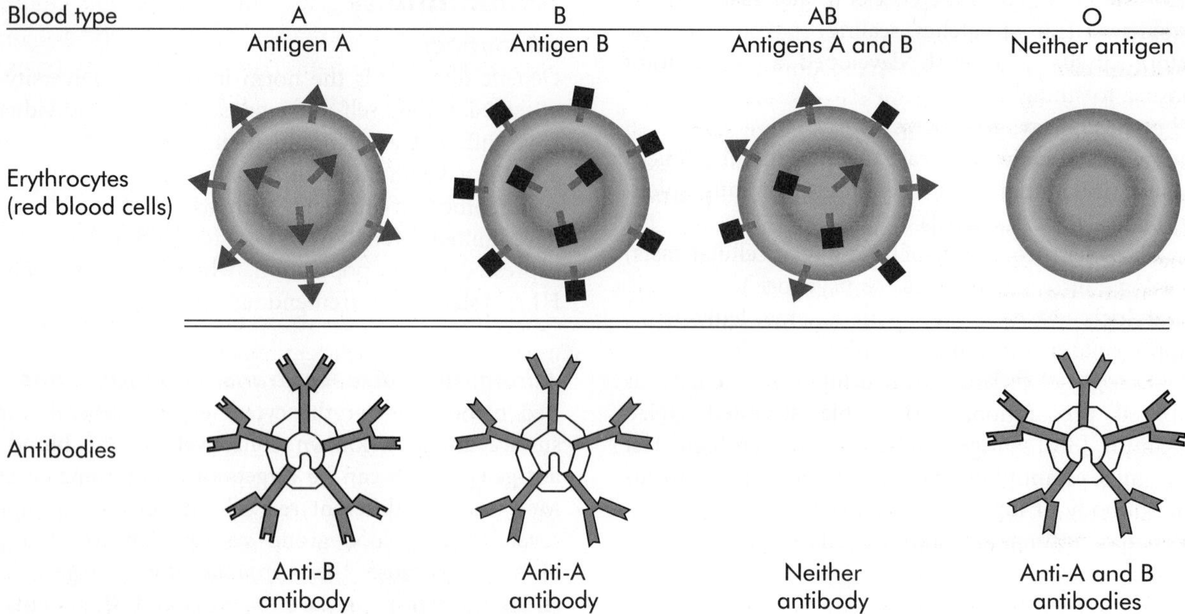

Figure 7-8 ■ **ABO Blood Types.** The relationship of antigens and antibodies associated with the ABO blood groups. The surfaces of erythrocytes of individuals with blood group A have the A antigenic carbohydrate. The blood of these individuals has IgM antibodies against the B antigen. In individuals with blood group B, the red blood cells have the B antigenic carbohydrate, and the blood contains IgM antibodies against the A antigen. In individuals of the blood group AB, the same cells have both the A and B antigens. These individuals do not have antibody to either A or B antigens. The erythrocytes of blood group O individuals have neither antigen, but their blood contains both antibodies to A and B.

individuals who do not express the D antigen are Rh-negative. When discussing the gene for the Rh antigen, the letter *d* is used to indicate lack of D. Rh-positive individuals can have either a *DD* or *Dd* genotype, whereas Rh-negative individuals have the *dd* genotype. About 85% of North Americans are Rh positive. Rh-negative individuals can make an IgG antibody to the D antigen (anti-D) if exposed to Rh-positive erythrocytes.

A disease called hemolytic disease of the newborn was most commonly caused by IgG anti-D alloantibody produced by Rh-negative mothers against erythrocytes of their Rh-positive fetuses (see Chapter 21). The mother's antibody crossed the placenta and destroyed the fetus' red blood cells. The occurrence of this particular form of the disease has decreased dramatically because of the use of prophylactic anti-D immunoglobulin (i.e., Rhogam). By mechanisms that are still not completely understood, administration of anti-D antibody within a few days of exposure to RhD-positive erythrocytes completely prevents sensitization against the D antigen. Because hemolytic disease of the newborn related to the D antigen has been controlled, alloantibodies against the other Rh antigens have become more important. In general, these alloantibodies are associated with a less severe hemolytic disease.

Alloimmune disease: transplant rejection

Major histocompatibility complex. Molecules of the **major histocompatibility complex (MHC)** were discussed in Chapter 6 as antigen-presenting molecules. MHC molecules are also a major target of transplant rejection. As a result of studies of transplantation, the human MHC molecules are also referred to as **human leukocyte antigens (HLA)** and the different MHC genetic loci are commonly called HLA-A, HLA-B, HLA-C, HLA-DR, HLA-DQ, and HLA-DP (Figure 7-9). Additional genes for complement components (e.g., C4, factor B) are also contained in the MHC and are referred to as class III loci. The class I (HLA-A, B, and C) and class II MHC loci (HLA-DR, DQ, and DP) are the most genetically diverse (polymorphic) of any human genetic loci. Within the human population, the numbers of possible different alleles (i.e., forms of the gene) expressed by each locus is astounding. For example, more than 300 different HLA-A antigens are expressed in the population. These numbers are based on the polymorphism of observed DNA sequences and may not reflect differences in function.

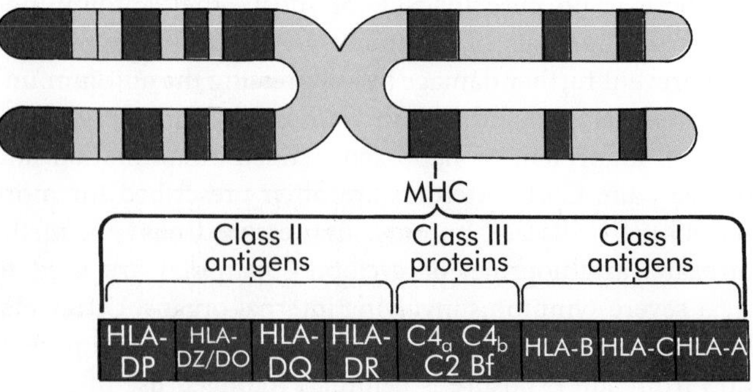

Figure 7-9 ■ **Human Leukocyte Antigens (HLA).** The major histocompatibility complex (MHC) is located on chromosome 6 and contains genes that code for class I antigens, class II antigens, and class III proteins (i.e., complement proteins and cytokines). (From Mudge-Grout C: *Immunologic disorders,* St Louis, 1992, Mosby.)

Clearly, not every allele is expressed in the same individual. Humans have two copies of each MHC locus (one inherited from each parent) that are codominant so that molecules encoded by each parent's genes are expressed on the cell surface. Within an individual, each locus will express only one allele. For instance, each person will have at most two different HLA-A proteins (one from each parent). However, with the tremendous number of possible alleles that can be expressed throughout the population, it is likely that any two unrelated individuals will have different MHC antigens and would reject organs transplanted from one to another.

Transplantation. The diversity of MHC molecules becomes clinically relevant during organ transplantation. The recipient of a transplant can mount an immune response against the foreign MHC antigens on the donor tissue, resulting in rejection. To minimize the chance of tissue rejection, the donor and recipient are often tissue-typed beforehand to identify differences in HLA antigens.[13] Because of the large number of different alleles, it is highly unlikely that a perfect match can be found between someone who needs a transplant and a potential donor from the general population. The more similar two individuals are in their HLA tissue type, the more likely a transplant from one to the other will be successful. Clearly, the most successful transplants would be between identical twins because they are identical genetically.

The specific combination of alleles at the six major HLA loci on one chromosome (A, B, C, DR, DQ, and DP) is termed a haplotype. Each individual has two HLA haplotypes, one from the paternal chromosome 6 and another from the maternal chromosome (Figure 7-10). Each parent passes on one set of HLA antigens to each of his or her offspring, meaning that children usually share half their HLA antigens with each parent. Odds dictate that children will share one haplotype with half their siblings and either no haplotypes or both haplotypes with a quarter of their siblings. Thus, the chance of finding a match among siblings is much higher (25%) than the general population.

Rejection. Transplant rejection may be classified as hyperacute, acute, or chronic, depending on the amount of time that elapses between transplantation and rejection. **Hyperacute rejection** is immediate and rare. When the circulation is reestablished to the grafted area, the graft may immediately turn white (the so-called *white graft*) instead of a normal pink color. Hyperacute rejection usually occurs because of preexisting antibody (type II reaction) to antigens on the vascular endothelial cells in the grafted tissue.

Acute rejection is a cell-mediated immune response that occurs within days to months after transplantation. This type of rejection occurs when the recipient develops an immune response against unmatched HLAs after transplantation. A biopsy of the rejected organ usually shows an infiltration of lymphocytes and macrophages characteristic of a type IV reaction.

Chronic rejection may occur after a period of months or years of normal function. It is characterized by slow, progressive organ failure. Chronic rejection may result from a weak cell-mediated (type IV) reaction against minor histocompatibility antigens on the grafted tissue.

QUICK CHECK 7-2

1. Why do certain drugs become immunogenic to the host?
2. Why is SLE considered an autoimmune disease?
3. Define the different types of graft rejection.

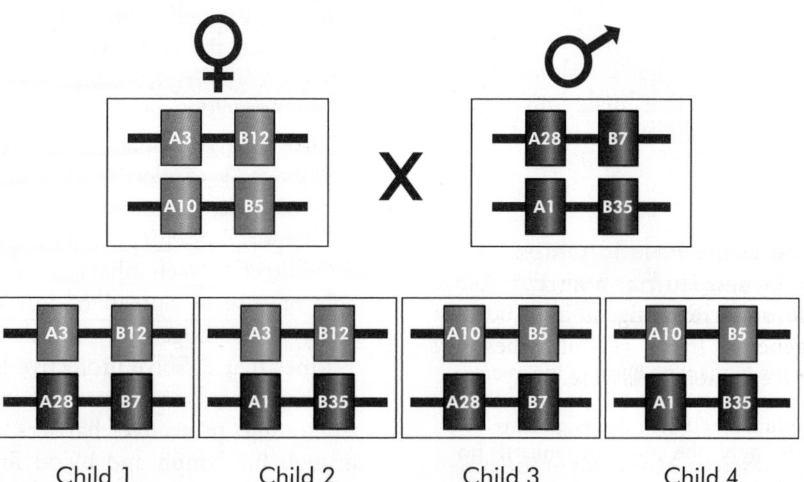

Figure 7-10 ■ **Inheritance of HLA.** HLA alleles are inherited in a codominant fashion; both maternal and paternal antigens are expressed. Specific HLA alleles are commonly given numbers to indicate different antigens. In this example, the mother has linked genes for HLA-A3 and HLA-B12 on one chromosome 6 and genes for HLA-A10 and HLA-B5 on the second chromosome 6. The father has HLA-A28 and HLA-B7 on one chromosome and HLA-A1 and HLA-B35 on the second chromosome. The children from this pairing may have one of four possible combinations of maternal and paternal HLA.

INFECTION

Modern health care has shown great progress in preventing and treating infectious diseases. In developed countries, sanitary living conditions, clean water, uncontaminated food, vaccinations, and antimicrobials make death from infectious disease most common only among those with debilitating diseases or immunosuppression. In the United States, heart disease and malignancies greatly surpass infectious disease as major causes of death.

However, infectious diseases remain the number one cause of death worldwide (causing 26% of all deaths in 2005).[14] In Africa, 62% of deaths in 2005 were attributable to infection. The infectious cause of death may be underestimated because many deaths related to cancer are the result of secondary infections because the immune system can be severely depressed both the cancer itself and by many of the treatments used to treat the cancer.

Developing countries with dense populations and poor sanitation are victims of plague, cholera, malaria, tuberculosis, leprosy, and schistosomiasis. Only smallpox has been eradicated worldwide by vaccination. Although vaccines and antimicrobials have altered the prevalence of some infectious diseases, mutant strains of bacteria and viruses have emerged with resistance to protection provided by drug therapy. The emergence of new diseases, such as West Nile virus, severe acute respiratory syndrome (SARS), Lyme disease, *Hantavirus,* and drug-resistant tuberculosis are examples of the current intense challenges being faced in the struggle to prevent and control infectious disease.

Microorganisms and Humans: A Dynamic Relationship

For many microorganisms, the human body is a very hospitable site to grow and flourish. The microorganisms are provided with nutrients and appropriate conditions of temperature and humidity. In many cases a mutual relationship exists, in which humans and the microorganisms benefit (Box 7-1). For instance, the human gut is colonized by a large variety of microorganisms that make up normal human flora. The normal floras of different body areas are summarized in Table 7-5. These bacteria are provided with nutrients from ingested food, and in exchange they produce enzymes that facilitate the digestion and utilization of many molecules in the human diet, produce antibacterial factors that prevent colonization by pathogenic microorganisms (see Chapter 5), and produce usable metabolites (e.g., vitamin K, B vitamins). This relationship normally is maintained through the physical integrity of the skin and mucosal epithelium and other mechanisms that guarantee that the immune and inflammatory systems do not attack these symbiotes (see Box 7-1). If those systems are compromised, many microorganisms will leave their normal sites and cause infection. Individuals with deficiencies in their immune system become easily infected with opportunistic microorganisms—those that normally would not cause disease but seize the opportunity provided by the person's decreased immune or inflammatory responses.

True pathogens have devised means to circumvent the normal controls provided by the host's main defensive barriers, the inflammatory system, and the immune system.[15] Infection by a pathogen is influenced by several factors:

- *Mechanism of action.* Direct damage of cells, interference with cellular metabolism, and rendering a cell dysfunctional because of the accumulation of pathogenic substances and toxin production
- *Infectivity.* Ability of the pathogen to invade and multiply in the individual—for example, coagulase (an enzyme) that causes coagulation and allows some microorganisms, such as *Staphylococcus,* to clot and form a sticky layer around themselves, protecting themselves against host defenses
- *Pathogenicity.* Ability of an agent to produce disease—success depends on its speed of reproduction, extent of tissue damage, and production of toxins
- *Virulence.* Potency of a pathogen measured in terms of the number of microorganisms or micrograms of toxin required to kill a host—for example, measles is of low virulence; the rabies virus is highly virulent
- *Immunogenicity.* Ability of pathogens to induce an immune response
- *Toxigenicity.* A factor important in determining a pathogen's virulence, such as production of soluble toxins or endotoxin

The portal of entry for pathogenic microorganisms may be by direct contact, inhalation, ingestion, or the bite of animals or insects. Spread of infection is facilitated by the ability of pathogens to attach to cell surfaces, release enzymes that dissolve protective barriers, escape the action of phagocytes, or resist the effect of low pH. After penetrating protective barriers, pathogens then spread through the lymph and blood for invasion of tissues and organs, where they multiply and cause disease. In humans the route of entrance of many pathogenic microorganisms also becomes the site of shedding of new infectious agents to other individuals, completing a cycle of infection (Figure 7-11).

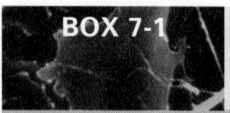

The Many Relationships Between Humans and Microorganisms

Symbiosis. Benefits only the human; no harm to the microorganism

Mutualism. Benefits the human and the microorganism

Commensalism. Benefits only the microorganism; no harm to the human

Pathogenicity. Benefits the microorganism; harms the human (*Opportunism* is the situation that occurs when benign microorganisms become pathogenic because of decreased human host resistance.)

TABLE 7-5

Normal Indigenous Flora of the Human Body

Location	Microorganisms
Skin	Predominantly gram-positive cocci and rods *Staphylococcus epidermidis,* corynebacteria, mycobacteria, and streptococci are primary inhabitants; *Staphylococcus aureus* in some people; also yeasts *(Candida, Pityrosporum)* in some areas of skin Numerous transient microorganisms may become temporary residents In moist areas, gram-negative bacteria Around sebaceous glands, *Propionibacteria* and brevibacteria The mite *Demodex folliculorum* lives in hair follicles and sebaceous glands around the face
Nose	Predominantly gram-positive cocci and rods, especially *S. epidermidis* Some people are nasal carriers of pathogenic bacteria, including *S. aureus*, β-hemolytic streptococci, and *Corynebacterium diphtheriae*
Mouth	A complex of bacteria that includes several species of streptococci, *Actinomyces,* lactobacilli, and *Haemophilus* Anaerobic bacteria and spirochetes colonize the gingival crevices
Pharynx	Similar to flora in mouth plus staphylococci, *Neisseria,* and diphtheroids Some asymptomatic persons also harbor the pathogens pneumococcus, *Haemophilus influenzae, Neisseria meningitidis,* and *C. diphtheria*
Distal intestine	Enterobacteria, streptococci, lactobacilli, anaerobic bacteria, and *C. albicans*
Colon	*Bacteroides,* lactobacilli, clostridia, *Salmonella, Shigella, Klebsiella, Proteus, Pseudomonas,* enterococci and other streptococci, bacilli, and *Escherichia coli*
Distal urethra	Typical bacteria found on the skin, especially *S. epidermidis* and diphtheroids; also lactobacilli and nonpathogenic streptococci
Vagina	Birth to 1 mo: similar to adult 1 mo to puberty: *S. epidermidis,* diphtheroids, *E. coli,* and streptococci Puberty to menopause: *Lactobacillus acidophilus,* diphtheroids, staphylococci, streptococci, and a variety of anaerobes Postmenopause: similar to prepubescence

From Grimes DE: *Infectious diseases,* Mosby's Clinical Nursing Series, St Louis, 1991, Mosby.

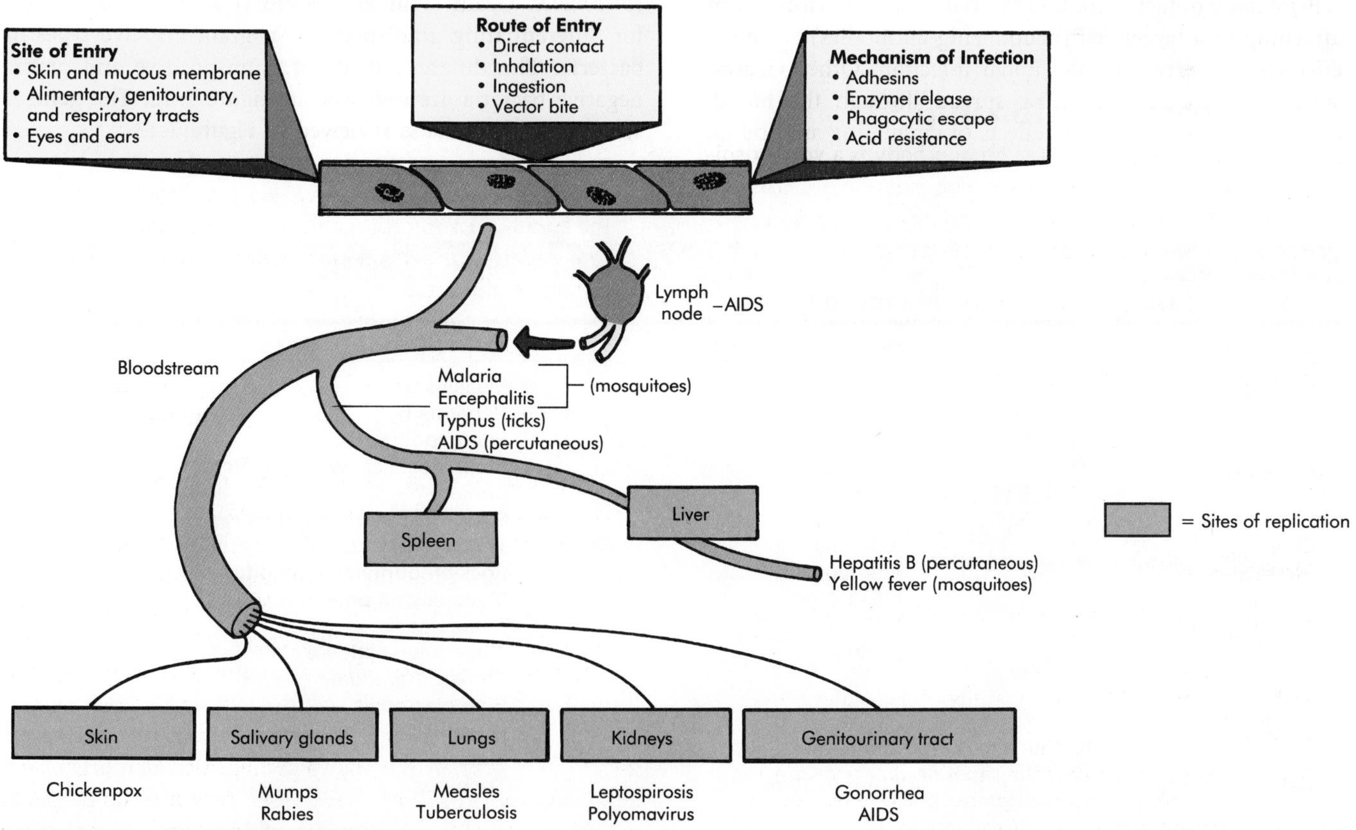

Figure 7-11 ■ The Spread of Infection. (Redrawn from Mims CA et al: *Medical microbiology,* St Louis, 1993, Mosby.)

Classes of Infectious Microorganisms

Infectious disease can be caused by microorganisms that range in size from 20 nanometers (nm) (poliovirus) to 10 meters (m) (tapeworm). Classes of pathogenic microorganisms and their characteristics are summarized in Table 7-6. Some mechanisms of tissue damage caused by microorganisms are summarized in Table 7-7.

Pathogenic Defense Mechanisms

Our multiple layers of defense against infection were described in Chapters 5 and 6. True pathogens have devised ways of circumventing these barriers. For example, some bacteria produce thick capsules of carbohydrate or protein that are antiphagocytic, preventing efficient phagocytosis. Others defend themselves by producing toxins that kill neutrophils. Because the primary immune response may take a week to develop adequately, some pathogens proliferate at rates that surpass the development of a protective response. Table 7-8 contains examples of microorganisms that fight off the immune system or cause it to attack the host.

Viral pathogens bypass many defense mechanisms by hiding within cells and away from normal inflammatory or immune responses. In many cases, however, because viral agents must spread from cell to cell, the developing immune response eventually cures the infection so the disease is self-limiting. However, many viruses (e.g., measles, herpes) are inaccessible to antibodies after initial infection because they do not circulate in the bloodstream but instead remain inside infected cells, spreading by direct cell-to-cell contact. Antibodies that block a virus from attaching to a target cell (neutralizing antibodies) are most effective in preventing the initial infection. Other viruses, such as polio and influenza, spread through the blood, are more susceptible to the effects of circulating antibodies, and can be controlled by antibodies even after the initial infection.

Some viruses can elude the immune response by undergoing antigenic variation. The virus can change its appearance by altering surface antigens. Influenza infection provides an example of how this occurs. The "flu" virus undergoes yearly **antigenic drift** resulting from mutations in key surface antigens, hemagglutinin (H antigen) and neuraminidase (N antigen), allowing the emergence of new strains of influenza virus. Thus, immunity against the previous year's viruses is no longer completely protective, thus creating the need for new vaccines every year. **Antigenic shifts** are major changes in antigenicity that occur from recombination of genes for H and N among different strains of viruses and can result in major worldwide pandemics. Other pathogens, such as some parasitic microorganisms, use a similar approach and change surface antigens by gene switching. A parasite (i.e., African trypanosomes) may carry thousands of genes for different surface molecules that the parasite can switch on and off at frequent intervals. Consequently, the immune system is always trying to catch up by generating new antibodies and T cells against the new antigens.

Infection and Injury

Bacterial disease

Bacteria are prokaryocytes (lacking a discrete nucleus) and are relatively small. They can be aerobic or anaerobic and motile or immotile. Spherical bacteria are called cocci, rodlike forms are called bacilli, and spiral forms are termed *spirochetes.* Gram stain and acid-fast stain are important for differentiating gram-positive or gram-negative types of bacteria. The different types of gram-positive and gram-negative bacteria are reviewed in Figure 7-12. The general structure of bacteria is reviewed in Figure 7-13.

TABLE 7-6
Classes of Human Infectious Microorganisms

Class	Size	Examples of Disease
Viruses	20–30 nm	Measles Hepatitis B Pneumonitis
Bacteria	0.8–15 μm	Staphylococcal wound infection Cholera Streptococcal pneumonia
Chlamydia	200–1000 nm	Trachoma
Rickettsiae	300–1200 nm	Rocky Mountain spotted fever
Mycoplasma	125–350 nm	Mycoplasma pneumonia
Mycobacterium	1–10 μm	Tuberculosis
Fungi	2–200 μm	Tinea pedis (athlete's foot) Thrush *(Candida)* Histoplasmosis
Protozoa	1–360 μm	Giardiasis Malaria
Helminths	3 mm to 10 m	Trichinosis Filariasis

TABLE 7-7

Summary of Some Mechanisms of Tissue Damage and the Microorganisms That Cause Them

PATHOGENS THAT DIRECTLY CAUSE TISSUE DAMAGE	
Infectious Agent	**Disease**
PRODUCE EXOTOXIN	
Streptococcus pyogenes	Tonsillitis, scarlet fever
Staphylococcus aureus	Boils, toxic shock syndrome, food poisoning
Corynebacterium diphtheriae	Diphtheria
Clostridium tetani	Tetanus
Vibrio cholerae	Cholera
PRODUCE ENDOTOXIN	
Escherichia coli	Gram-negative sepsis
Haemophilus influenzae	Meningitis, pneumonia
Salmonella typhi	Typhoid
Shigella	Bacillary dysentery
Pseudomonas aeruginosa	Wound infection
Yersinia pestis	Plague
CAUSE DIRECT DAMAGE WITH INVASION	
Variola	Smallpox
Varicella-zoster	Chickenpox, shingles
Hepatitis B virus	Hepatitis
Poliovirus	Poliomyelitis
Measles virus	Measles, subacute sclerosing panencephalitis
Influenza virus	Influenza
Herpes simplex virus	Cold sores

PATHOGENS THAT INDIRECTLY CAUSE TISSUE DAMAGE	
Infectious Agent	**Disease**
PRODUCE IMMUNE COMPLEXES	
Hepatitis B virus	Kidney disease
Malaria	Vascular deposits
S. pyogenes	Glomerulonephritis
Treponema pallidum	Kidney damage in secondary syphilis
Most acute infections	Transient renal deposits
PRODUCE ANTIBODY AGAINST AN INDIVIDUAL'S CELLS OR TISSUES (AUTOANTIBODY)	
S. pyogenes	Rheumatic fever
Mycoplasma pneumonia	Hemolytic anemia
CAUSE CELL-MEDIATED IMMUNITY	
Mycobacterium tuberculosis	Tuberculosis
Mycobacterium leprae	Tuberculoid leprosy
Lymphocytic choriomeningitis virus	Aseptic meningitis
Borrelia burgdorferi	Lyme arthritis
Schistosoma mansoni	Schistosomiasis
Herpes simplex virus	Herpes stromal keratitis

Data from Janeway CA et al: *Immunobiology: the system in health and disease,* ed 5, New York, 2001, Garland.

Bacterial survival and growth depend on the effectiveness of the body's defense mechanisms and on the bacterium's ability to resist these defenses. Many pathogens have devised ways of preventing destruction by the inflammatory and immune systems. For example, some bacteria produce thick capsules of carbohydrate or protein that are antiphagocytic, preventing efficient opsonization and phagocytosis. Such coatings include the thick polysaccharide covering of the pneumococcus and the waxy capsule surrounding the tubercle bacillus. The long M protein on the cell wall of the streptococcus suppresses complement activation.

Other bacteria survive and proliferate in the body by producing exotoxins and endotoxins that injure cells and tissues. **Exotoxins** are proteins released during bacterial growth. They are usually enzymes and have highly specific effects on host cells; they include cytotoxins, neurotoxins, pneumotoxins, enterotoxins, and hemolysins. Exotoxins can damage cell membranes, activate second messengers, and inhibit protein synthesis. Exotoxins are immunogenic

TABLE 7-8

Examples of Mechanisms Used by Pathogens to Resist the Immune System

Mechanisms	Effect on Immunity	Example
DESTROYS OR BLOCKS COMPONENT OF IMMUNE SYSTEM		
Produce toxins	Kills phagocyte or interferes with chemotaxis	*Staphylococcus* *Streptococcus*
	Prevents phagocytosis by inhibiting fusion between phagosome and lysosomal granules	*Mycobacterium tuberculosis*
Produce antioxidants (e.g., catalase, superoxide dismutase)	Prevents killing by O_2-dependent mechanisms	*Mycobacterium* sp. *Salmonella typhi*
Produce protease to digest IgA	Promotes bacterial attachment	*Neisseria gonorrhoeae* (urinary tract infection), *Haemophilus influenzae*, and *Streptococcus pneumoniae* (pneumonia)
Produce surface molecules that mimic Fc receptors and bind antibody	Prevents activation of complement system Prevents antibody functioning as opsonin	*Staphylococcus* Herpes simplex virus
MIMIC SELF-ANTIGENS		
Produce surface antigens (e.g., M protein, red blood cell antigens) that are similar to self-antigens	Pathogen resembles the individual's own tissue; in some individuals, antibodies can be formed against the self-antigen, leading to hypersensitivity disease (e.g., antibody to M protein also reacts with cardiac tissue, causing rheumatic heart disease; antibody to red blood cell antigens can cause anemia)	Group A streptococcus (M protein) *Mycoplasma pneumoniae* (red cell antigens)
CHANGE ANTIGENIC PROFILE		
Undergo mutation of antigens or activate genes that change surface molecules	Immune response delayed because of failure to recognize new antigen	Influenza HIV Some parasites

and elicit the production of antibodies known as **antitoxins**. Consequently, vaccines are available for many of the exotoxins (i.e., tetanus, diphtheria, and pertussis). Some strains of toxin-producing group A streptococci cause destructive skin infections (e.g., flesh-eating bacteria syndrome, or necrotizing fasciitis) and pneumonia that may kill an individual within 2 days.

Endotoxins (lipopolysaccharides [LPS]) are contained in the cell walls of gram-negative bacteria and are released during lysis, or destruction, of the bacteria. Endotoxin may be released also from the membrane of the bacteria during bacterial growth or during treatment with antibiotics, which therefore cannot prevent the toxic effects of the endotoxin. Bacteria that produce endotoxins are called pyrogenic bacteria because they activate the inflammatory process and produce fever. The innermost part of the lipopolysaccharide, lipid A, is made of polysaccharide and fatty acids and is responsible for the substance's toxic effects.

Inflammation is the body's initial response to the presence of the bacteria. Vascular permeability is increased, allowing blood-borne substances (i.e., the complement system) involved in bacterial destruction to access the site of infection. Endotoxins increase capillary permeability further by activating the anaphylatoxins (C5a and C3a) of the complement cascade. Capillary permeability may increase sufficiently to permit the escape of large volumes of plasma, contributing to hypotension and, in severe cases, cardiovascular shock (see Chapter 23). Endotoxin also can activate the coagulation cascade, leading to the syndrome of disseminated (or diffuse) intravascular coagulation (see Chapter 20).

Septicemia (bacteremia) is the presence of bacteria in the blood and is caused by a failure of the body's defense mechanisms. The usual cause is proliferation of gram-negative bacteria, although a few gram-positive bacteria and fungi can cause it. Symptoms of gram-negative septic shock are produced by endotoxins. Once in the blood, endotoxins cause the release of vasoactive peptides and cytokines that affect blood vessels, producing vasodilation, which reduces blood pressure, causes decreased oxygen delivery, and produces subsequent cardiovascular shock (see Chapter 23). Sepsis is diagnosed from evaluation of blood cultures.

Endotoxic shock is a complication of sepsis and can be fatal to the individual. The cytokine TNF-α plays a pivotal role in the pathogenesis of endotoxic shock. TNF-α is produced by activated macrophages on exposure to endotoxin from gram-negative bacterial infections. It is sometimes called cachectin because of its role in promoting cachexia in individuals with cancer. (Cachexia is discussed in Chapter 10; cytokines are discussed in Chapters 5 and 6; types of shock are discussed in Chapter 23.)

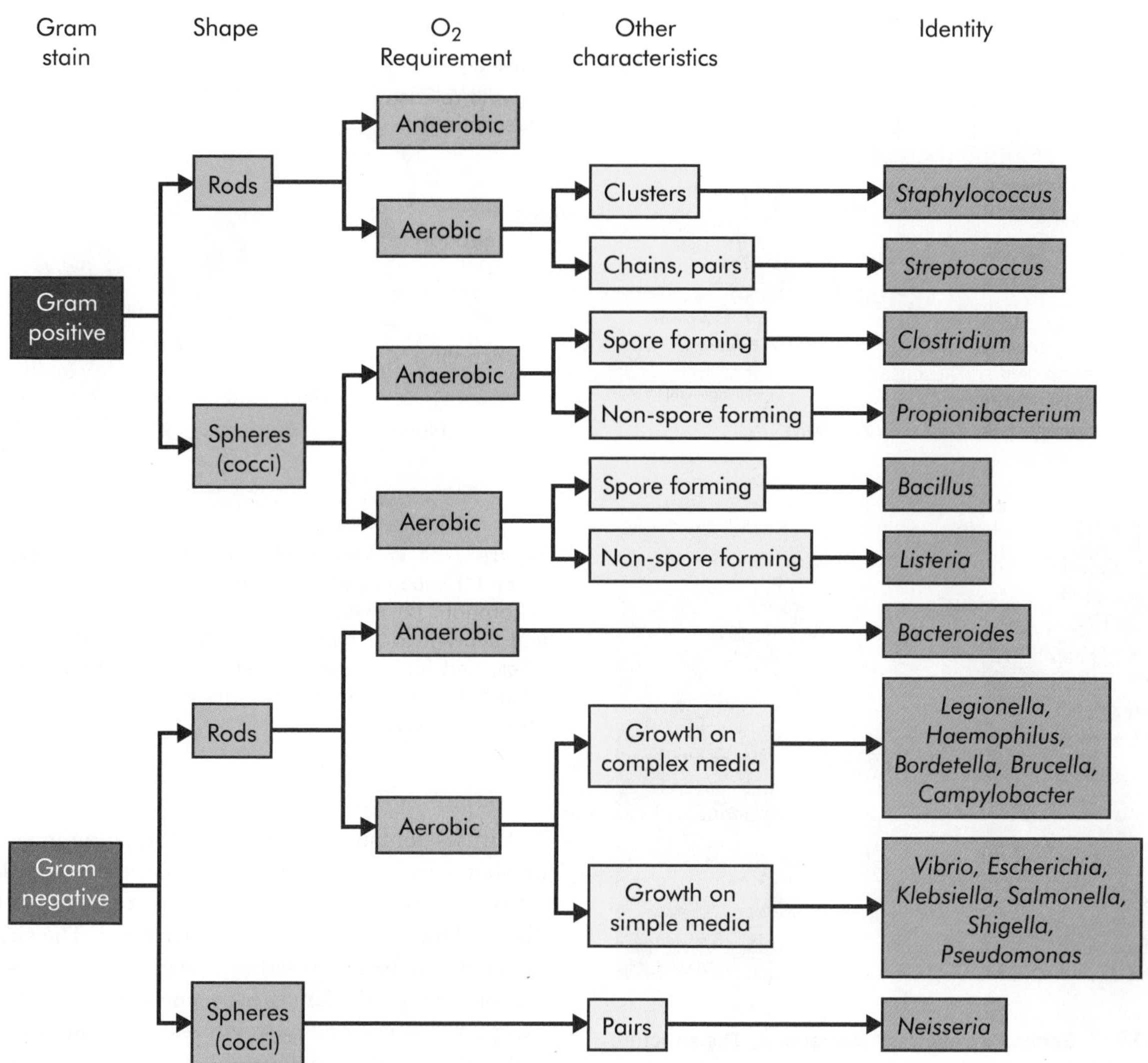

Figure 7-12 ■ **Types of Gram-Positive and Gram-Negative Bacteria.**

HEALTH ALERT

Antibiotic-Resistant Microorganisms Have Become the Primary Cause of Skin and Soft-Tissue Infections

The era of empirically prescribing an antibiotic for skin infections is past. In a recent study from 11 emergency rooms around the United States, *Staphylococcus aureus* was isolated from 320 of 422 adults with skin or soft-tissue infections (76%), and 249 (78%) of the isolates contained methicillin-resistant *Staphylococcus aureus* (MRSA). Thus, MRSA was isolated from 249 of 422 individuals (59%). In the past MRSA was observed primarily in hospitals and nursing homes. Now it is becoming the primary microorganism found in community acquired infections. If inadequately treated, MRSA can lead to severe complications, including sepsis, heart disease, and toxic shock syndrome. The MRSA isolated in this study were sensitive to other antibiotics, which suggests that antibiotic-susceptibility panels should routinely be performed on isolates from skin and soft-tissue infections.

From Moran GJ et al: Methicillin-resistant *S. aureus* infections among patients in the emergency department, *N Engl J Med* 355:666–674, 2006.

Viral disease

Viral diseases are the most common afflictions of humans and include a variety of diseases ranging from the common cold and the "cold sore" of herpes simplex to several types of cancers and AIDS. Viruses are very simple microorganisms consisting of nucleic acid (the viral genome) protected from the environment by a layer or layers of proteins. They are sensitive to many environmental factors and cannot survive for long outside a cell.

Viral replication

Virions (viral particles) do not possess any of the metabolic organelles found in prokaryotes (e.g., bacteria) or eukaryotes (e.g., human cells). Thus, viruses have no metabolism. Unlike bacteria, viruses are incapable of independent reproduction. Their replication depends totally on their ability to infect a permissive host cell—a cell that cannot resist viral invasion and replication. The replication cycle of most viruses can be divided into six distinct phases: adsorption, penetration, uncoating, replication, assembly, and release. Infection with a virus begins with a virion binding to a specific receptor on the plasma membrane of

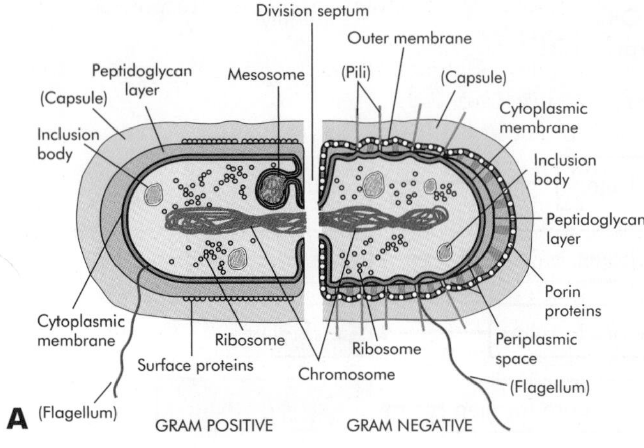

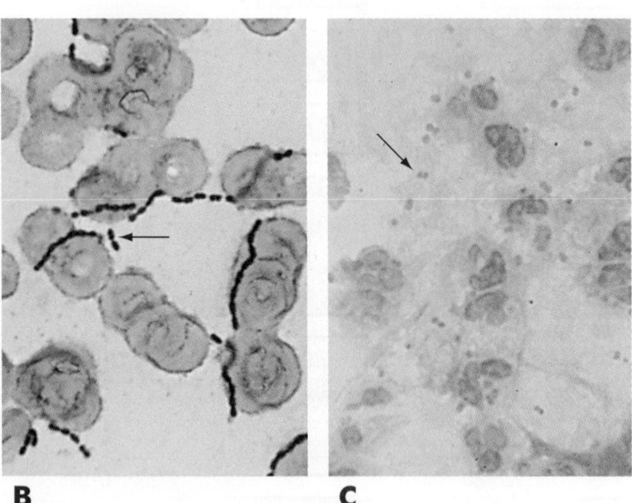

Figure 7-13 ■ **General Structure of Bacteria. A,** The structure of the bacterial cell wall determines its staining characteristics with gram stain. A gram-positive bacterium has a thick layer of peptidoglycan *(left)*. A gram-negative bacterium has a thick peptidoglycan layer and an outer membrane *(right)*. **B,** Example of a gram-positive (darkly stained microorganisms, *arrow*) group A *Streptococcus*. This microorganism consists of cocci that frequently form chains. **C,** Example of a gram-negative (pink microorganisms, arrow) *Neisseria meningitides* in cerebrospinal fluid. *Neisseria* form complexes of two cocci (diplococci). (From Murray PR et al: *Medical microbiology*, ed 4, St Louis, 2002, Mosby.)

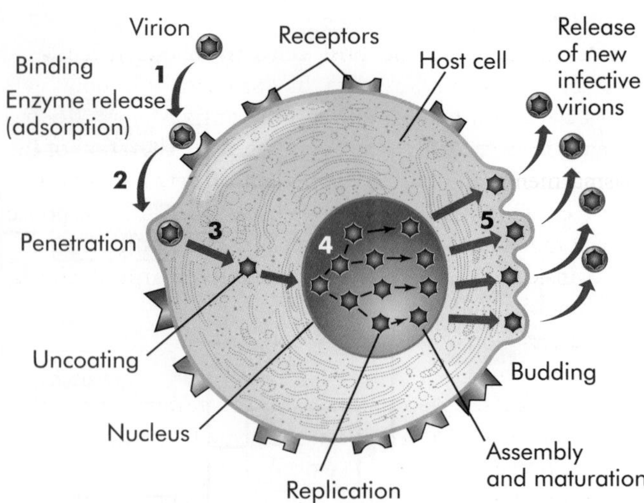

Figure 7-14 ■ **Stages of Viral Infection of a Host Cell.** The virion **(1)** becomes attached to the cell's plasma membrane by absorption; **(2)** releases enzymes that weaken the membrane and allow it to penetrate the cell; **(3)** uncoats itself; **(4)** replicates; and **(5)** matures and escapes from the cell by budding from the plasma membrane. The infection then can spread to other host cells.

a host cell (Figure 7-14). The specificity of this virus-receptor interaction dictates the range of host cells that a particular virus will infect and therefore the clinical symptoms, which reflect the alteration of the function of the infected cells. For example, the influenza virus binds to a receptor on respiratory epithelial cells, causing symptoms of an upper respiratory tract infection. Once bound, the virion penetrates the plasma membrane by one of several means: by receptor-mediated endocytosis, by viral envelope fusion with the plasma membrane, or by directly crossing the plasma membrane.

Viruses contain their genetic information in either DNA or ribonucleic acid (RNA). The viral genetic material is protected by a protein coat that must be removed in the cytoplasm of the infected host cell (uncoating). The viral genetic material may be processed by one of several paths, depending on the particular virus. Generally, all RNA viruses, except influenza and retroviruses, replicate their genetic material in the cytoplasm of the infected cell, and all DNA viruses, except poxviruses, require the DNA to enter the nucleus and use the cell's DNA polymerases to replicate. Poxviruses provide their own DNA polymerase and replicate their DNA in the cytoplasm of the infected cell. Retroviruses generally convert their RNA genetic information to DNA using an enzyme contained in the virion—reverse transcriptase.

After infection, viruses usually make multiple copies of their genetic material and produce the necessary viral proteins for replication. New virions are assembled in the host cell's cytoplasm and are released from the cell for transmission of the viral infection to other host cells. This cycle is referred to as the productive or lytic cycle because a large number of progeny are produced, and the result is often the destruction of the host cell.

Some viruses will not be productive initially but instead initiate a latency phase, during which the host cell is transformed. During this phase, the viral DNA may be integrated into the DNA of the host cell and become a permanent passenger in that cell and its progeny. In response to stimuli, such as stress, hormonal changes, or disease, the virus may exit latency and enter a productive cycle.

Cellular effects of viruses

Besides taking over the host cell's metabolic machinery, viral infection can injure cells. In some viral infections, cellular destruction results from large quantities of virus being released from the cell's plasma membrane. Alteration of the plasma membrane by the expression of new antigens as a result of viral infection can incite an immune response against the individual's infected cells (e.g., hepatitis B virus). Once inside the cell, virions have many harmful effects, including the following:

1. The cessation of DNA, RNA, and protein synthesis (e.g., herpes virus)
2. Disruption of lysosomal membranes, resulting in release of "digestive" lysosomal enzymes that can kill the cell (e.g., herpes virus)
3. Fusion of host cells, producing multinucleated giant cells (e.g., respiratory syncytial virus)
4. Alteration of the antigenic properties, or "identity" of the infected cell, causing the individual's immune system to attack the cell as if it were foreign (e.g., hepatitis B virus)
5. Transformation of host cells into cancerous cells, resulting in uninhibited and unregulated growth (e.g., human papilloma virus)
6. Promotion of secondary bacterial infection in tissues damaged by viruses

Examples of human diseases caused by specific viruses are listed in Table 7-9.

Viral pathogens bypass many defense mechanisms by developing intracellularly, thus hiding within cells and away from normal inflammatory or immune responses. In many cases, however, because viral agents must spread from cell to cell, the developing immune response eventually cures the infection so the disease is usually self-limiting, in that it resolves without the need for medications. Some viruses will persist, and a state of unapparent infection may result. In persistent infections, cellular injury may be minimal, and the virus persists until it is activated to replicate (e.g., the cold sores of herpesvirus infection). Immunity may limit recurrent outbreaks and protect the individual from an acute exacerbation only or may be sufficiently strong to prevent disease.

Fungal disease

Fungi are relatively large microorganisms with thick walls that grow as either single-celled yeasts (spheres) or multicelled molds (filaments or hyphae) (Figure 7-15). Some fungi can exist in either form and are called **dimorphic**

TABLE 7-9

List of DNA and RNA Viruses of Human Importance

DNA VIRUSES

Family	Viral Members
Adenoviridae	Human adenoviruses
Hepadnaviridae	Hepatitis B virus
Herpesvindae	Herpes simplex 1 and 2 varicella zoster virus cytomegalovirus, Epstein-Barr virus, human herpes-viruses 6, 7, and 8
Papillomaviridae	Human papilloma viruses
Parvoviridae	Parvovirus B-19
Polyomaviridae	BK and JC-polyomaviruses
Poxviridae	Variola, vaccinia, orf, molluscum contaglosum, monkeypox

RNA VIRUSES

Family	Viral Members
Arenaviridae	Lymphocytic choriomeningitis virus, Lassa fever virus
Astroviridae	Gastroenteritis-causing astroviruses
Bunyaviridae	Arboviruses including California encephalitis and Lacrosse viruses; nonarboviruses including sin nombre and related hantaviruses
Caliciviridae	Noroviruses and hepatitis E virus
Coronaviridae	Coronaviruses, including SARS coronavirus
Filoviridae	Ebola and Marburg hemorrhagic fever viruses
Flaviviridae	Arboviruses including yellow fever, dengue, West Nile, Japanese encephalitis, and St. Louis encephalitis viruses, nonarboviruses including hepatitis C virus
Orthomyxoviridae	Influenza A, B, and C viruses
Paramyxoviridae	Parainfluenza viruses, mumps virus, measles virus, respiratory syncytial virus, metapneumovirus, Nipah virus
Picornaviridae	Polio viruses, coxsackie A viruses, coxsackie B viruses, echoviruses, enteroviruses 68–71, enterovirus, 72 (hepatitis A virus), rhinoviruses
Reoviridae	Rotavirus, Colorado tick fever virus
Retroviridae	Human immunodeficiency viruses (HIV-1 and HIV-2), human T-lymphotropic viruses (HTLV-1 and HTLV-2)
Rhabdoviridae	Rabies virus
Togaviridae	Eastern, Western and Venezuela equine encephalitis, viruses, rubella virus

From Forbes BA et al: *Bailey & Scott's Diagnostic microbiology*, ed 12, St Louis, 2007, Mosby.

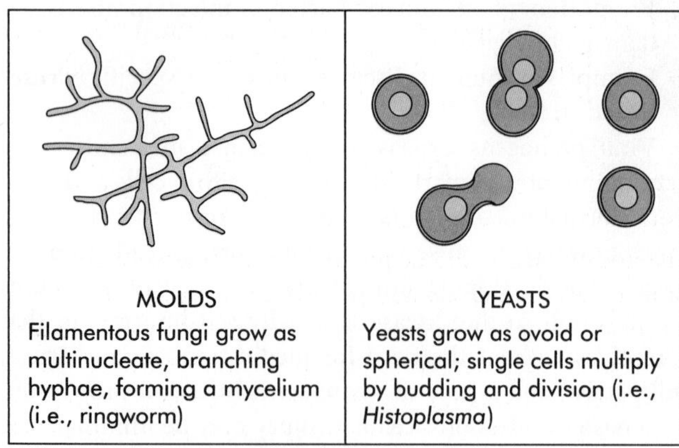

MOLDS
Filamentous fungi grow as multinucleate, branching hyphae, forming a mycelium (i.e., ringworm)
YEASTS
Yeasts grow as ovoid or spherical; single cells multiply by budding and division (i.e., Histoplasma)

Figure 7-15 ■ **Types of Fungi.** (From Mims CA et al: *Medical microbiology*, ed 3, London, 2004, Mosby.)

fungi. The cell walls of fungi are rigid and multilayered. The wall is composed of polysaccharides different from the peptidoglycans of bacteria. The lack of peptidoglycans allows fungi to resist the action of bacterial cell wall inhibitors such as penicillin and cephalosporin. In contrast to bacteria, the cytosols of fungi contain organelles: mitochondria, ribosomes, Golgi apparatus, microtubules, microvesicles, endoplasmic reticulum, and nuclei. Molds are aerobic, and yeasts are facultative anaerobes, which adapt to, but do not require, anaerobic conditions. They usually reproduce by simple division or budding.

Pathologic fungi cause disease by adapting to the host environment. Fungi that colonize the skin can digest keratin. Other fungi can grow with wide temperature variations in lower oxygen environments. Still other fungi have the capacity to suppress host immune defenses. Phagocytes and T lymphocytes are important in controlling fungi, and low white blood cell counts promote fungal infection. Fungi have two basic structures: hyphae and yeasts. Hyphae have branching, tubular filaments. Yeasts are singular spherical cells.

Diseases caused by fungi are called **mycoses.** Mycoses can be superficial, deep, or opportunistic. Superficial mycoses occur on or near skin or mucous membranes and usually produce mild and superficial disease. Fungi that invade the skin, hair, or nails are known as **dermatophytes.** The diseases they produce are called *tineas* (ringworm), for example, tinea capitis (scalp), tinea pedis (feet), and tinea cruris (groin). Superficial dermatophytes grow in a ringlike, erythematous patch with a raised border. Itching often is intense, and cracking of tissue can occur and lead to secondary bacterial infection. Infections of the scalp are accompanied by scaling and hair loss. (Chapter 39 discusses the various skin disorders caused by fungi.)

Deep infections involving internal organs can be life threatening and are most common in association with other diseases or as an opportunistic infection in immunosuppressed individuals. Fungi causing deep infection enter the body through inhalation or through open wounds. Filamentous forms can multiply extracellularly, but the spherical yeasts multiply within cells, including white blood cells. Some fungi are a part of the normal body flora and become pathologic only when immunity is compromised, allowing exaggerated growth and translocation. For example, *Candida albicans* is normally found in the mouth, gastrointestinal tract, and vagina of normal individuals. Changes in pH and use of antibiotics that kill bacteria that normally inhibit *Candida* growth permit rapid proliferation and overgrowth, which can lead to superficial or deep infection. Common pathologic fungi are summarized in Table 7-10.

Fungi are diagnosed by microscopic observation of specimens treated with potassium hydroxide and stained to enhance visualization of spheres and filaments. Specimens also can be cultured. Skin tests are available for species of *Aspergillus.* No vaccines are available to prevent fungal disease effectively. Many of the antifungal drugs (e.g., amphotericin B, ketoconazole, fluconazole) used to treat deep or systemic infections are toxic to the host because the fungal cell composition is similar to the host cell.

TABLE 7-10

Common Pathologic Fungi

Fungus	Growth Form	Mode or Site of Entry	Disease
SUPERFICIAL			
Microsporum spp.	Filament	Skin contact	Ringworm, jock itch, athlete's foot
Epidermophyton floccosum	Filament	Skin contact	Infects skin and nails
Malassezia furfur	Sphere	Skin contact	May infect skin, sweat glands, hair follicles, and other sites
DEEP			
Pneumocystis carinii	Sphere	Inhalation	Pneumonia
Histoplasma capsulatum	Sphere	Inhalation	Histoplasmosis (lungs)
Aspergillus fumigatus	Filament	Inhalation	Aspergillosis and pneumonia
Coccidioides immitis	Unusual form	Inhalation	Coccidioidomycosis
Candida albicans	Sphere	Normal flora of skin, mouth, intestine	Thrush, vaginal yeast infections, systemic infections

Clinical Manifestations of Infection

The progression from infection to infectious disease follows predictable stages (infection, incubation, symptoms, shedding of the microorganism) as demonstrated by the pathogenesis of measles illustrated in Figure 7-16. Clinical manifestations of infectious disease vary, depending on the pathogen and the organ system affected. Manifestations can arise directly from the infecting microorganism or its products; however, the majority of the clinical symptoms result from the host's inflammatory and immune responses (see Chapters 5 and 6). Infectious diseases typically begin with the nonspecific or general symptoms of fatigue, malaise, weakness, and loss of concentration. Generalized aching and loss of appetite are common complaints. However, the hallmark of most infectious diseases is fever.

Fever

Fever resulting from cytokines has been discussed in Chapter 5. Exogenous pyrogens produced by infectious agent may not cause fever directly but induce the production of endogenous pyrogens during inflammation. Endogenous pyrogens include interleukin-1 (IL-1), interleukin-6 (IL-6), interferon, tumor necrosis factor-alpha (TNF-α), and other cytokines. It is generally accepted that fever has a beneficial effect against infection, although the mechanisms have not been fully established.

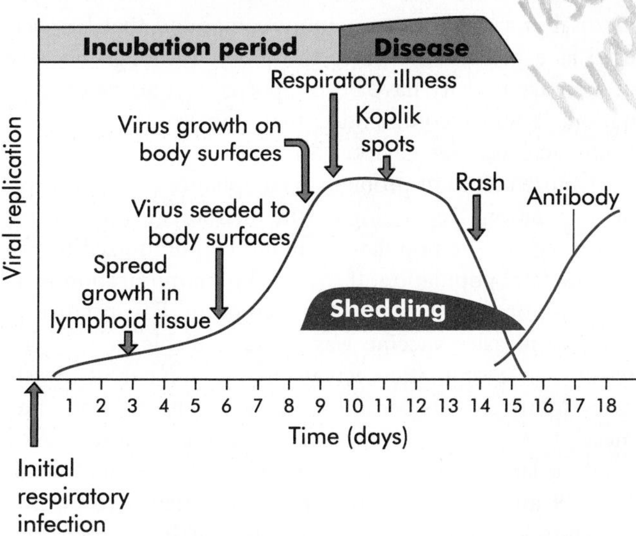

Figure 7-16 **Progression of Measles.** The pathogenesis of measles is representative of most viral infections in unimmunized individuals. The virus enters through the oropharynx, from where it infects the regional lymph nodes. After 5 to 7 days, virus enters the blood (viremia) and spreads to the body surfaces (respiratory, gastrointestinal, and urinary tracts, and the skin). The measles virus replicates in these tissues, leading to upper respiratory tract symptoms, with the appearance of red spots with bluish-white specks (Koplik spots) in the oral mucosa and later to an extensive rash involving most parts of the skin. At or near the onset of overt symptoms, the infected individual is shedding virus and is highly infectious to others. Antibodies against the measles virus are primarily responsible for resolving the infection. They are produced within 10 to 11 days but are immediately absorbed by viral particles in the blood so that free antibody is not measurable until about 2 weeks after the initial infection.

Countermeasures Against Pathogenic Defenses

The body's innate and acquired responses against microorganisms are numerous and involve an interaction between the immune and inflammatory systems. Pathogenic microorganisms, however, have developed means of circumventing the individual's protective defenses. Therefore, prophylactic or interventive procedures have been developed either to prevent the pathogen from initiating disease (vaccines) or to destroy the pathogen once the disease process has started (antimicrobials). Most vaccine development has focused on preventing the most severe and common infections. With the initial success of antibiotic therapy, there was no perceived need for vaccination against many common and non-life-threatening infections. The increasing problem of antibiotic-resistant pathogens, however, has forced a reappraisal of that strategy, and a greater emphasis now is being placed on the development of new vaccines.

Vaccines

The purpose of **vaccination** is to induce long-lasting protective immune responses under conditions that will not result in disease in a healthy recipient of the **vaccine.** The primary immune response from vaccination is generally short lived; therefore, booster injections are used to push the immune response through multiple secondary responses resulting in large numbers of memory cells and sustained protective levels of antibody or T cells, or both.

Development of a successful vaccine is costly and depends on several factors. These include identification of the protective immune response and the appropriate antigen to induce that response. For instance, individuals with ongoing HIV infection produce a great deal of antibody against several HIV antigens. But, for development of a successful vaccine, we must first understand which antibody will protect against an initial infection.

Once a good candidate antigen is identified, it must be developed into an effective, cost-efficient, stable, and safe vaccine. For instance, most vaccines against viral infection (measles, mumps, rubella, varicella [chickenpox]) contain live viruses that are weakened (attenuated) so they continue to express appropriate antigens but establish only a limited and easily controlled infection. For most common vaccines against viral infections, limited replication of the virus appears to afford better long-term protection than using viral antigen. One current exception is the hepatitis B vaccine, which uses a recombinant viral protein. The hepatitis A vaccine is an inactivated (killed) virus and normally should not cause an infection.

Even attenuated viruses can establish life-threatening infections in individuals whose immune system is congenitally deficient or suppressed.[16] The risk of infection by the vaccine strain of virus is extremely small, but it may affect the choice of recommended vaccines. For instance, two different vaccines were developed against polio. The Sabin vaccine was an attenuated virus that was administered orally. It provided systemic protection and induced a secretory immune response to prevent growth of the poliovirus in the intestinal tract. Being a live virus, the vaccine could cause polio in some children who had unsuspected immune deficiencies (about 1 case in 2.4 million doses). The Salk vaccine was a completely inactivated virus administered by injection. It induced protective systemic immunity but did not provide adequate secretory immunity. Therefore, even if the individual was protected from systemic infection by poliovirus, the virus could transiently infect their intestinal mucosa, be shed, and spread to others. When polio was epidemic, the oral vaccine was preferred. Vaccination has been extremely effective: 2525 cases of paralytic polio were reported in the United States in 1960, 61 cases were reported in 1965, and no cases of polio since 1979. In 1994, the disease polio was declared officially eradicated in all the Americas. The goal of the World Health Organization (WHO) is to eradicate polio worldwide in the next few years (Figure 7-17). However, the live attenuated vaccine itself caused about 8 cases of paralytic polio per year in the United States in individuals with inadequate immune systems. As a result, the current recommendation of the Centers for Disease Control and Prevention (CDC) is vaccination with the killed virus.

Some common bacterial vaccines are killed microorganisms or extracts of bacterial antigens. The vaccine against pneumococcal pneumonia consists of a mixture of capsular polysaccharides from 10 strains of *Streptococcus pneumoniae.* Of the more than 90 known strains of this microorganism, only these 10 cause the most severe illnesses.

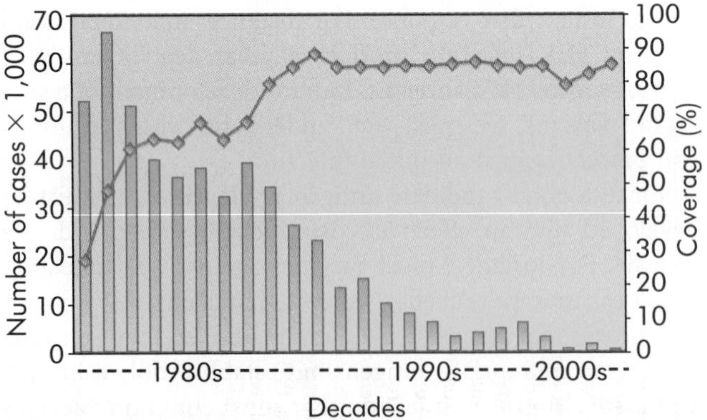

Figure 7-17 ■ The Effect of Vaccination on the Incidence of Polio Worldwide, 1980–2004. The number of global cases of polio has progressively decreased as the extent of immunization (coverage) has increased. The *coverage* is the percent of the world's population that has been reported to the World Health Organization (WHO) by 192 member countries as being immunized. (From World Health Organization: *WHO vaccine-preventable diseases: monitoring system, 2005 global summary,* Geneva, Switzerland, 2006; additional information is available at www.who.int/vaccines-documents.)

However, the capsular vaccine is not very immunogenic in young children. A *conjugated* vaccine is available that contains capsular polysaccharides from 7 strains that are conjugated to carrier proteins in order to increase immunogenicity. A similar vaccine is available for *Haemophilus influenzae* type b (Hib).

Some bacterial pathogens are not invasive, but do colonize mucosal membranes or wounds and release potent toxins that act locally or systemically. These include the bacteria that cause diphtheria, cholera, and tetanus. Vaccination against systemic toxins (e.g., diphtheria, tetanus) has been achieved using **toxoids**—purified toxins that have been chemically detoxified without loss of immunogenicity. Pertussis (whooping cough) vaccine has been changed from a killed whole-cell vaccine to cellular extract (acellular) vaccine that contains the pertussis toxin and additional bacterial antigens. This change has dramatically reduced adverse side effects (fever, local inflammatory reactions, and others).

Additional difficulties associated with vaccination include allergic reactions to the vaccine antigen itself or other components of the preparation. For instance, some viral vaccines are grown in chicken eggs and many elicit a reaction in individuals who are allergic to eggs. The preservative thimerosal has been removed from vaccines. Thimerosal is a mercury-containing compound that has been used as a preservative since the 1930s. Although no cases of mercury toxicity have been reported secondary to vaccination, it was recommended that thimerosal be removed from vaccines. (See Chapter 3.)

A more common problem is compliance of the susceptible population. Depending on the microorganism, a certain percentage of the population should be immunized to protect the total population. If this level of immunization is not achieved, outbreaks of infection can occur. For instance, an effective measles vaccine was made available in 1963 and resulted in a dramatic decrease in the number of measles cases. Many parents became complacent and did not obtain measles vaccination for their preschool children. As a result, a large increase in the number of cases and deaths in 1989 and 1990 occurred, which initiated a reemphasis on complete immunization before children could start school. Even with successful development of a vaccine, however, a certain percentage of the population will be genetically unresponsive to vaccination and therefore will not produce a protective immune response. With most vaccines, the percentage of unresponsive individuals is low, and they will benefit from successful immunization of the rest of the population.

Many vaccines are used in the United States to protect against pathogens. The vaccines recommended in childhood are listed in Table 7-11.

Antimicrobials

Since initiation of the widespread use of penicillin during World War II, antibiotics have had the greatest impact on successful resistance to infection. Antibiotics are natural products of fungi, bacteria, and related microorganisms

TABLE 7-11

Immunization Schedule: Range of Ages for Routine Immunizations

Vaccine	AGE (MONTHS [MO], YEARS [YR])												
	Birth	1 Mo	2 Mo	4 Mo	6 Mo	12 Mo	15 Mo	18 Mo	24 Mo	4 to 6 Yr	11 to 12 Yr	13 to 14 Yr	15 Yr	16 to 18 Yr
HBV	1	2			3									
DTaP			1	2	3		4			5	DT			
Hib			1	2	3	4								
IPV			1	2	3					4				
MMR						1				2				
VAR						1								
MCV4											1			
PCV			1	2	3	4								
FLU					Yearly									
HepA						1		2						
HPV*											1 2 3			
RV*			1	2	3									

Modified from Centers for Disease Control and Prevention: *Recommended childhood and adolescent immunization schedule, United States, 2006*; available at www.cdc.gov/nip/recs/child-schedule.htm.

*Provisional recommendation. *HBV,* hepatitis B virus: causes cirrhosis of the liver and liver cancer; the vaccine is a recombinant viral protein. *DTaP,* combination of (*D*), Diphtheria: a bacterial infection of the throat; produces a toxin that can lead to heart failure or paralysis; the vaccine is an inactivated form of diphtheria toxin (toxoid); (*T*), tetanus: a bacterial infection that produces a toxin that attacks the nervous system and may cause death; the vaccine is an inactivated form of the tetanus toxin (toxoid); and (*aP*), pertussis (acellular pertussis), or whooping cough: a bacterial infection that causes severe coughing in children younger than 5 years; the vaccine is an inactivated toxin and other bacterial antigens. *Hib, Haemophilus influenzae* type b: a bacterial infection that is commonly contracted by children younger than 5 years and infects the blood, joints, bones, and membrane covering the heart; most common cause of serious bacterial meningitis in children; the vaccine is an extracted bacterial antigen conjugated to a protein carrier. *IPV,* polio: polio is a viral infection that causes paralysis and death; the vaccine is an inactivated virus. *MMR,* combination of (MM), measles and mumps viruses that cause fever and rash (measles) or inflammation of the salivary glands (mumps); mumps also may cause meningitis; both vaccines are attenuated live viruses; and (R), rubella or German measles: a viral infection that causes fever and rash; may cause severe birth defects in pregnant women infected in the first trimester. *VAR,* varicella-zoster: a virus that causes chickenpox; vaccine is an attenuated live virus. *MCV4,* meningococcal: *Neisseria meningitides* is a major bacterial cause of meningitis, particularly in young adults; the vaccine contains four different extracted capsular polysaccharides. *PCV,* pneumococcal: *Streptococcus pneumoniae* is a bacteria that causes pneumonia, particularly in the elderly; the childhood vaccine is a protein conjugate with 7 different capsular antigens; the adult vaccine is a mixture of 10 extracted capsular polysaccharides. *FLU,* influenza: a virus that causes severe upper respiratory tract infections; the most common vaccine is an injected inactivated virus. HepA, Hepatitis A virus: a virus that causes liver disease; recommended in selected states and regions; vaccine is an inactivated virus. *HPV,* Human papillomavirus: a virus that causes genital warts and cervical cancer, (*) provisional recommendation for females, vaccine is quadrivalent non-infectious HPV-like particles made from capsid antigen. *RV,* Rotavirus: a virus that causes diarrheal disease, (*) provisional recommendation, vaccine is an attenuated live virus.

and kill or inhibit the growth of other microorganisms. Numerous chemicals or antimicrobials have been identified that either prevent the growth of microorganisms or directly destroy them (Table 7-12). Antibiotics generally act by preventing the function of enzymes or cell structures that are unique to the infecting agent. Because viruses use the enzymes of the host's cells, there has been far less success in developing antiviral antibiotics.

Recent pathogenic adaptations

Microbial pathogens have emerged that have developed mechanisms for circumventing the most modern techniques for destroying or controlling infection.[17,18] These include microorganisms that attack the immune system (e.g., HIV) and those that are resistant to multiple antibiotics (e.g., *Mycobacterium tuberculosis*). HIV is one of the few microorganisms that directly attacks the central processes involved in the development of an immune response and will be discussed later in this chapter.

Many pathogens have mutated and developed resistance to particular antibiotics. Resistance occurs primarily through inactivation of the drug, alteration of the bacterial membrane that prevents the antibiotic from being taken up, alteration of the target molecule, or reduced uptake or active efflux of the antibiotic. These changes result from genetic mutations and can be transmitted directly to neighboring microorganisms. Penicillin resistance, for example, results from the production of an enzyme (β-lactamase) that breaks down the antibiotic. Zidovudine (azidothymidine, AZT) is an antibiotic that suppresses the enzymatic activity of reverse transcriptase, a viral-specific enzyme responsible for the replication of viral RNA and a DNA strand. HIV frequently mutates and produces an AZT-resistant reverse transcriptase.

A rapid emergence of multiple antibiotic–resistant bacteria has been observed. These microorganisms are resistant to almost all currently available antibiotics. For example, *Streptococcus pneumoniae*, which causes pneumonia, meningitis, and acute otitis media (ear infections), was once routinely susceptible to penicillin. Since the 1980s, however, the incidence of penicillin-resistant microorganisms has risen to 30% or more in some populations. Many of these are resistant also to multiple antibiotics. In some areas, more than 20% of tuberculosis cases are caused by multiple antibiotic–resistant *M. tuberculosis*. Also, the incidence of drug-resistant gonorrhea, malaria, pneumococcal disease, salmonellosis, shigellosis, and staphylococcal infections has increased dramatically.

Why have multiple antibiotic–resistant microorganisms appeared? Overuse of antibiotics can lead to the destruction of the normal flora, allowing the selective overgrowth of antibiotic-resistant strains or pathogens that had previously been kept under control. For example, after treatment with the antibiotic clindamycin, the normal intestinal flora can become compromised, allowing the overgrowth of *Clostridium difficile* and the development of pseudomembranous colitis. Also, individuals commonly do not comply with the instructions of health care providers concerning the necessity of completing the therapeutic regimen with antibiotics. This practice allows the selective resurgence of microorganisms that are relatively resistant to the antibiotic.

✔ QUICK CHECK 7-3

1. How do antigenic changes in viral pathogens promote disease?
2. What are three mechanisms pathogens use to block the immune system?
3. What is the difference between endotoxin and exotoxin?

DEFICIENCIES IN IMMUNITY

An **immune deficiency** is the failure of the immune or inflammatory response to function normally, resulting in increased susceptibility to infections. **Primary (congenital) immune deficiency** is caused by a genetic defect, whereas **secondary (acquired) immune deficiency** is caused by another condition, such as cancer, infection, or normal physiologic changes, such as aging. Acquired forms of immune deficiency are far more common than the congenital forms.

TABLE 7-12
Chemicals or Antimicrobials Identified That Prevent Growth of or Destroy Microorganisms

Mechanism of Action	Agent
Inhibits synthesis of cell wall	Penicillins, cephalosporins, monobactams, carbapenems, vancomycin, bacitracin, cycloserine, fosfomycin
Damages cytoplasmic membrane	Polymyxins, polyene antifungals, imidazoles
Alters metabolism of nucleic acid	Quinolones, rifampin, nitrofurans, nitroimidazoles
Inhibits protein synthesis	Aminoglycosides, tetracyclines, chloramphenicol, macrolides, clindamycin, spectinomycin, sulfonamides
Alters energy metabolism	Trimethoprim, dapsone, isoniazid

Modified from Ellner PD, Neu HCP: *Understanding infectious disease,* St Louis, 1992, Mosby.

Initial Clinical Presentation

The clinical hallmark of immune deficiency is a tendency to develop unusual or recurrent, severe infections.[19,20] Preschool and school-age children normally may have 6 to 12 infections per year, and adults may have 2 to 4 infections per year. Most of these are not severe and are limited to viral infections of the upper respiratory tract, recurrent streptococcal pharyngitis, or mild otitis media (ear infections).

Potential immune deficiencies should be considered if the individual has had severe, documented bouts of pneumonia, otitis media, sinusitis (sinus infection), bronchitis, septicemia (blood infection), or meningitis or infections with opportunistic microorganisms that normally are not pathogenic (e.g., *Pneumocystis carinii*). Infections are generally recurrent with only short intervals of relative health, and multiple simultaneous infections are common. Individuals with immune deficiencies often have eight or more ear infections, two or more serious sinus infections, and two or more pneumonias, recurrent abscesses, or persistent fungal infections (particularly thrush) within a year. Recurrent internal infections, such as meningitis, osteomyelitis, or sepsis, are common. Prolonged antibiotic use is commonly ineffective by oral or injected routes and may necessitate intravenous administration. A familial history of immune deficiency may be found in some types of primary deficiency.

The type of recurrent infections may indicate the type of immune defect. Deficiencies in T cell immune responses are suggested when recurrent infections are caused by certain viruses (e.g., varicella, vaccinia, herpes, cytomegalovirus), fungi and yeasts (e.g., *Candida, Histoplasma*), or certain atypical microorganisms (e.g., *P. carinii*). B cell deficiencies and phagocyte deficiencies, however, are suggested if the individual has documented, recurrent infections with microorganisms that require opsonization (e.g., encapsulated bacteria) or viruses against which humoral immunity is normally effective (e.g., rubella). Some complement deficiencies resemble defects in antibody or phagocyte function, but others are commonly associated with disseminated infections with bacteria of the genus *Neisseria* (*Neisseria meningitides* and *Neisseria gonorrhoeae*).

Primary (Congenital) Immune Deficiencies

Most primary immune deficiencies are the result of a single gene defect (Table 7-13).[21] Generally, the mutations are sporadic and not inherited: a family history exists in only about 25% of individuals. The sporadic mutations occur before birth, but the onset of symptoms may be early or later, depending on the particular syndrome. In some instances, symptoms of immune deficiency appear within the first 2 years of life. Other immune deficiencies are progressive, with the onset of symptoms appearing in the second or third decade of life.

Many immune deficiencies also are associated with other characteristic defects, some of which appear to be unrelated to the immune system yet may be life threatening by themselves. Examples are given in the following discussion. These associated symptoms can be useful diagnostically and can clarify the pathophysiology of the disease.

Individually, primary immune deficiencies are rare. For instance, only 30 to 50 new cases of severe combined immune deficiency (SCID) are diagnosed in the United States yearly. However, more than 70 different deficiencies have been identified. Together, primary immune deficiencies are more common than cystic fibrosis, hemophilia, childhood leukemia, or many other well-know diseases. The distribution of male and female is about even, although some specific diseases have a male or female predominance. The three most commonly diagnosed deficiencies are common variable immune deficiency (34%), selective IgA deficiency (24%), and IgG subclass deficiency (17%).

Primary immune deficiencies are classified into five groups, based on which principal component of the immune or inflammatory systems is defective: defects of B lymphocytes, T lymphocytes, both B and T lymphocytes (combined), phagocytes, or complement.

B lymphocyte deficiencies

B lymphocyte deficiencies result from defects in B cell immune responses.[22] Because T cell immunity rarely depends on competent B cell responses, T cell immune responses are not affected in pure B lymphocyte deficiencies. The results are lower levels of circulating immunoglobulins **(hypogammaglobulinemia)** or occasionally totally or nearly absent immunoglobulins **(agammaglobulinemia).**

Some defects may involve a particular class of antibody, such as **selective IgA deficiency.** This occurs in 1 in 700 to 1 in 400 individuals. Individuals with this deficiency produce other classes of immunoglobulins but not IgA. This suggests a failure to class-switch to IgA and mature into IgA-producing plasma cells. Many individuals are asymptomatic, although others have a history of severe, recurring sinus, lung, and gastrointestinal infections. Individuals with IgA deficiency often have chronic intestinal candidiasis (infection with *C. albicans*). (The secretory, or mucosal, immune system is described in Chapter 6.) Complications of IgA deficiency include severe atopic disease and autoimmune diseases. Studies of these individuals show that secretory IgA normally may prevent the uptake of allergens from the environment. Therefore, IgA deficiency may lead to increased allergen uptake and a more intense challenge to the immune system because of prolonged exposure to environmental antigens.

Stem cells mature in the central or primary lymphoid organs (thymus and bursal-equivalent tissue). **Bruton agammaglobulinemia** is caused by blocked development of mature B cells in bursal-equivalent tissue. There are few or no circulating B cells, although T cell number and function are normal, resulting in repeated infections, such as otitis media, sore throat, and conjunctivitis, and more serious conditions, such as septicemia.

T lymphocyte deficiencies

T lymphocyte deficiencies are defects in the development and function of T lymphocytes.[22] Because helper T cells

TABLE 7-13

Examples of Primary Immune Deficiencies

Classification	Example	Immune Deficiency	Outcome
B LYMPHOCYTE DEFICIENCIES			
Defective development of B cells in central lymphoid organ (bone marrow)	Bruton agammaglobulinemia	Lack of B cells, little or no antibody production	Recurrent, life-threatening bacterial infections
Defect in class switch	Selective IgA deficiency	Little or no production of IgA, with normal production of other classes of antibody	Mild infections of gastrointestinal and respiratory tracts
T LYMPHOCYTE DEFICIENCIES			
Defective development of T cells in central lymphoid organ (thymus)	DiGeorge syndrome	Lack of T cells	Recurrent, life-threatening fungal and viral infections
Defect in development of cellular immunity against a specific antigen	Chronic mucocutaneous candidiasis	Lack of T cell response to *Candida*	Recurrent and disseminated infections with the fungus *Candida albicans*
COMBINED IMMUNE DEFICIENCIES			
Defective development of both B and T cells	Severe combined immunodeficiencies (SCID)	Lack of both T and B cells, little or no antibody production or cellular immunity	Recurrent, life-threatening infections with a variety of microorganisms
Defects in cooperation among B cells, T cells, and antigen-presenting cells	Bare lymphocyte syndrome	No antigen presentation because of lack of MHC class I or MHC class II molecules on the cell surface	Recurrent, life-threatening infections with a variety of microorganisms
A large variety of defects that affect the function of B or T cells	Wiskott-Aldrich syndrome	Cytoskeletal defect resulting in selective decrease in IgM production	Recurrent infections with select groups of microorganisms; in this example bacteria with polysaccharide capsules
COMPLEMENT DEFICIENCIES			
Defective production of one early component of the complement system	C3 deficiency	Little or no C3 produced	Recurrent, life-threatening bacterial infections
Defective production of a component of the membrane attack complex	C6 deficiency	Little or no C6 produced	Recurrent disseminated infections with *Neisseria gonorrhoeae* or *N. meningitidis*
PHAGOCYTE DEFICIENCIES			
Defects in production of neutrophils	Severe congenital neutropenia	Lack of neutrophils	Recurrent, life-threatening bacterial infections
Defects in bacterial killing	Chronic granulomatous disease	Lack of production of oxygen products (e.g., hydrogen peroxide)	Recurrent infections with bacteria that are sensitive to killing by oxygen-dependent mechanisms

are obligatory in the development of many B lymphocyte responses, antibody production is often diminished, although the B cells are fully capable of producing an adequate antibody response. Immunodeficiency of T cell function contributes to failure to thrive, oral infections (e.g.,candidiasis), chronic diarrhea, pneumonia, and skin rashes.

Some immune deficiencies are characterized by a defect in the capacity to produce an immune response against a particular antigen. In **chronic mucocutaneous candidiasis,** the T lymphocytes cannot respond to a specific infectious agent, *C. albicans.* These individuals usually have mild to extremely severe recurrent *Candida* infections involving the mucous membranes and skin.

DiGeorge syndrome (congenital thymic aplasia or hypoplasia and diminished parathyroid gland development) is caused by the lack or partial lack of the thymus, resulting in greatly decreased T cell numbers and function. The cause is defective development of several tissues originating from the third and fourth pharyngeal pouches during embryo development. Lack of the parathyroid gland causes inability to regulate calcium. Low blood calcium levels cause the development of tetany or involuntary rigid muscular contraction. DiGeorge syndrome is frequently associated with abnormal facial development, including low set ears, fish-shaped mouth, and other altered features (Figure 7-18).

Combined deficiencies

Combined deficiencies result from defects that directly affect the development of both T and B lymphocytes. Some combined deficiencies result in major defects in both the

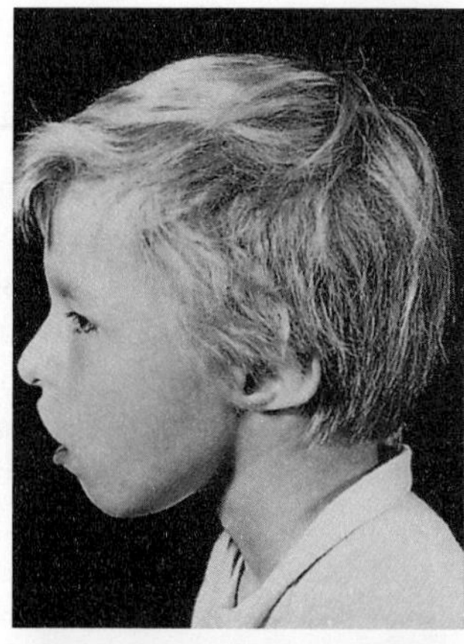

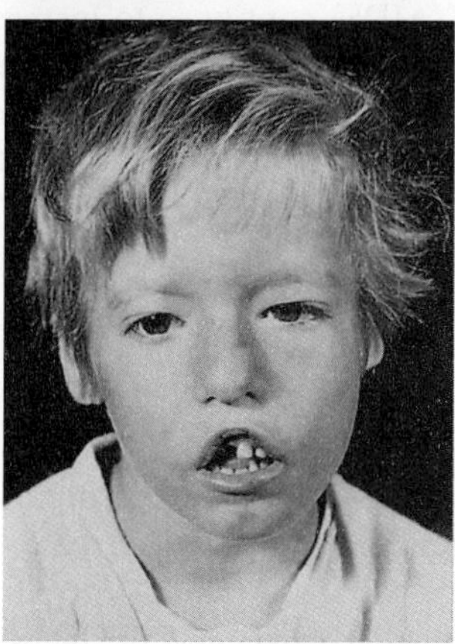

Figure 7-18 ■ **Facial Anomalies Associated With DiGeorge Syndrome.** Note the wide-set eyes, low-set ears, and shortened structure of the upper lip. (From Male D, et al: *Immunology,* ed 7, St Louis, 2006, Mosby.)

T and B cell immune responses, whereas others are "partial" and more adversely affect T cells than B cells. The most severe are called **severe combined immunodeficiencies (SCID).** Most individuals with SCID have few detectable lymphocytes in the circulation and secondary lymphoid organs (spleen, lymph nodes). The thymus usually is underdeveloped because of the absence of T cells. Immunoglobulin levels, especially IgM and IgA, are absent or greatly reduced. Several forms of SCID are caused by autosomal recessive enzymatic defects that result in the accumulation of toxic metabolites to which rapidly dividing cells, such as lymphocytes, are especially sensitive. Deficiency of **adenosine deaminase (ADA deficiency)** results in the accumulation of toxic purines.

Even if nearly adequate numbers of B and T cells are produced, their cooperation may be defective. The **bare lymphocyte syndrome** is an immune deficiency characterized by an inability of lymphocytes and macrophages to produce MHC class I or class II molecules. Without MHC molecules, antigen presentation and intercellular cooperation cannot occur effectively. Children with this deficiency develop serious, life-threatening infections and usually die before the age of 5 years.

Some combined immune deficiencies result in depressed development of a small portion of the immune system. For instance, an individual can be unable to produce a certain class of antibody, as in **Wiskott-Aldrich syndrome** (an X-linked recessive disorder). Here IgM antibody production is greatly depressed, and therefore antibody responses against antigens that elicit primarily an IgM response, such as polysaccharide antigens from bacterial cell walls (e.g., of *P. aeruginosa, S. pneumoniae, Haemophilus influenzae,* and other microorganisms with polysaccharide outer capsules), are deficient. In addition, there are defects in platelets presumably because of the absence of certain glycoproteins. Clinical manifestations include bleeding because of decreases in circulating platelets, eczema, and recurrent infections (e.g., otitis media, pneumonia, herpes simplex, cytomegalovirus).

Complement deficiencies

Many **complement deficiencies** have been described. **C3 deficiency** is the most severe defect.[23] C3 unites all pathways of complement activation, and complement component C3b is a major opsonin. Persons with C3 deficiency are at risk for recurrent life-threatening infections with encapsulated bacteria (e.g., *Hemophilus influenzae* and *Streptococcus pneumoniaea*) at an early age. Deficiencies of terminal components of the complement cascade (C5, C6, C7, C8, or C9 deficiencies) are associated with increased infections with only one group of bacteria; those of the genus *Neisseria (Neisseria meningitides* or *N. gonorrhoeae). Neisseria* usually cause localized infections (meningitis or gonorrhea), but those with terminal pathway defects have more than an 8000-fold increased risk for systemic infections with atypical strains of these microorganisms.

Phagocytic deficiencies

Phagocytic deficiencies usually result in recurrent infections with the same group of microorganisms (encapsulated bacteria) associated with antibody and complement deficiencies. A variety of defects in killing of microorganisms have been described. **Chronic granulomatous disease (CGD)** is a severe defect in the myeloperoxidase-hydrogen peroxide system. A major means of bacterial killing uses the enzyme myeloperoxidase, halides (e.g., chloride ion), and hydrogen peroxide (H_2O_2). As a result of phagocytosis, neutrophils and other phagocytes switch much of their glucose metabolism to the hexose-monophosphate shunt. A by-product of this pathway is the conversion of molecular oxygen by nicotinamide adenine dinucleotide phosphate (NADPH) oxidase into highly reactive oxygen derivatives, including hydrogen peroxide. Mutations in NADPH oxidase result in deficient production of hydrogen peroxide and other oxygen products. Thus, individuals have adequate myeloperoxidase and halide but lack the necessary hydrogen peroxide. Individuals with CGD have recurrent severe pneumonias, tumor-like granulomas in lungs, skin, and bones, and other infections with some normal, relatively innocuous microorganisms, such as *Staphylococcus aureus, Serratia marcescens, Aspergillus* spp., and others.

Secondary (Acquired) Immune Deficiencies

Secondary, or acquired, immune and inflammatory deficiencies are far more common than primary deficiencies. These deficiencies are not related to genetic defects but are complications of other physiologic or pathophysiologic conditions. Some conditions that are known to be associated with acquired deficiencies include the following:

Normal physiologic conditions
- Pregnancy
- Infancy
- Aging

Psychologic stress
- Emotional trauma
- Eating disorders

Dietary insufficiencies
- Malnutrition caused by insufficient intake of large categories of nutrients, such as protein or calories
- Insufficient intake of specific nutrients, such as vitamins, iron, or zinc
- Infections
- Congenital infections, such as rubella, cytomegalovirus, hepatitis B
- Acquired infections, such as AIDS

Malignancies
- Malignancies of lymphoid tissues, such as Hodgkin disease, acute or chronic leukemia, or myeloma
- Malignancies of nonlymphoid tissues, such as sarcomas and carcinomas

Physical trauma
- Burns

Medical treatments
- Stress caused by surgery
- Anesthesia
- Immunosuppressive treatment with corticosteroids or antilymphocyte antibodies
- Splenectomy
- Cancer treatment with cytotoxic drugs or ionizing radiation

Other diseases or genetic syndromes
- Diabetes
- Alcoholic cirrhosis
- Sickle cell disease
- SLE
- Chromosome abnormalities, such as Down syndrome

Although secondary deficiencies are common, many are not clinically relevant. In many cases, the degree of the immune deficiency is relatively minor and without any apparent increased susceptibility to infection. Alternatively, the immune system may be substantially suppressed, but only for a short duration, thus minimizing the incidence of clinically relevant infections. Some secondary immune deficiencies, however, are extremely severe and may result in recurrent life-threatening infections.

Acquired immunodeficiency syndrome (AIDS)

The human immune deficiency virus (HIV) infects and destroys the helper T cell, which is necessary for the development of both plasma cells and cytotoxic T cells. Therefore, HIV suppresses the immune response against itself and secondarily creates a generalized immune deficiency by suppressing the development of immune responses against other pathogens and opportunistic microorganisms, leading to the development of **acquired immunodeficiency syndrome (AIDS).**

Despite major efforts by health care agencies around the world, the number of cases and deaths from HIV infection and AIDS (HIV/AIDS) continues to increase. The number of people living with HIV/AIDS worldwide is estimated at 40 million, of which 2.5 million are under the age of 15. The rate of spread of the disease is still out of control: the number of people newly infected with HIV is estimated at 5 million yearly, with 700,000 being under the age of 15. Deaths from AIDS are about 3 million yearly. Since the end of 1998, more than 13 million people have died of HIV/AIDS.

The majority of cases are still in sub-Saharan Africa, but the epidemic is worldwide, and the number of new cases is increasing rapidly, particularly in Asia. As an example of the prevalence of HIV/AIDS, in the African country of Zambia it is estimated that 30% of the women age 30 to 34 years are HIV infected. In South Africa, about 35% of the pregnant women age 25 to 29 are HIV infected.

In the United States, the spread of HIV/AIDS remains somewhat stable.[24] The Centers for Disease Control and Prevention (CDC) estimates that since the year 2000 the rate of new cases of HIV/AIDS has remained at about 31,000 per year. The number of deaths related to HIV/AIDS continues at about 18,000 per year (Figure 7-19). The total number of HIV/AIDS-related deaths in the United States is in excess of 550,000, and more than 400,000 individuals are currently living with AIDS.

Before the implementation of massive public health campaigns and the use of antiviral drugs in the United States, the progression from HIV infection to AIDS and death was unrelenting. In 1995, AIDS became the number one killer of individuals between the ages of 25 and 44 years of age. With the advent of effective therapy in the mid-1990s, HIV infection has become a chronic disease in the United States, with many fewer deaths.

EPIDEMIOLOGY HIV is a blood-borne pathogen with the typical routes of transmission: blood or blood products, intravenous drug abuse, both heterosexual and homosexual activity, and maternal-child transmission before or during birth (Figure 7-20). Although the disease first gained attention in the United States as being related to sexual transmission between males, the most common route worldwide is through heterosexual activity. Worldwide, women make up more than half of those living with HIV/AIDS. In the United States, as in the rest of the world,

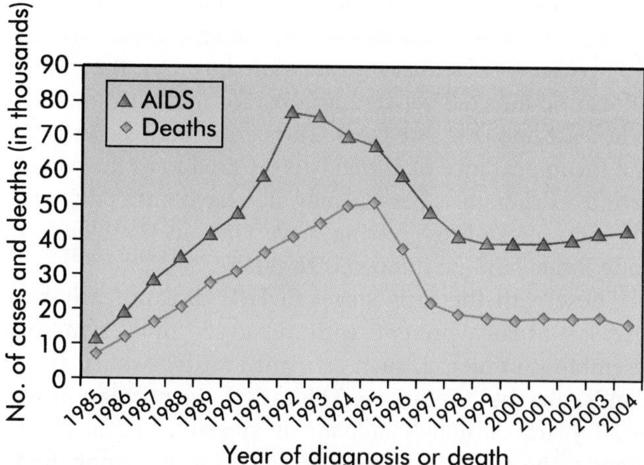

Figure 7-19 ■ Estimated Incidence of AIDS and Deaths Among Adults and Adolescents With AIDS in the United States (1985–2004). The incidence of AIDS and deaths related to AIDS rose almost linearly until about 1994. The introduction of effective antiviral treatments in the mid-1990s slowed the progression of the disease from HIV infection to AIDS and has maintained the number of AIDS-related deaths at about 17,000 per year. (From Centers for Disease Control website, 2005; available at www.cdc.gov/hiv/topics/surveillance/resources/slides/index.htm.)

the predominant means of transmission to women is through heterosexual contact, and the incidence of HIV/AIDS is increasing faster in women than men, particularly in the adolescent age groups. Hundreds of thousands of cases of HIV/AIDS have been reported in children who contracted the virus from their mothers across the placenta, through contact with infected blood during delivery, or through the milk during breastfeeding.

PATHOGENESIS HIV is a member of a family of viruses called retroviruses, which carry genetic information in the form of RNA rather than DNA (Figure 7-21). Retroviruses use a viral enzyme, **reverse transcriptase,** to convert RNA into double-stranded DNA. Using a second viral enzyme, an **integrase,** the new DNA is inserted into the infected cell's genetic material, where it may remain dormant. If the cell is activated, translation of the viral information may be initiated, resulting in the formation of new virions, lysis and death of the infected cell, and shedding of infectious HIV particles. If, however, the cell remains relatively dormant, the viral genetic material may remain latent for years and is probably present for the life of the individual.

The primary surface receptor on HIV is the envelope protein gp120, which binds to the molecule CD4 on the surface of helper T cells. Several other necessary coreceptors have been identified on target cells. Thus, the major immunologic finding in AIDS is the striking decrease in the number of CD4+ Th cells (Figure 7-22). Individuals who are not HIV-infected typically have 800 to 1000 CD4+ cells per cubic millimeter of blood, with a range from 600/mm^3 to 1200/mm^3.

HEALTH ALERT

Risk of HIV Transmission Associated With Sexual Practices

High Risk (in descending order of risk)

- Receptive anal intercourse with ejaculation (no condom)
- Receptive vaginal intercourse with ejaculation (no condom)
- Insertive anal intercourse (no condom)
- Insertive vaginal intercourse (no condom)
- Receptive anal intercourse with withdrawal before ejaculation
- Insertive anal intercourse with withdrawal before ejaculation
- Receptive vaginal intercourse (with spermicidal foam but no condom)
- Insertive vaginal intercourse (with spermicidal foam but no condom)
- Receptive anal or vaginal intercourse (with a condom)*
- Insertive anal or vaginal intercourse (with a condom)*

Some Risk (in descending order of risk)

- Oral sex with men with ejaculation
- Oral sex with women
- Oral sex with men with preejaculation fluid (precum)
- Oral sex with men, no ejaculation or precum
- Oral sex with men (with a condom)

Some Risk (depending on situation, intactness of mucous membranes, etc.)

- Mutual masturbation with external or internal touching
- Sharing sex toys
- Anal or vaginal fisting

No Risk

- Masturbating with another person without touching one another
- Hugging/massage/dry kissing
- Frottage (rubbing genitals while remaining clothed)
- Masturbating alone
- Abstinence

Unresolved Issues

- The role of precum in transmission
- The protection offered by covering female genitals with a dental dam during oral sex on the women
- The risk of transmission from wet kissing

Data from Grimes DE, Grimes RM: *HIV infection: progression and management. Mosby's clinical nursing series,* St Louis, 1994, Mosby; modified from Schram NR: Refusing safer sex, *Focus* 5 (7):3–4, 1990.

*Risk lower if no ejaculation or if spermicidal foam is used.

CLINICAL MANIFESTATIONS Depletion of CD4+ cells has a profound effect on the immune system, causing a severely diminished response to a wide array of infectious pathogens and malignant tumors (Box 7-2). At the time of diagnosis, the individual may present with one of several different conditions: serologically negative (no detectable antibody), serologically positive (positive for antibody against HIV) but asymptomatic, early stages of HIV disease, or AIDS (Figure 7-23).

The presence of circulating antibody against the HIV indicates infection by the virus, although many of these

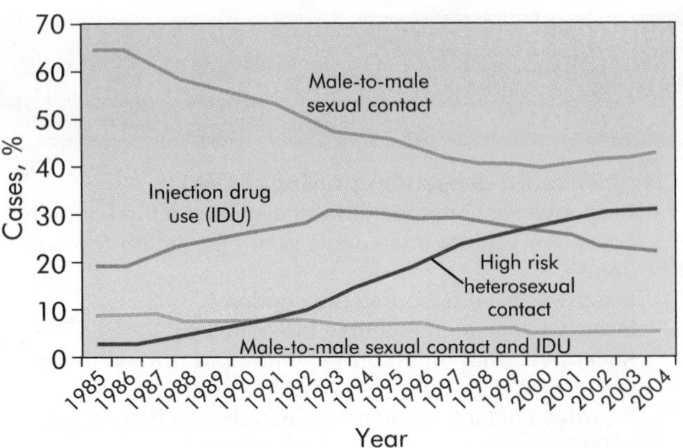

Figure 7-20 ■ Proportion of AIDS Cases Among Adults and Adolescents, by Exposure Category and Year of Diagnosis, in the United States (1985–2004). Worldwide, AIDS is primarily spread by heterosexual transmission. In the United States, the predominant route was by male-to-male sexual contact. The trend, however, is toward increasing heterosexual transmission. Transmission by injected drug use has remained relatively stable, as has the number of cases where both male-to-male sexual activity and injected drug use risk factors occur in the same individual. (Redrawn from Centers for Disease Control website, 2005; available at www.cdc.gov/hiv/topics/surveillance/resources/slides/index.htm.)

individuals are asymptomatic. Antibody appears rather rapidly after infection through blood products, usually within 4 to 7 weeks. After sexual transmission, however, the individual can be infected yet seronegative for 6 to 14 months or, in at least one case, for years. The period between infection and the appearance of antibody is referred to as the window period. Although a person may not have antibody, he or she may have virus growing, have virus in the blood and body fluids, and be infectious to others.

Those with the early stages of HIV disease (early-stage disease) usually present with relatively mild symptoms resembling influenza, such as night sweats, swollen lymph glands, diarrhea, or fatigue. The early stage may last as long as 10 years. Although individuals appear to be in clinical latency, the virus is actively proliferating in lymph nodes (Figure 7-24).

The currently accepted definition of AIDS relies on both laboratory tests and clinical symptoms. The most common laboratory test is for antibodies against HIV. If the individual is seropositive, the diagnosis of AIDS is made in association with various clinical symptoms (see Box 7-2) (Figure 7-25). The symptoms include atypical or opportunistic infections and cancers, as well as indications of

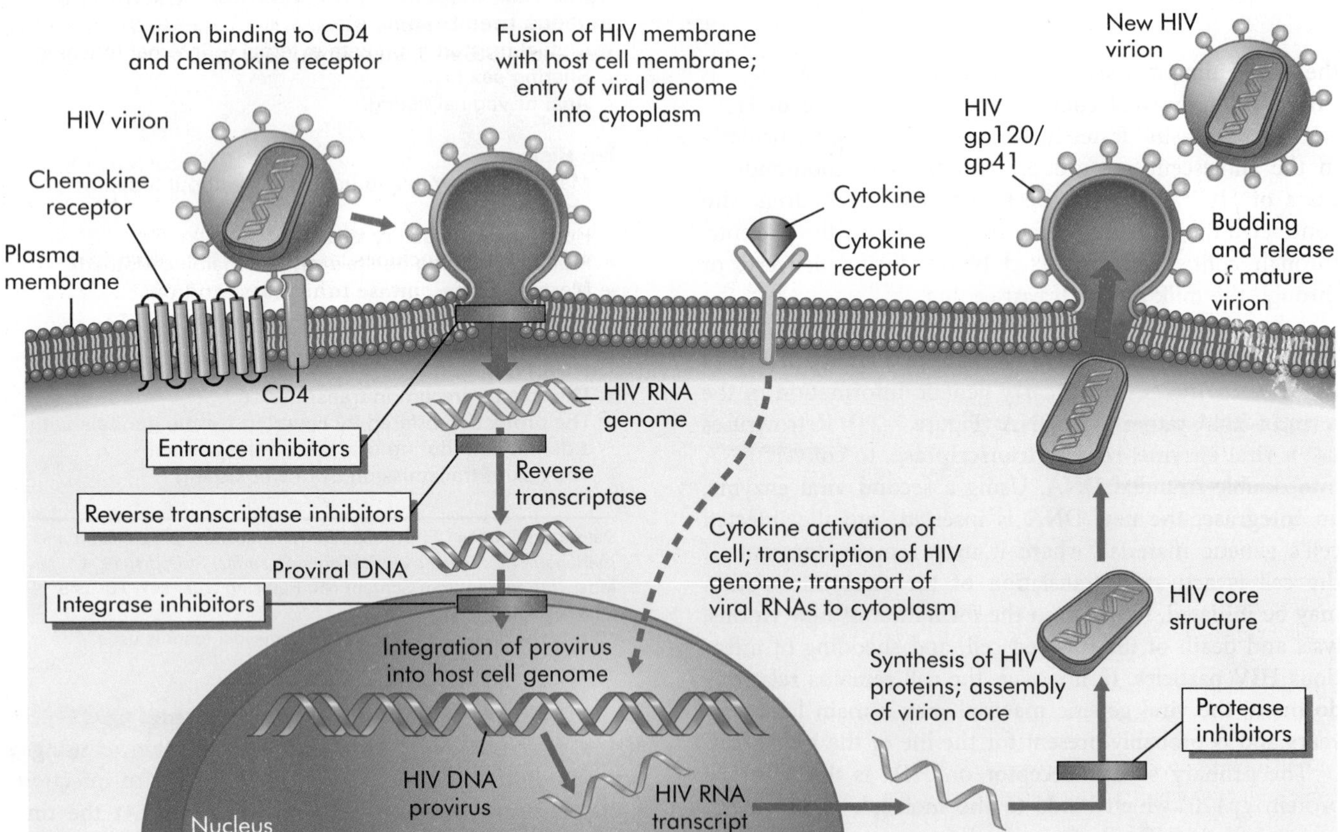

Figure 7-21 ■ Life Cycle and Possible Sites of Therapeutic Intervention of Human Immunodeficiency Virus (HIV). The HIV virion consists of a core of two identical strands of viral RNA encoated in a protein structure with viral proteins gp41 and gp120 on its surface (envelope). HIV infection begins when a virion binds to CD4 and chemokine coreceptors on a susceptible cell and follows the process described here. The provirus may remain latent in the cell's DNA until it is activated (e.g., by cytokines). The HIV life cycle is susceptible to blockage at several sites (see the text for further information), including entrance inhibitors, reverse transcriptase inhibitors, integrase inhibitors, and protease inhibitors. (Modified from Kumar V, Abbas A, Fausto N: *Robbins and Cotran pathologic basis of disease,* ed 7, Philadelphia, 2005, Saunders.)

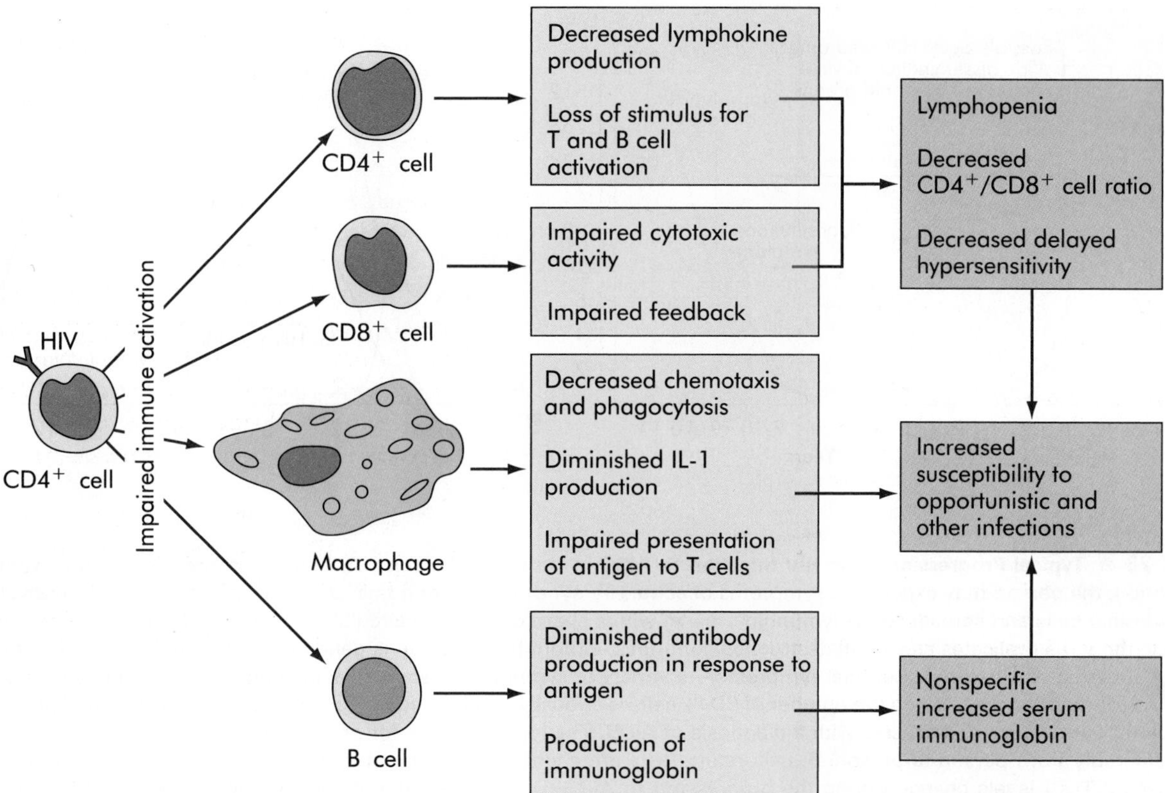

Figure 7-22 ■ **Summary of Human Immunodeficiency Virus (HIV) Infection on the Immune System.** (Redrawn from Morse SA, Ballard RC, Holmes KK, et al, editors: *Atlas of sexually transmitted diseases and AIDS,* ed 3, Edinburgh, 2003, Mosby.)

debilitating chronic disease (e.g., wasting syndrome, recurrent fevers). Most commonly, new cases of AIDS are diagnosed initially by decreased CD4+ T cell numbers. The average time from infection to development of AIDS has been estimated at just over 10 years. Some estimates are that approximately 99% of untreated HIV-infected individuals would eventually progress to AIDS.

TREATMENT AND PREVENTION The current regimen for treatment of HIV infection is a combination of drugs, termed **highly active antiretroviral therapy (HAART).** The combination includes inhibitors of reverse transcriptase **(reverse transcriptase inhibitors)** and of the viral protease **(protease inhibitors)** (see Figure 7-21). The clinical benefits of HAART are profound and durable. Death from

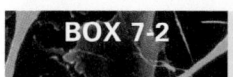

BOX 7-2 AIDS-Defining Opportunistic Infections and Neoplasms Found in Individuals With HIV Infection

Infections

Protozoal and Helminthic Infections
Cryptosporidiosis or isosporiasis (enteritis)
Pneumocystosis (pneumonia or disseminated infection)
Toxoplasmosis (pneumonia or CNS infection)

Fungal Infections
Candidiasis (esophageal, tracheal, or pulmonary)
Cryptococcosis (CNS infection)
Coccidioidomycosis (disseminated)
Histoplasmosis (disseminated)

Bacterial Infections
Mycobacteriosis (atypical, e.g., *M. avium-intracellulare,* disseminated or extrapulmonary; *M. tuberculosis,* pulmonary or extrapulmonary)
Nocardiosis (pneumonia, meningitis, disseminated)
Salmonella infections (disseminated)

Viral Infections
Cytomegalovirus (pulmonary, intestinal, retinitis, or CNS infections)
Herpes simplex virus (localized or disseminated)
Varicella-zoster virus (localized or disseminated)
Progressive multifocal (leukoencephalopathy)

Neoplasms

Kaposi sarcoma
B cell non-Hodgkin lymphomas
Primary lymphoma of the brain
Invasive cancer of the uterine cervix

From Kumar V, Abbas A, Fausto N: *Robbins and Cotran pathologic basis of disease,* ed 7, Philadelphia, 2005, Saunders.
CNS, Central nervous system.

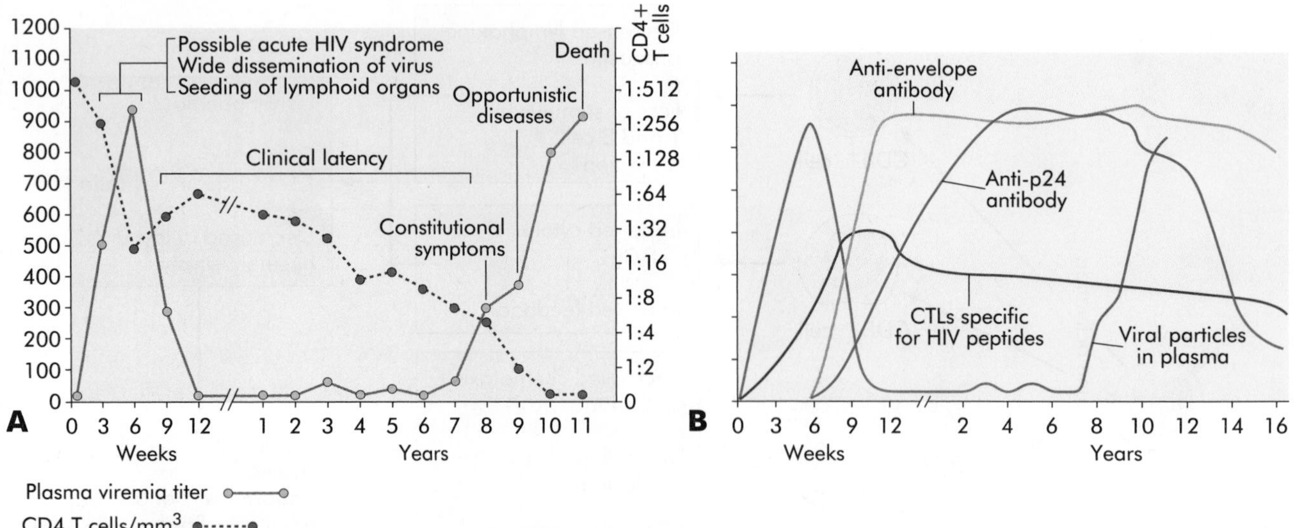

Figure 7-23 ■ **Typical Progression From HIV Infection to AIDS in Untreated Persons. A,** Clinical progression begins within weeks after infection; the person may experience symptoms of acute HIV syndrome. During this early period, the virus progressively infects T cells and other cells and spreads to the lymphoid organs, with a sharp decrease in circulating CD4+ T cells. During a period of clinical latency, the virus replicates and T cell destruction continues, although the person is generally asymptomatic. The individual may develop HIV-related disease (constitutional symptoms)—a variety of symptoms of acute viral infection that do not involve opportunistic infections or malignancies. When the number of CD4+ cells is critically suppressed, the individual becomes susceptible to a variety of opportunistic infections and cancers with a diagnosis of AIDS. The length of time for progression from HIV infection to AIDS may vary considerably from person to person. **B,** Laboratory tests are changing throughout infection. Antibody and Tc cell (cytotoxic T lymphocytes [CTLs]) levels change during the progression to AIDS. During the initial phase, antibodies against HIV-1 are not yet detectable (window period), but viral products, including proteins and RNA, and infectious virus, may be detectable in the blood a few weeks after infection. Most antibodies against HIV are not detectable in the early phase. During the latent phase of infection, antibody levels against p24 and other viral proteins, as well as HIV-specific CTLs, increase, then remain constant until the development of AIDS. (**A** redrawn from Fauci AS, Lane HC: Human immunodeficiency virus disease: AIDS and related conditions. In Fauci AS et al, editors: *Harrison's principles of internal medicine,* ed 14, New York, 1997, McGraw-Hill. **B** from Kumar V, Abbas A, Fausto N: *Robbins and Cotran pathologic basis of disease,* ed 7, Philadelphia, 2005, Saunders.)

AIDS-related diseases has been reduced significantly since the introduction of HAART. However, resistant variants to these drugs have been identified. Drug therapy for AIDS is difficult because, like most retroviruses, the AIDS virus incorporates into the genetic material of the host and may never be removed by antimicrobial therapy. Therefore, drug administration to control the virus may have to continue for the lifetime of the individual. Additionally, HIV may persist in regions where the antiviral drugs are not as effective, such as the CNS. Inhibitors of the initial viral entrance into the target cell **(entrance inhibitors)** and inhibitors of the viral integrase **(integrase inhibitors)** have undergone clinical trials and are being added to the combination.

Vaccine development is probably the most effective means of preventing HIV infection and may be useful in treating preexisting infection.[25] Most of the common viral vaccines (e.g., rubella, mumps, influenza) induce protective antibodies that block the initial infection. Only one vaccine (rabies) is used after the infection has occurred. That approach is successful because the rabies virus proliferates and spreads very slowly. Whether an HIV vaccine would either successfully prevent or treat HIV infection is questionable for several reasons. First, the AIDS virus is genetically and antigenically variable, like the influenza virus, so that a vaccine created against one variant may not provide protection against another variant. Second, although individuals with AIDS have high levels of circulating antibodies against the virus, these antibodies do not appear to be protective. Therefore, even if a circulating antibody response can be induced by vaccination, that response might not be effective. A vaccine may have to induce both circulating and secretory (to prevent initial infection of the mucosal T cell) antibody and Tc cells.

Evaluation and Care of Those With Immune Deficiency

Routine care of individuals with primary or secondary immune deficiencies must be tempered with the knowledge that the immune system may be totally ineffective. It may be unsafe to administer conventional immunizing agents or blood products to many of these individuals because of the risk that the immunizing agent will cause an uncontrolled infection. Uncontrolled infection is a problem when attenuated vaccines that contain live but weakened microorganisms are used (e.g., live polio vaccine, vaccines against measles, mumps, and rubella).

The most common presenting symptom of immune deficiencies is recurrent severe infections. Significant information on the specific immune deficiency can be obtained by noting certain characteristics of the individual, including the presence of any associated anomalies, age, gender, the types of infections (bacterial, viral, or fungal, and the specific microorganisms involved), family history, and risk factors associated with secondary immune deficiencies.[26]

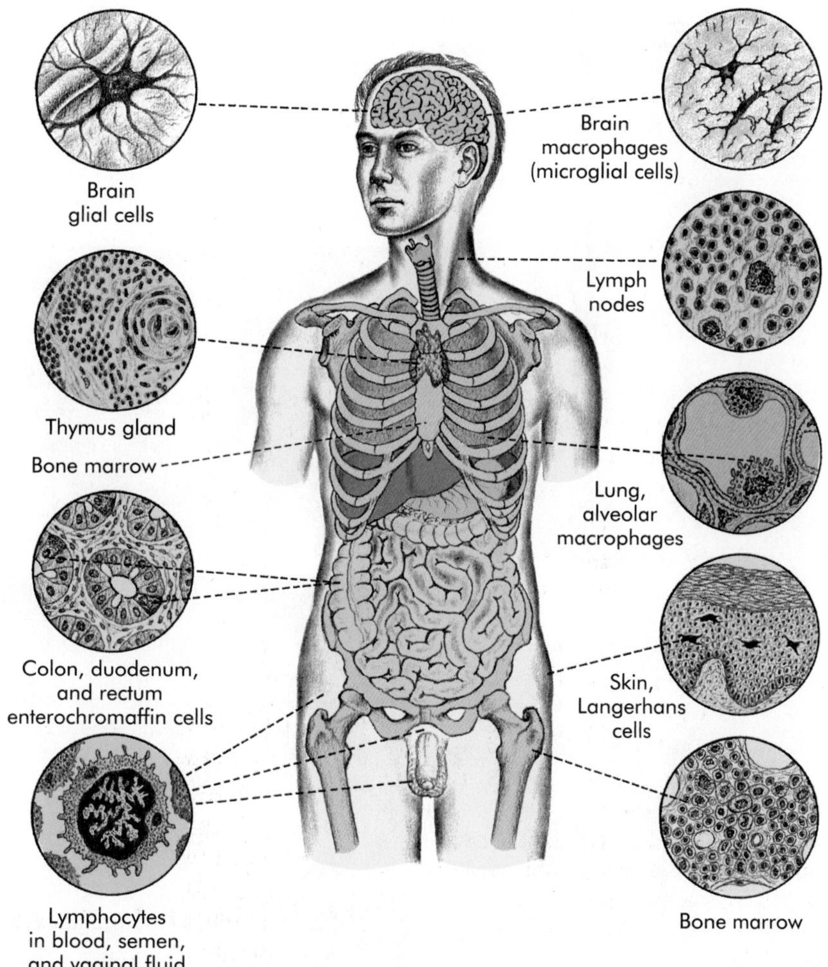

Figure 7-24 ■ **Distribution of Tissues That Can Be Infected by HIV.** Infection is closely linked to the presence of CD4 receptors or chemokine coreceptors on host tissue, particularly T cells and macrophages. (Modified from Weber JN, Weiss RA: HIV infection: the cellular picture, in the science of AIDS: readings from *Scientific American,* New York, 1989, Freeman.)

A variety of laboratory tests are available to evaluate specific immune deficiencies (Table 7-13). The choice of which particular tests to perform is determined on the characteristics described here. A basic screening test is a complete blood count (CBC) with a differential. The CBC provides information on the numbers of red cells, white cells, and platelets, and the differential indicates the quantities of lymphocytes, granulocytes, and monocytes in the blood. Quantitative determination of immunoglobulins (IgG, IgM, IgA) is a screening test for antibody production, and an assay for total complement (total hemolytic complement, CH_{50}) is useful if a complement defect is suspected. Further testing is described in Table 7-14.

Replacement Therapies for Immune Deficiencies

Many immune deficiencies can be successfully treated by replacing the missing component of the immune system.[27,28] Individuals with B cell deficiencies that cause hypogammaglobulinemia or agammaglobulinemia usually are treated with administration of gamma globulins, which are antibody-rich fractions prepared from plasma pooled from large numbers of donors. Administration of gamma globulin temporarily replaces the individual's antibodies. Antibodies from these preparations are removed slowly from the person's blood, with half of the antibodies being removed by 3 to 4 weeks. Thus, individuals must be treated repeatedly to maintain a protective level of antibodies in the blood.

Defects in lymphoid cell development in the primary lymphoid organs (e.g., SCID, Wiskott-Aldrich syndrome, leukocyte adhesion defect) can sometimes be treated by replacement of stem cells through transplantation of bone marrow, umbilical cord cells, or other cell populations that are rich in stem cells. Thymic defects (e.g., DiGeorge syndrome, ataxia-telangiectasia, or chronic mucocutaneous candidiasis) may be treated with transplantation of fetal thymus tissue or thymic epithelial cells (the cells that produce the thymic hormones). However, in most cases improvement is only temporary.

Enzymatic defects that cause SCID (e.g., adenosine deaminase deficiency) have been treated successfully with transfusions of glycerol frozen-packed erythrocytes. The donor erythrocytes contain the needed enzyme and can, at least temporarily, provide sufficient enzyme for normal

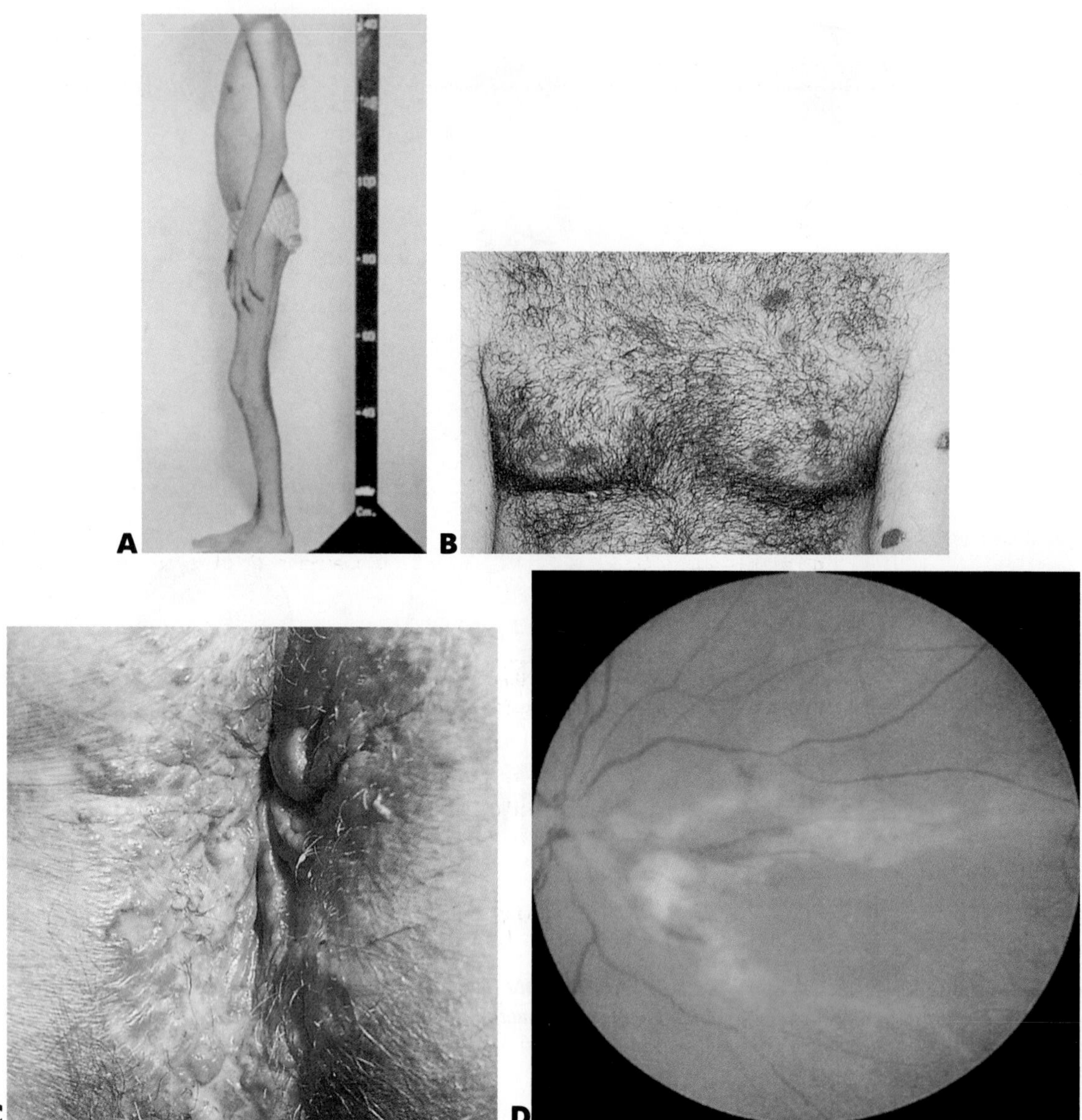

Figure 7-25 ■ **Clinical Symptoms of AIDS. A,** Severe weight loss and anorexia. **B,** Kaposi sarcoma lesions. **C,** Perianal lesions of herpes simplex infection. **D,** Deterioration of vision from cytomegalovirus retinitis leading to areas of infection, which can lead to blindness. (**A** and **D** from Taylor PK: *Diagnostic picture tests in sexually transmitted diseases,* London, 1995, Mosby; **B** and **C** from Morse SA, Ballard RC, Holmes KK, et al, editors: *Atlas of sexually transmitted diseases and AIDS,* ed 3, Edinburgh, 2003, Mosby.)

lymphocyte function. The first successful gene therapy was performed in ADA deficiency, resulting in reconstitution of the immune systems.

Individuals with immune deficiencies are at risk for **graft-versus-host disease (GVHD).** This occurs if T cells in a transplanted graft (e.g., transfused blood, bone marrow transplants) are mature and therefore capable of the cell-mediated immunity against the recipient's HLA. The primary targets for GVHD are the skin (e.g., rash, loss or increase of pigment, thickening of skin), liver (e.g., damage to bile duct, hepatomegaly), mouth (e.g., dry mouth, ulcers, infections), eyes (e.g., burning, irritation, dryness), and gastrointestinal tract (e.g., severe diarrhea), and the disease may lead to death from infections. GVHD is not a problem when the recipient is immunocompetent—that is, has an immune system that can control the donor's lymphocytes. If, however, the recipient's immune system is deficient, the grafted T cells remain unchecked and attack the recipient's tissues. Most GVHD should be prevented by the current practices of treating blood with irradiation to kill white blood cells before transfusion or removal of mature T cells from tissue used to treat individuals with immune deficiencies.

QUICK CHECK 7-4

1. Why is the development of recurrent or unusual infections the clinical hallmark of immunodeficiency?
2. Compare and contrast the most common infections in individuals with defects in cell-mediated immune response and those with defects in humoral immune response.
3. What are the new treatments for HIV?

TABLE 7-14
Laboratory Evaluation of Immunodeficiencies

Function Tested	Laboratory Test	Significance of Test
TESTS OF HUMORAL IMMUNE FUNCTION		
Antibody production	Total immunoglobulin levels, including IgG, IgM, and IgA.	Decrease or absence of total antibody production or of specific classes of antibody, which is associated with many B cell and combined deficiencies
	Levels of isohemagglutinins	Production of specific IgM antibodies, which is decreased in some combined deficiencies; not useful with persons who are blood type AB and do not have naturally occurring isohemagglutinins
	Levels of antibodies against vaccines—especially diphtheria and tetanus toxoids	Production of specific IgG antibodies, which is decreased when B cells are deficient or class-switch is blocked
B cell numbers	Numbers of lymphocytes with surface immunoglobulin	Production of circulating B cells, which is decreased in many severe B cell or combined deficiencies
Antibody subclasses	Levels specific subclasses, particularly IgG1, IgG2, and IgG3.	Decrease or absence of a particular subclass, which is characteristic of several immune deficiencies
TESTS OF CELLULAR IMMUNE FUNCTION		
Delayed hypersensitivity skin test	Skin test reaction against previously encountered antigens—especially *Candida albicans* or tetanus toxoid	Defects in antigen-responsive T cells and skin test cellular interactions (e.g., lymphokine activity and macrophage function)
T cell numbers	Numbers of T cells expressing characteristic membrane antigens (CD3 or CD11)	Defects in production of circulating T cells
T cell proliferation in vitro	Proliferative response to nonspecific mitogens (e.g., phytohemagglutinin)	General T cell defects in response to nonspecific stimulation (mitogens)
	Proliferative response to antigens (e.g., tetanus toxoid)	Defects in the response of T cells to specific antigens
T cell subpopulations	Quantify the percentage of T cells with specific markers for total T cells (CD3), Th cells (CD4), Tc cells (CD8)	Decrease in the numbers of CD4 cells, which is related to AIDS progression

Did You Understand?

Hypersensitivity: Allergy, Autoimmunity, and Alloimmunity

1. Hypersensitivity is an inappropriate immune response misdirected against the host's own tissues (autoimmunity) or directed against beneficial foreign tissues, such as transfusions or transplants (alloimmunity); or it can be exaggerated responses against environmental antigens (allergy).
2. Mechanisms of hypersensitivity are classified as type I (IgE-mediated) reactions, type II (tissue-specific) reactions, type III (immune-complex-mediated) reactions, and type IV (cell-mediated) reactions.
3. Hypersensitivity reactions can be immediate (developing within seconds or hours) or delayed (developing within hours or days).
4. Anaphylaxis, the most rapid immediate hypersensitivity reaction, is an explosive reaction that occurs within minutes of reexposure to the antigen and can lead to cardiovascular shock.
5. Allergens are antigens that cause allergic responses.
6. Type I (IgE-mediated) reactions are occur after antigen reacts with IgE on mast cells, leading to mast cell degranulation and the release of histamine and other inflammatory substances.
7. Type II (tissue-specific) reactions are caused by four possible mechanisms: complement-mediated lysis, opsonization and phagocytosis, antibody-dependent cell-mediated cytotoxicity, and modulation of cellular function.
8. Type III (immune complex–mediated) reactions are caused by the formation of immune complexes that are deposited in target tissues, where they activate the complement cascade, generating chemotactic fragments that attract neutrophils into the inflammatory site.

(Continued)

Did You Understand?—Cont'd

9. Immune-complex disease can be a systemic reaction, such as serum sickness (e.g., Raynaud phenomenon), or localized, such as the Arthus reaction.
10. Type IV (cell-mediated) reactions are caused by specifically sensitized T cells, which either kill target cells directly or release lymphokines that activate other cells, such as macrophages.
11. Allergies can be mediated by any of the four mechanisms of hypersensitivity.
12. Clinical manifestations of allergic reactions are usually confined to the areas of initial intake or contact with the allergen. Ingested allergens induce gastrointestinal symptoms, airborne allergens induce respiratory or skin manifestations, and contact allergens induce allergic responses at the site of contact.
13. Atopic individuals are genetically predisposed to the development of allergies.
14. Alloimmunity is the immune system's reaction against antigens on the tissues of other members of the same species.
15. Alloimmune disorders include transient neonatal disease, in which the maternal immune system becomes sensitized against antigens expressed by the fetus, and transplant rejection and transfusion reactions, in which the immune system of the recipient of an organ transplant or blood transfusion reacts against foreign antigens on the donor's cells.

Infection

1. Bacteria injure cells by producing exotoxins or endotoxins. Exotoxins are enzymes that can damage the plasma membranes of host cells or can inactivate enzymes critical to protein synthesis, and endotoxins activate the inflammatory response and produce fever.
2. Septicemia is the proliferation of bacteria in the blood. Endotoxins released by blood-borne bacteria cause the release of vasoactive enzymes that increase the permeability of blood vessels. Leakage from vessels causes hypotension that can result in septic shock.
3. Viruses enter host cells and use the metabolic processes of host cells to proliferate.
4. Viruses that have invaded host cells may decrease protein synthesis, disrupt lysosomal membranes, form inclusion bodies where synthesis of viral nucleic acids is occurring, fuse with host cells to produce giant cells, alter antigenic properties of the host cell, and transform host cells into cancerous cells.
5. Diseases caused by fungi are called mycoses, and they occur in two forms: yeasts (spheres) and molds (filaments or hyphae).
6. Dermatophytes are fungi that infect skin, hair, and nails with diseases such as ringworm and athlete's foot.
7. Fungi release toxins and enzymes that are damaging to tissue.

Deficiencies in Immunity

1. Immunodeficiency is the failure of mechanisms of self-defense to function in their normal capacity.
2. Immunodeficiencies are either congenital (primary) or acquired (secondary). Congenital immunodeficiencies are caused by genetic defects that disrupt lymphocyte development, whereas acquired immunodeficiencies are secondary to disease or other physiologic alterations.
3. The clinical hallmark of immunodeficiency is a propensity to unusual or recurrent severe infections. The type of infection usually reflects the immune system defect.
4. The most common infections in individuals with defects of cell-mediated immune response are fungal and viral, whereas infections in individuals with defects of the humoral immune response or complement function are primarily bacterial.
5. Severe combined immunodeficiency (SCID) is a total lack of T cell function and a severe (either partial or total) lack of B cell function.
6. DiGeorge syndrome (congenital thymic aplasia or hypoplasia) is characterized by complete or partial lack of the thymus (resulting in depressed T cell immunity), the parathyroid glands (resulting in hypocalcemia), and cardiac anomalies.
7. Defects in B cell function are diverse, ranging from a complete lack of the human bursal equivalent, the lymphoid organs required for B cell maturation (as in Bruton agammaglobulinemia), to deficiencies in a single class of immunoglobulins (e.g., selective IgA deficiency).
8. Acquired immunodeficiencies are caused by superimposed conditions, such as malnutrition, medical therapies, physical or psychologic trauma, or infections.
9. AIDS is an acquired dysfunction of the immune system caused by a retrovirus (HIV) that infects and destroys $CD4^+$ lymphocytes (helper T cells).
10. Immunodeficiency syndromes usually are treated by replacement therapy. Deficient antibody production is treated by replacement of missing immunoglobulins with commercial gamma-globulin preparations. Lymphocyte deficiencies are treated with the replacement of host lymphocytes with transplants of bone marrow, fetal liver, or fetal thymus from a donor.

Key Terms

ABO blood group, 179
Acquired immunodeficiency syndrome (AIDS), 198
Acute rejection, 181
Adenosine deaminase (ADA) deficiency, 197
Agammaglobulinemia, 195
Allergen, 177
Allergy, 169
Alloimmune disease, 169
Anaphylaxis, 190
Antibody-dependent cell-mediated cytotoxicity (ADCC), 174
Antigenic drift, 184
Antigenic shift, 184
Antitoxin, 186
Arthus reaction, 176
Atopic, 172
Autoimmune disease, 169
Autoimmunity, 169
Bare lymphocyte syndrome, 197
Blood group antigen, 179
B-lymphocyte deficiency, 195
Bruton agammaglobulinemia, 195
C3 deficiency, 197
Chronic granulomatous disease (CGD), 197
Chronic mucocutaneous candidiasis, 196
Chronic rejection, 181
Combined deficiency, 196
Complement deficiency, 197
Contact dermatitis, 176
Cryoglobulins, 175
Delayed hypersensitivity reaction, 170
Delayed hypersensitivity skin test, 176
Dermatophyte, 190
Desensitization, 172
DiGeorge syndrome, 196
Dimorphic fungus (*pl.*, fungi), 189
Endotoxic shock, 186
Endotoxin (lipopolysaccharide [LPS]), 186
Entrance inhibitor, 202
Erythema, 176
Exotoxin, 185
Graft-versus-host disease (GVHD), 204
Highly active antiretroviral therapy (HAART), 201
Human leukocyte antigen (HLA), 180
Hyperacute rejection, 181
Hypersensitivity, 169
Hypogammaglobulinemia, 195
Immediate hypersensitivity reaction, 170
Immune deficiency, 194
Induration, 176
Integrase inhibitor, 202
Integrase, 199
Isohemagglutinin, 179
Major histocompatibility complex (MHC), 180
Mycosis (*pl.*, mycoses), 190
Phagocytic deficiency, 197
Primary (congenital) immune deficiency, 194
Protease inhibitor, 201
Raynaud phenomenon, 175
Reverse transcriptase inhibitor, 201
Reverse transcriptase, 199
Rh blood group, 179
Secondary (acquired) immune deficiency, 194
Selective IgA deficiency, 195
Septicemia (bacteremia), 186
Serum sickness, 175
Severe combined immune deficiency (SCID), 197
Systemic lupus erythematosus (SLE), 178
Tissue-specific antigen, 172
T-lymphocyte deficiency, 195
Tolerance, 178
Toxoid, 192
Universal donor, 179
Universal recipient, 179
Urticaria (hives), 172
Vaccination, 191
Vaccine, 191
Wheal and flare reaction, 172
Wiskott-Aldrich syndrome, 197

References

1. Prussin C, Metcalfe DD: IgE, mast cells, basophils, and eosinophils, *J Allergy Clin Immunol* 117:S450–S456, 2006.
2. Nelson HS: Advances in upper airway diseases and allergen immunotherapy, *J Allergy Clin Immunol* 117:1047–1053, 2006.
3. Romi F, Gilhus NE, Aarli JA: Myasthenia gravis: clinical, immunologic, and therapeutic advances, *Acta Neurol Scand* 111:134–141, 2005.
4. Reid JR, Wheeler SF: Hyperthyroidism: diagnosis and treatment, *Am Fam Physician* 72:635–636, 2005.
5. Jancar S, Crespo MS: Immune complex-mediated tissue injury: a multistep paradigm, *Trends Immunol* 26:48–55, 2005.
6. Bianco P et al: Cytotoxic T lymphocytes and autoimmunity, *Curr Opin Rheumatol* 17:731–734, 2005.
7. Sicherer SH, Leung DYM: Advances in allergic skin disease, anaphylaxis, and hypersensitivity reactions to foods, drugs, and insects, *J Allergy Clin Immunol* 118:170–177, 2006.
8. Cunningham MW: Pathogenesis of group A streptococcal infections, *Clin Microbiol Rev* 13:470–511, 2000.
9. Riemekasten G, Hahn BH: Key autoantigens in SLE, *Rheumatol* 44:975–982, 2005.
10. American College of Rheumatology: Systemic lupus erythematosus, available at www.rheumatology.org/public/factsheets/sle_new.asp?aud=pat#4.
11. Burt RK et al: Nonmyeloablative hematopoietic stem cell transplantation for systemic lupus erythematosus, *JAMA* 295:527–535, 2006.
12. Nydegger UE et al: Histo-blood group antigens as allo- and autoantigens, *Ann N Y Acad Sci* 1050:40–51, 2005.
13. Sheldon S, Poulton K: HLA typing and its influence on organ transplantation, *Methods Mol Biol* 333:157–174, 2006.
14. World Health Organization: *World Health Report*, Geneva, 2005, World Health Organization.
15. Musher DM: How contagious are common respiratory tract infections? *N Eng J Med* 348:1256–1266, 2003.
16. Amanna I, Slifka MK: Public fear of vaccination: separating fact from fiction, *Viral Immunol* 18:307–315, 2005.
17. Macias AE, Ponce-de-León S: Infection control: old problems and new challenges, *Arch Med Res* 36:637–645, 2005.
18. Nucci M, Marr KA: Emerging fungal diseases, *Clin Infect Dis* 41:521–526, 2005.
19. Cooper MA, Pommering TL, Korányi K: Primary immunodeficiencies, *Am Fam Physician* 68:2001–2008, 2003.
20. Notarangelo L et al: Primary immunodeficiency diseases, *J Allergy Clin Immunol* 117:883–896, 2006.
21. Bonilla FA, Geha RS: Update on primary immunodeficiency diseases, *J Allergy Clin Immunol* 117:S435–S441, 2006.
22. Cunningham-Rundles C, Ponda PP: Molecular defects in T- and B-cell primary immunodeficiency diseases, *Nat Rev Immunol* 5:880–892, 2005.
23. Sjöholm AG et al: Complement deficiency and disease: an update, *Molec Immunol* 43:78–85, 2006.
24. Piot P: AIDS: from crisis management to sustained strategic response, *Lancet* 368:526–530, 2006.
25. Duerr A, Wasserheit JN, Corey L: HIV vaccines: new frontiers in vaccine development, *Clin Infect Dis* 43:500–511, 2006.
26. Buckley RH: Primary immunodeficiency or not? Making the correct diagnosis, *J Allergy Clin Immunol* 117:756–758, 2006.
27. Buckley RH: Molecular defects in human severe combined immunodeficiency and approaches to immune reconstitution, *Ann Rev Immunol* 22:625–655, 2004.
28. Puck JM, Malech HL: Gene therapy for immune disorders: good news tempered by bad news, *J Allergy Clin Immunol* 117:865–869, 2006.

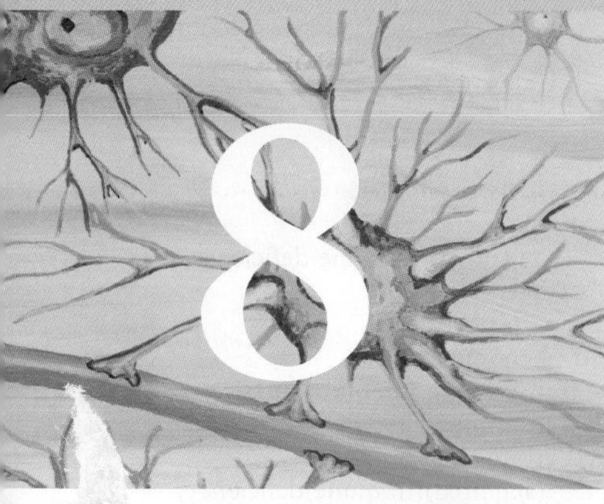

8 STRESS AND DISEASE

Beth A. Forshee ▪ Kathryn L. McCance

CHAPTER OUTLINE

ELECTRONIC RESOURCES

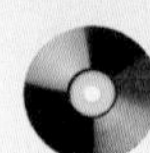

Companion CD
- Review Questions and Answers
- Animations

evolve Website
http://evolve.elsevier.com/Huether/
- Quick Check Answers
- Key Terms Exercises
- Critical Thinking Questions with Answers
- Algorithm Completion Exercises
- WebLinks

Walter B. Cannon used the term *stress* in both a physiologic and a psychologic sense as early as 1914.[1] He applied the engineering concept of stress and strain in a physiologic context and believed that emotional stimuli were also capable of causing stress. In 1946, Hans Selye popularized these same findings, viewing stress as a biologic phenomenon.[2] The concept that stress may influence immunity and resistance to disease has been investigated since the 1950s. In the 1970s, studies found that life changes or emotions resulting from life changes and occurring over a prolonged time were associated with decreased immune function. More recently, studies have been conducted to investigate the interactions among social, psychologic, and biologic factors and their role in causing and prolonging or shortening the course of disease. What is emerging from the various disciplines involved—molecular biology, immunology, neurology, endocrinology, and behavioral science—is a more holistic and complex model that involves biochemical relationships of the central nervous system (CNS), autonomic nervous system (ANS), endocrine system, and immune system. Thus, a new field—psychoneuroimmunology—has developed.

CONCEPTS OF STRESS

Psychologic stress may cause or exacerbate (worsen) several disease states, including many of the diseases (cardiovascular disease, cancer, and infectious diseases) implicated as the leading causes of death in the United States (Table 8-1). There is also evidence that stress is directly related to the cause of or affects the severity of symptoms and outcomes in a number of diseases and conditions, including irritable bowel syndrome, ulcers, asthma, autoimmune disorders, delayed wound healing, reproductive dysfunction, diabetes (worsening of symptoms), and depression. Chronic inflammation, which can be stimulated by stress, is suggested as being important in the functional decline that leads to frailty, disability, and untimely death.[3] As evidence has mounted concerning the important role that stress plays in many disease processes, research has focused on the mechanisms responsible for these mind-body interactions. Along with a greater understanding of the relationship between the human stress response and disease, new strategies for treatment of stress-related disorders are emerging. This chapter describes definitions of stress, the history of stress research, and findings on the role of stress in disease.

The term *stress* was used persistently and widely in the past in specialties such as biology, health sciences, and social sciences despite the lack of agreement over how it should be defined. Now stress has come to be defined by most as a *transactional* or *interactional concept.* Transactionally, stress is viewed as the state of affairs that arises when a person relates to (i.e., interacts or transacts with) situations in certain ways. People are not disturbed by situations per se but by the ways that they appraise and react to situations. In general, a person experiences stress when a demand exceeds that person's coping abilities, thereby resulting in reactions such as disturbances of cognition, emotion, and behavior that can adversely affect well-being.

TABLE 8-1

Examples of Stress-Related Diseases and Conditions

Target Organ or System	Disease or Condition	Target Organ or System	Disease or Condition
Cardiovascular system	Coronary artery disease Hypertension Stroke Disturbances of heart rhythm	Gastrointestinal system	Ulcer Irritable bowel syndrome Diarrhea Nausea and vomiting Ulcerative colitis
Muscle	Tension headaches Muscle contraction backache	Genitourinary system	Diuresis Impotence Frigidity
Connective tissues	Rheumatoid arthritis (autoimmune disease) Related inflammatory diseases of connective tissue	Skin	Eczema Neurodermatitis Acne
Pulmonary system	Asthma (hypersensitivity reaction) Hay fever (hypersensitivity reaction)	Endocrine system	Type 2 diabetes mellitus Amenorrhea
Immune system	Immunosuppression or deficiency Autoimmune diseases	Central nervous system	Fatigue and lethargy Type A behavior Overeating Depression Insomnia

General Adaptation Syndrome

Selye originally sought to discover a new sex hormone when he discovered the biologic syndrome of stress.[2] In his attempts to discover the new hormone, Selye injected crude ovarian extracts into rats. Repeatedly he found that the following triad of structural changes occurred: (1) enlargement of the cortex of the adrenal gland, (2) atrophy of the thymus gland and other lymphoid structures, and (3) development of bleeding ulcers of the stomach and duodenal lining. Selye soon discovered that this triad of manifestations was not specific to injected ovarian extracts but also occurred after he exposed the rats to other noxious stimuli, such as cold, surgical injury, and restraint. He called these stimuli **stressors.** Selye concluded that this triad or syndrome of manifestations represented a nonspecific response to noxious stimuli. Because many diverse agents caused the same syndrome, Selye suggested that it be called the **general adaptation syndrome (GAS).**

Three successive stages in development of the GAS were identified: (1) the **alarm stage** or reaction, in which the central nervous system (CNS) is aroused and the body's defenses are mobilized (e.g., "fight or flight") (Figure 8-1); (2) the **stage of resistance** or **adaptation,** during which mobilization contributes to "fight or flight"; and (3) the **stage of exhaustion,** in which continuous stress causes the progressive breakdown of compensatory mechanisms (acquired adaptations) and homeostasis. The stage of exhaustion marks the onset of certain diseases **(diseases of adaptation).**

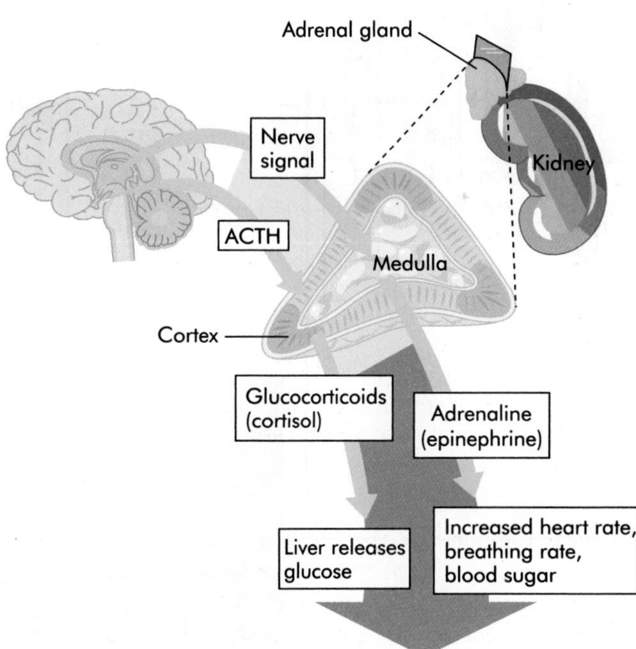

Figure 8-1 ■ **The Alarm Reaction.** The alarm reaction includes increased secretion of glucocorticoids (cortisol) by the adrenal cortex and increased secretion of epinephrine and small amounts of norepinephrine from the adrenal medulla. The response to the release of cortisol and sympathetic nerve activation is summarized in Figure 8-2. *ACTH,* Adrenocorticotropic hormone. (From Thibodeau GA, Patton KT: *Anatomy & physiology,* ed 6, St Louis, 2007, Mosby.)

Interactions among the sympathetic branch of the ANS and the hypothalamus, pituitary, and adrenal glands (HPA axis) produce the nonspecific physiologic responses identified by Selye. The alarm phase begins when a stressor activates the hypothalamus and sympathetic nervous system (Figures 8-1 and 8-2). The resistance or adaptation phase begins with the actions of the adrenal hormones

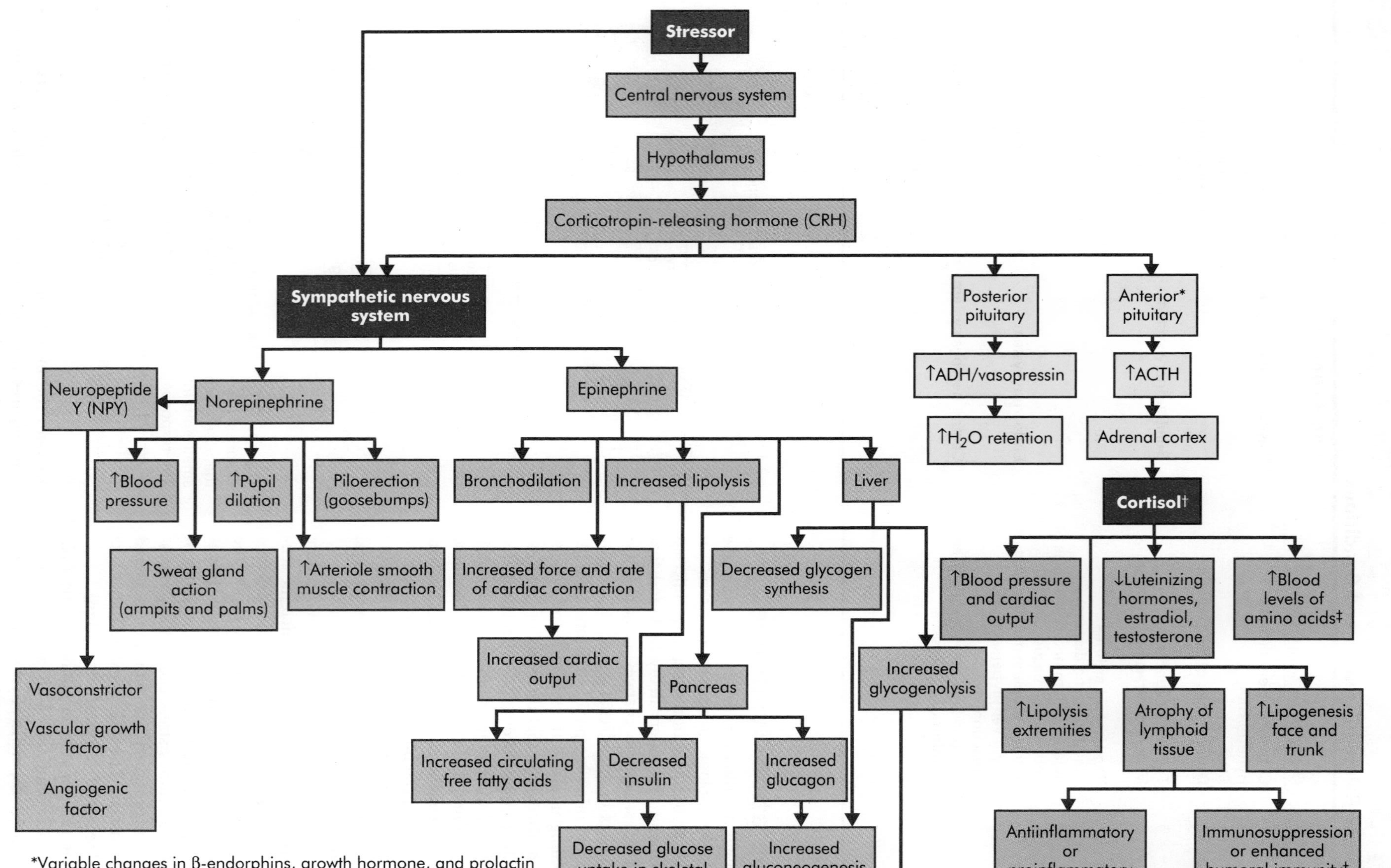

*Variable changes in β-endorphins, growth hormone, and prolactin (see text).
†Effects may be dependent on *amount* of cortisol and nature of the stressor.
‡Caused by protein catabolism in muscle, adipose tissue, skin, bones, lymphoid tissue.
ADH, Antidiuretic hormone; *ACTH*, adrenocorticotropic hormone.

Figure 8-2 ■ **The Stress Response.**

cortisol, norepinephrine, and epinephrine. Exhaustion occurs if stress continues and adaptation is not successful, ultimately causing impairment of the immune response, heart failure, and kidney failure leading to death.

Physiologic stress is a chemical or physical disturbance in the cells or tissue fluid produced by a change, either in the external environment or within the body itself, that requires a response (i.e., begins the GAS) to counteract the disturbance. Selye identified three components of physiologic stress: (1) the exogenous or endogenous stressor initiating the disturbance, (2) the chemical or physical disturbance produced by the stressor, and (3) the body's counteracting (adaptational) response to the disturbance.[2]

Psychologic Mediators and Specificity

Although Selye's identification of the GAS is regarded as tremendously important and the cornerstone of stress research, the idea that stress is a purely physiologic response is oversimplified. Activation of the adrenal cortex occurs in humans in response to psychologic stressors too. Several factors, including degrees of discomfort, unpleasantness, or suddenness of the stress, can account for the presence or absence of the physiologic stress response.

Selye believed that stressors cause a general or nonspecific response. However, research done since the 1970s has shown remarkable sensitivity of the CNS and endocrine system to emotional, psychologic, and social influences. Thus, it may be the way an individual thinks and feels about a physical stressor or the stressor itself that produces the neuroendocrine responses. Psychologic stressors can elicit a reactive or anticipatory stress response. The **reactive response** is a physiologic response derived from psychologic stressors. For example, the stress of an examination may produce an increased heart rate and dry mouth in the unprepared individual. Although there is no physical stressor, the psychologic stress of an examination elicits a reactive physiologic response. **Anticipatory response** occurs when the body mounts a physiologic response in anticipation of disruption of the optimal steady state, also known as **homeostasis.** These anticipatory responses can be generated either by innate fears, such as predators and unfamiliar situations, or by exercise-dependent memories.[4] In a conditioned response, the person learns that specific stimuli (such as objects or situation context) are associated with danger, and anticipation of subsequent encounters with the stimulus produces a physiologic stress response. For example, a child who is abused by a parent may experience a physiologic stress response in anticipation of further abuse when that parent enters the room.

QUICK CHECK 8-1

1. Define the term *stressor.*
2. Briefly describe the three stages of the general adaptation syndrome.
3. Describe the reactive and anticipatory responses to psychologic stressors.

THE STRESS RESPONSE

Neuroendocrine Regulation

The sympathetic nervous system is aroused during the **stress response,** releasing norepinephrine (adrenergic stimulation) and causing the medulla of the adrenal gland to release catecholamines (80% epinephrine and 20% norepinephrine) into the bloodstream. New data reveals that sympathetic nerves also contain nonadrenergic mediators that amplify or antagonize these catecholamines (see *Health Alert,* p. 215). Simultaneously, hypothalamic corticotropin-releasing hormone (CRH) stimulates the pituitary gland to release a variety of hormones, including antidiuretic hormone (ADH) from the posterior pituitary gland and prolactin, growth hormone, and adrenocorticotropic hormone (ACTH) from the anterior pituitary gland. ACTH stimulates the cortex of the adrenal gland to release cortisol (see Figure 8-2).

Catecholamines

Epinephrine goes to the liver and skeletal muscle but is then rapidly metabolized. Very little adrenal norepinephrine reaches distal tissue; thus, its effects during the stress response are primarily from the sympathetic nervous system. Catecholamines cannot cross the blood-brain barrier and are synthesized locally in the brain.

The catecholamines stimulate two major classes of receptors: α-adrenergic receptors (α_1 and α_2) and β-adrenergic receptors (β_1 and β_2). Table 12-7 summarizes the actions of the two subclasses of adrenergic receptors. (A thorough discussion of receptors can be found in Chapters 1, 17, and 22.) Epinephrine binds to and activates both α and β receptors. Norepinephrine at physiologic concentrations binds primarily to α-receptors.

The circulating catecholamines essentially mimic direct sympathetic stimulation. Norepinephrine regulates blood pressure because it is the primary constrictor of smooth muscle in all blood vessels. During stress, norepinephrine raises blood pressure by constricting peripheral vessels, dilates the pupils, causes piloerection, and increases sweat gland action in the armpits and palms (see Figure 8-2). Epinephrine has greater influence on cardiac action and is the principal catecholamine involved in metabolic regulation. The physiologic effects of the catecholamines are summarized in Table 8-2.

Cortisol

During stress, ACTH activates the adrenal cortex, increasing adrenocortical secretion of glucocorticoid hormones, primarily cortisol (see Figure 8-2). (Cortisol is known also as *hydrocortisone.*) Cortisol circulates in the plasma, both protein bound and free. The unbound, or free, fraction is approximately 8% of the total plasma cortisol and is the most biologically active fraction of cortisol. Cortisol mobilizes substances needed for cellular metabolism and stimulates gluconeogenesis, or the formation of glucose from noncarbohydrate sources, such as amino or free fatty acids

TABLE 8-2

Physiologic Effects of the Catecholamines*

Organ	Process of Result
Brain	Increased blood flow Increased glucose metabolism
Cardiovascular system	Increased rate and force of contraction Peripheral vasoconstriction
Pulmonary system	Bronchodilation Increased ventilation
Muscle	Increased glycogenolysis Decreased glucose uptake and utilization (decreases insulin release) Increased contraction Increased dilation of skeletal muscle vasculature
Liver	Increased glucose production Increased glycogenolysis
Adipose tissue	Increased lipolysis Decreased glucose uptake and utilization (decreases insulin release)
Skin	Decreased blood flow
Gastrointestinal and genitourinary tracts	Decreased protein synthesis genitourinary tracts Decreased smooth muscle contraction
Lymphoid tissue	Acute and chronic stress inhibits several components of cellular immunity, particularly decreasing natural killer cells†
Macrophages	Inhibit and stimulate macrophage activity; depends on availability of type 1/proinflammatory cytokines, the presence or absence of antigenic stressors, and peripheral corticotropin-releasing hormone (CRH)

Adapted from Granner DK: Hormones of the adrenal medulla. In Murray RK et al, editors: *Harper's biochemistry*, ed 23, New York, 1999, McGraw-Hill; Elenkov IJ, Chrousos GP: Stress hormones, proinflammatory and antiinflammatory cytokines, and autoimmunity, *Ann N Y Acad Sci* 966:290–303, 2002.

*Some of these responses require glucocorticoids (e.g., cortisol) for maximal activity (see text for explanation).

†Natural killer cells appear to be the most "sensitive" cells to the suppressive effect of stress and, thus, have become an important index of stress-induced suppression of cellular immunity.

in the liver. In addition, cortisol enhances the elevation of blood glucose promoted by other hormones, such as epinephrine, glucagon, and growth hormone. This action is said to be **permissive** for the actions of other hormones. Cortisol also inhibits the uptake and oxidation of glucose by many body cells. Overall, cortisol's actions on carbohydrate metabolism result in increased blood glucose levels, thereby energizing the body to combat the stressor. The physiologic effects of cortisol are summarized in Table 8-3.

Cortisol and the immune system

Stress hormones, especially glucocorticoids (cortisol) have been used therapeutically as powerful anti-inflammatory/immunosuppressive agents. This has lead to the conclusion that stress, in general, decreases immunity and inflammation. Data suggest, however, that glucocorticoids and catecholamines (epinephrine and norepinephrine) at concentration levels reached during stress may paradoxically decrease cellular immunity and increase autoimmune (humoral) responses. These data may help explain the seemingly contradictory response to stress of immunosuppression and increased risk of infection (decreased cellular immunity), and a heightened antibody response and autoimmune disease (increased humoral immunity).

Immune responses are regulated by cells of *innate immunity* called antigen-presenting cells (APCs), such as monocyte/macrophages (see Chapter 6), by dendritic cells and other phagocytic cells, and by lymphocyte Th1 and Th2 cells of *adaptive immunity*. These cells regulate the immune system by secreting chemicals called *cytokines*. Cytokines are a group of chemicals, such as interferons, interleukins, and tumor necrosis factors that can stimulate or inhibit various components of the immune system. Antigen-presenting cells release cytokines that induce T cells to differentiate into Th1 cells. Th1 cells and APC cytokines work together to stimulate the immune activity of cytotoxic T cells, natural killer cells and activated macrophages—the major components of cellular immunity. These cytokines also stimulate the synthesis of nitrous oxides and other inflammatory mediators that increase chronic delayed-type inflammatory responses. Because of this effect, these cytokines are considered to be the major *proinflammatory cytokines*.[5–7] The cytokines secreted by the Th2 cells act to inhibit Th1 cells and can promote humoral immunity by stimulating growth and activation of mast cells and eosinophils, as well as the differentiation of B-cell immunoglobulins. Thus, these cytokines are considered to be the major *anti-inflammatory cytokines* (Figure 8-3).[5]

Stress influences immunity by stimulating cortisol and epinephrine secretion from the adrenal glands and norepinephrine from the sympathetic nervous system. Cortisol suppresses the activity of Th1 cells, which leads to a

TABLE 8-3
Physiologic Effects of Cortisol

Functions Affected	Physiologic Effects
Carbohydrate and lipid metabolism	Diminishes peripheral uptake and utilization of glucose; promotes gluconeogenesis in liver metabolism cells; enhances the gluconeogenic response to other hormones; promotes lipolysis in adipose tissue
Protein metabolism	Increases protein synthesis in the liver and decreased protein synthesis (including immunoglobulin synthesis) in muscle, lymphoid tissue, adipose tissue, skin, and bone; increases plasma level of amino acids; stimulates deamination in the liver
Anti-inflammatory effects (systemic effects)	High levels of cortisol used in drug therapy suppress the inflammatory response; inhibit proinflammatory activity of many growth factors and cytokines; however, over time some patients may develop tolerance to glucocorticoids causing an increased susceptibility to both inflammatory and autoimmune disease
Proinflammatory effects (possible local effects)	Cortisol levels released during the stress response may increase proinflammatory effects
Lipid metabolism	Lipolysis in the extremities and lipogenesis in the face and trunk
Immune effects	*Treatment* levels of glucocorticoids are immunosuppressive, thus they are valuable agents used in numerous diseases; the T cell or cellular immunity system is particularly affected by these larger doses of glucocorticoids with suppression of Th1 function or cellular immunity; *stress* can cause a different pattern of immune response; these nontherapeutic levels can suppress cellular (Th1) and increase humoral (Th2) immunity—the so-called Th2 shift; several factors influence this complex physiology and include long-term adaptations, reproductive hormones (i.e., overall, androgens suppress and estrogens stimulate immune responses), defects of the hypothalamic-pituitary-adrenal axis, histamine-generated responses, and acute versus chronic stress; thus stress seems to cause a Th2 shift *systemically* whereas *locally*, under certain conditions, it can induce proinflammatory activities and by these mechanisms may influence the onset or course of infections, autoimmune/inflammatory, allergic, and neoplastic disease
Digestive function	Promotes gastric secretion
Urinary function	Enhances excretion of calcium
Connective tissue function	Decreases proliferation of fibroblasts in connective tissue (thus delaying healing)
Muscle function	Maintains normal contractility and maximal work output for skeletal and cardiac muscle
Bone function	Decreases bone formation
Vascular system/ myocardial function	Maintains normal blood pressure; permits increased responsiveness of arterioles to the constrictive action of adrenergic stimulation; optimizes myocardial performance
Central nervous system function	Somehow modulates perceptual and emotional functioning, essential for normal arousal and initiation of daytime activity
Possible synergism with estrogen in pregnancy?	Suppresses maternal immune system to prevent rejection of fetus?

decrease in cellular immunity and to the proinflammatory response. Cortisol also stimulates the activity of the Th2 cells, which leads to an increase in humoral immunity and the anti-inflammatory response. Epinephrine and norepinephrine have a similar effect, to decrease Th1 activity and increase Th2 activity. This decrease in Th1 activity and increase in Th2 activity is sometimes called the **Th2 shift.**

Corticotropin-releasing hormone (CRH) influences the immune system indirectly by the activation of cortisol (glucocorticoids) and catecholamines. CRH is secreted by the hypothalamus and also peripherally at inflammatory sites and called peripheral or immune CRH.[8,9] **Peripheral (immune) CRH** is proinflammatory, causing an increase in vasodilation and vascular permeability. Therefore, it appears that mast cells are the target of peripheral CRH. Mast cells release histamine, which is a well-known mediator of acute inflammation and allergic reactions (see Figure 8-3). Evidence has indicated that immune cells may have histamine receptors and that histamine may have an effect similar to the catecholamines. This would indicate that histamine would induce acute inflammation and allergic reactions while suppressing Th1 activity (decreasing cellular immunity) and promoting Th2 activity (increasing humoral immunity).[10–13]

In summary, stress can activate an excessive immune response and, through cortisol and the catecholamines, suppress the Th1 response and cause a Th2 shift. Locally, stress can exert proinflammatory or anti-inflammatory effects depending on what chemicals are released in the local environment and how the cells of the local environment respond to those chemicals. Finally, some evidence indicates that stress is not a uniform, nonspecific reaction.[14] Different types of stressors might have variable effects on the immune response. Thus, *systemically* stress may cause a decrease in cellular immunity and enhance humoral immunity, whereas *locally*, under certain conditions, it can induce proinflammatory activities that may influence the onset and cause of infection, autoimmune/inflammatory, allergic, and neoplastic disease.

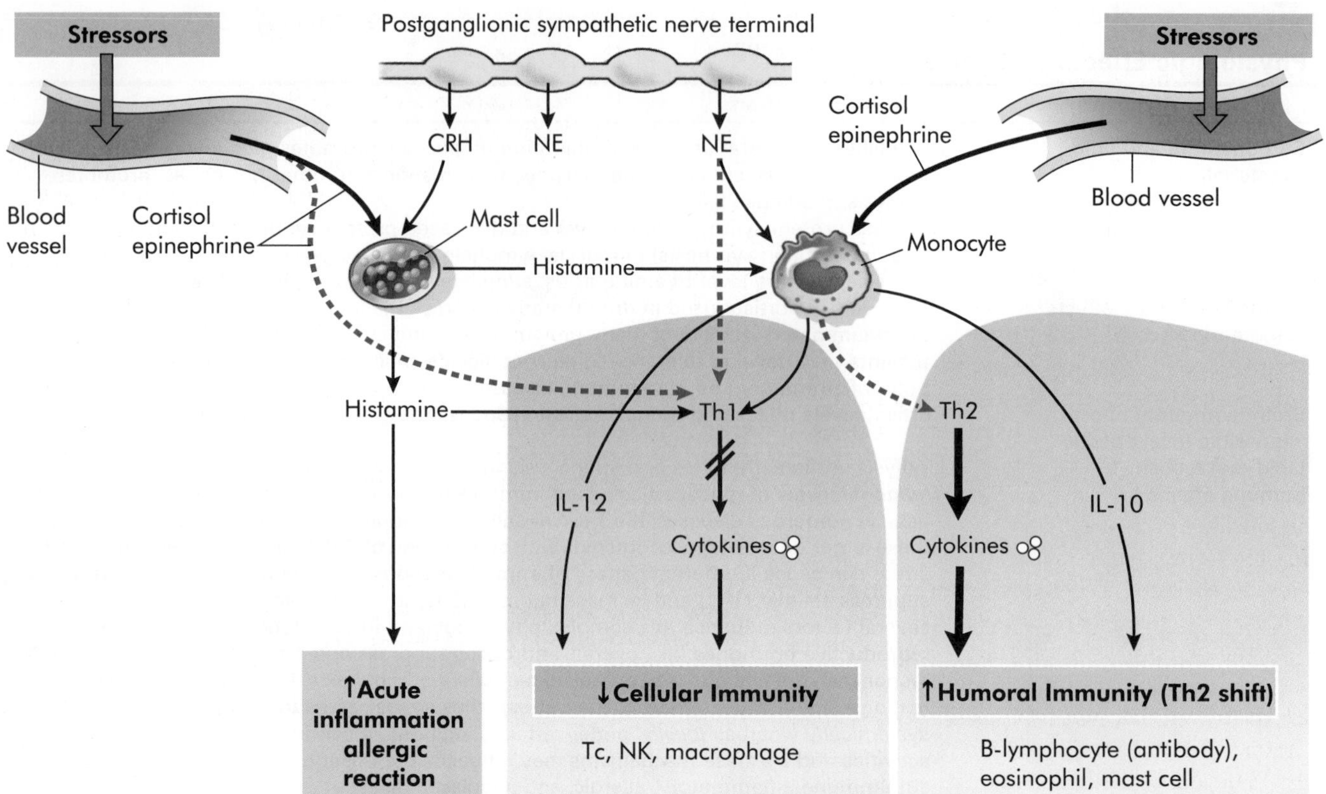

Figure 8-3 ■ Effect of Corticotropin-Releasing Hormone (CRH)—Mast Cell—Histamine Axis, Cortisol, and Catecholamines on the Th1/Th2 Balance—Cellular and Humoral Immunity. Humoral immunity provides protection against multicellular parasites, extracellular bacteria, some viruses, soluble toxins, and allergens. Cellular immunity provides protection against intracellular bacteria, fungi, protozoa, and several viruses. Type 1 cytokines or proinflammatory cytokines include IL-12, interferon-gamma (IFN-γ), and tumor necrosis factor-alpha (TNF-α). Type 2 cytokines or anti-inflammatory cytokines include IL-10 and IL-4. Solid lines *(black)* represent stimulation, whereas dashed lines *(blue)* represent inhibition (i.e., Th1 and Th2 are mutually inhibitory, IL-12 and IFN-γ inhibit Th2, and vice versa; IL-4 and IL-10 inhibit Th1 responses). Stress and CRH modulate inflammatory/immune and allergic responses by stimulating cortisol (glucocorticoid), catecholamines, and peripheral (immune) CRH secretion and by changing the production of regulatory cytokines and histamines. *CRH* (peripheral, immune), corticotropin-releasing hormone; *NE,* norepinephrine; *Th,* helper T cell; *IL,* interleukin; *Tc,* cytotoxic T cell; *NK,* natural killer cell; ↓, decreased (inhibited); ↑, increased (stimulation). (Redrawn from Elenkov IJ, Chrousos GP: Stress hormones, Th1/Th2 patterns, pro/anti-inflammatory cytokines and susceptibility to disease, *Trends Endocrinol Metab* 10[9]:359–368, 1999.)

Other hormones

Endorphins

β-Endorphins (endogenous opiates) are released into the blood as part of the response to stressful stimuli, including traumatic injury and an acute, intense stress situation, such as first-time parachute jumping. In inflamed tissue, immune cell–derived endorphins activate endorphin (opiate) receptors on peripheral sensory nerves leading to pain relief or analgesia. Hemorrhage increases β-endorphin levels that appear to *inhibit* blood pressure increase or delay compensatory changes that would increase blood pressure.[15] Thus, endogenous opiates modulate blood pressure instability and neuroendocrine and cytokine responses to blood losses.[16,17]

Growth hormone

Growth hormone (somatotropin) is released from the anterior pituitary gland and affects protein, lipid, and carbohydrate metabolism. Growth hormone levels increase in the blood after a variety of stressful stimuli, such as cardiac catheterization, electroshock therapy, gastroscopy, surgery, fever, and physical exercise. Immune cells are affected directly by growth hormone. Growth hormone receptors are present on lymphocytes. Prolonged activation of the stress response (chronic stress) suppresses growth hormone and leads to other growth factor effects on target tissues.

Prolactin

Prolactin is released from the anterior pituitary gland as well as numerous extrapituitary tissue sites.[18] Prolactin is necessary for lactation and breast development. Prolactin levels in plasma increase as a result of a variety of stressful stimuli, including procedures such as gastroscopy, proctoscopy, pelvic examination, and surgery.[19] Prolactin also rises during parachute jumping, motion sickness, after examinations,[20] and after various sexual stimuli, for example, stimulation of the nipple or areola in women. Like growth hormone, prolactin appears to require more intense stimuli than those leading to increases in catecholamine or cortisol levels. Immune cells also are affected by prolactin—several classes of lymphocytes have prolactin receptors.

Oxytocin

Oxytocin is well known as a hormone produced in high levels by the hypothalamus during childbirth and lactation. It is also produced during orgasm in both sexes and has been shown to promote bonding and social attachment. Oxytocin also has antistress properties, as has been shown in animal experiments where elevations in endogenous oxytocin were associated with reduced hypothalamic-pituitary-adrenal (HPA) activation levels and reduced anxiety.[21] Oxytocin in some tissues works in concert with estrogen; these two hormones have a calming effect during stressful situations.[22] In contrast, another hormone closely resembling oxytocin, vasopressin/ADH, acts in concert with testosterone to increase blood pressure and heart rate, thus enhancing the "fight or flight" stress response. One proposal is that the oxytocin-mediated stress response may promote the "tend and befriend" response, more commonly experienced by women because estrogen is a co-mediator.[23] Studies in animals have identified a wide group of affiliative behaviors involving social encounters, pair bonding, and attachment as being increased by oxytocin. Thus, different effects of stress on males and females may be explained, in part, by gender-related hormonal profiles that dictate to some extent the characteristics, quality, and outcomes of the stress response.

Sex steroids

Testosterone, a hormone secreted by Leydig cells in the testes, regulates male secondary sex characteristics and libido. Levels decrease after stressful stimuli, including anesthesia, surgery, marathon running, and mountain climbing.[24] In addition, psychologic stimuli decrease testosterone levels, and individuals with respiratory failure, burns, and congestive heart failure show a marked reduction in plasma testosterone.[25] Decreased levels of testosterone also occur during aging and is associated with a lower cortisol responsiveness to stress-induced inflammation, suggesting a dysregulation of adaptive physiologic responses to chronic stress in older men.[26] In acute, severe physical stress situations, males may be at a disadvantage because of the presence of testosterone. Males have a higher risk for morbidity after injury, and testosterone exhibits immunosuppressive activity.[25] Estrogen is thought to mediate the more robust immunologic profiles of females,[27] resulting in enhanced resistance to infection but risk for autoimmune diseases.

✔ QUICK CHECK 8-2

1. How does cortisol suppress the inflammatory response?
2. What predictable physiologic abnormalities would be expected in persons with high levels of stress hormones?

Psychoneuroimmunologic Regulation

Psychoneuroimmunology (PNI) is the study of how the consciousness *(psycho)*, brain and spinal cord *(neuro)*, and body's defense against external infection and abnormal cell division *(immunology)* interact. Psychoneuroimmunology assumes that all immune-mediated disease results from interrelationships among psychosocial, emotional, genetic, neurologic, endocrine, and immune systems and behavioral factors. Sufficient data now exists to conclude that immune modulation by psychosocial stressors or interventions leads directly to health outcomes, with the strongest data in the studies of infectious disease and wound healing.[28–32]

The immune system is integrated with other physiologic processes and is sensitive to changes in CNS and endocrine functioning, such as those that accompany psychologic states.[33,34] Stressors can elicit the stress response or **stress system** through the action of the nervous and endocrine systems, specifically corticotropin-releasing hormone (CRH) from the hypothalamus, the sympathetic nervous system, the pituitary gland, and the adrenal gland (see Figure 8-2). CRH is also released peripherally at inflammatory sites and called peripheral or immune CRH. Adaptive energy is redirected to the CNS and stressed body sites. The sympathetic system stimulates the release of norepinephrine throughout the brain, promoting arousal, increased vigilance, increased anxiety, and other protective emotional responses. Reproduction, growth, and thyroid hormone are suppressed during stress and may conserve energy during stress. Emerging is neuropeptide Y (NPY), a sympathetic neurotransmitter, as a stress mediator. Because NPY is a growth factor for many cells, it is implicated in atherosclerosis and tissue remodeling (see *Health Alert:* Chronic Stress, NPY, and Atherosclerosis). The adrenocortical hormones and the sympathetic nervous system may mediate enhancement or suppression of immune functioning.[33–41]

HEALTH ALERT
Chronic Stress, NPY, and Atherosclerosis

Neuropeptide Y (NPY) is a sympathetic neurotransmitter and a stress mediator with multiple activities. Recent is the implication of NPY in atherosclerosis because it not only induces vasoconstriction but also growth promotion, angiogenesis, and tissue remodeling. Various receptors are present on the vascular endothelium, including Y2 receptors specific for NPY. In addition, Y1 receptors present on vascular smooth muscle, when stimulated by NPY, cause angiogenic and proatherosclerotic activities. Unlike norepinephrine, NPY is released after more intense and prolonged nerve activation, such as chronic stress. Animal studies have shown that a low physiologic dose of NPY induces a rapid occlusion of a vessel after angioplasty.

Data from Li L et al: Neuropeptide Y-induced acceleration of postangioplasty occlusion in rat carotid artery, *Arterioscler Thromb Vasc Biol* 23:1204–1210, 2003; Li L et al: Chronic stress induces rapid occlusion of angioplasty-injured rat carotid artery by activating neuropeptide Y and its Y1 receptors, *Arterioscler Thromb Basc Biol* 24:2075–2080, 2005.

Role of the Immune System

Several conditions with variable pathophysiologic characteristics appear to have a common origin[26,42] relating to chronic inflammatory processes. These conditions include cardiovascular disease, osteoporosis, arthritis, type 2 diabetes mellitus, chronic obstructive pulmonary disease (COPD), other diseases associated with aging, and some cancers; all are characterized by the prolonged presence of proinflammatory cytokines.[26,42] (Inflammation is discussed in Chapter 5.) Stress and negative emotions are associated directly with the production of increased levels of proinflammatory cytokines, providing a possible link between stress, immune function, and disease.[43–45] More recent research is focused on the regulatory interactions between the immune system (including cell-derived cytokines) and the nervous and endocrine systems.

The immune, nervous, and endocrine systems communicate through similar pathways involving hormones, neurotransmitters, neuropeptides, and immune cell products. Various components of immune system responses can be affected by neuroendocrine-produced factors involved in the stress reaction. Conversely, immune cell–derived cytokines and other products affect neurocrine and endocrine cells.[33,40,46] Several pathways regulate communication among these systems (Figure 8-4).

The stress response directly influences the immune system through hypothalamic and pituitary peptides and through products of the sympathetic branch of the ANS. Immune cells have surface receptors for ACTH, CRH, endorphins, norepinephrine, growth hormone, steroids, and other products of the stress response.[34] There is direct innervation of the thymus, spleen, lymph nodes, and bone marrow.[40] Cholinergic, adrenergic, and peptidergic nerve terminals are present in the lymphoid organs and tissues. Endogenous opiates are released during stress and have concentration-dependent, enhancing, and suppressive effects on various immune cells.[40,47–50]

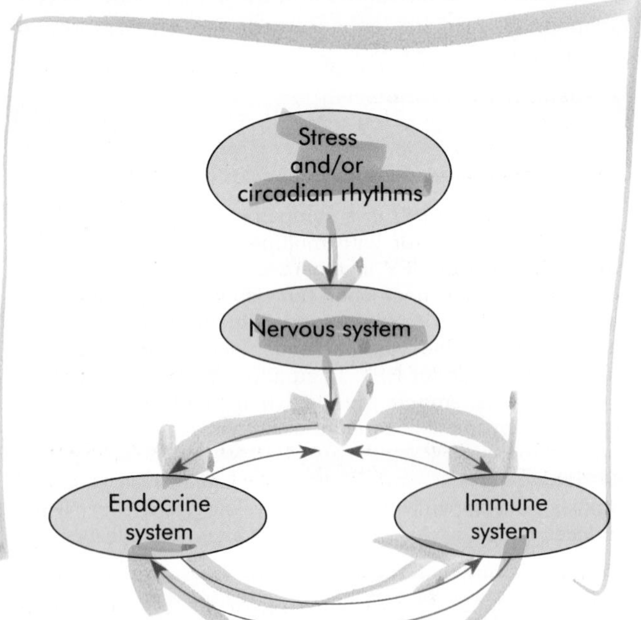

Figure 8-4 ■ Nervous System/Endocrine System/Immune System Interactions. Interconnections or pathways of communication among the immune, nervous, and endocrine systems.

The pineal gland regulates immune response and mediates the apparent effects of circadian rhythm on immunity. When melatonin production is blocked (by continuous light or by pharmacologic means), the immune response is suppressed, whereas administration of melatonin reverses these effects.[51] This immunomodulation pathway may effect immune changes found with sleep disturbance and dysregulated circadian rhythm,[52] which are common among acutely ill and stressed patients.

The hypothalamic-pituitary-adrenal (HPA) axis may produce indirect effects on the CNS that modulate immune responses. The result is profound with prolonged severe stress,[33] including enlargement of the adrenal gland with simultaneous involution of the thymus and lymph nodes. Increased levels of circulating glucocorticosteroids (GCSs) may be an important mechanism in stress-related immune structure alterations and in suppression of the immune response.[33] The GCS level increases are attributable to pituitary ACTH production—a result of increased hypothalamic CRH. A number of stress factors initiate CRH production, including high levels of interleukin-1 (IL-1) and interleukin-6 (IL-6). Production of IL-1 by activated macrophages and monocytes is inhibited by GCS, suggesting a feedback loop with IL-1, CRH, ACTH, and GCS secretion.[40,53]

Lymphocytes also produce ACTH and endorphins in small amounts, which probably influences immune response in an autocrine (same cell stimulation) or paracrine (cell to cell) manner in ongoing immune responses.[40,54] The T cell growth factor, IL-2, can up-regulate pituitary ACTH. Immune-derived cytokines have significant influence on neuroendocrine function, with evidence for direct and indirect cytokine effects on nervous and adrenal cell functions. Thus, the immune system has an adaptive role as a *signal* organ to alert other systems of inner threatening stimuli (e.g., infection, tissue damage, tumor cells) that may upset the dynamic steady state. The release of immune inflammatory mediators (IL-6, tumor necrosis factor-β [TNF-β], interferon) is triggered by bacterial or viral infections, cancer, tissue injury, and other stressors that in turn initiate a stress response through the HPA pathway. Enhanced systemic production of these cytokines also induces other CNS and behavior changes during an acute infectious episode (see p. 213).[55–58]

Neuropeptides and hormones have a significant effect on the immune response. Whether this impact on immune function is suppressive or potentiating depends on the type of factor secreted, with some factors enhancing, some suppressing, and some doing both, depending on the concentration and length of exposure, the target cell, and the specific immune function studies.[55] Neuropeptides and neuroendocrine hormones may directly control biochemical events affecting cell proliferation, differentiation, and function or may indirectly control immune cell behavior by affecting the production or activity of cytokines.[40,46]

Thus, stress-induced immune changes affect many immune cell functions, including decreased natural killer cell and T cell cytotoxicity and impaired B cell function.[59] These impairments in immune function may have dire health consequences for stressed individuals, including increased risk of infection and cancer.[60,61]

STRESS, PERSONALITY, COPING, AND ILLNESS

It is not entirely clear why cortisol secretion during stress is beneficial. Perhaps gluconeogenesis promoted by cortisol ensures an adequate source of glucose (energy) for body tissues, and nerve cells in particular. The pooling of amino acids from catabolized proteins may ensure amino acid availability for protein synthesis in certain cells. The redistribution of protein to sites where replacement is critical, such as muscle or cells of damaged tissue, is beneficial. Short-term, cortisol-induced alterations in immune cell distribution (e.g., traffic) patterns may be adaptive (see p. 213). In addition, with high concentrations of cortisol, decreased immune cell activity (both T cell and B cell) may prevent immune-mediated tissue damage by prolonged cell exposure to high levels of certain cytokines. Whether cortisol-induced effects are adaptive or destructive may depend on the intensity, type, and duration of the stressor and the subsequent concentration and length of cortisol exposure that target cells of the individual experience.

Extreme physiologic stressors, such as severe burn injury, represent a predictable stimulus for stress responses. A less severe and defined event or situation, however, can be a stressor for one person and not for another. Many stressors, such as fasting or temperature changes, do not necessarily cause a physiologic stress response if psychologic factors are minimized. Stress itself is not an independent entity but a system of interdependent processes moderated by the nature, intensity, and duration of the stressor and the perception, appraisal, and coping efficacy of the affected individual, all of which in turn mediate the psychologic and physiologic response to stress.

Psychosocial distress may be predictive of psychologic, social, and physical health outcomes. In **psychologic distress,** the individual feels a general state of unpleasant arousal after life events that manifests as physiologic, emotional, cognitive, and behavior changes. Periods of depression and emotional upheaval often are associated with adverse life events and place the affected individual at risk for immunologic deficits, increasing the risk of ill health.[33] Examples of triggering circumstances include bereavement, academic pressures, and marital conflict. Aging also may increase psychosocial distress and is associated with immune changes (see *AGING & The Stress-Age Syndrome*).[62,63]

HEALTH ALERT
Partner's Survival and Spouse's Hospitalizations and/or Death

A Harvard study shows that a spouse's chances of dying increase not only when the partner dies but when that partner becomes seriously ill. The 9-year follow-up study consisted of 518,240 elderly couples. Mortality after the partner's hospitalization varied according to the spouse's diagnosis. For elderly people whose spouse had been hospitalized, the short-term risk of dying approaches that of an elderly person after his or her spouse's death. A wife's hospitalization increased her husband's chances of dying within 1 month by 35%; a husband's hospitalization increased his wife's chances of dying by 44%. Likewise, a wife's death increased her partner's 1-month mortality risk by 53%, and a husband's death raised his partner's risk by 61%. The researchers commented that a spouse's illness or death can increase a partner's mortality by causing severe stress and removing a primary source of emotional, psychologic, practical, and financial support.

Data from Christakis NA, Allison PD: Mortality after the hospitalization of a spouse, *N Engl J Med* 354(7):719–730, 2006.

AGING &
The Stress-Age Syndrome

With aging, sometimes a set of neurohormonal and immune alterations, as well as tissue and cellular changes, develops. These changes have been defined as stress-age syndrome and include the following:

- Alterations in the excitability of structures of the limbic system and hypothalamus

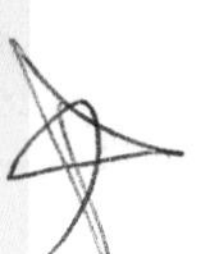

- Rise of the blood concentration of catecholamines, ADH, ACTH, and cortisol
- Decrease of testosterone, thyroxine, and others
- Alterations of opioid peptides
- Immunodepression and pattern of chronic inflammation
- Alterations in lipoproteins
- Hypercoagulation of the blood
- Free radical damage of cells

Some of the alterations are adaptational, whereas others are potentially damaging. These stress-related alterations of aging can influence the course of developing stress reactions and lower adaptive reserve and coping.

Data from Frolkis VV: Stress-age syndrome, *Mech Ageing Dev* 69(1–2):93–107, 1993.
ADH, Antidiuretic hormone; *ACTH,* adrenocorticotropic hormone.

Stressful life events and mood have been reported as important factors preceding the onset or exacerbation of symptoms in acquired immune deficiency syndrome (AIDS) infection, diabetes, and multiple sclerosis.[64–66] In addition, the interaction with health care providers in a clinical setting, the diagnosis of a major illness, and various clinical procedures (e.g., blood sampling, injections, examinations, surgical procedures) may represent significant negative life events to many individuals (Figure 8-5). These additional stresses may interfere with the efficacy of the

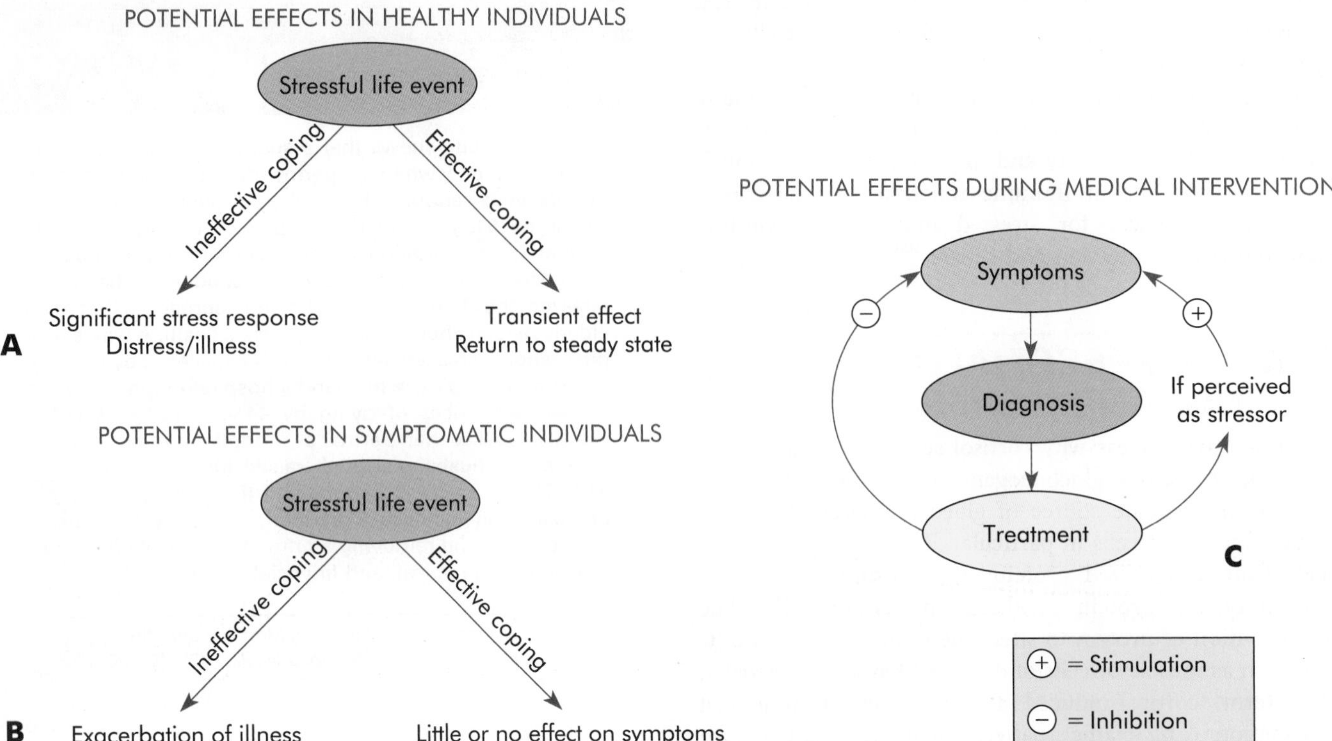

Figure 8-5 ■ **Health Outcome Determination in Stressful Life Situations Is Moderated by Numerous Factors.** Whether a life-challenged individual experiences distress or illness depends on the subject's appraisal of the event and the coping strategies used during the stressful period. Models **A** and **B** reflect possible outcomes in stressed healthy and symptomatic individuals. Model **C** illustrates the dynamic clinical setting in which the diagnosis of a serious illness and subsequent medical interventions may be perceived as stressful challenges and have potentially detrimental influences on physical outcome.

medical intervention. Identifying and reducing stress in the clinical setting have particular applicability for both preventing disease and managing illness.

Personality characteristics are associated with individual differences in appraisal and response to stressors.[34] Specific personality characteristics, such as academic achievement, motivation, and aggression, are correlated with immunologic alterations. For example, aggression was positively associated with changes in T and B cell numbers in male military personnel.[67]

A beneficial influence during stress has been shown with adaptive coping strategies, especially if they are problem focused and involve social support.[68–73] **Coping** is the process of managing stressful challenges that tax the individual's resources.[68] Adverse consequences of stress may be minimized by coping styles. Coping styles associated with altered immunity include repression, denial, escape-avoidance, and concealment.[34] Repression was associated with lower monocyte counts, higher eosinophil counts, higher serum glucose, and more self-reported medication reactions in medical outpatients[74] and with higher Epstein-Barr virus (EBV) antibody titers in students.[75] A prospective long-term study found increased markers of accelerated human immunodeficiency virus (HIV) infection in gay men who concealed their homosexual identity.[76]

Mediating factors that may influence stress susceptibility or resilience include age, socioeconomic status, gender, social support, religious or spiritual factors, personality, self-esteem, genetics, past experiences, and current health status. Evidence suggests that effective intervention may result in greater stress resilience and improved psychologic and physiologic outcomes.[77] For example, women with recurrent metastatic breast cancer who were provided weekly group counseling in addition to routine medical treatment lived an average of 19 months longer than control subjects.[73,78]

The importance of social support for seriously ill individuals has focused attention also on the health of caregivers. Significant stress manifested as depression, anxiety, and fatigue has been noted in family caregivers of those with cancer, Alzheimer disease, and burn trauma. Patients and caregivers exhibited suppression of various measures of immune function, with improved function associated with better perceived social support.[69–73] Gender-based coping differences may be attributed, in part, to the hormonal milieu of the individual, with females more likely to offer social support, a behavior with an oxytocin/estrogen association.[23]

Interventions to potentially prevent or manage stress-related psychologic or physical problems include both short- and long-term coping strategies. Educational components are specific to the individual's problems. Relaxation techniques may include meditation, imagery, massage, and biofeedback. These approaches may be used on an individual or support group basis. Incorporation of these approaches into clinical training facilitates their use in the clinical arena. Future research should focus on the efficacy of such approaches with various populations.

QUICK CHECK 8-3

1. Define psychoneuroimmunology.
2. How does the immune system participate in stress-related diseases?
3. Why are stress-related diseases a problem?
4. Why do stress-related diseases occur?
5. What intervention or prevention activities reduce stress-related diseases?

Did You Understand?

Concepts of Stress

1. Stress recently has been defined as the state of affairs arising when a person relates to (i.e., interacts or transacts with) situations in a certain way. How he or she appraises and reacts to situations is important.
2. Hans Selye identified three structural changes in rats subjected repeatedly to noxious stimuli (stressors): (1) enlargement of the cortex of the adrenal gland, (2) atrophy of the thymus gland and other lymphoid tissues, and (3) gastrointestinal ulceration.
3. Selye believed that the three changes were caused by a nonspecific physiologic response to any long-term stressor. He called this response the general adaptation syndrome (GAS).
4. The GAS occurs in three stages: (1) the alarm stage, (2) the stage of resistance or adaptation, and (3) the stage of exhaustion. Diseases of adaptation develop if the stage of resistance or adaptation does not restore homeostasis.
5. Selye identified three components of physiologic stress: the stressor, the physiologic or chemical disturbance produced by the stressor, and the body's adaptational response to the stressor.
6. Other investigators have shown that the physiologic stress response also occurs in response to psychologic or emotional stress.
7. Psychologic stressors can be anticipatory and triggered by anticipation of an upcoming stressor or it can be reactive to a stressor. Both of these psychologic stressors are capable of eliciting a physiologic stress response.

The Stress Response

1. The stress response involves the nervous system (sympathetic branch of the autonomic nervous system), the endocrine system (pituitary and adrenal glands), and the immune system.
2. The stress response is initiated when a stressor is present in the body or perceived by the mind.
3. The neuroendocrine response to stress consists of sympathetic stimulation of the adrenal medulla to secrete catecholamines (norepinephrine, epinephrine, neuropeptide Y) and stressor-induced stimulation of the pituitary to secrete ACTH, which in turn stimulates the adrenal cortex to secrete steroid hormones, particularly cortisol.
4. In general, the catecholamines prepare the body to act, and cortisol mobilizes energy (glucose) and other substances needed to fuel the action.
5. Epinephrine exerts its chief effects on the cardiovascular system. Epinephrine increases cardiac output and increases blood flow to the heart, brain, and skeletal muscles by dilating vessels that supply these organs. It also dilates the airways, thereby increasing delivery of oxygen to the bloodstream.
6. Norepinephrine's chief effects complement those of epinephrine. Norepinephrine constricts blood vessels of the viscera and skin; this has the effect of shifting blood flow to the vessels dilated by epinephrine. Norepinephrine also increases mental alertness.
7. Cortisol's chief effects involve metabolic processes. By inhibiting the use of metabolic substances while promoting their formation, cortisol mobilizes glucose, amino acids, lipids, and fatty acids and delivers them to the bloodstream. Cortisol at low levels consistent with stress increase humoral immunity, may activate proinflammatory mediators, and decrease cellular immunity. Cortisol at high levels (e.g., therapeutic levels) decreases both humoral and cellular immunity and is anti-inflammatory.
8. The nervous, endocrine, and immune systems communicate through the common use of signal molecules and their receptors, which in turn regulate the behavior of cells in each system during stress challenge.
9. There are direct and indirect pathways of influence among the nervous, endocrine, and immune systems. Neuropeptides have direct effects on immune cells, as well as indirect influences through neurologically mediated endocrine modulation of immune function. Endocrine products (cortisol) also influence neurologic cell behavior. Immune cell products affect both nervous and endocrine cell function, reflecting an adaptive role for the immune system as a "signal" organ to alert other systems of threatening stimuli.
10. Other hormones are affected by the stress response; these include increased circulating levels of β-endorphins, growth hormone, prolactin, oxytocin, and antidiuretic hormone. Testosterone decreases during the stress response.

Stress, Personality, Coping, and Illness

1. Stress is a system of interdependent processes that are moderated by the nature, intensity, and duration of the stressor and coping efficacy of the affected individual, all of which in turn mediate the psychologic and physiologic response to stress.

(Continued)

Did You Understand?—Cont'd

2. Personality characteristics are associated with individual differences in appraisal and response to stressors.
3. Coping styles associated with altered immunity include repression, denial, escape-avoidance, and concealment.
4. Many studies have linked psychologic distress with altered immune function, and there is now evidence that strengthens the association of stress with potential for illness in humans.

AGING & Stress-Age Syndrome

1. With aging, often a set of neurohormonal and immune alterations including tissue and cellular changes occur. These changes are collectively called stress-age syndromes.
2. The changes are numerous, with some being adaptational whereas others are potentially damaging.

Key Terms

Alarm stage, 209
Anticipatory response, 211
Coping, 218
Corticotrophin-releasing hormone (CRH), 213
Diseases of adaptation, 209
General adaptation syndrome (GAS), 209
Homeostasis, 211
Peripheral (immune) CRH, 213
Permissive, 212
Physiologic stress, 211
Psychologic distress, 217
Psychoneuroimmunology (PNI), 215
Psychosocial distress, 217
Reactive response, 211
Stage of exhaustion, 209
Stage of resistance or adaptation, 209
Stress response, 211
Stress system, 215
Stressor, 209
Th2 shift, 213

References

1. Cannon WB, Bringer CAL, Fritz R: Experimental hyperthyroidism, *Am J Physiol* 36:363, 1914.
2. Selye H: The general adaptation syndrome and the diseases of adaptation, *J Clin Endocrinol* 6:117–230, 1946.
3. Bruunsgard H, Pedersen BK: Age-related inflammatory cytokines and disease, *Immunol Allergy Clin North Am* 23(1): 15–39, 2003.
4. Herman JP et al: Central mechanisms of stress integration: hierarchical circuitry controlling hypothalamo-pituitary-adrenocortical responsiveness, *Front Neuroendocrinol* 24 (3):151–158, 2003.
5. Elenkov IJ et al: Cytokine dysregulation, inflammation, and well-being, *Neuroimmunomodulation* 12(5):255–269, 2005.
6. Fearon DT, Locksley RM: The instructive role of innate immunity in the acquired immune response (review), *Science* 272(5258):50–53, 1996.
7. Mosmann TR, Sad S: The expanding universe of T-cell subsets: Th1, Th2, and more (review), *Immunol Today* 17(3): 138–146, 1996.
8. Calcagni E, Elenkov I: Stress system activity, innate and T helper cytokines, and susceptibility to immune-related diseases (review), *Ann NY Acad Sci* 1069:62–76, 2006.
9. Lagier B et al: Different modulation by histamine of IL-4 and interferon-gamma (IFN-gamma) release according to the phenotype of human Th0, Th1, and Th2 clones, *Clin Exp Immunol* 108(3):545–551, 1997.
10. In: Rocklin RE (Ed. (1990). *Histamine and H_2 antagonists in inflammation and immunodeficiency* New York, 1990, Mercel Dekker.
11. Molina PE: Stress-specific opioid modulation of haemodynamic counter-regulation, *Clin Exp Pharmacol Physiol* 29(3): 248–253, 2002.
12. Jochem J, Josko J, Gwozdz B: Endogenous opioid peptides system in haemorrhagic shock—central cardiovascular regulation, *Med Sci Monit* 7(3):545–549, 2001.
13. Molina PE: Opiate modulation of hemodynamic, hormonal, and cytokine responses to hemorrhage, *Shock* 15(6):471–478, 2001.
14. Burguera B et al: Dual and selective actions of glucocorticoid upon basal and stimulated growth hormone release in man, *Neuroendocrinology* 51(1):51–58, 1990.
15. Amico JA, Mantella RC, Vollmer RR, Li X:*Anxiety and stress responses in female oxytocin deficient mice* 16(4):319–324, 2004(review).
16. Liu Y et al: Differential expression of vasopressin, oxytocin, and corticotropin-releasing hormone messenger RNA in the paraventricular nucleus of the prairie vole brain following stress, *J Neuroendocrinol* 13(12):1059–1065, 2001.
17. Taylor SE et al: Biobehavioral responses to stress in females: tend-and-befriend, not fight-or-flight, *Psychol Rev* 107(3): 411–429, 2000.
18. Angele MK, Chaudry IH: Surgical trauma and immunosuppression: pathophysiology and potential immunomodulatory approaches (review), *Langenbecks Arch Chir* 390(4):333–341, 2005.
19. Rohleder N et al: Age and sex steroid-related changes in glucocorticoid sensitivity of proinflammatory cytokine production after psychosocial stress, *J Neuroimmunol* 126 (1–2):69–77, 2002.
20. Bone RC: Toward an epidemiology and natural history of SIRS (systemic inflammatory response syndrome), *JAMA* 268(24):3452–3455, 1992.
21. Marucha PT, Kiecolt-Glaser JK, Favagehi M: Mucosal wound healing is impaired by examination stress, *Psychosom Med* 60(3):362–365, 1998.
22. Repka-Ramirez MS, Baraniuk JN: Histamine in health and disease, *Clin Allergy Immunol* 17:1–17, 2002.
23. Kiecolt-Glaser JK et al: Psychoneuroimmunology and psychosomatic medicine: back to the future (review), *Psychosom Med* 64(1):15–28, 2002.
24. Chesnokova V, Melmed S: Mini review: neuro-immmunoendocrine modulation of the hypothalamic-pituitary-adrenal axis (HPA) by gp130 signaling molecules (review), *Endocrinology* 143(5):1571–1574, 2002.
25. Bauer-Wu SM: Psychoneuroimmunology. Part I: physiology, *Clin J Oncol Nurs* 6(3):167–170, 2002.

References—Cont'd

26. Bauer-Wu SM: Psychoneuroimmunology. Part II: mind-body interventions, *Clin J Oncol Nurs* 6(4):243–246, 2002.
27. Chambers DA, Cohen RL, Perlman RL: Neuroimmune modulation: signal transduction and catecholamines, *Neurochem Int* 22(2):95–110, 1993.
28. Cacioppo JT et al: Autonomic, neuroendocrine, and immune responses to psychological stress: the reactivity hypothesis, *Ann N Y Acad Sci* 840:664–673, 1998.
29. Calcagni E, Elenkov I: Stress system activity, innate and T helper cytokines, and susceptibility to immune-related diseases (review), *Annal NY Acad Sci* 1069:62–76, 2006.
30. Maier SF, Watkins LR: Cytokines for psychologists: implications of bidirectional immune-to-brain communication for understanding behavior, mood, and cognition, *Psychol Rev* 105(1):83–107, 1998.
31. Charmandari E, Tsigos C, Chrousos G: Endocrinology of the stress response (review), *Annual Review of Physiology* 67:259–284, 2005.
32. Carrillo-Vico A, Guerrero JM, Lardone PJ, Reiter RJ: A review of the multiple actions of melatonin on the immune system (review), *Endocrine* 27(2):189–200, 2005.
33. Shelby J, Ku WW, Nielson HC: Neurohormone and neuropeptide regulation of the post-traumatic immune response, In: Faist E, Ed.. *Host defense alterations of trauma, shock, and sepsis: multi-organ failure/immunotherapy of sepsis,* Berlin, 1996, Pabst.
34. Sundar SK et al: Brain IL-1-induced immunosuppression occurs through activation of both pituitary-adrenal axis and sympathetic nervous system by corticotropin-releasing factor, *J Neurosci* 10(11):3701–3706, 1990.
35. Weigent DA, Carr DJ, Blalock JE: Bidirectional communication between the neuroendocrine and immune systems: common hormones and hormone receptors, *Ann N Y Acad Sci* 579:17–27, 1990.
36. Kusnecov AW, Goldfarb Y: Neural and behavioral responses to systemic immunologic stimuli: a consideration of bacterial T cell superantigens (review), *Current Pharmaceutical Design* 11(8):1039–1046, 2005.
37. Hori T et al: Immune cytokines and regulation of body temperature, food intake, and cellular immunity, *Brain Res Bull* 27(3-4):309–313, 1991.
38. Navarra P et al: Interleukins-1 and -6 stimulate the release of corticotropin-releasing hormone-41 from rat hypothalamus in vitro via the eicosanoid cyclooxygenase pathway, *Endocrinology* 128(1):37–44, 1991.
39. Kiecolt-Glaser JK et al: Psychoneuroimmunology: psychological influences on immune function and health, *J Consult Clin Psychol* 70(3):537–547, 2002.
40. Reiche EMV, Nunes SOV, Morimoto HK: Stress, depression, the immune system, and cancer (review), *Lancet Oncology* 5 (10):617–625, 2004.
41. Teicher MH et al: Developmental neurobiology of childhood stress and trauma, *Psych Clin North Am* 25(2):297–426, vii-viii, 2002.
42. Frolkis VV: Stress-age syndrome, *Mech Ageing Dev* 69(1-2): 93–107, 1993.
43. Hirokawa K: Reversing and restoring immune functions, *Mech Ageing Dev* 93(1-3):119–124, 1997.
44. Kopnisky KL, Stoff DM, Rausch DM: Workshop report: The effects of psychological variables on the progression of HIV-1 disease, *Brain, Behavior, & Immunity* 18(3):246–261, 2004.
45. Wellen KE, Hotamisligil GS: Inflammation, stress, and diabetes, *Journal of Clinical Investigation* 115(5):1111–1119, 2005.
46. Coyle PK: The neuroimmunology of multiple sclerosis, *Adv Neuroimmunol* 6(2):143–154, 1996.
47. Granger DA, Booth A, Johnson DR: Human aggression and enumerative measures of immunity, *Psychosomc Med* 62 (4):583–590, 2000.
48. Folkman S, Lazarus RS: The relationship between coping and emotion: implications for theory and research, *Soc Sci Med* 26(3):309–317, 1988.
49. Baron RS et al: Social support and immune function among spouses of cancer patients, *J Pers Soc Psychol* 59(2):344–352, 1990.
50. Fawzy FI et al: Malignant melanoma: effects of an early structured psychiatric intervention, coping, and affective state on recurrence and survival 6 years later, *Arch Gen Psychiatry* 50(9):681–689, 1993.
51. Spiegel D et al: Effects of psychosocial treatment in prolonging cancer survival may be mediated by neuroimmune pathways, *Ann N Y Acad Sci* 840:674–683, 1998.
52. Jamner LD, Schwartz GE, Leigh H: The relationship between repressive and defensive coping styles and monocyte, eosinophil, and serum glucose levels: support for the opioid peptide hypothesis of regression, *Psychosom Med* 50(6): 567–575, 1988.
53. Esterling B et al: Emotional repression, stress disclosure responses, and Epstein-Barr viral capsid antigen titers, *Psychosom Med* 52(4):397–410, 1990.
54. Cole SW et al: Accelerated course of human immunodeficiency virus infection in gay men who conceal their homosexual identity, *Psychosom Med* 58(3):219–231, 1996.
55. Spiegel D: Psychosocial aspects of breast cancer treatment, *Semin Oncol* 24(1, suppl 1):S1-36–S1-47, 1997.

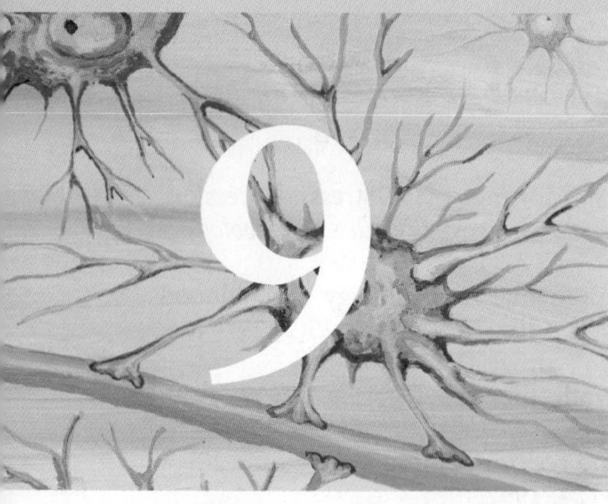

9 BIOLOGY OF CANCER AND TUMOR SPREAD

David M. Virshup ▪ Kathryn L. McCance

CHAPTER OUTLINE

ELECTRONIC RESOURCES

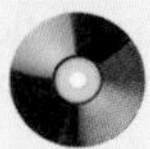

Companion CD
- Review Questions and Answers
- Animations

evolve Website
http://evolve.elsevier.com/Huether/
- Quick Check Answers
- Key Terms Exercises
- Critical Thinking Questions with Answers
- Algorithm Completion Exercises
- WebLinks

Cancer is a leading disease of adults in the Western world. The risk of developing cancer increases markedly with age. Since the 1970s, intensive research has led to a much improved understanding of this complex and frightening disease. We now understand that cancer is a collection of many different diseases, all caused by an accumulation of genetic alterations. Environment and heredity interact to modify both the risk of developing cancer and the response to treatment. Increased understanding of the basic pathophysiology of cancer has contributed to the number of effective therapies available to treat this dreaded disorder.

CANCER CHARACTERISTICS AND TERMINOLOGY

Any discussion of cancer must start with a definition of what it is and what it is not. Although most readers may have an intuitive understanding of this disorder, an exact definition that encompasses this broad category is more challenging. A definition from 1922 may summarize cancer as well as any:

The most generally accepted definition of a tumor is that it is a tissue overgrowth that is independent of the laws governing the remainder of the body. It is usual to add as a qualifying phrase to separate tumors from reparative processes, such as bone callus, that the neoplasm overgrowth serves no useful purpose to the organism.[1]

The term **cancer** derives from the Greek word for crab, *Karkinoma*, which the physician Hippocrates used to describe the appendage-like projections extending from tumors. The word **tumor** originally referred to any swelling—for example, that caused by inflammation—but is now generally reserved for a new growth, or **neoplasm**. Not all tumors or neoplasms, however, are cancer. The term *cancer* refers to any malignant tumor, or neoplasm, and is not used to refer to benign growths such as lipomas, meningiomas, or hypertrophy of an organ. Yet it is important to recognize that benign neoplasms also can cause life-threatening symptoms if they enlarge in critical locations. For example, a benign meningioma at the base of the skull may cause devastating symptoms by compressing the adjacent normal brain. The definitions of benign versus malignant are presented next and in Table 9-1.

Tumor Classification and Nomenclature

Benign tumors are not called cancers. **Benign tumors** are usually well encapsulated and well differentiated, retain some normal tissue structure, and do not invade the capsule, nor do they spread to regional lymph nodes or distant locations. Benign tumors are generally named according to the tissues from which they arise, with the suffix *oma*. For example, a benign tumor of the smooth muscle of the uterus is a leiomyoma, and a benign tumor of fat cells is a lipoma. Some benign tumors can progress to cancer, however.

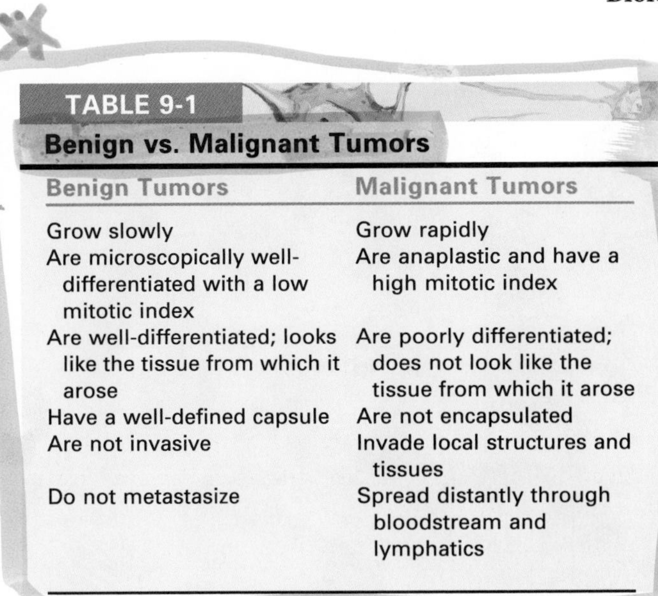

TABLE 9-1
Benign vs. Malignant Tumors

Benign Tumors	Malignant Tumors
Grow slowly	Grow rapidly
Are microscopically well-differentiated with a low mitotic index	Are anaplastic and have a high mitotic index
Are well-differentiated; looks like the tissue from which it arose	Are poorly differentiated; does not look like the tissue from which it arose
Have a well-defined capsule	Are not encapsulated
Are not invasive	Invade local structures and tissues
Do not metastasize	Spread distantly through bloodstream and lymphatics

Malignant tumors are distinguished from benign tumors by more rapid growth rates and specific microscopic alterations, including loss of differentiation; absence of normal tissue organization; lack of a capsule; invasion into blood vessels, lymphatics, and surrounding structures; and distant spread *(metastasis)*. One of the hallmarks of malignant cells is anaplasia, the loss of differentiation, nuclear irregularities, and loss of normal tissue structure. Table 9-1 and Figures 9-1 and 9-2 explain and illustrate some key differences between benign and malignant tumors.

Cancers are named according to the cell type of origin (Table 9-2). Cancers arising in epithelial tissue are called **carcinomas,** and those that arise from ductal or glandular epithelium are named **adenocarcinomas.** Hence, a malignant tumor arising from breast glandular tissue is a mammary adenocarcinoma. Cancers arising from connective tissue usually have the suffix **sarcoma.** For example, malignant cancers of skeletal muscle are termed *rhabdomyosarcomas.* Cancers of lymphatic tissue are **lymphomas,** whereas cancers of blood-forming cells are known as **leukemias.** However, there are many other cancers named for historical reasons (e.g., Hodgkin disease, Ewing sarcoma) that do not follow this naming convention.

Carcinoma in situ (often abbreviated CIS) (see Figure 9-1) refers to preinvasive epithelial tumors of glandular or squamous cell origin. These early stage tumors have not broken through basement membranes of the epithelium. Carcinoma in situ can be found in the cervix, skin, oral cavity, esophagus, and bronchus. In glandular

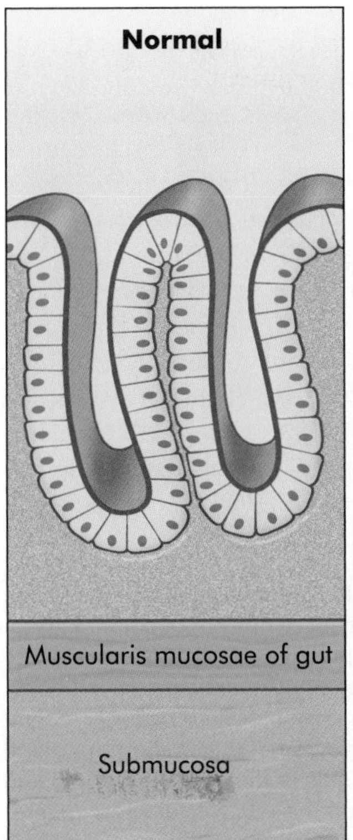

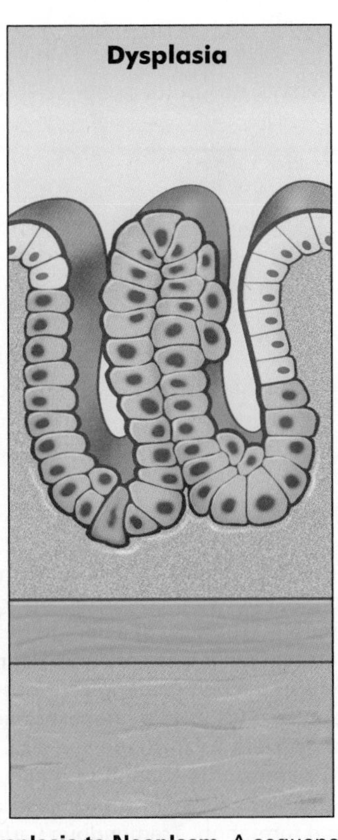

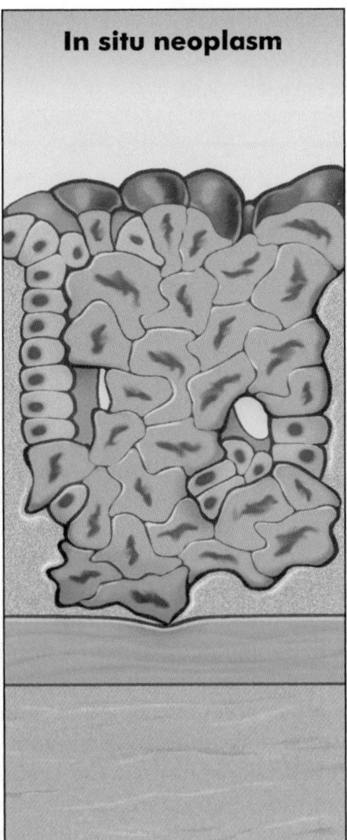

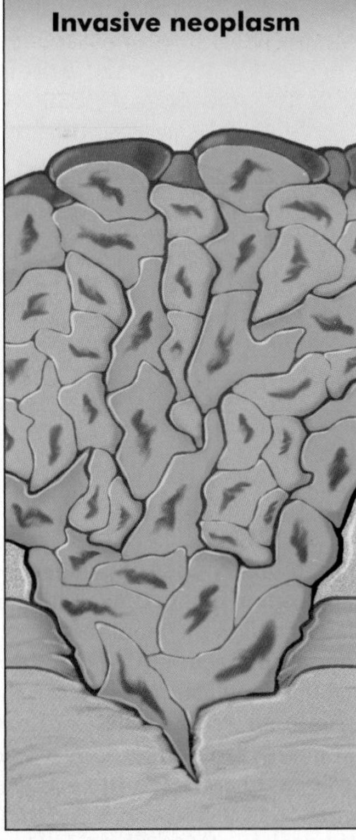

Figure 9-1 ■ **Progression of Dysplasia to Neoplasm.** A sequence of cellular and tissue changes progressing from dysplasia to in situ neoplasia and then to invasive neoplasia is seen often in the development of cancer. In this diagram, as in real life, distinguishing between dysplasia and in situ neoplasia is difficult. Loss of normal tissue architecture signifies development of neoplasia. The in situ neoplasms are most commonly found in the squamous epithelium of the uterine cervix, the epidermis of sun-exposed skin, and colonic and gastric mucosa after long-standing inflammation. The altered cell turnover during inflammation probably allows local environmental factors to cause genetic abnormalities leading to neoplasia. (Modified from Stevens A, Lowe J: *Pathology: illustrated review in color,* ed 2, Edinburgh, 2000, Mosby.)

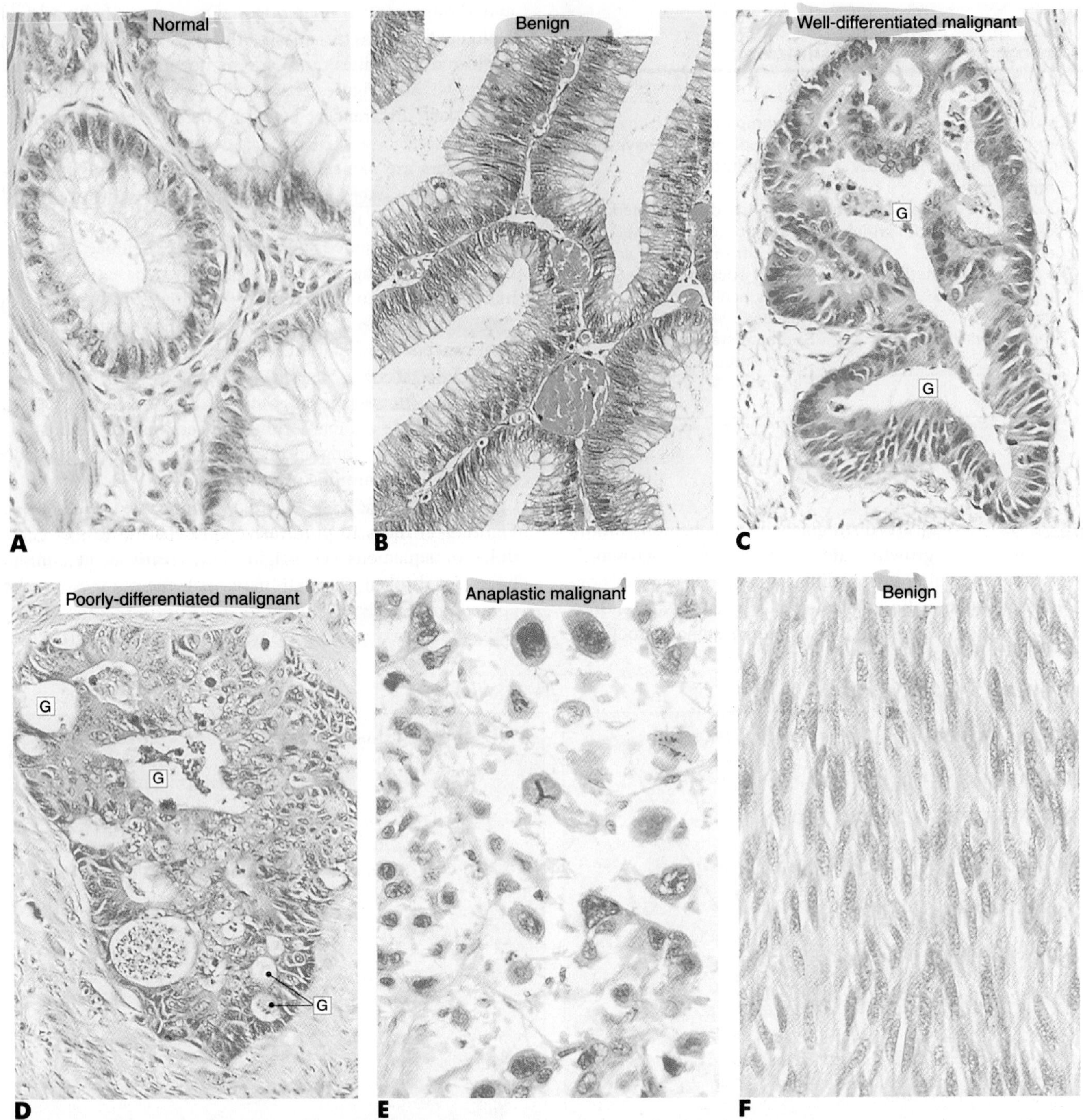

Figure 9-2 ■ **Loss of Cellular and Tissue Differentiation During the Development of Cancer. A,** Normal colonic epithelium. **B,** Benign neoplasm of colon. **C,** Well-differentiated malignant neoplasm of colon. **D,** Poorly differentiated malignant neoplasm of colon. **E,** Anaplastic malignant neoplasm of colon. **F,** Benign neoplasm of smooth muscle. The cells of a benign neoplasm **(B)** resemble those of the normal epithelium **(A)** in that they are columnar and have an orderly arrangement. Loss of some degree of differentiation is evident in that the neoplastic cells do not show much mucin vacuolation. The cells of the benign neoplasm of smooth muscle **(F)** closely resemble normal muscle cells. Cells of the well-differentiated malignant neoplasm **(C)** have a haphazard arrangement, and although gland lumina *(G)* are formed, they are architecturally abnormal and irregular. Nuclei vary in shape and size. Cells in the poorly differentiated malignant neoplasm **(D)** have an even more haphazard arrangement, with poor formation of gland lumina *(G)*. Nuclei show greater variation in shape and size compared with the well-differentiated malignant neoplasm **(C)**. Cells in anaplastic malignant neoplasms **(E)** bear no relation to the normal epithelium, with no attempt at gland formation. Tremendous variation is found in the size of cells and nuclei, with intense staining *(nuclear hyperchromatism)* of the latter. Not knowing the site of origin would make it impossible to tell what sort of tumor this was by microscopic appearance alone. Well-differentiated tumors often resemble their cell of origin, as shown in the example of a benign tumor of smooth muscle **(F)**. (From Stevens A, Lowe J: *Pathology: illustrated review in color,* ed 2, Edinburgh, 2000, Mosby.)

TABLE 9-2

Examples of Tumor Nomenclature

Cell/Tissue	Origin
Carcinomas	Arise from endothelial and epithelial tissues, such as hepatocellular carcinoma
Sarcomas	Arise from mesenchymal (connective) tissues, such as osteogenic sarcoma, leiomyosarcoma
Adenocarcinomas	Carcinomas arising from glandular or ductal epithelium, such as mammary adenocarcinoma
Terato-	Arise from germ cells (teratocarcinoma)

epithelium, in situ lesions occur in the stomach, endometrium, breast, and large bowel. These lesions may erroneously be confused with benign tumors, but both the squamous and glandular cell types show cellular disorganization and atypia. The length of time that such lesions remain in situ before becoming invasive is unknown. Some carcinomas of the cervix are known to be preinvasive lesions in situ for several years before they progress to invasive carcinoma or metastatic tumors (see Figure 9-1).

Stages of Cancer Spread

Staging the cancer is an important component of diagnosis and treatment planning (Box 9-1). Diverse schemes are employed for staging different tumors. In general, a four-stage system is used, with carcinoma in situ regarded as a special case. Cancer confined to the organ of origin is stage 1; cancer that is locally invasive is stage 2, or B; cancer that has spread to regional structures such as lymph nodes is stage 3, or C; and cancer that has spread to distant sites, such as a liver cancer spreading to lung or a prostate cancer spreading to bone, is stage 4, or D (Figure 9-3). In general, the earlier the stage, the more amenable the cancer is to treatment and the better the chance for cure.

Cell Differentiation

Cancer cells are defined by two heritable properties: autonomy and anaplasia. **Autonomy** refers to the cancer cell's independence from normal cellular controls. Anaplasia is the loss of differentiation, which is the process of developing specialized functions and organization (see

BOX 9-1 **Diagnosis and Clinical Staging of Cancer**

Diagnosis

Cancer is an uncontrolled clonal proliferation of cells that can arise from virtually any cell type in the body. Because of the large variety of cell types in the body, cancer is a diverse set of different diseases that can come to medical attention by a number of routes. Some cancers can be detected at early stages by screening procedures such as skin inspection, blood tests (e.g., prostate-specific antigen, or PSA), and routine colonoscopy. Others come to attention because of symptoms. The symptoms a person develops depend on where the cancer occurs. Benign tumors in the brain may cause neurologic disturbances despite being quite small, whereas malignant cancers in the abdomen (e.g., ovarian, pancreatic, kidney, and liver cancers) may not be detected until they are quite advanced. Symptoms can be caused by the size of the tumor, whether it presses on a nearby vital structure (e.g., pressure on nerves may cause pain and erosion of bone can led to pathologic fractures), or by loss of function of an organ. For example, individuals with leukemia seek medical attention when their bone marrow has been replaced by leukemia cells and no longer functions normally. This physiologic change leads to pallor and fatigue resulting from anemia, bleeding caused by low platelets, and infection related to loss of white blood cells. Sometimes cancers are detected when symptoms are caused by metastasis rather than the primary tumor or when a small tumor secretes hormones (e.g., insulin, epinephrine) that cause symptoms.

Cancers must be diagnosed correctly to provide useful information to the individual and to the treating medical team. Accurate and in-depth diagnosis allows a better understanding of the causes of cancer, as well as optimizing the therapy. Finally, an accurate diagnosis allows predictions about how the cancer will behave over time, including how likely it is to respond to treatment (the prognosis), and where it might spread (metastasis). With rare exceptions, the diagnosis of cancer requires that the pathologist examine tissue (a biopsy) obtained from the patient. Tissue can be obtained by diverse means, including brushings (e.g., the Pap smear), fine needle aspirations (e.g., of a thyroid or breast mass), core needle or open biopsies that sample a small part of a mass, or complete excision of a mass. To examine the tissue, the pathologist first inspects stained sections under the light microscope to determine whether the tissue is benign or malignant. More sophisticated testing may include immunostaining to identify the tissue of origin, various DNA tests to determine specific genetic lesions, analysis of chromosome number and integrity, and gene expression profiling. For example, a tumor arising from muscle will react with antibodies against muscle-specific proteins, whereas a tumor arising from nerves will react with nerve-specific antibodies. In some cases, specific chromosomal or genetic alterations can be detected that help classify the tumor.

Clinical Staging

The information obtained from the pathologic diagnosis is combined with clinical information to determine the extent of the cancer. **Clinical staging** refers to the combination of physical findings, laboratory testing, and imaging studies that reveal whether the cancer has spread locally or to distant locations. The final diagnosis and clinical staging is therefore based on a broad range of information including the organ and tissue of origin (e.g., medullary thyroid versus papillary thyroid carcinoma); whether it is benign or malignant, and if it is malignant, whether it is well, moderately well, or poorly differentiated; and whether it has spread beyond the site of origin to distant sites (see Figure 9-3).

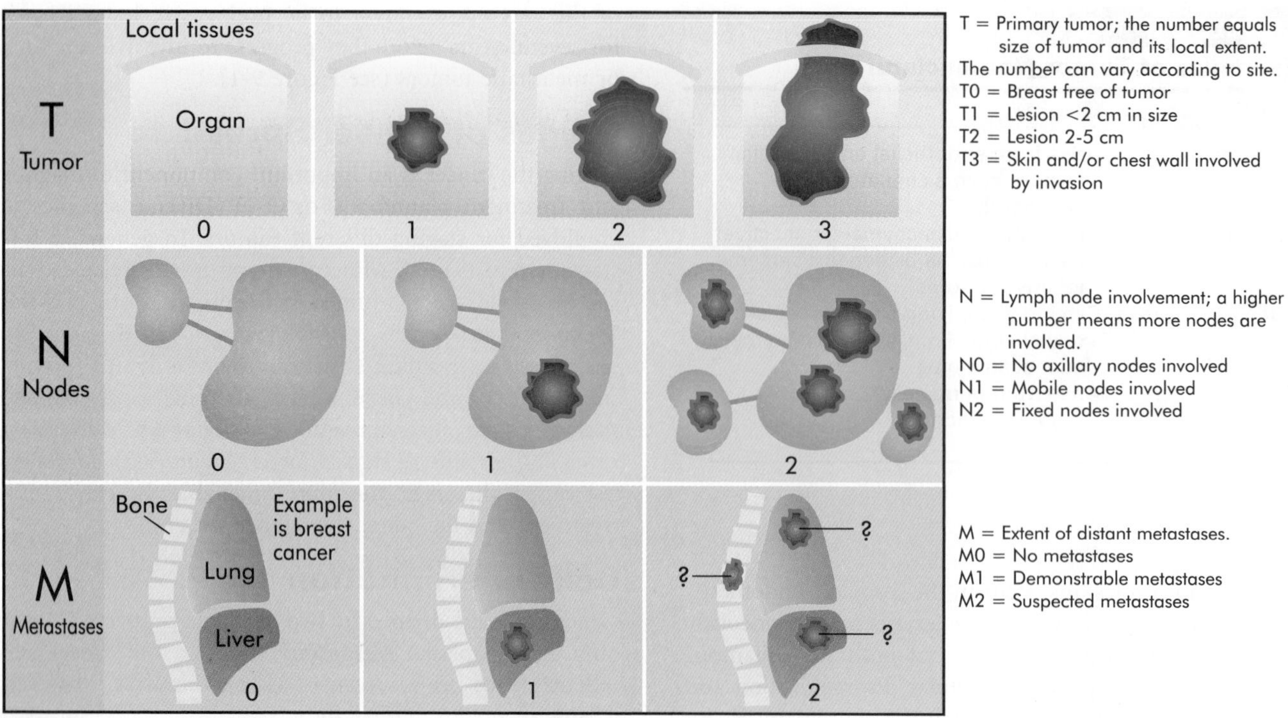

Figure 9-3 ■ **Tumor Staging by the TNM System.** Example of staging for breast cancer. (See the figure for explanation of the abbreviations.)

Figure 9-2). **Anaplasia** means literally "without form." In clinical specimens, anaplasia is recognized by a marked increase in nuclear size, with evidence of ongoing proliferation such as mitotic figures. In contrast to normal cells, which are uniform in size and shape, anaplastic cells are of variable size and shape, or **pleomorphic** (Figure 9-4). For example, a benign bone tumor retains the ability to make bone, whereas in a malignant bone tumor, new bone formation is seen only rarely. Thus, the bone cancer cells are undifferentiated as compared with the tissue they originated from. The most malignant tumors tend to have the most *anaplasia.* Figures 9-2 and 9-4 illustrate the loss of differentiation and cellular heterogeneity seen in anaplastic cancers of the colon and skeletal muscle.

As cells mature, they differentiate to perform the specific functions of the tissue they constitute. In comparison, cells within a developing embryo display the least amount of differentiation. In the adult, *undifferentiated cells* (not totally committed to a specific function) are known as *pluripotent cells, precursor cells,* or *stem cells* (Figure 9-5). As a cell becomes more differentiated, it loses its ability to replicate. Cancer cells act more like embryonic or precursor cells; they are less differentiated and divide more frequently. In some tissues, rapid growth and differentiation occurs in a matter of days. For example, in the epidermis, the intestinal epithelium, and the blood cells produced in the bone marrow, terminally differentiated cells die within several days to months and are regularly replaced by a new crop of cells arising from the local stem cells. A block in the ability to terminally differentiate may contribute to many of the cancers arising in these rapidly proliferating tissues.

Tumor Markers

Tumor markers (biologic markers) are substances produced by cancer cells that are found on tumor plasma membranes or in the blood, spinal fluid, or urine (Table 9-3). Tumor markers have been associated with cancer for many decades. For diseases that have a blood-based tumor marker, there is indeed a blood test for cancer. Tumor markers include hormones, enzymes, genes, antigens, and antibodies. For example, the adrenal medulla normally secretes catecholamines, such as epinephrine (adrenaline). Benign tumors of the adrenal medulla can produce catecholamines in vast excess, leading to rapid pulse, high blood pressure, sweats, and tremors. Elevated blood or urine levels of epinephrine and related compounds in someone with this set of symptoms strongly suggest the presence of an adrenal medullary tumor (pheochromocytoma). Liver and germ cell tumors secrete a protein known as alpha fetoprotein (AFP) into the blood, and prostate tumors secrete prostate-specific antigen (PSA) into the blood. These tumor markers can be used in three ways: (1) to screen and identify individuals at high risk for cancer; (2) to help diagnose the specific type of tumor in individuals with clinical manifestations relating to cancer, as in adrenal tumors; and (3) to follow the clinical course of cancer. For example, a falling PSA after therapy for prostate cancer indicates successful treatment, and a later rise in the PSA may indicate a recurrence.

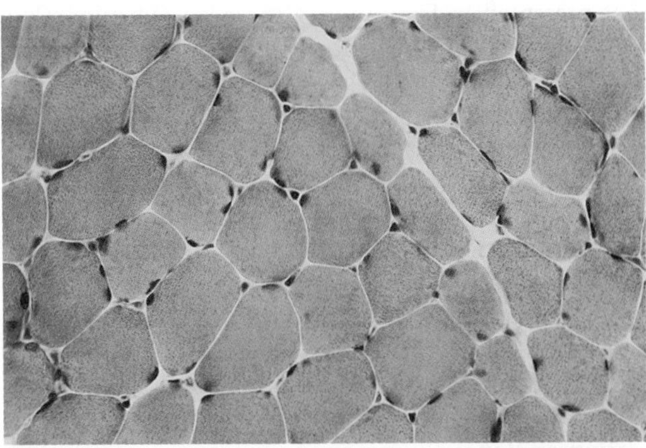

A

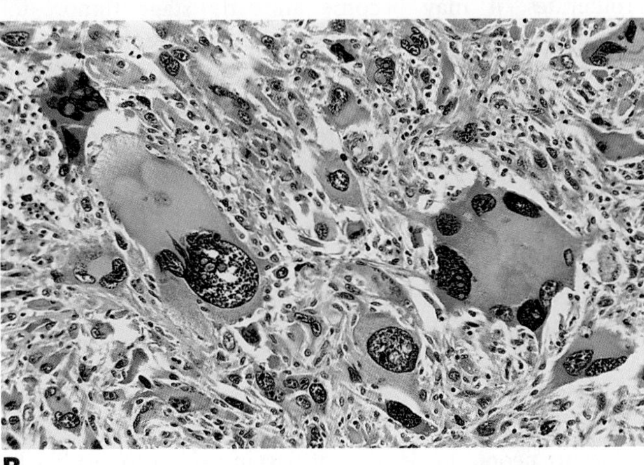

B

Figure 9-4 ■ Normal and Anaplastic Skeletal Muscle Cells. **A,** Normal skeletal muscle cells. **B,** Anaplastic tumor of the skeletal muscle (rhabdomyosarcoma). Note the marked cellular and nuclear pleomorphism (cellular and nuclear variation in size and shape) hyperchromatic nuclei, and giant tumor cells. The prominent cell in the center field has an abnormal tripolar spindle. Often the tissue of origin of an anaplastic tumor can only be established by the use of molecular markers such as immunohistochemical stains and chromosome analysis. (**A** from Damjanov I, Linder J, editors: *Anderson's pathology,* ed 10, St Louis, 1996, Mosby; **B** from Kumar V, Abbas AK, Fausto N: *Pathologic basis of disease,* ed 7, Philadelphia, 2005, Saunders, courtesy Dr. Trace Worrell, Department of Pathology, University of Texas Southwestern Medical School.)

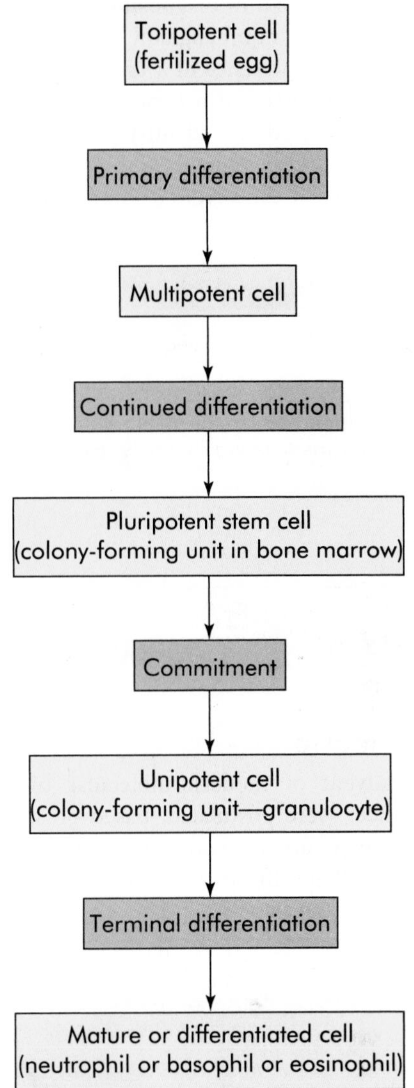

Figure 9-5 ■ Example of Differentiation. There often is a block in differentiation in cancer. Differentiation occurs several times in the lifetime of a granulocyte, with each step further limiting the cell's potential. Eventually, the cell terminally differentiates and can no longer divide, and the mature cell dies.

TABLE 9-3

Examples of Tumor Markers

Marker Name	Nature	Type of Cancer
α-Fetoprotein (AFP)	70 kDa plasma protein	Hepatic, germ cell
Carcinoembryonic antigen (CEA)	200 kDa glycoprotein	Colon, liver, pancreas, lung, breast, others.
β-Human chorionic gonadotropin (β-hCG)	Glycopeptide hormone	Germ cell, teratomas, islet cell
Prostate-specific antigen (PSA)	33 kDa glycoprotein	Prostate
Catecholamines	Epinephrine and precursors	Pheochromocytoma (adrenal medulla)
Homovanillic acid/vanillylmandilic acid (HVA/VMA)	Catecholamine metabolites	Neuroblastoma
Urinary Bence-Jones protein	Ig light chain	Multiple myeloma
Adrenocorticotropic hormone (ACTH)	Peptide hormone	Pituitary adenomas

A significant problem in diagnosing cancer using tumor marker assays is that nonmalignant diseases also produce tumor markers. The presence of a tumor marker may suggest a specific diagnosis, but it is not used alone as a diagnostic test. The need to identify ideal sensitive and specific tumor markers remains a high priority because the early detection of cancer often improves the treatment outcome.

QUICK CHECK 9-1

1. Identify the differences between benign and malignant tumors.
2. Define *anaplasia.*
3. How are tumor markers used?
4. What tumor markers are routinely used as a screening test?

THE GENETIC BASIS OF CANCER

Cancer Is Caused by Mutations in Genes

Clonal selection

Before the advent of modern molecular biology, many causes of cancer were postulated, based on epidemiologic observations, experiments with carcinogens, and studies with viruses. Perhaps the most telling epidemiologic data is that presented in Figure 9-6. Cancer is predominantly a disease of aging. The incidence of cancer—that is, the fraction of individuals in each age group who develop cancer—increases dramatically with age. The best explanation for this epidemiologic data is that each individual acquires a number of genetic "hits," or mutations, over time. When sufficient mutations have occurred, cancer develops. As an individual mutation occurs in a single cell, it may acquire some of the characteristics of a cancer, for example, increased growth rate or, alternatively, decreased apoptosis or death rate. That cell may then have a selective advantage over its neighbors; its progeny can accumulate faster than its nonmutant neighbors. This is referred to as **clonal proliferation** or **clonal expansion.** As a clone with a mutation proliferates, it may become an early stage tumor, for example, a carcinoma in situ or a benign colonic polyp. Additional mutations (or in modern videogame terminology, *hits*) then occur in these early lesions, permitting progression to more advanced tumors. The process of tumor development is a perverse form of Darwinian evolution: cells with a genetic change that confers a survival advantage outcompete their neighbors. The progressive accumulation of distinct advantageous (from the point of view of the cancer cell, *not* the individual) mutations leads from normal to fully malignant cancers.

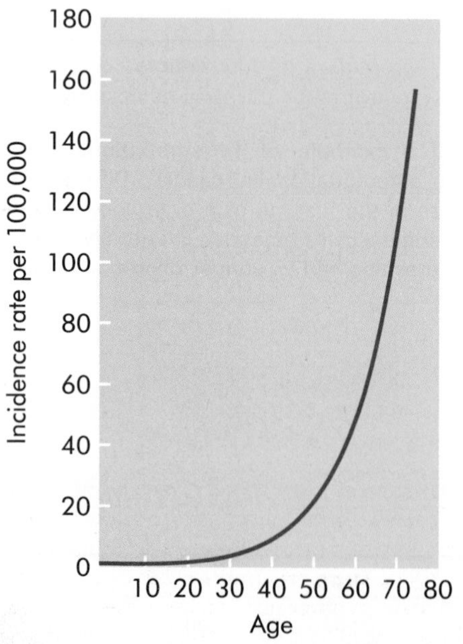

Figure 9-6 ■ Cancer Incidence Increases Markedly With Age. The graph depicts the number of cases of colon cancer diagnosed in women in England and Wales in 1 year. The incidence of cancer increases dramatically with advancing age. This type of data suggests that accumulation of genetic mutations over time increases the risk of developing cancer. The slope of the curve suggests that five to seven mutations must occur before a full-blown cancer develops. (Modified from Alberts B et al: *Molecular biology of the cell,* ed 4, New York, 2002, Garland.)

One organ in which this correlation of genetic and clinical progression has been especially well studied is the colon.[2] The colon is accessible to inspection with a colonoscope, so neoplastic lesions of varying size can readily be detected and removed. Intestinal polyps are benign neoplasms and the first stage in development of colon cancer. Small polyps tend to have only a few mutations that are detectable. Large polyps have more mutations, whereas frank colon cancers have even more mutations. This type of genetic data also strongly supports the notion that the accumulation of mutations in specific genes is required for the development of cancer (Figure 9-7).

Types of Gene Mutations in Cancer

Alteration of progrowth and antigrowth signals

It has been established that multiple mutations are required to develop cancer. One key question is, what types of genes must be mutated to cause a cancer? The prevailing view is that a number of cellular control pathways must be altered for a cell to become fully malignant[3] (Figure 9-8). First, cancer cells must have mutations that enable them to proliferate in the absence of external growth signals. To achieve this, some cancers secrete growth factors that stimulate their own growth, a process known as **autocrine stimulation** (also see Chapter 1). Other cancers have an increase in growth factor receptors; for example, in breast cancer the epidermal growth factor receptor HER2/*neu* is upregulated and likely sends growth signals into the cell even when external growth factors are at very low levels. Alternatively, the signal cascade from the cell surface receptor to the nucleus may be mutated in the "on" position.

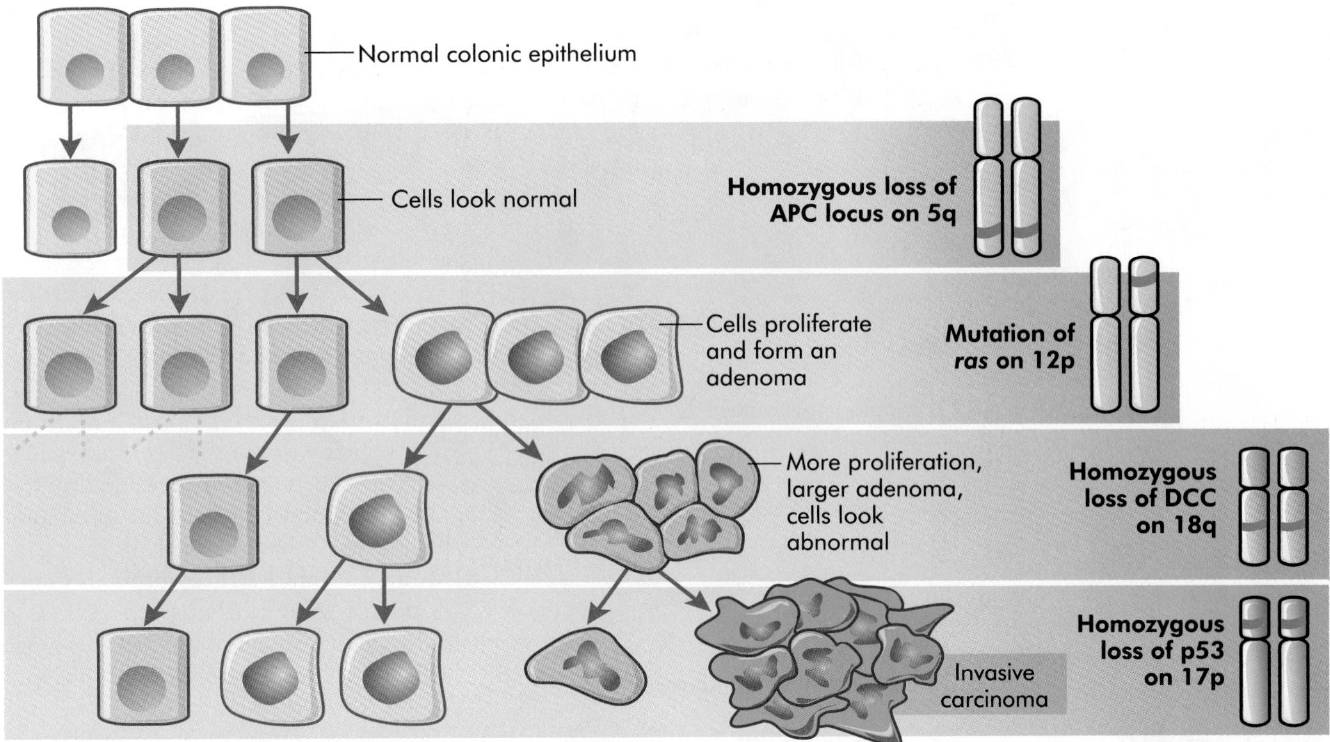

Figure 9-7 ■ **Sequential Acquisition of Genetic Changes.** Progression from benign to malignant colon cancer is accompanied by an accumulation of mutations. One of the earliest mutations in colon cancer is loss of the tumor suppressor gene *APC.* Additional mutations, often in the oncogene *ras,* and loss of the tumor suppressors *DCC* and *p53* occur as the lesion progresses from a benign polyp to an invasive carcinoma. APC, adenomatosis polyposis coli; DCC, deleted in colon cancer. (Modified from Kumar V, Cotran RS, Robbins SL: *Basic pathology,* ed 6, Philadelphia, 1997, Saunders.)

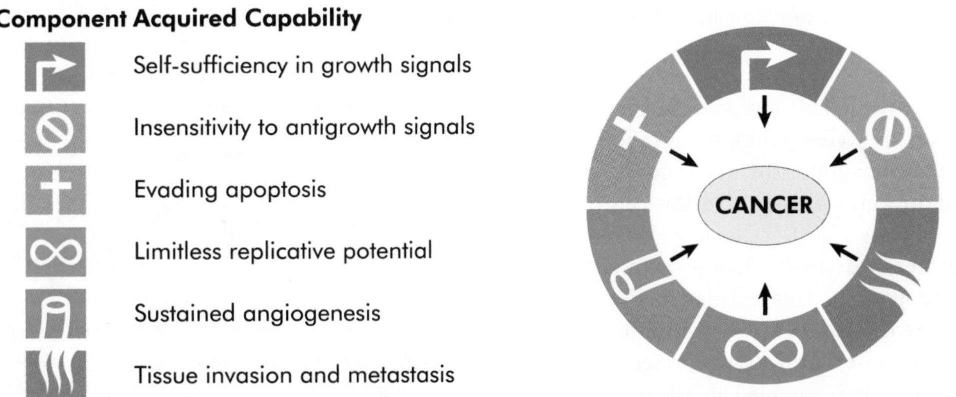

Figure 9-8 ■ **Six Hallmarks of Cancer.** Most cancers acquire mutations in six distinct areas of cell control during their development. All cancers must acquire the same six hallmark mutations, but their means of doing so varies mechanistically and chronologically. The order in which these capabilities are acquired is variable across different cancers. In some tumors, a particular mutation may confer several capabilities simultaneously, decreasing the number of intermediate mutational steps required for full development. Loss of the *p53* tumor-suppressor gene may facilitate angiogenesis and resistance to apoptosis. In other tumors, by comparison, a collaboration of two or more distinct genetic changes may be needed to acquire a given trait. (Modified from Hanahan D, Weinbert, RA: The hallmarks of cancer. *Cell* 100(1):57, 2000.)

For example, many cancers have an *activating mutation* in an intracellular signaling protein called ***ras***. Mutant *ras* stimulates cell growth even when growth factors are missing (Figure 9-9).

Cells usually receive diverse antigrowth signals from their normal milieu. Contact with other cells, with basement membranes, and soluble factors all normally signal cells to stop proliferating. These mechanisms can put a halt

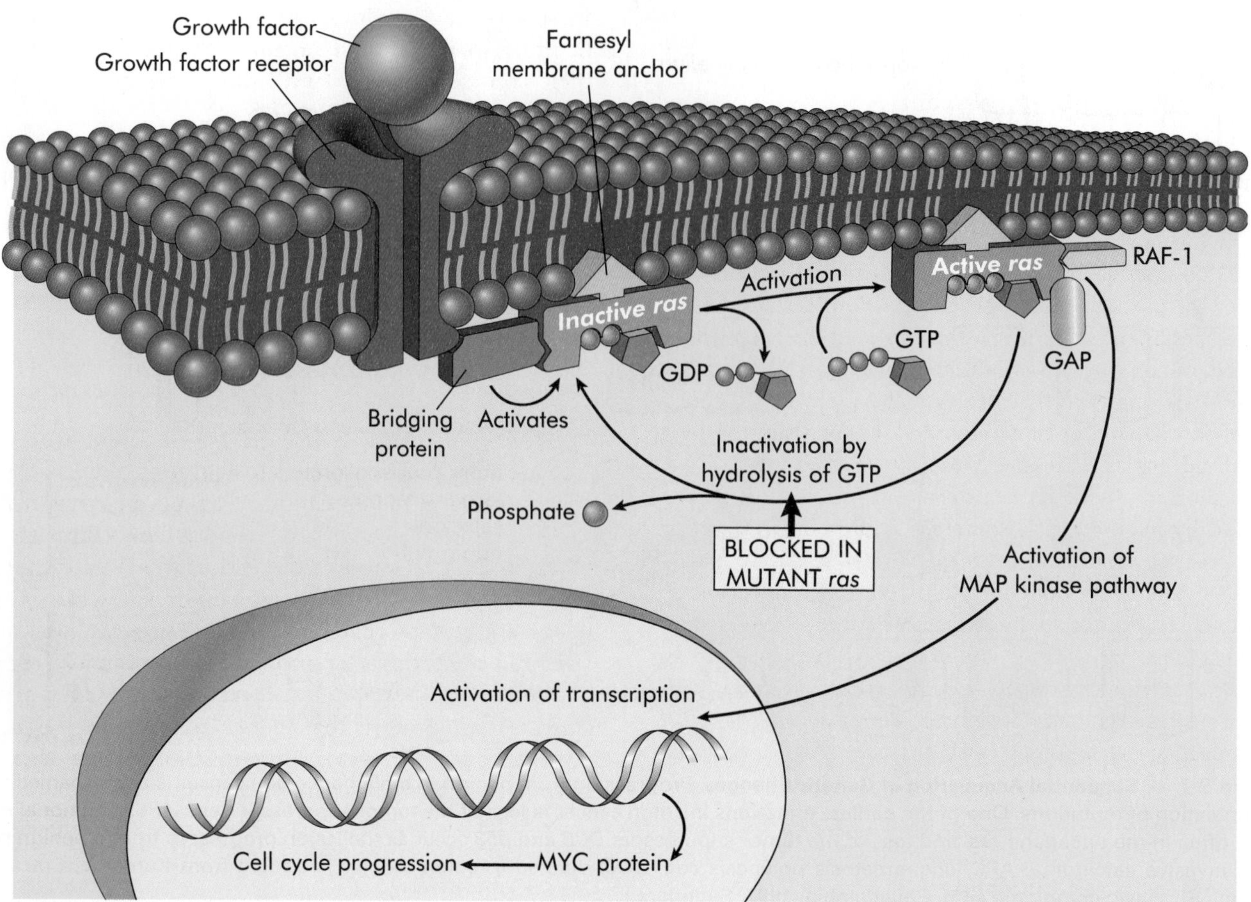

Figure 9-9 ■ Model for Action of *ras* Genes. When a normal cell is stimulated through a growth factor receptor, inactive (GDP-bound) *ras* is activated to a GTP-bound state. Activated *ras* sends growth signals to the nucleus through cytoplasmic kinases. The mutant *ras* protein is permanently activated because of its inability to hydrolyze GTP, leading to continual stimulation of the cell without any external trigger. *GDP,* Guanosine diphosphate; *GTP,* guanosine triphosphate; *GAP,* GTPase activating protein. (From Kumar V, Cotran RS, Robbins SL: *Basic pathology,* ed 7, Philadelphia, 2003, Saunders.)

to unregulated cell growth. This antigrowth signal must be inactivated in cancer as well. Common mutations include inactivation of the tumor suppressor *Rb*, or conversely, activation of the protein kinases that drive the cell cycle, the cyclin-dependent kinases. Next, cells have a mechanism that induces them to self-destruct when growth is excessive and checkpoints are ignored. This self-destruct mechanism, called **apoptosis**, is triggered by diverse stimuli, including normal development and excessive growth (see Chapter 3). The pathway to apoptosis is disabled in advanced cancers. The most common mutations conferring resistance to apoptosis occur in the **p53** gene (see Figure 9-8).

Angiogenesis

As cancers grow beyond a minimal size, they need their own blood supply to deliver oxygen and nutrients (Figure 9-10). However, in adults, new blood vessel growth (**angiogenesis**) is limited to wound healing and the female uterus during the proliferative phase of the menstrual cycle. Small cancers lack the ability to grow new blood vessels. More advanced cancers can secrete factors that stimulate new blood vessel growth. These **angiogenic factors,** such as *vascular endothelial growth factor* (VEGF), are required in small cancers to permit continued tumor expansion. The first antiangiogenesis drug to be approved, bevacizumab (Avastin), is a monoclonal antibody that binds to and

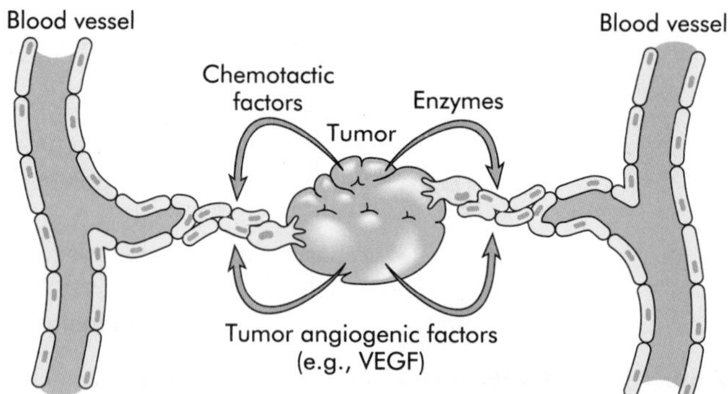

Figure 9-10 ■ Tumor-Induced Angiogenesis. Malignant tumors, especially those in metastatic sites, induce formation of blood vessels, which serve as routes for the transport of nutrients into the tumor. The approved drug bevacizumab blocks VEGF. *VEGF,* Vascular endothelial growth factor. (From Damjanov I: *Pathology for the health professions,* ed 3, St Louis, 2006, Saunders.)

inactivates VEGF. It is now used to treat metastatic colon cancer and may soon find additional uses.[4,5]

Telomeres and immortality

A hallmark of cancer cells is **immortality.** The only cells in the body that are usually "immortal" are germ cells (those that generate sperm and eggs) and some stem cells. Other cells in the body are not immortal and can divide only a limited number of times before they either cease dividing or die. One block to unlimited cell division (i.e., immortality) is a specialized structure at the end of each chromosome called the telomere. A **telomere** is a specialized, multicopy repeat DNA sequence that protects and maintains the ends of the chromosomes, and telomeres are maintained by a specialized enzyme called **telomerase** (Figure 9-11). Telomeres shorten after each cell division cycle and need to be restored by telomerase. Telomerase is present primarily in germ cells (in ovaries and testes) and in some stem cells. All other cells of the body lack telomerase. Therefore, when nongerm cells begin to proliferate abnormally, their telomere caps become shorter and shorter with each cell division. When the telomeres become critically small, they cannot protect the ends of chromosomes, which therefore become unstable, fragment, and the cells die. Cancer cells, when they reach a critical age, somehow activate telomerase in order to restore and maintain their telomeres, protect their chromosomes, and accordingly retain the ability to divide over and over again.[6–8]

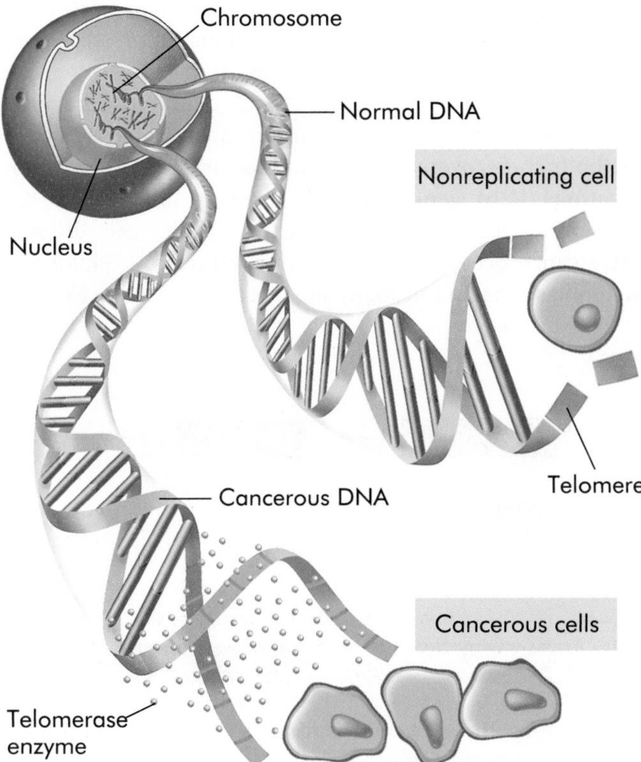

Figure 9-11 ■ **Control of Replication: Telomeres.** Normal cells cannot divide indefinitely. The ends of their chromosomes are capped by telomeres. In the absence of the telomerase enzyme, telomeres get shorter with each division until the cells finally stop dividing. In cancer cells, telomerase is switched on, producing an enzyme that rebuilds the telomeres. Thus, the cancer cell can divide indefinitely.

Finally, there appear to be genetic differences between cells that successfully metastasize and those that do not.[9] Specific mutations activate the ability of cancer cells to metastasize. Decreased cell-to-cell adhesion, the secretion of various proteases that digest surrounding barriers, and the ability to grow in new locations all contribute to successful metastasis.

Oncogenes and Tumor-Suppressor Genes: Accelerators and Brakes

The previous discussion refers to activating and inactivating various genes in the development of cancer. What types of mutations actually occur in cancer? Table 9-4 illustrates the types of cancer genes. It is first useful to distinguish between oncogenes and tumor-suppressor genes. **Oncogenes** are mutant genes that in their normal nonmutant state direct synthesis of proteins that positively regulate (accelerate) proliferation. Conversely, **tumor-suppressor genes** encode proteins that in their normal state negatively regulate (put the brakes on) proliferation. Hence, they also have been referred to as antioncogenes.

Mutations that create oncogenes

Point mutations

There are several types of genetic events that can activate oncogenes (Box 9-2). Perhaps the most common are small-scale changes in DNA, such as **point mutations,**

TABLE 9-4
Types of Cancer Genes

Dominant Oncogenes	Tumor Suppressors
Gene products that normally promote growth (i.e., proto-oncogenes)	Genes and proteins that normally inhibit growth or protect the genome
Activated by overexpression, increased copy number or gain of function mutations	Inactivated by loss of function mutation, loss of heterozygosity

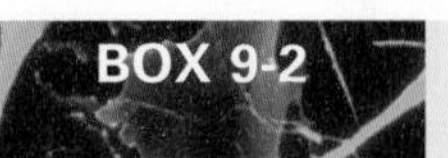

BOX 9-2 Types of Genetic Lesions in Cancers

1. Point mutations
2. Subtle alterations (insertions, deletions)
3. Chromosome changes (aneuploidy and loss of heterozygosity)
4. Amplifications
5. Gene silencing
6. Exogenous sequences (tumor viruses)

the alteration of one or a few nucleotide base pairs (see Chapter 2). This type of mutation can have profound effects on the activity of proteins. A point mutation in *ras* converts it from a regulated proto-oncogene to an unregulated oncogene, an accelerator of cellular proliferation. Activating point mutations in *ras* are found in many cancers, especially pancreatic and colorectal cancer.[10] Such point mutations can be difficult to detect without specialized tests.

Chromosome translocations

Another genetic lesion often found in cancer, **chromosome translocations,** can activate oncogenes by either of two distinct mechanisms. First, a translocation can cause excess and inappropriate production of a proliferation factor. One of the best examples is the *t(8;14)* translocation found in many Burkitt lymphomas.[11] Burkitt lymphoma is an aggressive cancer of B lymphocytes (see Chapter 20) (t[8;14] means a chromosome with a piece of chromosome 8 fused to a piece of chromosome 14). The *myc* proto-oncogene found on chromosome 8 is normally turned on at low levels in proliferating lymphocytes and is turned off in mature lymphocytes. The **MYC protein** is part of the positive signal for cell proliferation. If there is an accidental formation of t(8;14), the myc gene is aberrantly placed under the control of an immunoglobulin (Ig) gene present on chromosome 14. The Ig gene is turned on high in maturing B lymphocytes. The t(8;14) alters the control of MYC from its normal low level to high levels, directed by an Ig gene promoter. MYC, when inappropriately high, drives proliferation. Hence, the t(8;14) translocation causes cancers of maturing B cells (Figure 9-12).

Chromosome translocations also can lead to production of novel proteins with growth-promoting properties. In a different type of leukemia, chronic myeloid leukemia (CML), a specific translocation is found almost invariably. This translocation, t(9;22), was first identified in association with CML in Philadelphia in 1960 and so is often referred to as the Philadelphia chromosome.[12] This translocation fuses two chromosomes right in the middle of two genes, *bcr* on chromosome 9 and *abl* on chromosome 22. The result is production of a BCR-ABL fusion protein containing the first half of bcr and the second half of abl. BCR-ABL is a misregulated protein tyrosine kinase that promotes growth of myeloid cells. Notably, imatinib (Gleevec) and several other novel drugs that specifically inhibit this tyrosine kinase have shown great efficacy in the treatment of CML and lack the side effects noted with nonspecific antileukemia drugs.[13,14]

Chromosome amplification

Another type of genetic abnormality that turns on oncogenes is **chromosome amplifications** (Figure 9-13). Amplifications are the result of duplication of a small piece of a chromosome over and over again, so that instead of the normal two copies of a gene, there are tens or even hundreds of copies (see Chapter 3). Gene amplification results in increased expression of an oncogene or, in some cases, drug-resistant genes. The *N-myc* oncogene is amplified in 25% of childhood neuroblastomas and confers a poor prognosis,[15] whereas the epidermal growth factor receptor *erbB2* is amplified in 20% of breast cancers.[16]

Tumor suppressor genes

Tumor suppressor genes are genes whose major function is to negatively regulate cell growth. Tumor suppressors slow the cell cycle, inhibit proliferation from growth signals, and stop cell division when cells are damaged. Examples of several tumor suppressors are given in Table 9-5. One of the first discovered tumor suppressor genes, the **retinoblastoma (Rb) gene,** normally strongly inhibits the cell division cycle. When it is inactivated, the cell division cycle can proceed unchecked. *Rb* is mutated in childhood retinoblastoma and in many lung, breast, and bone cancers.

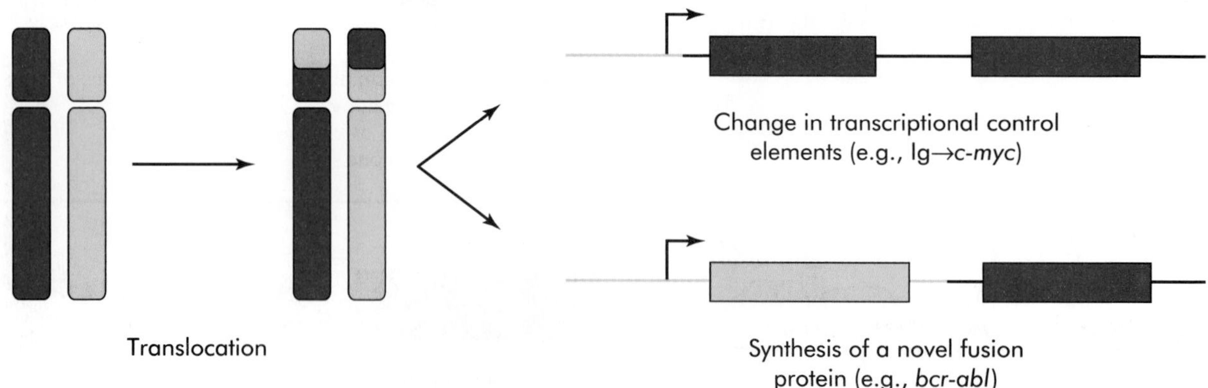

Figure 9-12 ■ Chromosome Translocations Are Oncogenic in Two Ways. Chromosome translocations can lead to inappropriate activation of an oncogene by fusing the transcriptional control elements of one gene, for example, the immunoglobulin (Ig) heavy chain promoter to the coding sequence for an oncogene, in this example, the *c-myc* oncogene. This leads to high-level expression of *c-myc* in B lymphocytes as they make immunoglobulins (antibodies). This type of translocation is found in B cell lymphomas. Chromosome translocations also can fuse two genes right in the middle, leading to synthesis of novel chimeric proteins. The fusion often creates a protein that either has new cancer-promoting properties or has lost the ability to regulate a protein kinase. A novel activated protein tyrosine kinase is created in chronic myeloid leukemia.

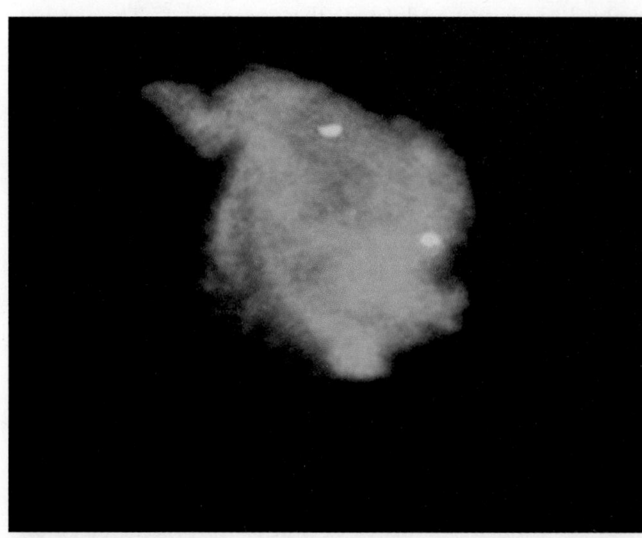

A

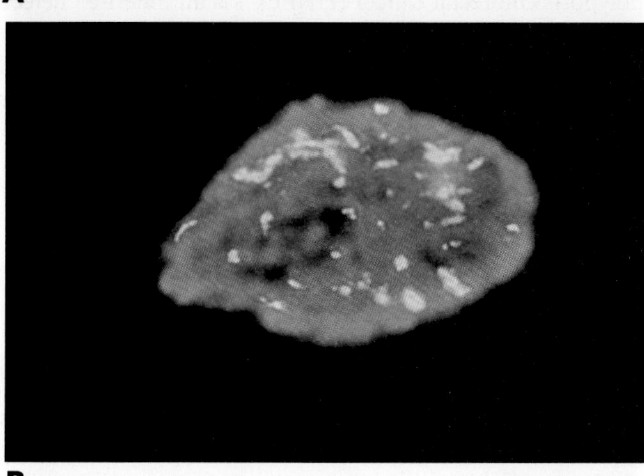

B

Figure 9-13 ■ *N-myc* Gene Amplification in Neuroblastoma. The *N-myc* gene is detected in human neuroblastoma cells using a technique called FISH (fluorescent in situ hybridization). **A,** A single pair of *N-myc* genes is detected in normal cells and in low-grade neuroblastoma. **B,** Multiple, amplified copies of the *N-myc* gene are detected in some cases of neuroblastoma. Amplification of *N-myc* is strongly associated with a poor prognosis in childhood neuroblastoma. (Courtesy Arthur R. Brothman, PhD, University of Utah School of Medicine.)

Although oncogenes are activated by mutation, tumor suppressors must be inactivated to allow cancer to occur (see Box 9-2 and Figure 9-14). A single genetic event can activate an oncogene. However, there are two copies, or alleles, of each gene, one from each parent. It therefore takes two "hits" to inactivate both copies of a tumor suppressor gene. The first copy of a tumor suppressor is often inactivated by point mutations. For example, the retinoblastoma gene may be inactivated on one chromosome by a point mutation (e.g., the copy inherited from the father). Because the other copy of the retinoblastoma gene (in this example, the one from the mother) is intact, however, a functional *Rb* protein can still be made and therefore the cell division cycle can be regulated appropriately. If the remaining gene is mutated, then all *Rb* function is lost and another step toward cancer occurs.

Loss of heterozygosity

For the function of a tumor suppressor to be lost, both chromosomal copies (alleles) of the gene must be inactivated, that is, they act in a recessive manner at the level of the cell. Although it may seem intuitive that simple inactivating mutations might disrupt both alleles, in fact this is not what usually happens.[17] Instead, the first allele (in the example above, the paternal copy) is inactivated by simple mutation, but the second allele (in this example, the maternal allele) is lost because entire regions of the maternal chromosome are lost (see Figure 9-14). Because you have two chromosomes, one from each parent, you can be *heterozygous* for nearby genetic markers; loss of a chromosome region in a tumor is referred to as **loss of heterozygosity,** or **LOH.** Loss of heterozygosity unmasks mutations in recessive tumor suppressor genes. For example, the *Rb* gene resides on chromosome 13, in a region referred to as q14 (13q14). Most individuals with *Rb* mutations have a subtle mutation in one allele and have lost the normal copy of *Rb* through loss of the 13q14 chromosome region on the other chromosome.

TABLE 9-5

Familial Cancer Syndromes Caused by Tumor-Suppressor Gene Function Loss

Syndrome	Gene
Retinoblastoma	*Rb*
Li-Fraumeni syndrome	*p53, CHEK2*
Familial melanoma	*p16*^{INK4a}, CDK4
Neurofibromatosis	Neurofibromin
Familial adenomatous polyposis	*APC*
Breast cancer	*BRCA1, BRCA2*

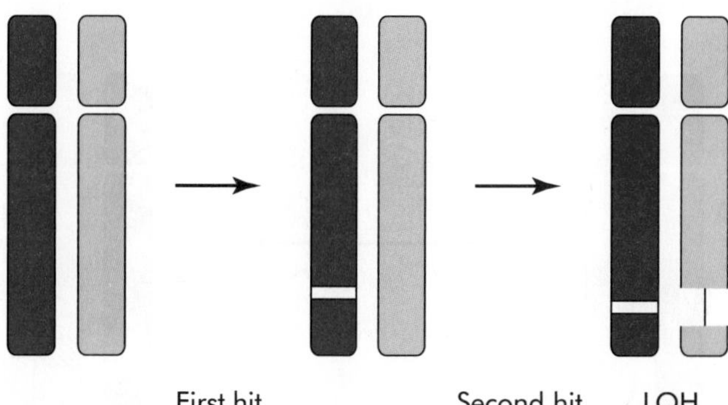

Figure 9-14 ■ Two Distinct Hits Are Required to Inactivate a Tumor Suppressor Gene. Tumor suppressor genes are often inactivated by a mutation (first hit) followed by complete loss of an entire region of chromosome encompassing the remaining normal allele (second hit, also known as loss of heterozygosity). *LOH,* Loss of heterozygosity.

QUICK CHECK 9-2

1. Define clonal proliferation.
2. What types of genes are mutated in cancer?
3. What is the significance of telomeres in cancer?
4. Define loss of heterozygosity.
5. What is imatinib, and how does it work?

Gene silencing

Gene expression can be regulated in a heritable manner (i.e., passed from a parent to a child or from a single cell to its progeny) by an **epigenetic** mechanism called **silencing** that does not require mutations or changes in DNA sequence (see Chapter 2). Silencing normally shuts off whole regions of chromosomes, so the pattern of gene expression is different in one tissue than in another tissue with the same genes. The boundaries of the silenced regions can spread in cancer cells, shutting off previously active genes. Silencing can shut off critical tumor suppressor genes in the absence of mutations in the gene. This epigenetic silencing is associated with methylation of the DNA and modification of associated chromatin. How silencing works, and how it is passed on from one generation of cells to the next, is an area of active research, but it is clear that silencing is one important way to inactivate tumor suppressor gene expression in cancers.[18,19] Certain chemotherapeutic drugs, such as 5-azacytidine, can reverse methylation and may prove useful in reactivating or turning tumor suppressor genes "back on again" in cancer[20,21] (Figure 9-15).

Guardians of the Genome

The previous discussion of mutations leads naturally to the question of how mutations occur in the first place. The integrity of genetic information can be compromised at several points: during each round of DNA synthesis, during each mitosis when chromosomes are segregated to daughter cells, and when external mutagens (chemicals and radiation) alter or disrupt DNA. Multiple mechanisms have evolved to protect and repair the genome.[22,23] These repair mechanisms are directed by **caretaker genes,** genes that are responsible for the maintenance of genomic integrity. Caretaker genes encode proteins that are involved in repairing damaged DNA, such as occurs with errors in DNA replication, mutations caused by ultraviolet or ionizing radiation, and mutations resulting from chemicals and drugs. Loss of function of caretaker genes leads to increased mutation rates. If DNA damage is severe, the cell undergoes programmed cell death, or apoptosis, rather than divide with damaged DNA.

Inherited mutations can disrupt the caretaker genes that protect the integrity of the genome. Examples include the disorder xeroderma pigmentosum (XP); affected individuals have defects in the repair of ultraviolet light–induced DNA damage and should avoid direct sunlight exposure. They have a high incidence of skin cancer. Hereditary nonpolyposis colorectal cancer (HNPCC) is an inherited defect in the repairing of DNA base pair mismatches that occurs from time to time during DNA replication. Affected individuals have an increased rate of small insertions and deletions in DNA, leading to a high rate of colon and other cancers.[24] Finally, there are inherited mutations that threaten the integrity of entire chromosomes. Bloom syndrome and Fanconi aplastic anemia are two autosomal recessive disorders in which affected individuals demonstrate marked chromosomal instability. Chromosome breaks, aberrant fusions, and loss are common. As a consequence, there is a high rate of cancer at an early age.

The rate of individual gene mutation is probably too low to account for the acquisition of many new mutations during the evolution of a malignant cancer clone. Instead, **chromosome instability** appears to be increased in malignant cells.[25] The underlying mechanism of this instability is not clear. Chromosome instability results in a high rate of chromosome loss, as well as loss of heterozygosity and chromosome amplification. Each of these events can accelerate the loss of tumor suppressor genes and the overexpression of oncogenes.

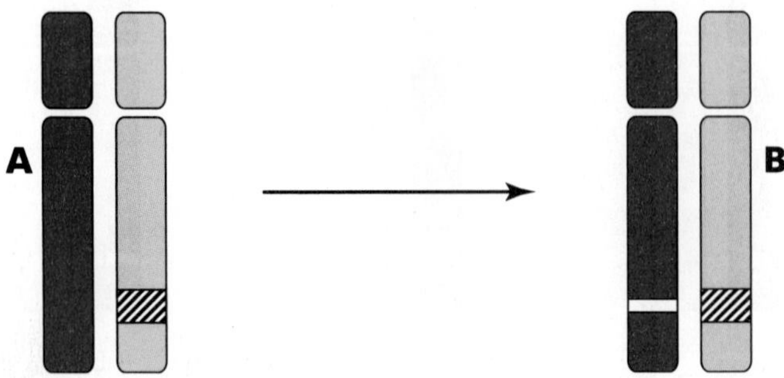

Figure 9-15 ■ Silencing of Tumor Suppressor Genes. **A,** Paternal allele methylated and inactivated. In this example, the first copy of a gene is turned off by gene silencing without mutation. **B,** Mutation of maternal allele results in no functional protein production. In this example, the remaining normal gene can be inactivated by mutation.

Genetics and Cancer-Prone Families

Genetic events are the primary basis of carcinogenesis.[26] Most of the genetic alterations that cause cancer occur during the lifetime of the individual, in the somatic tissues. The frequency of these events can be altered by exposure to **mutagens**—that is, agents causing mutations—and by defects in DNA repair that increase the rate of mutations. Because these genetic events occur in somatic cells as opposed to germ cells, they are not transmitted to future generations. Even though they are genetic events, they are not inherited! It is possible, however, for cancer-predisposing mutations to occur in germline cells (cells that produce gametes) (Figure 9-16). Mutations present in germline cells result in the vertical transmission of cancer-causing genes from one generation to the next, producing families with a high incidence of specific cancers. These inherited mutations that predispose to cancer are almost invariably in tumor-suppressor and caretaker genes (see Table 9-5).

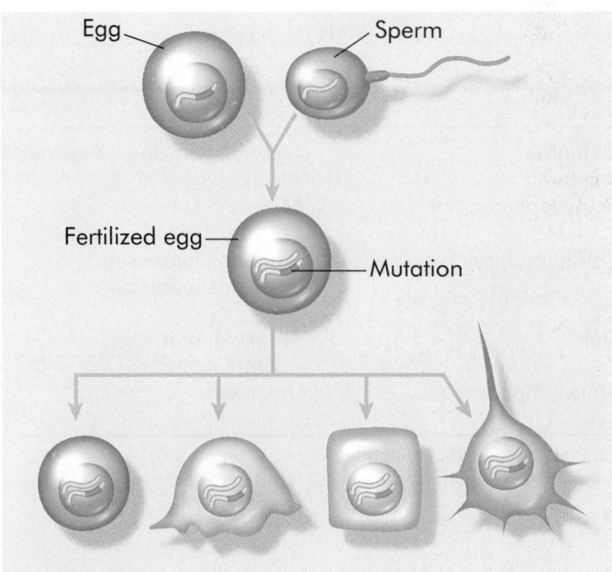

Figure 9-16 ■ **Germline Mutation.** Inherited mutations are carried in the DNA of reproductive cells. When reproductive cells containing mutations combine to produce offspring, the mutation will be present in *all* of the offspring's body cells. (Modified from Lea DN, Jenkins JF, Francomano CA: *Genetics in clinical practice,* Boston, 1998, Bartlett.)

Although rare, such "cancer-prone families" demonstrate that inheritance of a mutated gene can cause cancer (Figure 9-17). In these families, inheritance of one mutant allele predisposes to a specific form of cancer: individuals who inherit the germline mutant allele will inevitably suffer loss of the normal allele by loss of heterozygosity in some cells and go on to develop the tumor. Examples of human cancers that can be inherited are retinoblastoma, a childhood cancer of the eye, which can be caused by germline mutations in one allele of the *Rb* gene; Wilms tumor, a childhood cancer of the kidney *(Wt1)*; neurofibromatosis *(Nf1)*; inherited breast cancer *(BRCA1)*; and familial polyposis coli or adenomas of the colon *(APC)*. A specific tumor-suppressor gene has been isolated for each of these cancers and, in many cases, these tumor-suppressor genes are then found to be inactivated in sporadic (as opposed to inherited) cancers as well. For example, inherited mutations in the *APC* gene are rare and account for only a few percent of all colon cancers. However, 85% of sporadic colon cancers have acquired mutations of *APC*, mutations that developed over time specifically in the colon in the individual. Characterization of cancer-causing genes and other genetic factors helps identify individuals prone to developing cancer (see Figure 2-29 in Chapter 2) and contributes to our understanding of sporadic cancers. Individuals known to carry mutations in tumor suppressor genes (for example, women with a germline BRCA1 mutation) are targeted for cancer screening to facilitate early cancer detection and therapy.[27]

QUICK CHECK 9-3

1. What is gene silencing?
2. Cancer-prone families often have mutations in what type of genes?

INFECTION, IMMUNITY, INFLAMMATION, AND CANCER

Viral Causes of Cancer

A number of viruses have been associated with human cancer (Table 9-6).[28,29] An even broader spectrum of viruses have been associated with cancer in animals. In humans, hepatitis B and C viruses (HBV, HCV), Epstein-Barr virus (EBV), Kaposi sarcoma–associated herpesvirus (KSHV) (also known as human herpes virus [HHV8]), and human papillomavirus (HPV) are associated with about 15% of all human cancers worldwide. Cancer of the cervix and hepatocellular carcinoma account for about 80% of virus-linked cancer. The initial acute infection with hepatitis B or C is not associated with cancer; instead, it is acquisition of a chronic viral hepatitis that markedly increases cancer

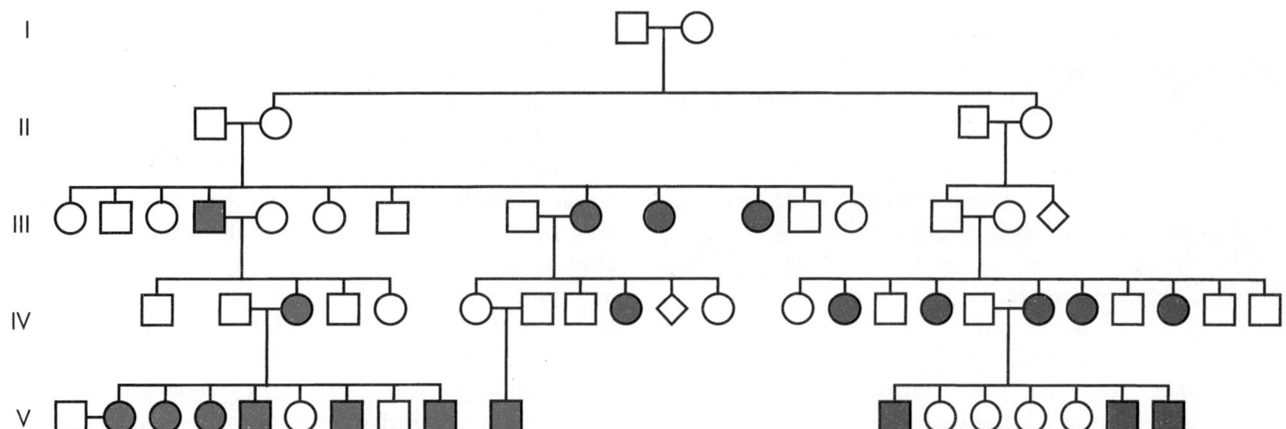

Figure 9-17 ■ **A Familial Colon Cancer Pedigree.** Darkened symbols represent individuals diagnosed with cancer. (From Jorde LB et al: *Medical genetics,* ed 3, updated, St Louis, 2006, Mosby.)

TABLE 9-6
Human Viruses Associated With Cancer

Virus Family	Type	Human Cancer	Cofactors
Hepatitis viruses	Hepatitis B	Hepatocellular carcinoma	Alcohol, smoking, aflatoxins
Flaviviruses	Hepatitis C	Hepatocellular carcinoma	Alcohol
Herpes viruses	Epstein-Barr	Burkitt lymphoma, nasopharyngeal carcinoma	Malaria
		Post-transplant lymphoproliferative disease	Immunosuppression
	KSHV/HHV-8 Immunodeficiency	Kaposi sarcoma	Immunosuppression
Papillomaviruses	HPV-16, -18, -31, -33, other	Cervical, anogenital	Smoking, oral contraceptives
Retroviruses	HTLV-1	Adult T cell leukemia/lymphoma	Unknown

Modified from Mendelsohn J et al, editors: *The molecular basis of cancer*, ed 2, Philadelphia, 2001, Saunders.
KSHV/HHV-8, Kaposi sarcoma–associated herpesvirus/human herpes virus-8; *HPV,* human papillomavirus; *HTLV-1,* human T-cell leukemia/lymphoma virus-1.

risk. Chronic hepatitis B infections are common in parts of eastern Asia and sub-Saharan Africa and confer up to a 200-fold increased risk of developing liver cancer. Chronic hepatitis C infections have become increasingly recognized in Western countries. Up to 80% of liver cancer worldwide is associated with chronic hepatitis caused either by HBV or HCV. In both cases, it appears that a lifetime of chronic liver inflammation predisposes to the development of hepatocellular carcinoma. Widespread use of the HBV vaccine is expected to significantly decrease the incidence of chronic hepatitis B and hence hepatocellular carcinoma. Unfortunately, a vaccine for HCV is not yet available.

Virtually all human cervical cancer is due to infection with specific subtypes of human papillomavirus (HPV). HPV infects basal skin cells and many subtypes cause warts. There are more than 70 types of HPV, but only a few (HPV 16, 18, 31, 45, and a few others) are associated with cervical, anogenital, and penile cancer. HPV is spread primarily through sexual contact; thus, cervical cancer is rare in populations with high rates of abstinence (e.g., nuns) or monogamy and is common in populations with high rates of sexual promiscuity.[30] HPV causes cancer when the viral DNA becomes accidentally integrated into the infected cervical basal cell chromosome and directs the production of viral oncogenes. Early oncogenic HPV infection is readily detected by Papanicolaou (Pap) smear, an examination of cervical epithelia scrapings. Early detection of cellular atypia in a Pap smear often leads to detection of cervical carcinoma in situ (see Figure 9-1 and p. 223), which can be easily and effectively treated. In parts of the world where routine Pap smears are common, cervical cancer is rare. In poor countries, cervical cancer is one of the leading causes of cancer death. Vaccines against HPV (Gardasil™, Cervarix™) have proven effective in preventing infection and have the potential to significantly reduce cancer mortality.[31]

Epstein-Barr virus (EBV) and Kaposi sarcoma herpesvirus (KSHV) are both members of the *Herpesvirus* family.[28] EBV, the cause of infectious mononucleosis, infects B lymphocytes and stimulates their proliferation. Individuals who are immunosuppressed, because of HIV infection or use of antirejection drugs after a heart or kidney transplant, can have persistent EBV infection that can lead to the development of B cell lymphomas. These lymphomas are known as post-transplant lymphoproliferative disorder (PTLD) in individuals after organ transplant. One effective therapy, where possible, for PTLD is to decrease or stop immunosuppressant drugs. EBV infection also is associated with Burkitt lymphoma in areas of endemic malaria and with nasopharyngeal carcinoma in parts of Asia. Kaposi sarcoma herpesvirus, also known as human herpesvirus 8 (KSHV/HHV-8), is the cause of Kaposi sarcoma, a cancer that occurs in elderly men and in a markedly more virulent form in immunocompromised individuals, especially those infected with HIV. HHV-8 also has been linked to several rare lymphomas.

Human T cell leukemia-lymphoma virus (HTLV) is an oncogenic retrovirus linked to the development of adult T cell leukemia and lymphoma (ATLL).[29] HTLV is transmitted both vertically—that is, inherited by children from infected parents—and horizontally by breastfeeding, sexual intercourse, blood transfusions, and exposure to infected needles. Infection with HTLV may be asymptomatic, and only a small fraction of infected individuals develop ATLL, often many years after acquiring the virus. It is clear that infection by an oncogenic virus is far from sufficient to cause cancer. For example, in some industrialized regions, Epstein-Barr virus can infect 90% of the adolescent and young adult population, yet only a very small percentage of these individuals develop EBV-related cancer. For each of these infections, there are important cofactors that increase the risk that an infection will develop into cancer.

Bacterial Cause of Cancer

Helicobacter pylori (H. pylori) is a bacterium that infects more than half of the world's population, making it one of the most prevalent infections.[30,32] *H. pylori* is now accepted as the most common cause of gastric infection and is responsible for the majority of cases of peptic ulcer disease, gastric lymphomas, and gastric carcinomas.[30,33,34] The association is stronger with B cell lymphoma of the stomach than with carcinomas. The high prevalence of *H. pylori* infection has been documented most notably in blacks and Hispanics, who also are at high risk for gastric cancer.[33] Treatment of *H. pylori* with antibiotics results in regression of the lymphoma in most cases.[35] The tumors arise in mucosa-associated lymphoid tissue (MALT) and are therefore sometimes called MALTomas. The mechanisms proposed for *H. pylori*–associated tumor development include (1) dysregulation of the gastric epithelial cell cycle, (2) the formation of DNA adducts (addition of a small chemical group to DNA bases), (3) the generation of free radicals, (4) alterations in growth factor secretion and cytokines, and (5) the effects of decreased gastric secretion. (For further discussion, see Chapter 34.)

Immunity and Cancer

The immune system reacts to infection and tissue damage. It also recognizes nonself and new antigens (see Chapter 6). The immune system plays a complex role in the development and progression of cancer. Historically, it has been suggested that immune surveillance might recognize some early cancers as nonself and suppress or eliminate them before they can develop further. This still appears to be true for viral-induced cancers (e.g., PTLD, Kaposi sarcoma) where we know the immune system recognition of viral antigens is important. Defects of the immune system (for instance, because of HIV infection or immunosuppressant drugs) increase the incidence of lymphomas, herpesvirus-caused cancers such as Kaposi sarcoma and EBV-induced posttransplant lymphoproliferative disease, and HPV-induced vulvar and cervical cancer up to 190-fold.[36,37] However, patients receiving immunosuppression after an organ (e.g., kidney, liver) transplant have little or no increase in the most prevalent cancers, such as breast, prostate, and colon cancers, strongly suggesting immune surveillance is not important in preventing these common cancers. Inherited defects in DNA repair (syndromes such as Fanconi aplastic anemia and ataxia-telangiectasia) can cause both immune defects and predispose to cancer, but in these immune defects the increased risk of cancer is probably due to the defect in DNA repair and increased mutation rates rather than the defect in immunity.

An Active Immune Response Causes Cancer

Chronic inflammation is a form of an immune response that has been recognized since the 1860s as an important contributing factor to the development of cancer.[38,39] Epidemiologic studies indicate that individuals with ulcerative colitis, a chronic inflammation of the large bowel, of over 10 years' duration have up to a 30-fold increase in the risk of developing colon cancer. Chronic inflammation of the liver as a result of HBV or HCV hepatitis markedly increases the risk of liver cancer. One large study found a 66% increase in risk of lung cancer among women with chronic asthma, an inflammatory disease of the airways.[40] The reasons for the positive association of inflammation and cancer are complex. After injury, inflammatory cells release cytokines and growth and survival factors that stimulate local cell proliferation, vascular growth, and wound healing. In chronic inflammation, these factors combine to promote continued proliferation (Figure 9-18). In addition, inflammatory cells release compounds such as reactive oxygen species and other reactive molecules that can both promote mutations and block the cellular response to DNA damage. Notably, increased abundance of the enzyme cyclooxygenase 2 (COX-2), which generates prostaglandins during acute inflammation, has been associated with colon and other cancers. Importantly, nonsteroidal anti-inflammatory drugs, such as aspirin and ibuprofen that inhibit COX-2 and prevent formation of inflammatory mediators, protect against colon cancer development. Studies in experimental animals further support the idea that inflammatory mediators released by immune cells accelerate the development of cancer. Cancer cells and macrophages also may secrete inflammatory mediators such as interleukin-8 that then stimulate immune and other cells

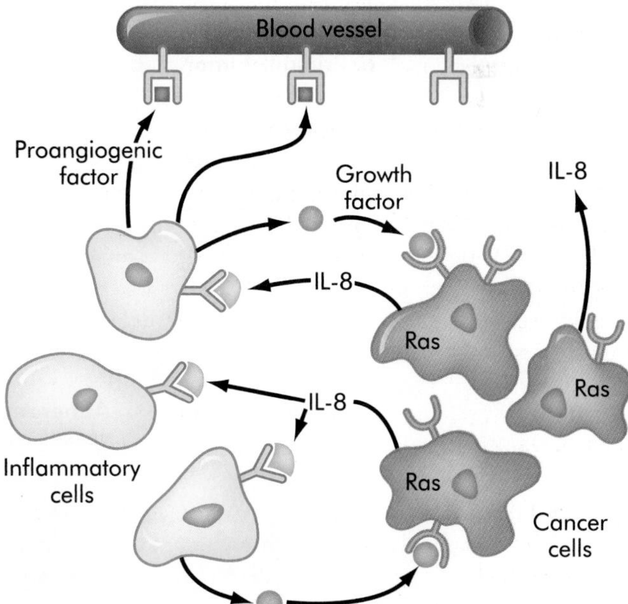

Figure 9-18 ■ The intimate association of inflammation and cancer. Cancers attract inflammatory cells by a number of methods. Cancer cell hypoxia and death releases factors that activate stromal and tumor-infiltrating macrophages. The activated Ras protein in many cancer cells also drives secretion of cytokines such as interleukin 8 (IL-8) that then stimulates inflammatory cells to secrete growth factors and pro-angiogenic factors. (Redrawn from Karin M: Inflammation and cancer: the long reach of Ras. *Nature Med* 11(1):20–21, 2005.)

to increase vascular permeability, tissue breakdown, and angiogenesis.[41,42] Studies using mice engineered to have immune cells unable to response to inflammation found this caused a 50% *decrease* in the rate of colitis-associated cancers.[43,44] In summary, the role of the immune system in cancer is complex. The concept that the immune system protects us against cancer is true for a limited number of cancers. Chronic activation of the immune system also promotes cancer growth, angiogenesis, and cancer progression. This is an area under active investigation (see Figure 9-18).

QUICK CHECK 9-4

1. What viruses cause cancer?
2. For which viral-induced cancers are there effective vaccinations?
3. How does the immune system prevent cancer?
4. How does the immune system contribute to cancer?
5. How does aspirin protect against cancer?

CANCER PROGRESSION AND METASTASIS

Metastasis is the spread of cancer cells from the site of the original tumor to distant tissues and organs throughout the body. Metastasis is a defining characteristic of cancer, contributes significantly to the pain and suffering from cancer, and is the major cause of death from cancer. While localized, low-stage cancers can often be cured by a combination of surgery, chemotherapy, and radiation, these same therapies are frequently ineffective against cancer that has metastasized. For example, in appropriately treated women with low-stage breast cancer the 5-year survival rate is often greater than 90%.[45] Tragically, less than 30% of women with metastatic breast cancer are alive 5 years after diagnosis.[46] An increasing body of basic and clinical research is defining the biologic principles of metastasis, with the hope that this improved understanding will lead to both novel diagnostic approaches and better therapies for metastatic cancers.

Local spread is a prerequisite for metastasis and the first step in the metastatic process. In its earliest stages, local invasion may occur as a function of direct tumor extension.[47] Eventually, however, cells migrate away from the primary tumor and invade the surrounding interstitial spaces. Mechanisms important in local invasion include (1) cellular proliferation, (2) angiogenesis and perhaps lymphatogenesis, (3) digestion of capsules and other structural barriers, (4) changes in cell-to-cell adhesion (making cancer cells slippery), and (5) increased motility of individual tumor cells.[47] These mechanisms are not mutually exclusive, and successful local invasion requires the successful completion of each step (Figure 9-19).

Patterns of Spread

Two distinct mechanisms give rise to patterns of metastatic spread. First, cancer cells spread through vascular and lymphatic pathways, as well as natural tissue planes. Blood vessels and lymphatic vessels within tumors offer malignant cells direct access into the blood and lymph circulation.

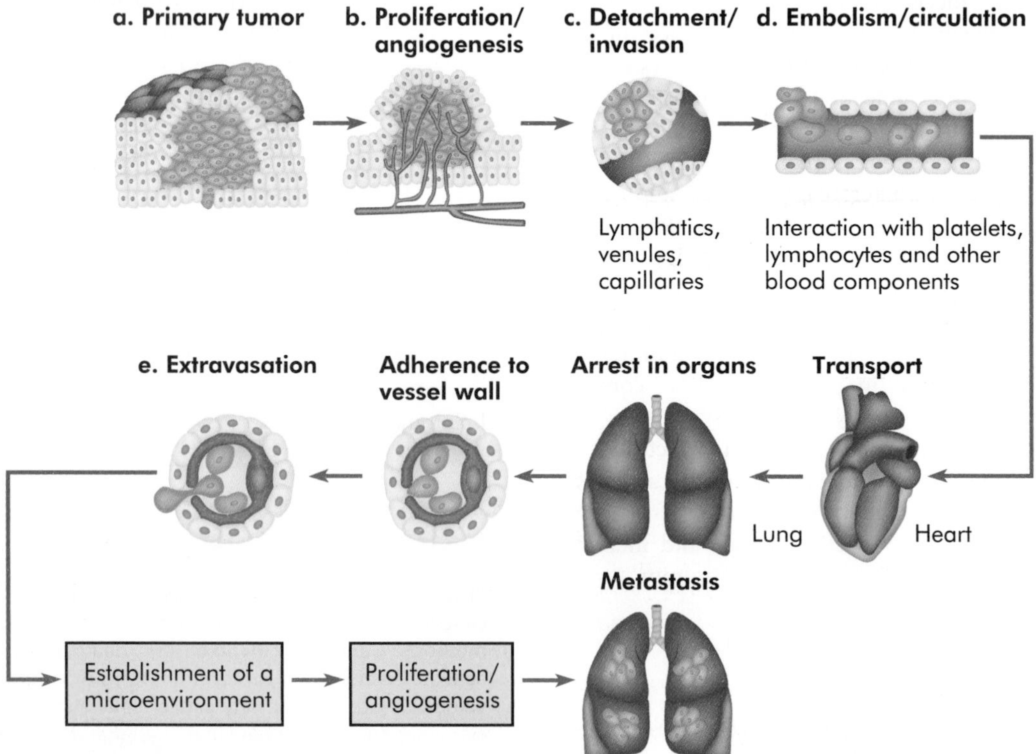

Figure 9-19 ■ **Multistep Nature of Metastasis.** (From Fidler IT: The pathogenesis of cancer metastasis: the "seed and soil" hypothesis revisited. *Nat Rev Ca* 3:453–458, 2003.)

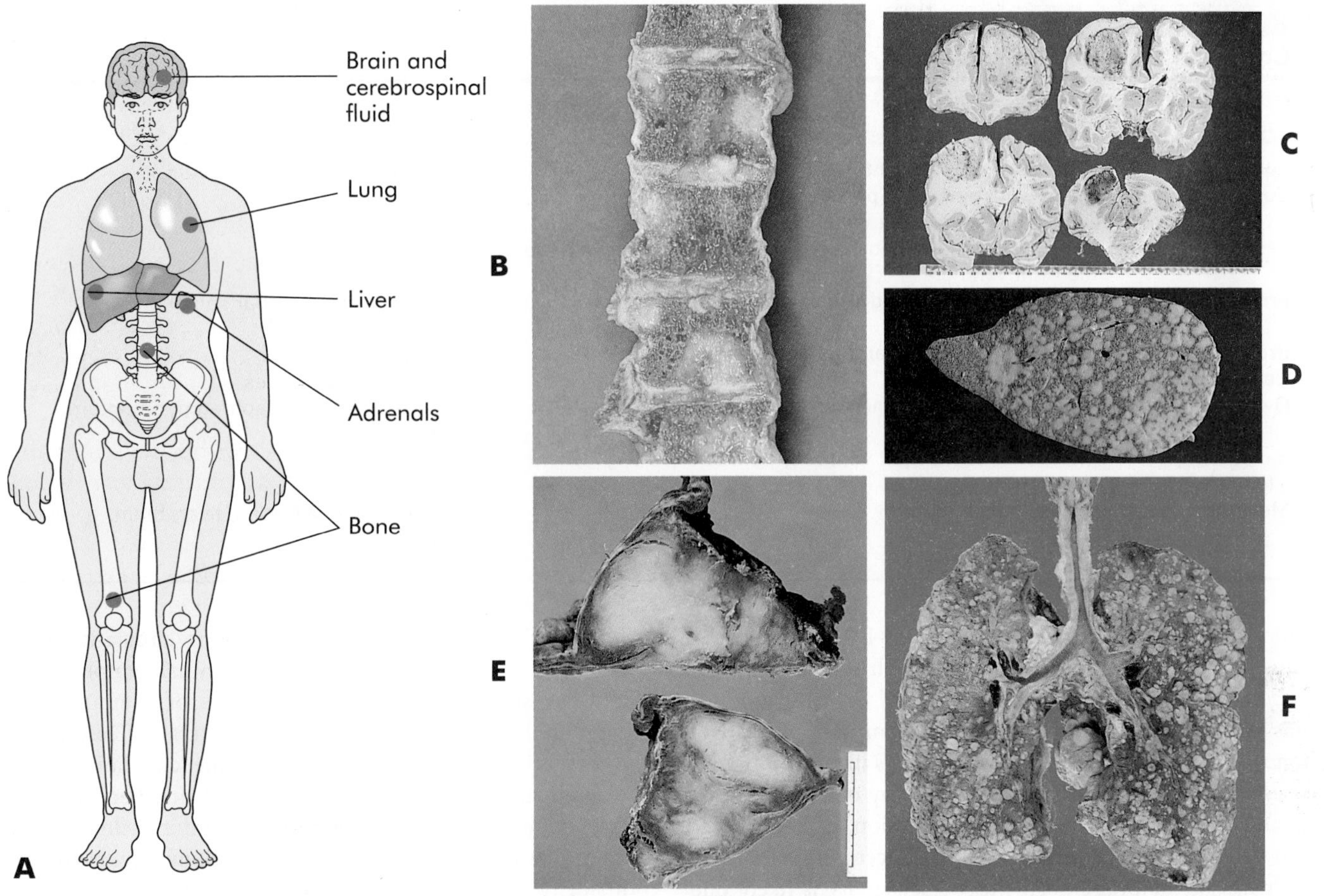

Figure 9-20 ■ **Main Sites of Blood-Borne Metastasis. A,** Sites of hematogenous metastasis. **B,** Metastasis in bone. **C,** Metastasis in brain. **D,** Metastasis in liver. **E,** Metastasis in adrenals. **F,** Metastasis in lung. Blood-borne tumor metastasis leads to growth of secondary tumors in several main sites. The macroscopic appearances of bone metastasis are shown in **B,** where lesions are seen in vertebrae. Numerous metastases from a neoplasm of the stomach are seen in the brain in **C.** The liver is the most common site for metastases from tumors in the gastrointestinal tract, as seen in **D,** which arose from a colonic neoplasm. In **E,** metastatic tumor has replaced both adrenal glands, as is commonly seen with spread from lung and breast tumors. The lung, **F,** is the most common site for blood-borne metastases from tumors outside the spinal tract, particularly mesenchymal tumors. (From Stevens A, Lowe J: *Pathology: illustrated review in color,* ed 2, Edinburgh, 2000, Mosby.)

Clusters, single cells, and fragments of tumor can disseminate by these routes. Therefore, liver tumors spread through the portal vein to the lungs, and breast cancer spreads through lymphatics to axillary lymph nodes (Figures 9-20 and 9-21). Second, there is a major yet poorly

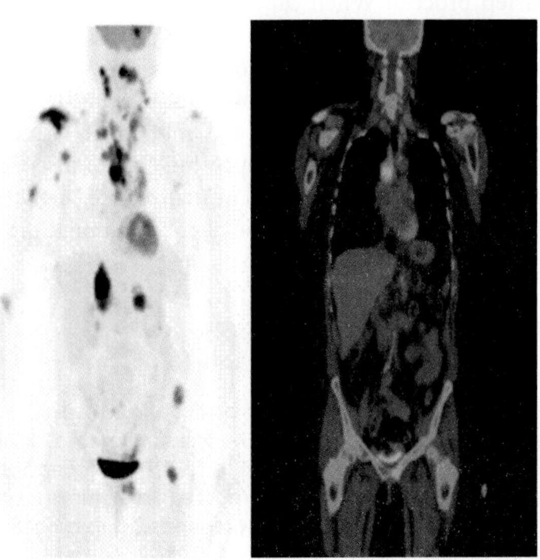

Figure 9-21 ■ **Metastatic Nonsmall Cell Lung Cancer (NSCLC).** This 54-year-old woman had a NSCLC resected from the left upper lobe. Five years later, these studies were obtained. The positron emission tomography (PET) scan using 18fluoro-deoxyglucose shows metastatic lesions in the brain, right shoulder, mediastinal and cervical lymph nodes, as well as the liver, left pelvis, and proximal femur. *(Left)* PET whole body image. *(Right)* Representative coronal image from the whole body FDG-PET/CT fused image of the same patient. The fused image consists of the CT image with the metabolic information superimposed in color. The pattern of spread is most likely from the primary tumor to the large mediastinal lymph nodes, followed by lymphatic spread to cervical nodes. Blood-borne spread produced the bone, brain, and liver metastases. Normally, only the heart, brain, and bladder show strong signal in PET scan. (Images courtesy John Hoffman, MD, Huntsman Cancer Institute.)

TABLE 9-7

Common Sites of Metastasis

Primary Tumor	Major Anatomic Pathway	Common Site of Distant Metastasis
Lung	Pulmonary vein, left ventricle	Multiple organs, including brain
Colorectal	Mesenteric lymphatics, portal venous system	Liver
	Inferior vena cava, right ventricle, pulmonary artery	Lungs
Testicular	Lymphatics to the periaortic area to the subclavian veins to the right ventricle	Lungs, liver, brain
Prostate	Regional lymphatics and veins, which drain to Batson plexus of presacral veins	Bones (especially lumbar spine), liver
Breast	Axillary, transpectoral, and internal mammary lymphatics	Bone, lung, brain, liver
Head and neck	Direct extension	Lymphatics, liver, bones
Ovarian	Direct extension, peritoneal seeding, mesenteric veins	Peritoneal surfaces, diaphragm, omentum, liver
Sarcoma (extremity)	Inferior vena cava, right ventricle, pulmonary artery	Lungs
Melanoma	Regional lymphatics	Intransit lymphatics, lung, liver, brain, gastrointestinal tract

understood selectivity of different cancers for different sites. Thus, breast cancer often spreads through the bloodstream to bones but rarely to kidney or spleen, whereas lymphomas often spread to the spleen but uncommonly spread to bone. In a key study, Fidler and coworkers injected different types of cancer cells into the carotid artery of mice. Despite identical blood flow-mediated distribution of the cancer cells, each cancer cell type produced cancers in very different parts of the brain.[48] This tissue selectivity is likely due to specific interactions between the cancer cells and specific receptors on the small blood vessels in different organs (Table 9-7). Molecular studies have identified specific factors secreted from cancers that are associated with specific site metastases.[49,50] For example, a factor that blocks bone growth, Dickkopf 1, was associated with bone lesions in multiple myeloma.

Distant Metastasis

What we have learned so far is that the invasion and metastasis of cancers is a complex and surprisingly difficult multistep process. When cancer cells are directly injected into the bloodstream of experimental animals, less than 0.01% of the cells survive. The most telling study is that of Tarin and coworkers, who followed a group of women with advanced ovarian cancer and malignant ascites.[51] These unfortunate women developed huge amounts of peritoneal fluid filled with malignant ovarian cancer cells. To relieve the pressure caused by the fluid accumulation, the fluid was surgically shunted into the venous circulation. This palliative procedure relieved the abdominal symptoms but had the side effect of moving millions of ovarian cancer cells an hour directly into the bloodstream. Despite this direct injection of cancer cells into the circulation, these women unexpectedly had no increased number of metastases when they died. Several important conclusions can be drawn from this surprising observational study: the vast majority of cancer cells do *not* have the ability to form a metastasis, and simple anatomic arrest of cancer cells in the first tissue they arrive at is not sufficient for them to establish a metastatic lesion. From this and many other studies, we now know that formation of a metastatic lesion requires a cancer cell to detach and migrate from its primary location, survive a passage through the body, and then successfully attach, invade, multiply, and stimulate angiogenesis in a new location. Thus, metastasis requires both an appropriate cancer cell, or "seed," and a permissive destination, or "soil."[47] Interruption of any of these steps may stop the establishment of metastatic disease.

QUICK CHECK 9-5

1. What steps are required for formation of distant metastasis?
2. Does the presence of circulating cancer cells in the blood mean a metastasis will happen?
3. What factors influence where a metastasis occurs?

Did You Understand?

Cancer Characteristics and Terminology

1. Benign tumors are usually encapsulated, well differentiated, and do not spread to distant locations.
2. Malignant tumors, compared to benign tumors, have more rapid growth rates, specific microscopic alterations (anaplasia and loss of differentiation), absence of normal tissue organization, and no capsule; they invade into blood vessels and lymphatics and have distant spread.

Did You Understand?—Cont'd

3. Carcinomas arise from epithelial tissue, sarcomas arise from connective tissue, lymphomas arise from lymphatic tissue, and leukemias are cancers of blood-forming cells. Carcinoma in situ (CIS) refers to preinvasive epithelial tumors of glandular or squamous cell origin.
4. Localized cancer is considered low stage, whereas cancers that have spread regionally or distantly are termed stage 3 and stage 4, respectively.
5. Cancer cells are characterized by anaplasia, or loss of differentiation, and autonomy, or independence from normal cellular controls.
6. Tumor markers are substances (i.e., hormones, enzymes, genes, antigens, antibodies) found in blood, spinal fluid, or urine. They are used to screen and identify individuals at high risk for cancer, to help diagnose specific types of tumors, and to follow the clinical course of cancer.
7. In the adult, undifferentiated cells (not totally committed to a specific function) are known as pluripotent cells, precursor cells, or stem cells. Cancer cells become more like embryonic cells and are less differentiated. Cancerous growth depends on derangements of cell differentiation.

The Genetic Basis of Cancer

1. Three main genetic mechanisms have a role in human carcinogenesis: (a) mutation of genes resulting in hyperactivity of growth-related gene products (such genes are called *oncogenes*); (b) mutation of genes resulting in loss or inactivity of gene products that normally would inhibit growth (such genes are called *tumor suppressor genes*); and (c) mutation of genes resulting in overexpression of products that prevent normal cell death, or apoptosis, thus allowing continued growth of tumors.
2. Genetic events are the primary basis of carcinogenesis. Mutations in cancer-causing genes accumulate with age, causing the increasing risk of cancer with advanced age.
3. Epidemiologic and molecular data suggest it takes five or six distinct mutations in different signaling pathways to produce cancer. Mutations activate growth-promotion pathways, block antigrowth signals, prevent apoptosis, turn on telomerase and new blood vessel growth (angiogenesis), and allow tissue invasion and distant metastasis.
4. In rare families, cancer is inherited in an autosomal dominant fashion as a result of mutations in tumor suppressor genes.
5. Proto-oncogenes encode for growth factors, growth-factor receptors, signal transducers, and nuclear growth-promoting proteins.
6. Tumor suppressor genes encode for proteins that act as inhibitors of growth. Tumor suppressor gene proteins block specific phases of the cell cycle, induce end-stage (e.g., terminal) differentiation, and stimulate cell senescence or death. Carcinogenesis, or the development of cancer, involves inactivation of tumor suppressor genes (usually by loss of heterozygosity, or by "silencing") and activation of oncogenes.

Infection, Immunity, Inflammation, and Cancer

1. A number of viruses can cause cancer. Human cervical cancer is caused by papillomavirus infection. Kaposi sarcoma is caused by infection with a member of the herpesvirus family. Chronic hepatitis B or C infection can cause liver cancer.
2. Immune system defects, such as those caused by immunosuppressant drugs or HIV infection, increase the risk of viral-associated cancers, such as EBV-associated lymphomas and cervical cancer.
3. Chronic inflammation contributes to the development of cancer by stimulating increased proliferation and angiogenesis. Chronic hepatitis and colitis are two examples where chronic inflammation markedly increases the risk of cancer.

Cancer Progression and Metastasis

1. Cancers metastasize through veins and lymphatics, first regionally and then distantly. Most cancer cells are not capable of successful metastasis; however, when metastasis does occur, it often portends a poor prognosis.
2. Most cancer cells are not capable of successful metastasis. Multiple steps, including invasion, survival in the circulation, attachment, and growth, and induction of angiogenesis at a favorable distant site are required. Thus, both the seed and the soil must be matched for metastasis to occur.

Key Terms

Adenocarcinoma, 223
Anaplasia, 226
Angiogenesis, 230
Angiogenic factor, 230
Apoptosis, 230
Autocrine stimulation, 228
Autonomy, 225
Benign tumor, 222
Cancer, 222
Carcinoma, 223
Carcinoma in situ (CIS), 223
Caretaker gene, 234
Chromosome amplification, 232
Chromosome instability, 234
Chromosome translocation, 232
Chronic inflammation, 237
Clinical staging, 225
Clonal expansion, 228
Clonal proliferation, 228
Epigenetic, 234
Human T cell leukemia virus (HTLV), 236
Immortality, 231
Leukemia, 223
Local spread, 238
Loss of heterozygosity (LOH), 233
Lymphoma, 223
Malignant tumor, 223
Metastasis, 238
Mutagen, 234
MYC protein, 232
Neoplasm, 222
Oncogene, 231
p53, 230
Pleomorphic, 226
Retinoblastoma *(Rb)* gene, 232
Point mutation, 231
Ras, 229
Sarcoma, 223
Silencing, 234
Telomerase, 231
Telomere, 231
Tumor, 222
Tumor marker, 226
Tumor-suppressor gene, 231

References

1. Kern SE: Progressive genetic abnormalities in human neoplasia, In Mendelsohn J et al, editors: *The molecular basis of cancer*, ed 2, Philadelphia, 2001, Saunders, p. 41.
2. Kinzler KW, Vogelstein B: Lessons from hereditary colorectal cancer, *Cell* 87:159–170, 1996.
3. Hanahan D, Weinberg RA: The hallmarks of cancer, *Cell* 100 (1):57–70, 2000.
4. Folkman J: Role of angiogenesis in tumor growth and metastasis, *Sem Oncol* 29(suppl 16):15–18, 2002.
5. Folkman J: Antiangiogenesis in cancer therapy—endostatin and its mechanisms of action, *Experi Cell Res* 312:594–607, 2006.
6. Mathon NF, Lloyd AC: Cell senescence and cancer, *Nat Rev Cancer* 1(3):203–213, 2001.
7. Shay JW, Wright WE: Telomerase: a target for cancer therapeutics, *Cancer Cell* 2(4):257–265, 2002.
8. Blasco MA: Telomeres and human disease: ageing, cancer, and beyond, *Nat Rev Genet* 6(8):611–622, 2005.
9. van't Veer LJ et al: Gene expression profiling predicts clinical outcome of breast cancer, *Nature* 415(6871):530–536, 2002.
10. Bos JL: *ras* oncogenes in human cancer: a review, *Cancer Res* 49(17):4682–4689, 1989.
11. Goldsby RE, Carroll WL: The molecular biology of pediatric lymphomas, *J Pediatr Hematol Oncol* 20(4):282–296, 1998.
12. Nowell P, Hungerford D: A minute chromosome in human granulocytic leukemia, *Science* 132:1497, 1960.
13. Druker BJ: Circumventing resistance to kinase-inhibitor therapy, *N Engl J Med* 354:2594–2596, 2006.
14. Druker BJ et al: Efficacy and safety of a specific inhibitor of the BCR-ABL tyrosine kinase in chronic myeloid leukemia, *N Engl J Med* 344(14):1031–1037, 2001.
15. Brodeur GM et al: Amplification of *N-myc* in untreated human neuroblastomas correlates with advanced disease stage, *Science* 224:1121–1124, 1984.
16. Berns EM et al: Prevalence of amplification of the oncogenes *c-myc*, HER2/*neu*, and int-2 in one thousand human breast tumours: correlation with steroid receptors, *Eur J Cancer* 28 (2–3):697–700, 1992.
17. Cavenee WK et al: Expression of recessive alleles by chromosomal mechanisms in retinoblastoma, *Nature* 305 (5937):779–784, 1983.
18. Esteller M et al: A gene hypermethylation profile of human cancer, *Cancer Res* 61(8):3225–3229, 2001.
19. Herman JG, Baylin SB: Gene silencing in cancer in association with promoter hypermethylation, *N Engl J Med* 349:2042–2054, 2003.
20. Karpf AR, Jones DA: Reactivating the expression of methylation silenced genes in human cancer, *Oncogene* 21(35): 5496–5503, 2002.
21. Feinberg AP, Ohlsson R, Henikoff S: The epigenetic progenitor origin of human cancer, *Nat Rev Genet* 7:21–33, 2006.
22. Rouse J, Jackson SP: Interfaces between the detection, signaling, and repair of DNA damage, *Science* 297(5581):547–551, 2002.
23. Mills KD, Ferguson DO, Alt FW: The role of DNA breaks in genomic instability and tumorigenesis, *Immunolog Rev* 194:77–95, 2003.
24. Liu B et al: Analysis of mismatch repair genes in hereditary *non-polyposis colorectal cancer patients, Nature Med* 2(2): 169–174, 1996.
25. Lengauer C, Kinzler KW, Vogelstein B: Genetic instability in colorectal cancers, *Nature* 386(6625):623–627, 1997.
26. Jorde LB et al: *Medical genetics*, ed 3, St Louis, 2003, Mosby.
27. Schneider K: *Counseling about cancer: strategies for genetic counseling*, ed 2, Hoboken, NJ, 2001, Wiley.
28. Howley PM, Ganem D, Kieff E: Etiology of cancer: DNA viruses, In Vincent J et al, editors: *Cancer: principles and practice*, Philadelphia, Lippincott, 2001, Williams, & Wilkins.
29. Poeschla EM et al: Etiology of cancer: RNA viruses, In Vincent J et al, editors: *Cancer: principles and practice of oncology*, Philadelphia, Lippincott, 2001, Williams & Wilkins.
30. Sepulveda AR et al: Molecular identification of main cellular lineages as a tool for the classification of gastric cancer, *Hum Pathol* 31(5):566–574, 2000.
31. Steinbrook R: The potential of human papillomaviruses, *N Engl J Med* 354:1109–1112, 2006.
32. Ando T et al: Causal role of *Helicobacter pylori* infection in gastric cancer, *World J Gastroenterol* 12:181–186, 2006.
33. Alexander GA, Brawley OW: Association of *Helicobacter pylori* infection with gastric cancer, *Mil Med* 165(1):21–27, 2000.
34. Smith VC, Genta RM: Role of *Helicobacter pylori* gastritis in gastric atrophy, intestinal metaplasia, and gastric neoplasia, *Microsc Res Tech* 48(6):313–320, 2000, review.
35. Byrd JC et al: Inhibition of gastric mucin synthesis by *Helicobacter pylori*, *Gastroenterology* 119(6):1072–1079, 2000.
36. Clifford GM et al: Cancer risk in the Swiss HIV cohort study: associations with immunodeficiency, smoking, and highly active antiretroviral therapy, *J Natl Ca Inst* 97:425–432, 2005.
37. Buell JF, Gross TG, Woodle ES: Malignancy after transplantation, *Transplant* 80:S254–S264, 2005.
38. Balkwill F, Coussens LM: Cancer: an inflammatory link, *Nature* 431:405–406, 2004.
39. Fitzpatrick FA: Inflammation, carcinogenesis and cancer, *Int Immunopharmacol* 1:1651–1667, 2001.
40. Vesterinen E et al: Cancer incidence among 78,000 asthmatic patients, *Int J Epidemiol* 22:976–982, 1993.
41. Karin M: Inflammation and cancer: the long reach of *ras*, *Nat Med* 11:20–21, 2005.
42. Sparmann A, Bar-Sagi D: *ras* oncogene and inflammation: partners in crime, *Cell Cycle* 4:735–736, 2005.
43. Greten FR et al: IKKbeta links inflammation and tumorigenesis in a mouse model of colitis-associated cancer, *Cell* 118:285–296, 2004.
44. Karin M: Nuclear factor-[kappa]B in cancer development and progression, *Nature* 441:431–436, 2006.
45. Fyles AW et al: Tamoxifen with or without breast irradiation in women 50 years of age or older with early breast cancer, *N Engl J Med* 351:963–970, 2004.
46. Carrick S et al: Single agent versus combination chemotherapy for metastatic breast cancer, *Cochrane Database Syst Rev* CD003372, 2005.
47. Fidler IJ: The pathogenesis of cancer metastasis: the "seed and soil" hypothesis revisited, *Nat Rev Cancer* 3:453–458, 2003.
48. Schackert G, Fidler IJ: Site-specific metastasis of mouse melanomas and a fibrosarcoma in the brain or meninges of syngeneic animals, *Cancer Res* 48:3478–3484, 1988.
49. Tian E et al: The role of the Wnt-signaling antagonist DKK1 in the development of osteolytic lesions in multiple myeloma, *N Engl J Med* 349:2483–2494, 2003.
50. Kang Y et al: Breast cancer bone metastasis mediated by the Smad tumor suppressor pathway, *PNAS* 102:13909–13914, 2005.
51. Tarin D et al: Mechanisms of human tumor metastasis studied in patients with peritoneovenous shunts, *Cancer Res* 44:3584–3592, 1984.

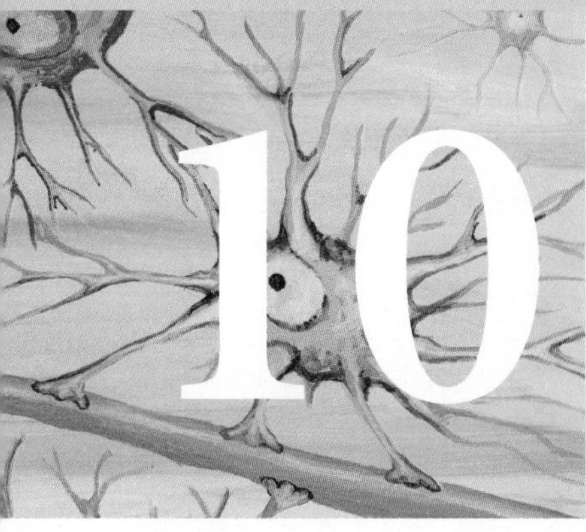

CANCER EPIDEMIOLOGY, MANIFESTATIONS, AND TREATMENT

Kathryn L. McCance ▪ Phillip Barnette

CHAPTER OUTLINE

ELECTRONIC RESOURCES

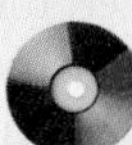

Companion CD
- Review Questions and Answers
- Animations

evolve Website
http://evolve.elsevier.com/Huether/
- Quick Check Answers
- Key Terms Exercises
- Critical Thinking Questions with Answers
- Algorithm Completion Exercises
- WebLinks

Cancer is fundamentally genetic. Tumors occur when certain changes, or mutations, occur in genes. The frequency and consequences of these genetic changes can, however, be altered by environmental factors. For example, certain chemicals can cause genetic mutations and induce tumor development in experimental animals. In addition, environmental factors may increase the growth of genetically altered cells without directly causing new mutations. Thus environmental factors interacting with genes play important roles in cancer development and progression.

Current treatment approaches are based on cell molecular alterations inherent in the initiation and progressive development of cancer invasion and metastases. The side effects and complications of cancer therapy can be troublesome, often rivaling the disease of cancer itself.

GENE-ENVIRONMENT INTERACTION AND RISK FACTORS

Research since the 1980s has led to a greater understanding of the genetic basis of neoplastic development. At the level of the cell, cancer is genetic. The frequency and consequences of these genetic mutations can be altered by a number of environmental factors. Two lines of evidence support the idea that exposure to environmental agents can increase an individual's risk of cancer. The first is based on the identification of environmental agents that have carcinogenic properties. In experimental animals, many agents cause cancer; thus, they are called **carcinogens.** Evidence from both epidemiologic and laboratory studies show, for example, that cigarette smoke causes lung cancer and other types of cancer. Many specific risk factors for cancer are now known, the most significant being smoking, radiation, obesity, a few oncogenic viruses, and *Helicobacter pylori* (*H. pylori*) bacteria (see Chapter 9 for a discussion of viruses and bacteria).[1,2]

The second line of evidence is based on comparisons of populations who have different lifestyles or different cancer rates of incidence (Figure 10-1). Important also is to understand that these rates include control factors such as access to health care, screening, and medical practice. Breast cancer, for example, is prevalent among northern Europeans

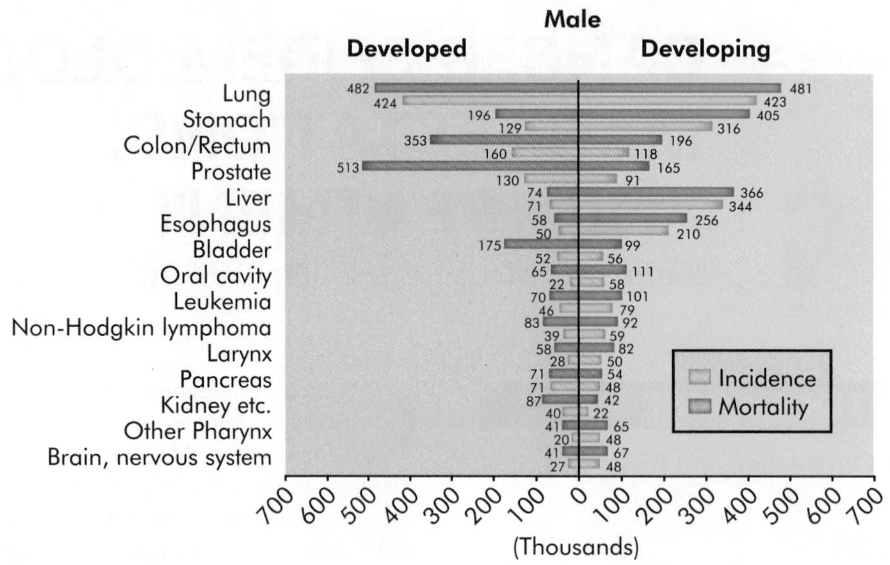

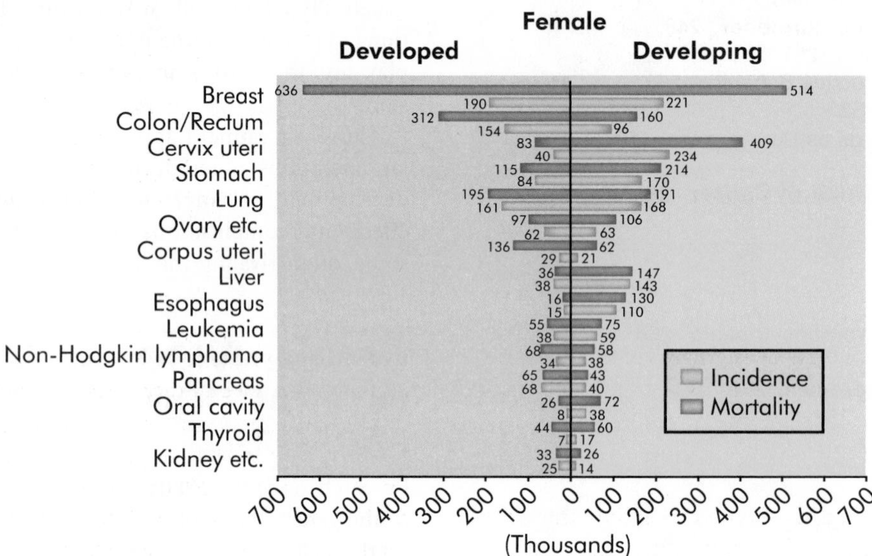

Figure 10-1 ■ **Estimated Numbers of New Cancer Cases (Incidence) and Deaths (Mortality) in 2002.** Data shown in thousands for developing and developed countries by cancer site and sex. (From Parkin DM et al: *CA Cancer J Clin* 55:74–108, 2005. © American Cancer Society.)

and Americans, but it is relatively rare among women in developing countries. The difficulty lies in determining whether these differences between populations are attributable to lifestyle factors, to genetics, or to both. The influence of environmental agents was demonstrated in studies of Japanese who immigrated to Hawaii and the U.S. mainland. Researchers studied the changes in incidence of colon and stomach cancer after emigration. Until recently, colon cancer was a relatively rare form of cancer in Japan. Among the first Japanese immigrants (first-generation) in Hawaii, colon cancer incidence rose several-fold but not as high as overall incidence on the U.S. mainland. Among second-generation Japanese on the U.S. mainland, colon cancer rates rose to the U.S. average. Conversely, stomach cancer is common in Japan but relatively rare in the United States. Japanese on the United States mainland have the same low incidence of stomach cancer as the U.S. average. Although these observations strongly implicate environment and lifestyle in the development of colon and stomach cancer, they do not rule out genetic factors. The difference in incidence rates could be the result of predisposing genes. One could argue that these genes are less penetrating for colon cancer in Japan because of environmental differences.[3] The incidence of colon cancer in Japan has increased dramatically, which is consistent with the Japanese adoption of a more Western diet (i.e., high fat, low fiber).

Environmental factors play important roles in cancer development. Because some individuals within the same environment develop cancer and others do not, cancer risk seems to depend on interaction between inherited factors

TABLE 10-1

Estimated New Cancer Cases and Deaths by Gender, United States, 2007*

	ESTIMATED NEW CASES			ESTIMATED DEATHS		
	Both Sexes	Male	Female	Both Sexes	Male	Female
All sites	1,444,920	766,860	678,060	559,650	289,550	270,100
Oral cavity and pharynx	34,360	24,180	10,180	7,550	5,180	2,370
Esophagus	15,560	12,130	3,430	13,940	10,900	3,040
Stomach	21,260	13,000	8,260	11,210	6,610	4,600
Colon†	112,340	55,290	57,050	52,180	26,000	26,180
Rectum	41,420	23,840	17,580	†	†	†
Pancreas	37,170	18,830	18,340	33,370	16,840	16,530
Lung and bronchus	213,380	114,760	98,620	160,390	89,510	70,880
Bones and joints	2,370	1,330	1,040	1,330	740	590
Melanoma-skin	59,940	33,910	26,030	8,110	5,220	2,980
Breast	180,510	2,030	178,480	40,910	450	40,460
Uterine cervix	11,150	—	11,150	3,670	—	3,670
Uterine corpus	39,080	—	39,080	7,400	—	7,400
Ovary	22,430	—	22,430	15,280	—	15,280
Prostate	218,890	218,890	—	27,050	27,050	—
Testis	7,920	7,920	—	380	380	—
Urinary bladder	67,160	50,040	17,120	13,750	9,630	4,120
Brain and other nervous system	20,500	11,170	9,330	12,740	7,150	5,590
Thyroid	33,550	8,070	25,480	1,530	650	880
Hodgkin lymphoma	8,190	4,470	3,720	1,070	770	300
Leukemia	44,240	24,800	19,440	21,790	12,320	9,470

From American Cancer Society: *Cancer facts and figures 2007,* Atlanta, 2007, The Society.
*Excludes basal and squamous cell skin cancers and in situ carcinomas except urinary bladder. About 62,030 female carcinoma in situ of the breast and 48,290 melanoma in situ will be newly diagnosed in 2007.
†Estimated deaths for colon and rectum cancers are combined.

and environmental agents. Table 10-1 summarizes the estimated new cases and deaths caused by cancer, by gender, for specified sites.

Tobacco Use

Cigarette smoke is carcinogenic and remains the most important cause of cancer. The risk is greatest in those who begin to smoke when young and continue throughout life.[1] Cigarette smoking remains the leading preventable cause of death in the United States, accounting for 1 of every 5 deaths each year.[4] An estimated 20.9% of all adults (44.5 million) smoke cigarettes in the United States.[4] Estimates of cigarette smoking by age include the following: 18 to 24 years (23.6%), 25 to 44 years (23.8%), 45 to 64 years (22.4%), and 65 years or older (8.8%).[4] Cigarette smoking is more common among men (23.4%) than women (18.5%). The Global Youth Tobacco Survey (GYTS), however, found no differences by gender showing an increase use of tobacco among young women in developing countries.[5] Prevalence of cigarette smoking is highest among American Indians/Alaskan Natives (33.4%), then whites (22.2%), African Americans (20.2%), Hispanics (15%), and Asians (11.3%).[4] Cigarette smoking is more common among adults living below the poverty level (29.1%) than those above the poverty level (20.6%).[4]

Tobacco smoking is responsible for 30% of all cancer deaths in developed countries, and an epidemic of cancer deaths is expected in developing countries.[6] Tobacco use is associated primarily with squamous and small cell carcinomas of the lung and pulmonary adenocarcinomas. It has been linked to cancers of the lower urinary tract (renal, penis, and bladder), upper aerodigestive tract (including the oral cavity, pharynx, larynx, nasal cavities, paranasal sinuses, esophagus, and stomach), liver, kidney, pancreas, cervix uteri, and myeloid leukemia.[6] Current evidence is not convincing for cancer of the large bowel and is inconsistent with breast cancer. In addition, smoking causes *even more* deaths from vascular, respiratory, and other diseases than from cancer; in total it accounts for an astonishing 4 to 5 million deaths a year worldwide.[6]

Secondhand smoke, also called **environmental tobacco smoke (ETS),** is the combination of sidestream smoke (burning end of a cigarette, cigar, or pipe) and mainstream smoke (exhaled by the smoker). More than 4000 chemicals have been identified in mainstream tobacco smoke, of which 60 are considered carcinogenic.[7] Measuring secondhand smoke is difficult. Nonsmokers who live with smokers are at greatest risk for lung cancer as well as numerous noncancerous conditions.[7]

Cigar or pipe smoking is strongly and causally related to cancers of the oral cavity, oropharynx, hypopharynx, larynx, esophagus, and lung.[6] Pipe smokers have a lower risk of dying from tobacco than cigarette smokers, but it is as harmful as, and perhaps more harmful, than cigar smoking.[8] Bidi smoking (a small amount of tobacco wrapped in the leaf of another plant—used in South Asia) delivers higher amounts of nicotine per gram of tobacco and comparable or greater amounts of tar compared to cigarettes.[6] Research case-control studies indicate bidi smoking can cause cancers of the respiratory and digestive tracts.

Measures that prevent young adults from starting smoking would substantially avoid the future disease burden. Therefore, an important public health approach is needed that *prevents* young people from *starting* smoking and helps others *stop* smoking.

Ionizing Radiation

Much of the knowledge of the effects of ionizing radiation on human cancer has stemmed from observations of the Hiroshima and Nagasaki atomic bomb exposures, particularly the Life Span Study. These data provide the best estimate of human cancer risk over the dose range from 20 to 250 cGy for low linear energy transfer (LET) radiation, such as x-rays or γ-rays. The horrible atomic bomb exposures in Japan caused acute leukemias in adults and children and increased frequencies of thyroid and breast carcinomas. Lung, stomach, colon, esophageal, and urinary tract cancers and multiple myeloma have lately been added to the list. These risks are apparently not heritable—offspring of both atomic bombs and cancer survivors do not have an increased risk of malformations, cancer, or chromosome abnormalities.[9–11]

Human exposure to ionizing radiation includes emissions from x-rays, radioisotopes, and other radioactive sources. Health risks involve not only neoplastic diseases but also somatic mutations that may contribute to other diseases (e.g., birth defects and eye maladies) and inherited mutations that may affect the incidence of diseases in future generations. The cancer risk of loss of life expectancy at doses below 20 cGy is uncertain and contentious and has been the subject of controversy for decades[12] (see below). Heritable mutations are of particular concern for women because the number of oocytes are presumably fixed at birth and mutations, if not repaired, are cumulative.[12]

Presently, radiobiologists, geneticists, physicists, and others are debating the risks of low-dose radiation because of the potential impact on the health of current and future generations.[12] Two opposing hypotheses have emerged: (1) there is no dose of radiation considered safe and the use of radiation must always be considered on the basis of risk versus benefit, and (2) the health risks of diagnostic doses less than 10 cGy are not now measurable and may be nonexistent. Limiting is that general findings on the health risks of low-dose radiation are made by analyses of data on the risk of cancer alone.[12] The expression of radiation-induced damage depends not only on dose, fractionation, and protraction but also on repair mechanisms, bystander effects, radioprotective substances such as antioxidants, and how it is delivered.[12]

Radiation-induced cancer

Human cancers result from the accumulation of multiple hits (overexpression of genes, deletion of genes, or gene mutations), some of which occur in critical genes that regulate proliferation and differentiation (see Biology of Cancer). Radiation-induced cancer in humans seems to have long latent periods: 10 years for leukemia and over 30 years for solid tumors.[13] This implies that radiation-induced gene mutations or chromosomal alterations that can be detected early (within 24 hours of radiation exposure) are not *solely* responsible for tumor development in normal human cells. Such mutations, however, provide a critical hit or induce genetic instability that make cells more susceptible to accumulation of genetic alterations caused by other spontaneous or induced mutations. The accumulation of mutations leads to full transformation and cancer.[12]

Carcinogenesis: genomic instability

Biologic consequences of exposure to ionizing radiation include cell death, gene mutations, and chromosome aberrations (Figure 10-2). Many in vitro studies have demonstrated chromosome aberrations and mutations not only exist in the clonal progeny of irradiated cells but in other cells (noncolonal) not directly radiated. These *innocent cells* are referred to as **bystander effects** and are considered manifestations of genomic instability[14] (see the discussion that follows and Figure 10-2, *C*). Radiobiologists, geneticists, physicists, and others have known for many years that radiation-induced cellular alterations (cytotoxicity), identified as a loss of reproductive potential, might be delayed for several generations of cell replication, with death occurring randomly among the progeny cells.[14] This delayed cell death phenotype is known as *lethal mutation* and *delayed reproductive death.*

The genome is constantly challenged by destabilizing factors, including normal DNA replication and cell division, intracellular and extracellular environmental stresses, such as oxidative metabolism, exposure to genotoxic chemical agents, and background radiation. Cells have complex mechanisms for trying to maintain genomic stability. Failure of any of these processes can result in destabilization of the genome, deleterious mutations, and alterations in cell proliferation.

Although similar to alterations to the chromosome instability syndromes, the radiation-induced genomic instability seems to reflect epigenetic phenomena rather than mutation of genome genes.[15] Experiments have shown that irradiation can induce growth factors and extracellular matrix (microenvironment) remodeling. A major function of the microenvironment is to control cell differentiation and proliferation, and its disruption is required for the establishment of cancer.[16] Some genotypes, however, may be more susceptible than others.

Bystander effects

Low-dose ionizing radiation causes significantly different biologic responses than does high-dose radiation. Two important findings concerning the biologic effects of a low dose of radiation occur in both the irradiated cells and in cells that are not, themselves, radiated—the so-called

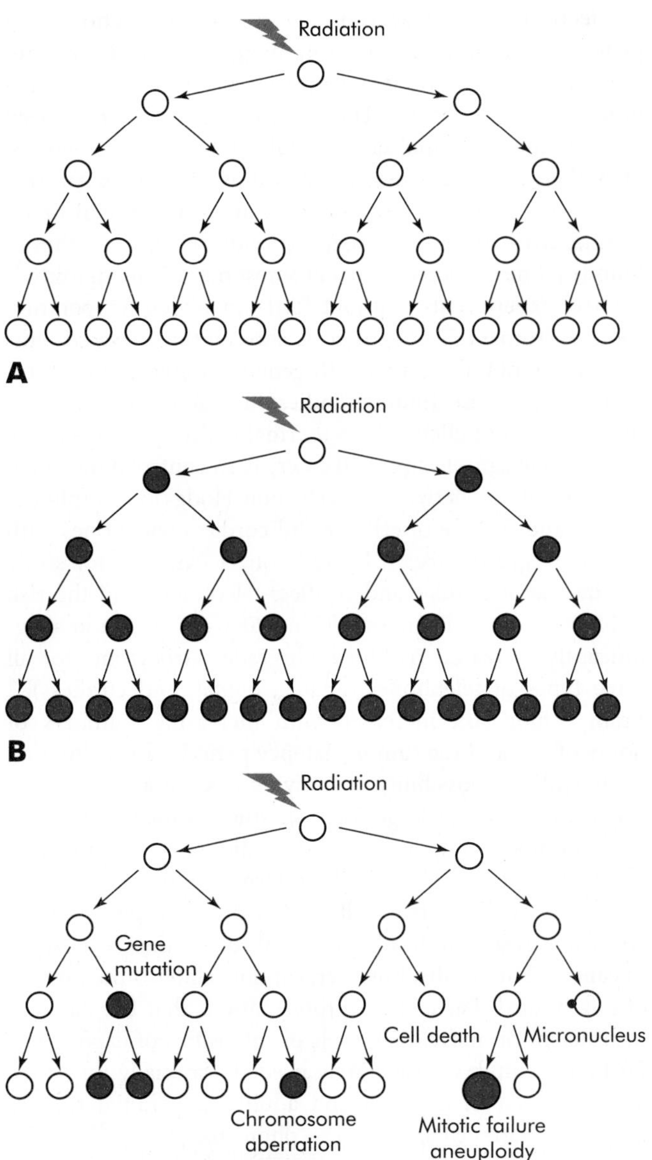

Figure 10-2 ■ **Models of the Responses of Clonogenic Cells to Ionizing Radiation.** Mutations or chromosomal aberrations are shown as filled circles and apparently normal cells as open circles. **A,** If a cell faithfully repairs DNA damage, then its clonal descendents will appear normal. **B,** If a cell is directly mutated by radiation, then all its descendents will express the same mutation. **C,** Radiation-induced genomic instability is characterized by nonclonal effects in descendant cells. (From Lorimore SA, Coates PJ, Wright EG: Radiation-induced genomic instability and bystander effects: inter-related nontargeted effects of exposure to ionizing radiation. *Oncogene* 22[45]:7058–7069, 2003.)

bystander effect: (1) radiation-induced genomic instability occurs in the descendant cells of the irradiated cell after several generations of cell division, and (2) radiation-induced bystander effects are caused as a consequence of damage signals transmitted from neighboring irradiated cells whereby transmission may be mediated by either direct or intercellular communication through gap junctions or by factors released into the surrounding medium.[17] In both findings, the biologic effects appear to be associated with oxidative stress and the generation of reactive oxygen species (ROS) (e.g., super oxide and hydrogen peroxide; see Chapter 3). Nitric oxide, however, may initiate intercellular signaling pathways that influence the bystander effects.[17,18]

Gap junction function

Confluent cell cultures respond as an integrated whole rather than separate individual cells that have been irradiated, indicating a critical role for cell-to-cell communication in mediating the bystander effect. This mediation could be controlled by gap junctions. Gap junctions consist of a cell-to-cell channel spanning two plasma membranes; they result from the bridging of two half channels, or connexons, contributed separately by each of the two participating cells (see Figure 1-8, in Chapter 1).[19] Exposure of cells to low levels of radiation ($\leq$0.16 cGy) significantly induces the expression of connexin 43, suggesting that oxidizing mediators increase expression of proteins involved in gap junction intercellular communication (GJIC).[20]

In conclusion, emerging data support a role for both oxidative stress and GJIC in the radiation-induced bystander effects. Further, studies of the molecular mechanisms underlying bystander cells should increase our understanding of the overall risk caused by ionizing radiation.

Ultraviolet Radiation

Ultraviolet sunlight *causes* basal cell carcinoma and squamous cell carcinoma (i.e., photocarcinogenesis), two common skin cancers found in white individuals. Exposure to ultraviolet radiation (UVR) can emanate from both natural and artificial sources; however, the principal source of exposure for most people is sunlight. With further depletion of the stratospheric ozone layer, people and the environment will be exposed to higher intensities of UVR. The degree of damage in skin depends on the intensity and wavelength content (i.e., ultraviolet A [UVA] or ultraviolet B [UVB]) and the depth of penetration. UV radiation is now known to cause specific gene mutations. In addition, UV light induces the release of tumor necrosis factor-α (TNF-α) in the epidermis, which may reduce immune surveillance against skin cancer.[21]

Inflammation is a critical component of tumor progression. The observed inflammatory response following acute and chronic UV radiation may contribute to skin carcinogenesis by releasing free radicals.[22]

Basal cell carcinoma commonly occurs on the head and neck. Individuals with these tumors generally have light complexions, light eyes, and fair hair. They tend to sunburn rather than tan and live in areas of high sunlight exposure. Usually these cancers arise on areas of the body that receive the greatest sun exposure, although they are not necessarily restricted to these skin sites. Squamous cell carcinoma is found more commonly in men who work outdoors. These tumors are distributed over the head, neck, and exposed areas of the upper extremities (see Chapter 39).

The incidence and mortality rates of those with melanoma have increased annually at rates of 2% to 3% since the 1970s.[23] Sun exposure and the risk of melanoma, a malignant pigmented mole, remain complex. Epidemiologic and case control studies suggest that UVR exposure is the most significant factor for the development of melanoma. Other evidence, however, reports that rates of melanoma are uncommon in persons with outdoor occupations.[24] Although the nonmelanoma skin cancers are related to cumulative exposure to UV radiation, melanoma is related to episodes of intense, intermittent exposure (measured as history of sunburn).[23] Sunburn reflects an overdose of UV light, triggering inflammation with an increase in cytokine production. Melanomas more commonly occur in areas less continuously exposed to sunlight, like the trunks in men and back of the legs in women. Family history (i.e., genetic factors), skin type, and the density of moles are important in determining the risk of developing melanoma. Traits associated with a high risk of melanoma are light-colored hair, eyes, and skin; an inability to tan; and a tendency to freckle, sunburn, and develop nevi.[25]

Electromagnetic Fields

Health risks associated with electromagnetic fields (EMF) are controversial. Exposure to electric and magnetic fields is widespread. EMFs are a type of nonionizing radiation, low-frequency radiation without enough energy to break off electrons from their orbits around atoms and ionize (charge) the atoms. Microwaves, radar, and power frequency radiation associated with electricity and radio waves, fluorescent lights, computers, and other electric equipment all create EMFs of varying strength. The major debate since the 1960s has focused on the association of exposure to EMF and resultant health consequences, including cancer. Currently, no consistent body of evidence exists in support of an association between EMF and childhood cancer, albeit it warrants further investigation.[26] Evidence of an association between EMF and adult cancers, derived largely from occupational settings, is also inconsistent. In addition, little evidence indicates an association between EMF and noncancer health effects. Scientific evidence, however, is hampered by methods to accurately measure exposure, the lack of a clear dose/response relationship, and the difficulty in reproducing effects.

In 1998, however, a National Institute of Environmental Health Sciences EMF working group recommended that low-frequency EMFs be classified as possible carcinogens.[27] A population-based study ($N = 5400$ women) linked residential EMF exposure from high-voltage power lines to a 60% increased risk of breast cancer in Norwegian women of all ages.[28]

The controversy about potential health hazards associated with the exposure of electromagnetic fields has been stimulated by the increased use of mobile telecommunication devices and emissions from cell towers. Cellular telephones emit electromagnetic radiation in the range of 800 to 2000 MHz, which is in the microwave range (300 MHz to 300 GHz).

Electromagnetic radiation from a cellular phone can penetrate the skull and deposit energy 4 cm to 6 cm into the brain.[29] This energy can potentially result in thermal heating of the tissue. The debate, therefore, has been whether these thermal effects could induce carcinogenesis. One thermal mechanism proposed is change in protein phosphorylation.[30,31] Exposure of human peripheral blood lymphocytes to EMFs associated with cellular telephones found a linear increase in chromosome 17 aneuploidy.[32] Control experiments (without EMF) involving temperature changes from 24.5° C to 38.5° C showed that elevated temperature is not associated with genetic or epigenetic alterations. Thus, these findings indicated a genotoxic effect of the EMFs is not elicited by a thermal pathway.[32] One study with a small sample size (910 cases, 1016 controls) indicated an association between T-cell non-Hodgkin lymphoma (NHL) and the use of cellular and cordless telephones with 5-year or greater use.[33] In addition, a case-control study on the use of cellular and cordless telephones and the risk of brain tumors (diagnosed during 2000–2003) found a significantly increased risk for high-grade astrocytoma for all three types of telephones (analog, digital, and cordless).[34] Brain tumor risk increased with increasing numbers of hours of use and the tumor's latency period. This is the first study with the possibility of studying risk among long-term users. Contrarily, a large Swedish study, which included a large number of long-term users, did not find any risk increases for either short- or long-term exposures.[35] In summary, the evidence from all studies does not give clear or consistent results indicating a causal role of EMF exposures in cancer. The results, however, cannot establish the *absence* of any hazard. Particularly problematic is that the data are insufficient on individual levels or intensities of exposure.[36] Further research is desperately needed, especially for EMFs and leukemia in children and adults and cranial tumors associated with cell and cordless phone use.

Diet and Endogenous Hormones

Understanding dietary factors that increase the risk for cancer is complex and challenging. It is complex because of the variety of foods consumed, the many constituents of foods, the metabolic consequences of eating, the temporal changes in the patterns of food use, and accurate recall and response. Cancer risks in the elderly may also depend as much on diet in early life as on current eating practices.[1,37]

People are constantly exposed to a variety of compounds termed **xenobiotics** (Greek *xenos,* foreign; *bios,* life) that include toxic, mutagenic, and carcinogenic chemicals. Many of these chemicals are found in the human diet. Most xenobiotics are transported in the blood by lipoproteins and penetrate through lipid membranes. These chemicals can react with cellular macromolecules, such as proteins and DNA, or can react directly with cell structures to cause cell damage.[38] The body has two defense systems for counteracting these effects: (1) detoxification enzymes and (2) antioxidant systems (see Chapter 3). Enzymes that activate xenobiotics are called **phase I activation enzymes** and are represented by the multigene cytochrome P450 family, aldehyde oxidase, xanthine oxidases, and peroxidases. **Phase II detoxification enzymes** then protect further against a large array of reactive intermediates and nonactivated xenobiotics.[38] These enzymes are located predominantly in the liver and provide clearance of compounds through the portal circulation, thereby preventing the potentially carcinogenic agent(s) from entering the body through the gastrointestinal tract and portal circulation. These enzymes also occur in the skin epithelia and can be induced in other extrahepatic tissue, such as the lung.

Dietary sources of potentially toxic carcinogenic substances include compounds produced in the cooking of fat, meat, or protein, and naturally occurring carcinogens associated with plant food substances, such as alkaloids or mold by-products.[38] The most studied and most relevant carcinogens produced by cooking are the polycyclic aromatic hydrocarbons benzo[a]pyrene and heterocyclic aromatic amines generated by meat protein. The greatest levels are found in well-done, charbroiled beef. People, likewise, ingest xenobiotics that are found in environmental or industrial contaminants (e.g., particulate matter of diesel exhaust, contaminating pesticides in food and water supplies) and in certain prescribed and over-the-counter medicines.

The strongest, most consistent and unequivocal support for diet playing a role in carcinogenesis comes from data related to consumption of alcohol; aflatoxin (produced by mold), which can contaminate corn, peanuts, and rice stored in hot, humid environments; and Chinese-style salted fish that has been fed to infants, which causes nasopharyngeal cancer.[1,39–41] Abundant research since the 1980s has shown that rates for various cancers correlate fairly consistently with certain dietary factors, but opinions differ on the strength of the evidence.[1,42,43] Table 10-2 shows the relationship between dietary factors and cancer risk. Emerging is an emphasis on dietary patterns. The Western pattern includes a higher intake of red and processed meats, refined grains, sweets and desserts, and high-fat dairy products. This pattern is opposed to a prudent pattern of fruits, vegetables, whole grains, low-fat diary products, fish, and poultry and may prove to increase cancer risk.

Obesity

The prevalence of overweight and obesity in most developed countries (and in urban areas of many less developed countries) has been increasing greatly since the 1980s. The only globally accepted criteria for overweight and obesity are based on body-mass index (BMI).

A large prospective study of 900,000 American adults showed obesity is linked to cancer. Starting with a mean age of 57 years, individuals were followed for 16 years and cancer mortality data were collected during that interval.[44] Compared with men whose body mass index was in the normal range (18.5 to 24.9), men with substantial obesity (BMI ≥40.0) had significant increases in cancer mortality. Women had a similar risk. Although significant, people with lesser degrees of obesity had lesser increases in cancer mortality. In men with higher BMI, there were higher rates of death from esophageal, stomach, colorectal, liver, gallbladder, pancreatic, prostate, and kidney cancers and non-Hodgkin lymphoma, multiple myeloma, and leukemia.[44] Among women, high BMI was correlated with greater morbidity from colorectal, liver, gallbladder, pancreatic, breast, uterine, cervical, ovarian, and kidney cancers and from non-Hodgkin lymphoma and multiple myeloma. Thus, the American Cancer Society estimates that obesity accounts for 14% of cancer deaths in men and 20% in women.

Biologic mechanisms

Adipose tissue is *active* endocrine and metabolic tissue and can have even more effects on the physiology of other tissue (see Chapter 34). In response to endocrine and metabolic signals from other organs, adipose tissue responds by increasing or decreasing the release of free fatty acids—fuel for skeletal muscle and other tissues. When triglycerides, the main storage lipid, are metabolically hydrolyzed, they release free fatty acids into the blood. Abdominal visceral adipocytes are more metabolically active than abdominal subcutaneous adipocytes and because visceral adipocytes have high lipolytic activity and release large amounts of free fatty acids, accurate measurements of adiposity needs to consider both the *amount* and the *site* of deposition of the adipose tissue. Adipose tissue is very important in the regulation of energy balance and lipid metabolism through the release of peptide hormones, including leptin, adiponectin, resistin, and tumor necrosis factor-γ (TNF-γ). Increased release of free fatty acids, resistin, and TNF-γ by adipose tissue and *reduced* release of adiponectin give rise to *insulin resistance*—a state characterized by reduced metabolic response of tissues (muscle, liver, adipose) to insulin and to compensatory hyperinsulinemia.[45] In addition to its role in regulating energy balance, lipid metabolism, and insulin sensitivity, adipose tissue cells produce various steroid-hormone-metabolizing enzymes and are an important source of circulating estrogens in postmenopausal women (also see breast cancer and prostate cancer in Chapter 32).

Excess weight, increased plasma triglyceride levels, low levels of physical activity, and certain dietary factors can all contribute to chronic hyperinsulinemia. Chronically increased insulin levels have been correlated with the pathogenesis of colon, breast, pancreatic, and endometrial cancers (Figure 10-3).[46] These cancer-causing effects of insulin might be mediated by insulin receptors in the preneoplastic or neoplastic target cells or could be caused by alterations in endogenous hormone metabolism secondary to hyperinsulinemia. For example, insulin promotes the synthesis and biologic activity of the growth factor **insulin-like growth factor–1 (IGF-1).** IGF-1 is a peptide hormone with a molecular structure similar to insulin that regulates cellular proliferation in response to available

TABLE 10-2

Relationship of Dietary Factors With Risk of Major Cancers*

Diet	Colorectal	Breast	Prostate	Lung	Stomach	Esophageal	Oral	Pancreatic	Bladder	Kidney	Endometrial
MICRONUTRIENTS/ENERGY BALANCE											
OBESITY	↑↑	↑↑			↑†	↑†		↑		↑	↑↑
GI/GL,‡ IGF, height, or metabolic syndrome	↑↑	↑	↑					↑		↑	↑
Animal fat			↑								↑
NUTRIENTS											
Folic acid	↓↓	↓		↓							
Alcohol	↑↑	↑↑				↑↑	↑				
Calcium	↓		↑								
Vitamin D	↓		↓								
β-carotene supplements				↑↑§	↓						
Lycopene-containing foods			↓	↓	↓						
Vitamin C				↓							
Vitamin E			↓								
Selenium			↓	↓							
FOODS											
Red or processed meat	↑		↑								
Fruits¶	↓		↓	↓	↓	↓	↓				↓
Vegetables¶	↓	↓	↓	↓	↓	↓	↓		↓		↓
OTHER											
Grilled meat	↑	↑									
Western diet pattern	↑										
High-fiber diet	↓										
Salt, preserved foods					↑						
Hot beverages						↑	↑				

From McCullough ML, Giovannucci EL: *Oncogene* 23(38):6349–6364, 2004.

IGF, Insulin-like growth factor.

*Two arrows indicate more consistent evidence.

†Cancers of the gastric cardia.

‡*GI/GL,* glycemic index/glycemic load.

§Increased risk limited to smokers.

¶Evidence for a potential benefit from some components of fruits and vegetables (not necessarily blanket effect).

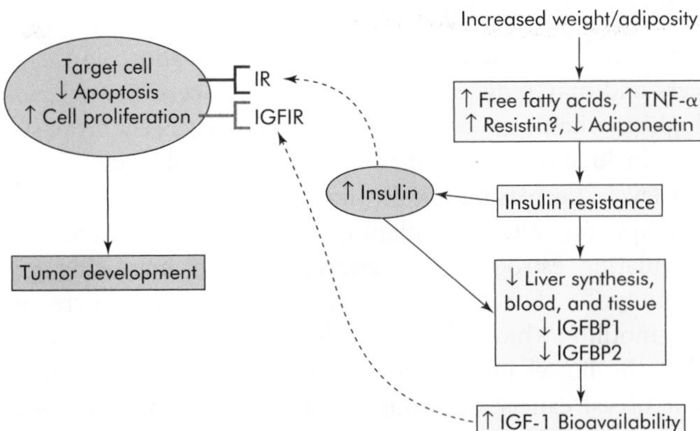

Figure 10-3 ■ Energy Balance, Lipid Metabolism, and Insulin Sensitivity and Tumor Development. In obesity, increased release from adipose tissue of free fatty acids (FFA), tumor necrosis factor alpha (TNF-α) and resistin, and reduced release of adiponectin lead to insulin resistance and compensatory chronic hyperinsulinemia. Increased insulin levels ultimately lead to decreased liver synthesis and blood levels of insulin-like growth factor-binding protein 1 (IGFBP1) and, theoretically, also decrease IGFBP1 synthesis locally in other tissues. Increased fasting levels of insulin in plasma are also correlated with decreased levels of IGFBP2 in the blood leading to increased levels of bioavailable IGF-1. Insulin and IGF-1 signal through the insulin receptors (IRs) and IGF-1 receptor (IGF1R) to stimulate cellular proliferation and inhibit apoptosis in many tissue types. These effects could promote tumor development. (Adapted from Calle EE, Kaaks R: Overweight, obesity and cancer: epidemiological evidence and proposed mechanisms. *Nat Rev Cancer* 4(8):579–591, 2004.)

energy and nutrients from diet and body constituents (see Figure 10-3). In addition, insulin promotes the synthesis and biologic availability of the male and female sex hormones, including estrogens, progesterone, and androgens.[5] The IGF-binding proteins (IGBPs) regulate the availability of IGF-1 because they stabilize the large pool of IGF-1 in the circulation, the efflux of IGF-1 from this circulation pool toward target tissues and binding of IGF-1 to its receptor.[45] IGBP3 increases tissue apoptosis, so decreased amounts may contribute to carcinogenesis.

Endogenous hormones

Three mechanisms are known involving how adiposity influences the synthesis and bioavailability of endogenous sex steroids, the estrogens, progesterone, and androgens.

1. Adipose tissue expresses various sex-steroid metabolizing enzymes that promote the formation of estrogens from androgenic precursors (secreted by the gonads and adrenal glands).
2. Adipose cells increase the circulating levels of insulin and increase IGF-1 biologic activity. This results in reduced liver synthesis and blood levels of sex hormone–binding globulin (SHBG), a binding hormone with affinity for estradiol and testosterone. The adiposity-related decrease in SHBG increases bioavailable estradiol in both men and women. In women, decreased SHBG also leads to increased levels of testosterone; in men, contrarily, decreases in SHBG generally lead to reduction in total testicular testosterone production and *no* increase in bioavailable testosterone.
3. High insulin levels can increase ovarian and, possibly, adrenal androgen synthesis and in some genetically susceptible, premenopausal women cause the development of polycystic ovary syndrome (PCOS) (see Chapter 32).[47]

Epidemiologic evidence shows that adiposity-induced alterations in blood levels of sex steroids could explain the correlation noted between indices of excess weight and risks of breast cancer (postmenopausal only) and endometrium cancer (both premenopausal and postmenopausal).[45] Among men, prostate carcinogenesis is thought to be related to endogenous hormone metabolism, including androgen production, and, possibly, estrogens.

Alcohol Consumption

Chronic alcohol consumption is a strong risk factor for cancer of the oral cavity, pharynx, hypopharynx, larynx, esophagus, and liver. Cirrhosis resulting from alcohol increases the risk of liver cancer. Although a statistical relationship is found consistently, alcohol consumption is less strongly related to breast cancer and colorectal cancer; however, it is known to increase cell growth of human breast cancer cells in vitro.[48] A meta-analysis showed no consistent relationship between alcohol and cancers of the pancreas, lung, prostate, or bladder.[49] Alcohol interacts with smoke, increasing the risk of malignant tumors, possibly by acting as a solvent for the carcinogenic chemicals in smoke products. In addition, inherited genetic factors put some individuals at increased risk. Genetic mechanisms may include differences in DNA repair ability, carcinogen metabolism, and cell cycle control.[50] Mechanisms that may promote carcinogenic action include (1) local cellular toxicity that affects the mucosal permeability; (2) reactive oxygen species resulting from ethanol metabolism; (3) presence of low levels of carcinogens in alcoholic beverages, oils, nitrosamines, and polycyclic aromatic hydrocarbons; (4) induction of enzymes that activate procarcinogens in target tissues; (5) alcoholic liver injury that may affect important mechanisms of chemical detoxification; (6) nutritional deficiencies (e.g., vitamins A and C, folate, riboflavin, and iron) that give rise to altered mucosal integrity, enzyme and metabolic dysfunction, and structural abnormalities; and (7) decreased immune responsiveness.[51]

Women have a greater sensitivity to alcohol, progress to alcohol toxicity faster, and have increased mortality at lower levels of consumption as compared with men.[52] The relationship between cancer risk and alcohol consumption is difficult to determine because of problems in accurately measuring the amount of alcohol ingested and in defining other behavioral habits, such as smoking, that further complicate or confound the clinical picture.

HEALTH ALERT

Possible Components of a Cancer-Prevention Diet

Some foods increase the risk of cancer, whereas other foods decrease the risk. Observing the following dietary guidelines might reduce the risk of cancer:

Increase
- Fiber (limiting glycemic index)
- Fruits and vegetables (especially broccoli, cabbage, and Swiss chard)
- Foods containing vitamins A, C, D, and E; mineral selenium (not to exceed 200 mcg/day)
- Epigallocatechin gallate (found in green tea)

Decrease
- Fat (especially large amounts of omega-6 fatty acids)
- High glycemic index carbohydrates, foods with high amounts of preservatives
- Alcohol
- Grilled, blackened foods
- Fried foods
- High levels of calcium (≥2000 mg)*

*Influences cancer risk in a complex way; lower levels (≤1000 mg/day may) confer protection.

Sexual and Reproductive Behavior

Research since the 1990s has demonstrated that sexually transmitted infection with carcinogenic types of human papilloma virus (HPV), called *high-risk types of HPV*, are required for the development of most cervical cancers. HPV infections, however, are common in sexually active women and the majority of these infections will resolve or only cause transient minor problems.[53] Eighty HPV types have been sequenced; 30 of these infect both the female and male genital tract, and two-thirds are classified as high-risk types. In most countries, HPV-16 accounts for 50% to 60% of cervical cancer cases, followed by HPV-18 (10% to 12%) and HPV-31 and HPV-45 (4% to 5% each). *Low-risk types of HPV* (HPV-2 and HPV-11) are correlated with genital warts and are rarely associated with cancer. Persistence of infection with high-risk HPV is a prerequisite for the development of cervical intraepithelial neoplasia (CIN) 3 (see Figure 32-13 in Chapter 32), lesions, and invasive cervical cancers.[53]

Biologic factors related to persistence include older age, 5 or more years of oral contraceptive use, five or more pregnancies, smoking, and human immunodeficiency virus (HIV) infection.[53,54] Earlier reported factors, such as number of sexual partners, are probable indicators of HPV exposure rather than an independent risk factor. HPV can be transmitted by genital contact (oral, touching, or sexual intercourse); therefore, condoms are not necessarily protective.

Newborn babies can be exposed to cervical HPV infection of the mother. The modes of transmission in children, however, are controversial.[55]

Physical Activity

Physical activity reduces the risk of breast and colon cancers and may reduce the risk of other cancers. Several biologic mechanisms causing this effect have been proposed and include decreasing insulin and insulin-like growth factor levels, decreasing obesity, increasing free radical scavenger systems, altering inflammatory mediators, decreasing circulating estrogens and androgens, and increasing gut motility.[56,57] For colon cancer, physical activity increases gut motility, which reduces the length of time (transit time) that the bowel lining is exposed to potential mutagens.[58] For breast cancer, vigorous physical activity may decrease exposure of breast tissue to ovarian hormones, insulin, and insulin-like factor. Decreased tissue exposure to growth factors may also improve outcomes for those with prostate cancer. A randomized trial found that after 12 months of moderate-intensity exercise, postmenopausal women had significantly decreased serum estrogens.[59] Physical activity also helps prevent type 2 diabetes that has been associated with risk of cancer of the colon and pancreas, as well as cancer-related fatigue.[59–61]

Many questions are unanswered regarding frequency, intensity, and duration of exercise. Much of the literature suggests between 3.5 and 4 hours of vigorous activity per week are necessary to optimize protection for colon cancer.[57] There is likely a dose-response relationship for colon cancer and breast cancer, and 30 to 60 minutes per day of moderate to vigorous intensity is proposed to decrease breast cancer risk.[62]

Occupational Hazards as Carcinogens

A substantial percentage of cancers of the upper respiratory passages, lung, bladder, and peritoneum are attributed to occupational factors; however, fewer studies of nonsmokers exist.[63] One notable occupational factor is **asbestos,** which increases the risk of mesothelioma and lung cancer. Asbestos was used in homes and buildings built before the 1970s to insulate ceiling tiles, flooring, and pipe covers. In western Europe, the epidemic of mesothelioma in building workers and other workers born after 1940 did not become apparent until the 1990s (i.e., because of long latency). Carcinoma of the bladder has been linked with the manufacture of dyes, rubber, paint, and aromatic amines, especially β-naphthylamine and benzidine. Benzol inhalation is linked to leukemia in shoemakers and in workers in the rubber cement, explosives, and dyeing industries. Other notable occupational hazards include heavy metals (e.g., high-nickel alloy, chromium VI compounds, inorganic arsenic), silica, polycyclic aromatic hydrocarbons, sulfuric acid, and chloromethyl ether. Studies of occupational exposure to diesel exhaust indicate an increased risk of lung cancer.[64] Disentangling data related to lung cancer, air pollution, and occupational risks is complex, especially in combination with active and passive smoking and the interplay of environmental factors and genetic polymorphisms at multiple loci.

Air Pollution

A person inhales about 20,000 L of air in 1 day; thus even modest contamination of the atmosphere can result in inhalation of appreciable doses of pollutants. Contaminants include outdoor and indoor air pollutants. Concerns include industrial emissions, including arsenicals, benzene, chloroform, formaldehyde, sulfuric acid, mustard gas, vinyl chloride, and acrylonitrite.[65] Living close to certain industries is a recognized cancer risk factor, although it is difficult to determine cancer risk from outdoor pollution *alone* because investigators must accurately control for smoking and radon. Studies that controlled or stratified for smoking demonstrated associations between excess lung cancer rates and heavy metal and aromatic hydrocarbon emissions in polluted air. Evidence for cancers, other than lung cancer and childhood cancer, is inconsistent.[66]

Indoor pollution generally is considered worse than outdoor pollution, partly because of cigarette smoke. Environmental tobacco smoke (ETS; passive smoking) can cause the formation of reactive oxygen-free radicals and, thus, DNA damage. The International Agency for Research on Cancer (IARC) has classified ETS as a human carcinogen. A meta-analysis of studies found a relative risk of 1.22 (95% confidence interval) in women and 1.36 (95% confidence interval) in men resulting from workplace exposure.[66] Other meta-analyses report similar results.[67] Another significant indoor air pollutant is radon gas. **Radon** is a natural radioactive gas derived from the radioactive decay of uranium that is ubiquitous in rock and soil; it can become trapped in houses and gives rise to radioactive decay products known to be carcinogenic to humans. The most hazardous houses can be identified by testing and then modified to prevent further radon contamination. Exposure levels are greater from underground mines than from houses. Most of the lung cancers associated with radon are bronchogenic; however, small-cell carcinoma does occur with greater frequency in underground miners. Radon increases the risk of lung cancer in underground miners whether they smoke or not.

In China, some regions report high levels of lung cancer in women who spend much of their time indoors. Exposures from heating and cooking combustion sources (e.g., oil vapors) are identified as risk factors for lung cancer.[67]

Inorganic arsenic (known as a carcinogen since the late 1960s), found principally in underground water (from 1000 to 4000 μg/L), is found in many regions of the world. According to the IARC, strong evidence indicates an increased risk of bladder, skin, and lung cancers following consumption of water with high levels of arsenic (generally above 200 μg/L).[68] Evidence for cancers of the liver, colon, and kidney is weaker. Other sources of inorganic arsenic are related to occupational exposures.

The central hypothesis, based on rat studies, for the mechanisms related to particle-induced lung carcinogenesis is that insoluble particles cause pulmonary inflammation (e.g., cytokine release, ROS), which leads to genotoxic stress, proliferative response, and tissue remodeling progressing toward fibrosis and tumor development. Much additional research is needed to understand the surface chemistry and lung tissue remodeling in relation to insoluble particles and lung carcinogenesis.

CLINICAL MANIFESTATIONS OF CANCER

Pain

Usually little or no pain is associated with the early stages of malignant disease, but pain does occur in 60% to 80% of those individuals who are terminally ill with cancer. Pain is strongly influenced by fear, anxiety, sleep loss, fatigue, and overall physical deterioration. It occurs as a result of the interaction among psychogenic, cultural, and physiologic components. (The neurophysiology of pain is discussed in Chapter 13.) New data suggest that many of the symptoms experienced by individuals with cancer may be mediated by cytokines acting on the peripheral and central nervous systems (Figure 10-4).

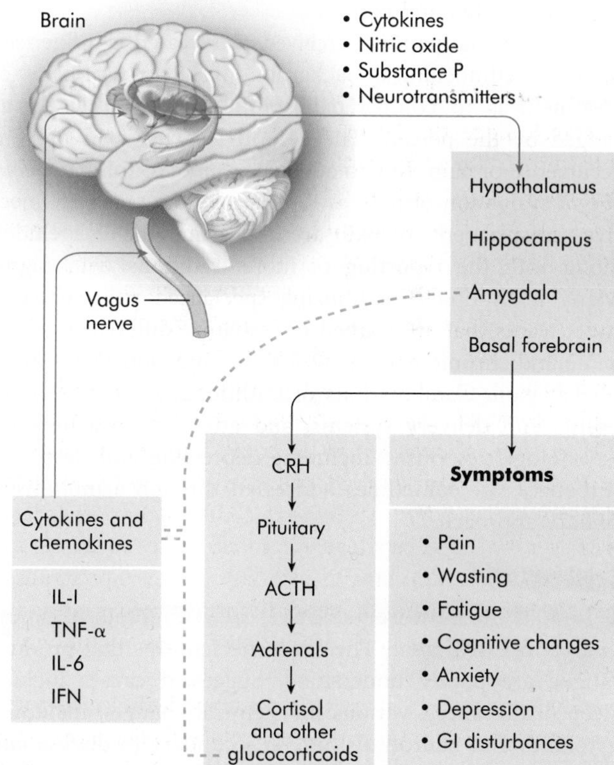

Figure 10-4 ■ Theoretical Framework for Cytokine-Induced Cancer Symptoms. Solid blue lines proinflammatory cytokines and chemokines (IL-1, TNF-α, IL-6, IFN) are released by immune cells. They exert their effect on peripheral nerves and the brain. Neurotransmitter responses by the brain are affected. The hypothalamic-pituitary-adrenal axis is activated with increased release of corticosteroids, which provide feedback *(dotted red lines)* to decrease cytokine production. (Adapted from Cleeland CS et al: Actytokine-immunologic model of cancer symptoms, *Cancer* 97(11):2919–2925, 2003.)

General mechanisms that cause pain associated with cancer include pressure, obstruction, invasion of a sensitive structure, stretching of visceral surfaces, tissue destruction, and inflammation. The pain may be directly related to the malignancy or can result from other problems, such as infection. Bone metastasis causes pain that may be referred away from the involved bone and manifested, for example, as back pain. Bone pain can be caused by periosteal irritation, medullary pressure, and pathologic fractures.

Abdominal pain often is caused by severe stretching from the tumor invasion of the hollow viscus. Tumors that obstruct and distend the bowel cause pain. Small bowel obstructions in persons with known malignant disease commonly result from recurrent cancer, surgical adhesions, or new primary tumors. Surgery often is needed to obtain relief. Hepatic malignancies stretch the liver, resulting in a dull pain or a feeling of fullness over the right upper abdominal quadrant.

Tumors that compress nerve endings create pain. Brain tumors, in particular, have little space to grow without compressing blood vessels and nerve endings between the tumor and the cranial vault. Infection and necrosis can destroy tissue and cause pain. The oral area, which often is the site of ulcerative lesions resulting from cancer, can become infected and painful.

The way that pain is perceived and treated is influenced by one's ethnocultural background. The first priority of treatment is to control pain rapidly and completely as judged by the person. The second priority is to prevent recurrence of pain. Key to adequate pain control is the *continual* evaluation of pain as reported by the person. Objective measurements of pain are increasingly being included along with the reporting of more traditional vital signs. Many institutions are utilizing specialized pain management teams that are trained to recognize different types of acute and chronic pain, as well as the individual's response to that pain. Combinations of traditional analgesics, novel agents and delivery systems, and attention to a person's psychologic responses, including depression and sleep disturbances, are sometimes addressed through a multidisciplinary approach.[69]

Fatigue

Fatigue is the most frequently reported symptom of cancer and cancer treatment. The exact mechanisms that produce fatigue are poorly understood. Suggested causes include sleep disturbances, various biochemical changes, including cytokines and neurotransmitters, secondary to disease and treatment, numerous psychosocial factors, level of activity, nutritional status, and other environmental and physical factors.

The physiologic understanding of fatigue probably includes mechanisms for decreased muscle contractility. Other areas of research include muscle function consequences from metabolic products of cancer treatment and associated muscle loss from circulating cytokines (e.g., tumor necrosis factor [TNF] and interleukin-1 [IL-1]).

Similar to pain, fatigue is a subjective clinical manifestation. Individuals with cancer describe *fatigue* as tiredness, weakness, lack of energy, exhaustion, lethargy, inability to concentrate, depression, sleepiness, boredom, lack of motivation, and decreased mental status.

Cachexia

The syndrome of **cachexia** (Greek *kakos,* bad; *lexis,* condition) includes anorexia, early satiety (filling), weight loss, anemia, asthenia (marked weakness), poor performance, taste alterations, and altered protein, lipid, and carbohydrate metabolism (Figure 10-5). Cachexia is the most severe form of malnutrition associated with cancer and results in wasting, extensive loss of adipose tissue, altered liver glucose and lipid metabolism, emaciation, and decreased quality of life. The **anorexia,** or loss of appetite-cachexia syndrome, is one of the most common causes of death among individuals with cancer.[70] The anorexia-cachexia syndrome results from a multifactorial process involving hormones (e.g., leptin), neuropeptides (e.g., neuropeptide Y and others), and proinflammatory cytokines (e.g., interleukins [IL-1 and IL-6], tumor necrosis factor [TNF-α], and interferon [INF-α]). Close interaction of these factors in the hypothalamus is hypothesized to decrease food intake and lead to cachexia.[71] The dysregulated production of proinflammatory cytokines are thought to induce an **acute phase (protein) response (APR)** that has been linked to accelerated weight loss and is a key marker of *systemic inflammation.* Systemic inflammation has been found in association with many cancers and has correlated with weight loss, hypermetabolism, anorexia, and a poor prognosis.[72,73] Although alterations in taste also can account for the anorexia in individuals with cancer by making foods seem bland or distasteful, it does not appear to be responsible for tissue wasting, especially skeletal muscle.

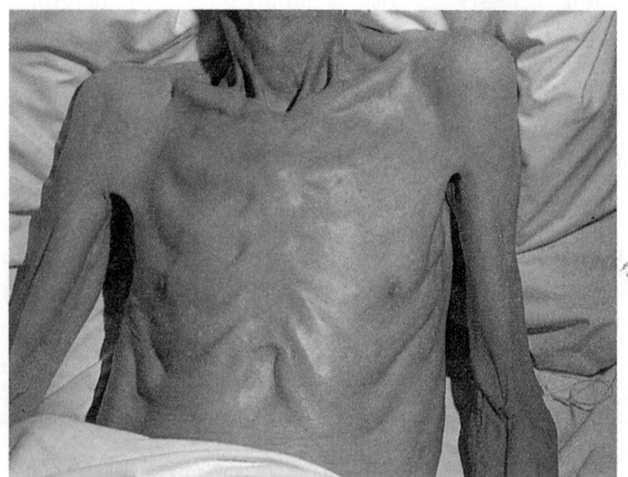

Figure 10-5 ■ **Cachexia.** This severe form of malnutrition results in wasting and extensive loss of adipose tissue. (From Kamal A, Brockelhurst JC: *Color atlas of geriatric medicine,* ed 2, St Louis, 1991, Mosby:)

Progressive weight loss in the person with cancer occurs despite normal or increased food intake. Weight loss can be massive, up to 80% of both adipose tissue and skeletal muscle mass.[74] Resting energy expenditure or metabolism is increased in individuals with lung and pancreatic cancer but not in those with gastric and colorectal cancer.[74] Increased energy expenditure is possibly related to the increase of uncoupling proteins (UCPs)—particularly in skeletal muscle.[74] The decrease in skeletal muscle arises from both a decrease in protein synthesis and an increase in protein degradation. The decrease in protein synthesis is possibly secondary to host inactivity together with a reduction in the supply or balance of amino acids because of proinflammatory cytokines.[70,74,75] Increased protein degradation is possibly the result of an increased expression of the **ubiquitin-proteasome protein degradation pathway** (i.e., tagging of proteins by the protein ubiquitin causes their disposal by the adenosine triphosphate [ATP]-dependent protease or proteasome) in skeletal muscle.[74,76]

Altered carbohydrate metabolism causes a syndrome resembling diabetes mellitus. Individuals show hyperinsulinemia, insulin resistance, hyperglycemia, and abnormal glucose tolerance test results. These disturbances cause increased gluconeogenesis, which produces glucose from amino acids. In starvation, protein usually is spared to protect vital structures, but in cancer, protein and fatty acids are used to meet energy needs.

An unusual and frustrating component of cancer care is the person's early **satiety,** or a sense of being full after only a few mouthfuls of food. One of the most significant proinflammatory involved cytokines is the activated macrophage-produced tumor necrosis factor-alpha (TNF-α), also called *cachectin* because of its role in the cachexia syndrome. TNF plays an important role in the defense against viral, bacterial, and parasitic infections; in autoimmune responses; and in the selective destruction of malignant cells.[77] Its overproduction, however, may be detrimental to the host as well as the cytokines mentioned earlier. (Cytokines are discussed in detail in Chapter 6.)

Clinical practice to date has mostly focused on increasing caloric intake to slow weight loss. With the new understanding about proinflammatory mediators and systemic inflammation, new interventions targeting the mediators of inflammation are needed.[78]

Anemia

Anemia is commonly associated with malignancy, with 20% of individuals having hemoglobin concentrations below 8 g/dl (normal value = 15 g/dl). Mechanisms that cause anemia in persons with cancer include chronic bleeding resulting in iron deficiency, severe malnutrition, medical therapies, or malignancy in blood-forming organs. Several of these mechanisms may cause suppression of the action of erythropoietin on the bone marrow, presumably by the release of cytokines.[79] Erythropoietin acts in progenitor cells in the bone marrow to stimulate the release of immature red blood cells (e.g., reticulocytes). Erythropoietin is effective in correcting the anemia associated with cancer. In addition, anemias that occurred after chemotherapy or radiation therapy also have been treated successfully by erythropoietin.[80,81] Chronic bleeding and iron deficiency can accompany colorectal or genitourinary malignancy. Iron also is malabsorbed in persons with gastric, pancreatic, or upper intestinal cancer. Often there is a defect in the reutilization of iron because of lack of transfer of iron from the storage pool to blood cell precursors. This defect may be caused by increased secretion of cytokines, such as IL-1, or alterations in nitric oxide regulation. Defects in erythropoietin production and shortened red cell survival also have been documented. Anorexia can cause iron deficiency, although folate deficiency is more common with anorexia.

Anemia can result from chemotherapy but normochromic (normal hemoglobin concentration) and normocytic (average red cell size) anemias can occur after prolonged administration of alkylating agents or nitrosoureas, both classes of chemotherapeutic agents.[82] Megaloblastic (large red cell) anemias may develop after treatment with methotrexate, which causes abnormal folate metabolism.

Malignancy of the blood-forming organs is associated with several hemolytic anemias. An autoimmune hemolytic anemia occasionally develops in persons with chronic lymphocytic leukemia. (Anemia associated with leukemia is discussed in Chapter 20.)

Chemotherapy often worsens anemia in individuals with cancer. The administration of recombinant human erythropoietin (r-HuEPO) can significantly improve the hematocrit and quality of life of anemic individuals receiving myelosuppressive chemotherapy.[81]

Leukopenia and Thrombocytopenia

Direct tumor invasion of the bone marrow causes both leukopenia (a decreased leukocyte count) and thrombocytopenia (a decreased number of platelets). Chemotherapeutic drugs are toxic to the bone marrow, often causing granulocytopenia and thrombocytopenia. Leukopenia can result from chemotherapy or radiotherapy of areas of the bone marrow. Thrombocytopenia is a major cause of hemorrhage in persons with cancer. It usually results from chemotherapy or bone marrow involvement by the malignancy. Thrombocytopenia is an accompanying disorder of disseminated intravascular coagulation that occurs in persons with acute promyelocytic leukemia (see Chapter 20) and prostate cancer (see Chapter 32).

Infection

Infection is the most significant cause of complications and death in persons with malignant disease. When the absolute granulocyte or lymphocyte count falls, the risk of infection increases and persons with cancer have reduced immunologic functions, debility with advanced disease, and immunosuppression from radiotherapy and chemotherapy. (Factors that predispose persons with cancer to infection are summarized in Table 10-3.) Surgery also can lower resistance to infection because removal of large quantities of tissue, together with hemorrhage, dead spaces, and poor tissue perfusion, creates favorable sites for infection. Hospital-related (nosocomial) infections increase because of indwelling medical devices, inadequate wound care, and the introduction of microorganisms from visitors and other persons.

Leukopenia resulting from bone marrow radiation dramatically increases the risk of infection. Mucous membranes and other rapidly dividing cells in the radiation field are prone to irritation and ulceration. Radiation, particularly of the cervix, bladder, and intestinal tract, also can lead to fistula formation or abnormal passages between tissue cavities. Surgery often is required to repair the fistula and eliminate continuous infectious cross contaminations.

Paraneoplastic Syndromes

Paraneoplastic syndromes are symptom complexes that cannot be explained by the local or distant spread of the tumor or by the effects of hormones released by the tissue from which the tumor arose. About 10% of individuals with malignancy are affected. Although infrequent, paraneoplastic syndromes are significant because (1) they may be the earliest symptom of an unknown cancer, (2) in affected individuals they may represent serious and life-threatening problems, and (3) they may mimic progression and therefore interfere with appropriate treatment. Table 10-4 presents the classifications of paraneoplastic syndromes.

QUICK CHECK 10-1

1. What are the most common clinical manifestations of cancer?
2. Discuss the role of cytokines and systemic inflammation in the clinical manifestations of cancer.
3. Identify some mechanisms of anemia in individuals with cancer.

TABLE 10-3

Factors Predisposing Individuals With Cancer to Infection

Factor	Basis
Age	Many common malignancies occur mostly in older age. Immunologic functions decline with age. General debility reduces immunocompetence. Immobility predisposes to infection. Far-advanced cancer often results in immobility and general debility that worsens with age. Elderly persons are predisposed to nutritional inadequacies. Malnutrition impairs immunocompetence.
Tumor	Nutritional derangements can be caused. Sites and circumstances favorable to growth of microorganisms (obstruction, serous or blood effusion, ulceration) can be created. Far-advanced disease predisposes patients to debility and immobility. Humoral or cellular immune defects may be caused. Metastasis to bone marrow may cause leukopenia or other defects in immunity.
Leukemias	Inadequate granulocyte production (impaired phagocytosis) results. Thrombocytopenia (bleeding, breaks in skin integrity) can occur. *Late effect*: Chronic lung disease from *Pneumocystis carinii* pneumonia can develop during therapy.
Lymphomas and other reticuloendothelial malignancies	Humoral and cellular immune defects (anergy, altered immunoglobulin production) result. *Late effect*: Splenectomy in children can cause increased susceptibility to infection.
Treatment surgery	Invasive procedure interrupts first lines of defense. Radical nature of surgery (removal of large blocks of tissue in lengthy procedures) causes hemorrhage, decreased tissue perfusion, creation of dead spaces, devitalization of tissues. Procedure may be "dirty" surgery (bowel, infected or contaminated areas). Surgery patients are often older and at poor risk. Long preoperative hospitalization often precedes surgery. Patients may have had previous adrenocorticosteroid therapy. Patients may have infections at sites remote from operative area. Nutritional derangements (especially important in head and neck surgery) may result. Lymph nodes dissection may predispose patient to local infection and impair containment to area. Gynecologic surgery may result in fistulas. Debility and immobility may be caused.

Data from Donovan MI, Girton SF: *Cancer care nursing,* ed 2, New York, 1984, Appleton-Century-Crofts; Murphy GP, Lawrence W, Lenhard RE: *Clinical oncology,* ed 2, New York, 1994, American Cancer Society.

TABLE 10-4
Paraneoplastic Syndromes

Clinical Syndromes	Major Forms of Underlying Cancer	Causal Mechanism
ENDOCRINOPATHIES		
Cushing syndrome	Small cell carcinoma of lung Pancreatic carcinoma Neural tumors	ACTH or ACTH-like substance
Syndrome of inappropriate antidiuretic hormone secretion	Small cell carcinoma of lung, intracranial neoplasms	Antidiuretic hormone or atrial natriuretic hormones
Hypercalcemia	Squamous cell carcinoma of lung Breast carcinoma Renal carcinoma Adult T-cell leukemia/lymphoma Ovarian carcinoma	Parathyroid hormone–related protein (PTHRP), TGF-α, TNF, IL-1
Hypoglycemia	Fibrosarcoma Other mesenchymal sarcomas Heptaocellular carcinoma	Insulin or insulin-like substance
Carcinoid syndrome	Bronchial adenoma (carcinoid) Pancreatic carcinoma Gastric carcinoma	Serotonin, bradykinin
Polycythemia	Renal carcinoma Cerebellar hemangioma Hepatocellular carcinoma	Erythropoietin
NERVE AND MUSCLE SYNDROMES		
Myasthenia	Bronchogenic carcinoma	Immunologic
Disorders of the central and peripheral nervous systems	Breast carcinoma	
DERMATOLOGIC DISORDERS		
Acanthosis nigricans	Gastric carcinoma Lung carcinoma Uterine carcinoma	Immunologic, secretion of epidermal growth factor
Dermatomyositis	Bronchogenic, breast carcinoma	Immunologic
OSSEOUS, ARTICULAR, AND SOFT TISSUE CHANGES		
Hypertrophic osteoarthropathy and clubbing of the fingers	Bronchogenic carcinoma	Unknown
VASCULAR AND HEMATOLOGIC CHANGES		
Venous thrombosis (Trousseau phenomenon)	Pancreatic carcinoma Bronchogenic carcinoma Other cancers	Tumor products (mucins that activate clotting)
Nonbacterial thrombotic endocarditis	Advanced cancers	Hypercoagulability
Anemia	Thymic neoplasms	Unknown
OTHERS		
Nephrotic syndrome	Various cancers	Tumor antigens, immune complexes

From Kumar V, Abbas AK, Fausto N: *Robbins and Cotran pathologic basis of disease,* ed 7, Philadelphia, 2005, Saunders.
ACTH, Adrenocorticotropic hormone; *TGF,* transforming growth factor; *TNF,* tumor necrosis factor; *IL,* interleukin.

CANCER TREATMENT

Cancer currently is treated with chemotherapy, radiotherapy, surgery, immunotherapy, and combinations of these modalities (Table 10-5).

Chemotherapy

Although technically it includes any medicinal agent having antitumor effect, *chemotherapy* actually denotes the use of relatively nonselective cytotoxic drugs that target vital

TABLE 10-5

Examples of Treatment of Site-Specific Cancers

Usual Treatment	Site
Surgery	Colon Breast Ovary Lung Thyroid Skin Uterus
Chemotherapy	Lymphoma Leukemia Choriocarcinoma Ovary Breast
Radiation	Breast (all have been combined with surgery) Uterus or cervix Lymphomas Lung Combined with surgery in many sites
Hormones	Breast Prostate Endometrium
Immunotherapy	Melanoma Prostate Breast? Leukemias Others?

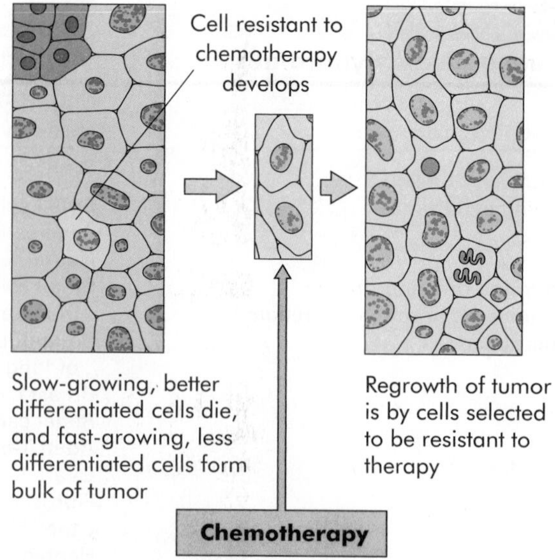

Figure 10-6 ■ **Chemotherapy and Resistant Cells.** A cell resistant to single-agent chemotherapy can develop from the pool of fast-growing tumor cells. Combination therapy helps prevent the development of resistant cells. (From Stevens A, Lowe J: *Pathology: illustrated review in color,* ed 2, Edinburgh, 2000, Mosby.)

cellular machinery or metabolic pathways critical to both malignant and normal cell growth and replication. To be curative, chemotherapy must eradicate enough tumor cells so that the body's own defenses can eradicate any remaining cells. Historically, initial attempts to treat cancer centered on **single-agent chemotherapy.** These agents were known to have significant early response rates, but the duration of response was short lived. Continued clinical studies have discovered several key points in chemotherapy use.

Combination chemotherapy is the synergistic use of several agents, each of which individually has an effect against a certain cancer. The primary rationale to this approach is to avoid single-agent drug resistance, which may be present even in previously untreated tumors (Figure 10-6). In addition, combination chemotherapy also may prevent acquired drug resistance. An added benefit of using lower doses of each drug in a combined manner is that the harmful effects to normal cells may be reduced. For example, much of the progress made in treating childhood acute lymphoblastic leukemia is the result of using combination chemotherapy. Whereas single-agent therapy produced remission rates of 60% with relapse within 6 to 9 months, combination therapy has led to nearly 95% remission rates with long-term remissions and cures approaching 75% to 80%.[83]

The **principle of dose intensity** implies there is a direct correlation between dose of a chemotherapeutic agent and killing of tumor cells. This relationship is often evident in a logarithmic fashion, in which small dose increases can significantly enhance the antitumor effect.[84,85] Use of maximal doses of chemotherapeutic agents is tempered by the increasing toxicities associated with their use as defined by the therapeutic index of the drug. The **therapeutic index**—that is, the relative effective dose needed to kill cancer cells as compared to the dose that would be harmful to normal cells—is generally quite low and is one of the limiting factors in the escalation of chemotherapy use.

A final key principle is the use of adjuvant chemotherapy after local treatment or removal of the primary tumor. It is in this context that chemotherapy has proven most useful—that is, useful to individuals who have minimal or no residual disease but who are at high risk for metastasis. Chemotherapy prevents the growth of micrometastatic deposits that are not clinically detectable at diagnosis. A variation of this approach, termed **primary,** or **neoadjuvant, chemotherapy,** is the early use of agents before definitive local control surgery or irradiation to decrease initial tumor size.[86] This approach allows for less extensive local control measures, as well as the opportunity to begin treatment early for micrometastatic disease.

Several classes of chemotherapeutic agents are used concurrently to treat different types of tumors (Table 10-6). The mechanism by which each drug acts to eradicate tumor cells depends largely on its effect on the cell cycle (described in Chapter 1). The use of drugs acting at different points in the cell cycle may confer a synergistic response against the tumor.

TABLE 10-6
Examples of Chemotherapeutic Drugs

Drug	Major Toxicity
ALKYLATING AGENTS	
Mechlorethamine	*Therapeutic doses:* moderate depression of peripheral blood cell count; *excessive doses:* severe bone marrow depression, leukopenia, thrombocytopenia, and bleeding; maximum toxicity may occur 2–3 wk after last dose; alopecia; nausea and vomiting
Chlorambucil	
Melphalan	
Thiotepa	
Busulfan	
Cyclophosphamide	
Ifosfamide	
ANTIMETABOLITES	
Methotrexate	Oral and digestive tract ulcerations; bone marrow depression with leukopenia, thrombocytopenia, and bleeding; toxicity enhanced by impaired kidney function; alopecia
6-Mercaptopurine	
6-Thioguanine	
5-Fluorodeoxyuridine	
Cytarabine	
Fludarabine	
2-Chlorodeoxyadenosine	
2′-Deoxycoformycin	
Gemcitabine	
ANTIBIOTICS	
Doxorubicin	Stomatitis, gastrointestinal injury; bone marrow depression; alopecia; cardiac toxicity at cumulative doses over 500 mg/m^2 (doxorubicin, daunorubicin); pneumonitis and pulmonary fibrosis at cumulative doses over 400 U (bleomycin); hypocalcemia; hepatic toxicity (plicamycin); nausea and vomiting
Bleomycin	
Dactinomycin	
Plicamycin	
Mitomycin-C	
Mitoxantrone	
STEROIDS AND HORMONALLY ACTIVE AGENTS	
Androgen	Fluid retention; masculinization/feminization; hot flashes (sex hormones); hypertension; diabetes; adrenal insufficiency
Fluoxymesterone	
Antiandrogen	
Flutamide	
Estrogen	
Ethinyl estradiol	
Diethylstilbestrol	
Antiestrogen	
Tamoxifen	
Progestin	
Megestrol acetate	
Luteinizing hormone–releasing hormone agonist	
Leuprolide	
Aromatase inhibitor	
Aminoglutethimide	
Adrenocortical compound	
Dexamethasone	
MISCELLANEOUS DRUGS	
Asparaginase	Anorexia, weight loss, somnolence, lethargy, confusion; hypoproteinemia (including albumin and fibrinogen); hyperlipidemia, abnormal liver function tests, fatty metamorphosis of liver; pancreatitis (rare); azotemia; granulocytopenia, lymphopenia, and thrombocytopenia (usually mild and transient)
Altretamine	Bone marrow depression; peripheral neuropathy
m-AMSA	Bone marrow depression; stomatitis; hepatic dysfunction; nausea and vomiting
Carmustine	Bone marrow depression; thrombocytopenia; nausea and vomiting
Lomustine	Bone marrow depression; thrombocytopenia; nausea and vomiting
Streptozocin	Hypoglycemia; nausea and vomiting
Mitotane	Skin eruptions; diarrhea; mental depression; muscle tremors; adrenal insufficiency; nausea and vomiting
Dacarbazine	Bone marrow depression; nausea and vomiting
Hydroxyurea	Bone marrow depression; nausea and vomiting

(Continued)

TABLE 10-6
Examples of Chemotherapeutic Drugs—Cont'd

Drug	Major Toxicity
Etoposide	Alopecia; nausea and vomiting
Cisplatin	Bone marrow depression; renal tubular damage; deafness; nausea and vomiting
Carboplatin	Bone marrow depression; nausea and vomiting
Procarbazine	Bone marrow depression with leukopenia and thrombocytopenia; mental depression; nausea and vomiting
Vinblastine	Alopecia; areflexia; bone marrow depression
Vincristine	Areflexia; muscular weakness; peripheral neuritis; paralytic ileus; mild bone marrow depression
Levamisole	None
Cis-retinoic acid	Cheilitis; stomatitis; conjunctivitis
Paclitaxel	Leukopenia; peripheral neuropathy
Docetaxel	Leukopenia; peripheral neuropathy

The development of resistance to one chemotherapeutic agent often results in the coincident development of resistance to other drugs despite being structurally unrelated. Research is currently isolating and characterizing genes responsible for multidrug resistance. Table 10-7 summarizes the mechanisms of action of certain common chemotherapeutic drugs.

Radiation

The goals of ionizing radiation are (1) to eradicate cancer without producing excessive toxicity during treatment and (2) to avoid damage to normal structures. Ionizing radiation damages important macromolecules, especially deoxyribonucleic acid (DNA) and components of the microenvironment (stroma). The damage may be (1) *lethal,* in which the cell is killed by radiation; (2) *potentially lethal,* in which the cell is so severely affected by radiation that modifications in its environment will cause it to die; or (3) *sublethal,* in which the cell can subsequently repair itself. Cellular compartments with rapidly renewing cells are, in general, more radiosensitive. (Cellular effects of ionizing radiation are discussed in Chapter 3 and p. 247.)

TABLE 10-7
Mechanisms of Action of Common Chemotherapeutic Drugs

Drug	Mechanism
Actinomycin D	Prevents transcription; inhibits tRNA, mRNA synthesis
Bleomycin	Breaks and fragments single strands of DNA
	Damages nonproliferating as well as proliferating cells
Cytosine arabinoside	Decreases production of DNA replicating units
	Inhibits transcription
	Prematurely terminates nucleic acid chains
Doxorubicin	Binds to DNA
	Uncoils DNA helix
	Inhibits DNA-directed RNA polymerase
Mitomycin	Produces cross-linking of DNA strand

Surgery

Surgical therapy of cancer has several objectives. Surgical biopsy of a tumor often begins the treatment process, and intraoperative staging and sampling of adjacent lymph node regions define further therapy.

Sentinel nodes are a limited set of lymph nodes that are first to receive drainage from any given location. Presumably, cancer metastasizes to these nodes before other nodes. Therefore, new techniques, such as sentinel node localization and biopsy, may allow less invasive tumor staging. A randomized clinical trial found sentinel lymph node biopsy is associated with reduced arm morbidity and better quality of life than standard axillary treatment.[87]

Surgery can be completely curative, where the tumor is removed with an adequate margin of normal tissue, thus alleviating the need for additional therapy. If the tumor cannot be completely excised because of fear of causing undue morbidity, **debulking surgery** may be performed in which the majority of the tumor is removed, thereby allowing for increased success of adjuvant chemotherapy or irradiation. Surgery also may take on a palliative role when cure is not possible, allowing for the relief of current symptoms or the prevention or delaying of anticipated symptoms as the tumor grows. Surgery also is indicated for benign tumors that could progress into malignant tumors. Premalignant and in situ tumors (see Chapter 9) of epithelial tissues, such as skin, mouth, and cervix, therefore are removed.

Hormonal Therapy

Hormonal therapy has been in use for a long time. Table 10-8 lists the commonly used hormonal agents and their primary indications. Their mechanism of action is presumed to include receptor activation or blockade, which interferes with intercellular growth and proliferation signaling cascades.

TABLE 10-8

Common Hormonal Agents and Types of Tumors

Agents	Types of Tumors
Corticosteroids	Leukemias Hodgkin disease Malignant lymphomas Breast cancer Multiple myeloma
Androgens	Breast cancer
Estrogens	Breast cancer Prostate cancer
Antiestrogens	Endometrial cancer Breast cancer
Aromatase inhibitors	Adrenal tumors Breast cancer
LH-RH analogs	Breast cancer Prostate cancer
Antiandrogens	Prostate cancer

LH, Luteinizing hormone; *RH,* releasing hormone.

Immunotherapy

Because cancer is a dynamic disease in which the transformed cells in a tumor mass can adapt to changes in their environment, a single form of cancer therapy that is effective against all types of cancer may not be possible. In this regard, immunotherapy (immunologic treatment) holds promise. (The immune system is discussed in Chapter 5.)

Immunotherapy is a specific method of treatment used to eliminate cancer cells without damaging normal tissues. The immune system recognizes antigens and is highly regulated; thus, theoretically antitumor immune rejection responses (described in Chapter 9) can selectively eliminate cancer cells while sparing normal tissues. Immune memory cells are long lived and can provide extended protection against the emergence of recurrent primary tumor cells and foci of metastatic cancer cells. Numerous immunologic mechanisms are able to cause rejection of various types of cancer. Research efforts in anticancer immunotherapies focus on characterizing the immunogenic properties of various tumor-specific antigens and developing methods to selectively enhance tumor rejection immune responses, including the development of new vaccines and monoclonal antibodies.

Development of tumor-specific vaccines has been most notable with malignant melanoma. Melanoma-specific antigens are genetically manipulated in an attempt to develop a T-cell-based immune response against the tumor. Although early clinical results show promise in decreasing tumor size in small numbers of individuals tested, the ideal means of maximally stimulating the immune system is yet to be developed.

Monoclonal antibodies have been most successful in use against hematologic and lymphatic malignancies. Certain acute myelogenous leukemia cells express the surface protein CD33, which is targeted by the antibody gemtuzumab.[88] Non-Hodgkin lymphomas expressing the CD20 surface antigen have been successfully targeted with rituximab.[89] This work is now expanding into solid-tumor immunotherapy with encouraging trials of trastuzumab for breast cancer cells expressing the Her-2 antigen.[90] The majority of these antibodies are being used in protocols incorporating standard, cytotoxic chemotherapy. A current focus of research involves **conjugated antibodies,** in which radioisotopes or toxins are attached to the antibody, thus delivering very specific doses of radiation or toxic agents to involved tissues.[91-93]

An additional type of immunotherapy involves the nonspecific enhancement of the immune system through the use of **biologic response modifiers (BRMs).** BRMs are mammalian gene products, agents, and clinical protocols that modify biologic responses in host-tumor interactions. BRMs have the following actions: (1) a direct cytotoxic effect on cancer cells, (2) the initiation or augmentation of the host's tumor-immune rejection response, and (3) the modification of cancer cell susceptibility to the lytic or tumor-static effects of the immune system. BRMs include immunomodulating agents, interferons and interferon inducers, thymosins, antigens (e.g., vaccines), effector cells (e.g., macrophages, NK cells, cytotoxic T cells), lymphokines, cytokines, and monoclonal antibodies.

Sentinel node biopsy is widely used in the initial staging of cancer and surgical treatments. A dye or radioactive tracer is injected into the primary tumor, for example, a breast cancer, or melanoma, and then allowed to be taken up by the regional lymph nodes draining the tumor. Lymphatic mapping allows for those specifically identified lymph nodes to be selectively biopsied, resulting in more accurate staging and decreased morbidity associated with a more radical dissection.

HEALTH ALERT

L-Glutamine

The amino acid L-glutamine, when administered orally during and shortly after cytotoxic chemotherapy or radiation therapy, has been shown to *significantly* decrease the severity and duration of mucositis. It is believed to support the metabolic response to injury and infection in enterocytes, lymphocytes, and fibroblasts. Recent studies reveal mechanisms of action of glutamine including tissue protection, antioxidant capacity, preservation of metabolism, immunomodulation, and decreased intestinal apoptosis.

Data from Anderson PM et al: Oral glutamine reduces the duration and severity of stomatitis after cytotoxic cancer chemotherapy. *Cancer* 83:1433–1439, 1998, and Neu J, Li N: Pathophysiology of glutamine and glutamate metabolism in premature infants. *Curr Opin Clin Nutr Metab Care* 10(1):75–79, 2007.

SIDE EFFECTS OF CANCER TREATMENT

To many individuals, the side effects and complications of cancer therapy can be quite troublesome, often rivaling the diagnosis of cancer itself. Special care needs to be directed toward addressing and alleviating these effects because individual compliance with therapy is directly linked to a person's perception of discomfort and treatment-related complications. Key to enhancing this compliance is education regarding expected side effects and treatments to alleviate them.

With the exception of surgery, most side effects can be attributed to the relatively nonspecific nature of cancer therapy—the targeting of the rapidly growing cell. Therefore, organ systems consisting of rapidly dividing cells are targeted as well as the cancer. Knowing which systems will be affected allows prediction of some of the more common general therapy-related side effects.

Gastrointestinal Tract

The entire gastrointestinal (GI) tract relies on rapidly growing cells to produce an effective barrier to trauma and infection and to provide an absorptive surface for nutrients. Both chemotherapy and radiation therapy may cause a decreased cell turnover, thereby leading to oral ulcers (stomatitis), malabsorption, and diarrhea. The disruption of barrier defenses also increases the risk for infection, especially invasion by a person's own GI flora. Therapy-induced nausea, thought to be caused by an agent's direct action upon the central nervous system's vomiting centers, historically has been a major obstacle in therapy.

Aggressive antinausea (antiemetic) therapy—including the centrally acting serotonin 5-HT3 antagonists, such as ondansetron or zolasetron—has allowed better tolerance of highly emetogenic protocols. Other popular antiemetics include steroids and phenothiazines. Synthetic cannabinoids, the active ingredients in marijuana, increase appetite in addition to having antinausea properties. Analgesia often includes opiate agents, vital in treating severe cases of mucosal lesions. Supplemental nutrition through enteral or parenteral routes may be needed to combat malnutrition. Good orâl care and close attention to hygiene may help prevent complications arising from mucosal membrane breakdown.

Bone Marrow

Chemotherapy is the usual offending agent causing bone marrow suppression, although radiation therapy also may contribute to suppression, especially if the two therapies are used together. The timing of suppression often can be predicted based on what agent is used. All three cell lines are usually affected (i.e., red blood cells, white blood cells, and platelets) (see anemia, p. 256). The anemia caused by red cell suppression may contribute to the generalized fatigue of the person with cancer and may require transfusion depending on the severity of the anemia or other comorbid medical conditions. Decreased platelet numbers may increase a person's tendency to spontaneously bleed and require transfusion as well. Perhaps the most potentially serious side effect is that of white blood cell suppression (neutropenia), creating for the person who already has weakened host immune defenses an even greater risk of infection. The risk of infection increases with both greater degrees of and prolonged durations of neutropenia. This infection risk mandates immediate evaluation of fever and initiation of antibiotic medication until the infection is disproved.

Red blood cell and platelet transfusions are routinely used in supportive care of marrow suppression; white cell transfusions are not. The development of recombinant human stimulatory cytokines are often used to stimulate the body's own regeneration of cells. These parenterally administered medications include granulocyte colony-stimulating factor (G-CSF) or granulocyte-macrophage colony-stimulating factor (GM-CSF) to aid in recovery of white blood cells, erythropoietin to stimulate red cell production, and thrombopoietin to stimulate platelet recovery (see Chapter 19).

Hair and Skin

Alopecia (hair loss) results from chemotherapy effects on hair follicles. Alopecia is usually temporary, although hair may grow back with a different texture initially. Not all chemotherapeutic agents cause alopecia. Decreased renewal rates of the epidermal layers in the skin may lead to skin breakdown and dryness, altering the normal barrier protection against infection. Radiation therapy may cause skin erythema (redness) and contribute to breakdown.

Reproductive Tract

Radiation therapy and chemotherapy may affect the gametes, leading to varying degrees of decreased fertility and premature menopause. These effects are dose and age dependent, with the prepubertal gonad thought to be more resistant to damage. The potential for harm is also dependent on the agent used, with the alkylating category of chemotherapies carrying the greatest risk. Craniospinal irradiation for central nervous system tumors also may affect the hypothalamus or pituitary gland, with subsequent secondary gonadal failure because of lack of production of gonadotropin-releasing hormone, luteinizing hormone, and follicle-stimulating hormone. The potential for reproductive harm should be addressed before therapy, if possible, with provisions made for sperm or embryo banking.

✔ QUICK CHECK 10-2

1. What are the advantages of combination chemotherapy versus single-agent chemotherapy?
2. What are the main treatment modalities for cancer?
3. What are the side effects of cancer treatment?

Did You Understand?

Gene-Environment Interaction

1. The frequency and consequences of genetic mutations can be altered by a number of environmental factors. The most significant factors include smoking, radiation, obesity, a few oncogenic viruses, and *Helicobactor pylori (H. pylori).*
2. Cigarette smoke is carcinogenic and is the most important cause of cancer.
3. Tobacco use is associated primarily with squamous and small cell carcinomas of the lung and pulmonary adenocarcinomas. It has been linked to cancers of the lower urinary tract, upper aerodigestive tract, liver, kidney, pancreas, cervix uteri, and myeloid leukemia.
4. Environmental tobacco smoke (ETS) or involuntary smoking has also been linked to lung cancer.
5. Health risks from ionizing radiation involve neoplastic diseases but also birth defects and eye maladies.
6. Presently the risks of low-dose radiation are being debated.
7. Radiation-induced damage depends on dose response, fractionation, protraction, repair mechanisms, bystander effects, and antioxidants.
8. Biologic consequences of exposure to ionizing radiation include cell death, gene mutations, and chromosome aberrations.
9. Progeny of irradiated cells can exhibit an increased death rate and loss of reproductive potential.
10. Low levels of radiation can induce bystander effects and genomic instability. Both findings appear to be associated with oxidative stress and cell-to-cell intercellular communication.
11. Ultraviolet (UV) sunlight and reactive oxygen species (ROS) (oxidative stress) are involved in skin carcinogenesis from ultraviolet light (UVL).
12. UVL causes basal cell carcinoma and squamous cell carcinoma.
13. UV radiation is now known to cause specific gene mutations.
14. Understanding dietary factors that increase the risk for cancer is complex because of the variety of foods consumed, the constituents of food, the metabolic consequences of eating, changes in patterns of food use, and accurate recall and response.
15. Toxic carcinogenic substances include compounds produced in the cooking of fat, meat, or protein; and naturally occurring carcinogens associated with plant foods.
16. The strongest and most consistent support for diet and cancer is data related to alcohol, aflatoxin, and Chinese-style salted fish fed to infants.
17. Table 10-2 is a comprehensive table showing the relationship between dietary factors and cancer risk.
18. Obesity is linked to cancer. High BMI is associated with higher rates of death from esophageal, stomach, colorectal, liver, breast, gallbladder, pancreatic, prostate, kidney, and cervical cancers; non-Hodgkin lymphoma; multiple myeloma; and leukemia.
19. Adipose tissue is active endocrine and metabolic tissue. Increased release of free fatty acids, resistin, TNF-α, and reduced release of adiponectin give rise to insulin resistance. Adipose tissue cells produce steroid-hormone-metabolizing enzymes and are an important source of estrogens in postmenopausal women. Insulin-like growth factor–1 (IGF-1) regulates cell proliferation and inhibits apoptosis and the synthesis and biologic availability of female and male sex hormones.
20. Chronic alcoholism is a strong risk factor for cancer of the oral cavity, pharynx, hypopharynx, larynx, esophagus, and liver. It is less strongly related to breast cancer and colorectal cancer; however, breast carcinogenesis can be enhanced with relatively low daily amounts.
21. Multiple mechanisms are involved in alcohol-related carcinogenesis and include acetaldehyde, induction of cytochrome P-450, and ROS, increased procarcinogen activation, cell cycle effects, and nutritional deficiencies.
22. Sexually transmitted infection with high-risk types of HPV is required for the development of virtually all cervical cancers.
23. Physical activity reduces the risk of breast and colon cancers and may reduce the risk of other cancers.
24. A substantial percentage of cancers of the upper respiratory passages, lung, bladder, and peritoneum are attributed to occupational factors.
25. Air pollution is a concern in regard to cancer because of inhalation of emissions, including arsenicals, benzene, chloroform, vinyl chloride, and acrylonitrile. Indoor pollution is considered worse than outdoor pollution because of cigarette smoke and possibly radon gas.
26. The relationship between electromagnetic fields (EMFs) and carcinogenesis is controversial. The evidence does not provide clear or consistent results; however, the results cannot establish the absence of any hazard.

Clinical Manifestations of Cancer

1. Clinical manifestations of cancer include pain, fatigue, cachexia, anemia, leukopenia, thrombocytopenia, and infection.
2. Pain generally is associated with the late stages of cancer. It can be caused by pressure, obstruction, invasion of a structure sensitive to pain, stretching, tissue destruction, and inflammation.
3. Key to adequate pain control is the continual evaluation of pain as reported by the individual.
4. Fatigue is the most frequently reported symptom of cancer and cancer treatment.
5. Cachexia (loss of appetite, weakness, inability to maintain weight, taste alterations, altered metabolism) leads to protein-calorie malnutrition and progressive wasting.
6. Anemia associated with cancer usually occurs because of malnutrition, long-term bleeding and resultant iron deficiency, chemotherapy, and malignancies in the blood-forming organs.
7. Leukopenia is usually a result of chemotherapy, which is toxic to bone marrow, or radiation, which kills circulating leukocytes.
8. Thrombocytopenia is usually the result of chemotherapy or malignancy in the bone marrow.
9. Infection may be caused by leukopenia, immunosuppression, or debility associated with advanced disease.

Did You Understand?—Cont'd

Cancer Treatment

1. Cancer is treated with surgery, radiotherapy, chemotherapy, immunotherapy, and combinations of these modalities.
2. The theoretic basis of chemotherapy is the vulnerability of tumor cells in various stages of the cell cycle. The goal of chemotherapy is to eradicate enough tumor cells so that the body's natural defenses can eradicate remaining cells.
3. Combination chemotherapy is the synergistic use of several agents. This approach helps decrease single agent drug resistance and reduce harmful effects on normal cells.
4. Ionizing radiation causes cell damage, so the goal of radiotherapy is to damage the tumor without causing excessive toxicity or damage to nondiseased structures.
5. Surgical therapy is used for nonmetastatic disease, for which cure is possible by removing the tumor, and as a palliative measure to alleviate symptoms.
6. Immunotherapy is appropriate for cancers that cannot be managed effectively by chemotherapy or radiation, usually because enough tumor cells are inactive and invulnerable to these modalities.
7. Forms of immunotherapy, such as vaccines and biologic response modifiers, include immunomodulating agents, interferons, antigens, effector cells, lymphokines, and monoclonal antibodies.

Side Effects of Cancer Treatment

1. Special care is needed to address and alleviate side effects because individual compliance with therapy is directly linked to a person's perception of discomfort and complications.
2. Key to increasing compliance is appropriate education about the side effects and treatments.
3. Most side effects are directly related to the targeting of the rapidly growing cell.
4. Both chemotherapy and radiation therapy may cause a decreased cell turnover leading to oral ulcers, malabsorption, and diarrhea.
5. Disruption of barrier defenses in the gastrointestinal tract increases risk for infection.
6. Nausea is thought to be caused by an agent's direct action on the vomiting center in the central nervous system. Thus aggressive treatment with antiemetic therapy is mandated.
7. Chemotherapy can cause bone marrow suppression of all three cell lines, red, white, and platelets. Anemia is common with red cell suppression, decreased platelet numbers can increase bleeding, and decreased white blood cells increases the risk of infection.
8. Hair loss (alopecia) results from chemotherapy effects on hair follicles. Alopecia is usually temporary and not all agents cause it.
9. Radiation and chemotherapy may affect the gametes, leading to varying degrees of decreased fertility and premature menopause. These effects are dose- and age-dependent, with the prepubertal gonad thought to be more resistant to damage.
10. Craniospinal irradiation for central nervous system tumors may affect the hypothalamus or pituitary gland resulting in gonadal failure.

Key Terms

Acute phase (protein) response (APR), 255
Anorexia, 255
Asbestos, 253
Biologic response modifier (BRM), 262
Bystander effect, 247
Cachexia, 255
Carcinogen, 244
Combination chemotherapy, 259
Conjugated antibody, 262
Debulking surgery, 261
Environmental tobacco smoke (ETS), 246
Fatigue, 255
Insulin-like growth factor–1 (IGF-1), 250
Paraneoplastic syndrome, 257
Phase I activation enzyme, 249
Phase II detoxification enzyme, 250
Primary (neoadjuvant) chemotherapy, 259
Principle of dose intensity, 259
Radon, 254
Satiety, 256
Sentinel node, 261
Single-agent chemotherapy, 259
Therapeutic index, 259
Ubiquitin-proteasome protein degradation pathway, 256
Xenobiotic, 249

References

1. Peto J: Cancer epidemiology in the last century and the next decade, *Nature* 411(6835):390–395, 2001.
2. Munger K et al: Viral carcinogenesis and genomic instability, *EXS* 96:170–199, 2006.
3. Jorde LB et al: *Medical genetics*, ed 3, St Louis, 2003, Mosby.
4. Centers for Disease Control: Cigarette smoking among adults—United States, 2004, *MMWR Morb Mortal Wkly Rep* 54(44):1121–1124, 2005.
5. Global Youth Tobacco Survey Collaborating Group: Differences in worldwide tobacco use by gender: findings from the Global Youth Tobacco Survey, *J School Health* 73 (6):207–215, 2003.
6. Vineis P et al: Tobacco and cancer: recent epidemiological evidence, *J Natl Cancer Inst* 96(2):99–106, 2004.
7. National Cancer Institute: *Secondhand smoke: questions and answers*, 2005; www.cancer.gov/cancertopics/factsheet/tobacco/ETS.
8. Henley SJ et al: Association between exclusive pipe smoking and mortality from cancer and other diseases, *J Natl Cancer Inst* 96(11):853–861, 2004.

References—Cont'd

9. Tawn EJ et al: Chromosome analysis in childhood cancer survivors and their offspring—no evidence for radiotherapy-induced persistent genome instability, *Mutat Res* 583(2): 198–206, 2005.
10. Byrne J et al: Genetic disease in offspring of long-term survivors of childhood and adolescent cancer, *Am J Hum Genet* 62(1):45–52, 1998.
11. Winther JF et al: Chromosomal abnormalities among offspring of childhood-cancer survivors in Denmark: a population-based study, *Am J Hum Genet* 74(6):1282–1285, 2004.
12. Prasad KN, Cole WC, Hasse GM: Health risks of low dose ionizing radiation in humans: a review, *Exp Biol Med* 229(5): 378–382, 2004.
13. Committee on the Biological Effects of Ionizing Radiation: *Biological effects of ionizing radiation BEIR V*, Washington, DC, 1990, National Academy Press.
14. Lorimore SA, Coates PJ, Wright EG: Radiation-induced genomic instability and bystander effects: inter-related nontargeted effects of exposure to ionizing radiation, *Oncogene* 22(45): 7058–7069, 2003.
15. Nagar S, Smith LE, Morgan WF: Mechanisms of cell death associated with death-inducing factors from genomically unstable cell lines, *Mutagenesis* 18(6):549–560, 2003.
16. Park CC et al: Ionizing radiation induces heritable disruption of epithelial cell interactions, *Proc Natl Acad Sci U S A* 100 (19):10728–10733, 2003.
17. Little JB: Genomic instability and bystander effects: a historical perspective, *Oncogene* 22(45):6978–6987, 2003.
18. Shao C et al: Targeted cytoplasmic irradiation induces bystander responses, *Proc Natl Acad Sci U S A* 101(37): 13495–13500, 2004.
19. Spitz DR et al: Metabolic oxidation/reduction reactions and cellular responses to ionizing radiation: a unifying concept in stress response biology, *Cancer Metastasis Rev* 23(3–4): 311–322, 2004.
20. Little JB: Cellular radiation effects and the bystander response, *Mutat Res* 597(1–2):113–118, 2006.
21. Streilein JW et al: Immune surveillance and sunlight-induced skin cancer, *Immunol Today* 15(4):174–179, 1994.
22. Sander CD et al: Role of oxidative stress and the antioxidant network in cutaneous carcinogenesis, *Intl J Dermatol* 43(5): 326–335, 2004.
23. Perlis C, Herlyn M: Recent advances in melanoma biology, *Oncologist* 9(2):182–187, 2004.
24. Polsky D et al: Molecular biology of melanoma. In Mendelsohn J et al, editors: *The molecular basis of cancer*, ed 2, Philadelphia, 2001, Saunders.
25. Rees JL: The melanocortin 1 receptor (MC1R): more than just red hair, *Pigment Cell Res* 13(3):135–140, 2000.
26. Habash RW et al: Health risks of electromagnetic fields. Part I: evaluation and assessment of electric and magnetic fields, *Crit Rev Biomed Eng* 31(3):141–195, 2003.
27. National Institute of Environmental Health Sciences (NIEHS) Working Group Report: *Assessment of health effects from exposure to power-line frequency electric and magnetic fields*, Washington, DC, 1998, US Government Printing Office.
28. Kliukiene J, Tynes T, Andersen A: Residential and occupational exposure to 50-Hz magnetic fields and breast cancer in women: a population-based study, *Am J Epidemiol* 159(9): 852–861, 2004.
29. Christensen HC et al: Cellular telephone use and risk of acoustic neuroma, *Am J Epidemiol* 159(3):277–283, 2004.
30. Independent Expert Group on Mobile Phones: Mobile phones and health (the Stewart report), Didcot, Oxon, United Kingdom, 2000, National Radiological Protection Board www.iegmp.org.uk/report/text.htm.
31. Repacholi MH: Radiofrequency field exposure and cancer: what do the laboratory studies suggest? *Environ Health Perspect* 105(suppl 6):1565–1568, 1997.
32. Mashevich M et al: Exposure of human peripheral blood lymphocytes to electromagnetic fields associated with cellular phones leads to chromosomal instability, *Bioelectromagnetics* 24(2):82–90, 2003.
33. Hardell L et al: Use of cellular or cordless telephones and the risk for non-Hodgkin's lymphoma, *Int Arch Occup Environ Health* 78(8):625–632, 2005.
34. Hardell L et al: Case-control study of the association between the use of cellular and cordless telephones and malignant brain tumors diagnosed during 2000–2003, *Environ Res* 100 (2):232–241, 2006.
35. Lönn S et al: Long-term mobile phone use and brain tumor risk, *Amer J Epid* 16(6):526–535, 2005.
36. Elwood JM: Epidemiological studies of radio frequency exposures and human cancer, *Bioelectromagnetics* 6:S63–73, 2003.
37. Working Group on Diet and Cancer of the Committee on Medical Aspects of Food and Nutrition Policy: *Nutritional aspects of the development of cancer*, London, 1998, Department of Health Rep Health Social Subjects 48, The Stationery Office.
38. Jones DP, Delong MJ: Detoxification and protective functions of nutrients. In Stipanuk M, editor: *Biochemical and physiological aspects of nutrition*, Philadelphia, 2000, Saunders.
39. International Agency for Research on Cancer (IARC): Some naturally occurring substances: food items and constituents, heterocyclic aromatic amines, and mycotoxins. In *IARC monographs on the evaluation of carcinogenic risks to humans*, 56, Lyon, 1993, Author.
40. Mucci L, Adami H: Oral and pharyngeal cancer, In Adami H, Hunter R, Trichopoulos D, editors: *Textbook of cancer epidemiology*, New York, 2002, Oxford University Press.
41. World Cancer Research Fund in association with the American Institute for Cancer Research: *Food, nutrition, and the prevention of cancer: a global perspective*, 96–106, Washington, DC, 1997, American Institute for Cancer Research.
42. Doll R, Peto R: Epidemiology of cancer. In Warrell DA et al, editors: *Oxford textbook of medicine*, ed 4, 2003, Oxford Medical Publications.
43. Parkin DM et al: Cancer burden in the year 2000. The global picture, *Eur J Cancer* 37(suppl 8):S4–S66, 2001, review.
44. Calle EE et al: Overweight, obesity, and mortality from cancer in a prospectively studied cohort of U.S. adults, *N Engl J Med* 348(17):1625–1638, 2003.
45. Calle EE, Kaaks R: Overweight, obesity and cancer: epidemiological evidence and proposed mechanisms, *Nat Rev Cancer* 4(8):579–591, 2004.
46. Khandwala HM et al: The effects of insulin-like growth factors on tumorigenesis and neoplastic growth, *Endocr Rev* 21(3): 215–244, 2000.
47. Dunaif A: Insulin resistance and the polycystic ovary syndrome: mechanism and implications for pathogenesis, *Endocr Rev* 18(6):774–800, 1997.
48. Izevbigie EB et al: Ethanol modulates the growth of human breast cancer cells in vitro, *Exp Biol Med* 227(4):260–265, 2002.
49. Bagnardi V et al: A meta-analysis of alcohol drinking and cancer risk, *Br J Cancer* 85(11):1700–1705, 2001.
50. Sturgis EM, Wei Q: Genetic susceptibility—molecular epidemiology of head and neck cancer, *Curr Opin Oncol* 14(3): 310–317, 2002.
51. Bagnardi V et al: Alcohol consumption and the risk of cancer: a meta-analysis, *Alcohol Res Health* 25(4):263–270, 2001.

References—Cont'd

52. Brienza RS, Stein MD: Alcohol use disorders in primary care: do gender-specific differences exist? *J Gen Intern Med* 17(5): 387–397, 2002.
53. Anhang R, Goodman A, Goldie SJ: HPV communication: review of existing research and recommendation for patient education, *CA Cancer J Clin* 54(5):248–259, 2004.
54. Palefsky JM, Holly EA: Chapter 6: Immunosuppression and co-infection with HIV, *J Natl Cancer Inst Monogr* 31:41–46, 2003.
55. Syrjanen S, Puranen M: Human papillomavirus infections in children: the potential role of maternal transmission, *Crit Rev Oral Biol Med* 11(2):259–274, 2000.
56. Eyre H et al: Preventing cancer, cardiovascular disease, and diabetes: a common agenda for the American Cancer Society, the American Diabetes Association, and the American Heart Association, *Stroke* 35(8):1999–2010, 2004.
57. Haydon AM et al: Physical activity, insulin-like growth factor 1, insulin-like growth factor binding protein 3, and survival from colorectal cancer, *Gut* 55(5):689–694, 2006.
58. McTiernan A et al: Physical activity and cancer etiology: associations and mechanisms, *Cancer Causes Control* 9(5): 487–509, 1998, review.
59. McTiernan A et al: Effect of exercise on serum estrogens in postmenopausal women: a 12-month randomized clinical trial, *Cancer Res* 64(8):2923–2928, 2004.
60. Calle EE et al: Diabetes mellitus and pancreatic cancer mortality in a prospective cohort of United States Adults, *Cancer Causes Control* 9(4):403–410, 1998.
61. Hewett JA et al: Exercise for breast cancer survival: the effect on cancer risk and cancer-related fatigue (CRF), *Int J Fertil Med* 50(5 Pt 1):231–239, 2005.
62. Lee IM: Physical activity and cancer prevention…data from epidemiologic studies, *Med Sci Sports Exerc* 35(11): 1823–1827, 2003.
63. Neuberger JS, Field RW: Occupation and lung cancer in non-smokers, *Rev Environ Health* 18(4):251–267, 2003, review.
64. Vineis P et al: Outdoor air pollution and lung cancer: recent epidemiologic evidence, *Int J Cancer* 111(5):647–652, 2004.
65. Blair A, Kazerouni N: Reactive chemicals and cancer, *Cancer Causes Control* 8(3):473–490, 1997.
66. Boffetta P et al: Mortality among workers employed in the titanium dioxide production industry in Europe, *Cancer Causes Control* 15(7):697–706, 2004.
67. Boffetta P: Involuntary smoking and lung cancer, *Scand J Work Environ Health* 28(suppl 2):30–40, 2002.
68. International Agency for Research on Cancer (IARC): *Cancer epidemiology*, Lyon, France, 2004, IARC Press.
69. Haigh C: Contribution of a multidisciplinary team to pain management, *Br J Nurs* 10(6):370–374, 2001.
70. Inui A: Cancer anorexia-cachexia syndrome: are neuropeptides the key? *Cancer Res* 59(18):4493–4501, 1999.
71. Ramos EJ et al: Cancer anorexia-cachexia syndrome: cytokines and neuropeptides, *Curr Opin Clin Nutr Metab* 7(4):427–434, 2004.
72. Deans C, Wigmore SJ: Systemic inflammation cachexia and prognosis in patients with cancer, *Curr Opin Clin Nutr Metab* 8(3):265–269, 2005.
73. Delano MJ, Moldawer LL: The origins of cachexia in acute and chronic inflammatory diseases, *Nutr Clin Pract* 21(1):68–81, 2006.
74. Tisdale MJ: Cachexia in cancer patients, *Nature Rev Cancer* 2 (11):862–871, 2002.
75. Sharma R, Akner SD: Cytokines, apoptosis, and cachexia: the potential for TNF antagonism, *Int J Cardiol* 85(1):161–167, 2002.
76. DeJong CH et al: Systemic inflammation correlates with increased expression of skeletal muscle ubiquitin but not uncoupling proteins in cancer cachexia, *Oncol Rep* 14(1): 257–263, 2005.
77. Fiers W: Review: tumor necrosis factor: characterization of the molecular, cellular, and in vivo level, *FEBS Lett* 285(2): 199–212, 1991.
78. McCarthy DO: Rethinking nutritional support for persons with cancer cachexia, *Biol Res Nurs* 5(1):3–17, 2003.
79. Erslev AJ: Erythropoietin and anemia of cancer, *Eur J Haematol* 64(6):353–358, 2000.
80. Bragga M et al: Erythropoiesis after therapy with recombinant human erythropoietin: a dose-response study in anemic cancer surgery patients, *Vox Sang* 76(1):38, 1999.
81. Gargano G et al: The utility of a growth factor: rHuEPO as a treatment for preoperation autologous blood donation in gynecological tumor surgery, *Int J Oncol* 14(1):157–160, 1999.
82. Sabatini P: The relationship between anemia and quality of life in cancer patients, *Oncologist* 5(suppl 2):19, 2000.
83. Henderson EH, Samaha RJ: Evidence that drugs in multiple combinations have materially advanced the treatment of human malignancies, *Cancer Res* 29:2272–2275, 1969.
84. Hryniuk W, Bush H: The importance of dose intensity in chemotherapy of metastatic breast cancer, *J Clin Oncol* 2:1281–1285, 1984.
85. Young RC: Mechanisms to improve chemotherapy effectiveness, *Cancer* 65(suppl):815–818, 1990.
86. Trimble EL et al: Neoadjuvant therapy in cancer treatment, *Cancer* 72:3515–3521, 1993.
87. Mansel RE et al: Randomized multicenter trail of sentinel node biopsy versus standard axillary treatment in operable breast cancer: the ALMANAC Trial, *J Natl Cancer Inst* 98 (9):599–609, 2006.
88. Bernstein ID: Monoclonal antibodies to the myeloid stem cells: therapeutic implications of CMA-676, a humanized anti-CD33 antibody calicheamicin conjugate, *Leukemia* 14 (3):474–475, 2000.
89. Maloney DG et al: IDEC-C2B8 (rituximab) anti-CD20 monoclonal antibody therapy in patients with relapsed low-grade non-Hodgkin's lymphoma, *Blood* 90(6):2188–2195, 1997.
90. Goldenberg MM: Trastuzumab, a recombinant DNA-derived humanized monoclonal antibody, a novel agent for the treatment of metastatic breast cancer, *Clin Ther* 21(2):309–318, 1999.
91. Hursey M et al: Specifically targeting the CD22 receptor of human B-cell lymphomas with RNA damaging agents: a new generation of therapeutics, *Leuk Lymphoma* 43(5):953–959, 2002.
92. Krasner C, Joyce RM: Zevalin: 90yttrium labeled anti-CD20 (ibritumomab tiuxetan), a new treatment for non-Hodgkin's lymphoma, *Curr Pharmaceutical Biotechnol* 2(4):341–349, 2001.
93. Kreitman RJ: Toxin-labelled monoclonal antibodies, *Curr Pharm Biotechnol* 2(4):313–325, 2001.

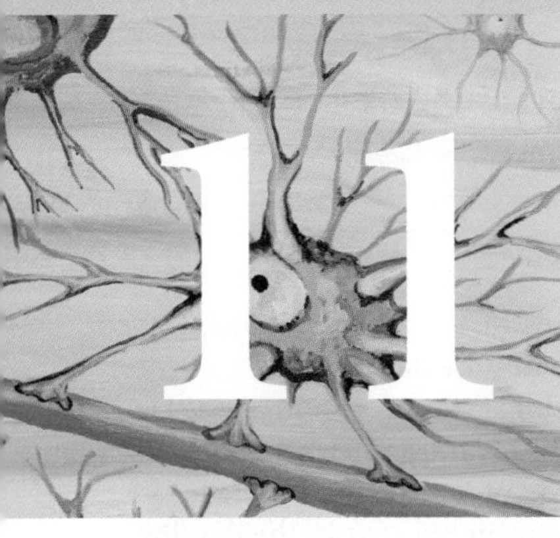

11 CANCER IN CHILDREN

Nancy E. Kline

CHAPTER OUTLINE

ELECTRONIC RESOURCES

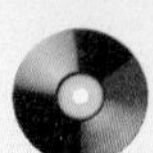

Companion CD
- Review Questions and Answers
- Animations

evolve Website
http://evolve.elsevier.com/Huether/
- Quick Check Answers
- Key Terms Exercises
- Critical Thinking Questions with Answers
- Algorithm Completion Exercises
- WebLinks

Cancer in children is rare, but it remains the second leading cause of death as the result of disease in children who have survived their first year.[1] The unique feature of childhood cancer is the short latency time, which contrasts sharply with the long latency period common in adults. Additionally, adult tumors are characterized by the anatomic sites of the primary tumor, whereas cancers in children are categorized by histology. Table 11-1 summarizes the differences between childhood and adult cancers.

INCIDENCE AND TYPES OF CHILDHOOD CANCER

Both incidence rates and types of cancer that develop vary between children and adults. For example, approximately 9500 children up to the age of 15 years are diagnosed with cancer each year, whereas approximately 1,400,000 adults are diagnosed with cancer during the same year. The incidence of cancer in children between birth and the age of 14 years is estimated to be 128 children per million per year.[1] Approximately 1 in every 900 persons between the ages of 15 and 45 years will be a survivor of childhood cancer. This is expected to increase to as many as 1 in every 250 persons in the year 2010.[2]

Most childhood cancers originate from the **mesodermal germ layer** that gives rise to connective tissue, bone, cartilage, muscle, blood, blood vessels, gonads, kidney, and the lymphatic system. Thus, the more common childhood cancers are leukemias, sarcomas, and embryonic tumors. Embryonic tumors originate during intrauterine life and contain abnormal cells that appear to be immature embryonic tissue unable to mature or differentiate into fully developed functional cells. **Embryonic tumors** are diagnosed early in life (usually by 5 years of age) and therefore are rare in adults.

Sarcomas and lymphoreticular cancers seen in childhood also occur in adults, but most adult cancers involve epithelial tissue (and are therefore carcinomas). Carcinomas rarely occur in children because these cancers most commonly result from environmental carcinogens and require a long period from exposure to the appearance of the carcinoma. Carcinomas begin to increase in incidence between the ages of 15 and 19 years, becoming the most common cancer tissue type seen after adolescence.

By far the most common malignancy in children is leukemia, which accounts for more than one third of childhood cancers. The second most common group of cancers is tumors of the nervous system, primarily brain tumors. All other pediatric malignancies occur much less often. Neuroblastoma is a tumor of the sympathetic nervous system. Wilms tumor is a malignancy of the kidney (named after Max Wilms, who identified the tumor); the histologic name is *nephroblastoma*. Rhabdomyosarcoma is a soft tissue sarcoma of striated muscle. Two major bone tumors also occur in children. These are osteosarcoma and Ewing sarcoma.

Childhood cancers usually are diagnosed during peak times of physical growth and maturation. In general, they are extremely fast-growing cancers. Many childhood cancers have a peak incidence before the child is 5 years of age. Among these are the leukemias, neuroblastoma, Wilms tumor, and retinoblastoma. Bone tumors, soft tissue sarcomas, and lymphomas are more likely to occur in children aged 15 to 19 years (see Table 11-1). Cancer is more common in white children than in Hispanic or black children (Table 11-2). In the United States, childhood cancer also

TABLE 11-1

Childhood Age-Adjusted Invasive Cancer Incidence Rates by Primary Site and Age, United States*

Site	0–14 Years	0–19 Years
All sites	14.5	16.1
Leukemia	4.5	4.1
Acute lymphocytic	3.4	3.0
Acute myeloid	0.6	0.7
Brain and other nervous system	3.2	2.9
Soft tissue	1.0	1.0
Kidney and renal	0.8	0.6
Bones and joints	0.7	0.9
Non-Hodgkin lymphoma	0.9	1.1
Hodgkin lymphoma	0.5	1.2
Other	2.9	4.3

Data modified from US Cancer Statistics Working Group: *United States cancer statistics: 1999–2002 incidence and mortality web-based report,* Atlanta, 2005, US Department of Health and Human Services, Centers for Disease Control and Prevention, and National Cancer Institute; www.cdc.gov/cancer/npcr/uscs.

*Rates are per 100,000 persons and are age-adjusted to the 2000 U.S. standard population (19 age groups–Census P25–1130).

TABLE 11-2

Childhood Age-Adjusted Cancer Incidence Rates for Children 0–19 Years of Age by Primary Site and Race and Ethnicity, United States*

Site	White	Black	Hispanic†	Other
All sites	18.3	11.0	17.8	13.7
Leukemia	4.8	2.4	5.8	8.0
Brain and other CNS	3.5	2.2	2.8	1.5
Soft tissue	1.1	0.6	1.0	1.2
Kidney and Renal	0.7	0.7	0.5	~
Bones and joints	1.1	0.8	1.2	~
Non-Hodgkin lymphoma	1.5	1.0	1.7	1.0
Hodgkin lymphoma	1.2	0.9	1.1	~
Other	4.5	2.5	3.7	6.3

Data modified from U.S. Cancer Statistics Working Group: *United States cancer statistics: 1999–2002 incidence and mortality web-based report.* Atlanta, 2005, U.S. Department of Health and Human Services, Centers for Disease Control and Prevention and National Cancer Institute; www.cdc.gov/cancer/npcr/uscs.

*Rates are per 100,000 persons and are age-adjusted to the 2000 US standard population (19 age groups–Census P25–1130)

†Hispanic origin is not mutually exclusive from race categories (white, black, other)

~Rates are suppressed if fewer than 16 cases were reported in a specific category (site, race, ethnicity)

is slightly more common in boys than in girls. The male/female ratio for childhood cancers is 1.2:1.0.[1]

ETIOLOGY

As in adult cancer, the causes of cancer in childhood are largely unknown. Some environmental and host factors are known to predispose a child to cancer, but causal factors have not been established for most childhood cancers. Table 11-3 lists host factors, many of which are genetic risk factors or congenital conditions, implicated in the development of childhood cancer. Childhood cancer most likely can be attributed to the complex interaction of both genetic and environmental factors called **ecogenetics.**

Most childhood cancers, however, do not lend themselves to early cancer warning signs. Certainly the American Cancer Society's seven warning signs of cancer do not apply because they describe adult, environmentally caused carcinomas. Although host factors are important in identifying populations of children at risk for cancer, most children who are diagnosed with cancer do not demonstrate any predisposing environmental or host factors.

Genetic Factors

Genetic factors may involve chromosome aberrations or single-gene defects. These chromosome abnormalities include aneuploidy, deletions, amplifications, translocations, and fragility (see Chapter 2). Some congenital malformations herald the onset of pediatric malignancies. Several syndromes with diagnosed abnormalities are known to be related to a higher incidence of cancer development. Children identified with certain congenital syndromes can then be carefully followed and screened for tumor development. One of the more recognized syndromes is the association of trisomy 21 (Down syndrome) with an increased susceptibility to acute leukemia. For children with Down syndrome, the risk of developing leukemia is 10 to 20 times greater than the risk in healthy children. The risk is greatest for children under 5 years of age.[3]

Wilms tumor is particularly recognized for its association with a number of other abnormalities, including genitourinary anomalies, aniridia (congenital absence of the iris), hemihypertrophy (muscular overgrowth of half of the body or face), and mental retardation. Approximately 10% of children diagnosed with Wilms tumor demonstrate one of these congenital abnormalities.[4] Retinoblastoma, a malignant embryonic tumor of the eye, occurs either as an inherited defect or as an acquired mutation.

More than 150 single-gene defects, oncogenes and tumor-suppressor genes, have been associated with the subsequent development of both childhood and adult cancers (Table 11-4). Two autosomal recessive disorders have been associated with pediatric malignancies. Children with Fanconi anemia have a high risk of developing acute myeloid leukemia,[5] and the development of other solid tumors has been associated with Bloom syndrome.[6,7]

TABLE 11-3

Congenital Factors Associated With Childhood Cancer

Syndrome	Associated Risk Factors
CHROMOSOME ALTERATIONS	
Down syndrome	Acute leukemia
13q syndrome	Retinoblastoma
CHROMOSOME INSTABILITY	
Ataxia-telangiectasia	Lymphoma
Bloom syndrome	Acute leukemia, lymphoma, Wilms tumor
Fanconi anemia	Nonlymphocytic leukemia, myelodysplastic syndrome, hepatic tumors
HEREDITARY SYNDROMES	
Beckwith-Wiedmann syndrome	Wilms tumor, sarcoma, brain tumors, neuroblastoma, hepatoblastoma
Neurofibromatosis	Brain tumor, sarcomas, neuroblastomas, Wilms tumor, nonlymphocytic leukemia
Li-Fraumeni syndrome	Sarcoma, adrenocortical carcinoma
Von Hippel-Lindau disease	Cerebellar hemangioblastoma, retinal angioma, renal cell, carcinoma, pheochromocytomas
Ataxia-telangiectasia	Leukemia, lymphoma
Tuberous sclerosis	Brain tumors
IMMUNODEFICIENCY DISORDERS	
Congenital	
Agammaglobulinemia	Lymphoma, leukemia, brain tumors
Immunoglobulin A (IgA) deficiency	Lymphoma, leukemia, brain tumors
Wiskott-Aldrich syndrome	Leukemia, lymphoma
Acquired	
Aplastic anemia	Leukemia
Organ transplantation	Leukemia, lymphoma
CONGENITAL MALFORMATION SYNDROMES	
Aniridia, hemihypertrophy, hamartoma, genitourinary anomalies	Wilms tumor
Cryptorchidism	Testicular tumor
Gonadal dysgenesis	Gonadoblastoma
FAMILY SUSCEPTIBILITY	
Twin or sibling with leukemia	Leukemia

The relative ineffectiveness of the immune surveillance system during intrauterine life may explain the occurrence of embryonic tumors. (The immune surveillance system is discussed in Chapter 9.) Because this period requires rapid proliferation and differentiation of cells in the developing fetus, cell mutation theoretically could result in embryonic tumors. Children with immunodeficiencies, congenital or acquired, have an increased risk of developing lymphoproliferative disorders and malignancies.[7,8]

Children with immunodeficiencies experience a striking increased risk of subsequent cancer over that of healthy children. These conditions may be either congenital, generally involving X-linked recessive inheritance, or acquired, generally caused by therapeutic immunosuppression after organ transplantation or treatment for aplastic anemia.

Although not determined to be genetically transmitted, a few malignancies seem to demonstrate a familial tendency, suggested by the clustering of specific cancers in a particular family. A child who has a twin who develops leukemia has a higher risk of developing acute lymphoblastic leukemia (ALL) him or herself. This association is not true when considering other types of affected first-degree relatives.[9]

Environmental Factors

Finding the cause of any disease is typically a long, slow process. It may take years for an epidemiologic study to determine whether a risk factor is possibly related to the development of a disease. No one factor determines whether an individual will develop cancer, even if a specific environmental exposure explains a high proportion of the occurrence of a specific cancer. Childhood cancer is no different. No single study, or even multiple epidemiologic studies, will tell a parent why his or her child developed cancer. The many factors that may play a role in the development of cancer include genetics, nutrition and diet, immune function, occupational exposure, hormonal variations, viral illnesses, and

TABLE 11-4

Selected Oncogenes and Tumor-Suppressor Genes Associated With Childhood Cancer

Gene	Associated Pediatric Tumor
ONCOGENES	
BCR-abl	Acute lymphoblastic leukemia
N-myc	Neuroblastoma
c-myb	Neural tumors, leukemia, lymphomas, rhabdomyosarcoma, Wilms tumor, neuroblastoma
Erb	Glioblastoma
N-ras	Neuroblastoma, leukemia
H/K-ras	Rhabdomyosarcoma, neuroblastoma, leukemia
ATM	Acute lymphoblastic leukemia
TUMOR-SUPPRESSOR GENES	
NF1	Meningiomas, primitive neuroectodermal tumor, juvenile chronic myelocytic leukemia
NF2	Brain tumors, melanoma
Rb1	Retinoblastoma
WT1, WT2, WT3	Wilms tumor
FWT1	Wilms tumor
p53	Soft tissue sarcoma, osteosarcoma, adrenocortical carcinoma, brain tumors, leukemia

Data from Dome JS, Coppes MS: Recent advances in Wilms tumor genetics, *Curr Opin Pediatr* 14(1):5–11, 2002; Lamorte L, Park M: The receptor tyrosine kinases: role in cancer progression, *Surg Oncol Clin North Am* 10(2):271–288, 2001; Lindblom A, Nordenskjold M: The biology of inherited cancer, *Semin Cancer Biol* 10(4):251–254, 2002; Sandberg AA, Chen Z: Some cytogenetic and molecular aspects of cancer therapy, *Compr Ther* 22 (2):76–80, 1996.

other individual characteristics such as biologic, social, or physical environments.

Prenatal exposure

Prenatal exposure to some drugs and to ionizing radiation has been linked to subsequent cancers. Perhaps the most well known of these is diethylstilbestrol (DES), a drug taken to avert early abortion. In 1971, DES was identified as a transplacental chemical carcinogen. Adenocarcinoma of the vagina developed in a small percentage of the daughters of mothers who had taken DES while pregnant.

Several associations have been found linking parental factors (both nonoccupational and occupational) to the risk of childhood cancer. Exposure to hazardous materials, such as petroleum products, solvents, chemicals, and radiation, could lead to genetic changes of the egg or sperm or to transplacental transfer of the carcinogen.[10]

Intrauterine exposure to radiation during pregnancy may be associated with an increased risk for all types of childhood cancers. However, studies of children exposed to atomic fallout in uteri show no increase in childhood cancer.[11] Thus, it is suggested that women who require prenatal radiologic studies may have some other cancer risks that predispose the fetus to the development of cancer. Children who develop cancer may have causative factors other than the exposure to radiation in utero.

Childhood exposure

Childhood exposures to drugs, secondhand smoke, ionizing radiation, and viruses have been implicated as risk factors that increase susceptibility to specific cancers. In addition to those drug and environmental agents that are known to cause cancer in adults and therefore also are risks for exposure during childhood, a few drugs in particular may increase cancer risk during childhood. These drugs include (1) anabolic androgenic steroids, which are used in the treatment of aplastic anemia or used illegally by teenage athletes for body development and have been associated with subsequent hepatocellular carcinoma; (2) cytotoxic agents used in the treatment of pediatric cancers, which may predispose the child to leukemia in later years; and (3) immunosuppressive agents, particularly those used in conjunction with transplant surgeries, which have been shown to increase the risk of lymphoma.

Although viruses have been implicated in childhood cancers, the association is not strong. (The viral causes of carcinogenesis are discussed in Chapter 9.) In children, the strongest carcinogenic relationship has been shown between the Epstein-Barr virus (EBV) and Burkitt lymphoma[12] and between EBV and Hodgkin lymphoma.[13] Research has shown that children with AIDS have an increased risk of developing certain cancers, predominantly non-Hodgkin lymphoma and Kaposi sarcoma.[8,14]

PROGNOSIS

Today, childhood cancer should not be considered an inevitably fatal illness. Since the mid-1980s, death rates have declined dramatically and the rate of survival has increased for most childhood cancers. For example, the 5-year survival rates for all childhood cancers combined increased from 55.7% in 1974 to 1976 to nearly 80% in 1998.[15] This improvement in survival rates is due to significant advances in treatment. Overall, children have a more favorable prognosis than adults. Children appear to be more responsive to therapies and more tolerant of the immediate side effects of treatment. More children than adults are enrolled in clinical trials, from which improved clinical therapy is derived. This may contribute to the higher survival rates observed in children.

Survivors of childhood cancer are at increased risk of developing a second malignancy later in life. This risk may be associated with a variety of factors, including previous chemotherapy or radiotherapy, genetic factors, and type of primary cancer (e.g., soft tissue sarcoma, neuroblastoma).[16]

Because childhood cancer should be viewed as a chronic disease instead of a fatal illness, the focus of treatment is on the quality of life. Even those cancers that cannot be cured generally can be treated, resulting in significantly improved quality of life. Although they may be cured, these children still face residual and late effects of their treatment. These late effects are more significant in children than in adults because treatment given in childhood occurs in a physically immature, growing individual. Late effects that need further study include physical impairments, reproductive dysfunction, soft tissue and bone atrophy, learning disabilities, secondary cancers, and psychologic sequelae. More must be learned about the genetic factors associated with childhood malignancies and about the genetic consequences of treatment. Genetic counseling is appropriate for children cured of cancers known to be transmitted genetically (e.g., retinoblastoma).

HEALTH ALERT
Late Effects of Childhood Cancer

Because of significant advances in treatment, nearly 80% of children treated for cancer survive 5 years or more, an increase of almost 45% since the early 1960s. It has become apparent that the effects of childhood cancer treatment may affect a child's health later in life. This result is known as the *late effects* of childhood cancer. Late effects are caused by the injury that cancer treatment causes to the healthy cells in the body and may occur as a result of surgery, radiation therapy, chemotherapy, or bone marrow transplant. Late effects may impair the brain, heart, lungs, breasts, muscle and bone, vision and hearing, growth and development, and fertility. One of the most serious late effects is the development of a second malignancy later in life. Each child receiving cancer therapy is unique. Late effects vary and depend largely on the type and doses of therapy received. The very young child may be at the greatest risk. Regular follow-up examinations are extremely important during and after treatment. Health providers involved in the care of childhood cancer survivors watch for short- and long-term effects of treatment, as well as signs of recurrent disease.

Data from Bhatia S, Blatt, J, Meadows A: Late effects of childhood cancer and its treatment. In Pizzo PA, Poplack DG, editors: *Principles and practice of pediatric oncology*, ed 5, pp 1490–1514, Philadelphia, 2006, Lippincott, Williams, & Wilkins.

✔ QUICK CHECK 11-1

1. What are the most common childhood cancers?
2. Why are children less likely to get carcinomas?
3. How are different etiologic factors associated with the development of childhood cancer?

Did You Understand?

Incidence and Types of Childhood Cancers

1. Childhood cancer is a rare disease, but it remains the second leading cause of death in children.
2. The most common type of childhood cancer is leukemia, and the second most common type of pediatric malignancy is a tumor involving the brain or central nervous system.

Etiology

1. Because most carcinomas are caused by environmental exposure, these cancers are extremely rare in children because they have not lived long enough to be exposed to carcinogens.
2. Children with immunodeficiencies are at increased risk for developing cancer because of an ineffective immune system.
3. Children with Down syndrome are at increased risk for developing leukemia.
4. Risk factors that may be associated with the development of childhood cancer include genetic, nutrition and diet, immune function, occupational exposure, hormonal variations, and viral illnesses, as well as other individual characteristics such as biologic, social, or physical environments.

Prognosis

1. Survivors of childhood cancer are at increased risk for developing a second cancer during their lifetime, compared with the general population.
2. Improved survival for children with cancer has led to research aimed at discovering less toxic treatments that will minimize residual effects.

Key Terms

Ecogenetics, 268
Embryonic tumors, 267
Mesodermal germ layer, 267

References

1. American Cancer Society: *Cancer facts and figures 2006*, Atlanta, 2006, American Cancer Society.
2. Stam H et al: Young adult patients with a history of pediatric disease: impact on course of life and transition into adulthood, *J Adolesc Health* 39(1):4–13, 2006.
3. Kurkjian C et al: Acute promyelocytic leukemia and constitutional trisomy 21, *Cancer Genet Cytogenet* 165(2):176–179, 2006.
4. Cook A, Farhat W, Khoury A: Update on Wilms' tumor in children, *J Med Liban* 53(2):85–90, 2005.
5. Meyer S et al: Spectrum and significance of variants and mutations in Fanconi anaemia group G gene in children with sporadic acute myeloid leukemia, *Br J Haematol* 133(3): 284–292, 2006.
6. Farris I et al: Risk factors for pediatric malignant bone tumors, *An Pediatr (Barc)* 63(6):537–547, 2005.
7. Varan A et al: Malignant solid tumors associated with congenital immunodeficiency disorders, *Pediatr Hematol Oncol* 21(5): 441–451, 2004.
8. Kest H et al: Malignancy in perinatally human immunodeficiency virus-infected children in the United States, *Pediatr Infect Dis J* 24(3):237–242, 2005.
9. Couto E, Chen B, Hemminiki K: Association of childhood acute lymphoblastic leukaemia with cancers in family members, *Br J Cancer* 93(11):1307–1309, 2005.
10. Smulevich VB, Solionova LG, Belyakova SV: Prenatal occupation and other factors and cancer risk in children. II. Occupational factors, *Int J Cancer* 83(6):718–722, 1999.
11. Boice JD Jr, Miller RW: Childhood and adult cancer after intrauterine exposure to ionizing radiation, *Teratology* 59(4): 227–233, 1999.
12. McNally RJ, Parker L: Environmental factors and childhood acute leukemias and lymphomas, *Leuk Lymphoma* 47(4): 583–598, 2006.
13. Andersson J: Epstein-Barr virus and Hodgkin's lymphoma, *Herpes* 13(1):12–16, 2006.
14. Mgulaiteye SM: Spectrum of cancer among HIV-infected persons in Africa: the Uganda AIDS-Cancer Registry Match Study, *Int J Cancer* 118(4):985–990, 2006.
15. Reis M et al: *SEER cancer statistics review 1973–1999*, Bethesda, MD, 2001, National Cancer Institute.
16. Bassal LA et al: Risk of selected subsequent carcinomas in survivors of childhood cancer: a report from the Childhood Cancer Survivor Study, *J Clin Oncol* 24(3):476–483, 2006.

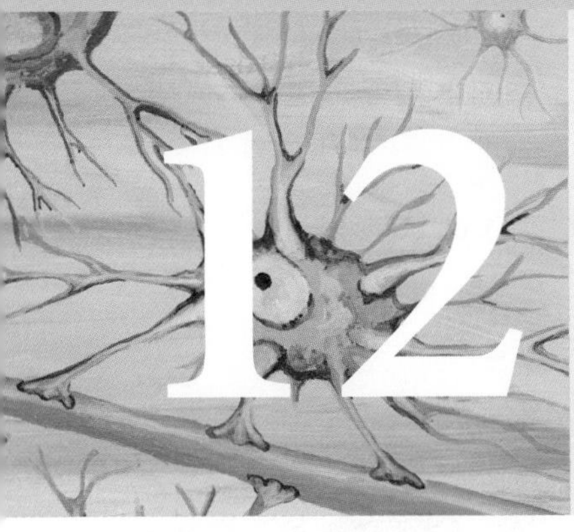

12 STRUCTURE AND FUNCTION OF THE NEUROLOGIC SYSTEM

Richard A. Sugerman

CHAPTER OUTLINE

ELECTRONIC RESOURCES

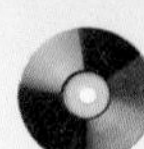

Companion CD
- Review Questions and Answers
- Animations

evolve Website
http://evolve.elsevier.com/Huether/
- Quick Check Answers
- Key Terms Exercises
- Critical Thinking Questions with Answers
- Algorithm Completion Exercises
- WebLinks

The human nervous system is a remarkable structure responsible for the body's ability to interact with the environment and for the regulation of activities involving internal organs. The nervous system literally drives the other systems of the body. It is a network composed of complex structures that transmit signals—both electrically and chemically—between the body's many organs and tissues and the brain.

OVERVIEW AND ORGANIZATION OF THE NERVOUS SYSTEM

Although the nervous system functions as a unified whole, structures and functions have been divided here to facilitate understanding. Structurally, the nervous system is divided into the central nervous system and the peripheral nervous system. The **central nervous system (CNS)** consists of the brain and spinal cord, enclosed within the protective cranial vault and vertebrae, respectively. The **peripheral nervous system (PNS)** is composed of the **cranial nerves** and the **spinal nerves.** Peripheral nerve pathways are differentiated into **afferent pathways (ascending pathways),** which carry sensory impulses toward the CNS, and **efferent pathways (descending pathways),** which innervate skeletal muscle or effector organs by transmitting motor impulses away from the CNS.

Functionally, the PNS can be divided into the somatic nervous system and the autonomic nervous system. The **somatic nervous system** consists of pathways that regulate voluntary motor control (e.g., skeletal muscle). The **autonomic nervous system (ANS)** is involved with regulation of the body's internal environment (viscera) through involuntary control of organ systems. The ANS is further divided into sympathetic and parasympathetic divisions. Organs innervated by specific components of the nervous system are called **effector organs.**

CELLS OF THE NERVOUS SYSTEM

Two basic types of cells constitute nervous tissue: neurons and supporting cells. The **neuron** is the primary cell of the nervous system, whereas cells such as **neuroglial cells** (in the CNS) and **Schwann cells** (in the PNS) provide structural support and nutrition for the neurons.[1]

The Neuron

Working alone or in units, neurons detect environmental changes and initiate body responses to maintain a dynamic steady state. Neuronal structure varies markedly, so that each neuron is adapted to perform specialized functions.

HEALTH ALERT
Neuroimaging Techniques

Functional and structural neuroimaging techniques have reached a level of sophistication where they can be used in diagnosing brain dysfunctions by looking at levels of brain activity in specific areas. The technologies include positron emission tomography (PET), functional magnetic resonance imaging (fMRI), single-photon emission computed tomography (SPECT), and magnetic resonance spectroscopy (MRS). In dyslexia, autism, and attention-deficit-hyperactivity disorder, abnormal brain symmetry or abnormal interactions between or within lobes are evident. Presently researchers are starting to apply these techniques and others to psychiatry and cognitive neuroscience problems. They are evaluating problems such as how brain areas interact in individuals with psychoses or hallucinations, recover from neurotrauma and the advancement of neurodegenerative diseases.

Data from Gore JC et al: Integration of fMRI, NIROT and ERP studies of human brain function, *Magn Reson Imaging* 24:507-513, 2006; Weiller C, May A, Sach M, Buhmann C, Rijntjes M: Role of functional imaging in neurological disorders, *J Magn Reson Imaging* Jun;23(6):840-850, 2006; Roffman JL, Weiss AP, Goff DC, Rauch SL, Weinberger DR: Neuroimaging-genetic paradigms: a new approach to investigate the pathophysiology and treatment of cognitive deficits in schizophrenia, *Harv Rev Psychiatry* Mar-Apr;14 (2):78-91, 2006.

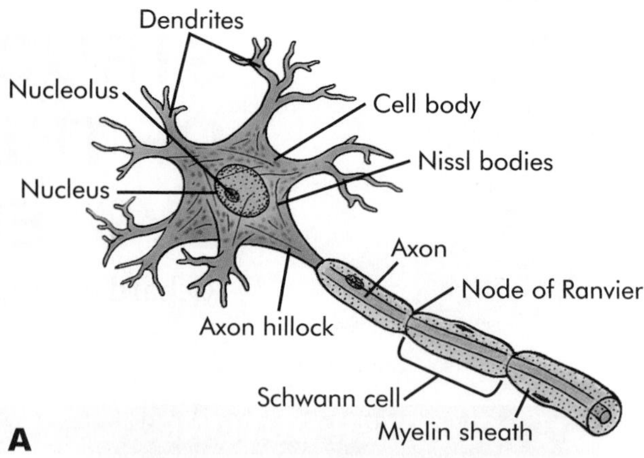

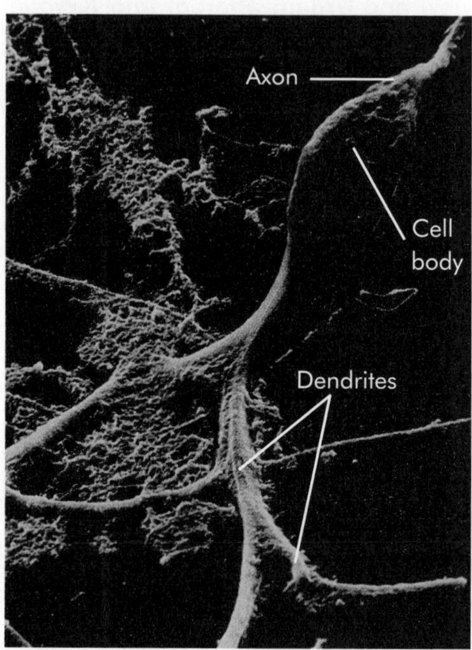

Figure 12-1 ■ **Neuron With Composite Parts. A,** Multipolar neuron: neuron with multiple extensions from the cell body. **B,** Scanning electron micrograph. (Modified from Thibodeau GA, Patton KT: *Anatomy & physiology,* ed 6, St Louis, 2007, Mosby.)

The fuel source for the neuron is predominantly glucose; insulin, however, is not required for cellular glucose uptake in the CNS. Among the cellular constituents of neurons are **microtubules, neurofibrils, microfilaments** (thought to be involved in transport of cellular products), and **Nissl substances** (involved in protein synthesis).

A neuron (Figure 12-1) has three components: a cell body (soma) and the thin processes of the cell, the dendrites, and the axons. Most cell bodies are located within the CNS; those in the PNS usually are found in groups called **ganglia** (or **plexuses**). The **dendrites** are extensions that carry nerve impulses toward the cell body. The **dendritic zone** receives a stimulus and continues further conduction. **Axons** are long, conductive projections from the cell body that carry nerve impulses away from the cell body. The **axon hillock** is the cone-shaped process where the axon leaves the cell body. The first part of the axon hillock has the lowest threshold for stimulation, so action potentials begin there. A typical neuron has only one axon, which may be covered with a segmented layer of lipid material called **myelin,** an insulating substance. This entire membrane is referred to as the **myelin sheath** (see Figure 12-22, *B*). The myelin sheaths are interrupted at regular intervals by the **nodes of Ranvier.** Axons branch extensively at the nodes of Ranvier.

The principle of *divergence* refers to the ability of axonal branches to influence many different neurons. *Convergence* applies when branches of various numbers of neurons "converge" on and influence a single neuron. Nutrient exchange is not possible through the myelin sheath, although it can occur at the nodes of Ranvier. Where there is myelin, the velocity of nerve impulses increases. Myelin acts as an insulator that allows ions to flow between segments rather than along the entire length of the membrane, yielding the increased velocity. This mechanism is referred to as **saltatory conduction.** Disorders of the myelin sheath (demyelinating diseases), such as multiple sclerosis and Guillain-Barré syndrome, demonstrate the important role myelin plays in nerve function (see Chapter 15). Conduction velocities depend not only on the myelin coating but also on the diameter of the axon. Larger axons transmit impulses at a faster rate.

Neurons are structurally classified on the basis of the number of processes (projections) extending from the cell body. There are four basic types of cell configuration: (1) unipolar, (2) pseudounipolar, (3) bipolar, and (4) multipolar.

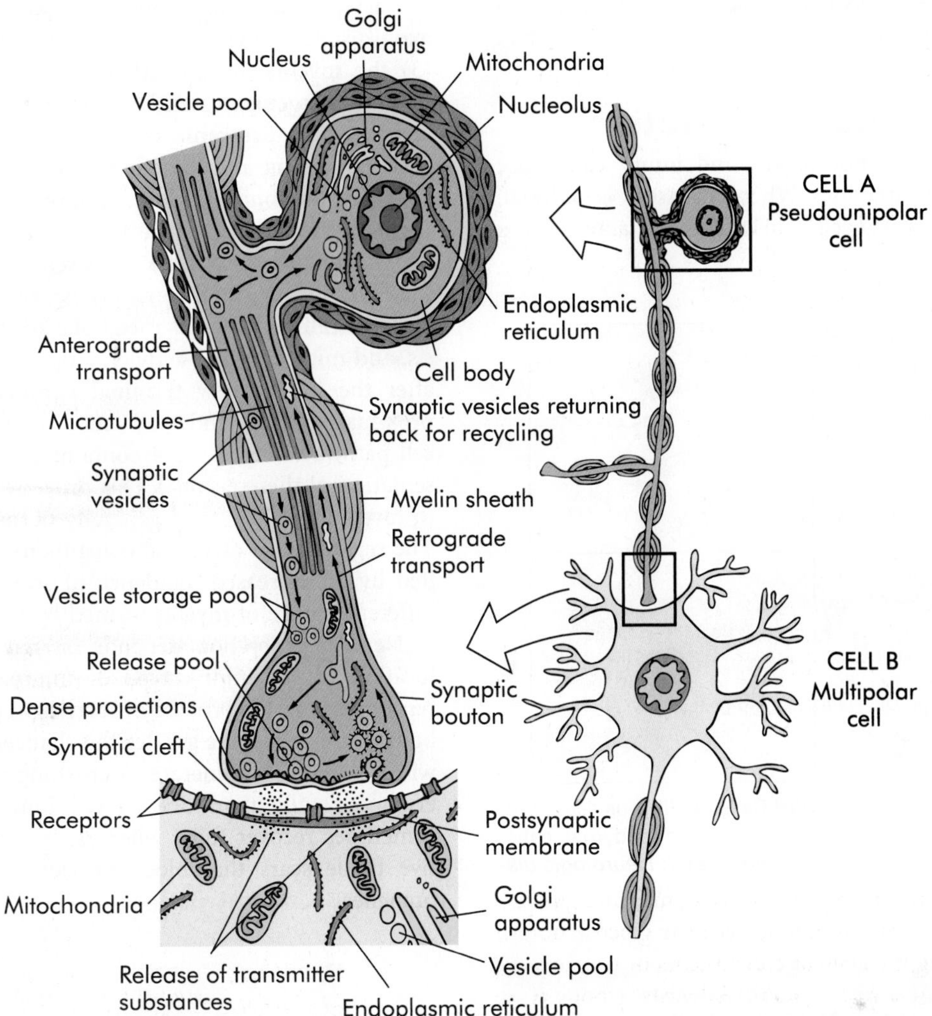

Figure 12-2 ■ **Neuronal Transmission and Synaptic Cleft.** Electrical impulse travels along axon of first neuron to synapse. Chemical transmitter is secreted into synaptic space to depolarize membrane (dendrite or cell body) of next neuron in pathway. *Cell A* represents unipolar cell; *cell B* represents multipolar cell.

Unipolar neurons have one process that branches shortly after leaving the cell body. One example is found in the retina. **Pseudounipolar neurons** (some authors call them *unipolar*) also have one process; the dendritic portion of each of these neurons extends away from the CNS and the axon portion projects into the CNS (Figure 12-2). This configuration is typical of sensory neurons in both cranial and spinal nerves. **Bipolar neurons** have two distinct processes arising from the cell body. This type of neuron connects the rod and cone cells of the retina. **Multipolar neurons** are the most common and have multiple processes capable of extensive branching. A motor neuron is typically multipolar (see Figure 12-2).

Functionally, there are three types of neurons (their direction of transmission and typical configuration are noted in parentheses): (1) sensory (afferent, mostly pseudounipolar), (2) associational (interneurons, multipolar), and (3) motor (efferent, multipolar). **Sensory neurons** carry impulses from peripheral sensory receptors to the CNS. **Associational neurons (interneurons)** transmit impulses from neuron to neuron—that is, sensory to motor neurons. They are located solely within the CNS. **Motor neurons** transmit impulses away from the CNS to an effector (i.e., skeletal muscle or organ). In skeletal muscle the end processes form a **neuromuscular (myoneural) junction.**

Neuroglia and Schwann Cells

Neuroglia ("nerve glue") are the general classification of cells that support the neurons of the CNS. They comprise approximately half of the total brain and spinal cord volume and are 5 to 10 times more numerous than neurons. Different types of neuroglia serve different functions. **Astrocytes,** for example, fill the spaces between neurons and surround blood vessels in the CNS; **oligodendroglia (oligondendrocytes)** deposit myelin within the CNS. Oligondendroglia are the CNS counterpart of the Schwann cells. Ependymal cells line the cerebrospinal fluid (CSF)-filled cavities of the CNS. **Microglia** remove debris (phagocytosis) in the CNS. (Characteristics of neuroglia and Schwann cells are summarized in Figure 12-3 and Table 12-1.)

Nerve Injury and Regeneration

Mature nerve cells do not divide, and injury can cause permanent loss of function. When an axon is severed, wallerian degeneration occurs in the distal axon: (1) a characteristic swelling appears within the portion of the axon distal to the cut; (2) the neurofilaments hypertrophy; (3) the myelin sheath shrinks and disintegrates; and (4) the axon degenerates and disappears. The myelin sheaths re-form into Schwann cells that line up in a column between the cut and the effector organ.

At the proximal end of the injured axon, similar changes occur but only back to the next node of Ranvier. The cell body responds to trauma by swelling and by dispersing the Nissl substance (chromatolysis). During the repair process, the cell increases its metabolic activity, protein synthesis, and mitochondrial activity. Approximately 7 to 14 days after the injury, new terminal sprouts project from the proximal segment and may enter the remaining Schwann cell pathway. (Figure 12-4 contains a more detailed representation of these events.) This process, however, is limited to myelinated fibers and generally occurs only in the PNS. The regeneration of axonal constituents in the CNS is limited by an increased incidence of scar formation and the different nature of myelin formed by the oligodendrocyte.

Nerve regeneration depends on many factors, such as location of the injury, type of injury, the inflammatory responses, and the process of scarring. The closer to the cell body of the nerve, the greater the chances that the nerve cell will die and not regenerate. A crushing injury allows recovery more fully than does a cut injury. Crushed nerves sometimes recover fully, whereas cut nerves form connective tissue scars that block or slow regenerating axonal branches.

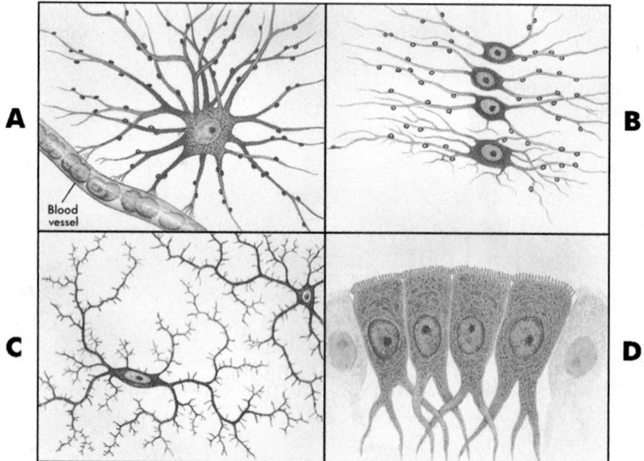

Figure 12-3 ■ Types of Neuroglial Cells. A, Fibrous astrocyte; **B,** oligodendrocytes; **C,** microglia cells; **D,** ependymal cells. (Modified from Chipps E, Clanin N, Campbell V: *Neurologic disorders,* St Louis, 1992, Mosby.)

TABLE 12-1

Support Cells of the Nervous System

Cell Type	Primary Functions
Astrocytes	Form specialized contacts between neuronal surfaces and blood vessels Provide rapid transport for nutrients and metabolites Believed to form an essential component of the blood-brain barrier Appear to be the scar-forming cells of CNS, which may be the foci for seizures Appear to work with neurons in processing information and memory storage
Oligodendroglia (oligodendrocytes)	Formation of myelin sheath in CNS
Schwann cells	Formation of myelin sheath in PNS
Microglia	Responsible for clearing cellular debris (phagocytic properties)
Ependymal cells	Serve as a lining for ventricles and choroid plexuses involved in production of cerebrospinal fluid

Some data from Martinez Banaclocha MA: Magnetic storage of information in the human cerebral cortex: a hypothesis for memory, *Int J Neurosci* 115(3):329-337, 2005.

CNS, Central nervous system; *PNS,* peripheral nervous system.

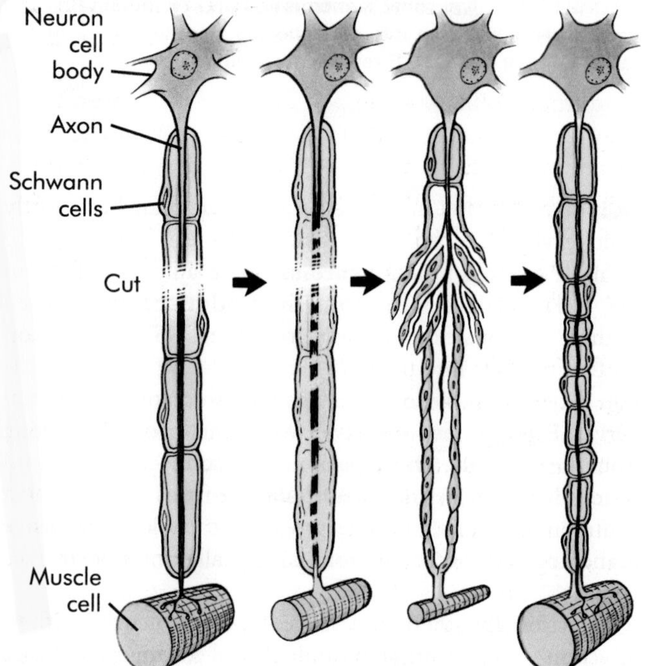

Figure 12-4 ■ Repair of a Peripheral Nerve Fiber. When cut, a damaged motor axon can regrow to its distal connection only if the Schwann cells remain intact (to form a guiding tunnel) and if scar tissue does not block its way.

QUICK CHECK 12-1

1. How do the functions of the somatic and autonomic nervous systems differ?
2. What are the three components of a neuron?
3. How does myelin affect nerve impulses?
4. Name the process through which injured axons are repaired, and describe the process.

THE NERVE IMPULSE

Neurons generate and conduct electrical and chemical impulses by selectively changing the electrical potential of the plasma membrane and influencing other nearby neurons by releasing chemicals **(neurotransmitters).** An unexcited neuron maintains a resting membrane potential (see Chapter 1). When the membrane potential is raised, an action potential is generated and the nerve impulse then flows to all parts of the neuron. The action potential response occurs only when the stimulus is strong enough; if it is too weak, the membrane remains unexcited. This property is termed the *all-or-none response* (see Chapter 1 for a discussion of electrical impulse conduction).

Synapses

Neurons are not physically continuous with one another. The region between adjacent neurons is called a **synapse** (see Figure 12-2). Impulses are transmitted across the synapse by chemical and electrical conduction (see Figure 12-2); only chemical conduction is discussed here. The neurons that conduct a nerve impulse are named according to whether they relay impulses toward **(presynaptic neurons)** or away from **(postsynaptic neurons)** the synapse.

Impulses are transmitted across the synapse by chemical conduction. When an impulse originates in a presynaptic neuron, the impulse reaches the vesicles, where chemicals (neurotransmitters) are stored in the **synaptic bouton.** Once released from the vesicles, the neurotransmitters diffuse across the **synaptic cleft** (the space between the neurons) and bind to receptor sites on the plasma membrane of the postsynaptic neuron[2] (see Figure 12-2).

Neurotransmitters

More than 30 substances are thought to be neurotransmitters, including norepinephrine, acetylcholine, dopamine, histamine, and serotonin. Many of these transmitters have more than one function.[3] For example, norepinephrine in the brain probably helps regulate mood, functions in dreaming sleep, and maintains arousal. Some neurotransmitters are amino acids, including gamma (γ)-aminobutyric acid (GABA), glutamic acid, and aspartic acid. Small chains of amino acids, such as enkephalins and endorphins, also function as neurotransmitters. Neurotransmitter and neuromodulator substances are listed in Table 12-2.

Because the neurotransmitter is normally stored on one side of the synaptic cleft and the receptor sites are on the other side, chemical synapses operate in one direction. Therefore, action potentials are transmitted along a multineuronal pathway in one direction. The binding of the neurotransmitter at the receptor site changes the permeability of the postsynaptic neuron and, consequently, its membrane potential. Two possible scenarios can then follow: (1) the postsynaptic neuron may be excited (depolarized; **excitatory postsynaptic potentials** [EPSPs]) or (2) the postsynaptic neuron's plasma membrane may be inhibited (hyperpolarized; **inhibitory postsynaptic potentials [IPSPs]**). Cannabinoid transmitters have been discovered that are released from postsynaptic neurons that modulate neurotransmitter release from the presynaptic neurons.[3,4] (Chapter 1 reviews electrical impulses and membrane potentials.)

Usually a single EPSP cannot induce a neuron's action potential and the propagation of the nerve impulse. Whether this occurs depends on the number and frequency of potentials the postsynaptic neuron receives—a concept known as **summation. Temporal summation** (time relationship) refers to the effects of successive, rapid impulses received from a single neuron at the same synapse. **Spatial summation** (spacing effect) is the combined effects of impulses from a number of neurons onto a single neuron at the same time. **Facilitation** refers to the effect of EPSP on the plasma membrane potential. The plasma membrane is facilitated when summation brings the membrane closer to the threshold potential and decreases the stimulus required to induce an action potential. The effect that a chemical neurotransmitter has on the plasma membrane potential depends on the balance of these effects.

QUICK CHECK 12-2

1. Explain the process of the chemical conduction of impulses.
2. What are neurotransmitters? Give several examples.
3. Compare summation and facilitation.

THE CENTRAL NERVOUS SYSTEM

The Brain

The human brain enables a person to reason, function intellectually, express personality and mood, and interact with the environment. This pinkish gray organ weighs approximately 3 pounds and receives 15% to 20% of the total cardiac output. The three major divisions of the brain are (1) the forebrain, formed by the two cerebral hemispheres; (2) the midbrain, which includes the corpora quadrigemina and cerebral peduncles; and (3) the hindbrain, which includes the cerebellum, pons, and medulla (Table 12-3). The midbrain, medulla, and pons make up the **brain stem,** which connects the hemispheres of the brain, cerebellum, and spinal cord. A collection of nerve cell bodies (nuclei) within the brain stem makes up the

TABLE 12-2

Substances That Are Neurotransmitters or Neuromodulators

Substance	Location	Effect	Clinical Example
Acetylcholine	Many parts of the brain, spinal cord, neuromuscular junction of skeletal muscle, and many ANS synapses	Excitatory or inhibitory	Alzheimer disease (a type of dementia) is associated with a decrease in acetylcholine-secreting neurons. Myasthenia gravis (weakness of skeletal muscles) results from a reduction in acetylcholine receptors.
MONOAMINES			
Norepinephrine	Many areas of the brain and spinal cord; also in some ANS synapses	Excitatory or inhibitory	Cocaine and amphetamines,* resulting in overstimulation of postsynaptic neurons.
Serotonin	Many areas of the brain and spinal cord	Generally inhibitory	Involved with mood, anxiety, and sleep induction. Levels of serotonin are elevated in schizophrenia (delusions, hallucinations, withdrawal).
Dopamine	Some areas of the brain and ANS synapses	Generally excitatory	Parkinson disease (depression of voluntary motor control) results from destruction of dopamine-secreting neurons. Drugs used to increase dopamine production induce vomiting and schizophrenia.
Histamine		Generally inhibitory	No clear indication of histamine-associated pathologic conditions. Histamine apparently is involved with arousal, pituitary hormone secretion, control of cerebral circulation, and thermoregulation.
AMINO ACIDS			
γ-Aminobutyric acid (GABA)	Most neurons of the CNS have GABA receptors	Majority of postsynaptic inhibition in the brain	Drugs that increase GABA function have been used to treat epilepsy (excessive discharge of neurons).
Glycine	Spinal cord	Most postsynaptic inhibition in the spinal cord	Glycine receptors are inhibited by strychnine.
Glutamate and aspartate	Widespread in the brain and spinal cord	Excitatory	Drugs that block glutamate or aspartate such as riluzole, used to treat amyotrophic lateral sclerosis. These drugs might prevent seizures and neural degeneration from overexcitation.
NEUROPEPTIDES			
Endorphins and enkephalins	Widely distributed in the CNS and PNS	Generally inhibitory	The opiates morphine and heroin bind to endorphin and enkephalin receptors on presynaptic neurons and reduce pain by blocking the release of neurotransmitter.
Substance P	Spinal cord, brain, and sensory neurons associated with pain, GI tract	Generally excitatory	Substance P is a neurotransmitter in pain transmission pathways. Blocking the release of substance P by morphine reduces pain.

From Seeley R, Stephens TD, Tate P: *Anatomy and physiology,* ed 6, New York, 2003, McGraw-Hill.
*Increase the release and block the reuptake of norepinephrine.
ANS, Autonomic nervous system; *CNS,* central nervous system; *PNS,* peripheral nervous system; *GI,* gastrointestinal.

reticular formation (Figure 12-5). The reticular formation is a large network of connected tissue that contains portions of vital reflexes, such as those controlling cardiovascular function and respiration. It is essential for maintaining wakefulness and therefore is referred to as the **reticular activating system** (see Figure 12-5). Some nuclei within the reticular formation cause specific motor movements.[3]

Divisions of the brain are associated with different functions, but attributing specific functions to definite regions of the brain is not entirely accurate. However, for clinical considerations functional specificity is very useful for localizing pathologic conditions in various nervous system regions. A neuropsychiatrist (Brodmann) is credited with postulating that various activities are correlated to many

TABLE 12-3

Divisions of the Central Nervous System

Primary Vesicles	Secondary Vesicles	Associated Structures
Forebrain (prosencephalon)	Telencephalon	Cerebral hemispheres Cerebral cortex Rhinencephalon Basal ganglia
	Diencephalon	Epithalamus Thalamus Hypothalamus Subthalamus
Midbrain (mesencephalon)	Mesencephalon	Corpora quadrigemina Cerebral peduncles
Hindbrain (rhombencephalon)	Metencephalon	Cerebellum Pons
Spinal cord	Myelencephalon Spinal cord	Medulla oblongata Spinal cord

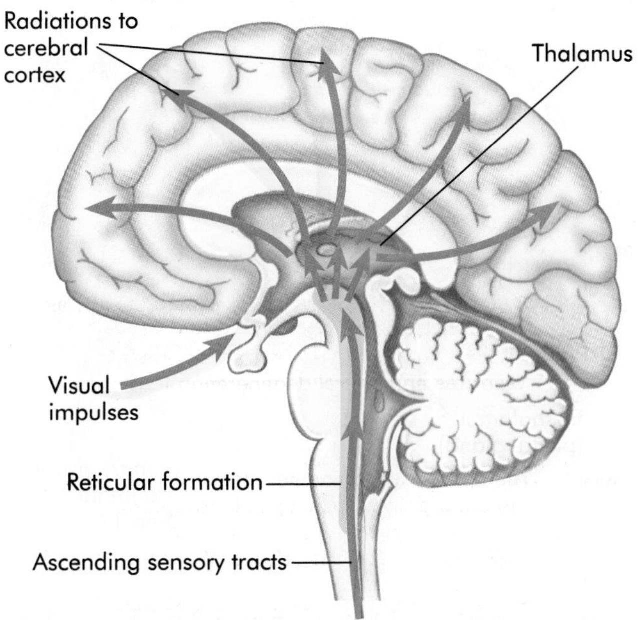

Figure 12-5 ■ **Reticular Activating System.** System consists of nuclei in the brain stem reticular formation plus fibers that conduct to the nuclei from below and fibers that conduct from the nuclei to widespread areas of the cerebral cortex. Functioning of the reticular activating system is essential for consciousness.

regions of the cerebral cortex. (Figure 12-6 illustrates these regions and describes some of the areas.)[5]

Forebrain

Telencephalon

The **telencephalon** consists of the **cerebrum** (the largest portion of the brain), the limbic system, and some basal ganglia (composed of several *nuclei*). The surface of the cerebrum (cerebral cortex) is covered with convolutions called *gyri* (see Figure 12-6), which greatly increases the cortical surface area and the number of neurons. Grooves between adjacent gyri are termed **sulci;** deeper grooves are **fissures.** The **cerebral cortex** contains the cell bodies of neurons **(gray matter). White matter** lies beneath the cerebral cortex and is composed of myelinated nerve fibers.

The two cerebral hemispheres are separated by the longitudinal fissure. The surface of each hemisphere is divided into lobes named after the region of the skull under which each lies. The **frontal lobe's** posterior margin is on the **central sulcus (fissure of Rolando),** and it borders inferiorly on the **lateral sulcus (sylvian fissure, lateral fissure)** (see Figure 12-6). The **prefrontal area** is responsible for goal-oriented behavior (e.g., ability to concentrate), short-term or recall memory, the elaboration of thought, and inhibition on the limbic areas of the CNS. The **premotor area (Brodmann area 6)** (see Figure 12-6, *C*) is involved in programming motor movements. This area contains the cell bodies that form part of the **basal ganglia system (extrapyramidal system**—efferent pathways outside the pyramids of the medulla oblongata). The frontal eye fields (the lower portion of Brodmann area 8), which are involved in controlling eye movements, area located on the middle frontal gyrus.

The **primary motor area (Brodmann area 4)** is located along the **precentral gyrus** forming the **primary voluntary motor area,** which has a somatotopic organization that is often referred to as a *homunculus* (little man) (Figure 12-7). Electrical stimulation of specific areas of this cortex causes specific muscles of the body to move. The medial part of the longitudinal fissure affects the lower limb and foot, whereas on the lateral surface, the superior third controls the torso and arm, the middle third of the hand, and the lowest third of the face and mouth/throat. The axons traveling from the cell bodies in and on either side of this gyrus project fibers (axons) that form the **corticospinal tracts (pyramidal system)** that descend into the spinal

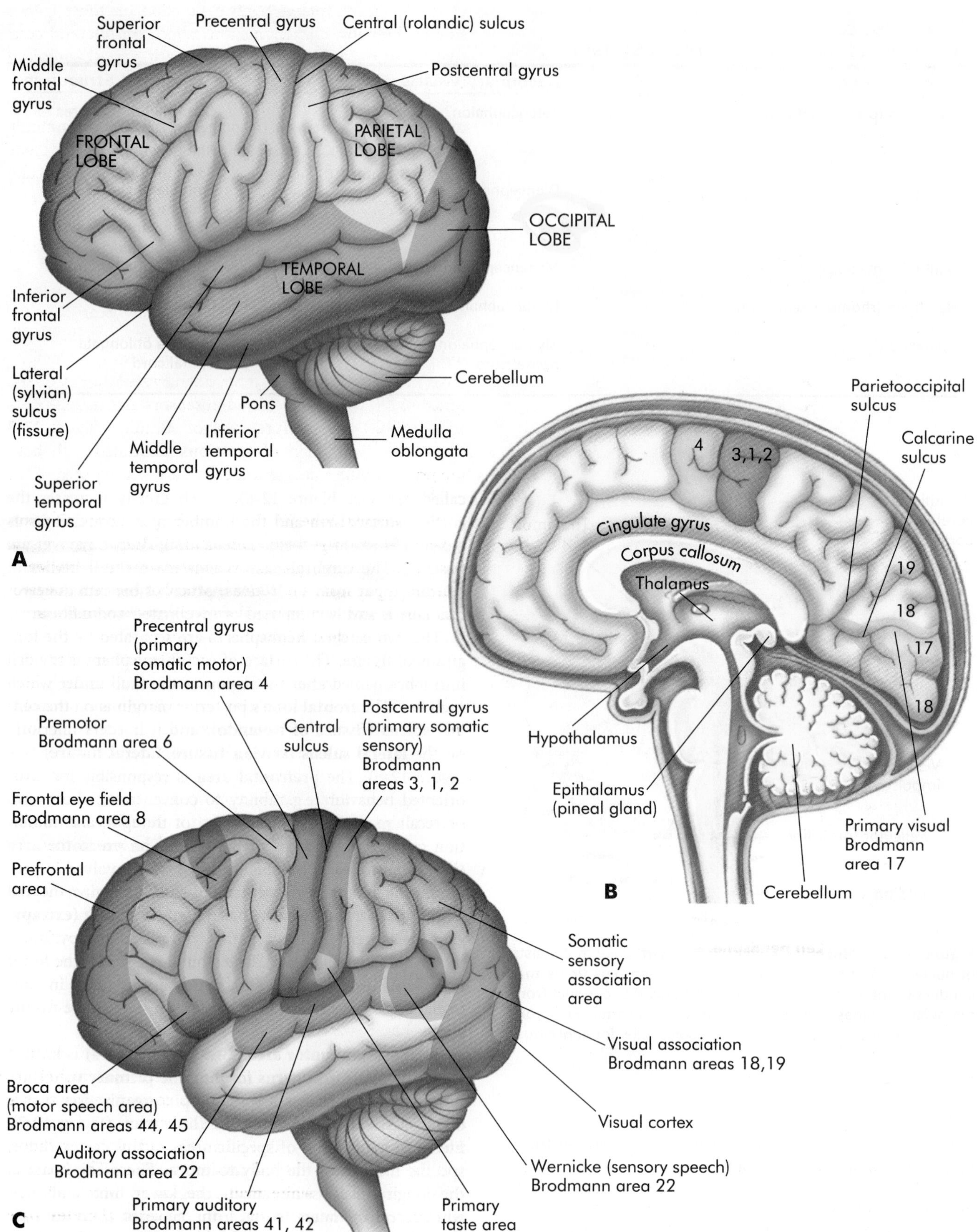

Figure 12-6 ■ **The Cerebral Hemispheres. A,** Left hemisphere of cerebrum, lateral view. **B,** Functional areas of the cerebral cortex, midsagittal view. **C,** Functional areas of the cerebral cortex, lateral view.

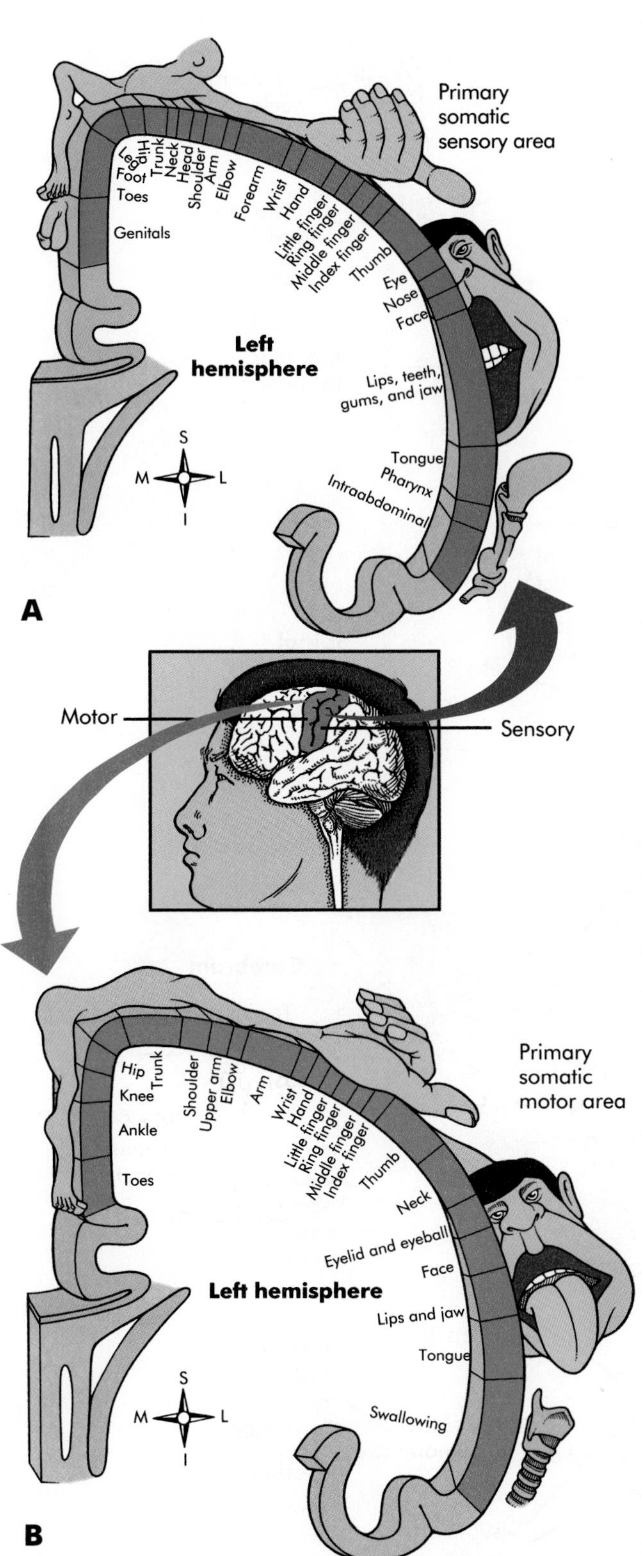

Figure 12-7 ■ Primary Somatic Sensory (A) and Motor (B) Areas of the Cortex. The body parts illustrated here show which parts of the body are "mapped" to specific areas of each cortical area. The exaggerated face indicates that more cortical area is devoted to processing information to and from the many receptors and motor units of the face than for the leg or arm, for example. (From Thibodeau GA, Patton KT: *Anatomy & physiology,* ed 6, St Louis, 2007, Mosby.)

cord. Cerebral impulses control function on the opposite side of the body, a phenomenon called **contralateral control** (Figure 12-8, *A*). The **Broca speech area (Brodmann areas 44, 45)** is rostral on the inferior frontal gyrus. It is usually on the left hemisphere and is responsible for the motor aspects of speech. Damage to this area, commonly as a result of a cerebrovascular accident (stroke), results in the inability to form words or at least some difficulty in forming words (expressive aphasia or dysphasia) (see Chapter 15).

The **parietal lobe** lies within the borders of the central, parietooccipital, and lateral sulci. This lobe contains the major area for somatic sensory input, located primarily along the **postcentral gyrus** (Brodmann's areas 3, 1, 2), which is adjacent to the primary motor area. Communication between the motor and sensory areas (and among other regions in the cortex) is provided by **association fibers.** Much of this region is involved in sensory association (storage, analysis, and interpretation of stimuli). (Figure 12-7 shows the distribution of functions associated with both the primary motor area and the primary sensory area of the cerebral cortex.)

The **occipital lobe** lies caudal to the parietooccipital sulcus and is superior to the cerebellum. The primary visual cortex (Brodmann area 17) is located in this region and receives input from the retinas. Much of the remainder of this lobe is involved in visual association (Brodmann areas 18, 19). The **temporal lobe** lies inferior to the lateral fissure and is composed of the superior, middle, and inferior temporal gyri. The primary auditory cortex (Brodmann's area 41) and its related association area (Brodmann area 42) lie deep within the lateral sulcus on the superior temporal gyrus. The **Wernicke area,** along with adjacent portions of the parietal lobe, constitutes a *sensory speech area.* This area is responsible for reception and interpretation of speech, and dysfunction may result in receptive aphasia or dysphasia. The temporal lobe also is involved in memory consolidation and smell.

Another lobe, the **insula,** lies hidden from view in the lateral sulci (see Figure 12-6). Lying directly beneath the longitudinal fissure is a mass of white matter pathways called the **corpus callosum (transverse** or **commissural fibers).** This structure connects the two cerebral hemispheres and is essential in coordinating activities between hemispheres (see Figure 12-6).

Inside the cerebrum are numerous tracts (white matter) and nuclei (gray matter). The major **cerebral nuclei** are called **basal ganglia** and include the **corpus striatum** and **amygdala.** The corpus striatum consists of the **lentiform nucleus** (lens-shaped), the putamen and globus pallidus, and the ram's horn-shaped **caudate nucleus.** The **internal capsule** is a thick white matter region in which afferent and efferent pathways, to and from the cerebral cortex, pass through the center of the cerebral hemispheres. The corpus striatum appears striped because of the rostral connections between its gray matter and the white matter of the internal capsule.

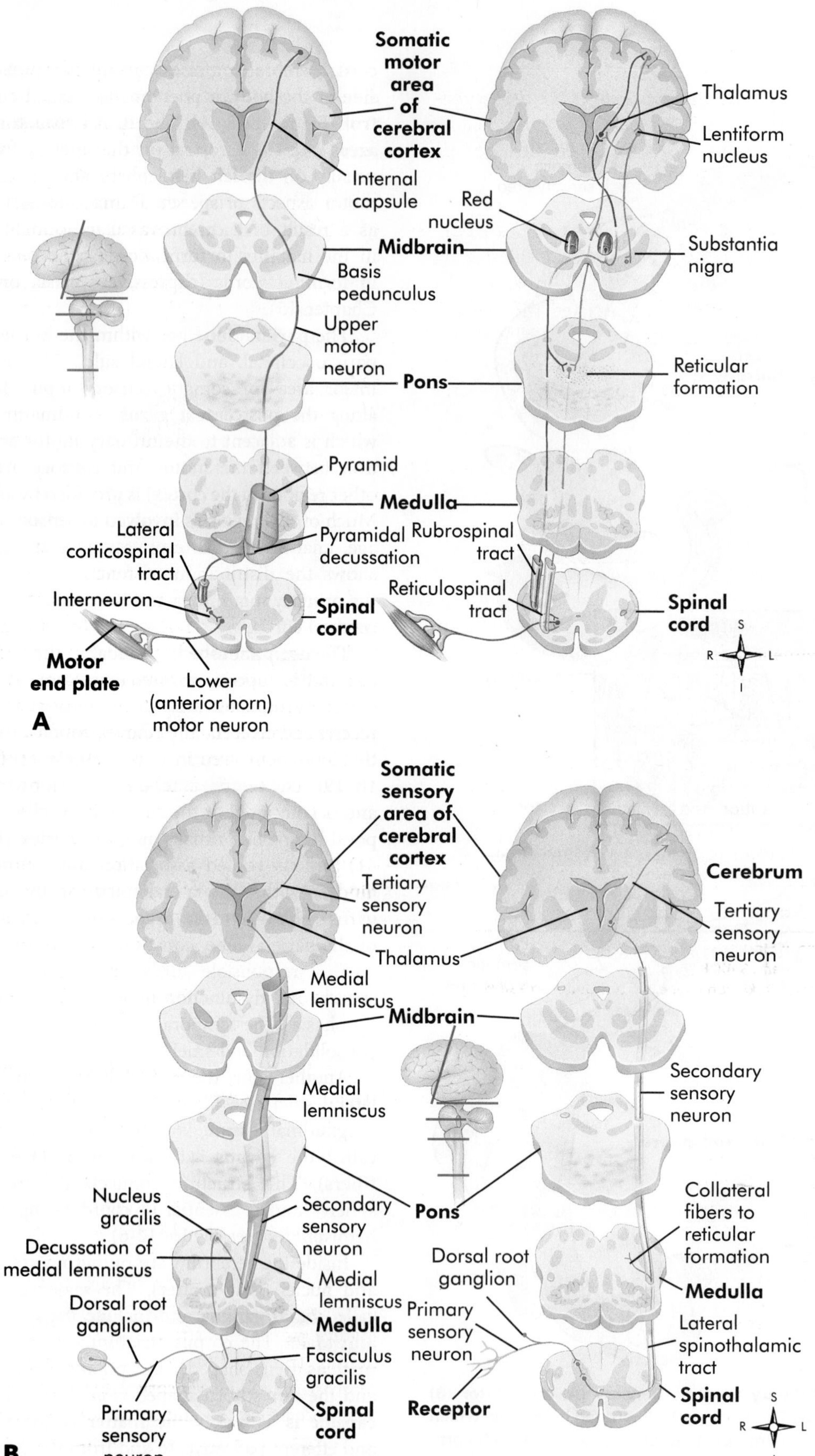

Figure 12-8 ■ **Examples of Somatic Motor and Sensory Pathways. A,** Motor: The pyramidal pathway illustrated by the lateral corticospinal tract and the extrapyramidal pathways illustrated by the rubrospinal and reticulospinal tracts. **B,** Sensory: pathways of the medial lemniscal system that conducts information about discriminating touch and kinesthesis and the spinothalamic pathway that conducts information about pain and temperature. (Modified from Thibodeau GA, Patton KT: *Anatomy & physiology,* ed 6, St Louis, 2007, Mosby.)

Functionally, basal ganglia include, in addition to the corpus striatum, the subthalamic nucleus of the diencephalon and the substantia nigra of the mesencephalon. The basal ganglia plus their direct and indirect interconnections with the thalamus, premotor cortex, red nucleus, reticular formation, and spinal cord have been considered part of the basal ganglia system (extrapyramidal system). The basal ganglia system is believed to exert a fine-tuning effect on motor movements. Parkinson disease and Huntington disease are conditions associated with defects of the basal ganglia (see the *Health Alert:* Surgery for Parkinson Disease box). They are characterized by various involuntary or exaggerated motor movements (see Chapter 14).

HEALTH ALERT
Surgery for Parkinson Disease

Surgery to reduce parkinsonian motor symptoms has been an effective treatment procedure for more than 40 years. Precise lesions are made in the subthalamic nucleus, globus pallidus, and thalamus, resulting in rapid reduction of symptoms in a high number of individuals with Parkinson disease. The use of concise imaging techniques allows precision in the placement of therapeutic lesions. Advances in new technologies, including gamma knife radiosurgery and deep brain stimulation from implanted electrodes, provide relief for individuals with advanced disease. Gene therapy to promote dopaminergic neurons and implantation of genetically engineered and stem cells are also being explored.

Data from Jankovic J: Update on the treatment of Parkinson's disease, *Mt Sinai J Med* 73(4):682-689, 2006; Pereira EA, Aziz TZ: Surgical insights into Parkinson's disease, *J R Soc Med* 99(5): 238-244, 2006.

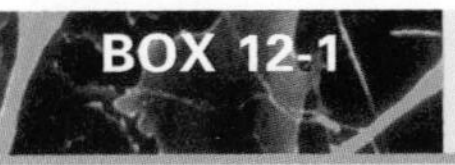

BOX 12-1 Functions of the Hypothalamus

- Visceral and somatic responses
- Affectual responses
- Hormone synthesis
- Sympathetic and parasympathetic activity
- Temperature regulation
- Feeding responses
- Physical expression of emotions
- Sexual behavior
- Pleasure-punishment centers
- Level of arousal or wakefulness

Data from Purves D et al: *Neuroscience*, ed 3, Sunderland, 2004, Sinauer Associates; Kiernan JA: *Barr's the human nervous system: an anatomical viewpoint*, ed 8, Philadelphia, 2005, Lippincott Williams & Wilkins.

The **limbic system** is a group of structures surrounding the corpus callosum that mediate emotion through connections in the prefrontal cortex. It is composed of the **Papez circuit** (amygdala, parahippocampal gyrus, **hippocampus,** fornix, mamillary body of the hypothalamus, thalamus, and cingulate gyrus), septal area, habenula, other portions of the hypothalamus, and related autonomic nuclei. It is an extension or modification of the olfactory system. Its principal effects are believed to be involved in primitive behavioral responses, visceral reaction to emotion, feeding behaviors, biologic rhythms, and the sense of smell.

Diencephalon

The **diencephalon,** surrounded by the cerebrum, has four divisions: **epithalamus, thalamus, hypothalamus,** and **subthalamus** (see Table 12-3 and Figure 12-6). The epithalamus forms the roof of the third ventricle (a brain cavity) and composes the most superior portion of the diencephalon. Its connections and functions are closely associated with those of the limbic system.

The thalamus borders and surrounds the third ventricle. It is a major integrating center for afferent impulses to the cerebral cortex. Various sensations are perceived at this level, but cortical processing is required for interpretation. The thalamus serves also as a relay center for information from the basal ganglia and cerebellum to the appropriate motor area.

The hypothalamus forms the base of the diencephalon. The hypothalamus functions to (1) maintain a constant internal environment and (2) implement behavioral patterns. Integrative centers control autonomic nervous system (ANS) function, regulate body temperature and endocrine function, and regulate emotional expression. The hypothalamus exerts its influence through the endocrine system, as well as through neural pathways (Box 12-1).

The subthalamus flanks the hypothalamus laterally. It serves as an important basal ganglia center for motor activities.

Midbrain

The **midbrain (mesencephalon)** is composed of three structures: the **corpora quadrigemina (tectum)** (composed of the superior and inferior colliculi), the **tegmentum** (containing the red nucleus and substantia nigra), and the basis pedunculi. (The tegmentum and basis pedunculi are called, collectively, the **cerebral peduncles.**)

The **superior colliculi** are involved with voluntary and involuntary visual motor movements (e.g., the ability of the eyes to track moving objects in the visual field). The **inferior colliculi** accomplish similar motor activities but involve movements affecting the auditory system (e.g., positioning the head to improve hearing). The **red nucleus** receives ascending sensory information from the cerebellum and projects a minor motor pathway to the cervical spinal cord. The last portion of the basal ganglia is the **substantia nigra,** which synthesizes **dopamine,** a neurotransmitter and precursor of norepinephrine. Its dysfunction is associated with Parkinson disease. The **basis pedunculi** are made up of efferent fibers of the corticospinal, corticobulbar, and corticopontocerebellar tracts.

Other notable structures of this region are the nuclei of the third and fourth cranial nerves. The **cerebral aqueduct (aqueduct of Sylvius),** which carries cerebrospinal fluid, also traverses this structure. Plugging of this aqueduct is often the cause of hydrocephalus.

Hindbrain

Metencephalon

The major structures of the **metencephalon** are the cerebellum and the pons. The **cerebellum** (see Figure 12-6) is composed of gray and white matter, and its cortical surface is convoluted like the surface of the cerebrum. It also is divided by a central fissure into two lobes connected by the **vermis.**

The cerebellum is responsible for reflexive, involuntary fine-tuning of motor control and for maintaining balance and posture through extensive neural connections with the medulla through the inferior cerebellar peduncle and with the midbrain through the superior cerebellar peduncle. The two hemispheres are connected to the pons by the middle cerebellar peduncles. These connections allow extensive sampling of visual, vestibular, and proprioceptive data from other regions of the CNS and periphery.

The **pons** (bridge) is easily recognized by its bulging appearance below the midbrain and above the medulla. Primarily it transmits information from the cerebellum to the brain stem and between the two cerebellar hemispheres. The nuclei of the fifth through eighth cranial nerves are located in this structure.

Myelencephalon

The **myelencephalon** usually is called the **medulla oblongata** and forms the lowest portion of the brain stem. Reflex activities, such as heart rate, respiration, blood pressure, coughing, sneezing, swallowing, and vomiting, are controlled in this area. The nuclei of cranial nerves IX through XII also are located in this region.

A major portion of the descending motor pathways (i.e., corticospinal tracts) cross to the other side, or decussate, at the medulla (see Figure 12-8). These pathways, together with other areas of decussation in the CNS, are the basis for the phenomenon of contralateral control. Sleep-wake rhythms also are processed by neural influences from lower brain centers and are associated with a complex group of diffuse structures and functions (see Chapter 13), including the reticular activating system (cells that receive collateral signals from the afferent sensory pathways and project the signals to the higher brain centers, thus controlling CNS activity).

✓ QUICK CHECK 12-3

1. Name the three major divisions of the brain and their component parts.
2. Describe the limbic system's functions.
3. What are the two major functions of the hypothalamus?

The Spinal Cord

The **spinal cord** is the portion of the CNS that lies within the vertebral canal and is surrounded and protected by the **vertebral column.** The spinal cord has many functions, which include a long nerve cable that connects the brain and body, somatic and autonomic reflexes, motor pattern control centers, and sensory and motor modulation. It continues from the medulla oblongata and ends at the level of the first or second lumbar vertebra in adults (Figure 12-9). The end of the spinal cord, **conus medullaris,** is cone shaped. Spinal nerves continue from the end of the spinal cord and form a nerve bundle called the **cauda equina.** The filament anchor from the conus medullaris to the coccyx is the **filum terminale** (see Figure 12-9).

Grossly, the spinal cord is divided into vertebral sections (8 cervical, 12 thoracic, 5 lumbar, 5 sacral, and 1 coccygeal) that correspond to paired nerves (see Figure 12-9). A cross section of the spinal cord (Figure 12-10) is characterized by a butterfly-shaped inner core of gray matter (containing nerve cell bodies). The **central canal** lies in the center of this region and extends through the spinal cord from its origin in the fourth ventricle. The gray matter of the spinal cord is divided into three regions and displays specific functional characteristics. These regions include the **posterior horn,** or **dorsal horn** (composed primarily of interneurons and axons from sensory neurons whose cell bodies lie in the **dorsal root ganglion**). At the tip of the posterior horn is the **substantia gelatinosa,** a structure involved in pain transmission (see Chapter 13). The **lateral horn** contains cell bodies involved with the ANS. The **anterior horn,** or **ventral horn,** contains the nerve cell bodies for efferent pathways that leave the spinal cord by way of spinal nerves.

Surrounding the gray matter is white matter that forms ascending and descending pathways called **spinal tracts.** Spinal tracts are named to denote their beginning and ending points. For example, the **spinothalamic tract** (see Figure 12-8, *B*) carries nerve impulses from the spinal cord to the thalamus in the diencephalon. Numerous spinal tracts are grouped into columns according to their location within the white matter. These include the **anterior columns, lateral columns,** and **posterior (dorsal) columns** (Figure 12-11).

Neural circuits in the spinal cord, when activated, display specific sets of motor responses. **Reflex arcs** form basic units that respond to stimuli and provide protective circuitry for motor output. Structures needed for a reflex arc are a receptor, an **afferent (sensory) neuron,** an **efferent (motor) neuron,** and an effector muscle or gland. A simple reflex arc may contain only two neurons (Figure 12-12).

The motor effects of reflex arcs generally occur before the event is perceived in the brain's higher centers. Much internal environmental regulation is mediated by reflex activity involving the ANS.

Afferent pathways transmit information from peripheral receptors and eventually terminate in the cerebral or cerebellar cortex or both. Efferent pathways primarily relay information from the cerebrum to the brain stem or spinal

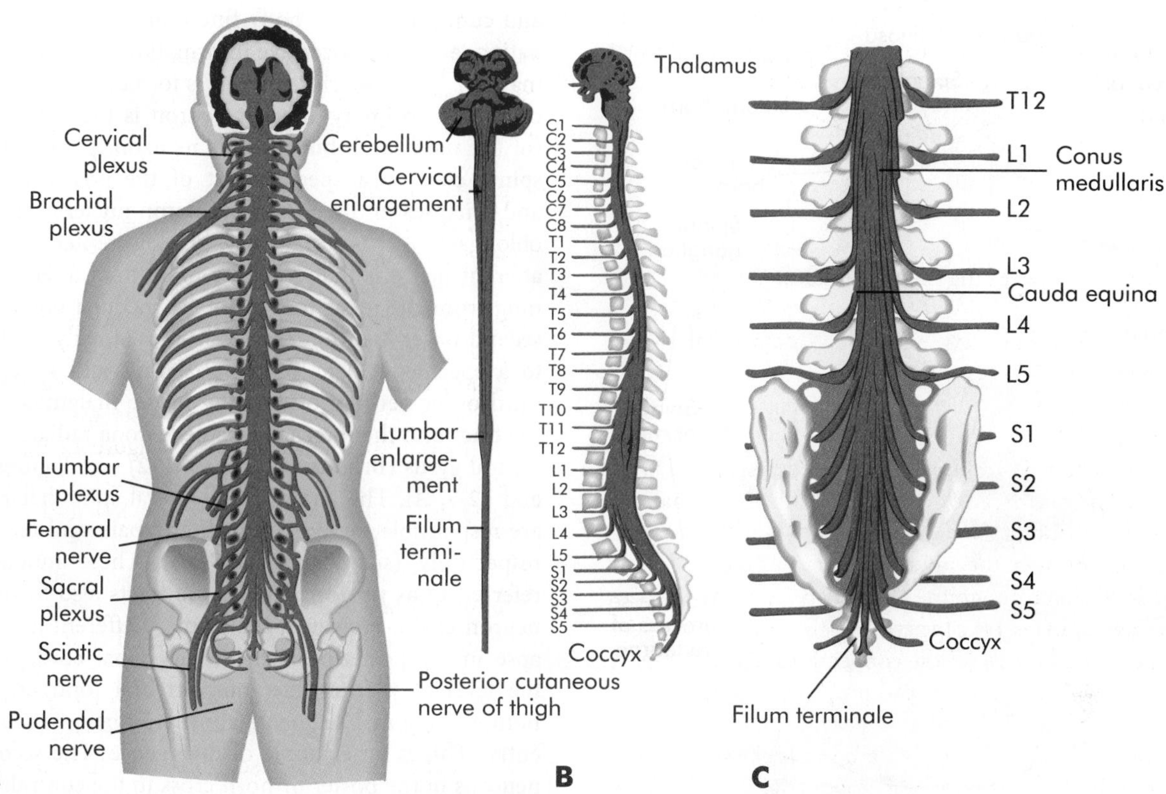

Figure 12-9 ■ **Spinal Cord Within Vertebral Canal and Exiting Spinal Nerves. A,** Posterior view of brain stem and spinal cord in situ with spinal nerves and plexus. **B,** Lateral view of brain stem and spinal cord. **C,** Enlargement of caudal area showing termination of spinal cord (conus medullaris) and group of nerve fibers constituting the cauda equina. (Redrawn from Rudy EB, editor: *Advanced neurological and neurosurgical nursing,* St Louis, 1984, Mosby.)

cord. **Upper motor neurons** are completely contained within the CNS. Their primary roles are controlling fine motor movement and influencing/modifying spinal reflex arcs and circuits. Generally, upper motor neurons form synapses with interneurons, which then form synapses with lower motor neurons before projecting into the periphery. **Lower motor neurons** directly influence muscles. Their cell bodies lie in the gray matter of the brain stem and spinal cord, but their processes extend out of the CNS and into the PNS. Destruction of upper motor neurons usually results in initial paralysis followed within days or weeks by partial recovery, whereas destruction of the lower motor neurons can lead to permanent paralysis. Peripheral nerve damage may be followed by nerve regeneration and recovery.

Muscle activity (i.e., stimulation and contraction) is regulated by nerve impulses. Motor neurons innervate one or more muscle cells, forming **motor units,** which consist of a neuron and the skeletal muscles it stimulates. The junction between the axon of the motor neuron and the plasma membrane of the muscle cell is called the neuromuscular (myoneural) junction (Figure 12-13). (Injury to motor neurons is discussed in Chapter 15.)

Motor Pathways

The four clinically relevant motor pathways are the **lateral corticospinal, corticobulbar, reticulospinal,** and **vestibulospinal tracts.**[5] The corticospinal (see Figure 12-8, *A*) and corticobulbar pathways are essentially the same tract and consist of a two-neuron chain. The cell bodies originate in and around the precentral gyrus; pass through the corona radiata of the cerebrum, the internal capsule, middle three fifths of the cerebral pedunculus, pons, and pyramid; and decussate (cross contralaterally) in the medulla oblongata and form the lateral corticospinal tract of the spinal cord (see Figure 12-11). The **corticobulbar tract** synapses on motor cranial nuclei within the brain stem. The lateral corticospinal tract axons (upper motor neurons) leave the tract to go to specific interneurons or motor neurons in the anterior horn. The lateral corticospinal tract has the same somatropic organization as the body (see Figures 12-7 and 12-8, *A*). These motor neurons project to specific motor units and are lower motor neurons. These tracts are involved in precise motor movements. The **reticulospinal tract** (see Figure 12-11) modulates motor movement by inhibiting and exciting spinal activity. The vestibulospinal tract arises from a vestibular nucleus in the pons and causes the extensor muscles of the body to rapidly contract, most dramatically witnessed when a person starts to fall backward.

Sensory Pathways

The three clinically important spinal afferent pathways are the posterior (dorsal) column, **anterior spinothalamic tract,** and **lateral spinothalamic tract** (see Figures 12-7 and 12-8, *B*). The posterior column (fasciculus gracilis

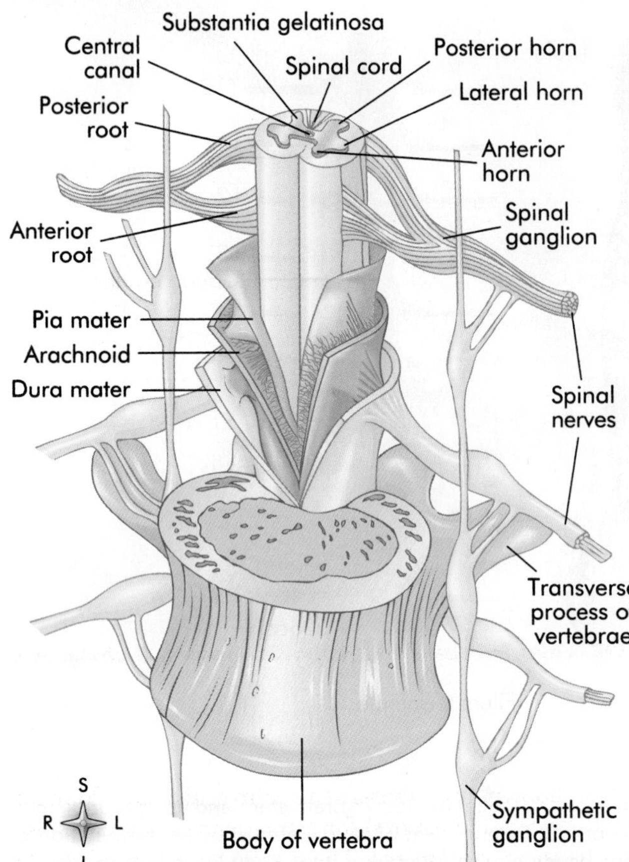

Figure 12-10 ■ Coverings of the Spinal Cord. The dura mater is shown in natural color. Note how it extends to cover the spinal nerve roots and nerves. The arachnoid is highlighted in blue and the pia mater in pink. (Modified from Thibodeau GA, Patton KT: *Structure and function of the human body*, ed 12, St Louis, 2004, Mosby.)

and cuneatus) carries body fine touch, two-point discrimination, and proprioceptive information (i.e., **epicritic** information). The posterior column is formed by a three-neuron chain. The primary afferent neuron is the sensory neuron (of the reflex arc), but it sends its axon ipsilaterally up the spinal cord to a specific part of the posterior funiculus and synapses in the posterior column nuclei in the medulla oblongata. A basketball star playing center has primary afferent neurons that could be more than 6 feet long, running from the great toe up to the medulla oblongata. The second-order neuron crosses contralaterally and ascends to a specific nucleus of the thalamus and synapses. The third-order neuron, originating in the thalamus, continues the tract into the internal capsule, corona radiata, and postcentral gyrus (Brodmann areas 3, 1, 2) (see Figures 12-6, *B*, and 12-7, *A*). The anterior and lateral spinothalamic tracts are responsible for vague touch and pain and temperature, respectively (see Figure 12-8, *B*). These modalities are referred to as **protopathic.** These tracts also form a three-neuron chain. However, the primary afferent neurons synapse in the posterior horn of the spinal cord, not just at the level they enter the intervertebral foramen but in a number of spinal segments above and below their point of entry. This is an example of divergence. The second-order neurons in the posterior horn cross to the contralateral side in the spinal cord and ascend to the same thalamic nucleus as the posterior column pathway and continue on with the posterior column pathway to the postcentral gyrus.

Protective Structures of the Central Nervous System

Cranium

The cranium is composed of eight bones. The cranial vault encloses and protects the brain and its associated structures.

Cranium bones: frontal, occipital, temporal 2, parietal 2, sphenoid, ethmoid.

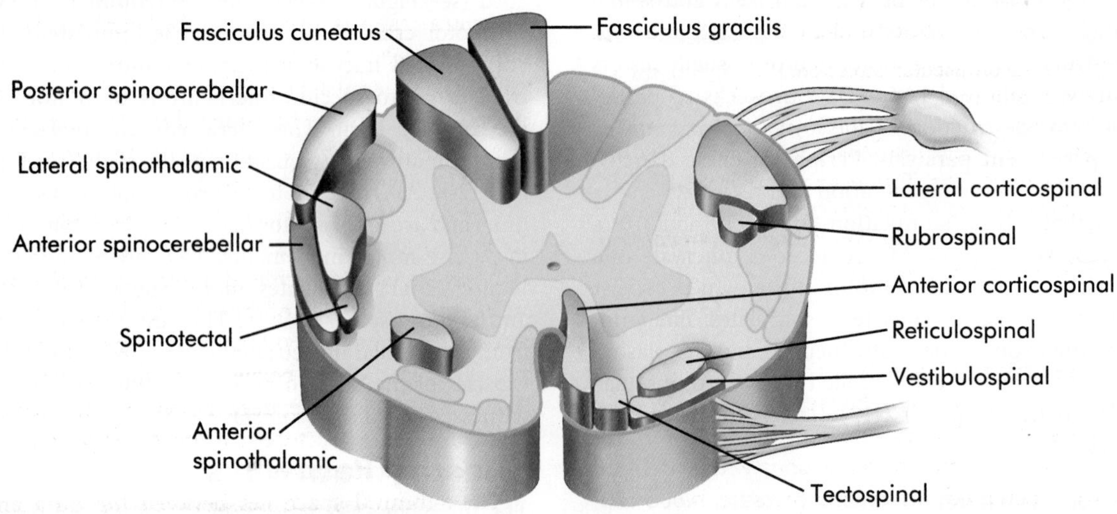

Figure 12-11 ■ Major Tracts of the Spinal Cord. The major ascending (sensory) tracts, shown only on the left here, are highlighted in blue. The major descending (motor) tracts, shown only on the right, are highlighted in red. (From Thibodeau GA, Patton KT: *Anatomy & physiology*, ed 6, St Louis, 2007, Mosby.)

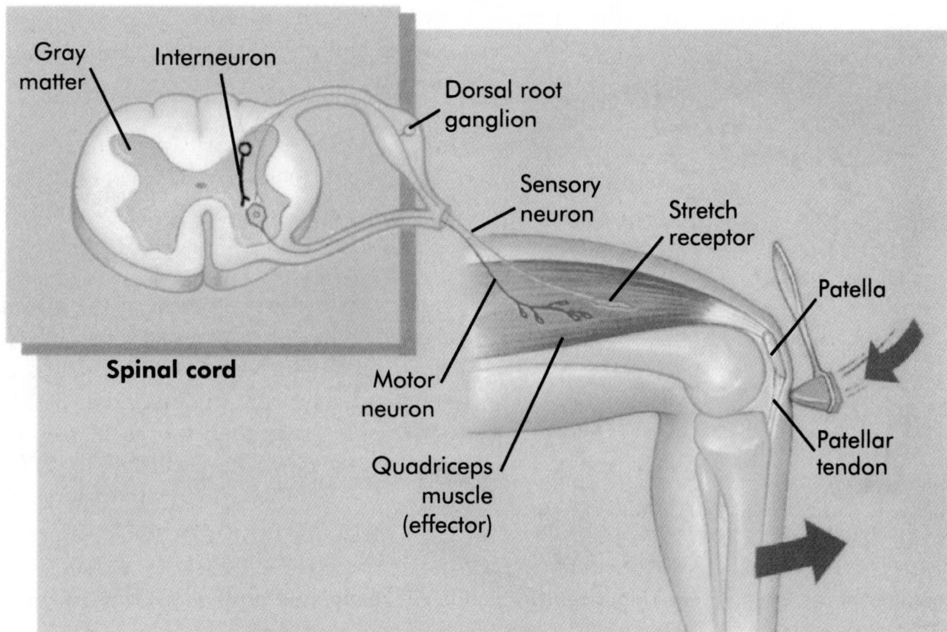

Figure 12-12 ■ **Cross Section of Spinal Cord Showing Simple Reflex Arc.** (From Thibodeau GA, Patton KT: *Anatomy & physiology,* ed 6, St Louis, 2007, Mosby.)

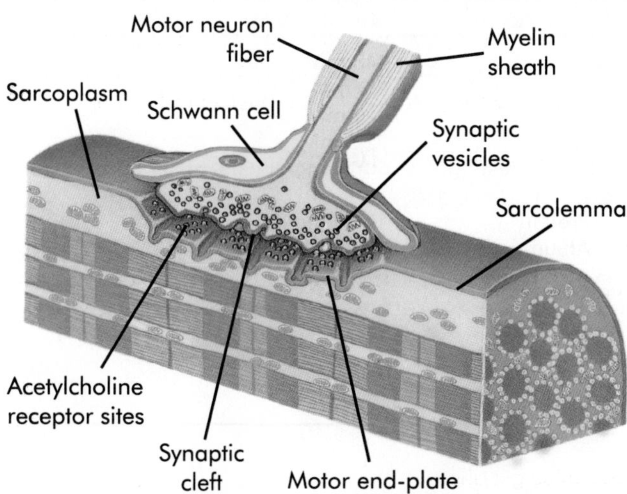

Figure 12-13 ■ **Neuromuscular Junction.** This figure shows how the distal end of a motor neuron fiber forms a synapse, or "chemical junction," with an adjacent muscle fiber. Neurotransmitters (specifically, acetylcholine) are released from the neuron's synaptic vesicles and diffuse across the synaptic cleft. There they stimulate receptors in the motor end-plate region of the sarcolemma. (From Thibodeau GA, Patton KT: *Anatomy & physiology,* ed 5, St Louis, 2003, Mosby.)

The **galea aponeurotica,** which is a thick, fibrous band of tissue overlying the cranium between the frontal and occipital muscles, affords added protection to the skull. The subgaleal space has venous connections with the dural sinuses, and with increased intracranial pressure, blood can be shunted to the space, thus reducing pressure in the intracranial cavity. The subgaleal space is also a common site for wound drains after intracranial surgery.

The floor of the cranial vault is irregular and contains many foramina (openings) for cranial nerves, blood vessels, and the spinal cord to exit. The cranial floor is divided into three fossae (depressions). The frontal lobes lie in the **anterior fossa,** the temporal lobes and base of the diencephalon lie in the **middle fossa (temporal fossa),** and the cerebellum lies in the **posterior fossa.** These terms are commonly used anatomic landmarks to describe the location of intracranial lesions.

Meninges

Surrounding the brain and spinal cord are three protective membranes: the dura mater, the arachnoid, and the pia mater. Collectively they are called the **meninges** (Figure 12-14, *B*). The **dura mater** (meaning literally "hard mother") is composed of two layers, with the venous sinuses formed between them. The outermost layer forms the **periosteum (endosteal layer)** of the skull. The **inner dura (meningeal layer)** is responsible for forming rigid membranes that support and separate various brain structures.

One of these membranes, the **falx cerebri,** dips between the two cerebral hemispheres along the longitudinal fissure. The falx cerebri is anchored anteriorly to the base of the brain at the crista galli of the ethmoid bone. The **tentorium cerebelli,** a common landmark, is a membrane that separates the cerebellum below from the cerebral structures above. Internal to the dura mater lies the **arachnoid,** a spongy, weblike structure that loosely follows the contours of the cerebral structures.

The **subdural space** lies between the dura and arachnoid. Many small bridging veins that have little support traverse the subdural space. Their disruption results in a subdural hematoma (see Chapter 15). The **subarachnoid**

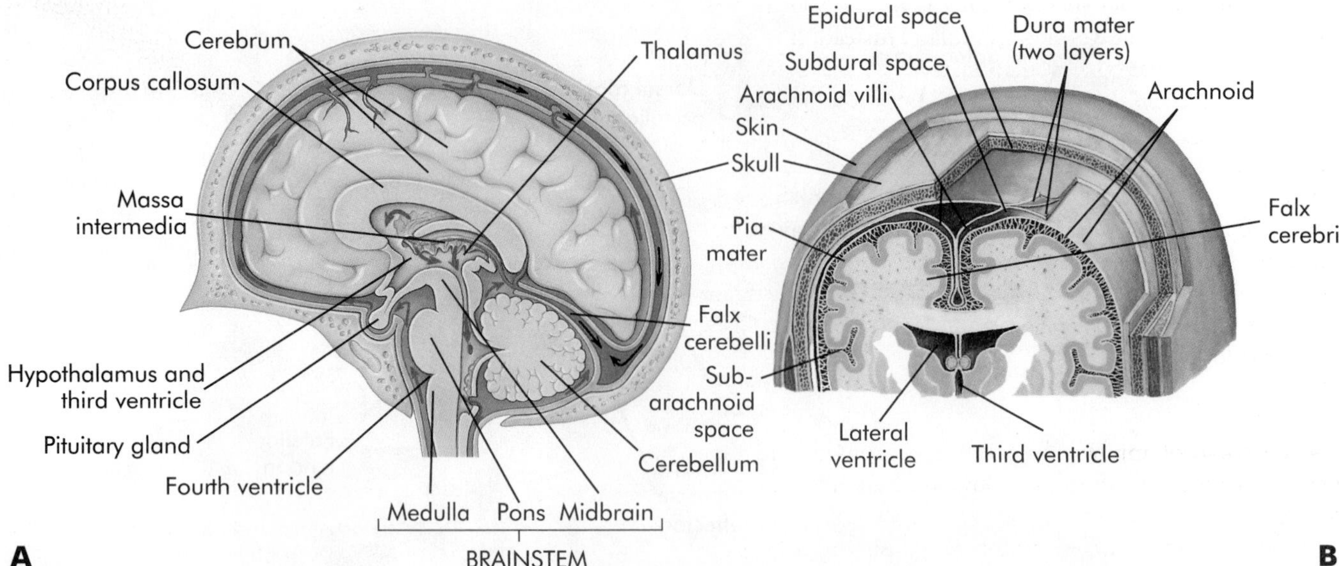

Figure 12-14 ■ **Meninges of the Brain.** (From Thibodeau GA, Patton KT: *Anatomy & physiology,* ed 6, St Louis, 2007, Mosby.)

space lies between the arachnoid and the **pia mater** and contains cerebrospinal fluid (CSF) (see Figure 12-14, *A* and *B*).

Unlike the dura mater and arachnoid, the delicate pia mater adheres to the contours of the brain and spinal cord. It provides support for blood vessels serving brain tissue. The **choroid plexuses,** structures that produce CSF, arise from the pial membrane (see Figure 12-14, *B*). The spinal cord is anchored to the vertebrae by extension of the meninges. The meninges continue beyond the end of the spinal cord to the lower portion of the sacrum. CSF contained within the subarachnoid space also circulates down to about the second sacral vertebra.

The meninges form potential and real spaces important to understanding functional and pathologic mechanisms. For example, between the dura mater and skull lies a potential space termed the **epidural space** (see Figure 12-14, *B*). The arterial supply to the meninges consists of blood vessels that lie within grooves in the skull. A skull fracture can cut one of these vessels and produce an epidural hematoma.

TABLE 12-4

Composition of Cerebrospinal Fluid

Constituent	Normal Value
Na^+	148 mM
K^+	2.9 mM
Cl^-	125 mM
HCO^3_-	22.9 mM
Glucose (fasting)	50-75 mg/dl (60% of serum glucose)
pH	7.3
Protein	15-45 mg/dl
Albumin	80%
Globulin	6%-10%
Cells	
White (lymphocyte)	0-6/mm^3
Red	0

Cerebrospinal fluid and the ventricular system

Cerebrospinal fluid (CSF) is a clear, colorless fluid similar to blood plasma and interstitial fluid. The intracranial and spinal cord structures float in CSF and are thereby protected from jolts and blows. The buoyant properties of the CSF also prevent the brain from tugging on meninges, nerve roots, and blood vessels. (Constituents of CSF are listed in Table 12-4.) Between 125 and 150 ml of CSF is circulating within the **ventricles** (small cavities) and subarachnoid space at any given time. Approximately 600 ml of CSF is produced daily.

The choroid plexuses in the lateral, third, and fourth ventricles produce the major portion of CSF. (Ventricles are illustrated in Figure 12-14.) These plexuses are characterized by a rich network of blood vessels, supplied by the pia mater, that lie close to the ependymal cells of the ventricles.

The CSF exerts pressure within the brain and spinal cord. With a person lying down, CSF pressure is about 80 to 180 mm of water pressure, or approximately 5 to 14 mm of mercury pressure, but doubles when the person sits up. CSF flow results from the pressure gradient between the arterial system and the CSF-filled cavities. Beginning in the lateral ventricles, the CSF flows through the **interventricular foramen (foramen of Monro)** into the third ventricle and then passes through the cerebral aqueduct (aqueduct of Sylvius) into the fourth ventricle. From the fourth ventricle the CSF may pass through either the paired **lateral apertures (foramen of Luschka)** or the **median aperture (foramen of Magendie)** before communicating with the subarachnoid spaces of the brain and spinal cord. The CSF does not, however, accumulate. Instead, it is reabsorbed into the venous circulation through the arachnoid villi. The **arachnoid villi** protrude from the arachnoid space, through the dura mater, and lie within the blood flow of the venous sinuses. CSF is reabsorbed through a pressure gradient between the arachnoid villi and the cerebral venous sinuses. The villi function as one-way valves directing CSF outflow into the blood but preventing blood flow into the subarachnoid space. Thus, CSF is formed from the blood, and after circulating throughout the CNS, it returns to the blood.

Vertebral column

The vertebral column (Figure 12-15) is composed of 33 vertebrae: 7 cervical, 12 thoracic, 5 lumbar, 5 fused sacral, and 4 fused coccygeal. Between each interspace (except for the fused sacral and coccygeal vertebrae) is an **intervertebral disk** (Figure 12-16). At the center of the intervertebral disk is the **nucleus pulposus,** a pulpy mass of elastic fibers. The intervertebral disk absorbs shocks, preventing damage to the vertebrae. The intervertebral disk is also a common source of back problems. If too much stress is applied to the vertebral column, the disk contents may rupture and protrude into the spinal canal, causing compression of the spinal cord or nerve roots.

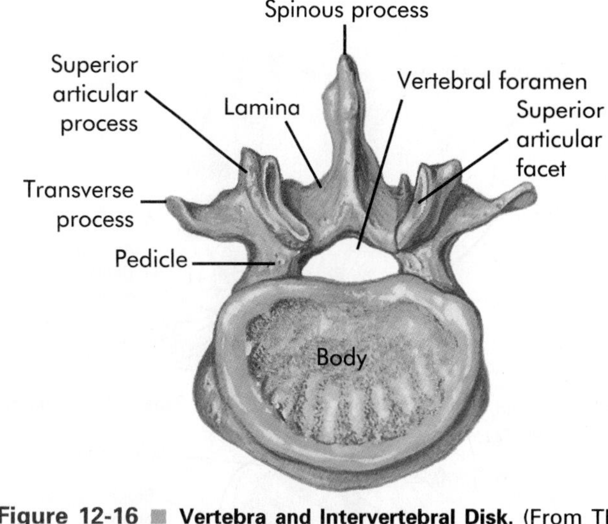

Figure 12-16 ■ **Vertebra and Intervertebral Disk.** (From Thibodeau GA, Patton KT: *Anatomy & physiology,* ed 5, St Louis, 2003, Mosby.)

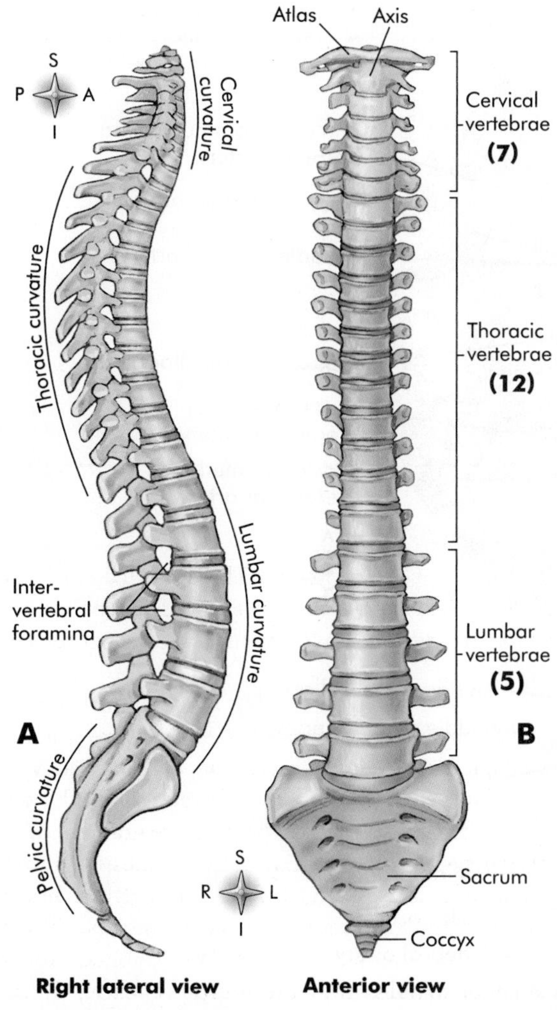

Figure 12-15 ■ **Vertebral Column. A,** Right lateral view. **B,** Anterior view. (From Thibodeau GA, Patton KT: *Anatomy & physiology,* ed 6, St Louis, 2007, Mosby.)

QUICK CHECK 12-4

1. What information is conveyed in the ascending and descending spinal tracts?
2. Contrast the functions of upper and lower motor neurons.
3. Name the protective structures of the central nervous system, and briefly describe each one.

Blood Supply of the Central Nervous System

Blood supply to the brain

The brain receives approximately 20% of the cardiac output, or 800 to 1000 ml of blood flow per minute. Carbon dioxide is a primary regulator for blood flow within the CNS. It is a potent vasodilator, and its effects ensure an adequate blood supply.

The brain derives its arterial supply from two systems: the **internal carotid arteries** and the **vertebral arteries** (Figure 12-17). The internal carotid arteries supply a proportionately greater amount of blood flow. They take their origin from the common carotid arteries, enter the cranium through the base of the skull, and pass through the **cavernous sinus.** After giving rise to some small branches, these arteries divide into the anterior and middle cerebral

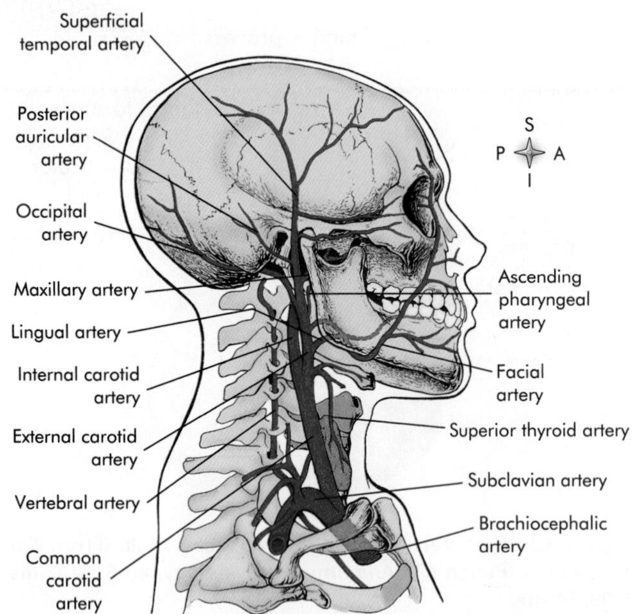

Figure 12-17 ■ Major Arteries of the Head and Neck. (From Thibodeau GA, Patton KT: *Anatomy & physiology,* ed 6, St Louis, 2007, Mosby.)

arteries. The vertebral arteries originate at the subclavian arteries and pass through the transverse foramina of the cervical vertebrae, entering the cranium through the foramen magnum. They join at the junction of the pons and medulla to form the **basilar artery.** The basilar artery divides at the level of the midbrain to form paired posterior cerebral arteries.

The **circle of Willis** (Figure 12-18) provides an alternative route for blood flow when one of the contributing arteries is obstructed (collateral blood flow). The circle of Willis is formed by the posterior cerebral arteries, posterior communicating arteries, internal carotid arteries, anterior cerebral arteries, and anterior communicating artery. The anterior cerebral, middle cerebral, and posterior cerebral arteries leave the circle of Willis and extend to various brain structures. (Table 12-5 and Figure 12-19 illustrate structures served, functional relationships, and pathologic considerations related to occlusion of cerebral arteries.)

Cerebral venous drainage does not parallel (lie side by side with) its arterial supply, whereas the venous drainage of the brain stem and cerebellum does parallel the arterial supply of these structures. The cerebral veins are classified

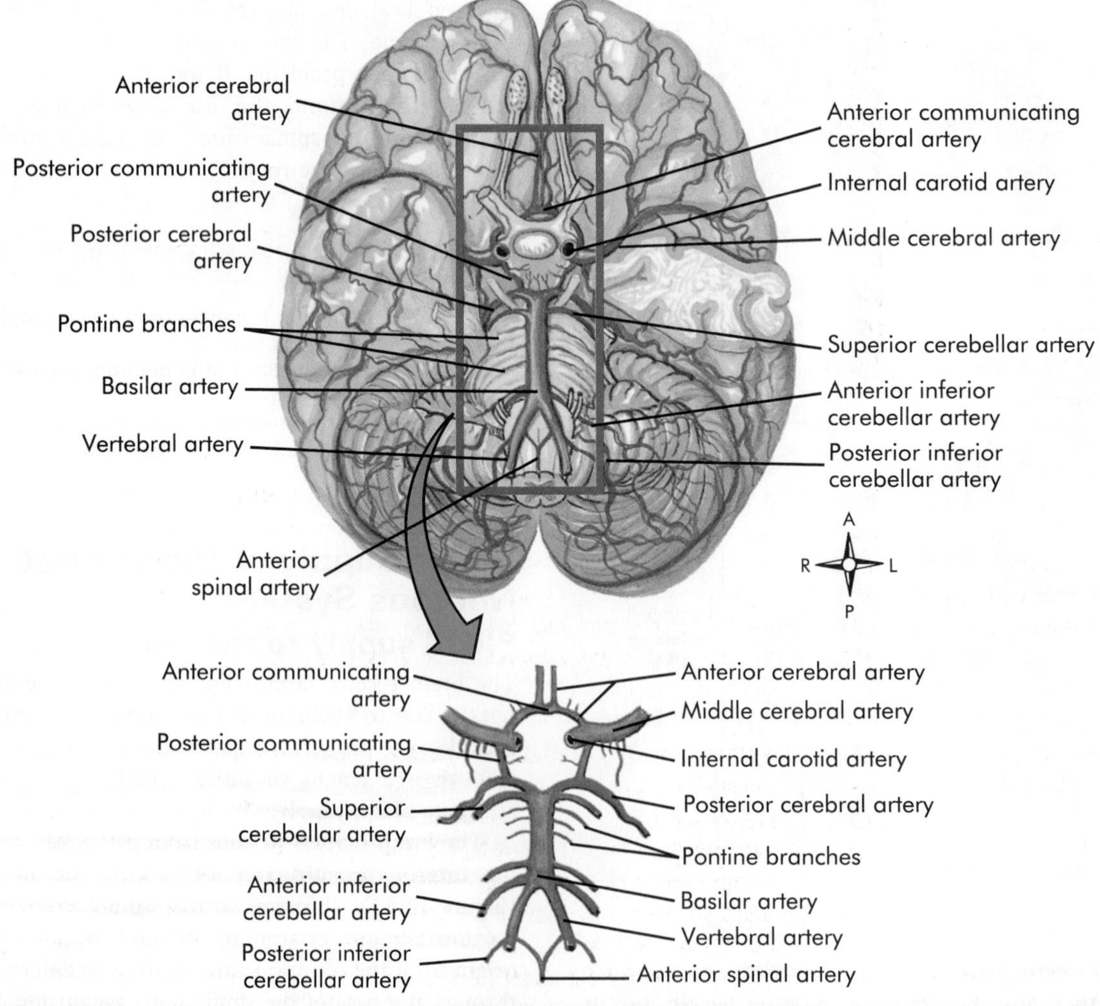

Figure 12-18 ■ Arteries at the Base of the Brain. The arteries that compose the circle of Willis are the two anterior cerebral arteries, joined to each other by the anterior communicating artery and two short segments of the internal carotids, off of which the posterior communicating arteries connect to the posterior cerebral arteries. (From Thibodeau GA, Patton KT: *Anatomy & physiology,* ed 5, St Louis, 2003, Mosby.)

TABLE 12-5

Arterial Systems Supplying the Brain

Arterial Origin	Structures Served	Conditions Caused by Occlusion
Anterior cerebral artery	Basal ganglia; corpus callosum; medial surface of cerebral hemispheres; superior surface of frontal and parietal lobes	Hemiplegia on the contralateral side of the body, greater in the lower than in the upper extremities
Middle cerebral artery	Frontal lobe; parietal lobe; temporal lobe (primarily the cortical surfaces)	Aphasia in dominant hemisphere and contralateral hemiplegia (see Chapter 14)
Posterior cerebral artery	Part of the diencephalon and temporal lobe; occipital lobe	Visual loss; sensory loss; contralateral hemiplegia if cerebral peduncle affected

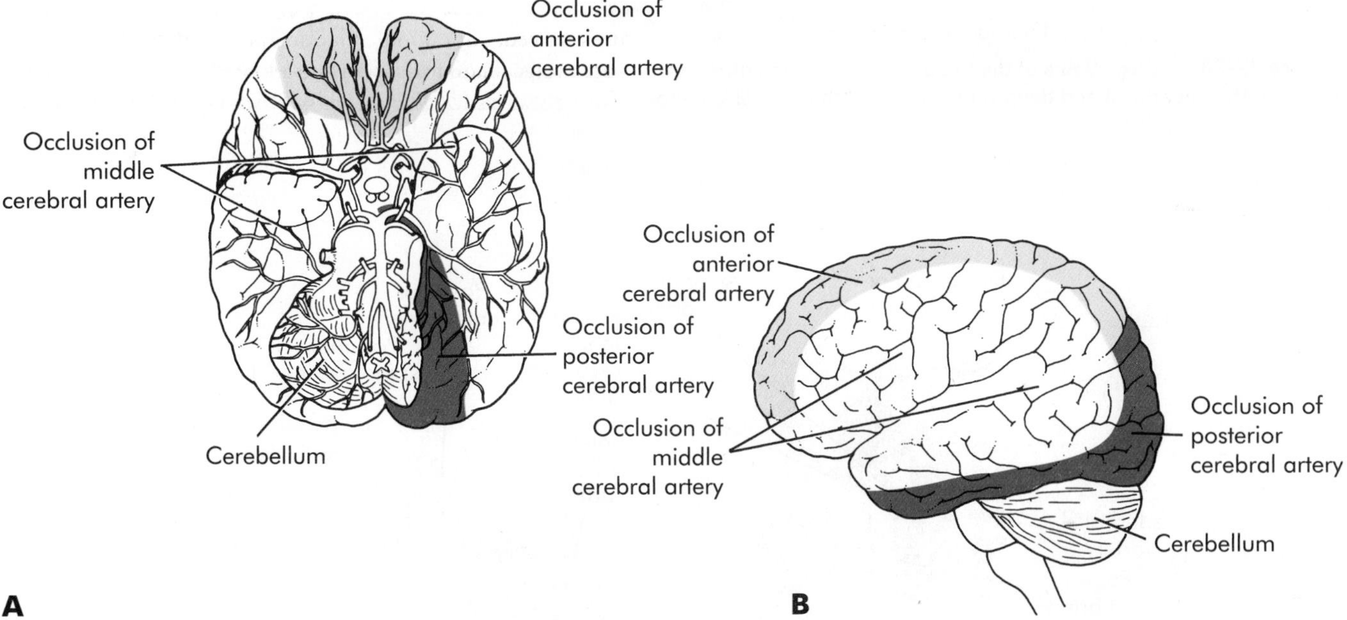

Figure 12-19 ■ **Areas of the Brain Affected by Occlusion of the Anterior, Middle, and Posterior Cerebral Artery Branches. A,** Inferior view. **B,** Lateral view.

as superficial and deep veins. The veins drain into venous plexuses and dural sinuses (formed between the dural layers) and eventually join the internal jugular veins at the base of the skull (Figure 12-20). Adequacy of venous outflow can significantly affect intracranial pressure. For example, head-injured individuals who turn or let their heads fall to the side partially occlude venous return, and the intracranial pressure can increase then because of decreased flow through the jugular veins.

Blood-brain barrier

The **blood-brain barrier** describes cellular structures that selectively inhibit certain potentially harmful substances in the blood from entering the interstitial spaces of the brain or CSF. Supporting cells (neuroglia), particularly the astrocytes, and tight junctions between endothelial cells of brain cell capillaries (see Chapter 1) are likely involved in forming this barrier. The exact nature of this mechanism is controversial, but it appears that certain metabolites, electrolytes, and chemicals can cross into the brain to varying degrees. This has substantial implications for drug therapy because certain types of antibiotics and chemotherapeutic drugs show a greater propensity than others for crossing this barrier.

Blood supply to the spinal cord

The spinal cord derives its blood supply from branches off the vertebral arteries and from branches from various regions of the aorta (Figure 12-21). The **anterior spinal artery** and the paired **posterior spinal arteries** branch off of the vertebral artery at the base of the cranium and descend alongside the spinal cord. Arterial branches from vessels exterior to the spinal cord follow the spinal nerve through the intervertebral foramina, pass through the dura, and divide into the anterior and posterior radicular arteries.

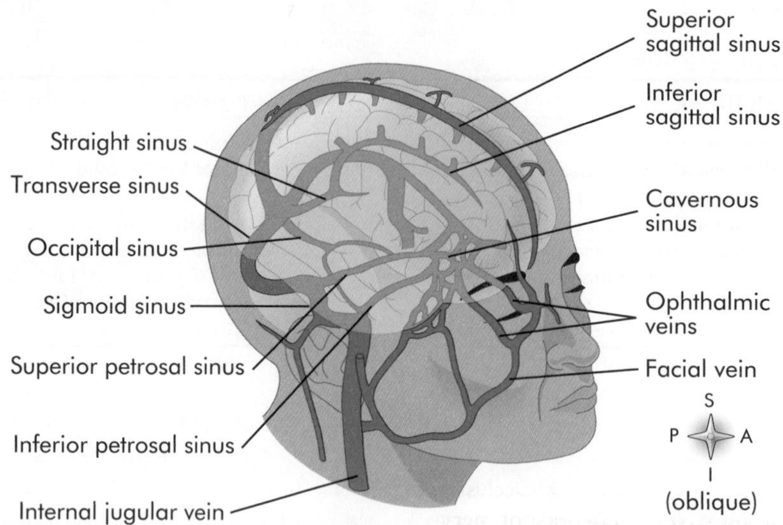

Figure 12-20 ■ **Large Veins of the Head.** Deep veins and dural sinuses are projected on the skull. Note connections (emissary veins) between the superficial and deep veins. (From Thibodeau GA, Patton KT: *Anatomy & Physiology,* ed 6, St Louis, 2007, Mosby.)

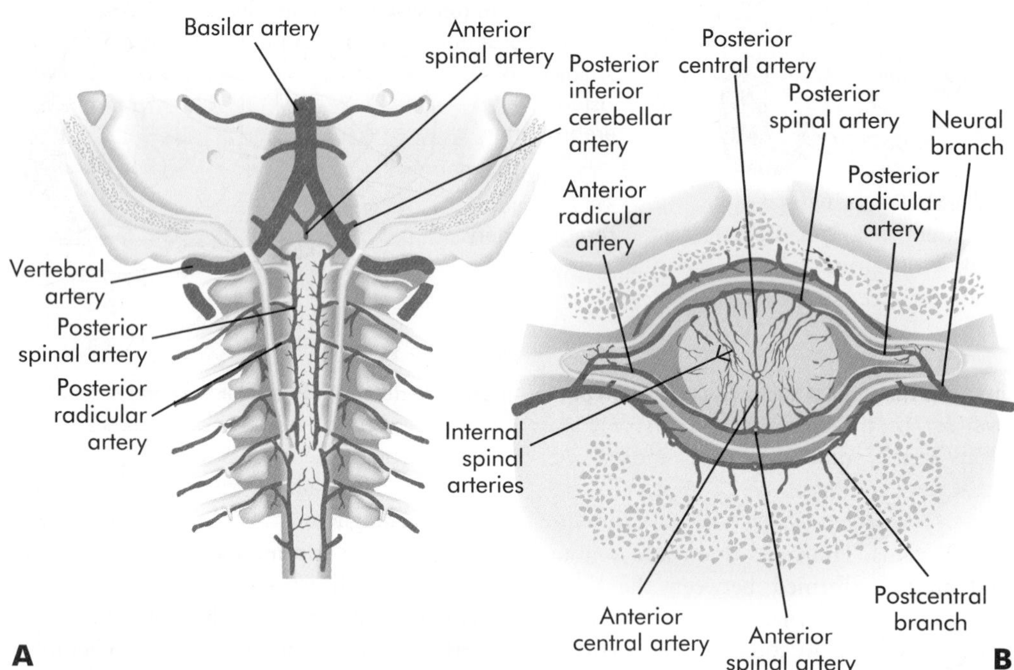

Figure 12-21 ■ **Arteries of the Spinal Cord. A,** Arteries of cervical cord exposed from the rear. **B,** Arteries of spinal cord diagrammatically shown in horizontal section. (Redrawn from Rudy EB, editor: *Advanced neurological and neurosurgical nursing,* St Louis, 1984, Mosby.)

The radicular arteries eventually connect to the spinal arteries. Branches from the radicular and spinal arteries form plexuses whose branches penetrate the spinal cord, supplying the deeper tissues. Venous drainage parallels the arterial supply closely and drains into venous sinuses located between the dura and periosteum of the vertebrae.

THE PERIPHERAL NERVOUS SYSTEM

The cranial and spinal nerves, including their branches and ganglia, constitute the peripheral nervous system (PNS). A peripheral nerve (cranial or spinal) is composed of individual axons wrapped in a myelin sheath. These individual fibers are arranged in bundles called **fascicles** (Figure 12-22, *B*).

The 31 pairs of spinal nerves derive their names from the vertebral level from which they exit. There are eight cervical spinal nerves. The first cervical nerve exits above the first cervical vertebra, and the rest of the spinal nerves exit below their corresponding vertebrae. From the thoracic region (and inferiorly), nerves correspond to the vertebral level above their exit.

Spinal nerves contain both sensory and motor neurons and are called **mixed nerves.** They arise as rootlets lateral to anterior and posterior horns of the spinal cord. These two spinal nerve roots converge in the region of the intervertebral foramen to form the spinal nerve trunk. Shortly after converging, the spinal nerve divides into anterior and posterior rami (branches). The anterior rami (except the thoracic) initially form **plexuses** (networks of nerve fibers), which then branch into the peripheral nerves. Instead of forming plexuses, the thoracic nerves pass through the intercostal spaces and innervate regions of the thorax.

The main spinal nerve plexuses innervate the skin and the underlying muscles of the limbs. The **brachial plexus,** for example, is formed by the last four cervical nerves (C5 to C8) and the first thoracic nerve (T1). The brachial plexus innervates the nerves of the arm, wrist, and hand. The **lumbar plexus** (L2 to L4) and **sacral plexus** (L5 to S5) contain nerves that innervate the anterior and posterior portions of the lower body, respectively.

The posterior rami of each spinal nerve, with their many processes, are distributed to a specific area in the body. Sensory signals thus arise from specific sites associated with a specific spinal cord segment. Specific areas of cutaneous innervation at these spinal cord segments are called **dermatomes.**

Like spinal nerves, cranial nerves are categorized as peripheral nerves. Most of these are mixed nerves (like the spinal nerves), although some are purely sensory or purely motor. Cranial nerves (Figure 12-22, *A*) connect to nuclei in the brain and brain stem. (Figure 12-22 illustrates their structure, and Table 12-6 describes structural and functional characteristics.)

✔ QUICK CHECK 12-5

1. Describe the circle of Willis and its role in supplying blood to the brain.
2. Where does the spinal cord's blood supply come from?
3. What are the plexuses? Give two examples in the PNS.
4. What are the cranial nerves? Give three examples.
5. Describe the anatomy and function of the PNS.

THE AUTONOMIC NERVOUS SYSTEM

Components of the autonomic nervous system (ANS) are located in both the CNS and the PNS; however, the ANS is considered to be part of the efferent division of the PNS, even though visceral afferent neurons are certainly an important part of this system. Many neurons of the ANS travel in the spinal nerves and certain cranial nerves. The widespread activity of this system indicates that its components are distributed all over the body. The peripheral autonomic nerves carry mainly efferent fibers. The motor component of the ANS is a two-neuron system consisting of **preganglionic neurons** (myelinated) and **postganglionic neurons** (unmyelinated) (Figure 12-23). This arrangement contrasts with the somatic nervous system, where a single motor neuron travels from the CNS to the innervated structure. Visceral afferent neurons have their cell bodies in some sensory and cranial ganglia and their fiber processes traveling in peripheral nerves. The CNS has autonomic areas in the intermediolateral horns of the spinal cord, cardiovascular and respiratory centers in the reticular formation, and both sympathetic and parasympathetic areas in the hypothalamus. CNS pathways interconnect all these areas.

The ANS coordinates and maintains a steady state among visceral (internal) organs, such as regulation of cardiac muscle, smooth muscle, and the glands of the body. This system is considered an involuntary system because one generally cannot *will* these functions to happen. The ANS is separated both structurally and functionally into two divisions: (1) the **sympathetic nervous system** (Figure 12-24) and (2) the **parasympathetic nervous system** (Figure 12-25).

Anatomy of the Sympathetic Nervous System

The sympathetic nervous system mobilizes energy stores in times of need (e.g., in the "fight or flight" response) (see Figure 8-1; see also Chapter 8.) The sympathetic division is innervated by cell bodies located from the first thoracic (T1) through the second lumbar (L2) regions of the spinal cord and therefore is called the **thoracolumbar division.** The preganglionic axons of the sympathetic division form synapses shortly after leaving the cord in the **sympathetic (paravertebral) ganglia.** At this point the impulse may travel several ways: (1) directly across the same ganglion level to form a synapse with the cell bodies of the postganglionic neuron, (2) up or down the sympathetic chain before forming synapses with a higher or lower postganglionic neuron, or (3) through the chain ganglion without synapsing (see Figure 12-24). Some preganglionic axons form pathways called **splanchnic nerves,** which lead to **collateral ganglia** on the front of the aorta. The collateral ganglia are named according to the branches of the aorta nearest them, namely, the **celiac, superior mesenteric,** and **inferior mesenteric.** The preganglionic neurons synapse with postganglionic neurons within the collateral ganglia. These postganglionic neurons leave the collateral ganglia and innervate the viscera below the diaphragm.

Preganglionic sympathetic neurons that innervate the adrenal medulla also travel in the splanchnic nerves

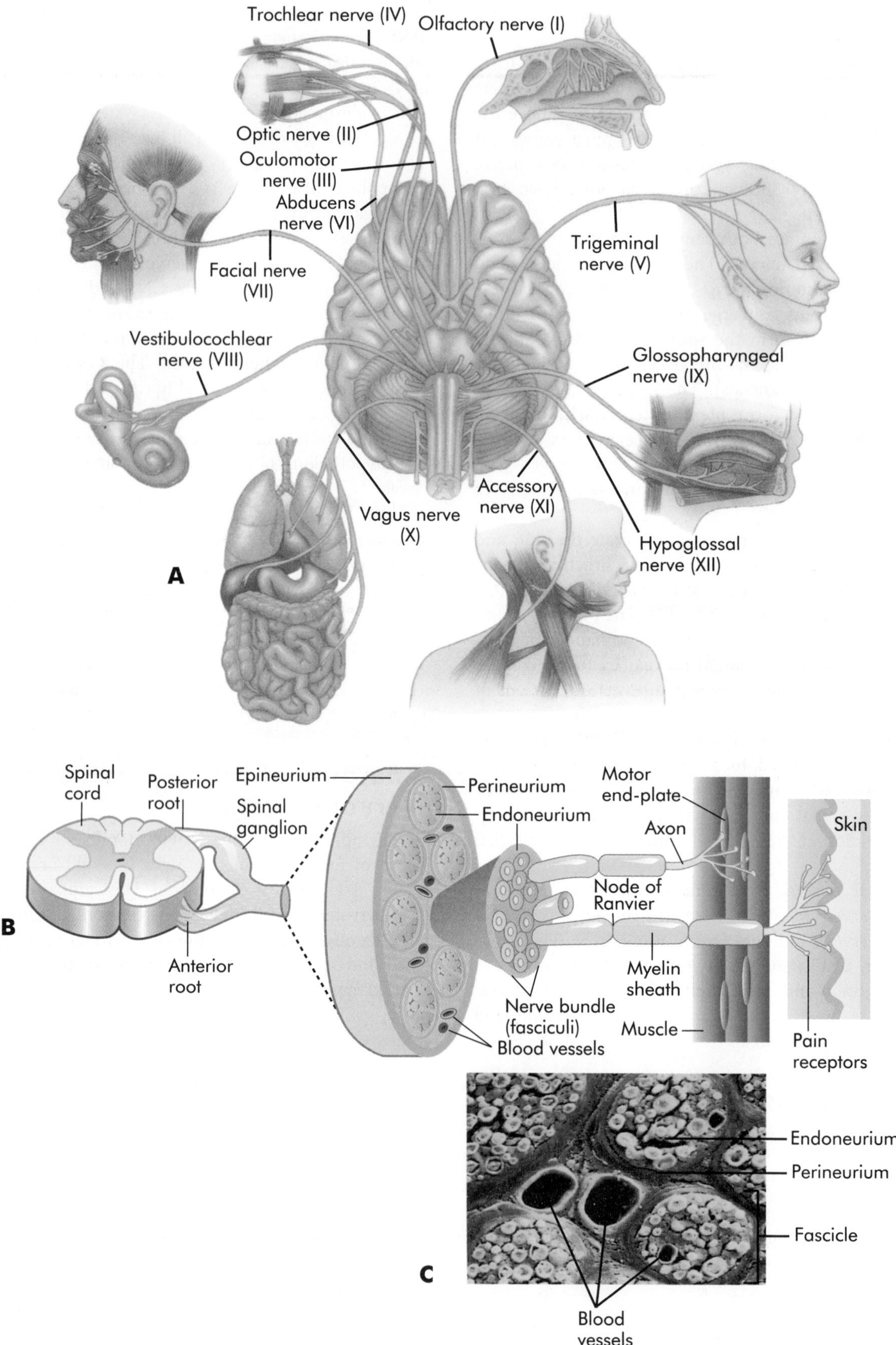

Figure 12-22 ■ **Cranial and Peripheral Nerves. A,** Ventral surface of the brain showing attachment of the cranial nerves. **B,** Peripheral nerve trunk and coverings. **C,** Scanning electron micrograph of a freeze-fractured preparation of peripheral nerve. (**A** and **C** from Thibodeau GA, Patton KT: *Anatomy & physiology,* ed 6, St Louis, 2007, Mosby.)

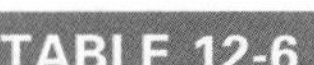

TABLE 12-6

The Cranial Nerves

Number and Name	Origin and Course	Function	How Tested
I. Olfactory	Fibers arise from nasal olfactory epithelium and form synapses with olfactory bulbs, which transmit impulses to temporal lobe	Purely sensory; carries impulses for sense of smell	Person is asked to sniff aromatic substances, such as oil of cloves and vanilla, and to identify them
II. Optic	Fibers arise form retina of eye to form optic nerve, which passes through sphenoid bone; two optic nerves then form optic chiasma (with partial crossover of fibers) and eventually end in occipital cortex	Purely sensory; carries impulses for vision	Vision and visual field tested with an eye chart and by testing point at which person first sees an object (finger) moving into visual field; inside of eye is viewed with ophthalmoscope to observe blood vessels of eye interior
III. Oculomotor	Fibers emerge from midbrain and exit from skull to run to eye	Contains motor fibers to inferior oblique, superior, inferior, and medial rectus extraocular muscles that direct eyeball; levator muscles of eyelid; smooth muscles of iris and ciliary body; and proprioception (sensory) to brain from extraocular muscles	Pupils examined for size, shape, and equality; pupillary reflex tested with a pen light (pupils should constrict when illuminated); ability to follow moving objects
IV. Trochlear	Fibers emerge from posterior midbrain and exit from skull to run to eye	Proprioceptor and motor fibers for superior oblique muscle of eye (extraocular muscle)	Tested in common with cranial nerve III relative to ability to follow moving objects
V. Trigeminal	Fibers emerge from pons and form three divisions that exit from skull and run to face and cranial dura mater	Both motor and sensory for face; conducts sensory impulses from mouth, nose, surface of eye, and dura mater; also contains motor fibers that stimulate chewing muscles	Sensations of pain, touch, and temperature tested with safety pin and hot and cold objects; corneal reflex tested with a wisp of cotton; motor branch tested by asking subject to clench teeth, open mouth against resistance, and move jaw from side to side
VI. Abducens	Fibers leave inferior pons and exit from skull to run to eye	Contains motor fibers to lateral rectus muscle and proprioceptor fibers from same muscle to brain	Tested in common with cranial nerve III relative to ability to move each eye laterally
VII. Facial	Fibers leave pons and travel through temporal bone to reach face	Mixed: (1) supplies motor fibers to muscles of facial expression and to lacrimal and salivary glands and (2) carries sensory fibers from taste buds of anterior part of tongue	Anterior two thirds of tongue tested for ability to taste sweet (sugar), salty, sour (vinegar), and bitter (quinine) substances; symmetry of face checked; subject asked to close eyes, smile, whistle, and so on; tearing tested with ammonia fumes
VIII. Vestibulocochlear (acoustic)	Fibers run from inner ear (hearing and equilibrium receptors in temporal bone) to enter brain stem just below pons	Purely sensory; vestibular branch transmits impulses for sense of equilibrium; cochlear branch transmits impulses for sense of hearing	Hearing checked by air and bone conduction by use of a tuning fork; vestibular tests: Brny and caloric tests
IX. Glossopharyngeal	Fibers emerge from midbrain and leave skull to run to throat	Mixed: (1) motor fibers serve pharynx (throat) and salivary glands, and (2) sensory fibers carry impulses from pharynx, posterior tongue (taste buds), and pressure receptors of carotid artery	Gag and swallow reflexes checked; subject asked to speak and cough; posterior one third of tongue may be tested for taste

(Continued)

TABLE 12-6

The Cranial Nerves—Cont'd

Number and Name	Origin and Course	Function	How Tested
X. Vagus	Fibers emerge from medulla, pass through skull, and descend through neck region into thorax and abdominal region	Fibers carry sensory and motor impulses for pharynx; a large part of this nerve is parasympathetic motor fibers, which supply smooth muscles of abdominal organs; receives sensory impulses from viscera	Same as for cranial nerve IX (IX and X are tested in common) because they both serve muscles of throat
XI. Spinal accessory	Fibers arise from medulla and superior spinal cord and travel to muscles of neck and back	Provides sensory and motor fibers for sternocleidomastoid and trapezius muscles and muscles of soft palate, pharynx, and larynx	Sternocleidomastoid and trapezius muscles checked for strength by asking subject to rotate head and shrug shoulders against resistance
XII. Hypoglossal	Fibers arise from medulla and exit from skull to travel to tongue	Carries motor fibers to muscles of tongue and sensory impulses from tongue to brain	Subject asked to stick out tongue, and any position abnormalities are noted

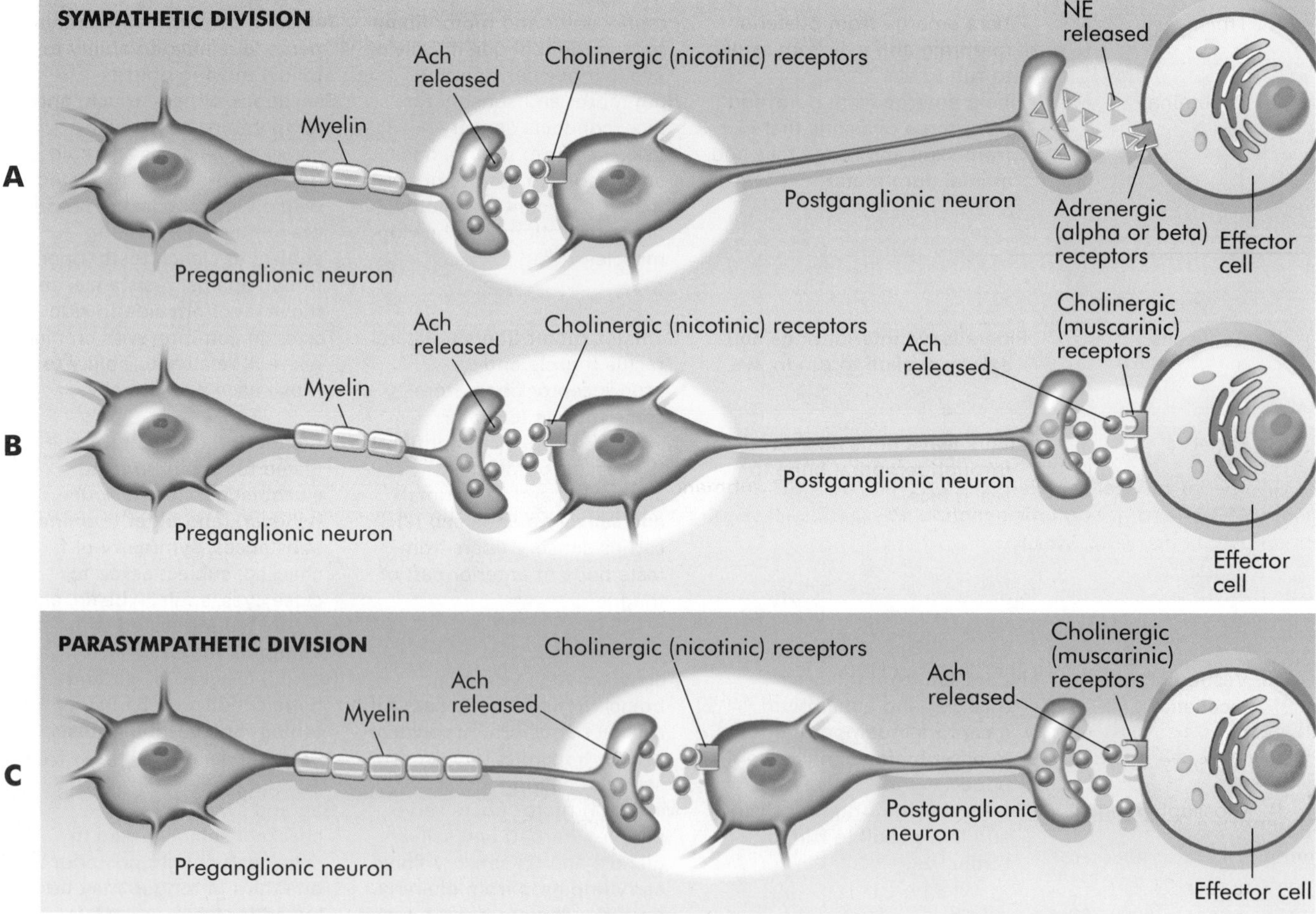

Figure 12-23 ■ **Locations of Neurotransmitters and Receptors of the Autonomic Nervous System.** In all pathways, preganglionic fibers are cholinergic, secreting acetylcholine (Ach), which stimulates nicotinic receptors in the postganglionic neuron. Most sympathetic postganglionic fibers are adrenergic, **A,** secreting norepinephrine (NE), thus stimulating α- or β-adrenergic receptors. A few sympathetic postganglionic fibers are cholinergic, stimulating muscarinic receptors in effector cells, **B.** All parasympathetic postganglionic fibers are cholinergic, **C,** stimulating muscarinic receptors in effector cells. (From Thibodeau GA, Patton KT: *Anatomy & physiology,* ed 6, St Louis, 2007, Mosby.)

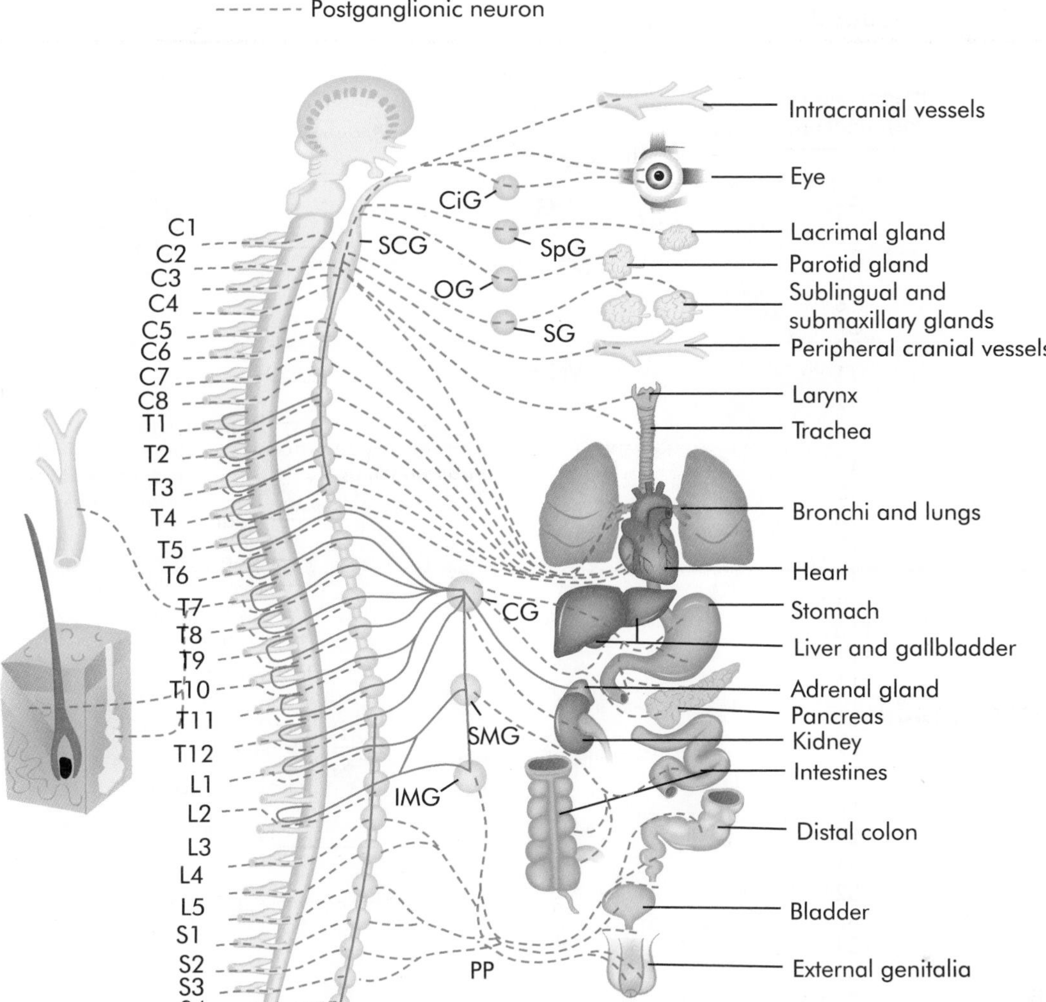

Figure 12-24 ■ **Sympathetic Division of the Autonomic Nervous System.** *CiG,* Ciliary ganglion; *SpG,* sphenopalatine ganglion; *SCG,* superior cervical ganglion; *OG,* otic ganglion; *SG,* submandibular ganglion; *CG,* celiac ganglion; *SMG,* superior mesenteric ganglion; *IMG,* inferior mesenteric ganglion; *PP,* pelvic plexus. (Redrawn from Rudy EB, editor: *Advanced neurological and neurosurgical nursing,* St Louis, 1984, Mosby.)

and *do not* synapse before reaching the gland. The secretory cells in the adrenal medulla are considered modified postganglionic neurons. Because preganglionic sympathetic fibers are all myelinated, travel to the adrenal medulla is quick, and innervation causes the rapid release of epinephrine and norepinephrine. Epinephrine and norepinephrine are mediators of the fight or flight response (see Chapter 8).

Anatomy of the Parasympathetic Nervous System

The parasympathetic nervous system conserves and restores energy. The nerve cell bodies of this division are located in the cranial nerve nuclei and in the sacral region of the spinal cord and therefore constitute the **craniosacral division.** Unlike the sympathetic branch, the preganglionic fibers in the parasympathetic division travel close to the organs they innervate before forming synapses with the relatively short postganglionic neurons (see Figure 12-25). Parasympathetic nerves arising from nuclei in the brain stem travel to the viscera of the head, thorax, and abdomen within cranial nerves—including the oculomotor (III), facial (VII), glossopharyngeal (IX), and vagus (X) nerves.

Preganglionic parasympathetic nerves that originate from the sacral region of the spinal cord run either separately or together with some spinal nerves. The preganglionic axons join together to form the **pelvic nerve,**

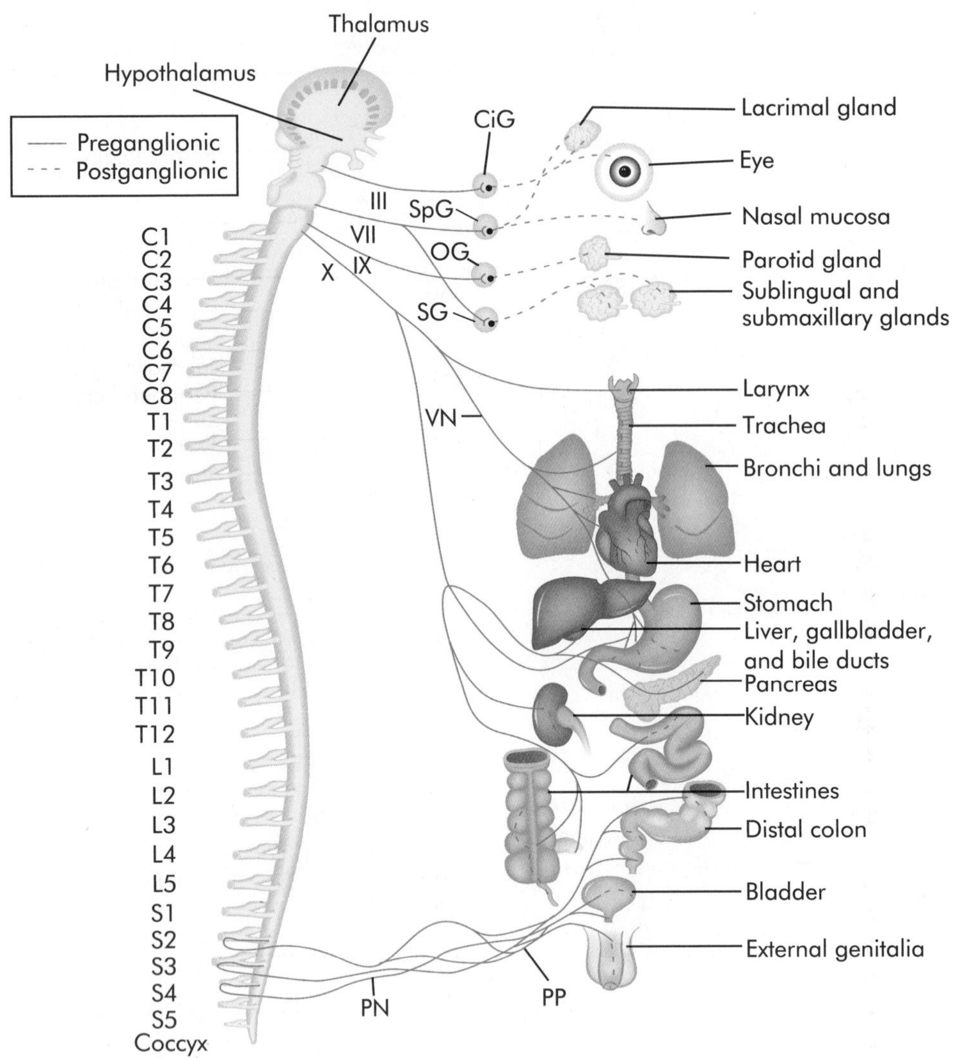

Figure 12-25 ■ **Parasympathetic Division of the Autonomic Nervous System.** *CiG,* Ciliary ganglion; *SpG,* sphenopalatine ganglion; *OG,* otic ganglion; *SG,* submandibular ganglion; *VN,* vagus nerve; *PP,* pelvic plexus; *PN,* pelvic nerve. (Redrawn from Rudy EB, editor: *Advanced neurological and neurosurgical nursing,* St Louis, 1984, Mosby.)

which innervates the viscera of the pelvic cavity. These preganglionic axons synapse with postganglionic neurons in terminal ganglia located close to the organs they innervate.

Neurotransmitters and Neuroreceptors

Sympathetic preganglionic fibers and parasympathetic preganglionic and postganglionic fibers release **acetylcholine**—the same neurotransmitter released by somatic efferent neurons (see Figures 12-23 and 12-26). These fibers are characterized by **cholinergic transmission.** Most postganglionic sympathetic fibers release **norepinephrine** (adrenaline) and thus are considered to function by **adrenergic transmission.** A few postganglionic sympathetic fibers, such as those that innervate the sweat glands, release acetylcholine.

The action of catecholamines varies with the type of neuroreceptor stimulated. It should be remembered that catecholamines also are released by the adrenal medulla gland that physiologically and biochemically resembles the sympathetic nervous system. Two types of adrenergic receptors exist, α and β. Cells of the effector organs may have only one or both types of adrenergic receptors. The **α-adrenergic receptors** have been further subdivided according to the action produced. α_1-Adrenergic activity is associated mostly with excitation or stimulation; α_2-adrenergic activity is associated with relaxation or inhibition. Most of the α-adrenergic receptors on effector organs belong to the α_1 class. The **β-adrenergic receptors** are classified as β_1-adrenergic receptors (which facilitate increased heart rate and contractility and cause the release of renin from the kidney) and β_2-adrenergic receptors (which facilitate all remaining effects attributed to β receptors).[6] Norepinephrine stimulates all α_1 and β_1 receptors and only

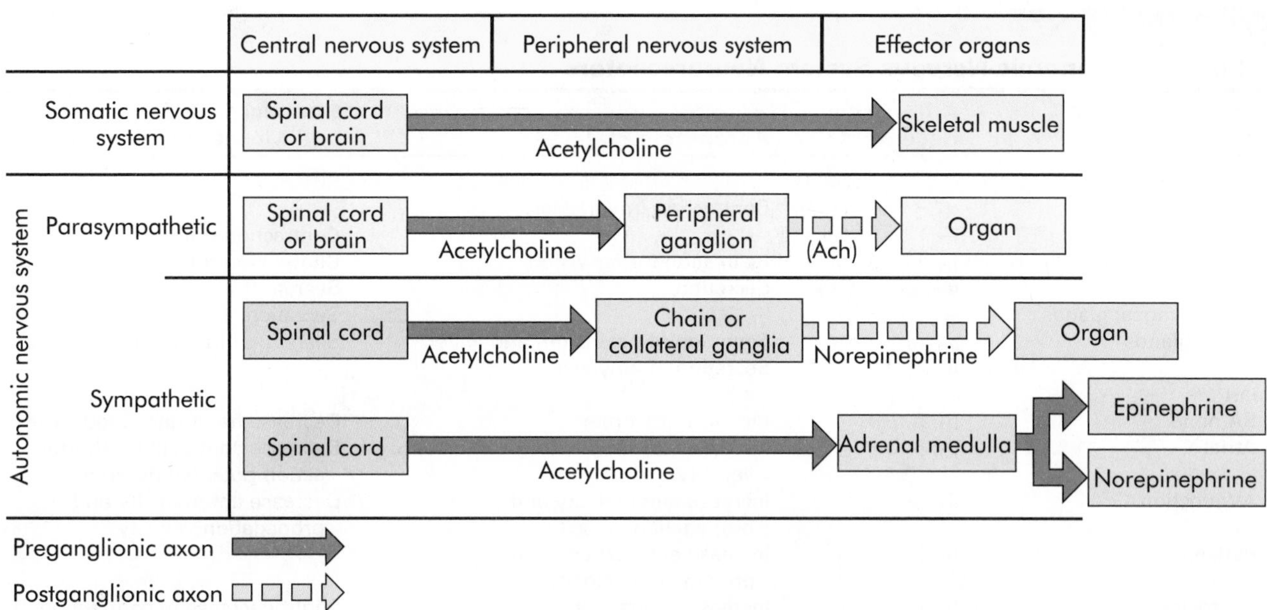

Figure 12-26 ■ **The Autonomic Nervous System and the Type of Neurotransmitters Secreted by Preganglionic and Postganglionic Fibers.** Note that all preganglionic fibers are cholinergic (Ach). A somatic nerve is used for comparison.

certain β_2 receptors. The primary response from norepinephrine, however, is stimulation of the α_1-adrenergic receptors that cause vasoconstriction. Epinephrine strongly stimulates all four types of receptors and induces general vasodilation because of the predominance of β receptors in muscle vasculatures. (Table 12-7 summarizes the effects of neuroreceptors on their effector organs.)

Functions of the Autonomic Nervous System

Many body organs are innervated by both the sympathetic and parasympathetic nervous systems. The two divisions often cause opposite responses; for example, sympathetic stimulation of the stomach causes decreased peristalsis, whereas parasympathetic stimulation of the intestine increases peristalsis. In general, sympathetic stimulation promotes responses for the protection of the individual. For example, sympathetic activity increases blood sugar levels and temperature and raises the blood pressure. In emergency situations, a generalized and widespread discharge of the sympathetic system occurs. This is accomplished by an increased firing frequency of sympathetic fibers and by activation of sympathetic fibers normally silent and at rest (fibers to the sweat glands, pilomotor muscles, and the adrenal medulla, as well as vasodilator fibers to muscle). Regulation of vasomotor tone is considered the single most important function of the sympathetic nervous system. (Figure 12-27 illustrates some of the most important functions of the sympathetic nervous system.)

Increased parasympathetic activity promotes rest and tranquility and is characterized by reduced heart rate and enhanced visceral functions concerned with digestion. Stimulation of the vagus nerve (cranial nerve X) in the gastrointestinal tract increases peristalsis and secretion, as well as the relaxation of sphincters. Activation of parasympathetic fibers in the head, provided by cranial nerves III, VII, and IX, causes constriction of the pupil, tear secretion, and increased salivary secretion. Stimulation of the sacral division of the parasympathetic system contracts the urinary bladder and facilitates the process of genital erection.

The parasympathetic system lacks the generalized and widespread response of the sympathetic system. Specific parasympathetic fibers are activated to regulate particular functions. Although the actions of the parasympathetic and sympathetic systems are usually antagonistic, there are exceptions. Peripheral vascular resistance, for example, is increased dramatically by sympathetic activation but is not altered appreciably by activity of the parasympathetic system. Most blood vessels involved in the control of blood pressure are innervated by sympathetic nerves. To decrease blood pressure, therefore, it is more important to block or paralyze the continuous (tonic) discharge of the sympathetic system than to promote parasympathetic activity.

✔ QUICK CHECK 12-6

1. What are the structural and functional divisions of the ANS?
2. Compare cholinergic and adrenergic transmission.
3. What does the ANS do?

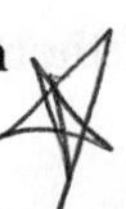

TABLE 12-7

Actions of Autonomic Nervous System Neuroreceptors

Effector Organ or Tissue	Adrenergic Receptors	Adrenergic Effects	Cholinergic Effects (Nicotine and Muscarinic Receptors)
Eye, iris			
Radial muscle	α_1	Contraction (mydriasis)	
Sphincter muscle	—	—	Contraction (miosis)
Eye, ciliary muscle	β_2	Relaxation for far vision	Contraction for near vision
Lacrimal glands	α	Secretion	Secretion
Nasopharyngeal glands	—	—	Secretion
Salivary glands	α_1	Secretion of potassium and water	Secretion of potassium and water
	β	Secretion of amylase	—
Heart			
SA node	β_1, β_2	Increase heart rate	Decrease heart rate; vagus arrest
Atrial	β_1, β_2	Increase contractility and conduction velocity	Decrease contractility; shorten action potential duration
AV junction	β_1, β_2	Increase automaticity and propagation velocity	Decrease automaticity and propagation velocity
Purkinje system	β_1, β_2	Increase automaticity and propagation velocity	—
Ventricles	β_1, β_2	Increase contractility	Slight decrease in contraction
Arterioles			
Coronary	α_1, α_2, β_2	Constriction, dilation	Dilation
Skin and mucosa	α_1, α_2	Constriction	Dilation
Skeletal muscle	α, β_2	Constriction, dilation	Dilation
Cerebral	α_1	Constriction (slight)	—
Pulmonary	α_1, β_2	Constriction, dilation	—
Mesenteric	α_1	Constriction	—
Renal	α_1, β_1, β_2, D	Constriction, dilation	—
Salivary glands	α_1, α_2	Constriction	Dilation
Veins, systemic	α_1, β_2	Constriction, dilation	
Lung			
Bronchial muscle	β_2	Relaxation	Contraction
Bronchial glands	α_1, β_2	Decreased secretion; increased secretion	Stimulation
Stomach			
Motility	α_1, α_2, β_2	Decrease (usually)	Increase
Sphincters	α_1	Contraction (usually)	Relaxation (usually)
Secretion	—	Inhibition (?)	Stimulation
Liver	α_1, β_2	Glycogenolysis and gluconeogenesis	Glycogen synthesis
Gallbladder and ducts	—	Relaxation	Contraction
Pancreas			
Acini	α	Decrease secretion	Secretion
Islet cells	α_2, β_2	Decreased secretion; increased secretion	
Intestine			
Motility and tone	α_1, α_2, β_1, β_2	Decrease	Increase
Sphincters	α_1	Contraction (usually)	Relaxation (usually)
Secretion	α_2	Inhibition (?)	Stimulation
Adrenal medulla	—	Secretion of epinephrine and norepinephrine (nicotinic effect)	
Kidney			
Renin secretion	α_1, β_1	Decrease; increase	—
Ureter			
Motility and tone	α_1	Increase	Increase
Urinary bladder			
Detrusor	β_2	Relaxation (usually)	Contraction
Trigone and sphincter	α_1	Contraction	Relaxation
Sex organs, male	α_1	Ejaculation	Erection
Skin			
Pilomotor muscles	α_1	Contraction	—
Sweat glands	α_1	Localized secretion	Generalized secretion
Fat cells	α_2, β_1, β_2	Inhibition of lipolysis; stimulation of lipolysis	—
Pineal gland	β	Melatonin synthesis	—

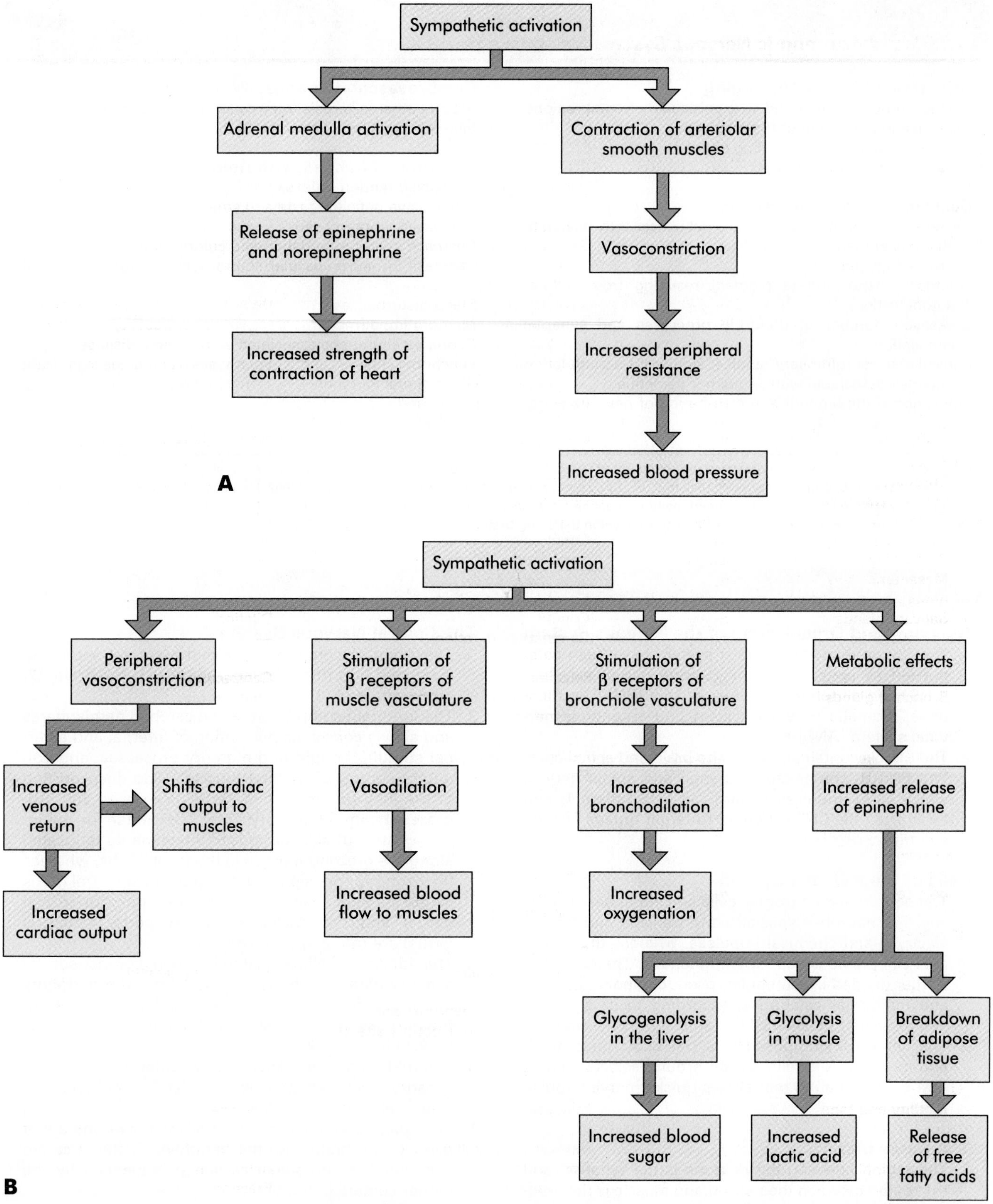

Sympathetic activation

Adrenal medulla activation

Release of epinephrine and norepinephrine

Increased strength of contraction of heart

Contraction of arteriolar smooth muscles

Vasoconstriction

Increased peripheral resistance

Increased blood pressure

A

Sympathetic activation

Peripheral vasoconstriction

Increased venous return

Shifts cardiac output to muscles

Increased cardiac output

Stimulation of β receptors of muscle vasculature

Vasodilation

Increased blood flow to muscles

Stimulation of β receptors of bronchiole vasculature

Increased bronchodilation

Increased oxygenation

Metabolic effects

Increased release of epinephrine

Glycogenolysis in the liver

Increased blood sugar

Glycolysis in muscle

Increased lactic acid

Breakdown of adipose tissue

Release of free fatty acids

B

Figure 12-27 ■ **Some Important Functions of the Sympathetic Nervous System. A,** Regulation of vasomotor tone. **B,** Regulation of strenuous muscular exercise ("fight or flight" response). (See also Chapter 8 and Figure 8-1 for more detail on the stress response.)

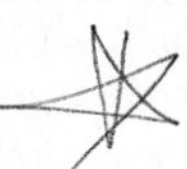

AGING & The Nervous System

Structural Changes With Aging

Decreased brain weight and size, particularly frontal regions
Fibrosis and thickening of the meninges
Narrowing of gyri and widening of sulci
Increase in size of ventricles

Cellular Changes With Aging

Decrease in the number of neurons not consistently related to changes in mental function
Decreased myelin
Lipofuscin deposition (a pigment resulting from cellular autodigestion)
Decreased number of dendritic processes and synaptic connections
Intracellular neurofibrillary tangles; significant accumulation in cortex associated with Alzheimer dementia
Imbalance in the amount and distribution of neurotransmitters

Cerebrovascular Changes With Aging

Arterial atherosclerosis (may cause infarcts and scars)
Increased permeability of the blood-brain barrier

Functional Changes With Aging

Decreased tendon reflexes
Progressive deficit in taste and smell
Decreased vibratory sense
Decrease in accommodation and color vision
Decrease in neuromuscular control with change in gait and posture
Sleep disturbances
Memory impairments
Cognitive alterations associated with chronic disease
Functional changes and nervous system aging has significant individual variation

Data from Hof PR, Mobbs CV: *Functional neurobiology of aging,* San Diego, 2001, Academic Press; Lambert K, Kinsley CH: *Clinical neuroscience,* ed 3, New York, 2005, Worthy; Sirven, JI, Malamut, BL: *Clinical neurology of the older adult,* Philadelphia, 2002, Lippincott Williams & Wilkins; Raz N, Rodrigue KM: Differential aging of the brain: patterns, cognitive correlates and modifiers, *Neurosci Biobehav* Rev 30(6):730–748, 2006; Friedman D, Nessler D, Johnson R Jr: Memory encoding and retrieval in the aging brain, *Clin EEG Neurosc* (1):2–7, 2007.

Did You Understand?

Overview and Organization of the Nervous System

1. The divisions of the nervous system have been categorized as either structural (central nervous system [CNS] and peripheral nervous system [PNS]) or functional (somatic nervous system and autonomic nervous system [ANS]).
2. The CNS is contained within the brain and spinal cord.
3. The PNS is composed of cranial and spinal nerves, which carry impulses toward the CNS (afferent) and away from the CNS (efferent) to target organs or skeletal muscle.

Cells of the Nervous System

1. The neuron and neuroglial cells constitute nervous tissue. The neuron is specialized to transmit and receive electrical and chemical impulses, whereas the neuroglial cell provides supportive functions. The neuron is further divided into unipolar, pseudounipolar, bipolar, and multipolar categories, according to its structure and particular mechanics of impulse transmission.
2. The neuron is composed of a cell body, dendrite(s), and an axon. A myelin sheath around selected axons forms an insulation that allows quicker nerve impulse conduction.

The Nerve Impulse

1. The region between the neurons is the synapse, and the region between the neuron and muscle is the myoneural junction.
2. Neurotransmitters are responsible for chemical conduction across the synapse, and myoneural junction nerve impulse is regulated predominantly by a balance of inhibitory postsynaptic potentials (IPSPs) and excitatory postsynaptic potentials (EPSPs), temporal and spatial summation, and convergence and divergence.

The Central Nervous System

1. The brain is contained within the cranial vault and is divided into three distinct regions: (1) forebrain, (2) hindbrain, and (3) midbrain.
2. The forebrain comprises the two cerebral hemispheres and allows conscious perception of internal and external stimuli, thought and memory processes, and voluntary control of skeletal muscles. The deep portion of the forebrain is termed the *diencephalon* and processes incoming sensory data. The center for voluntary control of skeletal muscle movements is located along the precentral gyrus in the frontal lobe, whereas the center for perception is along the postcentral gyrus in the parietal lobe. The Broca area (inferior frontal gyrus) and the Wernicke area (superior temporal gyrus) are major speech centers.
3. The hindbrain allows sampling and comparison of sensory data, which are received from the periphery and motor impulses of the cerebral hemispheres, for the purpose of coordination and refinement of skeletal muscle movement.
4. The midbrain is primarily a relay center for motor and sensory tracts, as well as a center for auditory and visual reflexes.
5. The spinal cord contains most of the nerve fibers that connect the brain with the periphery. Reflex arcs are completed in the spinal cord and influenced by the higher centers in the brain.
6. The CNS is protected by the scalp, bony cranium, meninges, vertebral column, and cerebrospinal fluid (CSF). CSF is formed from blood components in the choroid plexuses of the ventricles and is reabsorbed in the arachnoid villi (located in the dural venous sinuses) after circulating through the brain and subarachnoid space.

(Continued)

Did You Understand?—Cont'd

7. The paired carotid and vertebral arteries supply blood to the brain and connect to form the circle of Willis. The major branches projecting from the circle of Willis are the anterior, middle, and posterior cerebral arteries. Drainage of blood from the brain is accomplished through the venous sinuses and jugular veins.
8. The blood-brain barrier is provided by tight junctions between the cells of brain capillaries and surrounding supporting cells.
9. Blood supply to the spinal cord originates from the vertebral arteries and branches arising from the aorta.

The Peripheral Nervous System

1. The PNS relays information from the CNS to muscle and effector organs through cranial and spinal nerve tracts arranged in fascicles (multiple fascicles bound together form the peripheral nerve).

The Autonomic Nervous System

1. The ANS is responsible for maintaining a steady state in the internal environment. Two opposing systems make up the ANS: (1) the sympathetic nervous system responds to stress by mobilizing energy stores and prepares the body to defend itself, and (2) the parasympathetic nervous system conserves energy and the body's resources. Both systems function, more or less, at the same time.

AGING & the Nervous System

1. Major structural changes with aging include a decrease in number of neurons and a decrease in brain weight and size.
2. Deposition of lipofuscin and the presence of multiple neurofibrillary tangles are common cellular changes with aging.
3. A progressive slowing of neurologic function occurs with advancing age.

Key Terms

α-Adrenergic receptor, 298
Acetylcholine, 298
Adrenergic transmission, 298
Afferent (sensory) neuron, 284
Afferent pathway (ascending pathway), 273
Amygdala, 281
Anterior column, 284
Anterior fossa, 287
Anterior horn (ventral horn), 284
Anterior spinal artery, 291
Anterior spinothalamic tract, 285
Arachnoid villi, 289
Arachnoid, 287
Association fiber, 281
Associational neuron (interneuron), 275
Astrocyte, 275
Autonomic nervous system (ANS), 273
Axon, 274
Axon hillock, 274
β-Adrenergic receptor, 298
Basal ganglia system (extrapyramidal system), 279
Basal ganglia, 281
Basilar artery, 290
Basis pedunculi, 283
Bipolar neuron, 275
Blood-brain barrier, 291
Brachial plexus, 293
Brain stem, 277
Broca speech area (Brodmann areas 44, 45), 281
Cauda equina, 284
Caudate nucleus, 281
Cavernous sinus, 289
Celiac, 293
Central canal, 284
Central nervous system (CNS), 273
Central sulcus (fissure of Rolando), 279
Cerebellum, 284
Cerebral aqueduct (aqueduct of Sylvius), 284
Cerebral cortex, 279
Cerebral nuclei, 281
Cerebral peduncle, 283
Cerebrospinal fluid (CSF), 288
Cerebrum, 279
Cholinergic transmission, 298
Choroid plexus, 288
Circle of Willis, 290
Collateral ganglia, 293
Contralateral control, 281
Conus medullaris, 284
Corpora quadrigemina (tectum), 283
Corpus callosum (transverse fibers or commissural fibers), 281
Corpus striatum, 281
Corticobulbar tract, 285
Corticospinal tract (pyramidal system), 279
Cranial nerve, 273
Craniosacral division, 297
Dendrite, 274
Dendritic zone, 274
Dermatome, 293
Diencephalon, 283
Dopamine, 283
Dorsal root ganglion, 284
Dura mater, 287
Effector organ, 273
Efferent (motor) neuron, 284
Efferent pathway (descending pathway), 273
Epicritic, 286
Epidural space, 288
Epithalamus, 283
Excitatory postsynaptic potential (EPSP), 277
Facilitation, 277
Falx cerebri, 287
Fascicle, 293
Filum terminale, 284
Fissure, 279
Frontal lobe, 279
Galea aponeurotica, 287
Ganglia (plexus), 274
Gray matter, 279
Hippocampus, 283
Hypothalamus, 283
Inferior colliculi, 283
Inferior mesenteric, 293
Inhibitory postsynaptic potential (IPSP), 277
Inner dura (meningeal layer), 287
Insula, 281
Internal capsule, 281
Internal carotid artery, 289
Interventricular foramen (foramen of Monro), 288
Intervertebral disk, 289
Lateral aperture (foramen of Luschka), 288
Lateral column, 284
Lateral corticospinal tract, 285
Lateral horn, 284
Lateral spinothalamic pathway, 285
Lateral sulcus (sylvian fissure, lateral fissure), 279
Lentiform nucleus, 281
Limbic system, 283
Lower motor neuron, 285
Lumbar plexus, 293
Median aperture (foramen of Magendie), 288

Key Terms—Cont'd

Meninges, 287
Metencephalon, 284
Microfilament, 274
Microglia, 275
Microtubule, 274
Midbrain (mesencephalon), 283
Middle fossa (temporal fossa), 287
Mixed nerve, 293
Motor neuron, 275
Motor unit, 285
Multipolar neuron, 275
Myelencephalon (medulla oblongata), 284
Myelin, 274
Myelin sheath, 274
Neurofibril, 274
Neuroglia, 275
Neuroglial cell, 273
Neuromuscular (myoneural) junction, 275
Neuron, 273
Neurotransmitter, 277
Nissl substance, 274
Node of Ranvier, 274
Norepinephrine, 298
Nucleus pulposus, 289
Occipital lobe, 281
Oligodendroglia (oligodendrocyte), 275
Papez circuit, 283
Parasympathetic nervous system, 293
Parietal lobe, 281
Pelvic nerve, 297
Periosteum (endosteal layer), 287
Peripheral nervous system (PNS), 273
Pia mater, 288
Plexus, 293
Pons, 284
Postcentral gyrus, 281
Posterior (dorsal) column, 284
Posterior fossa, 287
Posterior horn (dorsal horn), 284
Posterior spinal artery, 291
Postganglionic neuron, 293
Postsynaptic neuron, 277
Precentral gyrus, 279
Prefrontal area, 279
Preganglionic neuron, 293
Premotor area (Brodmann area 6), 279
Presynaptic neuron, 277
Primary motor area (Brodmann area 4), 279
Primary voluntary motor area, 279
Protopathic, 286
Pseudounipolar neuron, 275
Red nucleus, 283
Reflex arc, 284
Reticular activating system, 278
Reticular formation, 278
Reticulospinal tract, 285
Sacral plexus, 293
Saltatory conduction, 274
Schwann cell, 273
Sensory neuron, 275
Somatic nervous system, 273
Spatial summation, 277
Spinal cord, 284
Spinal nerve, 273
Spinal tract, 284
Spinothalamic tract, 284
Splanchnic nerve, 293
Subarachnoid space, 287
Subdural space, 287
Substantia gelatinosa, 284
Substantia nigra, 283
Subthalamus, 283
Sulci, 279
Summation, 277
Superior colliculi, 283
Superior mesenteric, 293
Sympathetic (paravertebral) ganglia, 293
Sympathetic nervous system, 293
Synapse, 277
Synaptic bouton, 277
Synaptic cleft, 277
Tegmentum, 283
Telencephalon, 279
Temporal lobe, 281
Temporal summation, 277
Tentorium cerebelli, 287
Thalamus, 283
Thoracolumbar division, 293
Unipolar neuron, 275
Upper motor neuron, 285
Ventricle, 288
Vermis, 284
Vertebral artery, 289
Vertebral column, 284
Vestibulospinal tract, 285
Wernicke area, 281
White matter, 279

References

1. Martin JH: *Neuroanatomy: text and atlas*, ed 3, New York, 2003, McGraw-Hill.
2. 2. Purves D et al: *Neuroscience*, ed 3, Sunderland, 2004, Sinauer Assoc.
3. Kolb B, Whishaw IQ: *An introduction to brain and behavior*, ed 2, New York, 2006, Worth.
4. Szabo B, Schlicker E: Effects of cannabinoids on neurotransmission, *Handb Exp Pharmacol* (168):327–365, 2005.
5. Kiernan JA: *Barr's the human nervous system: an anatomical viewpoint*, ed 8, Philadelphia, 2005, Lippincott Williams & Wilkins.
6. Siegel R et al: *Basic neurochemistry: molecular, cellular, and medical aspects*, ed 7, Philadelphia, 2005, Academic Press.

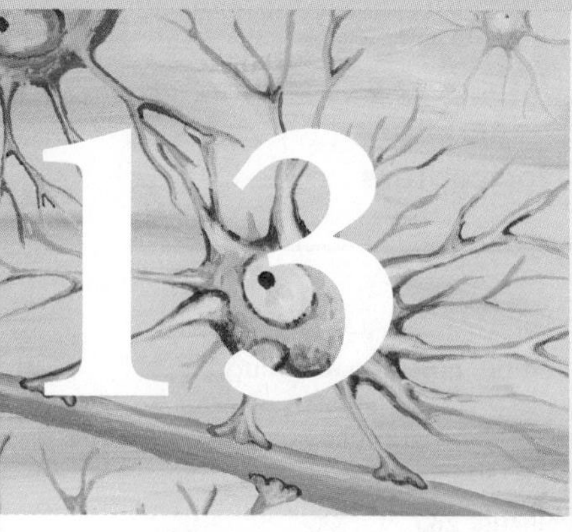

13 PAIN, TEMPERATURE, SLEEP, AND SENSORY FUNCTION

Curtis B. DeFriez ■ Sue E. Huether

CHAPTER OUTLINE

ELECTRONIC RESOURCES

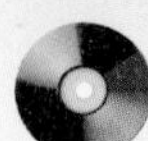

Companion CD
- Review Questions and Answers
- Animations

evolve Website
http://evolve.elsevier.com/Huether/
- Quick Check Answers
- Key Terms Exercises
- Critical Thinking Questions with Answers
- Algorithm Completion Exercises
- WebLinks

Alterations in sensory function may involve dysfunctions of the general or the special senses. Dysfunctions of the general senses include chronic pain, abnormal temperature regulation, and tactile or proprioceptive dysfunction. Pain is an unpleasant but protective phenomenon that is uniquely experienced by each individual and it cannot be adequately defined, identified, or measured by an observer. Like pain, variations in temperature can signal disease. Fever is a common manifestation of dysfunction and is often the first symptom observed in an infectious or inflammatory condition.

Sleep is a normal cyclic process that restores the body's energy and maintains normal functioning. Sleep is so essential to both physiologic and psychologic function that sleep deprivation causes a wide range of clinical manifestations. The special senses of vision, hearing, touch, smell, and taste are the means by which individuals perceive stimuli that are essential in interacting with the environment. Dysfunctions of the special senses include visual, auditory, vestibular, olfactory, and gustatory (taste) disorders.

PAIN

The Experience of Pain

Phantom limb

Pain is one of the body's most important adaptive mechanisms, and all definitions suggest it is a complex phenomenon and cannot be characterized as only a response to injury. McCaffery defined pain as "whatever the experiencing person says it is, existing whenever he says it does."[1] The International Association for the Study of Pain and the American Pain Society defined pain as "an unpleasant sensory and emotional experience associated with actual or potential tissue damage or described in terms of such damage."[2]

Three systems interact to produce pain.[3] The **sensory/discriminative system** processes information about the strength, intensity, and temporal and spatial aspects of pain. These sensations are mediated through afferent nerve fibers, the spinal cord, the brain stem, and the higher brain centers, and they result in prompt withdrawal from the painful stimulus. The **motivational/affective system** determines the individual's conditioned or learned approach/avoidance behaviors. These behaviors are mediated through the interaction of the reticular formation, limbic system, and brain stem. The **cognitive/evaluative system** overlies the individual's learned behavior concerning the experience of pain. The individual's interpretation of appropriate pain behavior is learned through cultural preferences, male and female roles, and life experience, among other ways. The influence of the cognitive/evaluative system may block, modulate, or enhance the perception of pain. Numerous instruments are available for the assessment and experience of pain.[4]

Neuroanatomy of Pain

The portions of the nervous system responsible for the sensation and perception of pain may be divided into the following three areas:

1. The *afferent pathways,* which begin in the peripheral nervous system (PNS), travel to the spinal gate in the dorsal horn and then ascend to higher centers in the central nervous system (CNS).
2. The *interpretive centers* located in the brainstem, midbrain, diencephalon, and cerebral cortex.
3. The *efferent pathways* that descend from the CNS back to the dorsal horn of the spinal cord.

The sensory process leading to the perception of pain is called **nociception. Nociceptors** are free nerve endings and respond to chemical, mechanical, and thermal stimuli (Table 13-1). Nociceptors are found under the epidermis and within joint and bone surfaces, the deep tissues, muscles, tendons, and subcutaneous tissue. They are not evenly distributed in the body, so the relative sensitivity to pain differs according to the area of the body. There are two major types of nociceptors, the small unmyelinated (C fibers) and lightly myelinated (Aδ fibers) afferent neurons. The small unmyelinated C polymodal nociceptor neurons are responsible for the transmission of diffuse burning or aching sensations. Because C fibers are small and lack a myelin sheath, transmission is relatively slow (slow pain) and poorly localized. Transmission through the slightly larger, myelinated Aδ nociceptors transmit pain more quickly and carry well-localized, sharp pain sensations.

TABLE 13-1

Stimuli that Activate Nociceptors (Pain Receptors)

Location of Receptor	Provoking Stimuli
Skin	Pricking, cutting, crushing, burning, freezing
Gastrointestinal tract	Engorged or inflamed mucosa, distention or spasm of smooth muscle, traction on mesenteric attachment
Skeletal muscle	Ischemia, injuries of connective tissue sheaths, necrosis, hemorrhage, prolonged contraction, injection of irritating solutions
Joints	Synovial membrane inflammation
Arteries	Piercing, inflammation
Head	Traction, inflammation, or displacement of arteries, meningeal structures, and sinuses; prolonged muscle contraction
Heart	Ischemia and inflammation

As Figure 13-1 illustrates, stimulated nociceptors produce impulses that are transmitted through the small, myelinated Aδ fibers and C fibers to the spinal cord. There they form synapses with interneurons primarily in the dorsal horn, cross over to the contralateral spinothalamic tract, and then ascend to the cerebral cortex (see Figure 12-8). The sensory reflex arc to and from the spinal cord is much faster than the transmission of sharp pain sensations by the

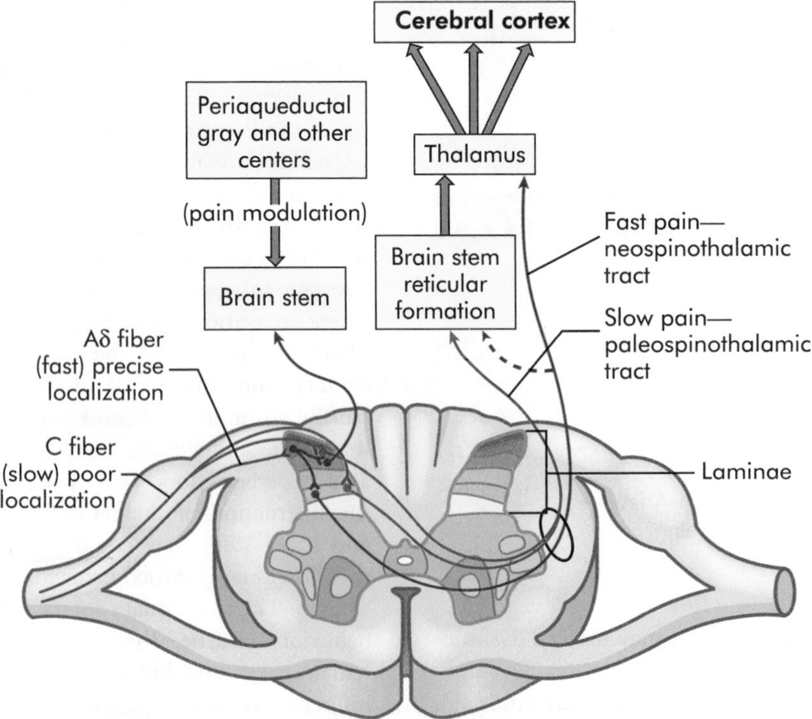

Figure 13-1 ■ **Transmission of Pain Sensations.** The Aδ and C fibers synapse in the laminae of the dorsal horn cross over to the contralateral spinothalamic tract then ascend to synapse in the midbrain through the neospinothalamic and paleospinothalamic tracts. Impulses are then conducted to the sensory cortex.

Aδ fibers, so the injured body part may retract before it perceives pain.

Two divisions of the spinothalamic tract carry pain information to the brain: (1) the lateral neospinothalamic tract (acute pain) and (2) the medial paleospinothalamic tract (dull and burning pain). The **neospinothalamic tract** carries information to the lateral thalamus and then projects to the somatosensory cortex which provides specific pain information. The **paleospinothalamic tract** carries information to the midbrain (medial thalamus, brain stem reticular formation, and hypothalamus) and is responsible for reflex responses to pain with changes in autonomic function, respiration, circulation, and endocrine function. Pain information is transmitted to the somatosensory cortex from the midbrain. Descending inhibitory pathways and nuclei modulate pain. Afferent stimulation of particularly the **ventromedial medulla** and **periaqueductal gray (PAG)** (gray matter surrounding the cerebral aqueduct) in the midbrain stimulates efferent pathways, which modulate or inhibit afferent pain signals at the dorsal horn.[5]

Theories of Pain

The **specificity theory of pain** was described by DesCartes in the seventeenth century and proposes that the intensity of pain is directly related to the amount of associated tissue injury. For instance, pricking one's finger with a needle causes minimal pain whereas cutting one's hand with a knife produces more tissue injury and thus is more painful. The specificity theory is useful for pain associated with specific injury and acute pain but does not account for chronic pain or cognitive and psychologic contributions to pain.

Melzack and Wall proposed the **gate control theory** in 1965 (Figure 13-2). According to this theory, pain transmission is modulated by a balance of impulses transmitted to the spinal cord by large Aδ and small C fibers (see Figure 13-2). These fibers terminate on inhibitory interneurons in the substantia gelatinosa (laminae in the dorsal horn of the spinal cord). Cells in the substantia gelatinosa function as a gate, regulating transmission of impulses to the CNS. Stimulation of non-nociceptive larger A fibers, such as touch, vibration or thermal stimulation, causes the cells in the substantia gelatinosa to "close the gate," which diminishes pain perception. This is why rubbing a pinched finger can reduce pain. Small fiber input inhibits cells in the substantia gelatinosa and opens the gate, enhancing pain perception. The CNS, through efferent pathways, may also close, partially close, or open the gate. The gate control theory is inadequate to explain some chronic pain problems, such as phantom limb pain, and the neuromatrix theory was proposed to explain such pain. The **neuromatrix theory of pain** proposes that when there is no discernable cause for chronic pain, such as phantom limb pain and some neuropathies, the brain produces patterns of nerve impulses from a widely distributed neural network with multidimensional inputs including genetic, affective, cognitive, evaluative, and other components.[6] The patterns may be triggered by sensory inputs from the periphery or originate *independently* in the brain with no external input. The theory represents the plasticity of the brain and provides a holistic, integrated, dynamic consideration of pain.

Neuromodulation of pain

Neuromodulators of pain are found in the pathways that mediate information about painful stimuli throughout the nervous system.[7] Some of the triggering mechanisms that initiate release of neuromodulators are tissue injury (prostaglandins, bradykinin) and chronic inflammatory lesions (lymphokines). Excitatory neuromodulators include such substances as substance P, glutamate, somatostatin, vasoactive intestinal polypeptide, and calcitonin-gene-related peptide. Inhibitory neuromodulators include gamma-aminobutyric acid (GABA), glycine, 5-hydroxytryptamine (serotonin), norepinephrine, and endorphins.

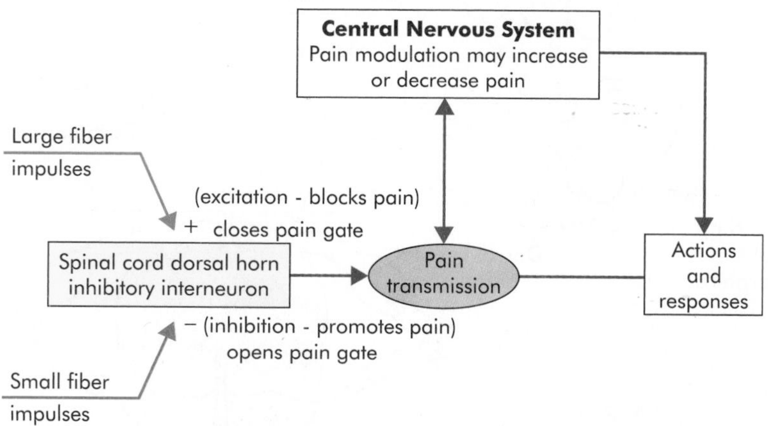

Figure 13-2 ■ **Gate Control Theory of Pain.** Schematic diagram of the gate control theory of pain mechanism. Large fiber non-nociceptor impulses (i.e., mechanical and thermal) activate inhibitory interneuron in spinal cord dorsal horn and decrease pain transmission (close pain gate). Small fiber impulses block the inhibitory interneuron and promote pain transmission (open pain gate).

Endorphins (endogenous morphines) are a family of neuropeptides that inhibit transmission of pain impulses in the spinal cord and brain by binding to **mu, kappa,** or **delta opioid receptors. β-endorphin** is a potent endorphin released from the hypothalamus and the pituitary gland. It may also be responsible for general sensations of well-being. **Enkephalin,** found in the neurons of the brain and spinal cord, is a weaker analgesic than other endorphins but is more potent and longer lasting than morphine. Dynorphin is 50 times more potent than β-endorphin. Dynorphins are found in the hypothalamus, periaqueductal gray, and spinal dorsal horn. **Dynorphin** generally impedes pain signals but can incite pain.[8] Midbrain stimulation in the area of the periaqueductal gray alleviates pain such as that associated with emergency situations.[9] **Endomorphins** are a relatively new group of peptides formed in the brain. They are highly antinociceptive with a high affinity for morphine receptors and cause vasodilation by release of nitric oxide from endothelial cells.[10]

All endorphins attach to **opiate receptors** on the plasma membrane of the afferent neuron (Figure 13-3), and the combination inhibits the release of excitatory neurotransmitters. Opiate drugs relieve pain by attaching to the opiate receptors and enhancing the natural endorphin response. Stress, excessive physical exertion, acupuncture, sexual intercourse, and other factors increase the levels of circulating endorphins, serotonin, norepinephrine, and other neurotransmitters, thereby raising the pain threshold.

Common Clinical Descriptions of Pain

The most widely used pain classifications are based on its temporal aspects, the inferred neurophysiologic mechanisms, etiology, and region affected. Temporal descriptions of pain as either acute or chronic are helpful and usually applied. The etiologic basis or region affected, or both, also can be useful descriptions under certain circumstances. These broad descriptions are summarized in Box 13-1.

Somatogenic pain, such as the pain of a crushed finger or the pain of a heart attack, is pain with a cause. In contrast, **psychogenic pain** is pain for which no physical cause can be diagnosed and the pain does not match the person's symptoms. Psychogenic pain, however, is not imaginary pain and the associated psychologic factors may cause, intensify, or prolong pain. Psychogenic pain may manifest as headaches or as muscle or back pain.

Acute pain is a protective mechanism that alerts the individual to a condition or experience that is immediately harmful to the body. Acute pain begins suddenly and is relieved after the chemical mediators that stimulate pain receptors are removed. Acute anxiety is always associated with acute pain and also is associated with the threat inherent in the painful experience, including its cause, treatment, and prognosis. Hope of recovery also is associated with acute pain. Acute pain mobilizes the individual to take prompt action to relieve it.[11]

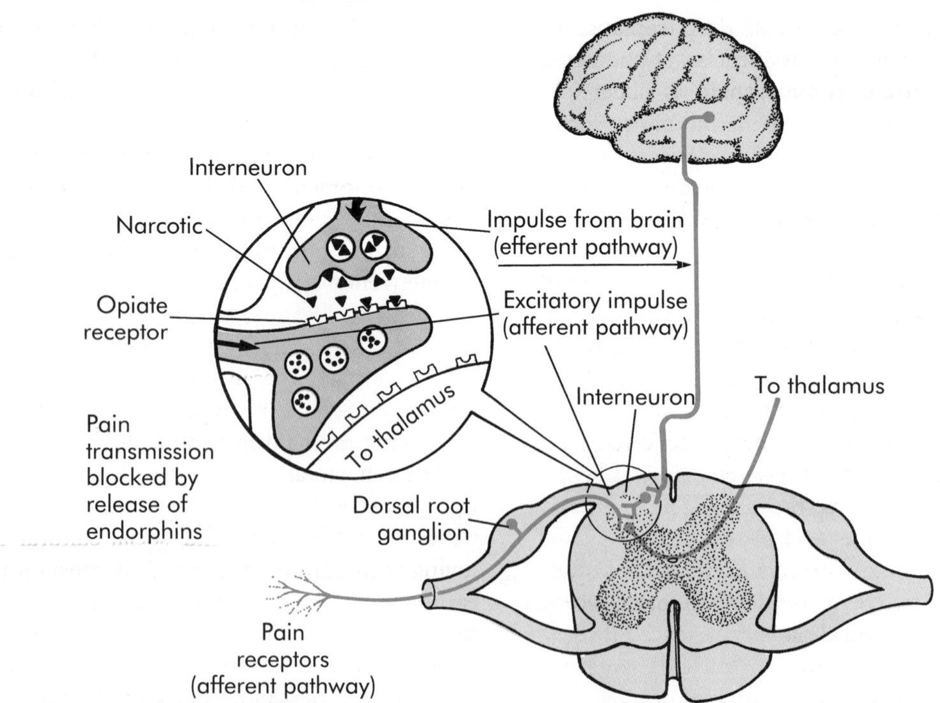

Figure 13-3 ■ **Descending Pathway and Endorphin Response.** Endorphin receptors are located close to known pain receptors in the periphery and ascending and descending pain pathways.

BOX 13-1 Categories of Pain

I. Neurophysiologic pain
  A. Nociceptive pain
    1. Somatic (i.e., skin, muscle, bone)
    2. Visceral (i.e., intestine, liver, stomach)
  B. Neuropathic (non-nociceptive)
    1. Central pain (lesion in brain or spinal cord)
    2. Peripheral pain (lesion in PNS)
II. Neurogenic pain
  A. Neuralgia (pain in the distribution of a nerve)
  B. Constant
    1. Sympathetically independent
    2. Sympathetically dependent
III. Temporal pain (time related)
  A. Acute pain
    1. Somatic
    2. Visceral
  B. Chronic
IV. Regional pain
  A. Abdominal pain
  B. Chest pain
  C. Headache
  D. Low back pain
  E. Orofacial pain
  F. Pelvic pain
V. Etiologic pain
  A. Cancer pain
  B. Dental pain
  C. Inflammatory pain
  D. Ischemic pain
  E. Vascular pain

Adapted from Derasari MD: Taxonomy of pain syndromes: classification of chronic pain syndromes. In Raj PP, editor: *Practical management of pain*, ed 3, St Louis, 2000, Mosby.

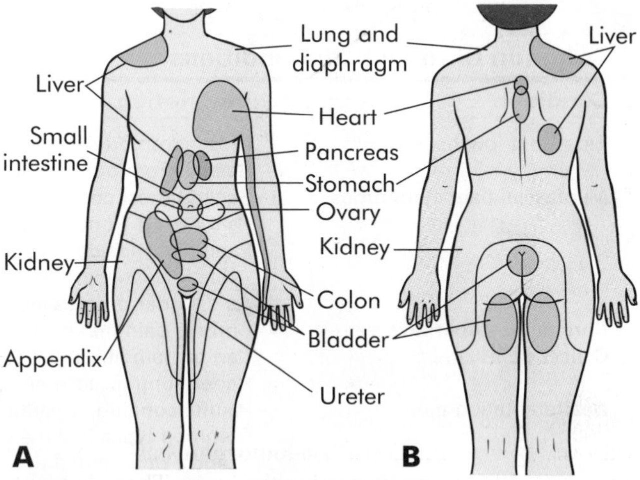

Figure 13-4 ■ **Sites of Referred Pain. A,** Front. **B,** Back.

Acute pain arises from cutaneous, deep somatic, or visceral structures and can be classified as (1) somatic, (2) visceral, or (3) referred. **Somatic pain** is superficial (coming from the skin or close to the surface of the body) and is either sharp and well localized or dull, aching, and poorly localized and accompanied by nausea and vomiting. Somatic pain is carried by sensory nerves. **Visceral pain** is pain in internal organs, the abdomen, or skeleton.[12] It is poorly localized and is associated with nausea and vomiting, hypotension, restlessness, and, in some cases, shock. Visceral pain often radiates (spreads away from the actual site of the pain) or is referred. Visceral pain is carried by sympathetic nerve fibers. **Referred pain** is pain that is present in an area removed or distant from its point of origin. Referred pain can be acute or chronic. The area of referred pain is supplied by the same spinal segment as the actual site of pain. Impulses from many cutaneous and visceral neurons converge on the same ascending neuron, and the brain cannot distinguish between the two. Because there are more receptors in the skin, the painful sensation is experienced there.[13] Figure 13-4 illustrates common areas of referred pain and their associated sites of origin.

Chronic pain is persistent—usually defined as lasting at least 3 to 6 months—and is related to tissue damage, inflammation, or injury of the nervous system. It may be persistent (e.g., low back pain) or intermittent (e.g., migraines). Causes or aggravating influences include a decreased level of endorphins or a predominance of C neuron stimulation. Changes in nerve terminals, afferent fibers, and the CNS may contribute to chronicity of pain.[14]

In contrast, the physiologic responses to chronic pain depend on the persistent or intermittent nature of the pain. Intermittent pain produces responses similar to those of acute pain, whereas persistent pain allows for physiologic adaptation, producing normal heart and respiratory rates and normal blood pressure. However, even though the physiologic responses are normal, the pain is not relieved.

Neuropathic pain is chronic pain and is characterized by increased sensitivity to painful stimuli (hyperalgesia), the perception of innocuous stimuli as painful (allodynia), and spontaneous pain. Neuropathic pain results from abnormal processing of sensory information by the peripheral and central nervous systems. **Peripheral pain** is the result of trauma or disease to peripheral nerves, such as nerve entrapment or diabetic neuropathy. **Central pain** is caused by a lesion or dysfunction in the brain or spinal cord, such as phantom pain or complex regional pain syndrome (reflex sympathetic dystrophy syndrome or causalgia), which is intense burning and swelling with extremity pain after an injury. Neuropathic pain requires individualized treatment because different mechanisms cause the hypersensitivity (or hyperalgesia) and identifying the underlying mechanism is difficult.[15]

The behavioral and psychologic changes of chronic pain include depression, difficulty sleeping and eating, preoccupation with the pain, and social-cultural influences.[16–18] Living with chronic pain requires constant attention to its earliest signs so the pain-provoking stimuli can be identified and avoided. Persons with chronic pain generally try to keep pain-related behavior to a minimum so they appear as normal as possible. The desire to relieve pain and the need to hide it are usually conflicting drives for those with chronic pain, who fear being labeled complainers. Table 13-2 lists some common chronic pain conditions.

TABLE 13-2
Common Chronic Pain Conditions

Condition	Description
Persistent low back pain	Most common chronic pain condition Results from poor muscle tone, inactivity, muscle strain, or sudden, vigorous exercise
Myofascial pain syndromes	Second most common chronic pain condition Pain results from muscle spasm, tenderness, and stiffness Examples include myositis, fibrositis, myofibrositis, myalgia, and muscle strain—conditions that involve injury to the muscle and fascia As disorder progresses, pain becomes increasingly generalized
Chronic postoperative pain	Chronic pain that can occur with disruption or cutting of sensory nerves
Cancer pain	Can be pain attributed to advance of disease, associated with treatment, or attributed to coexisting disease entities
Deafferentation pain	Painful condition resulting from injury to a peripheral nerve Common types include severe burning pain triggered by various stimuli, such as cold, light touch, or sound, and complex regional pain syndrome (occur after peripheral nerve injury and are characterized by continuous, severe, burning pain associated with vasomotor changes and muscle wasting)
Hyperesthesias	Increased sensitivity and decreased pain threshold to tactile and painful stimuli Pain is diffuse, modified by fatigue and emotion and mixed with other sensations May result from chronic irritations of CNS areas
Hemiagnosia	Loss of ability to identify source of pain on one side of the body Painful stimuli on that side produce discomfort, anxiety, moaning, agitation, and distress but no attempt to withdraw from the stimulus Associated with stroke
Phantom limb pain	Pain experience in amputated limb after stump has completely healed; may be immediate or occur months later Influenced by emotions/sympathetic stimulation Trigger points—small hypersensitive regions in muscle or connective tissues that, when stimulated, produce pain in a specific area

The pain frequently does not respond to usual therapy even when the cause is known. The onset may be sudden but chronic pain often develops insidiously. Individual behavior is adaptive and directed toward modifying the pain. Chronic pain is often associated with a sense of hopelessness and helplessness when no cure seems possible and more time elapses. The pain is perceived as meaningless; depression often results. Table 13-3 compares acute and chronic pain.[19]

Pain threshold and pain tolerance

The **pain threshold** is the lowest intensity at which a stimulus is perceived as pain and may be influenced by genetics.[20] Intense pain at one location may increase the threshold in another location. For example, a person with severe pain in one knee is less likely to experience chronic back pain that is less intense (called **perceptual dominance**). Because of perceptual dominance, an individual with many painful sites may report only the most painful one. Then when the dominant pain is diminished, the individual identifies other painful areas.

Pain tolerance is the amount of time or intensity of pain that an individual will endure before initiating overt pain responses. Pain tolerance varies greatly among people and in the same person over time because of the body's ability to respond differently to noxious stimuli (Table 13-4). Pain tolerance is influenced by the person's cultural perceptions, expectations, role behaviors, gender, and physical and mental health.[21] It generally decreases with repeated exposure to pain, fatigue, anger, boredom, apprehension, and sleep deprivation. Tolerance increases with alcohol consumption, medication, hypnosis, warmth, distracting activities, and strong beliefs or faith.

QUICK CHECK 13-1

1. Define the major categories of pain.
2. What portions of the nervous system are responsible for the sensation and perception of pain?
3. What physiologic responses are seen in acute pain?
4. List three common chronic pain conditions.

TEMPERATURE REGULATION

In all homeothermic animals, temperature regulation is achieved through precise balancing of heat production, heat conservation, and heat loss. In humans, body temperature is maintained in a range around 37° C (98.6° F). The normal range is considered to be 36.2° to 37.7° C (96.2° to 99.4° F) overall, but a person's individual body parts will vary in temperature. Body temperature rarely exceeds 41° C. The extremities are generally cooler than the trunk

TABLE 13-3

Comparison of Acute and Chronic Pain

Characteristic	Acute Pain	Chronic Pain
Experience	An event	A situation; state of existence
Source	External agent or internal disease, injury or inflammation	Unknown; if known, treatment is prolonged or ineffective
Onset	Usually sudden	May be sudden or develop insidiously
Duration	Transient (up to 6 months); usually of short duration Resolves with treatment and healing.	Prolonged (months to years)
Pain identification	Painful and nonpainful areas generally well identified	Painful and nonpainful areas less easily differentiated; change in sensations becomes more difficult to evaluate
Clinical signs	Typical response pattern with more visible signs Anxiety and emotional distress common	Response patterns vary; fewer overt signs (adaptation) Can interfere with sleep, productivity and quality of life
Significance	Significant (informs person something is wrong); protective	Person looks for significance
Pattern	Self-limiting or readily corrected	Continuous or intermittent; intensity may vary or remain constant
Course	Suffering usually decreases over time	Suffering usually increases over time
Actions	Leads to actions to relieve pain	Leads to actions to modify pain experience
Prognosis	Likelihood of eventual complete relief	Complete relief usually not possible

Data from Black RG: *Surg Clin North Am* 55(4):999, 1975.

TABLE 13-4

Pain Perception in Infants, Children, and Elderly Persons

	Infants	Children	Elderly Persons
Pain threshold	Painful neonatal experiences increase pain sensitivity	Lower or the same as adults	No increased change compared with middle age
Physiologic symptoms	Increased heart rate, blood pressure, and respiratory rate; flushing or pallor, sweating, and decreased oxygen saturation	Same as infants; nausea and vomiting	Same as infants and children; nausea and vomiting
Behavioral responses	Changes in facial expression, crying, and body movements, with lowered brows drawn together; vertical bulge and furrows in the forehead between the brows; broadened nasal root; tightly closed eyes; angular, square-shaped mouth, chin quiver; withdrawal of affected limbs, rigidity, flailing	Individual responses vary	Individual responses vary and may be influenced by presence of painful chronic diseases

Data from Gibson SJ, Farrell M: A review of age differences in the neurophysiology of nociception and the perceptual experience of pain, *Clin J Pain* 20(4):227-239, 2004; Kinouchi K: Anaesthetic considerations for the management of very low and extremely low birth weight infants, *Best Pract Res Clin Anaesthesiol* 18(2):273-290, 2004; Rustoen T et al: Age and the experience of chronic pain: differences in health and quality of life among younger, middle-aged, and older adults, *Clin J Pain* 21(6):513-523, 2005.

and the temperature at the core of the body (as measured by rectal temperature) is generally 0.5° C higher than at the surface (as measured by oral temperature). Internal temperature varies in response to activity, environmental temperature, and daily fluctuation **(circadian rhythm).** Oral temperatures fluctuate within 0.2° C to 0.5° C during a 24-hour period. Women tend to have wider fluctuations that follow the menstrual cycle with a sharp rise in temperature just before ovulation. The daily fluctuating temperature in both genders peaks around 6 PM and is at its lowest during sleep. Maintenance of body temperature within the normal range is necessary for life.

Hypothalamic Control of Temperature

Temperature regulation is mediated primarily by the hypothalamus. Peripheral thermoreceptors in the skin and central thermoreceptors in the hypothalamus, spinal cord, abdominal organs, and other central locations provide the hypothalamus with information about skin and core temperatures. If these temperatures are low, the hypothalamus triggers heat production and heat conservation mechanisms. The endocrine system also operates in increased heat production. The heat-producing mechanism begins with hypothalamic thyrotropin-stimulating hormone-releasing hormone (TSH-RH), which stimulates the anterior pituitary to release thyroid-stimulating hormone (TSH), which acts on the thyroid gland stimulating release of thyroxine. This hormone then acts on the adrenal medulla causing the release of epinephrine into the bloodstream. Epinephrine causes vasoconstriction, stimulates glycolysis, and increases metabolic rates thus increasing heat production.[22]

The hypothalamus also triggers heat conservation by stimulating the sympathetic nervous system, which stimulates the adrenal cortex increasing skeletal muscle tone, initiating the shivering response and producing vasoconstriction. The hypothalamus relays information to the cerebral cortex about cold, and voluntary responses result, such as increased body movement. The hypothalamus responds to warmer core and peripheral temperatures by reversing the same mechanisms.

Mechanisms of heat production and loss

Body heat is produced by the chemical reactions of metabolism, skeletal muscle tone and contraction, and chemical thermogenesis. Heat is distributed by the circulatory system. Heat loss is achieved through (1) radiation, (2) conduction, (3) convection, (4) vasodilation, (5) decreased muscle tone, (6) evaporation, (7) increased respiration, (8) voluntary measures, and (9) adaptation to warmer climates. For further explanation, see Table 13-5.

Mechanisms of heat conservation

The body conserves heat and protects core temperature through two important mechanisms: (1) involuntary vasoconstriction and (2) voluntary mechanisms. By constricting peripheral blood vessels, centrally warmed blood is shunted away from the periphery to the core of the body, where heat can be retained. This involuntary mechanism takes advantage of the insulating layers of the skin and subcutaneous

TABLE 13-5
Mechanisms of Heat Production and Loss

Condition	Description
HEAT PRODUCTION	
Chemical reactions of metabolism	Occur during ingestion and metabolism of food and while maintaining the body at rest (basal metabolism); occur in body core (liver)
Skeletal muscle contraction	Gradual increase in muscle tone or rapid muscle oscillations (shivering)
Chemical thermogenesis	Epinephrine is released and produces rapid, transient increase in heat production by raising basal metabolic rate; quick, brief effect that counters heat lost through conduction and convection; involves brown adipose tissue, which decreases markedly in older adults. Thyroid hormone increases metabolism.
HEAT LOSS	
Radiation	Heat loss through electromagnetic waves emanating from surfaces with temperature higher than the surrounding air
Conduction	Heat loss by direct molecule-to-molecule transfer from one surface to another, so that warmer surface loses heat to cooler surface
Convection	Transfer of heat through currents of gases or liquids; exchanges warmer air at body's surface with cooler air in surrounding space
Vasodilation	Diverts core-warmed blood to surface of body, with heat transferred by conduction to skin surface and from there to the surrounding environment; occurs in response to autonomic stimulation under control of hypothalamus
Decreased muscle tone	Washed out feeling caused by moderately reduced muscle tone and curtailed voluntary muscle activity
Evaporation	Body water evaporates from surface of skin and linings of mucous membranes; major source of heat reduction connected with increased sweating in warmer surroundings
Increased respiration	Air is exchanged with environment through normal process; minimal effect
Voluntary mechanisms	"Stretching out" and "slowing down" in response to high body temperatures, increasing the body surface area available for heat loss; dressing in light-colored, loose-fitting garments
Adaptation to warmer climates	Gradual process beginning with lassitude, weakness, and faintness, proceeding through increased sweating, lowered sodium content, decreased heart rate, increased stroke volume and extracellular fluid volume, and terminating in improved warm weather functioning and decreased symptoms of heat intolerance (work output, endurance, and coordination increase, and subjective feelings of discomfort decrease)

fat to protect core temperature. Chemical thermogenesis is produced by the release of thyroxine and epinephrine that increase metabolism.[23]

In response to lower body temperatures, individuals typically bundle up, keep moving, or curl up in a ball. These types of voluntary physical activity provide insulation, increase skeletal muscle activity, and decrease the amount of skin surface available for heat loss through radiation, convection, and conduction.[24] Muscle shivering also increases heat production.

Temperature Regulation in Infants and Elderly Persons

Infants and elderly persons require special attention to maintenance of body temperature. Infants produce sufficient body heat, primarily through metabolism of brown fat, but cannot conserve heat produced because of their small body size, greater ratio of body surface to body weight, and inability to shiver. Infants also have little subcutaneous fat and thus are not as well insulated as adults.[25] Elderly persons respond poorly to environmental temperature extremes because of their slowed blood circulation, structural and functional skin changes, and overall decreased heat-producing activities. In addition, they have a decreased shivering response (delayed onset and decreased effectiveness), slowed metabolic rate, decreased vasoconstrictor response, diminished or absent sweating, decreased peripheral sensation, desynchronized circadian rhythm, decreased perception of heat and cold, decreased thirst, undernutrition, and decreased brown adipose tissue.[26,27]

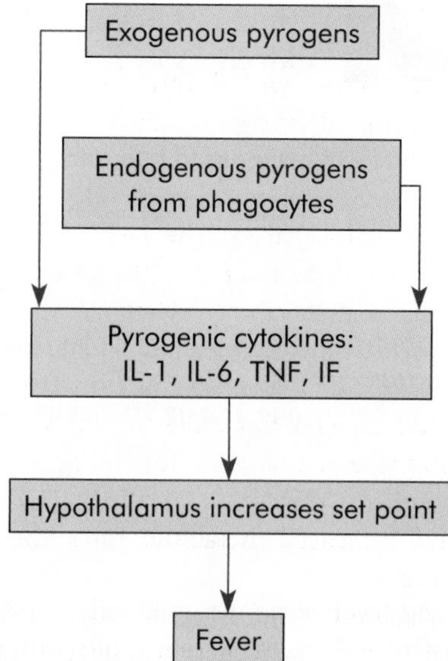

Figure 13-5 ■ **Production of Fever.** When monocytes/macrophages are activated, they secrete endogenous pyrogenic cytokines such as interleukin-1 (IL-1), interleukin-6 (IL-6) , tumor necrosis factor (TNF) and interferon (IF) which reach the hypothalamic temperature-regulating center. These cytokines promote the synthesis and secretion of prostaglandin E_2 (PGE_2) in the anterior hypothalamus. PGE_2 increases the thermostatic set point, and the autonomic nervous system is stimulated, resulting in shivering, muscle contraction, and peripheral vasoconstriction. (Adapted from Lewis SM, Heitkemper MM, Dirksen SR: *Medical-surgical nursing: assessment and management of clinical problems,* ed 5, St Louis, 2000, Mosby.)

Pathogenesis of Fever

Fever (febrile response) is a temporary "resetting of the hypothalamic thermostat" to a higher level in response to endogenous or exogenous pyrogens. The thermoregulatory mechanisms adjust heat production, conservation, and loss to maintain body core temperature at a normal level. During fever, this level is raised so that the thermoregulatory center now adjusts heat production, conservation, and loss to maintain the core temperature at the new, higher temperature, which functions as a new set point.[28] **Exogenous pyrogens,** or endotoxins produced by pathogens (see Chapter 7) (Figure 13-5), stimulate the release of substances such as tumor necrosis factor-alpha (TNF-α), interleukin-1 (IL-1), interleukin-6 (IL-6), and interferon (IF), which raise the set point by inducing the synthesis of prostaglandins. In response, the hypothalamus signals an increase in heat production and conservation to raise body temperature to the new level. The individual feels colder, dresses more warmly, decreases body surface area by curling up, and may go to bed in an effort to get warm. Body temperature is maintained at the new level until the fever "breaks," when the set point begins to return to normal. This response is mediated in part by cytokines associated with the inflammatory response.[29] There are decreased heat production and increased heat reduction mechanisms. The individual feels very warm, dons cooler clothes, throws off the covers, and stretches out. Once the body has returned to a normal temperature the individual feels more comfortable and the hypothalamus adjusts thermoregulatory mechanisms to maintain the new temperature.

Benefits of Fever

Fever helps the body respond to infectious processes through several mechanisms[30,31]:

1. Simple raising of body temperature kills many microorganisms and adversely affects their growth and replication.
2. Higher body temperatures decrease serum levels of iron, zinc, and copper—minerals needed for bacterial replication.
3. Increased temperature causes lysosomal breakdown and autodestruction of cells, preventing viral replication in infected cells.
4. Heat increases lymphocytic transformation and motility of polymorphonuclear neutrophils, facilitating the immune response.
5. Phagocytosis is enhanced, and production of antiviral interferon is augmented.

Suppression of fever by treatment with antipyrogenic medications should be used only if a fever produces or is high enough to produce serious side effects, such as cardiovascular stress nerve damage or convulsion.[32]

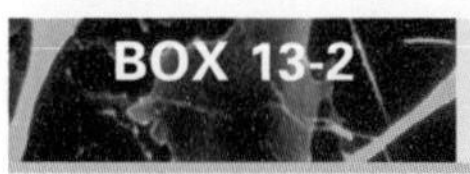

BOX 13-2 Effects of Fever at the Extremes of Age

Elderly Persons

Decreased or no fever response to infection so benefits are decreased

High morbidity and mortality result from lack of beneficial aspects

Children

Develop higher temperatures than adults for relatively minor infections

Febrile seizures before age 5 years are not uncommon

Infection and fever responses in elderly persons and children may vary from those in normal adults. Box 13-2 lists the principal features associated with fever at these extremes of age.[33]

Disorders of Temperature Regulation

Hyperthermia

Hyperthermia (marked warming of core temperature) can produce nerve damage, coagulation of cell proteins, and death. At 41° C (105.8° F), nerve damage produces convulsions in the adult. Death results at 43° C (109.4° F). Hyperthermia is not mediated by pyrogens and the hypothalamic set point is not reset. Hyperthermia may be therapeutic, accidental, or associated with stroke or head trauma. Prevention of hyperthermia in stroke and head trauma assists in limiting brain injury.[34] Therapeutic hyperthermia, a controversial therapy, is a form of local or general body-induced hyperthermia used to destroy pathologic microorganisms or tumor cells by facilitating the host's natural immune process or tumor blood flow.[35] The four forms of accidental hyperthermia are summarized as follows[36]:

1. **Heat cramps**—severe, spasmodic cramps in the abdomen and extremities that follow prolonged sweating and associated sodium loss. Usually occur in those not accustomed to heat or those performing strenuous work in very warm climates. Symptoms include fever, rapid pulse, and increased blood pressure.
2. **Heat exhaustion**—results from prolonged high core or environmental temperatures, which cause profound vasodilation and profuse sweating, leading to dehydration, decreased plasma volumes, hypotension, decreased cardiac output, and tachycardia. Symptoms include weakness, dizziness, confusion, nausea, and fainting.
3. **Heat stroke**—a potentially lethal result of overstressed thermoregulatory center. With very high core temperatures (≥40° C), the regulatory center ceases to function and the body's heat loss mechanisms fail. Symptoms include cerebral edema, degeneration of the CNS, swollen dendrites, renal tubular necrosis, and eventually death if treatment is not undertaken.
4. **Malignant hyperthermia**—a potentially lethal complication of a rare inherited muscle disorder that may be triggered by inhaled anesthetics and depolarizing muscle relaxants.[37] The syndrome involves altered calcium function in muscle cells with hypermetabolism, uncoordinated muscle contractions, increased muscle work, increased oxygen consumption, and a raised level of lactic acid production. Acidosis develops, and body temperature rises, with resulting tachycardia and cardiac dysrhythmias, hypotension, decreased cardiac output, and cardiac arrest. Symptoms resemble those of coma—unconsciousness, absent reflexes, fixed pupils, apnea, and a flat electroencephalogram (sometimes). Oliguria and anuria are common. It is most common in children and adolescents.

Hypothermia

Hypothermia (marked cooling of core temperature) produces depression of the central nervous and respiratory systems, vasoconstriction, alterations in microcirculation, coagulation, and ischemic tissue damage. Most tissues can tolerate low temperatures in controlled situations, such as surgery. However, in severe hypothermia, ice crystals form on the inside of the cell, causing cells to rupture and die. Tissue hypothermia slows cell metabolism, increases the blood viscosity, slows microcirculatory blood flow, facilitates blood coagulation, and stimulates profound vasoconstriction. Hypothermia may be accidental or therapeutic (Box 13-3).

Trauma and temperature

Major body trauma can affect temperature regulation through various mechanisms. Damage to the CNS, inflammation, increased intracranial pressures, or intracranial bleeding typically produces a fever of greater than 39° C (102.2° F). This sustained temperature, often referred to as a "central fever," appears with or without bradycardia. A central fever does not induce sweating and is very resistant to antipyretic therapy.

Other traumatic mechanisms that produce temperature alterations include accidental injuries, hemorrhagic shock, major surgery, and thermal burns. The severity and type of alteration (hyperthermia or hypothermia) vary with the severity of the cause and the body system affected.

QUICK CHECK 13-2

1. Why is temperature regulation important?
2. What are the principal heat production methods? Heat loss methods?
3. How does the hypothalamus alter its set point to change body temperature?
4. Compare and contrast hyperthermia and hypothermia and their effects on the body.

BOX 13-3 Defining Characteristics of Hypothermia

Accidental Hypothermia*

- Results from sudden immersion in cold water or prolonged exposure to cold environments
- Especially common among young and elderly persons, who have altered thermoregulatory mechanisms
- Factors that increase risk:
  1. Hypothyroidism
  2. Hypopituitarism
  3. Malnutrition
  4. Parkinson disease
  5. Rheumatoid arthritis
  6. Chronic increased vasodilation
  7. Decreased thermoregulatory control resulting from cerebral injury, ketoacidosis, uremia, and drug overdose
- Mechanisms
  1. Peripheral vasoconstriction—shunts blood away from cooler skin to core to decrease heat loss and produces peripheral tissue ischemia
  2. Intermittent reperfusion of extremities (Lewis phenomenon) helps preserve peripheral oxygenation until core temperature drops dramatically
  3. Hypothalamic center induces shivering; thinking becomes sluggish, and coordination is depressed
  4. Stupor; heart rate and respiratory rate decline; cardiac output diminishes; metabolic rate falls; acidosis; eventual ventricular fibrillation and asystole
- Treatment
  1. Passive rewarming for mild cases
  2. Core temperature greater than 30° C (86° F)—active rewarming (external)
  3. Core temperature less than 30° C (86° F) or with severe cardiovascular problems—active core rewarming (internal)

Therapeutic Hypothermia[†‡]

- Used to slow metabolism and preserve ischemic tissue during surgery, limb reimplantation, or neurologic emergencies
- Effects and cautions
  1. Stresses the heart, leading to ventricular fibrillation and cardiac arrest (may be desired outcome in open heart surgery when heart must be stopped)
  2. Exhausts liver glycogen stores by prolonged shivering
  3. Surface cooling may cause burns, frostbite, and fat necrosis
  4. May increase risk of pneumonia
  5. Slows drug metabolism

*From Wittmers LE Jr: Pathophysiology of cold exposure, *Minn Med* 84(11):30-36, 2001.
†From Gadkary CS, Alderson P, Signorini DF: Therapeutic hypothermia for head injury, *Cochrane Database System Review* (2)CD001048, 2000.
‡Insler SR, Sessler DI: Perioperative thermoregulation and temperature monitoring, *Anesthesiol Clin* 24(4):823-837, 2006.

SLEEP

Sleep is a temporary state of restful unconsciousness with spontaneous arousal. Normal sleep has two phases that can be documented by electroencephalogram (EEG): rapid eye movement (REM) sleep and slow wave (non-REM) sleep. Non-REM sleep is further divided into four stages (I-IV) from light to deep sleep.[38]

REM (rapid eye movement) sleep is initiated by *REM-on* and *REM-off* neurons in the pons and mesencephalon. REM sleep occurs about every 90 minutes beginning 1 to 2 hours after non-REM sleep begins. This sleep is known as *paradoxical sleep* because the EEG pattern is similar to the normal awake pattern and the brain is very active. REM and non-REM sleep alternate throughout the night, with lengthening intervals of REM sleep and fewer intervals of deeper stages of non-REM sleep toward morning. The changes associated with REM sleep include increased parasympathetic activity and variable sympathetic activity associated with rapid eye movement; muscle relaxation; loss of temperature regulation; altered heart rate, blood pressure, and respiration; penile erection in men and clitoral engorgement in women; release of steroids; and many memorable dreams. Respiratory control appears largely independent of metabolic requirements and oxygen variation. Loss of normal voluntary muscle control in the tongue and upper pharynx may produce some respiratory obstruction. Cerebral blood flow increases. About 20% to 25% of sleep time is represented by REM sleep in the adult.

Non-REM sleep (NREM) accounts for 75% to 80% of sleep time in adults and is initiated when inhibitory signals are released from the hypothalamus. Sympathetic tone is decreased and parasympathetic activity is increased during NREM sleep that creates a state of reduced activity. The basal metabolic rate falls by 10% to 15%; temperature decreases 0.5° to 1.0° C (0.9° to 1.8° F); heart rate, respiration, blood pressure, and muscle tone decrease; and knee jerk reflexes are absent. Pupils are constricted. During the various stages, cerebral blood flow to the brain decreases and growth hormone is released, with corticosteroid and catecholamine levels depressed. Box 13-4 summarizes sleep characteristics in infants and elderly persons.

Sleep is an active multiphase process with complex neural circuits, interacting hormones, and neurotransmitters involving the hypothalamus, thalamus, brainstem, and cortex. The hypothalamus is a major sleep center and the hypocretins (orexins) are neuropeptides secreted by the hypothalamus that promote wakefulness. Prostaglandin D_2, adenosine, melatonin, serotonin, L-tryptophan, and growth factors promote sleep.[39–41] The pontine reticular formation is primarily responsible for generating REM sleep, and projections from the thalamocortical network produce non-REM sleep.[42]

Sleep Disorders

The classification of sleep disorders is complex and a system has been established by the American Academy of Sleep Medicine and includes four classifications: (1) dyssomnias

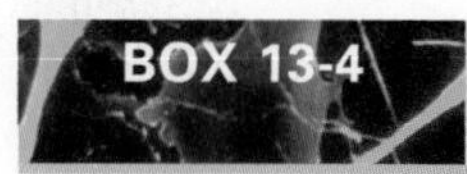

Sleep Characteristics of Infants and Elderly Persons

Infants

Sleep 16 to 17 hours per day; one half in REM sleep, one fourth in an indeterminate phase

Infant sleep cycles are 50 to 60 minutes in length; 20 minutes non-REM and 10 to 45 minutes of REM sleep

At 1 year, total sleep time decreases with about equal time in REM and non-REM sleep

Elderly Persons

Total sleep time is decreased with a longer time to fall asleep and poorer quality sleep

Total time in slow wave and final phase of non-REM sleep decreases by 15% to 30%

Alterations in sleep patterns occur about 10 years later in women than men

Sleep disordered breathing is common in the elderly

Older adults are less able to tolerate sleep deprivation than younger adults

Data from Anders TF, Keener M: Developmental course of nighttime sleep-wake patterns in full-term and premature infants during the first year of life, *Sleep* 8(3):173-192, 1985; Martin M, Shochat T, Ancoli-Israel S: Assessment and treatment of sleep disturbances in older adults, *Clin Psychol Rev* 20(6):783-805, 2000.

(disorders of initiating and maintaining sleep and disorders of excessive sleepiness), (2) parasomnias (disorders that primarily do not cause a complaint of insomnia or excessive sleepiness), (3) sleep disorders associated with medical/psychiatric disorders, and (4) proposed sleep disorders.[43] The most common dyssomnias and parasomnias are presented here.

Common dyssomnias

Insomnia

Insomnia is the inability to fall or stay asleep and may be mild, moderate, or severe. It may be transient, lasting a few days, and related to travel across time zones or caused by acute stress. Long-term insomnia can be idiopathic starting at an early age or associated with drug or alcohol abuse, chronic pain disorders, chronic depression, the use of certain drugs, obesity, and aging.[44]

Sleep disordered breathing

Obstructive sleep apnea syndrome generally results from upper airway obstruction recurring during sleep with excessive snoring and multiple apneic episodes that last 10 seconds or longer. The periodic breathing eventually produces arousal, which interrupts the sleep cycle, reducing total sleep time and producing sleep and REM deprivation.[45] Associated conditions include obesity, decreased sensitivity to carbon dioxide and oxygen tensions, and upper airway obstruction. Sleep apnea produces low oxygen saturation and eventually leads to polycythemia, pulmonary hypertension, right-sided congestive heart failure, liver congestion, cyanosis, and peripheral edema.[46] Systemic hypertension can be a response to repeated episodes of apnea and hypoxemia.[47] Cardiac dysrhythmias during sleep apnea are common. Treatments include nasal continuous positive airway pressure and dental devices, upper airway and jaw surgeries in selected individuals, and management of obesity.[48] Adenotonsillar hypertrophy is the major cause of obstructive sleep apnea in children and tonsillectomy and adenoidectomy are the treatments of choice.[49]

Primary hypersomnia (excessive daytime sleepiness) is an idiopathic disorder with an unknown etiology. Individuals may fall asleep while driving a car, working, or even while conversing,[50] with significant concerns for safety. Treatment is symptomatic with reinforcement of good sleeping habits. **Secondary hypersomnia** may be related to sleep disordered breathing and psychologic depression.

Disorders of the sleep-wake schedule

Common disorders of the sleep-wake schedule (circadian rhythm disorders) include rapid time-zone change (or jet-lag syndrome), changing sleep schedule involving 3 hours or more in sleep time, or changing total sleep time from day to day. These changes desynchronize circadian rhythm, which can depress the degree of vigilance, performance of psychomotor tasks, and arousal.[51]

Common parasomnias

Parasomnias are unusual behaviors occurring during sleep.[52] These behaviors include sleepwalking, night terrors, rearranging furniture, eating food, violent behavior, and restless leg syndrome. Sleepwalking and night terrors are discussed next. Information on restless leg syndrome is contained in Box 13-5.

Two dysfunctions of sleep (somnambulism and night terrors) are common in children and may be related to central nervous system immaturity. **Somnambulism (sleepwalking)** is a disorder primarily of childhood and appears to resolve within a few years. Sleepwalking is therefore not associated with dreaming, and the child has no memory of the event on awakening. Sleepwalking in adults is often associated with sleep disordered breathing.[53] **Night**

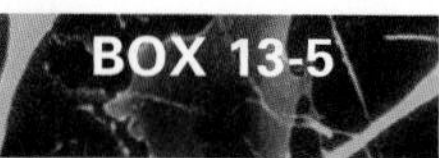

Restless Leg Syndrome (RLS)

A sensorimotor disorder associated with unpleasant sensations (prickling, tingling, or crawling) at rest and a compelling urge to move the legs for relief with a significant effect on sleep and quality of life

More common in women and the elderly

Associated with dopaminergic dysfunction, brain and spinal cord iron metabolism, abnormalities in supraspinal inhibition; may have a genetic origin

Dopamine agonists are used for treatment

Data from Winkelman JW: Considering the causes of RLS, *Eur J Neurol* 13(suppl 3):8-14, 2006.

terrors are characterized by sudden apparent arousals in which the child expresses intense fear or emotion. However, the child is not awake and can be difficult to arouse. Once awakened, the child has no memory of the night terror event. Night terrors are not associated with dreams. Although this problem occurs most often in children, adults also may experience it with corresponding daytime anxiety.

✔ QUICK CHECK 13-3

1. Describe REM and non-REM sleep.
2. What is the major difference between the dyssomnias and parasomnias?

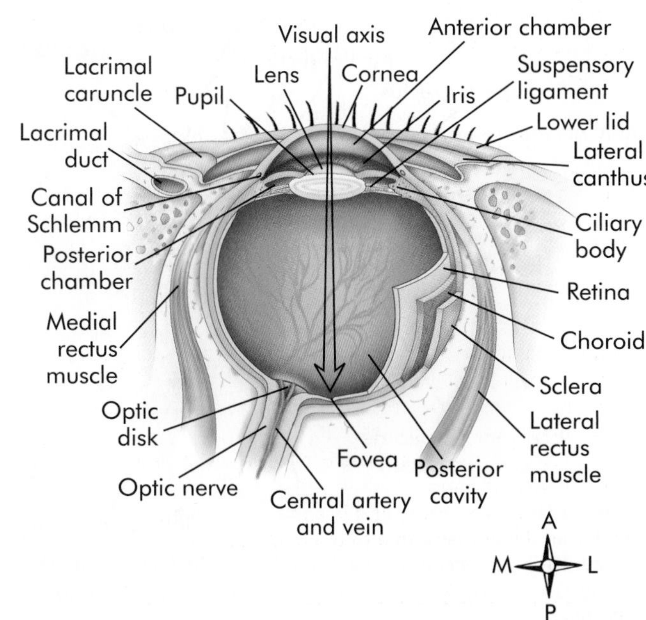

Figure 13-6 ■ Internal Anatomy of the Eye. (From Thibodeau GA, Patton KT: *Anatomy & physiology,* ed 6, St Louis, 2007, Mosby.)

THE SPECIAL SENSES

Vision

The eyes are complex sense organs responsible for vision. Within a protective casing, each eye has receptors, a lens system for focusing light on the receptors, and a system of nerves for conducting impulses from the receptors to the brain.[54] Visual dysfunction may be caused by abnormal ocular movements or alterations in visual acuity, refraction, color vision, or accommodation. Visual dysfunction also may be the secondary effect of another neurologic disorder.

The eye and its external structures

The wall of the eye is formed of three layers: (1) sclera, (2) choroid, and (3) retina (Figure 13-6). The **sclera** is the thick, white, outermost layer. It becomes transparent at the **cornea**—the portion of the sclera in the central anterior region that allows light to enter the eye. The choroid is the deeply pigmented middle layer that prevents light from scattering inside the eye. The **iris,** part of the choroid, has a round opening, the **pupil,** through which light passes. Smooth muscle fibers control the size of the pupil so that it adjusts to bright light or dim light and close or distant vision.

The innermost layer of the eye, the **retina,** contains millions of rods and cones—special photoreceptors that convert light energy into nerve impulses. **Rods** mediate peripheral and dim light vision and are densest at the periphery. **Cones,** densest in the center of the retina, are color and detail receptors. There are no photoreceptors where the optic nerve leaves the eyeball; this creates the **optic disc,** or blind spot. Lateral to each optic disc is the **fovea centralis**—a tiny area within the macula lutea that contains only cones and provides the greatest visual acuity (see Figure 13-6).

As shown in Figure 13-10 (p. 321), nerve impulses pass through the optic nerves to the optic chiasm. The nerves from the inner (nasal) halves of the retinas cross to the opposite side and join fibers from the outer (temporal) halves of the retinas to form the optic tracts. The fibers of the optic tracts synapse in the dorsal lateral geniculate nucleus and pass by way of the optic radiation (or geniculocalcarine tract) to the primary visual cortex in the occipital lobe of the brain.[55] Light entering the eye is focused on the retina by the **lens**—a flexible, biconvex, crystal-like structure. With age the lens becomes increasingly hard and opaque. The lens divides the anterior chamber into (1) the aqueous chamber and (2) the vitreous chamber. **Aqueous humor** fills the aqueous chamber and helps maintain pressure inside the eye, as well as provide nutrients to the lens and cornea. Aqueous humor is secreted by the ciliary processes and reabsorbed into the canal of Schlemm. If drainage is blocked, intraocular pressure increases (causing glaucoma). The vitreous chamber is filled with a gel-like substance called **vitreous humor.** Vitreous humor helps to prevent the eyeball from collapsing inward.

The central retinal artery provides blood to the inner retinal surface, and the choroid supplies nutrients to the outer surface of the retina. Six extrinsic eye muscles allow gross eye movements and permit eyes to follow a moving object (Figure 13-7).

The external structures protecting the eye include the eyelids (palpebrae), conjunctiva, and lacrimal apparatus (Figure 13-8). The eyelids are used to control the amount of light reaching the eyes, and the conjunctiva lines the eyelids. Tears released from the lacrimal apparatus bathe the surface of the eye and prevent friction, maintain hydration, and wash out foreign bodies and other irritants.

Visual dysfunction

Alterations in ocular movements

Abnormal ocular movements result from oculomotor, trochlear, or abducens cranial nerve dysfunction (see

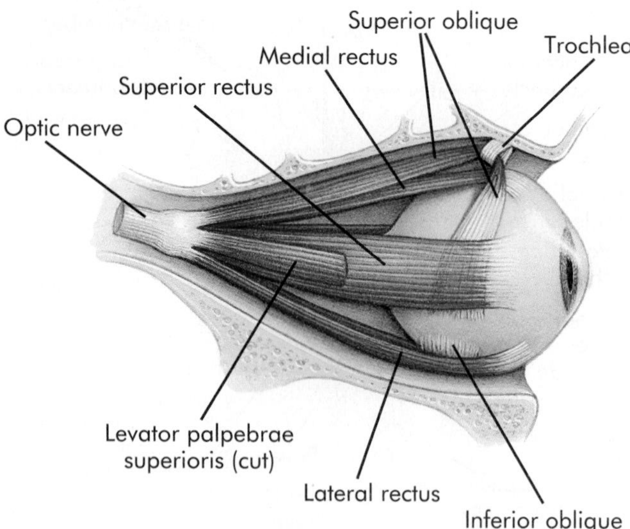

Figure 13-7 ■ **Extrinsic Muscles of the Right Eye.** (From Thibodeau GA, Patton KT: *Anatomy & physiology,* ed 6, St Louis, 2007, Mosby.)

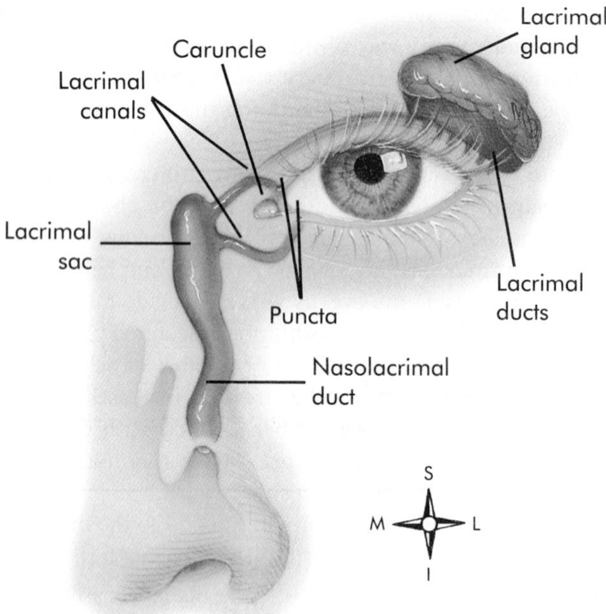

Figure 13-8 ■ **Lacrimal Apparatus.** Fluid produced by lacrimal glands (tears) streams across the eye surface, enters the canals, and then passes through the nasolacrimal duct to enter the nose. (From Thibodeau GA, Patton KT: *Anatomy & physiology,* ed 6, St Louis, 2007, Mosby.)

Table 12-6). The three types of eye movement disorders are (1) strabismus, (2) nystagmus, and (3) paralysis of individual extraocular muscles.

In **strabismus,** one eye deviates from the other when the person is looking at an object. This is caused by a weak or hypertonic muscle in one eye. The deviation may be upward, downward, inward (entropia), or outward (exotropia). Strabismus in children requires early intervention to prevent **amblyopia** (reduced vision in the affected eye caused by cerebral blockage of the visual stimuli). The primary symptom of strabismus is **diplopia** (double vision). Causes of strabismus include neuromuscular disorder of the eye muscle, diseases involving the cerebral hemispheres, or thyroid disease.

Nystagmus is an involuntary unilateral or bilateral rhythmic movement of the eyes. It may be present at rest or when the eye moves. **Pendular nystagmus** is characterized by a regular to-and-fro movement of the eyes. In **jerk nystagmus,** one phase of the eye movement is faster than the other. Nystagmus may be caused by an imbalanced reflex activity of the inner ear, vestibular nuclei, cerebellum, medial longitudinal fascicle, or nuclei of the oculomotor, trochlear, and abducens cranial nerves (see Table 12-6 and Figure 12-22). Drugs, retinal disease, and diseases involving the cervical cord also may produce nystagmus.

Paralysis of specific extraocular muscles may cause limited abduction, abnormal closure of the eyelid, ptosis (drooping of the eyelid), or diplopia (double vision) as a result of unopposed muscle activity. Trauma or pressure in the area of the cranial nerves or diseases such as diabetes mellitus and myasthenia gravis also paralyze specific extraocular muscles.

Alterations in visual acuity

Visual acuity is the ability to see objects in sharp detail. With advancing age, the lens of the eye becomes less flexible and adjusts slowly. In addition, the sclera changes shape, so that light falls on the macula. Thus, visual acuity declines with age. Table 13-6 contains a summary of changes in the eye caused by aging. Specific causes of visual acuity changes are (1) amblyopia, (2) scotoma, (3) cataracts, (4) papilledema, (5) dark adaptation, (6) glaucoma, (7) retinal detachment, and (8) macular degeneration (Table 13-7). **Glaucoma** is characterized by intraocular pressures greater than 12 to 20 mm Hg. There are three primary types of glaucoma:[56]

1. *Open angle.* Outflow obstruction of aqueous humor at trabecular meshwork or canal of Schlemm although there is adequate space for drainage; often is an inherited disease and a leading cause of blindness with few preliminary symptoms
2. *Angle closure.* Displacement of the iris toward the cornea with obstruction of the trabecular meshwork and obstruction of outflow of aqueous humor from the anterior chamber; may occur acutely with a sudden rise in intraocular pressure causing pain and visual disturbances
3. *Congenital closure.* A rare disease associated with congenital malformations and other genetic anomalies

Age-related macular degeneration (AMD) is a severe and irreversible loss of vision and a major cause of blindness in older individuals. Hypertension, cigarette smoking, and diabetes mellitus are risk factors. The degeneration

TABLE 13-6

Changes in the Eye Caused by Aging

Structure	Change	Consequence
Cornea	Thicker and less curved Formation of a gray ring at the edge of the cornea (arcus senilis)	Increase in astigmatism Not detrimental to vision
Anterior chamber	Decrease in size and volume caused by thickening of lens	Occasionally exerts pressure on Schlemm canal and may lead to increased intraocular pressure and glaucoma
Lens	Increase in opacity	Decrease in refraction with increased light scattering (blurring) and decreased color vision (green and blue); can lead to cataracts
Ciliary muscles	Reduction in pupil diameter, atrophy of radial dilation muscles	Persistent constriction (senile miosis); decrease in critical flicker frequency*
Retina	Reduction in number of rods at periphery, loss of rods and associated nerve cells	Increase in minimum amount of light necessary to see an object

*The rate at which consecutive visual stimuli can be presented and still be perceived as separate.

TABLE 13-7

Causes of Visual Acuity Changes

Disorder	Description
Amblyopia	Reduced or dimmed vision, cause unknown Accompanies such diseases as diabetes mellitus, renal failure, and malaria and the use of drugs such as alcohol and tobacco
Scotoma	Circumscribed defect of central field of vision Often associated with retrobulbar neuritis and multiple sclerosis, compression of optic nerve by tumor, inflammation of optic nerve, pernicious anemia, methyl alcohol poisoning, and use of tobacco
Cataract	Cloudy or opaque area in ocular lens Incidence increases with age because most commonly a result of degeneration; other causes are congenital
Papilledema	Edema and inflammation of optic nerve where it enters eyeball Caused by obstruction of venous return from retina from one of three main sources: increased intracranial pressure, retrobulbar neuritis, or changes in retinal blood vessels
Dark adaptation	With age, the eye does not adapt as readily to dark Also, changes in the quantity and quality of rhodopsin are causative; vitamin A deficiencies can produce this at any age
Glaucoma	Increased intraocular pressures (above 12 to 20 mm Hg) Loss of acuity results from pressure on the optic nerve, which blocks the flow of nutrients to optic nerve fibers, leading to their death; sixth leading cause of blindness
Retinal detachment	A tear or break in the retina with accumulation of fluid and separation from underlying tissue. Seen as floaters, flashes of light, or a curtain over visual field. Risks include extreme myopia, diabetic retinopathy, sickle cell disease

usually occurs after the age of 60 years. There are two forms: atrophic (dry) and neovascular (wet). The atrophic form may include limited night vision and difficulty reading. The neovascular form includes abnormal blood vessel growth, leakage of blood or serum, retinal detachment, fibrovascular scarring, and loss of photoreceptors. The neovascular form causes more severe loss of central vision. The neovascular form is treated by laser photocoagulation; antiangiogenic drugs are being developed.[57]

Alterations in accommodation

Accommodation refers to changes in the thickness of the lens. Accommodation is needed for clear vision and is mediated through the oculomotor nerve. Pressure, inflammation, age, and disease of the oculomotor nerve may alter accommodation, causing diplopia, blurred vision, and headache.

Loss of accommodation with advancing age is termed **presbyopia,** a condition in which the ocular lens becomes larger, firmer, and less elastic. The major symptom is reduced near vision, causing the individual to hold reading material at arm's length. Treatment includes corrective forward, contact, and intraocular lenses.[58]

Alterations in refraction

Alterations in refraction are the most common visual problem. Causes include irregularities of the corneal curvature, the focusing power of the lens, and the length of the eye. The major symptoms of refraction alterations are blurred vision and headache. Three types of refraction are as follows (Figure 13-9):

Myopia—nearsightedness. Light rays are focused in front of the retina when the person is looking at a distant object.

Hyperopia—farsightedness. Light rays are focused behind the retina when a person is looking at a near object.

Astigmatism—unequal curvature of the cornea. Light rays are bent unevenly and do not come to a single focus on the retina. Astigmatism may coexist with myopia, hyperopia, or presbyopia.

Alterations in color vision

Normal sensitivity to color diminishes with age because of the progressive yellowing of the lens that occurs with aging. All colors become less intense, although color discrimination for blue and green is greatly affected. Color vision deteriorates more rapidly for individuals with diabetes mellitus than for the general population.

Abnormal color vision also may be caused by **color blindness,** an inherited trait. Color blindness affects 8% of the male population and 0.5% of the female population. Although many forms of color blindness exist, most commonly the affected individual cannot distinguish red from green.[59]

Neurologic disorders causing visual dysfunction

Vision may be disrupted at many points along the visual pathway, causing various defects in the visual field. Visual changes may cause defects or blindness in the entire visual field or in half of a visual field (hemianopia). (Figure 13-10 illustrates the many areas along the visual pathway that may be damaged and the associated visual changes.)

Injury to the optic nerve causes same-side blindness. Injury to the **optic chiasm** (the X-shaped crossing of the optic nerves) can cause various defects, depending on the location of the injury.

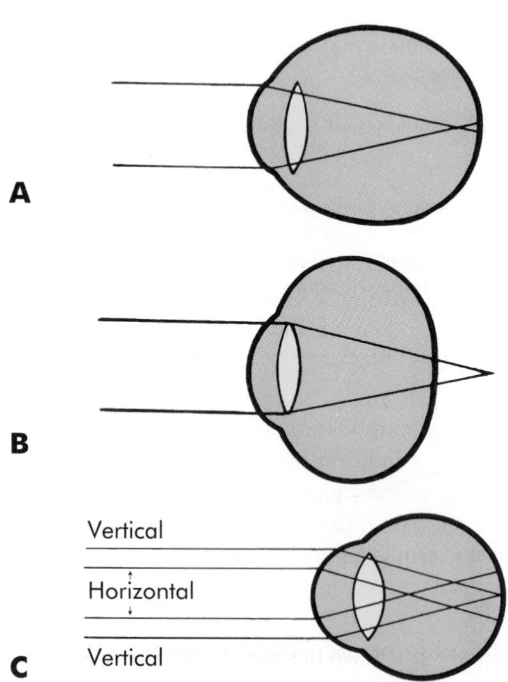

Figure 13-9 **Alterations in Refraction. A,** Myopic eye. Parallel rays of light are brought to a focus in front of the retina. **B,** Hyperopic eye. Parallel rays of light come to a focus behind the retina in the unaccommodative eye. **C,** Simple myopic astigmatism. The vertical bundle of rays is focused on the retina; the horizontal rays are focused in front of the retina. (From Stein HA, Slatt BJ, Stein RM: *The ophthalmic assistant: fundamentals and clinical practice,* ed 5, St Louis, 1998, Mosby.)

External eye structure disorders

Infection and inflammatory responses are the most common conditions affecting the supporting structures of the eyes. **Blepharitis** is an inflammation of the eyelids caused by staphylococcus or seborrheic dermatitis. A **hordeolum (stye)** is an infection of the sebaceous glands of the eyelids, and a **chalazion** is an infection of the meibomian (oil-secreting) gland. These conditions are treated symptomatically.

Conjunctivitis is an inflammation of the conjunctiva caused by bacteria, viruses, allergies, or chemical irritants.[60] **Acute bacterial conjunctivitis (pinkeye)** is highly contagious and often caused by *Staphylococcus, Haemophilus, Streptococcus pneumoniae,* and *Moraxella catarrhalis,* although other bacteria may be involved. In children younger than 6 years, *Haemophilus* infection often leads to otitis media (conjunctivitis-otitis syndrome). Preventing spread of the microorganism with meticulous handwashing and use of separate towels is important. The disease also is treated with antibiotics.

Viral conjunctivitis is caused by an adenovirus. Again, it is contagious, with symptoms of watering, redness, and photophobia. **Allergic conjunctivitis** is associated with a variety of antigens, including pollens. **Chronic conjunctivitis** results from any persistent conjunctivitis. **Trachoma** (chlamydial conjunctivitis) is caused by *Chlamydia trachomatis* and often is associated with poor hygiene. It is the leading cause of preventable blindness in the world.

Keratitis is an infection of the cornea caused by bacteria or viruses. Bacterial infections cause corneal ulceration, and type I herpes simplex virus can involve both the cornea and the conjunctiva. Severe ulcerations with residual scarring require corneal transplantation.

Hearing

The external auditory canal is surrounded by the bones of the cranium. The opening (meatus) of the canal is just above the **mastoid process.** The air-filled sinuses, called **mastoid air cells,** of the mastoid process promote conductivity of sound between the external and the middle ear.

The normal ear

The ear is divided into three areas: (1) the external ear, involved only with hearing; (2) the middle ear, involved only with hearing; and (3) the inner ear, involved with both hearing and equilibrium.

The external ear is composed of the **pinna** (auricle), which is the visible portion of the ear, and the **external auditory canal,** a tube that leads to the middle ear (Figure 13-11). Sound waves entering the external auditory

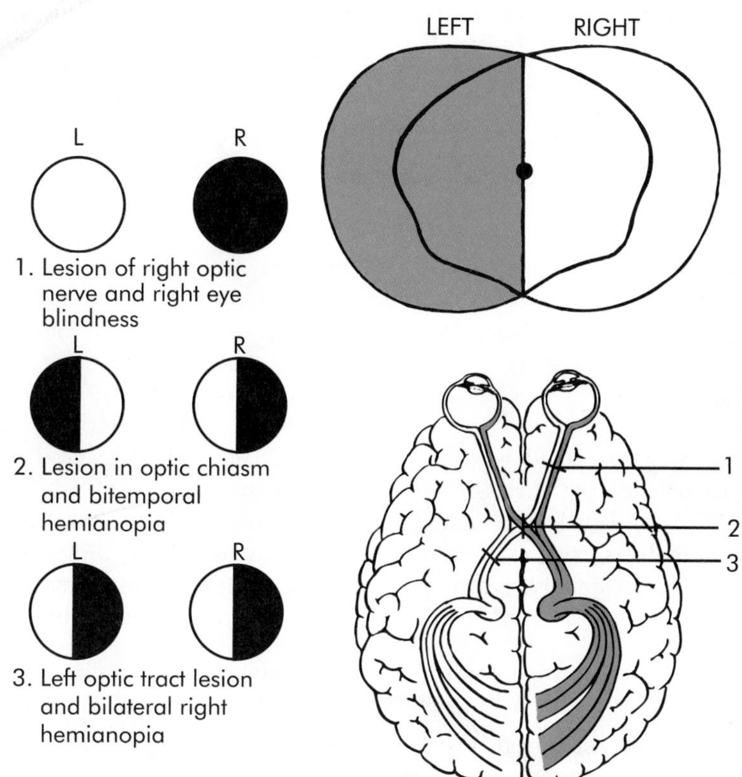

Figure 13-10 ■ **Visual Pathways and Defects.** (Modified from Thompson JM et al: *Mosby's clinical nursing,* ed 5, St Louis, 2002, Mosby.)

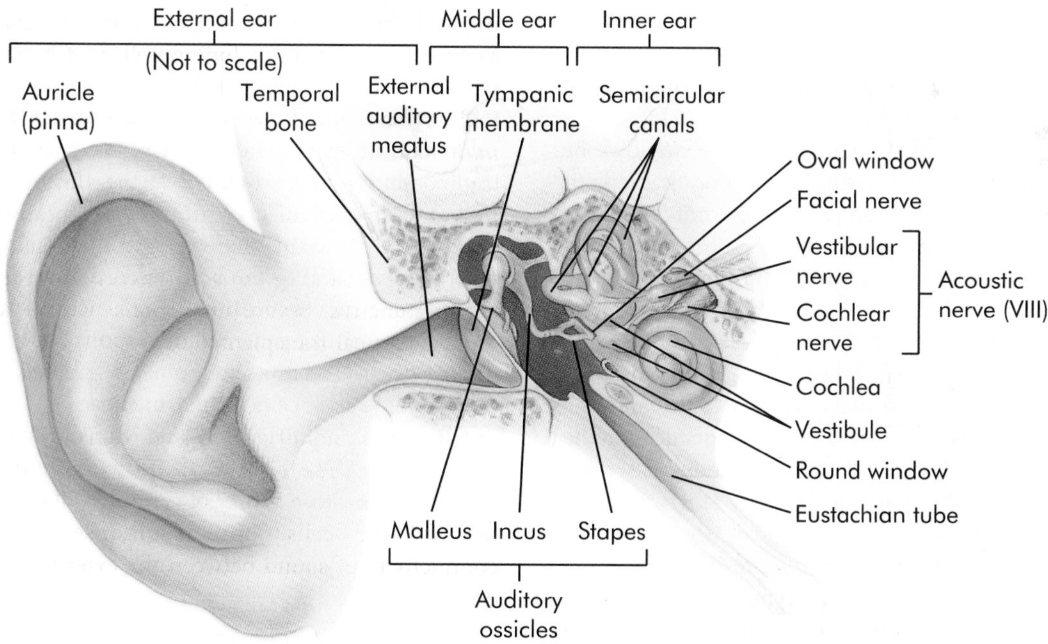

Figure 13-11 ■ **The Ear.** External, middle, and inner ears. (Anatomic structures are not drawn to scale.) (From Thibodeau GA, Patton KT: *Anatomy & physiology,* ed 6, St Louis, 2007, Mosby.)

canal hit the tympanic membrane (eardrum) and cause it to vibrate. The **tympanic membrane** separates the external ear from the middle ear.

The middle ear is composed of the **tympanic cavity,** a small chamber in the temporal bone. Three ossicles (small bones known as the **malleus [hammer], incus [anvil],** and **stapes [stirrup]**) transmit the vibration of the tympanic membrane to the inner ear. When the tympanic membrane moves, the malleus moves with it and transfers the vibration to the incus, which passes it on to the stapes. The

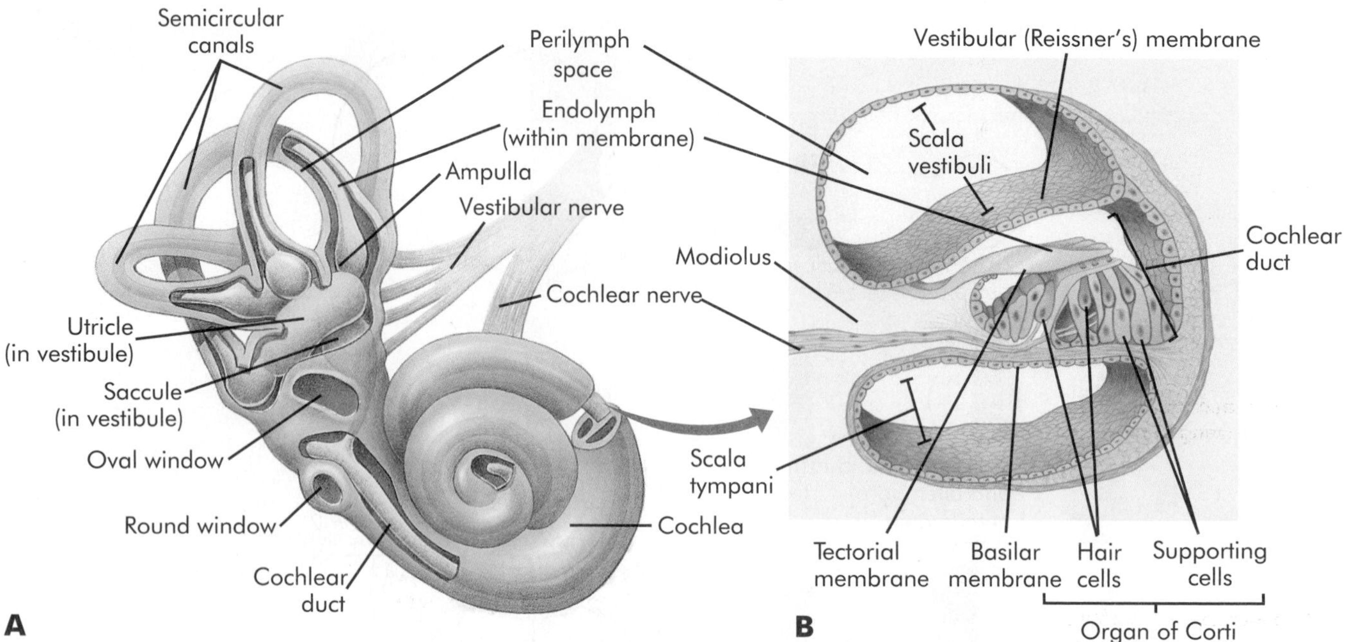

Figure 13-12 ■ **The Inner Ear. A,** The bony labyrinth *(orange)* is the hard outer wall of the entire inner ear and includes the semicircular canals, vestibule, and cochlea. Within the bony labyrinth is the membranous labyrinth *(purple),* which is surrounded by perilymph and filled with endolymph. Each ampulla in the vestibule contains a crista ampullaris that detects changes in head position and sends sensory impulses through the vestibular nerve to the brain. **B,** The inset shows a section of the membranous cochlea. Hair cells in the organ of Corti detect sound and send the information through the cochlear nerve. The vestibular and cochlear nerves join to form the eighth cranial nerve. (From Thibodeau GA, Patton KT: *Anatomy & physiology,* ed 6, St Louis, 2007, Mosby.)

stapes presses against the **oval window,** a small membrane of the inner ear. The movement of the oval window sets the fluids of the inner ear in motion (Figure 13-12).

The **eustachian (pharyngotympanic) tube** connects the middle ear with the thorax. Normally flat and closed, the eustachian tube opens briefly when a person swallows or yawns, and it equalizes the pressure in the middle ear with atmospheric pressure. Equalized pressure permits the tympanic membrane to vibrate freely. Through the eustachian tube the mucosa of the middle ear is continuous with the mucosal lining of the throat.

The inner ear is a system of osseous labyrinths (bony, mazelike chambers) filled with **perilymph.** The bony labyrinth is divided into the **cochlea,** the **vestibule,** and the **semicircular canals** (see Figure 13-11). Suspended in the perilymph is the endolymph-filled membranous labyrinth that basically follows the shape of the bony labyrinth.

Within the cochlea is the **organ of Corti,** which contains **hair cells** (hearing receptors). Sound waves that reach the cochlea through vibrations of the tympanic membrane, ossicles, and oval window set the cochlear fluids into motion. Receptor cells on the basilar membrane are stimulated when their hairs are bent or pulled by the movement. Once stimulated, hair cells transmit impulses along the cochlear nerve (a division of the vestibulocochlear nerve) to the auditory cortex of the temporal lobe in the brain (see Figure 13-12). There interpretation of the sound occurs.

The semicircular canals and vestibule of the inner ear contain **equilibrium receptors.** In the semicircular canals the dynamic equilibrium receptors respond to changes in direction of movement. Within each semicircular canal is the **crista ampullaris,** a receptor region composed of a tuft of hair cells covered by a gelatinous cupula. When the head is rotated, the endolymph in the canal lags behind and moves in the direction opposite to the head's movement. The hair cells are stimulated, and impulses are transmitted through the vestibular nerve (a division of the vestibulocochlear nerve) to the cerebellum.

The vestibule in the inner ear contains **maculae**—receptors essential to the body's sense of static equilibrium. As the head moves, **otoliths** (small pieces of calcium salts) move in a gel-like material in response to changes in the pull of gravity. The otoliths pull on the gel, which in turn pulls on the hair cells in the maculae. Nerve impulses in the hair cells are triggered and transmitted to the brain (see Figure 13-12). Thus, the ear not only permits the hearing of a large range of sounds but also assists with maintaining balance through the sensitive equilibrium receptors.

Auditory dysfunction

Between 5% and 10% of the general population have impaired hearing, and it is the most common sensory defect. The major categories of auditory dysfunction are conductive hearing loss, sensorineural hearing loss, mixed hearing loss, and functional hearing loss.[61] Hearing loss may range from mild to profound. Auditory changes caused by aging are common and incremental (see the *AGING & Changes in Hearing* box).

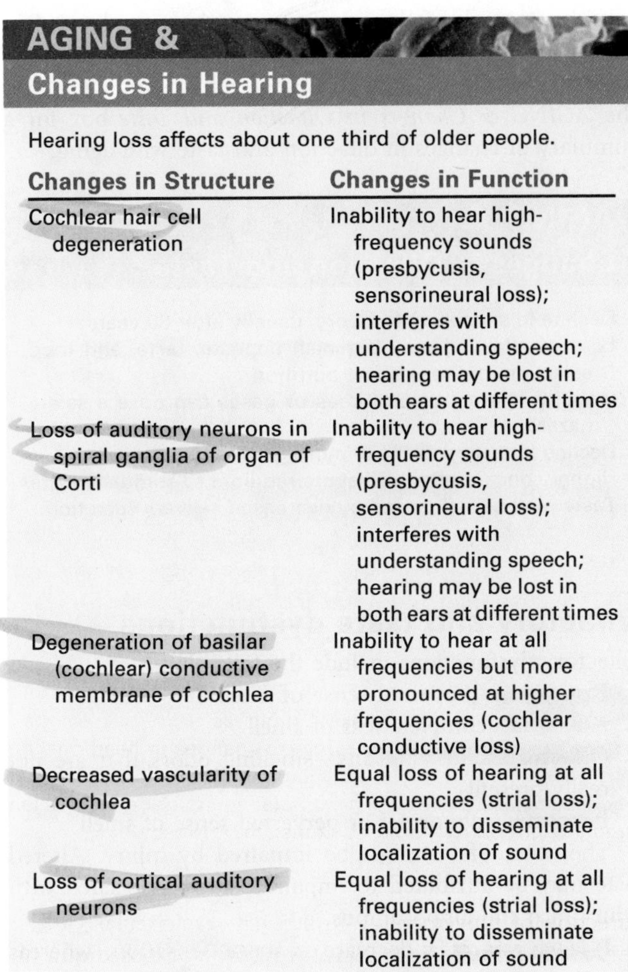

AGING &

Changes in Hearing

Hearing loss affects about one third of older people.

Changes in Structure	Changes in Function
Cochlear hair cell degeneration	Inability to hear high-frequency sounds (presbycusis, sensorineural loss); interferes with understanding speech; hearing may be lost in both ears at different times
Loss of auditory neurons in spiral ganglia of organ of Corti	Inability to hear high-frequency sounds (presbycusis, sensorineural loss); interferes with understanding speech; hearing may be lost in both ears at different times
Degeneration of basilar (cochlear) conductive membrane of cochlea	Inability to hear at all frequencies but more pronounced at higher frequencies (cochlear conductive loss)
Decreased vascularity of cochlea	Equal loss of hearing at all frequencies (strial loss); inability to disseminate localization of sound
Loss of cortical auditory neurons	Equal loss of hearing at all frequencies (strial loss); inability to disseminate localization of sound

Conductive hearing loss

A **conductive hearing loss** occurs when a change in the outer or middle ear impairs conduction of the sound from the outer to the inner ear. Conditions that commonly cause a conductive hearing loss include impacted cerumen, foreign bodies lodged in the ear canal, benign tumors of the middle ear, carcinoma of the external auditory canal or middle ear, eustachian tube dysfunction, otitis media, acute viral otitis media, chronic suppurative otitis media, cholesteatoma, and otosclerosis.

Symptoms of conductive hearing loss include diminished hearing and soft speaking voice. The voice is soft because often the individual hears his or her voice, conducted by bone, as loud.

Sensorineural hearing loss

A **sensorineural hearing loss** is caused by impairment of the organ of Corti or its central connections. The loss may occur gradually or suddenly. Conditions causing sensorineural loss include congenital and hereditary factors,[62] noise exposure, aging, Meniere disease, ototoxicity, systemic disease (syphilis, Paget disease, collagen diseases, diabetes mellitus), and neoplasms.[63] Congenital and neonatal sensorineural hearing loss may be caused by maternal rubella, ototoxic drugs, prematurity, traumatic delivery, erythroblastosis fetalis, and congenital hereditary malfunction. Diagnosis often is made when delayed speech development is noted.

Presbycusis is the most common form of sensorineural hearing loss and is especially common in elderly people. Its cause may be atrophy of the basal end of the organ of Corti, loss of auditory receptors, vascular changes, or stiffening of the basilar membranes. Drug ototoxicities (drugs that cause destruction of auditory function) have been observed after exposure to various chemicals; for example, antibiotics such as streptomycin, neomycin, gentamicin, and vancomycin; diuretics such as ethacrynic acid and furosemide; and chemicals such as salicylate, quinine, carbon monoxide, nitrogen mustard, arsenic, mercury, gold, tobacco, and alcohol. In most instances, the drugs and chemicals listed initially cause **tinnitus** (ringing in the ear), followed by a progressive high-tone sensorineural hearing loss that is permanent.

Mixed and functional hearing loss

A **mixed hearing loss** is caused by a combination of conductive and sensorineural losses. With **functional hearing loss,** which is rare, the individual does not respond to voice and appears not to hear. It is thought to be caused by emotional or psychologic factors.

Meniere disease

Meniere disease is a disorder of the middle ear with an unknown etiology. There is excessive endolymph and pressure in the membranous labyrinth that disrupts both vestibular and hearing functions. Recurring symptoms include profound vertigo, nausea and vomiting associated with deafness, and tinnitus (ringing in the ears). Treatment is symptomatic.[64]

Ear infections

Otitis externa

Otitis externa is the most common infection of the outer ear and may be acute or chronic.[65] The most common cause of acute infections are bacterial microorganisms including *Pseudomonas, Escherichia coli,* and *Staphylococcus aureus.* Fungal infections are less common. Infection usually follows prolonged exposure to moisture (swimmer's ear). The earliest symptoms are inflammation with pruritus, swelling and clear drainage progressing to purulent drainage with obstruction of the canal. Tenderness and pain with earlobe retraction accompany inflammation. Acidifying solutions are used for early treatment and topical antimicrobials usually provide effective treatment for later stages of disease.[66] Chronic infections are more often related to allergy or skin disorders.

Otitis media

Otitis media is the most common infection of infants and children.[67] Most children have one episode by 3 years of age. The most common pathogens are *Streptococcus pneu-*

moniae, Haemophilus influenzae, and *Moraxella catarrhalis.* Predisposing factors include allergy, sinusitis, submucous cleft palate, adenoidal hypertrophy, and immune deficiency. Breast-feeding is a protective factor. Recurrent acute otitis media may be genetically determined.[68]

Acute otitis media (AOM) is associated with ear pain, fever, irritability, inflamed tympanic membrane, and fluid in the middle ear. The tympanic membrane progresses from erythema to opaqueness with bulging as fluid accumulates. There is an increasing prevalence of AOM caused by penicillin-resistant microorganisms. **Otitis media with effusion (OME)** is the presence of fluid in the middle ear without symptoms of acute infection.

Treatment includes symptom management, particularly of pain, with watchful waiting, antimicrobial therapy for severe illness, and placement of tympanotomy tubes when there is persistent bilateral effusion and significant hearing loss.[69] Complications include mastoiditis, brain abscess, meningitis, and chronic otitis media with hearing loss. Persistent middle ear effusions may affect speech, language, and cognitive abilities. Multivalent vaccines (i.e., heptavalent pneumococcal conjugate vaccine) for prevention of otitis media are effective for reducing disease incidence.[70]

Olfaction and Taste

Olfaction (smell) is a function of cranial nerve I. Taste (gustation) is a function of multiple nerves in the tongue, soft palate, uvula, pharynx, and upper esophagus innervated by cranial nerves VII and IX. Dysfunctions of smell and taste may occur separately or jointly. The strong relationship between smell and taste creates the sensation of flavor. If either sensation is impaired, the perception of flavor is altered. (Olfactory structures are illustrated in Figure 13-13.)

Olfactory cells, located in the olfactory epithelium, are the receptor cells for smell. Seven different primary classes of olfactory stimulants have been identified: (1) camphoraceous, (2) musky, (3) floral, (4) peppermint, (5) ethereal, (6) pungent, and (7) putrid. The primary sensations of taste are (1) sour, (2) salty, (3) sweet, and (4) bitter. Taste buds sensitive to each of the primary sensations are located in specific areas of the tongue.[71]

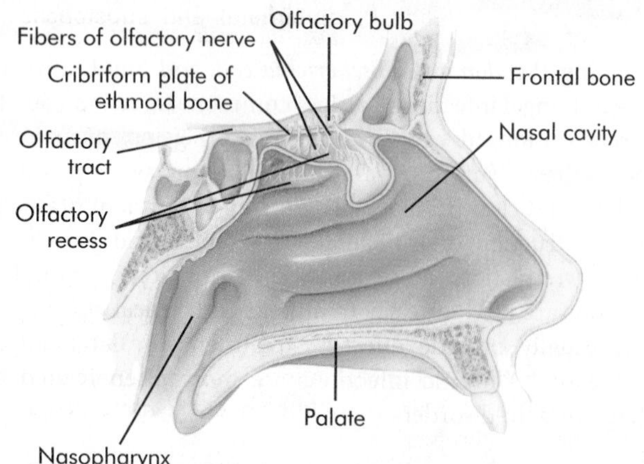

Figure 13-13 ■ **Olfaction.** Midsagittal section of the nasal area shows the location of major olfactory sensory structures. (From Thibodeau GA, Patton KT: *Anatomy & physiology,* ed 6, St Louis, 2007, Mosby.)

Sensitivity to odors declines steadily with aging. See the *AGING & Changes in Olfaction and Taste* box for a summary of changes in olfaction and taste with aging.

AGING & Changes in Olfaction and Taste

Decline in sensitivity to odors, usually after 80 years
Loss of olfaction may diminish appetite, taste, and food selection and may affect nutrition
Inability to smell toxic fumes or gases can pose a safety hazard
Decline in taste sensitivity more gradual than smell
Higher concentration of flavors required to stimulate taste
Taste may be influenced by decreased salivary secretion

Olfactory and taste dysfunctions

Olfactory dysfunctions include the following:

1. **Hyposmia**—impaired sense of smell
2. **Anosmia**—complete loss of smell
3. **Olfactory hallucinations**—smelling odors that are not really present
4. **Parosmia**—abnormal or perverted sense of smell

The sense of taste can be impaired by injury. Altered taste may be attributed to impaired smell associated with injury near the hippocampus.

Hypogeusia is a decrease in taste sensation, whereas **ageusia** is an absence of the sense of taste. These disorders result from cranial nerve injuries and can be specific to the area of the tongue innervated. **Dysgeusia** is a perversion of taste in which substances possess an unpleasant flavor (i.e., metallic). Alterations in taste may compromise adequate nutrition or cause anorexia.[72]

QUICK CHECK 13-4

1. List the major structures of the eye.
2. Visual disorders fall into several categories; name them.
3. How does fluid accumulate in the middle ear during otitis media?
4. What factors are involved in the sensation of flavor?

SOMATOSENSORY FUNCTION

Touch

The sensation of touch involves four afferent fiber types that mediate tactile sensation[73] with the fusion of several qualities, including modality, intensity, location, and duration of the sensory stimulus. Receptors sensitive to touch are present in the skin with high densities in the fingers and lips. **Meissner** and **pacinian corpuscles** are rapidly adapting receptors and sense movement across the skin and vibration respectively. The slowly adapting **Merkel disks** sense sustained light touch, and **Ruffini endings** respond to deep sustained pressure, stretch, and joint position. Specific sensory input is carried to the higher levels of the CNS by the dorsal column of the spinal cord and the anterior spinothalamic tract.

The cutaneous senses develop before birth, but structural growth continues into early adulthood. Then a gradual decline occurs, with loss in tactile sensitivity with advancing age.[74]

Abnormal tactile perception may be caused by alterations at any level of the nervous system, from the receptor to the cerebral cortex. Factors that interrupt or impair reception, transmission, perception, or interpretation of touch—including trauma, tumor, infection, metabolic changes, vascular changes, and degenerative diseases—may cause tactile dysfunction. In addition, most tactile sensations evoke affective responses that determine whether the sensation is unpleasant, pleasant, or neutral.

Proprioception

Awareness of the position of the body and its parts depends on impulses from the inner ear and from receptors in joints and ligaments. Sensory data are transmitted to higher centers, primarily through the dorsal columns and the spinocerebellar tracts, with some data passing through the medial lemnisci and thalamic radiations to the cortex. These stimuli are necessary for the coordination of movements, the grading of muscular contraction, and the maintenance of equilibrium.

A progressive loss of proprioception has been reported in elderly persons.[75] As with tactile dysfunction, any factor that interrupts or impairs the reception, transmission, perception, or interpretation of proprioceptive stimuli also alters proprioception and increases risk for falls and injury. Two common causes are vestibular dysfunction and neuropathy.

Specific vestibular dysfunctions are vestibular nystagmus and vertigo. **Vestibular nystagmus** is the constant, involuntary movement of the eyeball caused by ear disturbances. This condition occurs when the semicircular canal system is overstimulated. **Vertigo** is the sensation of spinning that occurs with inflammation of the semicircular canals in the ear. The individual may feel either that he or she is moving in space or that the world is revolving. Vertigo often causes loss of balance, and nystagmus may occur. Meniere disease can cause loss of proprioception during an acute attack, so that standing or walking is impossible.

Peripheral neuropathies also can cause proprioceptive dysfunction. They may be caused by several conditions and commonly are associated with renal disease and diabetes mellitus. Although the exact sequence of events is unknown, neuropathies cause a diminished or absent sense of body position or position of body parts. Gait changes often occur. (Neuropathies are discussed further in Chapter 14.)

QUICK CHECK 13-5

1. How are different touch receptors distributed over the body?
2. What are two causes of alterations in proprioception?

Did You Understand?

Pain

1. Pain is a complex phenomenon composed of sensory experiences (time, space, intensity) and emotion, cognition, and motivation.
2. The thalamus, cortex, and postcentral gyrus perceive, describe, and localize pain. The reticular formation and limbic system control the emotional and affective response to pain.
3. The portions of the nervous system responsible for the sensation and perception of pain may be divided into three areas: (a) the afferent fibers, (b) the central nervous system, and (c) the efferent pathways.
4. The afferent system is composed of nociceptors, Aδ and C fibers, the dorsal horn of the spinal column, and afferent neurons in the spinothalamic tract.
5. Efferent pathways from the ventromedial thalamus and periaqueductal gray are responsible for modulation or inhibition of afferent pain signals.
6. The specificity theory of pain proposes that the intensity of pain is directly related to the degree of associated tissue injury. According to the gate control theory, there are specialized cells within the substantia gelatinosa that act as a gate, opening and closing the afferent pathways to transmission of painful stimuli. The neuromatrix theory of pain proposes that chronic pain is related to multidimensional inputs triggered from the periphery or originating independently within the brain.
7. Modulators of pain include substances that stimulate pain receptors (i.e., prostaglandins, bradykinins, lymphokines, substance P, glutamate) and substances that suppress pain (i.e., endorphins, GABA, serotonin, norepinephrine).
8. Endorphins are endogenous opioids that attach to opiate receptors and inhibit transmission of pain impulses. Enkephalins and dynorphin are other opioid peptides. They are present in varying concentrations in the neurons of the brain, spinal cord, and gastrointestinal tract.
9. Clinical descriptions of pain include somatogenic pain (with a known physiologic cause), psychogenic pain (without a physiologic cause), acute pain (signal to the person of a harmful stimulus), and chronic pain (persistence of pain of unknown cause or unusual response to therapy).
10. Acute pain may be (a) somatic (superficial), (b) visceral (internal), or (c) referred (present in an area distant from its origin). The area of referred pain is supplied by the same spinal segment as the actual site of pain.

(Continued)

Did You Understand?—Cont'd

11. Chronic pain is persistent pain lasting at least 3 to 6 months and may be related to inflammation or injury to the nervous system or chronic inflammation.
12. Neuropathic pain is increased sensitivity to painful stimuli and results from abnormal processing of pain information in the peripheral or central nervous system.
13. Psychologic, behavioral, and physiologic responses to chronic pain include depression, difficulty in sleeping, preoccupation with pain, lifestyle changes, and physiologic adaptation.
14. Pain threshold is the point at which pain is perceived.
15. Pain tolerance is the duration of time or the intensity of pain that an individual will endure before initiating overt pain response.
16. Newborns and young children have the anatomic and functional ability to perceive pain. Older individuals tend to have a slightly higher pain threshold, probably because of changes in the thickness of the skin and peripheral neuropathies. Women appear to be more sensitive to pain than are men in all age groups.

Temperature Regulation

1. Temperature regulation is achieved through precise balancing of heat production, heat conservation, and heat loss. Body temperature is maintained in a range around 37° C (98.6° F).
2. Temperature regulation is mediated by the hypothalamus through thermoreceptors in the skin, hypothalamus, spinal cord, and abdominal organs.
3. Heat is produced through chemical reactions of metabolism, skeletal muscle contraction, chemical thermogenesis, and vasoconstriction.
4. Heat is lost through radiation, conduction, convection, vasodilation, decreased muscle tone, evaporation of sweat, increased respiration, and voluntary mechanisms.
5. Heat conservation is accomplished through vasoconstriction and voluntary mechanisms.
6. Infants do not conserve heat well because of their greater body surface/mass ratio and decreased subcutaneous fat. Elderly persons have poor responses to environmental temperature extremes as a result of slowed blood circulation, structural and functional changes in skin, and overall decrease in heat-producing activities.
7. Fever is triggered by the release of pyrogens from bacteria, leukocytes, and other cells involved in the immune response. Fever is both a normal immunologic mechanism and symptom of a disease.
8. Fever involves the "resetting of the hypothalamic thermostat" to a higher level. When the fever breaks, the set point returns to normal.
9. Fever production aids responses to infectious processes. Higher temperatures kill many microorganisms and decrease serum levels of iron, zinc, and copper that are needed for bacterial replication.
10. Hyperthermia (marked warming of core temperature) can produce nerve damage, coagulation of cell proteins, and death. Forms of accidental hyperthermia include heat cramps, heat exhaustion, heat stroke, and malignant hyperthermia. Heat stroke and malignant hyperthermia are potentially lethal.
11. Hypothermia (marked cooling of core temperature) slows the rate of chemical reaction (tissue metabolism), increases the viscosity of the blood, slows blood flow through the microcirculation, facilitates blood coagulation, and stimulates profound vasoconstriction. Hypothermia may be accidental or therapeutic.

Sleep

1. Sleep may be divided into REM and non-REM stages, each of which has its own series of stages. While asleep, an individual progresses through REM and non-REM (slow wave) sleep in a predictable cycle.
2. REM sleep is controlled by mechanisms in the pons and mesencephalon. Non-REM sleep accounts for 75% to 80% of sleep time and is controlled by release of inhibitory signals from the hypothalamus.
3. The sleep patterns of the newborn and young child vary from those of the adult in total sleep time, cycle length, and percentage of time spent in each sleep cycle. Elderly persons experience a total decrease in sleep time.
4. The restorative, reparative, and growth processes occur during slow wave (non-REM) sleep. Sleep deprivation can cause profound changes in personality and functioning.
5. Sleep disorders include (a) dyssomnias (disorders of initiating sleep [i.e., insomnia, sleep disordered breathing, hypersomnia, or disorders of the sleep-wake schedule]) and (b) parasomnias (i.e., sleepwalking or night terrors).

The Special Senses

1. The wall of the eye has three layers: sclera, choroid, and retina. The retina contains millions of baroreceptors known as rods and cones that receive light through the lens and then convey signals to the optic nerve and subsequently to the visual cortex of the brain.
2. The eye is filled with vitreous and aqueous humor, which prevent it from collapsing.
3. The eyelids, conjunctiva, and lacrimal apparatus protect the eye. Infections are the most common disorders; they include blepharitis, conjunctivitis, chalazion, and hordeolum.
4. Structural eye changes caused by aging result in decreased visual acuity.
5. The major alterations in ocular movement include strabismus, nystagmus, and paralysis of the extraocular muscles.
6. Alterations in visual acuity can be caused by amblyopia, scotoma, cataracts, papilledema, macular degeneration, and glaucoma.
7. Alterations in accommodation develop with increased intraocular pressure, inflammation, and disease of the oculomotor nerve. Presbyopia is loss of accommodation caused by loss of elasticity of the lens with aging.

Did You Understand?—Cont'd

8. Alterations in refraction, including myopia, hyperopia, and astigmatism, are the most common visual disorders.
9. Trauma or disease of the optic nerve pathways, or optic radiations, can cause blindness in the visual fields. Homonymous hemianopsia is caused by damage of one optic tract.
10. Conjunctivitis can be acute or chronic, bacterial, viral, or allergic. Redness, edema, pain, and lacrimation are common symptoms. Chlamydial conjunctivitis is the leading cause of blindness in the world and is associated with poor sanitary conditions.
11. Keratitis is a bacterial or viral infection of the cornea that can lead to corneal ulceration. Photophobia, pain, and tearing are common symptoms.
12. The ear is composed of external, middle, and inner structures. The external structures are the pinna, auditory canal, and tympanic membrane. The tympanic cavity (containing three bones: the malleus, the incus, and the stapes), oval window, eustachian tube, and fluid compose the middle ear and transmit sound vibrations to the inner ear.
13. The inner ear includes the bony and membranous labyrinths that transmit sound waves through the cochlea to the division of the eighth cranial nerve. The semicircular canals and vestibule help maintain balance through the equilibrium receptors.
14. Approximately one third of all people older than 65 years have hearing loss.
15. Hearing loss can be classified as conductive, sensorineural, mixed, or functional.
16. Conductive hearing loss occurs when sound waves cannot be conducted through the middle ear.
17. Sensorineural hearing loss develops with impairment of the organ of Corti or its central connections.
18. A combination of conductive and sensorineural loss is a mixed hearing loss.
19. Loss of hearing with no known organic cause is a functional hearing loss.
20. Meniere disease is a disorder of the middle ear that affects hearing and balance.
21. Otitis externa is an infection of the outer ear associated with prolonged exposure to moisture.
22. Otitis media is an infection of the middle ear that is common in children. Accumulation of fluid (effusion) behind the tympanic membrane is a common finding.
23. The perception of flavor is altered if olfaction or taste dysfunctions occur. Sensitivity to odor and taste decreases with aging.
24. Hyposmia is a decrease in the sense of smell, and anosmia is the complete loss of the sense of smell. Inflammation of the nasal mucosa and trauma or tumors of the olfactory nerve lead to a diminished sense of smell.
25. Hypogeusia is a decrease in taste sensation, and ageusia is the absence of the sense of taste. Loss of taste buds or trauma to the facial or glossopharyngeal nerves decreases taste sensation.

Somatosensory Function

1. Tactile sensation is a function of receptors present in the skin (pacinian corpuscles), and the sensory response is conducted to the brain through the dorsal column and anterior spinothalamic tract.
2. Alterations in touch can result from disruption of skin receptors, sensory transmission, or central nervous system perception.
3. Proprioception is the position and location of the body and its parts. Proprioceptors are located in the inner ear, joints, and ligaments. Proprioceptive stimuli are necessary for balance, coordinated movement, and grading of muscular contraction.
4. Disorders of proprioception can occur at any level of the nervous system and result in impaired balance and lack of coordinated movement.

Key Terms

Acute bacterial conjunctivitis (pinkeye), 320
Acute otitis media (AOM), 324
Acute pain, 308
Age-related macular degeneration (AMD), 318
Ageusia, 324
Allergic conjunctivitis, 320
Amblyopia, 318
Anosmia, 324
Aqueous humor, 317
Astigmatism, 320
β-endorphin, 308
Blepharitis, 320
Central pain, 309
Chalazion, 320
Chronic conjunctivitis, 320
Chronic pain, 309
Circadian rhythm, 311
Cochlea, 322
Cognitive/evaluative system, 305
Color blindness, 320
Conductive hearing loss, 323
Cone, 317
Conjunctivitis, 320
Cornea, 317
Crista ampullaris, 322
Delta opioid receptor, 308
Diplopia, 318
Dynorphin, 308
Dysgeusia, 324
Endomorphin, 308
Endorphin, 308
Enkephalin, 308
Equilibrium receptor, 322
Eustachian (pharyngotympanic) tube, 322
Exogenous pyrogen, 313
External auditory canal, 320
Fever, 313
Fovea centralis, 317
Functional hearing loss, 323
Gate control theory, 307
Glaucoma, 318
Hair cell, 322
Heat cramp, 314
Heat exhaustion, 314
Heat stroke, 314
Hordeolum (stye), 320
Hyperopia, 320
Hyperthermia, 314
Hypogeusia, 324
Hyposmia, 324
Hypothermia, 314
Incus (anvil), 321
Insomnia, 316
Iris, 317
Jerk nystagmus, 318
Kappa opioid receptor, 308
Keratitis, 320
Lens, 317
Macula, 322
Malignant hyperthermia, 314
Malleus (hammer), 321
Mastoid air cell, 320
Mastoid process, 320
Meissner corpuscle, 324
Meniere disease, 323
Merkel disk, 325
Mixed hearing loss, 323
Motivational/affective system, 305
Mu opioid receptor, 308
Myopia, 319
Neospinothalamic tract, 307
Neuromatrix theory of pain, 307
Neuropathic pain, 309
Night terrors, 316
Nociception, 306
Nociceptor, 306
Non-REM sleep (NREM), 315
Nystagmus, 318
Obstructive sleep apnea syndrome, 316
Olfactory hallucination, 324
Opiate receptor, 308
Optic chiasm, 320
Optic disc, 317
Organ of Corti, 322
Otitis externa, 323
Otitis media, 323
Otitis media with effusion (OME), 324
Otolith, 322
Oval window, 322
Pacinian corpuscle, 324
Pain threshold, 310
Pain tolerance, 310
Paleospinothalamic tract, 307
Parasomnia, 316
Parosmia, 324
Pendular nystagmus, 318
Perceptual dominance, 310
Periaqueductal gray (PAG), 307
Perilymph, 322
Peripheral pain, 309
Pinna, 320
Presbycusis, 323
Presbyopia, 319
Primary hypersomnia, 316
Psychogenic pain, 308
Pupil, 317
Referred pain, 309
REM (rapid eye movement) sleep, 315
Retina, 317
Rod, 317
Ruffini ending, 325
Sclera, 317
Secondary hypersomnia, 316
Semicircular canal, 322
Sensorineural hearing loss, 323
Sensory/discriminative system, 305
Somatic pain, 309
Somatogenic pain, 308
Somnambulism (sleepwalking), 316
Specificity theory of pain, 307
Stapes (stirrup), 321
Strabismus, 318
Temperature regulation, 311
Tinnitus, 323
Trachoma, 320
Tympanic cavity, 321
Tympanic membrane, 321
Ventromedial medulla, 307
Vertigo, 325
Vestibular nystagmus, 325
Vestibule, 322
Viral conjunctivitis, 320
Visceral pain, 309
Vitreous humor, 317

References

1. McCaffery M: Understanding your patient's pain, *Nursing* 80 (9):26–31, 1980.
2. International Association for the Study of Pain, American Pain Society: *IASP pain terminology*; www.iasp-pain.org/terms-p.html#Pain, updated November..
3. Melzak R: Toward a new concept of pain for the new millenium, In Waldman SD, editor: *Interventional pain management*, ed 2, Philadelphia, 2001, Saunders.
4. McCaffery M, Pasero C: Underlying complexities, misconceptions, and practical tools, In McCaffery M, Pasero C, , editors: *Pain: clinical manual*, ed 2, St Louis, 1999, Mosby.
5. Mason P: Deconstructing endogenous pain modulations, *J Neurophysiol* 94(3):1659–6316, 2005.
6. Melzack R: Toward a new concept of pain for the new millennium, In Waldman SD, editor: *Interventional pain management*, ed 2, Philadelphia, 2001, Saunders.
7. DeLeo JA: Basic science of pain, *J Bone Joint Surg Am* 88(suppl 2):58–62, 2006.
8. Hauser KF et al: Pathobiology of dynorphins in trauma and disease, *Front Biosci* 10:216–235, 2005.
9. Willis WD, Westlund KN: Neuroanatomy of the pain system and of the pathways that modulate pain, *J Clin Neurophysiol* 14(1):2–31, 1997.
10. Horvath G: Endomorphin-1 and endomorphin-2: pharmacology of the selective endogenous mu-opioid receptor agonists, *Pharmacol Ther* 88(3):437–463, 2000.
11. Wall PD, Melzack R: *Textbook of pain*,, Edinburgh, 1994, Churchill Livingstone.
12. Joshi SK, Gebhart GF: Visceral pain, *Curr Rev Pain* 4 (6):499–506, 2000.
13. Seeley RR, Stephens TD, Tate P: *Anatomy and physiology*,, ed 2, St Louis, 1992, Mosby.

References—Cont'd

14. Pace MC et al: Neurobiology of pain, *J Cell Physiol* 209 (1):8–12, 2006.
15. Baron R: Mechanisms of disease: neuropathic pain—a clinical perspective, *Nat Clin Pract Neurol* 2(2):95–106, 2006.
16. Kanner R: *Pain management secrets,*, ed 2, Philadelphia, 2003, Hanley & Belfus.
17. Cano A et al: Coping, pain severity, interference, and disability: the potential mediating and moderating roles of race and education, *J Pain* 7(11):869–870, 2006.
18. Turk DC, Okifuji A: Psychological factors in chronic pain: evolution and revolution, *J Consult Clin Psychol* 70(3): 678–690, 2002.
19. Derasari MD: Taxonomy of pain syndromes: classification of chronic pain syndromes, In Raj PP, editor: *Practical management of pain,*, ed 3, St Louis, 2001, Mosby.
20. Tegeder I et al: GTP cyclohydrolase and tetrahydrobiopterin regulate pain sensitivity and persistence, *Nat Med* 12 (11):1269–1277, 2006.
21. Fillingim RB: Individual differences in pain responses, *Curr Rheumatol Rep* 7(5):342–347, 2005.
22. Leppaluoto J et al: Pituitary and autonomic responses to cold exposures in man, *Acta Physiol Scand* 184(4):255–264, 2005.
23. Silva JE: Thermogenic mechanisms and their hormonal regulation, *Physiol Rev* 86(2):435–464, 2006.
24. Rothwell NJ: CNS regulation of thermogenesis, *Crit Rev Neurobiol* 8(1-2):1–10, 1994.
25. Sherman TI et al: Optimizing the neonatal thermal environment, *Neonatal Netw* 25(4):251–260, 2006.
26. Smolander J: Effect of cold exposure to older humans, *Int J Sports Med* 23(2):86–92, 2002.
27. Vogelaere P, Pereira C: Thermoregulation and aging, *Rev Port Cardiol* 24(5):747–761, 2005.
28. Netea MG, Kullberg BJ, Van der Meer JW: Circulating cytokines as mediators of fever, *Clin Infect Dis* 31(suppl 5): S178–S184, 2000.
29. Biddle C: The neurobiology of the human febrile response, *AANA J* 74(2):145–150, 2006.
30. Hanson DF: Fever, temperature, and the immune response, *Ann NY Acad Sci* 15(813):453–464, 1997.
31. Schulman CI et al: The effect of antipyretic therapy upon outcomes in critically ill patients: a randomized, prospective study, *Surg Infect (Larchmt)* 6:369–375, 2005.
32. Greisman LA, Mackowiak PA: Fever: beneficial and detrimental effects of antipyretics, *Curr Opin Infect Dis* 15(3):241–245, 2002.
33. Roghmann MC, Warner J, Mackowiak PA: The relationship between age and fever magnitude, *Am J Med Sci* 322 (2):68–70, 2001.
34. De Keyser J et al: Neuroprotection in acute ischemic stroke, *Acta Neurol Belg* 105(3):144–148, 2005.
35. Horsman MR: Tissue physiology and the response to heat, *Int J Hyperthermia* 22(3):197–203, 2006.
36. Wexler RK: Evaluation and treatment of heat-related illnesses, *Am Fam Physician* 65(11):2307–2314, 2002.
37. Litman RS, Rosenberg H: Malignant hyperthermia: update on susceptibility testing, *JAMA* 293(23):2918–2924, 2005.
38. Harris CD: Neurophysiology of sleep and wakefulness, *Respir Care Clin North Am* 11(4):567–586, 2005.
39. Bauman CR, Bassetti CL: Hypocretins (orexins) and sleep-wake disorders, *Lancet Neurol* 4(10):673–682, 2005.
40. Dugovic C: Role of serotonin in sleep mechanisms, *Rev Neurol (Paris)* 157(11 pt 2):S16–S19, 2001.
41. Sutcliffe JG, de Lecea L: The hypocretins: setting the arousal threshold, *Natural Rev Neurosci* 3(5):339–349, 2002.
42. Dan B, Boyd SG: A neurophysiological perspective on sleep and its maturation, *Dev Med Child Neuro*l 48(9):773–779, 2006.
43. American Academy of Sleep Medicine: *The international classification of sleep disorders, revised: diagnostic and coding manual,* Westchester, IL, 2001, Author; also available at www.absm.org/PDF/ICSD.pdf#search=%22International%20Classification%20of%20Sleep%20Disorders%22.
44. Summers MO, Crisostomo MI, Stepanski EJ: Recent developments in the classification, evaluation, and treatment of insomnia, *Chest* 130(1):276–286, 2006.
45. Wiegand L, Zwillich CW: Obstructive sleep apnea, *Disease-a-Month* 40(4):197–252, 1994.
46. Khalil MM, Rifaie OA: Electrocardiographic changes in obstructive sleep apnoea syndrome, *Respir Med* 92(1):25–27, 1998.
47. Coccagna G, Pollini A, Provini F: Cardiovascular disorders and obstructive sleep apnea syndrome, *Clin Exp Hypertens* 28(3-4):217–224, 2006.
48. White DP: Sleep apnea, *Proc Am Thorac Soc* 3(1):124–128, 2006.
49. Tauman R, Gulliver TF, Krishma J, Montgomery-Downs HE, O'Brien LM, Ivaneko A, Gozal D: Persistence of obstructive sleep apnea syndrome in children after adenotonsillectomy, *J Pediatr* 149(6):803–808, 2006.
50. Dauvilliers Y: Differential diagnosis in hypersomnia, *Curr Neurol Neurosci Rep* 6(2):156–162, 2006.
51. Richardson GS: The human circadian system in normal and disordered sleep, *J Clin Psychiatry,* 66(suppl 9)3–9 quiz 43–43, 2005.
52. Plante DT, Winkelman JW: Parasomnias, *Psychiatr Clin North Am* 29(4):969–987, 2006.
53. Guilleminault C et al: Adult chronic sleepwalking and its treatment based on polysomnography, *Brain* 128(Pt 5):1062–1069, 2005.
54. Thibodeau GA, Patton KT: *Anatomy & physiology,*, ed 6, St Louis, 2007, Mosby.
55. Crossman AR, Neary D: *Neuroanatomy: an illustrated color text,* ed 3, London, 2005, Churchill Livingstone, p. 157.
56. International Glaucoma Association: *Glaucoma—types of classification of the various types of glaucoma,* Available at www.glaucomaassociation.com/nqcontent.cfm?a_id=705&=fromcfc&tt=article&lang=en&site_id=483.
57. Arden GB: Age-related macular degeneration, *J Br Menopause Soc* 12(2):64–70, 2006.
58. Callina T, Reynolds TP: Traditional methods for the treatment of presbyopia: spectacles, contact lenses, bifocal contact lenses, *Ophthalmol Clin North Am* 19(1):25–33, 2006.
59. Deeb SS: The molecular basis of variation in human color vision, *Clin Genet* 67(5):369–377, 2005.
60. Wirbelauer C: Management of the red eye for the primary care physician, *Am J Med* 119(4):302–306, 2006.
61. Zadeh MH, Selesnick SH: Evaluation of hearing impairment, *Compr Ther* 27(4):302–310, 2001.
62. Willems PJ: Genetic causes of hearing loss, *N Engl J Med* 342 (15):1101–1109, 2000.
63. Davidson HC: Imaging evaluation of sensorineural hearing loss, *Semin Ultrasound CT MR* 22(3):229–249, 2001.
64. Gates GA: Meniere's disease review 2005, *J Am Acad Audio*l 17 (1):16–26, 2006.
65. Osguthorpe JD, Nielsen DR: Otitis externa: Review and clinical update, *Am Fam Physician 1* 74(9):1510–1516, 2006.
66. Rosenfeld RM et al: Systematic review of topical antimicrobial therapy for acute otitis externa, *Otolaryngol Head Neck Surg* 134(4 suppl):S24–S48, 2006.

References—Cont'd

67. Bernius M, Perlin D: Pediatric ear, nose, and throat emergencies, *Pediatr Clin North Am* 53(2):195–214, 2006.
68. Casselbrant ML, Mandel EM: Genetic susceptibility to otitis media, *Curr Opin Allergy Clin Immunol* 5(1):1–4, 2005.
69. American Academy of Pediatrics, Subcommittee on Management of Acute Otitis Media: Diagnosis and management of acute otitis media, *Pediatrics* 113(5):1451–1465, 2004.
70. Aliphas A, Prufer N, Grundfast KM: Emerging therapies for the treatment and prevention of otitis media, *Exp Opin Emerg Drugs* 11(2):251–264, 2006.
71. Breslin PA, Huang L: Human taste: peripheral anatomy, taste transduction, and coding, *Adv Otorhinolaryngol* 63:152–190, 2006.
72. Landis BN, Lacroix JS: Postoperative/posttraumatic gustatory dysfunction, *Adv Otorhinolaryngol* 63:242–254, 2006.
73. FitzGerald MJT, Folan-Curran J: *Clinical neuroanatomy and related neuroscience,* London, Saunders, 2002, p. 79.
74. Wickremaratchi MM, Llewelyn JG: Effects of ageing on touch, *Postgrad Med J* 82(967):301–304, 2006.
75. Snijders AH, van de Warrenburg BP, Giladi N, Bloem BR: Neurological gait disorders in elderly people: clinical approach and classification, *Lancet Neurol* 6(1):63–74, 2007.

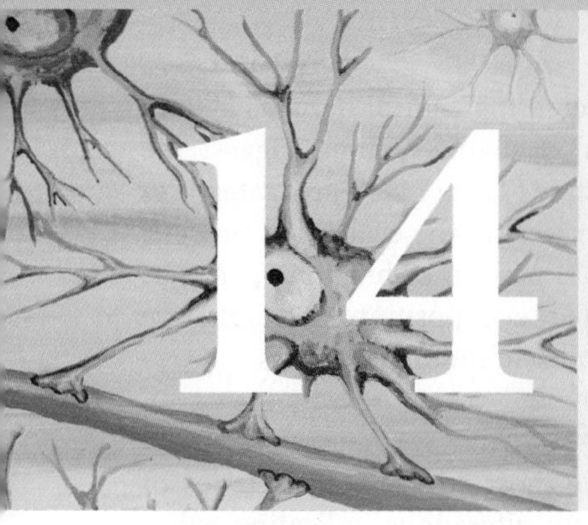

14 CONCEPTS OF NEUROLOGIC DYSFUNCTION

Barbara J. Boss

CHAPTER OUTLINE

ELECTRONIC RESOURCES

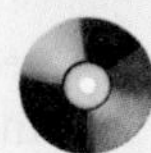

Companion CD
- Review Questions and Answers
- Animations

evolve Website at
http://evolve.elsevier.com/Huether/
- Quick Check Answers
- Key Terms Exercises
- Critical Thinking Questions with Answers
- Algorithm Completion Exercises
- WebLinks

A person achieves functional adequacy (competence) through complex integrated processes. Three major neural networks account for this functional adequacy: cognitive networks, sensory networks, and motor networks. Alterations in any or all of these affect functional adequacy. This chapter discusses alterations in cognitive and motor networks.

The neural networks that are basic (core) to cognitive function are (1) attentional networks that provide arousal and maintenance of attention over time, (2) memory and language networks by which information is communicated, and (3) affective or emotive networks that mediate feeling tone. These core networks are fundamental to the processes of abstract thinking and reasoning. The products of abstraction and reasoning are organized and made operational through the executive attentional networks. The normal functioning of these networks manifests through the motor network in a behavioral array viewed by others as appropriate to human activity and successful living.

ALTERATIONS IN COGNITIVE NETWORKS

Full consciousness is a state of awareness of oneself and the environment and a set of responses to that environment. The fully conscious individual responds to external stimuli with a wide array of responses. Any decrease in this state of awareness and varied responses is a decrease in consciousness.

Consciousness involves arousal and content of thought. **Arousal** is an individual's state of awakeness. It is mediated by the reticular activating system. When a person loses cerebral function, the reticular activating system and brain stem can maintain a crude waking state known as a **vegetative state.** Cognitive cerebral functions, however, cannot occur without a functioning reticular activating system. Content of thought encompasses all cognitive functions, including awareness of self, environment, and affective states (i.e., moods). **Content of thought** is mediated by all of the core networks under the guidance of executive attention networks.

Alterations in Arousal

An altered level of arousal (awareness) with acute onset may be caused by various factors (i.e., **structural arousal alteration, metabolic arousal alteration, psychogenic arousal alteration**). Structural causes are divided according to whether the original location of the pathologic condition is above or below the tentorial plate. Pathologic processes include infectious, vascular, neoplastic, traumatic, congenital (developmental), degenerative, polygenic, and metabolic causes. Metabolic causes are further divided into hypoxia, electrolyte disturbances, hypoglycemia, drugs, and toxins (both endogenous and exogenous). All the systemic diseases that eventually produce nervous system dysfunction are part of this metabolic category. Alterations in arousal range from slight drowsiness to coma.

PATHOPHYSIOLOGY *Processes above the tentorial plate* (supratentorial) produce changes in arousal by either diffuse or localized dysfunction. Disease processes may produce diffuse dysfunction (e.g., encephalitis) and may affect the cerebral cortex or the underlying subcortical white matter. Localized dysfunction generally is caused by masses that directly impinge on deep diencephalic structures or that secondarily compress these structures in the process of herniation. Such localized destructive processes directly impair function of the thalamic or hypothalamic activating systems.

Disorders outside the brain but within the cranial vault can produce diffuse dysfunction. Examples include neoplasms, closed-head trauma with subsequent subdural bleeding, and accumulation of pus in the subdural space. Disorders within the brain substance—bleeding, infarcts and emboli, tumors—function primarily as masses.

With *processes below the tentorial plate,* arousal declines by direct destruction of the reticular activating system and its pathways or of the entire brain stem either by direct invasion or by indirect impairment of its blood supply. In addition, decreased awareness may result from compression of the reticular activating system by a disease process. This compression may result from direct pressure or compression as structures either expand or herniate. Causes include accumulations of blood or pus, neoplasms, and demyelinating disorders.

Psychogenic unresponsiveness, although uncommon, may signal general psychiatric disorders. Despite apparent unconsciousness, the person actually is physiologically awake.

CLINICAL MANIFESTATIONS AND EVALUATION The cause of an altered level of arousal may be organic or functional. Further distinction is then made between metabolic and structural factors (Table 14-1).

Patterns of clinical manifestations help in determining the extent of brain dysfunction and serve as indexes for identifying increasing or decreasing central nervous system (CNS) function. The types of manifestations suggest the cause of the altered arousal state (Table 14-2). Five categories of neurologic function are critical to the evaluation process: (1) level of consciousness, (2) pattern of breathing, (3) size and reactivity of pupils, (4) eye position and reflexive responses, and (5) skeletal muscle motor responses.

Level of consciousness

Level of consciousness is the most critical clinical index of nervous system function, with alterations indicating either improvement or deterioration of the individual's condition. A person who is alert and oriented to self, others, place, and time is considered to be functioning at the highest level of consciousness, which implies full use of all the person's cognitive capacities. From this normal alert state, levels of consciousness diminish in stages, each of which is clinically defined (Table 14-3).

Pattern of breathing

Characteristic respiratory patterns help evaluate the level of brain dysfunction and coma (Figure 14-1). Rate, rhythm, and pattern should be evaluated. Breathing patterns can be categorized as hemispheric or brain stem patterns (Table 14-4).

With normal breathing, a neural center in the forebrain (cerebrum) produces a rhythmic pattern. When consciousness decreases, lower brain stem centers regulate the breathing pattern, responding only to changes in $PaCO_2$ levels. The result is the irregular breathing associated with posthyperventilation apnea (PHVA).

Cheyne-Stokes respirations result from an increased ventilatory response to carbon dioxide stimulation, causing hypercapnia and diminished ventilatory stimulus. Changes

TABLE 14-1

Clinical Manifestations of Metabolic and Structural Causes of Comas

Manifestations	Metabolically Induced Coma	Structurally Induced Coma
Blink to threat (cranial nerves II, VII)	Equal	Asymmetric
Optic discs (cranial nerve II)	Flat, good pulsation	Papilledema
Extraocular movement (cranial nerves III, IV, VI)	Roving eye movements; normal doll's eyes and calorics	Gaze paresis, nerve palsy
Pupils (cranial nerves II, III)	Equal and reactive, may be dilated (e.g., atropine), pinpoint (e.g., opiates), or midposition and fixed (e.g., glutethimide [Doriden])	Asymmetric or nonreactive; may be midposition (midbrain injury), pinpoint (pons injury), large (tectal injury)
Corneal reflex (cranial nerves V, VII)	Symmetric response	Asymmetric response
Grimace to pain (cranial nerve VII)	Symmetric response	Asymmetric response
Motor function movement	Symmetric	Asymmetric
Tone	Symmetric	Paratonic, spastic, flaccid, especially if asymmetric
Posture	Symmetric	Decorticate, especially if symmetric; decerebrate, especially if asymmetric
Deep tendon reflexes	Symmetric	Asymmetric
Babinski sign	Absent or symmetric response	Present
Sensation	Symmetric	Asymmetric

TABLE 14-2

Differential Characteristics of States Causing Coma

Mechanism	Manifestations
Supratentorial mass lesions compressing or displacing the diencephalons or brain stem	Initiating signs usually of focal cerebral dysfunction compressing or displacing Signs of dysfunction progress rostral to caudal Neurologic signs at any given time point to one anatomic area (e.g., diencephalon, mesencephalon, medulla) Motor signs often asymmetric
Infratentorial mass of destruction causing coma	History of preceding brain stem dysfunction or sudden onset of coma Localizing brain stem signs precede or accompany onset of coma and always include oculovestibular abnormality Cranial nerve palsies usually manifest "bizarre" respiratory patterns that appear at onset
Metabolic coma	Confusion and stupor commonly precede motor signs Motor signs usually are symmetric Pupillary reactions usually are preserved Asterixis, myoclonus, tremor, and seizures are common Acid-base imbalance with hyperventilation or hypoventilation is common
Psychiatric unresponsiveness	Lids close actively Pupils reactive or dilated (cycloplegics) Oculocephalic reflexes are unpredictable; oculovestibular reflexes are physiologic (nystagmus is present) Motor tone is inconsistent or normal Eupnea or hyperventilation is usual No pathologic reflexes are present Electroencephalogram (EEG) is normal

TABLE 14-3

Levels of Altered Consciousness

State	Definition
Confusion	Loss of ability to think rapidly and clearly; impaired judgment and decision making
Disorientation	Beginning loss of consciousness; disorientation to time followed by disorientation to place and impaired memory; lost last is recognition of self
Lethargy	Limited spontaneous movement or speech; easy arousal with normal speech or touch; may or may not be oriented to time, place, or person
Obtundation	Mild to moderate reduction in arousal (awakeness) with limited response to the environment; falls asleep unless stimulated verbally or tactilely; answers questions with minimum response
Stupor	A condition of deep sleep or unresponsiveness from which the person may be aroused or caused to open eyes only by vigorous and repeated stimulation; response is often withdrawal or grabbing at stimulus
Coma	No verbal response to the external environment or to any stimuli, noxious stimuli such as deep pain or suctioning do not yield motor movement
Light coma	Associated with purposeful movement on stimulation
Coma	Associated with nonpurposeful movement only on stimulation
Deep coma	Associated with unresponsiveness or no response to any stimulus

in $PaCO_2$ produce irregular breathing, contributing to overbreathing with carbon dioxide stimulation. The $PaCO_2$ level then decreases to below normal, and breathing stops until the carbon dioxide reaccumulates to bring the $PaCO_2$ level to normal. With opiate or sedative drug overdose, the respiratory center is depressed so the rate of breathing gradually decreases until respiratory failure occurs.

Pupillary changes

Anatomically, brain stem areas that control arousal are adjacent to areas that control the pupils. Pupillary changes thus indicate the presence and level of brain stem dysfunction (Figure 14-2). For example, severe ischemia and hypoxia usually produce dilated, fixed pupils. Hypothermia also may cause fixed pupils.

Some drugs affect pupils and must be considered in evaluating individuals in comatose states. Large concentrations of atropine and scopolamine fully dilate and fix pupils. Glutethimide doses sufficient to produce a coma cause the pupils to become midposition or moderately dilated, unequal, and commonly fixed to light. Opiates cause pinpoint pupils. Severe barbiturate intoxication may produce fixed pupils.

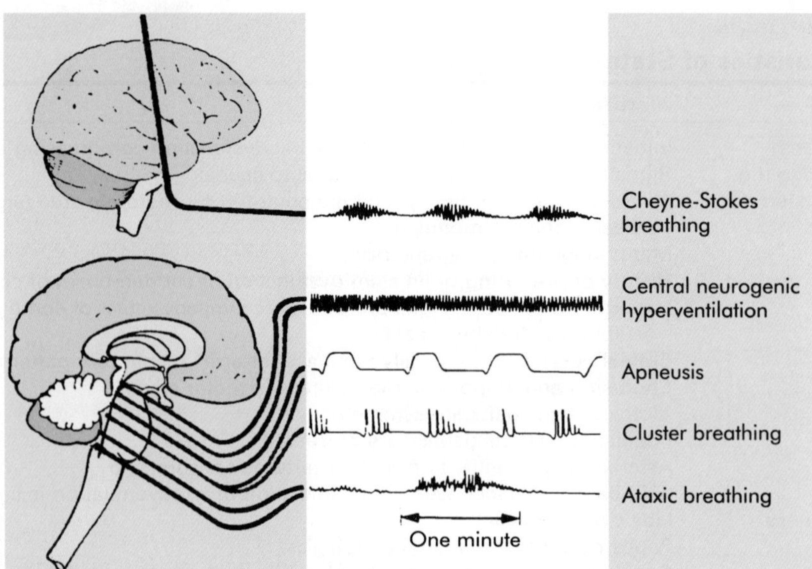

Figure 14-1 ■ **Abnormal Respiratory Patterns With Corresponding Level of Central Nervous System Activity.** (From Urden LD, Davie JK, Lough ME: *Thelan's critical care nursing: diagnosis and management,* ed 5, St Louis, 2006, Mosby.)

TABLE 14-4

Patterns of Breathing

Breathing Pattern	Description	Location of Injury
HEMISPHERIC BREATHING PATTERNS		
Normal	After a period of hyperventilation that lowers the arterial carbon dioxide pressure ($PaCO_2$), the individual continues to breathe regularly but with a reduced depth.	Response of the nervous system to an external stressor—not associated with injury to the CNS
Posthyperventilation apnea	Respirations stop after hyperventilation has lowered the Pco_2 level below normal. Rhythmic breathing returns when the Pco_2 level returns to normal.	Associated with diffuse bilateral metabolic or structural disease of the cerebrum
Cheyne-Stokes respirations	The breathing pattern has a smooth increase (crescendo) in the rate and depth of breathing (hyperpnea), which peaks and is followed by a gradual smooth decrease (decrescendo) in the rate and depth of breathing to the point of apnea, when the cycle repeats itself. The hyperpneic phase lasts longer than the apneic phase.	Bilateral dysfunction of the deep cerebral or diencephalic structures, seen with supratentorial injury and metabolically induced coma states
BRAIN STEM BREATHING PATTERNS		
Central neurogenic hyperventilation	A sustained, deep, rapid, but regular pattern (hyperpnea) occurs, with a decreased $PaCO_2$ and a corresponding increase in pH and PO_2.	May result from CNS damage or disease that involves the midbrain and upper pons; seen after increased intracranial pressure and blunt head trauma
Apneusis	A prolonged inspiratory cramp (a pause at full inspiration) occurs; a common variant of this is a brief end-inspiratory pause of 2 or 3 sec, often alternating with an end-expiratory pause.	Indicates damage to the respiratory control mechanism located at the pontine level; most commonly associated with pontine infarction but documented with hypoglycemia, anoxia, and meningitis
Cluster breathing	A cluster of breaths has a disordered sequence with irregular pauses between breaths.	Dysfunction in the lower pontine and high medullary areas
Ataxic breathing	Completely irregular breathing occurs, with random shallow and deep breaths and irregular pauses. Often the rate is slow.	Originates from a primary dysfunction of the medullary neurons controlling breathing
Gasping breathing pattern (agonal gasps)	A pattern of deep "all-or-none" breaths is accompanied by a slow respiratory rate.	Indicative of a failing medullary respiratory center

CNS, Central nervous system.

Oculomotor responses

Resting, spontaneous, and reflexive eye movements change at various levels of brain dysfunction. Persons with metabolically induced coma, except with barbiturate-hypnotic and phenytoin poisoning, generally retain ocular reflexes even when other signs of brain stem damage are present. If brisk oculocephalic reflexes and roving eye movements are present without nystagmus when cold or warm water is instilled into the external ear canal, decreased consciousness but an intact brain stem may be seen (Figures 14-3 and 14-4). Destructive or compressive injury to the brain stem causes specific abnormalities of the oculocephalic and oculovestibular reflexes. Those that involve an oculomotor nucleus or nerve cause the involved eye to deviate outward, producing a resting dysconjugate lateral position of the eye.

Motor responses

Motor responses help evaluate the level of brain dysfunction and determine the most severely damaged side of the brain. The pattern of response noted may be (1) purposeful; (2) inappropriate, generalized motor movement; or (3) not present. Motor signs indicating loss of cortical inhibition that are commonly associated with decreased consciousness include reflex grasping, reflex sucking, snout reflex, palmomental reflex, and rigidity (paratonia) (Figure 14-5). Abnormal flexor and extensor responses in the upper and lower extremities are defined in Table 14-5 and illustrated in Figure 14-6.

Vomiting

Yawning, vomiting, and hiccups are complex reflex-like motor responses that are integrated by neural mechanisms in the lower brain stem. These responses may be produced by compression or diseases involving tissues of the medulla oblongata (e.g., infection, neoplasm, infarct) but also occur relative to other more benign stimuli to the vagal nerve.

Most CNS disorders produce nausea and vomiting. Vomiting without nausea indicates direct involvement of the central neural mechanism (or pyloric obstruction; see Chapters 34 and 35). Vomiting often accompanies CNS injuries that (1) involve the vestibular nuclei or its immediate projections, particularly when double vision (diplopia) also is present; (2) impinge directly on the floor of the fourth ventricle; or (3) produce brain stem compression secondary to increased intracranial pressure.

QUICK CHECK 14-1

1. Why are structural as well as metabolic factors capable of producing coma?
2. Why is level of consciousness the most critical index of central nervous system function?
3. Why do Cheyne-Stokes respirations appear in coma?
4. Why are oculomotor changes associated with levels of coma?

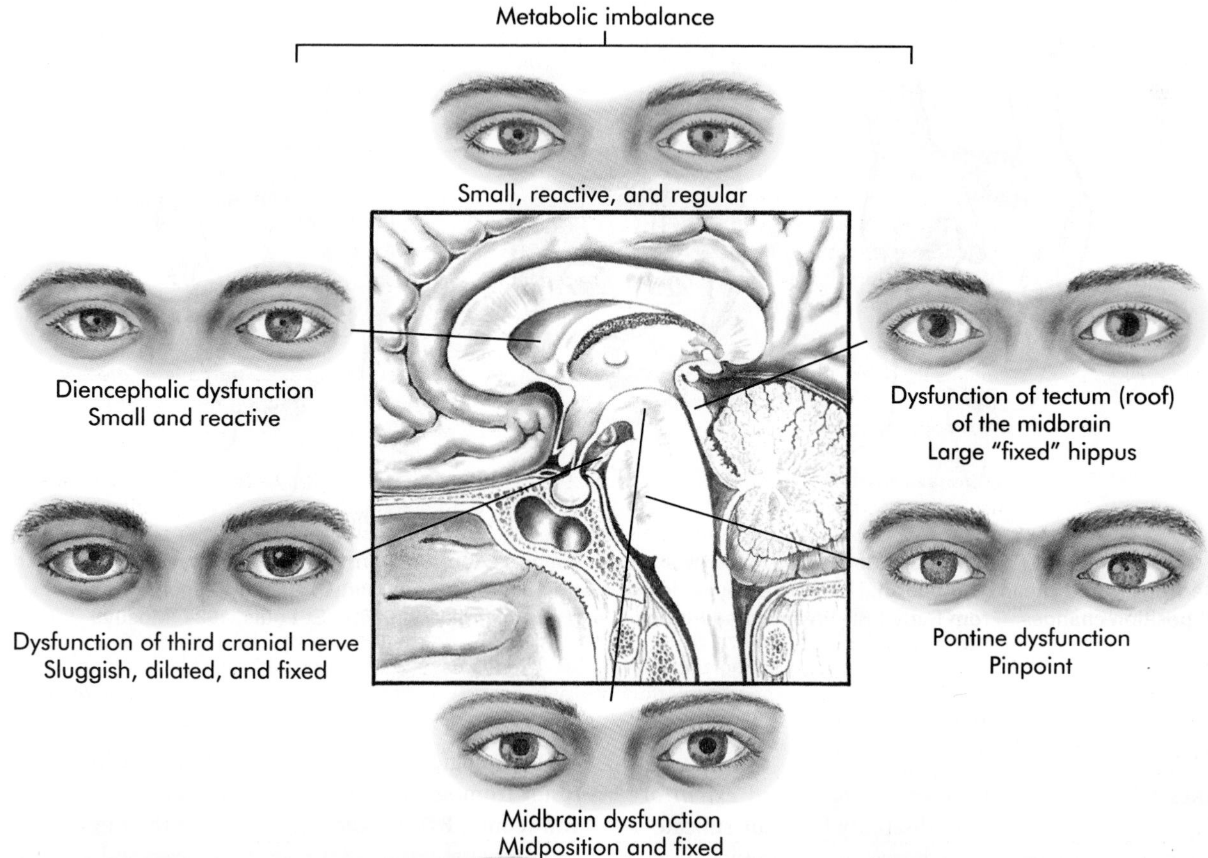

Figure 14-2 ■ **Pupils at Different Levels of Consciousness.**

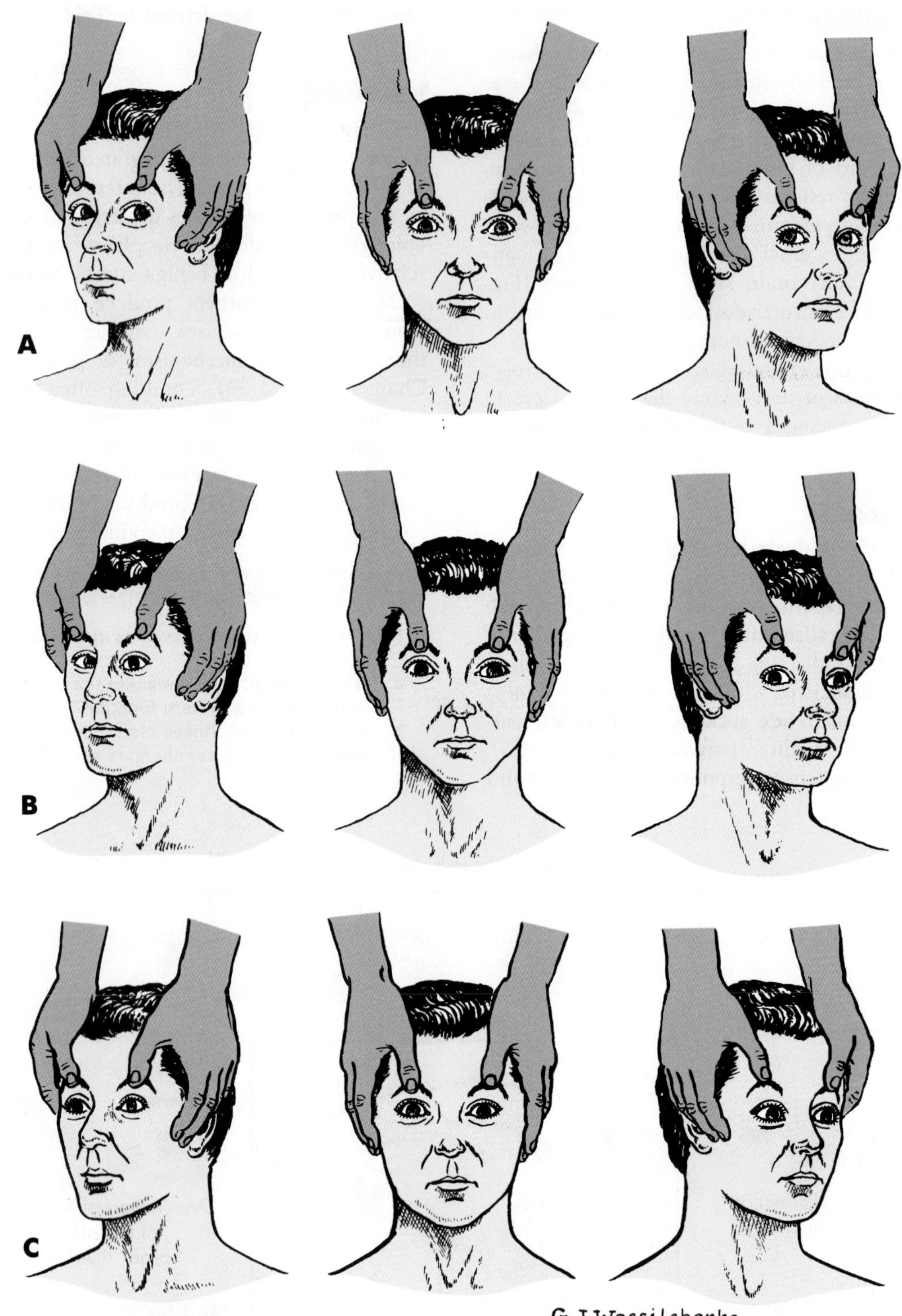

Figure 14-3 ■ **Test for Oculocephalic Reflex Response (Doll's Eyes Phenomenon). A,** Normal response—eyes turn together to side opposite from turn of head. **B,** Abnormal response—eyes do not turn in conjugate manner. **C,** Absent response—eyes do not turn as head position changes. (From Rudy EB: *Advanced neurological and neurosurgical nursing,* St Louis, 1984, Mosby.)

Outcomes

Outcomes fall into two categories: *mortality* and *extent of disability (morbidity)*. Extent of disability has four subcategories: recovery of consciousness, residual cognitive function, psychologic (functional), and vocational. Two forms of neurologic death—brain death and cerebral death—result from severe pathologic conditions and are associated with coma. **Brain death** occurs when the brain is damaged so completely that it can never recover and cannot maintain the body's internal homeostasis. State laws define brain

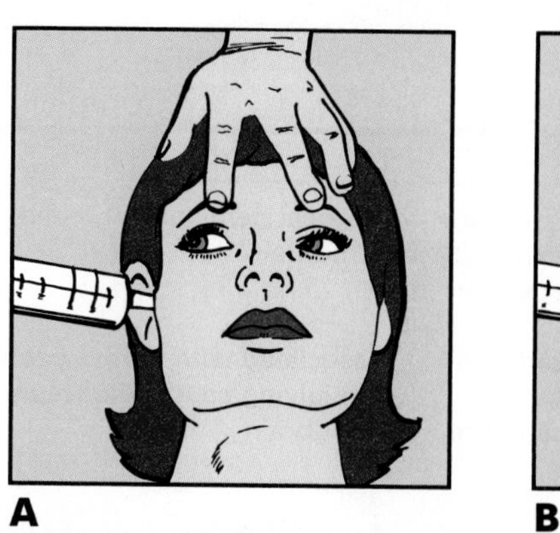

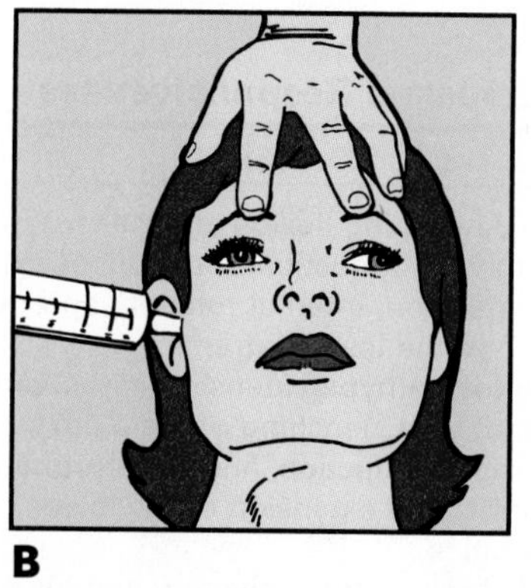

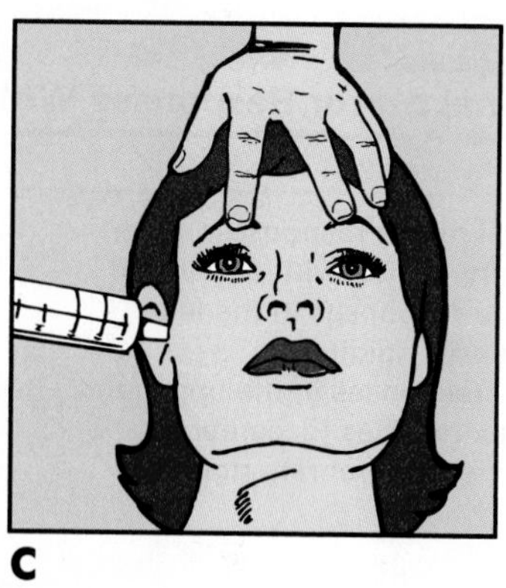

Figure 14-4 ■ **Test for Oculovestibular Reflex (Caloric Ice Water Test). A,** Normal response—conjugate eye movements. **B,** Abnormal response—dysconjugate or asymmetric eye movements. **C,** Absent response—no eye movements.

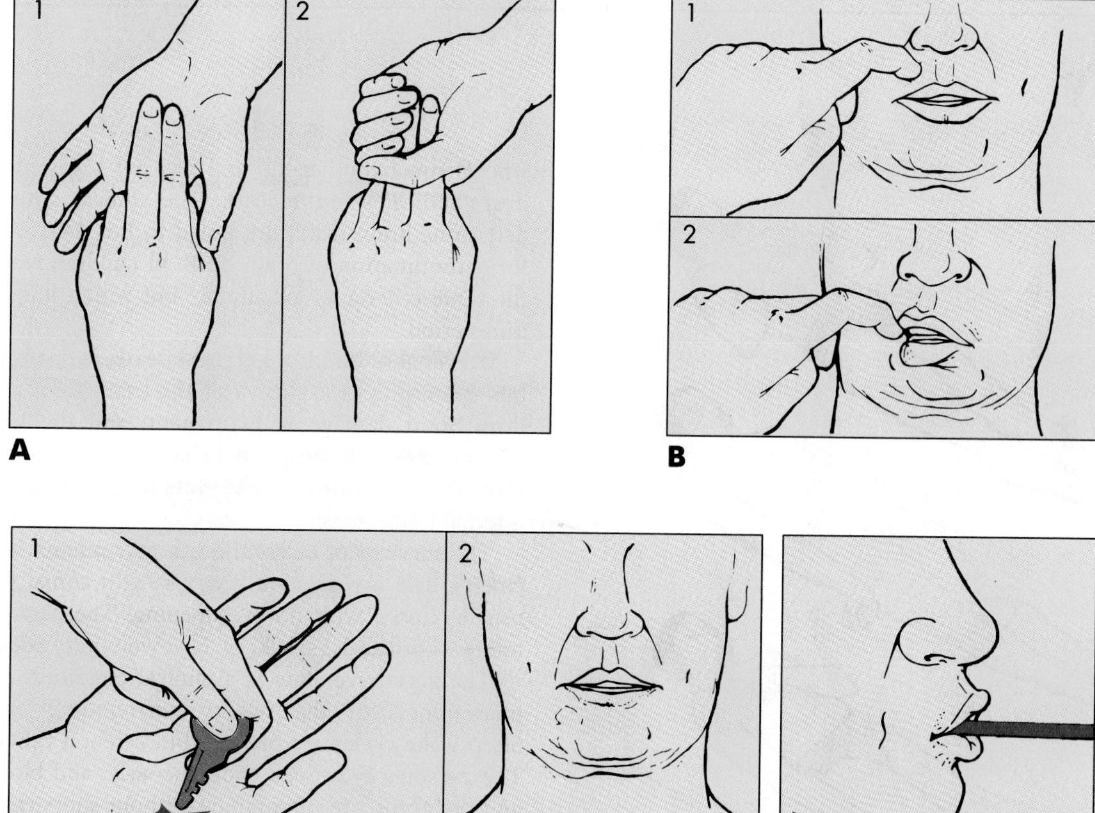

Figure 14-5 ■ **Pathologic Reflexes. A,** Grasp reflex. **B,** Snout reflex. **C,** Palmomental reflex. **D,** Suck reflex.

death as irreversible cessation of function of the entire brain.[1] Destruction includes the brain stem and cerebellum. On postmortem examination, the brain is autolyzing (self-digesting) or already autolyzed.

Brain death has occurred when there is no evidence of function above the foramen magnum[1]—that is, in the cerebral hemispheres or brain stem—for an extended period. The abnormality of brain function must result from structural or known metabolic disease and must *not* be caused by a depressant drug, alcohol poisoning, or hypothermia. An isoelectric, or flat, electroencephalogram (EEG) (electrocerebral silence) for 6 to 12 hours in a person

TABLE 14-5

Abnormal Motor Responses With Decreased Responsiveness

Motor Response	Description	Location of Injury
Abnormal motor responses, upper extremity flexion with or without extensor responses in the leg (decorticate rigidity)	Slowly developing flexion of the arm, wrist, and fingers with adduction in the upper extremity and extension, internal rotation, and plantar flexion of the lower extremity	Suggest hemispheric damage above midbrain
Extensor responses in the upper and lower extremities (decerebrate posturing, decerebrate rigidity)	Opisthotonos (hyperextension of the vertebral column) with clenching of the teeth; extension, abduction, and hyperpronation of the arms; and extension of the lower extremities	Associated with severe damage involving caudal diencephalon or midbrain
	In acute brain injury, shivering and hyperpnea may accompany unelicited recurrent decerebrate spasms	Acute injury often causes limb extension regardless of location
Extensor responses in the upper extremities accompanied by flexion in the lower extremities		Indicates pontine level dysfunction
Flaccid state with little or no motor response to stimuli		Damage to lower pons and upper myelencephalon

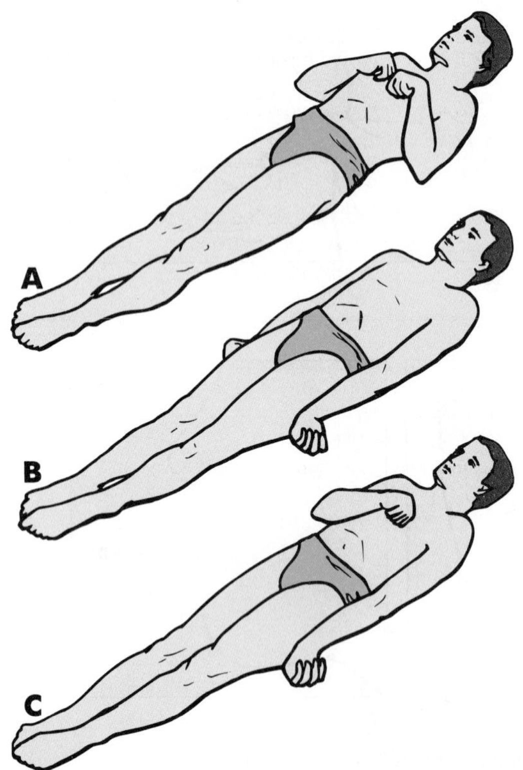

Figure 14-6 ■ Decorticate and Decerebrate Responses. **A,** Decorticate response. Flexion of arms, wrists, and fingers with adduction in upper extremities; extension, internal rotation, and plantar flexion in lower extremities. **B,** Decerebrate response. All four extremities in rigid extension, with hyperpronation of forearms and plantar extension of feet. **C,** Decorticate response on right side of body and decerebrate response on left side of body. (From Rudy EB: *Advanced neurological and neurosurgical nursing,* St Louis, 1984, Mosby.)

who is not hypothermic and has not ingested depressant drugs indicates brain death. The clinical criteria used to determine brain death are noted in Box 14-1. A task force for determination of brain death in children recommended the same criteria as for adults,[2] but with a longer observation period.[3]

Irreversible coma, or **cerebral death,** is death of the cerebral hemispheres exclusive of the brain stem and cerebellum. Brain damage is permanent, and the individual is forever unable to respond behaviorally in any significant way to the environment. The brain may continue to maintain internal homeostasis.

The survivor of cerebral death may remain in a coma or emerge into a vegetative state (VS). In coma, the eyes are usually closed with no eye opening. The person does not follow commands, speak, or have voluntary movement.[4]

The vegetative state is a clinical condition of complete unawareness of the self or surrounding environment. Sleep-wake cycles are present, but cerebral function is lost. The person's eyes open spontaneously, and blood pressure and breathing are maintained without support. Brain stem reflexes (pupillary, oculocephalic, chewing, swallowing) are intact. There is bowel and bladder incontinence. The individual does not speak any comprehensible words or follow commands. Recovery is unlikely if the state persists for 12 months.

Some survivors of coma progress to a **minimally conscious state (MCS).**[4] These persons may follow simple commands, manipulate objects, gesture or give yes/no responses, have intelligible speech, and have movements such as blinking or smiling.[4]

A **locked-in syndrome** differs in that both the content of thought and level of arousal are intact, but the efferent

BOX 14-1 Criteria for Brain Death

1. Completion of all appropriate and therapeutic procedures
2. Unresponsive coma (no motor or reflex movements)
3. No spontaneous respiration
4. No ocular responses to head turning or caloric stimulation; dilated, fixed pupils
5. Isoelectric (flat) EEG (electrocerebral silence)
6. Persistence of these signs for 30 minutes to 1 hour and for 6 hours after onset of coma and apnea
7. Confirming test indicating absence of cerebral circulation (optional)

Modified from Plum F, Posner JB: *The diagnosis of stupor and coma*, Philadelphia, 1980, FA Davis; Walker AE: *Cerebral death*, ed 3, Baltimore, 1985, Urban & Schwarzenberg.

pathways are disrupted. Thus, the individual cannot communicate through speech or body movement but is fully conscious, with intact cognitive function. The person retains vertical eye movement and blinking as a means of communication.

Seizures

A **seizure** results from a sudden, explosive, disorderly discharge of cerebral neurons and is characterized by a sudden, transient alteration in brain function, usually involving motor, sensory, autonomic, or psychic clinical manifestations and altered level of arousal. A seizure produces a brief disruption in the brain's electrical functions.[5] Seizure disorders represent a syndrome, however, and not a specific disease entity. The alteration in level of arousal is temporary.

Convulsion, a term sometimes applied to seizures, refers to the jerky, contract-relax (tonic-clonic) movement associated with some seizures. **Epilepsy** is a condition for which no underlying correctable cause for the seizure can be found; therefore, seizure activity recurs without treatment. The prevalence of epilepsy is 5 to 10 persons per 1000.[6]

TABLE 14-6 Causes of Recurrent Seizures in Different Age-Groups

Age at Onset	Probable Cause
Neonates (<1 month)	Perinatal hypoxia and ischemia Intracranial hemorrhage and trauma Acute CNS infection Metabolic disturbances (hypoglycemia, hypocalcemia, hypomagnesemia, pyridoxine deficiency) Drug withdrawal Developmental disorders Genetic disorders
Infants and children (>1 month and >12 yr)	Febrile seizures Genetic disorders (metabolic, degenerative, primary epilepsy syndromes) Developmental disorders Trauma Idiopathic
Adolescents (12–18 yr)	Trauma Genetic disorders Infection Brain tumor Illicit drug use Idiopathic
Young adults (18–35 yr)	Trauma Alcohol withdrawal Illicit drug use Brain tumor Idiopathic
Older adults (<35 yr)	Cerebrovascular disease Brain tumor Alcohol withdrawal Metabolic disorders (uremia, hepatic failure, electrolyte abnormalities, hypoglycemia) Alzheimer disease and other degenerative CNS diseases Idiopathic

From Lownstein DH: Seizures and epilepsy. In Kasper DL et al, editors: *Harrison's principles of internal medicine*, ed 16, vol 2, New York, 2005, McGraw-Hill.
CNS, Central nervous system.

PATHOPHYSIOLOGY

Conditions associated with seizure disorders

Any disorder that alters the neuronal environment may cause seizure activity, so, theoretically, anyone may experience a seizure. The seizure threshold of some persons, however, apparently is genetically lower.

Diseases or other processes that involve the nervous system can produce a seizure disorder. The onset may indicate the presence of an ongoing primary neurologic disease. Etiologic factors in seizures generally include (1) cerebral lesions, (2) biochemical disorders, (3) cerebral trauma, and (4) epilepsy, which can result from the following conditions:

- Metabolic defects
- Congenital malformation
- Genetic predisposition
- Perinatal injury
- Postnatal trauma
- Myoclonic syndromes
- Infection
- Brain tumor
- Vascular disease
- Fever
- Drug or alcohol abuse

Causes of recurrent seizures are age related (Table 14-6).

Seizures may be precipitated by hypoglycemia, fatigue or lack of sleep, emotional or physical stress, febrile illness, large amounts of water ingestion, constipation, use of stimulant drugs, withdrawal from depressant drugs (including alcohol), hyperventilation (respiratory alkalosis), and some environmental stimuli, such as blinking lights, a poorly adjusted television screen, loud noises, certain music, certain odors, or merely being startled. Women may have increased seizure activity immediately before or during menses.

Types of seizure disorders

Seizures are classified in different ways: by clinical manifestations, site of origin, EEG correlates, or response to therapy. A simplified version of the international classification of epileptic seizures is presented in Table 14-7. Terms used to describe seizure activity are defined in Table 14-8.

Epilepsy now is thought to be the result of complex genetic mutations with environmental effects that cause abnormalities in brain wiring or an imbalance in chemicals that the brain uses to send signals, or abnormal nerve connections made while attempting to repair itself after injury.[5] A group of neurons may exhibit a paroxysmal depolarization shift and function as an **epileptogenic focus.** These neurons are hypersensitive and are more easily activated by hyperthermia, hypoxia, hypoglycemia, hyponatremia, repeated sensory stimulation, and certain sleep phases.

Epileptogenic neurons fire more and more often and with greater amplitude. When the intensity reaches a threshold point, cortical excitation spreads. Excitation of the subcortical, thalamic, and brain stem areas corresponds to the **tonic phase** (muscle contraction with increased muscle tone) and is associated with loss of consciousness.

TABLE 14-7

International Classification of Epileptic Seizures

Traditional Terminology	New Nomenclature
	I. Partial seizures (seizures beginning locally)
Focal motor; jacksonian seizures (occasionally become secondarily generalized)	A. Simple (without impairment of consciousness) 1. With motor signs 2. With special sensory or somatosensory symptoms 3. With autonomic symptoms or signs 4. With psychic symptoms
Temporal lobe or psychomotor seizures	B. Complex (with impairment of consciousness) 1. Simple partial onset followed by impaired consciousness 2. Impaired consciousness at onset—with or without automatisms
	C. Secondarily generalized (partial onset evolving to generalized tonic-clonic seizures)
	II. Generalized seizures (bilaterally symmetric and without local onset)
Petit mal	A. Absence 1. Typical 2. Atypical
	B. Myoclonic
	C. Clonic
	D. Tonic
Grand mal	E. Tonic-Clonic
Drop attack	F. Atonic (astatic, akinetic)
	III. Unclassified epileptic seizures

TABLE 14-8

Terminology Applied to a Seizure Disorder

Term	Definition
Aura	A partial seizure experienced as a peculiar sensation preceding the onset of generalized seizure that may take the form of gustatory, visual, or auditory experience or a feeling of dizziness, numbness, or just "a funny feeling"
Prodroma	Early clinical manifestations, such as malaise, headache, or a sense of depression, that may occur hours to a few days before the onset of a seizure
Tonic phase	A state of muscle contraction in which there is excessive muscle tone
Clonic phase	A state of alternating contraction and relaxation of muscles
Postictal phase	The time period immediately following the cessation of seizure activity

The **clonic phase** (alternating contraction and relaxation of muscles) begins when inhibitory neurons in the cortex, anterior thalamus, and basal ganglia react to the cortical excitation. The seizure discharge is interrupted, producing intermittent muscle contractions that gradually decrease and finally cease. The epileptogenic neurons are exhausted.

During seizure activity, oxygen is consumed at a high rate—about 60% over normal. Although cerebral blood flow also increases, oxygen is rapidly depleted, along with glucose, and lactate accumulates in brain tissue. Continued, severe seizure activity holds the potential for progressive brain injury and irreversible damage. In addition, if a seizure focus is active for a prolonged period, a **mirror focus** may develop in normal tissue.

HEALTH ALERT

Epilepsy Surgery Stands the Test of Time

Theodore and Kelley, researchers at the National Institute of Neurological Disorders and Stroke (NINDS), obtained information from 48 persons and families about individuals who had right or left temporal lobe surgery for seizures between 1965 and 1974. Twenty-one persons were free of seizures that caused loss of consciousness, and three persons had been free of these types of seizures for 19 years. The others died or were never completely free of seizures causing loss of consciousness. Theodore and Kelley believe this type of surgery is underutilized because individuals shy away from brain surgery as a treatment option. The decision to pursue surgical treatment must balance the potential benefit of seizure control and the effect on cognitive function.

Data from Hamberger MJ, Drake EB: Cognitive functioning following epilepsy surgery, *Curr Neurol Neurosci Rep* 6(4):319–326, 2006; Kelley K, Theodore WH: Prognosis 30 years after temporal lobectomy, *Neurology* 64:1974–76, 2005.

CLINICAL MANIFESTATIONS The clinical manifestations associated with seizure depend on its type (see Table 14-7). Two types of symptoms signal a generalized tonic-clonic seizure: an **aura,** a partial seizure that immediately precedes the onset of a generalized tonic-clonic seizure, and a **prodroma,** an early manifestation occurring hours to days before a seizure. Both may become familiar to the person experiencing recurrent generalized seizures and may enable the person to prevent injuries during the seizure.

EVALUATION AND TREATMENT The health history, physical examination, and laboratory tests of blood and urine (blood glucose, serum calcium, blood urea nitrogen, urine sodium, creatinine clearance) can identify systemic diseases known to promote seizures. Radiographic studies and cerebrospinal fluid (CSF) examination help identify neurologic diseases associated with seizures. The EEG is used to assess the type of seizure and determine its focus.

Treatment involves correcting or controlling the cause and, if none is identified, administering antiseizure medications to suppress seizure activity. Counseling also may be of value. Prevention of epilepsy is the direction research has taken.[5a]

✔ QUICK CHECK 14-2

1. Why is irreversible coma different from brain death?
2. Why is a seizure different from epilepsy?
3. Why can so many conditions precipitate seizures?
4. Why is continued seizing dangerous? How does an epileptogenic focus differ from a mirror focus?

Cognitive Disorders

Selective attention (orienting) refers to the ability to select from available environmental and internal stimuli specific information to be processed. Certain midbrain and thalamic structures contribute to selective attention, so the etiologic factors for coma potentially can alter selective attention. Selective attention also is mediated by the right parietal lobe. An isolated (pure) **selective attention deficit** rarely occurs clinically. Causes of temporary, permanent, or progressive deficits include seizure activity, parietal lobe contusions, subdural hematomas, stroke, gliomas or metastatic tumor, and late Alzheimer and Pick diseases (see pp. 347–348).

There are two types of memory disorders: loss of domain-specific memories (that is, past memories; this disorder is known as **retrograde amnesia**) and an inability to form domain-independent memories (that is, new memories; this disorder is known as **anterograde amnesia**). These memory disorders may be temporary (e.g., after a seizure) or permanent (e.g., after severe head injury or in Alzheimer disease). There may be only the memory disorder, or the memory disorder may be associated with other cognitive disorders.

Executive attention deficits include the inability to maintain sustained attention, inability to set goals and recognize when an object meets a goal, and a working memory deficit (inability to remember instructions and information needed to guide behavior). Executive attention deficits may be temporary, progressive, or permanent. Table 14-9 summarizes cognitive networks deficits.

PATHOPHYSIOLOGY Very generally, the primary pathophysiologic mechanisms that operate in disorders of cognitive networks are (1) direct destruction caused by direct ischemia and hypoxia or indirect destruction resulting from compression and (2) the effects of toxins and chemicals. Disorders of selective attention, at least as they relate to visual orienting behavior, are produced by disease that involves portions of the midbrain. Disease affecting the superior colliculi manifests as a slowness in orienting

TABLE 14-9

Clinical Manifestations of Cognitive Network Deficits

Deficit	Clinical Signs	Symptoms
ATTENTION		
Selective attention (orienting)	Inability to focus attention; decreased eye, head, and body movements associated with focusing on the stimuli; decreased search and scanning; faulty orientation to stimuli, causing safety problems	Person reports inability to focus attention, failure to perceive objects and other stimuli (history of injuries, falls, safety problems)
MEMORY		
Domain-independent declarative memory	*Left hemisphere*: disorientation to time, situation, place, name, person (verbal identification); impaired language memory (e.g., names of objects); impaired semantic memory *Right hemisphere*: disorientation to self, person (visual), place (visual); impaired episodic memory (personal history); impaired emotional memory Either or both hemispheres: confusion; behavioral change	Person reports disorientation, confusion, "not listening," "not remembering"; reports by others of person being disoriented, not able to remember, not able to learn new information
Domain-specific declarative memory	*Left hemisphere*: inability to retrieve personal history, past medical history; unaware of recent current events *Right hemisphere*: inability to recognize persons, places, objects, music, and so on from the past	Person reports remote memory problems; others report that person cannot recall formerly known information
Image (semantic) processing	Inability to categorize (identify similarities and differences), sort; inability to form concepts; inability to analyze relationships; misinterpretations; inability to interpret proverbs	Reports by others of frequent misinterpretation of data, failure to conceptualize or generalize information
	Inability to perform deductive reasoning (convergent reasoning); inability to perform inductive reasoning (divergent reasoning); inability to abstract; concrete reasoning demonstrated; delusions	Reports by others of predominantly concrete thinking; lack of understanding of everyday situations, health care regimens, and such; delusional thinking
EXECUTIVE ATTENTIONAL NETWORKS		
Vigilance	Failure to stay alert and orient to stimuli	Person reports decreased alertness or ability to orient
Detection	Lack of initiative (anergy); lack of ambition; lack of motivation; flat affect; no awareness of feelings; appears depressed, apathetic, and emotionless; fails to appreciate deficit; disinterested in appearance; lacks concern about childish or crude behavior	Reports by others of laziness or apathy, flat affect or lack of emotional expression, failing to exhibit or be aware of feelings
Mild	Responds to immediate environment but no new ideas; grooming and social graces are lacking	Reports by others of lack of ambition, motivation, or initiative, failure to carry out adult tasks, lack of social graces and new ideas
Severe	Motionless, lack of responding to even internal cues, does not respond to physical needs, does not interact with surroundings	Reports by others of failure to groom or toilet self, unawareness of surroundings and own physical needs
	Inability to use feedback regarding behavior; failure to recognize omissions and errors in self-care, speech, writing, and arithmetic; impaired cue utilization; overestimation of performance	Reports by others of not changing behavior when requested; unawareness of limitations; does not recognize and correct errors in dressing, grooming, toileting, eating, and such; fails to recognize speech and arithmetic errors; careless speech
	Failure to shift response set; failure to change behavior when conditions change; cue utilization may be impaired	Reports by others of failure to use feedback; inability to incorporate feedback (does not correct when feedback is given)
Working memory	Inability to set goals or form goals; indecisiveness	Reports by others of failure to set goals, indecisiveness
	Failure to make plans; inability to produce a complete line of reasoning; inability to make up a story; appears impulsive	Reports by others of failure to plan, impulsiveness, "does not think things through"
	Failure to initiate behavior; failure to maintain behavior; failure to discontinue behavior; slowness to alternate response for the next step; motor perseveration	Reports by others of not knowing where to begin, inability to carry out sequential acts (maintain a behavior), inability to cease a behavior

attention. Parietal lobe disease may produce disengagement from a stimulus or unilateral neglect syndrome. **Sensory inattentiveness** is a form of neglect. The person is able to recognize individual sensory input from the dysfunctional side when called on to do so but ignores the sensory input from the dysfunctional side when stimulated from both sides **(extinction)**. The entire complex of denial of dysfunction, loss of recognition of one's own body parts, and extinction sometimes is referred to as the **neglect syndrome.** A disorder in vigilance may be produced by disease in the prefrontal areas. Right dysfunction in the anterior cingulate gyrus and basal ganglia may cause detection problems, whereas problems with working memory may be produced with left lateral frontal injury. Domain-independent memory disorders originate from pathology in the hippocampus and related temporal lobe structures. Domain-specific memory disorders originate from pathology in the association areas of the cerebral cortex.

CLINICAL MANIFESTATIONS Clinical manifestations of selective attention deficits, memory deficits, and executive attention function deficits are presented in Table 14-9.

EVALUATION AND TREATMENT Immediate medical management is directed at diagnosing the cause and treating reversible factors. Rehabilitative measures generally focus on compensatory or restorative activities and recently have been greatly facilitated by computer technology and other electronic devices.

Attention deficits and executive attention deficits masquerade as other cognitive deficits. Differential diagnosis is blocked and learning potential is largely obscured when an attention deficit is present. Therefore, the diagnosis and treatment of attention deficits are fundamental.

Data Processing Deficits

Agnosia

Agnosia is a defect of pattern recognition—a failure to recognize the form and nature of objects. Agnosia can be tactile, visual, or auditory, but generally only one sense is affected. For example, an individual may be unable to identify a safety pin by touching it with a hand but is able to name it when looking at it. Agnosia may be as minimal as a finger agnosia (failure to identify by name the fingers of one's hand) or more extensive, such as a color agnosia.

Although agnosia is associated most commonly with cerebrovascular accidents, it may arise from any pathologic process that injures specific areas of the brain.

Dysphasia

Dysphasia is impairment of comprehension or production of language (semantic processing). Comprehension or use of symbols, in either written or verbal language, is disturbed or lost. **Aphasia** is loss of the comprehension or production of language.

Dysphasias usually are associated with cerebrovascular accident involving the middle cerebral artery or one of its many branches. Language disorders, however, may arise from a variety of injuries and diseases—vascular, neoplastic, traumatic, degenerative, metabolic, or infectious causes. Dysphasia results from dysfunction in the left cerebral hemisphere, usually the frontotemporal region (Figure 14-7; see also Figure 12-6). Most language disorders result from acute processes or a chronic residual deficit of the acute process. Some progressive language disorders are the result of degenerative disorders. Genes located on chromosomes 3, 7, 13, 15, 16, and 19 have been linked to language development and disorders.[7–8]

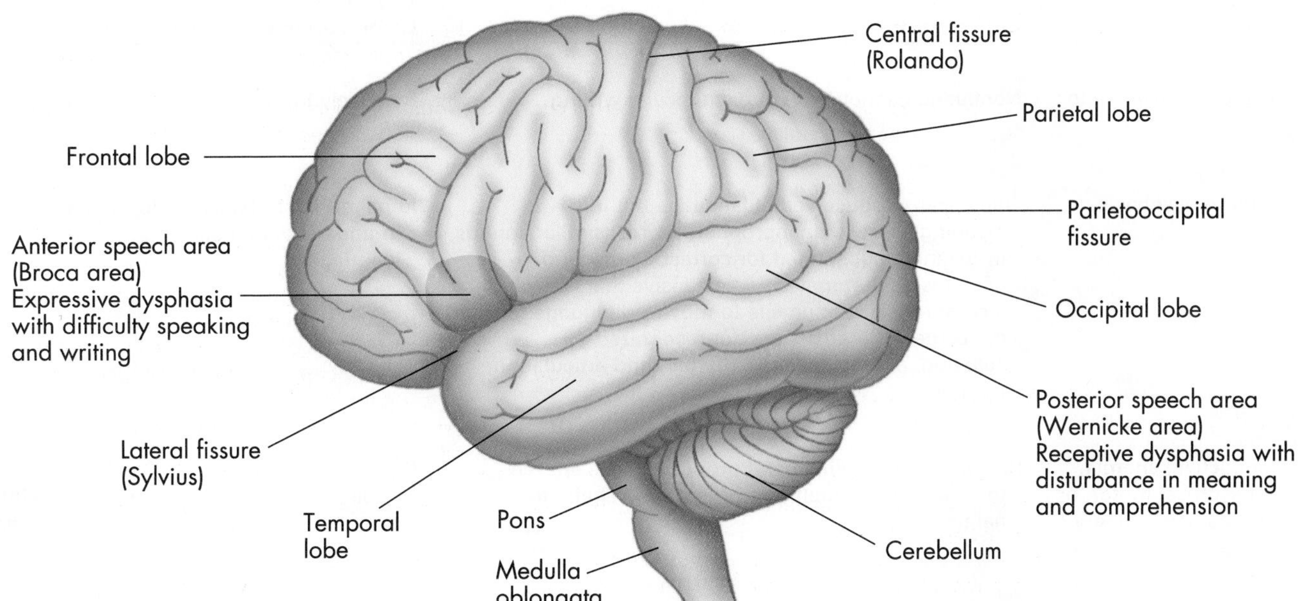

Figure 14-7 ■ **Development of Dysphasia.** Portion of the left cerebral hemisphere considered most important in the development of dysphasia.

Dysphasias have been classified both anatomically and functionally. Other classifications describe fluency, volume, or quantity of speech, although pure forms of any language dysfunction are rare. **Expressive dysphasias** involve primarily expression deficits, but verbal comprehension deficit also may be present. **Receptive dysphasias** may have expressive deficits. (Table 14-10 compares types of dysphasias; Table 14-11 illustrates some of the language disturbances.)

Some dysphasias are referred to as **transcortical dysphasias** and involve the ability to repeat **(echolalia)** and to recite. Speech is fluent but with striking paraphrases. The individual cannot read or write and has impaired comprehension. These dysphasias are caused by hypoxia or other mechanisms that destroy the border zone between the cerebral arteries (see Figure 12-19). The sensory and motor speech areas are functional, but connections with other sensory or motor areas are impaired. Information cannot be transmitted to Wernicke area and transformed into language.

Acute confusional states

Acute confusional states (ACS) result from cerebral dysfunction secondary to drug intoxication, metabolic disorder, or nervous system disease. Withdrawal from alcohol, barbiturate, or other sedative drug ingestion is a common cause. Acute confusional states may begin either suddenly or gradually, depending on the amount of exposure to the toxin. These states often occur with febrile illnesses, systemic diseases (e.g., heart failure), head injury, anesthesia, or certain focal cerebral lesions and are seen postnatally.

✔ QUICK CHECK 14-3

1. Why are there so many cognitive disorders?
2. Why can so many disorders cause dysphasia?
3. Why is impaired detection the most common feature of acute confusional states (ACS)?
4. How is an ACS different from dementia?

PATHOPHYSIOLOGY Acute confusional states arise from disruption of a widely distributed neural network involving the reticular activating system of the upper brain stem and its projections into the thalamus, basal ganglion, and specific association areas of the cortex and limbic areas. Delirium (hyperkinetic confusional states) is associated with right-upper middle-temporal gyrus or left temporal-occipital junction disruption. Hypokinetic confusional states are more likely to be associated with right-sided frontal-basal ganglion disruption.

Most metabolic disturbances that produce an acute confusional state interfere with neuronal metabolism or synaptic transmission. Many drugs and toxins also interfere with neurotransmission function at the synapse.

CLINICAL MANIFESTATIONS The predominant feature of an acute confusional state is impaired or lost detection. The person is highly distractible and unable to concentrate on incoming sensory information or on any one particular mental or motor task.

TABLE 14-10
Major Types of Dysphasia

Type	Expression	Verbal Comprehension	Repetition
EXPRESSIVE			
Broca dysphasia, motor	Nonfluent; cannot find words, difficulty writing	Relatively intact	Impaired
RECEPTIVE			
Wernicke dysphasia, sensory	Fluent; can produce verbal language but it is meaningless, with inappropriate words, similar sounds or meaning substituted for correct words, and neologisms that may be so extensive that speech is incomprehensible; unable to monitor language for correctness, so errors are not recognized Intonation, accent, cadence, rhythm, and articulation normal	Impaired (disturbance in understanding all language)	Impaired
OTHERS			
Global, conductive, anomia, transcortical motor, or transcortical sensory	Ranges from nonfluent and producing little speech to fluent with paraphrasia or impaired ability for naming	Can be relative intact, impaired, or completely lost	Can be intact or impaired with an inability to repeat

The onset of an ACS usually is abrupt. The first clinical manifestations are difficulty in concentration, restlessness, irritability, tremulousness, insomnia, and poor appetite. Later there are misperceptions, illusions, hallucinations, and delirium. Obsessions, compulsive behavior, and rituals may be evident.

In acute confusional states with associated underactivity, the individual exhibits decreases in mental function, specifically alertness, attention span, accurate perception, interpretation of the environment, and reaction to the environment. Forgetfulness is prominent, and the individual dozes frequently.

Delirium, an ACS associated with overactivity, typically develops over 2 to 3 days and is seen initially as difficulty in concentrating, restlessness, irritability, insomnia, tremulousness, and poor appetite. Some persons experience seizures. Unpleasant, even terrifying, dreams may occur.

In a fully developed delirium state, the individual is completely inattentive and perceptions are grossly altered, with extensive misperception and misinterpretation. Hallucinations may be present. The person appears distressed and often perplexed; conversation is incoherent. Frank tremor and high levels of restless movement are common. Violent behavior may be present. The individual cannot sleep, is flushed, and has dilated pupils, a rapid pulse (tachycardia), temperature elevation, and profuse sweating (diaphoresis). Delirium typically abates suddenly or gradually in 2 to 3 days, although occasionally delirium states persist for weeks.

EVALUATION AND TREATMENT The initial goal is to establish (1) that the individual is confused and (2) the cause (organic or functional) (Table 14-12). Next, is the confusion a delirium, an ACS with associated underactivity, or an underlying dementia? A complete history and physical examination as well as laboratory tests (electrocardiogram and blood, urine, cerebrospinal fluid, and radiologic studies) are needed. Once the cause is established, treatment is directed at controlling the primary disorder, with supportive measures used as appropriate.

Dementia

Dementia is a progressive failure of many cerebral functions not caused by impaired level of consciousness.[9] The result may be a decrease in orienting, memory, language and executive attentional networks. Because of declining intellectual ability, the individual exhibits alterations in behavior.

PATHOPHYSIOLOGY Mechanisms leading to dementia include degeneration, compression, atherosclerosis, and trauma. Genetic predisposition is associated with the degenerative diseases, including Alzheimer and Huntington diseases. CNS infections, including the human immunodeficiency virus (HIV) and slow-growing viruses associated with Creutzfeldt-Jakob disease, are associated with dementia in addition to changes in motor function (i.e., ataxia, rigidity, and spiru). Progressive dementias produce nerve cell degeneration and brain atrophy.

Reading Comprehension	Writing	Location of Lesion	Cause of Lesion
Variable	Impaired	Left posteroinferior frontal lobe (Broca area)	Occlusion of one or several branches of the left middle cerebral artery supplying the inferior frontal gyrus
Impaired	Impaired	Left posterosuperior temporal lobe (Wernicke area)	Occlusion of inferior division of left middle cerebral artery
Variable; may be impaired or completely lost	Variable or impaired	Various areas including frontotemporal lobe; arcuate fasciculus, supramarginal gyrus, bundle of fibers from the temporal lobe that project anteriorly to the premotor area; angular gyrus, and anterior or posterior presylvian fissures	Occlusion of the left middle cerebral artery of the left internal carotid artery, tumors, other mass lesions, hemorrhage, embolic occlusion of the ascending parietal or posterior temporal branch of the middle cerebral artery

TABLE 14-11

Examples of Language Disturbances

Disorder	Example
Verbal paraphrasia	Question: What did the car do? Patient: The car would spit sweetly down the road. (The car sped swiftly down the road.)
Literal paraphrasia	Request: Say "persistence is essential to success." Patient: Mesastence is instans to success.
Neologism	Question: What do you call this? (Pointing to a plant.) Patient: It's a logper.
Circumlocution	Question: What do you call this? (Pointing to a plant.) Patient: Something that grows.
Anomia	Question: What do you call this? (Pointing to a plant.) Patient: It's . . . Or Question: What did you do this morning? Patient: Reading. Question: Were you reading a book or newspaper? Patient: One of those.
Telegraphic style	Question: Where is your daughter? Patient: New Orleans . . . home . . . Monday.

From Boss BJ: Dysphasia, dyspraxia, and dysarthria: distinguishing features (part I), *J Neurosurg Nurs* 16(3):151–160, 1984.

TABLE 14-12

Differences Between Organic and Functional Confusion

Factor	Organic Confusion	Functional Confusion
Memory impairment	Recent, more impaired than remote	No consistent difference between recent and remote
Disorientation		
Time	Within own lifetime or reasonably near future	May not be related to patient's lifetime
Place	Familiar place or one where patient might easily be	Bizarre or unfamiliar places
Person	Sense of identity usually preserved Misidentification of others as familiar	Sense of identity diminished Misidentification of others based on delusion system
Hallucinations	Visual, vivid Animals and insects common	Auditory more frequent Bizarre and symbolic
Illusions	Common	Not prominent
Delusions	Concern everyday occurrences and people	Bizarre and symbolic
Confused	Spotty confusion Clear intervals mixed with confused episodes Worse at night	More consistent No tendency to become worse at night

From Morris M, Rhodes M: Guidelines for the care of confused patients, *Am J Nurs* 72(9):1632, 1972.

HEALTH ALERT

Exercising the Body Can Benefit the Mind

Exercise prompts nerve cells to multiply and strengthens their connections, and it protects them from harm. Benefits seem to extend to brains and nerves that are diseased or damaged in persons with Alzheimer disease, Parkinson disease, and spinal cord injury. Release of neurotrophic factors appears to account for exercise effect.

Data from Brownee C: Buff and brainy exercising the body can benefit the mind, *Sci News* 169(8):122–124, 2006; Dishman RK et al: Neurobiology of exercise, *Obesity (Silver Spring)* 14(3):345–356, 2006.

CLINICAL MANIFESTATIONS Symptoms of dementia may be categorized as cortical, subcortical, or both (Table 14-13).

EVALUATION AND TREATMENT Establishing the cause for dementia may be complicated, but individuals with clinical manifestations of dementia should be evaluated with laboratory and neuropsychologic testing to identify underlying conditions that may be treatable. Unfortunately, no specific cure exists for most progressive dementias. Therapy is directed at maintaining and maximizing use of the remaining capacities, restoring functions if possible, and accommodating to lost abilities. Helping

TABLE 14-13
Clinical Manifestations of Dementia

Type	Manifestation
Cortical dementia	Agnosias
	Apraxia
	Difficulty with naming
	Decreased language comprehension
	Loss of recent memory
	Loss of remote memory
	Decreased mathematical skill
	Altered visuospatial relationships
Subcortical dementia	Forgetfulness
	Apathy
	Depression
	Slowed thought processes
	Accident prone
	Personality changes and inappropriate affect
	Loss of motor function: wide shuffling gait with small steps, muscle rigidity, flexion posturing, tendency to fall, abnormal reflexes, bowel and bladder incontinence, immobility

the family to understand the process and to learn ways to assist the individual is essential.

Alzheimer disease

Alzheimer disease (AD) (dementia of Alzheimer type [DAT], senile disease complex) has been demonstrated to be one of the most common causes of severe cognitive dysfunction in older persons. Its more prevalent forms are late-onset familial Alzheimer dementia (FAD) and nonhereditary or sporadic, late-onset AD (70% of cases).

PATHOPHYSIOLOGY The exact cause of Alzheimer disease is unknown, but current theories include loss of neurotransmitter stimulation by choline acetyltransferase; mutation for encoding amyloid precursor protein; and alteration in apolipoprotein E, which binds beta amyloid.[10] Early-onset FAD has been linked to mutations on chromosomes 14 and 21, whereas late-onset FAD and sporadic AD are associated with chromosome 19 involved with apolipoprotein E (APOE-IV).[9,11] Accumulation of amyloid occurs with these disorders. Studies have correlated steady brain activity, such as daydreaming and idle thinking in young persons, with increased amyloid in those parts of the brain that are affected in AD.[10] Alzheimer disease also has been linked to abnormalities in a lysosomal pathway that yields a neurotoxic substance. A link between the pathologic findings of Alzheimer disease and aluminum has not been established, nor has a viral cause been proved, but submicroscopic proteinaceous infectious particles (prions) have been isolated. An autoimmune cause also is being investigated, as are the effects of aging and injury. APOE-IV predisposes to familial late-onset as well as sporadic late-onset cases.

Microscopically, the protein in the neurons becomes distorted and twisted, forming a **neurofibrillary tangle** (Figures 14-8 and 14-9). Tangles are composed of a microtubule-binding protein called *tau protein.* Groups of nerve

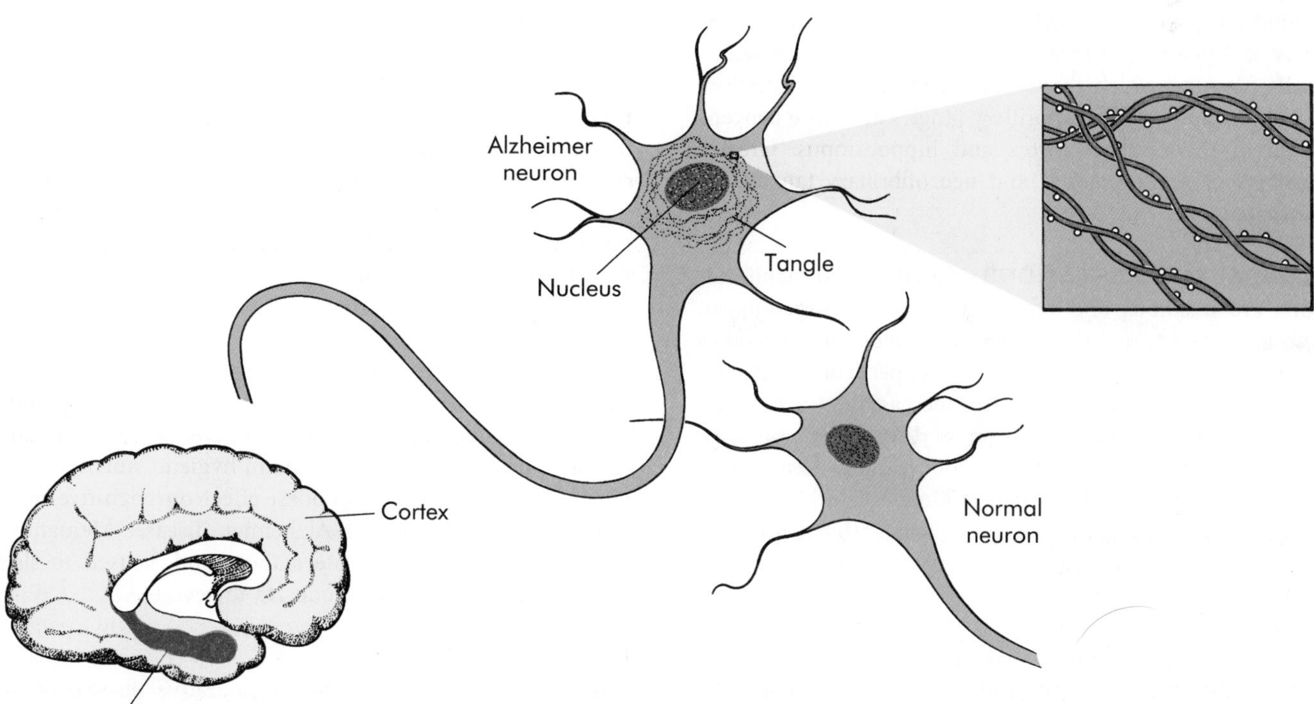

Figure 14-8 ■ Common Pathologic Findings in Alzheimer Disease. (From Beare PG, Myers JL: *Principles and practice of adult health nursing*, ed 3, St Louis, 1998, Mosby.)

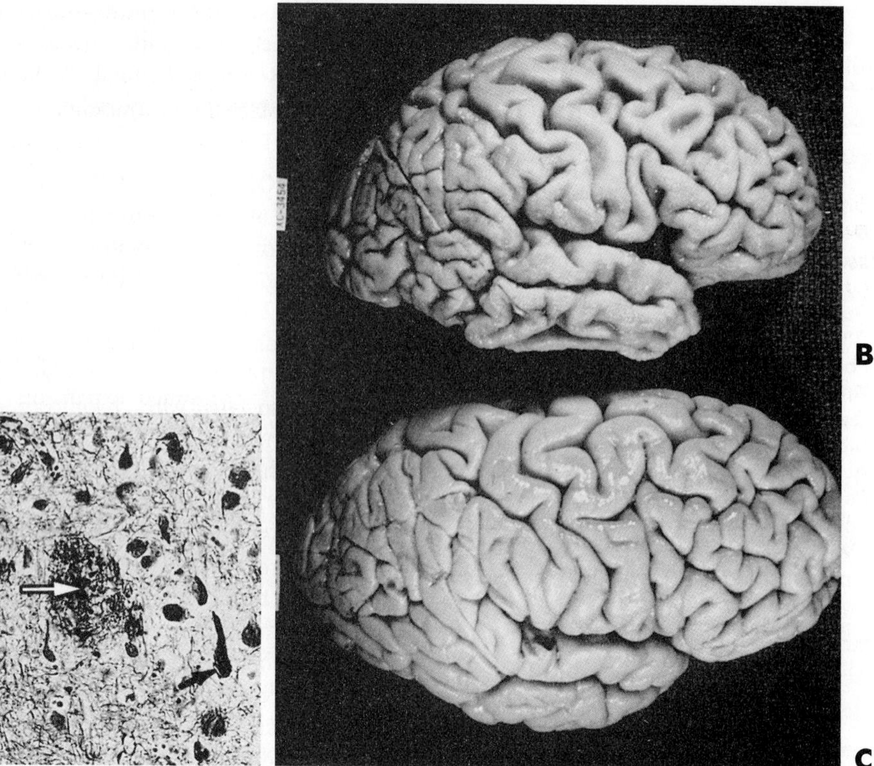

Figure 14-9 ■ **Pathologic Changes in Alzheimer Disease. A,** A neuritic (mature) plaque with central amyloid core *(white arrow)* next to a neurofibrillary tangle *(white arrow)*. Alzheimer disease **(B)** compared with age-matched and sex-matched control **(C)**: reduced size, narrow gyri, and wide sulci, notably in frontal and temporal lobes. (From Damjanov I, Linder J, editors: *Anderson's pathology,* ed 10, St Louis, 1996, Mosby.)

cells, especially terminal axons, degenerate and coalesce around an amyloid core. Microscopic examination of these areas of degeneration reveals plaquelike material known as **senile plaques,** which disrupt nerve-impulse transmission. Senile plaques and neurofibrillary tangles are more concentrated in the cerebral cortex and hippocampus. Greater numbers of senile plaques and neurofibrillary tangles are associated with AD.

CLINICAL MANIFESTATIONS Initial clinical manifestations are insidious and often attributed to forgetfulness, emotional upset, or other illness. The individual becomes progressively more forgetful over time, particularly in relation to recent events. Memory loss increases as the disorder advances, and the person becomes disoriented and confused and loses the ability to concentrate. Abstraction, problem solving, and judgment gradually deteriorate, with failure in mathematic calculation ability, language, and visuospatial orientation. Dyspraxia may appear. The mental status changes induce behavioral changes, including irritability, agitation, and restlessness. Mood changes also result from the deterioration in cognition. The person may become anxious, depressed, hostile, emotionally labile, and prone to mood swings. Motor changes may occur if the posterior frontal lobes are involved, causing rigidity (paratonia, gegenhalten), with flexion posturing, propulsion, and retropulsion. Great variability in age of onset, intensity and sequence of symptoms, and location and extent of brain abnormalities is common.

EVALUATION AND TREATMENT The diagnosis of Alzheimer disease is made by ruling out other causes. The history, including a mental status examination and the course of the illness, which may span 5 years or more, is used for diagnosis. Tests that are available to screen the genes for Alzheimer disease are presenilin 1 (PSEN1), presenilin 2 (PSEN2), amyloid precursor protein (APP), and apolipoprotein E (APOE-IV).[11]

Treatment is directed at using devices to compensate for the impaired cognitive function, such as memory aids; maintaining unimpaired cognitive functions; and maintaining or improving the general state of hygiene, nutrition, and health. Aricept has had a modest effect on cognitive function in the early stage of Alzheimer disease. Memantine (Namenda) blocks glutamate activity and is used to slow progression of disease in moderate to severe AD.[12–14]

Pick disease

Pick disease is a rare, severe degenerative disease of the frontal and anterior frontal lobes that produces death of tissue and dementia. It is difficult to distinguish clinically and pathologically from Alzheimer disease.

ALTERATIONS IN CEREBRAL HOMEOSTASIS

Cerebral Hemodynamics

Cerebral blood flow (CBF) to the brain is normally maintained at a rate that matches local metabolic needs of the brain. **Cerebral perfusion pressure (CPP)** is the pressure required to perfuse the cells of the brain, whereas **cerebral blood volume (CBV)** is the amount of blood in the intracranial vault at a given time. **Cerebral oxygenation** is the critical factor and is measured by oxygen saturation in the internal jugular vein.

Three injury states are possibly related to cerebral blood flow: too little cerebral perfusion (cerebral oligemia), normal cerebral perfusion but an elevated intracranial pressure exists, and too much cerebral blood volume (cerebral hyperemia). Treatments for these injury states are directed at improving or maintaining CPP, as well as controlling intracranial pressure. An injured brain requires a CPP of greater than 70 mm Hg.

Increased Intracranial Pressure

Intracranial pressure (ICP) normally is 5 to 15 mm Hg, or 60 to 180 cm H_2O. **Increased intracranial pressure (IICP)** may result from an increase in intracranial content (as occurs with tumor growth), edema, excess CSF, or hemorrhage. It necessitates an equal reduction in volume of the other cranial contents. The most readily displaced content is CSF. If intracranial pressure remains high after CSF displacement out of the cranial vault, cerebral blood volume is altered.

In stage 1 of intracranial hypertension, vasoconstriction and external compression of the venous system occur in an attempt to further decrease the intracranial pressure. Thus, during the first stage of intracranial hypertension, ICP may not change because of the effective compensatory mechanisms, and there may be few symptoms (Figure 14-10). Small increases in volume, however, cause an increase in pressure, and the pressure may take longer to return to baseline. This can be detected with ICP monitoring.

With continued expansion of the intracranial content, the resulting increase in ICP may exceed the brain's compensatory capacity to adjust. The pressure begins to compromise neuronal oxygenation, and systemic arterial vasoconstriction occurs in an attempt to elevate the systemic blood pressure sufficiently to overcome the IICP (stage 2 of intracranial hypertension). Clinical manifestations at this stage usually are subtle and transient, including episodes of confusion, restlessness, drowsiness, and slight pupillary and breathing changes (see Figure 14-10).

As ICP begins to approach arterial pressure, the brain tissues begin to experience hypoxia and hypercapnia and the individual's condition rapidly deteriorates. Clinical manifestations include decreasing levels of arousal or central neurogenic hyperventilation, widened pulse pressure, bradycardia, and pupils that become small and sluggish (stage 3 of intracranial hypertension) (see Figure 14-10).

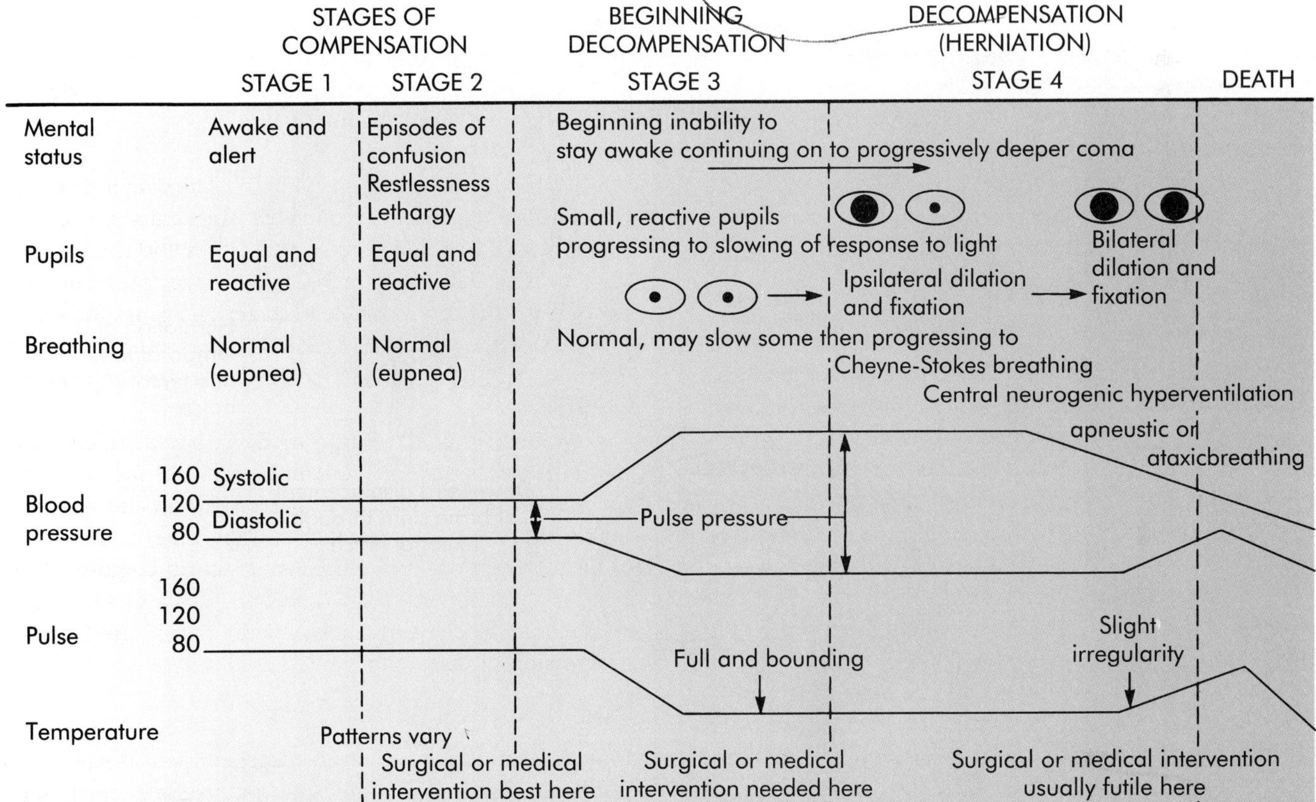

Figure 14-10 ■ **Clinical Correlates of Compensated and Uncompensated Phases of Intracranial Hypertension.** (From Beare PG, Myers JL: *Principles and practice of adult health nursing*, ed 3, St Louis, 1998, Mosby.)

Dramatic sustained rises in ICP are not seen until all compensatory mechanisms have been exhausted. Then dramatic rises in ICP occur over a very short period. **Autoregulation,** the compensatory alteration in the diameter of the intracranial blood vessels designed to maintain a constant blood flow during changes in cerebral perfusion pressure, is lost with progressively increased ICP. Accumulating carbon dioxide may still cause vasodilation locally, but without autoregulation this vasodilation causes the hydrostatic (blood) pressure in the vessels to drop and blood volume to increase. The brain volume is thus further enhanced, and ICP continues to rise. Small increases in volume cause dramatic increases in ICP, and the pressure takes much longer to return to baseline. As the ICP begins to approach systemic blood pressure, cerebral perfusion pressure falls and cerebral perfusion slows dramatically. The brain tissues experience severe hypoxia and acidosis.

IICP in one compartment of the cranial vault is not evenly distributed throughout the other vault compartments. In stage 4 of intracranial hypertension, brain tissue shifts (herniates) from the compartment of greater pressure to a compartment of lesser pressure (see Figures 14-10 and 14-11). With this shift in brain tissue, the herniating brain tissue's blood supply is compromised, causing further ischemia and hypoxia in the herniating tissues. The volume of content within the lower pressure compartment increases, exerting pressure on the brain tissue that normally occupies that compartment and impairing its blood supply. Small hemorrhages often develop in the involved brain tissue. Obstructive hydrocephalus may develop. The herniation process markedly and rapidly increases intracranial pressure. Mean systolic arterial pressure soon equals ICP, and cerebral blood flow ceases at this point.

The types of herniation syndromes are outlined in Box 14-2.

Cerebral Edema

Cerebral edema is an increase in the fluid content of brain tissue (Figure 14-12). The result is increased extracellular or intracellular tissue volume. It occurs after brain insult from trauma, infection, hemorrhage, tumor, ischemia, infarct, or hypoxia. The harmful effects of cerebral edema are caused by distortion of blood vessels, displacement of brain tissues, and eventual herniation of brain tissue from one brain compartment to another.

Four types of cerebral edema are (1) vasogenic edema, (2) cytotoxic (metabolic) edema, (3) ischemic edema, and (4) interstitial edema. **Vasogenic edema** is clinically the most important type and is caused by the increased permeability of the capillary endothelium of the brain after injury to the vascular structure. The blood-brain barrier is disrupted, and plasma proteins leak into the extracellular spaces, drawing water to them and increasing the water content of the brain parenchyma. Vasogenic edema starts in the area of

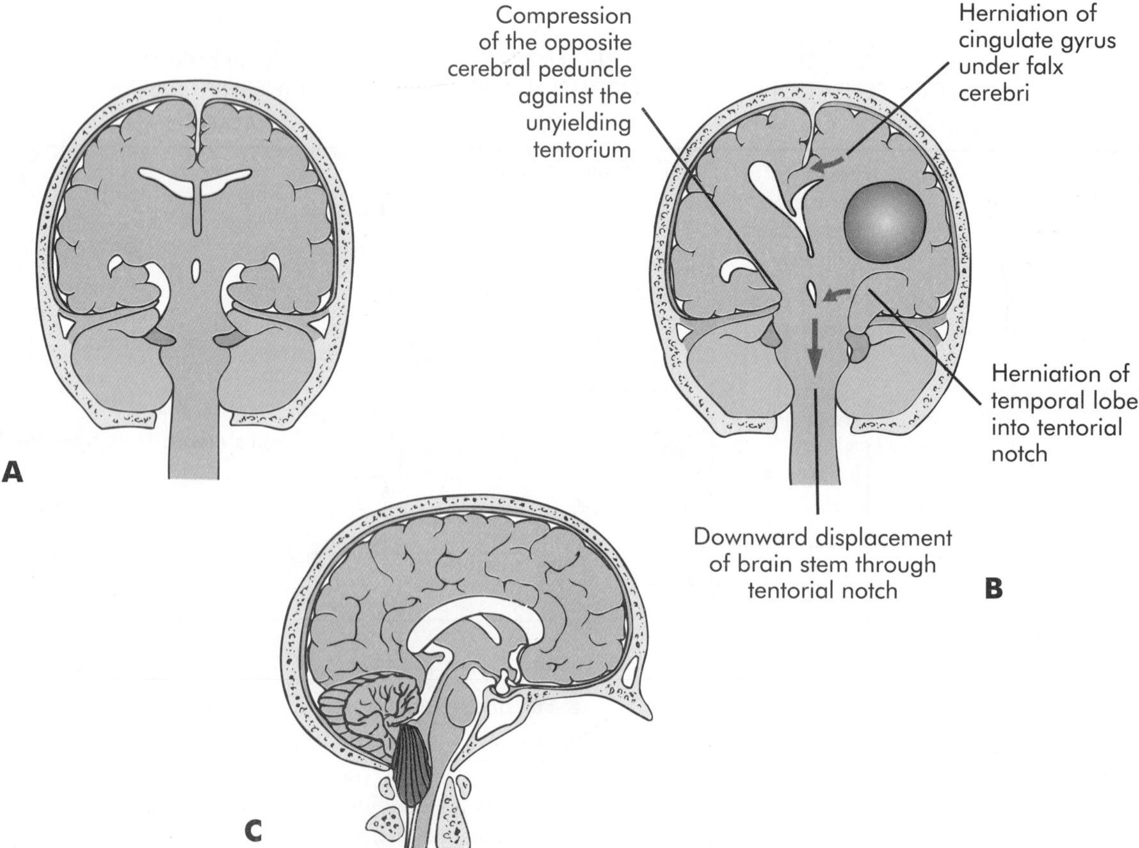

Figure 14-11 ■ **Herniation. A,** Normal relationship of intracranial structures. **B,** Shift of intracranial structures. **C,** Downward herniation of the cerebellar tonsils into the foramen magnum.

BOX 14-2 Herniation Syndrome

Supratentorial Herniation

1. *Uncal herniation.* Occurs when the uncus or hippocampal gyrus or both shift from the middle fossa through the tentorial notch into the posterior fossa, compressing the ipsilateral third cranial nerve, the contralateral third cranial nerve, and the mesencephalon. Uncal herniation generally is caused by an expanding mass in the lateral region of the middle fossa. The classic manifestations of uncal herniation are a decreasing level of consciousness, pupils that become sluggish before fixing and dilating (first the ipsilateral, then the contralateral pupil), Cheyne-Stokes respirations (which later shift to central neurogenic hyperventilation), and the appearance of decorticate and then decerebrate posturing.
2. *Central herniation.* The straight downward shift of the diencephalon through the tentorial notch. It may be caused by injuries or masses located around the outer perimeter of the frontal, parietal, or occipital lobes, extracerebral injuries around the central apex (top) of the cranium, bilaterally positioned injuries or masses, and unilateral cingulate gyrus herniation. The individual rapidly becomes unconscious; moves from Cheyne-Stokes respirations to apnea; develops small, reactive pupils and then dilated, fixed pupils; and passes from decortication to decerebration.
3. *Cingulate gyrus herniation.* Occurs when the cingulate gyrus shifts under the falx cerebri. Little is known about its clinical manifestations.

Infratentorial Herniation

In the most common syndrome the cerebellar tonsil shifts through the foramen magnum because of increased pressure within the posterior fossa. The clinical manifestations are an arched stiff neck, paresthesias in the shoulder area, decreased consciousness, respiratory abnormalities, and pulse rate variations. Occasionally the force produces an upward transtentorial herniation of a cerebellar tonsil or the lower brain stem. No specific set of clinical manifestations are associated with infratentorial herniation.

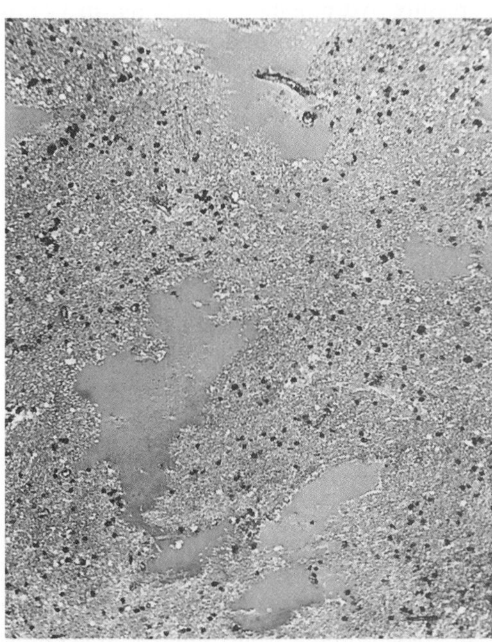

Figure 14-12 ■ **Brain Edema.** Intercellular lakes of high protein content fluid. (Hematoxylin-eosin stain; ×90.) (From Kissane JM, editor: *Anderson's pathology,* ed 9, St Louis, 1993, Mosby.)

injury and spreads, with fluid accumulating in the white matter of the ipsilateral side because the parallel myelinated fibers separate more easily. Edema promotes more edema because of ischemia from the increasing pressure.

Clinical manifestations of vasogenic edema include focal neurologic deficits, disturbances of consciousness, and a severe increase in ICP. Vasogenic edema resolves by slow diffusion.

In **cytotoxic (metabolic) edema,** toxic factors directly affect the cellular elements of the brain parenchyma (neuronal, glial, and endothelial cells), causing failure of the active transport systems. The cells lose their potassium and gain larger amounts of sodium. Water follows by osmosis into the cells, so that the cells swell. Cytotoxic edema occurs principally in the gray matter and may increase vasogenic edema.

Ischemic edema follows cerebral infarction. The ischemia has components of both vasogenic and cytotoxic edema. The initial edema is confined to the intracellular compartment, but over several days, brain cells begin to undergo necrosis and die, releasing lysosomes. In this autodigestive process, the blood-brain barrier's permeability increases.

Interstitial edema is seen most often with noncommunicating hydrocephalus (see Chapter 16). The edema is caused by transependymal movement of CSF from the ventricles into the extracellular spaces of the brain tissues. The brain fluid volume increases predominantly around the ventricles, with increased hydrostatic pressure within the white matter. The size of the white matter reduces because of the rapid disappearance of myelin lipids.

Hydrocephalus

The term **hydrocephalus** refers to various conditions characterized by excess fluid in the cranial vault, subarachnoid space, or both. Hydrocephalus occurs because of interference with CSF flow caused by increased fluid production, obstruction within the ventricular system, or defective reabsorption of the fluid. A tumor of the choroid plexus may, in rare instances, cause overproduction of CSF. The types of hydrocephalus are reviewed in Table 14-14.

Hydrocephalus may develop from infancy through adulthood. Congenital hydrocephalus (i.e., ventricular enlargement before birth) is rare. **Noncommunicating hydrocephalus (internal hydrocephalus, intraventricular**

TABLE 14-14
Types of Hydrocephalus

Type	Mechanism	Cause
Noncommunicating	Obstruction of CSF flow between ventricles	Congenital abnormality Aqueduct stenosis Arnold-Chiari malformation (brain extension through foramen magnum) Compression by tumor
Communicating	Impaired absorption of CSF within subarachnoid space	Infection with inflammatory adhesions Compression of subarachnoid space by a tumor High venous pressure in sagittal sinus Head injury Congenital malformation
	Increased CSF secretion by choroid plexus	Secreting tumor

CSF, Cerebrospinal fluid.

hydrocephalus)—obstruction within the ventricular system—is seen more often in children, and **communicating hydrocephalus**—defective resorption of CSF from the cerebral subarachnoid space—is found more often in adults.

Most cases of hydrocephalus develop gradually and insidiously over time. **Acute hydrocephalus,** however, may develop in a couple of hours in persons who have sustained head injuries. Acute hydrocephalus contributes significantly to IICP.

PATHOPHYSIOLOGY The obstruction of CSF flow associated with hydrocephalus produces dilation of the ventricles proximal to the obstruction. Obstructed CSF is under pressure, causing atrophy of the cerebral cortex and degeneration of the white matter tracts. There is selective preservation of gray matter. When excess CSF fills a defect caused by atrophy, a degenerative disorder, or a surgical excision, this fluid is not under pressure; therefore, atrophy and degenerative changes are not induced.

CLINICAL MANIFESTATIONS Acute hydrocephalus presents with signs of rapidly developing IICP. The person quickly deteriorates into a deep coma if not promptly treated. **Normal-pressure hydrocephalus** (dilation of the ventricles without increased pressure) develops slowly, with the individual or family noting declining memory and cognitive function. An unsteady, broad-based gait with a history of falling is common. Additional clinical manifestations are apathy, inattentiveness, and indifference to self, family, and the environment. Urinary incontinence is present.

EVALUATION AND TREATMENT The diagnosis is based on physical examination, computed tomography (CT) scan, and magnetic resonance imaging (MRI). A radioisotopic cisternogram may be performed to diagnose normal-pressure hydrocephalus. Hydrocephalus can be treated by surgery to resect cysts, neoplasms, or hematomas or by ventricular bypass into the normal intracranial channel or into an extracranial compartment using a shunting procedure, one of the three most common neurosurgical procedures. Excision or coagulation of the choroid plexus occasionally is needed when a papilloma is present. In normal-pressure hydrocephalus, reduction in CSF through a diuresis regimen often is used.

✔ QUICK CHECK 14-4

1. What are the four stages of intracranial hypertension (increased intracranial pressure)?
2. How does supratentorial herniation differ from infratentorial herniation?
3. What are the four different types of cerebral edema?
4. How is communicating hydrocephalus different from noncommunicating hydrocephalus?

ALTERATIONS IN MOTOR FUNCTION

Movements are complex patterns of activity controlled by the CNS. They are influenced by the cerebral cortex, the pyramidal system, the extrapyramidal system, and the motor units. Dysfunction in any of these areas can cause motor dysfunction. General motor dysfunctions may produce changes in muscle tone, movement, and complex motor performance.

Alterations in Muscle Tone

Normal muscle tone involves a slight resistance to passive movement. Throughout the range of motion, the resistance is smooth, constant, and even. The abnormalities of muscle tone are presented in Table 14-15.

Hypotonia

In **hypotonia** (decreased muscle tone), passive movement of a muscle occurs with little or no resistance. Causes include pure pyramidal tract damage (a rare occurrence)

TABLE 14-15
Alterations in Muscle Tone

Alterations	Characteristics	Cause
Hypotonia:	Passive movement of a muscle mass with little or no resistance Muscles may be moved rapidly without resistance	Thought to be caused by decreased muscle spindle activity as a result of decreased excitability of neurons
Flaccidity	Associated with limp, atrophied muscles and paralysis	Occurs typically when nerve impulses necessary for muscle tone are lost
Hypertonia:	Increased muscle resistance to passive movement May be associated with paralysis May be accompanied by muscle hypertrophy	Results when the lower motor unit reflex arc continues to function but is not mediated or regulated by higher centers
Spasticity	A gradual increase in tone causing increased resistance until tone suddenly reduces, which results in clasp-knife phenomenon	Exact mechanism unclear; appears to arise from an increased excitability of the alpha motor neurons to any input because of absence of the descending inhibition of the pyramidal systems
Gegenhalten (paratonia)	Resistance to passive movement, which varies in direct proportion to force applied	Exact mechanism unclear; associated with frontal lobe injury
Dystonia	Sustained involuntary twisting movement	Produced by slow muscular contraction
Rigidity	Muscle resistance to passive movement of a rigid limb that is uniform in both flexion and extension throughout the motion	Occurs as a result of constant, involuntary contraction of muscle
Plastic, or lead pipe	Increased muscular tone relatively independent of degree of force used in passive movement; does not vary throughout the passive movement	Associated with basal ganglion damage
Cogwheel	The uniform resistance may be interrupted by a series of brief jerks resulting in movements much like a rachet, "cogwheel" phenomenon	Associated with basal ganglion damage
Gamma	Characterized by extensor posturing (decerebrate rigidity)	Loss of excitation of extensor inhibitory areas by the cerebral cortex decreasing the inhibition of alpha and gamma motor neurons
Alpha	Impaired relaxation characterized by extensor rigidity of skeletal muscle after the contraction	Loss of cerebellum input to lateral vestibular nuclei

and cerebellar damage. A pure pyramidal tract injury produces hypotonia and weakness. The hypotonia contributes to the ataxia and intention tremor in cerebellar damage and manifests with minimal weakness and normal or slightly exaggerated reflexes. Hypotonia or flaccidity (a state in which the muscle may be moved rapidly without resistance) occurs when the nerve impulses needed for muscle tone are lost, such as in spinal cord injury or cerebrovascular accident.

Individuals with hypotonia tire easily (asthenia) or are weak. They may have difficulty rising from a sitting position, sitting down without using arm support, and walking up and down stairs, as well as an inability to stand on their toes. Because of their weakness, accidents during locomotion and self-care activities are common. The joints become hyperflexible, so persons with hypotonia may be able to assume positions that require extreme joint mobility. The joints may appear loose, and the knee jerks are pendulous.

The muscle mass atrophies because of decreased input entering the motor unit, and muscles appear flabby and flat. Muscle cells are gradually replaced by connective tissue and fat. Fasciculations may be present in some cases.

Hypertonia

In **hypertonia** (increased muscle tone), passive movement of a muscle occurs with resistance. Four types of hypertonia are described: spasticity, gegenhalten (paratonia), dystonia, and rigidity.

Spasticity results from hyperexcitability of the stretch reflexes and is associated with damage to the motor, premotor, and supplementary motor areas, as well as lateral corticospinal tract damage (Figure 14-13). Increased deep tendon reflexes (hyperreflexia) and the spread of reflexes (clonus) accompany it.

Gegenhalten (paratonia) manifests as resistance to passive movement that varies in direct proportion to the force applied and is associated with frontal lobe injury. **Dystonia** manifests as sustained, involuntary twisting movements caused by slow muscle contraction and may be caused by lack of appropriate reciprocal inhibition of the muscles (Figures 14-14 and 14-15). Injury to the putamen or its outflow tracts is associated with hemidystonia.

Rigidity produced by tonic reflex activity mediated by gamma motor neurons may be continuous or intermittent. The involved muscles are firm and tense; the increase in muscle movement is even and uniform throughout the range of passive movement. Four types of rigidity are described: plastic or lead-pipe rigidity, cogwheel rigidity, gamma rigidity, and alpha rigidity (see Table 14-15).

Individuals with hypertonia tire easily (asthenia) or are weak. Passive and active movement is affected equally, except in paratonia, in which more active than passive movement is possible. As a result of hypertonia and weakness, accidents occur during locomotion and self-care activities.

The muscles may atrophy because of decreased use. However, hypertrophy occasionally occurs as a result of the overstimulation of muscle fibers. Overstimulation occurs when the motor unit reflex arc remains intact and functioning but is not inhibited by higher centers. This causes continual muscle contraction, resulting in enlargement of the muscle mass and firm muscles (Figure 14-16).

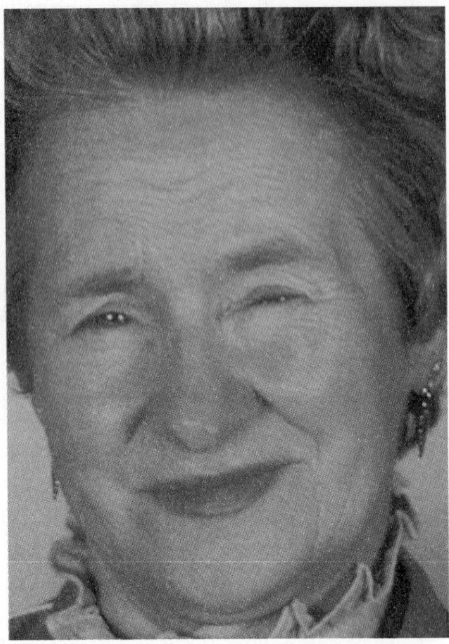

Figure 14-13 ■ **A Paroxysm of Left-Sided Hemifacial Spasm.** (From Perkin GD: *Mosby's color atlas and text of neurology,* ed 2, London, 2002, Mosby.)

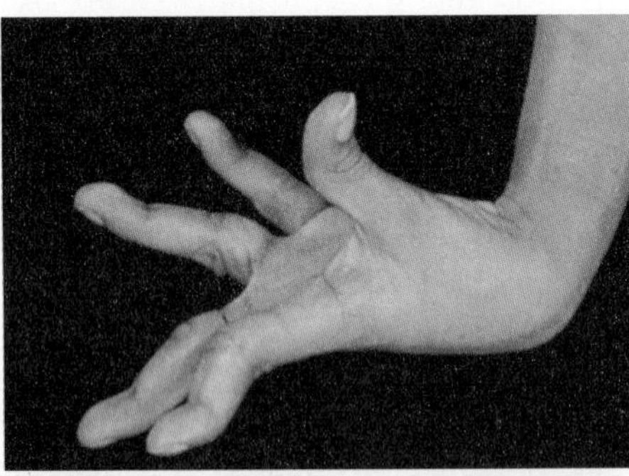

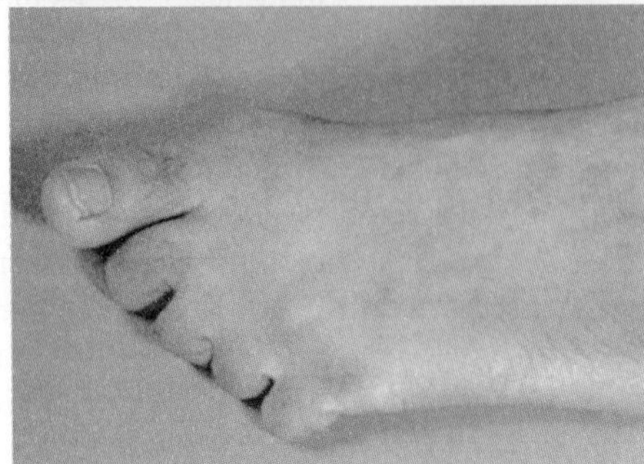

Figure 14-14 ■ **Dystonic Posturing of the Hand and Foot.** (From Perkin GD: *Mosby's color atlas and text of neurology,* ed 2, London, 2002, Mosby.)

Alterations in Movement

Movement requires a change in the contractile state of muscles. Abnormal movements occur when CNS dysfunctions alter muscle innervation. Currently, neuropharmacology and experimental therapeutics provide the knowledge base for movement disorders. Researchers have found that dopamine apparently functions in several movement disorders. Some (e.g., the akinesias) result from too little dopaminergic activity, whereas others (e.g., chorea, ballism, tardive dyskinesia) result from too much. Still others are not primarily related to dopamine function. Movement disorders are not necessarily associated with mass, strength, or

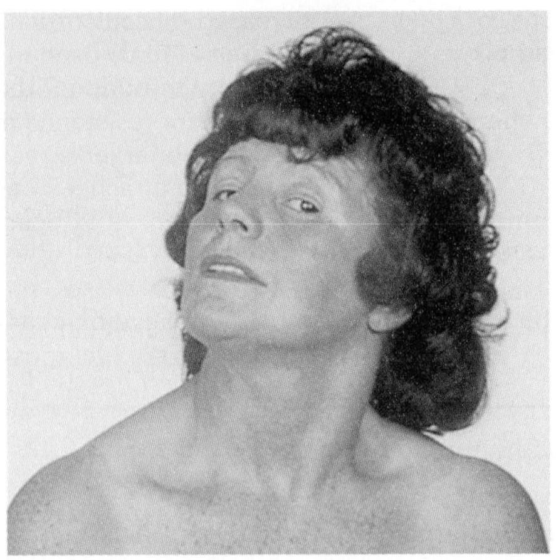

Figure 14-15 ■ **Spasmodic Torticollis.** A characteristic head posture. (From Perkin GD: *Mosby's color atlas and text of neurology,* ed 2, London, 2002, Mosby.)

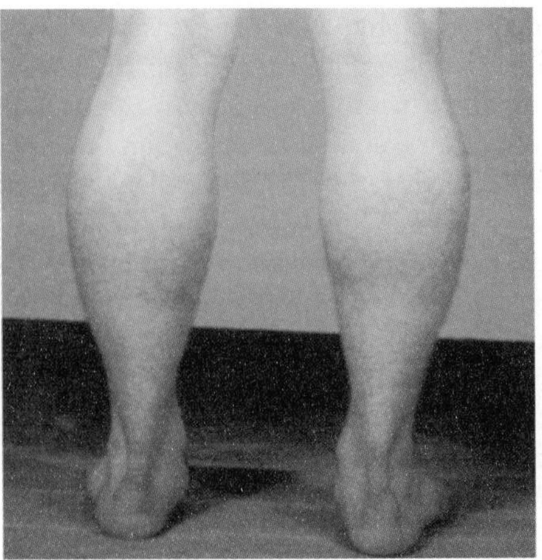

Figure 14-16 ■ **Pseudohypertrophy of the Calf Muscles.** (From Perkin GD: *Mosby's color atlas and text of neurology,* ed 2, London, 2002, Mosby.)

tone but are neurologic dysfunctions with either too little or too much movement. Muscle strength is quantitatively evaluated on a scale of 0 to 4+ or 5+, in which 4+ or 5+ is normal and 0 indicates an inability to move against gravity.

Paresis/paralysis

Paresis (weakness) is partial paralysis with incomplete loss of muscle power. **Paralysis** is loss of motor function so that a muscle group is unable to overcome gravity. Two subtypes of paresis/paralysis are described: upper motor neuron paresis/paralysis and lower motor neuron paresis/paralysis (Table 14-16).

Upper motor neuron syndromes

Upper motor neuron paresis/paralysis is known also as *spastic paresis/paralysis,* and many different terms are used to describe the specific disorder. **Hemiparesis/hemiplegia** is paresis/paralysis of the upper and lower extremities on one side. **Diplegia** is paralysis of both upper or lower extremities as a result of cerebral hemisphere injuries. **Paraparesis/paraplegia** refers to weakness/paralysis of the lower extremities. **Quadriparesis/quadriplegia** refers to paresis/paralysis of all four extremities. Both paraparesis/paraplegia and quadriparesis/quadriplegia may be caused by dysfunction of the spinal cord. Upper cord damage results in quadriparesis/quadriplegia, and lower cord damage preserves upper extremity function and causes paraparesis/paraplegia. (Spinal cord injury is discussed in Chapter 15.)

Upper motor neuron paresis/paralysis is associated with a **pyramidal motor syndrome,** which involves a series of motor dysfunctions resulting from interruption of the pyramidal system (Figures 14-17 and 14-18). The injury may be in the cerebral cortex, the subcortical white matter, the internal capsule, the brain stem, or the spinal cord. The clinical manifestations of a pure pyramidal injury are not known, but bilateral interruption of the pyramidal system in monkeys causes temporary hypotonic paralysis. In humans, however, injury generally involves more than interrupting the pyramidal system, so that an upper motor neuron paralysis occurs, indicating involvement of several motor pathways. Excessive movements, such as clonus and spasms, occur regularly as a result of loss of higher motor center control. There is great variation depending on the suddenness of onset and the age of the individual.

Spinal shock is the complete cessation of spinal cord functions below the lesion (below the level of the pons). It is characterized by complete flaccid paralysis, absence of reflexes, and marked disturbances of bowel and bladder function. A major factor in spinal shock is the sudden destruction of the efferent pathways. If destruction occurs more slowly, spinal shock may not develop (see Chapter 15).

If the pyramidal system is interrupted above the level of the pons, the hand and arm muscles are greatly affected. Paralysis rarely involves all the muscles on one side of the body, even when the hemiplegia results from complete damage to the internal capsule. Bilateral movements, such as those of the eye, jaw, and larynx, as well as those of the trunk, are affected only slightly if at all. Predominantly the limbs are influenced.

Paralysis associated with a pyramidal motor syndrome rarely remains flaccid for a prolonged time. After a few days or weeks, a gradual return of spinal reflexes marks the end of spinal shock. Reflexes then become hyperactive, and muscle tone increases significantly, particularly in antigravity muscles. Spasticity is common, although rigidity occasionally occurs. Most often, passive range-of-motion movements cause the "clasp-knife" phenomenon, probably by activating the stretch receptors in the muscle spindles and the Golgi tendon organ. (Muscle function is discussed in Chapter 36.) With pyramidal motor syndrome, predominantly the flexors of the arms and extensors of the legs are affected.

TABLE 14-16

Upper and Lower Motor Neuron Syndromes

Factor	Upper Motor Neuron Syndromes*	Lower Motor Neuron Syndromes†
Distribution of affected muscles	Muscle groups are affected; when movement is possible, the proper relationship among agonists, antagonists, synergists, and fixators is preserved Synkinesias (residual movements) are present; attempts to move paralyzed part cause a variety of associated movements; movements of normal limb may cause imitative or mirror movements in the paralyzed limb	Individual muscles may be affected
Muscle tone	Hypertonia, specifically spasticity	Hypotonia, flaccidity
Tendon reflexes	Hyperreflexia with extensor plantar reflex present	Hyporeflexia, no abnormal reflexes present
Atrophy	Slight, caused by disuse	Pronounced atrophy
Fasciculations	Absent	May be present

*Pyramidal motor syndromes.
†All are motor unit syndromes.

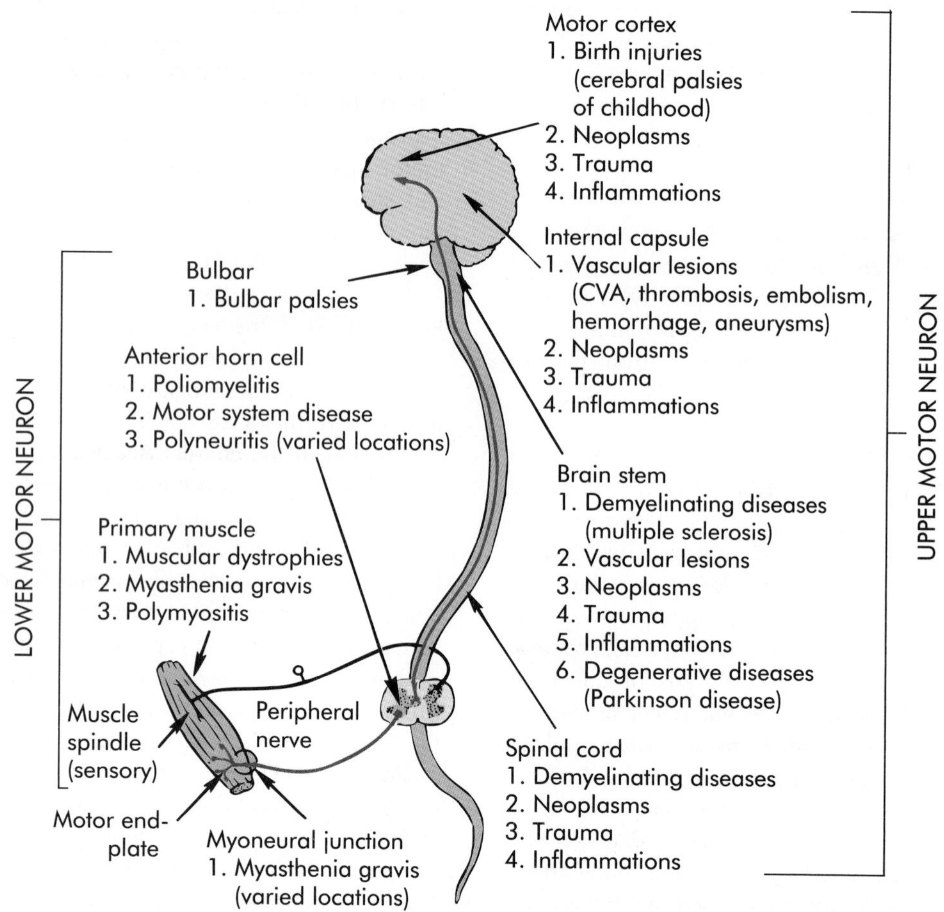

Figure 14-17 ■ **Disturbances in Motor Function.** Disturbances in motor function are classified pathologically along upper and lower motor neuron structures. It should be noted that the same pathologic condition occurs at more than one site in an upper motor neuron *(above right).* A few pathologic conditions involve both upper and lower motor neuron structures, as in amyotrophic lateral sclerosis, for example. Other lesion sites include myoneural junction and primary muscle, making it possible to classify conditions as neuromuscular and muscular, respectively.

Lower motor neuron syndromes

Lower (primary, alpha) motor neurons are the large motor neurons in the anterior (or ventral) horn of the spinal cord, the motor nuclei of the brain stem, and the axons that originate from these nerve cell bodies (to course in the anterior spinal roots or in the cranial nerves to reach skeletal muscles) (Figure 14-19). Dysfunction in this motor system impairs both voluntary and involuntary movement. The degree of paralysis or paresis is proportional to the number of lower motor neurons affected. If only some of the motor units that supply a muscle are affected, only partial paralysis (or paresis) results. If all motor units are affected, a complete paralysis results. Other clinical manifestations also are proportional to the degree of dysfunction, but the precise manifestations depend on the location of the dysfunction in the motor unit and in the CNS.

Small motor (gamma) neurons, which maintain muscle tone and protect the muscle from injury, are needed for normal motor movement. They depend on input from the muscle spindle (arriving through an afferent limb rising to the cord). Dysfunction in this motor system impairs tone and reduces the tendon reflexes, causing hyporeflexia. The muscles become susceptible to damage from hyperextensibility.

Generally, the large and small motor neuron systems are equally affected. Therefore, the muscle has reduced or absent tone and is accompanied by hyporeflexia or **areflexia** (loss of tendon reflexes) and **flaccid paresis/paralysis.**

Denervated muscles (i.e., muscles that have lost their nervous system input) atrophy over weeks to months, mostly from disuse, and demonstrate fasciculations (muscle rippling or quivering under the skin). Occasionally, denervated muscles cramp. **Fibrillation** (isolated contraction of a single muscle fiber) also may occur, although it is not visible clinically.

Amyotrophies

Lower motor neuron syndromes originating in the anterior horn cells or the motor nuclei of the cranial nerves are called **amyotrophies.** Paralytic **poliomyelitis** is the prototype of these disorders. It involves a severe inflammatory reaction in motor neurons, some of which do not survive, leaving a permanent lower motor neuron syndrome.

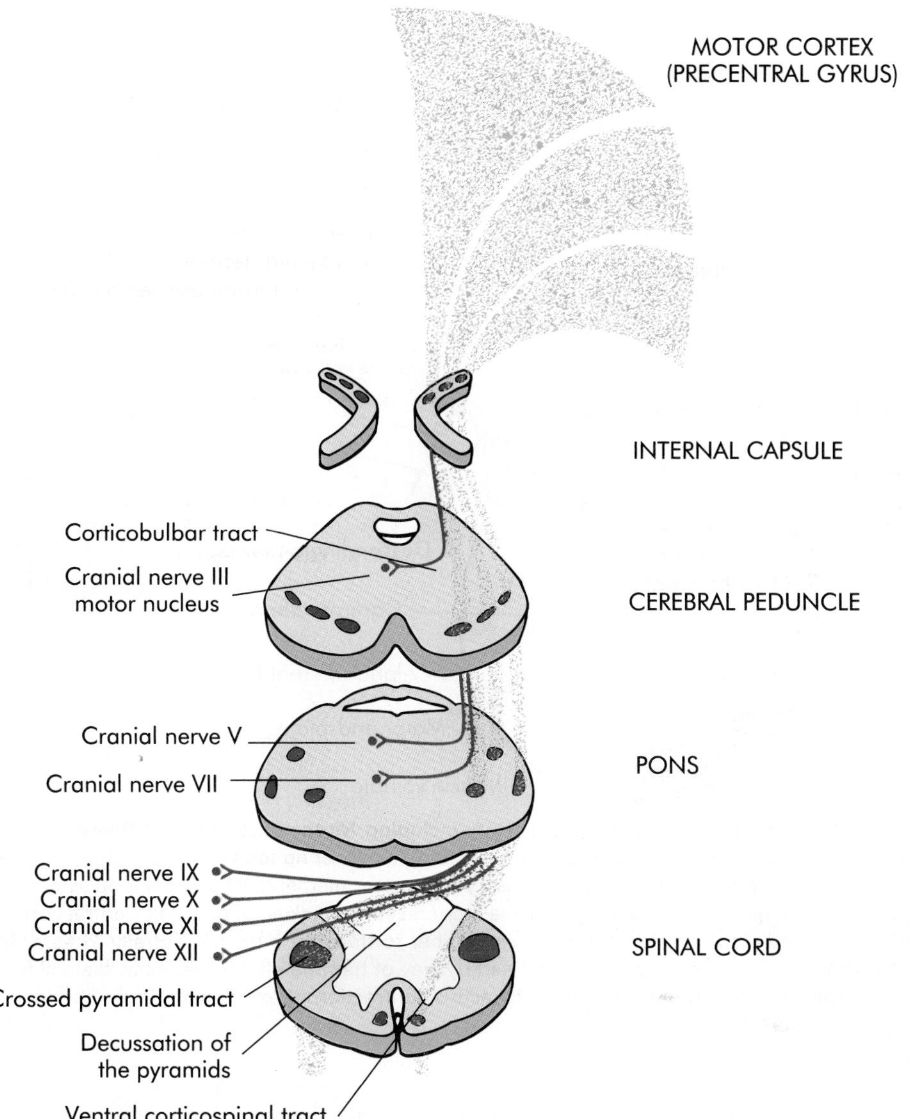

Figure 14-18 ■ **Structures Making up Upper Motor Neuron, or Pyramidal, System.** Pyramidal system fibers are shown to originate primarily in cells in precentral gyrus of motor cortex; to converge at internal capsule; to descend to form central third of cerebral peduncle; to descend further through pons, where small fibers are given off to cranial nerve motor nuclei along the way; to form pyramids at medulla, where most of the fibers decussate; and then to continue to descend in lateral column of white matter of spinal cord. A few fibers descend without crossing at medulla level (see Figure 12-8).

A virally induced or postinfectious/postvaccination inflammatory process may injure or destroy anterior horn cells or cranial nerve cell bodies. Most of these inflammatory processes are mild and are followed by rapid cellular recovery.

In the amyotrophies, muscle strength, muscle tone, and muscle bulk are affected in the muscles innervated by the involved motor neurons. The paresis and paralysis associated with anterior horn cell injury are segmental, but because each muscle is supplied by two or more roots, the segmental character may be difficult to see. When cranial nerve motor nuclei are affected (these lack nerve roots and have only small rootlets near the point of exit from the brain stem), the distribution of the motor weakness follows that of the cranial nerve. The weakness may involve distal muscles, proximal muscles, or the muscles of midline structures. Hypotonia and hyporeflexia/areflexia are present.

The atrophy associated with amyotrophy is segmental when the anterior horn cells of the spinal cord are involved and follows the distribution of the cranial nerve when the motor nuclei of the cranial nerves are affected. It may be in distal, proximal, or midline muscles. Fasciculations are associated particularly with primary motor neuron injury, and muscle cramps and mild fatigue are common. If the pathologic process is limited to the primary motor neuron, no sensory changes are evident.

Several brain stem syndromes, called **nuclear palsies,** involve damage to one or more of the cranial nerve nuclei. Causes include vascular occlusion, tumor, aneurysm, tuberculosis, and hemorrhage.

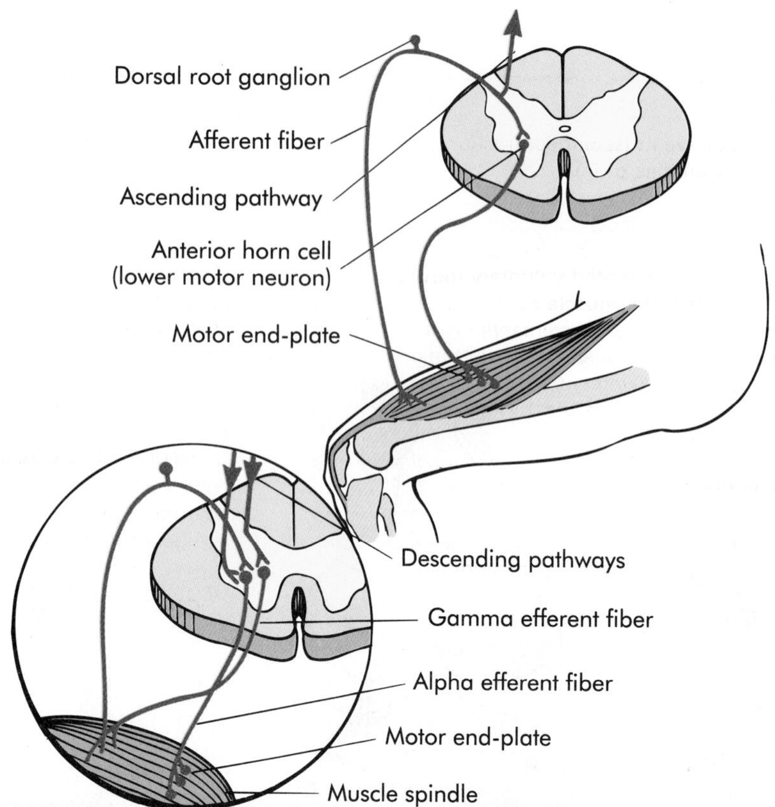

Figure 14-19 ■ **Structures Making up Lower Motor Neuron, Including Motor (Efferent) and Sensory (Afferent) Elements.** *(Top)* Anterior horn cell (in anterior gray column of spinal cord and its axon), terminating in motor end plate as it innervates extrafusal muscle fibers in quadriceps muscle. *(Detailed enlargement)* Sensory and motor elements of gamma loop system. Gamma efferent fibers shown innervating polar, or end, region of muscle spindle (sensory receptor of skeletal muscle). Contraction of muscle spindle fibers stretches central portion of spindle and causes afferent spindle fiber to transmit impulse centrally to cord. Muscle spindle afferent fibers in turn synapse on anterior horn cell and are transmitted by way of gamma efferent fibers to skeletal (extrafusal) muscle, causing it to contract. Muscle spindle discharge is interrupted by active contraction of extrafusal muscle fibers.

The anterior horn cells and the motor nuclei of the cranial nerves may be secondarily affected in many severe pathologic processes involving primarily the cranial nerves. The condition may extend proximally to affect the nerve roots or rootlets and the motor neurons themselves, a process commonly seen, for example, in **Guillain-Barré syndrome.** If enough motor neurons are destroyed, permanent loss of motor function results because regeneration of the damaged axons requires a living neuronal cell body.

In **progressive spinal muscular atrophy,** the anterior horn cells of the spinal cord are affected. This disorder occurs in adults and closely resembles the familial progressive muscular atrophies that occur in infants and children and are considered inherited metabolic disorders (see Chapter 38). If the motor nuclei of the cranial nerves are affected instead of the anterior horn cells, the disorder is called a **progressive bulbar palsy,** so named because the myelencephalon originally was called the *bulb* and a degenerative process causes a progressively more serious condition. When any lower motor neuron syndrome involves the cranial nerves that arise from the bulb (i.e., cranial nerves IX, X, XII), the dysfunction is called a **bulbar palsy.**

The clinical manifestations of bulbar palsy include paresis or paralysis of the jaw, face, pharynx, and tongue musculature. Articulation is affected, especially articulation of the lingual *(r, n, l)*, labial *(b, m, p, f)*, dental *(d, t)*, and palatal *(k, g)* consonants. Modulation is impaired, making the voice rasping or nasal. Pharyngeal reflexes are diminished or lost, palate and vocal cord movement during phonation is impaired, and chewing and swallowing are affected. The facial muscles are weak, and the face appears to droop, with decreased jaw jerk. Atrophy and fasciculations eventually become apparent. All these manifestations become progressively worse, leading to aspiration, malnutrition, possible dehydration, and an inability to communicate verbally.

Hyperkinesia

Hyperkinesia (excessive movements) represents the second broad category of abnormal movements. Within this category are a number of specific dysfunctions (Table 14-17). Also included under the general category of hyperkinesias are dyskinesias—that is, abnormal involuntary movements.

Paroxysmal dyskinesias are abnormal, involuntary movements that occur as spasms. The type of dyskinesia varies depending on the specific disorder.

TABLE 14-17

Types of Hyperkinesia

Type	Characteristics	Causes
Chorea*	Nonrepetitive muscular contractions, usually of the extremities of face; random pattern of irregular, involuntary rapid contractions of groups of muscles; disappears with sleep, decreases with resting; increases with emotional stress and attempted voluntary movement	Associated with excess concentration of or a supersensitivity to dopamine within basal ganglia
Athetosis*	Disorder of distal-muscle postural fixation; slow, sinuous, irregular movements most obvious in the distal extremities, more rhythmic than choreiform movements and always much slower; movements accompany characteristic hand posture; slowly fluctuating grimaces	Occurs most commonly as a result of injury to the putamen of the basal ganglion; exact pathophysiologic mechanism is not known
Ballism	Disorder of proximal-muscle postural fixation with wild flinging movement of the limbs; movement is severe and stereotyped, usually lateral; does not lessen with sleep; ballism is most common on one side of the body, a condition termed *hemiballism*	Results from injury to subthalamus nucleus (one of the nuclei that comprise the basal ganglia); thought to be caused by reduced inhibitory influence in the nucleus, a release phenomenon; hemiballism results from injury to the contralateral subthalamic nucleus
Hyperactivity	State of prolonged, generalized, increased activity that is largely involuntary but may be subject to some voluntary control; not highly stereotyped but rather manifests as continuous changes in total body posture or in excessive performance of some simple activity, such as pacing under inappropriate circumstances	May be caused by frontal and reticular activating system injury
Wandering	Tendency to wander without regard for environment	"Release phenomenon" associated with bilateral injury to globus pallidus or putamen
Akathisia	Special type of hyperactivity; mild compulsion to move (usually more localized to legs); severe frenzied motion possible; movements are partly voluntary and may be transiently suppressed; carrying out the movement brings a sense of relief; a frequent complication of antipsychotic drugs	Dopaminergic transmission may be involved
TREMOR AT REST	Rhythmic, oscillating movement affecting one or more body parts	Caused by regular contraction of opposing groups of muscles
Parkinsonian tremor	Regular, rhythmic, slower flexion-extension contraction; involves principally the metacarpophalangeal and wrist joints; alternating movements between thumb and index finger described as "pill rolling"; disappears during voluntary movement	Loss of inhibitory influence of dopamine in the basal ganglia, causing instability of basal ganglial feedback circuit within the cerebral cortex
POSTURAL TREMOR		
Asterixis (tremor of hepatic encephalopathy)	Irregular flapping movement of the hands accentuated by outstretching arms	Exact mechanisms responsible unknown; thought to be related to accumulation of products normally detoxified by the liver
Metabolic	Rapid, rhythmic tremor affecting fingers, lips, and tongue; accentuated by extending the body part; enhanced physiologic tremor	Occurs in conditions associated with disturbed metabolism or toxicity, as in thyrotoxicosis (hyperthyroidism), alcoholism, and chronic use of barbiturates; amphetamine, lithium amitriptyline [Elavil]; exact mechanism responsible unknown
Essential (familial)	Tremor of fingers, hands, and feet; absent at rest but accentuated by extension of body part, prolonged muscular activity, and stress	Not associated with any other neurologic abnormalities; cause unknown

*Choreoathetosis involves both chorea and athetosis; precise pathophysiology unknown.

(Continued)

TABLE 14-17

Types of Hyperkinesia—Cont'd

Type	Characteristics	Causes
INTENTION TREMOR		
Cerebellar	Tremor initiated by movement, maximal toward end of movement	Occurs in disease of the dentate nucleus (one of the deep cerebellar nuclei responsible for efferent output) and the superior cerebellar peduncle (a stalklike structure connected to the pons); caused by errors in feedback from the periphery and errors in preprogramming goal-directed movement
Rubral	Rhythmic tremor of limbs that originates proximally by movement	Results from lesions involving the dentatorubrothalamic tract (a spinothalamic tract connecting the red nucleus in the reticular formation and the dentate nucleus in the cerebellum)
Myoclonus	Series of shocklike nonpatterned contractions of portion of a muscle, entire muscle, or group of muscles that cause throwing movements of a limb; usually appear at random but frequently triggered by sudden startle; do not disappear during sleep	Associated with an irritable nervous system and spontaneous discharge of neurons; structures associated with myoclonus include the cerebral cortex, cerebellum, reticular formation, and spinal cord

Tardive dyskinesia is the involuntary movement of the face, trunk, and extremities. Although the condition occurs occasionally in individuals with Parkinson disease, it usually occurs as a side effect of prolonged phenothiazine drug therapy. The most common symptom of tardive dyskinesia is rapid, repetitive, stereotypic movements. Most characteristic is continual chewing with intermittent protrusions of the tongue, lip smacking, and facial grimacing.

Other movement disorders in this category are (1) complex repetitive movements, including automatism, stereotype, complex tics, compulsions, perseverations, and mannerisms; (2) positivism (excessive reactions to certain stimuli); and (3) paroxysmal excessive activity, including cataplexy and excessive startle reaction.

Huntington disease

Huntington disease (HD), also known as *chorea,* is a relatively rare, hereditary, degenerative disorder diffusely involving the basal ganglia and cerebral cortex. The onset of Huntington disease is usually between 30 and 50 years of age, when the trait may already have been passed to the person's children. The disorder has a prevalence rate of approximately 5 per 100,000 persons and occurs in all races.

PATHOPHYSIOLOGY Huntington disease is inherited as an autosomal dominant trait with high penetrance. The gene has been isolated and cloned on chromosome 4. (Mechanisms of genetic inheritance are discussed in Chapter 2.) The principal pathologic feature of Huntington disease is severe degeneration of the basal ganglia, particularly the caudate nucleus. Tangles of protein collect in the brain cells and chains of glutamine on the abnormal molecules stick to each other.[15] Early in the disease there is loss of the gamma-aminobutyric acid (GABA) pathway to the globus pallidus. Basal ganglia and nigral depletion of GABA, an inhibitory neurotransmitter, is the principal biochemical alteration in Huntington disease. It alters the integration of motor and mental function. Degeneration of the pallidus pathway to the substantia nigra causes GABA depletion in the substantia nigra with decreased inhibitory GABA activity on dopaminergic neurons in the substantia nigra and relative excess of dopaminergic activity in the basal ganglial feedback circuit with the cerebral cortex. Frontal cerebral atrophy occurs late in the disease. Symptoms progress slowly and include hypotonia and involuntary, fragmentary movements, such as chorea.

CLINICAL MANIFESTATIONS The classic manifestations of Huntington disease are abnormal movement and progressive dysfunction of intellectual and thought processes (dementia). Any one of these features may mark the onset of the disease. Chorea, the most common type of abnormal movement affecting these individuals, begins in the face and arms, eventually affecting the entire body. Cognitive deficits include loss of working memory and reduced capacity to plan, organize, and sequence. Thinking is slow, and apathy is present. Restlessness, disinhibition, and irritability are common. Euphoria or depression may be present.

EVALUATION AND TREATMENT The diagnosis of Huntington disease is based on family history and clinical presentation of the disorder. No known treatment is effective in halting the degeneration or progression of symptoms. Drug therapies are being explored.[16] Recombinant genetic techniques may someday prevent or control the disorder. Depression or psychosis is treated with drug therapy. Phenothiazines, which are antidopaminergic, may relieve some symptoms of chorea.

Hypokinesia

Hypokinesia (decreased movement) is loss of voluntary movement despite preserved consciousness and normal peripheral nerve and muscle function. Types of hypokinesia include akinesia, bradykinesia, and loss of associated movement.

Akinesia and bradykinesia

Akinesia is a decrease in associated and voluntary movements. It is related to dysfunction of the extrapyramidal system and caused by either a deficiency of dopamine or a defect of the postsynaptic dopamine receptors, which occurs in parkinsonism. **Bradykinesia** is slowness of voluntary movements. All voluntary movements become slow, labored, and deliberate, with difficulty in (1) initiating movements, (2) continuing movements smoothly, and (3) performing synchronous (at the same time) and consecutive tasks. Both akinesia and bradykinesia involve a disturbance in the time it takes to perform a movement.

Loss of associated neuron syndromes

In hypokinesia, the normal, habitually associated movements that provide skill, grace, and balance to voluntary movements are lost. Decreased associated movements accompanying emotional expression cause an expressionless face, a statue-like posture, absence of speech inflection, and absence of spontaneous gestures. Decreased associated movements accompanying locomotion cause reduction in arm and shoulder movements, in hip swinging, and in rotary motion of the cervical spine.

Parkinson disease

Parkinson disease is a commonly occurring degenerative disorder of the basal ganglia (corpus striatum) involving failure of the dopaminergic (dopamine-secreting) nigrostriatal pathway. Nigrostriatal disorders produce a syndrome of abnormal movement called **parkinsonism (Parkinson syndrome, parkinsonian syndrome, paralysis agitans)** (Figure 14-20).

Either primary Parkinson disease or secondary parkinsonism may occur. Secondary parkinsonism is parkinsonism caused by disorders other than Parkinson disease (i.e., trauma, infection, neoplasm, atherosclerosis, toxins, drug intoxication). Drug-induced parkinsonism, caused by neuroleptics, antiemetics, and antihypertensives, is the most common secondary form and usually is reversible.

Parkinson disease begins after the age of 40 years, with peak age of onset between 58 and 62 years. It is slightly more prevalent in males. This disease is one of the most prevalent of the primary CNS disorders and a leading cause of neurologic disability in individuals older than 60 years. The prevalence rate is 107 to 187 per 100,000 persons, with 40,000 new cases in the United States each year.

PATHOPHYSIOLOGY The pathogenesis of Parkinson disease is unknown. Epidemiologic data suggest genetic, viral, and environmental toxins as possible causes.

Nigral and basal ganglial loss of neurons with depletion of dopamine, an inhibitory neurotransmitter, is the principal biochemical alteration in Parkinson disease (see Figure 14-20, *B*). Symptoms in basal ganglial disorders result from an imbalance of dopaminergic (inhibitory) and cholinergic (excitatory) activity in the caudate and putamen of the basal ganglia. In Parkinson disease, degeneration of

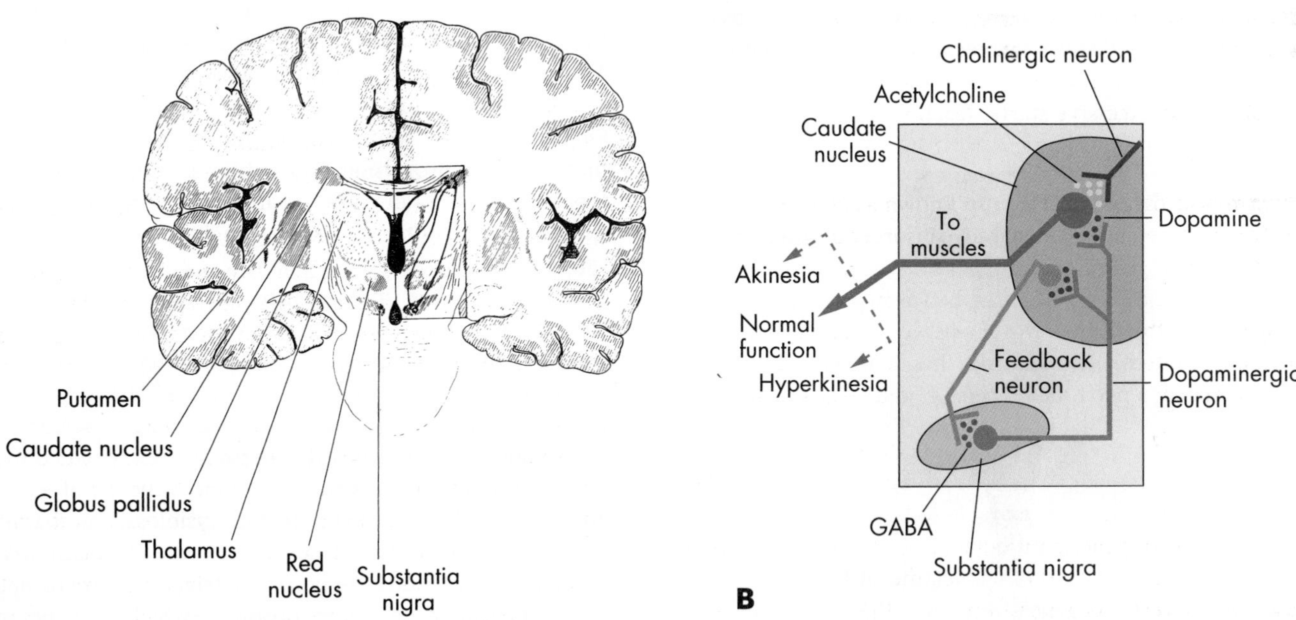

Figure 14-20 ■ **Nigrostriatal Disorders Produce the Parkinson Syndrome.** Coronal section of the brain shows the basal ganglia. Pathways controlling normal and abnormal motor function are depicted in a portion of the basal ganglia (caudate nucleus), **A;** they are shown enlarged in **B.** Dopaminergic synaptic activity is mediated by dopamine. Cholinergic synaptic activity is mediated by acetylcholine. A balance between the two kinds of activity produces normal motor function. A relative excess of cholinergic activity produces akinesia and rigidity. A relative excess of dopaminergic activity produces involuntary movements. Neurons in the caudate nucleus contain gamma-aminobutyric acid (GABA) and possibly control dopaminergic neurons in the substantia nigra through a feedback pathway. (**A** from Cutler WP: *Degenerative and hereditary diseases,* ed 7, Washington, DC, 1983, Scientific American Medicine.)

the dopaminergic nigrostriatal pathway causes dopamine depletion in the basal ganglia and relative excess cholinergic activity in the feedback circuit. This is manifested by hypertonia (tremor and rigidity) and akinesia.

CLINICAL MANIFESTATIONS The classic manifestations of Parkinson disease are tremor at rest (resting tremor), rigidity (muscle stiffness), bradykinesia/akinesia (poverty of movement), postural disturbance, dysarthria, and dysphagia. They may develop alone or in combination, but as the disease progresses, all are usually present. There is no true paralysis. The symptoms are always bilateral but usually involve one side early in the illness. Because the onset is insidious, the beginning of symptoms is difficult to document. Early in the disease, reflex status, sensory status, and mental status usually are normal. Postural abnormalities (flexed, forward leaning), difficulty walking, and weakness develop. Speech may be slurred. Autonomic-neuroendocrine symptoms include inappropriate diaphoresis, orthostatic hypotension, drooling, gastric retention, constipation, and urinary retention. Depression is also prevalent.

Disorders of equilibrium result from postural abnormalities (Figure 14-21). The person with Parkinson disease cannot make the appropriate postural adjustment to tilting or falling and falls like a post when starting to tilt. The festinating gait (short, accelerating steps) of the individual with Parkinson disease is an attempt to maintain an upright position while walking. Individuals are also unable to right themselves when changing from a reclining or crouching position to a standing position and when rolling over from a supine to a lateral or prone position. Excessive daytime sleepiness is experienced in over 50% of persons.[17] Postural instability, sleep disturbance, and difficulty concentrating are some of the most depressing symptoms to persons with Parkinson disease.[18]

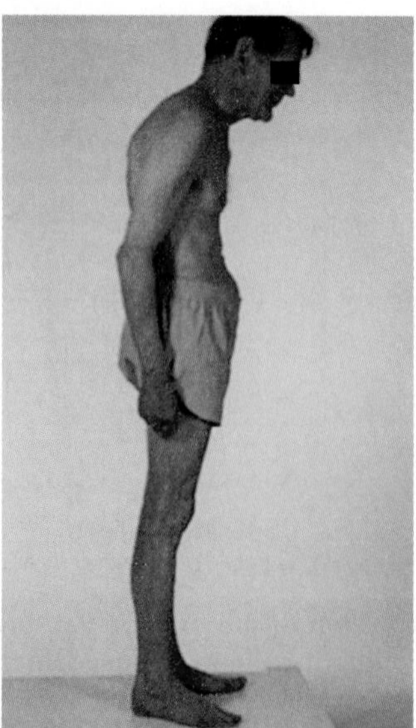

Figure 14-21 ■ **Stooped Posture of Parkinson Disease.** (From Perkin DG: *Mosby's color atlas and text of neurology,* ed 2, London, 2002, Mosby.)

Progressive dementia may be associated with the disease and is more common in persons older than 70 years. The person's mental status may be further compromised by the side effects of the medication taken to control symptoms.

EVALUATION AND TREATMENT The diagnosis of Parkinson disease is based on the history and physical examination. Causes of secondary parkinsonism are first excluded. No specific diagnostic tests are available, except positron emission tomography (PET). Treatment of Parkinson disease is symptomatic, involving drug therapy. The drugs used are to decrease akinesia. Because of troublesome side effects and loss of effectiveness, however, drug therapy may not be started until the symptoms become incapacitating. Surgical interventions, predominantly pallidotomy, thalamotomy, and thalamic stimulation are reemerging.[19,20] Research on transplants, both fetal and embryonic cells, is under way, as well as other species grafts. Parkinson disease progresses slowly for 15 to 20 years before producing severe immobility and dependence. Nutrition and exercise are important for maintaining energy and strength.

Alterations in Complex Motor Performance

The alterations in complex motor performance include disorders of posture (stance), disorders of gait, and disorders of expression.

Disorders of posture (stance)

When the tone in various muscle groups becomes unbalanced because of a loss of normal postural reflexes, posturing of limbs results. Equilibrium and balance are disrupted. Many reflex systems govern tone and posture, but the most important factor in posture control is the stretch reflex, in which extensor (antigravity) muscle stretching causes increased extensor tone and inhibited flexor tone. Four types of disorders of postures are (1) dystonic posture, (2) decerebrate posture, (3) basal ganglion posture, and (4) senile posture.

Dystonia is the maintenance of an abnormal posture through muscular contractions. When muscular contractions are sustained for several seconds, they are called **dystonic movements;** when contractions last for longer periods, they are called **dystonic postures.** Dystonic postures may last for weeks, causing permanent, fixed contractures. Dystonia has been associated with basal ganglia abnormality, but the exact pathophysiologic mechanisms are unknown. One dystonic posture already discussed in this chapter is decorticate posture (striatal posture or upper motor neuron dysfunction posture), which may be unilateral or bilateral. **Decorticate posture** (also referred to as **antigravity posture** or **hemiplegic posture**) is characterized by upper extremities flexed at the elbows and held close to the body and by lower extremities that are externally rotated and extended (see Figure 14-6). Decorticate posture is thought to occur when the brain stem is not inhibited by the cerebral cortex motor area. Upper motor neuron posture is more commonly described as the arm flexed at the elbow with a wrist drop, the leg inadequately bent at the knee, the hip excessively circumabducted, and presence of footdrop.

Decerebrate posture refers to increased tone in extensor muscles and trunk muscles, with active tonic neck reflexes. When the head is in a neutral position, all four limbs are rigidly extended. The decerebrate posture is caused by severe injury to the brain and brain stem, resulting in overstimulation of the postural righting and vestibular reflexes.

Basal ganglion posture refers to a stooped, hyperflexed posture with a narrow-based, short-stepped gait. This posture abnormality results from the loss of normal postural reflexes and not from defects in proprioceptive, labyrinthine, or visual function. Dysfunctional equilibrium results when the individual loses stability and cannot make the appropriate postural adjustment to tilting or loss of balance, falling instead. Dysfunctional righting is the inability to right oneself when changing from a lying or crouching to a standing position or when rolling from the supine to the lateral or prone position. Dysfunctional postural fixation is the involuntary flexion of the head and neck, causing the person difficulty in maintaining an upright trunk position while standing or walking. Basal ganglion dysfunction accounts for this posture.

Senile posture is characterized by an increasingly flexed posture similar to that caused by basal ganglion dysfunction. The posture is associated with frontal lobe dysfunction, but the primary pathophysiology is not known.

Disorders of gait

Four predominant types of gait are (1) upper motor neuron dysfunction gait, (2) cerebellar (ataxic) gait, (3) basal ganglion gait, and (4) senile gait (pseudoparkinsonian gait). As with posture, equilibrium and balance are affected with gait disturbances.

Several upper motor neuron gaits exist. With mild forms, the individual may have footdrop with fatigue and hip and leg pain. A **spastic gait,** which is associated with unilateral injury, manifests by a shuffling gait with the leg extended and held stiff, causing a scraping over the floor surface. The leg swings improperly around the body rather than being appropriately lifted and placed. The foot may drag on the ground, and the person tends to fall to the affected side. A **scissors gait** is associated with bilateral injury and spasticity. The legs are abducted so they touch each other. As the person walks, the legs are swung around the body but then cross in front of each other because of adduction. Injury to the pyramidal system accounts for these gaits.

A **cerebellar gait** is wide-based with the feet apart and often turned outward or inward for greater stability. The pelvis is held stiff, and the individual staggers when walking. Cerebellar dysfunction accounts for this particular gait.

A **basal ganglion gait** and a **senile gait** are both broad-based gaits in which the person walks with small steps and a decreased arm swing. The head and body are flexed and the arms semiflexed and abducted, whereas the legs are flexed and rigid in more advanced states. Basal ganglion and frontal lobe dysfunction, respectively, account for these two gaits.

Disorders of expression

Disorders of expression involve the motor aspects of communication and include (1) hypermimesis, (2) hypomimesis, and (3) dyspraxias/apraxias. Hypermimesis commonly manifests as pathologic laughter or crying. Pathologic laughter is associated with right hemisphere injury, and pathologic crying is associated with left hemisphere injury. The exact pathophysiology is not known. Hypomimesis manifests as aprosody—the loss of emotional language. Receptive aprosody involves an inability to understand emotion in speech and facial expression, whereas expressive aprosody involves the inability to express emotion in speech and facial expression. Aprosody is associated with right hemisphere damage.

Dyspraxia/apraxia is the inability to perform purposeful or skilled motor acts in the absence of paralysis, sensory loss, abnormal posture and tone, abnormal involuntary movement, incoordination, or inattentiveness. It is associated with vascular disorders, trauma, tumors, degenerative disorders, infections, and metabolic disorders. These are disorders of learned skilled movements.[21] Table 14-18 lists the types of disorders.

True dyspraxias occur when the connecting pathways between the left and right cortical areas are interrupted (Figure 14-22). Dyspraxias may result from any pathologic process that disrupts the cortical areas necessary for the conceptualization and execution of a complex motor act or the communication pathways within the left hemisphere or between the hemispheres.

Extrapyramidal Motor Syndromes

Because the extrapyramidal system encompasses all the motor pathways except the pyramidal system, two types of motor dysfunction make up the **extrapyramidal motor syndromes:** (1) the basal ganglia motor syndromes and (2) the cerebellar motor syndromes. Unlike pyramidal motor syndromes, both extrapyramidal motor syndromes result in movement or posture disturbance without significant paralysis, along with other distinctive symptoms (Table 14-19).

Basal ganglia motor syndromes

Basal ganglia motor syndromes involve either a paucity or an excess of movements. Stress and nervous tension typically worsen the symptoms, whereas relaxation improves motor performance. Akinesia may occur despite normal strength. Involuntary movements, such as tremor, chorea, ballism, athetosis, and dystonia, also may occur and probably are caused by loss of the normal modulating effects of the basal ganglia.

Basal ganglia motor syndromes also are characterized by alterations in muscle tone and posture. Rigidity and the cogwheel phenomenon are present in all muscle groups but are most prominent in those that maintain flexed

TABLE 14-18
Dyspraxias and Apraxias

Types	Description	Location
Ideomotor apraxia	Impairment in selecting, sequencing, and spatial orientation of movements involved in gestures (spatial and temporal production errors)	Left parietal cortex (angular gyrus or supramarginal gyrus)
Posterior form	Difficulty performing in response to command and imitation; cannot discriminate well between poorly performed and well performed acts	Left parietal cortex (angular gyrus or supramarginal gyrus) lesion
Anterior form	Performs poorly to command and imitation but comprehends and discriminates pantomime	Lesions anterior to the supramarginal gyrus, which disconnects visual kinesthetic motor engrams from premotor and motor areas
Conduction apraxia	Greater impairment in performance when imitating movements than when pantomiming to command; comprehends pantomime and gesture but cannot perform the movements	Location unknown at this time
Disassociation apraxia	Inability to gesture normally to command; has good performance with imitation and actual tools and objects	Callosal abnormalities but not all locations known
Ideational apraxia	Inability to carry out an ideational plan or a series of acts in the proper sequence	Location unclear at this time
Conceptual apraxia	Cannot recall type of action associated with specific tools, utensils, or objects (content and tool selection errors; may be unable to recall which tool is associated with a specific object or may have impaired mechanical knowledge)	Bilateral frontal and parietal dysfunction

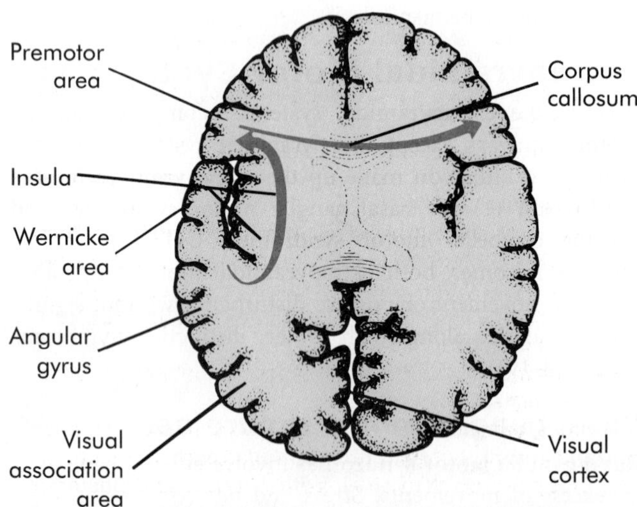

Figure 14-22 ■ Pathways Disrupted in Dyspraxias. Formulation of the idea of the motor act is thought to originate in the region of the supramarginal gyrus in the inferior left parietal lobe. This area is connected via associational pathways to the left premotor cortex. The left premotor cortex is connected through the corpus callosum to the right premotor and motor areas. An injury that interrupts the pathways between the left supramarginal gyrus and the premotor region produces a dyspraxia that involves the entire body. An injury that disrupts the callosal pathways produces a dyspraxia of the left side of the body only.

position. Postural abnormalities result from the loss of normal postural reflexes. Dysfunctional equilibrium results from the loss of postural stability.

Basal ganglia motor syndromes are caused by an imbalance of dopaminergic and cholinergic activity in the corpus striatum. A relative excess of cholinergic activity produces akinesia and hypertonia. A relative excess of dopaminergic activity produces hyperkinesia and hypotonia.

✓ QUICK CHECK 14-5

1. Why are there so many causes of hypertonia?
2. How is chorea different from athetosis?
3. Why is paresis/paralysis a type of hypokinesia?
4. What structures are involved in alterations of complex motor performance?

Cerebellar motor syndromes

Cerebellar motor syndromes involve the cerebellum and may result in (1) loss of muscle tone; (2) difficulty with coordination of voluntary movements; (3) minor degrees of muscle weakness, tendency toward fatigue, and impairment of associated movements; and (4) disorders of equilibrium, posture, and gait. Cerebellar effects primarily influence the same side of the body, so that damage to the right cerebellum generally causes symptoms on the right side of the body. Predominant symptoms depend on the area of damage within the cerebellum. It should be noted that the nervous system often can operate well despite destruction of parts of the cerebellum, although the mechanisms responsible for this retained function are not fully understood.

TABLE 14-19

Pyramidal vs. Extrapyramidal Motor Syndrome

Manifestations	Pyramidal Motor Syndrome	Extrapyramidal Motor Syndrome
Unilateral movement	Paralysis of voluntary movement	Little or no paralysis of voluntary movement
Tendon reflexes	Increased tendon reflexes	Normal or slightly increased tendon reflexes
Babinski sign	Present	Absent
Involuntary movements	Absence of involuntary movements	Presence of tremor, chorea, athetosis, or dystonia
Muscle tone	Spasticity in muscles (e.g., clasp-knife phenomenon)	Plastic (equal throughout movement) rigidity or intermittent (generalized but predominantly in flexors of limbs and trunk) rigidity (cogwheel rigidity)
	Hypertonia present in flexors of arms and extension of legs	Hypotonia in cerebellar disease

Did You Understand?

Alterations in Cognitive Networks

1. Full consciousness is an awareness of oneself and the environment with an ability to respond to external stimuli with a wide variety of responses.
2. Consciousness has two components: arousal and content of thought.
3. A decreased level of arousal occurs by diffuse bilateral cortical dysfunction, bilateral subcortical (reticular formation, brain stem) dysfunction, and localized hemispheric dysfunction.
4. An alteration in breathing pattern and level of coma reflect the level of brain dysfunction.
5. Pupillary changes reflect changes in level of brain stem function, drug action, and response to hypoxia and ischemia.
6. Abnormal eye movements, including nystagmus and divergent gaze, reflect alterations in brain stem function.
7. Level of brain function manifests by changes in generalized motor responses or no responses.
8. Loss of cortical inhibition associated with decreased consciousness produces abnormal flexor and extensor movements.
9. Cerebral death or irreversible coma represents permanent brain damage, with an ability to maintain cardiac, respiratory, and other vital functions.
10. Brain death results from irreversible brain damage, with an inability to maintain internal homeostasis.
11. Arousal returns in vegetative states, but content of thought is absent.
12. Seizures represent a sudden, chaotic discharge of cerebral neurons, with transient alterations in brain function. Seizures may be generalized or focal and can result from cerebral lesions, biochemical disorders, trauma, or epilepsy.
13. With a deficit in selective attention, mediated by midbrain, thalamus, and parietal lobe structures, the individual cannot focus on selective stimuli and thus neglects those stimuli.
14. In dysmnesia and amnesia, some past memories are lost and new memories cannot be stored.
15. Frontal areas mediate vigilance, detection, and working memory.
16. With vigilance deficits, the person cannot maintain sustained concentration.
17. With detection deficits, the person is unmotivated and unable to set goals and plan.
18. Some specific disorders of content of thought (cognition) are agnosias, dysphasias, acute confusional states, and dementias.
19. Agnosias are defects of recognition and may be tactile, visual, or auditory. They are caused by dysfunction in the primary sensory area or the interpretive areas of the cerebral cortex.
20. Dysphasia is an impairment of comprehension or production of language. Dysphasia may be expressive or sensory.
21. Aphasia is loss of language comprehension or production.
22. Wernicke dysphasia is a disturbance in understanding all language, both verbal and reading comprehension.
23. Conductive dysphasias result from disruption of temporal lobe fibers, with a failure to repeat words but an ability to initiate speech, writing, and reading aloud.
24. Anomic dysphasia is an inability to name objects, persons, or qualities.
25. Transcortical dysphasias involve an inability to repeat and recite.
26. Broca aphasia is an expressive dysphasia of speech and writing but with retention of comprehension.
27. Global aphasia involves both anterior and posterior speech areas, with both expressive and receptive aphasia.
28. Acute confusional states are characterized chiefly by a loss of detection and, in the case of delirium, an intense autonomic nervous system hyperactivity.
29. Alzheimer disease is a chronic irreversible dementia that may be related to beta-amyloid metabolism.
30. Pick disease is a rare degenerative disease similar to Alzheimer disease.

(Continued)

Did You Understand?—Cont'd

Alterations in Cerebral Homeostasis

1. Increased intracranial pressure may result from edema, excess cerebrospinal fluid, hemorrhage, or tumor growth. When intracranial pressure approaches arterial pressure, hypoxia and hypercapnia produce brain damage.
2. Cerebral edema is an increase in the fluid content of the brain resulting from infection, hemorrhage, tumor, ischemia, infarct, or hypoxia.
3. The shifting or herniation of brain tissue from one compartment to another disrupts the blood flow of both compartments and damages brain tissue.
4. Supratentorial herniation involves temporal lobe and hippocampal gyrus shifting from the middle fossa to posterior fossa; transtentorial herniation involves a downward shift of the diencephalon through the tentorial notch; and shifting of the cingulate gyrus can occur under the falx.
5. The most common infratentorial herniation is a shift of the cerebellar tonsils through the foramen magnum.
6. Hydrocephalus comprises a variety of disorders characterized by an excess of fluid within the cranial vault, subarachnoid space, or both. Hydrocephalus occurs because of interference with cerebrospinal fluid flow caused by increased fluid production or obstruction within the ventricular system or by defective reabsorption of the fluid.

Alterations in Motor Function

1. Motor dysfunction may be characterized as alterations of motor tone, movement, and complex motor performance.
2. Hypotonia and hypertonia are the main categories of altered tone.
3. The four types of hypertonia are spasticity, gegenhalten, dystonia, and rigidity.
4. Paresis, paraplegia, hyperkinesias, and hypokinesia are the main categories of altered movement.
5. Two subtypes of paresis/paralysis are described: upper motor neuron paresis/paralysis and lower motor neuron paresis/paralysis.
6. An upper motor neuron syndrome is characterized by paresis/paralysis, hypertonia, and hyperreflexia.
7. Interruption of the pyramidal tract below the pons results in spinal shock.
8. Lower motor neuron syndromes manifest by impaired voluntary and involuntary movements and flaccid paralysis.
9. Partial paralysis occurs with only partial loss of alpha motor neurons, and total paralysis is complete loss of alpha motor neurons. Loss of gamma motor neurons impairs muscle tone and decreases tendon reflexes.
10. Amyotrophy (e.g., poliomyelitis) is a lower motor neuron syndrome involving the anterior horn cells, with loss of muscle tone and strength resulting in segmental paresis and hyporeflexia.
11. Nuclear palsies involve damage to the cranial nerve nuclei.
12. Bulbar palsies involve cranial nerves IX, X, and XII.
13. Included in the category of hyperkinesias are chorea, athetosis, ballism, akathisia, tremor, and myoclonus.
14. Huntington disease (chorea) is a rare hereditary disease involving the basal ganglia and cerebral cortex. It is inherited as an autosomal dominant trait and commonly manifests between 30 and 50 years of age.
15. The major pathologic feature of Huntington disease is severe degeneration of the basal ganglia and the frontal cerebral cortex. The basal ganglia and the substantia nigra exhibit a depletion of gamma-aminobutyric acid (an inhibitory neurotransmitter) secreting neurons. This depletion leads to an excess of dopaminergic activity that causes involuntary, fragmentary movements.
16. Types of hypokinesia include akinesia, bradykinesia, and loss of associated movements.
17. Parkinson disease is a commonly occurring degenerative disorder of the basal ganglia (corpus striatum) involving degeneration of the dopamine-secreting nigrostriatal pathway. The pathogenesis of Parkinson disease is unknown, but researchers suggest genetic, viral, and environmental toxins as possible causes.
18. Degeneration of the dopaminergic nigrostriatal pathway causes dopamine depletion in the basal ganglia and excess of cholinergic activity in the cortex, basal ganglia, and thalamus. Tremor and rigidity are caused by the excess cholinergic activity. Progressive dementia may be associated with an advanced stage of the disease.
19. Treatment of Parkinson disease is symptomatic, involving levodpa (L-dopa), a precursor of dopamine. The disease takes a slowly progressive course for 15 to 20 years.
20. Alterations in complex motor performance include disorders of posture (stance), disorders of gait, and disorders of expression.
21. Disorders of posture include dystonic posture, decerebrate posture, basal ganglion posture, and senile posture.
22. Disorders of gait include upper motor neuron gait, cerebellar gait, basal ganglion gait, and senile gait.
23. Disorders of expression include hypermimesis, hypomimesis, and dyspraxia/apraxia.
24. Dyspraxia is an impairment of the conceptualization or execution of a complex motor act.
25. Extrapyramidal motor syndromes include basal ganglia and cerebellar motor syndromes.
26. Basal ganglia disorders manifest by alterations in muscle tone and posture, including rigidity, involuntary movements, and loss of postural reflexes.
27. Cerebellar motor syndromes result in loss of muscle tone, difficulty with coordination, and disorders of equilibrium and gait.

Key Terms

Acute confusional state (ACS), 344
Acute hydrocephalus, 352
Agnosia, 343
Akinesia, 361
Alzheimer disease (AD) (dementia of Alzheimer type [DAT], senile disease complex), 347
Amyotrophy, 356
Anterograde amnesia, 341
Antigravity posture, 362
Aphasia, 343
Apraxia, 363
Areflexia, 356
Arousal, 331
Aura, 341
Autoregulation, 350
Basal ganglia motor syndrome, 363
Basal ganglion gait, 363
Basal ganglion posture, 363
Bradykinesia, 361
Brain death, 336
Bulbar palsy, 358
Cerebellar gait, 363
Cerebellar motor syndrome, 364
Cerebral blood flow (CBF), 349
Cerebral blood volume (CBV), 349
Cerebral death, 338
Cerebral edema, 350
Cerebral oxygenation, 349
Cerebral perfusion pressure (CPP), 349
Clonic phase, 341
Communicating hydrocephalus, 352
Content of thought, 331
Cytotoxic (metabolic) edema, 351
Decerebrate posture, 363
Decorticate posture (antigravity posture, hemiplegic posture), 362
Diplegia, 355
Dysphasia, 343
Dyspraxia, 363
Dystonia, 353
Dystonic movement, 362
Dystonic posture, 362
Echolalia, 344
Epilepsy, 339
Epileptogenic focus, 340
Executive attention deficit, 341
Expressive dysphasia, 344
Extinction, 343
Extrapyramidal motor syndrome, 363
Fibrillation, 356
Flaccid paresis/paralysis, 356
Gegenhalten (paratonia), 353
Guillain-Barré syndrome, 358
Hemiparesis, 355
Hemiplegia, 355
Hemiplegic posture, 362
Huntington disease (HD), 360
Hydrocephalus, 351
Hyperkinesia, 358
Hypertonia, 353
Hypokinesia, 360
Hypotonia, 352
Increased intracranial pressure (IICP), 349
Interstitial edema, 351
Intracranial pressure (ICP), 349
Ischemic edema, 351
Locked-in syndrome, 338
Metabolic arousal alteration, 331
Minimally conscious state (MCS), 338
Mirror focus, 341
Neglect syndrome, 343
Neurofibrillary tangle, 347
Noncommunicating hydrocephalus (internal hydrocephalus, intraventricular hydrocephalus), 351
Normal-pressure hydrocephalus, 352
Nuclear palsy, 357
Paralysis, 355
Paraparesis, 355
Paraplegia, 355
Paresis, 355
Parkinson disease, 361
Parkinsonism (Parkinson syndrome, parkinsonian syndrome, paralysis agitans), 361
Paroxysmal dyskinesia, 358
Pick disease, 348
Poliomylitis, 356
Prodroma, 341
Progressive bulbar palsy, 358
Progressive spinal muscular atrophy, 358
Psychogenic arousal alteration, 331
Pyramidal motor syndrome, 355
Quadriparesis, 355
Quadriplegia, 355
Receptive dysphasia, 344
Retrograde amnesia, 341
Rigidity, 353
Scissors gait, 363
Seizure, 339
Selective attention deficit, 341
Senile gait, 363
Senile plaque, 348
Senile posture, 363
Sensory inattentiveness, 343
Spastic gait, 363
Spasticity, 353
Spinal shock, 355
Structural arousal alteration, 331
Tardive dyskinesia, 360
Tonic phase, 340
Transcortical dysphasia, 344
Upper motor neuron paresis/paralysis, 355
Vasogenic edema, 350
Vegetative state, 351

References

1. Bleck TP: Levels of consciousness and attention, In Goetz CG, editor: *Textbook of clinical neurology*, Philadelphia, 2003, Saunders.
2. Ropper AD, Brown RH: *Adam and Victor's principles of neurology*, ed 7, St Louis, 2001, Mosby.
3. Rakel RE: *Textbook of family practice*, ed 6, Philadelphia, 2002, Mosby.
4. Boss BJ, Fletcher A: Severe brain injury rehabilitation: what's going to happen after critical care? *Crit Care Nurs Clin North Am* 13(3):421–431, 2001.
5. Christensen D: Endgame for epilepsy? Researchers look toward a cure, *Sci News* 157:364–365, 2001.

5a. Herman ST: Clinical trials for prevention of epileptogenesis, *Epilepsy Res* 68(1):35–38, 2006.

6. Lownstein DH: Seizures and epilepsy. In Kasper DL et al, (editors): *Harrison's principles of internal medicine,* vol. 2. New York, 2005, McGraw-Hill.
7. Fisher S: On genes, speech, and language, *N Engl J Med* 353:1655–1657, 2005.
8. Haines J, Camarata S: Examination of candidate genes in language disorder: a model of genetic association for treatment studies, *Ment Retard Develop Disabilities Res Rev* 10: 1655–1657, 2005.
9. Drachman DA: Aging of the brain, entropy, and Alzheimer disease, *Neurology* 67(8):1340–1352, 2006.
10. Mele D: Cognitive, functional, and behavioral decline in Alzheimer disease: optimizing care for patients with Alzheimer disease: emerging treatment strategies, *J Acad Nurs Pract* (suppl) 16(1):6–7, 2004.
11. Bird TD: Alzheimer disease overview: gene reviews, latest revision 13 June 2007, available at: http://www.genetests.org/query?dz=alzheimer. Accessed 6/20/07.
12. Blennow K, de Leon MJ, Zetterberg H: Alzheimer's disease, *Lancet* 368(9533):387–403, 2006.
13. Molinuevo JL, Garcia-Gil V, Villar A: Memantine: an antiglutamateric option for dementia, *Am J Alzheimer Dis Other Dementia* 19(1):10–18, 2004.
14. Seppa N: Alzheimer drug shows staying power, *Sci News* 169(7): 110, 2006.

References—Cont'd

15. Jankovic J: Movement disorders, In Goetz CG, editor: *Textbook of clinical neurology*, Philadelphia, 2003, Saunders.
16. Bonelli RM, Wenning GK: Pharmacological management of Huntington's disease: an evidence- based review, *Curr Pharm Des* 12(21):2701–2720, 2006.
17. Dhawan V et al: Sleep-related problems of Parkinson's disease, *Age Ageing* 35(3):220–228, 2006.
18. Backer JH: The symptom experience of patients with Parkinson disease, *J Neursci Nurs* 38(1):51–57, 2006.
19. Petit JM: An update on Parkinson disease, *Long-term Care Interface* 6(12):48–52, 2005.
20. Jankovic J: An update on the treatment of Parkinson's disease, *Mt Sinai J Med* 73(4):682–689, 2006.
21. Heilman KM, Watson RT, Gonzalez-Roth LJ: Praxis, In Goetz CG, editor: *Textbook of clinical neurology*, Philadelphia, 2003, Saunders.

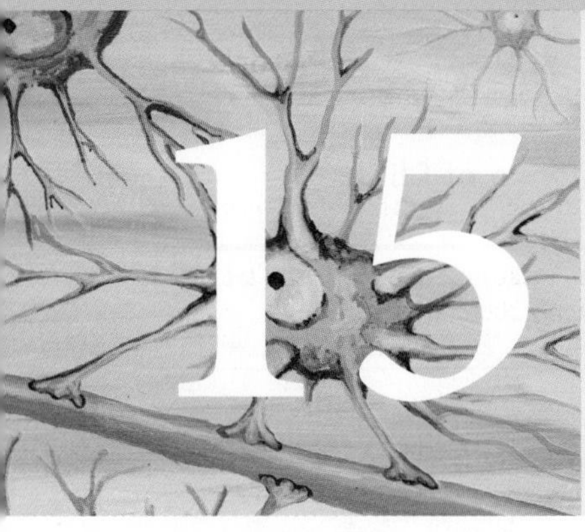

15 ALTERATIONS OF NEUROLOGIC FUNCTION

Barbara J. Boss

CHAPTER OUTLINE

ELECTRONIC RESOURCES

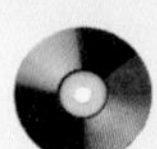

Companion CD
- Review Questions and Answers
- Animations

evolve Website
http://evolve.elsevier.com/Huether/
- Quick Check Answers
- Key Terms Exercises
- Critical Thinking Questions with Answers
- Algorithm Completion Exercises
- WebLinks

Alterations in central nervous system (CNS) function are caused by traumatic injury, vascular disorders, tumor growth, infectious and inflammatory processes, metabolic derangements (including those arising from nutritional deficiencies and drugs or chemicals), and degenerative processes. Alterations in peripheral nervous system function involve the nerve roots (radiculopathies), a nerve plexus, or the nerves themselves (neuropathies). Disorders of the neuromuscular junction occur also.

CENTRAL NERVOUS SYSTEM DISORDERS

Trauma

Brain trauma

Major head injury is defined by the National Head Injury Foundation as a traumatic insult to the brain capable of producing physical, intellectual, emotional, social, and vocational changes. Those at highest risk for traumatic brain injury (TBI) are young persons 15 to 24 years of age, infants 6 months to 2 years, young school-age children, and elderly persons. The male/female ratio for such injury is 2:1.[1] Traumatic brain injury is highest among blacks and in lower- and median-income families. Persons living in areas with high crime rates are at greater risk.

Head injuries are broadly categorized into **closed (blunt) trauma** and **open (penetrating) trauma.** Blunt trauma is more common and involves the head striking a hard surface or a rapidly moving object striking the head. The dura remains intact, and brain tissues are not exposed to the environment. Blunt trauma may result in both focal brain injuries and diffuse axonal injuries (Table 15-1). When a break in (penetration of) the dura results in exposure of the cranial contents to the environment, open trauma has occurred, which results in focal brain injuries.

The most common types of traumatic brain injury (75% to 90%) are mild concussion and classical cerebral concussion (Table 15-2). Focal brain injury and diffuse axonal injury (DAI) each account for half of all injuries. Focal brain injury accounts for more than two thirds of head injury deaths; DAI accounts for fewer than one third. However, more severely disabled survivors, including those in an unresponsive state or reduced level of consciousness, have DAI.

In recent years, the surviving traumatic brain injury population has changed, mostly because of focus on reducing the severity of injury (e.g., passive seat restraints, air bags), reduced transport time, and improved on-the-scene medical management. Improved management of secondary and tertiary injury also influences the situation; acute care health professionals focus more on morbidity than mortality. As a result, persons with more severe traumatic brain injuries are being admitted to rehabilitation programs.

TABLE 15-1

Severity of Trauma Related to Trauma State Induced and Onset and Persistence of Clinical Manifestations

Severity of Trauma	TRAUMA STATE INDUCED: Focal Injury	TRAUMA STATE INDUCED: DAI	Onset of Clinical Manifestations	Persistence of DAI Clinical Manifestations
Mild blunt trauma		Mild concussion	Immediate	Hours to days
Moderate blunt trauma		Classic cerebral concussion	Immediate	Up to 6 months or longer
	Paraplegia (associated with injury to top of head)		Immediate	
	Blindness (associated with occipital injury)		Immediate	
	Delayed development of unresponsiveness (vasomotor or vasovagal syncopal episode)		Delayed	
Severe blunt trauma		Mild DAI	Immediate	Permanent
		Moderate DAI	Immediate	Residual
		Severe DAI	Immediate	
	Acute epidural hemorrhage		Immediate to delayed (2–3 hours)	
	Acute contusional swelling		Delayed onset (few hours after injury)	
	Acute subdural hematoma		Delayed onset (few hours to 1 week after injury)	
	Subacute subdural hematoma*		Delayed onset (1 to few weeks)	
	Subdural hygroma (fluid accumulation)		Delayed onset	
	Traumatic cerebral hemorrhage*		Delayed onset (as late as 1 week after injury)	

*May be seen after moderate head injury, especially in elderly people.
DAI, Diffuse axonal injury.

TABLE 15-2

Categories of Diffuse Brain Injury

Type of Injury	Mechanism
Mild concussion	Temporary axonal disturbance affecting attentional and memory systems; consciousness not lost
Grade I	Confusion and disorientation with amnesia (momentary)
Grade II	Momentary confusion and retrograde amnesia after 5–10 min
Grade III	Confusion and retrograde amnesia from impact; also anterograde amnesia
Classic cerebral concussion	Same as grade IV mild concussion—diffuse cerebral disconnection from brain stem reticular activating system; physiologic neurologic dysfunction without substantial anatomic disruption; immediate loss of consciousness lasting less than 6 hr; retrograde and anterograde amnesia (posttraumatic); may be uncomplicated or complicated
Diffuse axonal injury (DAI)	Prolonged traumatic coma (longer than 6 hr)
Mild	Posttraumatic coma lasts 6–24 hr; death uncommon; persistent residual cognitive, psychologic, and sensorimotor deficits; rare—only 8% of severe head injuries
Moderate	Widespread physiologic impairment throughout the cerebral cortex and diencephalon; actual tearing of axons in both hemispheres; prolonged coma (longer than 24 hr); incomplete recovery among survivors; common—20% of severe head injuries
Severe	Formerly called *primary brain stem injury* or *brain stem contusion;* severe mechanical disruption of axons in both hemispheres, diencephalon, and brain stem; 16% of severe head injuries

Cause

Most traumatic brain injuries are caused by transportation-related events, falls, sports-related events, and violence. The causative mechanisms are summarized in Table 15-3.

PATHOPHYSIOLOGY Three mechanisms produce damage: primary, secondary, and tertiary injury. Primary injury is caused by the impact and involves neural injury, primary glial injury, and vascular response. Two types of primary injury may occur: focal and diffuse brain injury.

Focal brain injury. **Focal brain injuries** are specific, grossly observable brain lesions—cortical contusions, epidural hemorrhage, subdural hematoma, and intracerebral hematoma. The force of impact typically produces **contusions** from direct contact (as well as injury to the vault, vessels, and supporting structures) that, in turn, produces epidural hemorrhage and subdural and intracerebral hematomas. The mechanisms of injury are depicted in Figure 15-1. Damage results from compression of the skull at the point of impact and rebound effect. Contusion and bleeding occur from small tears in blood vessels caused by these forces. The severity of contusion varies with the amount of energy transmitted by the skull to underlying brain tissue. In addition, the smaller the area of impact, the greater the severity of injury because the force is concentrated into a smaller area. The focal injury may be coup or contrecoup. Brain edema forms around and in damaged neural tissues, contributing to the increasing intracranial pressure. Within the contused areas, infarction, necrosis, multiple hemorrhages, and edema occur. The tissue has a pulpy quality. The maximum effects of these injuries peak 18 to 36 hours after severe head injury.

Contusions are found most commonly in the frontal lobes, particularly at the poles and along the inferior orbital surfaces; in the temporal lobes, especially in the anterior poles and along the inferior surface; and at the frontotemporal junction. They result in changes in attention, memory, executive attention functions (see Chapter 14), affect, emotion, and behavior. Less commonly, contusions occur in the parietal and occipital lobes. Focal cerebral contusions are superficial, involving just the gyri. Hemorrhagic contusions may coalesce into a large confluent intracranial hematoma.

Extradural hematomas (epidural hematomas, epidural hemorrhages) represent 1% to 2% of major head injuries and occur in all age groups, but most commonly in 20- to 40-year-olds. An artery is the source of bleeding in 85% of extradural hematomas; 15% result from injury to the meningeal vein or dural sinus. The temporal fossa is the most common site of extradural hematoma caused by injury to the middle meningeal artery or vein. The temporal lobe shifts

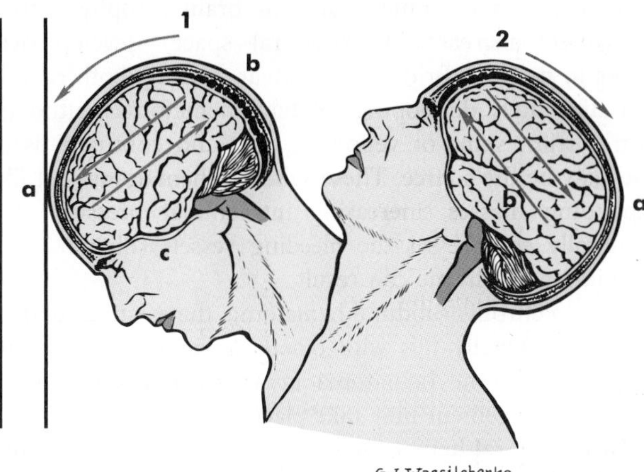

Figure 15-1 ■ **Coup and Contrecoup Head Injury After Blunt Trauma.** *1,* Coup injury: impact against object; *a,* site of impact and direct trauma to brain; *b,* shearing of subdural veins; *c,* trauma to base of brain. *2,* Contrecoup injury: impact within skull; *a,* site of impact from brain hitting opposite side of skull; *b,* shearing forces through brain. These injuries occur in one continuous motion—the head strikes the wall (coup) and then rebounds (contrecoup). (Modified from Rudy EB: *Advanced neurological and neurosurgical nursing,* St Louis, 1984, Mosby.)

TABLE 15-3

Causes of Brain Injuries

Type of Injury	Mechanism
Coup	Injury is directly below site of forceful impact
Contrecoup	Injury is on opposite side of brain from site of forceful impact
Extradural hematoma	Vehicular accidents, minor falls, sporting accidents
Subdural hematoma	Vehicular accidents or falls, especially in elderly persons or persons with chronic alcohol abuse
Intracerebral hemorrhage	Contusions caused by forceful impact, usually vehicular accidents or falls from a distance
Compound fracture	Objects strike head with great force or head strikes object forcefully; temporal blows, occipital blows, upward impact of cervical vertebrae (basilar skull fracture)
Penetrating injury	Missiles (bullets) or sharp projectiles (knives, ice picks, axes, screwdrivers)
Diffuse axonal injury	Moving head strikes hard, unyielding surface or moving object strikes stationary head; vehicular accidents (occupant or pedestrian); torsional head motion

medially, precipitating uncal and hippocampal gyrus herniation through the tentorial notch. Extradural hemorrhages are found occasionally in the subfrontal area, especially in the young and elderly populations, caused by injury to the anterior meningeal artery or a venous sinus, and in the occipital-suboccipital area, resulting in herniation of the posterior fossa contents through the foramen magnum.

Subdural hematomas arise in 10% to 20% of persons with traumatic brain injury. Acute subdural hematomas develop rapidly, commonly within hours, and usually are located at the top of the skull (the cerebral convexities). Bilateral hematomas occur in 15% to 20% of persons. Subacute subdural hematomas develop more slowly, often over 48 hours to 2 weeks. Chronic subdural hematomas (commonly found in elderly persons and persons who abuse alcohol and have some degree of brain atrophy with a subsequent increase in extradural space) develop over weeks to months. Bridging veins tear, causing both rapidly and subacutely developing subdural hematomas, although torn cortical veins or venous sinuses and contused tissue also may be the source. These subdural hematomas act like expanding masses, increasing intracranial pressure that eventually compresses the bleeding vessels (Figure 15-2). Herniation syndrome can result.

With a chronic subdural hematoma, the existing subdural space gradually fills with blood. A vascular membrane forms around the hematoma in approximately 2 weeks. Further enlargement may take place.

Intracerebral hematomas occur in 2% to 3% of persons with head injuries, may be single or multiple, and are associated with contusions. Although most commonly located in the frontal and temporal lobes, they may occur in the hemispheric deep white matter. Penetrating injury or shearing forces traumatize small blood vessels. The intracerebral hematoma then acts as an expanding mass, increasing intracranial pressure, compressing brain tissues, and causing edema (Figure 15-3). Delayed intracerebral hematomas may appear 3 to 10 days after the head injury.

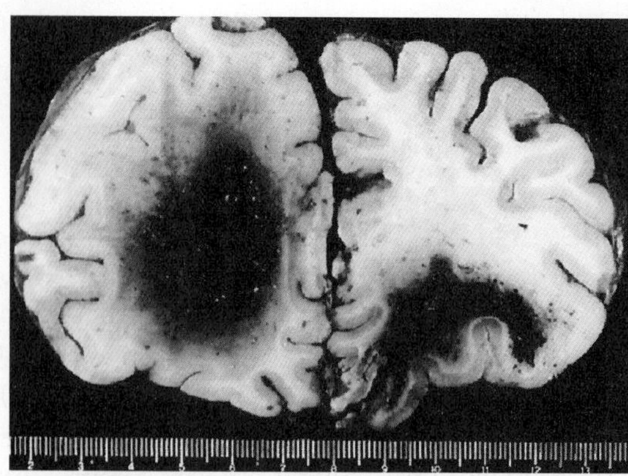

Figure 15-3 ■ **Hematomas.** Recent hematomas, resulting from trauma, in frontal lobes. (From Kissane JM, editor: *Anderson's pathology,* ed 9, St Louis, 1993, Mosby.)

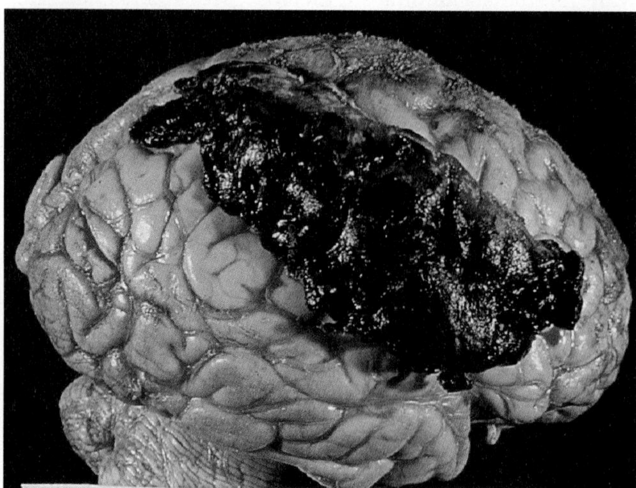

Figure 15-2 ■ **Acute Subdural Hematoma (Dura Removed).** Leptomeninges are intact. (From Damjanov I, Linder J: *Anderson's pathology,* ed 10, St Louis, 1996, Mosby.)

Open trauma produces discrete (focal) injuries and includes compound fractures and missile injuries. A compound fracture opens a communication between the cranial contents and the environment and should be investigated whenever lacerations of the scalp, tympanic membrane, sinuses, eye, or mucous membranes are present. Such fractures may involve the cranial vault or the base of the skull (basilar skull fracture). Bone fragments cause tangential injury (injury caused by direct contact) and, occasionally, penetrating injuries. Cranial nerves may be damaged with a basilar skull fracture.

Missiles include bullets, rocks, shell fragments, knives, and blunt instruments. The mechanisms of injury are crush injury (laceration and crushing of whatever the missile touches) and stretch injury (blood vessels and nerves damaged without direct contact as a result of stretching). The tangential injury is to the coverings and the brain (scalp and brain lacerations), skull fractures, laceration of the meninges, and cerebral lacerations. Projectiles and debris from scalp and skull injury, when driven into the brain substance, produce a penetrating brain injury. Occasionally, projectiles are so forceful that they pass completely through the cranial vault.

Diffuse brain injury. Immediately following concussion, all cells in the brain fire at once (a massive electrical discharge), releasing glutamate, which triggers brain cells to release potassium. Calcium in turn rushes into the cell, specifically into the mitochondria, which is then impaired. This mitochondrial dysfunction creates a cellular energy crisis, which prohibits the cell from restoring its electrolyte balance. Release of glutamine also causes overstimulation of the N-methyl-D-aspartate (NMDA) receptors essential for brain development and plasticity.[2]

Diffuse brain injury (diffuse axonal injury [DAI]) results from a shaking effect (inertial effects of mechanical input to the head associated with high levels of acceleration and deceleration). Rotational acceleration (twisting movement) is the primary mechanism of injury, producing strains and distortions within the brain (see Figure 15-1). The freely moving head is attached to the neck, allowing rotational forces to set up shearing forces on brain tissues. The most severe axonal injuries are located more peripheral to the brain stem, causing extensive cognitive and affective impairments, as seen in survivors of traumatic brain injury from vehicular crashes. Damage reduces the speed of informational processing and responding and disrupts attention.

Pathophysiologically, axonal damage can be seen only with an electron microscope and involves numerous axons, either alone or in conjunction with actual tissue tears. Areas where axons and small blood vessels are torn appear as small hemorrhages, particularly in the corpus callosum and dorsolateral quadrant of the rostral brain stem at the superior cerebellar peduncle. More and more damaged axons are visible 12 hours to several days after the injury. Severity of the diffuse injury correlates with how much shearing force was applied to the brain stem. DAI is not associated with intracranial hypertension immediately after injury, but acute brain swelling caused by increased intravascular blood within the brain, vasodilation, and increased cerebral blood volume is seen often.

Several categories of diffuse brain injury exist: mild concussion, classic concussion, mild DAI, moderate DAI, and severe DAI. An organic component is present within each category. These are summarized in Table 15-3.

CLINICAL MANIFESTATIONS, EVALUATION, AND TREATMENT

Focal brain injury. A contusion may be evidenced by immediate loss of consciousness (generally accepted to last no longer than 5 minutes), loss of reflexes (individual falls to the ground), transient cessation of respiration, brief period of bradycardia, and decreased blood pressure (lasting 30 seconds to a few minutes). Increased cerebrospinal fluid (CSF) pressure and electrocardiogram (ECG) and electroencephalogram (EEG) changes occur on impact. Vital signs may stabilize to normal values in a few seconds, and then reflexes return and the person regains consciousness over minutes to days. Residual deficits may persist, and some persons never regain a full level of consciousness.

Evaluation includes a complete history and physical examination. Skull and spinal x-ray films often are taken, and a computed tomography (CT) scan or magnetic resonance imaging (MRI) may be done. Large contusions and lacerations with hemorrhage may be surgically excised. Otherwise, treatment is directed at controlling intracranial pressure and managing symptoms.

Individuals with classic temporal extradural hematomas lose consciousness at injury, and then one third become lucid for a few minutes to a few days (if a vein is bleeding). As the hematoma accumulates, a headache of increasing severity, vomiting, drowsiness, confusion, seizure, and hemiparesis may develop. As temporal lobe herniation occurs, level of consciousness is rapidly lost, with ipsilateral pupillary dilation and contralateral hemiparesis.

A CT scan or MRI usually is needed to diagnose extradural hematoma. The prognosis is good if intervention is initiated before bilateral dilation of the pupils. Extradural hematomas are almost always medical emergencies, requiring surgical ligation of bleeding vessels.

In acute, rapidly developing subdural hematomas, the expanding clots directly compress the brain. As intracranial pressure rises, bleeding veins are compressed. Thus, bleeding is self-limiting, although cerebral compression and displacement of brain tissue can cause temporal lobe herniation.

An acute subdural hematoma classically begins with headache, drowsiness, restlessness or agitation, slowed cognition, and confusion. These symptoms worsen over time and progress to loss of consciousness, respiratory pattern changes, and pupillary dilation (i.e., the symptoms of temporal lobe herniation). Homonymous hemianopia (defective vision in either the right or the left field), disconjugate gaze, and gaze palsies also may occur.

Of persons affected by chronic subdural hematomas, 80% have chronic headaches and tenderness over the hematoma on palpation. Most persons appear to have a progressive dementia with generalized rigidity (paratonia). Chronic subdural hematomas require a craniotomy to evacuate the gelatinous blood. Percutaneous drainage for chronic subdural hematomas has proved successful. However, reaccumulation often occurs unless the surrounding membrane is removed.

Intracerebral hematomas cause a decreasing level of consciousness. Coma or a confusional state from other injuries, however, can make the cause of this increasing unresponsiveness difficult to detect. Contralateral hemiplegia also may occur, and as intracranial pressure rises, temporal lobe herniation may appear. In delayed intracerebral hematoma, the presentation is similar to that of a hypertensive brain hemorrhage: sudden, rapidly progressive decreased level of consciousness with pupillary dilation, breathing pattern changes, hemiplegia, and bilateral positive Babinski reflexes.

History and physical examination help to establish the diagnosis, and CT scan, MRI, and cerebral angiography confirm it. Evacuation of a singular intracerebral hematoma has only occasionally been helpful, mostly for subcortical white matter hematomas. Otherwise, treatment is directed at reducing the intracranial pressure and allowing the hematoma to reabsorb slowly.

With open-head injury, most persons lose consciousness. The depth and duration of the coma are related to the location of injury, extent of damage, and amount of bleeding.

Open-head injury often requires débridement of the traumatized tissues to prevent infection and to remove blood clots, thereby reducing intracranial pressure. Intracranial pressure is managed also with steroids, dehydrating agents, osmotic diuretics, or a combination of these drugs. Broad-spectrum antibiotics are administered.

A compound fracture may be diagnosed through physical examination, skull x-ray films, or both. Basilar skull fracture is determined based on clinical findings. Skull x-rays often do not demonstrate the fracture, although intracranial air or air in the sinuses on x-ray film, CT scan, or MRI is indirect evidence of a basilar skull fracture.

Bed rest and close observation for meningitis and other complications are prescribed for a basilar skull fracture. Prophylactic antibiotics are controversial and may or may not be given.

Diffuse brain injury. Diffuse axonal injury results in the following:

1. *Physical consequences:* spastic paralysis, peripheral nerve injury, swallowing disorders, dysarthria, visual and hearing impairments, taste and smell deficits
2. *Cognitive deficits:* disorientation and confusion, short attention span, memory deficits, learning difficulties, dysphasia, poor judgment, perceptual deficits
3. *Behavioral manifestations:* agitation, impulsiveness, blunted affect, social withdrawal, depression

Mild concussion is characterized by immediate but transitory clinical manifestations. CSF pressure rises, and ECG and EEG changes occur without loss of consciousness. The initial confusional state lasts for one to several minutes, possibly with amnesia for events preceding the trauma (retrograde amnesia). Anterograde amnesia may also exist transiently. Persons may experience head pain and complain of nervousness and "not being themselves" for up to a few days.

In **classic cerebral concussion,** consciousness is lost for up to 6 hours and reflexes fail, causing falls. Reflexes are regained as responsiveness returns. Transiently, breathing stops, bradycardia occurs, and blood pressure falls. Vital signs quickly stabilize to within normal limits. Retrograde and anterograde amnesia exist, along with a confusional state lasting for hours to days. Head pain, nausea, fatigue, attentional and memory system impairments (inability to concentrate and forgetfulness), and mood and affect changes (nervousness, anxiety reactions, depression, irritability, fatigability, insomnia) occur. A **postconcussive syndrome,** including headache, nervousness or anxiety, irritability, insomnia, depression, inability to concentrate, forgetfulness, and fatigability, may exist. Treatment entails reassurance and symptomatic relief in addition to 24 hours of close observation.

In *mild DAI,* 30% of persons display decerebrate or decorticate posturing, and they may experience prolonged periods of stupor or restlessness (see Figure 14-6).

In *moderate DAI,* the score on the Glasgow Coma Scale (GCS) is 4 to 8 initially and 6 to 8 by 24 hours. Thirty-five percent of victims have transitory decerebration or decortication, with unconsciousness lasting days or weeks. On awakening, the person is confused and suffers a long period of posttraumatic anterograde and retrograde amnesia. There is often permanent deficit in memory, attention, abstraction, reasoning, problem solving, executive functions, vision or perception, and language. Mood and affect changes range from mild to severe.

In *severe DAI,* the person experiences immediate autonomic dysfunction that disappears in a few weeks. Increased intracranial pressure appears 4 to 6 days after injury. Pulmonary complications occur often. Profound sensorimotor and cognitive system deficits are present. Severely compromised coordinated movements and verbal and written communication, inability to learn and reason, and inability to modulate behavior are found also.

High-resolution CT scan and MRI assist in the diagnosis of focal and diffuse injuries. Medical management must address endocrine and metabolic derangement. Early and late seizures must be prevented and controlled. Mortality associated with acute head injury is significantly higher in persons treated with corticosteroids within 8 hours of the injury.[3,4]

✓ QUICK CHECK 15-1

1. How is a concussion different from a contusion?
2. Why do extradural, subdural, and intracerebral hematomas act like expanding masses?
3. Why is head motion the principal causative mechanism of diffuse brain injury?

Spinal cord trauma

Each year, 10,000 persons experience serious spinal cord injury. Eighty-one percent are men with an average age of 33.4 years who sustain injuries from car and motorcycle crashes (44%), sports activities (18%), and violence (24%).[1] Elderly people, because of preexisting degenerative vertebral disorders, are particularly at risk for minor trauma that results in serious spinal cord injury; 22% of injuries are attributable to falls in the elderly population.[1]

PATHOPHYSIOLOGY Spinal cord injuries most commonly occur because of vertebral injuries that result from acceleration, deceleration, or deformation forces usually applied at a distance. These forces compress the tissues, pull or exert traction (tension) on the tissues, or shear tissues so that they slide into one another (Figures 15-4 to 15-7). The bones, ligaments, and joints of the vertebral column may be damaged through fracture and compression of one or more elements, dislocation of elements, or both fracture and dislocation. Vertebral injuries can be classified as (1) simple fracture—a single break usually affecting transverse or spinous processes; (2) compressed (wedged) vertebral fracture—vertebral body compressed anteriorly; (3) comminuted

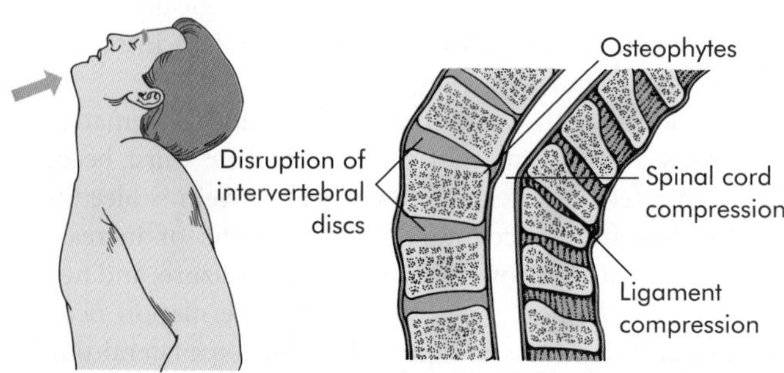

Figure 15-4 ■ Hyperextension Injuries of the Spine. Hyperextension injuries of the spine can result in fracture or nonfracture injuries with spinal cord damage.

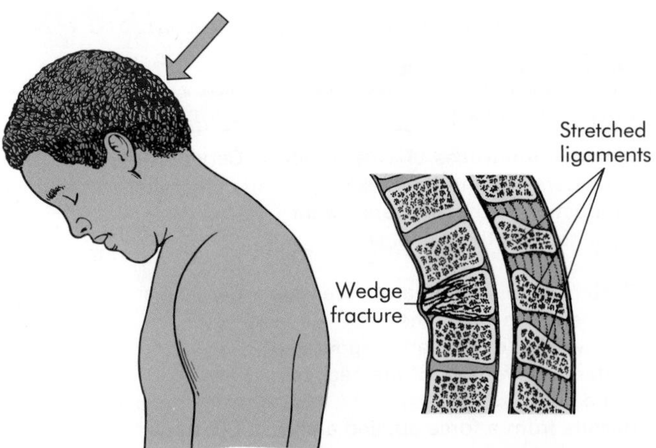

Figure 15-5 ■ **Flexion Injury of the Spine.** Hyperflexion produces translation (subluxation) of vertebrae that compromises the central canal and compresses spinal cord parenchyma or vascular structures.

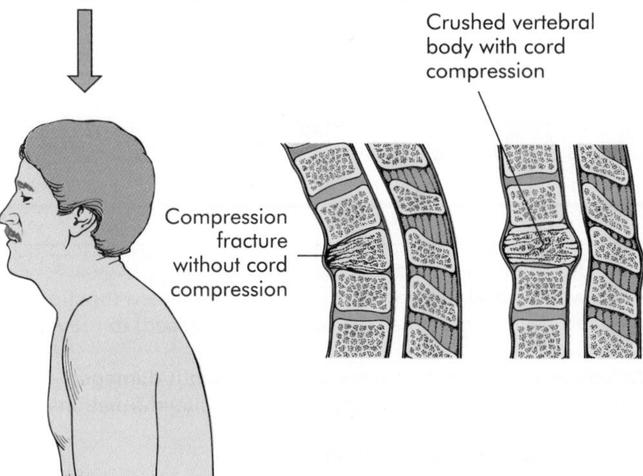

Figure 15-6 ■ **Axial Compression Injuries of the Spine.** In axial compression injuries of the spine, the spinal cord is contused directly by retropulsion of bone or disk material into the spinal canal.

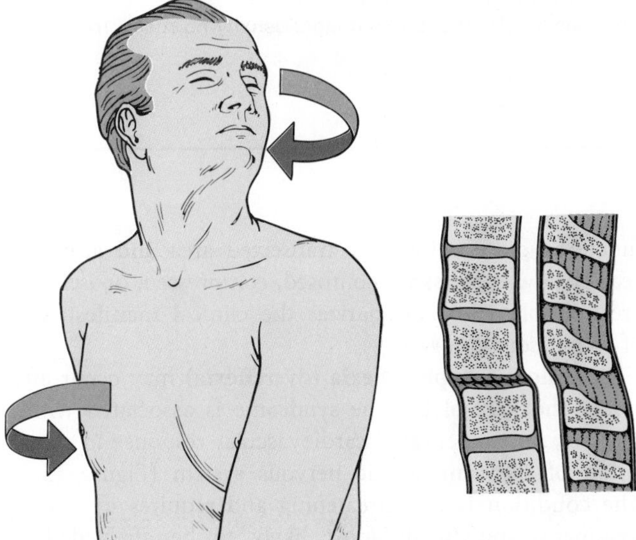

Figure 15-7 ■ **Flexion-Rotation Injuries of the Spine.**

(burst) fracture—vertebral body shattered into several fragments; and (4) dislocation.

The vertebrae fracture readily with both direct and indirect trauma. When the supporting ligaments are torn, the vertebrae move out of alignment and dislocations occur. A horizontal force moves the vertebrae straight forward; if the individual is in a flexed position at the time of injury, the vertebrae are then angulated. Flexion and extension injuries may result in dislocations. (Bone, ligament, and joint injuries are presented in Table 15-4.)

Vertebral injuries in adults occur most often at vertebrae C1 to C2 (cervical), C4 to C7, and T10 (thoracic) to L2 (lumbar) (see Figure 12-9), the most mobile portions of the vertebral column. The cord occupies most of the vertebral canal in the cervical and lumbar regions, so it is easily injured. (Injuries to the cord are summarized in Table 15-5.)

With injury, microscopic hemorrhages appear in the central gray matter and pia-arachnoid, increasing in size until the entire gray matter is hemorrhagic and necrotic. Edema in the white matter occurs, impairing the microcirculation of the cord. Localized hemorrhaging and edema are followed by reduced vascular perfusion and development of ischemic areas. Oxygen tension in the tissue at the injury site is decreased. The microscopic hemorrhages and edema are maximal at the level of injury and two cord segments above and below it.

Cellular and subcellular alterations and tissue necrosis occur. Cord swelling increases the individual's degree of dysfunction, so that it is hard to distinguish functions permanently lost from those temporarily impaired. In the cervical region, cord swelling may be life threatening because it may impair the diaphragm function (phrenic nerves exit at C3 to C5) and vegetative functions (mediated by the medulla oblongata).

Circulation in the white matter tracts of the spinal cord returns to normal in about 24 hours, but gray matter circulation remains altered. Phagocytes appear 36 to 48 hours after injury, and microglia proliferate with altered astrocytes. Red cells then begin to disintegrate, and resorption of hemorrhages begins. Degenerating axons are engulfed by macrophages in the first 10 days after injury. The traumatized cord is replaced by acellular collagenous tissue, usually in 3 to 4 weeks. Meninges thicken as part of the scarring process.

CLINICAL MANIFESTATIONS Normal activity of the spinal cord cells at and below the level of injury ceases because of loss of the continuous tonic discharge from the brain or brain stem and inhibition of suprasegmental impulses immediately after cord injury, thus causing spinal shock. In **spinal shock,** reflex function is completely lost in all segments below the lesion. This condition involves all skeletal muscles; bladder, bowel, and sexual function; and autonomic control. Severe impairment below the level of the lesion is obvious; it includes paralysis and flaccidity in muscles, absence of sensation, loss of bladder and rectal control, transient drop in blood pressure, and poor venous

TABLE 15-4

Mechanisms of Vertebral Injury Involving Bone, Ligaments, and Joints

Mechanism of Injury	Location of Vertebral Injury	Forces of Injury	Location of Injury
Hyperextension	Fracture and dislocation of posterior elements, such as spinous processes, transverse processes, laminae, pedicles, or posterior ligaments	Results from forces of acceleration-deceleration and the sudden reduction in the anteroposterior diameter of the spinal cord	Cervical area
Hyperflexion	Fracture or dislocation of the vertebral bodies, disks, or ligaments	Results from sudden and excessive force that propels the neck forward or causes an exaggerated lateral movement of the neck to one side	Cervical area
Vertical compression (axonal loading)	Shattering fractures	Results from a force applied along an axis from the top of the cranium through the vertebral bodies	T12 to L2
Rotational forces (flexion-rotation)	Rupture support ligaments in addition to producing fractures	Adds shearing force to acceleration forces	Cervical area

TABLE 15-5

Spinal Cord Injuries

Injury	Description
Cord concussion	Results in a temporary disruption of cord-mediated functions
Cord contusion	Bruising of the neural tissue causing swelling and temporary loss of cord-mediated functions
Cord compression	Pressure on the cord causing ischemia to tissues; must be relieved (decompressed) to prevent permanent damage to the spinal cord
Laceration	Tearing of the neural tissues of the spinal cord; may be reversible if only slight damage sustained by the neural tissues; may result in permanent loss of cord-mediated functions if spinal tracts are disrupted
Transection	Severing of the spinal cord, causing permanent loss of function
Complete	All tracts in the spinal cord completely disrupted; all cord-mediated functions below the transection are completely and permanently lost
Incomplete	Some tracts in the spinal cord remain intact, together with functions mediated by these tracts; has the potential for recovery although function is temporarily lost
Preserved sensation only	Some demonstrable sensation below the level of injury
Preserved motor nonfunctional	Preserved motor function without useful purpose; sensory function may or may not be preserved
Preserved motor functional	Preserved voluntary motor function that is functionally useful
Hemorrhage	Bleeding into the neural tissue as a result of blood vessel damage; usually no major loss of function
Damage or obstruction of spinal blood supply	Causes local ischemia

circulation. The condition also results in disturbed thermal control because the sympathetic nervous system is damaged. The hypothalamus cannot regulate body heat through vasoconstriction and increased metabolism; therefore, the individual assumes the temperature of the air (poikilothermia).

Spinal shock generally lasts 7 to 20 days, with a range of a few days to 3 months. It terminates with the reappearance of reflex activity, hyperreflexia, spasticity, and reflex emptying of the bladder.

Loss of motor and sensory function depends on the level of injury. All motor, sensory, reflex, and autonomic functions cease below any transected area and also may cease below concussive, contused, compressed, or ischemic areas. Table 15-6 summarizes the clinical manifestations of spinal cord injury.

Autonomic hyperreflexia (dysreflexia) may occur after spinal shock resolves. The syndrome is associated with a massive, uncompensated cardiovascular response to stimulation of the sympathetic nervous system (Figure 15-8). The condition is life threatening and requires immediate treatment. Individuals most likely to be affected have lesions at the T6 level or above. Characteristics include

TABLE 15-6

Clinical Manifestations of Spinal Cord Injury

Stage	Manifestations
SPINAL SHOCK STAGE Complete spinal cord transection	Loss of motor function 1. Quadriplegia with injuries of the cervical spinal cord 2. Paraplegia with injuries of the thoracic spinal cord Muscle flaccidity Loss of all reflexes below the level of injury Loss of pain, temperature, touch, pressure, and proprioception below the level of injury Pain at the site of injury caused by a zone of hyperesthesia above the injury Atonic bladder and bowel Paralytic ileus with distention Loss of vasomotor tone in the lower body parts; low and unstable blood pressure Loss of perspiration below the level of injury Loss or extreme depression of genital reflexes such as penile erection and bulbocavernous reflex Dry and pale skin; possible ulceration over bony prominences Respiratory impairment
Partial spinal cord transection	Asymmetric flaccid motor paralysis below the level of injury Asymmetric reflex loss Preservation of some sensation below the level of injury Vasomotor instability less severe than with complete cord transection Bowel and bladder impairment less severe than that seen with complete cord transection Preservation of ability to perspire in some portions of the body below the level of injury *Brown-Séquard syndrome* (associated with penetrating injuries, hyperextension and flexion, locked facets, and compression fractures) 1. Ipsilateral paralysis or paresis below level of injury 2. Ipsilateral loss of touch, pressure, vibration, and position sense below level of injury 3. Contralateral loss of pain and temperature sensations below level of injury *Central cervical cord syndrome* (acute cord compression between bony bars or spurs anteriorly and thickened ligamentum flavum posteriorly associated with hyperextension) 1. Motor deficits in upper extremities, especially hands, more dense than in lower extremities 2. Varying degrees of bladder dysfunction *Burning hand syndrome* (variant of central cord syndrome, half the time an underlying spine fracture/dislocation is present) 1. Severe burning paresthesias and dysesthesias in the hands or feet *Anterior cord syndrome* (compromise of anterior spinal artery by occlusion or pressure effect of disk) 1. Loss of motor function below level of injury 2. Loss of pain and temperature sensations below level of injury 3. Touch, pressure, position, and vibration senses intact *Posterior cord syndrome* (associated with hyperextension injuries with fractures of vertebral arch) 1. Impaired light touch and proprioception *Conus medullaris syndrome* (compression injury at T12 from disk herniation or burst fracture of body of T12) 1. Flaccid paralysis of legs 2. Flaccid paralysis of anal sphincter 3. Variable sensory deficits *Cauda equine syndrome* (compression of nerve roots below L1 caused by fracture and dislocation of spine or large posteriocentral intervertebral disk herniation) 1. Lower extremity motor deficits 2. Variable sensorimotor dysfunction 3. Variable reflex dysfunction 4. Variable bladder, bowel, and sexual dysfunction *Syndrome of neuropraxia* (seen postathletic injury, associated with congenital spinal stenosis) 1. Dramatic but transient neurologic deficits including quadriplegia *Horner syndrome* (injury to preganglionic sympathetic trunk or postganglionic sympathetic neurons of superior cervical ganglion) 1. Ipsilateral pupil smaller than contralateral pupil 2. Sunken ipsilateral eyeball 3. Ptosis of affected eyeball 4. Lack of perspiration on ipsilateral side of face

(Continued)

TABLE 15-6

Clinical Manifestations of Spinal Cord Injury—Cont'd

Stage	Manifestations
HEIGHTENED REFLEX ACTIVITY STAGE	Emergence of Babinski reflexes, possibly progressing to a triple reflex; possible development of still later flexor spasms Reappearance of ankle and knee reflexes, which become hyperactive Contraction of reflex detrusor muscle leading to urinary incontinence Appearance of reflex defecation Mass reflex with flexion spasms, profuse sweating, piloerection, and bladder and occasional bowel emptying may be evoked by an autonomic stimulation of skin or from a full bladder Episodes of hypertension Defective heat-induced sweating Eventual development of extensor reflexes, first in muscles of hip and thigh, later in leg Possible paresthesias below the level of transection: dull, burning pain in the lower back, abdomen, buttocks, and perineum

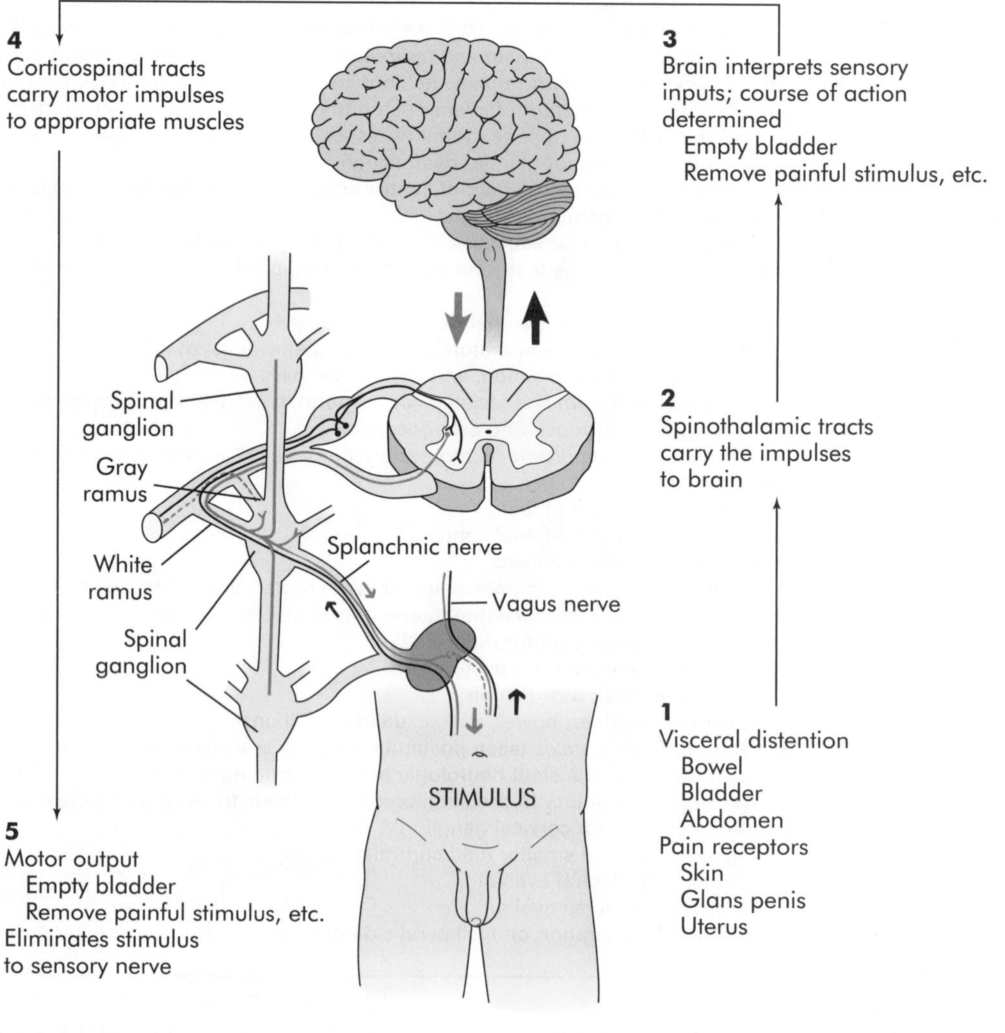

Figure 15-8 ■ **Autonomic Hyperreflexia. A,** Normal response pathway. (Modified from Rudy EB: *Advanced neurological and neurosurgical nursing,* St Louis, 1984, Mosby.)

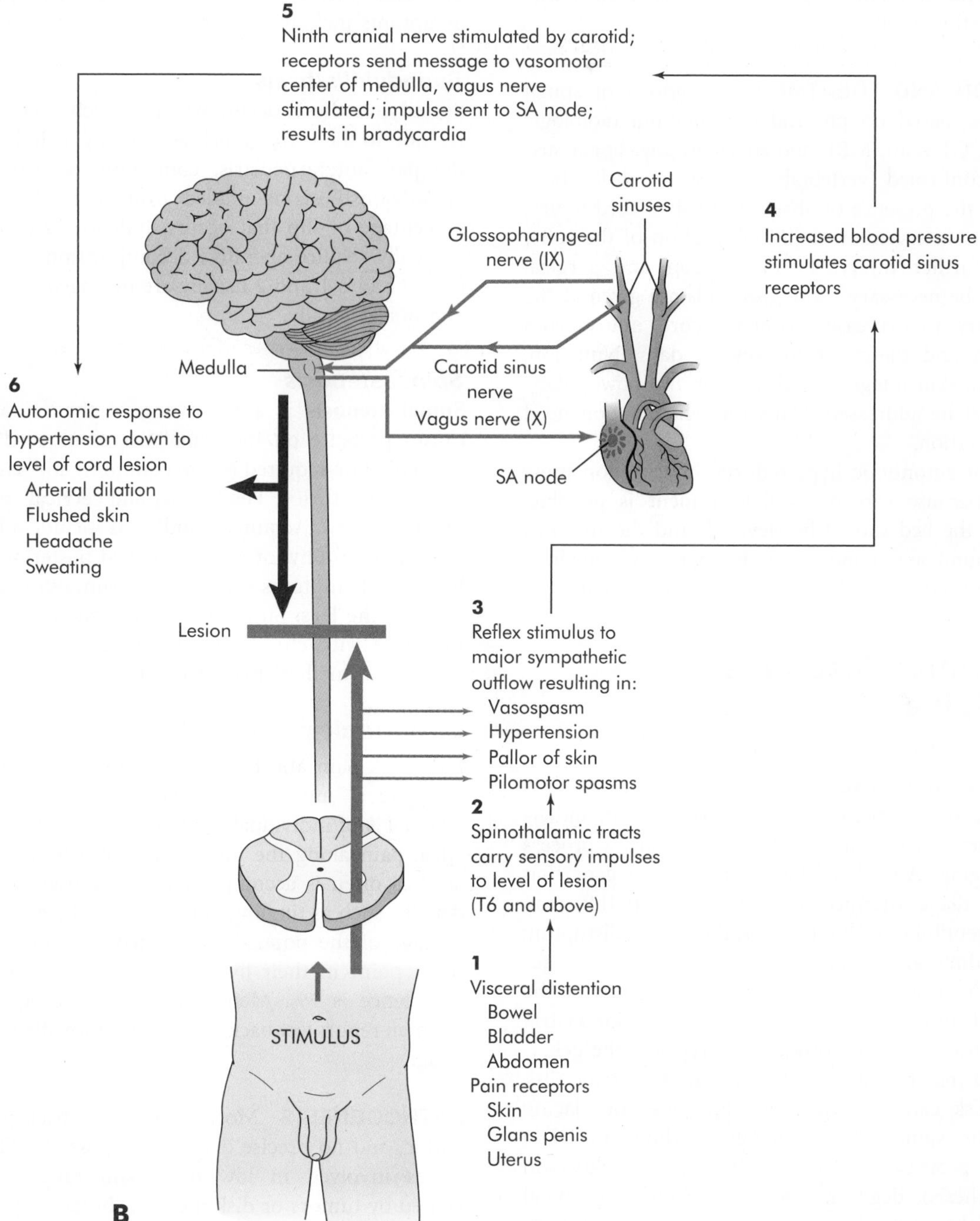
5
Ninth cranial nerve stimulated by carotid; receptors send message to vasomotor center of medulla, vagus nerve stimulated; impulse sent to SA node; results in bradycardia
Carotid sinuses
Glossopharyngeal nerve (IX)
4
Increased blood pressure stimulates carotid sinus receptors
Medulla
Carotid sinus nerve
Vagus nerve (X)
SA node
6
Autonomic response to hypertension down to level of cord lesion
Arterial dilation
Flushed skin
Headache
Sweating
Lesion
3
Reflex stimulus to major sympathetic outflow resulting in:
Vasospasm
Hypertension
Pallor of skin
Pilomotor spasms
2
Spinothalamic tracts carry sensory impulses to level of lesion (T6 and above)
1
Visceral distention
Bowel
Bladder
Abdomen
Pain receptors
Skin
Glans penis
Uterus
STIMULUS
B

Figure 15-8 cont'd ■ **B,** Autonomic dysreflexia pathway. *SA,* sinoatrial.

paroxysmal hypertension (up to 300 mm Hg, systolic), a pounding headache, blurred vision, sweating above the level of the lesion with flushing of the skin, nasal congestion, nausea, piloerection caused by pilomotor spasm, and bradycardia (30 to 40 beats/min). The symptoms may develop singly or in combination (syndrome) and often are associated with a distended bladder or rectum.

In autonomic hyperreflexia, sensory receptors below the level of the cord lesion are stimulated. The intact autonomic nervous system reflexively responds with an arteriolar spasm that increases blood pressure. Baroreceptors in the cerebral vessels, the carotid sinus, and the aorta sense the hypertension and stimulate the parasympathetic system. The heart rate decreases, but the visceral and peripheral vessels do not dilate because efferent impulses cannot pass through the cord.

The most common cause is a distended bladder or rectum, but any sensory stimulation can elicit autonomic hyperreflexia. Stimulation of the skin or pain receptors may cause autonomic hyperreflexia. Bladder or bowel emptying usually relieves the syndrome, and drugs such as phenoxybenzamine may facilitate this result.

EVALUATION AND TREATMENT Diagnosis of spinal cord injury is based on physical examination, radiologic examination, CT scan, MRI, and myelography. For a suspected or confirmed vertebral fracture or dislocation, regardless of the presence or absence of spinal cord injury, the immediate intervention is immobilization of the spine to prevent further injury. Decompression and surgical fixation may be necessary. Corticosteroids are given at the time of injury to decrease secondary cord injury from inflammation and thereafter for several days. Nutrition, lung function, skin integrity, and bladder and bowel management must be addressed. Plans for rehabilitation need early consideration.

In cases of autonomic hyperreflexia, intervention must be prompt because cerebrovascular accident is possible. The head of the bed should be elevated, and the stimulus should be found and removed. Antihypertensive medications may be used if blood pressure remains elevated.

Degenerative Disorders of the Spine

Degenerative joint disease (DJD)

Degenerative disk disease

Degenerative disk disease (DDD) is common in individuals 30 years of age and older and is, in part, a process of normal aging. An inheritable variation in a gene that codes the cartilage intermediate layer protein (CILP) may increase susceptibility to lumbar disk disease by disrupting normal building and maintenance of cartilage.[5] Causes include biochemical and biomechanical alterations of the intervertebral disk tissue. The spongy, soft interior matrix of the disk dries out and fibrocartilage replaces the gelatinous mucoid material of the nucleus pulposus as the disk ages. The disk can herniate pinching nerves or placing strain on the spine. The pathologic findings in DDD include disk protrusion, spondylolysis and/or subluxation (spondylolisthesis), degeneration of vertebrae, and spinal stenosis. Lumbar disk disease causes one third of all back pain that affects 70% to 90% of adults at some point in their lives. However, only a small percentage of people with degenerative disk disease have any functional incapacity because of pain.

Spondylolysis

Spondylolysis is a structural defect (degeneration or developmental defect) of the spine involving the lamina or neural arch of the vertebra. The lumbar spine is affected most often, particularly the portion of the lamina between the superior and inferior articular facets (pars interarticularis). Mechanical pressure may cause a forward displacement of the deficient vertebra (spondylolisthesis). Heredity plays a significant role, and spondylolysis is associated with an increased incidence of other congenital spinal defects. Symptoms include lower back and lower limb pain.

Spondylolisthesis

Spondylolisthesis occurs when a vertebra slides forward in relation to the vertebra below and may include a fracture of the pars interarticularis, commonly occurring at L5-S1. Spondylolisthesis is graded from 1 to 4 based on the percentage of slip that occurs. Individuals with grade 3 or 4 usually require operative decompression, stabilization, or both. Grades 1 and 2 usually are managed symptomatically and nonsurgically.

Spinal stenosis

Spinal stenosis is a narrowing of the spinal canal that causes pressure on the spinal nerves or cord and can be congenital or acquired (more common) and associated with trauma or arthritis. The lumbar and cervical spine are most often involved. Acquired conditions include a bulging disk, facet hypertrophy, or a thick ossified posterior longitudinal ligament. Symptoms can produce pain, numbness, and tingling in the legs. Surgical decompression is recommended for those with chronic symptoms and those who do not respond to medical management.

Low back pain

Low back pain affects the area between the lower rib cage and gluteal muscles and often radiates into the thighs. About 1% of individuals with acute low back pain have sciatica, pain along the distribution of a lumbar nerve root. Sciatica often is accompanied by neurosensory and motor deficits, such as tingling, numbness, and weakness. The percentage of the population affected with low back pain at some point in their lives is 60% to 80%, and the annual prevalence is 5%. Men and women are equally affected. Women report low back symptoms more often after 60 years of age.

PATHOGENESIS Most cases of low back pain are idiopathic, and no precise diagnosis is possible. The local processes involved in low back pain range from tension caused by tumors or disk prolapse, bursitis, synovitis, rising venous and tissue pressure (found in degenerative joint disease), abnormal bone pressures, problems with spinal mobility, inflammation caused by infection (as in osteomyelitis), bony fractures, or ligamentous sprains to pain referred from viscera or the posterior peritoneum. General processes resulting in low back pain include bone diseases, such as osteoporosis or osteomalacia, and hyperparathyroidism.

Risk factors include occupations that require repetitious lifting in the forward bent-and-twisted position; exposure to vibrations caused by vehicles or industrial machinery; obesity; and cigarette smoking. Osteoporosis increases the risk of spinal compression fractures and may be why elderly women report more symptoms than men. Genetic predispositions for low back pain include isthmic spondylolisthesis (vertebra slides forward or slips in relation to a vertebra below), spinal osteochondrosis, and spinal stenosis associated with achondroplasia.

The most commonly encountered causes of low back pain include lumbar disk herniation, degenerative disk disease, spondylolysis, spondylolisthesis, and spinal stenosis. Anatomically, low back pain must come from innervated structures, but deep pain is widely referred and varies. The nucleus pulposus has no intrinsic innervation, but when extruded or herniated through a prolapsed disk, it irritates the dural membranes and causes pain referred to the segmental area (Figure 15-9). The interspinous bursae can be a source of pain between L3, L4, L5, and S1 but also may affect L1, L2, and L3 spinous processes. The anterior and posterior longitudinal ligaments of the spine and the interspinous and supraspinous ligaments are abundantly supplied with pain receptors, as is the ligamentum flavum. All of these ligaments are vulnerable to traumatic tears (sprains) and fracture. Muscle injury may contribute to low back pain, with sprains and strains the most common diagnoses.

EVALUATION AND TREATMENT Diagnosis of low back injury is based on physical examination, electromyelography, CT with or without myelography, MRI, nerve conduction studies, diskography, and epidurography. Most individuals with acute low back pain benefit from a nonspecific short-term treatment regimen of bed rest, analgesic medications, exercises, physical therapy, and education. Surgical treatments, specifically diskectomy and spinal fusions, are used for individuals not responding to medical management. Individuals with chronic low back pain also are prescribed anti-inflammatory and muscle relaxant medications and are instructed to follow exercise programs. Aerobic exercises are a popular treatment and seem to be more effective than traction or low back exercises. Spinal surgery has a limited role in curing chronic low back pain.

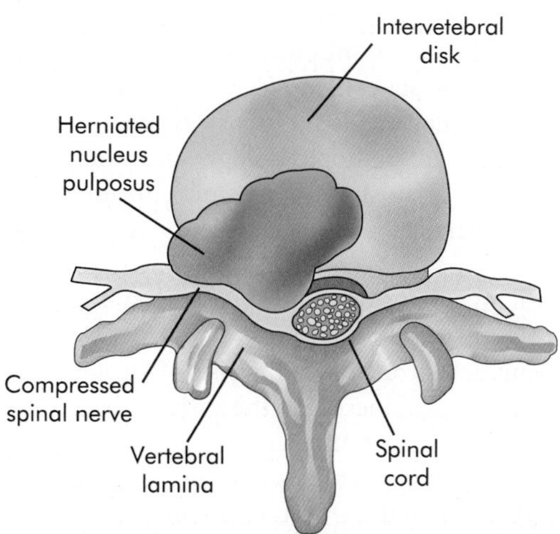

Figure 15-9 ■ **Herniated Nucleus Pulposus.** (Modified from Thompson JM et al: *Mosby's clinical nursing,* ed 5, St Louis, 2002, Mosby.)

HEALTH ALERT

Percutaneous Vertebroplasty

This relatively new, minimally invasive procedure has provided dramatic pain relief in selected persons with vertebral compression fractures (e.g., osteoporotic compression fracture, trauma, or metastatic disease). The procedure is relatively simple. The person under conscious sedation is placed in a prone position. Two needles are inserted into the fractured vertebra under fluoroscopy, and artificial bone cement is injected into the fractured vertebra filling in the spaces in the bone. The person stays prone until the cement hardens (about 2 hours) after which the individual can be discharged. Usually there is significant pain relief.

Data from Heran MK, Legiehn GM, Munk PL: Current concepts and techniques in percutaneous vertebroplasty, *Orthop Clin North Am* 37(3):409–434, vii, 2006; Satre TJ, Mackler L, Birch JT Jr: Clinical inquiries: Who should receive vertebroplasty? *J Fam Pract* 55 (7):637–638, 2006.

Herniated intervertebral disk

Herniation of an intervertebral disk is a protrusion of part of the nucleus pulposus through a tear in the posterior rim of the annulus fibrosus (the fibrous capsule enclosing the gelatinous center of the disk) (see Figure 15-5). Rupture of an intervertebral disk usually is caused by trauma, degenerative disk disease, or both. Lifting with the trunk flexed and sudden straining when the back is in an unstable position are the most common causes. Men are affected more often than women, with the highest incidence in the 30- to 60-year age group. Most commonly affected are the lumbosacral disks—that is, L5-S1 and L4-L5. Disk herniation occasionally occurs in the cervical area, usually at C5-C6 and C6-C7. Herniations at the thoracic level are extremely rare. The injury may occur immediately, within a few hours, or months to years after injury.

PATHOPHYSIOLOGY In a herniated disk, the ligament and posterior capsule of the disk are usually torn, allowing the gelatinous material (the nucleus pulposus) to extrude and compress the nerve root. Occasionally the injury tears the entire disk loose, and it protrudes onto the nerve root or compresses the spinal cord. Multiple nerve root compression may be found at the L5-S1 level, where the cauda equina may be compressed. Large amounts of extruded nucleus pulposus or complete disk herniation (i.e., of both the capsule and the nucleus pulposus) may compress the spinal cord.

CLINICAL MANIFESTATIONS The location and size of the herniation into the spinal canal, together with the amount of space in the canal, determine the clinical manifestations associated with the injury (Figure 15-10). A herniated disk in the lumbosacral area is associated with pain that radiates along the sciatic nerve course over the buttock

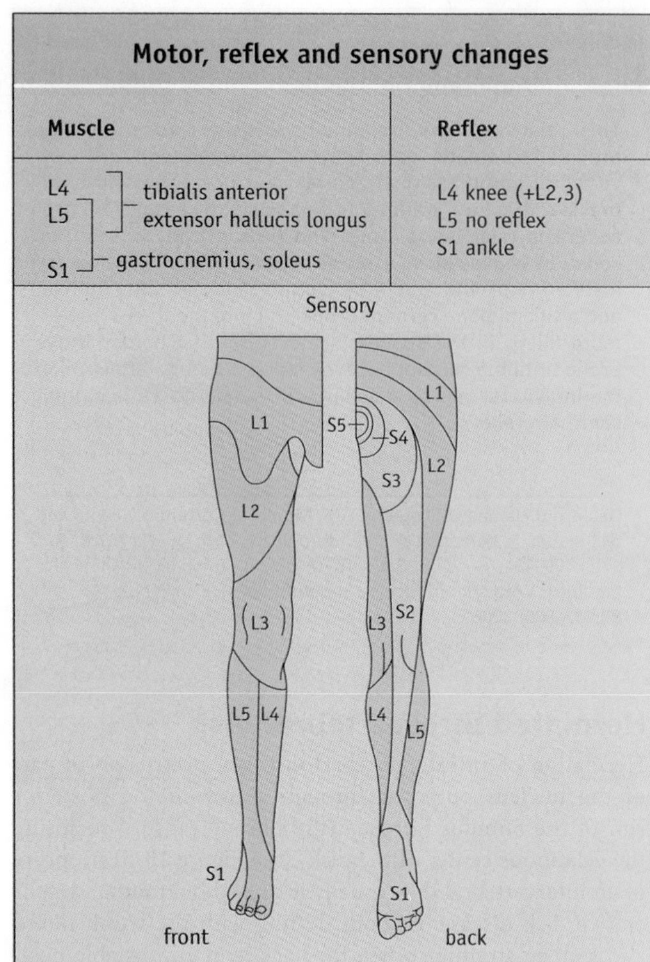

Figure 15-10 ■ Clinical Features of a Herniated Nucleus Pulposus.

and into the calf or ankle. The pain occurs with straining, including coughing and sneezing, and usually on straight leg raising. Other clinical manifestations include limited range of motion of the lumbar spine; tenderness on palpation in the sciatic notch and along the sciatic nerve; impaired pain, temperature, and touch sensation in the L5-S1 or L4-L5 dermatomes of the leg and foot; decreased or absent ankle jerk; and mild weakness of the foot.

With the herniation of a lower cervical disk, paresthesias and pain are present in the upper arm, forearm, and hand along the affected nerve root distribution. Neck motion and straining, including coughing and sneezing, may increase neck and nerve root pain. Neck range of motion is diminished. Slight weakness and atrophy of biceps or triceps may occur; the biceps or triceps reflex may decrease. Occasionally, signs of corticospinal and sensory tract impairments appear, including motor weakness of the lower extremities, sensory disturbances in the lower extremities, and presence of a Babinski reflex.

EVALUATION AND TREATMENT Diagnosis of a herniated intervertebral disk is made through the history and physical examination, spinal x-ray films, electromyelography, CT scan, MRI, myelography, diskography, and nerve conduction studies. Multiple avenues of therapy are available. The conservative approach comprises traction, bed rest, heat and ice to the affected areas, and an effective anti-inflammatory analgesic regimen. The surgical approach is indicated if there is evidence of severe compression (weakness or decreased deep tendon, bladder, or bowel reflexes) or if the conservative approach is unsuccessful.

Cerebrovascular Disorders

Cerebrovascular disease is the most frequently occurring neurologic disorder, accounting for more than 50% of the persons admitted to general hospitals with neurologic problems. Any abnormality of the brain caused by a pathologic process in the blood vessels is referred to as a *cerebrovascular disease.* Included in this category are lesions of the vessel wall, occlusion of the vessel lumen by thrombus or embolus, rupture of the vessel, and alteration in blood quality such as increased blood viscosity.

The brain abnormalities induced by cerebrovascular disease are either (1) ischemia with or without infarction (death of brain tissues) or (2) hemorrhage. The common clinical manifestation of cerebrovascular disease is a **cerebrovascular accident (CVA, stroke):** a sudden, nonconvulsive focal neurologic deficit.

Cerebrovascular accidents (stroke syndromes)

Cerebrovascular accidents are the leading cause of disability in the United States and the third cause of death.[6] Stroke occurs mainly among those older than 65 years, but 28% occur in individuals younger than 65 years. Stroke tends to run in families and is more common in men. The incidence is 2.5 times greater in blacks than whites. Blacks between the ages of 55 and 64 who live in the southern states are about 50% more likely to die of stroke than blacks of the same age who live in the north.[7] In addition, persons with both hypertension and type 2 diabetes mellitus have a fourfold increase in stroke incidence and an eightfold increase in stroke mortality.[8] In its mildest form, a cerebrovascular accident is so minimal as to be almost unnoticed. In its most severe state, hemiplegia, coma, and death result.

Cerebrovascular accidents (stroke syndromes) are classified according to pathophysiology and thus are global hypoperfusion (as in shock), ischemia (thrombotic, embolic), or hemorrhagic. Risk factors for stroke include the following:

- Arterial hypertension (both elevated systolic and diastolic blood pressures)
- Smoking, which increases the risk of stroke by 50%
- Diabetes, which increases the risk of ischemic stroke between 2½ and 3½ times
- Insulin resistance increases risk for ischemic stroke
- Polycythemia and thrombocythemia, which place the person at risk for ischemic stroke
- Presence of lipoprotein-a, which is a risk factor for ischemic stroke

- Impaired cardiac function, which increases risk for ischemic stroke
- Hyperhomocysteinemia increases risk for ischemic stroke
- Nonrheumatic atrial fibrillation, which is associated with a fivefold increase in the incidence of ischemic stroke
- *Chlamydia pneumoniae* can increase the risk of stroke by infiltrating and inflaming the vascular endothelium

Thrombotic stroke

Thrombotic strokes (cerebral thromboses) arise from arterial occlusions caused by thrombi formation in arteries supplying the brain or intracranial vessels. Cerebral thrombosis develops most often from atherosclerosis and inflammatory disease processes (arteritis) that damage arterial walls. Increased coagulation can lead to thrombus formation. Conditions causing inadequate cerebral perfusion (e.g., dehydration, hypotension, prolonged vasoconstriction from malignant hypertension) increase the risk of thrombosis. Over 20 to 30 years, atheromatous plaques (stenotic lesion) form at branchings and curves in the cerebral circulation. The smooth stenotic area can degenerate, forming an ulcerated area of the vessel wall. Platelets and fibrin adhere to the damaged wall, and a clot forms, gradually occluding the artery. The clot may enlarge both distally and proximally. Thrombotic strokes occur when parts of the clot break off and travel upstream.

Transient ischemic attacks (TIAs) are temporary decreases in brain blood flow resulting in brief changes in brain function including changes in vision, speech, motor function, or symptoms of dizziness or loss of consciousness. TIAs probably represent platelet clumps or vessel narrowing with spasm causing an intermittent blockage of circulation. In a true TIA, all the neurologic deficits are completely clear within 24 hours leaving no residual dysfunction and there is no permanent brain injury. Without definitive diagnosis and treatment, 80% of persons have a recurrence of symptoms by 1 year.

> **HEALTH ALERT**
>
> **Two New Warning Signs Found for Impending Stroke**
>
> A combined elevation of lipoprotein-associated phospholipase A2 (Lp-PLa2) (a proinflammatory enzyme secreted by macrophages which binds to LDL) and highly sensitive C-reactive protein (a protein produced by the liver during episodes of inflammation) has a significant increased risk for ischemic stroke. Persons with obstructive sleep apnea also have a greater risk for stroke independent of other risk factors.
>
> Data from Elkind MS, Tai W, Coates K, Paik MC, Sacco RL: High-sensitivity C-reactive protein, lipoprotein-associated phospholipase A2, and outcome after ischemic stroke, *Arch Intern Med* 166 (19):2073–2080, 2006; Munoz R et al: Severe sleep apnea and risk of ischemic stroke in the elderly, *Stroke* 37(9):2317–2321, 2006; Yaggi HK et al: Obstructive sleep apnea as a risk factor for stroke and death, *N Engl J Med* 353(19):2034–2041, 2005.

Embolic stroke

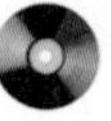

An **embolic stroke** involves fragments that break from a thrombus formed outside the brain or in the heart, aorta, or common carotid. The embolus usually involves small brain vessels and obstructs at a bifurcation or other point of narrowing, thus causing ischemia. An embolus may plug the lumen entirely and remain in place or break into fragments and move up the vessel. Risk factors for an embolic stroke include atrial fibrillation, myocardial infarction, endocarditis, rheumatic heart disease, valvular prostheses, atrial-septal defects, and disorders of the aorta, carotids, or vertebral-basilar circulation. Less common contributors to embolic stroke are air, fat, and tumors. Fat emboli sometimes develop with fractures of long bones. Air emboli also can develop after certain types of surgery. In persons who experience an embolic stroke, usually a second stroke follows because the source of emboli continues to exist. Embolization is usually in the distribution of the middle cerebral artery.

Hemorrhagic stroke

Hemorrhagic stroke (intracranial hemorrhage) is the third most common cause of cerebrovascular accident. Hypertension, ruptured aneurysms or vascular malformation, bleeding into a tumor, hemorrhage associated with bleeding disorders, anticoagulation, head trauma, and illicit drug use are common causes.

A hypertensive hemorrhage is associated with significantly increased systolic and diastolic pressure over several years and usually occurs in the brain tissue. A mass of blood is formed and grows, displacing and compressing adjacent brain tissue. Rupture or seepage into the ventricular system occurs in many cases. Hemorrhages are described as massive, small, slit, or petechial. Massive hemorrhages are several centimeters in diameter; small hemorrhages are 1 to 2 cm in diameter; a slit hemorrhage lies in the subcortical area; and a petechial hemorrhage is the size of a pinhead bleed. The most common sites for hypertensive hemorrhages are in the putamen of the basal ganglia (a portion of the lentiform nucleus) (55%), the thalamus (10%), the cortex and subcortex (15%), the pons (10%), and the cerebellar hemispheres (10%).

Lacunar stroke

Lacunar strokes (lacunar infarcts) are smaller than 1 cm in diameter and involve the small perforating arteries, predominantly in the basal ganglia, internal capsules, and pons. They are associated with smoking, hypertension, and diabetes mellitus.[9] Because of the subcortical location and small area of infarction, these strokes may have pure motor and sensory deficits.

PATHOPHYSIOLOGY

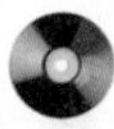

Cerebral infarction. Cerebral infarction results when an area of the brain loses its blood supply because of vascular occlusion. Causes include (1) abrupt vascular occlusion (e.g., embolus), (2) gradual vessel occlusion (e.g., atheroma), and

(3) vessels that are stenosed but not completely occluded. Cerebral thrombi and cerebral emboli most commonly produce occlusion, but atherosclerosis and hypotension are the dominant underlying processes.

Cerebral infarctions are ischemic or hemorrhagic. In ischemic infarcts, the affected area becomes slightly discolored and softens 6 to 12 hours after the occlusion. Necrosis, swelling around the insult, and mushy disintegration appear by 48 to 72 hours after infarction.

In hemorrhagic infarcts, bleeding occurs into the infarcted area when blood flow is restored. The embolic fragments may be moved or lysed, or compressive forces may lessen, allowing blood flow to be reestablished.

Cerebral hemorrhage. The primary cause of cerebral hemorrhage is hypertension. Hypertension involves primarily smaller arteries and arterioles, resulting in thickening of the vessel walls, and increased cellularity of the vessels and hyalinization. Necrosis may be present. Microaneurysms in these smaller vessels or arteriolar necrosis may precipitate the bleeding.

A mass of blood is formed as bleeding continues into the brain tissue. Adjacent brain tissue is displaced and compressed, producing ischemia, edema, and increased intracranial pressure. Rupture or seepage of blood into the ventricular system often occurs.

The cerebral hemorrhage resolves through reabsorption. Macrophages and astrocytes appear to clear away the blood. A cavity forms, surrounded by a dense gliosis after removal of the blood.

CLINICAL MANIFESTATIONS Because neurons surrounding the ischemic or infarcted areas undergo changes that disrupt plasma membranes, cellular edema results, causing further compression of capillaries. Cerebral edema reaches its maximum in about 72 hours and takes about 2 weeks to subside. Most persons survive an initial hemispheric ischemic stroke unless there is massive cerebral edema, which is nearly always fatal.

Clinical manifestations of thrombotic stroke vary, depending on the artery obstructed. Different sites of obstruction create different occlusion syndromes.

With hemorrhagic stroke, clinical manifestations vary, depending on the location and size of the bleed. Once a deep unresponsive state occurs, the person rarely survives. The immediate prognosis is grave. If the person survives, however, recovery of function often is possible.

Individuals experiencing intracranial hemorrhage from a ruptured or leaking aneurysm have one of three sets of symptoms: (1) onset of an excruciating generalized headache with an almost immediate lapse into an unresponsive state, (2) headache but with consciousness maintained, and (3) sudden lapse into unconsciousness. If the hemorrhage is confined to the subarachnoid space, there may be no local signs. If bleeding spreads into the brain tissue, hemiparesis/paralysis, dysphasia, or homonymous hemianopia may be present. Warning signs of an impending aneurysm rupture include headache, transient unilateral weakness, transient numbness and tingling, and transient speech disturbance. However, such warning signs often are absent.

EVALUATION AND TREATMENT MRI and magnetic resonance angiography (MRA) are used to diagnose stroke. In thrombotic stroke, thrombolytic therapy for acute ischemic stroke within 3 to 6 hours is desirable.[10] Treatment is directed at prevention of ischemic injury and supportive management to control cerebral edema and increased intracranial pressure. Arresting the disease process by control of risk factors is critical and aspirin therapy may be instituted.[11] In embolic strokes, treatment is directed at preventing further embolization by instituting anticoagulation therapy and correcting the primary problem. Rehabilitation is indicated in both thrombotic and embolic strokes. Treatment of an intracranial bleed, regardless of cause, focuses on stopping or reducing the bleeding, controlling the increased intracranial pressure, preventing a rebleed, and preventing vasospasm. Occasionally an attempt is made to evacuate or aspirate the blood.

Intravenous (IV) administration of recombinant activated factor VII (rFVIIa) within 4 hours of onset of a cerebral bleed is currently under study.[12] Some surgeons drain the blood, but the benefit is not documented in studies.

Intracranial aneurysm

Intracranial aneurysms may result from arteriosclerosis, congenital abnormality, trauma, inflammation, and cocaine. The size may vary from 2 mm to 2 or 3 cm. Most aneurysms are located at bifurcations in or near the circle of Willis, in the vertebrobasilar arteries, or within the carotid system (see Figures 12-17 and 12-18). Aneurysms may be single, but in 20% to 25% of the cases, more than one is present. In these instances, the aneurysms may be unilateral or bilateral. Peak incidence of rupture is in the decade of the 50s, and the incidence in women is slightly higher.

PATHOPHYSIOLOGY No single pathologic mechanism exists. Aneurysms may be classified on the basis of shape and form. **Saccular aneurysms (berry aneurysms)** occur frequently (in approximately 2% of the population) and probably result from congenital abnormalities in the media of the arterial wall and degenerative changes.[9] The sac gradually grows over time. A saccular aneurysm may be (1) round with a narrow stalk connecting it to the parent artery, (2) broad-based without a stalk, or (3) cylindrical (Figure 15-11). Saccular aneurysms are rare in childhood; their highest incidence of rupturing or bleeding is among persons 20 to 50 years of age (Figure 15-12).

Fusiform aneurysms (giant aneurysms) occur as a result of diffuse arteriosclerotic changes and are found most commonly in the basilar arteries or terminal portions of the internal carotid arteries (see Figure 15-11). They act as space-occupying lesions.

Aneurysms rupture through thin areas, causing hemorrhage into the subarachnoid space that spreads rapidly, producing localized changes in the cerebral cortex and focal irritation of nerves and arteries (see the discussion of the

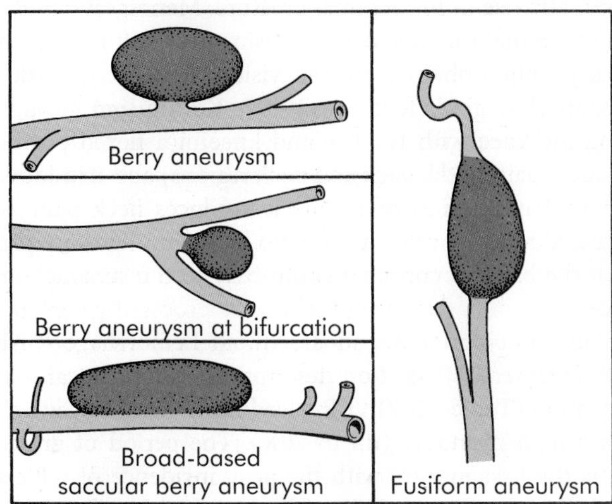

Figure 15-11 ■ **Types of Aneurysms.**

Laplace law in Chapter 22). Bleeding ceases when a fibrin-platelet plug forms at the point of rupture and as a result of compression. Blood undergoes reabsorption through arachnoid villi within 3 weeks.

CLINICAL MANIFESTATIONS Aneurysms often are asymptomatic. Of all persons undergoing routine autopsy, 5% are found to have one or more intracranial aneurysms. Clinical manifestations may arise from cranial nerve compression, but the signs vary, depending on the location and size of the aneurysm. Cranial nerves III, IV, V, and VI are affected most often (see Table 12-6). Unfortunately, the most common first indication of the presence of an aneurysm is an acute subarachnoid hemorrhage, intracerebral hemorrhage, or combined subarachnoid-intracerebral hemorrhage (see Subarachnoid Hemorrhage).

EVALUATION AND TREATMENT Diagnosis before a bleeding episode is made through arteriography. After a subarachnoid or intracerebral hemorrhage, a tentative diagnosis of an aneurysm is based on clinical manifestations, history, CT scan, and MRI. The treatment of choice for an aneurysm is surgical management. Use of coils is currently under study and appears to be a viable option and safer in terms of fever, heart problems, and infections for some persons.[13,14] The location and size of the aneurysm and the person's clinical status determine whether invasive therapy is feasible.

Vascular malformation

An **arteriovenous malformation (AVM)** is a tangled mass of dilated blood vessels creating abnormal channels between the arterial and venous systems (arteriovenous fistula). AVMs may occur in any part of the brain and vary in size from a few millimeters to large malformations extending from the cortex to the ventricle. AVMs occur equally in males and females and occasionally occur in families. Although AVMs are usually present at birth, symptoms

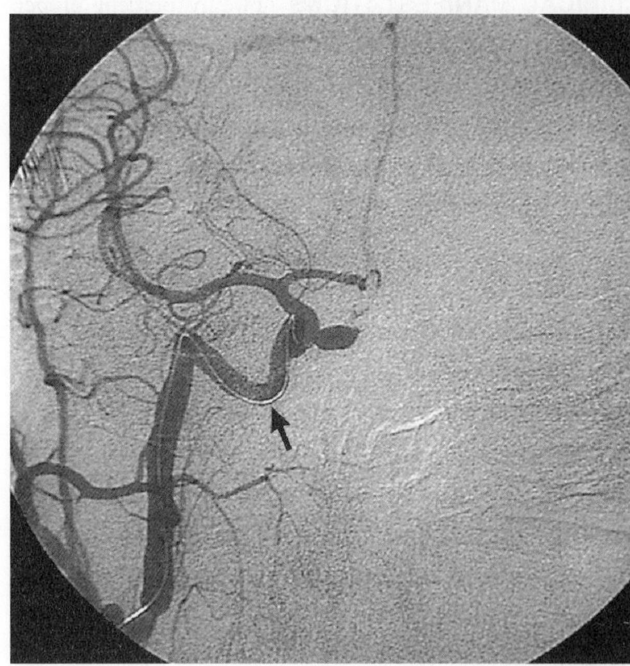

A

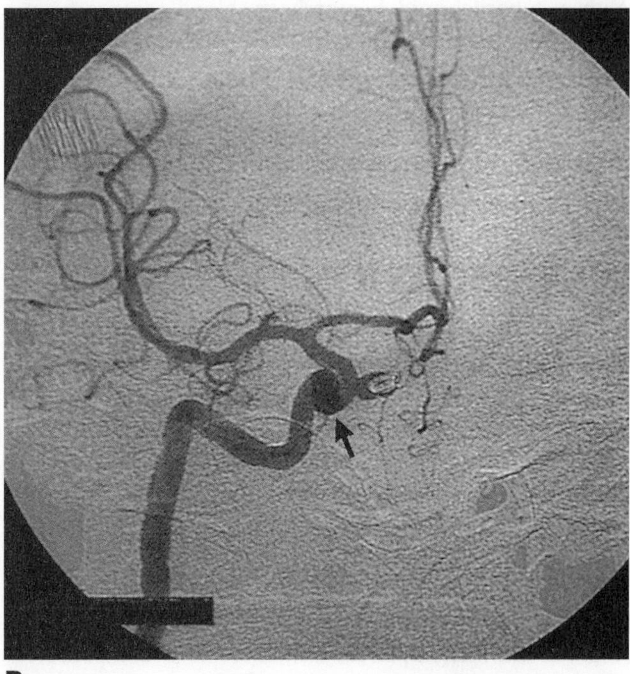

B

Figure 15-12 ■ **Ophthalamic Artery Aneurysm. A,** With endovascular coil; **B,** in situ. (From Perkin GD: *Mosby's color atlas and text of neurology,* London, 1998, Mosby-Wolfe.)

exhibit a delayed age of onset and commonly occur before 30 years of age.

PATHOPHYSIOLOGY AVMs do not have a normal blood vessel structure and are abnormally thin. One or several arteries may feed the AVM and become tortuous and dilated over time. With moderate to large AVMs, sufficient blood is shunted into the malformation to deprive surrounding tissue of adequate blood perfusion.

CLINICAL MANIFESTATIONS Twenty percent of persons with an AVM have a characteristic chronic, nondescript headache, although some experience migraine. Fifty percent of persons experience seizures caused by compression. The other 50% experience an intracerebral, subarachnoid, or subdural hemorrhage. Bleeding from an AVM into the subarachnoid space causes symptoms identical to those associated with a ruptured aneurysm. If bleeding is into the brain tissue, focal signs that develop resemble a stroke-in-evolution. Ten percent of persons experience hemiparesis or other focal signs. At times, noncommunicating hydrocephalus (see Chapter 16) develops with a large AVM that extends into the ventricular lining.

EVALUATION AND TREATMENT A systolic bruit over the carotid artery in the neck, the mastoid process, or the eyeball in a young person is almost diagnostic of an AVM. Confirming diagnosis is made by CT and MRI followed by MRA. Treatment options are direct surgical intervention, embolization, or radiotherapy.

Subarachnoid hemorrhage

With a **subarachnoid hemorrhage,** blood escapes from a defective or injured vessel into the subarachnoid space. Individuals at risk for a subarachnoid hemorrhage are those with intracranial aneurysm, intracranial arteriovenous malformation, or hypertension and those who have sustained head injuries. Subarachnoid hemorrhages often recur, especially from a ruptured intracranial aneurysm.

PATHOPHYSIOLOGY When a vessel is leaking, blood oozes into the subarachnoid space. When a vessel tears, blood under pressure is pumped into the subarachnoid space. The blood increases intracranial volume,[15] and it is also extremely irritating to the neural tissues and produces an inflammatory reaction. In addition, the blood coats nerve roots, clogs arachnoid granulations (impairing CSF reabsorption), and clogs foramina within the ventricular system (impairing CSF circulation). Intracranial pressure immediately increases to almost diastolic levels but returns to near baseline in about 10 minutes. Cerebral blood flow and cerebral perfusion pressure decrease. Autoregulation of blood flow is impaired, and there is a compensatory increase in systolic blood pressure.[16] The expanding hematoma acts like a space-occupying lesion, compressing and displacing brain tissue. Granulation tissue is formed, and meningeal scarring with impairment of CSF reabsorption and secondary hydrocephalus often results. Mortality in subarachnoid hemorrhage is 50% at 1 month.

CLINICAL MANIFESTATIONS Early manifestations associated with leaking vessels are episodic and include headache, changes in mental status or level of consciousness, nausea or vomiting, and focal neurologic defects. A ruptured vessel causes a sudden, throbbing, "explosive" headache, accompanied by nausea and vomiting, visual disturbances, motor deficits, and loss of consciousness related to a dramatic rise in intracranial pressure. Meningeal irritation and inflammation often occur, causing neck stiffness (nuchal rigidity), photophobia, blurred vision, irritability, restlessness, and low-grade fever. A positive **Kernig sign** (straightening the knee with the hip and knee in a flexed position produces pain in the back and neck regions) and **Brudzinski sign** (passive flexion of the neck produces neck pain and increased rigidity) may appear. No localizing signs are present if the bleed is confined completely to the subarachnoid space.

The Hunt and Hess subarachnoid hemorrhage (SAH) grading system is based on description of the clinical manifestations (Table 15-7).[17] Rebleeding is a significant risk with a high mortality (up to 70%). The period of greatest risk is the first month, with the peak incidence of rebleeding during the first 2 weeks after the initial bleed. Rebleeding is manifested by a sudden increase in blood pressure and intracranial pressure, along with a deteriorating neurologic status.

Delayed cerebral ischemia, a syndrome of progressive neurologic deterioration, is associated with cerebral artery vasospasm. From 40% to 60% of persons with a subarachnoid hemorrhage experience vasospasms in adjacent and, sometimes, in nonadjacent vessels. Vasospasm may occur because of the effects of vasoactive substances (e.g., calcium, prostaglandins, serotonin, catecholamines) on the arteries of the subarachnoid space. Edema, medial necrosis, and proliferation of the intima have been found. Vasospasm causes decreased cerebral blood flow, ischemia, and possibly infarct. The peak time of onset is 3 to 5 days with maximal narrowing at 5 to 14 days after the initial bleed, but it may persist for several weeks.

TABLE 15-7

Subarachnoid Hemorrhage Classification Scale

Category	Description
Grade I	Neurologic status intact; mild headache, slight nuchal rigidity
Grade II	Neurologic deficit evidenced by cranial nerve involvement; moderate to severe headache with more pronounced meningeal signs (e.g., photophobia, nuchal rigidity)
Grade III	Drowsiness and confusion with or without focal neurologic deficits; pronounced meningeal signs
Grade IV	Stuporous with pronounced neurologic deficits (e.g., hemiparesis, dysphasia); nuchal rigidity
Grade V	Deep coma state with decerebrate posturing and other brain stem functioning

From Cook HS: Aneurysmal subarachnoid hemorrhage: neuroscience frontiers and nursing challenges. In Winkelman C, editor: *AACN clinical issues in critical nursing,* Philadelphia, 1991, Lippincott.

Seizures occur in 25% of persons with an SAH, and hydrocephalus after a bleed occurs in 20% of cases. Hypothalamic dysfunction, manifested by salt wasting, hyponatremia, and ECG changes, is common.

EVALUATION AND TREATMENT The diagnosis of an SAH is based on the clinical presentation, a noncontrast CT scan, and a lumbar puncture. Arteriography is the definitive diagnostic measure for identifying an aneurysm or arteriovenous malformation. Treatment is directed at controlling intracranial pressure, preventing ischemia and hypoxia of neural tissues, and preventing rebleeding episodes. The primary problem must be diagnosed and corrected as well.

QUICK CHECK 15-2

1. Why is atherosclerosis a risk factor for thrombotic stroke?
2. Why do a TIA's signs and symptoms resolve completely?
3. Why do lacunar strokes involve small infarcts?
4. How is an AVM different from an aneurysm?

Infection and Inflammation of the Central Nervous System

Bacteria, viruses, fungi, protozoans, and rickettsiae can produce pyogenic, or pus-producing, disease in the CNS. The meninges, neural tissues, and vasculature may be involved in the inflammatory process.

Meningitis

The causes of **meningitis** (infection of the meninges) include bacteria, viruses, fungi, parasites, or toxins. The infection may be acute, subacute, or chronic, with the pathophysiology, clinical manifestations, and treatment differing for each type of organism.

Bacterial meningitis is primarily an infection of the pia mater and arachnoid, the subarachnoid space, the ventricular system, and the CSF. A systemic or bloodstream infection or a direct extension from an infected area is the access route to the subarachnoid space. Predisposing conditions are otitis or sinusitis (25%), immunocompromise (16%), and pneumonia (12%).[18,19] Meningococcus *(Neisseria meningitidis)* and pneumococcus *(Streptococcus pneumoniae)* are the most common causes of bacterial meningitis.[20] One in 100,000 persons are affected annually.

Meningococcus has been identified worldwide. Meningococcal meningitis occurs predominantly in men and boys and in the fall, winter, and spring of the year. Epidemics of meningococcal meningitis occur in approximately 10-year cycles, predominantly affecting children and adolescents. With pneumococcal meningitis, young persons and those over 40 years of age are mostly affected. Prognosis depends on the type of pathogen. In one series of studies, mortality was 30% with pneumococcal meningitis, 7% with meningococcal meningitis, and 20% for other pathogens.[18,19]

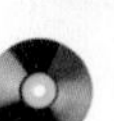

Aseptic meningitis (viral meningitis, nonpurulent meningitis) is believed to be limited to the meninges. It produces various symptoms and is caused by several infectious agents, usually viruses. Enteroviral viruses (echovirus, coxsackievirus, nonparalytic poliomyelitis), mumps, herpes simplex 1 and 2, California encephalitis virus, St. Louis encephalitis virus, West Nile virus, Venezuelan equine encephalitis, Colorado tick fever, lymphocytic choriomeningitis virus, Epstein-Barr virus, and influenza virus type A and B are the most common agents.[20] Bacterial infections not adequately treated also cause aseptic meningitis.

Fungal meningitis is a chronic, much less common condition than bacterial or viral meningitis. The most common fungal infections of the nervous system are histoplasmosis, cryptococcosis, coccidioidomycosis, mucormycosis, candidiasis, and aspergillosis. The infection occurs most often in persons with impaired immune responses or alterations in normal body flora. It develops insidiously, usually over days or weeks.

PATHOPHYSIOLOGY The bacteria that usually cause bacterial meningitis are common inhabitants of the nasopharynx, but a predisposing factor such as a prior upper respiratory infection must be present before the bacteria become blood borne. The method of CNS entry is thought to be through the choroid plexus or areas of altered blood-brain barrier. The bacteria or their toxins function as irritants and induce an inflammatory reaction by the meninges (pia and arachnoid), the CSF, and the ventricles. The meningeal vessels become hyperemic and increasingly permeable. Blood cells (neutrophils) migrate into the subarachnoid space, producing an exudate that thickens the CSF and interferes with normal CSF flow around the brain and spinal cord. The exudate can obstruct arachnoid villi and produce hydrocephalus. Further, inflammation occurs as the purulent exudate increases rapidly, especially around the base of the brain, and extends into the sheaths of the cranial and spinal nerves and into the perivascular spaces of the cortex. Meningeal cells become edematous, and the combined exudate and edematous cells increase intracranial pressure. Small and medium-size subarachnoid arteries, veins, and choroid plexuses become engorged, disrupting blood flow and potentially producing thrombosis. Secondary infection of the brain may occur.

Fungi in the nervous system usually produce a granulomatous reaction, forming granulomas or gelatinous masses in the meninges at the base of the brain. Fungi also may extend along the perivascular sites in the subarachnoid space and into the brain tissue, producing arteritis with thrombosis, infarction, and communicating hydrocephalus. Meningeal fibrosis develops later in the inflammatory process. Cranial nerve dysfunction, caused by compression, often results from the granulomas and fibrosis.

CLINICAL MANIFESTATIONS The clinical manifestations of a bacterial meningitis can be grouped into meningeal signs, infectious signs, and neurologic signs. Those clinical manifestations of systemic infection include fever, tachycardia, chills, and a petechial rash. The clinical manifestations that arise from the meningeal irritation are a generalized throbbing headache that becomes very severe, photophobia that becomes severe, nuchal rigidity, Kernig sign (inability to extend the leg with the hip flexed at a right angle), and Brudzinski sign (flexion of the legs and thighs with forceful flexion of the neck onto the chest). The neurologic signs include a decrease in consciousness, cranial nerve palsies, focal neurologic deficits (such as hemiparesis/hemiplegia and ataxia), and seizures. Often the vomiting center is irritated, causing projectile vomiting. With meningococcal meningitis, a petechial or purpuric rash covers the skin and mucous membranes. As intracranial pressure increases, papilledema develops and delirium may progress to unconsciousness.

The clinical manifestations of aseptic meningitis are mild compared with those associated with bacterial meningitis. Mild, generalized throbbing headache, mild photophobia, mild neck pain, stiffness, fever, and malaise accompany aseptic meningitis.

Fungal meningitis develops slowly and insidiously. The first manifestations are often those of dementia (see Chapter 14) or communicating hydrocephalus (see Chapter 14). The individual is characteristically afebrile.

EVALUATION AND TREATMENT Diagnosis of bacterial meningitis is based on physical examination, nasopharyngeal smear, and antigen tests. CSF cultures are required to diagnose fungal meningitis. Bacterial meningitis and fungal meningitis are treated with appropriate antibiotic therapy and other supportive measures. Aseptic meningitis is managed pharmacologically with antiviral drugs and steroids. There are vaccinations for meningococcal, pneumococcal, and *Haemophilus influenzae.* Treatment for persons exposed to meningococcal meningitis is chemoprophylaxis and vaccination.[21]

HEALTH ALERT

Meningococcal Vaccine and Guillain-Barré Syndrome

A joint alert has been issued by the Food and Drug Administration (FDA) and the Centers for Disease Control and Prevention (CDC) to consumers and health care providers concerning reports of Guillain-Barré syndrome diagnosed after the administration of meningococcal conjugate vaccine: "Because of the risk for meningococcal disease and the associated morbidity and mortality, CDC continues to recommend routine vaccination with MCV4 for adolescents, college freshmen living in dormitories, and other populations at increased risk."

Data from Centers for Disease Control and Prevention (CDC): Update: Guillain-Barré syndrome among recipients of Menactra meningococcal conjugate vaccine—United States, October 20, 2006, *MMWR Morb Mortal Wkly Rep* 55(41):1120–1124, 2006. Erratum in *MMWR Morb Mortal Wkly Rep* 55(43):1177, 2006. Available at http://www.cdc.gov/mmwr/preview/mmwrhtml/mm5541a2.htm.

Abscess

Abscesses are localized collections of pus within the parenchyma of the brain and spinal cord. They occur in about 1 of every 100,000 hospital admissions. Men experience abscesses twice as often as women. The median age for abscess formation is 30 to 40 years. They occur (1) after open trauma and during neurosurgery; (2) in association with a contiguous focus of infection, such as the middle ear, mastoid cells, nasal cavity, and nasal sinuses; (3) through metastatic or hematogenous spread from distant foci, such as the heart, lungs, pelvic organs, skin, tonsils, abscessed teeth, osteomyelitis in other than cranial bones, and dirty needles (especially in compromised hosts); and (4) cryptogenically, arising without other associated areas of infection. Streptococci, staphylococci, and *Bacteroides,* often combined with anaerobes, are the most common bacteria that cause abscesses; however, yeast and fungi have been found also. *Toxoplasma gondii* is producing an ever-increasing number of CNS abscesses in persons with acquired immunodeficiency syndrome (AIDS). Eighty percent of CNS abscesses are located in the cerebrum, and 20% are cerebellar, with the frontal and temporal lobes the most common sites. The abscesses are in more than one site in 5% to 20% of cases. Immunosuppressed persons are particularly at risk.

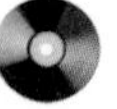

Brain abscesses are classified as extradural or intracerebral. **Extradural brain abscesses** are associated with osteomyelitis in a cranial bone. Unlike **intracerebral brain abscesses,** they rarely arise from a vascular source. **Spinal cord abscesses** are classified as epidural or intramedullary. Individuals with diabetes mellitus show an increased incidence of **spinal epidural abscesses** (which form in the epidural space), whereas debilitated individuals with sepsis more often develop **intramedullary spinal cord abscesses** (those within the spinal cord). Epidural spinal abscesses usually originate as osteomyelitis in a vertebra; the infection then spreads into the epidural space. (Osteomyelitis is discussed in Chapter 38.)

PATHOPHYSIOLOGY Organisms gain entrance to the CNS by direct extension or spread along the wall of a vein. Infective emboli carry organisms from distant sites. Brain abscesses evolve through four stages:

1. *Early cerebritis* (days 1 to 3) with localized inflammation with presence of inflammatory cells surrounding a core of necrosis, marked cerebral edema is present
2. *Late cerebritis* (days 4 to 9) with necrotic center surrounded by macrophages and fibroblasts, new blood vessels form rapidly around abscess, thin capsule develops, edema still persists
3. *Early capsule formation* (days 10 to 13) with necrotic center decreasing in size, more fibroblasts and macrophages are present, mature collagen evolves forming a capsule
4. *Late capsule formation* (days 14 and longer) with well-formed necrotic center surrounded by a dense collagen capsule (Figure 15-13)

Existing abscesses also tend to spread and form daughter abscesses.

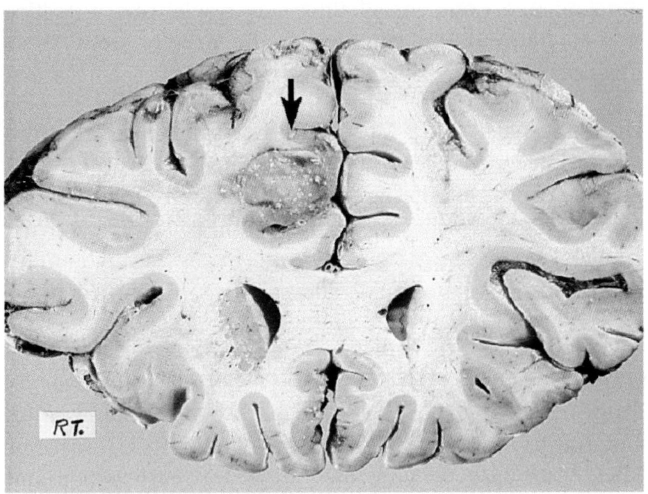

Figure 15-13 ■ **Brain Abscess.** Early brain abscess appearing as a poorly demarcated area *(arrow)* of cerebritis at the gray-white junction. (From Damjanov I, Linder J, editors: *Anderson's pathology,* ed 10, St Louis, 1996, Mosby.)

CLINICAL MANIFESTATIONS Clinical manifestations of brain abscesses are associated with (1) an intracranial infection or (2) an expanding intracranial mass. Early manifestations include low-grade fever, headache (most common symptom), neck pain and stiffness with mild nuchal rigidity, confusion, drowsiness, sensory deficits, and communication deficits. Later clinical manifestations include inattentiveness (distractibility), memory deficits, decreased visual acuity and narrowed visual fields, papilledema, ocular palsy, ataxia, and dementia. The development of symptoms may be very insidious, often making an abscess difficult to diagnose.

Extradural brain abscesses are associated with localized pain, purulent drainage from the nasal passages or auditory canal, fever, localized tenderness, and neck stiffness. Occasionally the individual experiences a focal seizure.

Clinical manifestations of spinal cord abscesses have four stages: (1) spinal aching; (2) severe root pain, accompanied by spasms of the back muscles and limited vertebral movement; (3) weakness caused by progressive cord compression; and (4) paralysis.

HEALTH ALERT

West Nile Virus

West Nile virus (WNV) is a potentially serious illness caused by arboviral infection spread by infected mosquitoes. The illness is seasonal in the summer and continues into the fall.

Symptoms: There may be no symptoms or there may be illness of varying severity with central nervous system involvement including fever, headache, stiff neck, vision loss, altered mental status ranging from confusion to coma with or without additional signs of brain dysfunction (e.g., paresis or paralysis, cranial nerve palsies, sensory deficits, abnormal reflexes, generalized convulsions, and abnormal movements). When the central nervous system is affected, clinical syndromes ranging from febrile headache to aseptic meningitis to encephalitis may occur, and these are usually indistinguishable from similar syndromes caused by other viruses. Symptoms usually develop between 3 and 14 days after a bite by an infected mosquito and may last for a few days to several weeks.

Laboratory criteria for diagnosis:

- Fourfold or greater change in virus-specific serum antibody titer, or
- Isolation of virus from or demonstration of specific viral antigen or genomic sequences in tissue, blood, cerebrospinal fluid (CSF), or other body fluid, or
- Virus-specific immunoglobulin M (IgM) antibodies demonstrated in CSF by antibody-capture enzyme immunoassay (EIA), or
- Virus-specific IgM antibodies demonstrated in serum by antibody-capture EIA and confirmed by demonstration of virus-specific serum immunoglobulin G (IgG) antibodies in the same or a later specimen by another serologic assay (e.g., neutralization or hemagglutination inhibition)

Transmission: Generally spread by the bite of an infected mosquito. Mosquitoes are WNV carriers that become infected when they feed on infected birds. Infected mosquitoes can then spread WNV to humans and other animals when they bite. In a very small number of cases, WNV also has spread through blood transfusions, organ transplants, breastfeeding, and even during pregnancy from mother to fetus, but the risk is low. WNV is not spread through casual contact such as touching or kissing a person with the virus.

Risk: Less than 20% of people who are bitten by mosquitoes develop any symptoms of the disease, and relatively few mosquitoes actually carry WNV. People older than age 50 and immunocompromised persons are more likely to develop serious symptoms.

Prevention: Prevent mosquito bites. Avoid outdoor activities dusk to dawn or wear protective clothing—long sleeves, long pants, and socks. Treat clothes with insect repellents containing DEET. Higher concentrations of active ingredients provide longer protection. Maintain good screens on windows and doors to keep mosquitoes out. Eliminate mosquito breeding sites by eliminating or treating standing water. Do not handle dead birds with bare hands. Contact your local health department for instructions on reporting and disposing of dead birds. No West Nile vaccine has been developed for humans. Since 2003, all blood banks use blood-screening tests for West Nile virus. In addition, blood banks will not take donations from people who had a fever and headache in the week before they volunteered to donate blood.

Treatment: There is no specific treatment for WNV infection. Severe symptoms require hospital care. A subset of persons remain profoundly weak and limited in daily functioning 1 year following acute illness. Work is in progress to develop a vaccine and antiviral therapy.

Data from Avalos-Bock SA: West Nile virus and the US blood supply: new tests substantially reduce the risk of transmission via donated blood products, *Am J Nurs* 105(12):34–37, 2005; Centers for Disease Control and Prevention, Division of Vector Borne Infectious Diseases: *West Nile Virus;* available at www.cdc.gov/ncidod/dvbid/westnile/surv&controlCase Count06_detailed.htm; Davis LE et al: West Nile virus neuroinvasive disease, *Ann Neurol* 60(3):286–300, 2006.

EVALUATION AND TREATMENT The diagnosis is suggested by clinical features and confirmed by CT scan. MRI is helpful when the CT scan does not show a strongly suggested abscess. Aspiration through a burr hole and excision through craniotomy accompanied by antibiotic therapy are treatment options. In addition, intracranial pressure may have to be managed.

Because decompression is necessary, spinal cord abscesses are treated with surgical excision or aspiration. Antibiotic therapy and support therapy also are instituted.

Encephalitis

Encephalitis is an acute febrile illness, usually of viral origin, with nervous system involvement. The most common forms are caused by arthropod-borne (mosquito-borne) viruses and herpes simplex type 1. Referred to as infectious viral encephalitides, encephalitis may occur also as a complication of systemic viral diseases such as poliomyelitis, rabies, or mononucleosis, or it may arise after recovery from viral infections such as rubella or rubeola. Encephalitis also may follow vaccination with a live attenuated virus vaccine if the vaccine has an encephalitis component, for example, measles, mumps, and rubella. Typhus, trichinosis, malaria, and schistosomiasis also are associated with encephalitis. **Toxoplasmosis** may acutely reactivate in immunosuppressed persons when the once-dormant parasite in cyst form disseminates in brain tissues.

With the exception of the California viral encephalitis, which is endemic, the arthropod-borne (mosquito-borne) encephalitides occur in epidemics, varying in geographic and seasonal incidence (Table 15-8). Eastern equine encephalitis is the most serious but least common of the encephalitides.

PATHOPHYSIOLOGY Meningeal involvement is present in all encephalitides. The various encephalitides may cause widespread nerve cell degeneration. Edema, necrosis with or without hemorrhage, and increased intracranial pressure develop. Infectious encephalitis may result from a postinfectious autoimmune response to the virus or from direct invasion of the CNS.

CLINICAL MANIFESTATIONS Encephalitis ranges from a mild infectious disease to a life-threatening disorder. Dramatic clinical manifestations include fever, delirium, or confusion progressing to unconsciousness, seizure activity, cranial nerve palsies, paresis and paralysis, involuntary movement, and abnormal reflexes. Signs of marked intracranial pressure may be present.

EVALUATION AND TREATMENT Diagnosis is made by history and clinical presentation aided by CSF examination and culture, serology, white blood cell count, CT scan, or MRI. Most cases of viral meningitis are self-limiting, and until recently no definitive treatment was available. However, herpes encephalitis in immunocompromised persons is now being treated with antiviral agents, such as acyclovir and steroids. Measures to control intracranial pressure are paramount.

Neurologic complications of AIDS

From 40% to 60% of all persons with AIDS have neurologic complications. On postmortem examination, 75% of AIDS victims have nervous system pathologic findings that result from (1) the primary human immunodeficiency virus (HIV) infection; (2) the immune dysregulation of early HIV infection and progressive immunosuppression in late HIV infection resulting in opportunistic infections, neoplasms, and systemic illness; and (3) complications of therapy.[22]

The most common neurologic disorder is HIV-associated cognitive dysfunction (HIV encephalopathy). Others are peripheral neuropathies, vacuolar (spongy softening) myelopathy, opportunistic infections of the CNS, and neoplasms.

HIV-infected macrophages and monocytes from blood accumulate in the brain by up-regulation of proinflammatory mediators that enable transendothelial migration of

TABLE 15-8

Classification and Characteristics of Viruses Causing Encephalitis

Viruses	Incubation Period (days)	Location	Season	Affected Population
Eastern equine encephalitis	5–15	Atlantic, Gulf Coast, and Great Lakes regions	Midsummer to early fall	Infants, children, and adults >50 yr
Western equine encephalitis	5–10	All parts of United States, especially western two thirds of country	Summer to early fall	Infants and young children
Venezuelan encephalitis	2–5	Texas, Florida, Mexico, Central and South America	Year round	Infants and young children
St. Louis encephalitis	4–21	United States and Canada, especially Mississippi River, Pacific Coast, Texas, and Florida	Summer and fall	Adults >40 yr; elderly more often affected than younger ages
California encephalitis	5–15	Midwestern United States, eastern seaboard, and Canada	Late summer and early fall	Children <15 yr
West Nile encephalitis	3–14	Lower 48 states of the United States	Summer and fall	Elderly most seriously

Modified from Barker E: *Neuroscience nursing,* ed 2, St Louis, 2002, Mosby.

the activated macrophages and monocytes. The virus can be isolated in the CSF at approximately the time of seroconversion.

Human immunodeficiency-associated cognitive dysfunction (HIV encephalopathy)

HIV-associated cognitive dysfunction (HIV encephalopathy, subacute encephalitis, HIV-associated dementia complex, HIV cognitive motor complex, AIDS encephalopathy, AIDS dementia complex, AIDS-related dementia) may affect adults or children and is characterized by progressive cognitive dysfunction with motor and behavioral alterations.[22] The syndrome typically develops later in the disease but may be an early or singular manifestation in some persons.

It is believed that HIV-associated cognitive dysfunction results from direct brain tissue infection by the virus. HIV is found mostly in white matter subcortical areas causing an immune demyelinating-mediated process, but some viral replication occurs in glial cells and, occasionally, neurons. Multiple small nodules containing inflammatory cells are found scattered throughout the white matter and in subcortical gray matter, such as the basal ganglia and thalami. Multinucleated giant cells and perivascular inflammation are present, with focal and diffuse demyelination of white matter and spongy changes of the spinal cord. Toxins, lymphokines, or other substances also are factors in this process.

HIV-associated cognitive dysfunction is insidious in onset and unpredictable in its course. Most persons experience a steady progression with abrupt accelerations of signs over several months to more than 1 year, although some individuals experience an abrupt onset or an accelerated course. Early clinical manifestations may be vague. Impaired concentration and memory deficits are common, and apathy, lack of motivation, social withdrawal, irritability, and emotional lability appear. Later, difficulties with language, spatial or temporal disorientation, and visual construction are present. Some persons manifest an organic psychosis with agitation, inappropriate behavior, and hallucinosis.

Generalized cognitive system deficits occur later in the course of HIV-associated cognitive dysfunction, often accompanied by psychomotor slowing and decreased speech spontaneity and fluency. Progressive loss of balance, gait ataxia, spastic paraparesis or paralysis, and generalized hyperreflexia are common motor signs, sometimes accompanied by decreased writing ability, tremor, myoclonus, and seizure.

Diagnosis is difficult, especially in early stages. History with physical examination findings and supporting CSF and CT scan and MRI data help establish the diagnosis. Treatment is antiviral agents and supportive measures.

HIV myelopathy

Myelopathy involving diffuse degeneration of the spinal cord may occur in persons with AIDS **(HIV myelopathy)**. **Vacuolar myelopathy** is believed to be a direct consequence of HIV. The lateral and posterior columns of the lumbar spinal cord are affected.

Progressive spastic paraparesis with ataxia is the predominant clinical manifestation. Leg weakness, upper motor neuron signs, incontinence, and posterior column sensory loss may be present. Diagnosis is made on the basis of history, physical findings, and supporting data from diagnostic procedures. Treatment is supportive. Vacuolar myelopathy is treated supportively because it does not respond to antivirals.

HIV neuropathy

The peripheral nervous system may sustain injury in AIDS, manifesting as a peripheral neuropathy **(HIV neuropathy)** or radiculopathy. The most common neuropathy is the sensory type and occurs later in the disease. It is unresponsive to treatment.

HIV has been isolated from peripheral nerves, so the virus may directly infect nerves. Persons experience painful, burning dysesthesias and paresthesias, typically in the extremities. Weakness and decreased or absent distal reflexes may be present. Diagnosis is established through history, physical findings, laboratory data, nerve conduction, and an electromyogram (EMG).

Aseptic viral meningitis

Some persons develop acute aseptic meningitis at approximately the time of seroconversion. This may represent the initial infection of the nervous system by the virus. Symptoms include headache, fever, and meningismus. Cranial nerve involvement, especially V and VII, may appear, but the disease is self-limiting and requires only symptomatic treatment.

Opportunistic infections

Opportunistic infections may be bacterial, fungal, or viral in origin and may produce disease. Typically, bacterial infections are caused by unusual microorganisms. Cryptococcal infection is the most common fungal disorder and the third leading cause of neurologic disease in persons with AIDS. The symptoms are vague, such as fever, headache, malaise, and meningismus. Herpes encephalitis and herpes varicella zoster radiculitis may develop. Papovavirus may produce a demyelinating disorder. Cytomegalovirus encephalitis is common in persons with AIDS. Toxoplasmosis (a protozoal infection) is a common CNS disorder associated with AIDS and occurs in one third of persons with AIDS. CNS toxoplasmosis typically manifests as a focal encephalitis that is difficult to diagnose but is treatable.

CNS neoplasms

CNS neoplasms associated with AIDS include CNS lymphoma, systemic non-Hodgkin lymphoma, and metastatic Kaposi sarcoma. Primary CNS lymphoma is a large-cell tumor that presents as rapidly developing and expanding multicentric intracranial mass lesions. The meninges and, possibly, the cranial nerves and spinal cord are invaded in systemic non-Hodgkin lymphoma. Metastasis of a Kaposi sarcoma to the CNS is uncommon.

Other CNS complications

Persons with AIDS may develop multifocal ischemic infarctions, hemorrhagic infarctions, hemorrhage into tumors, subdural hematomas, and epidural hemorrhage. Reported neurologic symptoms produced by AIDS therapeutics include extrapyramidal movements, myoclonus, dysphasia, delirium, and acute myelopathy.

Degenerative Diseases

Multiple sclerosis

Multiple sclerosis (MS) is a relatively common disorder involving destruction of CNS myelin, sparing the peripheral nervous system. Demyelinating disorders are acquired conditions and are characterized by degeneration of previously normal myelin with relative preservation of axons. CNS demyelinating disorders are subclassified as primary and secondary, with multiple sclerosis and its variants in the primary category. In secondary disorders, demyelination is caused by disorders other than multiple sclerosis.

The onset of MS is usually between 20 and 50 years of age. Five percent of persons are diagnosed before 18 years of age.[23] Male/female ratio is about 1:2. MS is the most prevalent CNS demyelinating disorder and a leading cause of neurologic disability in early adulthood. The disease is most prevalent in areas far from the equator. In the United States and Canada, the prevalence rate ranges from 30 to 80 per 100,000 persons, or about 250,000 to 350,000 persons.[24] MS occurs in all races but is more common in whites. Although the disorder does not exhibit a defined inheritance pattern, 15% of persons with MS have an affected relative.

PATHOPHYSIOLOGY MS involves an autoimmune process that develops when a previous viral insult to the nervous system has occurred in a genetically susceptible individual. The gene for syncytin is activated in astrocytes of persons with MS. It appears syncytin is produced and released along with inflammatory proteins and free radicals. This combination kills oligodendrites, the myelin-forming cells.[25] Glutamate is being studied as an agent of injury as are other proinflammatory cytokines.[26,27] Pathologic features of this process are (1) interaction between the systemic immune system and the CNS and (2) demyelinating lesions (plaques and diffuse lesions) in the white matter (Figure 15-14). (The systemic immune system is discussed in Chapter 6.)

Plaques characteristically involve the CNS white matter but occasionally extend into the adjacent gray matter. They often coalesce into larger plaques. In established disease the multifocal, multistaged feature of plaques produces symptoms that are multiple and variable.

The acute (early) stage of plaque formation is characterized by perivenular demyelination with inflammatory edema in and around the plaque and partial demyelination. Symptoms usually remit, partially or completely, weeks after the onset of an early episode.

The chronic stage of demyelination and plaque formation is characterized by **gliosis** (glial scarring with late degeneration of axons). Progressive loss of function leads to permanent disability, usually over 20 years or more.

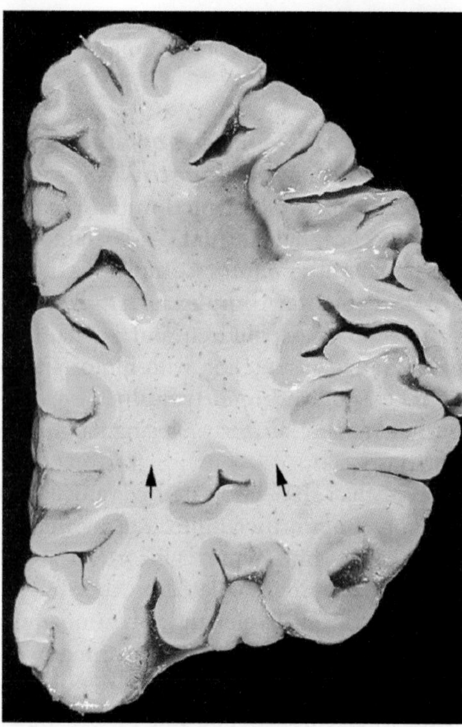

Figure 15-14 ■ Chronic Multiple Sclerosis. Demyelination plaque at gray-white junction and adjacent partially remyelinated shadow plaque *(arrows)*. (From Damjanov I, Linder J: *Anderson's pathology,* ed 10, St Louis, 1996, Mosby.)

Although plaques are considered diagnostic of MS, diffuse lesions are common pathologic findings in actively progressive cases. Diffuse lesions are small, widespread areas of perivenular demyelination that do not progress through gliosis. These lesions are sometimes accompanied by edema of surrounding normal brain tissue. The relationship of plaques to diffuse lesions is unknown.

CLINICAL MANIFESTATIONS Various events occur immediately before the onset or exacerbation of symptoms and are regarded as precipitating factors. Infection, trauma, and pregnancy are the least debated. Most of the pregnancy-related exacerbations occur 3 months postpartum, suggesting a relation to the stresses of labor and the increased fatigue during the postpartum period rather than to the pregnancy itself.

The major classifications of MS are remitting-relapsing (RR) MS, primary-progressive (PP) MS, secondary-progressive (SP) MS, and progressive-relapsing (PR). Initially, 90% of persons present with a remitting-relapsing course.

The major manifestations of MS are initial syndromes followed by remissions and established syndromes with no remissions. Usually persons with late MS predominantly have one of the following established syndromes: mixed (generalized), spinal, or cerebellar (pontobulbar cerebellar). The syndrome depends on the portion of the CNS most involved. Early cognitive changes are now being found on testing of asymptomatic persons. After years, 50% of individuals appear to have established syndromes of mixed involvement.

Short-lived attacks of neurologic deficits are the temporary appearance or worsening of symptoms. The mechanism of these attacks is complete, reversible conduction block in partially demyelinated axons. Conditions that cause short-lived attacks include (1) minor increases in body temperature or serum calcium (Ca^{++}) concentration and (2) functional demands exceeding conduction capacity. An increase in body temperature or serum Ca^{++} level increases current leakage through demyelinated neurons. Persons with MS may become dramatically worse when body temperature is raised. Other triggering events include hypercalcemia and physical and emotional stress.

Paroxysmal attacks are sensory or motor symptoms of abrupt onset and short duration (few seconds or minutes) and include paresthesias, dysarthria and ataxia, and tonic head turning. The mechanism of paroxysmal attacks is nonsynaptic transmission, in which nerve impulses are directly transmitted between adjacent demyelinated axons. A common paroxysmal symptom, called *Lhermitte sign,* is the momentary paresthesia (shocklike or tingling sensation) that shoots down the trunk or limbs during active or passive flexion of the neck. Bending the neck evokes nonsynaptic impulses in demyelinated axons of the dorsal column in the spinal cord. A person with MS may have many paroxysmal attacks each day. Inciting events include sensory stimulation, voluntary movement, hyperventilation, and emotional stress. Paroxysmal attacks tend to persist for weeks or months and may be followed by progressive symptoms of MS.

HEALTH ALERT

Neural Stem Cells Protect and Restore Brain Functions

Transplant of adult neural stem cells can protect and restore functions of the brain in animal models of ischemic and inflammatory brain injury. Some subsets of stem cells replace damaged tissue and also have modulated immune responses with potential benefit in diseases like multiple sclerosis. Progress toward the use of both embryonic and adult neural stem cells for neuroprotective and regenerative interventions holds much promise for the future.

Data from Leker RR: Manipulation of endogenous neural stem cells following ischemic brain injury, *Pathophysiol Haemost Thromb* 35(1–2):58–62, 2006; Sailor KA, Ming GL, Song H: Neurogenesis as a potential therapeutic strategy for neurodegenerative diseases, *Expert Opin Biol Ther* 6(9):879–890, 2006; Uccelli A et al: Stem cells in inflammatory demyelinating disorders: a dual role for immunosuppression and neuroprotection, *Expert Opin Biol Ther* 6(1):17–22, 2006.

EVALUATION AND TREATMENT There is no single test available to diagnose or rule out MS. The diagnosis of MS, possible MS or not MS is based on the history and physical examination supported by findings from CSF examination, evoked responses (ER) studies, CT scans of the head, and MRI. Signs of two separate attacks or flares with demyelination in the central nervous system supports the diagnosis. Persistently elevated CSF immunoglobulin G (IgG) is found in about two thirds of individuals with MS, and oligoclonal (IgG) bands on electrophoresis are found in more than 90%. Evoked response studies aid diagnosis by detecting decreased conduction velocity in visual, auditory, and somatosensory pathways. MRI is the most sensitive available method of detecting the disease.

MS is treated for three purposes: (1) acute managing of relapses to prevent disability, (2) reducing frequency of relapses, and disease progression (disease burden), and (3) managing symptoms.[28] Drugs with antiinflammatory properties and plasma exchange are used to treat acute episodes. Agents that affect the immune system by immunosuppression and immune modulation are used to reduce relapse rate. Symptom management is also part of treatment plans. Special problems requiring preventive and symptomatic management are fatigue; weakness; spasticity; bladder, bowel, and sexual dysfunction; pain; tremor and ataxia; depression; vertigo; sensory sensations; and heat intolerance. Supportive and rehabilitative management is directed toward relieving specific symptoms and preventing the complications of immobility—especially pressure sores and infections of the pulmonary and genitourinary systems.

Amyotrophic lateral sclerosis

Amyotrophic lateral sclerosis (ALS, sporadic motor neuron disease, sporadic motor system disease, motor neuron disease [MND]) is a worldwide degenerative disorder diffusely involving lower and upper motor neurons resulting in progressive muscle weakness. The term *amyotrophic* (without muscle nutrition or progressive muscle wasting) refers to the predominant lower motor neuron component of the syndrome. Lateral sclerosis, scarring of the corticospinal tract in the lateral column of the spinal cord, refers to the upper motor neuron component of the syndrome.

Classic ALS (Lou Gehrig disease) may begin at any time from the fourth decade of life; its peak occurrence is in the early 50s. The male/female ratio is 3:2, equalizing after menopause. Ten percent of persons with ALS have a familial form. Subtypes of ALS include primary lateral sclerosis, progressive bulbar palsy, and progressive muscular atrophy.

PATHOPHYSIOLOGY The cause of motor neuron death in ALS is unknown. Current data suggest a genetic factor is involved. Twenty percent of persons with familial ALS have a genetic mutation in copper-zinc superoxidase dismutase (SODI) on the glial cells surrounding the motor neuron.[29,30] This enzyme helps destroy free radicals. The reuptake of glutamate by glial cells also is diminished, and glutamate toxicity is now believed to cause or contribute to major neuron degeneration.

The principal pathologic feature of ALS is lower and upper motor neuron degeneration, although without inflammation. There are fewer large motor neurons in the spinal cord, brain stem, and cerebral cortex (premotor and motor areas), with ongoing degeneration in the remaining motor neurons. Death of the motor neuron results in axonal degeneration and secondary demyelination with glial proliferation and sclerosis (scarring).

Lower motor neuron degeneration denervates motor units. Adjacent, still viable lower motor neurons attempt to compensate by distal intramuscular sprouting, reinnervation, and enlargement of motor units. The initial symptoms of the disease may be related to lower or upper motor neuron dysfunction or to both.

CLINICAL MANIFESTATIONS Weakness may begin in any or all muscles of the body. Both flaccid paralysis and spastic paralysis occur with progressive muscle atrophy. No associated mental, sensory, or autonomic symptoms are present. Evidence is now emerging that there may be a comorbid frontotemporal dementia.[31] Sensory functions are sustained until death.

EVALUATION AND TREATMENT Diagnosis of the syndrome is based predominantly on the history and physical examination. Electromyography and muscle biopsy verify lower motor neuron degeneration and denervation. Little treatment is available to alter the overall course of the ALS syndrome. The drug riluzole (Rilutek) has extended time not requiring ventilatory assistance.[32] Supportive management and rehabilitative management are directed toward preventing complications of immobility. Psychologic support of the affected individual and the family is extremely important in this disorder.

The average duration of life is approximately 2 to 3 years from the appearance of symptoms, but the course of the disease may run from a few months to 15 years. Twenty percent of persons survive 5 years.

✓ QUICK CHECK 15-3

1. Why is multiple sclerosis an autoimmune disease?
2. Why is amyotrophic lateral sclerosis a motor neuron disease?

PERIPHERAL NERVOUS SYSTEM AND NEUROMUSCULAR JUNCTION DISORDERS

Peripheral Nervous System Disorders

Disease processes may injure the axons traveling to and from the brain stem and spinal cord neuronal cell bodies. The injury may affect a distinct anatomic area on the axon, or the spinal nerves may be injured at the roots, at the plexus before peripheral nerve formation, or at the nerves themselves. The cranial nerves do not have roots or plexuses and are affected only within themselves. Autonomic nerve fibers may be injured as they travel in certain cranial nerves and emerge through the ventral root and plexuses to travel in the peripheral nerves of the body. The injuries produced are summarized in Table 15-9.

TABLE 15-9

Peripheral Nervous System Disorders

Disorder	Pathology	Clinical Manifestations
Radiculopathies	Injury to spinal roots as they exit or enter the vertebral canal; caused by compression, inflammation, direct trauma	Affects strength, tone, and bulk of muscles innervated by involved roots; pattern similar to that seen in amyotrophies, with tone and deep-tendon reflexes decreased, rarely absent; fasciculations; mild fatigue; sensory alterations, pain
Plexus injuries	Involve nerve plexus distal to spinal roots but proximal to formation of peripheral nerves; caused by trauma, compression, infiltration, or iatrogenic (positioning or intramuscular injection)	Motor weakness, muscle atrophy, sensory loss in affected areas; paralysis common
Neuropathies	Called sensorimotor if sensory, motor, and reflex effects; pure sensory caused by leprosy, industrial solvents, chloramphenicol, and hereditary mechanisms; motor caused by Guillain-Barré syndrome, infectious mononucleosis, viral hepatitis, acute porphyria, lead, mercury, and triorthocresylphosphates (TCP)	Affects muscle strength, tone, and bulk; whole muscles or groups may be paretic or paralyzed; muscles of feet and legs first, then hands and arms; tone and deep tendon reflexes generally decreased with atrophy and fasciculation; mild fatigue; some specific symptoms of paresthesia and dysesthesia; altered reflexes; autonomic disturbances; deformities; metabolic changes
Guillain-Barré syndrome	Acute onset of motor paralysis (ascending); occurs throughout the world and in both genders and all age groups, at all seasons; mild respiratory or gastrointestinal viral infection 1 to 3 weeks or longer before symptoms appear is common	Paresis of legs to complete quadriplegia, respiratory insufficiency, autonomic nervous system instability; may progress to respiratory arrest or cardiovascular collapse

Neuromuscular Junction Disorders

Transmission of the nerve impulse at the neuromuscular junction requires the release of adequate amounts of neurotransmitter from the presynaptic terminals of the axon and effective binding of the released transmitter to the receptors on the membranes of muscle cells (see Figure 12-13). Nutritional deficits, certain drugs (e.g., reserpine, methyldopa [Aldomet]), and certain disorders that interfere with the synthesis or packaging of the neurotransmitter or its release into the synaptic cleft may result in weakness. Likewise, any pathologic process or drug that interferes with the binding of the neurotransmitter to the receptor may cause weakness.

Myasthenia gravis

Myasthenia gravis is a chronic autoimmune disease that affects the neuromuscular junction and is characterized by muscle weakness and fatigability. In 10% to 25% of persons with myasthenia gravis, thymic tumors are found, and in 70% to 80%, there are pathologic changes in the thymus.[33] Tumors are more common in males than in females. Myasthenia gravis is an autoimmune disease associated with an increased incidence of other autoimmune diseases, including systemic lupus erythematosus, rheumatoid arthritis, polymyositis, and thyrotoxicosis. (Autoimmune mechanisms are discussed in Chapter 7.)

The classifications for myasthenia gravis are neonatal myasthenia, congenital myasthenia (neonatal persistent myasthenia), juvenile myasthenia, ocular myasthenia, and generalized autoimmune myasthenia. In **neonatal myasthenia,** transitory signs of myasthenia gravis are present in 10% to 15% of infants born to mothers with myasthenia gravis. **Congenital myasthenia** presents in infancy and continues into adulthood. **Juvenile myasthenia** has a childhood onset, usually about 10 years of age. **Ocular myasthenia,** which is more common in males, involves weakness of the eye muscles and eyelids, and it also may include swallowing difficulties and slurred speech. **Generalized autoimmune myasthenia** involves the proximal musculature throughout the body and has several courses: (1) a course with periodic remissions, (2) a slowly progressive course, (3) a rapidly progressive course, and (4) a fulminating course.

PATHOPHYSIOLOGY Myasthenia gravis results from a defect in nerve impulse transmission at the neuromuscular junction. The postsynaptic acetylcholine receptors on the muscle cell's plasma membrane are no longer recognized as "self" and elicit the generation of autoantibodies. IgG antibody is produced against the acetylcholine receptors and fixes onto the receptor sites, blocking the binding of acetylcholine. Eventually the antibody action destroys receptor sites. This causes diminished transmission of the nerve impulse across the neuromuscular junction and lack of muscle depolarization. Why this autosensitization occurs is not known.

CLINICAL MANIFESTATIONS Myasthenia gravis typically has an insidious onset. Clinical manifestations may first appear during pregnancy, during the postpartum period, or in conjunction with the administration of certain anesthetic agents. The foremost complaints are muscle fatigue and progressive weakness. The person often complains of fatigue after exercise and has a recent history of recurring upper respiratory tract infections. The muscles of the eyes, face, mouth, throat, and neck usually are affected first. The extraocular (eye) muscles and the levator muscles are most affected. Manifestations include diplopia, ptosis, and ocular palsies.

The muscles of facial expression, mastication, swallowing, and speech are the next most involved. The results are facial droop and an expressionless face; difficulty chewing and swallowing associated with dietary changes and weight loss; drooling and episodes of choking and aspiration; and a nasal, low-volume, but high-pitched monotonous speech pattern.

The muscles of the neck, shoulder girdle, and hip flexors are less frequently affected. When these muscles do become involved, however, the person experiences fatigue requiring periods of rest, weakness of the arms and legs that improves with rest, and difficulty in maintaining head position. The respiratory muscles of the diaphragm and chest wall become weak, and ventilation is impaired. Deep breathing and coughing difficulties predispose the individual to atelectasis and congestion. In the advanced stage of the disease, all muscles are weak.

Myasthenic crisis occurs when severe muscle weakness causes extreme quadriparesis or quadriplegia, respiratory insufficiency with shortness of breath, and extreme difficulty in swallowing. The individual in myasthenic crisis is in danger of respiratory arrest.

Cholinergic crisis may arise from anticholinesterase drug toxicity. The clinical picture is like that of myasthenic crisis, but other symptoms are present also. Intestinal motility increases, with episodes of diarrhea and complaints of cramping, fasciculation, bradycardia, pupillary constriction, increased salivation, and increased sweating. These are caused by the smooth muscle hyperactivity secondary to excessive accumulation of acetylcholine at the neuromuscular junctions and excessive parasympathetic-like activity. As in myasthenic crisis, the individual is in danger of respiratory arrest.

EVALUATION AND TREATMENT The diagnosis of myasthenia gravis is made on the basis of a response to edrophonium chloride (Tensilon), an electromyogram (EMG), and antistriated muscle antibodies. With the intravenous administration of the drug, immediate demonstrable improvement in muscle strength usually persists for several minutes. On EMG, the amplitude of the action potentials of stimulated muscles rapidly declines. Mediastinal tomography and MRI help determine whether a thymoma is present. The progression of myasthenia gravis varies, appearing first as a mild case that spontaneously remits, with a series of relapses and symptom-free intervals ranging from weeks to months. Over time the disease can progress, leading to death. Ocular myasthenia has a very good prognosis.

Anticholinesterase drugs, steroids, and immunosuppressant drugs are used to treat myasthenia gravis and myasthenic crisis. Plasmapheresis may be lifesaving during myasthenic crisis, before and after thymectomy, and at the start of immunosuppressant therapy. For individuals with cholinergic crisis, anticholinergic drugs are withheld until blood levels fall out of the toxic range, while ventilatory support is provided and respiratory complications are prevented. Thymectomy is the treatment of choice in individuals with a thymoma.

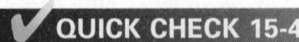

QUICK CHECK 15-4

1. Why do antibodies contribute to the development of myasthenia gravis?
2. Why is weakness the primary symptom of a myopathy?

Myopathies

Myopathy is the term applied to a primary muscle disorder. Many pathologic processes affect muscles and cause loss of functional muscle cells. In the presence of myopathies, muscle strength, tone, and bulk are affected.

Primary muscle disease invariably is associated with weakness—usually marked. The distribution of the weakness in myopathy is usually symmetric and proximal, although occasionally it is predominantly distal, as in myotonic dystrophy. Mild fatigue is noted. Tone is decreased, as are the tendon reflexes, and atrophy may be present. Some myopathies are associated with muscle hypertrophy (cretinism and the familial progressive muscular dystrophies of childhood), in which muscles are rubbery and weak. Fasciculations are not present with myopathy because no denervation is present. No sensory changes are found. (Specific myopathies are discussed in Chapter 37.)

TUMORS OF THE CENTRAL NERVOUS SYSTEM

No proven causative agents for CNS tumors have been established. Carcinogenesis is discussed in Chapter 9.

Cranial Tumors

Tumors within the cranium can be either primary or metastatic as follows:

- *Primary.* Intracerebral tumors originate from brain substance, including neuroglia, neurons, cells of blood vessels, and connective tissue. Extracerebral tumors originate outside substances of brain and include meningiomas, acoustic nerve tumors, and tumors of pituitary and pineal glands.
- *Metastatic.* Found inside or outside brain substance.

CNS tumors include both brain and spinal cord tumors. Primary brain tumors (both malignant and non-malignant) have an estimated incidence rate of 20,500 with 12,740 deaths in the United States.[34] The incidence of CNS tumors increases to age 70 years and then decreases. CNS tumors are the second most common group of tumors occurring in children. Approximately 70% to 75% of all intracranial tumors in children are located infratentorially, and in adults 70% are located supratentorially. Peripheral nerve tumors are rare in children and common in adults.

Local effects of cranial tumors are caused by the destructive action of the tumor itself on a particular site in the brain and by compression causing decreased cerebral blood flow. Effects include seizures, visual disturbances, unstable gait, and cranial nerve dysfunction. Generalized effects result from increased intracranial pressure caused by obstruction of the ventricular system, hemorrhages in and around the tumor, or cerebral edema (Figure 15-15).

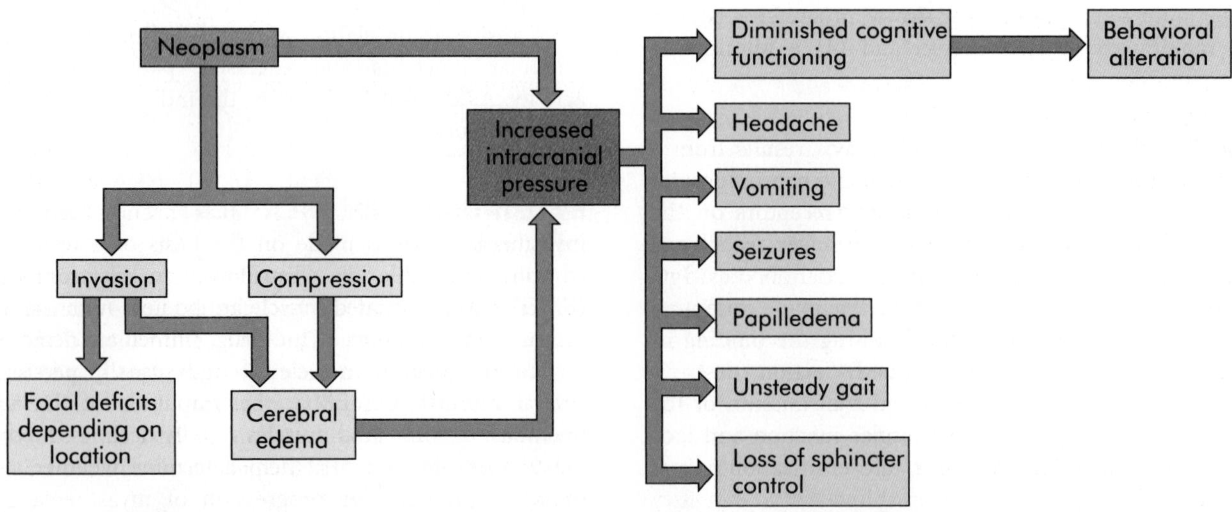

Figure 15-15 ■ **Origin of Clinical Manifestations Associated with an Intracranial Neoplasm.**

Intracranial brain tumors do not metastasize as readily as tumors in other organs because there are no lymphatic channels within the brain substance. If metastasis does occur, it is usually through seeding of cerebral blood or CSF during cranial surgery or through artificial shunts.

Primary intracerebral tumors

Primary intracerebral tumors **(gliomas)** comprise both encapsulated and nonencapsulated or invasive tumors (Table 15-10). Gliomas represent 42% of all primary brain tumors and 77% of malignant brain tumors.[35] Typically, invasive tumors invade and destroy adjacent normal CNS tissue, and more distal neural and vascular tissues are displaced and compressed, causing ischemia, edema, and increased intracranial pressure. Encapsulated tumors displace and compress adjacent and distal CNS tissues and vasculature. As with invasive tumors, encapsulated tumors produce ischemia, edema, and increased pressure. Both types impair the normal function of the neurons.

Surgical or radiosurgical excision, surgical decompression, chemotherapy, and radiotherapy are used for these tumors. Supportive treatment is directed at reducing edema. (Cancer treatment is discussed in Chapters 9 and 10.)

Astrocytoma

Astrocytomas are the most common glioma (about 40% of all tumors of the brain and spinal cord[35] and are graded by two classification systems (Table 15-11). Developed from astrocytes, astrocytomas expand and infiltrate into the normal surrounding brain tissues. These tumor cells are believed to have lost normal growth restraint and thus proliferate uncontrollably.

One third of astrocytomas are classified at diagnosis as grade I or grade II astrocytoma. These slow-growing but infiltrative gliomas tend to form cavities (pseudocysts); however, some are firm, noncavitating, avascular, gray-white masses that are difficult to distinguish from normal white matter. Although these tumors may occur anywhere in the brain or spinal cord, they generally are located in the cerebrum, hypothalamus, or pons. Low-grade astrocytomas in adults tend to be located laterally or supratentorially and in a midline or near midline position in children.

Headache and seizures may be early signs. Onset of a focal seizure disorder between the second and sixth decade of life suggests an astrocytoma. Other general or focal neurologic manifestations develop gradually, with increased intracranial pressure occurring late in the tumor's course.

Grade I astrocytomas are treated with surgery and follow-up CT scans. Grade II astrocytomas are treated surgically if accessible or by conventional external radiation, local radiation, or sterotactic radiosurgery. Twenty-five percent of persons survive 5 years following surgery alone. Fifty percent of persons survive 5 years when surgery is followed by radiation therapy (RT).[34] Grade I and II astrocytomas commonly progress to a higher-grade tumor.

Grades III and IV astrocytomas are found predominantly in the lobes and cerebral hemispheres, although they may occur in the brain stem, cerebellum, and spinal cord. Men are twice as likely to have them as women, and those 45 to 55 years old have the highest incidence.

Grade IV astrocytomas, **glioblastoma multiforme,** are highly vascular and extensively infiltrative. They may become large enough to extend from the meningeal surface through the ventricular wall. Fifty percent of glioblastomas are bilateral or at least occupy more than one lobe at the time of death.

The typical clinical presentation for a glioblastoma multiforme is that of diffuse, nonspecific clinical signs, such as headache, irritability, and "personality changes" that progress to more clear-cut manifestations of increased intracranial pressure, such as headache on position change, papilledema, or vomiting. Thirty percent to 40% of persons experience seizure activity. Symptoms may progress to include definite focal signs, such as hemiparesis, dysphasia, dyspraxia, cranial nerve palsies, and visual field deficits.

Diagnosis of high-grade astrocytomas most commonly takes 3 to 6 months from onset of the first clinical manifestations because the person does not recognize the need to consult a health care provider.

Grade III astrocytomas are treated surgically if they are accessible and with radiotherapy and chemotherapy. With treatment, 55% to 60% of persons survive 1 year, 30% to 35% survive 2 years, and 10% survive longer than 5 years. Grade IV astrocytomas are also treated with surgery, radiotherapy, and chemotherapy or placement of wafers. Median survival time is 1 year.[36]

Oligodendroglioma

Oligodendrogliomas constitute about 4% of all intracranial gliomas.[35] They are typically slow-growing tumors, and most oligodendrogliomas are macroscopically indistinguishable from other gliomas. The majority are found in the frontal and temporal lobes, often in the deep white matter, but they are found also in other parts of the cerebrum, third ventricle, brain stem, cerebellum, and spinal cord. Many are found in young adults with a history of temporal lobe epilepsy. Approximately half of tumors classified as oligodendrogliomas are actually a mixed type of oligodendroglioma and astrocytoma. Malignant degeneration occurs in approximately one third of persons with oligodendrogliomas, and the tumors are then referred to as **oligodendroblastomas.** If there is extension to the pia mater or ependymal wall (see Figure 12-14), oligodendrogliomas may metastasize to distant CNS sites through the ventriculoarachnoid spaces.

More than 50% of individuals experience a focal or generalized seizure as the first clinical manifestation. Only half of those with an oligodendroglioma have increased intracranial pressure at the time of diagnosis and surgery, and only one third develop focal manifestations. The time from first clinical manifestation to surgical intervention ranges from 2 to 6 years. Median survival time is 5 to 10 years.[34]

TABLE 15-10

Brain and Spinal Cord Tumors

Neoplasm	Location	Characteristics	Cell of Origin
GLIOMAS			
Astrocytoma	Anywhere in brain or spinal cord	Slow-growing, invasive	Astrocytes
Glioblastoma multiforme	Predominantly in cerebral hemispheres	Highly invasive and malignant	Thought to arise from mature astrocytes
Oligodendrocytoma	Most commonly in frontal lobes deep in white matter; may arise in brain stem, cerebellum, and spinal cord	Relatively avascular, tends to be encapsulated; more malignant form called an *oligodendroblastoma*	Oligodendrites
Ependymoma	Intramedullary: wall of the ventricles; may arise in caudal tail of the spinal cord	More common in children, variable growth rates; more malignant, invasive form is called *ependymoblastoma;* may extend into the ventricle or invade brain tissue	Ependymal cells
NEURONAL CELL			
Medulloblastoma	Posterior cerebellar vermis, roof of fourth ventricle	Well-demarcated but infiltrating, rapid-growing, fills fourth ventricle	Embryonic cells
MESODERMAL TISSUE			
Meningioma	Intradural, extramedullary: sylvian fissure region, superior parasagittal surface of frontal and parietal lobes, olfactory groove, wing of sphenoid bone, superior surface of cerebellum, cerebellopontine angle, spinal cord	Slow-growing, circumscribed, encapsulated, sharply demarcated from normal tissues, compressive in nature	Arachnoid cells, may be from fibroblast
CHOROID PLEXUS			
Papillomas	Choroid plexus of the ventricular system, lateral ventricle in children, fourth ventricle in adults	Usually benign, slow expansion inducing hemorrhage and hydrocephalus; malignant tumor is rare	Epithelial cells
CRANIAL NERVES AND SPINAL NERVE ROOTS			
Neurilemmoma	Cranial nerves (most commonly vestibular division of cranial nerve VIII)	Slow-growing	Schwann cells
Neurofibroma	Extramedullary—spinal cord	Slow-growing	Neurilemma, Schwann cells
PITUITARY TUMORS	Pituitary gland; may extend to or invade floor of the third ventricle	Age-linked, several types, slow-growing, macroadenomas and microadenomas	Pituitary cells, pituitary chromophobes, basophils, eosinophils
GERM CELL TUMORS	Neurohypophysis, hypothalamus, pineal region	Rare, 0.5% of all primary brain tumors Primarily in adolescents Male > female Variable prognosis	Several types—germinoma, embryonal carcinoma, yolk sac tumor, choriocarcinoma, teratoma, mixed germ cell tumor—with different cell origins
PINEAL REGION	Pineal region; pineal parenchyma	Several types (germinoma, pineocytoma, teratoma)	Several types with different cell origins
BLOOD VESSEL TUMORS			
Angioma	Predominantly in posterior cerebral hemispheres	Slow-growing	Arising from congenitally malformed arteriovenous connections
Hemangioblastomas	Predominantly in cerebellum	Slow-growing	Embryonic vascular tissue

TABLE 15-11
Classification Systems for Astrocytomas

	Kernohan et al System	Rigertz System	Criteria—Cellular Density, Atypia, Tumor Cell Mitosis
ASTROCYTOMA		Well-differentiated astrocytoma	Increased number of cells
Grade I	Well-differentiated astrocytoma		Least malignant, grow slowly, near normal appearance under microscope
Grade II	More cellular and anaplastic astrocytoma		Abnormal appearance under a microscope, infiltrated, and may recur at a higher grade
GLIOBLASTOMA		Malignant anaplastic astrocytoma	
Grade III	Poorly differentiated astrocytoma		Malignant, many cells undergoing mitosis, infiltrated, and may recur at a higher grade
Grade IV	Poorly differentiated astrocytoma (glioblastoma multiforme)	Glioblastoma multiforme	Increased number of cells undergoing cell division, bizarre appearance under a microscope, widely infiltrates, neovascularization, central necrosis

Ependymoma

Ependymomas are gliomas that arise from ependymal cells in the walls of the ventricles and grow either into the ventricle or into adjacent brain tissue; they are not encapsulated (Figure 15-16). They constitute about 3% of all primary brain tumors in adults and 10% in children and adolescents. About 70% occur in the fourth ventricle, with others found in the third ventricle, lateral ventricles, and caudal portion of the spinal cord. Approximately 40% of infratentorial ependymomas occur in children younger than 10 years. Cerebral (supratentorial) ependymomas occur at all ages.

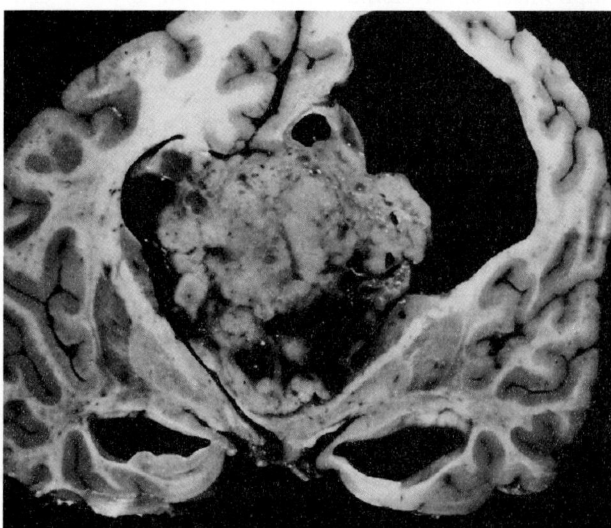

Figure 15-16 ■ **Large Septal Ependymoma.** This tumor represents the severity of tissue compression that occurs with a large brain tumor. The area in the upper-right part of the picture represents a secondary hydrocephalus that has further compressed brain tissue. (Courtesy Dr. JE Olivera-Rabiela, Mexico City, Mexico. From Rosai J: *Ackerman's surgical pathology,* ed 7, St Louis, 1989, Mosby.)

Fourth ventricle ependymomas present with difficulty in balance, unsteady gait, uncoordinated muscle movement, and difficulty with fine motor movement. The clinical manifestations of a lateral and third ventricle ependymoma that involves the cerebral hemispheres are seizures, visual changes, and contralateral weakness of a body part of one side of the body. Blockage of the CSF pathway by the tumor clinically results in the presence of headache, nausea, and vomiting related to the hydrocephalus produced.

The course of ependymomas may be short or long. The interval between first manifestations and surgery may be as short as 4 weeks or as long as 7 or 8 years.

Ependymomas are treated with radiotherapy, radiosurgery, and chemotherapy. Twenty percent to 50% of persons survive 5 years. Some persons benefit from a shunting procedure when the ependymoma has caused a noncommunicating hydrocephalus.

Primary extracerebral tumors

Meningioma

Meningiomas constitute about 30% of all intracranial tumors. They are considered benign because they are encapsulated and usually do not invade the surrounding brain. These tumors usually originate from the dura mater or arachnoid membranes and rarely from arachnoid cells of the choroid plexus of the ventricles. Meningiomas are located most commonly in the olfactory grooves, on the wings of the sphenoid bone (at the base of the skull), in the tuberculum sellae (a structure next to the sella turcica), on the superior surface of the cerebellum, and in the cerebellopontine angle and spinal cord.

Small meningiomas (less than 2 cm in diameter) often are found on postmortem examination in middle-aged and elderly individuals who experienced no clinical manifestations and died of totally unrelated causes. The cause of meningiomas is unknown.

A meningioma is sharply circumscribed and adapts to the shape it occupies. It may extend to the dural surface and erode the cranial bones or produce an osteoblastic reaction. A few meningiomas exhibit malignant, invasive qualities.

When meningiomas reach a certain size and begin to indent the brain parenchyma, clinical manifestations occur. Focal seizures are often the first manifestation. Because of the extremely slow-growing nature of these tumors, increased intracranial pressure is less common than with gliomas.

There is a 20% recurrence rate even with complete surgical excision. If only partial resection is possible, the tumor recurs. Radiation therapies also are used to slow growth.

Nerve sheath tumors

Nerve sheath tumors are either neurofibroma or schwannoma (neuroma, neurolemma). Five percent of all neuromas are attributable to neurofibromatosis,[37,38] an inherited disorder; the remainder are benign tumors that arise from the sheath of the Schwann cell surrounding the axons of the cranial nerves. These tumors most commonly affect persons in their 20s and 30s. Men and women are equally affected.[38] The vestibular division of cranial nerve VIII is most commonly affected, although neurilemmomas of the acoustic division of cranial nerve VIII, cranial nerve V, and cranial nerve IX are found.

The tumor generally originates just distal to the junction between the nerve root and the brain stem. As it grows, it extends into the posterior fossa to occupy the cerebellopontine angle and compress adjacent nerves. Eventually the brain stem is displaced, and the CSF flow is obstructed.

Initial clinical manifestations include headache, tinnitus, hearing loss, impaired balance, unsteady gait, facial pain, and loss of facial sensations. Later, vertigo with nausea and vomiting, a sense of pressure in the ear, and moderate to severe unsteadiness with rapid position changes may appear.

CT scan or MRI can establish the diagnosis. Posterior fossa dye studies may be required. Treatment is by surgical excision and radiotherapy of the neuroma.

Pituitary tumors are discussed in Chapter 18, and cerebral tumors in children are discussed in Chapter 16.

Metastatic carcinoma

Metastatic brain tumors from systemic cancers are the most common type of brain tumor and an estimated 10% to 15% of persons with cancer develop metastasis to the brain.[34] Fifty percent of metastatic brain tumors arise from the lung, 13% from melanomas, 6% from the breast, and 4% from the kidneys.[39] Carcinoma of the gallbladder, liver, thyroid, testes, uterus, ovary, and pancreas also may metastasize to the brain. Other tumors that metastasize only occasionally are rhabdomyosarcoma, Ewing tumor, chorioepithelioma, and lymphoma.

Carcinomas are disseminated to the brain through the circulation. In more than three fourths of persons, the metastases are multiple and found scattered throughout the cerebrum and cerebellum. Metastatic tumors often are located in the meninges and near the brain surface in the gray matter and subcortical white matter. These tumors produce little glial cell reaction in the brain tissue but do cause vasogenic edema in surrounding brain tissue.

Metastatic brain tumors produce signs resembling those of glioblastomas, although several unusual syndromes do exist. Carcinomatous encephalopathy causes headache, nervousness, depressed mood, trembling, confusion, and forgetfulness. In carcinomatosis of the cerebellum, headache, dizziness, and ataxia are found. Carcinomatosis of the craniospinal meninges (carcinomatous meningitis) manifests with headache, confusion, and manifestations of cranial or spinal nerve root dysfunction.

Metastatic brain tumors carry a poor prognosis. If a solitary tumor is found, surgery or radiation therapy is used, but if multiple tumors exist, symptomatic relief only is pursued.

Spinal Cord Tumors

Spinal cord tumors are named to reflect their cell type, growth rate, and structure of origin. They may be **intramedullary tumors** (originating within the neural tissues) or **extramedullary tumors** (originating from tissues outside the spinal cord). Extramedullary tumors arise from the meninges or roots (forming **intradural tumors**) or from epidural tissue or vertebral structure (forming **extradural tumors**). About 5% of spinal cord tumors seen in general hospital settings are intramedullary; 40% are intradural-extramedullary; and 55% are extradural.

Metastatic spinal cord tumors are usually carcinomas, lymphomas, or myelomas. Their location is often extradural, with 50% metastatic, having spread to the spine through direct extension from tumors of the vertebral structures or from extraspinal sources extending through the interventricular foramen or bloodstream.

The most common primary extramedullary spinal cord tumors are neurofibromas and meningiomas. These tumors are intradural more often than extradural. Neurofibromas generally are found in the thoracic and lumbar region, whereas meningiomas are more evenly distributed through the spine. Other extramedullary tumors in order of frequency of occurrence are sarcomas, vascular tumors, chordomas, and epidermoid and similar tumors. Of intradural-extramedullary tumors, 70% are meningiomas, neurofibromas, or sarcomas.

Intramedullary tumors have the same cellular origins as brain tumors. Ependymomas account for 40% of intramedullary spinal cord tumors. Astrocytomas, glioblastomas, oligodendrogliomas, ganglioneuromas, medulloblastomas, hemangiomas, and hemangioblastomas are more or less equally distributed in frequency of occurrence.

PATHOPHYSIOLOGY Extramedullary spinal cord tumors produce dysfunction by compressing adjacent tissue, not by direct invasion. Compression destroys the white matter tracts, and the spinal canal around the cord becomes filled by tumor.

Intramedullary spinal cord tumors produce dysfunction by both invasion and compression. The cord enlarges as the tumor grows inside the cord. Adjacent white matter tracts are then distorted. Metastases from spinal cord tumors occur from seeding through the CSF; medulloblastomas and ependymomas establish distant implants in this way.

CLINICAL MANIFESTATIONS The acute onset of clinical manifestations suggests a vascular insult caused by thrombosis of vessels supplying the spinal cord. Clinical manifestations that are gradual and progressive suggest compression. Three major categories of clinical manifestations have been distinguished: (1) a compressive syndrome, (2) an irritative syndrome, and (3) rarely, a syringomyelic syndrome.

The **compressive syndrome (sensorimotor syndrome)** occurs with compression or, less often, invasion and destruction of the spinal cord tracts. Symptoms are usually gradual and progressive, and initial manifestations may be asymmetric. Both motor function and sensory function are affected as the tumor grows and involves both the anterior and posterior spinal tracts.

The **irritative syndrome (radicular syndrome)** combines the clinical manifestations of a cord compression with radicular pain (occurs in the sensory root distribution and indicates root irritation). The segmental manifestations include segmental sensory changes (that is, paresthesias and impaired pain and touch perception); motor disturbances, including cramps, atrophy, fasciculations, and decreased or absent deep tendon reflexes; and ache in the spine.

EVALUATION AND TREATMENT The diagnosis of a spinal cord tumor is made through bone scan, PET, CT-guided needle biopsy, or open biopsy. Involvement of specific cord segments is established. Any metastases also are identified. Treatment varies, depending on the nature of the tumor and the person's clinical status.

QUICK CHECK 15-5

1. How is an encapsulated CNS tumor different from a nonencapsulated CNS tumor?
2. What are three types of spinal cord tumors?
3. What are some common signs and symptoms of compressive and irritative spinal cord tumor syndromes?

Did You Understand?

Central Nervous System Disorders

1. Motor vehicle crashes are the major cause of traumatic CNS injury. Traumatic injuries to the head are classified as closed-head trauma (blunt) or open-head trauma (penetrating). Closed-head trauma is the more common type of trauma.
2. Different types of focal brain injury include contusion (bruising of the brain), laceration (tearing of brain tissue), extradural hematoma (accumulation of blood above the dura mater), subdural hematoma (blood between the dura mater and arachnoid membrane), intracerebral hematoma (bleeding into the brain), and open-head trauma.
3. Open-head trauma involves a skull fracture with exposure of the cranial vault to the environment. The types of open-head trauma (compound fracture, perforated fracture) are linear, comminuted, compound, and basilar skull fracture (in the cranial vault or at the base of the skull).
4. Diffuse brain injury (diffuse axonal injury [DAI]) results from the effects of head rotation. The brain experiences shearing stresses resulting in axonal damage ranging from concussion to a severe DAI state.
5. Spinal cord injury involves damage to vertebral or neural tissues by compressing tissue, pulling or exerting tension on tissue, or shearing tissues so that they slide into one another.
6. Spinal cord injury may cause spinal shock with cessation of all motor, sensory, reflex, and autonomic functions below any transected area. Loss of motor and sensory function depends on the level of injury.
7. Paralysis of the lower half of the body with both legs involved is called *paraplegia*. Paralysis involving all four extremities is called *quadriplegia*.
8. Return of spinal neuron excitability occurs slowly. Reflex activity can return in 1 to 2 weeks in most persons with acute spinal cord injury. A pattern of flexion reflexes emerges, involving first the toes, then the feet and the legs. Eventually, reflex voiding and bowel elimination appear and mass reflex (flexor spasms accompanied by profuse sweating, piloerection, and automatic bladder emptying) may develop.
9. Degenerative disk disease is an alteration in intervertebral disk tissue and can be related to normal aging.
10. Spondylolysis is a structural defect of the spine with displacement of the vertebra.
11. Spondylolisthesis involves forward slippage of the vertebra and can involve a crack or fracture of the pars interarticularis, usually at the L5-S1 vertebra.
12. Low back pain is pain between the lower rib cage and gluteal muscles and often radiates into the thigh.
13. Most causes of low back pain are unknown; however, some secondary causes are disk prolapse, tumors, bursitis, synovitis, degenerative joint disease, osteoporosis, fracture, inflammation, and sprain.

(Continued)

Did You Understand?—Cont'd

14. Herniation of an intervertebral disk is a protrusion of part of the nucleus pulposus. Herniation most commonly affects the lumbosacral disks (L5-S1 and L4–5). The extruded pulposus compresses the nerve root, causing pain that radiates along the sciatic nerve course.
15. Cerebrovascular disease is the most frequently occurring neurologic disorder. Any abnormality of the blood vessels of the brain is referred to as a cerebrovascular disease.
16. Cerebrovascular disease is associated with two types of brain abnormalities: (a) ischemia with or without infarction and (b) hemorrhage.
17. Cerebrovascular accidents (stroke syndromes) are classified according to pathophysiology and include global hypoperfusion, ischemic (thrombotic or embolic), hemorrhagic (intracranial hemorrhage).
18. Transient ischemic attacks (TIAs) are temporary decreases in brain blood flow.
19. Intracranial aneurysms result from defects in the vascular wall and are classified on the basis of form and shape. They are often asymptomatic, but the signs vary depending on the location and size of the aneurysm.
20. An arteriovenous malformation (AVM) is a tangled mass of dilated blood vessels. Although sometimes present at birth, AVM exhibits a delayed age of onset.
21. A subarachnoid hemorrhage occurs when blood escapes from defective or injured vasculature into the subarachnoid space. When a vessel tears, blood under pressure is pumped into the subarachnoid space. The blood produces an inflammatory reaction in these tissues.
22. Infection and inflammation of the CNS can be caused by bacteria, viruses, fungi, protozoans, and rickettsiae. Bacterial infections are pyogenic or pus producing.
23. Meningitis (infection of the meninges) is classified as bacterial, aseptic (nonpurulent), or fungal. Bacterial meningitis primarily is an infection of the pia mater and arachnoid and of the fluid of the subarachnoid space. Aseptic meningitis is believed to be limited to the meninges. Fungal meningitis is a chronic, less common type of meningitis.
24. The meningeal vessels become hyperemic, and neutrophils migrate into the subarachnoid space with bacterial meningitis. An inflammatory reaction occurs, and exudate is formed and increases rapidly.
25. Brain abscesses often originate from infections outside the CNS. Organisms gain access to the CNS from adjacent sites or spread along the wall of a vein. A localized inflammatory process develops with exudate formation, thrombosis of vessels, and degenerating leukocytes. After a few days, the infection becomes delimited with a center of pus and a wall of granular tissue.
26. Clinical manifestations of brain abscesses include headache, nuchal rigidity, confusion, drowsiness, and sensory and communication deficits. Treatment includes antibiotic therapy and surgical excision or aspiration.
27. Encephalitis is an acute, febrile illness of viral origin with nervous system involvement. The most common encephalitides are caused by arthropod-borne (mosquito-borne) viruses and herpes simplex. Meningeal involvement appears in all encephalitides.
28. Clinical manifestations of encephalitis include fever, delirium, confusion, seizures, abnormal and involuntary movement, and increased intracranial pressure.
29. Herpes encephalitis is treated with antiviral agents. No definitive treatment exists for the other encephalitides.
30. The common neurologic complications of AIDS are HIV encephalopathy, HIV neuropathy, HIV myelopathy, opportunistic infections, cytomegalovirus, parasitic infection, and neoplasms. Pathologically, there may be diffuse CNS involvement, focal pathology, and obstructive hydrocephalus.
31. Multiple sclerosis (MS) is a relatively common degenerative disorder involving CNS myelin. Although the pathogenesis is unknown, the demyelination is thought to result from an immunogenetic-viral cause. A previous viral insult to the nervous system in a genetically susceptible individual yields a subsequent abnormal immune response in the CNS.
32. Amyotrophic lateral sclerosis (ALS) is a degenerative disorder diffusely involving lower and upper motor neurons. The pathogenesis of ALS is not fully known; however, there is lower and upper motor neuron degeneration.

Peripheral Nervous System and Neuromuscular Junction Disorders

1. Radiculopathies are disorders of the roots of spinal cord nerves. The roots may be compressed, inflamed, or torn. Clinical manifestations include local pain or paresthesias in the sensory root distribution. Treatment may involve surgery, antibiotics, steroids, radiation therapy, and chemotherapy.
2. Plexus injuries involve the plexus distal to the spinal roots. Paralysis can occur with complete plexus involvement.
3. Neuropathies are the resulting syndrome when the peripheral nerves are affected. Axon and myelin degeneration may be present. Neuropathies are classified as sensorimotor, sensory, or motor. The neuropathies are characterized by varying degrees of sensory disturbance, paresis, and paralysis. Secondary atrophy may be present.
4. Guillain-Barré syndrome is a demyelinating disorder caused by a humoral and cell-mediated immunologic reaction directed at the peripheral nerves. The clinical manifestations may vary from paresis of the legs to complete quadriplegia, respiratory insufficiency, and autonomic nervous system instability. Plasmapheresis is used during the acute phase and followed by aggressive rehabilitation.
5. Myasthenia gravis is a disorder of voluntary muscles characterized by muscle weakness and fatigability. It is considered an autoimmune disease and is associated with an increased incidence of other autoimmune diseases.

Did You Understand?—Cont'd

6. Myasthenia gravis results from a defect in nerve impulse transmission at the neuromuscular junction. IgG antibody is secreted against the "self" acetylcholine receptors and blocks the binding of acetylcholine. The antibody action destroys the receptor sites, causing decreased transmission of the nerve impulse across the neuromuscular junction.
7. Primary disorders of muscles with weakness and atrophy are known as myopathies.

Tumors of the Central Nervous System

1. Two main types of tumors occur within the cranium: primary and metastatic. Primary tumors are classified as intracerebral tumors (astrocytomas, oligodendrogliomas, and ependymomas) or extracerebral tumors (meningioma or nerve sheath tumors). Metastatic tumors can be found inside or outside the brain substance.
2. CNS tumors cause local and generalized manifestations. The effects are varied, and local manifestations include seizures, visual disturbances, loss of equilibrium, and cranial nerve dysfunction.
3. Spinal cord tumors are classified as intramedullary tumors (within the neural tissues) or extramedullary tumors (outside the spinal cord). Metastatic spinal cord tumors are usually carcinomas, lymphomas, or myelomas.
4. Extramedullary spinal cord tumors produce dysfunction by compression of adjacent tissue, not by direct invasion. Intramedullary spinal cord tumors produce dysfunction by both invasion and compression.
5. The onset of clinical manifestations of spinal cord tumors is gradual and progressive, suggesting compression. Specific manifestations depend on the location of the tumor; for example, there may be paresis and spasticity of one leg with thoracic tumors, followed by involvement of the opposite leg.

Key Terms

Amyotrophic lateral sclerosis (ALS, sporadic motor neuron disease, sporadic motor system disease, motor neuron disease [MND]), 393
Arteriovenous malformation (AVM), 385
Aseptic meningitis (viral meningitis, nonpurulent meningitis), 387
Autonomic hyperreflexia (dysreflexia), 376
Bacterial meningitis, 387
Brain abscess, 388
Brudzinski sign, 386
Cerebrovascular accident (CVA, stroke), 382
Cholinergic crisis, 395
Classic ALS (Lou Gehrig disease), 393
Classic cerebral concussion, 374
Closed (blunt) trauma, 369
Compressive syndrome (sensorimotor syndrome), 401
Congenital myasthenia, 395
Contusion, 371
Degenerative disk disease, 380
Diffuse brain injury, 372
Embolic stroke, 383
Encephalitis, 390
Ependymoma, 399
Extradural brain abscess, 388
Extradural hematoma, 371
Extradural tumor, 400
Extramedullary tumor, 400
West Nile virus, 389
Focal brain injury, 371
Fungal meningitis, 387
Fusiform aneurysm (giant aneurysm), 384
Generalized autoimmune myasthenia, 395
Glioblastoma multiforme, 397
Glioma, 397
Gliosis, 392
Guillain-Barré syndrome, 394
Hemorrhagic stroke (intracranial hemorrhage), 383
HIV myelopathy, 391
HIV neuropathy, 391
HIV-associated cognitive dysfunction (HIV encephalopathy, subacute encephalitis, HIV-associated dementia complex, HIV cognitive motor complex, AIDS encephalopathy, AIDS dementia complex, AIDS-related dementia), 391
Intracerebral brain abscess, 388
Intracerebral hematoma, 372
Intradural tumor, 400
Intramedullary spinal cord abscess, 388
Intramedullary tumor, 400
Irritative syndrome (radicular syndrome), 401
Juvenile myasthenia, 395
Kernig sign, 386
Lacunar stroke (lacunar infarct), 383
Meningioma, 399
Meningitis, 387
Multiple sclerosis (MS), 392
Myasthenia gravis, 395
Myasthenic crisis, 395
Myopathy, 396
Neonatal myasthenia, 395
Nerve sheath tumor, 400
Neuropathies, 394
Ocular myasthenia, 395
Oligodendroblastoma, 397
Oligodendroglioma, 397
Open (penetrating) trauma, 369
Plexus injuries, 394
Postconcussive syndrome, 374
Radiculopathies, 394
Saccular aneurysm (berry aneurysm), 384
Spinal cord abscess, 388
Spinal epidural abscess, 388
Spinal shock, 375
Spinal stenosis, 380
Spondylolisthesis, 380
Spondylolysis, 380
Subarachnoid hemorrhage, 386
Subdural hematoma, 372
Thrombotic stroke (cerebral thrombosis), 383
Toxoplasmosis, 390
Transient ischemic attack (TIA), 383
Vacuolar myelopathy, 391

References

1. Evans RW, Wilberger JE: Traumatic disorders, In Goetz CG, editor: *Textbook of clinical neurology*, Philadelphia, 2003, Saunders.
2. Yeoman B: Lights out, *Discover* 166:68–73, 2004.
3. Edwards P et al: Final results of MRC CRASH, a randomised placebo-controlled trial of intravenous corticosteroid in adults with head injury-outcomes at 6 months, *Lancet* 365(9475): 1957–1959, 2005.
4. Sauerlaud S, Maegele MA: CRASH landing in severe head injury, *Lancet* 364:729–782, 2004.
5. Moreira N: Back to genetics DNA variant may code for lumbar pain, *Sci News* 167:373, 2005.
6. American Heart Association: *Heart disease and stroke statistics: 2005 update*, Dallas, 2005, author.
7. Seppa N: Southern blacks face excess risk of stroke, *Sci News* 167:126, 2005.
8. Hu G et al: The impact of history of hypertension and type 2 diabetes at baseline on the incidence of stroke and stroke mortality, *Stroke* 36:2538–2543, 2005.
9. Chung CS, Caplan LR: Neurovascular disorders, In Goetz CG, editor: *Textbook of clinical neurology*, Philadelphia, 2003, Saunders.
10. Adams HP et al: Guidelines for the early management of patients with ischemic stroke: a statement for health care professionals from a special writing group of the Stroke Council of the AHA, *Stroke* 27:1711–1718, 2003.
11. Mohr JP et al: A comparison of warfarin and aspirin for the prevention of recurrent ischemic stroke, *N Engl J Med* 345 (20):1444–1451, 2001.
12. Seppa N: To stanch the flow, *Sci News* 167:133, 2005.
13. Gupta J: To clip or to coil, *Time* 159:9, 2002.
14. Seppa H: Head-to-head comparison coils top clips in brain aneurysm treatment, *Sci News* 168:180–181, 2005.
15. Manno EM: Subarachnoid hemorrhage, *Neuro Clin* 22:347–366, 2005.
16. Blissit PA et al: Cerebrovascular dynamics with head-of-bed elevation in patients with mild or moderate vasospasm after aneurismal subarachnoid hemorrhage, *Am J Crit Care* 15(2): 206–216, 2006.
17. Cavanaugh SJ, Gordon VL: Grading scales used in the management of aneurismal subarachnoid hemorrhage: a critical review, *J Neurosci Nurs* 34:288–295, 2002.
18. van de Beek D et al: Clinical features and prognostic factors in adults with bacterial meningitis, *N Engl J Med* 351(18): 1849–1859, 2004.
19. Swartz MN: Bacterial meningitis—a view of the past 90 years, *N Engl J Med* 351:1826–1828, 2004.
20. Roos KI: Viral infections, In Goetz CG, editor: *Textbook of clinical neurology*, Philadelphia, 2003, Saunders.
21. Roos KI: Nonviral infections, In Goetz CG, editor: *Textbook of clinical neurology*, Philadelphia, 2003, Saunders.
22. Belman AL, Marett-Savatic M: Human immunodeficiency virus and acquired immunodeficiency syndrome, In Goetz CG, editor: *Textbook of clinical neurology*, Philadelphia, 2003, Saunders.
23. Boyd JR, MacMillan LJ: Experiences of children and adolescents living with multiple sclerosis, *J Neurosci Nurs* 37(6): 334–342, 2005.
24. Calabresi PA: Diagnosis and management of multiple sclerosis, *Am Fam Physician* 70(10):1934–1944, 2004.
25. Seppa N: Adopted protein might be MS culprit, *Sci News* 166:237, 2004.
26. Seppa N: Glutamate glut linked to multiple sclerosis, *Sci News* 157(2):22, 2000.
27. Chabus D et al: The influence of the proinflammatory cytokine, osteopontin, on autoimmune demyelinating disease, *Science* 294(5547):1731–1735, 2001.
28. Pirko I, Noseworthy JH: Demyelinating disorders of the central nervous system, In Goetz CG, editor: *Textbook of clinical neurology*, Philadelphia, 2003, Saunders.
29. Carroll L: Researchers tease out cellular biology of ALS and it is not just motor neurons, *Neurology Today* 5(1):70–72, 2005.
30. Lui J et al: Toxicity of familial ALS-linked SODI mutants from selective recruitment to spinal mitochondria, *Neuron* 43 (1):5–15, 2004.
31. Moyer P: Can neuroimaging differentiate dementia in ALS from other types of dementia, *Neurology Today* 5(1):77–78, 2005.
32. Dib M: Amyotrophic lateral sclerosis: progress and prospects for treatment, *Drugs* 63(3):289–310, 2003.
33. Ragheb S, Lisak RP: The thymus and myasthenia gravis, *Chest Surg Clin N Am* 11(2):311–327, 2001.
34. American Cancer Society: *Cancer Facts and Figures, Estimated New Cancer Cases and Deaths by Sex for all Sites*, US, 2007, p. 4, Available at http://www.cancer.org/docroot/stt/stt_0.asp. Accessed 2/1/07.
35. Brain Tumor Society: *Brain Tumor Facts & Statistics.* Available at http://www.tbts.org/itemDetail.asp?categoryID=384&itemID=16535. Accessed 2/1/07.
36. Janus TJ, Yung KA: Primary neurological tumors, In Goetz CG, editor: *Textbook of clinical neurology*, Philadelphia, 2003, Saunders.
37. Evans DG, Sainio M, Baser ME: Neurofibromatosis type 2, *J Med Genet* 37(12):897–904, 2000.
38. Harris C: Neurofibromatosis type 2—living with the complications: a case study. *J Neurosci Nurs* 37(3):156–158.
39. Benjamin RK, Das A, Hockberg FH: Metastatic neoplasms and paraneoplasms, In Goetz CG, editor: *Textbook of clinical neurology*, Philadelphia, 2003, Saunders.

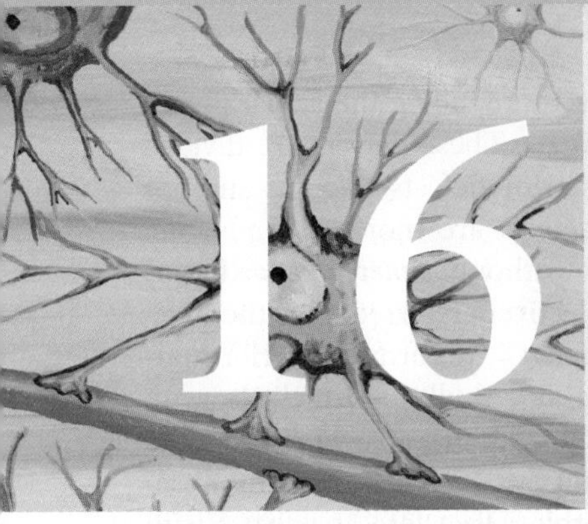

16 ALTERATIONS OF NEUROLOGIC FUNCTION IN CHILDREN

Robin R. Wilkerson ▪ Barbara J. Boss

CHAPTER OUTLINE

ELECTRONIC RESOURCES

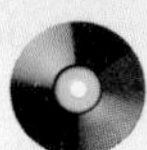

Companion CD

- Review Questions and Answers
- Animations

evolve Website
http://evolve.elsevier.com/Huether/

- Quick Check Answers
- Key Terms Exercises
- Critical Thinking Questions with Answers
- Algorithm Completion Exercises
- WebLinks

Neurologic disorders in children can occur from infancy through adolescence and include congenital malformations, genetic defects in metabolism, brain injuries, infection, tumors and other disorders that affect neurologic function. The symptoms, diagnosis, and management of neurologic disorders in children are often different from that of adults.

NORMAL GROWTH AND DEVELOPMENT OF THE NERVOUS SYSTEM

Environmental influences have a significant role in nervous system development. Nutrition, hormones, oxygen levels, and external stimulation all affect normal growth. The proper proportions of essential nutrients are necessary for proliferation of the nervous system tissue. Maternal lifestyle, nutrition, and state of health also have a crucial impact on nervous system development at certain critical periods of maturation.

The growth and development of the brain occurs rapidly during the fifteenth to twentieth weeks of gestation and again at 30 weeks of gestation through the first year of life, reflecting the development and multiplication of neurons. The head is the fastest growing body part during infancy. One half of postnatal brain growth is achieved by the first year and is 90% complete by age 6 years. The cortex thickens with maturation, and the sulci deepen as cortical functions develop. Cerebral blood flow and oxygen consumption is about twice that of the adult brain during these years.

The bones of the infant's skull are separated at the suture lines forming two **fontanelles** or "soft spots": one diamond-shaped anterior fontanelle and one triangular-shaped posterior fontanelle. The fontanelles allow for expansion of the rapidly growing brain. The posterior fontanelle may be open until 2 to 3 months of age; the anterior fontanelle normally does not fully close until 18 months of age (Figure 16-1). Abnormal intracranial conditions, such as those characterized by increased intracranial pressure, also may result in distention or bulging of the fontanelles and an increased head circumference in excess of that expected with normal growth. Health care providers carefully monitor the fontanelles for 2 years and head growth during the first 5 years by measuring head circumference and comparing the results with a standardized growth chart.

Human neurologic functioning is primarily at a subcortical level at birth (impulses are handled by the brain stem and spinal cord). Many reflex patterns mediated by brain stem and spinal cord mechanisms are present at birth and then disappear at predictable times during infancy. Table 16-1 summarizes the age at which reflexes appear and disappear.

Absence of expected reflex responses at the appropriate age indicates general depression of central or peripheral motor functions. Asymmetric responses may indicate lesions in the motor cortex or may occur with fractures of bones after traumatic delivery or postnatal injury. As the infant matures, the neonatal reflexes disappear in a predictable order as voluntary motor functions supersede them. Abnormal persistence of these reflexes is seen in infants with developmental delays or with central motor lesions.

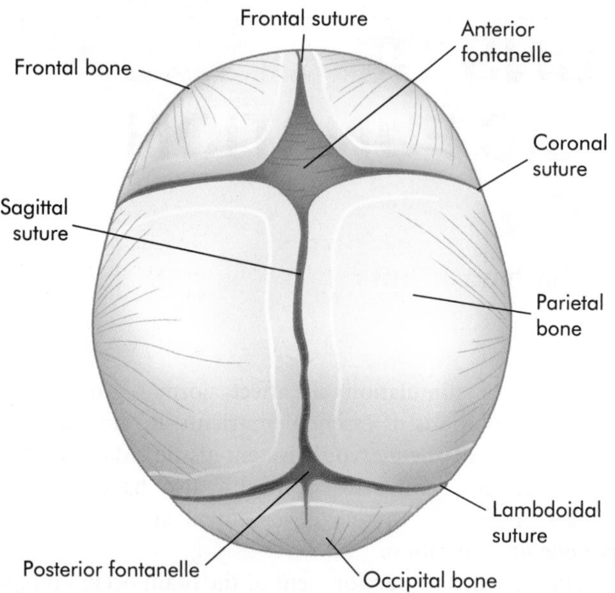

Figure 16-1 ■ Cranial Sutures and Fontanelles in Infancy. Fibrous union of suture lines and interlocking of serrated edges (occurs by 6 months; solid union requires approximately 12 years).

TABLE 16-1

Reflexes of Infancy

Reflex	Age of Appearance of Reflex	Age at Which Reflex Should No Longer Be Obtainable
Moro	Birth	3 mo
Stepping	Birth	6 wk
Sucking	Birth	4 mo awake 7 mo asleep
Rooting	Birth	4 mo awake 7 mo asleep
Palmar grasp	Birth	6 mo
Plantar grasp	Birth	10 mo
Tonic neck	2 mo	5 mo
Neck righting	4-6 mo	24 mo
Landau	3 mo	24 mo
Parachute reaction	9 mo	Persists indefinitely

STRUCTURAL MALFORMATIONS

Central nervous system (CNS) malformations are responsible for 75% of fetal deaths and 40% of deaths during the first year of life. During the perinatal period, CNS malformations account for one third of all apparent congenital malformations, and 90% of CNS malformations are defects of neural tube closure.

Defects of Neural Tube Closure

Neural tube defects occur in approximately 1.0 of every 1000 live births in the United States each year.[1] Fetal death often occurs as a result, thereby reducing the actual prevalence of neural defects at birth.[2] These defects are divided into two categories: (1) posterior defects and (2) anterior midline defects. Posterior defects are more common and include anencephaly (*an* = without; *enkephalos* = brain) and a group of disorders collectively referred to as the **myelodysplasias** (*dys* = bad; *plassein* = to form). Anterior midline defects may cause brain and skull abnormalities, with the most extreme form being **cyclopia,** in which the child has a single midline orbit and eye with a protruding nose-like appendage above the orbit. Disorders associated with embryonic development are summarized in Figure 16-2. The cause of neural tube defects is believed to be multifactoral (a combination of genes and environment). No single gene has been found to cause neural tube defects.[1,3] Folic acid deficiency during early stages of pregnancy increases the risk for neural tube defects,[1,2] but preconceptional supplementation assures adequate folate status. Other risk factors include heredity, maternal blood glucose concentrations, use of anticonvulsant drugs (particularly valproic acid), and maternal hyperthermia.[1,2]

In **anencephaly,** the soft, bony component of the skull and part of the brain are missing. This is a relatively common disorder, with an incidence of approximately 1 per 8000 total live births in the United States each year.[4] At birth the infant's head, viewed face-on, has a froglike appearance. These infants are stillborn or die within a few days after birth.

Encephalocele refers to a herniation or protrusion of brain and meninges through a defect in the skull, resulting in a saclike structure. The prevalence is approximately 1.4 per 10,000 live births in the United States each year.[5] Most encephaloceles occur in the occipital area, with the remainder found in the frontal, parietal, or nasopharyngeal regions.

Meningocele, which is a saclike cyst of meninges filled with spinal fluid, occurs when the neural tube fails to close completely (Figure 16-3). This cystic dilation of meninges protrudes through the vertebral defect and around the malformed tube but does not involve the spinal cord. Meningoceles occur with equal frequency in the cervical, thoracic, and lumbar spine areas.

Myelomeningocele (meningomyelocele; spina bifida cystica) is a hernial protrusion of a saclike cyst (containing meninges, spinal fluid, and a portion of the spinal cord with its nerves) through a defect in the posterior arch of a vertebra. Eighty percent of myelomeningoceles are located in the lumbar and lumbosacral regions, the last regions of the neural tube to close. Myelomeningocele is one of the most common developmental anomalies of the nervous system, with an incidence rate ranging from 0.2 to 0.4 per 1000 live births.[6]

CLINICAL MANIFESTATIONS A myelomeningocele is the failure of the neural tube to close, resulting in a cystic dilation of meninges and protuberance of the spinal cord through the vertebral defect. A myelomeningocele is evident at birth as a pronounced skin defect on the infant's

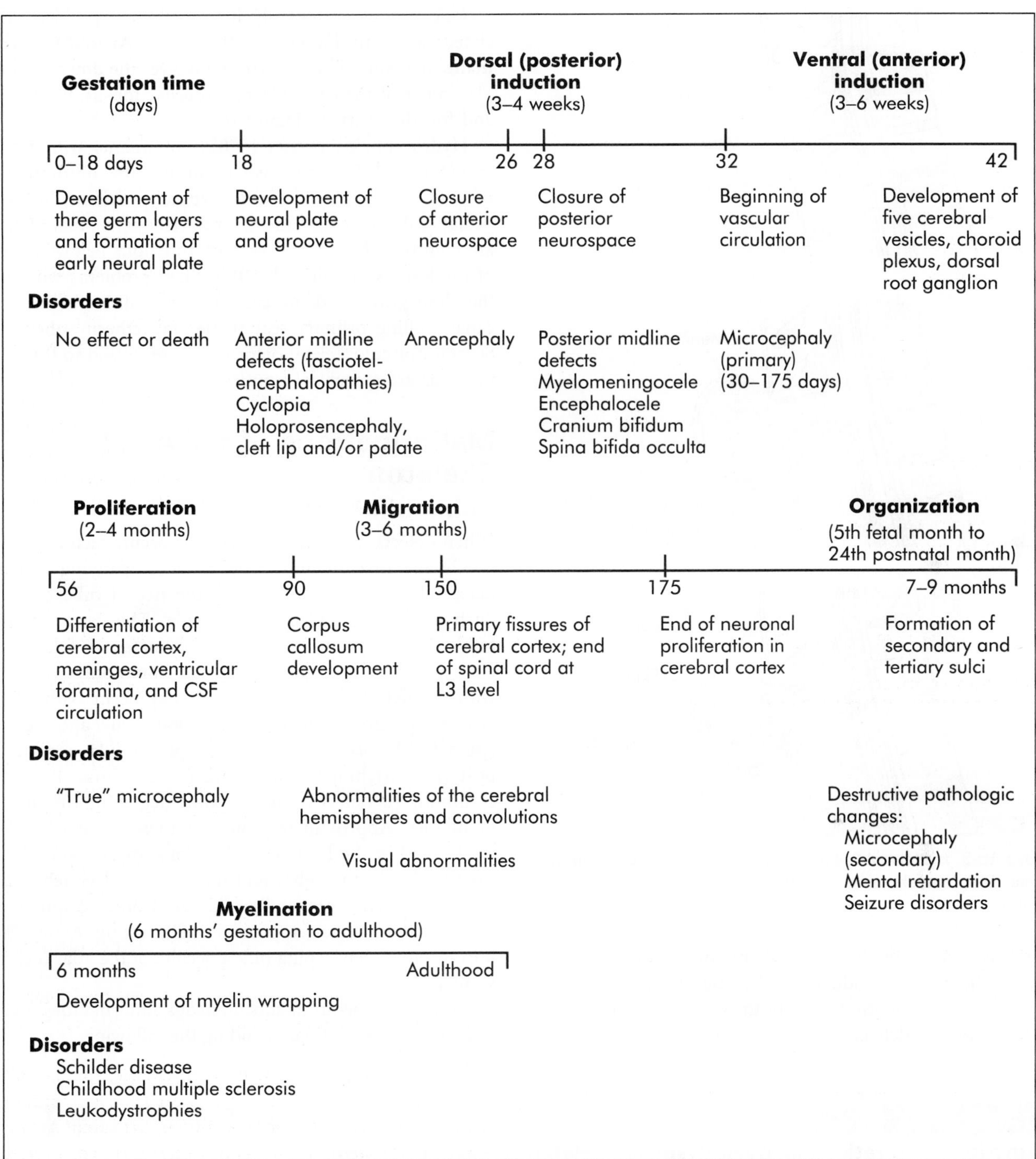

Figure 16-2 ■ **Disorders Associated With Specific Stages of Embryonic Development.**

back (see Figure 16-3). The bony prominences of the unfused neural arches can be palpated at the lateral border of the defect. The defect usually is covered by a transparent membrane that may have neural tissue attached to its inner surface. This membrane may be intact at birth or may leak cerebrospinal fluid (CSF), thereby increasing the risks of infection and neuronal damage. Until the defect is surgically closed, CSF may accumulate, resulting in further dilation and enlargement of the sac, which is a risk for further damage to neuronal function.

The actual involvement of the spinal cord has greater implications for the overall function of the infant throughout childhood (Table 16-2). Neurologic function may be absent in some infants with myelomeningocele. Function may be attained if underlying fluid or pus accumulation is prevented from stretching and applying pressure to the

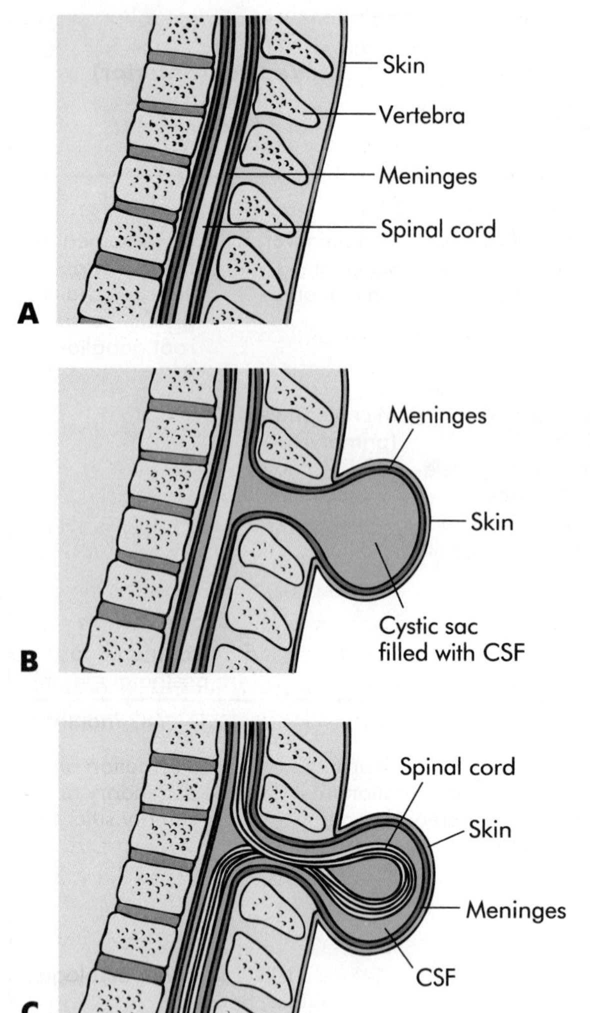

Figure 16-3 ■ **Normal Spine, Meningocele, and Myelomeningocele.** Diagram showing section through normal spine **(A)**, meningocele **(B)**, and myelomeningocele **(C)**.

neural tissue or if the biochemical alterations do not cause neural tissue to die. Residual neural tissue also may be temporarily or permanently lost at birth because of trauma to the tissue during delivery.

One serious, potentially life-threatening problem associated with myelomeningocele is the **Arnold-Chiari II malformation.**[7] This deformity involves the downward displacement of the cerebellum, cerebellar tonsils, brain stem, and fourth ventricle (Figure 16-4).

Hydrocephalus occurs in 85% of infants with myelomeningocele.[8] Seizures also occur in 30% of those with myelodysplasia. Visual and perceptual problems, including ocular palsies, astigmatism, and visuoperceptual deficits, are common. Motor and sensory functions below the level of the lesions are altered. Often these problems worsen as the child grows and the cord ascends within the vertebral canal, pulling primary scar tissue and tethering the cord.[9] Several musculoskeletal deformities are related to this diagnosis, as are spinal deformities.

Malformations of the Axial Skeleton

Spina bifida occulta

When defects of neural tube closure occur, such as meningocele and myelomeningocele, an accompanying vertebral defect allows the protrusion of the neural tube contents. Such a defect is called **spina bifida.** The cause of spina bifida is unknown. Periconceptual maternal folate deficiency and genetic alterations are commonly associated with the defect.[10] The defect also may occur without any visible exposure of meninges or neural tissue, and the term **spina bifida occulta** is used. In spina bifida occulta, the posterior vertebral laminae have failed to fuse. Extremely common, the defect occurs to some degree in 10% to 25% of infants. Approximately 80% of these vertebral defects are located in the lumbosacral regions, most commonly in the fifth lumbar vertebra and the first sacral vertebra; they may be detected prenatally with ultrasonic scanning and amniotic fluid alpha-fetoprotein (AFP) testing. About 3% of normal adults have spina bifida occulta of the atlas (cervical vertebra 1).

Certain cutaneous or subcutaneous abnormalities suggest underlying spina bifida, including the following:

TABLE 16-2

Functional Alterations in Myelodysplasia Related to Level of Lesion

Level of Lesion	Functional Implications
Thoracic	Flaccid paralysis of lower extremities; variable weakness in abdominal trunk musculature; high thoracic level may mean respiratory compromise; absence of bowel and bladder control
High lumbar	Voluntary hip flexion and adduction; flaccid paralysis of knees, ankles, and feet; may walk with extensive braces and crutches; absence of bowel and bladder control
Mid lumbar	Strong hip flexion and adduction; fair knee extension; flaccid paralysis of ankles and feet; absence of bowel and bladder control
Low lumbar	Strong hip flexion, extension, and adduction and knee extension; weak ankle and toe mobility; may have limited bowel and bladder function
Sacral	Normal function of lower extremities; normal bowel and bladder function

Modified from Farley JA, Dunleavy MJ: Myelodysplasia. In Allen PJ, Vessey JA, editors: *Primary care of the child with a chronic condition*, ed 4, St Louis, 2004, Mosby.

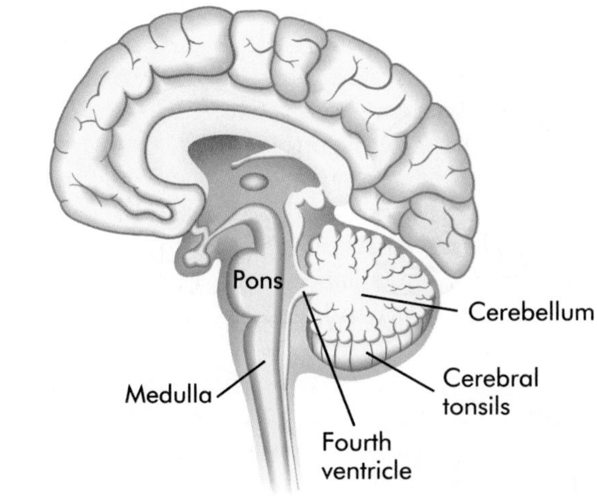

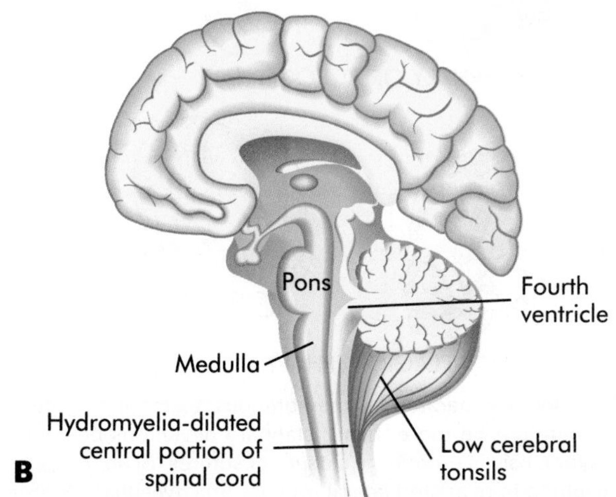

Figure 16-4 ■ Normal Brain and Arnold-Chiari II Malformation. Diagram showing normal brain **(A)** and brain with Arnold-Chiari II malformation **(B)**.

1. Abnormal growth of hair along the spine, which often is either very coarse or very silky
2. A midline dimple with or without a sinus tract
3. A cutaneous angioma, usually of the "port wine" variety
4. A subcutaneous mass, usually representing a lipoma or dermoid cyst

Spina bifida occulta usually causes no serious neurologic dysfunctions. When dysfunctions occur, the common lumbosacral defects cause gait abnormalities, positional deformities of the feet as a result of muscle weakness, or sphincter disturbances of the bladder and bowel. These dysfunctions become evident during periods of rapid growth. Surgical closure is usually completed in the neonatal period, and techniques are being developed for intrauterine closure.[11]

Cranial deformities

Skull malformations range from minor, insignificant defects to major defects that are incompatible with life. In **acrania,** the cranial vault is almost completely absent, and an extensive defect of the vertebral column often is present. Acrania associated with anencephaly (absence of brain and spinal column) occurs in approximately 1 per 1000 live births and is incompatible with life.

Craniosynostosis (craniostenosis) is the premature closure of one or more of the cranial sutures during the first 18 to 20 months of the infant's life. The incidence of craniosynostosis is 1 per 2100 live births.[12] Males are affected twice as often as females. Craniosynostosis prevents normal skull expansion and causes asymmetric skull growth. Brain growth may be restricted, and compression may cause neurologic dysfunction from brain damage after age 6 months (Figure 16-5).

Microcephaly is a defect in brain growth as a whole (see Figure 16-5). The word *microcephaly* is derived from the Greek (*mikro* = small; *kephale* = head). Cranial size is significantly below average for the infant's age, gender, race, and gestation. The condition is not treatable.

True (primary) microcephaly can be caused by an autosomal recessive disorder, a chromosomal abnormality, or toxin exposure during the period of induction and major cell migration. Secondary microcephaly is associated with various causes. Infection, trauma, metabolic disorders, and anoxia experienced during the third trimester of pregnancy, the perinatal period, or early infancy may be responsible. Table 16-3 summarizes the causes of microencephaly.

Congenital hydrocephalus is characterized by an increased volume of CSF. It may be caused by blockage within the ventricular system where the CSF flows, an imbalance in the production of CSF, or a reduced reabsorption of CSF. The pressure within the ventricular system pushes and compresses the brain tissue against the skull cavity. When hydrocephalus develops before fusion of the cranial sutures, the skull can accommodate this additional space-occupying volume and preserve neuronal function. The overall incidence of hydrocephalus is approximately 3 per 1000 live births. The incidence of hydrocephalus, excluding the hydrocephalus associated with myelomeningocele, is approximately 0.5 to 1 per 1000 live births.[13] (Types of hydrocephalus are discussed in Chapter 14.)

Dandy-Walker deformity is a congenital defect of midline cerebellar structures in which hydrocephalus is caused by cystic dilation of the fourth ventricle and aqueductal compression. Other causes of obstructions within the ventricular system that can result in hydrocephalus include brain tumors, cysts, trauma, arteriovenous malformations, blood clots, and infections.

Congenital hydrocephalus may cause fetal death in utero, or the increased head circumference may require cesarean delivery of the infant. Symptoms depend directly on the cause and rate of hydrocephalus development. When there is separation of the cranial sutures, a resonant note sounds when the skull is tapped, a manifestation termed **Macewen sign** or **"cracked pot" sign.** The eyes may assume a staring expression, with sclera visible above the cornea, called *sunsetting.*

Correlation between the degree of hydrocephalus and impaired cognitive function often is a result of additional

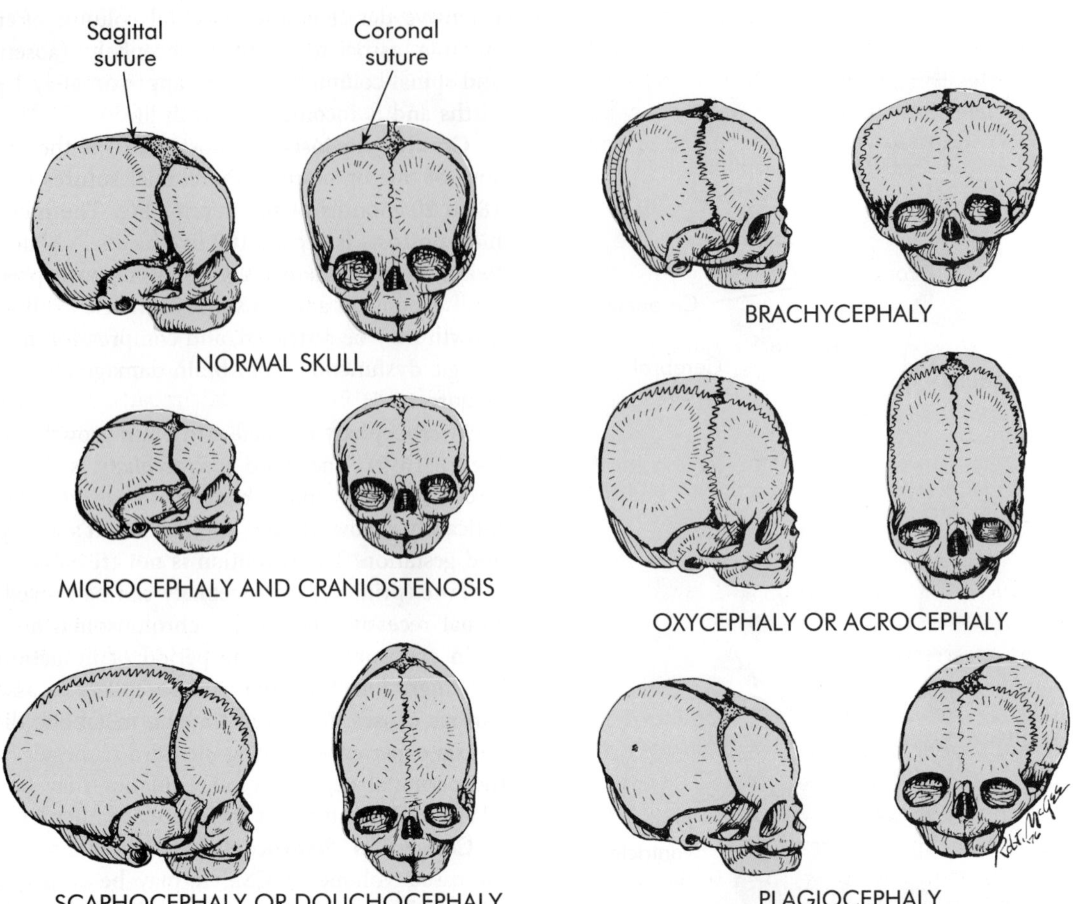

Figure 16-5 ■ Normal and Abnormal Head Configurations. *Normal skull:* Bones separated by membranous seams until sutures gradually close. *Microcephaly and craniostenosis:* Microcephaly is head circumference more than 2 standard deviations below the mean for age, gender, race, and gestation and reflects a small brain; craniosynostosis is premature closure of sutures. *Scaphocephaly or dolichocephaly* (frequency 56%): Premature closure of sagittal suture, resulting in restricted lateral growth. *Brachycephaly:* Premature closure of coronal suture, resulting in excessive lateral growth. *Oxycephaly or acrocephaly* (frequency 5.8% to 12%): Premature closure of all coronal and sagittal sutures resulting in accelerated upward growth and small head circumference. *Plagiocephaly* (frequency 13%): Unilateral premature closure of coronal suture, resulting in asymmetric growth. (From Hockenberry MJ: *Wong's nursing care of infants and children,* ed 7, St Louis, 2003, Mosby.)

TABLE 16-3

Causes of Microcephaly

Defects in Brain Development	Intrauterine Infections	Perinatal and Postnatal Disorders
Hereditary (recessive) microcephaly	Congenital rubella	Intrauterine or neonatal anoxia
Down syndrome and other trisomy syndromes	Cytomegalovirus infection	Severe malnutrition in early infancy
Fetal ionizing radiation exposure	Congenital toxoplasmosis	Neonatal herpesvirus infection
Maternal phenylketonuria		
Cornelia de Lange syndrome		
Rubinstein-Taybi syndrome		
Smith-Lemli-Opitz syndrome		
Fetal alcohol syndrome		
Angelman syndrome		
Seckel syndrome		

complications, such as severe congenital malformations, acute or chronic infections, or progressive brain tumors. Approximately two thirds of children with uncomplicated congenital hydrocephalus who have been treated successfully with shunting may have normal to borderline normal intelligence.[14]

QUICK CHECK 16-1

1. List two defects of neural tube closure.
2. Why do motor and sensory functions worsen with growth in a child with a neural tube defect?

ENCEPHALOPATHIES

Encephalopathy, a disorder involving the brain, is a general category that includes a number of syndromes and diseases (see Chapter 14). These disorders may be acute or chronic, as well as static or progressive.

Static Encephalopathies

Brain injury may occur during gestation or birth or at any time during childhood growth and development, causing a static, nonprogressive disorder. Varying degrees of impairment may result from diffuse or localized injury to the cortex. Prenatal factors that affect the developing nervous system may be endogenous or exogenous. The developing nervous system is most susceptible to injury during the first trimester of pregnancy. Anoxia, trauma, and infections are the most common factors that cause injury to the nervous system in the perinatal period. Infections, metabolic disturbances (acute or a result of inborn errors), trauma, toxins, and vascular disease may injure the nervous system in the postnatal period.

Cerebral palsy is the term given to a diverse group of nonprogressive syndromes that affect the brain and cause motor dysfunction beginning in early infancy. The cause may include prenatal cerebral hypoxia or trauma. It can be classified on the basis of neurologic signs and symptoms, with the major types involving spasticity, ataxia, dyskinesia, and a mix of one or more of the three. Cerebral palsy is one of the most common crippling disorders of childhood, affecting approximately 764,000 children and adults in the United States alone. Although the exact incidence is unknown, studies suggest that the incidence is 2 to 2.5 cases of cerebral palsy per 1000 live births.[15]

Spastic cerebral palsy is associated with increased muscle tone, prolonged primitive reflexes, exaggerated deep tendon reflexes, clonus, rigidity of the extremities, scoliosis, and contractures. This accounts for approximately 70% to 80% of cerebral palsy cases. **Dyskinetic cerebral palsy** is associated with extreme difficulty in fine motor coordination and purposeful movements. Movements are jerky, uncontrolled, and abrupt, resulting from injury to the basal ganglia or extrapyramidal tracts. This form of cerebral palsy accounts for approximately 10% to 20% of cases. **Ataxic cerebral palsy** manifests with gait disturbances and instability. The infant with this form of cerebral palsy may have hypotonia at birth, but stiffness of the trunk muscles develops by late infancy. Persistence of this increased tone in truncal muscles affects the child's gait and ability to maintain equilibrium. This form of cerebral palsy accounts for approximately 5% to 10% of cases. A child may have symptoms of each of these cerebral palsy types, which leads to a mixed disorder accounting for approximately 13% of cases.[15]

Children with cerebral palsy often have associated neurologic disorders, such as seizures (about 50%), and intellectual impairment ranging from mild to severe (about 67%). Other complications include visual impairment, communication disorders, respiratory problems, bowel and bladder problems, and orthopedic disabilities.[15]

Although the brain injury is static, the chemical picture of cerebral palsy may change with growth and development. Therefore, a fundamental component to an effective treatment regimen includes ongoing assessment, evaluation, and revision of the child's overall management plan. The use of baclofen pumps and botulinum toxin has shown some improvement in some children with cerebral palsy. Family-focused interdisciplinary team management provides the best treatment outcomes.[16,17]

Inherited Metabolic Disorders of the Central Nervous System

A large number of inherited metabolic disorders have been identified. Typically these metabolic disorders damage the entire CNS so extensively that these children do not survive to adulthood. Table 16-4 lists some of these inherited metabolic disorders. Defects in amino acid and lipid metabolism are among the most common.

Defects in amino acid metabolism

Biochemical defects in amino acid metabolism include (1) those in which the transport of amino acid is impaired, (2) those involving an enzyme or cofactor deficiency, and (3) those grouped around certain chemical components, such as sulfur-containing amino acids. Most disorders described to date suggest that the absence of enzymatic activity generally is caused by the genetically determined absence of the enzyme protein.

Phenylketonuria

Phenylketonuria (PKU) is an inborn error of metabolism characterized by the inability of the body to convert the essential amino acid phenylalanine to tyrosine (Figure 16-6). PKU is caused by phenylalanine hydroxylase deficiency and has an incidence of 1:14,000 worldwide.[18] Most natural food proteins contain about 15% phenylalanine, an essential amino acid. Phenylalanine hydroxylase controls the conversion of this essential amino acid to tyrosine in the liver. The body uses tyrosine in the biosynthesis of protein, melanin, thyroxine, and the catecholamines in the brain and adrenal medulla. Phenylalanine hydroxylase deficiency causes an accumulation of phenylalanine in the serum. Abnormalities occur, such as anomalous development of the CNS, defective myelination, cystic degeneration of the gray and white matter, and disturbances in cortical layers. Unfortunately, brain damage occurs before the metabolites can be detected in the urine, and damage continues as long as phenylalanine levels remain high. Nonselective newborn screening is used to detect PKU in the United States and in more than 30 other countries. Most children develop normally on a PKU diet.

Defects in lipid metabolism

Disorders of lipid metabolism are termed **lysosomal storage diseases** because each disorder in this group can be

TABLE 16-4

Inherited Metabolic Disorders of the Central Nervous System

Age of Onset	Disorder
Neonatal period	Pyridoxine dependency, galactosemia, maple syrup urine disease and its variant, phenylketonuria (PKU)
Early infancy	Tay-Sachs disease and its variants, infantile Gaucher disease, infantile Niemann-Pick disease, Krabbe disease (leukodystrophy), Farber lipogranulomatosis, Pelizaeus-Merzbacher disease and other sudanophilic leukodystrophies, spongy degeneration, Alexander disease, Alpers disease, Leigh disease (subacute necrotizing encephalomyelopathy), congenital lactic acidosis, Zellweger encephalopathy, Lowe disease (oculocerebrorenal disease)
Late infancy and early childhood	Disorders of amino acid metabolism, metachromatic leukodystrophy, late infantile GM, gangliosidosis, late infantile Gaucher and Niemann-Pick diseases, neuroaxonal dystrophy, mucopolysaccharidosis, mucolipidosis, fucosidosis, mannosidosis, aspartylglycosaminuria, amaurotic idiocy (Jansky-Bielschowsky disease, Batten disease, Vogt-Spielmeyer disease, neuronal ceroid lipofuscinosis), Cockayne syndrome
Later childhood and adolescence	Progressive cerebellar ataxias of childhood and adolescence, hepatolenticular degeneration (Wilson disease), Hallervorden-Spatz disease, Lesch-Nyhan syndrome and other uremic states, familial calcification of vessels in basal ganglia and cerebellum, familial polymyoclonus, chronic familial leukodystrophy, homocystinuria, Fabry disease

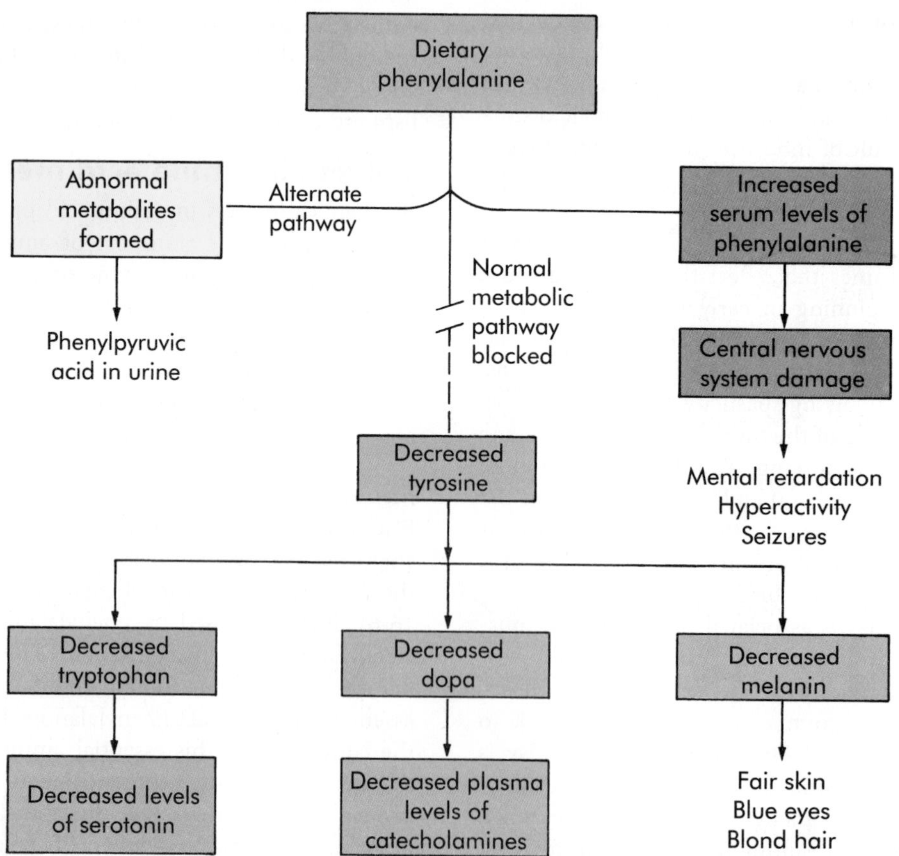

Figure 16-6 ■ **Metabolic Error and Consequences in Phenylketonuria.** (From Hockenberry MJ: *Wong's nursing care of infants and children,* ed 8, St Louis, 2007, Mosby.)

traced to a missing lysosomal enzyme. Lysosomal storage disorders include more than 40 known genetic disorders caused by an inborn error of metabolism. The incidence of lysosomal storage disorders is approximately 1 in 7500 live births.[19] This causes an excessive accumulation of a particular cell product, occurring in the brain, liver, spleen, bone, and lung and thus involving several organ systems. Therapy has been unsuccessful to date.

Perhaps the best known of the lysosomal storage disorders is **Tay-Sachs disease (gangliosidosis),** an autosomal recessive disorder related to a deficiency of the enzyme hexosaminidase A (HEXA). Approximately 80% of individuals diagnosed are of Jewish ancestry, although sporadic cases appear in the non-Jewish population. In Tay-Sachs disease, the pathologic progressive changes predominate in the CNS, but neurons throughout the body contain characteristic changes in the cytoplasm. Onset of this disease usually occurs when the infant is 4 to 6 months old. The symptoms of the disease include developmental retardation, paralysis, dementia, and blindness. Death from this disease is almost universal and occurs by 5 years of age. Screening for carriers of the gene is available for prevention of the disease.[20]

QUICK CHECK 16-2

1. List three types of cerebral palsy.
2. Why does failure to metabolize phenylalanine produce such widespread and devastating consequences?

Seizure Disorders

Epilepsy

Seizures are the abnormal discharge of electrical activity within the brain. Repeated recurrence of seizure activity is known as **epilepsy.** Seizures may result from an underlying disorder of the CNS or a disorder that directly or indirectly affects normal CNS function. Certain types of seizures may have a genetic component or familial predisposition, or they can result from maternal diseases or congenital structural anomalies of the CNS. From the newborn period through childhood, asphyxia, intracranial hemorrhage, CNS infections, injury, electrolyte imbalances, and inborn errors of metabolism may cause seizures. Often the cause of seizures is unknown.

The incidence of epilepsy varies greatly with age and is estimated to be 0.5% to 1% of children, with onset occurring during infancy or childhood.[21] It decreases with age; 75% to 80% of epilepsy cases initially occur before 20 years of age, with 30% of the cases initially occurring within the first 4 years of life. Approximately 181,000 individuals in the United States are newly affected each year.[22] Table 16-5 summarizes the major types of seizures.

Acute Encephalopathies

Reye syndrome

Reye syndrome is characterized by encephalopathy and fatty changes in various organs, especially the liver. The incidence of Reye syndrome has declined sharply since the 1980s, coinciding with increased public awareness of the association between ingestion of aspirin or aspirin-containing products during illness and subsequent development of Reye syndrome.[23]

An overview of Reye syndrome is important for the following reasons: (1) it may be considered a prototype for acute hepatic encephalopathies, (2) the potential for recurrence is a factor, and (3) the use of acetaminophen rather than aspirin should be considered important and discussed with the parents when obtaining a history.

Typically, Reye syndrome develops in a previously healthy child who is recovering from varicella, influenza B, upper respiratory infection, or gastroenteritis. The manifestations of the various clinical states are as follows:

Stage I: vomiting, lethargy, drowsiness

Stage II: disorientation, delirium, aggressiveness and combativeness, central neurologic hyperventilation, shallow breathing, hyperactive reflexes, stupor

Stage III: obtundation, coma, hyperventilation, decorticate rigidity

Stage IV: deepening coma, decerebrate rigidity, loss of ocular reflexes, large fixed pupils, divergent eye movements

Stage V: seizures, loss of deep tendon reflexes, flaccidity, respiratory arrest

Treatment and outcome depend on the stage of development at diagnosis and the individual child's symptoms.

Intoxications of the central nervous system

Drug-induced encephalopathies must always be considered a possibility in the child with unexplained neurologic changes. Such encephalopathies may result from accidental ingestion, therapeutic overdosage, intentional overdose, or ingestion of environmental toxins (the most commonly ingested poisons are listed in Table 16-6). About 1.5 million childhood poisonings that require medical attention occur each year. Approximately 100 children die each year of poisonings.[24]

High blood levels of lead occur in lead poisoning. If lead poisoning is untreated, lead encephalopathy results and is responsible for serious and irreversible neurologic damage (Figure 16-7). Those at greatest risk are 2- to 3-year-olds and children prone to **pica,** the habitual, purposeful, and compulsive ingestion of nonfood substances, such as clay, dirt, and paint chips. Lead intoxication also may occur from chronic exposure to smelters, sniffing of gasoline, and ingestion of airborne lead.[25]

An estimated 434,000 children aged 1 to 5 years in the United States (2.2% of children 1 month to 5 years of age) have excessive amounts of lead in their blood.[26] Black children have a five times greater incidence of symptoms than white children. Most lead exposures are preventable.

TABLE 16-5

Major Types of Seizure Disorders Found in Children

Disorder	Pathology
SEIZURE TYPES	First clinical manifestations indicate that seizure activity starts in or involves both cerebral hemispheres; consciousness may be impaired
CONVULSIVE ACTIVITY	
Tonic-clonic	Musculature stiffens, then intense jerking as trunk and extremities undergo rhythmic contraction and relaxation
Atonic	Sudden, momentary loss of muscle tone; drop attacks
Myoclonic	Sudden, brief contractures of a muscle or group of muscles
NONCONVULSIVE ACTIVITY	
Absence	Brief loss of consciousness with minimal or no loss of muscle tone; may experience 20 or more episodes a day lasting approximately 5-10 seconds each; may have minor movement, such as lip smacking, twitching of eyelids
EPILEPSY SYNDROMES	Seizure disorders that display a group of signs and symptoms that occur collectively and characterize or indicate a particular condition
Infantile spasm (West syndrome)	Form of epilepsy with episodes of sudden flexion or extension involving the neck, trunk, and extremities; clinical manifestations range from subtle head nods to violent body contractions (jackknife seizures); onset between 3 and 12 mo of age; may be idiopathic or in response to CNS insult; spasms occur in clusters of 5 to 150 times per day; increases with time
Lennox-Gastaut syndrome	Epileptic syndrome with onset in early childhood, 1-5 yr of age; includes various generalized seizures—tonic-clonic, atonic (drop attacks), akinetic, absence, and myoclonic; results in mental retardation and delayed psychomotor developments
PARTIAL SEIZURE TYPES	Seizure activity that begins and usually is limited to one part of the left or right hemisphere
Simple	Seizure activity that occurs without loss of consciousness
Complex	Seizure activity that occurs with impairment of consciousness
UNCLASSIFIED EPILEPTIC SEIZURES	Wide variety of abnormal clinical activity, including rhythmic eye movements, chewing, and swimming movements; common in neonatal seizures
Neonatal seizures	
Febrile seizures	
Pseudoseizures	
STATUS EPILEPTICUS	Continuing or recurring seizure activity in which recovery from the seizure activity is incomplete; unrelenting seizure activity can last 30 min or more; other forms can evolve into status epilepticus; medical emergency that requires immediate intervention
Nonconvulsive	
Convulsive	

TABLE 16-6

Commonly Ingested Poisons

Pharmacologic Agents	Heavy Metals	Miscellaneous Agents
Acetaminophen	Lead	Botulism toxin
Amphetamines	Acute	Alcohols
Anticonvulsants	Chronic	Ethyl
Antidepressants	Mercury	Isopropyl
Antihistamines	Thallium	Methyl
Atropine	Arsenic	Pesticides
Barbiturates		Organophosphates
Methadone		Chlorinated hydrocarbons
Phencyclidine		Mushrooms
Salicylates		Venoms
Tranquilizers		Snakebite
		Tick bites
		Ethylene glycol

From Swaiman KF: *Pediatric neurology: principles and practice*, ed 3, vol 2, St Louis, 1999, Mosby.

HEALTH ALERT

Iron and Cognitive Function

Iron deficiency is the single most significant nutrient deficiency, affecting 15% of the world population and causing anemia in 40% to 50% of children. Iron is essential for neurologic activity, including synthesis of dopamine, serotonin, catecholamine, and, possibly, myelin formation. Children with iron deficiency have decreased attentiveness, narrow attention spans, and perceptual restrictions. In some studies, cognitive deficits caused by iron deficiency can be reversed with iron supplements. Continued research is in progress to determine effects of acute versus chronic iron deficiency and the relationship between severity of deficiency and cognitive functioning.

Data from Lozoff B et al: Long-lasting neural and behavioral effects of iron deficiency in infancy, *Nutr Rev* 64(5 Pt 2):S34–S43, discussion S72–S91, 2006.

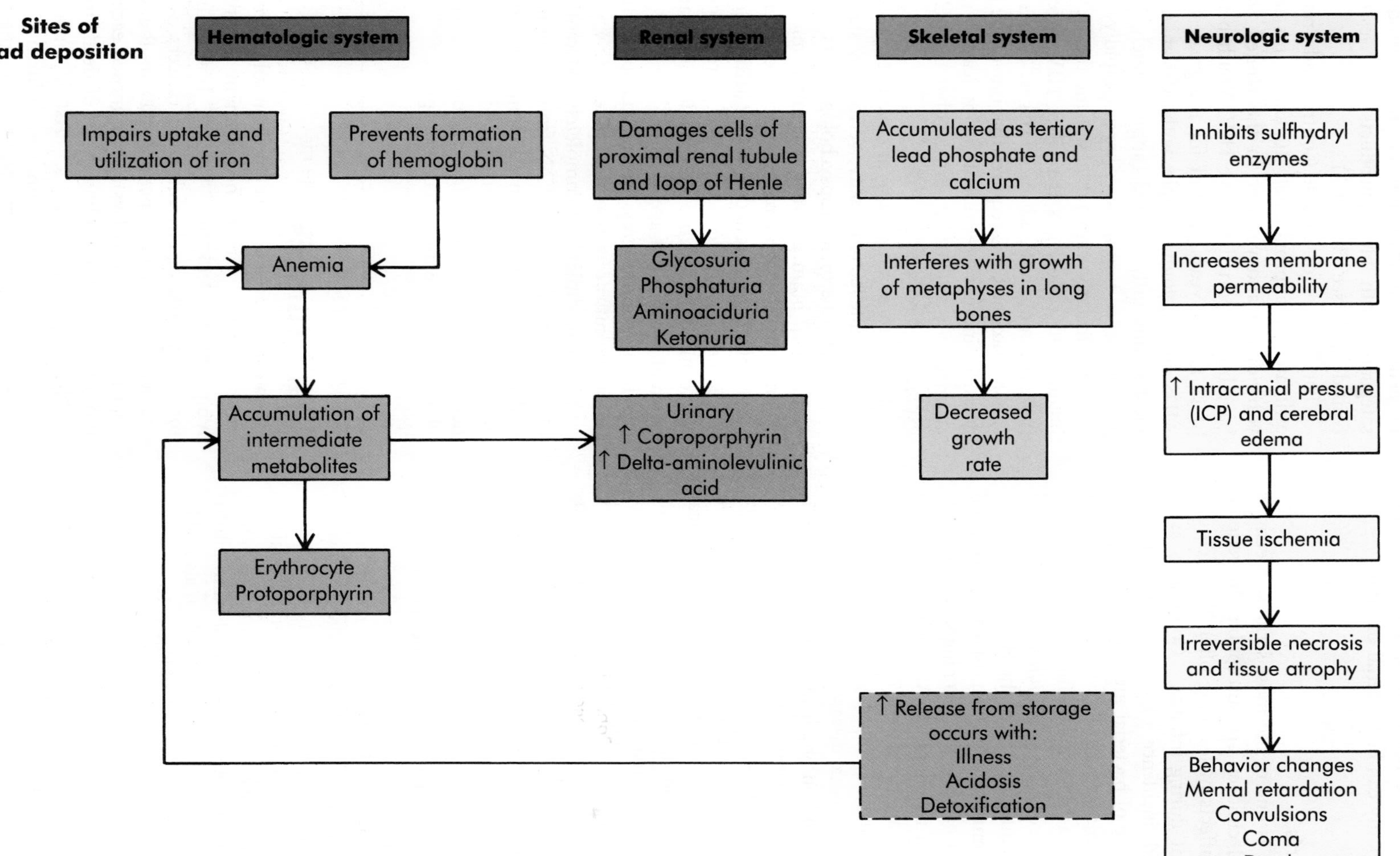

Figure 16-7 ■ **Systemic Effects of Increased Lead Absorption in Children.**

Meningitis

Meningitis refers to the inflammation of the meningeal coverings of the brain. The origin of such inflammation and acute encephalopathy can be bacterial or viral.

Bacterial meningitis

Bacterial meningitis is one of the most serious infections to which infants and children are susceptible. In general, bacterial meningitis affects males more often than females and is most prevalent during infancy.[27] Conditions associated with increased incidence of respiratory infection heighten the occurrence of bacterial meningitis.

Haemophilus influenzae type B was once the most common pathogen of bacterial meningitis in children younger than 5 years. The occurrence of *H. influenza* has declined dramatically since the introduction of the Hib vaccine.[28-32]

Now the most common organism to cause bacterial meningitis is *Neisseria meningitidis* (meningococcus)—60% of all pediatric cases of meningitis.[33] Approximately 2% to 5% of healthy children are carriers of *N. meningitidis.* The risk of developing meningitis from day-care center contact of children with meningococcal disease is 1 per 1000.[34]

The second most common organism that causes meningitis is *Streptococcus pneumoniae,* which is likely to be found in children older than 4 years. Staphylococcal or streptococcal meningitis shows a predilection for children who have had neurosurgery, skull fracture, or a complication of systemic bacterial infection. Infections that originate in the middle ear, sinuses, or mastoid cells also may lead to *S. pneumoniae* in children. In addition, 1 in every 24 children with sickle cell disease develops pneumococcal meningitis by the age of 4 years. *Escherichia coli* and group B β-hemolytic streptococci are the most common causes of meningitis in the newborn.

Viral meningitis

The hallmark of **viral meningitis,** or aseptic meningitis, is a mononuclear response in the CSF and the presence of normal sugar as well. Viral meningitis may result from a direct infection of a virus, or it may be secondary to disease, such as measles, mumps, herpes, or leukemia.

Onset of symptoms may be sudden or gradual. Malaise, fever, headache and stiff neck, abdominal pain, and nausea and vomiting are common. Sore throat, chest pain, photophobia, and maculopapular rash can develop also. The child usually recovers spontaneously within 3 to 10 days. Treatment is usually symptomatic.

HUMAN IMMUNODEFICIENCY VIRUS AND CENTRAL NERVOUS SYSTEM INVOLVEMENT

Infants and children have become infected with human immunodeficiency virus (HIV) through a variety of sources, including the placenta, exposure to infected maternal blood and vaginal secretions, and postpartum ingestion of breast milk.[35] Perinatal transmission accounts for up to 90% of pediatric acquired immunodeficiency syndrome (AIDS) cases in the United States. Infection also can occur as a result of being given contaminated blood products, although safeguards with blood products have lessened this risk considerably (see Chapter 7).

The Centers for Disease Control and Prevention (CDC) estimate that approximately 10,000 infants and children 13 years of age and younger in the United States currently have been reported to have HIV. Youth between the ages of 13 and 24 years account for the greatest proportion of AIDS among young people, with African-American youth most significantly affected (approximately 32,000 cases).[36] This incidence continues to increase rapidly (see Chapter 7).

A particularly vulnerable site for the HIV infection in infants and children is the CNS. HIV encephalopathy is more common in the advanced stages.[37] The revised classification from the CDC requires that one of the following progressive findings be present for at least 2 months in the absence of a concurrent illness other than HIV that could explain the findings:

1. Failure to attain or loss of developmental milestones or loss of intellectual ability, verified by standard developmental scale or neuropsychologic tests
2. Impaired brain growth or acquired microcephaly demonstrated by head circumference measurements or brain atrophy demonstrated by CT or MRI, with serial imaging required in children less than 2 years of age
3. Acquired symmetric motor deficits manifested by a child 1 month of age or older[38]

The onset of progressive encephalopathy may be a prognostic indicator of a poor outcome.

It may be difficult to completely differentiate the impact of HIV infection on the CNS from the impact of prenatal and perinatal exposure. In addition, other insults probably accompany HIV in a young child and affect growth and development, such as drug exposure, prematurity, chronic illness, and a chaotic social atmosphere.[39,40]

TUMORS

Brain Tumors

Brain tumors are the most common solid tumor and are the most common primary neoplasm in children, surpassing lymphoblastic leukemia. Overall, brain tumors account for nearly 20% of all childhood cancers, with an annual incidence of 2.4 to 4 per 100,000 in the United States; approximately 2000 cases are diagnosed each year.[41] Brain tumors remain the leading cause of death from disease in children ages 1 to 15 years.[42] Astrocytomas are the most common type of brain tumor in children.[43]

The cause of brain tumors is largely unknown, although genetic, environmental, and immune factors have been implicated in some tumor development. Factors that have been investigated as the cause of brain tumors include familial tendencies, radiation, oncologic viruses, and chemical carcinogens.[44] An important area of study has been investigation of the relationship of parental occupation to subsequent brain tumors in offspring. Associations have been found among children with tumors and parents exposed to hydrocarbons and employed in the aircraft and paper/pulp industries. Alterations in embryologic development also may play a part in the development of childhood brain tumors.

Two thirds of all pediatric brain tumors are found in the posterior fossa (infratentorial) region of the brain, and approximately one third of childhood brain tumors are located in the supratentorial space. Brain tumors can arise from any CNS cell, and tumors are classified by cell type. The types and characteristics of childhood brain tumors are summarized in Table 16-7.

Medulloblastoma, ependymoma, astrocytoma, brain stem glioma, craniopharyngioma, and optic nerve glioma make up approximately 75% to 80% of all pediatric brain tumors. Most brain tumors in children are located in the posterior fossa (Figure 16-8); treatment strategies and prognosis are listed in Table 16-8.

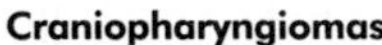

TABLE 16-7

Brain Tumors in Children

Type	Characteristics
Astrocytoma	Arises from astrocytes, often in the cerebellum or lateral hemisphere Slow growing, solid or cystic Often very large before diagnosed Varies in degree of malignancy
Optic nerve glioma	Arises from optic chiasm or optic nerve Slow growing, low-grade astrocytoma
Medulloblastoma (infiltrating glioma)	Often located in cerebellum, extending into fourth ventricle and spinal fluid pathway Rapidly growing malignant tumor Can extend outside CNS
Brain stem glioma	Arises from pons or myelencephalon Numerous cell types Compresses cranial nerves V through X
Ependymoma	Arises from ependymal cells lining ventricles Circumscribed, solid, nodular tumors
Craniopharyngioma	Arises near pituitary gland, optic chiasm, and hypothalamus Cystic and solid tumors that affect vision, pituitary, and hypothalamic functions

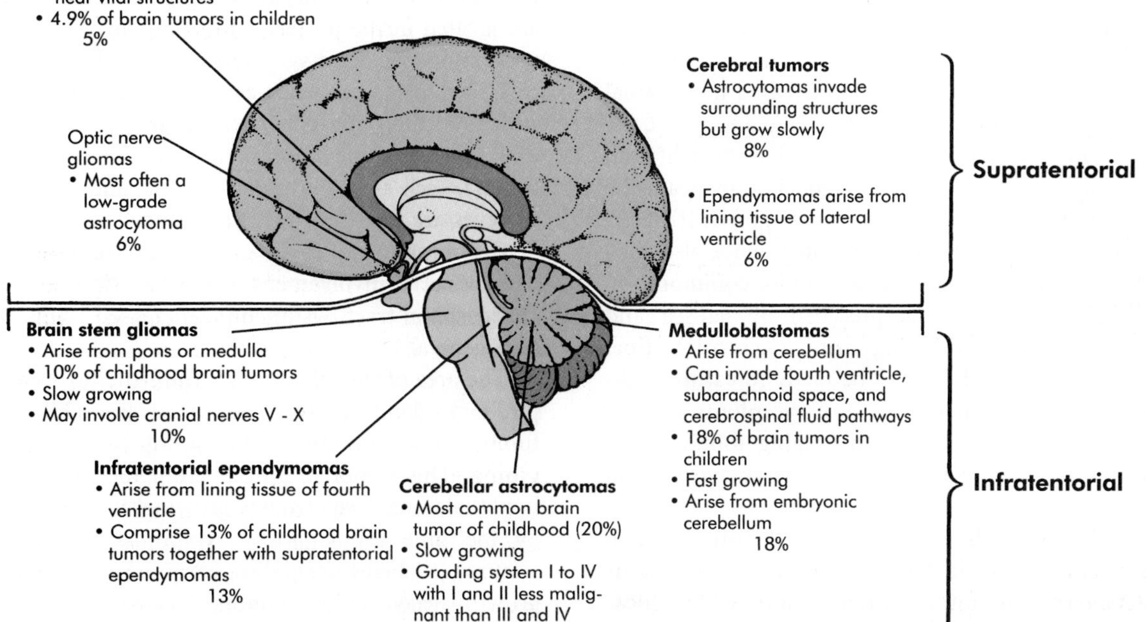
Craniopharyngiomas
• Located adjacent to the sella turcica (structure containing the pituitary gland), often considered to lie supratentorial
• Considered to have benign properties but is life threatening because of its location near vital structures
• 4.9% of brain tumors in children
5%
Optic nerve gliomas
• Most often a low-grade astrocytoma
6%
Cerebral tumors
• Astrocytomas invade surrounding structures but grow slowly
8%
• Ependymomas arise from lining tissue of lateral ventricle
6%
Supratentorial
Brain stem gliomas
• Arise from pons or medulla
• 10% of childhood brain tumors
• Slow growing
• May involve cranial nerves V - X
10%
Infratentorial ependymomas
• Arise from lining tissue of fourth ventricle
• Comprise 13% of childhood brain tumors together with supratentorial ependymomas
13%
Cerebellar astrocytomas
• Most common brain tumor of childhood (20%)
• Slow growing
• Grading system I to IV with I and II less malignant than III and IV
20%
Medulloblastomas
• Arise from cerebellum
• Can invade fourth ventricle, subarachnoid space, and cerebrospinal fluid pathways
• 18% of brain tumors in children
• Fast growing
• Arise from embryonic cerebellum
18%
Infratentorial

Figure 16-8 ■ **Location of Brain Tumors in Children.**

TABLE 16-8

Treatment Strategies for Childhood Brain Tumors

Tumor Type	Treatment and Prognosis
Cerebellar astrocytoma	Surgery; possibly curative Radiation and chemotherapy not proved successful but may delay recurrence Survival rate of more than 5 yr in 50%-75%; if tumor recurs, it does so very slowly
Medulloblastoma	Surgery, primarily as a partial resection to relieve increased intracranial pressure and "debulk" the tumor Type of treatment is age dependent Radiation as the primary treatment; may include spinal radiation Chemotherapy showing some promise in conjunction with craniospinal radiation* 35% 5-yr survival rate
Brain stem glioma	Surgery, resection occasionally possible Radiation, primarily palliative treatment Chemotherapy not yet proved beneficial, but new protocols being studied 20%-40% 5-yr survival rate
Ependymoma	Tumor possibly indolent for many years Surgery rarely curative; risk of resecting an infratentorial tumor too great Radiation for palliation (current controversy over whether local or craniospinal radiation is best) Chemotherapy used for recurrent disease but with disappointing results 20%-80% 5-yr survival rate dependent on total resection
Craniopharyngioma	Surgery possibly successful when a complete resection is performed (partial resection usually requires further treatment) Radiation after partial surgical resection Chemotherapy not commonly used 75%-85% 5-yr survival rate
Optic nerve glioma	Initial treatment controversial Surgery used for diagnosis or relief of hydrocephalus Radiation useful, particularly if tumor not treated by surgery
Cerebral astrocytoma	Surgery used if resection is possible Radiation useful for all grades of astrocytoma Chemotherapy beneficial in higher grade tumors but further study required

*Reddy AT, Packer RJ: Pediatric central nervous system tumors, *Curr Opin Oncol* 10(3):186–193, 1998.

Signs and symptoms of brain tumors in children vary from generalized and vague to localized and related specifically to an anatomic area. Signs of increased intracranial pressure may occur, including headache, vomiting, lethargy, and irritability. If a young child complains of repeated and worsening headache, a thorough investigation should take place because headache is an uncommon complaint in young children. Headache caused by increased intracranial pressure usually is worse in the morning and gradually improves during the day when the child is upright and venous drainage is enhanced. The frequency of headache and other symptoms worsens as the tumor grows. Irritability or possible apathy and increased somnolence also may result. Like headache, vomiting occurs more commonly in the morning. Often it is *not* preceded by nausea and may become projectile, differing from a gastrointestinal disturbance in that the child may be ready to eat immediately after vomiting. Other signs and symptoms include increased head circumference with bulging fontanelle in the child younger than 2 years, cranial nerve palsies, and papilledema (Box 16-1).

Localized findings relate to the degree of disturbance in physiologic functioning in the area where the tumor is located. Children with infratentorial tumors exhibit localized signs of impaired coordination and balance, including ataxia, gait difficulties, truncal ataxia, and loss of balance. **Medulloblastoma** occurs as an invasive malignant tumor that develops in the vermis of the cerebellum and may extend into the fourth ventricle. **Ependymoma** develops in the fourth ventricle and arises from the ependymal cells that line the ventricular system. Because both tumors are located in the posterior fossa region along the midline, presenting signs and symptoms are similar.

In contrast, **cerebellar astrocytomas** are located on the surface of the right or left cerebellar hemisphere and cause unilateral symptoms (occurring on the same side as the tumor), such as head tilt, limb ataxia, and nystagmus when the eyes are turned toward the tumor.

Brain stem gliomas often cause a combination of cranial nerve involvement, cerebellar signs of ataxia, and corticospinal tract dysfunction. Increased intracranial pressure generally does not occur.

The area of the sella turcica, the structure containing the pituitary gland, is the site of several childhood brain tumors; most common of this group is the **craniopharyngioma.** This tumor originates from the pituitary gland or hypothalamus. Usually slow growing, it may be quite large by the time of diagnosis. Symptoms include headache, seizures, diabetes insipidus, early onset of puberty, and growth delay. Other tumors located in this region of the brain include **optic gliomas.** Tumors that involve the optic tract may cause complete unilateral blindness and

BOX 16-1 Clinical Manifestations of Brain Tumors

Headache
Recurrent and progressive
In frontal or occipital areas
Worse on arising, less during the day
Intensified by lowering head and straining, such as during bowel movement, coughing, sneezing

Vomiting
With or without nausea or feeding
Progressively more projectile
More severe in morning
Relieved by moving about and changing position

Neuromuscular Changes
Incoordination or clumsiness
Loss of balance (use of wide-based stance, falling, tripping, banging into object)
Poor fine motor control
Weakness
Hyporeflexia or hyperreflexia
Positive Babinski sign
Spasticity
Paralysis

Behavioral Changes
Irritability
Decreased appetite
Failure to thrive
Fatigue (frequent naps)
Lethargy
Coma
Bizarre behavior (staring, automatic movements)

Cranial Nerve Neuropathy
Cranial nerve involvement varies according to tumor location
Most common signs
- Head tilt
- Visual defects (nystagmus, diplopia, strabismus, episodic "graying out" of vision, and visual field defects)

Vital Sign Disturbances
Decreased pulse and respiration
Increased blood pressure
Decreased pulse pressure
Hypothermia or hyperthermia

Other Signs
Seizures
Cranial enlargement*
Tense, bulging fontanelle at rest*
Nuchal rigidity
Papilledema (edema of optic nerve)

From Hockenberry MN: *Wong's essentials of pediatric nursing*, ed 7, St Louis, 2005, Mosby.
*Present only in infants and young children.

hemianopia of the other eye. Optic atrophy is another common finding. Supratentorial tumors of the cerebral hemispheres in children are uncommon.

Embryonal Tumors

Neuroblastoma

Neuroblastoma is an embryonal tumor originating in neural crest cells that normally give rise to the sympathetic ganglia and the adrenal medulla. Because neuroblastoma involves a defect of embryonal tissue, it most commonly is diagnosed during the first 2 years of life, and 75% of neuroblastomas are found before the child is 5 years old. Occasionally, these tumors have been diagnosed at birth with metastasis apparent in the placenta. It is seen more commonly in white children (9.6 per million) than in black children (7 per million). Although it accounts for only 8% to 10% of pediatric malignancies,[45] neuroblastoma causes 15% of cancer deaths in children.

Neuroblastoma is the most common and immature form of the sympathetic nervous system tumors. Areas of necrosis and calcification often are present in the tumor. More than with any other cancer, neuroblastoma has been associated with spontaneous remission, commonly in infants who have liver, bone marrow, or skin involvement in addition to the primary site.[46]

Although familial tendency has been noted in individual cases, a nonfamilial or sporadic pattern is found in most children with neuroblastoma. Familial cases of neuroblastoma are considered to have an autosomal dominant pattern of inheritance (mechanisms of inheritance are discussed in Chapter 2).

The most common location of neuroblastoma is in the retroperitoneal region (65% of cases), most often the adrenal medulla. The tumor is evident as an abdominal mass and may cause anorexia, bowel and bladder alteration, and sometimes spinal cord compression.

The second most common location of neuroblastoma is the mediastinum (area separating the lungs) (15% of cases). There the tumor may cause dyspnea or infection related to airway obstruction. Less commonly, neuroblastoma may arise from the cervical sympathetic ganglion (3% to 4% of cases). Cervical neuroblastoma often causes Horner syndrome, which consists of miosis (pupil contraction), ptosis (drooping eyelid), enophthalmos (backward displacement of the eyeball), and anhidrosis (sweat deficiency).

A number of systemic signs and symptoms are characteristic of neuroblastoma, including weight loss, irritability, fatigue, and fever. Intractable diarrhea occurs in 7% to 9% of children and is caused by tumor secretion of a hormone called *vasoactive intestinal polypeptide (VIP).*

More than 90% of children with neuroblastoma have increased amounts of catecholamines and associated metabolites in their urine. High levels of urinary catecholamines and serum ferritin are associated with a poorer prognosis.

Retinoblastoma

Retinoblastoma is a rare congenital eye tumor of young children that originates in the retina of one or both eyes

(Figure 16-9). Two forms of retinoblastoma are exhibited: inherited and acquired. The inherited form of the disease generally is diagnosed during the first year of life. The acquired disease most commonly is diagnosed in children 2 to 3 years of age and involves unilateral disease.

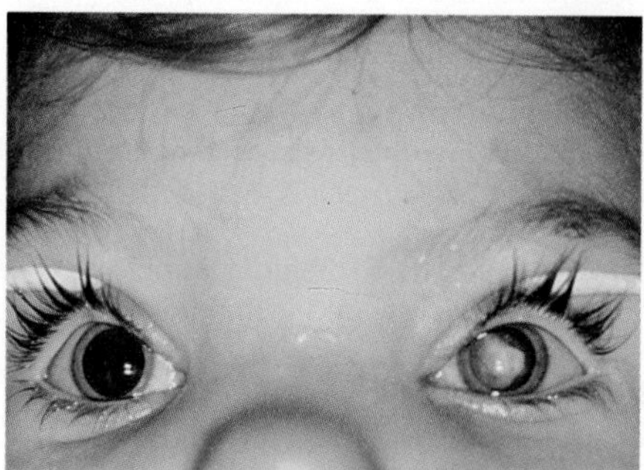

Figure 16-9 ■ **Retinoblastoma.** The tumor occupies a large portion of the inside of the eye bulbus. (From Damjanov I: *Pathology for the health professions,* ed 3, St Louis, 2006, Saunders. Courtesy Dr. Walter Richardson and Dr. Jamsheed Khan, Kansas City, Kansas.)

Approximately 40% of retinoblastomas are inherited as an autosomal dominant trait with incomplete penetrance (see Figure 2-2). The remaining 60% are acquired. In the early 1970s, Knudson proposed the "two-hit" hypothesis to explain the occurrence of both hereditary and acquired forms of the disease.[47] This hypothesis predicts that two separate transforming events or "hits" must occur in a normal retinoblast cell to cause the cancer. Further, it proposes that in the inherited form, the first hit or mutation occurs in the germ cell (inherited from either parent), and the mutation is contained in every cell of the child's body. Only a second, random mutation in a retinoblast cell is needed to transform that cell into cancer. Multiple tumors are observed in the inherited form because these second mutations are likely to occur in several of the approximately 1 to 2 million retinoblast cells. In contrast, the acquired form of retinoblastoma requires two independent hits or mutations to occur in the same somatic cell (after the egg is fertilized) for the transformation to cancer. This is much less likely to happen. Figure 16-10 illustrates the two-mutation model for these two patterns of mutation.

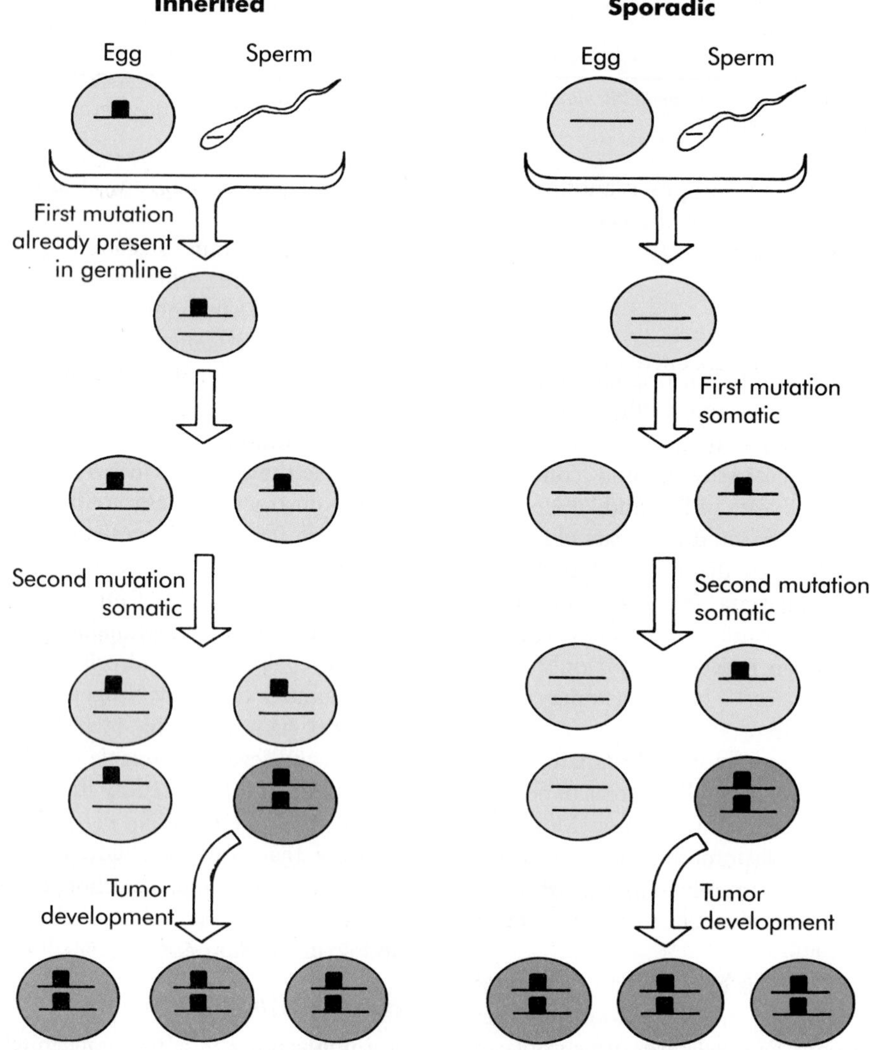

Figure 16-10 ■ **The Two-Mutation Model of Retinoblastoma Development.** In inherited retinoblastoma, the first mutation is transmitted through the germline of an affected parent. The second mutation occurs somatically in a retinal cell, leading to development of the tumor. In sporadic retinoblastoma, development of a tumor requires two somatic mutations.

The primary sign of retinoblastoma is leukokoria, a white pupillary reflex also called *cat's eye reflex,* which is caused by the mass behind the lens (see Figure 16-9). Other signs and symptoms include strabismus, a red, painful eye, and limited vision.

Because retinoblastoma is a treatable tumor, dual priorities are saving the child's life and restoring useful vision. The prognosis for most children with retinoblastoma is excellent, with a greater than 90% long-term survival.

QUICK CHECK 16-3

1. Why are the principal symptoms of brain tumors in children related to brain stem function?

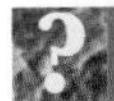

Did You Understand?

Normal Growth and Development of the Nervous System

1. Growth and development of the brain occur most rapidly during fetal development and during the first year of life.
2. The bones of the skull are joined by sutures, and the wide, membranous junctions of the sutures known as *fontanelles* allow for brain growth and close by 18 months of age.
3. At birth, neurologic function is primarily at the subcortical level with transition in reflexes as motor development progresses during the first year.

Structural Malformations

1. Defects of neural tube closure include anencephaly (absence of part of the skull and brain), encephalocele (herniation of the meninges and brain through a skull defect), meningocele (a saclike meningeal cyst that protrudes through a vertebral defect), and myelomeningocele also known as spina bifida (failure of the vertebrae to close and the resulting protrusion of neural tube contents).
2. Acrania is nearly complete absence of the cranial vault.
3. Premature closure of the cranial sutures causes craniosynostosis and prevents normal skull expansion, resulting in compression of growing brain tissue.
4. Microcephaly is lack of brain growth and retarded mental and motor development.
5. Congenital hydrocephalus results from an overproduction, impaired absorption, or blockage of circulation of cerebrospinal fluid. Dandy-Walker deformity is caused by cystic dilation of the fourth ventricle and aqueductal compression.

Encephalopathies

1. Static encephalopathies are nonprogressive disorders of the brain that can occur during gestation, birth, or childhood and can be caused by endogenous or exogenous factors.
2. Cerebral palsy can be caused by prenatal cerebral hypoxia or perinatal trauma, with symptoms of motor dysfunction including increased muscle tone, increased reflexes, and loss of fine motor coordination, mental retardation, seizure disorders, or developmental disabilities.
3. Inherited metabolic disorders that damage the nervous system include defects in amino acid metabolism (phenylketonuria) and lipid metabolism (Tay-Sachs disease) and result in abnormal behavior, seizures, and deficient psychomotor development.
4. Seizure disorders are abnormal discharges of electrical activity within the brain. They are associated with numerous nervous system disorders and more often are a generalized rather than a partial type of seizure.
5. Generalized forms of seizures include tonic-clonic, myoclonic, atonic, akinetic, and infantile spasms.
6. Partial seizures suggest more localized brain dysfunction.
7. Febrile seizures usually are limited to children ages 6 months to 3 years, with a pattern of one seizure per febrile illness.
8. Reye syndrome is an encephalopathy with fatty changes in the liver associated with influenza B, varicella viruses, and aspirin ingestion. Progressive manifestations include lethargy, stupor, rigidity, seizures, and respiratory arrest.
9. Accidental poisonings from a variety of toxins can cause serious neurologic damage.
10. Bacterial meningitis is commonly caused by *Neisseria meningitidis* or *Streptococcus pneumoniae* and may result from respiratory or gastrointestinal infections; symptoms include fever, headaches, photophobia, seizures, rigidity, and stupor.
11. Viral meningitis may result from direct infection or be secondary to a systemic viral infection (i.e., measles, mumps, herpes, or leukemia).

Human Immunodeficiency Virus and Central Nervous System Involvement

1. HIV may be transmitted to infants and children through the placenta, by exposure to infected blood or vaginal secretions, or by ingestion of infected breast milk.
2. The incidence of HIV among children is increasing. AIDS is most prevalent among youth ages 15 to 24 years.
3. The classic symptoms are related to progressive encephalopathy.

(Continued)

Did You Understand?—Cont'd

Tumors

1. Brain tumors are the most common tumors of the nervous system and the second most common type of childhood cancer.
2. Tumors in children most often are located below the tentorial plate.
3. Fast-growing tumors produce symptoms early in the disease, whereas slow-growing tumors may become very large before symptoms appear.
4. Symptoms of brain tumors may be generalized or localized. The most common general symptom is increased intracranial pressure (headache, irritability, vomiting, somnolence, bulging of fontanelles).
5. Localized signs of infratentorial tumors in the cerebellum include impaired coordination and balance. Cranial nerve signs occur with tumors in or near the brain stem.
6. Supratentorial tumors may be located near the cortex or deep in the brain. Symptoms depend on the specific location of the tumor.
7. Neuroblastoma is an embryonal tumor of the sympathetic nervous system and can be located anywhere there is sympathetic nervous tissue. Symptoms are related to tumor location and size of metastasis.
8. Retinoblastoma is a congenital eye tumor that has two forms: inherited and acquired.

Key Terms

References

1. Cabrera R et al: Investigations into the etiology of neural tube defects, *Birth Defects Res C Embryo Today* 72(4):330–344, 2004.
2. Kaufman B: Neural tube defects, *Pediatr Clin North Am* 51 (2):389–419, 2004.
3. Detrait E et al: Human neural tube defects: developmental biology, epidemiology, and genetics, *Neurotoxicol Teratol* 27 (3):515–524, 2005.
4. Quinn L, Thompson S, Ott MK: Application of the social ecological model; in folic acid public health initiatives, *J Obstet Gynecol Neonat Nurs* 34(6):672–681, 2005.
5. Rowland CA, Correa A, Cragan JD, Alverson CJ: Are encephaloceles neural tube defects? *Pediatrics* 118(3):916–923, 2006.
6. Behrman R, Kleigman R, Jenson H: *Nelson's textbook of pediatrics*, ed 17, Philadelphia, 2004, Saunders.
7. Stevenson K: Chiari type II malformation: past, present and future, *Neurosurg Focus* 16(2):E5, 2004.
8. Adzick N, Walsh D: Myelomeningocele: prenatal diagnosis, pathophysiology, and management, *Semin Pediatr Surg* 12 (2):168–174, 2003.
9. Wakhlu A, Ansari N: The predicting of postoperative hydrocephalus in patients with spina bifida, *Childs Nerv Syst* 20 (2):104–106, 2004.
10. Mitchell KE et al: Spina bifida, *Lancet* 364(9448):1885–1895, 2004.
11. Bruner JP et al: Intrauterine repair of spina bifida: preoperative predictors of shunt-dependent hydrocephalus, *Am J Obstet Gynecol* 190(5):1305–1312, 2004.
12. Cartwright C: Assessing asymmetrical infant head shapes, *Nurse Pract* 27(8):33, 35–36, 39, 2002.
13. Garton HJ, Piatt JH Jr: Hydrocephalus, *Pediatr Clin North Am* 51:305–325, 2004.
14. Kestle J: Pediatric hydrocephalus: current management, *Neurol Clin* 21(4):883–895, 2003.
15. Krigger KW: Cerebral palsy: an overview, *Am Fam Physician* 73(1):91–100, 2006.
16. Koman LA, Smith BP, Shilt JS: Cerebral palsy, *Lancet* 364 (9428):28, 2004.
17. Singhi PD: Cerebral palsy-management, *Indian J Pediatr* 71 (7):635–639, 2004.
18. Mijuskovic Z: Phenylketonuria. *Emedicine;* access Feb 2006 from www.emedicine.com/derm/topic712.htm.
19. Hodges BL, Cheng SH: Cell and gene-based therapies for the lysosomal storage diseases, *Curr Gene Ther* 6(2):227–241, 2006.
20. Edwards Q et al: Assessing ethnicity in preconception counseling: genetics—what nurse practitioners need to know, *J Am Acad Nurs Pract* 16(11):472–480, 2004.

References—Cont'd

21. Schmidt K: Phenylketonuria, In Jackson PL, Vessey JA, editors: *Primary care of the child with a chronic conditions*, ed 4, St Louis, 2003, Mosby.
22. Epilepsy Foundation of America: *Epilepsy and seizure stats;* accessed 2005 from www.epilepsyfoundation.org/answerplace/About-Epilepsy.cfm.
23. Monto AS: The disappearance of Reye's syndrome: a public health triumph, *N Engl J Med* 340(18):1423–1424, 1999.
24. Litovitz TL et al: 2001 Annual report of the American Association of Poison Control Centers Toxic Exposure Surveillance System, *Am J Emerg Med* 20(5):391–452, 2002.
25. Needleman H: Lead poisoning, *Annu Rev Med* 55:209–222, 2004.
26. Meyer PA et al: Surveillance for elevated blood lead levels among children—United States, 1997-2001, *MMWR Surveill Summ* 52(10):1–21, 2003.
27. Chang CJ et al: Bacterial meningitis in infants: the epidemiology, clinical features, and prognostic factors, *Brain Dev* 26 (3):168–175, 2004.
28. Progress toward elimination of *Haemophilus influenzae* type b invasive disease among infants and children—United States, 1998-2000, *MMWR* 51(11):234–237, 2000.
29. Hoekelman RA et al: *Primary pediatrics*, ed 4, St Louis, 2001, Mosby.
30. Victor M, Ropper AH: *Adam and Victor's principles of neurology*, ed 7, St Louis, 2001, Mosby.
31. Roos KL, Tyler KL: Bacterial meningitis and other suppurative infections, In Braunwald E, Fauci AS, Kasper DL et al, editors: *Harrison's principles of internal medicine* ed 15, vol. 2, New York, 2001, McGraw-Hill.
32. Rakel RE: *Textbook of family practice*,, ed 6, Philadelphia, 2002, Mosby.
33. Zimmer SM, Stephens DS: Meningococcal conjugate vaccines, *Expert Opin Pharmacother* 5(4):855–863, 2005.
34. Nigrovic LE, Kuppermann N, Malley R: Development and validation of a multivariable predictive model to distinguish bacterial from aseptic meningitis in children in post-*Haemophilus influenzae* era, *Pediatrics* 110(4):712–719, 2002.
35. Newell ML, Brahmbhatt HH, Ghys PD: Child mortality and HIV infection in Africa: a review, *AIDS* 18(suppl 2):S27–S34, 2004.
36. Centers for Disease Control and Prevention: *HIV/AIDS among youth*, Atlanta, GA, 2003, CDCwww.cdc.gov/hiv/pubs/facts/youth.htm.
37. Foster CJ et al: Neurodevelopmental outcomes in children with HIV infection under 3 years of age, *Dev Med Child Neurol* 48(8):677–682, 2006.
38. Centers for Disease Control and Prevention: Revised classification system for human immunodeficiency virus infection on children less than 13 years of age, *MMWR* 43(rr12):1–10, 1994.
39. Fahrner R: Pediatric HIV infections and AIDS. In Jackson PL, Vessey JA, editors: *Primary care of the child with a chronic condition*, ed 4, St Louis, 2003, Mosby.
40. Tardieu M et al: HIV-1 related encephalopathy in infants compared with children and adults, *Neurology* 54(5): 1089–1095, 2000.
41. Walter AW: Brain tumors in children, *Curr Oncol Rep* 6 (6):438–444, 2004.
42. Kline ME: Solid tumors in children, *J Pediatr Nurs* 18 (2):96–102, 2003.
43. Burzynski SR: Treatments for astrocytic tumors in children: current and emerging strategies, *Paediatr Drugs* 8(3): 167–178, 2006.
44. Pediatric Brain Tumor Foundation: *Facts about pediatric brain tumors*, North Carolina, 2006, Ashvillehttp://www.pbtfus.org/medcomm/research/facts.html.
45. Schwab M et al: Neuroblastoma: biology and molecular and chromosomal pathology, *Lancet Oncol* 41(8):472–489, 2004.
46. Weinstein JL, Katzenstein HM, Cohn SL: Advances in the diagnosis and treatment of neuroblastoma, *Oncologist* 8 (3):278–292, 2003.
47. Knudson AG Jr: Mutation and cancer: a statistical study of retinoblastoma, *Proc Natl Acad Sc U S A* 68(4):820–823, 1971.

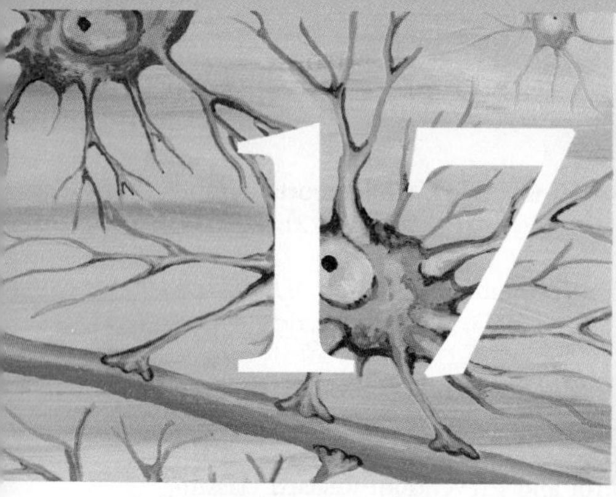

17 MECHANISMS OF HORMONAL REGULATION

Valentina L. Brashers ▪ Sue E. Huether

CHAPTER OUTLINE

ELECTRONIC RESOURCES

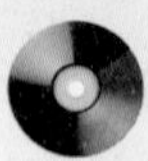

Companion CD
- Review Questions and Answers
- Animations

evolve Website
http://evolve.elsevier.com/Huether/
- Quick Check Answers
- Key Terms Exercises
- Critical Thinking Questions with Answers
- Algorithm Completion Exercises
- WebLinks

The endocrine system is composed of various glands located throughout the body (Figure 17-1). These glands can synthesize and release special chemical messengers called hormones. The endocrine system has five general functions: (1) differentiation of the reproductive and central nervous systems in the developing fetus; (2) stimulation of sequential growth and development during childhood and adolescence; (3) coordination of the male and female reproductive systems, which makes sexual reproduction possible; (4) maintenance of an optimal internal environment throughout life; and (5) initiation of corrective and adaptive responses when emergency demands occur. Hormones convey specific regulatory information among cells and organs and are integrated with the nervous system to maintain communication and control. The mechanisms of communication include autocrine (within cell), paracrine (between local cells), and endocrine (between remote cells).

MECHANISMS OF HORMONAL REGULATION

The endocrine glands respond to specific signals by synthesizing and releasing **hormones** into the circulation, which then trigger intracellular responses. All hormones share certain general characteristics:

1. Have specific rates and rhythms of secretion. Three basic secretion patterns are (a) diurnal patterns, (b) pulsatile and cyclic patterns, and (c) patterns that depend on levels of circulating substrates (e.g., calcium, sodium, potassium, or the hormones themselves). Diurnal, pulsatile, and cyclic patterns of hormone release involve consistent patterns of secretion.
2. Operate within feedback systems, either positive or negative, to maintain an optimal internal environment.
3. Affect only target cells with specific receptors for the hormone and then act on these cells to initiate specific cell functions or activities.
4. Are constantly excreted by the kidneys or are deactivated by the liver or cellular mechanisms.

Hormones may be classified according to structure, gland of origin, effects, or chemical composition. (Table 17-1 categorizes known hormones based on structure.) The secretion and mechanisms of action of hormones represent an extremely complex system of integrated responses. The endocrine and nervous systems work together to regulate responses to the internal and external environments.

Regulation of Hormone Release

Hormones are released either in response to an altered cellular environment or in the maintenance of a regulated level of another hormone or substance. One or more of the following mechanisms regulates hormone release: (1) chemical factors (such as blood sugar or calcium levels), (2) endocrine factors (a hormone from one endocrine gland controlling another endocrine gland), and (3) neural control. For example, insulin is secreted in response to increased glucose levels (a chemical stimulus), to direct stimulation of the insulin-secreting cells of the pancreas by the autonomic nervous system (a neural stimulus), and to the secretion of cortisol by the adrenal medulla, a form of endocrine regulation.

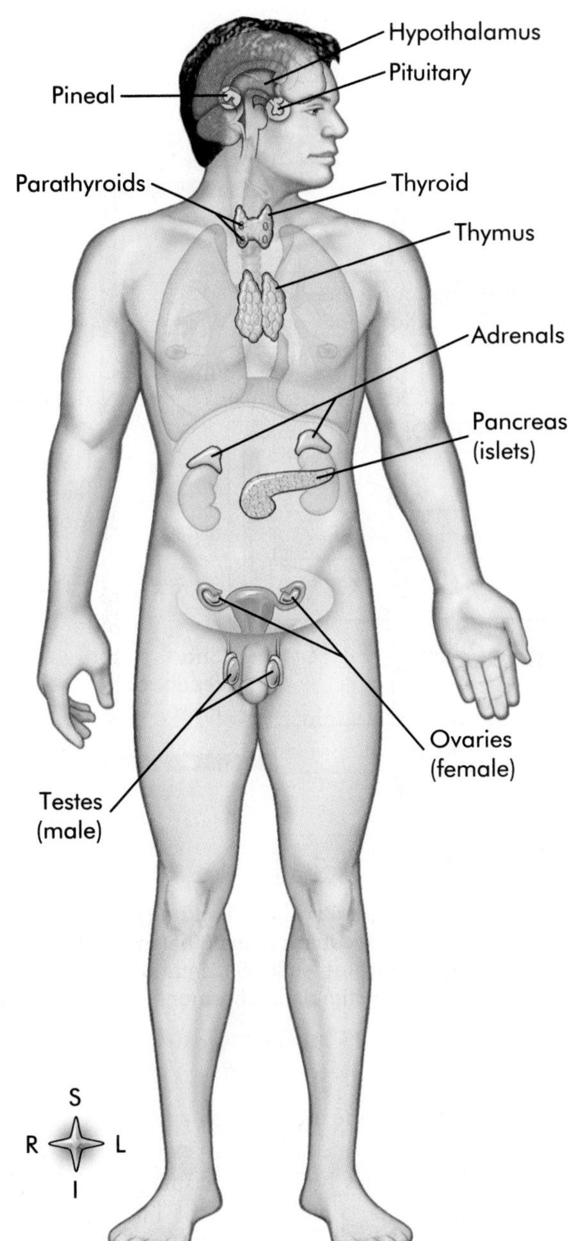

Figure 17-1 ■ **Principal Endocrine Glands.** (From Thibodeau GA, Patton KT: *Anatomy & physiology,* ed 6, St Louis, 2007, Mosby.)

Feedback systems provide precise monitoring and control of the cellular environment. The most common feedback system, **negative feedback,** occurs because the rising hormone level negates the initiating change that triggered the release of the hormone. An example of hormone negative feedback is shown in Figure 17-2, *A*. Increased anterior pituitary release of thyroid-stimulating hormone (TSH) stimulates the synthesis and secretion of thyroid hormones. TSH secretion is regulated by thyrotropin-releasing hormone primarily in the hypothalamus and by negative feedback inhibition from thyroid hormones. TSH is inhibited by thyroxine (T_4) and to a lesser extent by triiodothyronine (T_3). Negative-feedback systems are important in maintaining hormones within physiologic ranges. The lack of negative-feedback inhibition on hormonal release often results in pathologic conditions. As discussed in Chapter 18, various hormonal imbalances and related conditions are caused by excessive hormone production, which is the result of failure to "turn off" the system. These negative-feedback regulatory systems are diagrammed in Figure 17-2, *B*.

TABLE 17-1

Structural Categories of Hormones

Structural Category	Examples
WATER SOLUBLE	
Peptides	Growth hormone
	Insulin
	Leptin
	Parathyroid hormone
	Prolactin
Glycoproteins	Follicle-stimulating hormone
	Luteinizing hormone
	Thyroid-stimulating hormone
Polypeptides	Adrenocorticotropic hormone
	Antidiuretic hormone
	Calcitonin
	Endorphins
	Glucagon
	Hypothalamic hormones
	Lipotropins
	Melanocyte-stimulating hormone
	Oxytocin
	Somatostatin
	Thymosin
	Thyrotropin-releasing hormone
Amines	Epinephrine
	Norepinephrine
LIPID SOLUBLE	
Thyroxine (an amine but lipid soluble)	Both thyroxine [T_4] and triiodothyronine [T_3])
Steroids (cholesterol is a precursor for all steroids)	Estrogens
	Glucocorticoids (cortisol)
	Mineralocorticoids (aldosterone)
	Progestins (progesterone)
	Testosterone
Derivatives of arachidonic acid (autocrine or paracrine action)	Leukotrienes
	Prostacyclins
	Prostaglandins
	Thromboxanes

Hormone Transport

Once hormones are released into the circulatory system, they are distributed throughout the body. The protein (peptide) hormones (Table 17-1) are water soluble and generally circulate in free (unbound) forms. This process immediately exposes these water-soluble hormones to circulating catabolizing enzymes, giving them an expected half-life of seconds to minutes. Lipid-soluble hormones (Table 17-1) are transported bound to a carrier or transport protein.

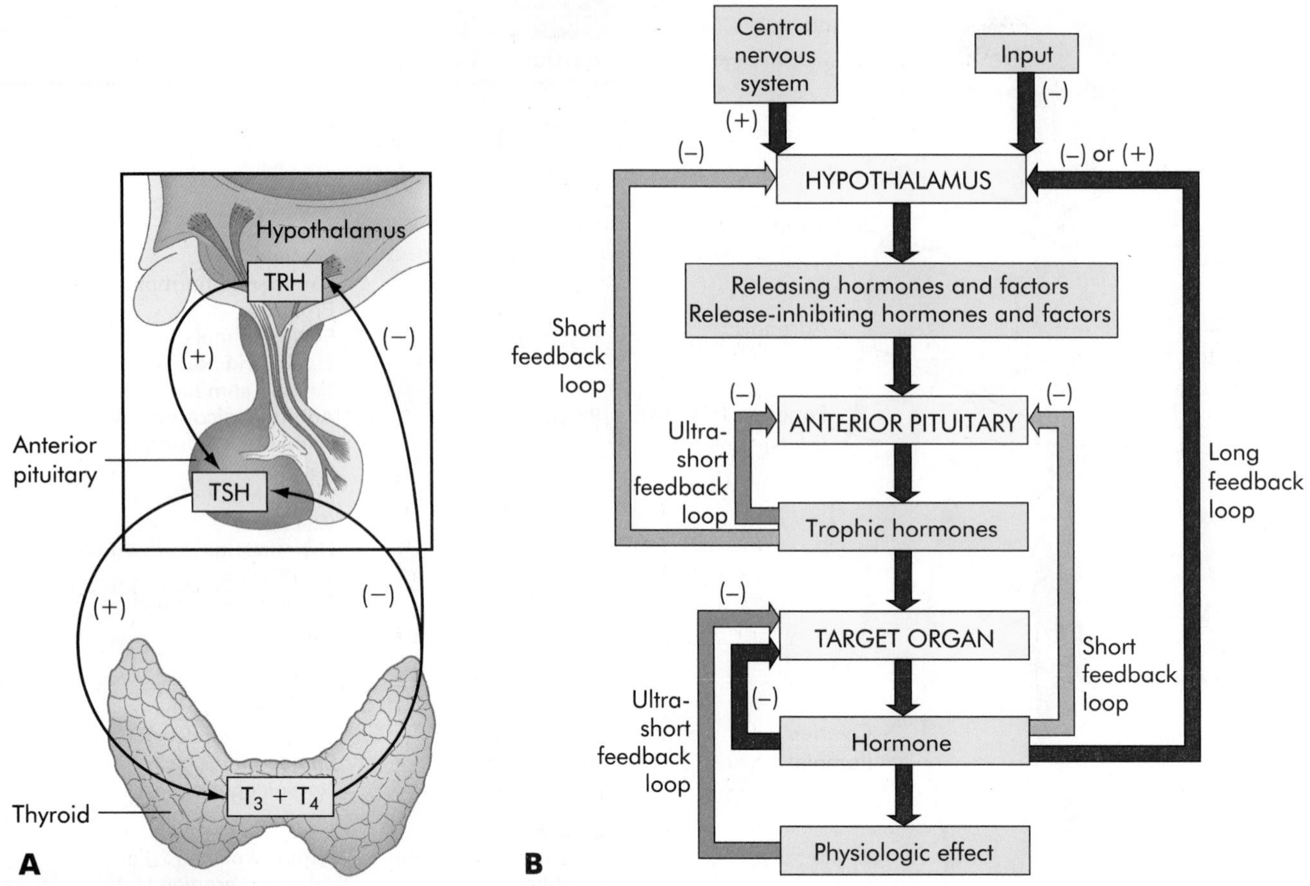

Figure 17-2 ■ **Feedback Loops. A,** Endocrine feedback loops involving the hypothalamus-pituitary gland and end organs, in this example, the thyroid gland (endocrine regulation). **B,** General model for control and negative feedback to hypothalamic–pituitary target organ systems. Negative-feedback regulation is possible at three levels: target organ (ultrashort feedback), anterior pituitary (short feedback), and hypothalamus (long feedback). *TRH,* Thyroid releasing hormone; *TSH,* thyroid stimulating hormone; T_3, triiodothyronine; T_4, tetraiodothyronine.

Lipid-soluble hormones can remain in the blood for hours to days. Water-soluble hormones mediate short-acting responses, and lipid soluble hormones mediate both rapid and long-acting responses.[1,2] Water-soluble hormones bind to cell surface receptors, and lipid-soluble hormones may bind to plasma membrane receptors or diffuse through the cellular plasma membrane and bind to cytosolic or nuclear receptors.[3–6] Because an equilibrium exists between free hormones and hormones bound to plasma proteins, a significant change in the concentration of binding proteins can affect the concentration of free hormones in the plasma (Table 17-2). Only free hormones can signal a target

TABLE 17-2

Binding Proteins, Their Hormones, and Variables That Affect Their Circulating Levels

Binding Protein	Hormone	Factors That Increase Binding Protein Levels	Factors That Decrease Binding Protein Levels
Corticosteroid-binding globulin	Cortisol Progesterone	Estrogen	Liver disease
Sex hormone–binding globulin	Dihydrotestosterone Testosterone Estradiol	—	Androgens Hypothyroidism Liver disease
Thyroid-binding globulin	Thyroxine (T_4) Triiodothyronine (T_3)	Estrogen Hyperthyroidism	Testosterone Glucocorticoids Liver disease
Albumin	All lipid-soluble hormones	Estrogen	Liver disease Malnutrition Renal disease

cell. (Mechanisms of hormone binding are discussed in Chapter 1.)

Mechanisms of Hormone Action

Although a hormone is distributed throughout the body, only those cells with appropriate receptors for that hormone are affected. *Hormone receptors* of the **target cell** have two main functions: (1) to recognize and bind specifically and with high affinity to their particular hormones and (2) to initiate a signal to appropriate intracellular effectors.

The sensitivity of the target cell to a particular hormone is related to the total number of receptors per cell: the more receptors, the more sensitive the cell. Low concentrations of hormone increase the number of receptors per cell; this is called **up-regulation**. High concentrations of hormone decrease the number of receptors; this is called **down-regulation** (Figure 17-3). Thus, the cell can adjust its sensitivity to the concentration of the signaling hormone. The receptors on the plasma membrane are continuously synthesized and degraded, so that changes in receptor concentration may occur within hours. Various physiochemical conditions can affect both the receptor number and the affinity at which the hormone binds to its receptor. Some of these physiochemical conditions are the fluidity and structure of the plasma membrane, pH, temperature, ion concentration, diet, and the presence of other chemicals (e.g., drugs).

Hormones affect target cells directly or permissively. **Direct effects** are the obvious changes in cell function that result specifically from stimulation by a particular hormone. **Permissive effects** are less obvious hormone-induced changes that facilitate the maximal response or functioning of a cell. For example, insulin via insulin receptors has a direct effect on skeletal muscle cells, causing increased glucose transport into these cells. Insulin also has a permissive effect on mammary cells, facilitating the response of these cells to the direct effects of prolactin.

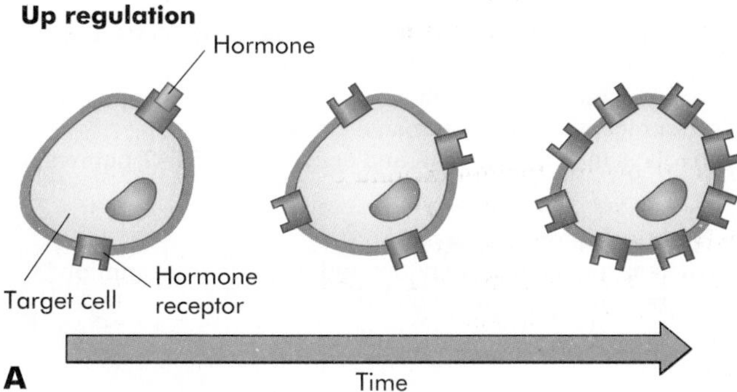

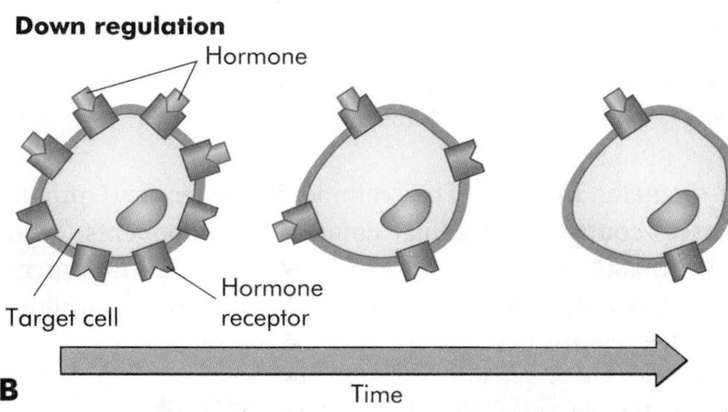

Figure 17-3 ■ **Regulation of Target Cell Sensitivity. A,** Low hormone level and up-regulation, or an increase in number of receptors. **B,** High hormone level and down-regulation, or a decrease in number of receptors. (From Thibodeau GA, Patton KT: *Anatomy & physiology,* ed 6, St Louis, 2007, Mosby.)

Some hormones have biphasic effects that are dependent on the concentration of the hormone. For example, low or physiologic levels of antidiuretic hormone (ADH), in response to dehydration, stimulate renal tubular reabsorption of sodium and water. However, at very high levels (i.e., achieved with exogenous administration), ADH acts as a vasoconstrictor.

Hormone receptors

Hormone receptors may be located in the plasma membrane or in the intracellular compartment of the target cell. Water-soluble (peptide) hormones, which include the protein hormones and the catecholamines, have a high molecular weight and cannot diffuse across the cell membrane. They interact or bind with receptors located in or on the cell membrane. Fat-soluble steroid, vitamin D, retinoic acid, and thyroid hormones diffuse freely across the plasma and nuclear membranes and bind with cytosolic or nuclear receptors (Figure 17-4). The hormone-receptor complex binds to a specific region in the deoxyribonucleic acid (DNA) and stimulates the expression of a specific gene. There is new evidence that some fat-soluble hormones (i.e., estrogen [see Chapter 31]) may bind with plasma membrane receptors and can have rapid cellular effects.[4,6,7] (Types of hormones, their corresponding receptors, and the mechanisms by which they affect the cell are summarized in Table 17-3.)

First and second messengers

Receptors for most water-soluble hormones and some steroid hormones are located in the plasma membranes of cells. The hormone is the **first messenger** and is secreted into the bloodstream and carries a message to the target cell. At the target cell it interacts with the receptor on the plasma membrane. The interaction initiates a signal that generates a **second messenger** inside the cell. The second messenger transduces the signal from the receptor to the cytoplasm and nucleus of the cell and mediates the effect of the hormone on the target cell, for example, membrane transport, contractile proteins, enzyme activation, protein synthesis, and cellular growth. The second messengers are small molecules, such as cyclic adenosine monophosphate (cAMP). Other second messengers include cyclic guanosine monophosphate (cGMP), inositol triphosphate, calcium or calcium-calmodulin, and the tyrosine kinase system (Figure 17-5).

Hormone-receptor binding increases the intracellular level of second messengers, such as cAMP and cGMP. cAMP activates protein kinase A or C, which leads to phosphorylation and enzyme activation. cGMP also activates enzymes that direct a number of cellular processes.

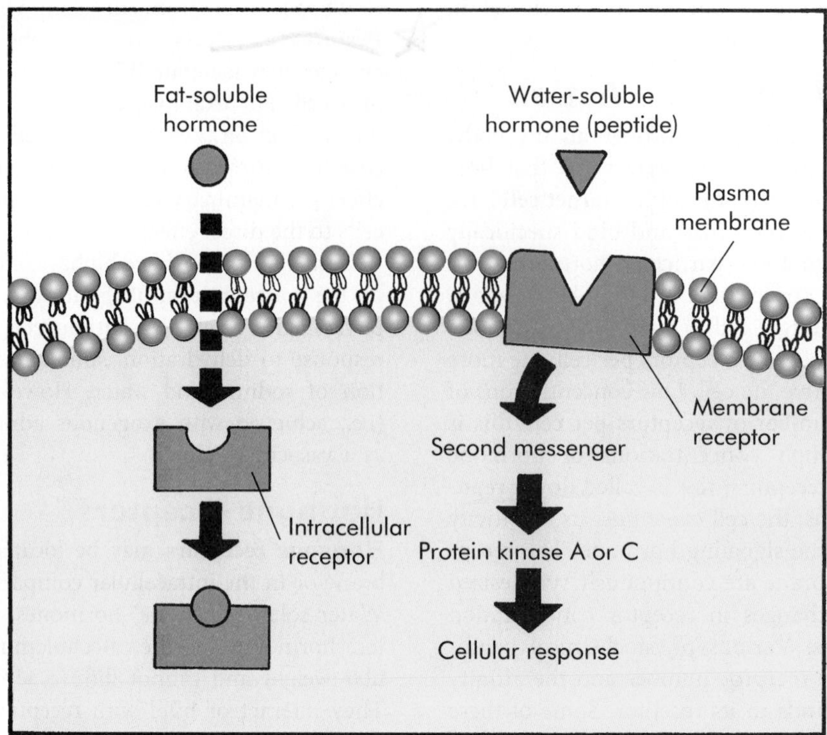

Figure 17-4 ■ **Hormone Binding at Target Cell.**

TABLE 17-3

Types of Hormones, Their Receptors, and Their Mechanisms of Action

Hormone	Type of Receptor	Mechanism of Action
WATER-SOLUBLE HORMONES		
Glycoproteins, amines, small peptides	Plasma membrane receptors	Second messengers; cAMP, cGMP, Ca^{++}, IP_3, DAG and proteins (except insulin)
Insulin	Plasma membrane receptors	Involves receptor autophosphorylation and activation of the receptor protein tyrosine kinase
Growth hormone, prolactin	Plasma membrane receptors	Involves intracellular JAK and activation of STAT pathway
LIPID-SOLUBLE HORMONES		
Steroid hormones	Plasma membrane receptors	Rapid nongenomic action
	Nuclear receptors	Nuclear translocation and altered genome transcription*
Thyroid hormones (iodothyronines)	Nuclear receptor	Altered genome transcription*
	Cytosolic receptors	

*Involves gene expression (i.e., protein hormone synthesis).

cAMP, Cyclic adenosine monophosphate; *cGMP*, cyclic guanosine monophosphate; *IP_3*, inositol triphosphate; *DAG*, diacylglycerol; *JAK*, Janus family of tyrosine kinases; *STAT*, signal transducers and activators of transcription.

Consequently, the second messengers direct the actions or products of specific cells.

Inositol triphosphate functions as a second messenger for nonsteroid hormones, such as angiotensin II and gonadotropin-releasing hormone (GnRH). Hormone receptor binds through a plasma membrane G protein and results in generation of inositol triphosphate. Inositol triphosphate triggers a cascade of chemical reactions that produce the cell's response.

The calcium-calmodulin complex mediates the effects of calcium on intracellular activities, particularly the activation of protein kinases. The calmodulin-dependent protein kinases control intracellular contractile components (myosin and actin, which cause contraction), alter plasma membrane permeability to calcium, and regulate the intracellular enzyme activity that promotes hormone secretion.

Steroid (lipid-soluble) hormone receptors

The lipid-soluble hormones are steroid hormones and are synthesized from cholesterol. They include androgens, estrogens, progestins, glucocorticoids, and mineralocorti-

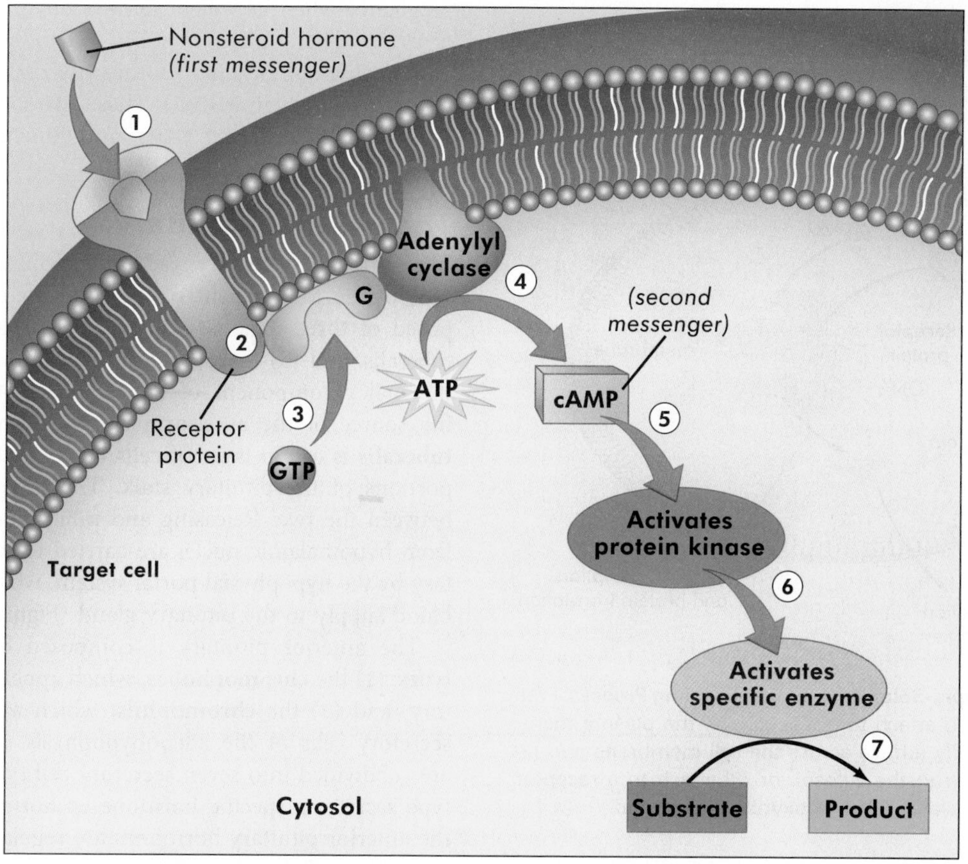

Figure 17-5 ■ **Example of First- and Second-Messenger Mechanisms.** A nonsteroid hormone *(first messenger)* binds to a fixed receptor in the plasma membrane of the target cell *(1)*. The hormone-receptor complex activates the G protein *(2)*. The activated G protein *(G)* reacts with guanosine triphosphate *(GTP)*, which in turn activates the membrane-bound enzyme adenylyl cyclase *(3)*. Adenylyl cyclase catalyzes the conversion of adenosine triphosphate *(ATP)* to cyclic adenosine monophosphate *(cAMP) (second messenger) (4)*. cAMP activates protein kinase A *(5)*. Protein kinases activate specific intracellular enzymes *(6)*. These activated enzymes then influence specific cellular reactions, thus producing the target cell's response to the hormone *(7)*. (From Thibodeau GA, Patton KT: *Anatomy & physiology,* ed 6, St Louis, 2007, Mosby.)

coids, thyroid hormones, vitamin D, and retinoid. Because these are relatively small, lipophilic, hydrophobic molecules, they can cross the lipid plasma membrane by simple diffusion (see Chapter 1). Receptors for steroid hormones are in the cytosol and nucleus and direct gene expression (Figure 17-6). Modulation of gene expression can take hours to days. Studies also reveal that steroid hormone receptors are in the plasma membrane and are associated with rapid responses that may have genomic and nongenomic effects.[6–9]

✔ QUICK CHECK 17-1

1. What are hormones? By what mechanisms do they function?
2. Describe a direct effect and a permissive effect of hormones on cells.
3. How do first messengers differ from second messengers?
4. Where are the receptors for steroid (lipid soluble) hormones located?

STRUCTURE AND FUNCTION OF THE ENDOCRINE GLANDS

Hypothalamic-Pituitary System

The hypothalamic-pituitary system (sometimes referred to as the hypothalamic pituitary axis [HPA]) produces a number of hormones that affect a number of diverse body functions. The hypothalamic-pituitary unit forms the structural and functional basis for central integration of the neurologic and endocrine systems.

The hypothalamus, which contains special neurosecretory cells and is located at the base of the brain, is connected to the pituitary gland by the pituitary stalk. The special cells of the hypothalamus are like other neurons in that they have similar electrical properties, organelles, membranes, and synapses. Neurosecretory cells, however, can synthesize and secrete the hypothalamic-releasing hormones and synthesize the hormones of the posterior portion of the pituitary gland. The hypothalamus synthesizes and releases hormones that regulate secretion by other glands, including **prolactin-inhibiting factor (PIF), thyrotropin-releasing**

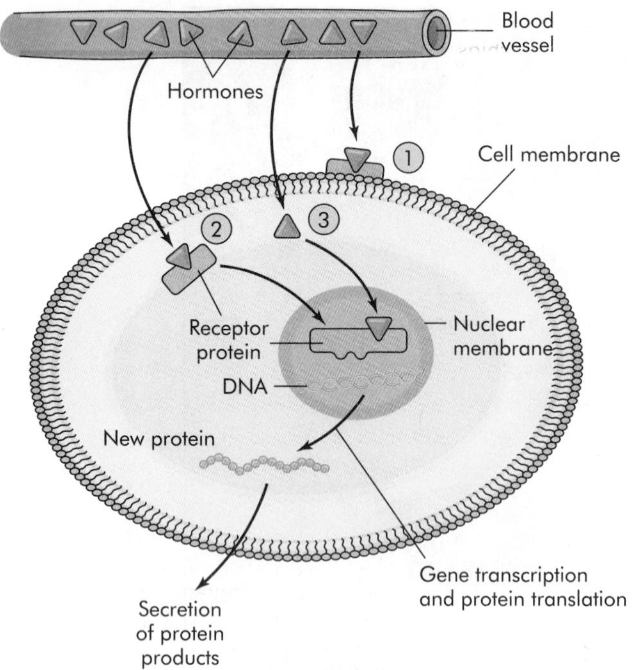

Figure 17-6 ■ **Lipid-Soluble Hormone Signaling Process.** Free hormones either *(1)* attach to a receptor on the plasma membrane, and or readily diffuse across the cell membrane and *(2)* attach to a receptor in the cytosol, or *(3)* attach to a receptor molecule in the nucleus. *DNA,* Deoxyribonucleic acid.

hormone (TRH), gonadotropin-releasing hormone (GnRH), somatostatin, **growth hormone–releasing factor (GRF), corticotropin-releasing hormone (CRH),** and **substance P.** These hormones are summarized in Table 17-4.

The **pituitary gland** is located in the sella turcica (a saddle-shaped depression of the sphenoid bone at the base of the skull). It weighs approximately 0.5 g, except during pregnancy when its weight approaches 1 g. It is composed of two distinctly different lobes: (1) the anterior pituitary, or adenohypophysis, and (2) the posterior pituitary, or neurohypophysis (Figure 17-7). These two lobes differ in their embryonic origins, cell types, and functional relationship to the hypothalamus.

The anterior pituitary

The **anterior pituitary** (adenohypophysis) accounts for 75% of the total weight of the pituitary gland. It is composed of three regions: (1) the pars distalis, (2) the pars tuberalis, and (3) the pars intermedia. The **pars distalis** is the major component of the anterior pituitary, which is the source of the anterior pituitary hormones. The **pars tuberalis** is a thin layer of cells on the anterior and lateral portions of the pituitary stalk. The **pars intermedia** lies between the two. Releasing and inhibiting factors secreted from hypothalamic nuclei are carried to the anterior pituitary by the hypophysial portal system, which is the primary blood supply to the pituitary gland (Figure 17-8).

The anterior pituitary is composed of two main cell types: (1) the **chromophobes,** which appear to be nonsecretory, and (2) the **chromophils,** which are considered the secretory cells of the adenohypophysis. The chromophils are subdivided into seven secretory cell types, and each cell type secretes a specific hormone or hormones. In general, the anterior pituitary hormones are regulated by: (1) secretion of hypothalamic peptide hormones or releasing factors, (2) feedback effects of the hormones secreted by target glands, and (3) direct effects of other mediating neurotransmitters. (These are summarized in Figure 17-2.)

The anterior pituitary secretes tropic hormones, including adrenocorticotropic hormone (ACTH), melanocyte-stimulating hormone (MSH), somatotropic hormones (growth hormone [GH], and prolactin), and the glycoprotein hormones (follicle-stimulating hormone [FSH], luteinizing

TABLE 17-4

Hypothalamic Hormones

Hormone	Target Tissue	Action
Thyrotropin-releasing hormone (TRH)	Anterior pituitary	Stimulates release of thyroid-stimulating hormones (TSH) Modulates prolactin secretion
Gonadotropin-releasing hormone (GnRH)	Anterior pituitary	Stimulates release of follicle-stimulating hormone (FSH) and luteinizing hormone (LH)
Somatostatin	Anterior pituitary Gastrointestinal tract	Inhibits release of growth hormone (GH) Decreases gastric motility, intestinal secretion, and secretion of TSH, parathyroid hormone, renin, glucagon, and insulin
Growth hormone–releasing factor (GRF)	Anterior pituitary	Stimulates release of GH factor (GRF)
Corticotropin-releasing hormone (CRH)	Anterior pituitary	Stimulates release of adrenocorticotropic hormone (ACTH) and β-endorphin
Substance P	Anterior pituitary	Inhibits synthesis and release of ACTH Stimulates secretion of GH, FSH, LH, and prolactin
Prolactin-inhibiting factor (PIF; possibly dopamine)	Anterior pituitary	Inhibits secretion of prolactin
Prolactin-releasing hormone (PRH)	Anterior pituitary	Stimulates secretion of prolactin

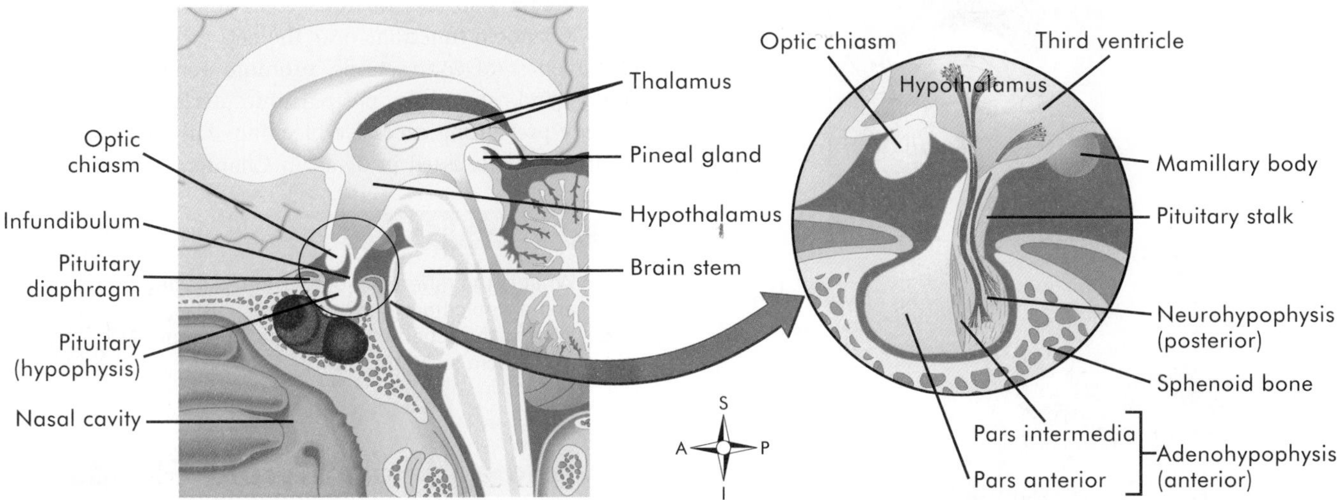

Figure 17-7 ■ **Location and Structure of the Pituitary Gland (Hypophysis).** The pituitary gland is located within the sella turcica of the skull's sphenoid bone and is connected to the hypothalamus by a stalklike infundibulum. The pituitary stalk passes through a gap in the portion of the dura mater that covers the pituitary (the pituitary diaphragm). The inset shows that the pituitary is divided into an anterior portion, the adenohypophysis, and a posterior portion, the neurohypophysis. The adenohypophysis is further subdivided into the pars anterior and pars intermedia. The pars intermedia is almost absent in the adult pituitary. (From Thibodeau GA, Patton KT: *Anatomy & physiology,* ed 6, St Louis, 2007, Mosby.)

hormone [LH] including the male analog of LH [interstitial cell-stimulating hormone—ICSH], and thyroid-stimulating hormone [TSH]). Each hormone affects the physiologic function of the specific target organ (Figure 17-9 and Table 17-5).

The posterior pituitary

The embryonic **posterior pituitary** (neurohypophysis) is derived from the hypothalamus and comprises three parts: (1) the median eminence located at the base of the hypothalamus, (2) the pituitary stalk, and (3) the pars nervosa or neural lobe. The **median eminence** is composed largely of the nerve endings of axons from the ventral hypothalamus. It often is designated as part of the posterior pituitary but contains at least 10 biologically active hypothalamic-releasing hormones, as well as the neurotransmitters dopamine, norepinephrine, serotonin, acetylcholine, and histamine, so it might be more appropriately considered part of the hypothalamus. The **pituitary stalk** contains the axons of neurons that originate in the supraoptic and paraventricular nuclei of the hypothalamus and connects the pituitary gland to the brain. Axons originating in the hypothalamus terminate in the **pars nervosa,** which secretes the hormones of the posterior pituitary (Figure 17-10).

The posterior pituitary secretes two polypeptide hormones: (1) **antidiuretic hormone (ADH),** also called arginine vasopressin, and (2) oxytocin. These hormones differ by only two amino acids. They are synthesized—along with their binding proteins, the neurophysins—in the supraoptic and paraventricular nuclei of the hypothalamus (see Figure 17-10). They are packaged in secretory vesicles and are moved down the axons of the pituitary stalk to the pars nervosa for storage. The posterior pituitary thus can be seen as a storage and releasing site for hormones synthesized in the hypothalamus.

The release of ADH and oxytocin is mediated by cholinergic and adrenergic neurotransmitters. Stimulation of the cholinergic receptors by acetylcholine, angiotensin II, and β-endorphins results in the release of ADH and oxytocin, whereas activation of β-adrenergic receptors inhibits hormone secretion. Before release into the circulatory system, ADH and oxytocin are split from the neurophysins and are secreted in unbound form.

Antidiuretic hormone

The major homeostatic function of the posterior pituitary is the control of plasma osmolality as regulated by ADH, or arginine vasopressin (see Chapter 4). At physiologic levels, ADH increases the permeability of the distal renal tubules and collecting ducts (see Chapter 28). This increased permeability leads to increased water reabsorption and more concentrated urine. Hypercalcemia, prostaglandin E, and hypokalemia can inhibit this action.

ADH was originally named *vasopressin* because in extremely high doses it causes vasoconstriction and increased arterial blood pressure. These levels are not reached physiologically, but high doses of ADH (as the drug vasopressin) may be administered to achieve hemostasis during hemorrhage.

The secretion of ADH is regulated primarily by the osmoreceptors of the hypothalamus, located near or in the supraoptic nuclei (osmoreceptors are stimulated by increased osmolality). As plasma osmolality increases, the rate of ADH secretion increases. ADH has no direct effect on electrolyte levels, but by increasing water reabsorption, serum electrolyte concentrations may decrease because of a dilutional effect.

ADH secretion also is increased by changes in intravascular volume, which are monitored by baroreceptors in the

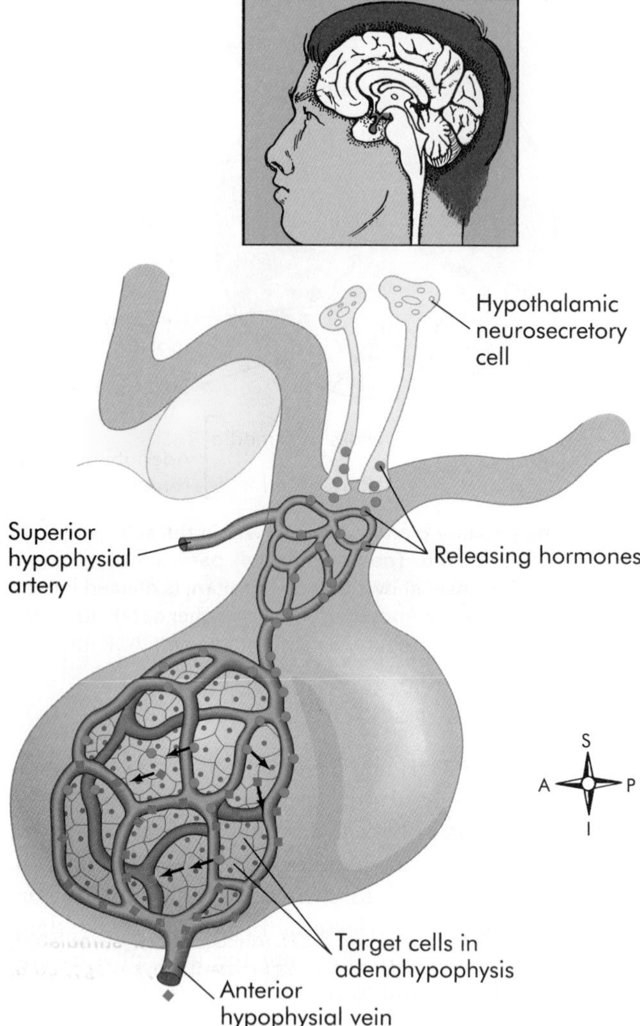

Figure 17-8 ■ **Hypophysial Portal System.** Neurons in the hypothalamus secrete releasing hormones into veins that carry the releasing hormones directly to the vessels of the adenohypophysis, thus bypassing the normal circulatory route. (From Thibodeau GA, Patton KT: *Anatomy & physiology,* ed 6, St Louis, 2007, Mosby.)

left atrium, in the carotid, and in the aortic arches. A volume loss of 7% to 25% stimulates ADH secretion. Stress, trauma, pain, exercise, nausea, nicotine, exposure to heat, and drugs such as morphine also increase ADH secretion. ADH secretion decreases with decreased plasma osmolality, increased intravascular volume, hypertension, and alcohol ingestion.

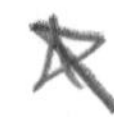

Oxytocin

Oxytocin is responsible for contraction of the uterus and milk ejection in lactating women and may affect sperm motility in men. In both genders, oxytocin has an antidiuretic effect similar to that of ADH.

In women, oxytocin is secreted in response to suckling and mechanical distention of the female reproductive tract. Oxytocin binds to its receptors on myoepithelial cells in the mammary tissues and causes contraction of those cells, which increases intramammary pressure and milk expression ("let-down" reflex).

Oxytocin also acts on the uterus to stimulate contractions. Oxytocin functions near the end of labor to enhance effectiveness of contractions, promote delivery of the placenta, and stimulate postpartum uterine contractions, thereby preventing excessive bleeding. The function of this hormone is discussed in detail in Chapter 31.

QUICK CHECK 17-2

1. What is the difference between a releasing hormone and a tropic hormone?
2. What is the action of antidiuretic hormone (ADH)? How is oxytocin similar to ADH?

Thyroid and Parathyroid Glands

The thyroid gland, located in the neck just below the larynx, produces hormones that control the rates of metabolic processes throughout the body. The four parathyroid glands are near the posterior side of the thyroid and function to control serum calcium levels (Figure 17-11).

Thyroid gland

The two lobes of the **thyroid gland** lie on either side of the trachea, inferior to the thyroid cartilage and joined by the **isthmus** (see Figure 17-11). The normal thyroid gland is not visible on inspection, but it may be palpated on swallowing, which causes it to be displaced upward.

The thyroid gland comprises **follicles** that contain follicular cells that surround a viscous substance called *colloid* (Figure 17-12). The follicular cells synthesize and secrete the thyroid hormones. Neurons terminate on blood vessels within the thyroid gland and on the follicular cells themselves, so neurotransmitters may directly affect the secretory activity of follicular cells.

Also found in the thyroid are parafollicular, or C cells (see Figure 17-12). **C cells** secrete various polypeptides, including calcitonin and somatostatin. **Calcitonin,** also called *thyrocalcitonin,* lowers serum calcium levels by inhibition of bone-resorbing osteoclasts (Table 17-6). (Bone resorption is explained in Chapter 37.) Calcitonin and parathyroid hormone together regulate calcium balance.

Synthesis of thyroid hormone

The thyroid gland produces thyroid hormone (TH) when stimulated by pituitary thyroid-stimulating hormone (TSH), low serum iodide levels, or drugs interfering with the thyroid gland's uptake of iodide from the blood. The first step in the synthesis of TH is the concentration of iodide (the inorganic ionic form of iodine that enters the thyroid gland) by the thyroid gland. Because there is an iodide concentration gradient of about 30:1 to 40:1 between the thyroid gland and the blood, iodide is moved by active transport from the extracellular fluid to the thyroid follicular cells. The iodide must be oxidated to iodine, which is facilitated by the enzyme thyroidal peroxidase inside the follicular cells.

Thyroglobulin (TG), a large glycoprotein synthesized within the follicular cell, is the precursor of thyroid

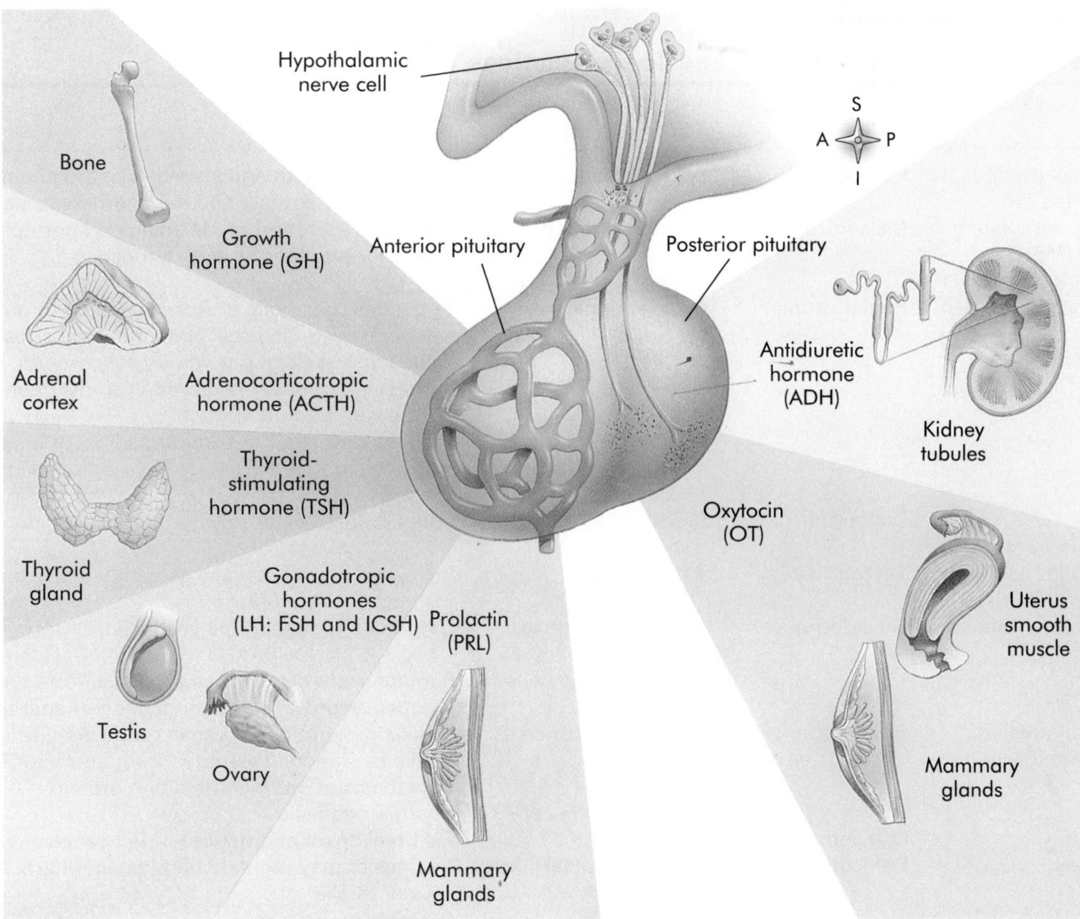

Figure 17-9 ■ **Anterior Pituitary Hormones and Their Target Hormones.** *LH,* Luteinizing hormone; *ICSH,* interstitial cell–stimulating hormone (male); *FSH,* follicle-stimulating hormone (female). (Modified from Thibodeau GA, Patton KT: *Anatomy & physiology,* ed 6, St Louis, 2007, Mosby.)

hormones. Uniodinated TG is released into the colloid, and iodine combines with tyrosine in the TG to form iodotyrosines. Triiodothyronine (T_3) has three iodine molecules and thyroxine (T_4) has four. Most T_4 is converted to T_3, which acts on the target cell. Thyroid hormones are stored in the colloid.

Thyroid hormone (TH) is available in the body as either thyroxine (T_4, 90% of thyroid hormone) or triiodothyronine (T_3, 10% of thyroid hormone). Thyroid hormones are transported in the blood in bound and free forms. Most of the TH is transported bound to **thyroxine-binding globulin (TBG)** and to a lesser extent by thyroxine-binding prealbumin or albumin. The free form is generally considered to be biologically active, and the bound form serves as a reservoir.

Regulation of thyroid hormone secretion

Thyroid hormone (TH) is regulated through a negative feedback loop involving the hypothalamus, the anterior pituitary, and the thyroid gland (see Figure 17-2). Thyrotropin-releasing hormone (TRH), which is synthesized and stored within the hypothalamus, initiates this loop. TRH is released into the hypothalamic-pituitary portal system and circulates to the anterior pituitary, where it stimulates the release of TSH. TRH levels increase with exposure to cold, stress, and decreased levels of T_4.

Thyroid-stimulating hormone (TSH) is a glycoprotein synthesized and stored within the anterior pituitary. Once TSH is secreted by the anterior pituitary, it circulates to bind with receptor sites on the outer side of the thyroid cell's plasma membrane. TSH's effects include (1) an immediate increase in the release of stored thyroid hormone, (2) an increase in iodide uptake and oxidation, (3) an increase in thyroid hormone synthesis, (4) an increase in the synthesis and secretion of prostaglandins by the thyroid, and (5) growth of the thyroid gland. Thyroid gland hormones and their regulation and function are summarized in Table 17-6.

TH acts on the thyroid gland, the anterior pituitary, and the median eminence to regulate further TH production. It operates in a negative feedback effect to inhibit TRH and TSH, which then results in decreased TH synthesis and secretion.

TH affects most body tissues by increasing the rate of protein, fat, and glucose metabolism and as a result increases heat production and body temperature. Normal linear growth requires TH, as does the central and autonomic nervous systems.[10]

TABLE 17-5

Hormones of the Anterior Pituitary and Their Functions

Hormone	Secretory Cell Type	Target Organ	Functions
Adrenocorticotropic hormone (ACTH)	Corticotropic	Adrenal gland	Regulates growth and secretion of the adrenal gland, particularly cortisol and the androgenic steroids
Melanocyte-stimulating hormone (MSH)	Melanotropic	Anterior pituitary	Promotes secretion of melanin and lipotropin by anterior pituitary; makes skin darker
Somatotropic hormones			
Growth hormone (GH)	Somatotropic	Muscle, bone, liver	Regulates metabolic processes related to growth and adaptation to physical and emotional stressors, including skeletal growth, muscle growth, increased protein synthesis, increased liver glycogenolysis, increased fat mobilization
		Liver	Induces formation of somatomedins, or insulin-like growth factors (IGFs) that have actions similar to insulin
Prolactin	Lactotropic	Breast	Milk production
Glycoprotein hormones			
Thyroid-stimulating hormone (TSH)	Thyrotropic	Thyroid gland	Increased production and secretion of thyroid hormone Increased iodine uptake
Luteinizing hormone (LH)	Gonadotropic	In women: ovarian follicle	Ovulation, progesterone production
		In men: Leydig cells	Regulates spermatogenesis, testosterone production, testicular growth, and production of androgens
Follicle-stimulating hormone (FSH)	Gonadotropic	In women: ovarian follicle	Follicle maturation, estrogen production; acts on Sertoli cells to stimulate estrogen from androgens and synthesis of androgen-binding protein
		In men: Leydig cell	Spermatogenesis
β-Lipotropin	Corticotropic	Adipose cells	Fat breakdown and release of fatty acids
β-Endorphins	Corticotropic	Brain and spinal cord	Analgesia; may regulate body temperature, food and water intake

Parathyroid glands

Normally two pairs of small parathyroid glands are present behind the upper and lower poles of the thyroid gland (see Figure 17-12). However, their number may range from two to six.

The parathyroid glands produce **parathyroid hormone (PTH),** which is the single most important factor in the regulation of serum calcium. The overall effect of PTH secretion is to increase serum calcium and decrease serum phosphate. A decrease in serum-ionized calcium stimulates PTH secretion, which acts directly on the bone to release calcium. PTH also acts on the kidney to increase calcium reabsorption and to decrease phosphate reabsorption. The resultant increase in serum calcium inhibits PTH secretion. Phosphate, magnesium, and vitamin D levels also affect PTH secretion. An increase in serum phosphate decreases serum calcium by causing calcium-phosphate precipitation into soft tissue and bone. This indirectly stimulates PTH secretion. Hypomagnesemia in persons with normal calcium acts as a mild stimulant to PTH secretion; but in persons with hypocalcemia, hypomagnesemia decreases PTH secretion. PTH decreases serum phosphate by decreasing renal tubular phosphate reabsorption. 1,25-Dihydroxyvitamin D_3 is the active form of vitamin D, and it promotes calcium and phosphate absorption in the gut, decreases PTH secretion, and promotes bone mineralization.

HEALTH ALERT
Recombinant PTH (rPTH)

Sustained PTH secretion leads to a reduction in bone density and increased bone fragility by stimulating osteoclasts to resorb bone and release calcium into the bloodstream. PTH stimulates bone resorption by first interacting with osteoblast receptors resulting in osteoblast release of inflammatory stimulants for osteoclast activation. However, intermittent administration of rPTH (teriparatide) can be used therapeutically to strengthen bone, especially in individuals with osteoporotic fractures. Intermittent exposures to rPTH (once a day) increase bone turnover such that osteoblasts are stimulated more than osteoclasts, and bone mineral density increases. Furthermore, there is improvement in bone architecture as well as density (bone quality as well as quantity).

Data from Bilezikian JP: Anabolic therapy for osteoporosis, *Int J Fertil Womens Med* 50(2):53–60, 2005; Deal C, Gideon J: Recombinant PTH 1–34 (Forteo): an anabolic drug for osteoporosis, *Cleve Clin J Med* 70(7):585–601, 2003; Eastell R: Management of bone health in postmenopausal women, *Horm Res* 64(suppl 2): 76–80, 2005; Ma YL, Zeng Q, Donley DW, Ste-Marie LG, Gallagher JC, Dalsky GP, Marcus R, Eriksen EF: Teriparatide increases bone formation in modeling and remodeling osteons and enhances IGF-II immunoreactivity in postmenopausal women with osteoporosis, *J Bone Miner Res* 21(6):855–864, 2006.

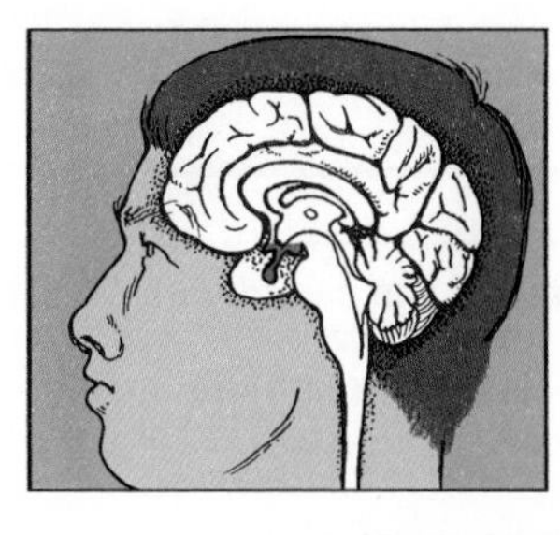

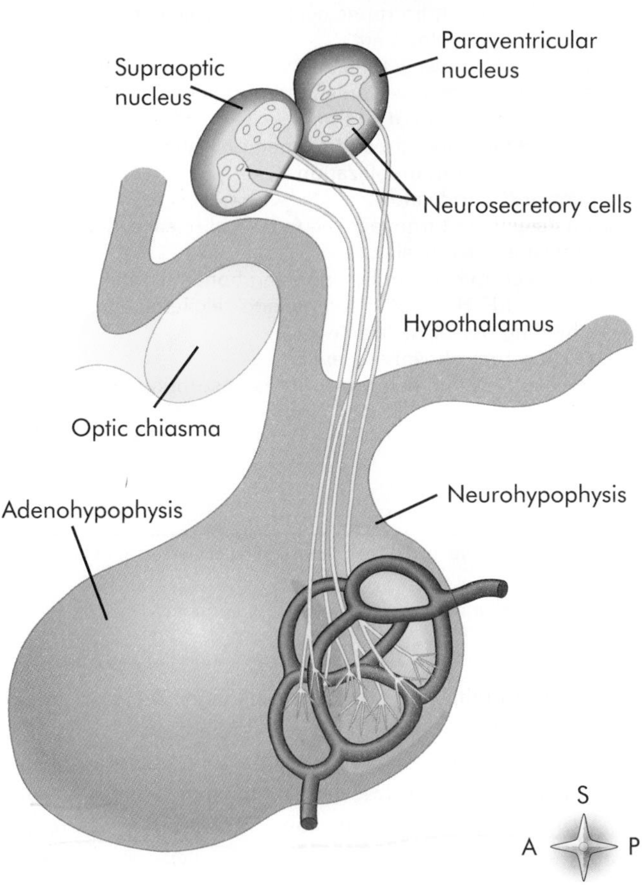

Figure 17-10 ■ **Relationship of the Hypothalamus and Neurohypophysis.** Neurosecretory cells have their cell bodies in the hypothalamus and their axon terminals in the neurohypophysis. Thus, hormones synthesized in the hypothalamus are actually released from the neurohypophysis. (From Thibodeau GA, Patton KT: *Anatomy & physiology,* ed 6, St Louis, 2007, Mosby.)

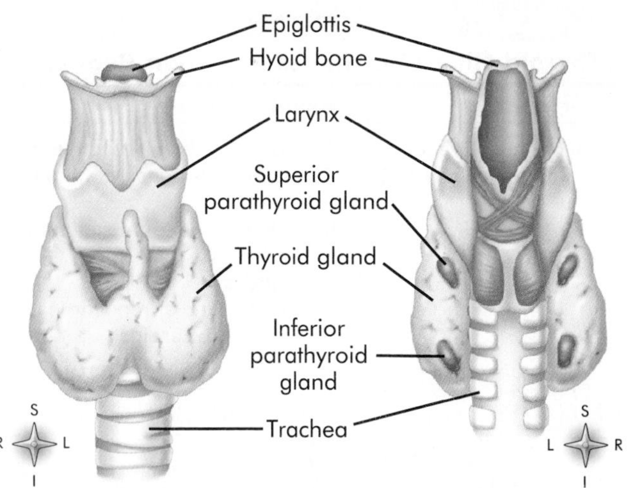

Figure 17-11 ■ **Thyroid and Parathyroid Glands.** Note their location in relation to each other and to the larynx and trachea. (From Thibodeau GA, Patton KT: *Anatomy & physiology,* ed 6, St Louis, 2007, Mosby.)

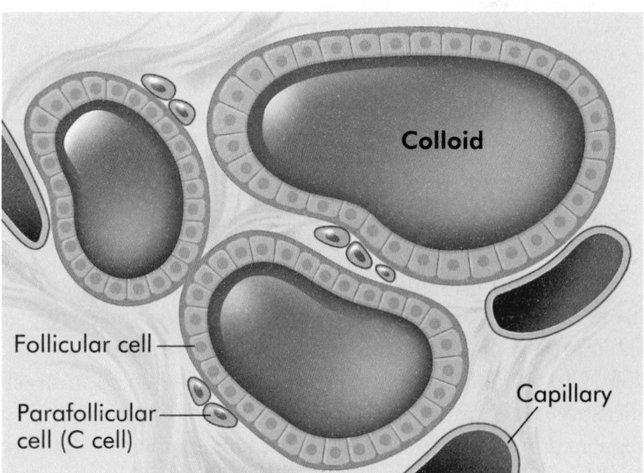

Figure 17-12 ■ **Thyroid Follicle Cells.**

QUICK CHECK 17-3

1. How does the anterior pituitary regulate the thyroid gland?
2. What form of thyroid hormone is biologically active?
3. What two organs are the sites of action of parathyroid hormone (PTH)?

Endocrine Pancreas

The **pancreas** is both an endocrine gland that produces hormones and an exocrine gland that produces digestive enzymes. (The exocrine function of the pancreas is discussed in Chapter 33.) The pancreas is located behind the stomach, between the spleen and the duodenum. It houses the **islets of Langerhans.** The islets of Langerhans have four types of hormone-secreting cells: **alpha cells,** which secrete glucagon; **beta cells,** which secrete insulin and amylin; **delta cells,** which secrete gastrin and somatostatin; and **F** (or **PP**) **cells,** which secrete pancreatic polypeptide. These hormones regulate most carbohydrate, fat, and protein metabolism. (The pancreas is illustrated in Figure 17-13.) Nerves from both the sympathetic and parasympathetic divisions of the autonomic nervous system innervate the pancreatic islets.

Insulin

The beta cells of the pancreas synthesize **insulin** from the precursor, proinsulin, which is formed from a larger precursor molecule, preproinsulin. Proinsulin is composed of

TABLE 17-6

Thyroid Gland Hormones and Their Regulation and Functions

Hormone	Regulation	Functions
Thyroxine (T_4) and triiodothyronine (T_3)	T_4 and T_3 levels are controlled by TSH Released in response to metabolic demand Influences on amount secreted: Gender Pregnancy Gonadal- and adrenocortical- increased steroids = ↑ levels Exposure to extreme cold = ↑ levels Nutritional state Chemicals GHIH = ↓ levels Dopamine = ↓ levels Catecholamines = ↑ levels	Regulates protein, fat, and carbohydrate catabolism in all cells Regulates metabolic rate of all cells Regulates body heat production Insulin antagonist Maintains growth hormone secretion, skeletal maturation Affects CNS development Necessary for muscle tone and vigor Maintains cardiac rate, force, and output Maintains secretion of GI tract Affects respiratory rate and oxygen utilization Maintains calcium mobilization Affects RBC production Stimulates lipid turnover, free fatty acid release, and cholesterol synthesis
Calcitonin	Elevated serum calcium—major stimulant for calcitonin Other stimulants Gastrin Calcium-rich foods (regardless of serum Ca^{++} levels) Pregnancy Lowered serum calcium—suppresses calcitonin release	Lowers serum calcium by opposing bone-resorbing effects of PTH, prostaglandins, and calciferols by inhibiting osteoclastic activity Lowers serum phosphate levels Decreases calcium and phosphorus absorption in GI tract

From Monohan FD, Sands JK, Neighbors M, Marek J, Green CJ: Phipps' *Medical-surgical nursing:* health and illness perspective, ed 8, St Louis, 2007, Mosby.

TSH, Thyroid-stimulating hormone; *CNS,* central nervous system; *GI,* gastrointestinal; *GHIH,* growth hormone-inhibiting hormone; *RBC,* red blood cell; *PTH,* parathyroid hormone.

A peptide and B peptide connected by a C peptide and two disulfide bonds. C peptide is cleaved by proteolytic enzymes leaving the bonded A and B peptides as the insulin molecule. C peptide can be measured in the blood as an indirect measure of serum insulin synthesis.[11] Secretion of insulin is regulated by chemical, hormonal, and neural control. Insulin secretion is promoted when blood levels of glucose, amino acids (arginine and lysine), and gastrointestinal hormones (glucagon, gastrin, cholecystokinin, secretin) increase, and when the beta cells are stimulated parasympathetically. Insulin secretion diminishes in response to low blood levels of glucose (hypoglycemia), high levels of insulin (through negative feedback to the beta cells), and sympathetic stimulation of the alpha cells in the islets. Prostaglandins also may inhibit insulin secretion.

At the target cell, insulin combines with an enzyme-linked plasma membrane receptor that contains tyrosine kinase on the cytosolic surface. Insulin receptor binding activates tyrosine kinase autophosphorylation and sends a cascade of signals to activate glucose transporters (GLUT) for entry of glucose into the cell, and to phosphorylate protein kinase.[12] Protein kinase then activates or deactivates target enzymes for glucose metabolism (Figure 17-14).

Insulin is an anabolic hormone that promotes glucose uptake and the synthesis of proteins, carbohydrates, lipids, and nucleic acids and functions mainly in the liver, muscle, and adipose tissue. Table 17-7 summarizes the actions of insulin. The net effect of insulin in these tissues is to stimulate protein and fat synthesis and decrease blood glucose. The brain, red blood cells, kidney, and lens of the eye do not require insulin for glucose transport. Insulin also facilitates the intracellular transport of potassium (K^+), phosphate, and magnesium. Increased K^+ increases insulin secretion.

Amylin

Amylin is a peptide hormone co-secreted with insulin in response to nutrient stimuli. It regulates blood glucose by delaying nutrient uptake and suppressing glucagon secretion after meals. Amylin also has a satiety effect. Through these mechanisms, amylin has an antihyperglycemic effect.[13]

Glucagon

Glucagon is produced by the alpha cells of the pancreas and by cells lining the gastrointestinal tract. Glucagon acts primarily in the liver and increases blood glucose by stimulating glycogenolysis and gluconeogenesis in muscle and lipolysis in adipose tissue.

Amino acids, such as alanine, glycine, and asparagine, stimulate glucagon secretion. Glucagon release is inhibited by high glucose levels and increased by low glucose levels and sympathetic stimulation, thus it is antagonistic to insulin.

Somatostatin

The **somatostatin** produced by delta cells of the pancreas is essential in carbohydrate, fat, and protein metabolism

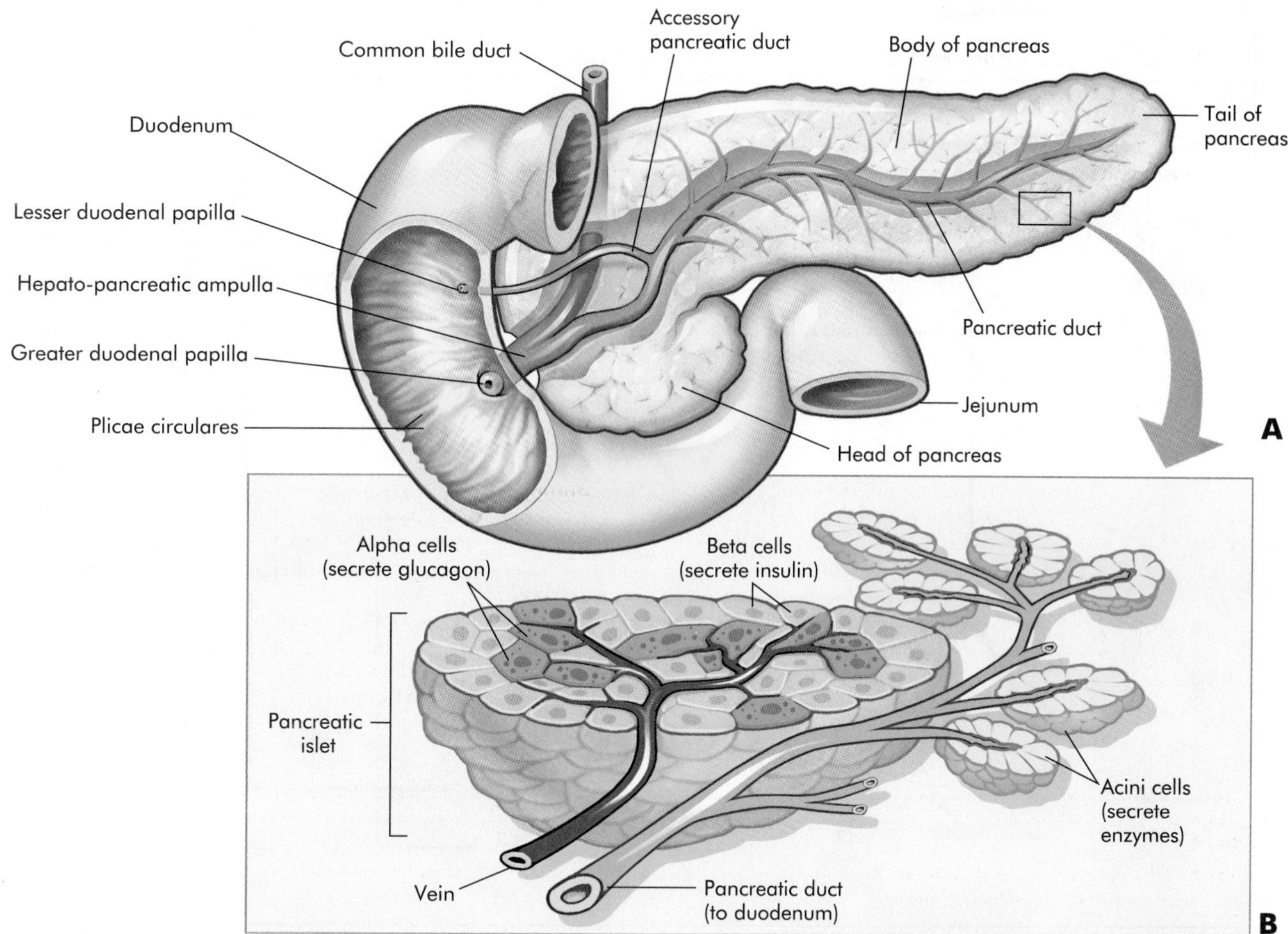

Figure 17-13 ■ **The Pancreas. A,** Pancreas dissected to show main and accessory ducts. The main duct may join the common bile duct, as shown here, to enter the duodenum by a single opening at the major duodenal papilla, or the two ducts may have separate openings. The accessory pancreatic duct is usually present and has a separate opening into the duodenum. **B,** Exocrine glandular cells (around small pancreatic ducts) and endocrine glandular cells of the pancreatic islets (adjacent to blood capillaries). Exocrine pancreatic cells secrete pancreatic juice, alpha endocrine cells secrete glucagon, and beta cells secrete insulin. (From Thibodeau GA, Patton KT: *Anatomy & physiology,* ed 6, St Louis, 2007, Mosby.)

(homeostasis of ingested nutrients). It is different from hypothalamic somatostatin, which inhibits the release of growth hormone and TSH. It is involved in regulating alpha-cell and beta-cell function within the islets by inhibiting secretion of insulin, glucagon, and pancreatic polypeptide.

Gastrin and pancreatic polypeptide

The function of pancreatic **gastrin** has not been established. It is postulated that fetal pancreatic gastrin secretion is necessary for adequate islet cell development.[14] **Pancreatic polypeptide** is released by F cells in response to hypoglycemia and protein-rich meals. It inhibits gallbladder contraction and exocrine pancreas secretion and is frequently increased in pancreatic tumors and in diabetes.

Adrenal Glands

The **adrenal glands** are paired, pyramid-shaped organs behind the peritoneum and close to the upper pole of each kidney. Each gland is surrounded by a capsule, embedded in fat, and well supplied with blood from the phrenic and renal arteries and the aorta. Venous return from the left adrenal gland is to the renal vein and from the right adrenal gland is to the inferior vena cava.

Each adrenal gland consists of two separate portions—an inner medulla and an outer cortex. These two portions have different embryonic origins, structures, and hormonal functions. In effect, each adrenal gland functions like two separate glands, although there are interrelationships (Figure 17-15).

The **adrenal cortex,** or outer region of the gland, accounts for 80% of the weight of the adult gland. The cortex is histologically subdivided into the following three zones:

1. The **zona glomerulosa,** the outer layer, which constitutes about 15% of the cortex and primarily produces the mineralocorticoid aldosterone
2. The **zona fasciculata,** the middle layer, which constitutes 78% of the cortex and secretes glucocorticoids: cortisol, cortisone, and corticosterone

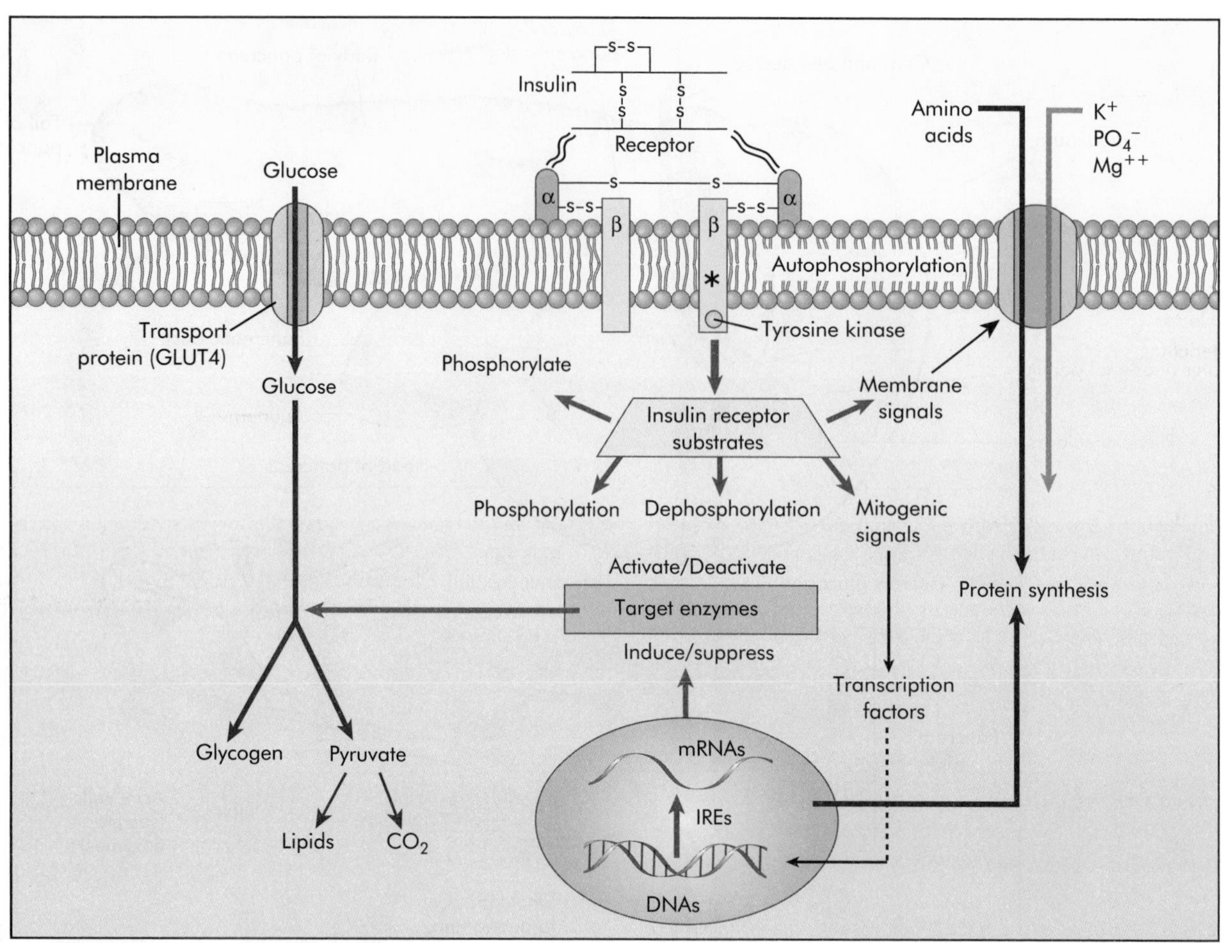

Figure 17-14 ■ **Insulin Action on Cells.** Binding of insulin to its receptor causes autophosphorylation of the receptor, which then itself acts as a tyrosine kinase that phosphorylates insulin receptor substrate 1 (IRS-1). Numerous target enzymes, such as protein kinase B and MAP kinase, are activated, and these enzymes have a multitude of effects on cell function. The glucose transporter, GLUT4, is recruited to the plasma membrane, where it facilitates glucose entry into the cell. The transport of amino acids, potassium, magnesium, and phosphate into the cell is also facilitated. The synthesis of various enzymes is induced or suppressed, and signal molecules that modulate gene expression regulate cell growth. *mRNA,* Messenger ribonucleic acid; *IREs,* insulin responsive elements. (From Berne RM, Levy MN: *Principles of physiology,* ed 3, St Louis, 2000, Mosby.)

TABLE 17-7

Insulin Actions

	SITES OF INSULIN ACTION		
Actions	**Liver Cells**	**Muscle Cells**	**Adipose Cells**
Glucose uptake	Increased	Increased	Increased
Glucose use	—	—	Increased glycerol phosphate
Glycogenesis	Increased	Increased	—
Glycogenolysis	Decreased	Decreased	—
Glycolysis	Increased	Increased	Increased
Gluconeogenesis	Increased	—	—
Other	Increased fatty acid synthesis Decreased ketogenesis Decreased urea cycle activity	Increased amino acid uptake Increased protein synthesis Decreased proteolysis	Increased fat esterification Decreased lipolysis Increased fat storage

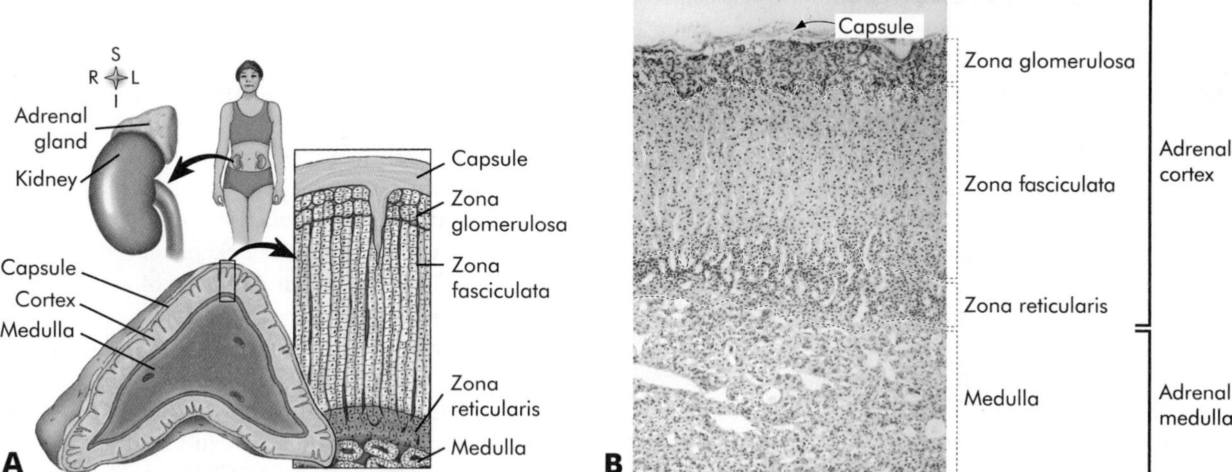

Figure 17-15 ■ Structure of the Adrenal Gland Showing Cell Layers (Zonae) of the Cortex. Zona glomerulosa secretes aldosterone. Zona fasciculata secretes abundant amounts of glucocorticoids, chiefly cortisol. Zona reticularis secretes minute amounts of sex hormones and glucocorticoids. A portion of the medulla is visible at the lower right in the photomicrograph (×35) and at the bottom of the drawing. (**A** from Thibodeau GA, Patton KT: *Anatomy & physiology,* ed 6, St Louis, 2007, Mosby; **B** from Kierszenbaum A: *Histology and cell biology,* St Louis, 2002, Elsevier.)

3. The **zona reticularis,** the inner layer, which constitutes 7% of the cortex and secretes mineralocorticoids (aldosterone), adrenal androgens and estrogens, and glucocorticoids

The **adrenal medulla,** which accounts for 20% of the gland's total weight, secretes the catecholamines epinephrine (adrenaline) and norepinephrine (noradrenaline). Both sympathetic and parasympathetic cholinergic fibers innervate the adrenal medulla.

Adrenal cortex

The adrenal cortex secretes several steroid hormones, including the glucocorticoids, the mineralocorticoids, and the adrenal androgens and estrogens. These hormones are all synthesized from cholesterol. The cells of the adrenal cortex are stimulated by **adrenocorticotropic hormone (ACTH)** from the pituitary gland.[15] The best known pathway of steroidogenesis involves the conversion of cholesterol to pregnenolone, which is then converted to the major corticosteroids. The adrenal cortex also contains a high concentration of ascorbic acid and vitamin A.

Glucocorticoids

Functions of the glucocorticoids. The **glucocorticoids** are steroid hormones that have metabolic, antiinflammatory, and growth-suppressing effects and influence levels of awareness and sleep patterns. (These functions are summarized in Box 17-1). Glucocorticoids have direct effects on carbohydrate metabolism. In hepatic tissue, glucocorticoids act primarily to stimulate glucose formation. In extrahepatic tissues, they stimulate protein catabolism and inhibit amino acid uptake and protein synthesis.

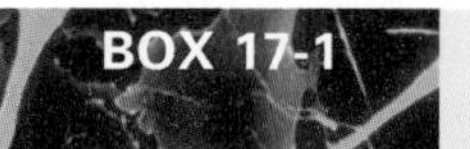

Major Functions of Glucocorticoids

Metabolic

- Increase blood glucose
  - Increase hepatic gluconeogenesis
  - Decease glucose use in muscle, adipose, and lymphatic tissue
  - Antagonize insulin
- Stimulate protein catabolism and decrease protein synthesis

Inflammatory and Immune

- Decrease cellular immunity
  - Decrease T lymphocyte proliferation
  - Decrease natural killer cell activity
  - Decrease macrophage activity
- Antiinflammatory
  - Decrease numbers of eosinophils
  - Decrease number of fibroblasts
  - Decrease inflammatory cytokines (interleukins, bradykinin, serotonin, and histamine)
  - Stimulate antiinflammatory cytokines (interleukin-10, transforming growth factor beta)
  - Stabilize lysosomal membranes

Other

- Inhibit bone formation
- Inhibit ADH and ACTH secretion
- Stimulate gastric acid secretion
- Potentiate the effects of catecholamines, thyroid hormone, and growth hormone on adipose tissue.
- Affect nerve function in the brain (affects mood and sleep)

The glucocorticoids act at several sites to influence immune and inflammatory reactions. One major immune suppressant effect is the glucocorticoid-mediated decrease in the proliferation of T lymphocytes, primarily T helper lymphocytes. There is a greater effect on T helper 1 cytokine production (including antiviral interferons) than there is T helper 2 cytokine production and therefore greater depression of cellular immunity than humoral immunity (see Chapter 8). Glucocorticoids also have antiinflammatory effects related to decreased natural killer cell function, suppression of inflammatory cytokines, and stabilization of lysosomal membranes, which decreases the release of proteolytic enzymes.[16]

Other effects of glucocorticoids include inhibition of bone formation, inhibition of ADH secretion, and stimulation of gastric acid secretion. Glucocorticoids appear to potentiate the effects of catecholamines, thyroid hormone, and growth hormone on adipose tissue. A metabolite of cortisol may act like a barbiturate and depress nerve cell function in the brain, accounting for the noted effects on mood associated with steroid fluctuation in disease or stress.

Pathologically high levels of glucocorticoids increase circulating erythrocytes (leading to polycythemia), increase the appetite, promote fat deposition in the face and cervical areas, increase uric acid excretion, decrease serum calcium levels (possibly by inhibiting gastrointestinal absorption of calcium), suppress the secretion and synthesis of ACTH, and interfere with the action of growth hormone so that somatic growth is inhibited. They also have important "permissive" effects, sensitizing arterioles to the vasoconstrictive effects of norepinephrine.

Cortisol. The most potent naturally occurring glucocorticoid is **cortisol**. It is the main secretory product of the adrenal cortex and is needed to maintain life and protect the body from stress (see Figure 8-1). Cortisol has a biologic half-life of approximately 90 minutes, with the liver primarily responsible for its deactivation.

Cortisol secretion is regulated primarily by the hypothalamus and the anterior pituitary gland (Figure 17-16). Corticotropin-releasing hormone (CRH) is produced by several nuclei in the hypothalamus and stored in the median eminence. Once released, CRH travels through the portal vessels to stimulate the production of ACTH, β-lipotropin, γ-lipotropin, endorphins, and enkephalins by the anterior pituitary. ACTH is the main regulator of cortisol secretion and adrenocortical growth.

ACTH is synthesized as part of a precursor called proopiomelanocortin (POMC). Three factors appear to be primarily involved in regulating the secretion of ACTH: (1) high circulating levels of cortisol and synthetic glucocorticoids suppress both CRH and ACTH, whereas low cortisol levels stimulate their secretion; (2) diurnal rhythms affect ACTH and cortisol levels (in persons with regular sleep-wake patterns, ACTH peaks 3 to 5 hours after sleep begins and declines throughout the day, and cortisol levels follow a similar pattern); and (3) stress increases ACTH secretion, leading to increased cortisol levels. (Neurologic mechanisms regulating sleep are discussed in Chapter 13.) A form of immunoreactive ACTH (ir ACTH) is produced by the cells of the immune system and may account, in part, for integration of the immune and endocrine systems.

Once ACTH is secreted, it binds to specific plasma membrane receptors on the cells of the adrenal cortex and on other extraadrenal tissues. Because both adrenal and extraadrenal tissues have ACTH receptors, a number of effects result from stimulation by ACTH. In addition to increasing adrenocortical secretion of cortisol, ACTH maintains the size and synthetic functions of the adrenal

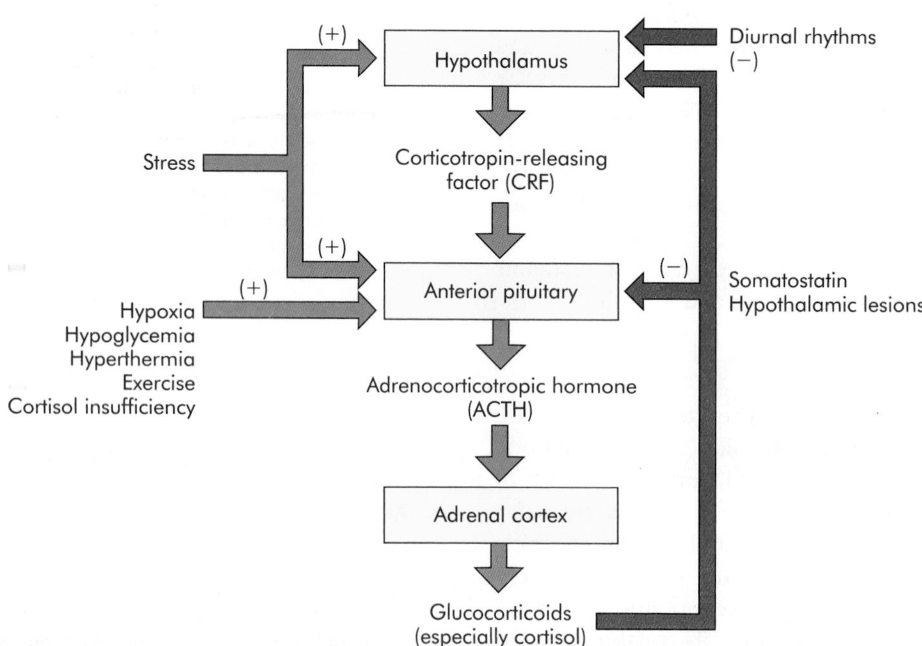

Figure 17-16 ■ **Feedback Control of Glucocorticoid Synthesis and Secretion.**

cortex through activation of crucial enzymes and storage of cholesterol for metabolism into steroid hormones. Extra-adrenal effects of ACTH include stimulation of melanocytes and activation of tissue lipase.

Once ACTH stimulates the cells of the adrenal cortex, cortisol synthesis and secretion immediately occur. In the healthy person, the secretory patterns of ACTH and cortisol are nearly identical. After secretion, some cortisol circulates in bound form attached to albumin but primarily it is bound to the plasma protein transcortin. A smaller amount circulates in the free form and diffuses into cells with specific intracellular receptors for cortisol. ACTH is rapidly inactivated in the circulation, and the liver and kidneys remove the deactivated hormone.

Mineralocorticoids: aldosterone

Mineralocorticoid steroids directly affect ion transport by epithelial cells, causing sodium retention and potassium and hydrogen loss. **Aldosterone** is the most potent naturally occurring mineralocorticoid and conserves sodium by increasing the activity of the sodium pump of epithelial cells. (The sodium pump is described in Chapter 1.)

The initial stages of aldosterone synthesis occur in the zona fasciculata and zona reticularis. The final conversion of corticosterone to aldosterone is confined to the zona glomerulosa. Aldosterone synthesis and secretion are regulated primarily by the renin-angiotensin system (described in Chapter 28). The renin-angiotensin system is activated by sodium and water depletion, increased potassium, and a diminished effective blood volume (Figure 17-17). Angiotensin II is the primary stimulant of aldosterone synthesis and secretion; however sodium and potassium levels also may directly affect aldosterone secretion. ACTH may transiently stimulate aldosterone synthesis but does not appear to be a major regulator of secretion.

When sodium and potassium levels are within normal limits, approximately 50 to 250 mg of aldosterone is secreted daily. Of the secreted aldosterone, 50% to 75% binds

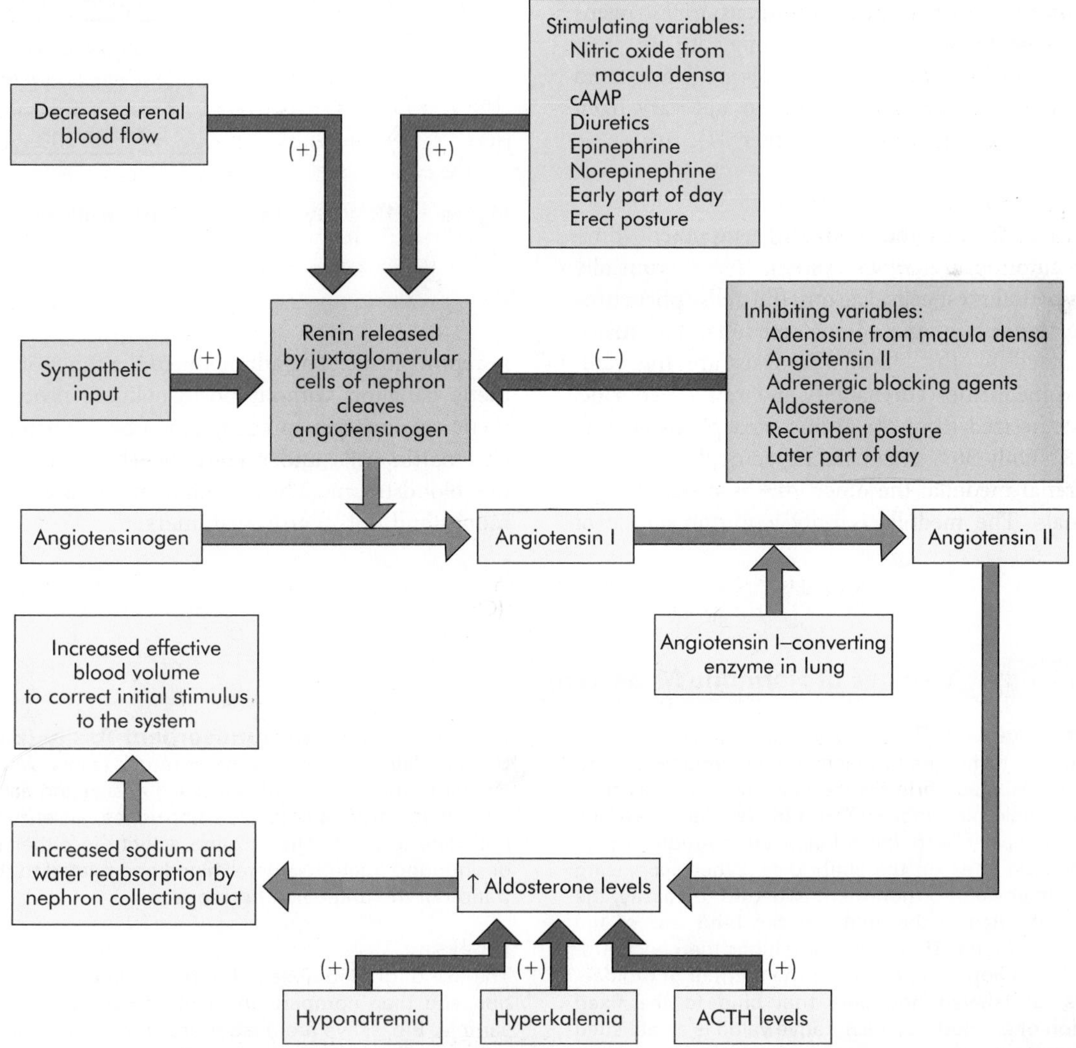

Figure 17-17 ■ **The Feedback Mechanisms Regulating Aldosterone Secretion.** *cAMP,* Cyclic adenosine monophosphate; *ACTH,* adrenocorticotropic hormone.

to plasma proteins. The large proportion of unbound aldosterone contributes to its rapid metabolic turnover in the liver, its low plasma concentration, and its short half-life (about 15 minutes). Aldosterone is degraded in the liver and is excreted by the kidney.

Aldosterone maintains extracellular volume by acting on distal nephron epithelial cells to increase sodium reabsorption and potassium and hydrogen excretion. This renal effect takes 90 minutes to 6 hours. Other effects of aldosterone include enhancement of cardiac muscle contraction, possible stimulation of ectopic ventricular activity through secondary cardiac pacemakers in the ventricles, stiffening of blood vessels and increased vascular resistance, and decreased fibrinolysis.[17–19]

Adrenal estrogens and androgens

The healthy adrenal cortex secretes minimal amounts of estrogen and androgens. ACTH appears to be the major regulator. Some of the weakly androgenic substances secreted by the cortex (dehydroepiandrosterone [DHEA], androstenedione) are converted by peripheral tissues to stronger androgens, such as testosterone, thus accounting for some androgenic effects initiated by the adrenal cortex. Peripheral conversion of adrenal androgens to estrogens is enhanced in some cases, including aging, obesity, liver disease, and hyperthyroidism.[20] The biologic effects and metabolism of the adrenal sex steroids do not vary from those produced by the gonads (see Chapter 31).

Adrenal medulla

The adrenal medulla, together with the sympathetic divisions of the autonomic nervous system, is embryonically derived from neural crest cells. Chromaffin cells (pheochromocytes) are the cells of the adrenal medulla. The major products secreted by the chromaffin cells are the catecholamines epinephrine (adrenaline) and norepinephrine, which are synthesized from the amino acid phenylalanine (Figure 17-18). Only 30% of circulating epinephrine comes from the adrenal medulla; the other 70% is released from nerve terminals. The medulla is only a minor source of norepinephrine. The adrenal medulla functions as a sympathetic ganglion without postganglionic processes. Sympathetic cholinergic preganglion fibers terminate on the chromaffin cells and secrete catecholamines directly into the bloodstream. The catecholamines are therefore hormones and not neurotransmitters.

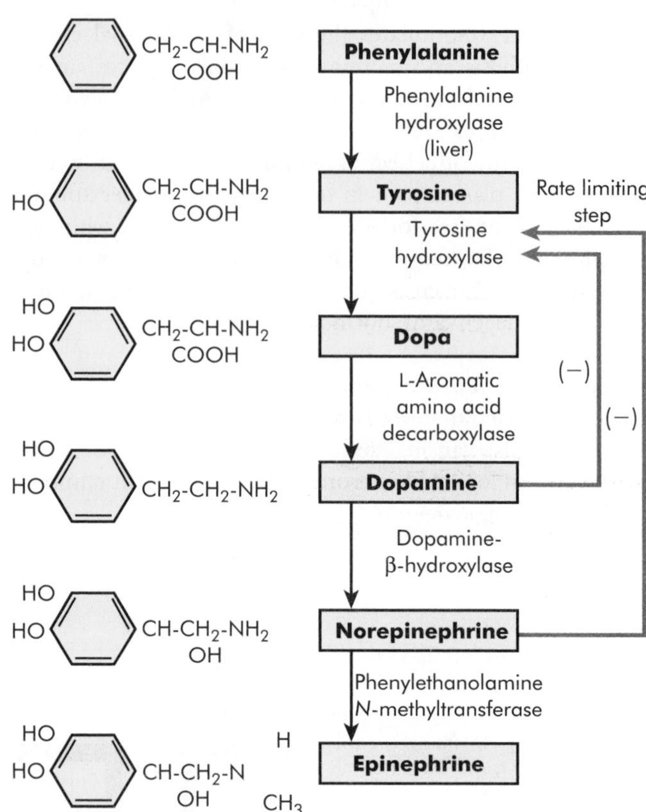

Figure 17-18 ■ **Synthesis of Catecholamines.**

BOX 17-2 Methods of Hormone Measurement

Radioimmunoassay (RIA)

An immunologic technique in which known amounts of antibody and radiolabeled hormone are placed in an assay tube with the unlabeled hormone. The radiolabeled hormone competes chemically with the nonlabeled hormone molecules for binding sites on the antibodies. When increasing amounts of unlabeled hormones are added to the assay, the limited binding sites of the antibody can bind less of the radiolabeled hormone. Therefore, the higher the concentration of unlabeled hormone, the fewer the number of radioactive *counts,* or labeled hormone, that bind to the fixed concentration of antibody. A quantitative value is established by use of standard reference curves.

Enzyme-Linked Immunosorbent Assay (Elisa)

Used to determine circulating hormone levels. The method is similar to that of RIA but is less expensive and easier to conduct. Instead of radiolabeled hormones, an enzyme-labeled hormone is used. The enzyme activity in either the bound or unbound fraction is determined and related to the concentration of the unlabeled hormone.

Bioassay

The use of graded doses of hormone in a reference preparation and then comparison of the results with an unknown sample. Bioassays are used more commonly in investigative endocrinology than in clinical laboratories.

Stimuli to adrenal medullary secretion include sympathetic nerve stimulation, hypoglycemia, hypoxia, hypercapnia, acidosis, hemorrhage, glucagon, nicotine, pilocarpine, histamine, and angiotensin II. In addition, ACTH and the glucocorticoids increase adrenal catecholamine secretion. On stimulation of the adrenal medullary cell, cytoplasmic storage granules that contain the catecholamines migrate to the cell surface and undergo exocytosis, a process that probably involves calcium. The catecholamines apparently directly inhibit their own secretion by decreasing the formation of tyrosine hydroxylase (the rate limiting step).

Catecholamines have diverse effects on the entire body. Their release and the body's response have been characterized as the fight-or-flight response (stress response see Figure 8-2 and Tables 8-3 and Table 8-4). Epinephrine is 10 times more potent than norepinephrine in exerting metabolic effects. The metabolic effects of catecholamines promote hyperglycemia through a variety of mechanisms including interference with the usual glucose regulatory feedback mechanisms.

QUICK CHECK 17-4

1. What are the islets of Langerhans? Where are they located?
2. Compare and contrast the actions of alpha, beta, delta, and F cells.
3. What is the most potent naturally occurring glucocorticoid, and how is its secretion related to that of adrenocorticotropic hormone (ACTH)?
4. How does aldosterone influence fluid and electrolyte balance?
5. What are catecholamines?

Neuroendocrine Response to Stressors

The endocrine system acts together with the nervous and immune systems to respond to stressors. Perception that an event is stressful may be essential to the emotional arousal and initiation of the stress response. Some events, such as bacterial invasion, can activate the stress response without emotional arousal. Details of the stress response are presented in Chapter 8. Methods of hormone measurement are given in Box 17-2.

AGING & Its Effects on Specific Endocrine Glands

General Endocrine Changes With Aging
Atrophy and weight loss with vascular changes; decreased secretion and clearance of hormones often occurs; variable change in receptor binding and intracellular responses.

Pancreas
Nearly half of older individuals have glucose intolerance or diabetes, and these disorders frequently go undiagnosed in aging adults. Mechanisms include decreased insulin receptor activity and decreased beta cell secretion of insulin.

Thyroid
Glandular atrophy, fibrosis, nodularity, and increased inflammatory infiltrates; possible changes in thyroid hormone (TH) are difficult to determine because of concurrent disease in elderly persons; may find decreased T_4 secretion and turnover, decline in T_3 (especially in men), diminished thyroid-stimulating hormone (TSH) secretion; reduced response of plasma TSH concentration to thyroid-releasing hormone (TRH) administration (especially in men)

Adrenal
Decreased DHEA leads to decreased synthesis of androgen-derived estrogen and testostesrone, decreased metabolic clearance of glucocorticoids, and cortisol, causes decreased cortisol secretion; there also are decreased levels of aldosterone.

Gonads
Women after the menopause have decreased estrogen and progesterone, increased follicle stimulating hormone, and relative increases in androgen levels; these changes have numerous physiologic and pathophysiologic consequences (see Chapter 32); in men, there is a gradual decrease in serum testosterone levels leading to decreased sexual activity, decreased muscle strength, and decreased bone mineralization.

Pituitary
Posterior: Decrease in size; reduced antidiuretic hormone (ADH) secretion
Anterior: Increased fibrosis and moderate increase in size of gland; decline in growth hormone release

See also Larsen SW: Endocrinology of aging. In *Williams Textbook of endocrinology*, ed 10, Philadelphia, 2003, Saunders.

Did You Understand?

Mechanisms of Hormonal Regulation

1. The endocrine system has diverse functions, including sexual differentiation, growth and development, and continuous maintenance of the body's internal environment.
2. Hormones are chemical messengers synthesized by endocrine glands and released into the circulation.
3. Hormones have specific negative and positive feedback mechanisms. Most hormone levels are regulated by negative feedback, in which hormone secretion raises the level of a specific hormone, ultimately causing secretion to subside.
4. Endocrine feedback is described in terms of short, long, and ultra-short feedback loops.
5. Water-soluble hormones circulate throughout the body in unbound form, whereas lipid-soluble hormones (i.e., steroid and thyroid hormones) circulate throughout the body bound to carrier proteins.
6. Hormones affect only target cells with appropriate receptors and then act on these cells to initiate specific cell functions or activities.
7. Hormones have two general types of effects on cells: (a) direct effects, or obvious changes in cell function, and (b) permissive effects, or less obvious changes that facilitate cell function.
8. Receptors for hormones may be located on the plasma membrane or in the intracellular compartment of a target cell.
9. Water-soluble hormones act as first messengers, binding to receptors on the cell's plasma membrane. The signals initiated by hormone-receptor binding are then transmitted into the cell by the action of second messengers.
10. Lipid-soluble hormones (including steroid and thyroid hormones) cross the plasma membrane by diffusion. These hormones diffuse directly into the cell nucleus and bind to nuclear receptors. Rapid responses of steroid hormones may be mediated by plasma membrane receptors.

Structure and Function of the Endocrine Glands

1. The pituitary gland, consisting of anterior and posterior portions, is connected to the central nervous system through the hypothalamus.
2. The hypothalamus regulates anterior pituitary function by secreting releasing hormones and releasing factors into the portal circulation.
3. Hypothalamic hormones include prolactin-inhibiting factor (PIF), which inhibits prolactin secretion; thyrotropin-releasing hormone (TRH), which affects release of thyroid hormones; gonadotropin-releasing hormone (GnRH), which facilitates release of adrenocorticotropic hormone (ACTH) and endorphins; and substance P, which inhibits ACTH release and stimulates release of a variety of other hormones.
4. The posterior pituitary secretes antidiuretic hormone (ADH), which also is called vasopressin, and oxytocin.
5. Hormones of the anterior pituitary are regulated by: (a) secretion of hypothalamic-releasing hormones or factors, (b) negative feedback from hormones secreted by target organs, and (c) mediating effects of neurotransmitters.
6. Hormones of the anterior pituitary include ACTH, melanocyte-stimulating hormone (MSH), somatotropic hormones (growth hormone [GH], prolactin), and glycoprotein hormones—follicle-stimulating hormone (FSH), luteinizing hormone (LH), and thyroid-stimulating hormone (TSH).
7. ADH controls serum osmolality, increases permeability of the renal tubules to water, and causes vasoconstriction when administered pharmacologically in high doses. ADH also may regulate some central nervous system functions.
8. Oxytocin causes uterine contraction and lactation in women and may have a role in sperm motility in men. In both men and women, oxytocin has an antidiuretic effect similar to that of ADH.
9. The two-lobed thyroid gland contains follicles, which secrete some of the thyroid hormones, and C cells, which secrete calcitonin and somatostatin.
10. Regulation of thyroid hormone (TH) levels is complex and involves the hypothalamus, anterior pituitary, thyroid gland, and numerous biochemical variables.
11. Thyroid hormone (TH) secretion is regulated by thyroid-releasing hormone (TRH) through a negative feedback loop that involves the anterior pituitary and hypothalamus.
12. Thyroid-stimulating hormone (TSH), which is synthesized and stored in the anterior pituitary, stimulates secretion of TH by activating intracellular processes, including uptake of iodine necessary for the synthesis of TH.
13. Once secreted, TH acts on the thyroid gland, the anterior pituitary, and the median eminence to regulate further TH production.
14. Synthesis of TH depends on the glycoprotein thyroglobulin (TG), which contains a precursor of TH, tyrosine. Tyrosine then combines with iodine to form precursor molecules of the thyroid hormones thyroxine (T_4) and triiodothyronine (T_3).
15. When released into the circulation, T_3 and T_4 are bound by carrier proteins in the plasma, which store these hormones and provide a buffer for rapid changes in hormone levels. The free form is the active form.
16. Thyroid hormones alter protein synthesis and have a wide range of metabolic effects on proteins, carbohydrates, lipids, and vitamins. TH also affects heat production and cardiac function.
17. The paired parathyroid glands normally are located behind the upper and lower poles of the thyroid. These glands secrete parathyroid hormone (PTH), an important regulator of serum calcium levels.
18. PTH secretion is regulated by levels of ionized calcium in the plasma and by cyclic adenosine monophosphate (cAMP) within the cell.
19. In bone, PTH causes bone breakdown and resorption. In the kidney, PTH increases reabsorption of calcium and decreases reabsorption of phosphorus and bicarbonate.
20. The endocrine pancreas contains the islets of Langerhans, which secrete hormones responsible for much of the carbohydrate metabolism in the body.

Did You Understand?—Cont'd

21. The islets of Langerhans consist of alpha cells, beta cells, delta cells, and F cells.
22. Alpha cells produce glucagon, which is secreted inversely to blood glucose concentrations.
23. Delta cells secrete somatostatin, which inhibits glucagon and insulin secretion.
24. Beta cells secrete preproinsulin, which is ultimately converted to insulin.
25. F cells secrete pancreatic polypeptide.
26. Insulin is a hormone that regulates blood glucose concentrations and overall body metabolism of fat, protein, and carbohydrates.
27. The paired adrenal glands are situated above the kidneys. Each gland consists of an adrenal medulla, which secretes catecholamines, and an adrenal cortex, which secretes steroid hormones.
28. The steroid hormones secreted by the adrenal cortex are synthesized from cholesterol. These hormones include glucocorticoids, mineralocorticoids, and adrenal androgens and estrogens.
29. Glucocorticoids directly affect carbohydrate metabolism by increasing blood glucose concentration through gluconeogenesis in the liver and by decreasing use of glucose. Glucocorticoids inhibit immune and inflammatory responses.
30. The most potent naturally occurring glucocorticoid is cortisol, which is necessary for the maintenance of life and for protection from stress. Secretion of cortisol is regulated by the hypothalamus and anterior pituitary.
31. Cortisol secretion is related to secretion of adrenocorticotropic hormone (ACTH), which is stimulated by corticotropin-releasing hormone (CRH). ACTH binds with receptors of the adrenal cortex, which activates intracellular mechanisms (specifically cyclic AMP) and leads to cortisol release.
32. Mineralocorticoids are steroid hormones that directly affect ion transport by renal tubular epithelial cells, causing sodium retention and potassium and hydrogen loss.
33. Aldosterone is the most potent of the naturally occurring mineralocorticoids. Its primary role is to conserve sodium.
34. Aldosterone secretion is regulated primarily by the renin-angiotensin system and serum sodium concentration.
35. Aldosterone acts by binding to a site on the cell nucleus and altering protein production within the cell. Its principal site of action is the kidney, where it causes sodium reabsorption and potassium and hydrogen excretion.
36. Androgens and estrogens secreted by the adrenal cortex act in the same way as those secreted by the gonads.
37. The adrenal medulla secretes the catecholamines epinephrine and norepinephrine. Epinephrine is 10 times more potent than norepinephrine in exerting metabolic effects. Their release is stimulated by sympathetic nervous system stimulation, ACTH, and glucocorticoids.
38. Catecholamines bind with various target cells and are taken up by neurons or excreted in the urine. They cause a range of metabolic effects characterized as the fight-or-flight response and include hyperglycemia and immune suppression.
39. The endocrine system acts together with the nervous system to respond to stressors.
40. The response to stressors involves (a) activation of the sympathetic division of the autonomic nervous system and (b) activation of the endocrine system.
41. Other hormones that are secreted in response to stress include growth hormone (GH), prolactin, testosterone, antidiuretic hormone (ADH), and insulin.
42. The adrenal glands and the sympathetic neurons that innervate these glands form the sympathoadrenal axis.

AGING & Its Effects on Specific Endocrine Glands

1. The general changes in the endocrine glands that occur with older age include atrophy and weight loss with vascular changes, decreased secretion and clearance of hormones, and variable change in receptor binding and intracellular responses.

Key Terms

Adrenal cortex, 437
Adrenal gland, 437
Adrenal medulla, 439
Adrenocorticotropic hormone (ACTH), 431
Aldosterone, 441
Alpha cell, 435
Amylin, 436
Anterior pituitary, 430
Antidiuretic hormone (ADH), 431
Beta cell, 435
C cell, 432
Calcitonin, 432
Chromophil, 430
Chromophobe, 430
Corticotropin-releasing hormone (CRH), 430
Cortisol, 440
Delta cell, 435
Direct effect, 427
Down-regulation, 427
F (or PP) cell, 435
First messenger, 427
Follicle, 432
Gastrin, 437
Glucagon, 436
Glucocorticoid, 439
Gonadotropin-releasing hormone (GnRH), 430
Growth hormone–releasing factor (GRF), 430
Hormone receptor, 427
Hormone, 424
Insulin, 435
Islet of Langerhans, 435
Isthmus, 432
Median eminence, 431
Mineralocorticoid, 441
Negative feedback, 425
Oxytocin, 432
Pancreas, 435

Key Terms—Cont'd

References

1. Cato AC, Nestl A, Mink S: Rapid actions of steroid receptors in cellular signaling pathways, *Sci STKE* Jun 25(138):RE9, 2002.
2. Watson CS, Lange CA: Steadying the boat: Integrating mechanisms of membrane and nuclear steroid signaling, *EMBO Reports* 6:116–119, 2005.
3. Levin ER: Cellular functions of plasma membrane estrogen receptors, *Steroids* 67(6):471–475, 2002.
4. Losel R, Wehling M: Nongenomic actions of steroid hormones, *Nat Rev Mol Cell Biol* 4(1):46–56, 2003.
5. Watson CS, Gametchu B: Proteins of multiple classes may participate in nongenomic steroid actions, *Exp Biol Med* 228:1272–1281, 2003.
6. Song IH, Buttgereit F: Non-genomic glucocorticoid effects to provide the basis for new drug developments, *Mol Cell Endocrinol* 246(1-2):142–146, 2006.
7. Manavathi B, Kumar R: Steering estrogen signals from the plasma membrane to the nucleus: two sides of the coin, *J Cell Physiol* 207(3):594–604, 2006.
8. Quirk CC, Nilson JH: Hormones and gene expression: basic principles, In DeGroot LJ, Jamerson JL, editors: *Endocrinology,* ed 5, St Louis, 2006, Elsevier Saunders.
9. Pietras RJ, Nemere I, Szego CM: Steroid hormone receptors in target cell membranes, *Endocrine* 14(3):417–427, 2001.
10. St. Germain DL: Thyroid hormone metabolism, In DeGroot LJ, Jamerson JL, editors: *Endocrinology,* ed 5, St Louis, 2006, Elsevier Saunders.
11. Marques RG, Fontaine MJ, Rogers J: C-peptide: much more than a byproduct of insulin biosynthesis, *Pancreas* 29(3): 231–238, 2004.
12. Fiory F et al: Tyrosine phosphorylation of phosphoinositide-dependent kinase 1 by the insulin receptor is necessary for insulin metabolic signaling, *Molec Cell Biol* 25(24): 10803–10814, 2005.
13. Ryan GJ, Jobe LJ, Martin R: Pramlintide in the treatment of type 1 and type 2 diabetes mellitus [journal article review], *Clin Ther* 27(10):1500–1512, 2005.
14. Bonner-Weir S, Weir G: New sources of pancreatic β-cells, *Nat Biotech* 12:857–861, 2005.
15. White A: Adrenocorticotropic hormone, In DeGroot LJ, Jamerson JL, editors: *Endocrinology,*, ed 5, St Louis, 2006, Elsevier Saunders.
16. Munck A, Naray-Fejes-Toth A: Glucocorticoid physiology, In DeGroot LJ, Jamerson JL, editors: *Endocrinology,* ed 5, St Louis, 2006, Elsevier Saunders.
17. Chai W et al: Nongenomic effects of aldosterone in the human heart: interaction with angiotensin II, *Hyperten* 46(4):701–706, 2005.
18. Fuller PJ, Young MJ: Mechanisms of mineralocorticoid action, *Hyperten* 46(6):12271235, 2005.
19. Losel R et al: Rapid effects of aldosterone on vascular cells: clinical implications, *Steroids* 69(8-9):575–578, 2004.
20. Larsen SW: Endocrinology of aging. In *Williams textbook of endocrinology,* ed 10, Philadelphia, 2003, Saunders.

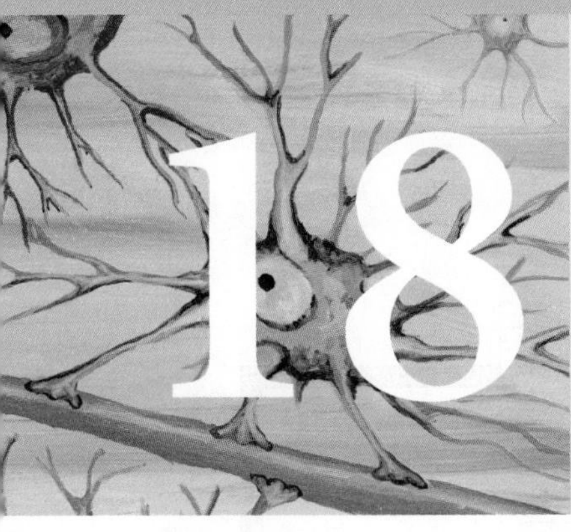

18 ALTERATIONS OF HORMONAL REGULATION

Robert E. Jones ▪ Valentina L. Brashers ▪ Sue E. Huether

CHAPTER OUTLINE

ELECTRONIC RESOURCES

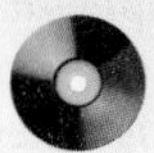

Companion CD
- Review Questions and Answers
- Animations

evolve Website
http://evolve.elsevier.com/Huether/
- Quick Check Answers
- Key Terms Exercises
- Critical Thinking Questions with Answers
- Algorithm Completion Exercises
- WebLinks

Function of the endocrine system involves complex interrelationships and interactions that maintain dynamic steady states and provide growth and reproductive capabilities. Dysfunction was initially described in terms of excessive or insufficient function of the endocrine gland with alterations in hormone levels. These alterations were thought to be caused by either hypersecretion or hyposecretion of the various hormones, leading to abnormal hormone concentrations in the blood. Evidence now shows that dysfunction may result from abnormal receptor function or from altered intracellular response to the hormone-receptor complex.

MECHANISMS OF HORMONAL ALTERATIONS

Significantly elevated or significantly depressed hormone levels may result from various causes (Figure 18-1). Feedback systems that recognize the need for a particular hormone may fail to function properly or may respond to inappropriate signals. Dysfunction of an endocrine gland may involve its failure to produce adequate amounts of biologically free or active hormone, or a gland may synthesize or release too much hormone. Once hormones are released into the circulation, they may be degraded at an altered rate or inactivated by antibodies before reaching the target cell. Hormones produced by nonendocrine tissues may cause abnormally elevated hormone levels. This mechanism operates without benefit of the normal feedback system for hormone control, and the ectopic hormone production is said to be autonomous.

Why do target cells fail to respond to hormones? The general types of abnormal target cell responses currently recognized are as follows:

1. *Cell surface receptor-associated disorders.* These have been identified primarily in water-soluble hormones, such as insulin. The disorders may involve a decrease in the number of receptors, leading to decreased or defective hormone-receptor binding; impaired receptor function, resulting in insensitivity to the hormone; presence of antibodies against specific receptors that either reduce available binding sites or mimic hormone action, suppressing or exaggerating target cell response; or unusual expression of receptor function, for example, tumor cells with abnormal receptor activity.
2. *Intracellular disorders.* These involve acquired defects in postreceptor signaling cascades or inadequate synthesis of a second messenger, such as cyclic adenosine monophosphate (cAMP), needed to transduce the hormonal signal into intracellular events. The target cell for water-soluble hormones may have a faulty response to hormone-receptor binding and thus fail to generate the required second messenger, or the cell may respond abnormally to the second messenger if levels of intracellular enzymes or proteins are altered. As a result, the target cell fails to express the usual hormonal effect.

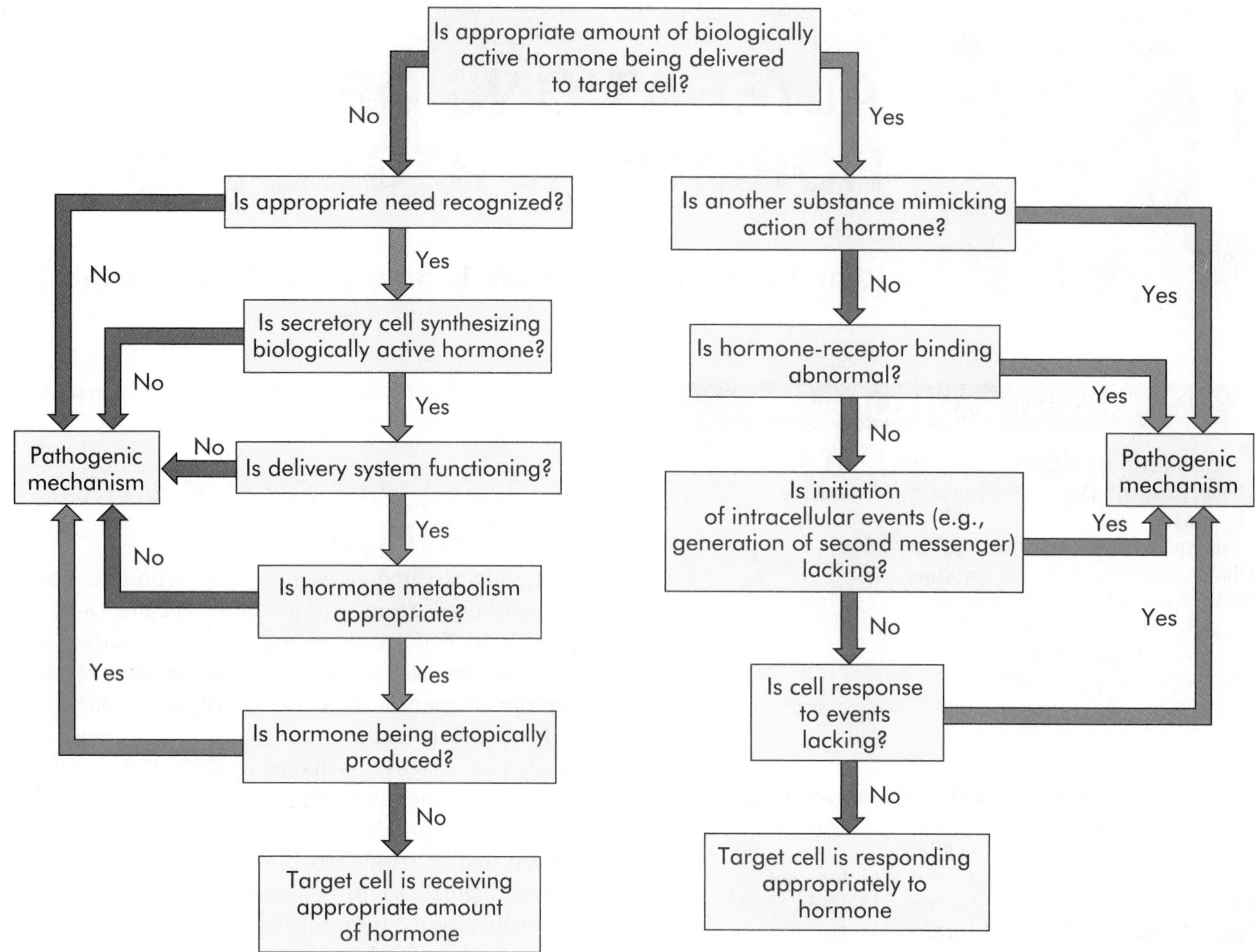

Figure 18-1 ■ **Hormone Delivery to Cells.** Phases at which pathogenic mechanisms may develop in delivering appropriate amounts of hormone to the cells.

3. *Circulating inhibitors.* Antibodies directed against a hormone, or nonimmune proteins that can bind a specific hormone, will impair the ability of that hormone to bind to and activate its receptor.

Pathogenic mechanisms affecting target cell response for lipid-soluble hormones either occur less often or are recognized less often than those affecting water-soluble hormones. The number of intracellular receptors may be decreased, or receptors may have an altered affinity for hormones, which would affect hormone-receptor binding. The generation of new messenger ribonucleic acid (RNA) may be altered or substrates for new protein synthesis may be altered, resulting in altered target cell response.

ALTERATIONS OF THE HYPOTHALAMIC-PITUITARY SYSTEM

Perhaps the most common cause of apparent hypothalamic dysfunction is interruption of the pituitary stalk caused by destructive lesions, rupture after head injury, surgical transection, or stem tumor. Interruption of the physical connections between the hypothalamus and the pituitary gland causes apparent pituitary disease. For example, diabetes insipidus (antidiuretic hormone insufficiency) may result, depending on where the pituitary stalk is interrupted. The farther away the lesion is from the hypothalamus, the less likely is the occurrence of diabetes insipidus.

Without hypothalamic hormones (Figure 18-2), women cease to menstruate and men experience impaired spermatogenesis. Adrenocorticotropic hormone (ACTH) response to low serum cortisol levels is decreased because of the absence of corticotropin-releasing hormone (CRH). Hypothalamic hypothyroidism is caused by the absence of thyrotropin-releasing hormone (TRH). Low levels of growth hormone (GH) cause the absence of GH regulatory hormones. Hyperprolactinemia is caused by an absence of usual inhibitory controls of prolactin secretion.

Diseases of the Posterior Pituitary

Syndrome of inappropriate antidiuretic hormone secretion

Diseases of the posterior pituitary are rare and are usually related to abnormal antidiuretic hormone (ADH/

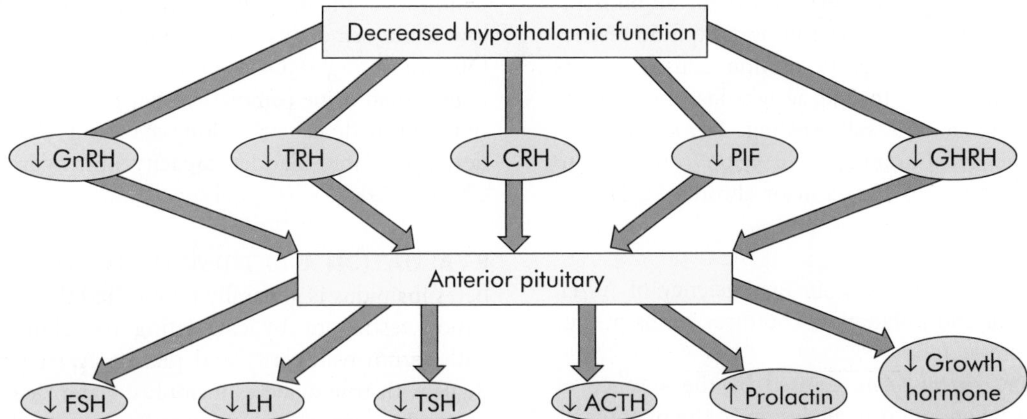

Figure 18-2 ■ **Loss of Hypothalamic Hormones.** *GnRH,* Gonadotropin-releasing hormone; *TRH,* thyrotropin-releasing hormone; *CRH,* corticotropin-releasing hormone; *PIF,* prolactin inhibitory factor (probably dopamine); *GHRH,* growth hormone releasing hormone; *FSH,* follicle-stimulating hormone; *LH,* luteinizing hormone; *TSH,* thyroid-stimulating hormone; *ACTH,* adrenocorticotropic hormone.

vasopressin) secretion. **Syndrome of inappropriate ADH secretion (SIADH)** is characterized by high levels of ADH without normal physiologic stimuli for its release.[1] The most common cause is ectopically produced ADH, associated with cancer, wherein tumor cells secrete ADH. Tumors associated with SIADH include samll cell carcinoma of the lung (the most common cause of SIADH), carcinoma of the duodenum and pancreas, leukemia, lymphoma, Hodgkin disease, sarcoma, and squamous cell carcinoma of the tongue. Another important cause of SIADH is brain injury or infection such as trauma, stroke, hemorrhage, or meningitis.[2]

Any surgery can result in postoperative fluid volume shifts that result in increased ADH secretion for as long as 5 to 7 days after surgery. Transient SIADH may also follow pituitary surgery, because stored ADH is released in an unregulated fashion. SIADH is seen also in individuals with infectious pulmonary diseases, where ADH is produced by infected lung tissue or posterior pituitary secretion of ADH is increased in response to a hypoxia-induced decrease in pulmonary perfusion.

Finally, SIADH may be associated with psychiatric disease and various drugs, including hypoglycemic medications (chlorpropamide), barbiturates, general anesthesia, vincristine, nicotine, morphine, diuretics, and synthetic ADH analogs. These drugs either simulate ADH release or enhance the physiologic effects of ADH or have a biologic action similar to ADH.[3]

PATHOPHYSIOLOGY The cardinal features of SIADH are symptoms of water intoxication resulting from enhanced renal water retention or increases in total body water, which leads to hyponatremia (low serum sodium), hypoosmolarity and urine that is inappropriately concentrated with respect to serum osmolarity.[4] In SIADH, ADH is released continually. Water retention results from the normal action of ADH on the renal tubules and collecting ducts, increasing their permeability to water and increasing water reabsorption by the kidneys. (Renal function is discussed in Chapter 28.)

Extracellular fluid volume expands, and a dilutional hyponatremia develops, suppressing renin and therefore aldosterone secretion, and decreasing proximal tubule reabsorption of sodium. This explains renal sodium loss during hyponatremia.

CLINICAL MANIFESTATIONS A diagnosis of SIADH requires the following signs: (1) serum hypoosmolality and hyponatremia, (2) urine hyperosmolarity (i.e., urine osmolality is greater than expected for the concomitant serum osmolality), (3) urine sodium excretion that matches sodium intake, (4) normal adrenal and thyroid function, and (5) absence of conditions that can alter volume status (e.g., congestive heart failure, hypovolemia from any cause, or renal insufficiency).

The symptoms of SIADH result from hyponatremia and are determined by its severity and sudden onset. Thirst, impaired taste, anorexia, dyspnea on exertion, fatigue, and dulled sensorium occur when the serum sodium decreases rapidly from 140 to 130 mEq/L. Severe gastrointestinal symptoms, including vomiting and abdominal cramps, occur with a drop in sodium from 130 to 120 mEq/L. Peripheral edema is absent. Symptoms usually resolve with correction of hyponatremia. Even if hyponatremia develops slowly, serum sodium levels below 110 mEq/L to 115 mEq/L cause confusion, lethargy, muscle twitching, and convulsions, and severe and sometimes irreversible neurologic damage may occur.

EVALUATION AND TREATMENT Serum electrolyte levels, serum osmolality, urine volume, urine electrolyte levels, and urine osmolality are adequate measures of the presence of SIADH. The treatment of SIADH involves the correction of any underlying causal problems, emergency correction of severe hyponatremia by careful administration of hypertonic saline, and, most important, fluid restriction with careful monitoring. Resolution usually occurs within 3 days, with a 2-kg to 3-kg weight loss and correction of hyponatremia and salt wasting. Demeclocycline, which causes the renal tubules to develop resistance to ADH, may be used to treat resistant or chronic SIADH.

Diabetes insipidus

Diabetes insipidus is related to an insufficiency of ADH, leading to polyuria and polydipsia. The three forms of diabetes insipidus are as follows:

1. *Neurogenic or central form.* Caused by the absence of ADH; occurs when any organic lesion of the hypothalamus, pituitary stalk, or posterior pituitary interferes with ADH synthesis, transport or release; lesions include primary brain tumors, hypophysectomy, aneurysms, thrombosis, infections, and immunologic disorders.
2. *Nephrogenic form.* Caused by inadequate response of the renal tubules to ADH, which is usually acquired or may be genetic.[5,6] Lesions in the collecting tubules are generally related to disorders and drugs that inhibit the generation of cAMP in the tubules. This is related to diseases that irreversibly damage the renal tubules, such as pyelonephritis, polycystic disease, or destructive uropathies. The use of methoxyflurane anesthesia, lithium, or demeclocycline can cause a reversible form of nephrogenic diabetes insipidus.
3. *Psychogenic form (primary polydipsia).* This condition may be confused with a partial deficiency of ADH and is caused by the chronic ingestion of extremely large quantities of fluid that wash out the renal medullary concentration gradient, which results in a partial resistance to ADH. This condition resolves with effective management.

PATHOPHYSIOLOGY Individuals with diabetes insipidus will have a partial to total inability to concentrate urine. Insufficient ADH secretion causes immediate excretion of large volumes of dilute urine, leading to increased plasma osmolality. In conscious individuals, the thirst mechanism is stimulated and induces polydipsia—usually a craving for cold drinks. The urine output varies. With profound ADH deficiency, output may be more than 12 L/day. The urine specific gravity is low. Dehydration develops rapidly without ongoing fluid replacement. In nephrogenic diabetes insipidus, ADH levels are normal or high but the collecting ducts do not increase their permeability to water in response to ADH.

Diabetes insipidus usually has an acute onset. With traumatic diabetes insipidus, a classic, three-phase syndrome has been observed related to progressive loss of nerve tissue with significant diuresis, then antidiuresis, and finally polyuria and polydipsia, reflecting a permanent loss of the ability to secrete adequate amounts of ADH.

CLINICAL MANIFESTATIONS The clinical manifestations of diabetes insipidus include polyuria, nocturia, continuous thirst, polydipsia, low urine specific gravity, low urine osmolality,[5] and high-normal plasma osmolality (300 mOsm/kg H_2O or more). Plasma osmolality is always higher than urine osmolality after 8 hours of water deprivation. Individuals with long-standing diabetes insipidus develop a large bladder capacity and hydronephrosis (see Chapter 29).

EVALUATION AND TREATMENT The diagnosis of diabetes insipidus is generally established through water deprivation testing or by correlating the clinical presentation with serum osmolarity and plasma ADH levels. In individuals with true diabetes insipidus, water deprivation testing can be hazardous. If the person loses more than 3% of their pretest body weight, circulatory collapse and shock can ensue. The diagnosis of psychogenic polydipsia can be extremely difficult, and differentiation from nephrogenic diabetes insipidus (caused by the washout of the renal concentrating gradient) is based on plasma ADH levels.

Treatment of neurogenic diabetes insipidus is based on the extent of the ADH deficiency and on age, endocrine and cardiovascular status, and lifestyle. Some individuals require ADH replacement, but oral hydration often is adequate.

Replacement therapy for symptomatic central or neurogenic diabetes insipidus includes intravascular or, more commonly, oral or intranasal administration of the synthetic vasopressin analog DDAVP (desmopressin). Drugs that potentiate the action of otherwise insufficient amounts of endogenous ADH may be used in individuals with incomplete ADH deficiency.

Diseases of the Anterior Pituitary

Hypopituitarism

Hypopituitarism involves a range of dysfunction from absence of selective pituitary hormones to the complete failure of hormonal functions. Primary hypopituitarism and secondary hypopituitarism are not usually distinguished. Secondary hypopituitarism (resulting from dysfunction of the hypothalamus) is difficult to document because the neurohormonal output of the hypothalamus does not lend itself to measurement.

Pituitary infarction causes hypopituitarism, and infarction may be seen with Sheehan syndrome (postpartum pituitary necrosis), pituitary apoplexy, shock, sickle cell disease, and diabetes mellitus. Other more common causes of hypopituitarism are pituitary tumors; head trauma; infections (e.g., meningitis, syphilis, tuberculosis); vascular malformations; surgical ablation related to tumor removal; and, rarely, granulomatous lesions.[7]

PATHOPHYSIOLOGY The pituitary gland is extremely vascular and therefore extremely vulnerable to infarction. The likelihood of infarction increases when the gland enlarges and becomes more vascular, which occurs during pregnancy. The primary pathologic mechanism in postpartum pituitary infarction is vasospasm of the artery supplying the anterior pituitary. If vasospasm is sustained for more than several hours, tissue necrosis occurs. The pituitary gland may be particularly susceptible because its blood supply, through the portal system, is already partially deoxygenated and, especially in the hyperplastic pituitary of pregnancy, oxygen demands increase.

After tissue necrosis, edema occurs. The pituitary expands within the fixed confines of the sella turcica, further impeding its blood supply. A second mechanism, which may be involved in Sheehan syndrome (postpartum pituitary infarction), is increased risk for intravascular coagulation. Excessive fibrin is deposited in the pituitary vessels, predisposing to decreased blood supply and infarction.[8]

CLINICAL MANIFESTATIONS The signs and symptoms of hypofunction of the anterior pituitary are highly variable and depend on the affected hormones. In **panhypopituitarism,** when all hormones are absent, the individual suffers from cortisol deficiency, thyroid deficiency, diabetes insipidus, gonadal failure, and loss of secondary sex characteristics. Low GH and insulin-like growth factor I may affect growth in children but generally do not cause symptoms in adults (Figure 18-3). In addition, postpartum women cannot lactate with decreased or absent prolactin.

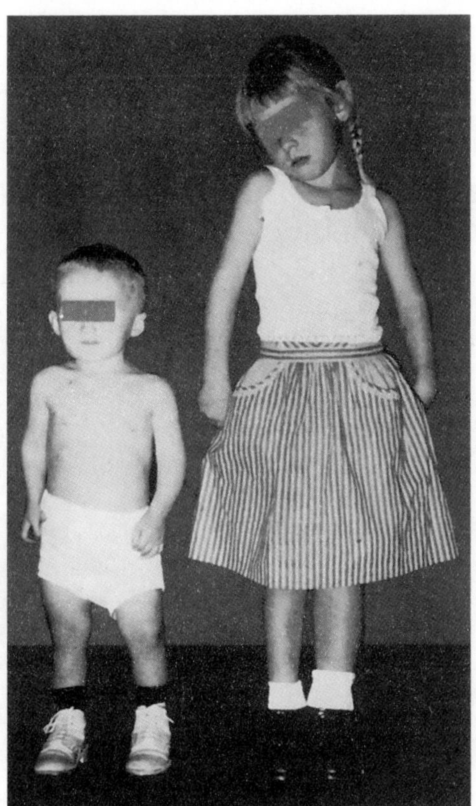

Figure 18-3 ■ **Hypopituitary Dwarfism.** A 4-year-old boy whose height is 25 inches. Girl is also 4 years old and has a normal height of 39 inches. Boy (dwarf) has a normal face, as well as head, trunk, and limbs of approximately normal proportions. (From Brashear HR, Raney RB: *Handbook of orthopaedic surgery,* ed 10, St Louis, 1986, Mosby.)

ACTH deficiency is a potentially life-threatening disorder, because cortisol is required for functional maintenance. ACTH deficiency usually is encountered with generalized pituitary hypofunction; it rarely occurs as an isolated event. Within 2 weeks of the complete absence of ACTH, symptoms of cortisol insufficiency develop, including nausea, vomiting, anorexia, fatigue, and weakness. The resulting hypoglycemia is caused by increased insulin sensitivity, decreased glycogen reserves, and decreased gluconeogenesis associated with hypocortisolism. ACTH deficiency also limits maximum aldosterone secretion, although the renin-angiotensin system can stimulate some aldosterone secretion. The glomerular filtration rate decreases, causing decreased urine output. (Renal function is described in Chapter 28.) This may be of some benefit in the individual who has diabetes insipidus, but the polyuria associated with diabetes insipidus worsens after correction of cortisol levels.

Thyroid-stimulating hormone (TSH) deficiency is rarely seen in isolation but often occurs with other pituitary hormone deficiencies. The effects of decreased TSH levels become apparent 4 to 8 weeks after hypothyrotropinemia occurs. Cold intolerance, skin dryness, mild myxedema, lethargy, and decreased metabolic rate occur as with hypothyroidism induced by decreased TSH levels. The symptoms usually are less severe than those of primary hypothyroidism.

The onset of follicle-stimulating hormone (FSH) and luteinizing hormone (LH) deficiencies in women of reproductive age is associated with amenorrhea and an atrophic vagina, uterus, and breasts. In postpubertal males, testicles atrophy and beard growth is stunted. Both men and women experience decreased body hair and diminished libido. FSH and LH deficiencies often occur with pressure on the pituitary from other sources, such as tumors. If there is enlargement caused by tumor, symptoms include headache and visual disturbances (blurring and field defects).

EVALUATION AND TREATMENT The diagnostic evaluation of suspected pituitary disease is often challenging and must be carefully interpreted together with the individual's signs and symptoms. Simultaneous measurements of the tropic hormones from the pituitary and target endocrine glands are crucial and, on occasions, dynamic testing of the various axes is undertaken. Imaging of the pituitary (magnetic resonance imaging [MRI] or computed tomography [CT] scans) is critical to assess for anatomic lesions, such as tumors. In hypopituitarism, the underlying disorder should be corrected as quickly as possible. Thyroid and cortisol replacement therapy must be maintained and sex steroid replacement therapy initiated, depending on the individual's needs and desires.

Hyperpituitarism: primary adenoma

Pituitary adenomas usually are benign, slow-growing tumors that arise from cells of the anterior pituitary. Most are microscopic and asymptomatic, found only on postmortem examinations. The cause of pituitary adenomas is not known. The mortality associated with pituitary tumors is usually attributable to alterations in hormone secretion or tissue changes caused by tumor expansion.

PATHOPHYSIOLOGY Local expansion of the adenoma may impinge on the optic chiasma and cause various visual disturbances, depending on the portion of the nerve compressed. If the tumor is locally aggressive, invasion of the oculomotor and trigeminal nerves can occur, with attending symptoms. Extension to the hypothalamus disturbs control of wakefulness, thirst, appetite, and temperature.

The adenomatous tissue secretes the hormone of the cell type from which it arose, without regard to the needs of the body and without benefit of regulatory feedback mechanisms. Because of the pressure exerted by the tumor in the unexpandable skull, those secreting cells that are most sensitive to pressure also may be affected (GH-, FSH-, and LH-secreting cells). The result is hyposecretion of these hormones.

CLINICAL MANIFESTATIONS The clinical manifestations of pituitary adenomas are related to tumor growth and hormone hypersecretion or hyposecretion. Increased tumor size causes headache, fatigue, neck pain or stiffness, and seizures. Visual changes include visual field impairments (often beginning in one eye and progressing to the other) and temporary blindness. If the tumor infiltrates other cranial nerves, neuromuscular function is affected.

Hyposecretion of pituitary hormones results in impaired pituitary function. Hyposecretion of GH almost always occurs, but in adults it is clinically asymptomatic. Gonadotropic hyposecretion often results in menstrual irregularity in women, decreased libido, and receding secondary sex characteristics in both men and women. If the tumor exerts sufficient pressure, thyroid and adrenal hypofunction may occur, resulting in hypothyroidism and hypocortisolism. Hypersecretion of hormones secreted by the adenoma itself leads to symptoms associated with the particular hormone affected.

EVALUATION AND TREATMENT Diagnosis of pituitary adenoma involves physical and laboratory evaluations, including pertinent hormone assays and radiographic examination of the skull (MRI or contrast-enhanced CT). The goal of treatment is to protect the individual from the effects of tumor growth and to control hormone hypersecretion while minimizing damage to appropriately secreting portions of the pituitary. Surgery and radiation therapy are used also, as appropriate.

QUICK CHECK 18-1

1. What is the mechanism of receptor-associated hormonal disorder?
2. Why do individuals with the syndrome of inappropriate antidiuretic hormone (SIADH) secrete concentrated urine?
3. Why may individuals with a pituitary adenoma develop visual disturbances?

Hypersecretion of growth hormone: acromegaly

Acromegaly is a relatively uncommon disease that occurs in adults exposed to continuously high levels of growth hormone (GH) and insulin-like growth factor 1 (IGF-1). The most common cause of acromegaly is a GH-secreting pituitary adenoma. Acromegaly occurs in adults in their 40s and 50s, although it is often present for years before diagnosis.[9] It is a slowly progressive disease and, if untreated, is associated with a decreased life expectancy. Deaths from acromegaly are caused by heart disease, secondary to hypertension and diabetes mellitus, or malignancy (colon or lung cancers).

PATHOPHYSIOLOGY With a GH-secreting adenoma, the usual GH baseline secretion pattern and sleep-related GH peaks are lost, and a totally unpredictable secretory pattern ensues. However, GH levels in acromegalics are never completely suppressed in contrast to normal individuals where GH levels are frequently unmeasurable. In children and adolescents whose epiphyseal plates have not yet closed, the effect of increased GH levels is termed **giantism** (Figure 18-4). Skeletal growth is excessive, with some individuals becoming 8 or 9 feet tall. In the adult, epiphyseal closure has occurred, and increased amounts of GH and IGF-1 cause connective tissue proliferation and increased

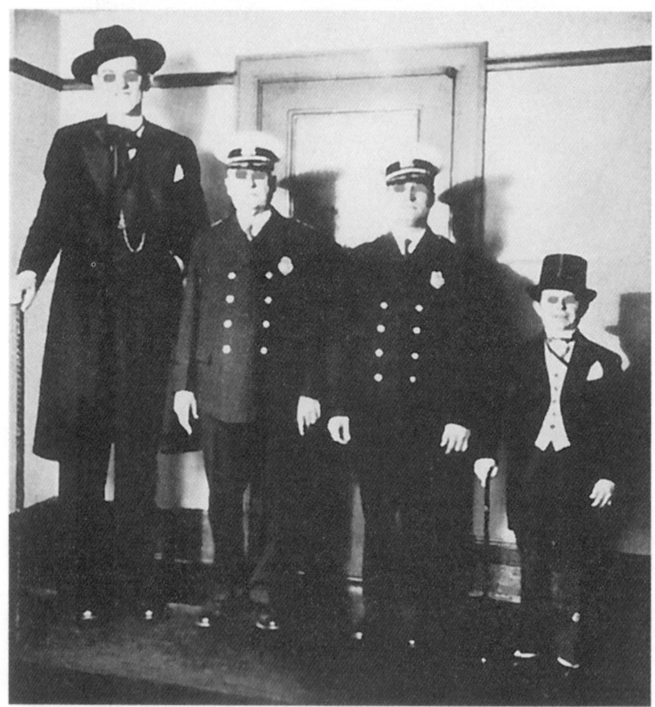

Figure 18-4 ■ **Giantism.** A pituitary giant and dwarf contrasted with normal-size men. Excessive secretion of growth hormone by the anterior lobe of the pituitary gland during the early years of life produces giants of this type, whereas deficient secretion of this substance produces well-formed dwarfs. (From Thibodeau GA, Patton KT: *Anatomy & physiology*, ed 6, St Louis, 2007, Mosby.)

cytoplasmic matrix, as well as bony proliferation that results in the characteristic appearance of acromegaly (Figure 18-5).

GH acts on the renal tubules to increase phosphate reabsorption, leading to mild hyperphosphatemia. The metabolic effects include impaired carbohydrate tolerance and increased metabolic rate. Hyperglycemia results from GH's inhibition of peripheral glucose uptake and increased hepatic glucose production, followed by compensatory hyperinsulinism and, finally, insulin resistance. Diabetes mellitus occurs when the pancreas cannot secrete enough insulin to offset the effects of GH. Coexisting hyperprolactinemia may lead to oligomenorrhea in women and erectile dysfunction or loss of libido in men.

CLINICAL MANIFESTATIONS With connective tissue proliferation, individuals with acromegaly have an enlarged tongue, interstitial edema, enlarged and overactive sebaceous and sweat glands (leading to increased body odor), and coarse skin and body hair. Bony proliferation involves periosteal vertebral growth and enlargement of the bones of the face, hands, and feet (see Figure 18-5). The lower jaw and forehead also protrude.

Increased IGF-1 levels cause ribs to elongate at the bone-cartilage junction, leading to a barrel-chested appearance and increased proliferation of cartilage in joints. This causes backache, arthralgia, and arthritis, the early manifestations of acromegaly. With bony and soft tissue overgrowth, nerve entrapment occurs, leading to peripheral nerve damage manifested by weakness, muscular atrophy, footdrop, and sensory changes in the hands.

Hypertension and left heart failure are seen in one third to one half of individuals with acromegaly.[10] Because the adenoma becomes increasingly a space-occupying lesion, central nervous system symptoms of headache, seizure activity, visual disturbances, papilledema, and compression hypopituitarism may occur.[11]

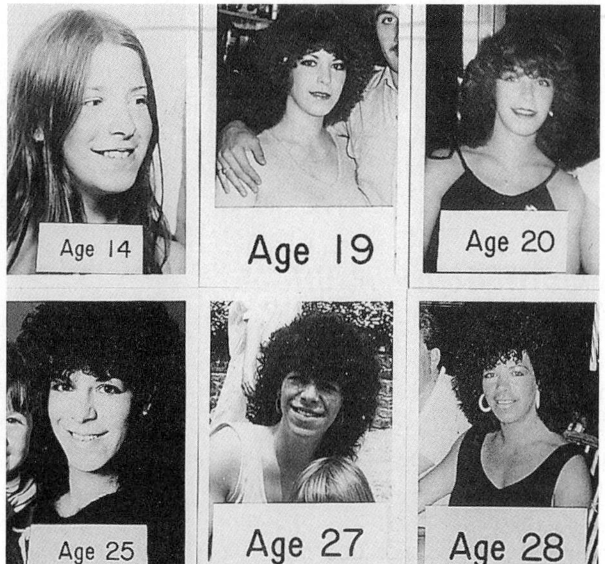

Figure 18-5 ■ **Acromegaly.** Chronologic sequence of photographs showing slow development of acromegaly. (From Belchetz P, Hammond P: *Mosby's color atlas and text of diabetes and endocrinology,* Edinburgh, 2003, Mosby.)

If compression hypopituitarism occurs, gonadotropin secretion may be affected, causing amenorrhea in women and sexual dysfunction in men. Approximately one third of people with acromegaly have impaired glucose tolerance, and one half of these are diabetic. There is an increased incidence of colon polyps and colon cancer.[12]

EVALUATION AND TREATMENT Diagnosis is confirmed by clinical features of the disease, MRI, and elevated levels of GH not suppressed by oral glucose. IGF-1 levels also are elevated. The goals of treatment are to normalize or reduce GH secretion, allowing normal pituitary function and relieving or preventing complications related to tumor expansion. The treatment of choice in acromegaly is surgical removal of the GH-secreting adenoma. Radiation therapy may be effective when rapid control of GH levels is not essential, when the individual is not a good surgical candidate, or when hyperfunction persists after subtotal resection. Somatostatin analogs normalize IGF-1 levels and lower growth hormone levels.[13]

Prolactinoma

Pituitary tumors that secrete prolactin, **prolactinomas,** are the most common hormonally active pituitary tumors.[14] Prolactin is under tonic inhibitory hypothalamic control through the secretion of dopamine. The physiologic actions of prolactin include breast development during pregnancy, postpartum milk production, and suppression of ovarian function in nursing women. Pathologic elevation of prolactin in women results in amenorrhea, nonpuerperal milk production (galactorrhea), hirsutism, and osteopenia resulting from estrogen deficiency. Hyperprolactinemia in men causes hypogonadism and erectile dysfunction.[15]

Approximately 30% of pituitary tumors secrete prolactin. Other conditions or medications can elevate prolactin in the absence of pituitary pathologic condition. For example, renal failure, polycystic ovarian disease, primary hypothyroidism, breast stimulation, or even venipuncture can increase prolactin levels. Medications that can increase prolactin block the effects of dopamine at the pituitary or stimulate proliferation of prolactin-secreting cells (lactotrophes) (i.e., antipsychotics [risperidone, chlorpromazine], metoclopramide, tricyclic antidepressants, methyldopa, and estrogens). Because TRH stimulates prolactin secretion in addition to enhancing TSH release, prolactin may be elevated in patients with primary hypothyroidism.

PATHOPHYSIOLOGY The hallmark of a prolactinoma is sustained increases in serum prolactin. Prolactin suppresses gonadotropin-releasing hormone (GnRH) pulses at the hypothalamus, impairs pulsatile pituitary gonadotropin release, and blunts the gonadal responsiveness to gonadotropins. In estrogen- and progesterone-primed breasts, milk production is stimulated.

CLINICAL MANIFESTATIONS Women with hyperprolactinemia generally present with galactorrhea (nonpuerperal milk production) and menstrual disturbances including amenorrhea. In susceptible women, hirsutism develops because of estrogen deficiency. If not detected until after many years, this estrogen deficiency also may result in osteoporosis. Men often present late with symptoms related to the increasing size of the adenoma (i.e., headache or visual impairment) because they may minimalize or overtly ignore symptoms of hypogonadism (erectile dysfunction or loss of libido).[16]

EVALUATION AND TREATMENT The diagnostic evaluation of hyperprolactinemia includes a careful history to exclude medications that may cause elevations in prolactin. Symptoms of hypothyroidism should be elicited, and screening with a serum TSH is mandatory. If serum prolactin is less than 50 ng/ml, a careful search for a nonpituitary cause should be pursued. Prolactin levels over 200 ng/ml are usually associated with a prolactinoma. MRI scanning of the pituitary is often helpful in detecting prolactinoma, but the chance of finding an unrelated and insignificant lesion must always be considered.

Dopaminergic agonists (bromocriptine and cabergoline) are the treatment of choice for prolactinomas.[17] Restoration of fertility in previously anovulatory women is common. In individuals resistant or intolerant to these medications, transsphenoidal surgery and radiotherapy are options.

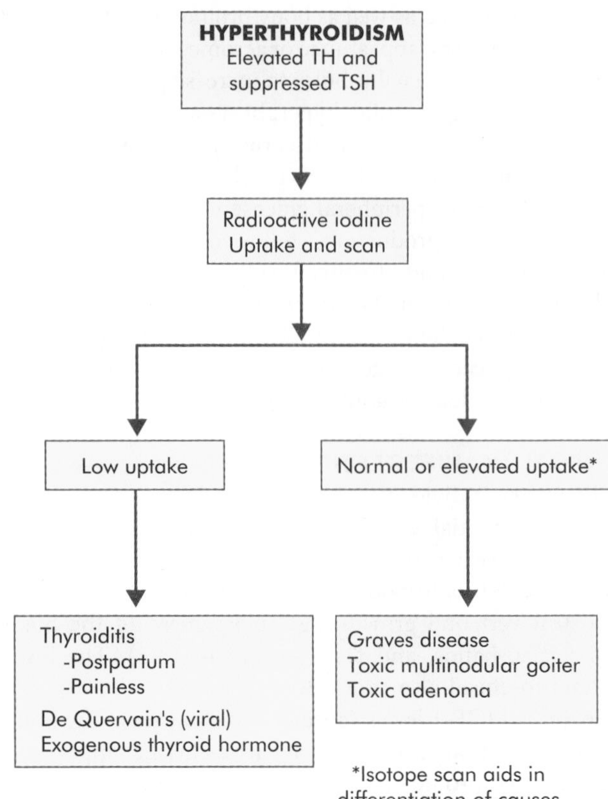

Figure 18-6 ■ **Evaluation of Hyperthyroidism.** Radioactive iodine is used in the differential diagnosis of hyperthyroidism.

ALTERATIONS OF THYROID FUNCTION

Hyperthyroidism

Thyrotoxicosis

Thyrotoxicosis is a condition that results from increased thyroid hormones (TH). Hyperthyroidism is a form of thyrotoxicosis in which excess amounts of TH are secreted from the thyroid gland. Common diseases that cause hyperthyroidism include Graves disease, toxic multinodular goiter, and a solitary toxic adenoma. Rare causes include thyroid cancer and TSH-secreting pituitary adenomas. Thyrotoxicosis not associated with hyperthyroidism includes subacute thyroiditis, ectopic thyroid tissue, and ingestion of excessive TH. Each condition is associated with a specific pathophysiology and manifestations, and the most commonly occurring ones are described in the following pages. All forms of thyrotoxicosis share some common characteristics.[18] Figure 18-6 illustrates the central role of a radioactive iodine uptake and scan in determining the underlying cause of thyrotoxicosis.

CLINICAL MANIFESTATIONS The metabolic effects of increased circulating levels of thyroid hormones cause clinical symptoms. The metabolic rate increases with heat intolerance and increased tissue sensitivity to sympathetic stimulation. The major manifestations are summarized in Table 18-1. Minimal or atypical symptoms are common in the elderly population.[19] **Goiter** (enlarged thyroid) is usually present.

EVALUATION AND TREATMENT Elevated serum thyroxine (T_4) and triiodothyronine (T_3) and suppressed serum TSH levels are diagnostic for hyperthyroidism. By contrast, TSH-secreting pituitary tumors are characterized by normal to increased TSH levels in the face of elevated thyroid hormone concentrations. Radioactive iodine is used to test for increased uptake in hyperthyroidism.[20] Treatment is directed at controlling excessive TH production, secretion, or action and employs drug therapy, radioactive iodine therapy, and surgery.

Hyperthyroid conditions

Graves disease

Graves disease is the most common cause of thyrotoxicosis and is the result of stimulation of the thyroid with antibodies against the TSH receptor. The antibodies stimulate the thyroid cells to produce high concentrations of triiodo-L-thyronine (T_3) and L-thyroxine (T_4). The combined action of the antibodies and increased serum levels of TH produce the symptoms of Graves disease: diffuse thyroid enlargement (goiter), ophthalmopathy, dermopathy (pretibial myxedema), and effects on the extremities in various combinations. The incidence is less than 1% in the U.S. population and is more common in women.

The many signs and symptoms of Graves disease can be divided into three components: (1) adrenergic stimulation (tachycardia, palpitations, nervousness, depression, tremor, lid lag, increased systolic blood pressure, increased cardiac contractility); (2) excess thyroid hormone (increased oxygen consumption, metabolic changes in protein metabolism); and (3) immunologic stimulation of diffuse goiter (see Table 18-1).[21]

Two categories of ocular manifestations are associated with Graves disease (Figure 18-7): (1) functional abnormalities resulting from hyperactivity of the sympathetic division of the autonomic nervous system (lag of the globe on upward gaze and of the upper lid on downward gaze) and (2) infiltrative changes involving the orbital contents with enlargement of the ocular muscles (edema of orbital contents, globe protrusion, paralysis of extraocular muscles, and damage to retina and optic nerve, leading to blindness). These changes result in exophthalmos (protrusion of the eyeball), periorbital edema, and extraocular muscle weakness leading to diplopia (double vision). The individual may experience irritation, pain, lacrimation, photophobia, blurred vision, decreased visual acuity, papilledema, visual field impairment, exposure keratosis, and corneal ulceration. Unfortunately, current treatment for Graves disease does not reverse the ocular changes and is palliative.[21]

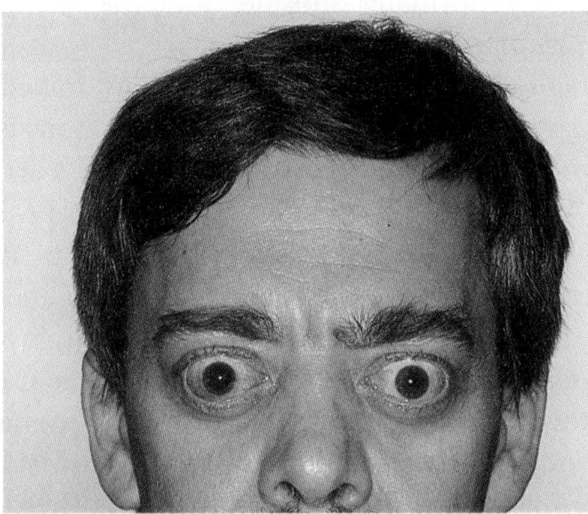

Figure 18-7 ■ **Graves Disease.** Note large and protruding eyeballs. (From Belchetz P, Hammond P: *Mosby's color atlas and text of diabetes and endocrinology,* Edinburgh, 2003, Mosby.)

TABLE 18-1

Systemic Effects of Hyperthyroidism

System	Manifestations	Mechanisms
Endocrine	Enlarged thyroid gland (97%-99% of cases), systolic or continuous bruit over thyroid, increased cortisol degradation, hypercalcemia and decreased PTH secretion, diminished sensitivity to exogenous insulin and increased hepatic glucose release	Hyperactivity of the thyroid gland, excess bone resorption leading to hypercalcemia and a disruption of PTH-regulating mechanisms, increased insulin degradation
Reproductive	Oligomenorrhea or amenorrhea in women, impotence and decreased libido in men, increased serum estradiol and estrone but lower than normal levels of free estradiol and estrone	Menstrual cycle alterations that may be related to hypothalamic or pituitary disturbances, increase in sex hormone-binding globulin with reduction in free sex steroid levels
Gastrointestinal	Weight loss and an associated increase in appetite; increased peristalsis leading to less formed and more frequent stools; nausea, vomiting, anorexia, abdominal pain; increased use of hepatic glycogen stores and of adipose and protein stores; decrease in serum lipid levels (including triglycerides, phospholipids, cholesterol); changes in vitamin metabolism leading to decrease in tissue stores of vitamins	Increased catabolism leading to the body's inability to meet its metabolic needs; malabsorption; increase in cholesterol excretion in feces and cholesterol conversion to bile salts; impaired conversion of B vitamins to their coenzymes, causing increased need for water-soluble and fat-soluble vitamins
Integumentary	Excessive sweating, flushing, and warm skin; heat intolerance; hair fine, soft, and straight; temporary hair loss; nails that grow away from nail beds, palmar erythema	Hyperdynamic circulatory state
Sensory (eyes)	Ocular manifestations, including elevated upper eyelid leading to decreased blinking and a staring quality, fine tremor of lid, infiltrative ocular changes associated with Graves disease	Overactivity of Müller muscle, inflammation of orbital contents (fat and ocular muscles)
Cardiovascular	Increased cardiac output and decreased peripheral resistance, tachycardia at rest, loud heart sounds, supraventricular dysrhythmias	Hypermetabolism and need to dissipate heat
Nervous	Restlessness, short attention span, compulsive movement, fatigue, tremor, insomnia, emotionally labile	Not clearly defined: alterations in cerebral metabolism resulting from excess thyroid hormone
Pulmonary	Dyspnea, reduced vital capacity	Weakness of respiratory muscles

PTH, Parathyroid hormone.

Hyperthyroidism resulting from nodular thyroid disease

The thyroid gland normally enlarges in response to the increased demand for TH that occurs in puberty, pregnancy, iodine deficiency, and immunologic, viral, or genetic disorders. When the condition requiring increased TH resolves, TSH secretion normally subsides and the thyroid gland returns to its original size.

Irreversible changes may occur in some follicular cells, however, so that they then function autonomously. Hyperthyroidism may or may not result from these irreversible changes. Autonomously functioning cells may produce less TH than the body requires. The remainder of the gland then functions to supply the remainder of the body's need, and a euthyroid state is achieved and maintained. If the autonomously functioning cells produce sufficient or excessive TH for the usual body requirement, the remainder of the gland undergoes involution, becoming normal but inactive tissue. This condition may result in euthyroidism or hyperthyroidism, depending on the amount of TH produced.

Hyperthyroidism can lead to a hypermetabolic state known as thyrotoxicosis or **toxic multinodular goiter.** If only one nodule is hyperfunctioning, it is termed **toxic adenoma.** Symptoms usually develop slowly and consist of rapid heart action; tremors; elevated basal metabolic rate; enlarged, multinodular goiter or a single, large nodule; and weight loss. Lid lag and proptosis may be seen, but exophthalmus and pretibial myxedema do not occur.

Thyrotoxic crisis

Thyrotoxic crisis (thyroid storm) is a rare but dangerous worsening of the thyrotoxic state, in which death occurs within 48 hours without treatment. The condition may develop spontaneously, but it usually occurs in individuals who have undiagnosed or partially treated Graves disease and are subjected to excessive stress, such as infection, pulmonary or cardiovascular disorders, emotional distress, physical stress, dialysis, plasmapheresis, or inadequate preparation for thyroid surgery.

The systemic symptoms of thyrotoxic crisis include hyperthermia; tachycardia, especially atrial tachydysrhythmias; high-output heart failure; agitation or delirium; and nausea, vomiting, or diarrhea contributing to fluid volume depletion. The symptoms may be attributed to increased β-adrenergic receptors and catecholamines.[22] The treatment is designed (1) to reduce both circulating TH levels by inducing a block of TH synthesis (i.e., propylthiouracil) and thereby reducing their effects to eliminate the precipitating disorder and (2) to provide symptomatic and supportive care.

Hypothyroidism

Deficient production of TH by the thyroid gland results in the clinical state termed **hypothyroidism.** It may be primary or secondary. Primary causes include (1) congenital defects, (2) defective hormone synthesis resulting from autoimmune thyroiditis endemic iodine deficiency, or antithyroid drugs, or (3) iatrogenic loss of thyroid tissue after surgical or radioactive treatment for hyperthyroidism. Causes of secondary hypothyroidism are less common and are related to either pituitary or hypothalamic failure. Hypothyroidism is the most common disorder of thyroid function and occurs more commonly in women.[23]

HEALTH ALERT

Subclinical Hypothyroidism

Subclinical hypothyroidism (isolated suppression of TSH with normal thyroid levels) is a condition that occurs in 1% to 2% of the aging population and is seen in approximately 10% of people taking thyroid hormone therapy. Risk factors for the spontaneous form of this condition include female gender and the presence of thyroid antibodies. The recognized complications of subclinical hyperthyroidism include osteoporosis, diminished arterial elasticity, reduced cognitive performance, diminished muscle strength, and increased risk of atrial fibrillation. Treatment decisions should be individualized, but there appears to be a trend for improvement in some of the complications with effective treatment.

Data from Brennan MD et al: The impact of overt and subclinical hyperthyroidism on skeletal muscle, *Thyroid* 16(4):375–380, 2006; Cappola AR et al: Thyroid status, cardiovascular risk, and mortality in older adults, *J Am Med Assoc* 295(9):1033–1041, 2006; Shargodsky M et al: Long-term thyrotropin-suppressive therapy with levothyroxine impairs small and large artery elasticity and increases left ventricular mass in patients with thyroid carcinoma, *Thyroid* 16(4): 381–386, 2006.

PATHOPHYSIOLOGY In primary hypothyroidism, loss of thyroid tissue leads to decreased production of TH, increased secretion of TSH, and goiter. Secondary hypothyroidism is usually caused by the pituitary's failure to synthesize adequate amounts of TSH. Pituitary tumors or the results of their treatment are the most common causes of secondary hypothyroidism.

CLINICAL MANIFESTATIONS Hypothyroidism generally affects all body systems and occurs insidiously over months or years. The decrease in TH lowers energy metabolism and heat production. The individual develops a low basal metabolic rate, cold intolerance, lethargy, tiredness, and slightly lowered basal body temperature (Table 18-2). The decrease in TH can lead to excessive TSH production and goiter.

The characteristic sign of severe or long-standing hypothyroidism is **myxedema,** which results from the altered composition of the dermis and other tissues. The connective fibers are separated by large amounts of protein and mucopolysaccharide. This complex binds water, producing nonpitting, boggy edema, especially around the eyes, hands, and feet and in the supraclavicular fossae (Figure 18-8). The tongue and laryngeal and pharyngeal mucous membranes thicken, producing thick, slurred speech and hoarseness.

TABLE 18-2

Systemic Manifestations of Hypothyroidism

System	Manifestations	Mechanisms
Neurologic	Confusion, syncope, slowed speech and thinking, memory loss; lethargy, headaches, hearing loss, night blindness; slow, clumsy movements; cerebellar ataxia, slow alpha wave activity and loss of amplitude in EEG; decreased tendon reflexes	Decreased cerebral blood flow leading to cerebral hypoxia; TH plays a role in the functional maintenance of the CNS; reduced intracellular processes caused by decreased β-adrenergic activity that may be related to a decrease in the number of β-adrenergic receptor sites
Endocrine	Increased TSH production in primary hypothyroidism; enlarged pituitary thyrotropes, increased serum prolactin levels with galactorrhea; decreased rate of cortisol turnover but with normal serum cortisol levels	Impaired TH synthesis or defects in iodide trapping leading to compensatory TSH production; chronic overstimulation of thyrotropes by TRH and by TSH synthesis; stimulation of lactotropes by TRH related to increased prolactin levels; decreased deactivation of cortisol
Reproductive	Anovulation, decreased libido, and a high incidence of spontaneous abortion in women; erectile dysfunction, decreased libido, and oligospermia in men	Altered metabolism of estrogens and androgens; decreased sex hormone–binding globulin, decreased androgen secretion in men, increased estriol formation in women; low total hormone values but with increased amounts of unbound hormone
Hematologic	Decrease in red cell mass leading to normocytic, normochromic anemia; macrocytic anemia associated with vitamin B_{12} deficiency and inadequate folate or iron absorption in the GI tract	Decreased basal metabolic rate and reduced oxygen requirements, decreased production of erythropoietin, possible relationship between TH and optimal hematologic response to vitamin B_{12}
Cardiovascular	Reduction in stroke volume and heart rate causing lowered cardiac output; increased peripheral vascular resistance to maintain systolic blood pressure; normal response to exercise but with alterations in circulatory system at rest (prolonged circulation time and decreased blood flow to tissues); cool skin and cold intolerance; enlarged heart; decreased intensity of heart sounds and variety of ECG changes (sinus bradycardia, prolonged PR interval, depressed P waves, flattened or inverted T waves, and low-amplitude QRS complexes); cardiac tamponade (although rare)	Decreased metabolic demands and loss of regulatory and rate-setting effects of TH, protein-mucopolysaccharide-rich fluid in the pericardial sac associated with enlarged heart; pericardial effusions associated with heart sounds and ECG changes
Pulmonary	Dyspnea; hypoventilation and carbon dioxide retention, which contributes to myxedema coma; hoarseness	Myxedematous changes in respiratory muscles; pleural effusions associated with dyspnea, although effusions may be asymptomatic
Renal	Decreased renal excretion of water; increased total body water and dilutional hyponatremia; reduced production of erythropoietin	Reduced renal blood flow and glomerular filtration rate; hemodynamic alterations associated with reduced blood flow and filtration; increased total body water related to decreased excretion and mucinous deposits in tissue
Gastrointestinal	Decreased appetite; constipation, weight gain, and fluid retention; decreased absorption of most nutrients; decreased protein metabolism leading to retarded skeletal and soft tissue growth and slightly positive nitrogen balance; edema; decreased glucose absorption and delayed glucose uptake; increased sensitivity to exogenous insulin; elevated serum lipid values	Reduced intake and reduced peristaltic activity that may progress to fecal impaction; water absorption related to prolonged transit time; fluid retention associated with myxedematous changes; edema associated with high concentrations of exchangeable albumin in the extravascular space caused by increased capillary permeability to proteins; depressed lipid synthesis and degradation
Musculoskeletal	Muscle aching and stiffness; slow movement and slow tendon jerk reflexes; decreased bone formation and resorption, increased bone density; aching and stiffness in joints	Decreased rate of muscle contraction and relaxation contributing to slow movement and reflexes; reduction in the number of fast-twitch fibers
Integumentary	Coarse, dry, flaky skin; dry, brittle head and body hair; reduced growth of nails and hair; slow wound healing	Reduced sweat and sebaceous gland secretion
	Myxedema	Accumulation of hyaluronic acid, which binds water and causes a puffy appearance
	Cool skin	Decreased circulation to skin

EEG, Electroencephalogram; *TSH*, thyroid-stimulating hormone; *TH*, thyroid hormone; *TRH*, thyroid-releasing hormone; *GI*, gastrointestinal; *ECG*, electrocardiogram.

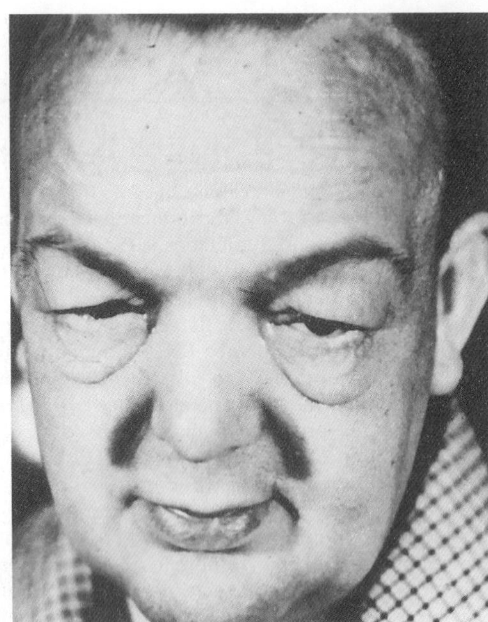

Figure 18-8 ■ **Myxedema.** Note edema around eyes and facial puffiness. (From Thibodeau GA, Patton KT: *Anatomy & physiology,* St Louis, 1987, Mosby.)

EVALUATION AND TREATMENT In addition to the clinical symptoms of hypothyroidism, a decrease in serum T_4 and free T_4 is nearly always present. TSH concentration increases from loss of negative feedback from TH.[24] When hypothyroidism is caused by pituitary deficiencies, serum TSH levels and basal metabolic rate (BMR) decrease. Hormone replacement therapy is the treatment of choice. The restoration of normal TH levels should be timed appropriately; a regimen of hormonal therapy depends on the individual's age, the duration and severity of the hypothyroidism, and the presence of other disorders, particularly cardiovascular disorders.

Hypothyroid conditions

Primary hypothyroidism

Primary hypothyroidism results from several disorders: acute thyroiditis, subacute thyroiditis, painless thyroiditis, postpartum thyroiditis, and autoimmune thyroiditis. **Acute thyroiditis** is caused by a bacterial infection of the thyroid gland and is rare. **Subacute thyroiditis** is a nonbacterial inflammation of the thyroid often preceded by a viral infection. Both conditions are accompanied by fever, tenderness, and enlargement of the thyroid gland. Symptoms may last for 2 to 4 months, and corticosteroids usually resolve symptoms. **Autoimmune thyroiditis (Hashimoto disease, chronic lymphocytic thyroiditis)** results in destruction of thyroid tissue by circulating thyroid antibodies and infiltration of lymphocytes. Autoimmune thyroiditis also may be caused by an inherited immune defect. Goiter formation is common. **Painless thyroiditis** has a course similar to subacute thyroiditis but is pathologically identical to Hashimoto disease. **Postpartum thyroiditis** generally occurs up to 6 months after delivery with a course similar to Hashimoto disease. Spontaneous recovery occurs in 95% of these hypothyroid conditions. A hyperthyroid phase (with a low thyroid ratio-iodine uptake) precedes the hypothyroid phase in typical cases of subacute, painless, or postpartum thyroiditis.

Myxedema coma

Myxedema coma, a medical emergency, is a diminished level of consciousness associated with severe hypothyroidism.[25] Symptoms include hypothermia without shivering, hypoventilation, hypotension, hypoglycemia, and lactic acidosis. Older patients with severe vascular disease and with moderate or untreated hypothyroidism are particularly at risk. The overuse of narcotics or sedatives or an acute illness in hypothyroid individuals also can be causative.

Congenital hypothyroidism

Hypothyroidism in infants occurs when thyroid tissue is absent (thyroid dysgenesis) and with hereditary defects in TH synthesis. Thyroid dysgenesis occurs more often in female infants, with permanent abnormalities in 1 of every 4000 live births.

Because TH is essential for embryonic growth, particularly of brain tissue, the infant will be mentally retarded if there is no thyroxine during fetal life. This can be partially reversed if thyroxine is given immediately after birth.

Hypothyroidism at birth involves high birth weight, hypothermia, delay in passing meconium, and neonatal jaundice. The newborn's blood can be examined in the first days of life for thyroxine and TSH levels.[26] Frequent monitoring of TSH and thyroxine is essential to guide treatment. Treatment is administration of thyroxine.

Without early screening, hypothyroidism may not be evident until after 4 months of age. Symptoms include difficulty eating, hoarse cry, and protruding tongue caused by myxedema of oral tissues and vocal cords; hypotonic muscles of the abdomen with constipation, abdominal protrusion, and umbilical hernia; subnormal temperature; lethargy; excessive sleeping; slow pulse; and cold, mottled skin. Skeletal growth is stunted because of impaired protein synthesis, poor absorption of nutrients, and lack of bone mineralization. The child will be dwarfed, with short limbs, if not treated (cretinism) (Figure 18-9). Dentition is often delayed. Mental retardation varies with the severity of hypothyroidism and the length of delay before treatment is initiated.

Thyroid Carcinoma

Thyroid carcinoma is the most common endocrine malignancy but is relatively rare, with only 33,550 new cases annually and approximately 0.25% of all cancer deaths per year.[28] Exposure to ionizing radiation, especially during childhood, is the most consistent causal factor.[27,29]

Most individuals with thyroid carcinoma have normal T_3 and T_4 levels and are therefore euthyroid. The cancer is typically discovered as a small thyroid nodule or metastatic tumor in the lungs, brain, or bone. Changes in voice and swallowing and difficulty breathing are related to tumor growth impinging on the trachea or esophagus.

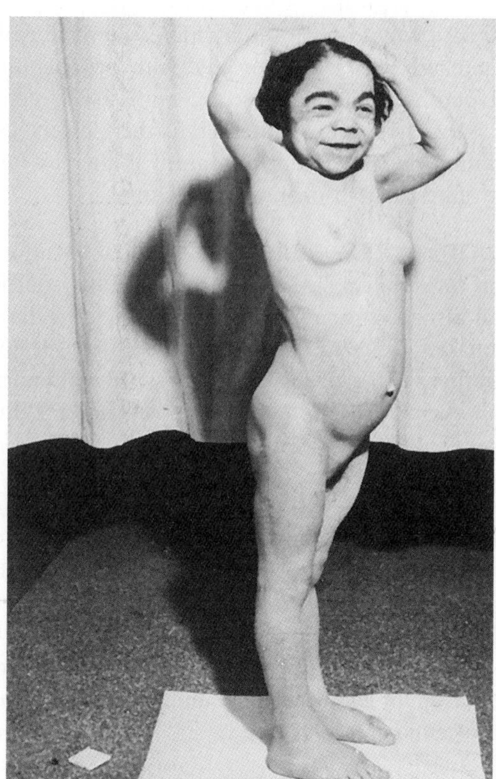

Figure 18-9 ■ **An Adult Cretin.** Note the characteristic facial features, dwarfism (44 inches), absent axillary and scant pubic hair, poorly developed breasts, potbelly, and small umbilical hernia. (From Schneeberg NG: *Essentials of clinical endocrinology,* St Louis, 1970, Mosby.)

Diagnosing a thyroid cancer is generally made by fine needle aspiration of a thyroid nodule. Ultrasonography and radioisotope scanning are less helpful in determining the malignant potential of the tumor. Treatment may include partial or total thyroidectomy, TSH suppression therapy (levothyroxine), radioactive iodine therapy (in iodine-concentrating tumors), postoperative radiation therapy, and chemotherapy (especially in anaplastic carcinoma).[30]

QUICK CHECK 18-2

1. What is thyrotoxicosis?
2. List three manifestations of Graves disease.
3. What is myxedema?

ALTERATIONS OF PARATHYROID FUNCTION

Hyperparathyroidism

Hyperparathyroidism is characterized by greater than normal secretion of parathyroid hormone (PTH). Hyperparathyroidism is classified as primary or secondary.

PATHOPHYSIOLOGY Estimates suggest that **primary hyperparathyroidism** occurs in 0.2% to 0.3% of the adult population, with twice as many cases in women. It is generally found in older adults.[31] Because postmenopausal women are at risk for developing osteoporosis, the effects of increased levels of PTH on bone disease can be significant. Most cases of hyperparathyroidism (approximately 80%) result from chief cell adenoma with an increased secretion of PTH.[32]

In primary hyperparathyroidism, PTH secretion is increased and is not under the usual feedback control mechanisms. Gastrointestinal absorption of calcium increases with increased extracellular calcium and reflects the kidney's increased generation of biologically active vitamin D in response to increased PTH levels.[33]

Secondary hyperparathyroidism is a compensatory response of the parathyroid glands to chronic hypocalcemia, which can be associated with decreased renal activation of vitamin D (renal failure) or malabsorption (see Chapters 4 and 29). Secretion of PTH is elevated, but PTH cannot achieve normal calcium levels because of insufficient levels of activated vitamin D.

Hyperplasia of the parathyroid glands and loss of sensitivity to circulating calcium levels can cause autonomous secretion of PTH, even with normal calcium levels. It often occurs in individuals with chronic renal failure. Signs and symptoms are similar to those of primary hyperparathyroidism.

CLINICAL MANIFESTATIONS PTH hypersecretion causes hypercalcemia and may be asymptomatic or present with excessive osteoclastic and osteocytic activity, resulting in bone resorption.[34] (Bone resorption is discussed in Chapter 37.) Pathologic changes include pathologic fractures, kyphosis of the dorsal spine, and compression fractures of the vertebral bodies. The increased renal filtration load of calcium leads to hypercalciuria.

Hypercalcemia also affects proximal renal tubular function, causing metabolic acidosis and production of an abnormally alkaline urine. PTH hypersecretion enhances renal phosphate excretion and results in hypophosphatemia and hyperphosphaturia (see Chapter 4). The combination of these three variables—hypercalciuria, alkaline urine, and hyperphosphaturia—predisposes the individual to the formation of calcium stones, particularly in the renal pelvis or renal collecting ducts. These may be associated with infections. Both kidney stones and renal infection can lead to impaired renal function. Hypercalcemia also impairs the concentrating ability of the renal tubule by decreasing its response to ADH.

Chronic hypercalcemia of hyperparathyroidism is associated with mild insulin resistance, necessitating increased insulin secretion to maintain normal glucose levels. Hypercalcemia also affects the muscular, nervous, and gastrointestinal systems, causing fatigue, headache, depression, anorexia, and nausea and vomiting.[33]

EVALUATION AND TREATMENT Hyperparathyroidism is generally diagnosed by excluding all other possible causes of hypercalcemia. A definitive diagnosis must be supported by at least a 6-month history of symptoms associated with hypercalcemia, including kidney stones, hypophosphatemia, hyperchloremia, and increased urinary calcium levels. With continued improvements in the ability to measure PTH, the evaluation of hyperparathyroidism has become simplified. Simultaneous measurements of serum PTH and calcium will document elevations of both, and diagnosis is confirmed by measuring urinary calcium excretion.

Definitive treatment involves surgical removal of the solitary adenoma or, in the case of hyperplasia, complete removal of three and partial removal of the fourth hyperplastic parathyroid glands. Observation of asymptomatic individuals with mild hypercalcemia also is an option. These individuals are advised to avoid dehydration and limit dietary calcium intake.[35]

Hypoparathyroidism

Hypoparathyroidism (abnormally low PTH levels) is most commonly caused by damage to the parathyroid glands during thyroid surgery. This occurs because of the anatomic proximity of the parathyroid glands to the thyroid.

PATHOPHYSIOLOGY A lack of circulating PTH causes depressed serum calcium levels and increased serum phosphate levels. In the absence of PTH, resorption of calcium from bone and regulation of calcium reabsorption from the renal tubules are impaired. Phosphate reabsorption by the renal tubules is therefore increased, causing hyperphosphatemia.

Hypoparathyroidism also may result from hypomagnesemia. Once serum magnesium levels return to normal, PTH secretion does likewise. Hypomagnesemia may be related to chronic alcoholism, malnutrition, malabsorption, increased renal clearance of magnesium caused by the use of aminoglycoside antibiotics or certain chemotherapeutic agents, or prolonged magnesium-deficient parenteral nutritional therapy.

CLINICAL MANIFESTATIONS Symptoms associated with hypoparathyroidism are primarily those of hypocalcemia. Hypocalcemia causes a lowered threshold for nerve and muscle excitation so that a nerve impulse may be initiated by a slight stimulus anywhere along the length of a nerve or muscle fiber. This creates muscle spasms, hyperreflexia, clonic-tonic convulsions, laryngeal spasms, and, in severe cases, death by asphyxiation. Other symptoms of hypocalcemia include dry skin, loss of body and scalp hair, hypoplasia of developing teeth, horizontal ridges on the nails, cataracts, basal ganglia calcifications (which may be associated with a parkinsonian syndrome), and bone deformities, including brachydactyly and bowing of the long bones.

Phosphate retention caused by increased renal reabsorption of phosphate is also associated with hypoparathyroidism. Hyperphosphatemia results from PTH deficiency and, in turn, hyperphosphatemia further lowers calcium by inhibiting the activation of vitamin D thereby lowering the gastrointestinal absorption of calcium.

EVALUATION AND TREATMENT A low-serum calcium and high phosphorus level in the absence of renal failure, intestinal disorders, or nutritional deficiencies is diagnostic of hypoparathyroidism. PTH levels are low in primary hypoparathyroidism. Daily doses of PTH can normalize serum and urine calcium levels, but this is not a therapeutic option.[36]

Treatment is directed toward alleviation of the hypocalcemia. In acute states, this involves parenteral administration of calcium, which corrects serum calcium within minutes. Maintenance of serum calcium is achieved with pharmacologic doses of an active form of vitamin D and oral calcium. Hypoplastic dentition, cataracts, bone deformities, and basal ganglia calcifications do not respond to the correction of hypocalcemia, but the other symptoms of hypocalcemia are reversible.

✓ QUICK CHECK 18-3

1. How does excessive parathyroid hormone (PTH) affect bones?
2. What are the results of a lack of circulating PTH?

DYSFUNCTION OF THE ENDOCRINE PANCREAS: DIABETES MELLITUS

Diabetes mellitus is not a single disease but a group of disorders with glucose intolerance in common. The term *diabetes mellitus* describes a syndrome characterized by chronic hyperglycemia and other disturbances of carbohydrate, protein, and fat metabolism. The American Diabetes Association classifies four categories of diabetes mellitus[37] (Table 18-3):

1. Type 1 (absolute insulin deficiency)
2. Type 2 (insulin resistance with an insulin secretory deficit)
3. Other specific types
4. Gestational diabetes

The diagnosis of diabetes mellitus is based on either fasting plasma glucose levels or the results of glucose tolerance testing and is supported by clinical manifestations (Box 18-1). Impaired glucose tolerance, a condition characterized by nondiabetic elevations in either fasting glucose or the 2-hour value during a glucose tolerance test, has been associated with a significantly increased risk for

TABLE 18-3

Classification and Characteristics of Diabetes Mellitus

Name	Previous Synonyms	Characteristics
TYPE 1 DIABETES MELLITUS Absolute insulin deficiency Primary B cell defect or failure	Insulin-dependent diabetes mellitus (IDDM) Juvenile diabetes Juvenile-onset diabetes Ketosis-prone diabetes Brittle diabetes Idiopathic diabetes	Long preclinical period with abrupt onset of clinical manifestations Individual prone to ketoacidosis Insulin dependent Several syndromes, both primary autoimmune and genetic environment Often affects young people around age of puberty; can occur at any age Immune infiltration of islets (insulitis)
TYPE 2 DIABETES MELLITUS Insulin resistance with an insulin secretory deficiency	Non–insulin-dependent diabetes mellitus (NIDDM) Adult-onset diabetes	Usually not insulin dependent at the time of diagnosis Individual not ketosis prone (but may form ketones under stress)
	Maturity-onset diabetes	Multiple syndromes; obese, nonobese, and maturity-onset diabetes of the young (MODY)
	Ketosis-resistant diabetes	Generally occurs in those over age 40 yr, but frequency is rapidly increasing in children Strong genetic predisposition
OTHER TYPES OF DIABETES MELLITUS	Secondary diabetes	Associated with other conditions or syndromes, such as pancreatic disease, hormonal disease, drugs, and chemical agents
GESTATIONAL DIABETES MELLITUS (GDM)		Glucose intolerance first recognized during pregnancy, most likely in the third trimester After pregnancy, glucose may normalize, remain impaired, or progress to diabetes mellitus Occurs in 2% of all pregnancies; 60% will develop diabetes mellitus within 15 yr of gestation
IMPAIRED FASTING GLUCOSE (IFG)		Fasting plasma glucose ≥100 and <126 mg/dl
IMPAIRED GLUCOSE TOLERANCE (IGT)		Abnormal response to oral glucose tolerance test: 2 hr PG ≥140 and <200 mg/dl 10%-25% will convert to type II diabetes within 10 yr Many with IGT are obese

PG, Plasma glucose.

cardiovascular disease. Impaired glucose tolerance (IGT) results from diminished insulin secretion, whereas impaired fasting glucose (IFG) is due to enhanced hepatic glucose output. Both conditions are now called *prediabetes.*

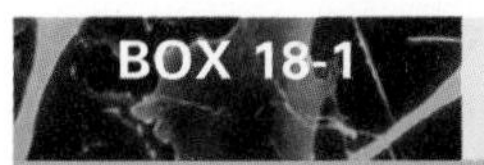

BOX 18-1 **Diagnostic Criteria for Diabetes Mellitus**

1. Symptoms of diabetes (polyuria, polydipsia, unexplained weight loss) plus a causal or random glucose concentration ≥200 mg/dl
2. Fasting plasma glucose ≥126 mg/dl (fasting defined as no caloric intake for 8 hours)
3. 2-hour plasma glucose ≥200 mg/dl during a 75-gram oral glucose tolerance test

From American Diabetes Association: Diagnosis and classification of diabetes mellitus, *Diabetes Care* 30(suppl 1):S42–S47, 2007.

Another mechanism used to measure plasma glucose levels over time is the measurement of **glycosylated hemoglobin.** Because of lack of standardization, it is not a diagnostic test for diabetes. In the normal 120-day life span of the red blood cell, glucose molecules join hemoglobin, forming glycosylated hemoglobin. In an individual with persistent hyperglycemia (poorly controlled diabetes), increases in the quantities of glycosylated hemoglobin (principally Hb A_{1c}) are noted. Once a hemoglobin molecule is glycosylated, it remains that way. A buildup of glycosylated hemoglobin within the red cell reflects the average level of glucose to which the cell has been exposed during its life cycle. Measuring glycosylated hemoglobin assesses the effectiveness of therapy by monitoring long-term serum glucose regulation.

For any diagnosis of diabetes mellitus, the goals of therapy are to maintain euglycemia, avoid hypoglycemia, and prevent severe cardiovascular and neurologic complications.

Types of Diabetes Mellitus

Type 1 diabetes mellitus

Type 1 diabetes mellitus accounts for approximately 10% of all diabetes mellitus in the Western world. Its incidence is increasing in some areas, with other areas showing no change in incidence.[38] Variations occur, however, even within individual countries. (Table 18-4 summarizes the epidemiology of diabetes mellitus.)

Type 1 diabetes mellitus results from autoimmune destruction of beta cells and is thought to be the result of a gene-environment interaction, with the strongest genetic risk markers in the human leukocyte antigen (HLA) region of chromosome 6. Genetic factors may increase susceptibility to environmental causes of diabetes.[38,39] There is a 50% concordance rate in twins. Between 10% and 13% of individuals with newly diagnosed type 1 diabetes have a first-degree relative (parent or sibling) with type 1 diabetes. Diagnosis is rare during the first 9 months of life and peaks at 12 years of age.

Historically, type 1 diabetes mellitus has been thought to have an abrupt onset. More recently, however, prospective studies show a distinctive natural history involving genetic susceptibility; a long preclinical period; immunologically mediated destruction of beta cells, eventually leading to insulin deficiency; and hyperglycemia.

PATHOPHYSIOLOGY Type 1 diabetes results from a severe, absolute lack of insulin caused by loss of beta cells. Destruction of islet cells is related to genetic susceptibility, autoimmunity, and environmental factors.[38,39] The most common type of type I diabetes is called type IA (80% to 90% of cases) and results from beta cell autoantibodies and antibodies to insulin and to glutamic acid decarboxylase that participate in damage to islet cells. Autoantibodies are often detected long before symptoms appear. Environmental factors that may trigger autoimmune injury are summarized in Box 18-2. Nonimmune type 1 diabetes occurs secondarily to other diseases such as pancreatitis.

Hyperglycemia and other symptoms

Before hyperglycemia occurs, 80% to 90% of the insulin-secreting beta cells of the islet of Langerhans must be destroyed. Beta cell abnormalities are present long before the acute clinical onset of type 1 diabetes. In addition to the decline in insulin secretion, the production of amylin, another beta cell hormone, also falls; amylin is co-secreted with insulin. One of the critical actions of amylin is to suppress glucagon release from the alpha cells.

Regardless of cause, a disequilibrium of hormones produced by the islets of Langerhans occurs in diabetes mellitus. Both beta cell function and alpha cell function are abnormal, with a lack of insulin and a relative excess of glucagon (produced by alpha cells).

Hyperglycemia and ketonemia can result from insulin deficiency alone, but a relative excess of glucagon clearly facilitates the metabolic alterations seen in diabetes. Elevated blood glucose levels fail to suppress the production of glucagon. Thus, both hormones cause the full metabolic syndrome.

CLINICAL MANIFESTATIONS Type 1 diabetes mellitus affects the metabolism of fat, protein, and carbohydrates. Glucose accumulates in the blood and spills into the urine as the renal threshold for glucose is exceeded. In addition, proteins and fats break down because of the lack of insulin, resulting in weight loss.

Initial clinical manifestations of type 1 diabetes are generally acute, with polyuria, polydipsia, and polyphagia (Table 18-5). Weight loss and wide fluctuations in blood glucose levels occur.

Ketoacidosis is caused by increased metabolism of fats and proteins resulting in high levels of circulating ketones. The pH drops, triggering the buffering systems associated with metabolic acidosis (see Chapter 4). Acetone (a volatile form of ketones) then is blown off, giving the breath a sweet or "fruity" odor. Occasionally, diabetic coma is the initial symptom of the disease.

EVALUATION AND TREATMENT The diagnosis of diabetes is not difficult when the symptoms of polydipsia, polyuria, polyphagia, weight loss, and hyperglycemia are present in fasting and postprandial states.

Currently, treatment regimens are designed to avoid high and low levels of glucose and insulin.[40] Management requires individual planning according to type of disease, age, and activity level, but all individuals require some combination of insulin, meal planning, and exercise. Hemoglobin A_{1c} testing is useful in confirming the diagnosis and in monitoring effectiveness of treatment and preventing complications. Islet cell transplantation is being explored for treatment of type 1 diabetes, and early results are promising.[41] Pancreas transplant is generally reserved for those individuals with type 1 diabetes and associated end-stage renal failure.[42]

Type 2 diabetes mellitus

Type 2 diabetes mellitus (non-insulin-dependent diabetes mellitus) is much more common than type 1 and has been rising in incidence since 1940. One case is undiagnosed for each known case in the United States. The condition is more common in Native Americans, Hispanics, and blacks. Interactions of metabolic, genetic, and environmental factors affect prevalence. It affects people primarily after 40 years of age, many of whom are obese. There is an increasing incidence of type 2 diabetes in children. The risk factors include obesity and increased body mass index, family history of type 2 diabetes, member of an ethnic minority, puberty, female gender, and metabolic syndrome.[43]

TABLE 18-4

Epidemiology and Etiology of Diabetes Mellitus

	Type 1 Diabetes: Primary Beta-Cell Defect or Failure	Type 2 Diabetes: Insulin Resistance with Inadequate Insulin Secretion
INCIDENCE		
Frequency	One of the most common childhood diseases (10% of all cases of diabetes mellitus) Affects approximately 1 in every 400–600 children in the United States	Accounts for most cases (~90%) Prevalence rate in United States (for age 18 yr and older): 9.6%*
Change in incidences	Increasing 2.5% per year worldwide, higher in some regions (e.g., Finland) and stable elsewhere	Incidence has risen in United States since 1940
CHARACTERISTICS		
Age at onset	Peak onset at age 11–13 yr (slightly earlier for girls than for boys) Rare in children younger than 1 yr and adults older than 30 yr	Risk of developing diabetes increases after age 40 yr; in general, incidence increases with age into the 70s; among Pima Indians, incidence peaks between age 40 and 50 yr, then falls
Gender	Similar in males and females	In the United States, more females than males
Racial distribution	Rates for whites 1.5–2 times higher than for nonwhites Higher rates for those of Scandinavian descent than for those of central or southern European descent	Certain racial groups may be more likely to develop type 2 diabetes when exposed to a particular environment Common in migrant groups encountering a different environment (e.g., Polynesians moving from traditional to Western lifestyle) Non-hispanic blacks, hispanic/Latino, American Indians, Alaska Natives, Asian Americans, and Pacific Islanders have between 1.5 and 2.2 times the risk of whites.
Socioeconomic status	Conflicting data	A disease of the affluent in developing nations but more common among those of lower incomes and less education in the United States
Seasonal distribution	More new cases documented during fall and winter in the northern hemisphere	No known association
Childbirth association	No association documented	Effect of parity on subsequent development of type 2 diabetes varies among different populations
Obesity	Generally normal or underweight	Frequent contributing factor to precipitate type 2 diabetes among those susceptible; a major factor in populations recently exposed to westernized environment Increased risk related to duration, degree, and distribution of obesity
ETIOLOGY		
Common theory	*Autoimmune*: genetic and environmental factors; resulting in gradual process of autoimmune destruction in genetically susceptible individuals *Nonautoimmune:* idiopathic without evidence of autoimmunity or, rarely, the result of environmental toxins Strong association with HLA-DR3 and HLA-DR4	Disease results from genetic susceptibility (although the precise gene or genes have not yet been determined) combined with environmental determinants and other risk factors Associated with long-duration obesity
Hereditary	Risk to sibling: 5%-10%; risk to offspring: 2%-5%	Risk to first-degree relative (child or sibling): 10%-15%
Presence of antibody	Islet cell autoantibodies (ICA) or autoantibodies to insulin, and autoantibodies to glutamic acid decarboxylase (GAD_{65}) are present in 85%-90% of individuals when fasting hyperglycemia is initially detected	Islet cell antibodies not present
Insulin resistance	Insulin resistance at diagnosis is unusual but insulin resistance may occur as the individual ages and gains weight	Increased insulin resistance caused by altered cellular metabolism and an intracellular postreceptor defect
Insulin secretion	Severe insulin deficiency or no insulin secretion at all	Typically increased at time of diagnosis; may be normal or decreased

Data from the American Diabetes Association 2007 (http://www.diabetes.org/diabetes-statistics.jsp), Daneman D: Type 1 diabetes, *Lancet* 367:847–858, 2006, and Brancati FL et al: Diabetes mellitus, race, and socioeconomic status: a population-based study *Ann Epidemiol* 6(1):67–73, 1996.

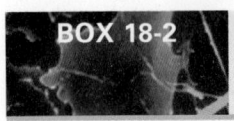

Specific Environmental Factors Linked to Type 1 Diabetes

Drugs and Chemicals
Alloxan
Streptozocin
Pentamidine
Vacor (a rodenticide)

Nutritional Intake
Bovine milk (controversial)
High levels of nitrosamines

Viruses
Mumps and Coxsackie—type 1 diabetes does occur rarely as a complication of viral infections, but no evidence of substantial relationship exists
Rubella—40% of individuals with congenital rubella infection develop type 1 diabetes later
Cytomegalovirus (CMV)—persistent CMV infections appear to be relevant to pathogenesis of some cases of type 1 diabetes

Data from Akerblom HK, Knip M: Putative environmental factors in Type 1 diabetes. *Diabetes Metab Rev* 14(1):31–67, 1998; Knip M, Akerblom HK: Environmental factors in the pathogenesis of Type 1 diabetes mellitus, *Exp Clin Endocrinol Diabetes* 107(suppl 3): S93–100, 1999.

TABLE 18-5

Clinical Manifestations and Mechanisms for Type 1 Diabetes Mellitus

Manifestation	Rationale
Polydipsia	Because of elevated blood sugar levels, water is osmotically attracted from body cells, resulting in intracellular dehydration and stimulation of thirst in the hypothalamus
Polyuria	Hyperglycemia acts as an osmotic diuretic; the amount of glucose filtered by the glomeruli of the kidney exceeds that which can be reabsorbed by the renal tubules; glycosuria results, accompanied by large amounts of water lost in the urine
Polyphagia	Depletion of cellular stores of carbohydrates, fats, and protein results in cellular starvation and a corresponding increase in hunger
Weight loss	Weight loss occurs because of fluid loss in osmotic diuresis and the loss of body tissue as fats and proteins are used for energy
Fatigue	Metabolic changes result in poor use of food products, contributing to lethargy and fatigue

HEALTH ALERT
The Metabolic Syndrome/Insulin Resistance Syndrome/Syndrome X

The metabolic syndrome is a clustering of clinical traits that when occurring together increase the risk for the development of cardiovascular disease. The diagnostic criteria for the metabolic syndrome have been recently revised and include (1) increased abdominal adiposity (waist circumference ≥40 inches in men and ≥35 inches in women), (2) elevated triglycerides (≥150 mg/dl), (3) reduced HDL cholesterol (≤50 mg/dl in women and ≤40 mg/dl in men), (4) increased blood pressure (≥130/≥85 mm Hg), and (5) hyperglycemia (fasting plasma glucose ≥100 mg/dl) or diabetes. The presence of three out of five criteria in an individual is diagnostic of the metabolic syndrome. Fibrinogen and plasminogen activator inhibitor type 1 are increased, leading to hypercoagulability and the risk of thrombosis. Decreased nitric oxide mediated vasodilation contributes to atherogenesis.

The syndrome occurs in up to 24% of the U.S. population between the ages of 20 to 70 years and older and is more common in men and Mexican Americans. The syndrome may have a genetic basis, but environmental factors including lack of exercise, excess nutrients, and obesity are influential. Early recognition and treatment are critical to reducing cardiovascular events and improving clinical outcomes. Treatment includes reducing environmental risk factors and enhancing insulin sensitivity with drugs, such as the thiazolidinediones.

Data from Grundy SM et al: Diagnosis and management of the metabolic syndrome, *Circulation* 112:2735–2752, 2005; Lopez-Candales A: Metabolic syndrome X: a comprehensive review of the pathophysiology and recommended therapy, *J Med* 32(5–6):283–300, 2001; Meigs JB: Epidemiology of the metabolic syndrome, *Am J Manag Care* 8(11 suppl):S283-S292, 2002; Johnson LW, Weinstock RS: The metabolic syndrome: concepts and controversy, *Mayo Clin Proc* 81(12):1615–1620, 2006.

PATHOPHYSIOLOGY The cause of the common form of type 2 diabetes mellitus is unknown, although it clearly runs in families and results from a combination of genetic susceptibility and environmental factors. Although the genetics of type 2 are complex and not clearly defined, numerous susceptibility genes have been identified.[44] The pathogenesis of type 2 diabetes involves genes that influence either cellular responses to insulin or beta cell function or viability or both.

There is a subset of type 2 diabetes called maturity-onset diabetes of the young (MODY), which is thought to be autosomal dominant because it affects 50% of first-degree relatives. There are at least six types of MODY, and each type is caused by specific mutation in a critical enzyme involved in beta cell function or insulin action. For example, MODY2 is characterized by a glucose-sensing defect (glucokinase mutation), and MODY3 results from a mutation in the hepatocyte nuclear factor alpha-1. It is estimated that only 2% to 5% of cases of diabetes are monogenic and therefore are classified as MODY.[45]

Cellular resistance is a factor for 60% to 80% of individuals with type 2 diabetes. Insulin resistance increases with obesity. Decreased beta cell responsiveness to plasma glucose levels is also an important part of the pathogenesis of type 2 diabetes, along with abnormal glucagon secretion. Islet dysfunction may be caused by a decrease in beta cell mass, abnormal function of the beta cells, alterations in the insulin receptor, or postreceptor events.[46] Although levels of insulin may increase (hyperinsulinemia) to compensate for insulin resistance in peripheral tissues, there is still a relative deficiency of insulin.

Pancreatic changes in individuals with type 2 diabetes mellitus are nonspecific and have been observed to a lesser degree in persons without diabetes. Amyloid deposits in the islets occur in 10% to 40% of the pancreases from individuals with type 2 diabetes. Amyloid formation is associated with islet cell destruction. The extent of amyloid deposits is positively correlated with the age of the individual and the duration and severity of the disease. In long-standing type 2 diabetes, beta cell mass is decreased by 20% to 40%,[46] but functional mass is considerably lower and inexorably declines over time.

The accumulation of fat in nonadipose tissue (ectopic fat) is common in type 2 diabetes and insulin-resistance states. Lipid accumulation in islets is associated with impaired insulin secretion, and excess fat in muscle has been correlated with insulin resistance. Fatty infiltration of the liver, called *nonalcoholic steatohepatitis,* is common and may result in hepatic failure and cirrhosis. The pathogenesis of ectopic fat is poorly understood but is clearly related to overnutrition. Pancreatic fibrosis, occurring in 33% to 66% of individuals with type 2 diabetes, also contributes to loss of beta cell function.

A progressive decrease in the weight and number of beta cells occurs in type 2 diabetes, and several different mechanisms have been implicated. Beta cells are extremely sensitive to high levels of both glucose and free fatty acids and, under these so-called glucolipotoxic conditions, beta cells undergo apoptotic cell death. A variety of cytokines, including tumor necrosis factor-alpha (TNF-α) and interleukin 1-beta (IL-1β), have also been shown to be toxic to beta cells. Interestingly, intra-abdominal fat, or its supporting tissue, has been demonstrated to produce these cytokines and have excessive rates of free fatty acid release. As mentioned previously, excess intra-abdominal fat is a major component of the metabolic syndrome. Most experts now believe that the combination of excess nutrients, obesity, inflammatory cytokines, and the production of obesity-related cytokines called adipokines are major contributors to insulin resistance and beta cell death in type 2 diabetes.[47–49]

The most powerful risk factor for type 2 diabetes is obesity, especially intra-abdominal obesity. The risk for developing type 2 diabetes mellitus increases 10 times with severe obesity.[48] Excessive caloric intake predisposes an individual to type 2 diabetes by contributing to obesity.

In obese persons, insulin is less able to facilitate the entry of glucose into the liver, skeletal muscles, and adipose tissue. Multiple theories have been presented to explain this phenomenon and are as follows:

1. A decreased number of insulin receptors in the plasma membrane causes decreased insulin binding.
2. Postreceptor insulin signaling is impaired by intracellular satiety signals (principally glucosamine).
3. Release of free fatty acids interferes with insulin signaling and impedes the cellular metabolism of glucose.
4. Inflammatory cytokines (TNF-α and interleukin 6) disrupt insulin signaling.
5. Hyperinsulinemia from overeating induces insulin resistance to protect from hypoglycemia.

In any event, the mechanism responsible for insulin receptor binding or postreceptor activity may be reversed through weight loss.

Amylin is a hormone co-secreted with insulin by the beta cells. There is a deficiency of amylin in type 1 diabetes that parallels insulin. Problems with glycemic control may be related to altered glucagon control or assimilation of nutrients in relation to amylin deficit. Amyloid deposition also may be related to amylin loss.[50]

CLINICAL MANIFESTATIONS Clinical manifestations of type 2 diabetes often are nonspecific. The individual often is overweight and hyperlipidemic. The onset often is slow and insidious, making diagnosis difficult. Some of the classic symptoms of diabetes may be present, but more often there will be nonspecific symptoms, such as pruritus, recurrent infections, visual changes, and paresthesias (Table 18-6).

TABLE 18-6

Clinical Manifestations and Mechanisms for Type 2 Diabetes Mellitus

Manifestations	Mechanisms
Recurrent infections (e.g., boils and carbuncles), skin infections and prolonged wound healing	Growth of microorganisms is stimulated by increased glucose levels; impaired blood supply hinders healing
Genital pruritus	Hyperglycemia and glycosuria favor fungal growth; candidal infections, resulting in pruritus, are a common presenting symptom in women
Visual changes	Blurred vision occurs as water balance in the eye fluctuates because of elevated blood glucose levels; diabetic retinopathy may ensue
Paresthesias	Paresthesias are common manifestations of diabetic neuropathies
Fatigue	Metabolic changes result in poor use of food products, contributing to lethargy and fatigue

EVALUATION AND TREATMENT Type 2 diabetes is underdiagnosed, but methods that can be used to diagnose it are similar to those used for type 1 (see p. 462). The goal of treatment is restoration of euglycemia (a normal blood glucose level) and correction of related metabolic disorders. Dietary measures, including the restriction of the total caloric intake, are of primary importance in the overweight individual. As in type 1 diabetes, the ratio of fats, carbohydrates, and protein is important, and both cholesterol and saturated fats are restricted. Some research suggests that high-fiber diets also improve diabetic control.[51] As the obese individual loses weight, the body's resistance to insulin often diminishes so that weight loss results in improved glucose tolerance. Oral hyperglycemic agents often are needed for optimal management, and exercise is an essential component of treatment. Insulin therapy is used when oral medications fail to maintain euglycemia.

Gestational diabetes

Gestational diabetes mellitus develops when glucose intolerance appears during pregnancy, and pregnant women at risk should be screened. Risk factors include a family history of diabetes, membership in a high-risk ethnic group, advanced maternal age (>25 years of age), prior history of gestational diabetes or polycystic ovary syndrome, overweight (BMI >25 kg/m^2), and history of obstetrical complications associated with gestational diabetes. Aggressive treatment is required to prevent morbidity and fetal mortality.[52]

Acute Complications of Diabetes Mellitus

The major acute complications of diabetes mellitus are hypoglycemia, diabetic ketoacidosis (Figure 18-10), and hyperosmolar hyperglycemic nonketotic syndrome (see comparison in Table 18-7). In addition, the Somogyi phenomenon and dawn phenomenon may be seen.

Hypoglycemia occurs in more than 90% of cases of type 1 diabetes and is related to insulin treatment. Hypoglycemia in diabetes is sometimes called *insulin shock* or *insulin reaction.* Symptoms result from decreased blood glucose (45 to 60 mg/dl) and neurogenic reactions. Symptoms include pallor, tremor, anxiety, tachycardia, palpitations, diaphoresis, headache, dizziness, irritability, fatigue, poor judgment, confusion, visual disturbances, hunger, seizures, and coma. The treatment is to provide an immediate replacement of glucose. Prevention is achieved with individualized treatment, blood glucose monitoring, and education.

Diabetic ketoacidosis (DKA) is a serious complication related to a deficiency of insulin and an increase in insulin counterregulatory hormones (catecholamines, cortisol, glucagon, growth hormone). Under these conditions, hepatic glucose production increases and peripheral glucose usage decreases. Fat is mobilized, and ketogenesis is stimulated[53] (see Figure 18-10). The frequency of DKA peaks in adolescence.[54]

Hyperosmolar hyperglycemic nonketotic syndrome is an uncommon but significant complication of type 2 diabetes mellitus with a high overall mortality. It occurs more often in elderly individuals who have other comorbidities, including infections or cardiovascular or renal disease. Poor glucose control results in high levels of serum glucose (more than 500 mg/dl) and high serum osmotic pressures that lead to severe dehydration, low blood volume, and low perfusion pressures. Concurrent ketosis is less common because there is enough insulin to prevent lipolysis and protein catabolism. Treatment is controversial but mandates aggressive fluid and electrolyte resuscitation and strict control of serum glucose levels.[55]

The **Somogyi effect** is a unique combination of hypoglycemia followed by rebound hyperglycemia. The rise in blood glucose occurs because of counterregulatory hormones (epinephrine, GH, corticosteroids), which are stimulated by hypoglycemia. They produce gluconeogenesis. Excessive carbohydrate intake may contribute to the rebound hyperglycemia. The clinical occurrence of Somogyi effect is controversial.

The **dawn phenomenon** is an early morning rise in blood glucose concentration with no hypoglycemia during the night. It is related to nocturnal elevations of GH, which decrease metabolism of glucose by muscle and fat. Increased clearance of plasma insulin also may be involved. Altering the time and dose of insulin administration manages the problem.

Chronic Complications of Diabetes Mellitus

A number of serious complications are associated with any type of long-term diabetes mellitus and include microvascular and macrovascular disease and neuropathies. Most complications are associated with metabolic alterations, primarily hyperglycemia.[56] Strict control of blood glucose significantly reduces complications. Several metabolic events are associated with chronic hyperglycemia and are believed to be involved in the pathogenesis of diabetic complications. They include shunting of glucose into the polyol pathway, activation of protein kinase C, overproduction of reactive oxygen species (oxidative stress), and production of advanced glycation end products or nonenzymatic glycosylation of proteins.

Hyperglycemia and nonenzymatic glycosylation

Nonenzymatic glycosylation is the reversible attachment of glucose to proteins, lipids, and nucleic acids without the action of enzymes. With recurrent or persistent hyperglycemia, glucose becomes irreversibly bound to collagen and other proteins in blood vessel walls and interstitial tissue. **Advanced glycosylation endproducts (AGEs)** result from the attachment of glucose metabolites onto proteins. AGEs have a number of properties that may cause tissue injury or pathologic conditions associated with diabetes[57]:

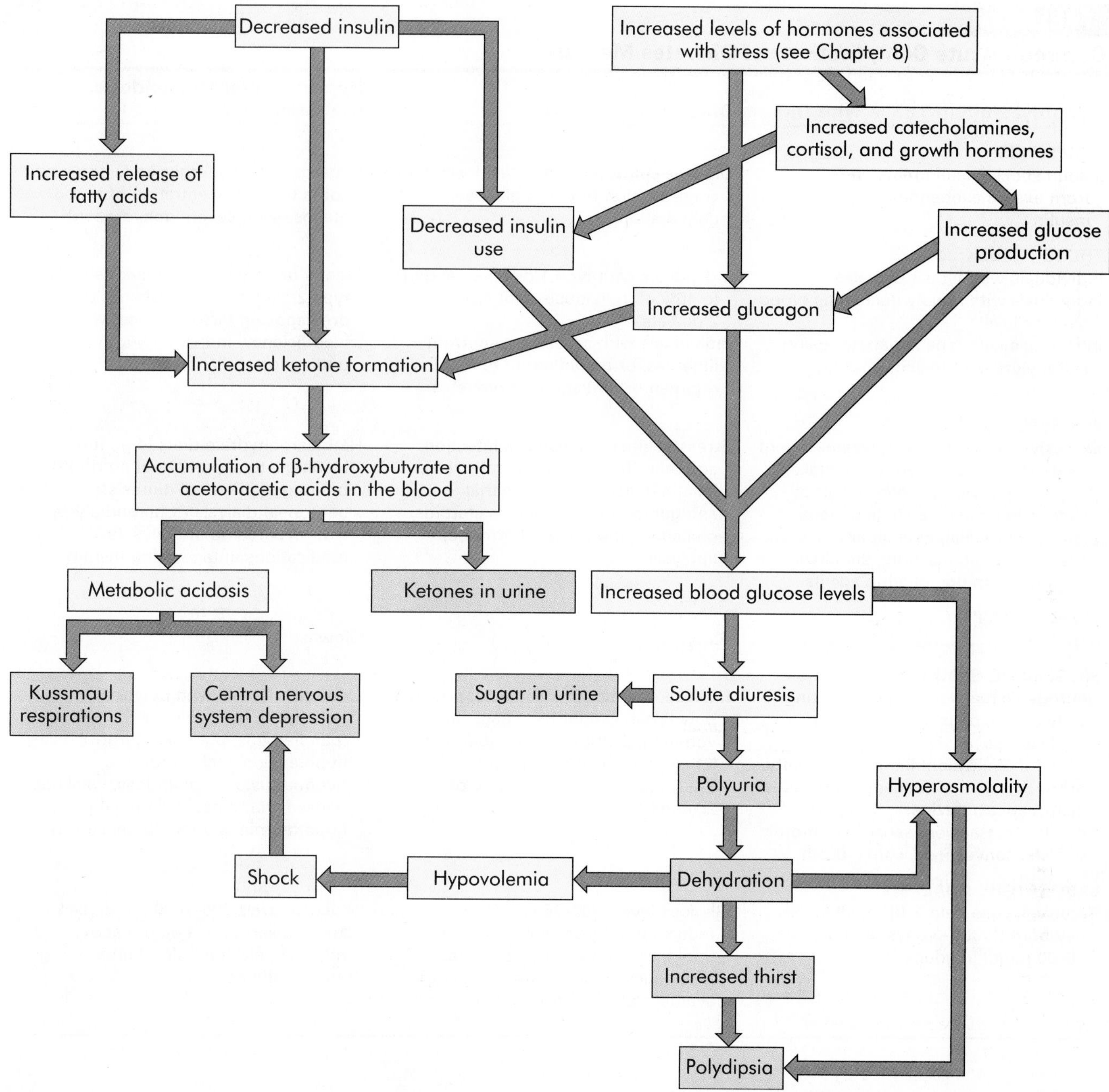

Figure 18-10 ■ **Diabetic Ketoacidosis.** Contributing causes of metabolic acidosis that result from ketosis and consequences of hyperglycemia.

1. Cross-linking and trapping of proteins, including albumin, low-density lipoprotein (LDL), immunoglobulin, and complement, with thickening of the basement membrane or increased permeability in blood vessels and nerves
2. Binding to cell receptors, such as macrophages, and inducing release of cytokines and growth factors that stimulate cellular proliferation in the glomeruli and smooth muscle of blood vessels
3. Induction of lipid oxidation and oxygen free radicals
4. Inactivation of nitric oxide with loss of vasodilation
5. Procoagulant changes on endothelial cells

Pharmacologic agents, such as aminoguanidine, inhibited AGE formation in animal studies but have been somewhat disappointing in clinical trials.

Hyperglycemia and the polyol pathway

Tissues that do not require insulin for glucose transport, such as kidney, red blood cells (RBCs), blood vessels, eye lens, and nerves, use an alternate metabolic pathway for glucose metabolism known as the **polyol pathway.** With hyperglycemia, glucose is shunted to this pathway and is converted to sorbitol (a polyol) by the enzyme aldose reductase. Sorbitol is then only very slowly converted to

TABLE 18-7

Common Acute Complications of Diabetes Mellitus

	Hypoglycemia in Those with DM	Diabetic Ketoacidosis	Hyperosmolar Nonacidotic Diabetes
SYNONYMS	Insulin shock, insulin reaction from excess exogenous insulin	Diabetic coma syndrome (acidosis, high concentration of blood glucose, dehydration)	Hyperosmolar hyperglycemia nonketotic coma (high concentration of blood glucose with severe dehydration)
THOSE AT RISK	Individuals with type 1 diabetes Individuals with rapidly fluctuating blood glucose levels Individuals with type 2 diabetes using sulfonylureas or insulin	Individuals with type 1 diabetes and up to 10% of individuals with type 2 diabetes Individuals with severe, intercurrent illnesses, or nonadherent to medical regimen or undiagnosed diabetes	Elderly or very young individuals with type 2 diabetes, nondiabetics with predisposing factors, those with renal insufficiency, individuals with undiagnosed diabetes
PREDISPOSING FACTORS	Excessive insulin or hypoglycemic agent intake, lack of sufficient food intake, excessive physical exercise, abrupt decline in insulin needs (e.g., renal failure; immediately postpartum, some cases of insulin reaction), simultaneous use of insulin-potentiating agents	Stressful situation, such as infection, accident, trauma, emotional stress; insulin deficiency; factors that antagonize insulin, such as steroids, glucagon, and growth hormone; lipolysis	High-carbohydrate diets (e.g., tube feedings, total parenteral nutrition), prolonged mannitol diuresis, peritoneal dialysis or hemodialysis with hyperosmolar dialysate, medications antagonizing insulin
TYPICAL ONSET	Rapid	Slow	Slowest
PRESENTING SYMPTOMS	Neurogenic reaction: pallor, sweating, tachycardia, palpitations, hunger, restlessness, anxiety, tremors Cellular malnutrition: fatigue, irritability, headache, loss of concentration, visual disturbances, dizziness, hunger, confusion, transient sensory or motor defects, convulsions, coma, death	Malaise, dry mouth, headache, polyuria, polydipsia, weight loss, nausea, vomiting, pruritus, abdominal pain, lethargy, shortness of breath, Kussmaul respirations, fruity or acetone odor to breath	Osmotic diuresis with polyuria, polydipsia, hypovolemia, dehydration (parched lips, poor skin turgor), hypotension, tachycardia, hypoperfusion, weight loss, weakness, nausea, vomiting, abdominal pain, hypothermia, stupor, coma, seizures
LABORATORY ANALYSIS	Serum glucose below 10 mg/dl in newborn (first 2–3 days) and below 55–60 mg/dl in adults	Glucose levels 300–750 mg/dl, pH <7.3, reduction in bicarbonate concentration, increased anion gap, increased plasma levels of β-hydroxybutyrate, acetoacetate, and acetone	Glucose levels 600–2000 mg/dl, lack of ketosis, serum osmolarity above 350 mOsm/L, elevated blood urea nitrogen and creatinine

fructose by sorbitol dehydrogenase. The resulting accumulation of sorbitol increases intracellular osmotic pressure and attracts water, leading to cell injury. This is particularly evident in the lens of the eye and leads to swelling with visual changes and cataracts. In nerves, sorbitol interferes with ion pumps, damages Schwann cells, and disrupts nerve conduction. RBCs become swollen and stiff and interfere with perfusion. Aldose reductase inhibitors have been studied in humans, but their clinical utility has been severely hampered by serious side effects.

Protein kinase C

Protein kinase C (PKC) is actually a family of different intracellular signaling proteins that can become inappropriately activated in different tissues by hyperglycemia. Various consequences have been observed, including insulin resistance, production of extracellular matrix and cytokines, vascular cell proliferation, enhanced contractility, and increased permeability. These effects may contribute to the macrovascular, microvascular, and neurologic complications of diabetes. Ruboxistaurin, a selective PKCβ inhibitor, has shown to be fairly effective in limiting or preventing neuropathy and nephropathy in experimental animals.[58] Human clinical trials are ongoing.

Diabetic neuropathies

Diabetic neuropathy is the most common cause of neuropathy in the Western world and is the most common complication of diabetes. The underlying pathologic mechanism includes both metabolic and vascular factors related to hyperglycemia. Advanced glycosylation end products and increased formation of polyols contribute to nerve degeneration and delayed conduction. Both somatic and peripheral nerve cells show diffuse or focal damage resulting in polyneuropathy. Sensory deficits and symptoms are more common than motor involvement.

Some neuropathies are progressive, but many—such as painful peripheral neuropathy, mononeuropathy (wristdrop, footdrop), diabetic amyotrophy, diabetic neuropathic cachexia, and visceral manifestations associated with autonomic neuropathy (e.g., delayed gastric emptying, diabetic diarrhea, altered bladder function, orthostatic hypotension)—may spontaneously appear to improve. Neuropathy may occur during periods of "good" glucose control and may be the initial clinical manifestation of diabetes. Chronic hyperglycemia also can cause cognitive dysfunction.[59]

Microvascular disease

Thickening of the capillary basement membrane, endothelial hyperplasia, thrombosis, and pericyte degeneration are characteristic of diabetic microangiopathy and emerge over a period of 1 to 2 years. Decreased tissue perfusion and hypoxia eventually result. Some degree of hyperglycemia is a necessary prerequisite for the vascular changes, and accumulation of AGEs may alter structural proteins. The frequency of the lesions appears to be proportional to the duration of the disease (more or less than 10 years) and blood glucose levels. Hypoxia and ischemia of various organs may result from microangiopathy, especially in the retina and kidney. If carefully evaluated at the time of presentation, many individuals with type 2 diabetes will be found to have microvascular complications because of the long duration of asymptomatic hyperglycemia that generally precedes diagnosis. This underscores the need to screen adults for diabetes.

Visual changes

Diabetic retinopathy appears to be a response to retinal ischemia resulting from blood vessel changes and RBC aggregation and is influenced by growth hormone and metabolic control. Activation of PKC also is important. The prevalence and severity of the retinopathy are strongly related to the age of the individual and duration of the diabetes. In comparison to type 1 diabetes, retinopathy appears to develop more rapidly in individuals with type 2 because of the likelihood of long-standing hyperglycemia before diagnosis. The majority of individuals with diabetes will eventually develop retinopathy.

The three stages of retinopathy are *nonproliferative* (stage I), characterized by an increase in retinal capillary permeability, vein dilation, microaneurysm formation, and superficial (flame-shaped) and deep (blot) hemorrhages; *preproliferative* (stage II), a progression of retinal ischemia with areas of poor perfusion that culminate in infarcts; and *proliferative* (stage III), the result of neovascularization and fibrous tissue formation within the retina or optic disc. Traction of the new vessels on the vitreous humor may cause retinal detachment or hemorrhage into the vitreous humor. Macular edema is the leading cause of decreased vision among persons with diabetes. Hard exudates and microaneurysms can result in loss of vision. Blurring of vision also can be a consequence of hyperglycemia and sorbitol accumulation in the lens. Cataract formation and dehydration of the lens, aqueous humor, and vitreous humor reduce visual acuity.

Diabetic nephropathy

Diabetes is the most common cause of end-stage renal disease. AGEs, activation of the polyol pathway, glucose toxicity, and protein kinase C all contribute to renal tissue injury; yet the exact process responsible for destruction of kidneys in diabetes is unknown. The glomeruli are injured by protein denaturation by high glucose levels, hyperglycemia with high renal blood flow (hyperfiltration), and intraglomerular hypertension exacerbated by systemic hypertension. Renal glomerular changes occur early in diabetes mellitus, occasionally preceding the overt manifestation of the disease. Progressive changes include glomerular enlargement, glomerular basement membrane thickening with proliferation of mesangial cells, and mesangial matrix. This results in diffuse intercapillary glomerulosclerosis and decreased blood flow. Alterations in glomerular membrane permeability occur with loss of negative charge and albuminuria.[60]

Microalbuminuria is the first manifestation of renal dysfunction. Continuous proteinuria generally heralds a life expectancy of less than 10 years. Before proteinuria, no clinical signs or symptoms of progressive glomerulosclerosis are likely to be evident. Later, hypoproteinemia, reduction in plasma oncotic pressure, fluid overload, anasarca (generalized body edema), and hypertension may occur. As renal function continues to deteriorate, individuals with type 1 diabetes may experience hypoglycemia (because of loss of renal insulin metabolism), which necessitates a decrease in insulin therapy. As the glomerular filtration rate drops below 10 ml/min, uremic signs, such as nausea, lethargy, acidosis, anemia, and uncontrolled hypertension, occur (see Chapter 29 for a discussion of renal failure). Impaired kidney function also accelerates retinopathy. Death from renal failure is much more common in individuals with type 1 diabetes mellitus than in those with type 2 diabetes because the appearance of proteinuria in these individuals is strongly correlated with death from cardiovascular disease.

Macrovascular disease

Macrovascular disease causes morbidity and mortality, particularly among individuals with type 2 diabetes mellitus. Unlike microangiopathy, atherosclerotic disease is unrelated to the severity of diabetes and often is present in those with merely an impaired glucose tolerance.[61] (Atherosclerosis is discussed in Chapter 23.) Children with poorly controlled type 2 diabetes have high risk for macrovascular complications within one to two decades.[62] Atherosclerosis has many contributing factors. Advanced glycosylated end products attach to cells in the walls of blood vessels and promote changes leading to atherosclerosis (Figure 18-11).[63]

Lipids may be deposited in the lesions, and triglyceride and serum cholesterol elevations are common. High-density lipoproteins (HDLs), which tend to protect vessels, are present in only low concentrations in individuals with diabetes. As in the nondiabetic person, the presence of

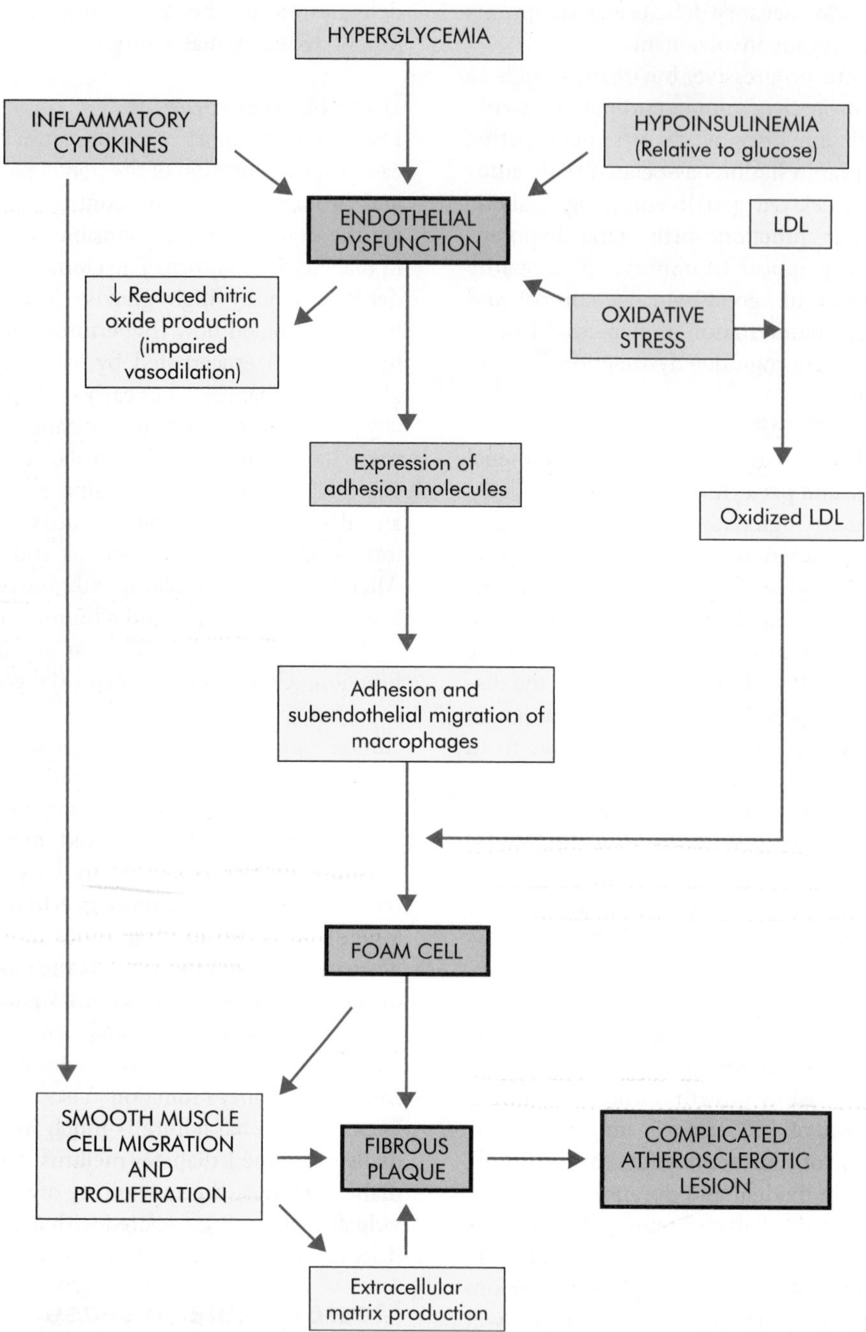

Figure 18-11 ■ **Diabetes Mellitus and Atherosclerosis.** Diabetes with its associated hyperglycemia, relative hypoinsulinemia, oxidative stress, and proinflammatory state contributes to atherogenesis by causing arterial endothelial dysfunction (impaired vasodilation and adhesion of inflammatory cells), dyslipidemia, and smooth muscle proliferation. (Data from Charo IF, Ransohoff RM: The many roles of chemokines and chemokine receptors in inflammation, *N Engl J Med* 354[6]:610–621, 2006; Heinecke JW: Lipoprotein oxidation in cardiovascular disease: chief culprit or innocent bystander? *J Exp Med* 203[4]:813–816, 2006; Kaperonis EA et al: Inflammation and atherosclerosis, *Eur J Vasc Endovasc Surg* 31[4]:386–393, 2006; Tedgui A, Mallat Z: Cytokines in atherosclerosis: pathogenic and regulatory pathways, *Physiol Rev* 86(2):515–581, 2006.)
LDL, Low-density liprotein.

other risk factors, including hypertension, increases vulnerability to atherosclerosis.

Coronary artery disease

The risk of coronary artery disease (CAD) for those with diabetes is higher than for the general population even when hypertension and hyperlipidemia are taken into account. CAD is the most common cause of death in individuals with type 2 diabetes because of insulin resistance, high levels of LDLs and triglycerides, low levels of HDLs, platelet abnormalities, and endothelial cell dysfunction.[64] Mortality is high for both men and women. In general, the prevalence of CAD increases with the duration but not the severity of diabetes.

Myocardial infarction causes death in 20% of those with diabetes. In addition, the incidence of congestive heart failure is higher in individuals with diabetes, even without myocardial infarction. This may be related to the presence of increased amounts of collagen in the ventricular wall, which reduces the mechanical compliance of the heart during filling. Increased platelet adhesion and decreased fibrinolysis promote thrombus formation in persons with diabetes.[65] (Heart disease is described in Chapter 23.) Guidelines have been developed to reduce the risk of CAD in individuals with diabetes.[66]

Stroke

Stroke is twice as common in those with diabetes as in the nondiabetic population.[67] The survival rate for individuals with diabetes after a massive stroke is typically shorter than for nondiabetic individuals. Hypertension and hyperglycemia are definite risk factors (see Chapter 23).

Peripheral vascular disease

The increased incidence of peripheral vascular disease (PVD), gangrene, and amputation in the individual with diabetes has been well documented. Many individuals with type 2 diabetes have evidence of PVD at the time of their initial diagnosis.[68] Individuals with diabetes are more likely to have atherosclerosis that appears at a younger age and advances more rapidly than vascular changes in nondiabetic persons. Age, duration of diabetes, genetics, and additional risk factors influence the development of PVD.

Because of occlusions of the small arteries and arterioles, most of the gangrenous changes of the lower extremities occur in patchy areas of the feet and toes.[69] The lesions begin as ulcers and progress to osteomyelitis or gangrene requiring amputation.[70] Significant morbidity and mortality are associated with major amputation.

Infection

The individual with diabetes is at an increased risk for infection throughout the body for at least five reasons:

1. *The senses.* Impaired vision caused by retinal changes and impaired touch caused by neuropathy diminish the prevention of breaks in the skin by decreasing the early warning systems.
2. *Hypoxia.* Once skin integrity is compromised, tissues' susceptibility to infection increases as a result of hypoxia. In addition, the glycosylated hemoglobin in the RBCs impedes the release of oxygen to tissues.
3. *Pathogens.* Some pathogens proliferate rapidly because of increased glucose in body fluids, which provides an excellent source of energy.
4. *Blood supply.* Decreased blood supply results from vascular changes and decreases the supply of white blood cells to the affected area.
5. *White cells.* These cells suffer impaired function, including abnormal chemotaxis and defective phagocytosis.

QUICK CHECK 18-4

1. What are the major differences between type 1 and type 2 diabetes in relation to insulin?
2. What are three metabolic alterations related to hyperglycemia that contribute to diabetic complications?
3. What is the single most important factor in the management of diabetes mellitus?

ALTERATIONS OF ADRENAL FUNCTION

Disorders of the Adrenal Cortex

Disorders of the adrenal cortex are related either to hyperfunction or to hypofunction. Hyperfunction that causes **hypercortisolism** leads to Cushing disease or Cushing syndrome; that which causes increased secretion of adrenal androgens and estrogens leads to virilization or feminization; and that which causes increased levels of aldosterone leads to hyperaldosteronism, which may be primary or secondary. Hypofunction of the adrenal cortex leads to Addison disease.

Hypercortical function (Cushing syndrome, Cushing disease)

Cushing disease is caused by excessive anterior pituitary secretion of ACTH. Cushing disease is more common in adults and is two to three times more common in women than in men. **Cushing syndrome** is an uncommon disorder and occurs whenever there is an excessive level of cortisol regardless of the cause and can be described as ACTH dependent and ACTH independent. ACTH-dependent Cushing syndrome can occur at any age but usually occurs between 30 and 50 years of age. Cushing syndrome is the most common complication of Cushing disease. Cushing syndrome resulting from ectopic ACTH secretion is more common in older adults, particularly men. ACTH-independent Cushing syndrome is usually the result of adrenal tumors and may occur in children, especially girls. In addition, a Cushing-like syndrome may develop as a result of the exogenous administration of glucocorticoids.[71]

PATHOPHYSIOLOGY Approximately 75% to 80% of individuals with hypercortisolism have Cushing disease. Autonomous, ectopic ACTH secretion by a tumor outside the pituitary (usually a malignant tumor such as a small cell carcinoma of the lung) is a far less common cause of ACTH-dependent hypercortisolism. Ectopic secretion of CRH has rarely been seen in neuroendocrine tumors. Whatever the cause, two observations consistently apply to individuals with Cushing syndrome: (1) they do not have diurnal or circadian secretion patterns of ACTH and cortisol, and (2) they do not increase ACTH and cortisol secretion in response to a stressor.[72] In individuals with ACTH-stimulated hypercorticoadrenalism, secretion of both cortisol and adrenal androgens is increased, and cortisol-releasing hormone is inhibited. Hormone-secreting tumors of the adrenal cortex, however, generally secrete only cortisol. When the secretion of cortisol by the tumor exceeds normal cortisol levels, symptoms of hypercortisolism develop.

CLINICAL MANIFESTATIONS Weight gain is the most common feature and results from the accumulation of adipose tissue in the trunk, facial, and cervical areas. These characteristic patterns of fat deposition have been described as "truncal obesity," "moon face," and "buffalo hump" (Figures 18-12 and 18-13). Transient weight gain from sodium and water retention also may be present.

Glucose intolerance occurs because of cortisol-induced insulin resistance and increased gluconeogenesis and glycogen storage by the liver. Overt diabetes mellitus develops in approximately 20% of individuals with hypercortisolism. Polyuria is a manifestation of hyperglycemia and resultant glycosuria.

Protein wasting is caused by the catabolic effects of cortisol on peripheral tissues. Muscle wasting leads to muscle weakness. In bone, loss of the protein matrix leads to osteoporosis, with pathologic fractures, vertebral compression fractures, bone and back pain, kyphosis, and reduced height. Cortisol interferes with the action of GH in long bones. Children who present with short stature may be experiencing growth retardation related to Cushing syndrome rather than GH deficiency. Bone disease may contribute to hypercalciuria and resulting renal stones, which are experienced by approximately 20% of individuals with disease. Loss of collagen also leads to thin, weakened integumentary tissues, through which capillaries are more visible and which are easily stretched by adipose deposits. Together, these changes account for the characteristic purple striae in the trunk area. Loss of collagenous support around small vessels makes them susceptible to rupture, leading to easy bruising, even with minor trauma. Thin, atrophied skin is also easily damaged, leading to skin breaks and ulcerations.

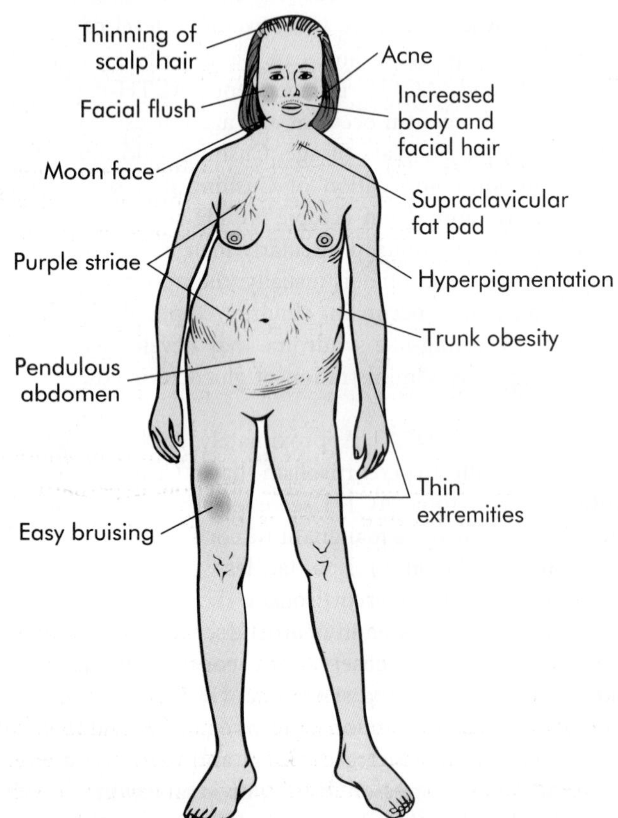

Figure 18-12 ■ **Symptoms of Cushing Disease.**

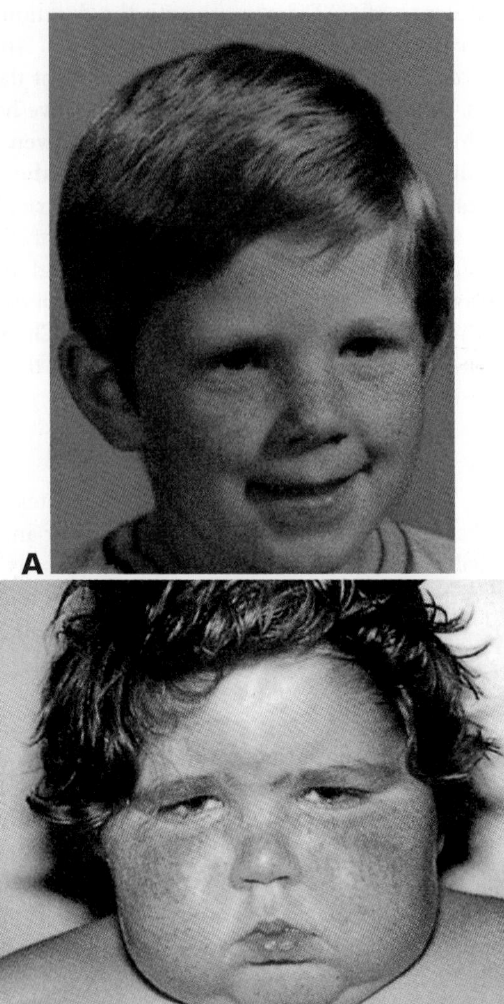

Figure 18-13 ■ **Cushing Syndrome. A,** Patient before onset of Cushing syndrome. **B,** Patient four months later. Moon facies is clearly demonstrated. (From Zitelli BJ, Davis HW: *Atlas of pediatric physical diagnosis,* ed 3, London, 1997, Gower.)

Hyperpigmentation in Cushing syndrome can occur when ectopic ACTH production leads to very high levels of ACTH. The pigmentation involves the mucous membranes, hair, and skin, all of which acquire a characteristic brownish or bronze color.

With elevated cortisol levels, vascular sensitivity to catecholamines increases significantly, leading to vasoconstriction and hypertension. Mineralocorticoid effects promote sodium retention and hypokalemia. Elevated blood pressure occurs in most individuals with Cushing syndrome. Suppression of the immune system and increased susceptibility to infections also occur.

Approximately 50% of individuals with Cushing syndrome experience alterations in their mental status that range from irritability and depression to severe psychiatric disturbances, such as schizophrenia.[72] Females may experience symptoms of increased adrenal androgen levels, increased hair growth (especially facial hair), acne, and oligomenorrhea. Rarely do androgen levels become high enough to cause changes of the voice, recession of the hairline, and clitoral hypertrophy unless an adrenal carcinoma is involved. Routine laboratory examinations may reveal hyperglycemia, glycosuria, hypokalemia, and metabolic alkalosis.

EVALUATION AND TREATMENT The diagnosis of Cushing syndrome is challenging, and various laboratory tests must be used, including urinary free cortisol (17-hydroxycorticosterol) higher than 100 mcg/24 hr and a dexamethasone suppression test. Visualizing procedures include pituitary MRI and abdominal scanning.[73]

Without treatment, approximately 50% of individuals with Cushing syndrome die within 5 years of onset as a result of overwhelming infection, suicide, complications from generalized arteriosclerosis, and hypertensive disease. Treatment is specific for the cause of hypercorticoadrenalism and includes medication, radiation, and surgery. Therefore, differentiation among pituitary, adrenal, and ectopic causes of the hypercortisolism is essential for effective treatment.

Congenital adrenal hyperplasia

Congenital adrenal hyperplasia results from the deficiency of an enzyme that is critical in cortisol biosynthesis. Because cortisol production is low, ACTH increases and causes adrenal hyperplasia, which results in the overproduction of either mineralocorticoids or androgens. The most common form is a 21-hydroxylase deficiency, which involves both mineralocorticoid and cortisol synthesis. Affected female infants are virilized, and infants of both genders exhibit salt wasting.

Hyperaldosteronism

Hyperaldosteronism is characterized by excessive aldosterone secretion by the adrenal glands. The excessive secretion can result from a primary adrenal disorder, such as an aldosterone-secreting adenoma, or from excessive stimulation of the normal adrenal cortex by angiotensin, ACTH, or elevated potassium. Hyperaldosteronism may be primary or secondary. In primary hyperaldosteronism, excessive secretion of aldosterone is caused by an abnormality of the adrenal cortex. In secondary hyperaldosteronism, excessive aldosterone secretion results from an extra-adrenal stimulus, most often a renin-angiotensin mechanism.

Primary hyperaldosteronism (Conn disease, primary aldosteronism) presents with hypertension, renal potassium wasting, hypokalemia, and neuromuscular manifestations.[74] The most common cause of primary aldosteronism is a benign, single adrenal adenoma. Bilateral adrenal nodular hyperplasia and adrenal carcinomas account for the remainder of cases. The incidence of primary hyperaldosteronism is estimated to be 1% to 2% of all hypertensive individuals.

Because aldosterone secretion normally is stimulated by the renin-angiotensin system, **secondary hyperaldosteronism** results from sustained elevated renin release and activation of angiotensin II. This occurs in various situations, including decreased circulating blood volume (e.g., in dehydration, shock, or hypoalbuminemia) and decreased delivery of blood to the kidneys (e.g., renal artery stenosis, heart failure, or hepatic cirrhosis). Here, the activation of the renin-angiotensin system and subsequent aldosterone secretion may be seen as compensatory, although in some instances (e.g., congestive heart failure), the increased circulating volume further worsens the condition. Other causes of secondary hyperaldosteronism are Bartter syndrome, in which the underlying disorder is a renal tubular defect leading to hypokalemia, and renin-secreting tumors of the kidney.

PATHOPHYSIOLOGY In primary hyperaldosteronism, pathophysiologic alterations are caused by excessive aldosterone secretion and the fluid and electrolyte imbalances that ensue. Hyperaldosteronism promotes (1) increased renal sodium and water reabsorption with corresponding hypervolemia (see Chapter 4) and hypertension and (2) renal excretion of potassium. The extracellular fluid volume overload, hypertension, and suppression of normal feedback mechanisms of renin secretion are characteristic of primary disorders. Edema usually does not occur with primary aldosteronism because hypervolemia-induced atrial natriuretic factor release results in loss of sodium and water.[75]

In secondary hyperaldosteronism, the effect of increased extracellular volume on renin secretion may vary. If renin secretion is being stimulated by variables other than pressure-initiated cellular changes at the juxtaglomerular apparatus (see Chapter 25), increased circulating blood volume may not decrease renin secretion through feedback mechanisms. This process occurs, for instance, in states of increased estrogen levels.

Potassium secretion is promoted by aldosterone, so that with excessive aldosterone, hypokalemia occurs (see Chapter 4). Hypokalemic alkalosis, changes in myocardial conduction, and skeletal muscle alterations may be seen, particularly with severe potassium depletion. The renal tubules may become insensitive to ADH, thus promoting excessive loss of free water. In this situation, hypernatremia also may occur because water is not able to follow the sodium that is reabsorbed.

CLINICAL MANIFESTATIONS Hypertension and hypokalemia are the hallmarks of primary hyperaldosteronism. With sustained hypertension, the chronic effects of elevated arterial pressure become evident, for example, left ventricular dilation and hypertrophy and progressive arteriosclerosis. Aldosterone-stimulated potassium loss can be substantial, resulting in typical manifestations of hypokalemia. Hypokalemic alkalosis may develop (see Chapter 4).

EVALUATION AND TREATMENT Various clinical and laboratory measurements are useful in assessing hyperaldosteronism. Tests include the following:

1. Blood pressure: elevated
2. Serum and urinary electrolyte levels: serum sodium is normal or elevated; serum potassium is depressed, but urinary potassium is elevated
3. Serum and urinary levels of aldosterone: increases
4. Aldosterone suppression testing: fludrocortisone acetate (Florinef) is used
5. Plasma renin activity: suppressed

Imaging techniques, including CT scans and nuclear magnetic resonance (NMR), may be used to localize an aldosterone-secreting adenoma.

Treatment includes management of hypertension and hypokalemia, as well as correction of any underlying causal abnormalities. If an aldosterone-secreting adenoma is present, it must be surgically removed.[76]

Hypersecretion of adrenal androgens and estrogens

Hypersecretion of adrenal androgens and estrogens may be caused by adrenal tumors, either adenomas or carcinomas, Cushing syndrome, or defects in steroid synthesis. The clinical syndrome that results depends on the hormone secreted, the gender of the individual, and the ages at which the hypersecretion is initiated. Hypersecretion of estrogens causes **feminization,** the development of female sex characteristics. Hypersecretion of androgens causes **virilization,** the development of male sex characteristics (Figure 18-14).

The effects of an estrogen-secreting tumor are most evident in males and result in gynecomastia (98% of cases), testicular atrophy, and decreased libido. In female children, such tumors may lead to early development of secondary sex characteristics. The changes caused by an androgen-secreting tumor are more easily observed in females and include excessive face and body hair growth, hirsutism, clitoral enlargement, deepening of the voice, amenorrhea, acne, and breast atrophy. In children, virilizing tumors promote precocious sexual development and bone aging. Treatment of androgen-secreting tumors usually involves surgical excision.

Hypocortical functioning

Hypocortisolism (low levels of cortisol secretion) develops because of either inadequate stimulation of the adrenal glands by ACTH or a primary inability of the adrenals to produce and secrete the adrenocortical hormones. Sometimes there is partial dysfunction of the adrenal cortex, so only synthesis of aldosterone or the adrenal androgens is affected. Hypofunction of the adrenal cortex may affect glucocorticoid or mineralocorticoid secretion or both.

Primary adrenal insufficiency is termed **Addison disease.** It is relatively rare, occurring most often in adults ages 30 to 60 years, although it may appear at any time. Addison disease is caused by autoimmune mechanisms that destroy adrenal cortical cells and is more common in women.

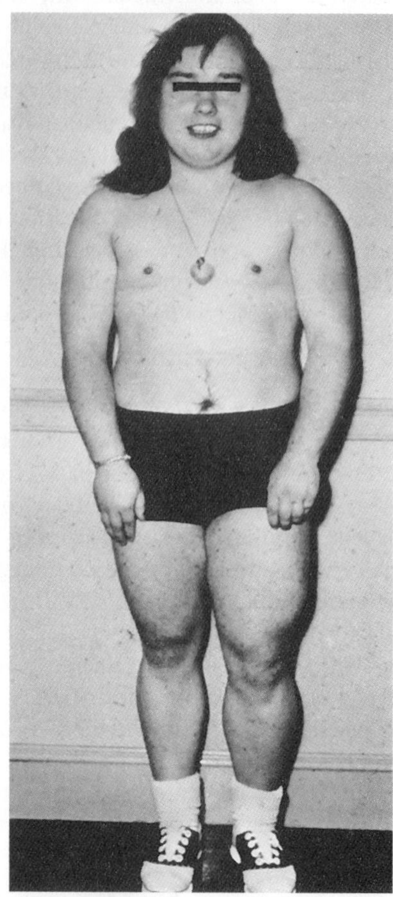

Figure 18-14 ■ **Virilization.** Virilization of a young girl by an androgen-secreting tumor of the adrenal cortex. Masculine features include lack of breast development, increased muscle bulk, and hirsutism (excessive hair). (From Thibodeau GA, Patton KT: *Anatomy & physiology,* St Louis, 1987, Mosby.)

PATHOPHYSIOLOGY Addison disease is characterized by inadequate corticosteroid and mineralocorticoid synthesis and elevated serum ACTH (loss of negative feedback). Before clinical manifestations of hypocortisolism are evident, more than 90% of total adrenocortical tissue must be destroyed.

Idiopathic Addison disease

Idiopathic Addison disease (organ-specific autoimmune adrenalitis) causes adrenal atrophy and hypofunction and is an organ-specific autoimmune disease. Autoantibodies specific to adrenal cortical cells are present in 50% to 70% of individuals with idiopathic Addison disease, and this percentage increases in younger persons and in those with other autoimmune diseases. Apparently, a genetic defect in immune surveillance mechanisms causes a deficiency of immune suppressor cells. This deficiency allows the proliferation of immunocytes directed against specific antigens within the adrenocortical cells.[77,78]

Idiopathic Addison disease is often associated with other autoimmune diseases, especially Hashimoto thyroiditis, pernicious anemia, and idiopathic hypoparathyroidism. In these cases, Addison disease may be inherited as an autosomal recessive trait. (Mechanisms of inheritance are described in Chapter 2.)

The adrenal glands in idiopathic Addison disease are smaller than normal and may be misshapen. Extensive diffuse cortical lymphocytic infiltrate supports the immune component of the disease process.

Secondary hypocortisolism

Secondary hypocortisolism is characterized by low to absent ACTH levels, causing inadequate adrenal stimulation, adrenal atrophy, and ultimately decreased corticosteroidogenesis. The prolonged administration of exogenous glucocorticoids for nonendocrine disease results in this form of hypocortisolism. Cortisol-secreting tumors also results in hypocortisolism. The increased glucocorticoid level from the tumor suppresses ACTH production. With decreased ACTH levels, cortisol synthesis by remaining adrenal tissue is suppressed. Pituitary hypofunction, as occurs in postpartum pituitary infarction (Sheehan syndrome) and panhypopituitarism, hypophysectomy, or isolated ACTH deficiency, causes inadequate ACTH production and secretion and absence of pituitary responsiveness to normal feedback mechanisms. In all instances of low ACTH levels, adrenal atrophy occurs and endogenous adrenal steroidogenesis is depressed.

Clinical manifestations of secondary hypocortisolism are similar to those of Addison disease, although hyperpigmentation usually does not occur. The renin-angiotensin system usually is normal, so aldosterone and potassium levels also tend to be normal.

CLINICAL MANIFESTATIONS The symptoms of Addison disease are primarily a result of hypocortisolism and hypoaldosteronism. They are summarized in Table 18-8.

EVALUATION AND TREATMENT Serum and urine levels of cortisol are depressed with hypocortisolism. ACTH levels may increase if there is adrenocortical insufficiency. ACTH levels are low in secondary adrenal insufficiency. ACTH levels can only be interpreted with simultaneous measurement of serum cortisol levels. Because of dehydration, blood urea nitrogen levels may increase. Serum glucose is low. Eosinophil and lymphocyte counts often are elevated. Hyperkalemia is seen in Addison disease and may cause mild alkalosis (see Chapter 4). The ACTH stimulation test may be used to evaluate serum cortisol levels.

The treatment of Addison disease involves glucocorticoid and possibly mineralocorticoid replacement therapy, together with dietary modifications. All individuals with hypocortisolism require lifetime daily glucocorticoid replacement therapy. With acute stressors, additional cortisol must be administered to approximate the amount of cortisol that might be expected if normal adrenal function were present (approximately 100 to 300 mg/day).

The individual's diet should include at least 150 mEq sodium per day, with sodium intake increased with excessive sweating or diarrhea. Treatment also must include correction of any underlying disorders.

Disorders of the Adrenal Medulla

Tumor of the adrenal medulla

Adrenomedullary hyperfunction is caused by chromaffin cell tumors of the adrenal medulla. These tumors, **pheochromocytomas,** secrete catecholamines on a continual basis. They are rare, and fewer than 10% are malignant. Those that are malignant metastasize to the lungs, liver, bones, or para-aortic lymph nodes.

PATHOPHYSIOLOGY Pheochromocytomas cause excessive production of catecholamines because of autonomous secretion of the tumor. Approximately 5% of people with pheochromocytomas have no symptoms, apparently

TABLE 18-8

Clinical Manifestations and Pathophysiologic Mechanisms of Addison Disease

Clinical Manifestations	Pathophysiologic Mechanisms
Weakness and easy fatigability that worsens as the day progresses, seen especially after exposure to stressors	Not known, may be related to hypoglycemia, decreased metabolism of proteins
Gastrointestinal disturbances: anorexia, nausea, vomiting, diarrhea, abdominal pain	Not known
Hypoglycemia, manifested by fatigue, mental confusion, apathy, psychosis	Absence of cortisol leads to decreased gluconeogenesis, decreased glycogen storage by liver, decreased metabolism of proteins, increased insulin sensitivity
Hyperpigmentation (seen only in cases of Addison disease with increased ACTH)	Increased secretion of ACTH is accompanied by increased secretion of beta-lipotropin and melanocyte-stimulating hormone; both hormones induce pigment changes in epithelial cells
Vitiligo: white patchy areas of depigmented skin	Autoimmune destruction of melanocytes
Hypotension	Decreased blood volume resulting from hypoaldosteronism causing increased renal sodium losses
Addisonian crisis: severe hypotension and vascular collapse	Combined effects of hypocortisolism, hypoaldosteronism, extracellular volume depletion, and some precipitating stressor (e.g., infection, vomiting, diarrhea); decreased vasomotor tone caused by cortisol deficiency

ACTH, Adrenocorticotropic hormone.

because the tumor is nonfunctioning. Such tumors can, however, release catecholamines, especially in response to a stressor, such as surgery.

CLINICAL MANIFESTATIONS The clinical manifestations of a pheochromocytoma are related to the chronic effects of catecholamine secretion and include persistent hypertension associated with headache, pallor, diaphoresis, tachycardia, and palpitations. Hypertension results from increased peripheral vascular resistance and may be sustained or paroxysmal. Headaches appear because of sudden changes in catecholamine levels in the blood, affecting cerebral blood flow. Hypermetabolism is related to chronic activation of sympathetic receptors in adipocytes, hepatocytes, and other tissues.[79] Glucose intolerance may occur because of catecholamine-induced inhibition of insulin release by the pancreas. Complaints of warmth, heat intolerance, and weight loss are common despite a normal-to-increased appetite. Other symptoms of catecholamine excess include excessive sweating, palpitations and tachycardia, and gastrointestinal alterations, especially constipation.

An acute episode of hypertension related to hypersecretion of catecholamines may follow specific events, such as exercise, excessive ingestion of tyrosine-containing foods (aged cheese, red wine, beer, yogurt), ingestion of caffeine-containing foods, external pressure on the tumor, and induction of anesthesia. These tumors tend to be extremely vascular and can rupture, causing massive and potentially fatal hemorrhage. Rupture is characterized by a sudden, unexplained decrease in blood pressure; sudden, severe abdominal pain; and a rigid abdomen.

EVALUATION AND TREATMENT A diagnosis of pheochromocytoma is made when increased catecholamine production is demonstrated in the blood or urine. After elevation of urinary or plasma catecholamines is documented, the site of the tumor is determined using abdominal imaging techniques. Because of the possibility of metastasis, whole-body scanning may be done.

The usual treatment of pheochromocytoma is laparoscopic surgical excision of the tumor, although open resection is still completed for large tumors or when metastasis is suspected. Medical therapy is used to stabilize blood pressure before, during, or after surgery.[80]

QUICK CHECK 18-5

1. What are the symptoms of hyperaldosteronism?
2. What major diseases are classified as hypocortisolism?

Did You Understand?

Mechanisms of Hormonal Alterations

1. Abnormalities in endocrine function may be caused by elevated or depressed hormone levels that result from (a) faulty feedback systems, (b) dysfunction of the gland, (c) altered metabolism of hormones, or (d) production of hormones from nonendocrine tissues.
2. Target cells may fail to respond to hormones because of (a) cell surface receptor-associated disorders, (b) intracellular disorders, or (c) circulating inhibitors

Alterations of the Hypothalamic-Pituitary System

1. Dysfunction in the release of hypothalamic hormones is probably related to interruption of the connection between the hypothalamus and pituitary, the pituitary stalk.
2. Disorders of the posterior pituitary include syndrome of inappropriate ADH secretion (SIADH) and diabetes insipidus. SIADH secretion is characterized by abnormally high ADH secretion; diabetes insipidus is characterized by abnormally low ADH secretion.
3. In SIADH, high ADH levels interfere with renal free water clearance, leading to hyponatremia and hypoosmolality, and is associated with brain injury and with certain forms of cancer, apparently because of ectopic secretion of ADH by tumor cells.
4. Diabetes insipidus may be neurogenic (caused by insufficient amounts of ADH) or nephrogenic (caused by an inadequate response to ADH). Its principal clinical features are polyuria and polydipsia.
5. Hypopituitarism can be primary (dysfunction of the pituitary) or secondary (dysfunction of the hypothalamus). Primary hypopituitarism can result from a pituitary tumor, trauma, infections, stroke, or surgical removal.
6. Hypopituitarism can affect any or all of the pituitary hormones and symptoms may range from mild to life threatening
7. Hyperpituitarism is caused by pituitary adenomas. These are usually benign, slow-growing tumors that arise from cells of the anterior pituitary.
8. Expansion of a pituitary adenoma causes both neurologic and secretory effects. Pressure from the expanding tumor causes hyposecretion of cells, dysfunction of the optic chiasma (leading to visual disturbances), and dysfunction of the hypothalamus and some cranial nerves.
9. Hypersecretion of growth hormone (GH) causes acromegaly, in which GH secretion becomes high and unpredictable. Pituitary adenoma is the most common cause of acromegaly.
10. Prolonged, abnormally high levels of GH lead to proliferation of body and connective tissue and slowly developing renal, thyroid, and reproductive dysfunction.
11. Prolactinomas result in galactorrhea, hirsutism, amenorrhea, hypogonadism, and osteopenia.

Alterations of Thyroid Function

1. Thyrotoxicosis is a general condition in which elevated thyroid hormone (TH) levels cause greater than normal physiologic responses. The condition can be caused by a variety of specific diseases, each of which has its own pathophysiology and course of treatment.

Did You Understand?—Cont'd

2. In general, hyperthyroidism has a range of endocrine, reproductive, gastrointestinal, integumentary, and ocular manifestations. These are caused by increased circulating levels of TH and by stimulation of the sympathetic division of the autonomic nervous system.
3. Graves disease, the most common form of hyperthyroidism, is caused by an autoimmune mechanism that overrides normal mechanisms for control of TH secretion and is characterized by thyrotoxicosis, ophthalmopathy, and circulating thyroid-stimulating immunoglobulins.
4. Toxic nodular goiter and toxic multinodular goiter occur when TH-regulating mechanisms and abnormal hypertrophy of the thyroid gland cause hyperthyroidism. Toxic multinodular goiter is caused by independently functioning follicular cell adenomas.
5. Thyrotoxic crisis is a severe form of hyperthyroidism that is often associated with physiologic or psychologic stress. Without treatment, death occurs quickly.
6. Primary hypothyroidism is caused by deficient production of TH by the thyroid gland. Secondary hypothyroidism is caused by hypothalamic or pituitary dysfunction. Symptoms depend on the degree of TH deficiency. Common manifestations include decreased energy metabolism, decreased heat production, and myxedema.
7. Acute thyroiditis is inflammation of the thyroid gland, often caused by a bacterium that can result in hypothyroidism.
8. Subacute thyroiditis is a self-limiting nonbacterial inflammation of the thyroid gland. The inflammatory process damages follicular cells, causing leakage of T_3 and T_4. Hyperthyroidism then is followed by transient hypothyroidism, which is corrected by cellular repair and a return to normal levels in the thyroid.
9. Autoimmune thyroiditis is associated with infiltration or fibrosis of the thyroid, circulating thyroid antibodies, and gradual loss of thyroid function. Autoimmune thyroiditis occurs in those individuals with genetic susceptibility to an autoimmune mechanism that causes thyroid damage and eventual hypothyroidism.
10. Myxedema is a sign of hypothyroidism caused by alterations in connective tissue with water-binding proteins that leads to edema and thickened mucous membranes.
11. Myxedema coma is a severe form of hypothyroidism that may be life threatening without emergency medical treatment.
12. Congenital hypothyroidism is absence of thyroid tissue during fetal development or defects in hormone synthesis.
13. Thyroid carcinoma is a relatively rare cancer. The most consistent causal risk factor associated with thyroid carcinoma is exposure to ionizing radiation, especially in childhood.

Alterations of Parathyroid Function

1. Hyperparathyroidism, which may be primary or secondary, is characterized by greater than normal secretion of parathyroid hormone (PTH).
2. Primary hyperparathyroidism is caused by an interruption of the normal mechanisms that regulate calcium and PTH levels. Manifestations include chronic hypercalcemia, increased bone resorption, and hypercalciuria.
3. Secondary hyperparathyroidism is a compensatory response to hypocalcemia and often occurs with chronic renal failure.
4. Hypoparathyroidism, defined by abnormally low PTH levels, is caused by thyroid surgery, autoimmunity, or genetic mechanisms.
5. The lack of circulating PTH in hypoparathyroidism causes depressed serum calcium levels, increased serum phosphate levels, decreased bone resorption, and eventual hypocalciuria.

Dysfunction of the Endocrine Pancreas: Diabetes Mellitus

1. Diabetes mellitus is a group of disorders characterized by glucose intolerance, chronic hyperglycemia, and disturbances of carbohydrate, protein, and fat metabolism.
2. A diagnosis of diabetes mellitus is based on elevated plasma glucose concentrations and measurement of glycosolated hemoglobin. Classic signs and symptoms are often present as well.
3. The two most common types of diabetes mellitus are type 1 and type 2.
4. Type 1 diabetes mellitus is characterized by loss of beta cells, islet cell antibody, a lack of insulin, and excess of glucagon, which causes improper metabolism of fat, protein, and carbohydrates.
5. Type 1 diabetes mellitus seems to be caused by a gradual process of autoimmune destruction of beta cells in genetically susceptible individuals.
6. In type 1 diabetes mellitus, hyperglycemia causes polyuria and polydipsia resulting from osmotic diuresis.
7. Ketoacidosis is caused by increased levels of circulating ketones without the inhibiting effects of insulin. Increased levels of circulating fatty acids and weight loss are all manifestations of type 1 uncontrolled diabetes mellitus.
8. Type 2 diabetes mellitus is caused by genetic susceptibility that is triggered by environmental factors. The most compelling environmental risk factor is obesity.
9. In the obese, insulin has a diminished ability to influence glucose uptake and metabolism.
10. Some insulin production continues in type 2 diabetes mellitus, but the weight and number of beta cells decrease. There are dysfunctional levels of both insulin and glucagon.
11. Gestational diabetes is glucose intolerance during pregnancy.

(Continued)

Did You Understand?—Cont'd

12. Acute complications of diabetes mellitus include hypoglycemia, diabetic ketoacidosis, hyperosmolar hyperglycemic nonketotic coma, the Somogyi effect, and the dawn phenomenon.
13. Hypoglycemia is a complication related to insulin treatment.
14. Diabetic ketoacidosis develops when there is an absolute or relative deficiency of insulin and an increase in the insulin counterregulatory hormones of catecholamines, cortisol, glucagon, and growth hormone.
15. Hyperosmolar hyperglycemic nonketotic syndrome is pathophysiologically similar to diabetic ketoacidosis, although levels of free fatty acids are lower in hyperosmolar nonacidotic diabetes and lack of ketosis indicates that some level of insulin is present.
16. The Somogyi effect is a combination of hypoglycemia with rebound hyperglycemia.
17. The dawn phenomenon is an early morning rise in glucose levels caused by nocturnal elevations in growth hormone.
18. Chronic sequelae of diabetes mellitus include diabetic neuropathies, microvascular disease (e.g., retinopathy, nephropathy), macrovascular disease (e.g., coronary artery disease, stroke, peripheral vascular disease), and infection.
19. Microangiopathy is caused by thickening of the capillary basement membrane and eventual decreased tissue perfusion affecting the microcirculation.
20. Macrovascular disease associated with diabetes mellitus is most often related to the proliferation of fibrous plaques in the arterial wall and to elevated lipid levels.
21. Incidence of coronary heart disease, peripheral vascular disease, and stroke is greater in those with diabetes than in nondiabetic individuals.
22. Individuals with diabetes are at risk for a variety of infections.
23. Infection may be related to sensory impairment and resulting injury, hypoxia, increased proliferation of pathogens in elevated concentrations of glucose, decreased blood supply associated with vascular damage, and impaired white cell function.

Alterations of Adrenal Function

1. Disorders of the adrenal cortex are related to hyperfunction or hypofunction. No known disorders are associated with hypofunction of the adrenal medulla, but medullary hyperfunction causes clinically defined syndromes.
2. Cortical hyperfunction, or hypercortisolism, causes Cushing syndrome, which may or may not involve the pituitary gland, and Cushing disease, which is hypercortisolism with pituitary involvement.
3. Hypercortisolism is usually caused by Cushing disease but can also be caused by ectopic production of cortisol or by adrenocortical tumors. Complications include obesity, diabetes, protein wasting, immune suppression, and mental status changes.
4. Excessive aldosterone secretion causes hyperaldosteronism, which may be primary or secondary. Primary hyperaldosteronism is caused by an abnormality of the adrenal cortex. Secondary hyperaldosteronism involves an extra-adrenal stimulus, often angiotensin.
5. Hyperaldosteronism promotes increased sodium reabsorption, corresponding hypervolemia, increased extracellular volume (which is variable), and hypokalemia related to renal reabsorption of sodium.
6. Hypersecretion of adrenal androgens and estrogens can be a result of adrenal tumors, either adenomas or carcinomas. Hypersecretion of estrogens causes feminization, the development of female sex characteristics. Hypersecretion of androgens causes virilization, the development of male sex characteristics.
7. Hypofunction of the adrenal cortex can affect glucocorticoid or mineralocorticoid secretion or both. Hypofunction can be caused by a deficiency of ACTH or by a primary deficiency in the gland itself.
8. Hypocortisolism, or low levels of cortisol, is caused by inadequate adrenal stimulation by ACTH or by primary cortisol hyposecretion. Primary adrenal insufficiency is termed Addison disease.
9. Addison disease is characterized by elevated ACTH levels with inadequate corticosteroid synthesis and output.
10. Manifestations of Addison disease are related to hypocortisolism and hypoaldosteronism. Symptoms include weakness, fatigability, hypoglycemia and related metabolic problems, lowered response to stressors, vitiligo, and manifestations of hypovolemia and hyperkalemia.
11. Hyperfunction of the adrenal medulla is usually caused by a pheochromocytoma, a catecholamine-producing tumor. Symptoms of catecholamine excess are related to their sympathetic nervous system effects and include hypertension, palpitations, tachycardia, glucose intolerance, excessive sweating, and constipation.

Key Terms

References

1. Terpstra TL, Terpstra TL: Syndrome of inappropriate antidiuretic hormone secretion: recognition and management, *Medsurg Nurs* 9(2):69–70, 2000.
2. Diringer MN, Zazulia AR: Hyponatremia in neurologic patients: consequences and approaches to treatment, *Neurologist* 12(3):117–126, 2006.
3. Chan TY: Drug-induced syndrome of inappropriate antidiuretic hormone secretion: causes, diagnosis, and management, *Drugs Aging* 11(1):27–44, 1997.
4. Miller M: Syndromes of excess antidiuretic hormone release, *Crit Care Clin* 17(1):11–23, 2001.
5. Morello JP, Bichet DG: Nephrogenic diabetes insipidus, *Annu Rev Physiol* 63:607–630, 2001.
6. Knoers NV, Deen PM: Molecular and cellular defects in nephrogenic diabetes insipidus, *Pediatr Nephrol* 16(12):1146–1152, 2001.
7. Geffner ME: Hypopituitarism in childhood, *Cancer Control* 9:212–222, 2002.
8. Kelestimur F: Sheehan's syndrome, *Pituitary* 6:181–189, 2003.
9. Ben-Shlomo A, Melmed S: Acromegaly, *Endocrinol Metab Clin North Am* 30(3):565–583, 2001.
10. Melmed S: Acromegaly. In Melmed S, editors: *The pituitary*, ed 2, Cambridge, Mass, 2002, Blackwell Scientific.
11. Ezzat S: Acromegaly, *Endocrinol Metab Clin North Am* 26 (4):703–723, 1997.
12. Bogazzi F et al: Peroxisome proliferator activated receptor gamma expression is reduced in the colonic mucosa of acromegalic patients, *J Clin Endocrinol Metab* 87(5):2403–2406, 2002.
13. Melmed S: Medical progress: Acromegaly, *N Engl J Med*, 355 (24):2558–2573, 2006.
14. Xu RK et al: Pituitary prolactin-secreting tumor formation: recent developments, *Biol Signals Recept* 9(1):1–20, 2000.
15. De Rosa M et al: Hyperprolactinemia in men: clinical and biochemical feature and response to treatment, *Endocrine* 20(1–2):75–82, 2003.
16. Luciano AA: Clinical presentation of hyperprolactinemia, *J Reprod Med* 44(12 suppl):1085–1090, 1999.
17. Gillam MP, Molitch ME, Lombardi G, Colao A: Advances in the treatment of prolactinomas, *Endocrinol Rev,* 27(5):485–534, 2006.
18. Meurisse M et al: Iatrogenic thyrotoxicosis: causal circumstances, pathophysiology, and principles of treatment: review of the literature, *World J Surg* 24(11):1377–1385, 2000.
19. Rehman SU et al: Thyroid disorders in elderly patients, *South Med J* 98:543–549, 2005.
20. Smith JR, Oates E: Radionuclide imaging of the thyroid gland: patterns, pearls, and pitfalls, *Clin Nucl Med* 29:181–193, 2004.
21. Ginsberg J: Diagnosis and management of Graves' disease, *CMAJ* 168(5):575–585, 2003.
22. Nayak B, Burman K: Thyrotoxicosis and thyroid storm, *Endocrinol Metab Clin North Am* 35(4):663–686, 2006.
23. Wartofsky L, Van Nostrand D, Burman KD: Overt and 'subclinical' hypothyroidism in women, *Obstet Gynecol Surv* 61(8):535–542, 2006.
24. Meier C et al: Serum thyroid stimulating hormone in assessment of severity of tissue hypothyroidism in patients with overt primary thyroid failure: cross sectional survey, *Br Med J* 326:311–312, 2003.
25. Wartofsky L: Myxedema coma. *Endocrinol Metab Clin North Am* 35(4):687–698, 2006.
26. Kempers MJ et al: Neonatal screening for congenital hypothyroidism based on thyroxine, thyrotropin, and thyroxine-binding globulin measurement: potentials and pitfalls, *J Clin Endocrinol Metab* 91(9):3370–3376, 2006.
27. Ronckers CM et al: Thyroid cancer in childhood cancer survivors: a detailed evaluation of radiation dose response and its modifiers, *Radiat Res* 166:618–628, 2006.
28. American Cancer Society: *Cancer facts and figures—2007*, Atlanta, 2007, Author. Available at: www.cancer.org/downloads/STT/CAFF2007PWSecured.pdf.
29. Saad AG, Kumar S, Ron E, Lubin JH, Stanek J, Bove KE, Nikiforov YE: Proliferative activity of human thyroid cells in various age groups and its correlation with the risk of thyroid cancer after radiation exposure, *J Clin Endocrinol Metab* 91(7):2672–2677, 2006.

References—Cont'd

30. Sherman SI: Thyroid carcinoma, *Lancet* 361(9356):501–511, 2003.
31. Conroy S, Moulias S, Wassif WS: Primary hyperparathyroidism in the older person, *Age Ageing* 32:571–578, 2003.
32. Carling T: Molecular pathology of parathyroid tumors, *Trends Endocrinol Metab* 12(2):53–58, 2001.
33. Levine MA: Primary hyperparathyroidism: 7,000 years of progress, *Clev Clin J Med* 72(12):1084–1085, 1088, 1091–1092 passim, 2005.
34. Painter SE, Kleerekoper M, Camacho PM: Secondary osteoporosis: a review of the recent evidence, *Endocr Pract* 12:436–445, 2006.
35. Silverberg SJ, Bilezikian JP: The diagnosis and management of asymptomatic primary hyperparathyroidism, *Nat Clinl Prac Endocrinol Metab* 2(9):494–503, 2006.
36. Winer KK et al: A randomized, cross-over trial of once-daily versus twice-daily parathyroid hormone 1–34 in treatment of hypoparathyroidism, *J Endocrinol Metab* 83(10):3480–3496, 1998.
37. American Diabetes Association: Diagnosis and classification of diabetes mellitus, *Diabetes Care* 30(suppl 1):S42–S47, 2007.
38. Daneman D: Type 1 diabetes, *Lancet* 367:847–858, 2006.
39. Sanjeevi CB: Genes influencing innate and acquired immunity in type 1 diabetes and latent autoimmune diabetes in adults, *Annals New York Acad Sci* 1079:67–80, 2006.
40. Vinik AI, Vinik E: Prevention of the complications of diabetes, *Am J Manag Care* 9(3 suppl):S63–S80, 2003.
41. Nanji SA, Shapiro AM: Advances in pancreatic islet transplantation in humans, *Diabetes Obes Metab* 8(1):15–25, 2006.
42. Ryan EA, Bigam D, Shapiro AM: Current indications for pancreas or islet transplant, *Diabetes Obes Metab* 8(1):1–7, 2006.
43. Arslanian S: Type 2 diabetes in children: clinical aspects and risk factors, *Hormone Res* 57(suppl 1):19–28, 2002.
44. McCarthy MI, Zeggini E: Genetics of type 2 diabetes, *Curr Diab Rep* 6(2):147–154, 2006.
45. Giuffrida FMA, Reis AF: Genetic and clinical characteristics of maturity-onset diabetes of the young, *Diabetes Obes Metab* 7:318–326, 2005.
46. Donath MY, Halban PA: Decreased beta-cell mass in diabetes: significance, mechanisms and therapeutic implications, *Diabetologica* 47(3):581–589, 2004.
47. Dandona P et al: Metabolic syndrome: a comprehensive perspective based on interactions between obesity, diabetes, and inflammation, *Circulation* 111(11):1448–1454, 2005.
48. Haslam DW, James WP: Obesity, *Lancet* 366:1197–1209, 2005.
49. Hutley L, Prins JB: Fat as an endocrine organ: relationship to the metabolic syndrome, *Am J Med Sci* 330(6):280–289, 2005.
50. Weyer C et al: Amylin replacement with pramlintide as an adjunct to insulin therapy in type 1 and type 2 diabetes mellitus: a physiological approach toward improved metabolic control, *Curr Pharmaceutical Design* 7(14):1353–1373, 2001.
51. Brennan CS: Dietary fiber, glycemic response, and diabetes, *Mol Nutr Food Res* 49:560–570, 2005.
52. Crowther CA et al: Effect of treatment of gestational diabetes mellitus on pregnancy outcomes, *N Engl J Med* 352: 2477–2486, 2005.
53. Eledrisi MS, Alshanti MS, Shah MF, Brolosy B, Jaha N: Overview of the diagnosis and management of diabetic ketoacidosis, *Am J Med Sci* 331(5):243–251, 2006.
54. Skinner TC: Recurrent diabetic ketoacidosis: causes, prevention and management, *Hormone Res* 57(suppl 1):78–80, 2002.
55. Kitabchi AE, Nyenwe EA: Hyperglycemic crises in diabetes mellitus: diabetic ketoacidosis and hyperglycemic hyperosmolar state, *Endocrinol Metab Clin North Am* 35(4):725–751, 2006.
56. Monnier L et al: Activation of oxidative stress by acute glucose fluctuations compared with sustained chronic hyperglycemia in patients with type 2 diabetes, *JAMA* 295:1681–1687, 2006.
57. Vlassara H, Palace MR: Diabetes and advanced glycation end-products, *J Intern Med* 251(2):87–101, 2002.
58. Avignon A, Sultan A: PKC-B inhibition: a new therapeutic approach for diabetic complications? *Diabetes Metab* 32(3): 205–213, 2006.
59. McCall AL: Altered glycemia and brain-update and potential relevance to the aging brain, *Neurobiol Aging* 26(suppl 1): 70–75, 2005.
60. Raptis AE, Viberti G: Pathogenesis of diabetic nephropathy, *Exp Clin Endocrinol Diabetes* 109(suppl 2):S424–S437, 2001.
61. Schnell O: The links between diabetes and cardiovascular disease, *J Intervent Cardiol* 18(6):413–416, 2005.
62. Chiarelli F, Mohn A: Angiopathy in children with diabetes, *Minerva Pediatr* 54(3):187–201, 2002.
63. Soldatos G, Cooper ME: Advanced glycation end products and vascular structure and function, *Curr Hypertens Rep* 8(6):472–478, 2006.
64. Beckman JA, Creager MA, Lippy P: Diabetes and atherosclerosis: epidemiology, pathophysiology and management, *J Am Med Assoc* 287(19):2570–2581, 2002.
65. Vinik A, Flemmer M: Diabetes and macrovascular disease, *J Diabetes Complications* 16(3):235–245, 2002.
66. Buse JB et al: Primary prevention of cardiovascular diseases in people with diabetes mellitus: A scientific statement from the American Heart Association and the American Diabetes Association, *Diabetes Care* 30:162–172, 2007.
67. Baliga SS, Weinberger J: Diabetes and stroke: part one—risk factors and pathophysiology, *Curr Cardiol Rep* 8:23–28, 2006.
68. Fujii S: Advances in the understanding of diabetic vascular disease, *J Cardiovasc Risk* 4(2):67–69, 1997.
69. Diamantopoulos EJ et al: Management and outcome of severe diabetic foot infections, *Exp Clin Endocrinol Diabetes* 106 (4):346–352, 1998.
70. Bowering CK: Diabetic foot ulcers: pathophysiology, assessment, and therapy, *Can Fam Physician* 47:1007–1016, 2001.
71. Hopkins RL, Leinung MC: Exogenous Cushing's syndrome and glucocorticoid withdrawal. *Endocrinol Metab Clin N Am* 34(2):371–384, ix, 2005.
72. Findling JW, Raff H: Cushing's syndrome: important issues in diagnosis and management, *J Clin Endocrinol Metab* 91 (10):3746–53, 2006.
73. Findling JW, Raff H: Diagnosis and differential diagnosis of Cushing's syndrome. *Endocrinol Metab Clin North Am* 30 (3):729–747, 2001.
74. Nishizaka MD, Calhoun DA: Primary aldosteronism: diagnostic and therapeutic considerations, *Curr Cardiol Rep* 7: 412–417, 2005.
75. Moneva MH, Gomez-Sanchez CE: Pathophysiology of adrenal hypertension, *Semin Nephrol* 22(1):44–53, 2002.
76. Bravo EL: Medical management of primary hyperaldosteronism, *Curr Hypertens Rep* 3(5):406–409, 2001.
77. Betterle C et al: Autoimmunity in isolated Addison's disease and in polyglandular autoimmune disease type 1, 2, and 4, *Ann Endocrinol (Paris)* 62:193–201, 2001.
78. Soderbergh A, Kampe O: Adrenal autoantibodies and organ-specific autoimmunity in patients with Addison's disease, *Clin Endocr (Oxf)* 45(4):453–460, 1996.
79. Daub KF: Pheochromocytoma: challenges in diagnosis and nursing care, *Nurs Clin North Am* 42(1):101–111, 2007.
80. Widimsky J Jr: Recent advances in the diagnosis and treatment of pheochromocytoma, *Kidney Blood Press Res* 29(5): 321–326, 2006.

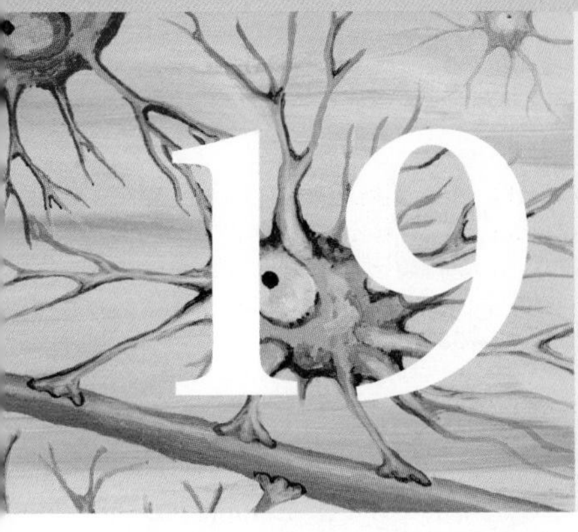

19 STRUCTURE AND FUNCTION OF THE HEMATOLOGIC SYSTEM

Neal S. Rote ▪ Kathryn L. McCance

CHAPTER OUTLINE

ELECTRONIC RESOURCES

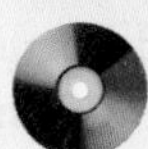

Companion CD
- Review Questions and Answers
- Animations

evolve Website
http://evolve.elsevier.com/Huether/
- Quick Check Answers
- Key Terms Exercises
- Critical Thinking Questions with Answers
- Algorithm Completion Exercises
- WebLinks

All the body's tissues and organs require oxygen and nutrients to survive. These essential needs are provided by the blood that flows through miles of vessels throughout the human body. The red blood cells provide the oxygen, and the fluid portion of the blood carries the nutrients. The blood also cleans discarded waste from the tissues and transports cells (white blood cells) and other ingredients that are necessary for protecting the entire body from injury and infection.

Thom J. Mansen, RN, PhD, contributed to this chapter in the previous edition.

COMPONENTS OF THE HEMATOLOGIC SYSTEM

Composition of Blood

Blood consists of various cells that circulate in the cardiovascular system suspended in a solution of protein and inorganic materials (plasma), which is approximately 90% water and 10% dissolved substances (solutes). The blood volume amounts to about 6 quarts (5.5 L) in adults. The continuous movement of blood guarantees that critical components are available to all parts of the body to carry out their chief functions: (1) delivery of substances needed for cellular metabolism in the tissues, (2) removal of the wastes of cellular metabolism, (3) defense against invading microorganisms and injury, and (4) maintenance of acid-base balance.

Plasma and plasma proteins

In adults, plasma accounts for 50% to 55% of blood volume (Figure 19-1). **Plasma** is a complex aqueous liquid containing a variety of organic and inorganic elements (Table 19-1). The concentration of these elements varies depending on diet, metabolic demand, hormones, and vitamins. Plasma differs from serum in that **serum** is plasma that has been allowed to clot in the laboratory in order to remove fibrinogen and other clotting factors that may interfere with some diagnostic tests.

The plasma contains a large number of proteins (**plasma proteins**). These vary in structure and function and can be classified into two major groups, albumin and globulins. Most plasma proteins are produced by the liver. The major exception is antibody, which is produced by plasma cells in the lymph nodes and other lymphoid tissues (see Chapter 6).

Albumin (about 60% of total plasma protein) serves as a carrier molecule for both normal components of blood and drugs. Its most essential role is regulation of the passage of water and solutes through the capillaries. Albumin molecules are large and do not diffuse freely through the vascular endothelium, and thus they maintain the critical colloidal osmotic pressure (or oncotic pressure) that regulates the passage of water and solutes into the surrounding tissues (see Chapters 1 and 3). Water and solute particles tend to diffuse out of the arterial portions of the capillaries because blood pressure is greater in arterial than in venous blood vessels. Water and solutes move from tissue cells into

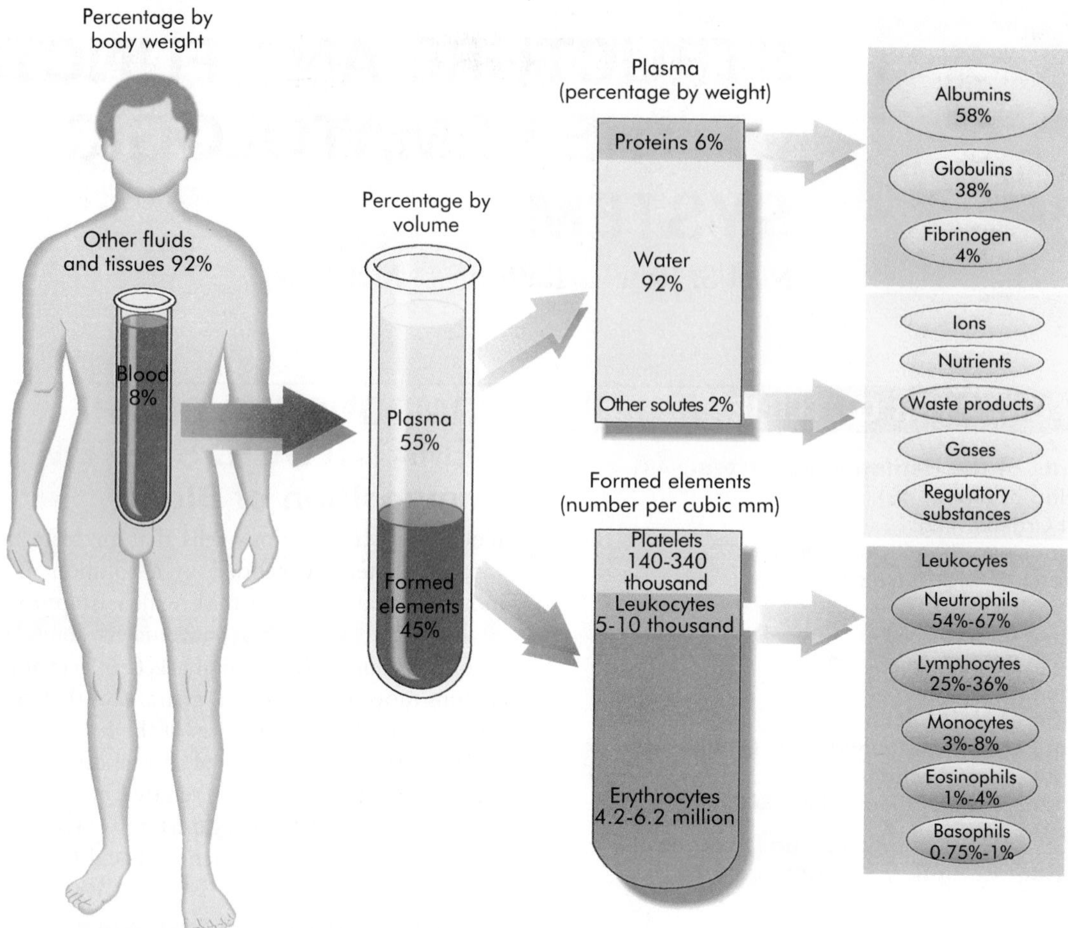

Figure 19-1 ■ **Composition of Whole Blood.** Approximate values for the components of blood in a normal adult. (From Thibodeau GA, Patton KT: *Anatomy & physiology,* ed 6, St Louis, 2007, Mosby.)

the venous portions of the capillaries where the pressures are reversed, oncotic pressure being greater than intravascular pressure or hydrostatic pressure. In the case of decreased production (e.g., cirrhosis, other diffuse liver diseases, protein malnutrition) or excessive loss of albumin (e.g., certain kidney diseases), the reduced oncotic pressure leads to excessive movement of fluid and solutes into the tissue and decreased blood volume.

The remaining plasma proteins, or **globulins,** are often classified by their properties in an electric field (serum electrophoresis). Under the normal conditions used to perform serum electrophoresis, albumin is the most rapidly moving protein. The globulins are classified by their movement relative to albumin: alpha globulins (those moving most closely to albumin), beta globulins, and gamma globulins (those with the least movement). The alpha- and beta-globulins may be subdivided into subregions (alpha-1, alpha-2, beta-1, or beta-2 globulins). Fibrinogen is a major plasma protein (about 4% of total plasma protein) that would move between the beta and gamma regions but is removed during the formation of serum. The gamma globulin region consists primarily of antibodies (see Chapter 6).

Plasma proteins can also be classified by function: clotting, defense, transport, or regulation. The **clotting factors** promote coagulation and stop bleeding from damaged blood vessels. Fibrinogen is the most plentiful of the clotting factors and is the precursor of the fibrin clot (see Figure 19-7). Proteins involved in defense, or protection, against infection include antibodies and complement proteins (see Chapters 5 and 6). Transport proteins specifically bind and carry a variety of inorganic and organic molecules, including iron (transferrin), copper (ceruloplasmin), lipids and steroid hormones (**lipoproteins**) (see Chapters 1 and 22), and vitamins (e.g., retinol-binding protein). Regulatory proteins include a variety of enzymatic inhibitors (e.g., alpha-1 antitrypsin) that protect the tissues from damage, precursor molecules (e.g., kininogen) that are converted into active biologic molecules when needed, and protein hormones (e.g., cytokines) that communicate between cells.

Plasma also contains several inorganic ions that regulate cell function, osmotic pressure, and blood pH. These include electrolytes, sodium, potassium, calcium, chloride, and phosphate. (Electrolytes are described in Chapters 1 and 3.)

Cellular components of the blood

The cellular elements of the blood are broadly classified as red blood cells (i.e., erythrocytes), white blood cells (i.e.,

TABLE 19-1

Organic and Inorganic Components of Arterial Plasma

Constituent	Amount/Concentration	Major Functions
Water	92% of plasma weight	Medium for carrying all other constituents
Electrolytes	Total >1% of plasma	Maintain H_2O in extracellular compartment; act as buffers; function in membrane excitability
Na^+	142 mEq/L (142 mM)	
K^+	4 mEq/L (4 mM)	
Ca^{++}	5 mEq/L (2.5 mM)	
Mg^{++}	3 mEq/L (1.5 mM)	
Cl^-	103 mEq/L (103 mM)	
HCO_3^-	27 mEq/L (27 mM)	
Phosphate (mostly HPO_4^{--})	2 mEq/L (1 mM)	
S_4^{--}	1 mEq/L (0.5 mM)	
Proteins	7.3 g/gl (2.5 mM)	Provide colloid osmotic pressure of plasma; act as buffers; see text for other functions
Albumins	4.5 g/dl	
Globulins	2.5 g/dl	
Fibrinogen	0.3 g/dl	
Transferrin	250 mg/dl	
Ferritin	15–300 mg/L	
GASES		
CO_2 content	22–20 mmol/L plasma	By-product of oxygenation, most CO_2 content is from HCO_3^- and acts as a buffer
O_2	PaO_2 80 torr or greater (arterial); Pvo_2 30–40 torr (venous)	Oxygenation
N_2	0.9 ml/dl	By-product of protein catabolism
NUTRIENTS		Provide nutrition and substances for tissue repair
Glucose and other carbohydrates	100 mg/dl (5.6 mM)	
Total amino acids	40 mg/dl (2 mM)	
Total lipids	500 mg/dl (7.5 mM)	
Cholesterol	150–250 mg/dl (4–7 mM)	
Individual vitamins	0.0001–2.5 mg/dl	
Individual trace elements	0.001–0.3 mg/dl	
Iron	50–150 mg/dl	
WASTE PRODUCTS		
Urea (BUN)	7–18 mg/dl (5.7 mM)	End product of protein catabolism
Creatinine (from creatine)	1 mg/dl (0.09 mM)	End product from energy metabolism
Uric acid (from nucleic acids)	5 mg/dl (0.3 mM)	End product from protein metabolism
Bilirubin (from heme)	0.2–1.2 mg/dl (0.003–0.018 mM)	End product of red blood cell destruction
Individual hormones	0.000001–0.5 mg/dl	Functions specific to target tissue

Data from Vander AJ, Sherman JH, Luchiano DS: *Human physiology: the mechanisms of body function*, New York, 2001, McGraw-Hill.

leukocytes), and platelets. The components of the blood are listed in Table 19-2.

Erythrocytes

Erythrocytes (red blood cells) are the most abundant cells of the blood, occupying approximately 48% of the blood volume in men and about 42% in women. Erythrocytes are primarily responsible for tissue oxygenation. The erythrocyte containing hemoglobin (Hb) carries the gases, and electrolytes regulate diffusion through the cell's plasma membrane. The mature erythrocyte lacks a nucleus and cytoplasmic organelles (e.g., mitochondria), so it cannot synthesize protein or carry out oxidative reactions. Because it cannot undergo mitotic division, the erythrocyte has a limited life span (approximately 120 days), ages, and is removed from the circulation to be replaced by new erythrocytes.

The erythrocyte's size and shape are ideally suited to its function as a gas carrier. It is a small disk with two unique properties: (1) a *biconcave* shape and (2) the capacity to be *reversibly deformed.* The flattened, biconcave shape provides a surface area/volume ratio that is optimal for gas diffusion into and out of the cell. During its life span, the erythrocyte, which is 6 to 8 μm in diameter, repeatedly circulates through splenic sinusoids (see Figure 19-5) and capillaries that are only 2 μm in diameter. Reversible deformity enables the erythrocyte to assume a more compact torpedo-like shape, squeeze through the microcirculation, and return to normal.

TABLE 19-2

Cellular Components of the Blood

Cell	Structural Characteristics	Normal Amounts of Circulating Blood	Function	Life Span
Erythrocyte (red blood cell)	Nonnucleated cytoplasmic disk containing hemoglobin	4.2–6.2 million/mm^3	Gas transport to and from tissue cells and lungs	80–120 days
Reticulocyte Absolute reticulocyte count		60,000 mm^3 0.5%–2.0% of erythrocytes	Immature erythrocyte	
Leukocyte (white blood cell)	Nucleated cell	5000–10,000/mm^3	Body defense mechanisms	See below
Lymphocyte	Mononuclear immunocyte	25%–36% of leukocyte count (leukocyte differential)	Humoral and cell-mediated immunity (see Chapter 6)	Days or years depending on type
Natural killer cell	Large granular lymphocyte	5%–10% circulatory pool (some in spleen)	Defense against some tumors and viruses (see Chapters 5 and 6)	Unknown
Monocyte and macrophage	Large mononuclear phagocyte	3%–8% of leukocyte differential	Phagocytosis; mononuclear phagocyte system	Months or years
Eosinophil	Segmented polymorphonuclear granulocyte	1%–4% of leukocyte differential	Control of inflammation, phagocytosis, defense against parasites, allergic reactions	Unknown
Neutrophil	Segmented polymorphonuclear granulocyte	54%–67% of leukocyte differential	Phagocytosis, particularly during early phase of inflammation	4 days
Basophil	Segmented polymorphonuclear granulocyte	0%–0.75% of leukocyte differential	Mast cell-like functions, associated with allergic reactions and mechanical irritation	Unknown
Platelet	Irregularly shaped cytoplasmic fragment (not a cell)	140,000–340,000/mm^3	Hemostasis after vascular injury; normal coagulation and clot formation/retraction	8–11 days

Leukocytes

Leukocytes (white blood cells) defend the body against organisms that cause infection and also remove debris, including dead or injured host cells of all kinds (Figure 19-2). The leukocytes act primarily in the tissues but are transported in the circulation. The average adult has approximately 5000 to 10,000 leukocytes/mm^3 of blood.

Leukocytes are classified according to structure as either **granulocytes** or **agranulocytes** and according to function as either **phagocytes** or **immunocytes**. The granulocytes, which include neutrophils, basophils, and eosinophils, are all phagocytes. (Phagocytic action is described in Chapter 5.) Of the agranulocytes, the monocytes and macrophages are phagocytes, whereas the lymphocytes are immunocytes (cells that create immunity; see Chapter 6).

Granulocytes. The granulocytes have many membrane-bound granules in their cytoplasm. These granules contain enzymes capable of killing microorganisms and catabolizing debris ingested during phagocytosis. The granules also contain powerful biochemical mediators with inflammatory and immune functions. These mediators, along with the digestive enzymes, are released from granulocytes in response to specific stimuli. The biochemical mediators have vascular and intercellular effects. Granulocytes are capable of ameboid movement, by which they migrate through vessel walls (diapedesis) and then to sites where their action is needed.

The **neutrophil (polymorphonuclear neutrophil [PMN])** is the most numerous and best understood of the granulocytes (Figure 19-3). Neutrophils constitute about 55% of the total leukocyte count in adults.

Neutrophils are the chief phagocytes of early inflammation. Soon after bacterial invasion or tissue injury, neutrophils migrate out of the capillaries and into the inflamed

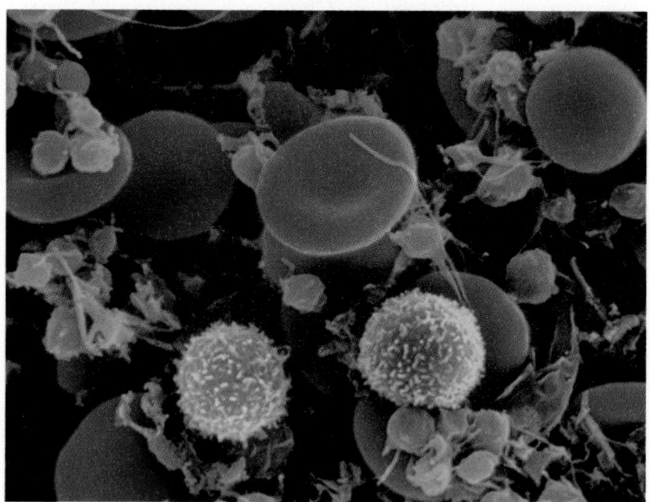

Figure 19-2 ■ **Blood Cells.** Leukocytes are spherical and have irregular surfaces with numerous extending pili. Leukocytes are the cotton candy–like cells in yellow. Erythrocytes are flattened spheres with a depressed center. (Copyright by Dennis Kunkel Microscopy, Inc.)

site, where they ingest and destroy microorganisms and debris and then die in 1 or 2 days. The dissolution of dead neutrophils releases digestive enzymes from their cytoplasmic granules. These enzymes dissolve cellular debris and prepare the site for healing.

Eosinophils, which have large, coarse granules, constitute only 1% to 4% of the normal leukocyte count in adults.[1] Like neutrophils, eosinophils are capable of ameboid movement and phagocytosis. Unlike neutrophils, eosinophils ingest antigen-antibody complexes and are induced by IgE-mediated hypersensitivity reactions to attack parasites (see Chapters 5 and 6). The eosinophil granules contain a variety of enzymes (e.g., histaminase) that help to control inflammatory processes. During type I hypersensitivity, allergic reactions and asthma are characterized by high eosinophil counts, which may be involved in control but may also contribute to the destructive inflammatory processes observed in the lungs of asthmatics.

Basophils, which make up less than 1% of the leukocytes, are structurally similar to the mast cells found throughout extravascular tissue (see Figure 19-3).[2] Like the mast cells, basophils have cytoplasmic granules that contain vasoactive amines (e.g., histamine) and an anticoagulant (heparin). Their function is similar to tissue mast cells (see Chapter 5).

Agranulocytes. The agranulocytes—monocytes, macrophages, and lymphocytes—contain relatively fewer granules than granulocytes. Monocytes and macrophages make up the mononuclear phagocyte system (or MPS, described on p. 487) Both monocytes and macrophages participate in the immune and inflammatory response, being powerful phagocytes. They also ingest dead or defective host cells, particularly blood cells.

Monocytes are immature macrophages (see Figure 19-3). Monocytes are formed and released by the bone marrow into the bloodstream. As they mature, monocytes migrate into a variety of tissues (e.g., liver, spleen, lymph nodes, peritoneum, gastrointestinal tract) and fully mature into tissue **macrophages.** Other monocytes may mature into macrophages and migrate out of the vessels in response to infection or inflammation.

Lymphocytes constitute approximately 36% of the total leukocyte count and are the primary cells of the immune response (see Figure 19-3) (see Chapter 6). Most lymphocytes transiently circulate in the blood and eventually reside in lymphoid tissues as mature T cells, B cells, or plasma

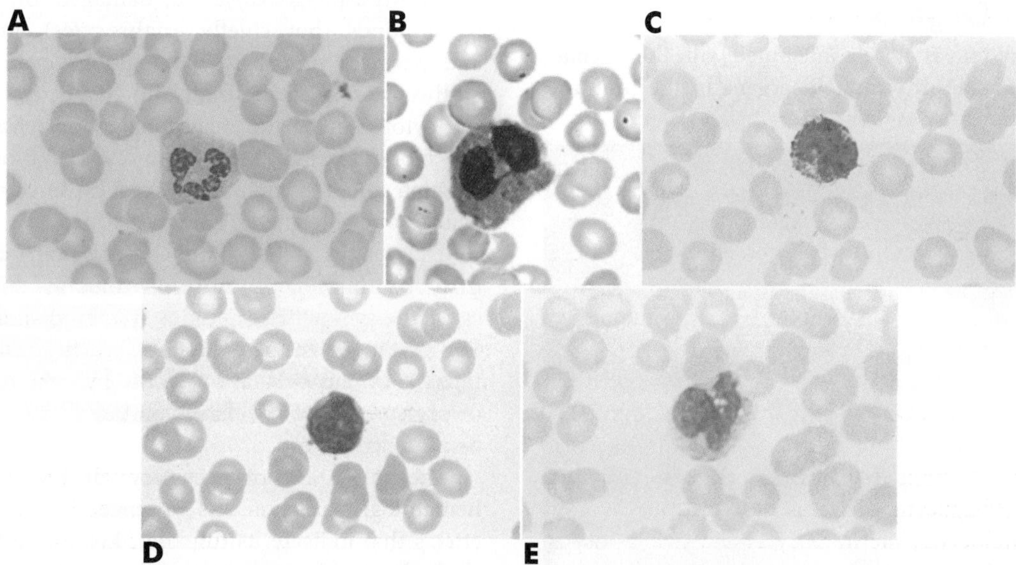

Figure 19-3 ■ **Leukocytes.** An example of leukocytes in human blood smear. **A,** Neutrophil. **B,** Eosinophil. **C,** Basophil with obscured nucleus. **D,** Lymphocyte. **E,** Typical monocyte showing vacuolated cytoplasm and cerebriform nucleus. (**A, C, D,** and **E** from Rodak, BF: *Hematology: clinical principles and applications,* ed 2, Philadelphia, 2002, Saunders; **B** from Carr JC, Rodak BF: *Clinical hematology atlas,* Philadelphia, 1999, Saunders.)

cells. (Lymphocyte function and dysfunction are described in detail in Unit 2.)

Natural killer (NK) cells, which resemble lymphocytes, kill some types of tumor cells (in vitro) and some virus-infected cells without prior exposure (see Chapter 6). They develop in the bone marrow and circulate in the blood.

Platelets

Platelets (thrombocytes) are not true cells but disk-shaped cytoplasmic fragments that are essential for blood coagulation and control of bleeding. They lack a nucleus, have no deoxyribonucleic acid (DNA), and are incapable of mitotic division. They do, however, contain cytoplasmic granules capable of releasing biochemical mediators when stimulated by injury to a blood vessel (Figure 19-4) (see Chapter 5).

There are approximately 140,000 to 340,000 platelets/mm^3 of circulating blood. An additional one third of the body's available platelets are in a reserve pool in the spleen. A platelet circulates for approximately 10 days, ages, and is removed by macrophages of the MPS, mostly in the spleen. **Thrombopoietin (TPO),** a hormone growth factor, is the main regulator of the circulating platelet mass. TPO is primarily produced by the liver and induces platelet production in the bone marrow. Platelets express receptors for TPO, and when circulating platelet levels are normal, TPO is adsorbed onto the platelet surface and prevented from accessing the bone marrow and initiation further platelet production. (Platelets are discussed below)

QUICK CHECK 19-1

1. Why are plasma proteins important to blood volume?
2. Which leukocytes are granulocytes?
3. Compare and contrast granulocytes, agranulocytes, phagocytes, and immunocytes.

Lymphoid Organs

The lymphoid system is closely integrated with the circulatory system. The role of lymphoid organs in the immune response was discussed in Chapter 6. Lymphoid organs are sites of residence, proliferation, differentiation, or a function of lymphocytes and mononuclear phagocytes (monocytes, macrophages). (The liver, which also has hematologic functions, is primarily a digestive organ and is described in Chapter 33.)

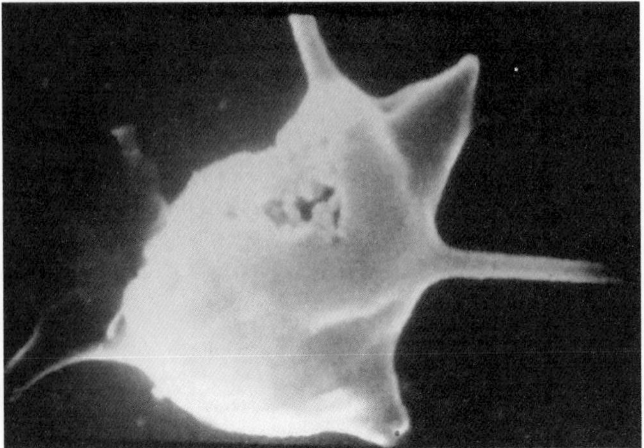

Figure 19-4 ■ Scanning Electron Micrograph of Moderately Active Platelet. (From Bick RL: *Hematology: clinical and laboratory practice,* St Louis, 1993, Mosby.)

Spleen

The **spleen** is one of the largest of the lymphoid organs. It is a site of fetal hematopoiesis, its mononuclear phagocytes filter and cleanse the blood, its lymphocytes mount an immune response to blood-borne microorganisms, and it serves as a blood reservoir.

The spleen is a concave, encapsulated organ that weighs about 150 g and is about the size of a fist (see Figure 6-2). It is located in the left upper abdominal cavity, curved around a portion of the stomach. Strands of connective tissue (trabeculae) extend throughout the spleen from the splenic capsule, dividing it into compartments that contain masses of lymphoid tissue called *splenic pulp.* The spleen is interlaced with many blood vessels, some of which can distend to store blood.

Blood that circulates through the spleen first encounters the white splenic pulp, which consists of masses of lymphoid tissue containing lymphocytes and macrophages. The white pulp forms clumps around the splenic arterioles and is the chief site of immune and phagocytic function within the spleen. Here blood-borne antigens encounter lymphocytes, initiating the immune response (see Chapter 6).

Some of the blood continues through the microcirculation and enters highly distensible storage areas called *venous sinuses.* Most of the blood, however, oozes through the capillary walls into the principal site of splenic filtration, the red pulp (Figure 19-5). Here the resident macrophages of the MPS phagocytose old, damaged, or old blood cells of all kinds (but chiefly erythrocytes), microorganisms, and particles of debris. Hemoglobin from phagocytosed erythrocytes is catabolized, and heme (iron) is stored in the cytoplasm of the macrophages or released back into the blood plasma (see Figure 19-13). Blood that filters through the red pulp then moves through the venous sinuses and into the portal circulation.

The venous sinuses (and the red pulp) can store more than 300 ml of blood. Sudden reductions in blood pressure cause the sympathetic nervous system to stimulate constriction of the sinuses and expel as much as 200 ml of blood into the venous circulation, helping to restore blood volume or pressure in the circulation and increasing the hematocrit by as much as 4%.

The spleen is not necessary for life or for adequate hematologic function. Its absence, however, has several effects that indicate its function. For example, leukocytosis (high levels of circulating leukocytes) often occurs after splenectomy, so the spleen must exert some control over the rate of proliferation of leukocyte cells. After splenectomy iron levels in the circulation are decreased, immune function

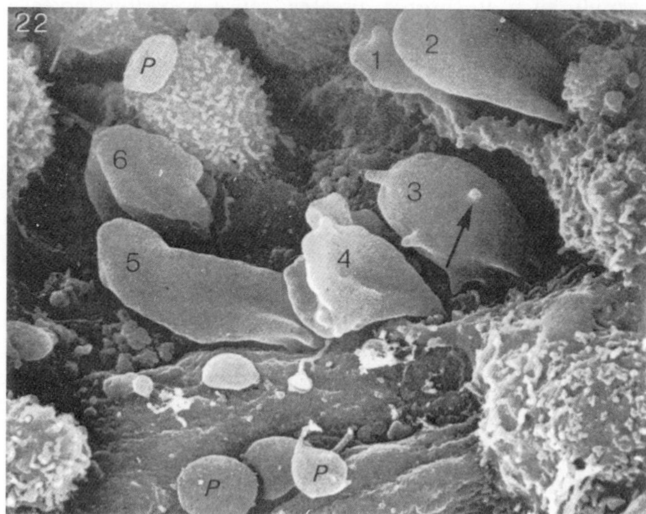

Figure 19-5 ■ **Red Cells in the Spleen.** Scanning electron micrograph of spleen, demonstrating erythrocytes (numbered 1–6) squeezing through the fenestrated wall in transit from the splenic cord to the sinus. The view shows the endothelial lining of the sinus wall, to which platelets *(P)* adhere, along with "hairy" white cells, probably macrophages. The arrow shows a protrusion on a red blood cell (×5000). (From Weiss L: A scanning electron microscope study of the spleen, *Blood* 1974;43;665; reprinted with permission.)

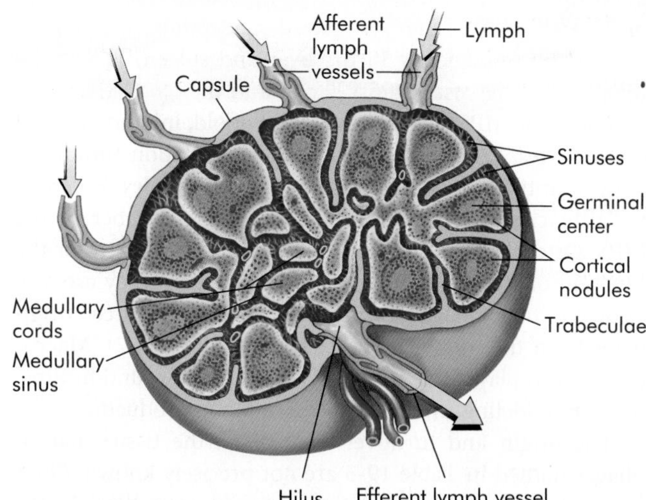

Figure 19-6 ■ **Cross Section of Lymph Node.** Several afferent valved lymphatics bring lymph to node. A single efferent lymphatic leaves the node at the hilus. *Note that the artery and vein also enter and leave at the hilus. Arrows show direction of lymph flow.* (From Thibodeau GA, Patton KT: *Anatomy & physiology,* ed 6, St Louis, 2007, Mosby.)

is diminished, and the blood contains more structurally defective blood cells than normal.

Lymph nodes

Structurally, **lymph nodes** are part of the lymphatic system. Thousands are clustered around the lymphatic veins, which collect interstitial fluid from the tissues and transport it, as lymph, back into the circulatory system near the heart. Functionally, however, lymph nodes are part of the hematologic and immune systems because large numbers of lymphocytes, monocytes, and macrophages develop or function within the lymph nodes. As the lymph filters through the bean-shaped lymph nodes clustered in the inguinal, axillary, and cervical regions of the body, it is cleansed of foreign particles and microorganisms by the monocytes and macrophages. The microorganisms in lymph stimulate the resident lymphocytes to develop into antibody-producing plasma cells. During an infection, the rate of proliferation of macrophages within the nodes is so great that the nodes enlarge and become tender.

Each lymph node is enclosed in a fibrous capsule (Figure 19-6), with strands of connective tissue (trabeculae) extending inward, dividing the node into several compartments. Reticular fibers divide the compartments into smaller sections and trap and store large numbers of lymphocytes, monocytes, and macrophages. The node has an outer cortex area and an inner medullary area. Within the cortex are germinal centers, or separate masses of lymphoid tissue (see Figure 6-14). Lymph enters the node, slowly filters through its sinuses, and leaves through efferent lymphatic vessels.

The Mononuclear Phagocyte System

The **mononuclear phagocyte system (MPS)** consists of a line of cells that originate in the bone marrow, are transported by the bloodstream, and after differentiation to blood monocytes, finally settle in the tissues as mature macrophages.[3] Table 19-3 lists the various names given to macrophages localized in specific tissues.

The cells of the MPS ingest and destroy (by phagocytosis) unwanted materials, such as foreign protein particles,

TABLE 19-3

Mononuclear Phagocyte System (Formerly Called the Reticuloendothelial System)

Name of Cell	Location
Monocytes macrophages	Bone marrow and peripheral blood
Kupffer cells (inflammatory macrophages)	Liver
Alveolar macrophages	Lung
Histiocytes	Connective tissue
Macrophages	Bone marrow
Fixed and free macrophages	Spleen and lymph nodes
Pleural and peritoneal macrophages	Serous cavities
Microglial cells	Nervous system
Mesangial cells	Kidney
Osteoclasts	Bone
Langerhans cells	Skin
Dendritic cells	Lymphoid tissue

microorganisms, debris from dead or injured cells, defective or injured erythrocytes, and dead neutrophils (see Figure 5-7). The MPS (mostly in the liver and spleen) is also the main line of defense against bacteria in the bloodstream. In addition, the MPS cleanses the blood of old, injured, or dead erythrocytes, leukocytes, platelets, coagulation products, antigen-antibody complexes, and macromolecules. Recently, the osteoclast cell was classified as a true member of the MPS. Osteoclasts are multinucleated cells specialized for the function of lacunar bone resorption; however, they are also known to have phagocytic abilities. The osteoclast cell originates from the monocyte cell lineage (Figure 19-7). Macrophages also play a role in blood coagulation, wound healing, tissue remodeling, and the control of blood production.

The origin and turnover time of all the tissue macrophages named in Table 19-3 are not precisely known. Once monocytes leave the circulation, they do not return. In the tissues, monocytes differentiate into macrophages without dividing and can survive for many months or perhaps even years. Under normal circumstances, macrophages show little evidence of mitotic division, but production can be rapidly elevated in response to need, as in infection.

QUICK CHECK 19-2

1. Why is the spleen considered a hematologic organ? Why can humans live without it?
2. Why are lymph nodes considered part of the hematologic system?
3. What is the MPS?

DEVELOPMENT OF BLOOD CELLS

Hematopoiesis

The typical human requires about 100 billion new blood cells per day. Blood cell production, termed **hematopoiesis,** is constantly ongoing, occurring in the liver and spleen of the fetus and only in bone marrow after birth, and is known as *medullary hematopoiesis.* This process involves the biochemical stimulation of populations of relatively undifferentiated cells to undergo mitotic division (i.e., proliferation) and maturation (i.e., differentiation) into mature hematologic cells.[4] Certain blood cells proliferate and differentiate simultaneously. Proliferation usually ceases after a number of doubling divisions, but differentiation continues. Erythrocytes and neutrophils generally differentiate fully before entering the blood, but monocytes and lymphocytes do not.

Hematopoiesis continues throughout life, increasing in response to proliferative disease, hemorrhage, hemolytic anemia (in which erythrocytes are destroyed), chronic infection, idiopathic thrombocytopenic purpura (bleeding caused by platelet insufficiency; see Chapter 20), and other disorders that deplete blood cells. In general, long-term stimuli, such as chronic diseases, cause a greater increase in hematopoiesis than acute conditions, such as hemorrhage. Abnormal proliferation of erythrocytes occurs in polycythemia vera, a myeloproliferative disease.

In adults, extramedullary hematopoiesis—blood cell production in tissues other than bone marrow—is usually a sign of disease, occurring in pernicious anemia, sickle cell anemia, thalassemia, hemolytic disease of the newborn (erythroblastosis fetalis), hereditary spherocytosis, and certain leukemias. Extramedullary hematopoiesis of apparently normal blood cells has been reported in the spleen, liver, and, less frequently, lymph nodes, adrenal glands, cartilage, adipose tissue, intrathoracic areas, and kidneys.

Bone marrow

Bone marrow is confined to the cavities of bone. It consists of blood vessels, nerves, mononuclear phagocytes, stromal cells, blood cells in various stages of differentiation, and fatty tissue. Adults have two kinds of bone marrow: red, or active (hematopoietic), marrow (also called **myeloid tissue**) and yellow, or inactive, marrow. The large quantities of fat in inactive marrow make it yellow. Not all bones contain active marrow. In adults, active marrow is found primarily in the flat bones of the pelvis (34%), vertebrae (28%), cranium and mandible (13%), sternum and ribs (10%), and in the extreme proximal portions of the humerus and femur (4% to 8%). Inactive marrow predominates in cavities of other bones. (Bones are discussed further in Chapter 36.)

Hematopoietic marrow receives oxygen and nutrients needed for cellular differentiation from the primary arteries of the bones. Branches of these arteries terminate in a capillary network that coalesces into large venous sinuses, which eventually drain into a central vein. Hematopoietic marrow and fat fill the spaces surrounding the network of venous sinuses. Newly produced blood cells traverse narrow openings in the venous sinus walls and thus enter the circulation. Normally, cells do not enter the circulation until they have differentiated to a certain extent, but premature release occurs in certain diseases.

Cellular differentiation

The hematologic system arises from the proliferation and differentiation of **hematopoietic stem cells.** All humans originate from a single cell (the fertilized egg) that has the capacity to proliferate and eventually differentiate into the huge diversity of cells of the human body. After fertilization, the egg divides over a 5-day period to form a hollow ball (blastocyst) that implants on the uterus. Until about 3 days after fertilization, each cell (blastomere) is undifferentiated and retains the capacity to differentiate into any cell type. In the 5-day blastocyst, the outer layer cells have undergone differentiation and commitment to become the placenta. Cells of the inner cell mass, however, continue to have unlimited differentiation potential (currently referred to as being *pluripotent*) and can grow into different kinds of tissue—blood, nerves, heart, bone, and so forth. After implantation, cells of the inner cell mass begin

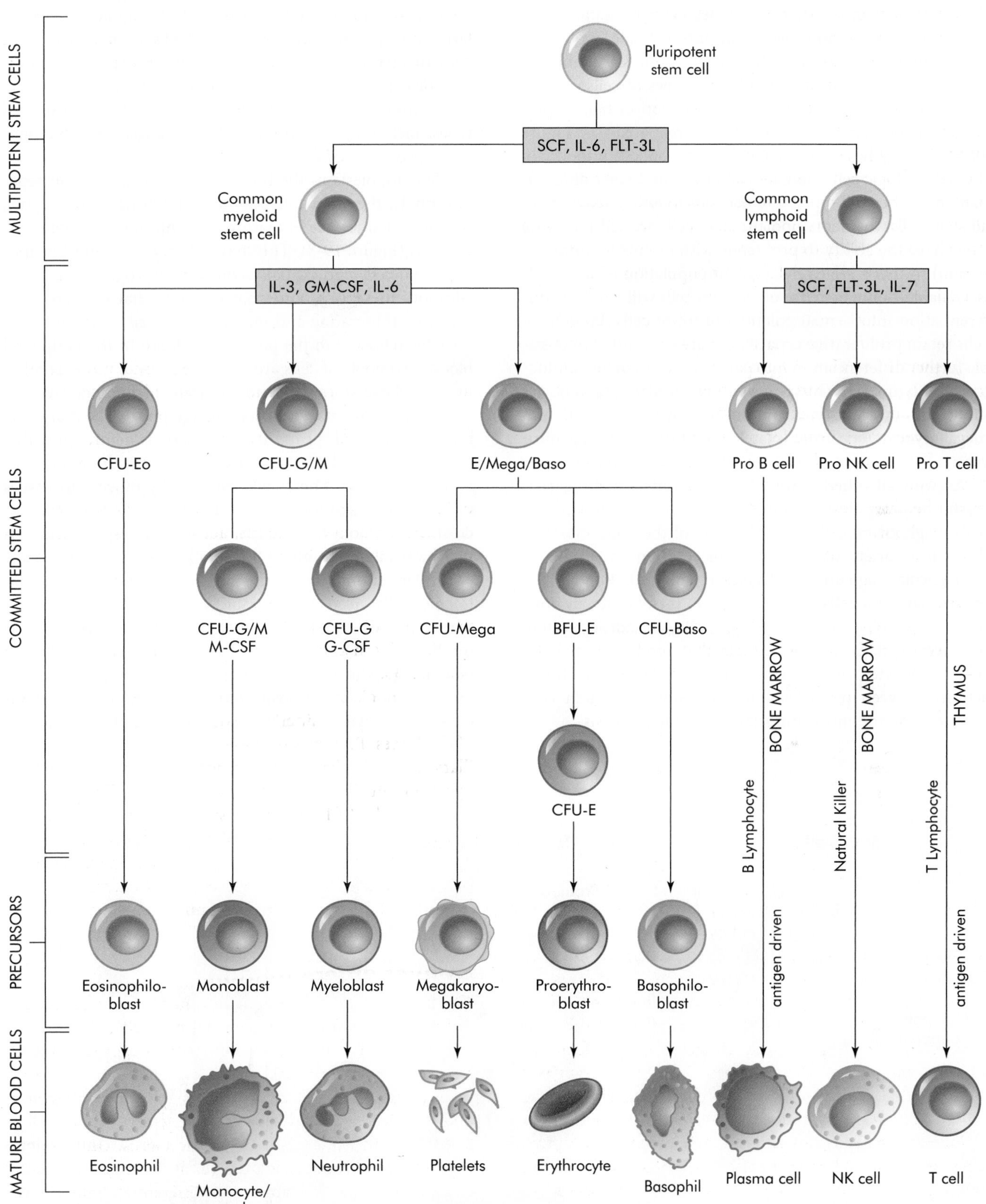

Figure 19-7 ■ **Differentiation of Hematopoietic Cells.** *SCF,* Stem cell factor; *FTL-3L,* fms-like tyrosine kinase 3 ligand; *GM-CSF,* granulocyte-macrophage colony-stimulating factor; *M-CSF,* macrophage colony-stimulating factor; *G-CSF,* granulocyte colony-stimulating factor; *CFU,* colony-forming unit; *Eo,* eosinophil; *G,* granulocyte; *M,* macrophage; *BFU,* burst-forming unit; *IL,* interleukin; *E,* erythrocyte; *Mega,* megakaryocyte; *Baso,* basophil. (Mast cells are discussed in Chapter 5.)

differentiation into other cell types. Differentiation is a multistep process and results in intermediate groups of stem cells with more limited, but still impressive, abilities to differentiation into many different types of cells.

The bone marrow contains a population of hematopoietic stem cells that have partially differentiated (see Figure 19-7).[5,6] They have the capacity to differentiate into any of the hematologic cell populations but can no longer differentiate into other cell types, like nerve or muscle cells. As with all stem cells, the hematopoietic stem cells are self-renewing (they have the ability to proliferate without further differentiation) so that a relatively constant population of stem cells is available. Some hematopoietic stem cells will continue differentiation into hematopoietic progenitor cells. Progenitor cells retain proliferative capacity but are committed to possible further differentiation into particular types of hematologic cells: lymphoid (lymphocytes, NK cells), granulocyte/monocyte (granulocytes, monocytes, macrophages), and megakaryocyte/erythroid (platelets, erythrocytes) progenitor cells.

As with all other forms of cellular differentiation, successful hematopoiesis requires that progenitor cells interact with neighboring cells (**stromal cells** of the bone marrow) through a variety of adhesion molecules and are exposed to particular signaling molecules (cytokines). Populations of **stromal stem cells** differentiate into many different bone marrow cell types, including bone cells (chondrocytes that produce cartilage and osteoblasts that produce bone), fat cells (adipocytes), muscle (myocytes), and fibroblasts. Interactions between osteoclasts and hematopoietic stem cells appear to be the most important for hematopoiesis.

Several cytokines participate in hematopoiesis, particularly **colony-stimulating factors (CSFs or hematopoietic growth factors),** which stimulate the proliferation of progenitor cells and their progeny and initiate the maturation events necessary to produce fully mature cells. Multiple cell types, including endothelial cells, fibroblasts, and lymphocytes, produce CSFs.

Hematopoiesis in the bone marrow occurs in two separate pools, the stem cell pool and the bone marrow pool, with eventual release of mature cells into the peripheral circulation (Figure 19-8). The stem cell pool contains pluripotent stem cells and partially committed progenitor cells. In addition, there is a bone marrow pool that contains cells that are proliferating and maturing and cells that are stored for later release into the peripheral blood. In the peripheral blood, two pools of cells are also categorized: those circulating and those stored around the walls of the blood vessels (often called the **marginating storage pool**). The marginating storage pool primarily consists of neutrophils that adhere to the endothelium in vessels where the blood flow is relatively slow. These cells can rapidly move into tissues and mucous membranes when needed. Cells from the circulating pool join the marginating pool to replace the cells that have migrated out of the capillaries.

Under certain conditions, the levels of circulating hematologic cells need to be rapidly replenished. Medullary hematopoiesis can be accelerated by any or all of three mechanisms: (1) conversion of yellow bone marrow, which does not produce blood cells, to red marrow, which does, by the actions of **erythropoietin** (a hormone that stimulates erythrocyte production); (2) faster differentiation of

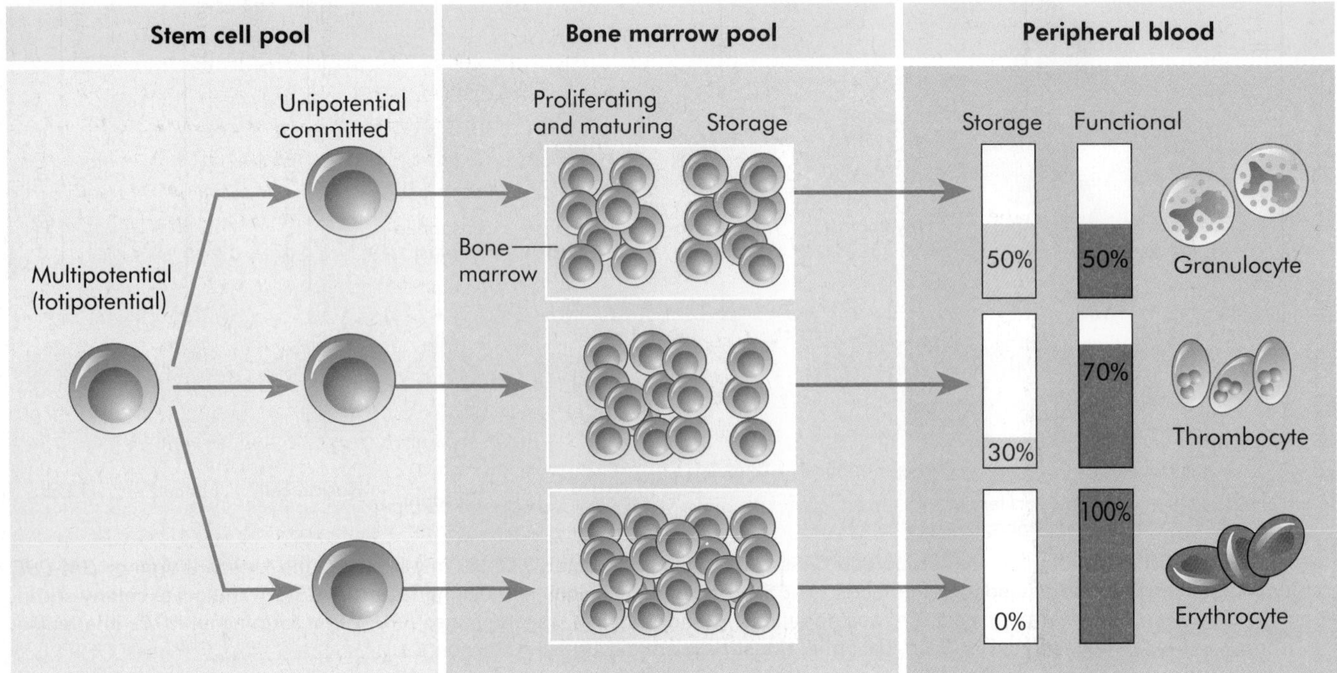

Figure 19-8 ■ **Hematopoiesis.** Hematopoiesis from the stem cell pool; activity mainly in the bone marrow and in the peripheral blood.

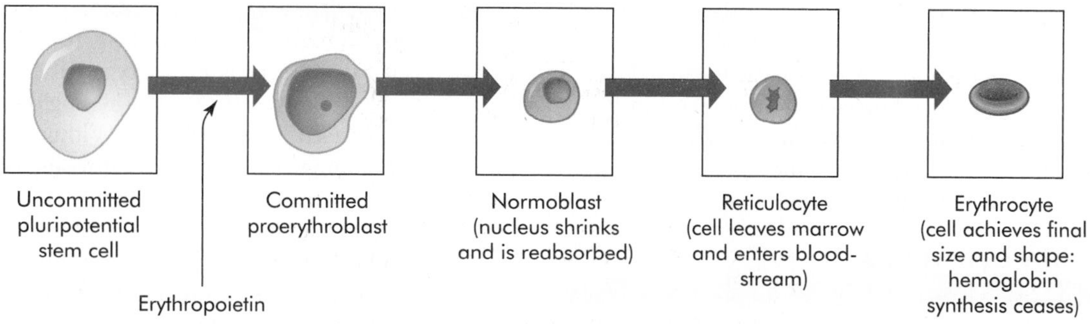

Figure 19-9 ■ **Erythrocyte Differentiation.** Erythrocyte differentiation from large, nucleated stem cell to small, nonnucleated erythrocyte.

daughter cells; and presumably (3) faster proliferation of stem cells.

QUICK CHECK 19-3

1. Why is the stem cell system important to hematopoiesis?
2. Why are some stem cells called pluripotent?
3. Why are CSFs necessary for blood cell proliferation?

Development of Erythrocytes

For almost 100 years it was believed that erythrocytes developed from lymphocytes that were transformed in the spleen. It was not until the 1950s that the bone marrow was identified as the site of **erythropoiesis,** or development of red blood cells (Figure 19-9).

Erythropoiesis

In the confines of the bone marrow erythroid progenitor cells proliferate and differentiate into large, nucleated **proerythroblasts,** which are committed into producing cells of the erythroid series. The proerythroblast differentiates through several intermediate form of **erythroblast** (sometimes called **normoblast**) while progressively eliminating most intracellular structures, including the nucleus, synthesizing hemoglobin, and becoming more compact, eventually taking on the shape and characteristics of an erythrocyte.

The last immature form is the **reticulocyte,** which contains a mesh-like (reticular) network of ribosomal RNA that is visible microscopically after staining with certain dyes. Reticulocytes remain in the marrow approximately 1 day and are released into the venous sinuses. They continue to mature in the bloodstream and may travel to the spleen for several days of additional maturation. The normal reticulocyte count is 1% of the total red blood cell count. Approximately 1% of the body's circulating erythrocyte mass normally is generated every 24 hours. Therefore, the reticulocyte count is a useful clinical index of erythropoietic activity and indicates whether new red cells are being produced.

Most steps of this process are primarily under the control of erythropoietin.[7] In healthy humans, the total volume of circulating erythrocytes remains surprisingly constant. In conditions of tissue hypoxia, erythropoietin is secreted by the kidney (Figure 19-10). It causes a compensatory increase in erythrocyte production if the oxygen content of blood decreases because of anemia, high altitude, or pulmonary

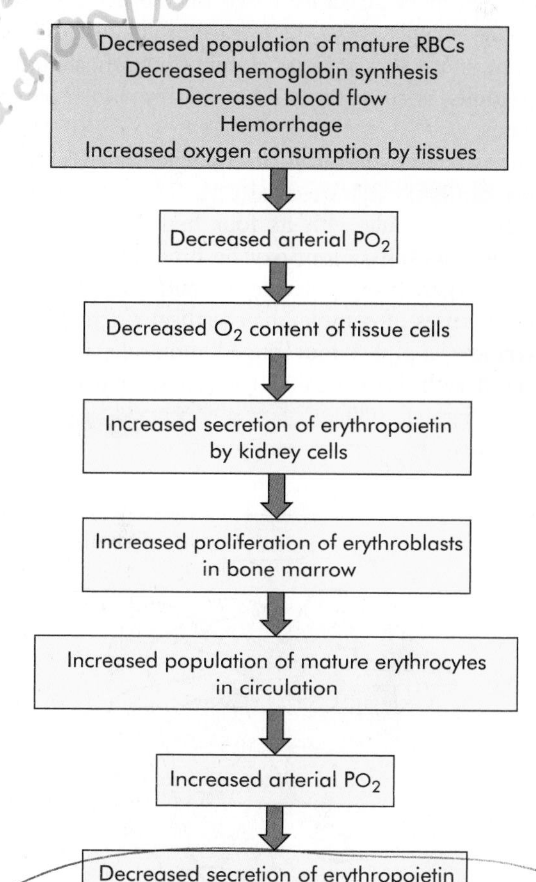

Figure 19-10 ■ **Role of Erythropoietin in Regulation of Erythropoiesis.** Decreased arterial oxygen levels stimulate production of erythropoietin, which in turn stimulates red cell production and expansion of the erythron. The increase in red cells frequently corrects the problem of low oxygen levels (hypoxia). This restoration to normal oxygen levels alerts the kidney to stop producing erythropoietin (negative feedback). Further erythrocyte production is not needed. *RBCs,* Red blood cells; PO_2, partial pressure of oxygen in the blood.

disease. The normal steady-state rate of production (2.5 million erythrocytes per second) can increase (to 17 million per second) under anemic or low-oxygen states. Thus, the body responds to reduced oxygenation of blood in two ways: (1) by increasing intake of oxygen through increased respiration and (2) by increasing the oxygen-carrying capacity of the blood through increased erythropoiesis.

Hemoglobin synthesis

Hemoglobin (Hb), the oxygen-carrying protein of the erythrocyte, constitutes approximately 90% of the cell's dry weight. Hemoglobin-packed blood cells take up oxygen in the lungs and exchange it for carbon dioxide in the tissues. A single erythrocyte can contain as many as 300 hemoglobin molecules. Hemoglobin increases the oxygen carrying capacity of blood by 100-fold. Each hemoglobin molecule is composed of two pairs of polypeptide chains (the **globins**) and four colorful complexes of iron plus protoporphyrin (the hemes) (Figure 19-11). Hemoglobin is responsible for blood's ruby-red color.

Several variants of hemoglobin exist, but they differ only slightly in primary structure based on the use of different polypeptide chains; alpha, beta, gamma, delta, epsilon, or zeta (α, β, γ, δ, ε, or ζ). Hemoglobin A, the most common type in adults, is composed of two α- and two β-polypeptide chains.

Heme is a large, flat, iron-protoporphyrin disk that can carry one molecule of oxygen (O_2). Thus, an individual hemoglobin molecule with its four hemes can carry four oxygen molecules. If all four oxygen-binding sites are occupied by oxygen, the molecule is said to be saturated. Through a series of complex biochemical reactions, **protoporphyrin,** a complex four-ringed molecule, is produced and bound with ferrous iron. It is crucial that the iron be correctly charged; reduced ferrous iron (Fe^{2+}) can bind oxygen, whereas ferric iron (Fe^{3+}) cannot. Binding of oxygen to ferrous iron temporally oxidizes Fe^{2+} to Fe^{3+} (**oxyhemoglobin**), but after the release of oxygen the body reduces the iron to Fe^{2+} and reactivates the hemoglobin (**deoxyhemoglobin** [reduced hemoglobin]). Without reactivation, the Fe^{3+}-containing hemoglobin (**methemoglobin**) cannot bind oxygen. An excess of ferric iron occurs with certain drugs and chemicals, such as nitrates and sulfonamides.

Several other molecules can competitively bind to deoxyhemoglobin. Carbon monoxide (CO) directly competes with oxygen for binding to ferrous ion with an affinity that is about 200-fold greater than oxygen. Thus, even a small amount of CO can dramatically decrease the ability of hemoglobin to bind and transport oxygen. Hemoglobin also binds carbon dioxide (CO_2), but at a binding site separate from where oxygen binds. In the lungs, CO_2 is released allowing hemoglobin to bind oxygen.

Erythrocytes may play a role in the maintenance of vascular relaxation. Nitric oxide (NO) produced by blood vessels is a major mediator of relaxation and dilation of the vessel walls. In the lungs, hemoglobin can concurrently bind oxygen to the ferrous ion and NO to cysteine residues in the globins (Figure 19-12). As hemoglobin transfers its oxygen to tissue, it may also shed small amounts of nitric oxide contributing to dilation of the blood vessels and helping get the oxygen into tissues.

Nutritional requirements for erythropoiesis

Normal development of erythrocytes and synthesis of hemoglobin depend on an optimal biochemical state and adequate supplies of the necessary building blocks, including protein, vitamins, and minerals (Table 19-4). If these

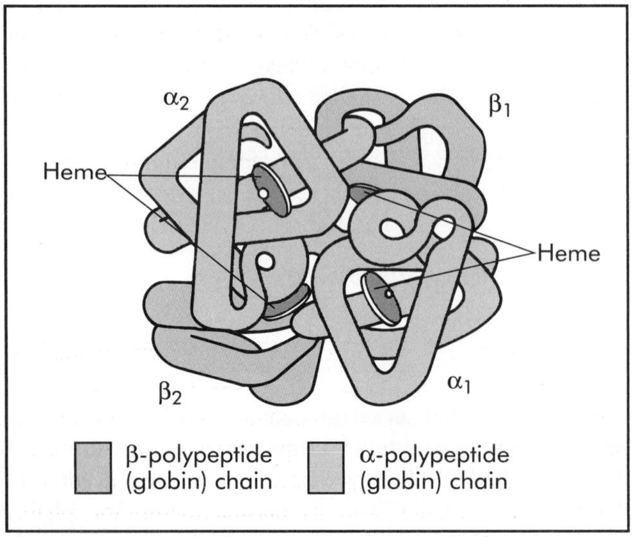

Figure 19-11 ■ **Molecular Structure of Hemoglobin.** Molecule is spherical tetramer weighing approximately 64,500 daltons. It contains a pair of α-polypeptide chains and a pair of β-polypeptide chains and several heme groups.

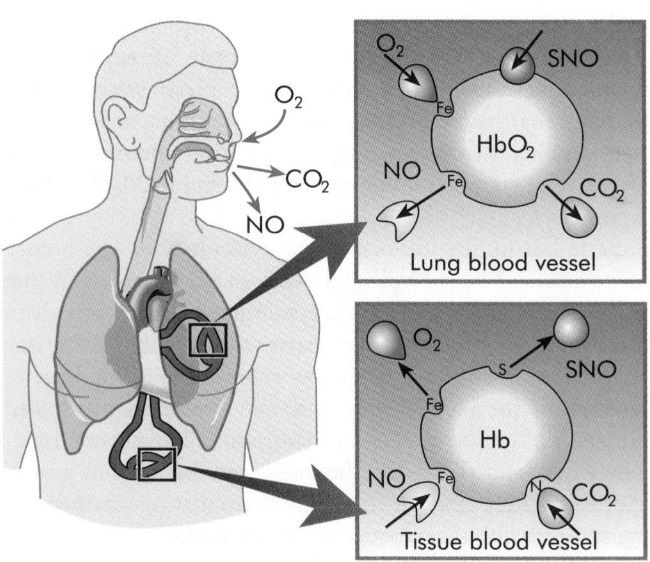

Figure 19-12 ■ **Hemoglobin (Hb) Binding to Nitric Oxide.** In the lungs, hemoglobin (Hb) binds to nitric oxide (NO) as S-nitrosothiol (SNO). In tissue, this SNO is released, and free, circulating NO is bound to a different site for exhalation. *Fe,* Iron; *N,* nitrogen.

TABLE 19-4

Nutritional Requirements for Erythropoiesis

Nutrient	Role in Erythropoiesis	Consequence of Deficiency (see Chapter 20)
Protein (amino acids)	Structural component of plasma membrane	Decreased strength, elasticity, and flexibility of membrane; hemolytic anemia
	Synthesis of hemoglobin	Decreased erythropoiesis and life span of erythrocytes
Intrinsic factor	Gastrointestinal absorption of vitamin B_{12}	Pernicious anemia
Cobalamin (vitamin B_{12})	Synthesis of DNA, maturation of erythrocytes, facilitator of folate metabolism	Macrocytic (megaloblastic) anemia
Folate (folic acid)	Synthesis of DNA and RNA, maturation of erythrocytes	Macrocytic (megaloblastic) anemia
Vitamin B_6 (pyridoxine)	Heme synthesis, possibly increases folate metabolism	Hypochromic-microcytic anemia
Vitamin B_2 (riboflavin)	Oxidative reactions	Normochromic-normocytic anemia
Vitamin C (ascorbic acid)	Iron metabolism, acts as a reducing agent to maintain iron in its ferrous (Fe^{++}) form	Normochromic-normocytic anemia
Pantothenic acid	Heme synthesis	Unknown in humans*
Niacin	None, but needed for respiration in mature erythrocytes	Unknown in humans
Vitamin E	Synthesis of heme; possible protection against oxidative damage in mature erythrocytes	Hemolytic anemia with increased cell membrane fragility; shortens life span of erythrocytes in individual with cystic fibrosis
Iron	Hemoglobin synthesis	Iron-deficiency anemia
Copper	Structural component of plasma membrane	Hypochromic-microcytic anemia

Data from Lee GR et al: *Wintrobe's clinical hematology*, ed 9, Philadelphia, 1993, Lee & Febiger; Harmening DM: *Clinical hematology and fundamentals of hemostasis*, ed 3, Philadelphia, 1997, FA Davis.
DNA, Deoxyribonucleic acid; *RNA*, ribonucleic acid.
*Although pantothenic acid is important for optimal synthesis of heme, experimentally induced deficiency failed to produce anemia or other hematopoietic disturbances.

components are lacking for a prolonged time, erythrocyte production slows and anemia (insufficient numbers of functional erythrocytes) may result (see Chapter 20).

Iron cycle

Approximately 67% of total body iron is bound to heme in erythrocytes (hemoglobin) and muscle cells (**myoglobin**), and approximately 30% is stored in mononuclear phagocytes (i.e., macrophages) and hepatic parenchymal cells as either ferritin or hemosiderin. The remaining 3% (less than 1 mg) is lost daily in urine, sweat, bile, and epithelial cells shed from the gut. Iron is transported in the blood bound to **transferrin,** a glycoprotein synthesized primarily by the liver but also by tissue macrophages, submaxillary and mammary glands, and ovaries or testes (Figure 19-13).

Iron for hemoglobin production is carried by transferrin to erythroblasts in the bone marrow, where it binds to transferrin receptors on erythroblasts. The iron is transported to the erythroblast's mitochondria (the site of hemoglobin production) and incorporated into protoporphyrin by the action of the enzyme heme synthetase.

Aged or damaged erythrocytes are removed from the bloodstream by macrophages of the MPS—chiefly in the spleen. Within the phagolysosomes (digestive vacuoles) of the macrophage, the erythrocyte is broken down, the hemoglobin molecule catabolized, and the iron stored as ferritin or hemosiderin. The stored iron is released into the bloodstream, where it binds to transferrin (see Figure 19-13).

Iron balance is maintained through controlled absorption rather than excretion. Regulation of iron transport across the plasma membrane of gastrointestinal epithelial cells is related to the cell's iron content and the overall rate of erythropoiesis. If the body's iron stores are low or the demand for erythropoiesis increases, iron is transported rapidly through the epithelial cell and into the plasma. If body stores are high and erythropoiesis is not increased, iron crosses the epithelial cell's plasma membrane passively and is stored as ferritin. Excretion of iron occurs when the epithelial cells of the intestinal mucosa slough off.

Normal destruction of senescent erythrocytes

Although mature erythrocytes lack nuclei, mitochondria, and endoplasmic reticulum, they do have cytoplasmic enzymes capable of glycolysis (anaerobic glucose metabolism) and production of small quantities of adenosine triphosphate (ATP). ATP provides the energy needed to maintain cell function and its plasma membrane pliable (see Figure 1-1). Metabolic processes diminish as the erythrocyte ages, so less ATP is available to maintain plasma membrane function. The senescent red cell becomes increasingly fragile and loses its reversible deformability,

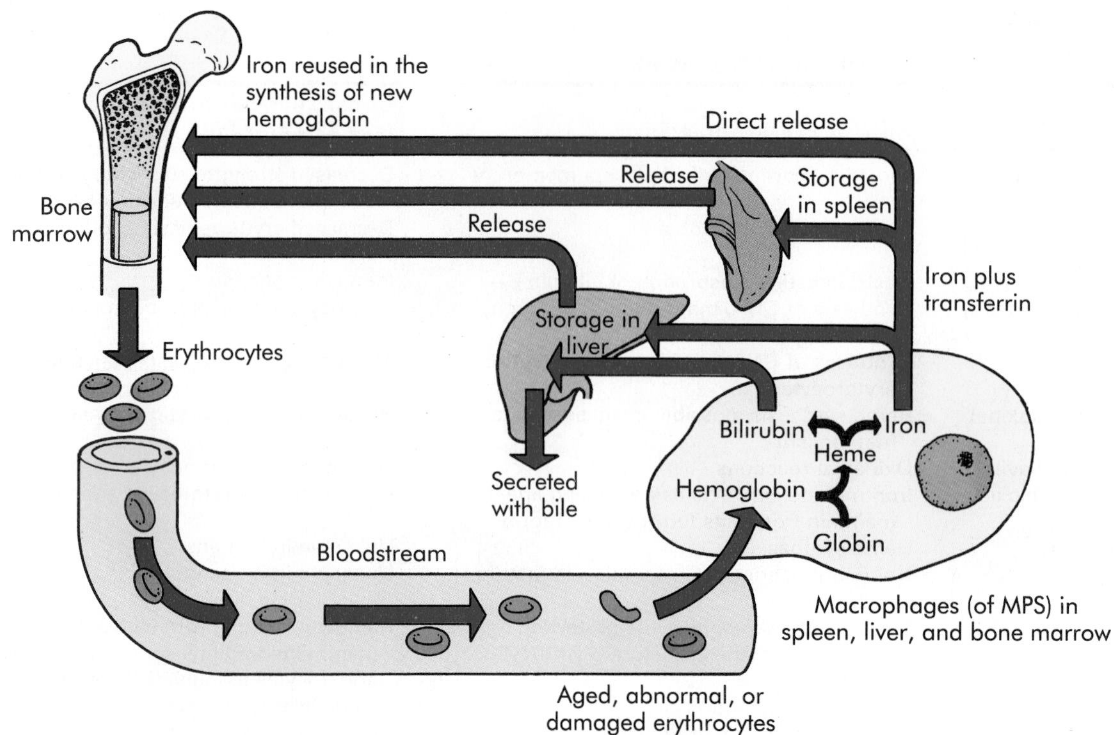

Figure 19-13 ■ **Iron Cycle.** Iron (Fe) released from gastrointestinal epithelial cells circulates in the bloodstream associated with its plasma carrier, transferrin. It is delivered to erythroblasts in bone marrow, where most of it is incorporated into hemoglobin. Mature erythrocytes circulate for approximately 120 days, after which they become senescent and are removed by mononuclear phagocyte system (MPS). Macrophages of MPS (mostly in spleen) break down ingested erythrocytes and return iron to the bloodstream directly or after storing it as ferritin or hemosiderin.

becoming susceptible to rupture while passing through narrowed regions of the microcirculation.

Additionally, the plasma membrane of senescent red cells undergoes phospholipid rearrangement that is recognized by receptors on macrophages (primarily in the spleen), which selectively remove and sequester the red cells. If the spleen is dysfunctional or absent, macrophages in the liver (Kupffer cells) take over. During digestion of hemoglobin in the macrophage, porphyrin reduces to bilirubin, which is transported to the liver, conjugated, and finally excreted in the bile as glucuronide (Figure 19-14). Bacteria in the intestinal lumen transform conjugated bilirubin into urobilinogen. Although a small portion is reabsorbed, most urobilinogen is excreted in feces.

Conditions causing accelerated erythrocyte destruction increase the load of bilirubin for hepatic clearance, leading to increased serum levels of unconjugated bilirubin and increased urinary excretion of urobilinogen. Gallstones (cholelithiasis) can result from a chronically elevated rate of bilirubin excretion.

QUICK CHECK 19-4

1. Why is the reticulocyte count important?
2. Why is iron important to erythropoiesis?
3. What happens to aging erythrocytes?

Development of Leukocytes

All leukocytes arise from stem cells in the bone marrow (their pathways of differentiation are shown in Figure 19-7). Lymphoid progenitor cells develop into lymphocytes, which are released into the bloodstream to undergo further maturation in the primary and secondary lymphoid organs (see Chapter 6). Monocyte progenitors develop into monocytic cells, which continue maturing into macrophages after release into the bloodstream and entrance into various tissues. Progenitor cells for granulocytes normally fully mature in the marrow into neutrophils, eosinophils, and basophils and are released into the blood.

The bone marrow selectively retains immature granulocytes as a reserve pool that can be rapidly mobilized in response to the body's needs. Further maturation is under the control of several hematopoietic growth factors, including interleukins, granulocyte-macrophage colony-stimulating factor (GM-CSF), and granulocyte colony-stimulating factor (G-CSF).

Leukocyte production increases in response to infection, to the presence of steroids, and to reduction or depletion of reserves in the marrow. It is also associated with strenuous exercise, convulsive seizures, heat, intense radiation, increased heart rates, pain, nausea and vomiting, and anxiety.

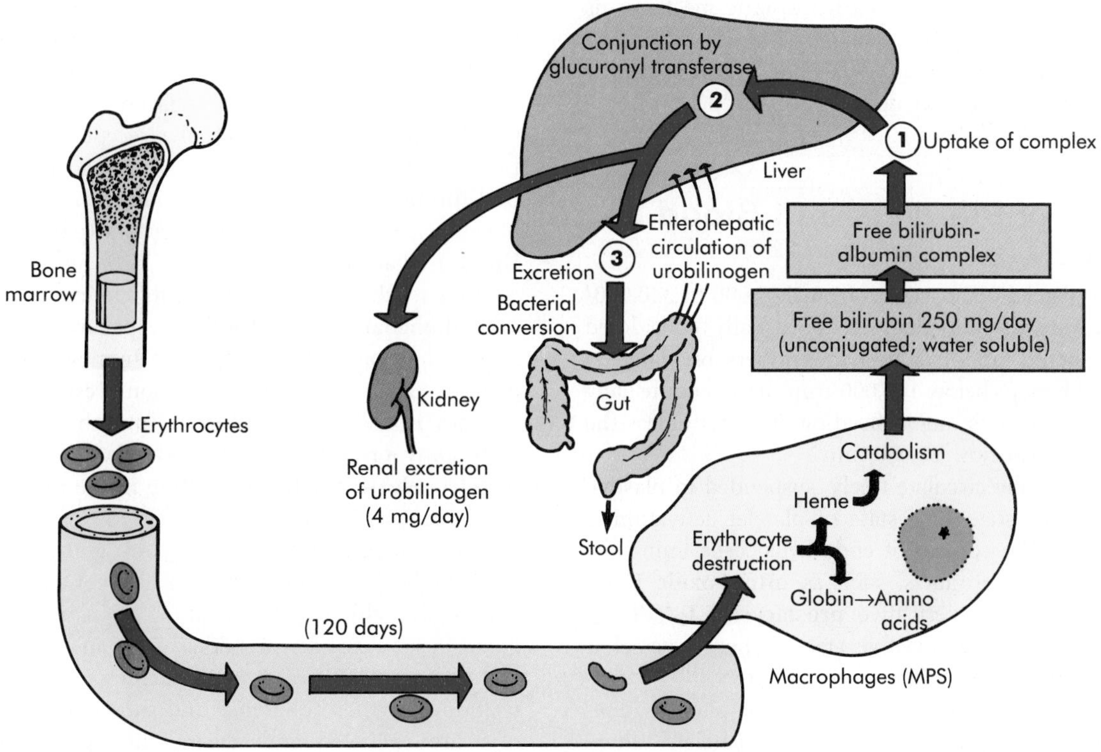

Figure 19-14 ■ **Metabolism of Bilirubin Released by Heme Breakdown.** *MPS,* Mononuclear phagocyte system.

Development of Platelets

Platelets (thrombocytes) are derived from stem cells and progenitor cells that differentiate into megakaryocytes.[8,9] During thrombopoiesis, the megakaryocyte progenitor is programmed to undergo an endomitotic cell cycle (**endomitosis**) during which DNA replication occurs, but anaphase and cytokinesis are blocked (see Chapter 1) (see Figures 19-4 and 19-7). Thus, the megakaryocyte nucleus enlarges and become extremely polyploidy (up to 100-fold or more of the normal amount of DNA) without cellular division. Concurrently, the numbers of cytoplasmic organelles (e.g., internal membranes, granules) increase, and the cell develops cellular surface elongations and branches that progressively fragment into platelets. Like erythrocytes, platelets released from the bone marrow lack nuclei.

An optimal number of platelets and committed platelet precursors (megakaryoblasts) in the bone marrow is maintained by primarily by thrombopoietin, with other factors such as GM-CSF, produced by the liver and kidney. These factors affect the rate of differentiation into megakaryocytes and the rate of platelet release. About two thirds of platelets enter the circulation, and the remainder reside in the splenic pool. Platelets circulate in the blood stream for about 10 days before beginning to lose their ability to carry out biochemical reactions. Senescent platelets are sequestered and destroyed in the spleen by mononuclear cell phagocytosis.

MECHANISMS OF HEMOSTASIS

Hemostasis means arrest of bleeding. As a result of hemostasis, damaged blood vessels may maintain a relatively steady state of blood volume, pressure, and flow. Three equally important components of the control of hemostasis are platelets, blood proteins (clotting factors), and the vasculature (endothelial cells and subendothelial matrix) (Figure 19-15).[10] The role of platelets is to (1) contribute to regulation of blood flow into a damaged site through induction of vasoconstriction (vasospasm), (2) initiate platelet-to-platelet interactions resulting in formation of a platelet plug to stop further bleeding, (3) activate the coagulation (or clotting) cascade to stabilize the platelet plug, and (4) initiate repair processes including clot retraction and clot dissolution (**fibrinolysis**) (see Figure 19-18).

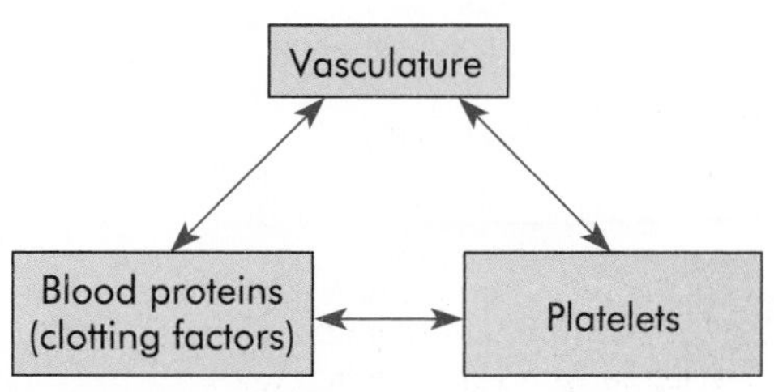

Figure 19-15 ■ **Three Hemostatic Compartments.**

The relative importance of the hemostatic mechanisms clearly varies with vessel size. Damage to large vessels cannot easily be controlled by hemostasis but requires vascular contraction and dramatically decreased blood flow into the damaged vessels (Table 19-5).

Function of Platelets and Blood Vessels

The normal platelet count ranges from 140,000 to 340,000/mm^3. However, an individual is not usually considered thrombocytopenic (abnormally low numbers of platelets) until the count drops below 100,000/mm^3 and is not usually at risk for spontaneous major bleeding episodes unless the platelet count falls below 20,000/mm^3.

Platelets normally circulate freely, suspended in plasma, in an unactivated state. The state of platelet activation is primarily under the control of endothelial cells lining the vessels. Endothelial products, such as **nitric oxide (NO)** and the prostaglandin derivative **prostacyclin I_2 (PGI_2)**, maintain platelets in an inactive state. When a vessel is damaged, platelet activation may be initiated.[11,12] Activation proceeds through a process of increasing platelet adhesion, aggregation, and activation. Initially, platelets adhere weakly to the vessel wall, followed by increased strength of adherence to the vessels, adherence between platelets (aggregation), and finally the development of an immobilizing meshwork of platelets and fibrin (Figure 19-16).

This process can begin in several ways. If the vessel lining remains intact in an area of inflammation, the endothelial cells may become activated and begin expressing new proteins on their surface. Several of these, particularly P-selectin, bind specifically yet weakly with receptors on the surface of inactive platelets (e.g., GPIb). As inflammation progresses, the platelets adhere more avidly through additional receptors that bind through a fibrinogen bridge to the endothelial cell surface. The principal fibrinogen receptor is the **integrin $\alpha_{IIb}\beta3$** (also known as **GPIIb/IIIa**).

During vessel damage, the endothelial layer is frequently compromised resulting in exposure of the underlying matrix that contains **collagen** and other components including fibronectin. The matrix also contains **von Willebrand factor (vWF),** and the exposed collagen can bind additional vWF from the circulation (see Figure 19-16). Platelets adhere strongly to collagen through the receptor GPVI and to vWF through the receptor complex GPIb/IX/V. Progressively the platelets undergo further aggregation through platelet-to-platelet adhesion involving further fibrinogen bridging between receptors (particularly GPIIb/IIIa) on adjacent platelets.

As a result of interactions with the endothelium or the subendothelial matrix, as well as exposure to inflammatory mediators produced by the endothelium and other cells, the platelets are activated. Activation results in dynamic changes in platelet shape from smooth spheres to those with spiny projections and degranulation (also called the **platelet-release reaction**) resulting in the release of various potent biochemicals.

Platelets contain three types of granules: lysosomes, dense bodies, and alpha granules. The contents of the dense bodies and alpha granules are particularly important in hemostasis. The dense bodies contain ADP, serotonin, and calcium. ADP reacts with specific receptors on platelets to induce further adherence and subsequent degranulation of nearby platelets and causing their plasma membranes to become ruffled and sticky. The new activated platelets cause a platelet plug to seal the injured endothelium. Serotonin is a vasoactive amine that functions like histamine and has immediate effects on smooth muscle in the vascular endothelium, causing an immediate temporary constriction of the injured vessel (see Chapter 5). Vasoconstriction reduces blood flow and diminishes bleeding. Vasodilation soon follows, permitting the inflammatory response to proceed (see Figures 23-2 and 23-3). Calcium is necessary for many of the intracellular signaling mechanisms that control platelet activation.

Alpha granules contain a large number of clotting factors (e.g., fibrinogen, factor V), growth factors (e.g., platelet-derived growth factor), and heparin-binding proteins (e.g., platelet factor 4). Many of these mediators either promote or inhibit platelet activity and the eventual process of clot formation (see Figure 19-16). Platelet-derived growth

TABLE 19-5

Types of Bleeding: Sources, Vessel Size, and Sealing Requirements

Types and Sources of Bleeding	Involved vessel	Size	Sealing Requirements
Pinpoint petechial hemorrhage (blood leakage from small vessels)	Capillary	Smallest	Generally direct-sealing
	Venule	↓	Mostly fused platelets
	Arteriole		Mostly fused platelets
Ecchymosis (large, soft tissue bleeding)	Vein		Vascular contraction, fused platelets, perivascular and intravascular hemostatic factor activation (see Figure 19-16)
Rapidly expanding "blowout" hemorrhage	Artery	Largest	Greater vascular contraction, more fused platelets, greater perivascular, and intravascular hemostatic factor activation

Modified from Harmening DM, editor: *Clinical hematology and fundamentals of hemostasis,* ed 3, Philadelphia, 1997, FA Davis.

I. Subendothelial exposure

- Occurs after endothelial sloughing
- Platelets begin to fill endothelial gaps
- Promoted by thromboxane A_2 (TXA_2)
- Inhibited by prostacyclin I_2 (PGI_2)
- Platelet function depends on many factors, especially calcium

Endothelial sloughing
Platelets
PGI_2
Collagen

II. Adhesion

- Adhesion is initiated by loss of endothelial cells (or rupture or erosion of atherosclerotic plaque) which exposes adhesive glycoproteins such as collagen and von Willebrand factor (VWF) in the subendothelium. VWF and, perhaps, other adhesive glycoproteins in the plasma deposit on the damaged area. Platelets adhere to the subendothelium through receptors that bind to the adhesive glycoproteins (GPIb, GPIa/IIa, GPIIb/IIIa).

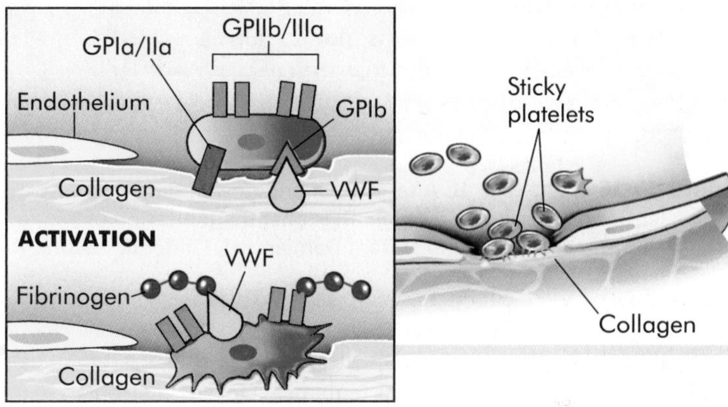

III. Activation

- After platelets adhere they undergo an activation process that leads to a conformational change in GPIIb/IIIa receptors, resulting in their ability to bind adhesive proteins, including fibrinogen and von Willebrand factor
- Changes in platelet shape
- Formation of pseudopods
- Activation of arachidonic pathway

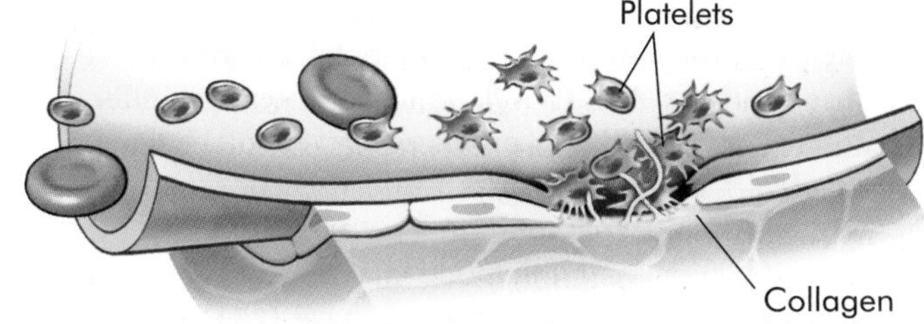

IV. Aggregation

- Induced by release of TXA_2
- Adhesive glycoproteins bind simultaneously to GPIIb/IIIa on two different platelets
- Stabilization of the platelet plug (blood clot) occurs by activation of coagulation factors, thrombin, and fibrin
- Heparin neutralizing factor enhances clot formation

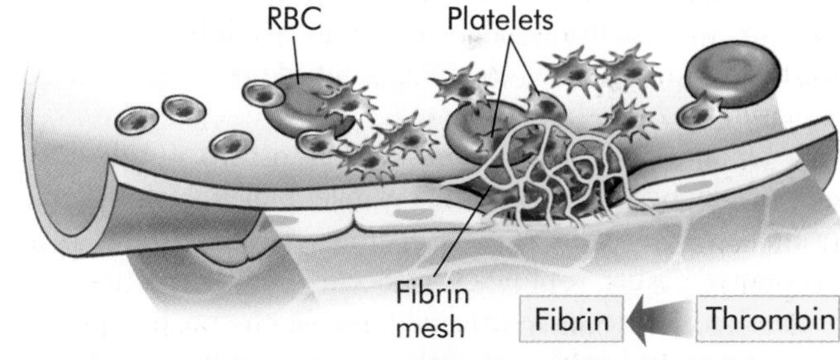

V. Platelet plug formation

- RBCs and platelets emeshed in fibrin

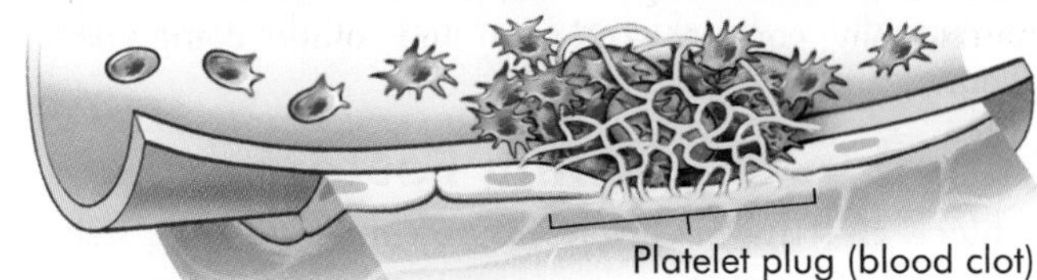

VI. Clot retraction and clot dissolution

- Clot retraction, using large number of platelets, joins the edges of the injured vessel
- Clot dissolution is regulated by thrombin and plasminogen activators

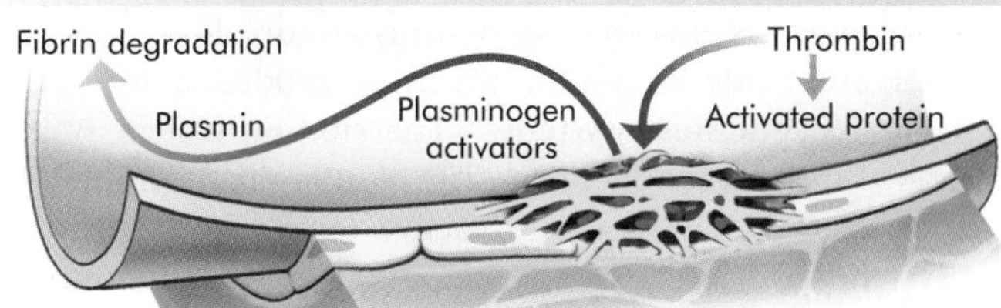

A

Figure 19-16 ■ **Platelet Degranulation. A,** Plug formation and clot dissolution.

(Continued)

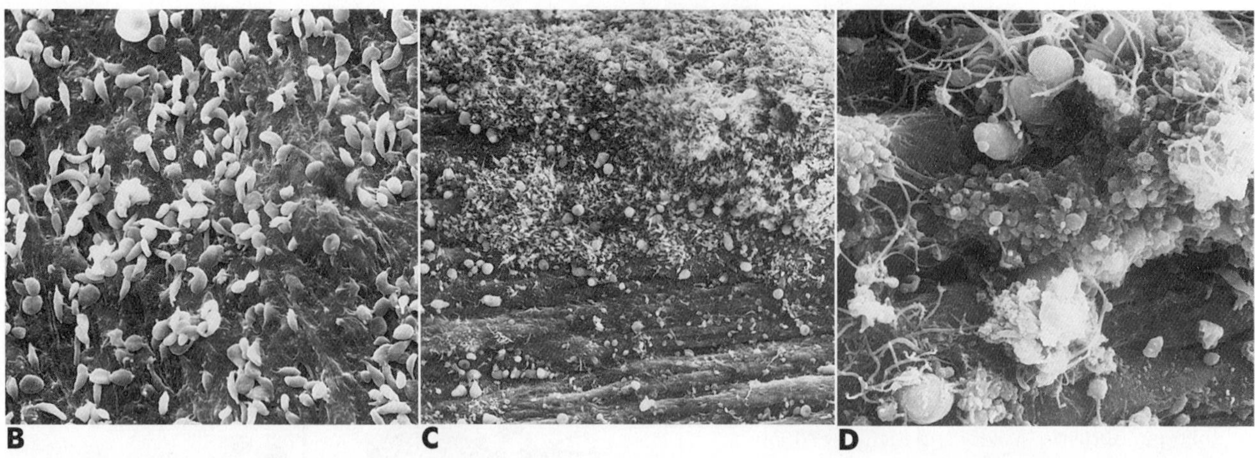

Figure 19-16, cont'd ■ **B,** After simple endothelial denudation, platelets adhere to the subendothelium in a monolayer fashion. **C,** Platelet-fibrin thrombus formation. **D,** Higher magnification of the thrombus shows a mixture of red cells and platelets incorporated into the fibrin meshwork. (**B** to **D** from Damjanov I, Linder J, editors: *Anderson's pathology,* ed 10, St Louis, 1996, Mosby.)

factor stimulates smooth muscle cells and promotes tissue repair. Heparin-binding proteins enhance clot formation at the site of injury.

Platelets also begin producing the prostaglandin derivative **thromboxane A_2 (TXA_2),** which counters the effects of prostacyclin I_2 (PGI_2), produced by endothelial cells (see Figure 19-18). TXA_2 causes vasoconstriction and promotes the degranulation of platelets, whereas PGI_2 promotes vasodilation and inhibiting platelet degranulation. In platelets, an isoform of **cyclooxygenase (COX-1)** converts arachidonic acid to TXA_2. Aspirin, particularly at low doses, specifically and irreversibly inhibits COX-1, decreasing production of TXA_2 and decreasing platelet activation.

If blood vessel injury is minor, hemostasis is achieved temporarily by formation of the platelet plug, which usually forms within 3 to 5 minutes of injury. Platelet plugs seal the many minute ruptures that occur daily in the microcirculation, particularly in capillaries. With too few platelets, numerous small hemorrhagic areas called *purpuras* develop under the skin and throughout the tissues (see Chapter 20).

Function of Clotting Factors

A **blood clot** is a meshwork of protein strands that stabilizes the platelet plug and traps other cells, such as erythrocytes, phagocytes, and microorganisms (Figure 19-17). The strands are made of fibrin, which is produced by the **clotting (coagulation) system.**[13] The clotting system was described in Chapter 5 and consists of a family of proteins that circulate in the blood in inactive forms. Initiation of the system results in sequential activation (cascade) of multiple members of the system until a fibrin clot is created. As was described for the clotting, complement, and kinin systems (see Chapter 5), each is usually diagrammed with multiple pathways of activation that come together in a common pathway. This organization is purely for convenience, and many members of each pathway may be activated by several alternative means and members of one system frequently activate members of another (e.g., activated members of the complement system can activate members of the clotting system).

The clotting system is usually presented as two pathways of initiation (intrinsic and extrinsic pathways) that join in a common pathway. The intrinsic pathway is activated when Hageman factor (factor XII) in plasma contacts negatively charged subendothelial substances exposed by vascular injury. The extrinsic pathway is activated when **tissue thromboplastin,** a substance released by damaged endothelial cells, reacts with clotting factors, particularly factor VII. Both pathways lead to the common pathway and activation of factor X (Stuart-Prower factor), which proceeds to clot formation. As with complement and kinin systems, the clotting system is complex with a large number of alternative activators and inhibitors. Also, there is interaction between the pathways so that an activated member of one pathway may activate a member of the other pathway.

Activated platelets are important participants in clotting. During activation, phospholipids in the platelet plasma membrane undergo redistribution so that a particular phospholipid, phosphatidylserine (PS), is greatly enriched on the platelet surface. PS provides a matrix for formation of several important complexes of clotting factors, including the tenase complex (factor X and activated factors VIII and IX) that activates factor X and the prothrombinase complex (prothrombin and activated factors X and V) that activated prothrombin into thrombin. Thrombin then converts fibrinogen into fibrin, which polymerizes into a fibrin clot (e.g., factor VIIa of the extrinsic pathway can directly activate factor IX of the intrinsic pathway).

A variety of substances, some of which are products of the coagulation system itself, control coagulation.[14] For example, excess thrombin is inactivated by antithrombin III. Other anticoagulants, most notably heparin, are produced and secreted locally by tissue mast cells and basophils activated by the injury (see Chapter 5).

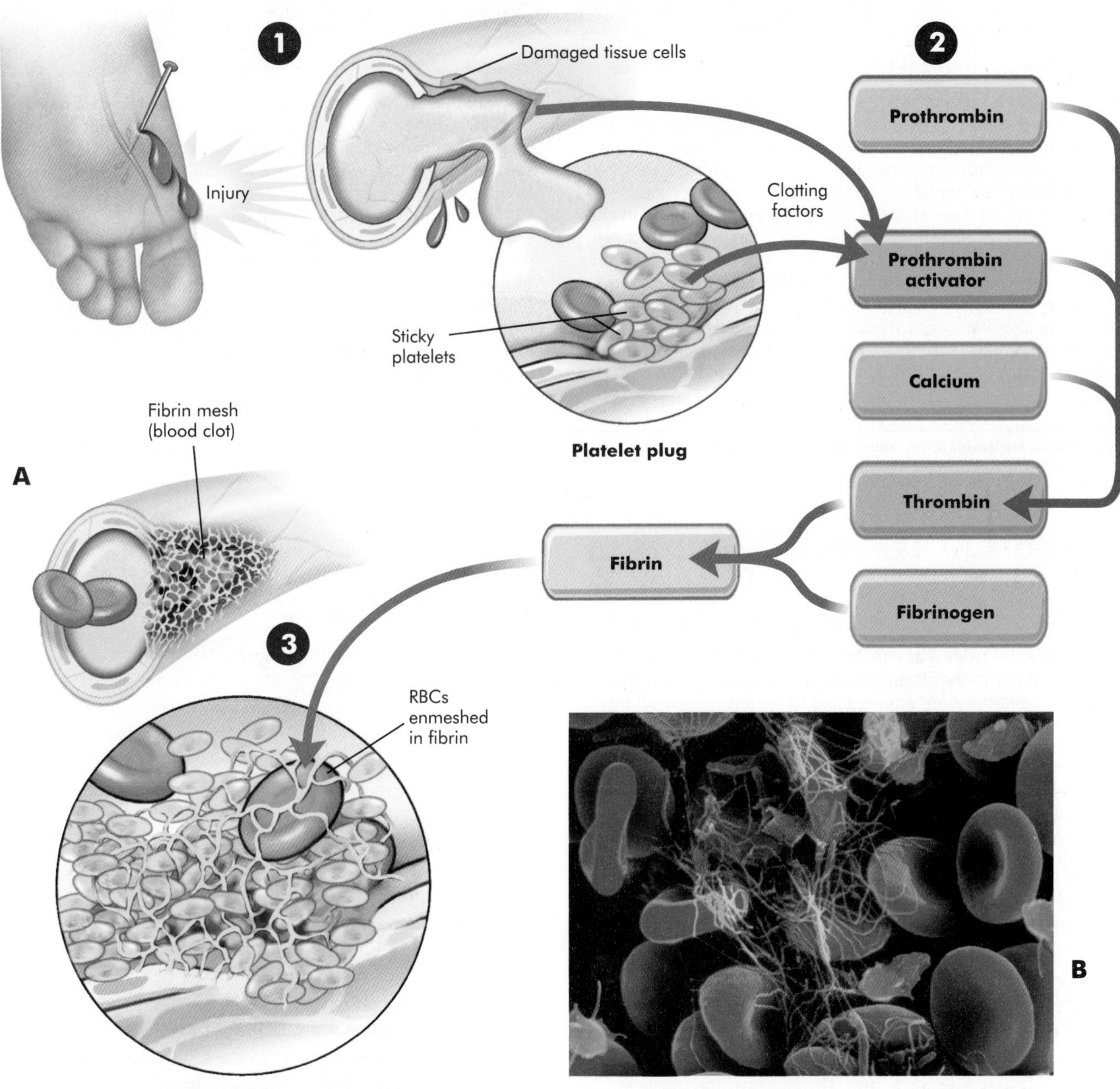

Figure 19-17 ■ **Blood Clotting Mechanism. A,** The clotting mechanism involves release of platelet factors at the injury site, formation of thrombin, and trapping of red blood cells (RBCs) in fibrin to form a clot. **B,** An electron micrograph showing entrapped RBCs in a fibrin clot. (**A** from Thibodeau GA, Patton KT: *Anatomy & physiology,* ed 6, St Louis, 2007, Mosby; **B** copyright by Dennis Kunkel Microscopy, Inc.)

HEALTH ALERT
Sticky Platelets, Genetic Variations, and Cardiovascular Complications

Investigators report that a genetic trait induces some people to make sticky platelets. People with platelets that tend to stick together have an increased risk of suffering complications from heart procedures. After individuals received angioplasty, in which a balloon-tipped catheter opens a blocked artery, investigators compared complications in the group with more sticky, or reactive, platelets with those with less reactive platelets. Of 112 participants, 3 months after the procedure, 15 individuals with sticky platelets experienced chest pain or a heart attack; 4 individuals with less reactive platelets experienced such complications. In addition, 10 people with sticky platelets needed another angioplasty, compared with only 2 from the less reactive platelet group.

In another study, investigators analyzed the receptor glycoprotein GP11b/111a for weaknesses that might direct attempts to prevent clotting, heart attack, and stroke. Blood samples from 1340 people revealed that 72% had inherited from both parents a gene for a version of GP11b/111a called $P1^{A1}$, whereas 28% had inherited one or two copies of a gene encoding a version called $P1^{A2}$. The blood from the group with two copies of $P1^{A1}$ clotted less readily than did the blood of the other group. The degree of clotting also depended on fibrinogen levels in the blood. In individuals with unusually high fibrinogen, the presence of $P1^{A1}$ glycoprotein seemed to increase clotting more than did $P1^{A2}$. Thus, testing for platelet stickiness and GP11b/111a status could determine which people need anticlotting drugs and for how long.

Data from Furlan M: Sticky and promiscuous plasma proteins maintain the equilibrium between bleeding and thrombosis, *Swiss Med Wkly* 132(15–16):181–189, 2002; Mammen EF: Sticky platelet syndrome, *Semin Thromb Hemost* 25(4):361–365, 1999.

HEALTH ALERT
Changes in the Management of Abnormalities in the Hemostatic System

Since the 1990s, new agents for the management of thrombotic and hemorrhagic disorders have been developed. For many years, the only agents used to inhibit procoagulant clotting factors was heparin and warfarin. New agents targeting factor Xa and factor IX, and thrombin, offer therapeutic alternatives for the management of arterial and venous thrombosis. The management of individuals with bleeding disorders has been advanced by the development of recombinant factor agents, the prolonged half-life of agents, or agents with reduced activation of immune responses. First introduced for hemophiliacs, recombinant factor VIIa (rFVIIa) is now used for several inherited and acquired bleeding disorders.

Data from Kempton CL, Harvey RD, Roberts HR: Novel therapeutic agents in the management of hemorrhage and thrombosis, *Cardoiovasc Hematol Agents Med Chem* 4(4):319–334, 2006.

Retraction and Lysis of Blood Clots

After a clot is formed, it retracts, or "solidifies." Fibrin strands shorten, becoming denser and stronger, which approximates the edges of the injured vessel wall and seals the site of injury. Retraction is facilitated by the large numbers of platelets trapped within the fibrin meshwork. The platelets contract and "pull" the fibrin threads closer together while releasing a factor that stabilizes the fibrin. Contraction expels protein-free serum from the fibrin meshwork (see Figure 19-17). This process usually begins within a few minutes after a clot has formed, and most of the serum is expressed within 20 to 60 minutes.

Lysis (breakdown) of blood clots is carried out by the **fibrinolytic system** (Figure 19-18).[15] Another plasma protein, plasminogen, is converted to **plasmin** by several products of coagulation and inflammation (e.g., activated factor XII, thrombin, lysosomal enzymes). Plasmin is an enzyme that dissolves clots (fibrinolysis) by degrading fibrin and fibrinogen into **fibrin degradation products (FDPs).** The fibrinolytic system removes clotted blood from tissues and dissolves small clots (thrombi) in blood vessels. A balance between the amounts of thrombin and plasmin in the circulation maintains normal coagulation and lysis.

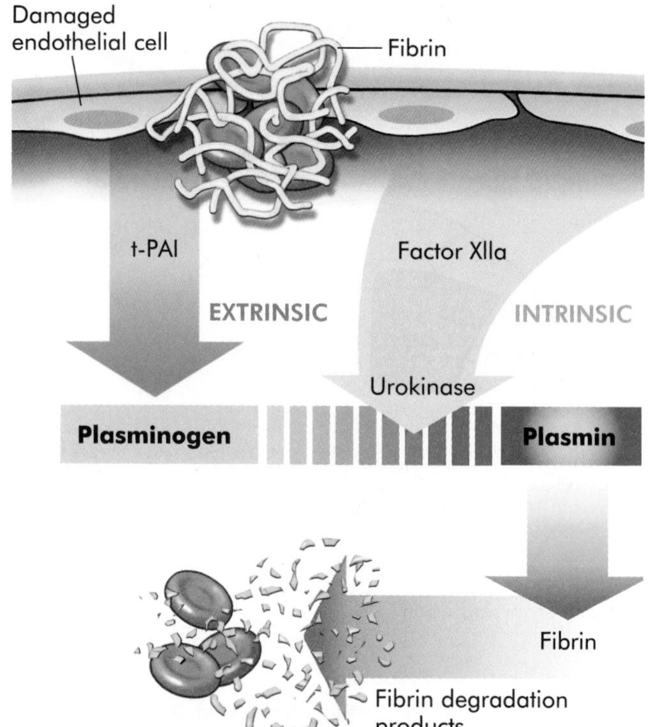

Figure 19-18 ■ **The Fibrinolytic System.** The central reaction is the conversion of plasminogen to the enzyme plasmin. Activity of plasminogen is achieved by the extrinsic pathway *(blue)* initiated by the release of tissue-type plasminogen activator t-PAI (also called T-PA) released from the endothelial cells and by the intrinsic pathway *(gold)* from factor XIIa and urokinase. Plasmin splits fibrin in the clot into fibrin degradation products.

Blood tests for evaluating the hematologic system are listed in Table 19-6.

TABLE 19-6

Common Blood Tests for Hematologic Disorders

Cell Type and Test	Properly Evaluated by Test	Possible Hematologic Cause of Abnormal Findings
ERYTHROCYTE		
Red cell count	Number (in millions) of erythrocytes/μl of blood	Altered erythropoiesis, anemias, hemorrhage, Hodgkin disease, leukemia
Mean corpuscle volume (MCV)	Size of erythrocytes	Anemias, thalassemias
Mean corpuscle hemoglobin (MCH)	Amount of hemoglobin in each erythrocyte (by weight)	Anemias, hemoglobinopathy
Mean corpuscular hemoglobin concentration (MCHC)	Concentration of hemoglobin in each erythrocyte (percentage of erythrocyte occupied by hemoglobin)	Anemias, hereditary spherocytosis
Hemoglobin determination	Amount of hemoglobin (by weight)/dl of blood	Anemias
Hematocrit determination	Percentage of a given volume of blood that is occupied by erythrocytes	Hemorrhage, polycythemia, erythrocytosis, anemias, leukemia
Reticulocyte count	Number of reticulocytes/μl of blood (also expressed as percentage of reticulocytes in total red blood cell count)	Hyperactive or hypoactive bone marrow function
Erythrocyte osmotic fragility test	Cellular shape (biconcavity), structure of plasma membrane	Anemias, hemolytic disease caused by ABO or Rh incompatibility, Hodgkin disease, polycythemia vera, thalassemia major
Hemoglobin electrophoresis	Relative percentage of different types of hemoglobin in erythrocytes	Sickle cell disease, sickle cell trait, hemoglobin C disease, hemoglobin C trait, thalassemias
Sickle cell test	Presence of hemoglobin S in erythrocytes	Sickle cell trait, sickle cell anemia
Glucose-6-phosphate dehydrogenase (G6PD) deficiency test	Deficiency of G6PD in erythrocytes	Hemolytic anemia
HEMOGLOBIN METABOLISM		
Serum ferritin determination	Depletion of body iron (potential deficiency of heme synthesis)	Iron deficiency anemias
Total iron-building capacity (TIBC)	Amount of iron in serum plus amount of transferrin available in serum (μγ/δγ)	Hemorrhage, iron deficiency anemia, hemochromatosis, hemosiderosis, iron overload, anemias, thalassemia
Transferrin saturation	Percentage of transferrin that is saturated with iron	Acute hemorrhage, hemochromatosis, hemosiderosis, sideroblastic anemia, iron deficiency anemia, iron overload, thalassemia
Porphyrin analysis (protoporphyrin analysis)	Concentration of protoporphyrin in erythrocytes (μg/dl); an indictor of iron-deficient erythropoiesis	Megaloblastic anemia, congenital erythropoietic porphyria
Direct antiglobulin test (DAT)	Antibody binding to erythrocytes	Hemolytic disease of the newborn, autoimmune hemolytic anemia, drug-induced hemolytic anemia, transfusion reaction
Antibody screen test (indirect Coombs test)	Detection of antibodies to erythrocyte antigens (other than the ABO antigens)	Same as for DAT
	See below	See below

(Continued)

TABLE 19-6

Common Blood Tests for Hematologic Disorders—cont'd

Cell Type and Test	Properly Evaluated by Test	Possible Hematologic Cause of Abnormal Findings
LEUKOCYTES: DIFFERENTIAL WHITE CELL COUNT (ABSOLUTE NUMBER OF A TYPE OF LEUKOCYTE/μl OF BLOOD)		
Neutrophil count	Neutrophils/μl	Myeloproliferative disorders, hematopoietic disorders, hemolysis, infection
Lymphocyte count	Lymphocytes/μl	Infectious lymphocytosis, infectious mononucleosis, hematopoietic disorders, anemias, leukemia, lymphosarcoma, Hodgkin disease
Plasma cell count	Plasma cells/μl	Infectious mononucleosis, lymphocytosis, plasma cell leukemia
Monocyte count	Monocytes/μl	Hodgkin disease, infectious mononucleosis, monocytic leukemia, non-Hodgkin lymphoma, polycythemia vera
Eosinophil count	Eosinophils/μl	Hematopoietic disorders
Basophil count	Basophils/μl	Chronic myelogenous leukemia, hemolytic anemias, Hodgkin disease, polycythemia vera
PLATELETS AND CLOTTING FACTORS		
Platelet count	Number of circulating platelets (in thousands)/μl of blood	Anemias, multiple myeloma, myelofibrosis, polycythemia vera, leukemia, disseminated intravascular coagulation (DIC), hemolytic disease of the newborn, transfusion reaction, lymphoproliferative disorders
Bleeding time	Duration of bleeding following a standardized superficial puncture wound of the skin, integrity of the platelet plug, measured in minutes following puncture	Leukemia, anemias, DIC, fibrinolytic activity, purpuras, hemorrhagic disease of the newborn, infectious mononucleosis, multiple myeloma, clotting factor deficiencies, thrombasthenia, thrombocytopenia, von Willebrand disease
Clot retraction test	Platelet number and function, fibrinogen quantity and use, measured in hours required for expression of serum from a clot incubated in a test tube	Acute leukemia, aplastic anemia, factor XIII deficiency, increased fibrinolytic activity, Hodgkin disease, hyperfibrinogenemia or hypofibrinogenemia, idiopathic thrombocytopenic purpura, multiple myeloma, polycythemia vera, secondary thrombocytopenia, thrombasthenia
Platelet adhesion studies	Ability of platelets to adhere to foreign surfaces	Anemia, macroglobulinemia, Bernard-Soulier syndrome, multiple myeloma, myeloid metaplasia, plasma cell dyscrasias, thrombasthenia, thrombocytopathy, von Willebrand disease
Platelet aggregation tests	Ability of platelets to adhere to one another	Afibrinogenemia, Bernard-Soulier syndrome, thrombasthenia, hemorrhagic thrombocythemia,

TABLE 19-6

Common Blood Tests for Hematologic Disorders—cont'd

Cell Type and Test	Properly Evaluated by Test	Possible Hematologic Cause of Abnormal Findings
		myeloid metaplasia, plasma cell dyscrasias, platelet release defects, polycythemia vera, preleukemia, sideroblastic anemia, von Willebrand disease, Waldenström macroglobulinemia, hypercoagulability
Whole blood clotting time (Lee-White coagulation time)	Overall ability of blood to clot, as measured in minutes in a test tube	Afibrinogenemia, clotting factor deficiencies, excessive fibrinolysis, hemorrhagic disease of the newborn, hypofibrinogenemia, hypoprothrombinemia, leukemia
Circulating anticoagulants (immunoglobulin G [IgG] antibodies that inhibit coagulation)	Presence of antibodies that neutralize clotting factors and inhibit coagulation, as indicated by prolonged clotting time, prothrombin time, or partial thromboplastin time	Afibrinogenemia, presence of fibrin-fibrinogen degradation products, macroglobulinemia, multiple myeloma, DIC, plasma cell dyscrasias
Partial thromboplastin time (PTT)	Effectiveness of clotting factors (except factors VII and VIII), effectiveness of intrinsic pathway of coagulation cascade, as measured by a test tube (in seconds)	Presence of circulating anticoagulants, DIC, clotting factor deficiencies, excessive fibrinolysis, hemorrhagic disease of the newborn, hypofibrinogenemia and afibrinogenemia, prothrombin deficiency, von Willebrand disease, acute hemorrhage
Prothrombin time	Effectiveness of activity of prothrombin, fibrinogen, and factors V, VII, and X; effectiveness of vitamin K–dependent coagulation factors of the extrinsic and common pathways of the coagulation cascade as measured in a test tube (in seconds)	Hypofibrinogenemia, dysfibrinogenemia, and afibrinogenemia; presence of circulating anticoagulants; DIC; deficiency of factors V, VII, or X; presence of fibrin degradation products, increased fibrinolytic activity, hemolytic jaundice, hemorrhagic disease of the newborn; acute leukemia, polycythemia vera, prothrombin deficiency, multiple myeloma
Thrombin time	Quantity and activity of fibrinogen as measured in a test tube (in seconds)	Hypofibrinogenemia, dysfibrinogenemia, and afibrinogenemia; presence of circulating anticoagulants; hemorrhagic disease of the newborn, polycythemia vera; increase in fibrinogen-fibrin degradation products; increased fibrinolytic activity
Fibrinogen assay	Amount of fibrinogen available for fibrin formation	Acute leukemia, congenital hypofibrinogenemia or afibrinogenemia, DIC, increased fibrinolytic activity, severe hemorrhage
Fibrin-fibrinogen degradation products (fibrin-fibrinogen split products)	Fibrinogenic activity as measured by levels of fibrin-fibrinogen degradation products (in μl/ml of blood)	Transfusion reactions, DIC, internal hemorrhage in the newborn, deep vein thrombosis, pulmonary embolism

Data from Bick RL, et al: *Hematology: clinical and laboratory practice*, St Louis, 1993, Mosby; Byrne CJ et al: *Laboratory tests: implications for nursing care*, Menlo Park, Calif, 1986, Addison-Wesley.

QUICK CHECK 19-5

1. Why are platelets necessary to stop bleeding?
2. Briefly describe the steps of platelet adhesion and aggregation.
3. How does plasminogen initiate fibrinolysis?

PEDIATRICS & Hematologic Value Changes

Blood cell counts tend to rise above adult levels at birth and then decline gradually throughout childhood. Table 19-7 lists normal ranges during infancy and childhood. The immediate rise in values is the result of accelerated hematopoiesis during fetal life, increased numbers of cells that result from the trauma of birth, and cutting of the umbilical cord.

Average blood volume in the full-term neonate is 85 ml/kg of body weight. The premature infant has a slightly larger blood volume of 90 ml/kg of body weight, with the mean increasing to 150 ml/kg during the first few days after birth. In both full-term and premature infants, blood volume decreases during the first few months. Thereafter the average blood volume is 75 to 77 ml/kg, which is similar to that of older children and adults.

The hypoxic intrauterine environment stimulates erythropoietin production in the fetus and accelerates fetal erythropoiesis, producing polycythemia (excessive proliferation of erythrocyte precursors) in the newborn. After birth, the oxygen from the lungs saturates arterial blood, and more oxygen is delivered to the tissues. In response to the change from a placental to a pulmonary oxygen supply during the first few days of life, levels of erythropoietin and the rate of blood cell formation decrease. The active rate of fetal erythropoiesis is reflected by the large numbers of immature erythrocytes (reticulocytes) in the peripheral blood of full-term neonates. After birth, the number of reticulocytes decreases about 50% every 12 hours, so it is rare to find an elevated reticulocyte count after the first week of life. During this period of rapid growth, the rate of erythrocyte destruction is greater than that in later childhood and adulthood. In full-term infants, the normal erythrocyte life span is 60 to 80 days; in premature infants, it may be as short as 20 to 30 days; and in children and adolescents, it is the same as that in adults—120 days.

The postnatal fall in hemoglobin and hematocrit values is more marked in premature infants than it is in full-term infants. In preschool and school-aged children, hemoglobin, hematocrit, and red blood cell counts gradually rise. Metabolic processes within the erythrocytes of neonates differ significantly from those found in erythrocytes of normal adults. The relatively young population of erythrocytes in newborns consumes greater quantities of glucose than do erythrocytes in adults.

The lymphocytes of children tend to have more cytoplasm and less compact nuclear chromatin than do the lymphocytes of adults. A possible explanation is that children tend to have more frequent viral infections, which are associated with atypical lymphocytes. Minor infections, in which the child fails to exhibit clinical manifestations of illness, and the administration of immunizations also may account for the lymphocyte changes.

At birth the lymphocyte count is high, and it continues to rise during the first year of life. Then it steadily declines until the lower value seen in adults is reached. It is unknown whether these developmental variations are physiologic or a pathologic response to frequent viral infection and immunizations in children.

The neutrophil count, like the lymphocyte count, is high at birth and rises during the first days of life. After 2 weeks, the neutrophil count falls to within or below the normal adult range. By approximately 4 years of age, the neutrophil count is the same as that of an adult.

The eosinophil count is high in the first year of life and higher in children than in teenagers or adults. Monocyte counts too are high in the first year of life but then decrease to adult levels. Platelet counts in full-term neonates are comparable with platelet counts in adults and remain so throughout infancy and childhood.

AGING & Hematologic Value Changes

Blood composition changes little with age. The erythrocyte life span in elderly persons is normal, although the erythrocytes are replenished more slowly after bleeding, probably because of iron depletion. Total serum iron, total iron-binding capacity, and intestinal iron absorption are all decreased somewhat in elderly persons. Iron deficiency is often responsible for the low hemoglobin levels noted in elderly persons. The plasma membranes of erythrocytes become increasingly fragile, with portions being lost, presumably because of physical trauma inflicted during circulation.

Lymphocyte function decreases with age (see Chapters 6 and 7), causing changes in cellular immunity and some decline in T cell function. The humoral immune system is less able to respond to antigenic challenge.

No changes in platelet numbers or structure have been observed in elderly persons, yet evidence shows that platelet adhesiveness probably increases. Although fibrinogen levels and factors V, VII, and IX tend to be increased in elderly people, evidence concerning hypercoagulability is inconclusive.

TABLE 19-7

Hematologic Values from Birth to Adulthood

				DIFFERENTIAL COUNTS					
Age	Hemoglobin (g/dl): Mean	Hematocrit (%): Mean	Reticulocytes (%): Mean	Leukocytes (WBC/mm^3): Mean	Neutrophils (%): Mean	Lymphocytes (%): Mean	Eosinophils (%): Mean	Monocytes (%): Mean	Platelets (10^3/mm^3): Mean
Newborn (cord blood)	16.8	55	5.0	18,000	61	31	2	6	290
2 wk	16.5	50	1.0	12,000	40	48	3	9	252
3 months	12.0	36	1.0	12,000	30	63	2	5	140–340
6 months–6 yr	12.0	37	1.0	10,000	45	48	2	5	140–340
7–12 yr	13.0	38	1.0	8000	55	38	2	5	140–340
Adult	13.0	40	1.0	8000	55	35	2	5	140–340
Female	14	41	0.8–4.1	7400	54–62	25–33	1–4	3–7	140–340
Male	16	47	0.8–2.5	7400	54–62	25–33	1–4	3–7	140–340

Did You Understand?

Components of the Hematologic System

1. Blood consists of a variety of components: about 90% water and 10% solutes. In adults, the total blood volume is approximately 5.5 L.
2. Plasma, a complex aqueous liquid, contains two major groups of plasma proteins: (a) albumins and (b) globulins.
3. The cellular elements of blood are the red blood cells (erythrocytes), white blood cells (leukocytes), and platelets.
4. Erythrocytes are the most abundant cells of the blood, occupying approximately 48% of the blood volume in men and approximately 42% in women. Erythrocytes are responsible for tissue oxygenation.
5. Leukocytes are fewer in number than erythrocytes and constitute approximately 5000 to 10,000 cells/mm^3 of blood. Leukocytes defend the body against infection and remove dead or injured host cells.
6. Leukocytes are classified as either granulocytes (neutrophils, basophils, eosinophils) or agranulocytes (monocytes/macrophages, lymphocytes).
7. Platelets are not cells but disk-shaped cytoplasmic fragments. Platelets are essential for blood coagulation and control of bleeding.
8. The lymphoid organs are sites of residence, proliferation, differentiation, or function of lymphocytes and mononuclear phagocytes.
9. The spleen is one of the largest lymphoid organs and functions as the site of fetal hematopoiesis, filters and cleanses the blood, and acts as a reservoir for lymphocytes and other blood cells.
10. The lymph nodes are the site of development or activity of large numbers of lymphocytes, monocytes, and macrophages.
11. The mononuclear phagocyte system (MPS) is composed of monocytes in bone marrow and peripheral blood and macrophages in tissue.
13. The MPS is the main line of defense against bacteria in the bloodstream and cleanses the blood by removing old, injured, or dead blood cells; antigen-antibody complexes; and macromolecules.

Development of Blood Cells

1. Hematopoiesis, or blood cell production, occurs in the liver and spleen of the fetus and in the bone marrow after birth.
2. Hematopoiesis involves two stages: (a) proliferation and (b) differentiation, or maturation. Each type of blood cell has parent cells called *stem cells.*
3. Hematopoiesis continues throughout life to replace blood cells that grow old and die, are killed by disease, or are lost through bleeding.
4. Bone marrow consists of blood vessels, nerves, mononuclear phagocytes, stem cells, blood cells in various stages of differentiation, and fatty tissue.
5. Hemoglobin, the oxygen-carrying protein of the erythrocyte, enables the blood to transport 100 times more oxygen than could be transported dissolved in plasma alone.
6. Erythropoiesis depends on the presence of vitamins (especially vitamin B_{12}, folate vitamin, vitamin B_6, riboflavin, pantothenic acid, niacin, ascorbic acid, and vitamin E).
7. Regulation of erythropoiesis is mediated by erythropoietin. Erythropoietin is secreted by the kidneys in response to tissue hypoxia and causes a compensatory increase in erythrocyte production if the oxygen content of the blood decreases because of anemia, high altitude, or pulmonary disease.
8. Maintenance of optimal levels of granulocytes and monocytes in the blood depends on the availability of pluripotential stem cells in the marrow, induction of these into committed stem cells, and timely release of new cells from the marrow.
9. Specific humoral colony-stimulating factors (CSFs) are necessary for the adequate growth of myeloid, erythroid, lymphoid, and megakaryocytic lineages.
10. Platelets develop from megakaryocytes by a process called *endomitosis.* In endomitosis, the megakaryocytes undergo DNA replication but not cell division; thus, the cell does not divide into two daughter cells.

Mechanisms of Hemostasis

1. Hemostasis, or arrest of bleeding, involves (a) vasoconstriction (vasospasm), (b) formation of a platelet plug, (c) activation of the clotting cascade, (d) formation of a blood clot, and (e) clot retraction and clot dissolution.
2. The normal vascular endothelium prevents clotting by producing factors such as nitric oxide (NO) and prostacyclin (PGI_2) that relax the vessels and prevent platelet activation.
3. Lysis of blood clots is the function of the fibrinolytic system. Plasmin, a proteolytic enzyme, splits fibrin and fibrinogen into fibrin degradation products that dissolve the clot.

PEDIATRICS & Hematologic Value Changes

1. Blood cell counts tend to rise above adult levels at birth and then decline gradually throughout childhood.
2. The lymphocytes of children tend to have more cytoplasm and less compact nuclear chromatin than do the lymphocytes of adults.

AGING & Hematologic Value Changes

1. Blood composition changes little with age. Erythrocyte replenishment may be delayed after bleeding, presumably because of iron deficiency.
2. Lymphocyte function appears to decrease with age. Particularly affected is a decrease in cellular immunity.
3. Platelet adhesiveness probably increases with age.

Key Terms

Agranulocyte, 484
Albumin, 481
Basophil, 485
Blood clot, 498
Bone marrow (myeloid tissue), 488
Clotting (coagulation), system, 498
Clotting factor, 482
Collagen, 496
Colony-stimulating factor (CSF hematopoietic growth factor), 490
Cyclooxygenase (COX-1), 498
Deoxyhemoglobin, 492
Endomitosis, 495
Eosinophil, 485
Erythroblast (normoblast), 491
Erythrocyte (red blood cell), 483
Erythropoiesis, 491
Erythropoietin, 490
Fibrin degradation product (FDP), 500
Fibrinolysis, 495
Fibrinolytic system, 500
Globin, 482
Globulin, 482
Granulocyte, 484
Hematopoiesis, 488
Hematopoietic stem cell, 488
Heme, 492
Hemoglobin (Hb), 492
Hemostasis, 495
Immunocyte, 484
Integrin $\alpha_{IIb}\beta_3$ (GPIIb/IIIa), 496
Leukocyte (white blood cell), 484
Lipoprotein, 482
Lymph node, 487
Lymphocyte, 485
Macrophage, 485
Marginating storage pool, 490
Methemoglobin, 492
Monocyte, 485
Mononuclear phagocyte system (MPS), 487
Myoglobin, 493
Natural killer (NK) cells, 486
Neutrophil (polymorphonuclear neutrophil [PMN]), 484
Nitric oxide (NO), 496
Oxyhemoglobin, 492
Phagocyte, 484
Plasma, 481
Plasma protein, 481
Plasmin, 500
Platelet (thrombocyte), 486
Platelet-release reaction, 496
Proerythroblast, 491
Prostacyclin I_2 (PGI_2), 496
Protoporphyrin, 492
Reticulocyte, 491
Serum, 481
Spleen, 486
Stromal cell, 490
Stromal stem cell, 490
Thrombopoietin (TPO), 486
Thromboxane A_2 (TXA_2), 498
Tissue thromboplastin, 498
Transferrin, 493
Von Willebrand factor (vWF), 496

References

1. Karikyawasam HH, Robinson DS: The eosinophil: the cell and its weapons, the cytokines, its locations., *Semin Respir Crit Care Med* 27(2):117–127, 2006.
2. Prussin C, Metcalfe DD: IgE, mast cells, basophils, and eosinophils, *J Allergy Clin Immunol* 117(2 suppl):S450–S456, 2006.
3. Hume DA: The mononuclear phagocyte system, *Curr Opin Immunol* 18(1):49–53, 2005.
4. Kaushansky K: Lineage-specific hematopoietic growth factors, *N Eng J Med* 354:2034–2045, 2006.
5. Yin T, Li L: The stem cell niches in bone, *J Clin Invest* 116(5):1195–1201, 2006.
6. Ross FP, Christiano AM: Nothing but skin and bones, *J Clin Invest* 116(5):1140–1149, 2006.
7. Eckardt KU, Kurtz A: Regulation of erythropoietin production, *Eur J Clin Invest* 35(suppl 3):13–19, 2005.
8. Kaushansky K: The molecular mechanisms that control thrombopoiesis, *J Clin Invest* 115(12):3339–3347, 2005.
9. Patel SR, Hartwig JH, Italiano JE Jr: The biogenesis of platelets from megakaryocyte proplatelets, *J Clin Invest* 115(12): 3348–3354, 2005.
10. Furie B, Furie BC: Thrombus formation in vivo, *J Clin Invest* 115(12), 2005.
11. Aird WC: Coagulation, *Crit Care Med* 33(12, suppl): S485–S487, 2005.
12. Gawaz M, Langer H, May AE: Platelets in inflammation and atherogenesis, *J Clin Invest* 115(12):3378–3384, 2005.
13. Moran TA, Viele CS: Normal clotting, *Sem Oncol Nurs* 21 (4):1–11, 2005.
14. Lasne D, Jude B, Susen S: From normal to pathological hemostasis, *Can J Anaesth* 53(6 suppl):S2–S11, 2006.
15. Laurens N, Koolwijk P, de Maat MP: Fibrin structure and wound healing, *J Thromb Haemost* 4(5):932–939, 2006.

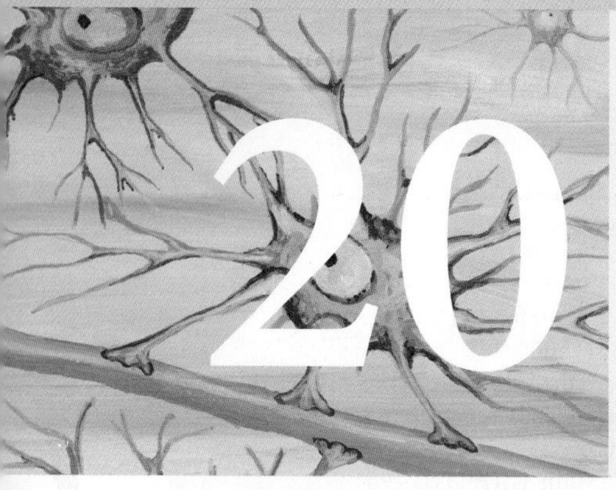

20 ALTERATIONS OF HEMATOLOGIC FUNCTION

Neal S. Rote ▪ Kathryn L. McCance ▪ Thom J. Mansen*

CHAPTER OUTLINE

ELECTRONIC RESOURCES

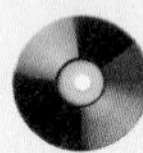

Companion CD
- Review Questions and Answers
- Animations

evolve Website
http://evolve.elsevier.com/Huether/
- Quick Check Answers
- Key Terms Exercises
- Critical Thinking Questions with Answers
- Algorithm Completion Exercises
- WebLinks

Alterations of erythrocyte function involve either insufficient or excessive numbers of erythrocytes in the circulation or normal numbers of cells with abnormal components. Anemias are conditions in which there are too few erythrocytes or an insufficient volume of erythrocytes in the blood. Polycythemias are conditions in which erythrocyte numbers or volume is excessive. Each condition has many causes and are pathophysiologic manifestations of a variety of disease states.

Many disorders involving leukocytes range from increased numbers of leukocytes, leukocytosis, in response to infections to proliferative disorders, such as leukemia. Many hematologic disorders are malignancies, and many nonhematologic malignancies metastasize to bone marrow, affecting leukocyte production. Thus, a large portion of this chapter is devoted to malignant disease.

The primary role of clotting (hemostasis) is to stop bleeding through an interaction of endothelium lining the vessels, platelets, and clotting factors. A large number of disease states may be associated with a clinically significant increase or decrease in clotting resulting from alterations in any of the three main components of the clotting process.

ALTERATIONS OF ERYTHROCYTE FUNCTION

Strictly speaking, anemia is a reduction in the total number of circulating erythrocytes or a decrease in the quality or quantity of hemoglobin. The causes of anemia are (1) altered production of erythrocytes, (2) blood loss, (3) increased erythrocyte destruction, or (4) a combination of all three.

Classification of Anemias

Anemias are classified by their causes or by the changes that affect the size, shape, or substance of the erythrocyte. The most common classification of anemias is based on the changes that affect the cell's size and hemoglobin content (Table 20-1). Terms used to identify anemias reflect these characteristics. Terms that end with *cytic* refer to cell size, and those that end with *chromic* refer to hemoglobin content. Additional terms describing erythrocytes found in some anemias are **anisocytosis** (assuming various sizes) and **poikilocytosis** (assuming various shapes).

CLINICAL MANIFESTATIONS The fundamental alteration of anemia is a reduced oxygen-carrying capacity of the blood resulting in tissue hypoxia. Symptoms of anemia vary, depending on the body's ability to compensate for the reduced oxygen-carrying capacity. Anemia that is mild and starts gradually is usually easier to compensate for and may cause problems for the individual only during physical exertion. As red cell reduction continues, symptoms become more pronounced and alterations in specific organs and compensation effects are more apparent.

*Thom J. Mansen, RN, PhD, contributed to this chapter in the previous edition.

TABLE 20-1
Morphologic Classification of Anemias

Morphology of Remaining Erythrocytes	Name and Mechanism of Anemia	Primary Cause
Macrocytic-normochromic anemia: large, abnormally shaped erythrocytes, normal hemoglobin concentrations	Pernicious anemia: lack of vitamin B_{12}; abnormal DNA and RNA synthesis in the erythroblast; premature cell death	Congenital or acquired deficiency of intrinsic factor (IF); genetic disorder of DNA synthesis
	Folate deficiency anemia: lack of folate; premature cell death	Dietary folate deficiency
Microcytic-hypochromic anemia: small, abnormally shaped erythrocytes and reduced hemoglobin concentration	Iron deficiency anemia: lack of iron for hemoglobin; insufficient hemoglobin	Chronic blood loss; dietary iron deficiency, disruption of iron metabolism or iron cycle (see Chapter 19)
	Sideroblastic anemia: dysfunctional iron uptake by erythroblasts and defective porphyrin and heme synthesis	Congenital dysfunction of iron metabolism in erythroblasts, acquired dysfunction of iron metabolism as a result of drugs or toxins
	Thalassemia: impaired synthesis of α- or β-chain of hemoglobin A; phagocytosis of abnormal erythroblasts in the marrow	Congenital genetic defect of globin synthesis
Normocytic-normochromic anemia: normal size, normal hemoglobin concentration	Aplastic anemia: insufficient erythropoiesis	Depressed stem cell proliferation
	Posthemorrhagic anemia: blood loss	Increased erythropoiesis; iron depletion
	Hemolytic anemia: premature destruction (lysis) of mature erythrocytes in the circulation	Increased fragility of erythrocytes
	Sickle cell anemia: abnormal hemoglobin synthesis, abnormal cell shape with susceptibility to damage, lysis, and phagocytosis	Congenital dysfunction of hemoglobin synthesis
	Anemia of chronic inflammation; abnormally increased demand for new erythrocytes	Chronic infection or inflammation; malignancy

DNA, Deoxyribonucleic acid; *RNA,* ribonucleic acid.

Compensation generally involves the cardiovascular, respiratory, and hematologic systems (Figure 20-1). Laboratory tests for various anemias are described in Table 20-2.

A reduction in the number of blood cells in the blood causes a reduction in the consistency and volume of blood. Initial compensation for cellular loss is movement of interstitial fluid into the blood causing an increase in plasma volume. This movement maintains an adequate blood volume, but the viscosity (thickness) of the blood decreases. The "thinner" blood flows faster and more turbulently than normal blood, causing a hyperdynamic circulatory state. This hyperdynamic state creates cardiovascular changes—increased stroke volume and heart rate. These changes may lead to cardiac dilation and heart valve insufficiency if the underlying anemic condition is not corrected.

Hypoxemia, reduced oxygen level in the blood, further contributes to cardiovascular dysfunction by causing dilation of arterioles, capillaries, and venules, thus increasing flow through them. Increased peripheral blood flow and venous return further contributes to an increase in heart rate and stroke volume in a continuing effort to meet normal oxygen demand and prevent cardiopulmonary congestion. These compensatory mechanisms may lead to heart failure.

Tissue hypoxia creates additional demands and effects on the pulmonary and hematologic systems. The rate and depth of breathing increases in an effort to increase oxygen availability accompanied by an increase in the release of oxygen from hemoglobin. All of these compensatory mechanisms may cause individuals to experience shortness of breath (dyspnea), a rapid and pounding heartbeat, dizziness, and fatigue. In mild chronic cases, these symptoms may be present only when there is an increased demand for oxygen (e.g., during physical exertion), but in severe cases, symptoms may be experienced even at rest.

Manifestations of anemia may be seen in other parts of the body. The skin, mucous membranes, lips, nail beds, and conjunctivae become either pale because of reduced hemoglobin concentration or yellowish (jaundiced) because of accumulation of end products of red cell destruction (**hemolysis**) if that is the cause of the anemia. Tissue hypoxia of the skin results in impaired healing and loss of elasticity, as well as thinning and early graying of the hair. Nervous system manifestations may occur where the cause

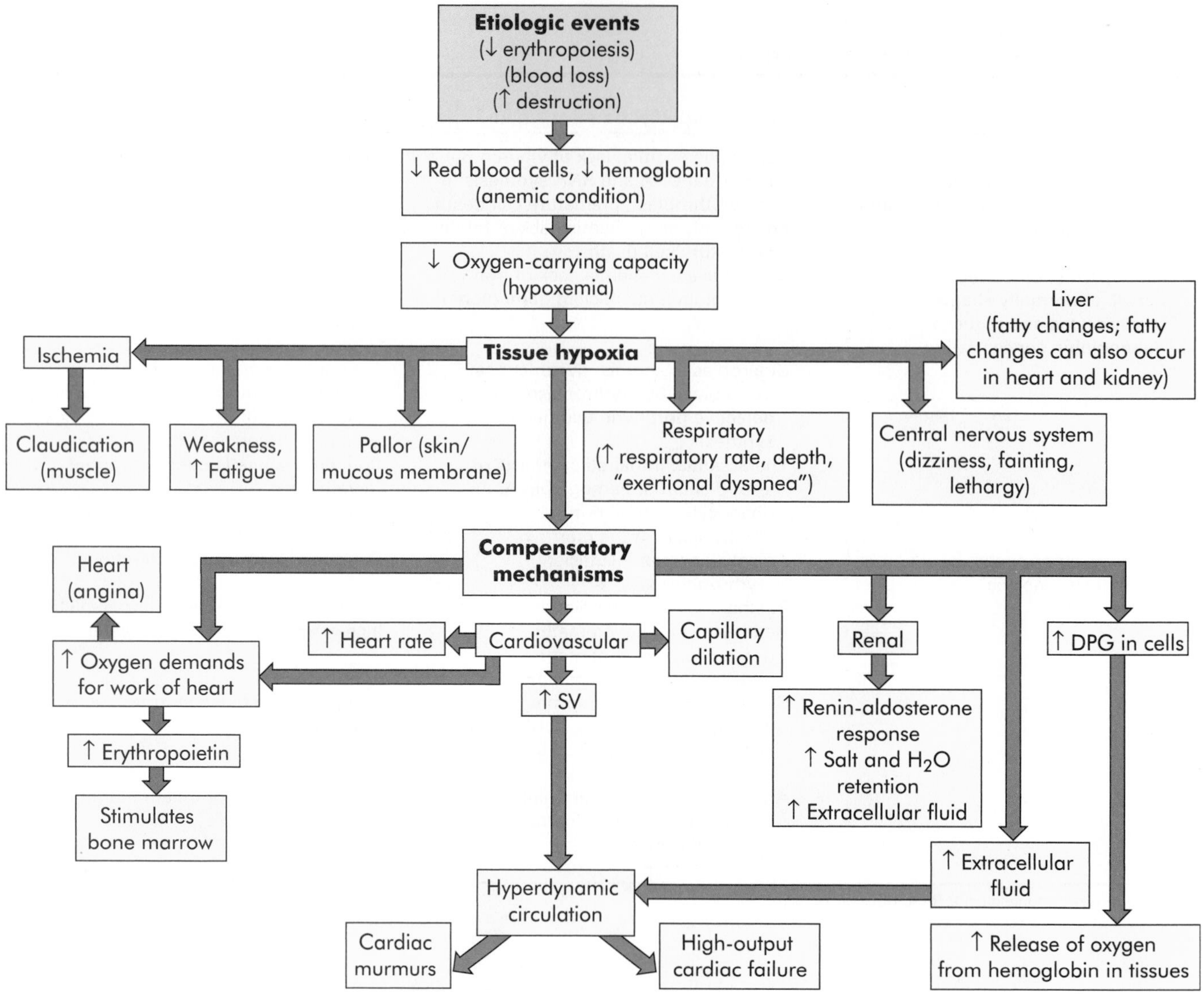

Figure 20-1 ■ **Progression and Manifestations of Anemia.** *SV,* Stroke volume; *DPG,* 2,3-diphosphoglycerate.

of anemia is a deficiency of vitamin B_{12}. Myelin degeneration occurs, causing a loss of nerve fibers in the spinal cord, resulting in paresthesias (numbness), gait disturbances, extreme weakness, spasticity, and reflex abnormalities. Decreased oxygen supply to the gastrointestinal (GI) tract often produces abdominal pain, nausea, vomiting, and anorexia. Low-grade fever (<101° F) occurs in some anemic individuals and may result from the release of leukocyte pyrogens from ischemic tissues.

When the anemia is severe or acute in onset (e.g., hemorrhage), the initial compensatory mechanism is peripheral blood vessel constriction, diverting blood flow to essential vital organs. Decreased blood flow detected by the kidneys activates the renin-angiotensin response, causing salt and water retention in an attempt to increase blood volume. These situations are considered to be emergencies and require immediate intervention to correct the underlying problem that caused the acute blood loss; therefore, long-term compensatory mechanisms do not develop.

Therapeutic interventions for slowly developing anemic conditions require treatment of the underlying condition and palliation of associated symptoms.[1] Therapies include transfusion, dietary correction, and administration of supplemental vitamins or iron.

Macrocytic-Normochromic Anemias

The **macrocytic (megaloblastic) anemias** are characterized by unusually large stem cells (megaloblasts) in the marrow that mature into erythrocytes that are unusually large in size (macrocytic), thickness, and volume.[2] The hemoglobin content is normal, thus allowing them to be classified as normochromic.

These anemias are the result of ineffective erythrocyte deoxyribonucleic acid (DNA) synthesis, commonly caused by deficiencies of vitamin B_{12} (cobalamin) or folate (folic acid). These defective erythrocytes die prematurely, which decreases their numbers in the circulation, causing anemia.

TABLE 20-2

Laboratory Tests for Various Anemias

Test	Pernicious Anemia	Folate Deficiency Anemia	Iron Deficiency Anemia	Sideroblastic Anemia	Aplastic Anemia	Posthemorrhagic Anemia	Anemia of Hemolytic Anemia	Chronic Inflammation
Hemoglobin	Low	Low	Low	Low	Low or normal	Normal or low	Low	Low
Hematocrit	Low	Low	Low	Low	Low or normal	Normal or low	Low	Low
Reticulocyte count	Low	Low	Normal or slightly high or low	Normal or slightly high	Low	Increased	High	Normal
Mean corpuscular volume (MCV)	High	High	Low	Low	Normal or slightly high	Slightly low	Normal or high	Normal or low
Plasma iron	High	High	Low	High	High	Normal	Normal or high	Low
Total iron-binding capacity	Normal	Normal	High	Normal	Normal	Normal	Normal	Low
Ferritin	High	High	Low	High	Normal	Normal	Normal	Normal
Serum B_{12}	Low	Normal	Normal	Normal	Normal	Normal	Normal	Normal
Folate	Normal	Low	Normal	Normal	Normal	Normal	Normal	Normal
Bilirubin	Slightly high	Slightly high	Normal	High	Normal	Normal	Slightly high	Normal
Free erythrocyte protoporphyrin	Normal	Normal	High	Increased or normal	High	Normal	Normal	Normal or slightly high
Transferrin	Slightly high	Slightly high	Low	High	Normal	Normal	Normal	Slightly low

Defective DNA synthesis in megaloblastic anemias causes red cell growth and development to proceed at unequal rates. DNA synthesis and cell division is blocked or delayed. However, ribonucleic acid (RNA) replication and protein (hemoglobin) synthesis proceed normally. Asynchronous development leads to an overproduction of hemoglobin during prolonged cellular division, creating a larger than normal erythrocyte with a disproportionately small nucleus. With each cell division, the disproportion between RNA and DNA becomes more apparent.

Pernicious anemia

Pernicious anemia (PA), the most common type of megaloblastic anemia, is caused by vitamin B_{12} deficiency, which often accompanies the end stage of type A chronic atrophic (autoimmune) gastritis (Figure 20-2, *C*).[3] *Pernicious* means highly injurious or destructive and reflects the fact that this condition was once fatal. It most commonly affects individuals over the age of 30 who are of Northern European descent, as well as blacks and Hispanics. Females are more prone to develop PA, with black females having an earlier onset.

PATHOPHYSIOLOGY The underlying alteration in PA is the absence of **intrinsic factor (IF),** an enzyme required for gastric absorption of dietary vitamin B_{12}, a vitamin essential for nuclear maturation and DNA synthesis in red blood cells. Deficiency of IF may be congenital or may be the result of adult-onset gastric mucosal atrophy in which the parietal cells are destroyed. Subsequently, all secretions of the stomach—hydrochloric acid, pepsin, and IF—are deficient. Gastric atrophy may be caused by type A chronic gastritis, an autoimmune disorder that causes destruction of parietal and zymogenic cells. These destroyed cells are replaced with mucus-containing cells (intestinal metaplasia). In addition, PA may be caused by heavy alcohol ingestion, hot tea, and cigarette smoking. PA is also associated with other autoimmune conditions, particularly those that affect the endocrine system. Complete or partial removal of the stomach (gastrectomy) causes IF deficiency and results in PA. Individuals with chronic gastritis are at risk for the development of gastric cancer and must be followed regularly to prevent this condition.

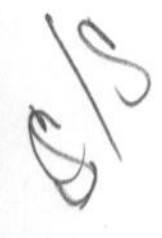

CLINICAL MANIFESTATIONS Pernicious anemia develops slowly (over 20 to 30 years), so by the time an individual seeks treatment, it is usually severe. Early symptoms are often ignored because they are nonspecific and vague and include infections, mood swings, and gastrointestinal, cardiac, or kidney ailments. When the hemoglobin has decreased to 7 to 8 g/dl, the individual experiences the classic symptoms of anemia: weakness, fatigue, paresthesias of feet and fingers, difficulty walking, loss of appetite, abdominal pain, weight loss, and a sore tongue that is smooth and beefy red. The skin may become "lemon yellow" (sallow), caused by a combination of pallor and jaundice. Hepatomegaly, indicating right-sided heart failure, may be present in the elderly along with splenomegaly, which is nonpalpable.

EVALUATION AND TREATMENT Evaluation is based on blood tests (see Table 20-2), bone marrow aspiration, serologic studies, gastric biopsy, clinical manifestations, and the Schilling test. The Schilling test determines cobalamin absorption. It is performed by administering radioactive cobalamin and then measuring its excretion in the urine. Low urinary excretion is significant for PA. Serologic studies reveal the presence of antibodies against gastric cells and gastric biopsy reveals achlorhydria, a total absence of hydrochloric acid (HCl).

Untreated PA is fatal, usually because of heart failure. With replacement therapy of vitamin B_{12}, mortality has decreased significantly. Death from PA is now rare and relapses are often the result of noncompliance with therapy. Initial replacement of vitamin B_{12} is accomplished by weekly injections until the deficiency is corrected. Monthly injections are then required for the remainder of an individual's life. Conventional wisdom and practice determined that oral preparations were ineffective because there was no IF to facilitate absorption of B_{12}. However, recent practice has shown that oral administration of higher doses of B_{12} is beneficial. Apparently, an alternative mechanism for B_{12} absorption exists that is independent of IF. PA is not curable; therefore, treatment must be continued throughout the individual's lifetime.

Folate deficiency anemias

Folate (folic acid) is an essential vitamin required for RNA and DNA synthesis within the erythrocyte. Humans are totally dependent on dietary intake to meet the daily requirement of 50 to 200 mg/day. Increased amounts are required for lactating and pregnant females. Folate is absorbed from the upper small intestine and does not require any other element (i.e., IF) to facilitate absorption. After absorption, folate circulates through and is stored in the liver. Folate deficiency occurs more often than B_{12} deficiency, particularly in alcoholics and individuals who are malnourished because of fad diets or diets low in vegetables. It is estimated that at least 10% of North Americans are folate deficient.

Clinical manifestations are similar to the malnourished appearance of individuals with PA, except for the absence of neurologic symptoms. Specific manifestations include cheilosis (scales and fissures of the mouth), stomatitis (inflammation of the mouth), and painful ulcerations of the buccal mucosa and tongue. Dysphagia, flatulence, and watery diarrhea also may be present, as well as histologic changes in the GI tract suggestive of sprue (chronic absorption disorder). Neurologic manifestations, if present, may be caused by thiamine deficiency, which often accompanies folate deficiency.

Evaluation of folate deficiency is based on blood tests, measurement of serum folate levels, and clinical manifestations. Treatment requires administration of oral folate preparations until adequate blood levels are obtained and manifestations are reduced or eliminated. Long-term therapy is not necessary except for maintenance of an adequate daily

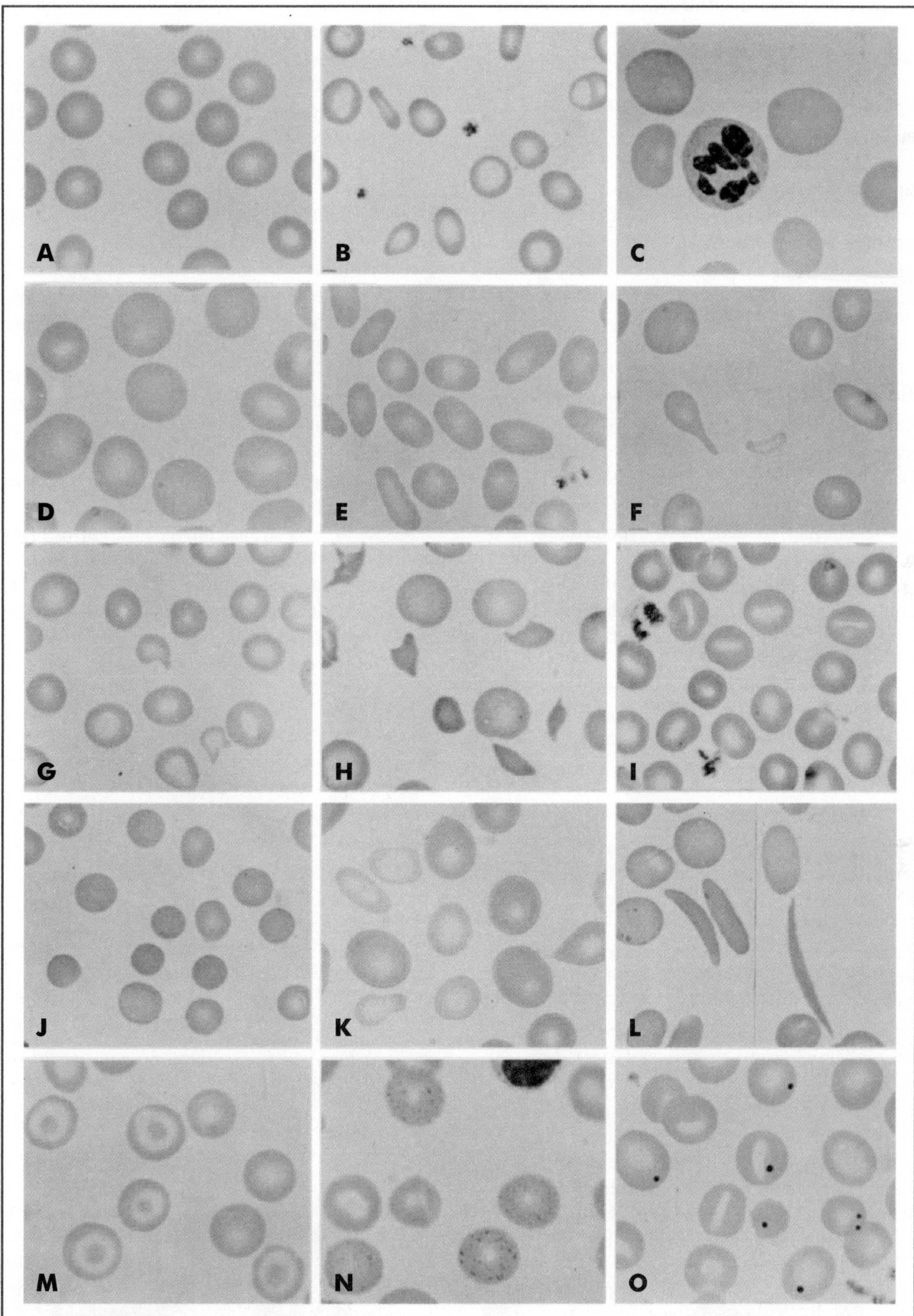

Figure 20-2 ■ **Appearance of Red Blood Cells in Various Disorders. A,** Normal blood smear. **B,** Hypochromic-microcytic anemia (iron deficiency). **C,** Macrocytic anemia (pernicious anemia). **D,** Macrocytic anemia in pregnancy. **E,** Hereditary elliptocytosis. **F,** Myelofibrosis (teardrop). **G,** Hemolytic anemia associated with prosthetic heart valve. **H,** Microangiopathic anemia. **I,** Stomatocytes. **J,** Spherocytes (hereditary spherocytosis). **K,** Sideroblastic anemia; note the double population of red blood cells. **L,** Sickle cell anemia. **M,** Target cells (after splenectomy). **N,** Basophil stippling in case of unexplained anemia. **O,** Howell-Jolly bodies (after splenectomy). (From Wintrobe MM et al: *Clinical hematology,* ed 8, Philadelphia, 1981, Lea & Febiger.)

intake of folate. Folate is essential for reducing blood levels of homocysteine, which has been recently recognized as a risk factor for the development of coronary artery disease.

Microcytic-Hypochromic Anemias

The **microcytic-hypochromic anemias** are characterized by abnormally small erythrocytes that contain abnormally reduced amounts of hemoglobin (Figure 20-2, *B*). Hypochromia occurs even in cells of normal size.

Microcytic-hypochromic anemia can result from (1) disorders of iron metabolism, (2) disorders of porphyrin and heme synthesis, or (3) disorders of globin synthesis. Specific conditions include iron deficiency anemia, sideroblastic anemia, and thalassemia.

Iron deficiency anemia

Iron deficiency anemia (IDA) is the most common type of anemia throughout the world, occurring in both developing and developed countries.[4] The overall incidence of IDA is difficult to establish because of the lack of standardized methods and techniques to determine hypoferremia and IDA. Certain populations are at high-risk for developing hypoferremia and IDA and include individuals living in poverty, women of childbearing age, and children. Females in the United States have a higher incidence than males for both hypoferremia and IDA, with the peak incidence occurring in the reproductive years and decreasing at menopause. Males have a higher incidence during childhood and adolescence. Children under 2 years of age are often affected because of their increased demand for iron during growth.

PATHOPHYSIOLOGY In developed countries, pregnancy and a continuous loss of blood are the most common causes of IDA. A blood loss of 2 to 4 ml/day (1 to 2 mg of iron) is enough to cause IDA. Males may experience bleeding as a result of ulcers, hiatal hernia, esophageal varices, cirrhosis, hemorrhoids, ulcerative colitis, or cancer. Menorrhagia (excessive menstrual bleeding) causes primary IDA in females. Other causes of blood loss for both genders include (1) use of medications that cause GI bleeding; (2) surgical procedures that decrease stomach acidity, intestinal transit time, and absorption; (3) insufficient dietary intake of iron; and (4) eating disorders such as pica—the craving and eating of nonnutritional substances.

Iron in the form of hemoglobin is in constant use in the body. An important attribute of iron is that it can be recycled; therefore, the body maintains a balance between iron that is in use as hemoglobin and iron that is stored and available for future hemoglobin synthesis. Blood loss disrupts this balance by creating a need for more iron, thus depleting the iron stores more rapidly to replace the iron lost from bleeding.

IDA develops slowly through three overlapping stages. In stage I, the body's iron stores for red cell production and hemoglobin synthesis are depleted. Red cell production proceeds normally with hemoglobin content of red cells also remaining normal. In stage II, insufficient amounts of iron are transported to the marrow, and iron-deficient red cell production begins. Stage III begins when the hemoglobin-deficient red cells enter the circulation to replace normal, aged erythrocytes that have been destroyed. The manifestations of IDA appear in stage III when there is an insufficient iron supply and diminished hemoglobin synthesis.

CLINICAL MANIFESTATIONS The onset of symptoms is gradual, and individuals usually do not seek medical attention until hemoglobin levels drop to 7 or 8 g/dl. Early symptoms are nonspecific and include fatigue, weakness, shortness of breath, and pale ear lobes, palms, and conjunctiva (Figure 20-3).

As the condition progresses and becomes more severe, structural and functional changes occur in epithelial tissue. The fingernails become brittle and "spoon shaped" or concave **(koilonychia)** (Figure 20-4). Tongue papillae atrophy and cause soreness along with redness and burning (Figure 20-5). These changes can be reversed within 1 to 2 weeks of iron replacement. The corners of the mouth become dry and sore (angular stomatitis), and an individual may experience difficulty with swallowing because of a "web" that develops from mucus and inflammatory cells at the opening of the esophagus. These lesions have the potential to become cancerous.

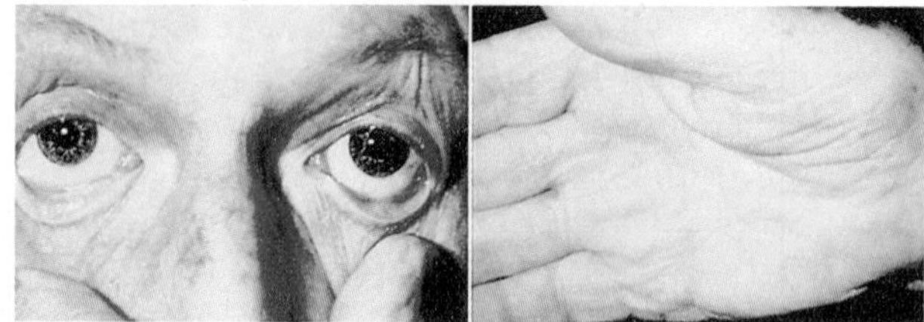

Figure 20-3 ■ **Pallor and Iron Deficiency.** Pallor of the skin, mucous membranes, and palmar creases in an individual with hemoglobin of 9 g/dl. Palmar creases become as pale as the surrounding skin when the hemoglobin level approaches 7 g/dl. (From Hoffbrand AV, Pettit JE: *Sandoz atlas of clinical hematology,* London, 1988, Gower Medical.)

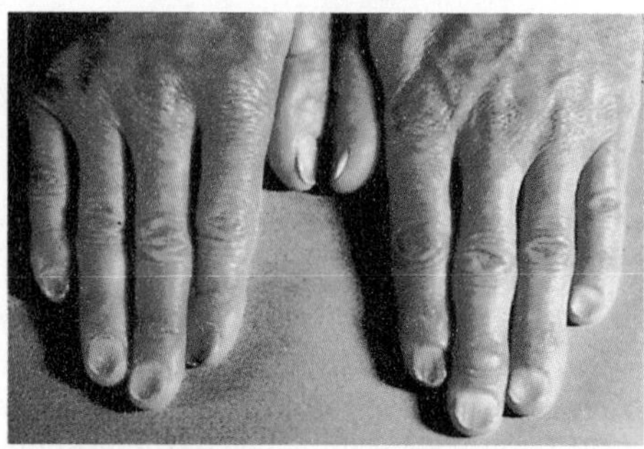

Figure 20-4 ■ **Koilonychia.** The nails are concave, ridged, and brittle. (From Hoffbrand AV, Pettit JE: *Sandoz atlas of clinical hematology,* London, 1988, Gower Medical.)

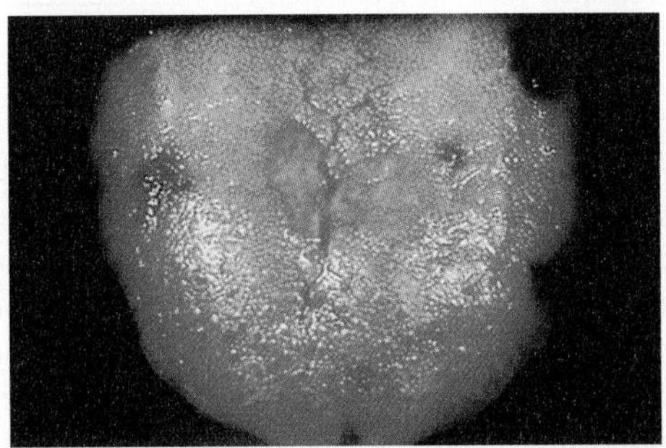

Figure 20-5 ■ **Glossitis.** Tongue of individual with iron deficiency anemia has bald, fissured appearance caused by loss of papillae and flattening. (From Hoffbrand AV, Pettit JE: *Sandoz atlas of clinical hematology,* London, 1988, Gower Medical.)

Iron is a component of many enzymes in the body, and lack of iron may alter other physiologic processes and contribute to the clinical manifestations. Individuals with IDA exhibit gastritis, neuromuscular changes, irritability, headache, numbness, tingling, and vasomotor disturbances. Gait disturbances are rare. In the elderly, mental confusion, memory loss, and disorientation may be wrongly perceived as normal events associated with aging.

EVALUATION AND TREATMENT Evaluation is based on clinical manifestations and laboratory tests (see Table 20-2). Iron stores are measured directly, by bone marrow biopsy, or indirectly, by tests that measure serum ferritin, transferrin saturation, or total iron-binding capacity. A sensitive indicator of heme synthesis is the amount of free erythrocyte protoporphyrin (FEP) within erythrocytes. A test that determines the concentration of soluble fragment transferrin receptor differentiates primary IDA from IDA that is associated with chronic disease.

The first step in treatment of IDA is to find and eliminate, or rule out, sources of blood loss. If this is not done, replacement therapy is ineffective. Iron replacement therapy is required and very effective. Initial doses are 150 to 200 mg/day and are continued until the serum ferritin level reaches 50 mg/L, indicating that adequate replacement has occurred. A rapid decrease in fatigue, lethargy, and other associated symptoms is generally seen within the first month of therapy. Replacement therapy usually continues for 6 to 12 months after the bleeding has stopped but may continue for as long as 24 months. Menstruating females may need daily therapy (325 mg/day) until menopause.

Sideroblastic anemia

Sideroblastic anemias (SAs) are a heterogeneous group of disorders characterized by anemia of varying severity because of inefficient iron uptake, resulting in abnormal hemoglobin synthesis. SA is characterized by the presence of ringed sideroblasts in the bone marrow. These are red cells that contain iron granules that have not been synthesized into hemoglobin but instead are arranged in a circle around the nucleus. Individuals with SA also have increased tissue levels of iron.

PATHOPHYSIOLOGY Sideroblastic anemias have various causes but all share the commonality of altered heme synthesis in the erythroid cells in bone marrow. SAs are either acquired or hereditary. **Acquired sideroblastic anemias,** which are the most common, occur as a primary disorder with no known cause (idiopathic) or are associated with other myeloproliferative or myeloplastic disorders. Another form is described as reversible SAs; these are secondary to various conditions such as alcoholism, drug reactions, copper deficiency, and hypothermia.

Hereditary sideroblastic anemias are rare and occur almost exclusively in males, supporting a recessive X-linked transmission; however, autosomal transmission affecting females has been reported. Other genetic, chromosomal, or enzyme dysfunctions also have been associated with hereditary SA. In all instances, SA anemia is present in infancy or childhood but may remain undetected until midlife, when other conditions, such as diabetes or cardiac failure from iron overload, cause it to be manifest.

Reversible sideroblastic anemia, associated with alcoholism, results from nutritional deficiencies of folate. Alcohol impairs heme synthesis by reducing the activity of specific enzymes along the biosynthetic pathway and also by direct effects of alcohol or acetaldehyde, or both, on the heme biosynthetic steps or mitochondrial metabolism. Some specific drugs also cause reversible SA and include antituberculous agents (isoniazid [INH], pyrazinamide, cycloserine, and chloramphenicol), which interfere with B_{12} metabolism or directly injure the mitochondria. Copper deficiency also causes reversible SA by interfering with conversion of ferric iron to ferrous iron. This is extremely rare and is associated with gastrectomy and prolonged parenteral nutrition without copper supplements. Hypothermia causes decreased heme synthesis and incorporation into hemoglobin.

CLINICAL MANIFESTATIONS Along with the cardiovascular and respiratory manifestations common to all anemias, individuals with SA may show signs of iron overload **(hemosiderosis),** including mild to moderate enlargement of the liver (hepatomegaly) and spleen (splenomegaly); however, liver function remains normal or only mildly affected. Occasionally the skin may become abnormally colored (bronze-tinted). Neurologic and skin alterations associated with other anemias are absent. Hemosiderosis of cardiac tissue may result in heart rhythm disturbances, which is a major but quite uncommon complication and generally occurs late in the course of the disease. Growth and development impairment may occur in infants and young children who are severely affected.

EVALUATION AND TREATMENT Initially, SA may be mistaken for deficiency of stem cells in the marrow **(hypoplastic anemia)** or iron deficiency anemia. (Laboratory findings are listed in Table 20-2.) The diagnosis of SA is established by bone marrow biopsy, which documents the presence of sideroblasts and confirms the diagnosis.

Hereditary SA is initially treated with pyridoxine therapy (50 to 200 mg/day), which is effective in approximately one third of individuals treated; however, response is variable. An optimal response is reticulocytosis with normal levels of hemoglobin and FEP returning within 1 to 2 months; cellular morphologic abnormalities do not disappear. A less optimal response is an elevated hemoglobin level that stabilizes at less than normal levels. A therapeutic response to pyridoxine may be maintained with lifelong administration of a reduced dosage. Nonresponse to pyridoxine requires blood transfusions for symptom relief and to promote growth and development.

Evidence of iron overload requires iron depletion therapy to prevent or minimize organ damage. **Phlebotomy,** or removal of blood from the circulation, is used in individuals with mild to moderate anemia without other complications (i.e., heart disease). After iron removal, maintenance phlebotomies are continued. Severely anemic individuals who may require transfusions become extremely iron overloaded, which mandates use of deferoxamine, an iron-chelating agent, to reduce iron levels.

Individuals with acquired SA are less likely to respond to pyridoxine, but SA rarely incapacitates them. When SA is secondary to an identifiable cause, treatment or removal of the cause is essential. In the absence of blood cell abnormalities and iron overload, progression takes place over years. Transfusion and iron overload therapy is the same as for hereditary SA when indicated.

Death from SA is rare and often secondary to complications such as infection, bone marrow failure, liver failure, or cardiac failure, or arrhythmias. Idiopathic SA has the potential to convert to **myelodysplastic syndrome,** or abnormal marrow proliferation, which may then convert to acute myeloblastic leukemia.

Normocytic-Normochromic Anemias

Normocytic-normochromic anemias (NNAs) are characterized by erythrocytes that are relatively normal in size and hemoglobin content but insufficient in number.[5] These anemias do not share any common etiology, pathologic mechanism, or morphologic characteristics. They are less common than the macrocytic-normochromic and the microcytic-hypochromic anemias. Five distinct anemias—aplastic, posthemorrhagic, hemolytic, sickle cell, and anemia of chronic inflammation—exemplify the diversity of the NNA characteristics and are summarized in Table 20-3. (Sickle cell anemia is discussed in Chapter 21.)

✔ QUICK CHECK 20-1

1. How do cell size and content determine classification of anemia?
2. Why is iron important to hemoglobin synthesis, and why is iron deficiency related to anemia?
3. How is anemia diagnosed?

MYELOPROLIFERATIVE RED CELL DISORDERS

Hematologic dysfunction results from an overproduction of cells, as well as a deficiency. One or more marrow elements may be produced in excess, responding to exogenous (radiation, drugs) or endogenous (physiologic compensatory response, immune disorder) signals. Excessive red cell production is classified as **polycythemia** (Table 20-4). Polycythemia exists in two forms: relative and absolute. **Relative polycythemia** results from hemoconcentration of the blood associated with dehydration. It is of minor consequence and resolves with fluid administration or treatment of underlying conditions.

Absolute polycythemia consists of two forms: primary and secondary. Secondary polycythemia, the most common of the two, is a physiologic response resulting from erythropoietin secretion caused by hypoxia. This hypoxia is noted in individuals living at higher altitudes (>10,000 ft), smokers with increased blood levels of CO, and individuals with chronic obstructive pulmonary disease or coronary heart failure, or both. Abnormal types of hemoglobin (San Diego, Chesapeake), which have a greater affinity for oxygen, also cause secondary polycythemia, as does inappropriate secretion of erythropoietin by certain tumors (renal cell carcinoma, hepatoma, and cerebellar hemiangioblastomas). The absolute primary form of polycythemia is referred to as *polycythemia vera.*

Polycythemia Vera

Polycythemia vera (PV) is a chronic, clonal alteration characterized by overproduction of red cells (frequently with increased white cells and platelets) accompanied by splenomegaly.[6] Hypercellularity of bone marrow, along with hyperplasia of myeloid, erythroid, and megakaryocytes, is a distinguishing feature. PV is quite rare, occurring mostly in white males of Eastern European Jewish origin between 55 to 80 years of age, with a median age of 55 to 60 years, but it has been observed in females and individuals less than 40 years of age. It is rarely seen in children or in multiple members of a single family; however, an autosomal dominant form exists that causes increased secretion of erythropoietin.

PATHOPHYSIOLOGY PV is a neoplastic, nonmalignant condition characterized by an abnormal proliferation of bone marrow stem cells with subsequent self-destructive expansion of red cells. This aberrant proliferation occurs despite normal to below normal erythropoietin levels. The underlying cause remains unknown, with the most likely etiology thought to be an acquired genetic stem cell alteration of the erythropoietin receptor that causes the abnormal proliferation. Laboratory studies have found red cell precursors that are capable of growth independent of erythropoietin. They also demonstrate sensitivity to other growth factors, such as interleukin-3 (IL-3), granulocyte-macrophage growth factor (GM-CSF), or insulin-like growth factor.

TABLE 20-3

Normocytic-Normochromic Anemias

Anemia	Pathophysiology	Clinical Manifestations	Evaluation and Treatment
Aplastic	Rare; may result from infiltrative disorders of bone marrow, autoimmune diseases, renal failure, splenic dysfunction, vitamin B_{12} or folate deficiency, parvovirus infection; or exposure to radiation, drugs, and toxins; also may be congenital Common stem cell population may be altered so it cannot proliferate or differentiate, or stem cell environment is altered to inhibit erythropoiesis Outcome ranges from death to minimal manifestations	Classic cardiovascular and respiratory manifestations with thrombocytopenia, hemorrhage into the tissues, leukopenia, and infection	Bone marrow biopsy determines whether anemia is caused by pure red cell aplasia or hypoplasia Treat underlying disorder or prevent further exposure to causative agent Blood transfusions, marrow transplant, and pharmacologic stimulation of bone marrow function
Posthemorrhagic	Caused by sudden blood loss with normal iron stores	Often obscured by cardiovascular manifestations of acute hemorrhage Severe shock, lactic acidosis, and death can occur if blood loss exceeds 40% to 50% of plasma volume	Restoration of blood volume by intravenous administration of saline, dextran, albumin, or plasma Transfusion of whole blood also required occasionally
Hemolytic	Acquired: caused by infection, systemic disease, drugs or toxins, liver disease, kidney disease, abnormal immune responses Hereditary: caused by abnormalities of the RBC membrane or cytoplasmic contents; present at birth Hemolysis: in blood vessels or lymphoid tissues that filter blood (e.g., spleen, liver) Erythrocytes: rigid, slowing their passage and making them vulnerable to phagocytosis Types: warm antibody disease (mediated by IgG antibody specific for erythrocyte antigens), cold antibody disease (mediated by IgM), and drug induced	Splenomegaly, jaundice, aplastic hemolytic, or megaloblastic crises can develop with viral infection With severe disease, bones become deformed and pathologic fractures occur Cardiovascular and respiratory manifestations correspond with severity of anemia	Blood and bone marrow studies Erythroid hyperplasia is found in marrow and blood smears Treatment of acquired disease involves removing the cause or treating the underlying disorder Other forms of treatment are transfusions, splenectomy, and steroids or folate
Anemia of chronic inflammation	Associated with chronic infections (e.g., AIDS), chronic inflammatory diseases (e.g., rheumatoid arthritis, SLE), and malignancies Causes are decreased erythrocyte life span, failure of mechanisms of compensatory erythropoiesis, or disturbance of the iron cycle	Manifestations fewer and milder than most other anemias Generally disability caused by chronic disease limits physical activity so hemoglobin levels adequate; if they drop, signs of iron deficiency anemia develop	Blood tests reveal iron deficiency in marrow despite normal or increased iron stores elsewhere No treatment is needed unless anemia becomes symptomatic Erythropoietin may be used

RBC, Red blood cell; *AIDS,* acquired immune deficiency syndrome; *SLE,* systemic lupus erythematosus.

CLINICAL MANIFESTATIONS Clinical manifestations of PV are due to increased blood volume, which increases blood viscosity, creating a hypercoagulable state resulting in clogging and occlusion of blood vessels. Tissue injury (ischemia) and death (infarction) is the outcome of blood vessel blockage, and this occurs about 40% of the time. These outcomes are directly correlated with hematocrit levels. Increases in numbers of thrombocytes, as well as production of dysfunctional platelets, also contribute to this hypercoagulable condition.

Circulatory alterations caused by the thick, sticky blood give rise to other manifestations, such as plethora (ruddy,

TABLE 20-4
Disorders Classified as Polycythemia

Type of Polycythemia	Mechanism of Increased Erythropoiesis	Cause of Associated Disorder
Primary polycythemia (polycythemia vera)	Excessive proliferation of erythroid precursors in marrow; increased sensitivity of stem cell to erythropoietin	Possible mutation in the erythropoietin receptor
Secondary polycythemia	Physiologic increase in erythropoietin secretion by the kidneys in response to underlying systemic disorder	Tissue hypoxia caused by cardiopulmonary disorders (chronic obstructive pulmonary disease, congestive heart failure), decreased barometric pressure, cardiovascular malformations causing mixing of arterial and venous blood, methemoglobinemia, carboxy-hemoglobinemia, smoking, obesity
	"Nonphysiologic"* increase in erythropoietin secretion	Renal disorders, cerebellar hemangioblastomas, hepatoma (liver tumor), ovarian carcinoma, uterine leiomyoma, pheochromocytoma, adrenocortical hypersecretion
Familial polycythemia	Genetically induced increase in erythroid precursors of the marrow Abnormal Hb with increased oxygen affinity Decreased 2,3-DPG Increased sensitivity of stem cells to erythropoietin Increased erythropoietin in secretion	Genetic defect

Hb, Hemoglobin; *2,3-DPG,* 2,3-diphosphoglycerate.
*Nonphysiologic means that there is no obvious physiologic explanation for hypersecretion of erythropoietin.

red color of the face, hands, feet, ears, and mucous membranes) and engorgement of retinal and cerebral veins. Other symptoms may include headache, drowsiness, delirium, mania, psychotic depression, chorea, and visual disturbances. Death from cerebral thrombosis is approximately five times greater in individuals with PV.[7]

Cardiovascular function, despite the vascular alterations, remains relatively normal. Cardiac workload and output remain constant; however, increased blood volume does increase blood pressure. Coronary blood flow may be affected, precipitating angina, although cardiovascular infarctions are uncommon. Other cardiovascular manifestations include Raynaud phenomenon and thromboangiitis obliterans.

A unique feature of PV, and helpful in diagnosis, is the development of intense, painful itching that appears to be intensified by heat or exposure to water (aquagenic pruritus) so that individuals avoid exposure to water, particularly warm water (baths, showers). The intensity of itching is related to the concentration of mast cells in the skin and is generally not responsive to antihistamines or topical lotions.

EVALUATION AND TREATMENT Blood and laboratory findings, characterized by an absolute increase in red blood cells and in total blood volume, confirm the diagnosis. Erythrocytes appear normal, but anisocytosis may be present. There also may be moderate increases in white blood cells and platelets. A bone marrow examination may be done; however, it cannot definitively confirm the diagnosis. Treatment of PV consists of reducing red cell proliferation and blood volume, controlling symptoms, and preventing clogging and clotting of the blood vessels. Phlebotomy (approximately 300 to 500 ml) is used to reduce red cell mass and blood volume. Initial phlebotomies are done two to three times a week until hematocrit levels drop sufficiently and then are repeated every 3 to 4 months to maintain appropriate hematocrit levels (<45). Frequent phlebotomies also reduce iron levels, a condition that impedes erythropoiesis, but they also may contribute to the development of thrombosis; thus, use of phlebotomies needs to be individualized. Smokers are urged to quit smoking, and individuals with congestive heart failure and chronic obstructive pulmonary disease require appropriate drug intervention.

Radioactive phosphorus (^{32}P) also is used as an effective and easily tolerated intervention to suppress erythropoiesis. Its effects may last up to 18 months. Side effects of ^{32}P include suppression of hematopoiesis resulting in anemia, leukopenia, and thrombocytopenia. Acute leukemia is also a side effect, although most often it occurs only after 7 or more years of treatment, making its use in elderly persons more common. Hydroxyurea, a nonalkylating myelosuppressive, is the drug of choice for myelosuppression because of its reduced incidence of causing leukemia and thrombosis. Interferon is gaining popularity as an effective drug therapy because of its ability to inhibit growth of the abnormal clone, which diminishes the clinical and laboratory manifestations of myeloproliferation. Interferon use for this purpose is still new, and long-term effects are as yet unknown.

Without proper treatment, 50% of individuals with PV die within 18 months of the onset of initial symptoms because of thrombosis or hemorrhage. A significant potential outcome of PV is the conversion to acute myeloid leukemia (AML), occurring spontaneously in 10% of individuals and generally being resistant to conventional therapy. Conversion to AML is most likely related to treatment methods associated with cytotoxic myelosuppressive agents, chlorambucil, and busulfan. Although PV is a chronic disorder, appropriate therapy results in remissions and prevention of significant pathologic outcomes. Survival for 10 to 15 years is common.

ALTERATIONS OF LEUKOCYTE FUNCTION

Leukocyte function is affected if too many or too few white cells are present in the blood or if the cells that are present are structurally or functionally defective. Phagocytic cells (granulocytes, monocytes, macrophages) may lose their ability to act as effective phagocytes, and the lymphocytes may lose their ability to respond to antigens. (Disruptions of inflammatory and immune processes caused by leukocyte disorders are described in Chapter 7.) Other leukocyte alterations include infectious mononucleosis and cancers of the blood—leukemia and multiple myeloma.

Quantitative Alterations of Leukocytes

Quantitative alterations are increases or decreases in numbers of leukocytes in the blood. **Leukocytosis** is present when the count is higher than normal; **leukopenia** is present when the count is lower than normal. Leukocytosis and leukopenia may affect a specific type of white blood cell and may result from a variety of physiologic conditions and alterations.

Leukocytosis occurs as a normal protective response to physiologic stressors, such as invading microorganisms, strenuous exercise, emotional changes, temperature changes, anesthesia, surgery, pregnancy, and some drugs, hormones, and toxins. It also is caused by pathologic conditions, such as malignancies and hematologic disorders. Unlike leukocytosis, leukopenia is never normal. When the leukocyte count falls to less than 1000/mm^3, the risk of infection increases drastically. With counts below 500/mm^3, the possibility for life-threatening infections is high. Leukopenia may be caused by radiation, anaphylactic shock, autoimmune disease (e.g., systemic lupus erythematosus), immune deficiencies (see Chapter 7), and certain chemotherapeutic agents.

Granulocyte and monocyte alterations

Increased levels of circulating granulocytes (neutrophils, eosinophils, basophils) and monocytes are chiefly a physiologic response to microbial invasion. Increased numbers also occur as a result of myeloproliferative disorders (polycythemia vera, chronic myelocytic leukemia [CML]) that increase stem cell proliferation in the bone marrow.

Decreases occur when infectious processes deplete the supply of circulating granulocytes and monocytes, drawing them out of the circulation and into infected tissues faster than they can be replaced. Decreases also can be caused by disorders that suppress marrow function.

Granulocytosis—an increase in granulocytes (neutrophils, eosinophils, or basophils)—begins when stored blood cells are released. **Neutrophilia** is another term that may be used to describe *granulocytosis* because neutrophils are the most numerous of the granulocytes (Table 20-5). Neutrophilia is seen in the early stages of infection or inflammation and is established when the absolute count exceeds 7500/mm^3. Release and depletion of stored neutrophils stimulates granulopoiesis to replenish neutrophil reserves. Specific conditions associated with neutrophilia are identified in Table 20-5.

When the demand for circulating mature neutrophils exceeds the supply, immature neutrophils (and other leukocytes) are released from the bone marrow. Premature release of the immature cells is responsible for the phenomenon known as a **shift-to-the-left** or **leukemoid reaction.** This refers to the microscopic detection of disproportionate numbers of immature leukocytes in peripheral blood smears. To understand this phenomenon, visualize cellular differentiation, maturation, and release (see Figure 19-7) as progressing from left to right instead of vertically. The early release of immature white cells prevents the completion of the sequence and shifts the distribution of leukocytes in the blood toward those on the left side of the diagram. This phenomenon is also seen in the blood smear of individuals with leukemia, hence the term *leukemoid reaction.* As infection or inflammation diminishes, and granulopoiesis replenishes circulating granulocytes, a **shift-to-the-right,** or return to normal, occurs.

Neutropenia is a condition associated with a reduction in circulating neutrophils and exists clinically when the neutrophil count is less than 2000/mm^3. Reduction in neutrophils occurs in severe prolonged infections when production of granulocytes cannot keep up with demand.[8]

Other causes of neutropenia, in the absence of overwhelming infection may be (1) decreased neutrophil production or ineffective granulopoiesis, (2) reduced neutrophil survival, and (3) abnormal neutrophil distribution and sequestration. Hematologic disorders that cause ineffective or decreased production include hypoplastic or aplastic anemia, megaloblastic anemias, leukemia, or drug-/toxin-induced neutropenia. Neutropenia also is seen in starvation and anorexia nervosa because of an inadequate supply of protein building blocks. Decreased neutrophil survival is seen in autoimmune disorders (e.g., systemic

TABLE 20-5

Other Conditions Associated With Neutrophils, Eosinophils, Basophils, Monocytes, and Lymphocytes

Condition	Cause	Example
NEUTROPHIL		
Neutrophilia (granulocytosis)	Inflammation or tissue necrosis	Surgery, burns, MI, pneumonitis, rheumatic fever, rheumatoid arthritis
	Infection	Bacterial: gram-positive (staphylococci, streptococci, pneumococci), gram-negative *(Escherichia coli, Pseudomonas species)*
	Physiologic	Exercise, extreme heat or cold, third-trimester pregnancy, emotional distress
	Hematologic	Acute hemorrhage, hemolysis, myeloproliferative disorder, chronic granulocytic leukemia
	Drugs or chemicals	Epinephrine, steroids, heparin, histamine, endotoxin
	Metabolic	Diabetes (acidosis), eclampsia, gout, thyroid storm
	Neoplasm	Liver, GI tract, bone marrow
Neutropenia	Decreased marrow production	Radiation, chemotherapy, leukemia, aplastic anemia, abnormal granulopoiesis
	Increased destruction	Splenomegaly, hemodialysis, autoimmune disease
	Infection	Gram-negative (typhoid), viral (influenza, hepatitis B, measles, mumps, rubella), severe infections, protozoal infections (malaria)
EOSINOPHIL		
Eosinophilia	Allergy	Asthma, hay fever, drug sensitivity
	Infection	Parasites (trichinosis, hookworm), chronic (fungal, leprosy, TB)
	Malignancy	CML, lung, stomach, ovary, Hodgkin disease
	Dermatosis	Pemphigus, exfoliative dermatitis (drug-induced)
	Drugs	Digitalis, heparin, streptomycin, tryptophan (eosinophilia-myalgia syndrome), penicillins, propranolol
Eosinopenia	Stress response	Trauma, shock, burns, surgery, mental distress
	Drugs	Steroids (Cushing syndrome)
BASOPHIL		
Basophilia	Inflammation	Infection (measles, chickenpox), hypersensitivity reaction (immediate)
	Hematologic	Myeloproliferative disorders (CML, polycythemia vera, Hodgkin lymphoma, hemolytic anemia)
	Endocrine	Myxedema, antithyroid therapy
Basopenia	Physiologic	Pregnancy, ovulation, stress
	Endocrine	Graves disease
MONOCYTE		
Monocytosis	Infection	Bacterial (subacute bacterial endocarditis, TB), recovery phase of infection
	Hematologic	Myeloproliferative disorders, Hodgkin disease, agranulocytosis
	Physiologic	Normal newborn
Monocytopenia	Rare	
LYMPHOCYTE		
Lymphocytosis	Physiologic	4 mo to 4 yr
	Acute infection	Infectious mononucleosis, CMV infection, pertussis, hepatitis, mycoplasma pneumonia, typhoid
	Chronic infection	Congenital syphilis, tertiary syphilis
	Endocrine	Thyrotoxicosis, adrenal insufficiency
	Malignancy	ALL, CLL, lymphosarcoma cell leukemia
Lymphocytopenia	Immunodeficiency syndrome	AIDS, agammaglobulinemia
	Lymphocyte destruction	Steroids (Cushing syndrome), radiation, chemotherapy
		Hodgkin lymphoma
		CHF, renal failure, TB, SLE, aplastic anemia

MI, Myocardial infarction, *GI,* gastrointestinal; *CML,* chronic myelogenous leukemia; *TB,* tuberculosis, *CMV,* cytomegalovirus; *ALL,* acute lymphocytic leukemia; *CLL,* chronic lymphocytic leukemia; *AIDS,* acquired immunodeficiency syndrome; *CHF,* congestive (left) heart failure; *SLE,* systemic lupus erythematosus.

lupus erythematosus, rheumatoid arthritis). Abnormal neutrophil distribution and sequestration are associated with hypersplenism and a pseudoneutropenia, which in the presence of rheumatoid arthritis constitute Felty syndrome. Viral infections (human immunodeficiency virus [HIV], Epstein-Barr virus [EBV]) also may cause neutropenia, as does chemotherapy and other toxic drugs received for cancer treatment and transplantation.

If neutrophils are drastically reduced (<500/mm^3) and the entire granulocyte count is extremely low, **granulocytopenia** or **agranulocytosis** results. Usually, when this occurs, hematopoiesis is arrested in the bone marrow or cell destruction increases in the circulation. Chemotherapeutic agents used to treat hematologic and other malignancies cause bone marrow suppression. Several other drugs cause agranulocytosis, which occurs rarely but carries a high mortality rate of 10% to 48%. Clinical manifestations of agranulocytosis include infection (particularly of the respiratory system), general malaise, septicemia, fever, tachycardia, and ulcers in the mouth and colon. If untreated, sepsis results in death within 3 to 6 days. Other conditions associated with neutropenia are identified in Table 20-5.

Eosinophilia is an absolute increase (>450/mm^3) in the total number of circulating eosinophils. Allergic disorders (type 1) associated with asthma, hay fever, and drug reactions often cause eosinophilia. Hypersensitivity reactions trigger the release of eosinophilic chemotaxic factor of anaphylaxis (ECF-A) and histamine from mast cells, attracting eosinophils to the area. Areas with abundant mast cells, such as the respiratory and GI tracts, are commonly affected. Eosinophilia also may occur in dermatologic disorders, eosinophilia-myalgia syndrome, and parasitic invasion. Other conditions that cause eosinophilia are detailed in Table 20-5.

Eosinopenia, a decrease in circulating eosinophils, generally is caused by migration of eosinophils into inflammatory sites. It may be seen in Cushing syndrome and as a result of stress caused by surgery, shock, trauma, burns, or mental distress. Other conditions that cause eosinopenia are detailed in Table 20-5.

Basophilia is a response to inflammation and immediate hypersensitivity reactions. Basophils contain histamine that is released during an allergic reaction. Increased basophils are seen in myeloproliferative disorders, such as chronic myeloid leukemia and myeloid metaplasia. Other conditions that are associated with basophilia are listed in Table 20-5.

Basopenia is seen in hyperthyroidism, acute infection, and long-term therapy with steroids. Other conditions associated with basopenia are listed in Table 20-5.

Monocytosis, an increase in monocytes, is often transient and correlates poorly with disease states. It is usually associated with neutropenia during bacterial infections, particularly in the late stages or recovery stage, when monocytes are needed to phagocytize surviving microorganisms and debris. Increased monocytes also may indicate marrow recovery from agranulocytosis. Monocytosis is often seen in chronic infections such as tuberculosis (TB) and subacute bacterial endocarditis (SBE), and it has been found to correlate with the extent of myocardial damage following myocardial infarctions. Other conditions associated with monocytosis are identified in Table 20-5. **Monocytopenia,** a decrease in monocytes, is rare but has been identified with hairy cell leukemia and prednisone therapy.

Lymphocyte alterations

Quantitative alterations of lymphocytes occur when lymphocytes are activated by antigenic stimuli, usually microorganisms (see Chapter 6). **Lymphocytosis** is rare in acute bacterial infections and is seen most commonly in acute viral infections, particularly those caused by the Epstein-Barr virus (EBV)—a causative agent in infectious mononucleosis. Other specific disorders associated with lymphocytosis are listed in Table 20-5.

Lymphocytopenia may be attributed to (1) abnormalities of lymphocyte production associated with neoplasias and immune deficiencies and (2) destruction by drugs, viruses, or radiation. It is also known to occur without any detectable cause. Conditions associated with lymphocytopenia are identified in Table 20-5. The lymphocytopenia associated with heart failure and other acute illnesses may be caused by elevated levels of cortisol. The most recent condition in which lymphocytopenia is a major problem is acquired immunodeficiency syndrome (AIDS). AIDS-related lymphocytopenia is caused by HIV, which destroys T-helper lymphocytes. (For a detailed discussion of AIDS, see Chapter 7.)

Infectious mononucleosis

Infectious mononucleosis (IM) is an acute infection of B lymphocytes (B cells) with Epstein-Barr virus (EBV).[9] Infections with EBV are common in children, particularly those from low socioeconomic environments. Approximately 50% to 85% of these children are infected with EBV by age 4, and more than 90% of adults have indications of exposure to EBV. These early infections are usually asymptomatic and provide immunity to EBV, thus children with an early infection rarely develop IM. Mononucleosis may arise when the initial infection with EBV occurs during adolescence or later, but it results in mononucleosis in only 35% to 50% of these individuals.

The incidence of IM is approximately 45 in 10,000 individuals and is most commonly seen in young adults between 15 and 35 years of age, with the peak incidence between 15 and 19 years. It is rarely seen in individuals over 40 years, and when it does occur, is more commonly caused by cytomegalovirus (CMV).

Transmission of EBV is usually through saliva from close personal contact (e.g., kissing, hence the term *kissing disease*). The virus also may be secreted in other mucosal secretions of the genital, rectal, and respiratory tract, as well as blood. Transmission through sneezing or coughing has not been documented. The infection begins with widespread invasion of the B lymphocytes, which have receptors for EBV. The virus initial infects the oropharynx, nasopharynx, and salivary epithelial cells with later extension into lymphoid tissues and B cells.

Unaffected B cells produce antibodies (IgG, IgA, IgM) against the virus. Cytotoxic T lymphocytes (Tc cells) are activated and multiply to assist the B cells in attacking the virus and virus-infected cells directly (see Chapter 6). The production of B and T cells and the process of removing dead and damaged leukocytes are largely responsible for lymphoid tissue swelling (lymph nodes, spleen, tonsils, and occasionally, liver). Sore throat and fever, two initial manifestations of IM, are caused by inflammation and infection at the site of initial viral entry—the mouth and throat.

CLINICAL MANIFESTATIONS The incubation period for IM is approximately 30 to 50 days. Early flulike symptoms, such as headache, malaise, joint pain, and fatigue, may appear during the first 3 to 5 days, although some individuals are without symptoms. At the time of diagnosis, the individual commonly presents with the classic group of symptoms: fever, sore throat, cervical lymph node enlargement, and fatigue. As the condition progresses, generalized lymph node enlargement also may develop as well as enlargement of the spleen and liver (25% to 75% of individuals). Splenic rupture is rare and can occur spontaneously or as a result of mild trauma, occurring primarily in males (90%) between day 4 and day 21 after symptom onset. It is the most common cause of death related to IM. Other causes of the rare fatalities associated with IM are hepatic failure, extensive bacterial infection, or viral myocarditis. Other organ systems are rarely involved, but such involvement may be present with characteristic manifestations, such as fulminant hepatitis with jaundice and anemia, encephalitis, meningitis, Guillain-Barré syndrome, and Bell palsy. Eye manifestations may include eyelid and periorbital edema, dry eyes, keratitis, uveitis, and conjunctivitis. Pulmonary involvement is rare, although incidences of pneumonia and respiratory failure have been documented in immunocompromised individuals. Reye syndrome has been known to develop in children with EBV infection.

IM is usually self-limiting, and recovery occurs in a few weeks; severe clinical complications are rare (5%). Fatigue may last for 1 to 2 months after resolution of other symptoms.

EVALUATION AND TREATMENT The blood of affected individuals contains an increased number of white blood cells with many atypical forms. Serologic tests to determine a heterophile antibody response are necessary to diagnose EBV infection.[10] Heterophilic antibodies are a heterogenous group of IgM antibodies that are agglutinins against nonhuman red blood cells (e.g., horse, sheep) and are detected by qualitative (monospot) or quantitative (heterophile antibody test) methods. Use of the monospot test is limited because other infections (e.g., CMV, adenovirus) and toxoplasmosis also produce heterophilic antibodies. Thus, 5% to 15% of monospot tests yield false-positive results. Heterophilic antibodies in the blood increase as the condition progresses, although some individuals and children under 4 years of age do not produce them. Diagnosis of EBV infection specifically may be increased with newer viral-specific tests that identify EBV-specific antibodies. These tests are more expensive and labor intensive so are reserved for instances when the monospot is not appropriate.

Treatment is supportive and consists of rest and alleviation of symptoms with analgesics and antipyretics. Aspirin is avoided with children because of its association with Reye syndrome. Streptococcal pharyngitis, which occurs in 20% to 30% of cases, is treated with penicillin or erythromycin, not ampicillin—ampicillin is known to cause a rash. Bed rest with avoidance of strenuous activity and contact sports is indicated. Steroids are used when severe complications, such as impending airway obstruction or other organ involvement (central nervous system [CNS] manifestations, thrombocytopenic purpura, myocarditis, pericarditis), is evident. Acyclovir has been used in immunocompromised individuals but is not considered standard therapy. IM and EBV infection were thought to be associated with chronic fatigue syndrome, but that is no longer the case.

QUICK CHECK 20-2

1. Explain the relationship between the early release of premature white blood cells and a "shift-to-the-left."
2. What is meant by "shift-to-the-right"?

Qualitative Alterations of Leukocytes

Leukemias

Leukemia is a clonal malignant disorder of the blood and blood-forming organs.[11] The common pathologic feature of all forms of leukemia is an uncontrolled proliferation of malignant leukocytes, causing an overcrowding of bone marrow and decreased production and function of normal hematopoietic cells.

The classification of leukemia is based on (1) the predominant cell of origin (either myeloid or lymphoid) and (2) the degree of differentiation that took place before the cell became malignant (acute, with a rapid growth of immature blood cells, or chronic, with a slow growth of more differentiated cells) (Figure 20-6). Thus, there are four types of leukemia: acute lymphocytic (ALL) or myelogenous (AML) and chronic lymphocytic (CLL) or myelogenous (CML).[12,13] Further classification of acute leukemias is based on characteristics that may provide significant therapeutic prognostic information, such as structure, number of cells, genetics, identification of surface markers, and histochemical staining.

Acute leukemia is characterized by undifferentiated or immature cells, usually a **blast cell.** The onset of disease is abrupt and rapid. Disease progression results in a short survival time. In chronic leukemia, the predominant cell is more mature but does not function normally. The onset of the disease is gradual, and the prolonged clinical course results in a relatively longer survival time.

Leukemia occurs with varying frequencies at different ages and is more common in adults than in children. It is estimated that more than 44,000 cases of leukemia will be newly diagnosed in 2007, with males having a slightly

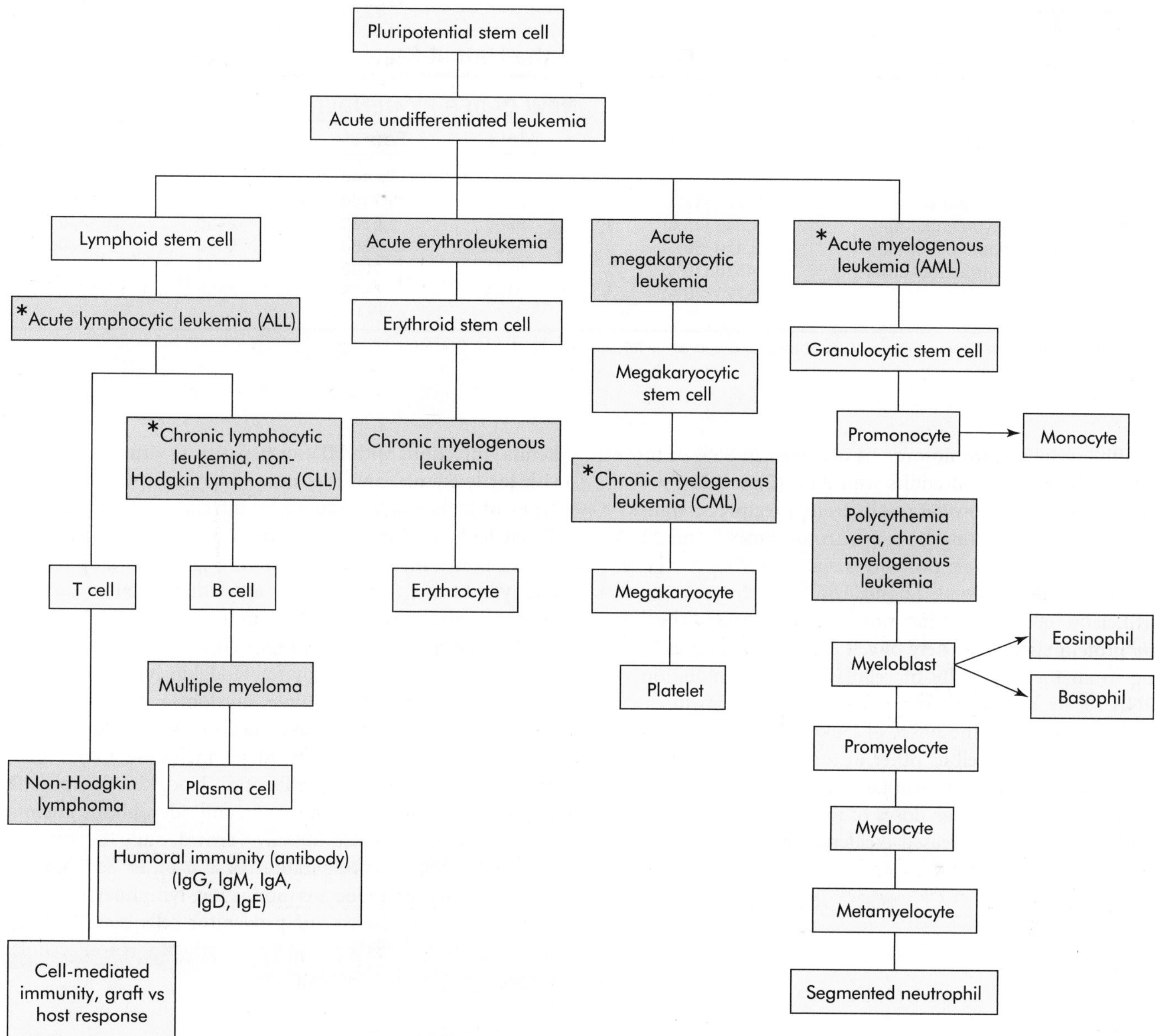

Figure 20-6 ■ **Cell-Specific Leukemias.** Differentiation pathways of blood-forming cells and reported sites of blockage resulting in cell-specific leukemias. *Ig,* Immunoglobulin.

higher incidence than females (Table 20-6). ALL is the least common type (12% of all leukemias) overall, but it is the most common in children. Leukemia accounts for about 30% of all childhood cancers; ALL accounts for almost 78% of all new cases of leukemia in children. CLL and AML (35% and 30% of leukemias, respectively) are the most common types in adults. CML (13% of leukemias) is found mostly in adults. The sites of highest overall incidence are the United States, Canada, Sweden, and New Zealand.

Over the past 2 decades, remission induction rate and survival in most forms of leukemia have increased. Current survival rates range from 20% for AML to 73% for CLL. This progress is the result of more effective chemotherapeutic agents, improved blood product and antimicrobial support, and specialized nursing care. Chemotherapy and bone marrow transplants have significantly increased the survival time for individuals with acute leukemia.

PATHOPHYSIOLOGY Although the exact cause of leukemia is unknown, several risk factors and related genetic aberrations are associated with the onset of malignancy. There is a statistically significant tendency for leukemia to reappear in families. There is also an increased incidence of leukemia in association with other hereditary abnormalities such as Down syndrome, Fanconi aplastic anemia, Bloom syndrome, trisomy 13, Patau syndrome, and some immune deficiencies (ataxia-telangiectasia, Wiskott-Aldrich syndrome, congenital X-linked agammaglobulinemia; see Chapter 7).

Several genetic translocations (mitotic errors) are observed in leukemic cells. One of these translocations,

TABLE 20-6

Estimated New Cases and Deaths from Leukemia in the United States—2007

Types of Leukemia	Total New Cases (Proportion of New Cases)	NEW CASES BY GENDER Male	NEW CASES BY GENDER Female	DEATHS BY GENDER Male	DEATHS BY GENDER Female
All types	44,240 (100%)	24,800	19,440	12,320	9470
Acute lymphocytic leukemia	5200 (12%)	3060	2140	820	600
Chronic lymphocytic leukemia	15,340 (35%)	8960	6380	2560	1940
Acute myelogenous leukemia	13,410 (30%)	7060	6350	5020	3970
Chronic myelogenous leukemia	4570 (10%)	2570	2000	240	250
Other	5720 (13%)	3150	2570	3680	2710

Data from American Cancer Society: *Cancer facts and figures—2007*, Atlanta, 2007, The Society.

the Philadelphia chromosome, is observed in 95% of those with CML and 30% of adults with ALL (Figure 20-7). The Philadelphia chromosome results from a reciprocal translocation between the long arms of chromosomes 9 and 22. A unique protein (*bcr-abl* protein) is encoded from two genes (*BCR* from chromosome 22 and *ABL* from chromosome 9) artificially linked at the junction of translocation. The *bcr-abl* protein affects a variety of cell cycle control genes leading to an increased rate of cellular division, inhibition of DNA repair, and other dysregulations of cell growth.

Risk factors for the onset of leukemia include environmental factors as well as other diseases. Increased risk has been linked to cigarette smoke, exposure to benzene, and ionizing radiation. Large doses of ionizing radiation particularly result in an increased incidence of myelogenous leukemia. Infections with HIV or hepatitis C virus increase the risk for leukemia, and it is now widely accepted that some types of leukemia are caused by infection with the human T-cell leukemia/lymphoma virus-1 (HTLV-1). Drugs that cause bone marrow depression (e.g., chloramphenicol, phenylbutazone, and certain alkylating agents, such as cytoxan) also can predispose an individual to leukemia. AML is the most frequently reported secondary cancer after high doses of chemotherapy for Hodgkin lymphoma, non-Hodgkin lymphoma, multiple myeloma, ovarian cancer, and breast cancer. Acute leukemia also may develop secondary to certain acquired disorders, including CML, CLL, polycythemia vera, myelofibrosis, Hodgkin lymphoma, multiple myeloma, ovarian cancer, and sideroblastic anemia.

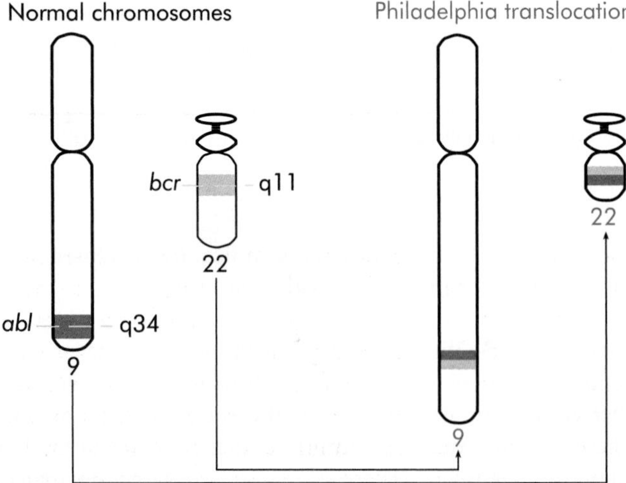

Figure 20-7 ■ Philadelphia Chromosome. Schema of the Philadelphia (Ph) translocation (+) seen in chronic myelocytic leukemia. The Ph^1 chromosome results from an exchange of materials between chromosomes 9 and 22—that is, t(9;22)(q34;q11). Because chromosome 22 gives up much more of its long arm than that translocated to it from chromosome 9, chromosome 22 becomes much abbreviated and is known as Ph^1. (From Damjanov I, Linder J, editors: *Anderson's pathology,* ed 10, St Louis, 1996, Mosby.)

The leukemia blasts literally "crowd out" the marrow and cause cellular proliferation of the other cell lines to cease. Normal granulocytic-monocytic, lymphocytic, erythrocytic, and megakaryocytic progenitor cells cease to function, resulting in **pancytopenia** (a reduction in all cellular components of the blood).

Acute leukemias

About 85% of ALL arise from the B cell line, and about 15% arise from T cell lineage. A small percentage of ALL cases have neither B nor T cell origination and are called *null cell.* Acute leukemias are seen in both genders and in all ages, with the incidence increasing dramatically in individuals older than 50 years. Mortality for all acute leukemias in the United States is about 7 per 100,000. In children younger than 15 years, leukemia accounts for a third of all deaths from cancer. North American and Scandinavian countries have the highest mortality; Eastern European countries, Asia (except Japan), and Central America have the lowest mortality. Japan's higher mortality is the result of the atomic bombs dropped in World War II. Blacks have consistently shown a lower mortality than whites.

CLINICAL MANIFESTATIONS The clinical manifestations of all varieties of acute leukemia are generally similar. Mechanisms associated with common manifestations are summarized in Table 20-7. Signs and symptoms related to bone marrow depression include fatigue caused by anemia,

TABLE 20-7

Clinical Manifestations and Related Pathophysiology in Leukemia

Clinical Manifestations	Laboratory Abnormalities	Cause	Comments
Anemia	Key is the relative *proportion* of erythroblasts to total count (decreased in anemia)	Decreased stem cell input or ineffective erythropoiesis or both	In acute leukemia, anemia is usually present from the beginning, often the first symptom noticed, and severe; mild form without symptoms is common in CML and CLL; hemorrhage common in acute forms, occasional in CML, but rare in CLL
Bleeding (purpura, petechiae, ecchymosis, hemorrhage)	Decreased and possibly abnormal platelets	Reduction in megakaryocytes leading to thrombocytopenia	Bleeding more common in acute than in chronic leukemia
Infection	Increased multisegmented neutrophils	Opportunistic organisms; decreased protection resulting from granulocytopenia or immune deficiency secondary to chemotherapy, corticosteroids, and the disease process	Major sites of infection: oral cavity, throat, lower colon, urinary tract, lungs, and skin; prevention of infection focuses on restoration of host defenses, decreasing invasive procedures, and reducing colonization of organisms
Weight loss	Decreased 24-hr urinary creatinine excretion; hypoalbuminemia	Condition can be attributed to pain, depression, chemotherapy, radiation therapy, loss of appetite, and alterations in taste	Severe weight loss may be related to excess production of TNFα
Bone pain	Often no radiographic evidence of bone problems	Result of bone infiltration by leukemic cells or intramedullary infection	If combination drug regimens are ineffective, radiation therapy is used
Liver, spleen, and lymph node enlargement	Biopsy abnormal for liver and spleen	Leukemic cell infiltration; lymph nodes also undergo leukemia proliferation in CLL	
Elevated uric acid	Normal excretion of uric acid is 300–500 mg/day; the leukemic individual can excrete 50 times more	Increased catabolism of protein and nucleic acid; urate precipitation increased from dehydration caused by anorexia or fever and drug therapy	Hyperuricemia is present in both acute leukemia and CML; increasing urine pH or decreasing acid production with the drug allopurinol

RBC, Red blood cell; *CML,* chronic myelocytic leukemia; *CLL,* chronic lymphocytic leukemia.

bleeding resulting from thrombocytopenia, and fever caused by infection. Bleeding may occur in the skin, gums, mucous membranes, and GI tracts. Visible signs include petechiae and ecchymosis, as well as discoloration of the skin, gingival bleeding, hematuria, and midcycle or heavy menstrual bleeding.

Infection sites include the mouth, throat, respiratory tract, lower colon, urinary tract, and skin and may be caused by gram-negative bacilli (*Escherichia coli*), *Pseudomonas*, and *Klebsiella*. Fever is an early sign often accompanied by chills.

Anorexia is accompanied by weight loss, diminished sensitivity to sour and sweet tastes, wasting of muscle, and difficulty swallowing. Liver, spleen, and lymph node enlargement occurs more commonly in ALL than in CML. Liver and spleen enlargement commonly occur together. The leukemic individual often experiences abdominal pain and tenderness and also breast tenderness.

Neurologic manifestations are common and may be caused by either leukemic infiltration or cerebral bleeding. Headache, vomiting, papilledema, facial palsy, blurred vision, auditory disturbances, and meningeal irritation can occur if leukemic cells infiltrate the cerebral or spinal meninges. Because chemotherapeutic agents do not penetrate the blood-brain barrier, leukemia cells can grow easily in these locations.

EVALUATION AND TREATMENT Because leukemia often is confused with other conditions, early detection is difficult. Persistent symptoms need intensive medical investigation. The diagnosis is made through blood tests and examination of bone marrow.

Chemotherapy, used in various combinations, is the treatment of choice for leukemia. Supportive measures include blood transfusions, antibiotics, antifungals, and antivirals. Allopurinol is used to prevent uric acid production and elevation that occurs because of cellular death caused by treatment. Bone marrow transplantation as a treatment has increased since the 1980s. Survival rates have dramatically increased because of improvements in donor matching, transfusion support, conditioning regimens, and antibiotics.

The 5-year survival rate for those with leukemia is 38%, largely because of poor survival rates of individuals with certain types of leukemia (e.g., acute myelogenous). Since the 1970s, 5-year survival rates for those with ALL have increased from 38% to 65% for adults and from 53% to 85% for children. Factors influencing increased survival rate include the use of combined and multimodality treatment methods, improved supportive services such as blood banking and nutritional support, and antimicrobial treatment. The presence of the Philadelphia chromosome (observed in about 5% of children with ALL, in 30% of adults with ALL, and occasionally in AML) is a poor prognostic indicator.

Stimulation of blood cell growth and development with hematopoietic drugs has increased neutrophil recovery during chemotherapy and bone marrow transplant. Blood granulocyte numbers (e.g., eosinophils, neutrophils, basophils/mast cells) are normally in the range of 4000 to 6000 cells/μl, and susceptibility to infection develops below 1000 cells/μl. During a natural response to a bacterial infection, granulocytes usually rise in number to 10,000 to 20,000 cells/μl. Leukemia itself as well as the chemotherapeutic agents used to treat the disease can result in dramatic decreases in circulating granulocytes. The administration of colony-stimulating factors (CSFs) can raise white cell numbers and afford protection from infections (Table 20-8).

Chronic leukemias

The two main types of chronic leukemia are (1) myelogenous (CML) and (2) lymphocytic (CLL). Several forms of CML can occur, depending on the lineage of the malignant cells (e.g., chronic neutrophilic leukemia [CNL], chronic eosinophilic leukemia [CEL]). Unlike cells in acute leukemia, chronic leukemic cells are well differentiated and can be readily identified. Individuals with chronic leukemia have a longer life expectancy, usually extending several years from the time of diagnosis.

The chronic leukemias account for the majority of cases in adults (see Table 20-6). The incidences of CLL and CML increase significantly in individuals over 40 years of age, with prevalence in the sixth through eighth decades. CML is a group of diseases called *myeloproliferative disorders,* which also include polycythemia vera, primary thrombocytosis, and idiopathic myelofibrosis (invasion of bone marrow by fibrous tissue).

PATHOPHYSIOLOGY AND CLINICAL MANIFESTATIONS Chronic leukemia advances slowly and insidiously. Individuals are generally unaware of the condition until symptoms appear. When symptoms do appear, they present as splenomegaly, extreme fatigue, weight loss, night sweats, and low-grade fever. Individuals with CML may progress through three phases of the disease; a chronic phase lasting 2 to 5 years during which symptoms may not be apparent, an accelerated phase of 6 to 18 months during which the primary symptoms develop, and a terminal blast phase with a survival of only 3 to 6 months. The accelerated phase is characterized by excessive proliferation and accumulation

TABLE 20-8

Some Examples of Human CSFs

CSF	Cell Origin	Cell Stimulated
M-CSF	Macrophage, fibroblast	Macrophage
GM-CSF	T cell, macrophage, fibroblast	Neutrophil, monocyte, macrophage, eosinophil
G-CSF	Macrophage, fibroblast	Neutrophil, eosinophil, basophil
IL-3	T cell	Neutrophil, macrophage
Erythropoietin	Kupffer and peritubular kidney cells	Erythrocyte

Morphologic Effects of Growth Factor. Marrow aspirate from a patient receiving granulocyte colony-stimulating factor (G-CSF) showing an early neutrophil response. There is a marked shift toward immaturity in the neutrophils with the majority at the promyelocyte and early myelocyte stages of maturation. (Wright-Giemsa stain.) (Courtesy Laura Schmitz, MD, Hennepin County Medical Center, Minn. From Damjanov I, Linder J, editors: *Anderson's pathology,* ed 10, St Louis, 1996, Mosby.)

of malignant cells. Splenomegaly is prominent and more painful, but lymphadenopathy generally is not present. Liver enlargement also occurs, but liver function is rarely altered. Hyperuricemia is common and produces gouty arthritis. Infections, fever, and weight loss also are seen often. The terminal blast phase is characterized by rapid and progressive leukocytosis with an increase in basophils. In the later stages of the terminal phase, which then resembles AML, blast cells or promyelocytes predominate, and the individual experiences a "blast crisis."

The Philadelphia chromosome is a useful diagnostic marker for CML and is observed in 95% of individuals with CML. The median age for persons with Philadelphia chromosome-positive CML is 40 to 45 years. The Philadelphia chromosome, although present in red cells, white cells, and platelets, appears to affect only white cell function and production. Although it is difficult to identify alterations within the cell's structure, absent or low levels of the enzyme neutrophil alkaline phosphatase, along with decreased phagocytic capabilities, indicate that cells fail to differentiate normally. There is no known specific cause for CML except exposure to ionizing radiation.

CLL involves predominantly malignant transformation of B cells; rarely (<5%) are T cells involved. The malignant transformation is thought to be caused by failure of the normal mechanisms of programmed cell destruction (apoptosis), allowing these cells to have an extended life, thus the chronic nature of the disease. These cells fail to develop into antibody-producing cells and fail to respond to stimulation by helper T cells.

Suppression of normal antibody production is the most significant effect in CLL. Individuals are thus at risk for recurrent bacterial and other infections that are commonly sensitive to antibodies. Anemia, thrombocytopenia, and neutropenia are typically present with overt CLL. Invasion of most organs by leukemic cells is uncommon, but infiltration of lymph nodes, liver, spleen, and salivary glands is observed. Central nervous system involvement and elevated blood levels of calcium are rare, whereas elevated levels of lactic dehydrogenase (LDH) and uric acid are common.

EVALUATION AND TREATMENT Therapeutic approaches include bone marrow transplantation, biologic response modifiers, and combination chemotherapy. Alone, state-of-the-art chemotherapy for CML does not cure the disease, prevent blastic transformation, or prolong the average survival time. New drugs, including Imatinib mesylate, which is highly specific for CML, are being utilized. Bone marrow transplantation, when compared with biologic response modifiers and combination chemotherapy, appears to increase the survival time more significantly. Allogeneic bone marrow transplant survival rates increase 20% to 30% with concurrent high-dose radiation, chemotherapy, and interferon therapy.

When to begin treatment for CLL is difficult to determine and is related to the degree of symptoms. Treatment consists of alkylating agent or purine analog chemotherapy. Steroids and, later, splenectomy also may be used to control leukocytosis and cytopenias. Radiation therapy may be used to alleviate lymphadenopathy. Late stages of the disease require combination chemotherapy. Regardless of the approach, cure rates for CLL are poor.

QUICK CHECK 20-3

1. How are leukemias classified?
2. What is the pathogenesis of ALL?
3. What is the significance of the Philadelphia chromosome, and how is it related to leukemia?

ALTERATIONS OF LYMPHOID FUNCTION

Lymphadenopathy

Lymphadenopathy is characterized by enlarged lymph nodes (Figure 20-8). Lymph node enlargement is caused by an increase in size and number of its germinal centers caused by proliferation of lymphocytes and monocytes (immature phagocytes) or invasion by malignant cells.

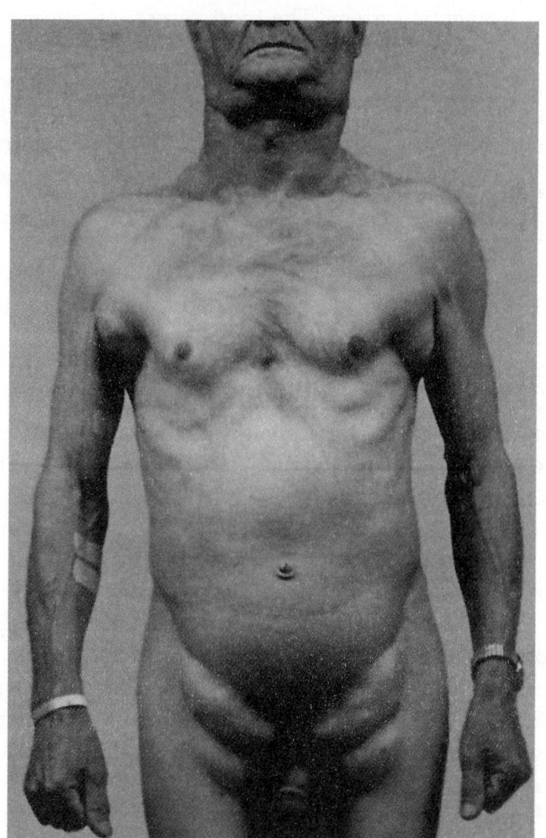

Figure 20-8 ■ **Lymphadenopathy.** Individual with lymphocyte leukemia with extreme but symmetric lymphadenopathy. (Courtesy Dr. AR Kagan, Los Angeles. From del Regato JA, Spjut HJ, Cox JD: *Cancer: diagnosis, treatment, and prognosis,* ed 6, St Louis, 1985, Mosby.)

Normally, lymph nodes are not palpable or are barely palpable. Enlarged lymph nodes are characterized by being palpable and often also may be tender or painful to touch, although not in all situations.

Localized lymphadenopathy (reactive lymph nodes) usually indicates drainage of an area associated with an inflammatory or infectious lesion. Generalized lymphadenopathy, associated with infection, occurs less often and is generally seen in the presence of malignant or nonmalignant disease. Lymphadenopathy is of more significance in adult disease than in children. The location and size of the enlarged nodes are important factors in diagnosing the cause of the lymphadenopathy, as are the individual's age, gender, and geographic location. Generalized lymphadenopathy occurs with non-Hodgkin lymphomas, chronic lymphocytic leukemia, histiocytosis, and disorders that produce lymphocytosis. In general, lymphadenopathy results from four types of conditions: (1) neoplastic disease, (2) immunologic or inflammatory conditions, (3) endocrine disorders, or (4) lipid storage diseases. Diseases of unknown cause, including autoimmune diseases and reactions to drugs, also may lead to generalized lymphadenopathy.

Malignant Lymphomas

Lymphomas consist of a diverse group of neoplasms that develop from the proliferation of malignant lymphocytes in the lymphatic system. The most recent classification of lymphomas was published by the World Health Organization (WHO) and is derived from the Revised European-American Lymphoma (REAL) Classification. This classification is based on the cell type from which the lymphoma probably originated. The groups include Hodgkin lymphoma and two that were previously classified as non-Hodgkin lymphoma (B-cell neoplasms, T-cell and NK-cell neoplasms). With the new classification, multiple myeloma, which was previously classified independently, is included as a B-cell lymphoma.

Incidence rates of lymphoma differ with respect to age, gender, geographic location, and socioeconomic class. The estimated new cases of lymphoma, including multiple myeloma, for 2007 are approximately 91,280 individuals. These consist of 8190 cases of Hodgkin lymphoma, 63,190 cases of non-Hodgkin lymphoma (except multiple myeloma), and 19,900 cases of multiple myeloma. It is estimated that about 30,520 people will have died from these diseases in 2007. Since the early 1970s, the incidence of non-Hodgkin lymphoma has nearly doubled. The exact reason for this increase remains a mystery; however, a modest portion of the increase had been attributed to lymphomas developing in association with immune deficiencies, including AIDS and organ transplants. Conversely, the incidence of Hodgkin lymphoma has declined over the same time period, especially among elderly persons. In children under 15 years, Hodgkin lymphoma accounts for about 4.3% of childhood cancer and non-Hodgkin lymphoma for 4.0%. Currently the 5-year survival rates for children are 79% for all childhood cancers and 96% for Hodgkin lymphoma.

Hodgkin lymphoma

PATHOPHYSIOLOGY **Hodgkin lymphoma (HL)** is characterized by its progression from one group of lymph nodes to another, the development of systemic symptoms, and the presence of **Reed-Sternberg (RS) cells** (Figure 20-9).[14] It is widely accepted that the RS cell represents the malignant transformation of lymph cells.[15] The RS cells are often large and binucleate, with occasional mononuclear variants. The RS cells are necessary for the diagnosis of HL; however, they are not specific to HL. In rare instances, cells resembling them can be found in benign illnesses, as well as in other forms of cancer, including non-Hodgkin lymphomas and solid tissue cancers and in infectious mononucleosis.

A

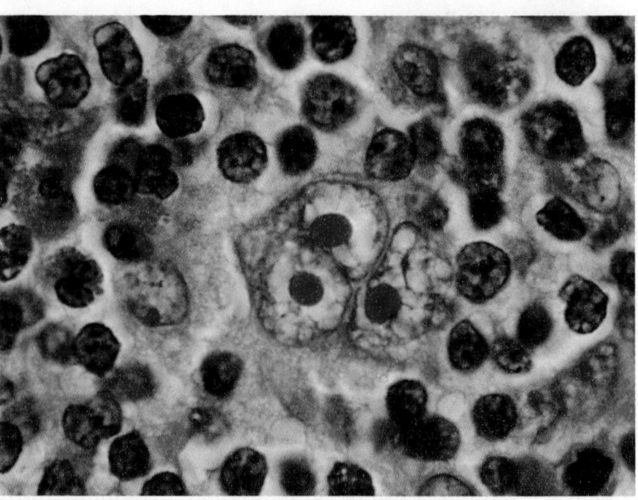

B

Figure 20-9 ■ **Lymph Nodes. A,** Lymphocytes and histiocytes of Hodgkin lymphoma, nodular type. Large nodules with small, round lymphocytes, histiocytes, and scattered lymphocyte and histiocyte cells. **B,** Diagnostic Reed-Sternberg cell. A large multinucleated or multilobed cell with inclusion body-like nucleoli surrounded by a halo of clear nucleoplasm. (From Damjanov I, Linder J, editors, *Anderson's pathology,* ed 10, St Louis, 1996, Mosby.)

The incidence of HL is approximately 3.0/100,000 males and 2.6/100,000 females and peaks at two different times—during the second and third decades of life and later during the sixth and seventh decades. The incidence is greater in whites than blacks, with Denmark, the Netherlands, and the United States having the highest incidence and Japan and Australia having the lowest. The overall incidence is lower in economically disadvantaged countries, although a greater proportion of HL is observed in the elderly in those countries.

The triggering mechanism for the malignant transformation of cells remains unknown. Classical HL appears to be derived from a B cell in the germinal center that has not undergone successful immunoglobulin gene rearrangement (see Chapter 6) and would normally be induced to undergo apoptosis. Survival of this cell may be linked to infection with Epstein-Barr virus (EBV). Laboratory and epidemiologic studies have linked HL with EBV infections and EBV DNA, RNA, and proteins are frequently observed in HL cells.[16] The RS cells secrete and release cytokines (e.g., IL-10, TGF-β) that result in the accumulation of inflammatory cells that produces the local and systemic effects. Classical HL is subclassified into four types (Table 20-9) based on the morphology of RS cells, and the characteristics of the inflammatory cell infiltrate in the tumor.

CLINICAL MANIFESTATIONS Many clinical features of HL can be explained by the complex action of cytokines and other growth factors that are secreted and released by the malignant cells. These substances induce infiltration and proliferation of inflammatory cell, resulting in an enlarged, painless lymph node in the neck (often the first sign of HL) (Figure 20-10). The discovery of an asymptomatic mediastinal mass on routine chest x-ray is not uncommon. The cervical, axillary, inguinal, and retroperitoneal lymph nodes are commonly affected in HL (Figure 20-11). Local symptoms caused by pressure and obstruction of the lymph nodes are the result of the lymphadenopathy.

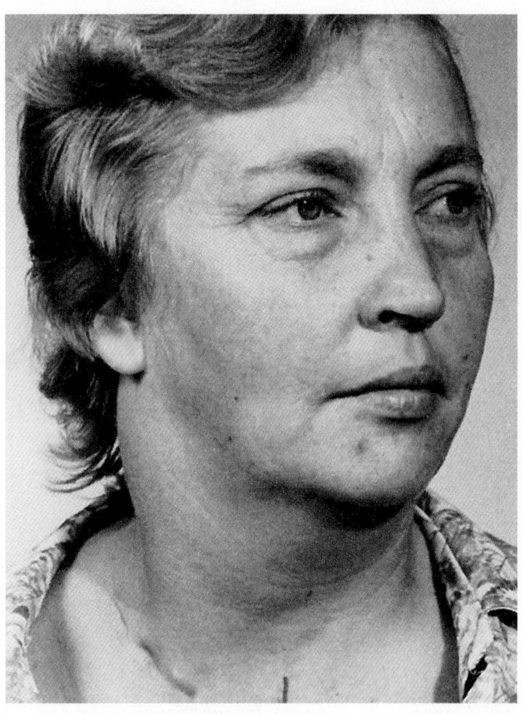

Figure 20-10 ■ Hodgkin Lymphoma and Enlarged Cervical Lymph Node. Typical enlarged cervical lymph node in the neck of a 35-year-old woman with Hodgkin lymphoma. (From del Regato JA, Spjut HJ, Cox JD: *Cancer: diagnosis, treatment, and prognosis,* ed 6, St Louis, 1985, Mosby.)

TABLE 20-9
Subtypes of Classical Hodgkin Lymphoma

Subtype	Incidence	Presentation
Nodular sclerosis HL	Most common subtype in developing countries Found in all ages but most common in adolescents and young adults (median age of onset is about 28 years) Incidence in females exceeds that in males	Large tumor nodules with RS cells surrounded by collagen and fibrous bands
Mixed cellularity HL	Second most common subtype Incidence in males exceeds that in females	RS cells with mixed inflammatory cell (lymphocytes, monocyte/macrophage, eosinophils, plasma cells) infiltrate
Lymphocyte-rich classical HL	Uncommon subtype Found in all ages but most common in adults Incidence in males exceeds that in females	Few RS cells and predominantly lymphocytic infiltration Usually localized at diagnosis Survival is long with or without treatment
Lymphocyte depletion HL	Uncommon subtype Most common type in elderly persons, human immunodeficiency virus (HIV)-positive individuals, and persons in nonindustrialized countries Incidence in males exceeds that in females	Large number of RS cells with less additional cellular infiltrate Usually widespread disease: abdominal lymphadenopathy; spleen, liver, and bone marrow involvement, without peripheral lymphadenopathy Stage is usually more advanced at diagnosis

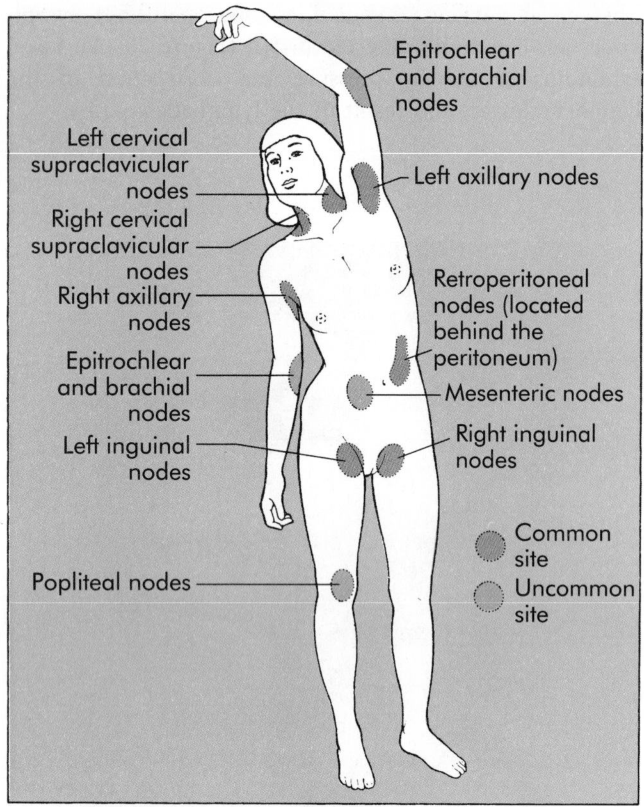

Figure 20-11 ■ Common and Uncommon Involved Lymph Node Sites for Hodgkin Lymphoma.

TABLE 20-10

Modified Cotswold Staging Classification System

Stage	Criteria
I	Involvement of a single lymph node region or single extranodal organ or site
II	Involvement of two or more lymph node regions on the same side of the diaphragm or a single extranodal organ or site and its regional lymph nodes
III	Involvement of lymph node regions or structures on both sides of the diaphragm
IV	Disseminated involvement of one or more extralymphatic organs or an isolated extralymphatic organ with distant nodal involvement
	Modifying characteristics for all four stages
	A: no B symptoms
	B: unexplained fever of >38°C, drenching night sweats, unexplained loss of >10% of body weight in the 6 months preceding diagnosis
	E: large mediastinal mass with direct extension into extranodal sites

Data from Lister TA, Crowther D: Staging for Hodgkin's disease, *Semin Oncol* 17:696, 1990.

About a third of individuals will have some degree of systemic symptoms. Intermittent fever, without other symptoms of infection, drenching night sweats, itchy skin (pruritus), and fatigue are relatively common. These constitutional symptoms accompanied by weight loss are associated with a poor prognosis. The Cotswold staging classification system used for HL is able to establish a correlation between the anatomic extent of the disease and prognosis (Table 20-10). This classification system is based on the individual's medical history, examination (presence of symptoms and palpable lymph nodes), and other radiologic and hematologic results. Prognostic indicators include clinical stage, histologic type, tumor cell concentration and tumor burden, constitutional symptoms, and age.

Although HL rarely arises in the lung, mediastinal and hilar node adenopathy can cause secondary involvement of the trachea, bronchi, pleura, or lungs. Retroperitoneal nodes can involve vertebral bodies and nerves and also can cause displacement of ureters. Spinal cord involvement is more common in the dorsal and lumbar regions than in the cervical region. Skin lesions, although uncommon, include psoriasis and eczematoid lesions, causing itching and scratching.

As a result of direct invasion from mediastinal lymph nodes, pericardial involvement can cause pericardial friction rub, pericardial effusion, and engorgement of neck veins. The GI tract and urinary tract are rarely involved. Anemia is often found in individuals with HL accompanied by a low serum iron and iron-binding capacity. Other laboratory findings include elevated sedimentation rate, leukocytosis, and eosinophilia. Leukopenia occurs in advanced stages of HL.

Splenic involvement in HL depends on histologic type. In mixed cellularity and lymphocytic deletion types of HL, the spleen is involved in 60% of cases. With lymphocyte and nodular sclerosis types, 34% of cases involve the spleen.

EVALUATION AND TREATMENT Because of the variability in symptoms, early definitive detection may be difficult. Asymptomatic lymphadenopathy can progress undetected for several years. Careful evaluation, including chest x-ray films, positron emission tomography (PET) scans, and biopsy, should be carried out for individuals with fever of unknown origin and peripheral lymphadenopathy. A lymph node biopsy with scattered RS cells and a cellular infiltrate is highly indicative of HL. The effectiveness of treatment is related to the age of the individual and the extent of the disease. Approximately 75% of individuals diagnosed with HL can be cured, largely because of successful treatment of HL with irradiation and chemotherapy. The 5-year survival rate is 83%.

Persons with stage III or IV disease, bulky disease (>10 cm mass or mediastinal disease with a transverse diameter exceeding 33% of the transthoracic diameter), or presence of B symptoms require combined chemotherapy with or without additional radiation treatment. Those with stage I or II disease are candidates for chemotherapy, combined, or radiation therapy alone. The survival rate depends on many factors, including the age of the individual, the stage of the disease, gender, and other variables. The 5-year survival rate with no additional factors is about 85%, but drops precipitously with each additional factor to about 42% with five or more factors.

Non-Hodgkin lymphomas

The previously used generic classification of **non-Hodgkin lymphoma** has been reclassified in the WHO/REAL scheme into **B-cell neoplasms,** which includes a variety of lymphomas including myelomas that originate from B cells at various stages of differentiation, and **T-cell** and **NK-cell neoplasms,** which includes lymphomas that originate from either T or NK cells. These cancers are differentiated from HL by lack of RS cells and other cellular changes not characteristic of HL.

Because malignant changes can occur at various stages of B-cell, T-cell, or NK-cell development, these cancers present with a variety of clinical states. In the following section, the types of tumors previously classified as non-Hodgkin lymphoma are considered together, and myeloma is described separately.

PATHOPHYSIOLOGY As with all cancers, lymphomas most likely originate from mutations in cellular genes (many of which are environmentally induced) in a single cell that lead to loss of control of proliferation and other aspects of cell growth. The most common type of chromosomal alteration in NHL is translocation, which disrupts the genes encoded at the breakpoints. Risk factors include a family history, exposure to a variety of mutagenic chemicals, irradiation, infection with certain cancer-related viruses (e.g., Epstein-Barr virus, human herpes virus-8, HIV, HTLV-1, hepatitis C), and immune suppression related to organ transplantation. Gastric infection with *Helicobacter pylori* increases the risk for gastric lymphomas. NHL is a disease of middle age, usually found in persons over 50 years old.

CLINICAL MANIFESTATIONS Clinical manifestations of NHL usually start out as localized or generalized lymphadenopathy, similar to HL. Differences in clinical features are noted in Table 20-11. The cervical, axillary, inguinal, and femoral chains are the most commonly affected sites. Generally, the swelling is painless and the nodes have enlarged and transformed over a period of months or years. Other sites of involvement are the nasopharynx, GI tract, bone, thyroid, testes, and soft tissue. Some individuals have retroperitoneal and abdominal masses with symptoms of abdominal fullness, back pain, ascites (fluid in the peritoneal cavity), and leg swelling.

EVALUATION AND TREATMENT Individuals with NHL can survive for extended periods. Survival with nodular lymphoma ranges up to 15 years. Individuals with diffuse disease generally do not survive as long. Overall, the survival rates for NHL are less than those for Hodgkin lymphoma. For NHL, the survival rates are 1-year, 77%; 5-year, 59%; and 10-year, 42%. Many investigators think that more aggressive treatment increases the cure rate. High-grade NHL is seen with increasing frequency in persons with AIDS and has an extremely poor prognosis.

Success of treatment is dependent on several parameters, including the type of lymphoma, stage of disease, cell type, involvement of organs outside the lymph nodes, age of the person, and the severity of the body's reaction to the disease (e.g., fever, night sweats, weight loss).[17] Treatment with chemotherapy alone may be adequate in many cases, although radiation therapy is frequently included. Low-dose chemotherapy has been followed by autologous stem cell transplantation in some NHLs or for recurrent disease. Treatment of B-cell lymphomas with rituximab has proven effective. Rituximab is a commercial monoclonal antibody against antigen CD20, which is expressed on the surface of all B cells, including malignant ones. Administration of rituximab depletes most B cells and allows the replenishment of normal B cells from the lymphoid stem cell pool. It has also proven useful in a variety of autoimmune diseases, including immune thrombocytopenia purpura, autoimmune anemias, systemic lupus erythematosus, and rheumatoid arthritis.

TABLE 20-11

Clinical Differences Between Non-Hodgkin Lymphoma and Hodgkin Lymphoma

Characteristics	Non-Hodgkin Lymphoma	Hodgkin Lymphoma
Nodal involvement	Multiple peripheral nodes	Localized to single axial group of nodes (i.e., cervical, mediastinal, paraaortic)
	Mesenteric nodes and Waldeyer ring commonly involved	Mesenteric nodes and Waldeyer ring rarely involved
Spread	Noncontiguous	Orderly spread by contiguity
B symptoms*	Uncommon	Common
Extranodal involvement	Common	Rare
Extent of disease	Rarely localized	Often localized

*Fever, weight loss, night sweats.

Burkitt lymphoma

Burkitt lymphoma is a B-cell tumor with unique clinical and epidemiologic features that accounts for 30% of childhood lymphomas worldwide. It occurs in children from east-central Africa and New Guinea and is characterized by a facial mass around the jaw (Figure 20-12). In the United States, Burkitt lymphoma is rare, usually involves the abdomen, and is characterized by extensive bone marrow invasion and replacement.

PATHOPHYSIOLOGY Epstein-Barr virus (EBV) is associated with almost all cases (>90%) of Burkitt lymphoma. It is suspected that suppression of the immune system by other illnesses (e.g., HIV infection, chronic malaria) increase the individual's susceptibility to EBV. B cells are particularly sensitive because of specific surface receptors for EBV. As a result, the B cell undergoes chromosomal translocations that result in overexpression of the *c-myc* protooncogene and loss of control of cell growth. The most common translocation (75% of individuals) is between chromosomes 8 (containing the *c-myc* gene) and 14 (containing the immunoglobulin heavy chain genes). Other translocations have been reported between chromosome 8 and chromosomes 2 or 22, which contain genes for immunoglobulin light chains.

CLINICAL MANIFESTATIONS In non-African Burkitt lymphoma the most common presentation is abdominal swelling. More advanced disease may involve other organs—eye, ovaries, kidneys, glandular tissue (breast, thyroid, tonsil)—and presents with type B symptoms (night sweats, fever, weight loss).

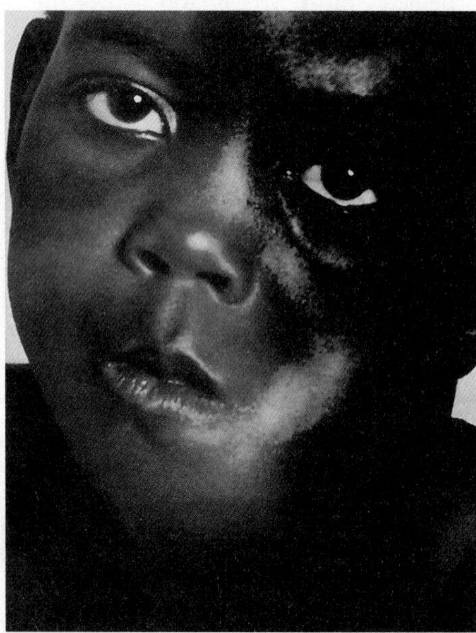

Figure 20-12 ■ **Burkitt Lymphoma.** Burkitt lymphoma involving the jaw in young African boy. (Courtesy Dr. JNP Davies, Albany, NY. From del Regato JA, Spjut HJ, Cox JD: *Cancer: diagnosis, treatment, and prognosis,* ed 6, St Louis, 1985, Mosby.)

EVALUATION AND TREATMENT The distribution of tumors and biopsies of enlarged lymph nodes or the bone marrow containing malignant B cells are usually indicative of Burkitt lymphoma. It is one of the most aggressive and quickly growing malignancies. However, the African variety in children has been successfully treated with radiotherapy and cyclophosphamide (60% survival overall; 90% survival with limited disease). The American type is more resistant to treatment.

Multiple myeloma

Multiple myeloma (MM) is a B-cell cancer characterized by the proliferation of malignant plasma cells that infiltrate the bone marrow and aggregate into tumor masses throughout the skeletal system (Figure 20-13).[18] The reported incidence of MM has doubled in the past 2 decades, possibly as a result of more sensitive testing used for diagnosis. The annual incidence rate in the United States is 5/100,000, with 16,570 new cases estimated for 2006. Multiple myeloma occurs in all races, but the incidence in blacks is about twice that of whites. It rarely occurs before the age of 40 years—the peak age of incidence is about 65 years. It is slightly more common in men (10,960 estimated new cases) than women (8940 new cases). It is estimated that almost 11,000 people in the United States will die of MM in 2007.

Neoplastic cells of multiple myeloma reside in the bone marrow and are usually not found in the peripheral blood. Occasionally, however, it may spread to other tissues, especially in very advanced disease. The basic defect is genetic, which may result from chronic stimulation of B cells with bacterial or viral antigens.

PATHOPHYSIOLOGY Most, if not all, multiple myelomas involve chromosomal translocations (break points), which recur in many individuals. In about half of MM cases, one of the chromosomal partners is 14 (site of genes

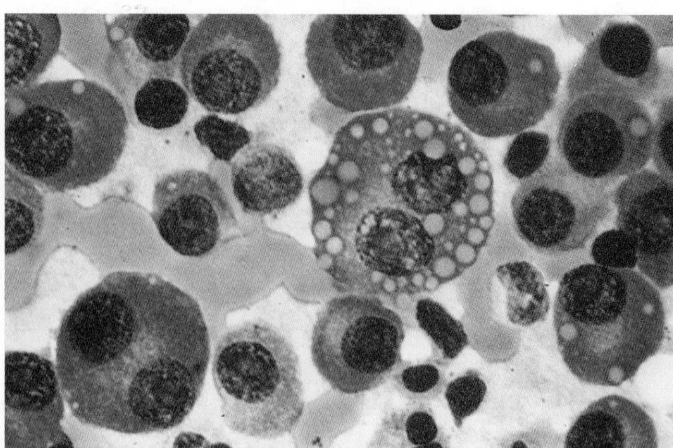

Figure 20-13 ■ **Multiple Myeloma, Bone Marrow Aspirate.** Normal marrow cells are largely replaced by plasma cells, including atypical forms with multiple nuclei, and cytoplasmic droplets containing immunoglobulin. (From Kumar V, Abbas AK, Fausto N: *Robbins and Cotran pathologic basis of disease,* ed 7, Philadelphia, 2005, Saunders.)

for the immunoglobulin heavy chain), which recombines with a number of other chromosomal sites of oncogenes, most commonly 11(q13), 4(p16), 16(q23), 20(q11), and 6(p25), resulting in probable dysregulation of the oncogenes. Breaks in 11q13 occur in about 25% of multiple myelomas and are associated with a more aggressive disease and a poorer prognosis. Deletions in chromosome 13 are observed in about 50% of cases. The molecular pathogenesis of multiple myeloma also involves proto-oncogene mutations and, more rarely, inactivation of tumor-suppressor genes. The precise timing and reason for the genetic alteration and accumulation is unknown.

Malignant plasma cells arise from one clone of B cells that produce abnormally large amounts of one class of immunoglobulin (usually IgG, occasionally IgA, and rarely IgM, IgD, or IgE). The malignant transformation may begin early in B cell development, possibly before encountering antigen in the secondary lymphoid organs. The myeloma cells return to either the bone marrow or other soft tissue sites. Their return is aided by cell adhesion molecules that help them target favorable sites that promote continued expansion and maturation. Cytokines, particularly interleukin-6 (IL-6), have been identified as essential factors that promote the growth and survival of multiple myeloma cells. (Lymphocytes and cytokines are described in Chapter 6.)

Myeloma cells in the bone marrow produce several cytokines themselves (e.g., IL-6, IL-1, TNFα). IL-6 in particular acts as an osteoclast-activating factor and stimulates osteoclasts to reabsorb bone. This process results in bone lesions and hypercalcemia (high calcium levels in the blood) resulting from release of calcium from the break down of bone.

The antibody produced by the transformed plasma cell is frequently defective, containing truncations, deletions, and other abnormalities, and is frequently referred to as a paraprotein (abnormal protein in the blood). Because of the large number of malignant plasma cells, the abnormal antibody, called the **M-protein,** becomes the most prominent protein in the blood (see Figure 20-15). Suppression of normal plasma cells by the myeloma results in diminished or absent normal antibodies. The excessive amount of M-protein may also contribute to many of the clinical manifestations of the disease. If the myeloma produces IgM (Waldenström macroglobulinemia), the excessive amount of large molecule weight proteins (about 900,000 daltons) can lead to abnormally high blood viscosity (hyperviscosity syndrome). Frequently, the myeloma produces free immunoglobulin light chain **(Bence Jones protein)** that is present in the blood and urine and contributes to damage of renal tubular cells.

CLINICAL MANIFESTATIONS The common presentation of MM is characterized by elevated levels of calcium in the blood (hypercalcemia), renal failure, anemia, and bone lesions. The hypercalcemia and bone lesions result from infiltration of the bone by malignant plasma cells and stimulation of osteoclasts to reabsorb bone. This process results in the release of calcium (hypercalcemia) and development of "lytic lesions" (round, "punched out" regions of bone) (Figure 20-14). Destruction of bone tissue causes pain, the most common presenting symptom, and pathologic fractures. The bones most commonly involved, in decreasing order of frequency, are the vertebrae, ribs, skull, pelvis, femur, clavicle, and scapula. Spinal cord compression, because of the weakened vertebrae, occurs in about 10% of individuals.

Proteinuria is observed in 90% of individuals. Renal failure may be either acute or chronic and is usually secondary to the hypercalcemia. Bence Jones protein is present in about 80% and may also lead to damage of the proximal tubules. Anemia is usually normocytic and normochromic and results from inhibited erythropoiesis caused by tumor cell infiltration of the bone marrow.

The high concentration of paraprotein in the blood, particularly associated with the large molecular weight IgM produced in Waldenström macroglobulinemia, may lead to hyperviscosity syndrome. The increased viscosity interferes with blood circulation to various sites (brain, kidneys, extremities). IgM paraprotein may also result in cryoglobulins (proteins that precipitate from the blood at lower than body temperature). Hyperviscosity syndrome is observed in up to 20% of persons. Additional neurologic symptoms (e.g., confusion, headaches, blurred vision) may occur secondary to hypercalcemia or hyperviscosity.

Suppression of the humoral (antibody-mediated) immune response results in repeated infections, primarily pneumonias and pyelonephritis. The most commonly involved organisms are encapsulated bacteria that are particularly sensitive to the effects of antibody; pneumonia

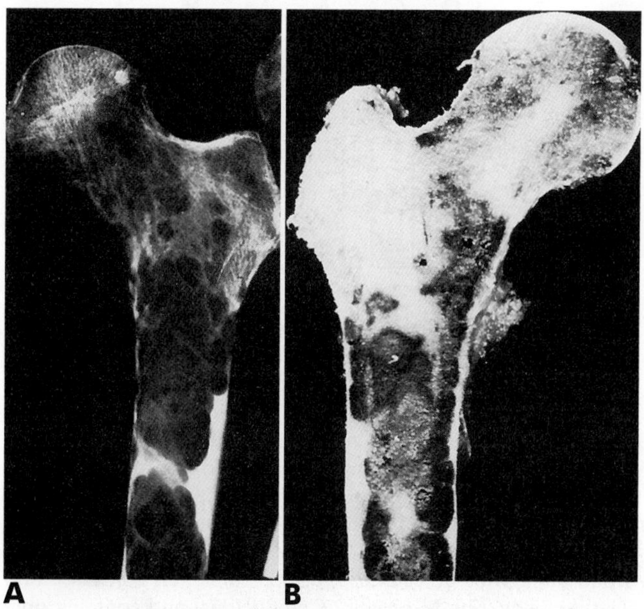

Figure 20-14 ■ **Multiple (Plasma Cell) Myeloma. A,** Roentgenogram of femur showing extensive bone destruction caused by tumor. Note absence of reactive bone formation. **B,** Gross specimen from same individual; myelomatous sections appear as dark granular sections. (From Kissane JM, editor: *Anderson's pathology,* ed 9, St Louis, 1990, Mosby.)

caused by *S. pneumoniae*, *S. aureus*, or *K. pneumoniae* or pyelonephritis caused by *E. coli* or other gram-negative organisms. Cell-mediated (T cell) function is relatively normal. Overwhelming infection is the leading cause of death from MM.

EVALUATION AND TREATMENT Diagnosis of MM is made by symptoms, radiographic and laboratory studies, and a bone marrow biopsy. Quantitative measurements of immunoglobulins (IgG, IgM, IgA) are usually performed. Typically, one class of immunoglobulin (the M protein produced by the myeloma cell) is greatly increased, while the others are suppressed. Serum electrophoretic analysis reveals increased levels of M protein (Figure 20-15).

Normal serum

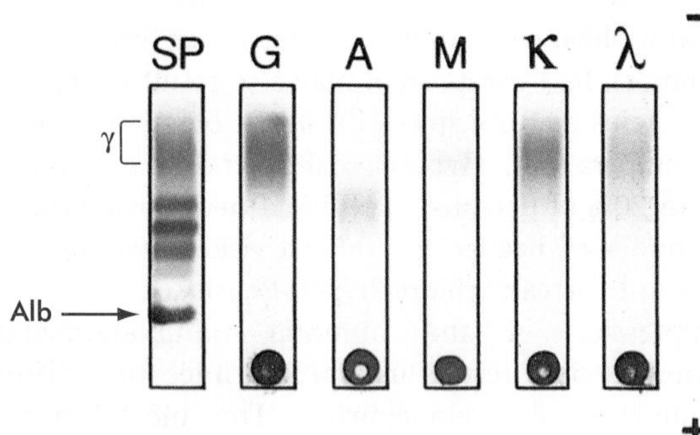

Patient serum

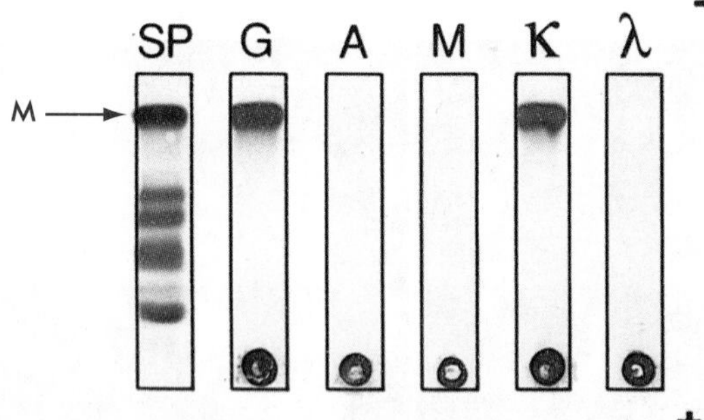

Figure 20-15 ■ **M Protein Detection.** Serum protein (SP) electrophoresis is used to screen for M proteins (M) in multiple myeloma. In normal serum the proteins separate into several regions between albumin (Alb) and a broad band in the gamma (γ) region, where most antibodies (γ-globulins) are found. Serum from an individual with multiple myeloma contains a sharp M protein (M) band. Using specific antibodies the location of specific types of heavy (G, A, M) and light (κ, λ) chains can be determined. In this example, normal serum contains a broad band with polyclonal IgG molecules that contain κ and λ light chains. The M protein is monoclonal and contains only one heavy chain and one light chain. The M protein in this example is an IgG that contains κ light chain. (Courtesy Dr. David Sacks, Department of Pathology, Brigham and Women's Hospital, Boston, MA. Modified from Kumar V, Abbas A, Fausto N: *Robbins and Cotran pathologic basis of disease,* ed 7, Philadelphia, 2005, Saunders.)

Because the M protein is monoclonal, each molecule has the same electric change and migrates at about the same site on electrophoresis, resulting in a highly concentrated protein (M spike). Bence Jones protein is observed in the urine or serum by immunoelectrophoresis or in the serum using newly available ELISA assays. Usually an intact antibody paraprotein coexists with Bence Jones protein. However, variants of MM include individuals in which free light chain only is produced and a rare variant that produces only free heavy chain. Measurement of another protein, free β_2-microglobulin, is used as an indicator of prognosis or effectiveness of therapy.

Although chemotherapy, radiation therapy, and marrow transplant have been used for treatment, the prognosis for persons with MM remains poor. Autologous peripheral blood stem cell transplantation is preferred to bone marrow transplantation. Individuals with multiple bone lesions, if untreated, rarely survive more than 6 to 12 months. Individuals with inactive (indolent) myeloma, however, can survive for many years. With chemotherapy and aggressive management of complications, the prognosis can improve significantly, with a median survival of 24 to 30 months and a 10-year survival rate of 3%. The median survival for all states of MM is 3 years.

A recent addition to treatment of MM in individuals who have a relapse after conventional chemotherapy is the drug thalidomide. The use of thalidomide in treating MM is based on its suppression of TNFα and its anti-angiogenesis ability.

✔ QUICK CHECK 20-4

1. Define multiple myeloma and discuss its pathogenesis.
2. Describe the features of a clonal disorder. Give an example.
3. How is lymphadenopathy related to infection?

Lymphoblastic lymphoma

Lymphoblastic lymphoma (LL) is a relatively rare variant of NHL overall (2% to 4%) but accounts for almost a third of cases of NHL in children and adolescents, with a male predominance. The vast majority of LL (>85%) is of T cell origin, and the remainder arises from B cells. LL is similar to acute lymphoblastic leukemia and may be considered a variant of that disease.

PATHOPHYSIOLOGY The disease arises from a clone of relatively immature T cells that becomes malignant in the thymus. As with most lymphoid tumors, LL is frequently associated with translocations, primarily of the chromosomes that encode for the T-cell receptor (chromosomes 7 and 14). These aberrations result in increased expression of a variety of transcription factors and loss of growth control.

CLINICAL MANIFESTATIONS The first sign of LL is usually a painless lymphadenopathy in the neck. Peripheral lymph nodes in the chest become involved in about 70% of individuals. Involved nodes are located mostly above the diaphragm. LL is a very aggressive tumor that presents as stage IV in most people. T cell LL is associated with a unique mediastinal mass (up to 75%) because of the apparent origin of the tumor in the thymus. The mass results in chest pain and may cause compression of bronchi or the superior vena cava. The tumor may infiltrate the bone marrow in about half of those affected, and suppression of bone marrow hematopoiesis leads to increased susceptibility to infections. Other organs, including the liver, kidney, spleen, and brain, may also be affected. Many individuals express type B symptoms: fever, night sweats, and significant weight loss.

EVALUATION AND TREATMENT The most common therapeutic approach is combined chemotherapy. In early disease, the response rate is high with increased survival; the 5-year survival in children is 80% to 90%, and it is 45% to 55% in adults. Although LL is easily treated, there is a high relapse rate: 40% to 60% of adults.

ALTERATIONS OF SPLENIC FUNCTION

In the past, **splenomegaly** (enlargement of the spleen) has been associated with various disease states. It is now recognized that splenomegaly is not necessarily pathologic; an enlarged spleen may be present in certain individuals without any evidence of disease. Splenomegaly may be, however, one of the first physical signs of underlying conditions, and its presence should not be ignored. In conditions where splenomegaly is present, the normal functions of the spleen may become overactive, producing a condition known as **hypersplenism.**

Current diagnostic criteria for hypersplenism include (1) anemia, leukopenia, thrombocytopenia, or combinations of these; (2) cellular bone marrow; (3) splenomegaly; and (4) improvement after splenectomy. Some individuals may seek treatment for problems even though they have not met all the above clinical criteria; therefore, the relevance and significance of hypersplenism are still uncertain. Primary hypersplenism is recognized when no etiologic factor has been identified; secondary hypersplenism occurs in the presence of another condition.

PATHOPHYSIOLOGY Overactivity of the spleen results in hematologic alterations that affect all three blood components. Splenic sequestering of red cells, white cells, and platelets results in a reduction of all circulating blood cells. Up to 50% of red cells may be sequestered; however, the rate of splenic pooling is directly related to spleen size and the degree of increased blood flow through it. Sequestering exposes the red cells to splenic activities, which accelerates their destruction, causing further reductions in red cell concentration. Anemia is the result of these combined actions. Anemia is further potentiated by an increased blood volume, producing a dilutional effect on the already reduced red cell concentration.

The white cells and platelets also are affected by sequestering, although not to the same degree as the red cell. The degree of red cell destruction and the diluting effect are determined by the degree of spleen enlargement.

CLINICAL MANIFESTATIONS Specific diseases or particular conditions related to the various classifications of splenomegaly are detailed in Box 20-1. Different pathologic processes that produce splenomegaly are briefly described here.

Acute inflammatory or infectious processes cause splenomegaly because of increased demand for defensive activities. An acutely enlarged spleen secondary to infection may become so filled with erythrocytes that its natural rubbery resilience is lost and becomes fragile and vulnerable to blunt trauma. Splenic rupture is a complication associated with infectious mononucleosis.

Congestive splenomegaly is accompanied by ascites, portal hypertension, and esophageal varices and is most commonly seen in hepatic cirrhosis. Splenic hyperplasia develops in any disorder in which splenic workload is increased and is most commonly associated with various types of anemias (hemolytic) and chronic myeloproliferative disorders (i.e., polycythemia vera).

Infiltrative splenomegaly is caused by engorgement of the macrophages with indigestible materials associated with various "storage diseases." Tumors and cysts are neoplastic disorders that cause actual growth of the spleen. Metastatic

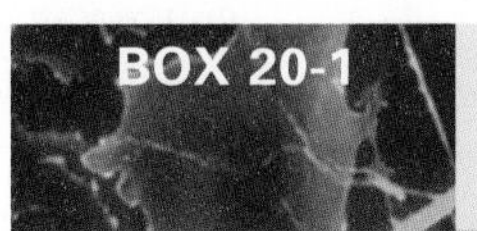

Diseases Related to Classification of Splenomegaly

Inflammation or Infection

Acute: viral (hepatitis, infectious mononucleosis, cytomegalovirus), bacterial (salmonella, gram negative), parasitic (typhoid)

Subacute or chronic: bacterial (subacute bacterial endocarditis, tuberculosis), parasitic (malaria), fungal (histoplasmosis), Felty syndrome, systemic lupus erythematosus, rheumatoid arthritis, thrombocytopenia

Congestive

Cirrhosis, heart failure, portal vein obstruction (portal hypertension), splenic vein obstruction

Infiltrative

Gaucher disease, amyloidosis, diabetic lipemia

Tumors or Cysts

Malignant: polycythemia rubra vera, chronic or acute leukemias, Hodgkin lymphoma, metastatic solid tumors

Nonmalignant: hamartoma

Cysts: true cysts (lymphangiomas, hemangiomas, epithelial, endothelial); false cysts (hemorrhagic, serous, inflammatory)

tumors of the spleen are rare and may result from skin, lungs, breast, and cervical primary sites.

EVALUATION AND TREATMENT Treatment for hypersplenism is splenectomy; however, it may not always be indicated. A splenectomy is performed when its removal is considered necessary, eliminating its destructive effects on red cells. Clinical indicators should determine the need for splenectomy, not necessarily specific conditions. Splenectomy for splenic rupture is no longer considered mandatory because of the possibility of overwhelming sepsis after removal. Repair and preservation should be considered before the decision to remove the spleen is made.

QUICK CHECK 20-5

1. Contrast the principal features of Hodgkin lymphoma with those of non-Hodgkin lymphoma.
2. What is Burkitt lymphoma?
3. Identify the major causes of splenomegaly. How does it differ from hypersplenism?

ALTERATIONS OF PLATELETS AND COAGULATION

Disorders of Platelet Function

Quantitative or qualitative abnormalities of platelets can interrupt normal blood coagulation and prevent hemostasis. The quantitative abnormalities are thrombocytopenia, a decrease in the number of circulating platelets, and thrombocythemia, an increase in the number of platelets. Qualitative disorders affect the structure or function of individual platelets and can coexist with the quantitative disorders. Qualitative disorders usually prevent platelet adherence and aggregation, thereby preventing formation of a platelet plug.

Thrombocytopenia

Thrombocytopenia is defined as a platelet count below 150,000/mm^3 of blood, although most individuals do not consider the decrease significant unless it falls below 100,000/mm^3, and the risk for hemorrhage associated with minor trauma does not appreciably increase until the count falls below 50,000/mm^3. Spontaneous bleeding without trauma can occur with counts ranging from 10,000/mm^3 to 15,000/mm^3. When this happens, skin manifestations (i.e., petechiae, ecchymoses, and larger purpuric spots) are observed or frank bleeding from mucous membranes occurs. Severe bleeding results if the count falls below 10,000/mm^3 and can be fatal if it occurs in the gastrointestinal, respiratory, or central nervous systems.

Before thrombocytopenia is diagnosed, the presence of a pseudothrombocytopenia must be ruled out. This phenomenon is seen in approximately 1 in 1000 to 10,000 samples and results from an error in platelet counting when a blood sample is analyzed by an automated cell counter. Platelets in the blood can become nonspecifically agglutinated by immunoglobulins in the presence of ethylenediaminetetraacetic acid (EDTA) and are not counted, thus giving an apparent, but false, thrombocytopenia. Thrombocytopenia also may be falsely diagnosed because of a dilutional effect observed after massive transfusion of platelet-poor packed cells to treat a hemorrhage. This is observed when more than 10 units of blood have been transfused within a 24-hour period. The precipitating hemorrhage also depletes platelets, contributing to the pseudothrombocytopenic state. Splenic sequestering of platelets in hypersplenism also stimulates thrombocytopenia. Hypothermia (<25° C) also predisposes to a thrombocytopenic state, which is reversed when temperatures return to normal, suggesting sequestering and release.

PATHOPHYSIOLOGY Thrombocytopenia results from decreased platelet production, increased consumption, or both. The condition may also be either congenital or acquired and may be either primary or secondary to other conditions.[19,20] Thrombocytopenia secondary to congenital conditions occurs in a large number of different diseases, although each is relatively rare.[21] These include thrombocytopenia with absent radii (TAR) syndrome, Wiskott-Aldrich syndrome (see Chapter 7), various forms of MYH9 gene mutation (e.g., May-Hegglin syndrome), X-linked thrombocytopenia, and many other examples.

Acquired thrombocytopenia is more common and may occur in relationship to acute viral infections (EBV, rubella, CMV, and HIV), drug reactions, autoimmune diseases, nutritional deficiencies, anemia (e.g., aplastic anemia), or cancer. Thrombocytopenia that results from decreased platelet production is usually the result of nutritional deficiencies (vitamin B_{12} or folic acid, in particular), some infections (e.g., HIV), drugs (e.g., thiazides, estrogens), quinine-containing medications, chemotherapeutic agents, ethanol), radiation therapy, bone marrow infiltration by some cancers, bone marrow hypoplasia (aplastic anemia), or chronic renal failure.

Most common forms of thrombocytopenia are the result of increased platelet consumption. Examples include heparin-induced thrombocytopenia, idiopathic (immune) thrombocytopenia purpura, thrombotic thrombocytopenia purpura, and disseminated intravascular coagulation (discussed later in this chapter).

Heparin-induced thrombocytopenia

Heparin is the most common cause of drug-induced thrombocytopenia.[22] Approximately 4% of individuals treated with unfractionated heparin develop **heparin-induced thrombocytopenia (HIT).** The incidence is lower (about 0.1%) with the use of low-molecular-weight heparin. The onset of HIT is most common in people undergoing surgery. HIT is an immune mediated, adverse drug reaction caused by IgG antibodies primarily against the heparin-platelet factor 4 complex. The IgG binds to platelet Fc receptors and activates platelet aggregation, release of additional platelet factor 4, and activation of thrombin, resulting in decreased platelet counts 5 to 10 days after heparin administration. If HIT is not recognized and treated, intravascular aggregation of platelets causes rapid development of arterial and venous thrombosis.

CLINICAL MANIFESTATIONS The hallmark of HIT is thrombocytopenia. However, 30% or more of those with thrombocytopenia are also at risk for thrombosis. Venous thrombosis is more common and results in deep venous thrombosis and pulmonary emboli. Arterial thrombosis affects the lower extremities causing limb ischemia. Cardiovascular accidents and myocardial infarctions also may be experienced. Other major arteries (renal, mesenteric, upper limb) may be affected too.

EVALUATION AND TREATMENT Diagnosis is primarily based on clinical observations. The individual presents with dropping platelet counts after 5 days or longer of heparin treatment. On average, platelet counts may reach 60,000/mm^3. The onset of symptoms, including thrombosis, may be delayed until after release from the hospital. Most people are postsurgery, therefore other possible causes of thrombocytopenia (e.g., infection, other drugs) must be considered. ELISAs and other tests are available to measure anti-heparin-platelet factor 4 antibodies. The sensitivity of this test is extremely high (>90%), but the specificity is less because of false-positive reactions (e.g., those on dialysis).

Treatment is the withdrawal of heparin and use of alternative anticoagulants. A switch to low-molecular-weight heparin is not indicated, and warfarin should not be used until the symptoms of HIT have resolved because of an increased risk of initiating skin necrosis. The thrombocytopenia should then progressively resolve. The chance of blood clots can be diminished using thrombin inhibitors (e.g., argatroban, lepirudin).

Idiopathic (immune) thrombocytopenia purpura

Most of the literature refers to thrombocytopenic purpura as **idiopathic** (no known cause) **thrombocytopenia purpura (ITP),** although the majority of cases are immune in nature.[23] ITP may be acute or chronic. The acute form is frequently observed in children and typically lasts 1 to 2 months with a complete remission. In some instances it may last for up to 6 months, and some children (7% to 28%) may progress to the chronic condition. Acute ITP is usually secondary to infections (particularly viral) or other conditions that lead to large amounts of antigen in the blood, such as some drugs or systemic lupus erythematosus (SLE). Under these conditions, the antigen usually forms immune complexes with circulating antibody, and it is thought that the immune complexes bind to Fc receptors on platelets, leading to their destruction in the spleen. The acute form of ITP usually resolves as the source of antigen is removed.

Chronic ITP is the primary form of the disease associated with the presence of autoantibodies against platelet-associated antigens. This form is more commonly observed in adults, being most prevalent in women between 20 and 40 years old, although it can be found in all age categories. The chronic form tends to get progressively worse. The autoantibodies are generally of the IgG class and are against one or more of several platelet glycoproteins (e.g., GPIIb/IIIa, GPIIb/IX, GPIa/IIa). The antibodies bind directly to the platelet antigens, after which the antibody-coated platelets are recognized and removed from the circulation by macrophages in the spleen.

CLINICAL MANIFESTATIONS Initial manifestations range from minor bleeding problems (development of petechiae and purpura) over the course of several days to major hemorrhage from mucosal sites (epistaxis, hematuria, menorrhagia, bleeding gums). Rarely will an individual present with intracranial bleeding or other sites of internal bleeding.

EVALUATION AND TREATMENT Diagnosis is based on a history of bleeding and associated symptoms (weight loss, fever, headache). Physical examination includes notations on the types of bleeding, location, and severity of bleeding. In addition, evidence of infections (bacterial, HIV and other viral), medication history, family history, and evidence of thrombosis are assessed. Other diagnostic tests include complete blood count (CBC) and peripheral blood smear. Unlike some other forms of thrombocytopenia, there is usually no evidence of splenectomy. Testing for antiplatelet antibodies is usually not helpful. Although most cases of ITP are associated with elevated levels of IgG on platelets, other forms of thrombocytopenia also have a high incidence of platelet-associated IgG; thus, the sensitivity is low (50% to 65%). In addition, some cases of ITP will not present with elevated platelet-associated antibodies; the specificity is 75% to 94%, so that a negative test does not rule out ITP.

Treatment is palliative, not curative, focusing on prevention of platelet destruction (spleen). Initial therapy for ITP is glucocorticoids (e.g., prednisone), which suppresses the immune response and prevents sequestering and further destruction of platelets. If steroid therapy is ineffective, other reagents have been used. Treatment with intravenous immunoglobulin (IVIg) is used to prevent major bleeding. The response rate is 80%, but the effects are transient lasting only days to a few weeks. Anti-(Rh)D (Rhogam) has been used with limited success to treat individuals who are Rh+.

If platelet counts do not increase appropriately, splenectomy is considered to remove the site of platelet destruction. However, splenectomy is not without risks, and approximately 10% to 20% of individuals who undergo a splenectomy suffer a relapse and require further treatment. In that situation, it is thought that the liver has become the site for platelet destruction. If splenectomy is unsuccessful, more aggressive immunosuppressive medications (e.g., azathioprine, cyclophosphamide) are usually recommended. Because of potential complications, these medications are reserved for individuals who are severely thrombocytopenic and refractive to other therapies.

Thrombotic thrombocytopenia purpura

Thrombotic thrombocytopenia purpura (TTP) is characterized by thrombotic microangiopathy, which includes microangiopathic hemolytic anemia and occlusion of arterioles and capillaries by aggregated platelets within the microcirculation.[24] Aggregation may lead to increased platelet consumption and organ ischemia. TTP is relatively uncommon, occurring in about 5:1,000,000 individuals per year. The incidence of TTP is increasing and does appear to be an actual increase and not just the result of improved recognition.

There are two types of TTP: familial and acquired idiopathic. The familial type is the more rare type and is usually chronic, relapsing, and usually seen in children. When recognized and treated early, the child experiences predictable recurring episodes approximately every 3 weeks that are responsive to treatment. Acquired TTP is more common and more acute and severe. It occurs mostly in females in their 30 s and is rarely observed in infants and the elderly.

Most cases of TTP are related to a dysfunction of the plasma metalloprotease ADAMTS13. This enzyme is responsible for cutting large precursor molecules of von Willebrand factor (vWF) produced by endothelial cells into smaller molecules. Defects in ADAMTS13 result in expression of large molecular weight vWF on the endothelial cell surface and the formation of large aggregates of platelets, which can break off and form occlusions in smaller vessels. People with TTP (about 80%) have <5% of normal plasma ADAMTS13 levels. Most individuals with familial TTP are homozygous for mutations in ADAMTS13. Acquired TTP of unexplained origin is associated in most (44% to 94%) people with an IgG autoantibody against ADAMTS13 that is able to neutralize the enzymes activity and accelerate its clearance from the plasma.

CLINICAL MANIFESTATIONS TTP is clinically related to and must be distinguished from other thrombotic microangiopathic conditions, including hemolytic uremic syndrome, malignant hypertension, preeclampsia, and pregnancy-induced HELLP (hemolysis, elevated liver enzymes, low platelet count) syndrome. Early diagnosis and treatment is essential because TTP may prove fatal within 90 days of onset if untreated.

Acute idiopathic TTP is characterized by a pentad of symptoms, including extreme thrombocytopenia (<20,000/mm^3), intravascular hemolytic anemia, ischemic signs and symptoms most often involving the central nervous system (about 65% present with memory disturbances, behavioral irregularities, headaches, or coma), kidney failure (65%), and fever (33%).

EVALUATION AND TREATMENT A routine blood smear usually reveals fragmented red cells (*schizocytes*) produced by shear forces when red cells are in contact with the fibrin mesh in clots that form in the vessels. As a result of tissue injury, serum levels of lactate dehydrogenase (LDH) may be very high, and low-density lipoprotein [LDL] levels may be elevated. Tests for antibody on red cells are negative, excluding immune hemolytic anemia.

Plasma exchange with fresh frozen plasma, which replenishes functional ADAMTS13, is the treatment of choice, achieving a 70% to 80% response rate. Additionally, steroids (glucocorticoids) are administered. Nonresponse to conventional therapy may require a splenectomy; however, postoperative hemorrhage remains a dangerous complication. Immunosuppressive (azathioprine) therapy has been successful in some individuals.

Thrombocythemia

Thrombocythemia (also called **thrombocytosis**) is defined as a platelet count greater than 400,000/mm^3 of blood.[25] Thrombocythemia may be primary or secondary (reactive) and is usually asymptomatic until the count exceeds 1 million/mm^3. Then intravascular clot formation (thrombosis), hemorrhage, or other abnormalities can occur.

PATHOPHYSIOLOGY **Essential (primary) thrombocythemia (ET)** is a myeloproliferative disorder in which platelet production increases, resulting in platelet counts in excess of 600,000/mm^3. It can occur in individuals at most any age. Manifestations include increased numbers of bone marrow megakaryocytes, splenomegaly, and periodic episodes of hemorrhage or thrombosis, or both. The thrombocythemia is secondary to increased plasma thrombopoietin levels resulting from defects in the thrombopoietin receptor. The defective receptor cannot adequately bind and remove thrombopoietin from the blood, thus circulating levels remain high. Along with increased platelets, there may be a concomitant increase in red cells, indicating a myeloproliferative disorder; however, the increase in red cells is not to the extent seen in polycythemia vera.

Secondary thrombocythemia may occur after splenectomy because platelets that normally would be stored in the spleen remain in circulating blood. The increase in platelets may be gradual, with thrombocythemia not occurring for up to 3 weeks after splenectomy. Reactive thrombocythemia may occur during some inflammatory conditions, such as rheumatoid arthritis and cancers. In these conditions, excessive production of some cytokines (e.g., IL-6, IL-11) may induce increased production of thrombopoietin in the liver resulting in increased megakaryocyte proliferation. Reactive thrombocythemia may also occur during a variety of physiologic conditions, such as after exercise.

CLINICAL MANIFESTATIONS Clinical manifestations vary among individuals. Those with ET are at risk for large-vessel arterial or venous thrombosis, and ischemia in the fingers, toes, or cerebrovascular regions is common. Digital ischemia is characterized by warm, congested red extremities with a burning sensation, particularly on the forefoot sole and toes. The lower extremities are affected more often, and only one side may be involved. Standing, exercise, or warmth precipitates the pain, which is relieved by elevation and cooling. In extreme situations, acrocyanosis and gangrene may result.

Thrombosis of arteries is more common than of veins, and myocardial and renal arteries may be involved. The carotid, mesenteric, and subclavian arteries also may be affected. Myocardial ischemia and infarction have occurred without clear evidence of coronary artery disease.

Involvement of the nervous system is manifested by headache and dizziness, with paresthesias, transient ischemic attacks, strokes, visual disturbances, and seizures also being reported. Major thrombotic events, not directly related to platelet count, occur in about 20% to 30% of individuals with ET. Other risk factors (prior thrombosis, age, and duration of ET) are better predictors of future thrombosis.

Although thrombosis is the more common symptom, hemorrhage can also occur. Sites for bleeding include the GI tract, skin, urinary tract, gums, joints, and brain. GI bleeding may be mistaken for a duodenal ulcer. Hemorrhage is not severe and generally occurs in the presence of very high platelet counts; transfusions are required only occasionally. Bleeding and clotting may occur simultaneously, and individuals are not necessarily prone to one or the other.

EVALUATION AND TREATMENT Initial diagnosis is not difficult; as many as two thirds of cases are diagnosed from a routine complete blood cell count (CBC). Secondary thrombocytosis also may occur as a moderate rise in the platelet count that resolves with treatment or resolution of the underlying condition.

Essential thrombocythemia is diagnosed by a platelet count that exceeds 600,000/mm^3 and remains elevated, with no other indicated cause, such as arthritis, iron deficiency anemia, cancer, or splenectomy. Many individuals present with a mild anemia and a slightly elevated white blood cell count.

Hydroxyuria (HU), a nonalkylating myelosuppressive agent, is used to suppress platelet production and at one time was the drug of choice for treating ET; however, long-term therapy with this drug may cause progression to other myeloplastic disorders, particularly acute myeloid leukemia. Other drugs used to treat ET include aspirin and interferon-alpha (IFNα). IFNα may not be effective for everyone and aspirin, with its blood thinning properties, may cause hemorrhage. Anagrelide is now the drug of choice. Anagrelide interferes with platelet maturation rather than production, thus not interfering with red and white cell growth and development.

Alterations of Platelet Function

Qualitative alterations in platelet function are characterized by an increased bleeding time in the presence of a normal platelet count. Associated clinical manifestations include spontaneous petechiae and purpura, bleeding from the GI tract, genitourinary tract, pulmonary mucosa, and gums. Congenital alterations in platelet function (thrombocytopathies) are quite rare and may be categorized into several types of disorders: (1) platelet-vessel wall adhesion (e.g., defect in GPIb expression [Bernard-Soulier syndrome]), (2) platelet-platelet interactions (e.g., defect in GPIIb-IIIa expression [Glanzmann thrombasthenia]), (3) platelet granules and secretion (e.g., receptor defects [ADP, collagen]), (4) arachidonic acid pathways (e.g., thromboxane synthase deficiency), (5) cytoskeletal function (e.g., Wiskott-Aldrich syndrome [see Chapter 7]), and (6) membrane phospholipid regulation (coagulation protein-platelet interactions) (e.g., Scott syndrome).

HEALTH ALERT

Dark Chocolate, Wine, and Platelet-Inhibitory Functions

An increasing number of foods have been reported to have platelet-inhibitory functions. Recent studies showed flavanol-rich cocoa inhibited several measures of platelet activity. Dark chocolate contains much more cocoa than does light chocolate. Additional cardioprotective effects may include antioxidant properties and activation of nitric oxide (NO). Low to moderate consumption of red wine reportedly has a greater benefit than other alcoholic beverages on cardioprotective mechanisms. Emerging are the effects of the polyphenol resveratrol known to be abundant in red wine. Investigators documented that the polyphenolic antioxidants, resveratrol, and proanthocyanidins provide cardioprotection by their function in vivo as antioxidants.

Data from Pearson DA et al: Flavanols and platelet reactivity, *Clin Dev Immunol* 12(1):1–9, 2005; Holt RR et al: Chocolate consumption and platelet function, *JAMA* 287(17):2212–2213, 2002; Engler MB: Flavonoid-rich dark chocolate improves endothelial function and increases plasma epicatechin concentrations in healthy adults, *J Am Coll Nutr* 23(3):197–204, 2004; Sato M, Maulik N, Das DK: Cardioprotection with alcohol: role of both alcohol and polyphenolic antioxidants, *Annals N Y Acad Sci* 957:122–135, 2002.

Acquired disorders of platelet function are more common than the congenital disorders and may be categorized into three principal causes: (1) drugs, (2) systemic conditions, and (3) hematologic alterations.

Multiple drugs are known to affect platelet function by interfering with platelet function in three ways: (1) inhibition of platelet membrane receptors, (2) inhibition of prostaglandin pathways, and (3) inhibition of phosphodiesterase activity. Aspirin is the most commonly used drug that affects platelets. It irreversibly inhibits cyclooxygenase function for several days after administration. Nonsteroidal anti-inflammatory drugs also affect cyclooxygenase, although in a reversible fashion.

Systemic disorders that affect platelet function are chronic renal disease, liver disease, cardiopulmonary bypass surgery, and severe deficiencies of iron or folate. Hematologic disorders associated with platelet dysfunction include chronic myeloproliferative disorders, multiple myeloma, leukemias, and myelodysplastic syndromes.

Disorders of Coagulation

Disorders of coagulation are usually caused by defects or deficiencies of one or more of the clotting factors. (Normal function of the clotting factors is described in Chapter 19.) Qualitative or quantitative abnormalities interfere with or prevent the enzymatic reactions that transform clotting factors, circulating as plasma proteins, into a stable fibrin clot (see Figure 19-16).

Some clotting factor defects are inherited and involve one single factor, such as the hemophilias, and von Willebrand disease, caused by deficiencies of clotting factors. Other coagulation defects are acquired and tend to result from deficient synthesis of clotting factors by the liver. Causes include liver disease and dietary deficiency of vitamin K.

Other coagulation disorders are attributed to pathologic conditions that trigger coagulation inappropriately, engaging the clotting factors and causing detrimental clotting within blood vessels. For example, any cardiovascular abnormality that alters normal blood flow by speeding it up, slowing it down, or obstructing it can create conditions in which coagulation proceeds within the vessels. An example of this is thromboembolic disease, in which blood clots obstruct blood vessels. Coagulation is also stimulated by the presence of tissue factor that is released by damaged or dead tissues. **Vasculitis,** or inflammation of the blood vessels, along with vessel damage activates platelets, which in turn activates the coagulation cascade. In extensive or prolonged vasculitis, blood clot formation can suppress mechanisms that normally control clot formation and breakdown, leading to clogging of the vessels. In each of these acquired conditions, normal hemostatic function proves detrimental to the body by consuming coagulation factors excessively or by overwhelming normal control of clot formation and breakdown (fibrinolysis) (see Figure 19-18).

Impaired hemostasis

Impaired hemostasis, or the inability to promote coagulation and the development of a stable fibrin clot, is commonly associated with liver dysfunction, which may be caused by either specific liver disorders or lack of vitamin K.

Vitamin K deficiency

Vitamin K, a fat-soluble vitamin, is required for the synthesis of prothrombin; the procoagulant factors II, VII, IX, and X; and the anticoagulant factors (proteins C and S). Parenteral administration of vitamin K is the treatment of choice and usually results in correction of the deficiency. Fresh frozen plasma also may be administered but is usually reserved for individuals with life-threatening hemorrhages or those who require emergency surgery.

Liver disease

Individuals who have liver disease present with a broad range of hemostatic derangements that may be characterized by defects in the clotting or fibrinolytic system and by platelet function. The usual sequence of events is an initial reduction in clotting factors, which parallels the degree of liver cell damage or destruction. Factor VII is the first to decline because of its rapid turnover, followed by declines in factors II and X. Factor IX levels are less affected and do not decline until the liver destruction is well advanced. Protein C (an antithrombin) levels decline early, similar to levels of factor VII, and protein S (also an antithrombin) levels decline in the later stages of liver disease. Declines of factor V are of special importance because factor V plasma levels appear to be a direct reflection of liver cell damage.

Other alterations of hemostasis in liver disease include an increase in fibrinolytic activity that is either primary in origin or a manifestation that is secondary to disseminated intravascular coagulation (DIC). This increased fibrinolysis results from excessive fibrinolytic activators and decreased levels of inhibitors, such as alpha-2 (α2)-antiplasmin.

Thrombocytopenia and thrombocytopathies are manifestations of liver disease. Thrombocytopenia is caused by splenomegaly, which often accompanies liver disease. Splenic pooling of platelets is the major cause of thrombocytopenia. Thrombocytopathies are associated with elevated levels of fibrin split products, ethanol, or drugs.

Treatment of hemostasis alterations in liver disease must be comprehensive to cover all aspects of dysfunctions. Fresh frozen plasma (FFP) administration is the treatment of choice; however, not all individuals tolerate the volume needed to adequately replace all deficient factors. Alternative modalities include the addition of exchange transfusions and platelet concentration to FFP administration.

Consumptive thrombohemorrhagic disorders

Consumptive thrombohemorrhagic disorders are a heterogeneous group of conditions that demonstrate the entire spectrum of hemorrhagic and thrombotic pathologic findings. The symptoms of these disorders also range from the subtle to the devastating and are generally considered to be intermediary disease processes that complicate a vast number of primary disease states. These disorders are also characterized by confusion and controversy related to their diagnosis, treatment, and management. No one term is capable of covering all the possible varieties of these disorders; however, DIC is most commonly used in the clinical setting to describe a pathologic condition that is associated with hemorrhage and thrombosis.

Disseminated intravascular coagulation

Disseminated intravascular coagulation (DIC) is an acquired clinical syndrome characterized by widespread activation of coagulation resulting in formation of fibrin clots in medium and small vessels throughout the body.[26] Widespread clotting may lead to blockage of blood flow to organs, resulting in multiple organ failure. The magnitude of clotting may result in consumption of platelets and clotting factors leading to severe bleeding.

The clinical course of DIC is largely determined by the intensity of the stimulus, host response, and comorbidities and range from an acute, severe, life-threatening process that is characterized by massive hemorrhage and thrombosis to a chronic, low-grade condition. The chronic condition is characterized by subacute hemorrhage and diffuse microcirculatory thrombosis. DIC may be localized to one specific organ or generalized, involving multiple organs.

PATHOPHYSIOLOGY Coagulation is designed to function at local areas of vascular damage, resulting in cessation of bleeding and activation of repair to the vessels. DIC results from abnormally widespread and ongoing activation of clotting.

A variety of conditions are associated with DIC (Box 20-2). Infectious disease, particularly involving sepsis, is the most common condition associated with DIC. Although all types of infections may cause DIC, bacterial infections (both gram-negative and gram-positive) are the most commonly observed underlying causes. DIC may occur in up to 50% of persons with gram-negative sepsis. Most solid tumors and hematologic cancers may trigger DIC. Approximately 15% of those with metastatic cancer or acute leukemia have symptoms of DIC. Severe trauma, especially to the brain, can induce DIC. DIC occurs in about two-thirds of individuals with a systemic inflammatory response to the trauma. Some complications of pregnancy are also associated with DIC; incidences range from 50% for women with placental abruptions to less than 10% for severe preeclampsia.

Regardless of the underlying disease that initiates DIC, the common pathway appears to be excessive and widespread exposure of tissue factor (TF or tissue thromboplastin) (Figure 20-16). This may occur by several mechanisms. Widespread damage to vascular endothelium results in exposure of subendothelial tissue factor. Several types of

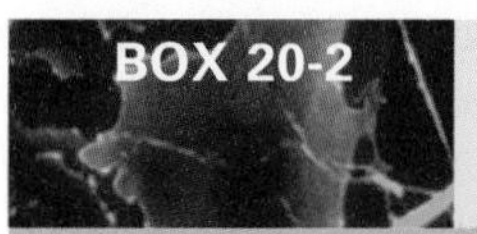

Acute Disseminated Intravascular Coagulation (DIC)

- Malignancy: acute leukemias, metastatic solid malignancies
- Infections: bacterial (gram-negative endotoxin, gram-positive mucopolysaccharides), viral (hepatitis, varicella, cytomegalovirus), fungal, parasitic
- Pregnancy complications: eclampsia/preeclampsia, placental abruption, amniotic fluid embolism
- Severe trauma: head injury, burns, crush injuries, tissue necrosis
- Liver disease: obstructive jaundice, acute liver failure
- Intravascular hemolysis: transfusion reactions, drug-induced hemolysis
- Medical devices: aortic balloon, prosthetic devices
- Hypoxia and low blood flow states: arterial hypotension secondary to shock, cardiopulmonary arrest

Data from Bick, RL et al: *Hematology: clinical and laboratory practice*, St Louis, 1993, Mosby.

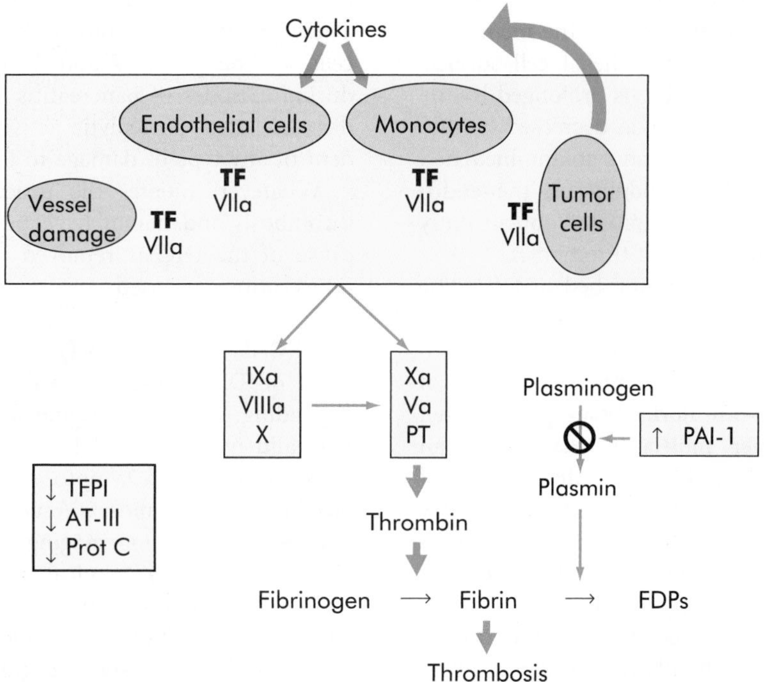

Figure 20-16 ■ **Pathophysiology of Disseminated Intravascular Coagulation (DIC).** DIC is initiated by exposure of tissue factor (TF) after vessel damage, on tumor cells, or on the surface of endothelial cells or monocytes after exposure to cytokines, some of which may be produced by cytokines. TF reacts with and activates factor VII to produce a TF-VIIa complex, which can directly activate clotting factors IX and X. Activated factor IX (IXa) can interact with factors VIIIa and X to activate factor X to Xa. Factor Xa complexes with factor Va and prothrombin (PT) to form the prothrombinase complex that produces thrombin, which in turn activates fibrinogen to fibrin. Fibrin polymerizes to form clots. In DIC, natural regulators of the clotting system (tissue factor pathway inhibitor [TFPI], antithrombin-III [AT-III], and protein C [Prot C]) are decreased resulting in increased thrombin formation. Clots are normally broken down by plasmin, which is produced from plasminogen and degrades fibrin into fibrin degradation products (FDPs). In DIC, fibrinolysis is prevented by high levels of plasminogen-activator inhibitor type 1 (PAI-1), which inhibits the production of plasmin. The summation of these changes is greatly increased deposition of fibrin clots in the vessels and thrombosis.

cells either after induction by cytokines or constitutively express TF on their surface. Endothelial cells and monocytes do not normally express surface TF unless stimulated by inflammatory cytokines (particularly IL-6 and TNFα). These cytokines are abundantly produced during many of the conditions listed in Box 20-2. Many tumors express surface TF or produce cytokines that can stimulate TF expression by endothelium, monocytes, or both.

TF binds clotting factor VII, which undergoes activation to factor VIIa (also see Figure 19-17). The TF-VIIa complex is a potent activator of clotting factors IX and X, which leads to conversion of prothrombin to thrombin and formation of fibrin clots. This pathway appears to be the primary route by which DIC is initiated; in animal models of DIC, inhibition of TF or factor VIIa completely prevents the generation of thrombi by gram-negative bacterial endotoxin.

Not only is the clotting system extensively activated in DIC, but the predominant natural anticoagulants (tissue factor pathway inhibitor, antithrombin III, protein C) are also greatly diminished. Tissue factor pathway inhibitor (TFPI) in association with factor Xa inactivates the TF-VIIa complex, preventing further activation of clotting. Antithrombin III (AT-III) is the principal inhibitor of thrombin, preventing further activation of fibrinogen to fibrin. Protein C is activated by thrombin to form activated protein C, which uses protein S as a cofactor to degrade factors Va and VIIIa. The rate of protein C activation increases dramatically if thrombin has first bound to the membrane protein thrombomodulin on the endothelial cell surface. During DIC, the activation of clotting is prolonged by the increased rate of consumption, as well as decreased synthesis, of these inhibitors and protein S and cytokine-mediated decreased expression of thrombomodulin on the endothelial cell surface. Thus, clotting is initiated concurrently with loss of regulation of the extent of thrombosis.

The rate of fibrinolysis is also diminished in DIC. The primary component of the fibrinolysis is **plasmin,** which exists in the circulation as an inactive precursor, plasminogen. Plasminogen is activated to plasmin by a variety of substances, including thrombin, fibrin, tissue plasminogen activator (t-PA), and other molecules. Plasmin is an enzyme that digests fibrin clots, thus controlling the extent of fibrin deposition in the vessels. During DIC, the activity of plasmin is diminished by increased production of its natural inhibitor, plasminogen-activator inhibitor type I. Although some fibrinolytic activity remains, the level is inadequate to control the systemic deposition of fibrin. The slow breakdown of fibrin by plasmin produces fibrin degradation products that are released into the blood. These are potent anticoagulants that are normally removed from blood by fibronectin and macrophages. During DIC, the presence of fibrin degradation products is prolonged, probably because of diminished production of fibronectin. Low levels of fibronectin suggest a poor prognosis.

Although thrombosis is generalized and widespread, individuals with DIC are paradoxically at risk for hemorrhage. Hemorrhage is secondary to the abnormally high consumption of clotting factors and platelets, as well as the anticoagulant properties of fibrin degradation products. Thrombin causes platelet activation and aggregation—an event that occurs early in the development of DIC—which facilitates microcirculatory coagulation and obstruction in the initial phase. However, platelet consumption exceeds production, resulting in a thrombocytopenia that increases bleeding.

Activation of clotting also leads to activation of other inflammatory pathways, including the kallikrein-kinin and complement systems (see Chapter 5). Factor XIIa, generated in DIC, converts prekallikrein to kallikrein, ultimately resulting in conversion to circulating kinins. Activation of these systems contributes to increased vascular permeability, hypotension, and shock. Activated complement components also induce platelet destruction, which initially contributes to the thrombosis and later to the thrombocytopenia.

The deposition of fibrin clots in the circulation interferes with blood flow, causing widespread organ hypoperfusion. This condition may lead to ischemia, infarction, and necrosis, further potentiating and complicating the existing DIC process by causing further release of TF and eventually organ failure.

In addition to initiation of clotting by tissue factor, DIC may be precipitated by direct proteolytic activation of factor X. This has been described as thrombin mimicry and is the result of proteases directly converting fibrinogen to fibrin. These proteases may come from snake venom, some tumor cells, or the pancreas and liver where they are released during episodes of pancreatitis and various stages of liver disease. Direct proteolytic activity appears to be independent of any type of damage to the endothelium or tissue.

Whatever initiates the process of DIC, the cycle of thrombosis and hemorrhage persists until the underlying cause of the DIC is removed or appropriate therapeutic interventions are used.

CLINICAL MANIFESTATIONS Clinical signs and symptoms of DIC present a wide spectrum of possibilities, depending on the underlying disease process that initiates DIC and whether the DIC is acute or chronic in nature (Box 20-3). Most symptoms are the results of either bleeding or thrombosis. Acute DIC presents with rapid development of hemorrhaging (oozing) from venipuncture sites, arterial lines, surgical wounds, or development of ecchymotic lesions (purpura, petechiae) and hematomas. Other sites of bleeding include the eyes (sclera, conjunctiva), the nose, and the gums. Most individuals with DIC demonstrate bleeding at three or more unrelated sites, and any combination may be observed. Shock of variable intensity, out of proportion to the amount of blood loss, also may be observed. Hemorrhaging into closed compartments of the body also can occur and may precede the development of shock.

Manifestations of thrombosis are not always as evident, even though it is often the first pathologic alteration to occur. Several organ systems are susceptible to microvascular

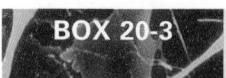

BOX 20-3 Clinical Manifestations Associated With DIC

Integumentary System
Widespread hemorrhage and vascular lesions
Oozing from puncture sites, incisions, mucous membranes
Acrocyanosis (irregular-shaped cyanotic patches)
Gangrene

Central Nervous System
Subarachnoid hemorrhage
Altered state of consciousness (slight confusion to convulsions and coma)

Gastrointestinal System
Occult bleeding to massive gastrointestinal bleeding
Abdominal distention
Malaise
Weakness

Pulmonary System
Pulmonary infarctions
ARDS
Cyanosis
Tachypnea
Hypoxemia

Renal System
Hematuria
Oliguria
Renal failure

Modified from Bailes BK: Disseminated intravascular coagulation. Principles, treatment, nursing management, *AORN J* 55(2):517–529, 1992.
DIC, Disseminated intravascular coagulation; *ARDS,* adult respiratory distress syndrome.

thrombosis associated with dysfunction: cardiovascular, pulmonary, central nervous, renal, and hepatic systems. Acute and accurate clinical interpretations are critical to preventing progression of DIC that may lead to multisystem organ dysfunction and failure. (Multiple organ dysfunction and failure are discussed further in Chapter 23.) Indicators of multisystem dysfunction include changes in level of consciousness, behavior, and confusion, seizure activity, oliguria, hematuria, hypoxia, hypotension, hemoptysis, chest pain, and tachycardia. Symmetric cyanosis of fingers and toes (blue finger/toe syndrome), nose, and breast may be observed and indicates macrovascular thrombosis. This may lead to infarction and gangrene that may require amputation. Jaundice also is observed and most likely results from red cell destruction rather than liver dysfunction.

Individuals with chronic or low-grade DIC do not present with the overt manifestations of hemorrhaging and thrombosis but instead have subacute bleeding and diffuse thrombosis and are described as having compensated DIC. The major characteristic of this state is an increased turnover and decreased survival time of the components of hemostasis: platelets and clotting factors. Occasionally, diffuse or localized thrombosis develops, but this is infrequent.

EVALUATION AND TREATMENT No single laboratory test can be used to effectively diagnosis DIC. Diagnosis is based primarily on clinical symptoms and confirmed by a combination of laboratory tests. The person must present with a clinical condition that is known to be associated with DIC. The most commonly used combination of laboratory tests usually confirm thrombocytopenia or a rapidly decreasing platelet count on repeated testing, prolongation of clotting times, the presence of fibrin degradation products, and decreased levels of coagulation inhibitors.

Platelet counts below 100,000/mm^3 or a progressive decrease in platelet counts is very sensitive for DIC, although not greatly specific. These changes usually indicate consumption of platelets.

The standard coagulation tests (e.g., prothrombin time [PT], activated partial thromboplastin time [aPTT]) also have a high degree of sensitivity, but they are not highly specific for DIC. As a result of consumption of circulating clotting factors, these tests are usually abnormal, ranging from shortened to prolonged times. However, conditions other than DIC may prolong clotting times.

Detection of fibrin degradation products is more specific for DIC. Detection of D-dimers is a widely used test for DIC. A D-dimer is a molecule produced by plasmin degradation of cross-linked fibrin in clots. D-dimers in the blood can be quantified using ELISA tests that include commercially available and highly specific monoclonal antibody against the D-dimer. Agglutination tests for other fibrin degradation products are available. Fibrin degradation products are elevated in the plasma in 95% to 100% of cases; however, they are less specific for DIC than D-dimers and only document the presence of plasmin and its action of fibrin. ELISAs for markers of thrombin activity are sometimes used. For instance, ELISAs for fibrinopeptide A, a breakdown product of fibrinogen produced during activation by thrombin, are available. However, these assays are also less specific for DIC.

Levels of coagulation inhibitors (e.g., antithrombin III [AT-III], protein C) can be measured by assays that rely on function or by ELISAs that quantify the amount of the specific inhibitor. AT-III levels can provide key information for diagnosing and monitoring therapy of DIC. Initial levels of functional AT-III are low in DIC because thrombin is irreversibly complexed with activated clotting factors and AT-III.

Treatment of DIC is directed toward (1) eliminating the underlying pathology, (2) controlling ongoing thrombosis, and (3) maintaining organ function. Elimination of the underlying pathology is the initial intervention in the treatment phase in order to eliminate the trigger for activation of clotting. Once the stimulus is gone, production of coagulation factors in the liver leads to restoration of normal plasma levels within 24 to 48 hours.

Control of thrombosis is more difficult to attain. Heparin has been used for this; however, its use is controversial because its mechanism of action is binding to and activating AT-III, which is deficient in many types of DIC.

Currently, heparin is only indicated in certain types of situations related to DIC. For instance, heparin seems to be effective in DIC caused by a retained dead fetus or associated with acute promyelocytic leukemia. Organ function is compromised by microthrombi, and there is a risk of losing an extremity because of vascular occlusion; thus, heparin is also indicated in these conditions. Heparin's usefulness, however, for DIC that is precipitated by septic shock has not been established and so is contraindicated in that instance; heparin is also contraindicated when there is evidence of postoperative bleeding, peptic ulcer, or central nervous system bleeding.

Replacement of deficient coagulation factors, platelets, and other coagulation elements is gaining recognition as an effective treatment modality. Their use is not without controversy, however, because a major concern with replacement therapy is the possible risk of adding components that will increase the rate of thrombosis. Clinical judgment is the key factor in determining whether replacement is to be used as a treatment modality.

Several clinical trials are evaluating replacement of anticoagulants (i.e., AT-III, protein C). Replacement of AT-III appears to be effective in DIC caused by sepsis. Low levels of AT-III correlate with sepsis-initiated DIC, which makes a case for its use. AT-III inactivates thrombin, factor Xa, factor IXa, and other activated components of the clotting system. Heparin augments AT-III, but the combination of heparin with AT-III replacement has not been established. Antifibrinolytic drugs also are used in treatment but are limited to instances of life-threatening bleeding that have not been controlled by blood component replacement therapy.

Maintenance of organ function is achieved by fluid replacement to sustain adequate circulating blood volume and maintain optimal tissue and organ perfusion. Fluids may be required to restore blood pressure, cardiac output, and urine output to normal parameters.

Thromboembolic disorders

Certain conditions within the blood vessels predispose an individual to develop clots spontaneously. A clot attached to the vessel wall is called a **thrombus** (Figure 20-17). A thrombus is composed of fibrin and blood cells and can develop in either the arterial or venous system. Arterial clots form under conditions of high blood flow and are composed mostly of platelet aggregates held together by fibrin strands. Venous clots form in conditions of low flow and are composed mostly of red cells with larger amounts of fibrin and few platelets.

A thrombus eventually reduces or obstructs blood flow to tissues or organs, such as the heart, brain, or lungs, depriving them of essential nutrients critical to survival. A thrombus also has the potential of detaching from the vessel wall and circulating within the bloodstream (referred to as an **embolus**). The embolus may become lodged in smaller blood vessels, blocking blood flow into the local tissue or organ and leading to ischemia. Whether episodes of thromboembolism are life threatening depends on the site of vessel occlusion.

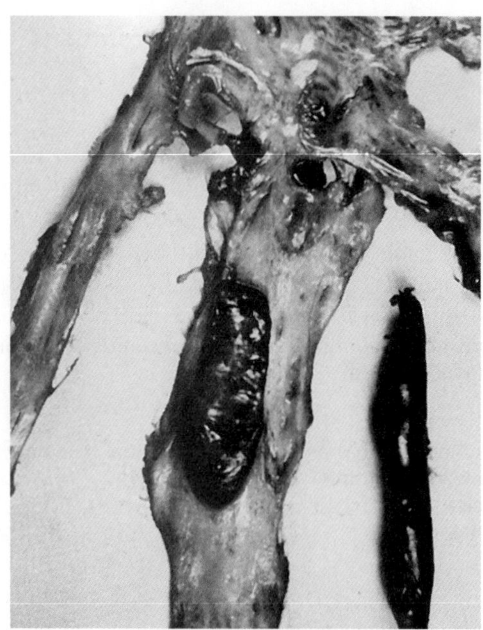

Figure 20-17 ■ **Thrombus.** Thrombus arising in valve pocket at upper end of superficial femoral vein. Postmortem clot on the right is shown for comparison. (From McLachlin J, Paterson JC: Some basic observations on venous thrombosis and pulmonary embolism, *Surg Gynecol Obstet* 93(1):1–8, 1951.)

Therapy consists of removal or breakdown of the clot and supportive measures. Anticoagulant therapy is effective in treating or preventing venous thrombosis; it is not as useful in treating or preventing arterial thrombosis. Parenteral heparin is the major anticoagulant used to treat thromboembolism. Oral coumarin drugs also are widely used, particularly for individuals not hospitalized. More aggressive therapy may be indicated for such conditions as pulmonary embolism, coronary thrombosis, or thrombophlebitis. Streptokinase and urokinase activate the fibrinolytic system and are administered to accelerate the lysis of known thrombi. Thrombolytic therapy has limited uses and is prescribed with a high degree of caution because it can cause hemorrhagic complications.

The risk for developing spontaneous thrombi is related to several factors, referred to as the **Virchow triad:** (1) injury to the blood vessel endothelium, (2) abnormalities of blood flow, and (3) hypercoagulability of the blood.

Endothelial injury to blood vessels can result from atherosclerosis (plaque deposits on arterial walls) (see Chapter 23). Atherosclerosis initiates platelet adhesion and aggregation, promoting the development of atherosclerotic plaques that enlarge, causing further damage and occlusion. Other causes of vessel endothelial injury may be related to hemodynamic alterations associated with hypertension and turbulent blood flow. Injury also is caused by radiation injury, exogenous chemical agents (toxins from cigarette smoke), endogenous agents (cholesterol), bacterial toxins or endotoxins, or immunologic mechanisms. Whatever the precipitating cause of endothelial injury, it is a potent thrombogenic agent.

Sites of turbulent blood flow in the arteries and stasis of blood flow in the veins are at risk for thrombus formation. In areas of turbulence, platelets and endothelial cells may be activated, leading to thrombosis. In sites of stasis, platelets may remain in contact with the endothelium for prolonged lengths of time, and clotting factors that would normally be diluted with fresh flowing blood are not diluted and may become activated. The most common clinical conditions that predispose to venous stasis and subsequent thromboembolic phenomena are major surgery (e.g., orthopedic surgery), acute myocardial infarction, congestive heart failure, limb paralysis, spinal injury, malignancy, advanced age, the postpartum period, and bed rest longer than 1 week. Turbulence and stasis occur with ulcerated atherosclerotic plaques (myocardial infarction), hyperviscosity (polycythemia), and conditions with deformed red cells (sickle cell anemia).

Hypercoagulability is the condition in which an individual is at risk for thrombosis, but by itself it is a rare cause of thrombosis. Hypercoagulability is differentiated according to whether it results from primary (hereditary) or secondary (acquired) causes.

Hereditary hypercoagulability and thrombosis

Hereditary thrombophilias that increase the risk to develop thrombosis include factor V Leiden mutation; prothrombin mutation; methylenetetrahydrofolate reductase (MTHFR) mutation leading to high homocysteine levels; and deficiencies in protein C, protein S, and antithrombin III (AT-III).[27] Most are autosomal dominant. Factor V Leiden results from a single nucleotide mutation that confers partial resistance to inactivation by activated protein C, resulting in prolonged high levels of activated factor V (factor Va) and overproduction of thrombin. It is the most common hereditary thrombophilias and is primarily observed in individuals of European ancestry. It is observed in about 5% of whites in the United States and in about 30% of individuals presenting with deep venous thrombosis (DVT) or pulmonary embolism.

Other hereditary thrombophilias are less common. Prothrombin mutation is observed in about 5% of individuals and leads to high levels of circulating prothrombin. More than 100 different known mutations lead to defects of proteins C, protein S, and AT-III and increase the risk of venous thrombosis. Mutations may lead to either quantitative (low levels of protein) or qualitative (production of defective protein) changes. MTHFR mutation leads to alterations in the metabolism of the amino acid homocysteine into methionine and abnormally elevated levels of that amino acid in the blood (hyperhomocysteinemia). Acquired hyperhomocysteinemia may result from deficiencies in vitamins B_6 or B_{12}, endocrine diseases (e.g., diabetes mellitus, hypothyroidism), pernicious anemia, inflammatory bowel disease, renal failure, and therapy with some drugs. The mechanism of hypercoagulability conferred by hyperhomocysteinemia is unclear but may be related to direct injury of endothelial cells or platelets or alteration of some components of the clotting system.

Tests to diagnosis-inherited thrombophilias include prothrombin time, partial thromboplastin time, levels of protein C, protein S, and AT-III. More elaborate tests to detect precise mutations in factor V, prothrombin, or MTHFR may be indicated.

Acquired hypercoagulability and thrombosis

Acquired hypercoagulable states include the antiphospholipid syndrome (APS).[28] The APS is an autoimmune syndrome characterized by autoantibodies against plasma membrane phospholipids and phospholipid-binding proteins. As with most autoimmune diseases, the predominate individual is female and of reproductive age. Those with APS are at risk for both arterial and venous thrombosis and a variety of obstetrical complications, including pregnancy loss and preeclampsia/eclampsia. The pathophysiology is related to autoantibodies directly reacting with platelets or endothelial cells (increasing the risk for thrombosis) or the placental surface (resulting in damage to the placenta). The predominant diagnostic tests measure prolongation of laboratory blood coagulation tests related to an antibody inhibitor (lupus anticoagulant) and specific ELISAs for antibodies against phospholipids (e.g., anticardiolipin antibody) or proteins that bind to phospholipids (e.g., β_2-glycoprotein I). Highly effective therapy (i.e., unfractionated or low-molecular-weight heparin with low-dose aspirin) is available to prevent the obstetrical complications.

✓ QUICK CHECK 20-6

1. Identify the three pathologic causes of DIC, and describe the manifestations associated with it.
2. Compare and contrast thrombocytopenia with thrombocytosis.
3. Why does vitamin K deficiency predispose an individual to coagulation disorder?
4. Compare and contrast a thrombus with an embolus.

Did You Understand?

Alterations of Erythrocyte Function

1. Anemia is generally defined as a reduction in the number or volume of circulating red cells or an alteration in hemoglobin.
2. The most common classification of anemias is based on changes in the cell size—represented by the suffix *cytic*—and changes in the cell's hemoglobin content—represented by the suffix *chromic.*
3. Clinical manifestations of anemia can be found in all organs and tissues throughout the body. Decreased oxygen delivery to tissues causes fatigue, dyspnea, syncope, angina, compensatory tachycardia, and organ dysfunction.
4. Macrocytic (megaloblastic) anemias are caused most commonly by deficiency of vitamin B_{12}. Pernicious anemia can be fatal unless vitamin B_{12} replacement is given.
5. Microcytic-hypochromic anemias are characterized by abnormally small red cells with insufficient hemoglobin content. The most common cause is iron deficiency.
6. Iron deficiency anemia usually develops slowly, with a gradual insidious onset of symptoms, including fatigue, weakness, dyspnea, alteration of various epithelial tissues, and vague neuromuscular complaints.
7. Iron deficiency anemia is usually a result of a chronic blood loss or decreased iron intake. Once the source of blood loss is identified and corrected, iron replacement therapy can be initiated.
8. Sideroblastic anemia results from impaired iron metabolism and abnormal sequestration of iron within the red cell. Treatment varies depending on the cause.
9. Normocytic-normochromic anemias are characterized by insufficient numbers of normal erythrocytes. Included in this category are aplastic, posthemorrhagic, and hemolytic anemia and anemia of chronic inflammation.
10. In aplastic anemia, erythrocyte stem cells are underdeveloped, defective, or absent. Unless the cause is determined, bone marrow aplasia results in death.
11. Posthemorrhagic anemia results from a sudden blood loss. Restoration of blood volume by plasma expanders or transfusions may diminish subjective symptoms of anemia. Hemoglobin restoration may take 6 to 8 weeks.
12. Hemolytic anemia results from premature destruction of red cells and may be acquired or hereditary. Of the acquired forms, autoimmune reaction and drug-induced hemolysis are the most common causes.
13. Anemia of chronic inflammation is associated with chronic infections, chronic inflammatory diseases, and malignancies.

Myeloproliferative Red Cell Disorders

1. Polycythemia vera is characterized by excessive proliferation of erythrocyte precursors in the bone marrow. Signs and symptoms result directly from increased blood volume and viscosity. Therapeutic phlebotomy to remove excessive blood volume and use of radioactive phosphorus have been helpful in decreasing the excessive red cell pool.
2. Polycythemia vera may spontaneously covert to acute myelogenous leukemia.

Alterations of Leukocyte Function

1. Quantitative alterations of leukocytes (too many or too few) can be caused by bone marrow dysfunction or premature destruction of cells in the circulation. Many quantitative changes in leukocytes occur in response to invasion by microorganisms.
2. Leukocytosis is a condition in which the leukocyte count is higher than normal and is usually a response to stress and invasion of microorganisms.
3. Leukopenia is a condition in which the leukocyte count is lower than normal and is caused by pathologic conditions, such as malignancies and hematologic disorders.
4. Granulocytosis (particularly as a result of an increase in neutrophils) occurs in response to infection. The marrow releases immature cells, causing a shift-to-the-left, when responding to an infection that has created a demand for neutrophils that exceeds the supply in the circulation.
5. Eosinophilia results most commonly from parasitic invasion and ingestion or inhalation of toxic foreign particles.
6. Basophilia is seen in hypersensitivity reactions because of the high content of histamine and subsequent release.
7. Monocytosis occurs during the late or recuperative phase of infection when macrophages (mature monocytes) phagocytose surviving microorganisms and debris.
8. Granulocytopenia, a significant decrease in neutrophils, can be a life-threatening condition if sepsis occurs; it is often caused by chemotherapeutic agents, severe infection, and radiation.
9. Infectious mononucleosis is an acute infection of B lymphocytes most commonly associated with the Epstein-Barr virus (EBV), a type of herpes virus. Transmission of EBV is through close personal contact, commonly through saliva, thus its nickname, the *kissing disease.*
10. Two of the earliest manifestations of infectious mononucleosis are sore throat and fever caused by inflammation at the primary site of viral entry.
11. Most causes of EBV infectious mononucleosis include fever lasting 7 to 10 days, sore throat, and enlargement and tenderness of the cervical lymph nodes. It is self-limiting and treatment consists of rest and symptomatic treatment.
12. The common pathologic feature of all forms of leukemia is an uncontrolled proliferation of leukocytes, overcrowding the bone marrow and resulting in decreased production and function of the other blood cell lines.
13. All leukemias are classified by the cell type involved, (a) lymphocytic or (b) myelogenous, and are differentiated by onset, acute or chronic. Thus, there are four major types of leukemia: acute lymphocytic leukemia (ALL), chronic lymphocytic leukemia (CLL), acute myelogenous leukemia (AML), and chronic myelogenous leukemia (CML).

Did You Understand?—Cont'd

14. Although the exact cause of leukemia is unknown, it is considered a clonal disorder. A high incidence of acute leukemias and CLL is reported in certain families, suggesting a genetic predisposition.
15. The major clinical manifestation of leukemia includes fatigue caused by anemia, bleeding caused by thrombocytopenia, fever secondary to infection, anorexia, and weight loss.
16. Chemotherapy is the treatment of choice for leukemia. Acute leukemias are associated with an increasing survival rate of 80% to 90%, with long-term survival of 30% to 40%. Chronic leukemias are associated with a longer life expectancy than are acute leukemias.
17. Chronic leukemias progress differently than acute leukemias, advancing slowly and without warning. The presence of the Philadelphia chromosome is a diagnostic marker for CML.

Alterations of Lymphoid Function

1. The number of lymphocytes is decreased (lymphocytopenia) in most acute infections and in some immunodeficiency syndromes.
2. Lymphocytosis occurs in viral infections (infectious mononucleosis and infectious hepatitis, in particular), leukemia, lymphomas, and some chronic infections.
3. Lymphomas are tumors of primary lymphoid tissue (thymus, bone marrow) or secondary lymphoid tissue (lymph nodes, spleen, tonsils, intestinal lymphoid tissue). The two major types of malignant lymphomas are Hodgkin lymphoma and non-Hodgkin lymphoma.
4. Distinctive abnormal chromosomes are present in multiple cells of the lymph nodes of an individual with Hodgkin lymphoma. The abnormal cell is called the Reed-Sternberg cell.
5. A virus might be involved in the pathogenesis of Hodgkin lymphoma. Some familial clustering suggests an unknown genetic mechanism.
6. An enlarged, painless mass or swelling, most commonly in the neck, is an initial sign of Hodgkin lymphoma. Local symptoms are produced by lymphadenopathy, usually caused by pressure or obstruction.
7. Treatment of Hodgkin lymphoma includes radiation therapy and chemotherapy. A cure is possible regardless of the stage of Hodgkin lymphoma; however, individuals treated with chemotherapy who relapse in less than 2 years have a poor prognosis.
8. The cause of lymph node enlargement and cancerous transformation in non-Hodgkin lymphoma is unknown. Immunosuppressed persons have a higher incidence of non-Hodgkin lymphoma, suggesting an immune mechanism.
9. Generally, with non-Hodgkin lymphoma, the swelling of lymph nodes is painless, and the nodes enlarge and transform over a period of months or years.
10. Individuals with non-Hodgkin lymphoma can survive for long periods. The treatment used is chemotherapy.
11. Burkitt lymphoma involves the jaw and facial bones and occurs in children from east-central Africa and New Guinea.
12. Multiple myeloma is a neoplasm of B cells (immature plasma cells) and mature plasma cells. It is characterized by multiple malignant tumor masses of plasma cells scattered throughout the skeletal system and sometimes found in soft tissue.
13. The exact cause of multiple myeloma is unknown, but genetic factors and chronic stimulation of the mononuclear phagocyte system by bacteria, viral agents, and chemicals have been suggested.
14. The major clinical manifestations for multiple myeloma include recurrent infections caused by suppression of the humoral immune response and renal disease as a result of Bence Jones proteinuria.
15. Chemotherapy is the treatment of choice for multiple myeloma. Survival is still only 2 to 3 years with chemotherapy, however. Treatment with thalidomide is showing promise as an effective therapeutic agent in producing long-term remissions.

Alterations of Splenic Function

1. Splenomegaly (enlargement of the spleen) may be considered normal in certain individuals, but its presence should not be ignored.
2. Splenomegaly results from (a) acute inflammatory or infectious processes, (b) congestive disorders, (c) infiltrative processes, and (d) tumors or cysts.
3. Hypersplenism (overactivity of the spleen) results from splenomegaly. Hypersplenism results in sequestering of the blood cells, causing increased destruction of red blood cells, which leads to the development of anemia.

Alterations of Platelets and Coagulation

1. Thrombocytopenia is characterized by a platelet count below 100,000/mm^3 of blood; a count below 50,000/mm^3 increases the potential for hemorrhage associated with minor trauma.
2. Thrombocytopenia exists in primary or secondary forms and is commonly associated with autoimmune diseases and viral infections; bacterial sepsis with DIC also results in thrombocytopenia.
3. Thrombocythemia is characterized by a platelet count more than 400,000 platelets/mm^3 of blood and is symptomatic when the count exceeds 1,000,000/mm^3, at which time the risk for intravascular clotting (thrombosis) is high.
4. Thrombocythemia is caused by accelerated platelet production in the bone marrow.
5. Qualitative alterations in normal platelet adherence or aggregation prevent platelet plug formation and may result in prolonged bleeding times.
6. Platelet dysfunction results from changes in the cellular contents and integrity.
7. Disorders of coagulation are usually caused by defects or deficiencies of one or more clotting factors.
8. Coagulation is impaired when there is a deficiency of vitamin K because of insufficient production of prothrombin and synthesis of clotting factors II, VII, IX, and X, often associated with liver diseases.

(Continued)

Did You Understand?—Cont'd

9. Disseminated intravascular coagulation (DIC) is a complex syndrome resulting from a variety of clinical conditions that release tissue factor causing an increase in fibrin and thrombin activity in the blood producing augmented clot formation and accelerated fibrinolysis. Sepsis is a condition that is often associated with DIC.
10. DIC is characterized by a cycle of intravascular clotting followed by active bleeding caused by the initial consumption of coagulation factors and platelets and diffuse fibrinolysis.
11. Diagnosis of DIC is based on measurement in the blood of end products characteristic of dysfunctional coagulation activity. Treatment is complex and nonstandardized and focused on removing the primary cause, restoring hemostasis, and preventing further organ damage.
12. Thromboembolic disease results from a fixed (thrombus) or moving (embolus) clot that blocks flow within a vessel, denying nutrients to tissues distal to the occlusion; death can result when clots obstruct blood flow to the heart, brain, or lungs.
13. Hypercoagulability is the result of deficient anticoagulation proteins. Secondary causes are conditions that promote venous stasis.
14. The term *Virchow triad* refers to three factors that can cause thrombus formation: (a) loss of integrity of the vessel wall, (b) abnormalities of blood flow, and (c) alterations in the blood constituents.

Key Terms

Absolute polycythemia, 516
Acquired sideroblastic anemia, 515
Agranulocytosis, 521
Anemia, 508
Anisocytosis, 508
Basopenia, 521
Basophilia, 521
B-cell neoplasm, 531
Bence Jones protein, 533
Blast cell, 522
Burkitt lymphoma, 532
Consumptive thrombohemorrhagic disorder, 540
Disseminated intravascular coagulation (DIC), 540
Embolus, 544
Eosinopenia, 521
Eosinophilia, 521
Essential (primary) thrombocythemia (ET), 538
Folate, 510
Granulocytopenia, 521
Granulocytosis, 519
Hemolysis, 509
Hemosiderosis, 515
Heparin-induced thrombocytopenia (HIT), 536
Hereditary sideroblastic anemia, 515
Hodgkin lymphoma (HL), 528
Hypercoagulability, 545
Hypersplenism, 535
Hypoplastic anemia, 515
Hypoxemia, 509
Idiopathic thrombocytopenia purpura (ITP), 537
Impaired hemostasis, 540
Infectious mononucleosis (IM), 521
Intrinsic factor (IF), 512
Iron deficiency anemia (IDA), 514
Koilonychia, 514
Leukemia, 522
Leukocytosis, 519
Leukopenia, 519
Lymphoblastic lymphoma (LL), 534
Lymphocytopenia, 521
Lymphocytosis, 521
Macrocytic (megaloblastic) anemia, 510
Microcytic-hypochromic anemia, 514
Monocytopenia, 521
Monocytosis, 521
M-protein, 533
Multiple myeloma (MM), 532
Myelodysplastic syndrome, 516
Neutropenia, 519
Neutrophilia, 519
NK-neoplasm, 531
Non-Hodgkin lymphoma (NHL), 531
Normocytic-normochromic anemia (NNA), 516
Pancytopenia, 524
Pernicious anemia (PA), 512
Phlebotomy, 516
Plasmin, 542
Poikilocytosis, 508
Polycythemia vera (PV), 548
Polycythemia, 516
Reed-Sternberg (RS) cell, 528
Relative polycythemia, 516
Reversible sideroblastic anemia, 515
Secondary thrombocythemia, 538
Shift-to-the-left (leukemoid reaction), 519
Shift-to-the-right, 519
Sideroblastic anemia (SA), 515
Splenomegaly, 535
T-cell neoplasm, 531
Thrombocythemia (thrombocytosis), 538
Thrombocytopenia, 536
Thrombotic thrombocytopenia purpura (TTP), 538
Thrombus, 544
Vasculitis, 540
Virchow triad, 544

References

1. Weiss G, Goodnough LT: Anemia of chronic disease, *N Engl J Med* 352:1011–1023, 2005.
2. Aslinia F, Mazza JJ, Yale SH: Megaloblastic anemia and other causes of macrocytosis, *Clin Med Res* 4(3):236–241, 2006.
3. Toh BH, Alderuccio F: Pernicious anaemia, *Autoimmunity* 37 (4):357–361, 2004.
4. Morris CR, Singer ST, Walters MC: Clinical hemoglobinopathies: iron, lungs, and new blood, *Curr Opin Hematol* 13 (6):407–418, 2006.
5. Young NS, Calado RT, Scheinberg P: Current concepts in the pathophysiology and treatment of aplastic anemia, *Blood* 108 (8):2509–2519, 2006.
6. Michiels JJ et al: Clinical and laboratory features, pathobiology of platelet-mediated thrombosis and bleeding complications, and the molecular etiology of essential thrombocythemia and polycythemia vera: therapeutic implications, *Semin Thromb Hemost* 32(3):174–207, 2006.

References—Cont'd

7. Harrison CN: Platelets and thrombosis in myeloproliferative diseases, *Hematology Amer Soc Hematol Educ Program* 2005:409–415, 2005.
8. Marris JA: Care of patients with neutropenia, *Clin J Oncol Nurs* 10(2):164–166, 2006.
9. Ebell MH: Epstein-Barr virus infectious mononucleosis, *Am Fam Physician* 70(7):1279–1287, 2004.
10. Bell AT, Fortune B, Sheeler R: Clinical inquiries: what test is the best for diagnosing infectious mononucleosis? *J Fam Pract* 55(9):799–802, 2006.
11. Jordan CT, Guzman ML, Noble M: Cancer stem cells, *N Engl J Med* 355:1253–1261, 2006.
12. Estey E, Dohner H: Acute myeloid leukemia, *Lancet* 368 (9550):1894–1907, 2006.
13. Chiorazzi N, Rai KR, Ferrarini M: Chronic lymphocytic leukemia, *N Engl J Med* 353:804–815, 2005.
14. Poppema S: Immunobiology and pathophysiology of Hodgkin lymphoma, *Hematology Amer Soc Hematol Educ Program* 2005:231–238, 2005.
15. Kuppers R, Hansmann ML: The Hodgkin and Reed/Sternberg cell, *Int J Biochem Cell Biol* 37(3):511–517, 2005.
16. Thorley-Lawson DA, Gross A: Persistence of the Epstein-Barr virus and the origins of associated lymphomas, *N Engl J Med* 350:1328–1337, 2004.
17. Cairo MS et al: Childhood and adolescent non-Hodgkin lymphoma: new insights in biology and critical challenges for the future, *Pediatr Blood Cancer* 45(6):753–769, 2005.
18. Yasui H et al: Recent advances in the treatment of multiple myeloma, *Curr Pharm Biotechnol* 7(5):381–393, 2006.
19. Hassan AA, Kroll MH: Acquired disorders of platelet function, *Hematology Amer Soc Hematol Educ Program* 2005:403–408, 2005.
20. Cines DB et al: Congenital and acquired thrombocytopenia, *Hematology Amer Soc Hematol Educ Program* 2004:390–406, 2004.
21. Handin RI: Inherited platelet disorders, *Hematology Amer Soc Hematol Educ Program* 2005:396–402, 2005.
22. Warkentin TE, Sheppard, J-A I: Testing for heparin-induced thrombocytopenia antibodies, *Transfus Med Rev* 20 (4):259–272, 2006.
23. Bennett CM, de Jong JLO, Neufeld EJ: Targeted ITP strategies: do they elucidate the biology of ITP and related disorders? *Pediatr Blood Cancer* 47(5 suppl):706–709, 2006.
24. Sadler JE et al: Recent advances in thrombotic thrombocytopenia purpura, *Hematology Amer Soc Hematol Educ Program* 2004:407–423, 2004.
25. Schafer AI: Thrombocytosis, *N Engl J Med* 350:1211–1219, 2004.
26. Levi M, Cate HT: Disseminated intravascular coagulation, *N Engl J Med* 341:586–592, 1999.
27. Franchini M et al: Inherited thrombophilia, *Crit Rev Clin Lab Sci* 43(3):249–290, 2006.
28. Merrill JT, Asherson RA: Catastrophic antiphosholipid syndrome, *Nat Clin Pract Rheumatol* 2(2):81–89, 2006.

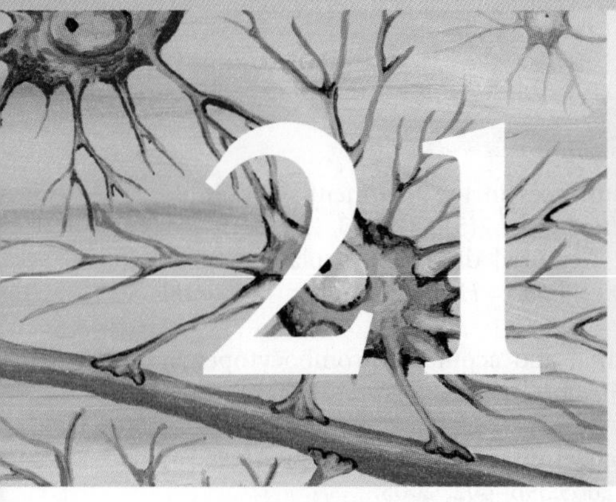

21 ALTERATIONS OF HEMATOLOGIC FUNCTION IN CHILDREN

Nancy E. Kline

CHAPTER OUTLINE

ELECTRONIC RESOURCES

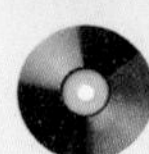

Companion CD
- Review Questions and Answers
- Animations

evolve Website
http://evolve.elsevier.com/Huether/
- Quick Check Answers
- Key Terms Exercises
- Critical Thinking Questions with Answers
- Algorithm Completion Exercises
- WebLinks

Among the diseases that affect erythrocytes are acquired disorders, such as iron deficiency anemia and hemolytic disease of the newborn, and inherited disorders, such as glucose-6-phosphate dehydrogenase deficiency, sickle cell disease, and the thalassemias.

Childhood disorders of coagulation and platelets include inherited hemorrhagic diseases, such as the hemophilias, and antibody-mediated hemorrhagic diseases, including idiopathic thrombocytopenic purpura. Finally, leukocyte disorders, such as leukemia and the lymphomas (both Hodgkin lymphoma and non-Hodgkin lymphoma) are discussed in this chapter.

DISORDERS OF ERYTHROCYTES

Anemia is the most common blood disorder in children. Like the anemias of adulthood, the anemias of childhood are caused by ineffective erythropoiesis or premature destruction of erythrocytes. The most common cause of insufficient erythropoiesis is iron deficiency, which may result from insufficient dietary intake or chronic loss of iron caused by bleeding. The **hemolytic anemias** of childhood may be divided into (1) disorders that result from premature destruction caused by intrinsic abnormalities of the erythrocytes and (2) disorders that result from damaging extraerythrocytic factors. The hemolytic anemias are either inherited or acquired.

The most dramatic form of acquired congenital hemolytic anemia is **hemolytic disease of the newborn (HDN),** also termed **erythroblastosis fetalis.** HDN is an alloimmunity (isoimmunity) disease in which maternal blood and fetal blood are antigenically incompatible, causing the mother's immune system to produce antibodies against fetal erythrocytes. Fetal erythrocytes attacked by (i.e., bound to) maternal antibodies are recognized as foreign or defective by the fetal mononuclear phagocyte system and are removed from the circulation by phagocytosis, usually in the fetal spleen. (For a complete examination of HDN, see discussion that follows.) Other acquired hemolytic anemias—some of which begin in utero—include those caused by infections or the presence of toxic chemicals.

The inherited forms of hemolytic anemia result from intrinsic defects of the child's erythrocytes, any of which can lead to erythrocyte removal by the mononuclear phagocyte system. Structural defects include abnormal cellular size or shape and abnormalities of plasma membrane structure (spherocytosis). Intracellular defects include enzyme deficiencies, the most common of which is **glucose-6-phosphate dehydrogenase (G6PD) deficiency,** and defects of hemoglobin synthesis, which manifest as sickle cell disease or thalassemia, depending on which component of hemoglobin is defective. These and other causes of childhood anemia are listed in Table 21-1.

Acquired Disorders

Iron deficiency anemia

Iron deficiency anemia is the most common blood disorder of infancy and childhood, with the highest incidence occurring between 6 months and 2 years of age. Incidence is not related to gender or race, but socioeconomic factors are important because they affect nutrition. Iron deficiency anemia is common in children because they need an extremely high amount of iron for normal growth to occur.

Between 4 years of age and the onset of puberty, dietary iron deficiency is uncommon. During adolescence, however, it is relatively common, especially in menstruating females.

TABLE 21-1

Anemias of Childhood

Cause	Anemic Condition
DEFICIENT ERYTHROPOIESIS OR HEMOGLOBIN SYNTHESIS	
Decreased stem cell population in marrow (congenital or acquired pure red cell aplasia)	Normocytic-normochromic anemia
Decreased erythropoiesis despite normal stem cell population in marrow (infection, inflammation, cancer, chronic renal disease, congenital dyserythropoiesis)	Normocytic-normochromic anemia
Deficiency of a factor or nutrient needed for erythropoiesis	
Cobalamin (vitamin B_{12}), folate	Megaloblastic anemia
Iron	Microcytic-hypochromic anemia
INCREASED OR PREMATURE HEMOLYSIS	
Alloimmune disease (maternal-fetal Rh, ABO, or minor blood group incompatibility)	Autoimmune hemolytic anemia
Autoimmune disease (idiopathic autoimmune hemolytic anemia, symptomatic systemic lupus erythematosus, lymphoma, drug-induced autoimmune processes)	Autoimmune hemolytic anemia
Inherited defects of plasma membrane structure (spherocytosis, elliptocytosis, stomatocytosis) or cellular size or both (pyknocytosis)	Hemolytic anemia
Infection (bacterial sepsis, congenital syphilis, malaria, cytomegalovirus infection, rubella, toxoplasmosis, disseminated herpes)	Hemolytic anemia
Intrinsic and inherited enzymatic defects (deficiencies) of glucose-6-phosphate dehydrogenase [G-6-PD], pyruvate kinase, 5-nucleotidase, glucose phosphate isomerase	Hemolytic anemia
Inherited defects of hemoglobin synthesis	Sickle cell anemia Thalassemia
Disseminated intravascular coagulation (see Chapter 20)	Hemolytic anemia
Galactosemia	Hemolytic anemia
Prolonged or recurrent respiratory or metabolic acidosis	Hemolytic anemia
Blood vessel disorders (cavernous hemangiomas, large vessel thrombus, renal artery stenosis, severe coarctation of the aorta)	Hemolytic anemia

Rapid growth, together with the average teenager's dietary habits, causes iron depletion.

PATHOPHYSIOLOGY Blood loss is a common cause of iron deficiency anemia in childhood. Chronic iron deficiency anemia from occult (hidden) blood loss may be caused by a gastrointestinal lesion, parasitic infestation, or hemorrhagic disease. As many as one third of infants with severe iron deficiency anemia have chronic intestinal blood loss induced by exposure to a heat-labile protein in cow's milk. Such exposure causes an inflammatory gastrointestinal reaction that damages the mucosa and results in diffuse hemorrhage.

CLINICAL MANIFESTATIONS The symptoms of mild anemia—listlessness and fatigue—usually are not present or are undetectable in infants and young children, who are unable to describe these symptoms. Therefore, parents generally do not note any change in the child's behavior or appearance until moderate anemia has developed. General irritability, decreased activity tolerance, weakness, and lack of interest in play are nonspecific indications of anemia. When hemoglobin levels fall below 5 g/dl, pallor, anorexia, tachycardia, and systolic murmurs may occur.

Other symptoms and signs include splenomegaly, widened skull sutures, decreased physical growth and developmental delays, pica (a behavior in which nonfood substances are eaten), and altered neurologic and intellectual functions, especially those involving attention span, alertness, and learning ability.

EVALUATION AND TREATMENT The most definitive test for differentiating iron deficiency from other microcytic states is the absence of iron stores in the bone marrow. However, measurement of serum ferritin concentration, transferrin saturation, and free erythrocyte protoporphyrin prevent having to proceed to actual bone marrow evaluation to make a diagnosis.[1] Evaluation and treatment of iron deficiency anemia in children are similar to those in adults. Dietary modification is required to prevent recurrences of iron deficiency anemia.

Hemolytic disease of the newborn

The most common cause of hemolytic anemia in newborns is alloimmune disease (HDN). HDN can occur only if antigens on fetal erythrocytes differ from antigens on maternal erythrocytes. Maternal-fetal incompatibility exists if mother and fetus differ in ABO blood type or if the fetus is Rh-positive and the mother is Rh-negative. Some minor blood antigens also may be involved. (The antigenic properties of erythrocytes are described in Chapter 7.)

ABO incompatibility occurs in about 20% to 25% of all pregnancies, but only 1 in 10 cases of ABO incompatibility results in HDN. Rh incompatibility occurs in fewer than 10% of pregnancies and rarely causes HDN in the first incompatible fetus. Even after five or more pregnancies, only 5% of women have babies with hemolytic disease. Usually erythrocytes from the first incompatible fetus cause the mother's immune system to produce antibodies that affect the fetuses of subsequent incompatible pregnancies. Only one in three cases of HDN is caused by Rh incompatibility; most cases are caused by ABO incompatibility.

PATHOPHYSIOLOGY HDN will result (1) if the mother's blood contains preformed antibodies against fetal erythrocytes or produces them on exposure to fetal erythrocytes, (2) if sufficient amounts of antibody (usually immunoglobulin G [IgG]) cross the placenta and enter fetal blood, and (3) if IgG binds with sufficient numbers of fetal erythrocytes to cause widespread antibody-mediated hemolysis or splenic removal. (Antibody-mediated cellular destruction is described in Chapter 7.

Maternal antibodies may be formed against type B erythrocytes if the mother is type A or against type A if the mother is type B. Usually, however, the mother is type O and the fetus is A or B. ABO incompatibility can cause HDN even if fetal erythrocytes do not escape into the maternal circulation during pregnancy. This occurs because the blood of most adults already contains anti-A or anti-B antibodies, which are produced on exposure to certain foods or infection by gram-negative bacteria. (Anti-O antibodies do not exist because type O erythrocytes are not antigenic.) Therefore, IgG against type A or B erythrocytes usually is preformed in maternal blood and can enter the fetal circulation throughout the first incompatible pregnancy.

Anti-Rh antibodies, on the other hand, are formed only in response to the presence of incompatible (Rh-positive) erythrocytes in the blood of an Rh-negative mother. Sources of exposure include fetal blood that is mixed with the mother's blood at the time of delivery, transfused blood, and, rarely, previous sensitization of the mother by her own mother's incompatible blood (Figure 21-1).

The first Rh-incompatible pregnancy generally presents no difficulties because few fetal erythrocytes cross the placental barrier during gestation. When the placenta detaches at birth, however, a large number of fetal erythrocytes usually enter the mother's bloodstream. If the mother is Rh-negative and the fetus is Rh-positive, the mother produces anti-Rh antibodies. Anti-Rh antibodies persist in the bloodstream for a long time, and if the next offspring is

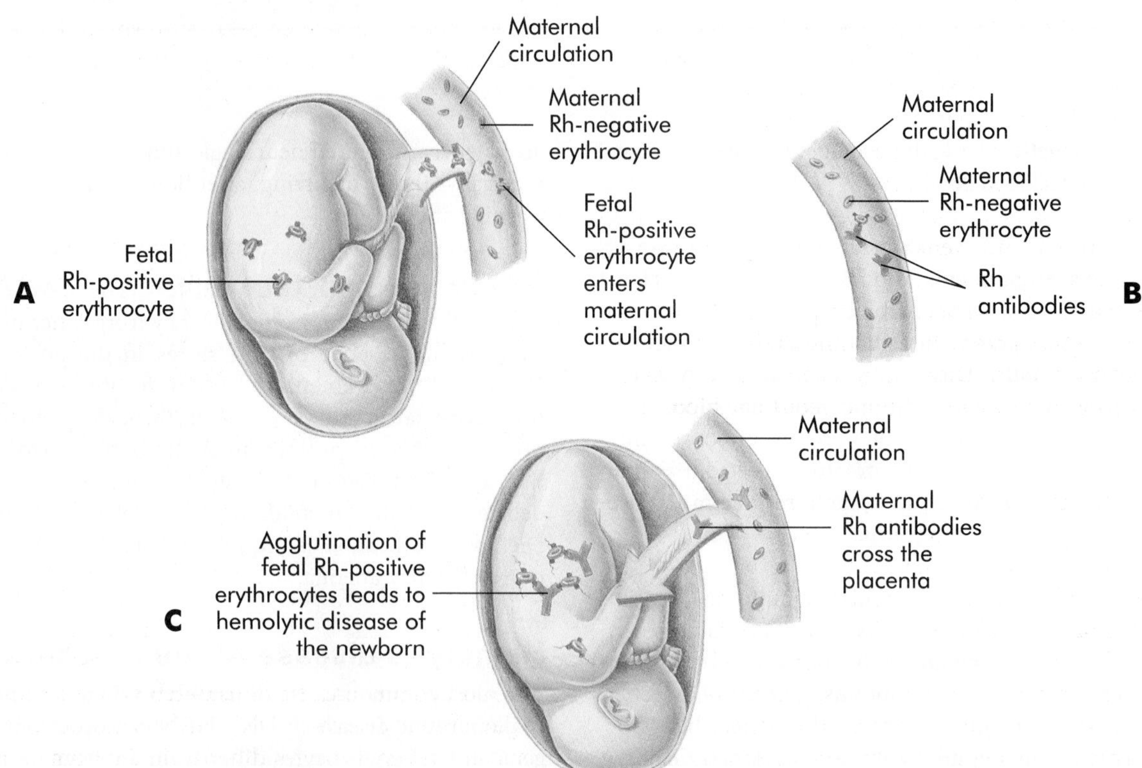

Figure 21-1 ■ Hemolytic Disease of the Newborn (HDN). A, Before or during delivery, Rh-positive erythrocytes from the fetus enter the blood of an Rh-negative woman through a tear in the placenta. **B,** The mother is sensitized to the Rh antigen and produces Rh antibodies. Because this usually happens after delivery, there is no effect on the fetus in the first pregnancy. **C,** During a subsequent pregnancy with an Rh-positive fetus, Rh-positive erythrocytes cross the placenta, enter the maternal circulation, and stimulate the mother to produce antibodies against the Rh antigen. The Rh antibodies from the mother cross the placenta, using agglutination and hemolysis of fetal erythrocytes, and HDN develops. (Modified from Seeley RR, Stephens TD, Tate P: *Anatomy and physiology,* ed 3, St Louis, 1995, Mosby.)

Rh-positive, the mother's anti-Rh antibodies can enter the fetus's bloodstream and destroy the erythrocytes. Antibodies against Rh antigen D are of the IgG class and easily cross the placenta.

IgG-coated fetal erythrocytes usually are destroyed in the spleen. As hemolysis proceeds, the fetus becomes anemic. Erythropoiesis accelerates, particularly in the liver and spleen, and immature nucleated cells (erythroblasts) are released into the bloodstream (hence the name *erythroblastosis fetalis*). The degree of anemia depends on the length of time the antibody has been in the fetal circulation, antibody concentration, and the ability of the fetus to compensate for increased hemolysis. Unconjugated (indirect) bilirubin, which is formed during breakdown of hemoglobin, is transported across the placental barrier into the maternal circulation and is excreted by the mother. Hyperbilirubinemia occurs in the neonate after birth because excretion of lipid-soluble unconjugated bilirubin through the placenta no longer is possible.

The pathophysiologic effects of HDN are more severe in Rh incompatibility than in ABO incompatibility. ABO incompatibility may resolve after birth without life-threatening complications. Maternal-fetal incompatibility in which a mother with type O blood has a child with type A or B blood usually is so mild that it does not require treatment.

Rh incompatibility is more likely than ABO incompatibility to cause severe or even life-threatening anemia, death in utero, or damage to the central nervous system. Severe anemia alone can cause death as a result of cardiovascular complications. Extensive hemolysis also results in increased levels of unconjugated bilirubin in the neonate's circulation. If bilirubin levels exceed the liver's ability to conjugate and excrete bilirubin, some of it is deposited in the brain, causing cellular damage and eventually, if the neonate does not receive exchange transfusions, death.

Fetuses that do not survive anemia in utero usually are stillborn, with gross edema in the entire body, a condition called **hydrops fetalis.** Death can occur as early as 17 weeks' gestation and results in spontaneous abortion.

CLINICAL MANIFESTATIONS Neonates with mild HDN may appear healthy or slightly pale, with slight enlargement of the liver or spleen. Pronounced pallor, splenomegaly, and hepatomegaly indicate severe anemia, which predisposes the neonate to cardiovascular failure and shock. Life-threatening Rh incompatibility is rare today, largely because of the routine use of Rh immunoglobulin.

Because the maternal antibodies remain in the neonate's circulatory system after birth, erythrocyte destruction can continue. This causes **hyperbilirubinemia** and **icterus neonatorum (neonatal jaundice)** shortly after birth. Without replacement transfusions, in which the child receives Rh-negative erythrocytes, the bilirubin is deposited in the brain, a condition termed **kernicterus.** Kernicterus produces cerebral damage and usually causes death **(icterus gravis neonatorum).** Infants who do not die may have mental retardation, cerebral palsy, or high-frequency deafness.

EVALUATION AND TREATMENT Routine evaluation of fetuses at risk for HDN (i.e., fetuses resulting from Rh- or ABO-incompatible matings) includes the Coombs test. The indirect Coombs test measures antibody in the mother's circulation and indicates whether the fetus is at risk for HDN. The direct Coombs test measures antibody already bound to the surfaces of fetal erythrocytes and is used primarily to confirm the diagnosis of antibody-mediated HDN. With a prior history of fetal hemolytic disease, diagnostic tests are done to determine risk with the current pregnancy. These tests include maternal antibody titers, fetal blood sampling, amniotic fluid spectrophotometry, and ultrasound fetal assessment.

The key to treatment of HDN resulting from Rh incompatibility lies in prevention (immunoprophylaxis). One of the success stories of immunology has been the result obtained with Rh immune globulin (RhoGAM), a preparation of antibody against Rh antigen D. If an Rh-negative woman is given Rh immune globulin within 72 hours of exposure to Rh-positive erythrocytes, she will not produce antibody against the D antigen, and the next Rh-positive baby she conceives will be protected.

If antigenic incompatibility of the mother's erythrocytes is not discovered in time to administer prophylactic immune globulin (RhoGAM) and a child is born with HDN, treatment consists of exchange transfusions in which the neonate's blood is replaced with new Rh-positive blood that is not contaminated with anti-Rh antibodies. Phototherapy also is used to reduce the toxic effects of unconjugated bilirubin.

Inherited Disorders

Sickle cell disease

Sickle cell disease is a group of disorders characterized by the production of abnormal **hemoglobin S (Hb S)** within the erythrocytes. Hb S is formed by a genetic mutation in which one amino acid (valine) replaces another (glutamic acid) (Figure 21-2). Hb S, the so-called sickle hemoglobin, reacts to deoxygenation and dehydration by solidifying and stretching the erythrocyte into an elongated sickle shape, producing hemolytic anemia.

Sickle cell disease is an inherited, autosomal recessive disorder expressed as sickle cell anemia, sickle cell–thalassemia disease, or sickle cell–hemoglobin C disease, depending on mode of inheritance (Table 21-2). (See Chapter 2 for a discussion of genetic inheritance of disease.) **Sickle cell anemia,** a homozygous form, is the most severe. **Sickle cell–thalassemia** and **sickle cell–Hb C disease** are heterozygous forms in which the child simultaneously inherits another type of abnormal hemoglobin from one parent. **Sickle cell trait,** in which the child inherits Hb S from one parent and normal hemoglobin (Hb A) from the other, is a heterozygous carrier state that rarely has clinical manifestations. All forms of sickle cell disease are lifelong conditions and have no known cure.

Sickle cell disease tends to occur in persons with origins in equatorial countries, particularly central Africa, the Near

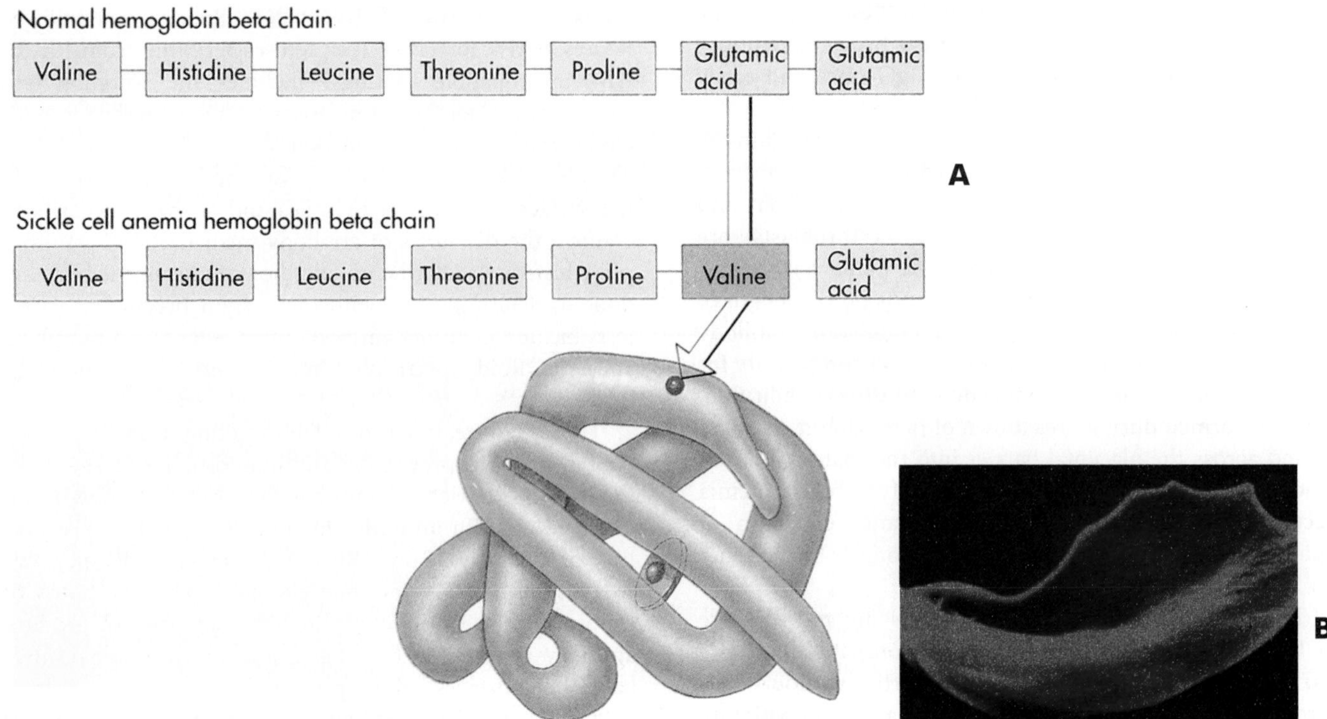

Figure 21-2 ■ **Sickle Cell Hemoglobin. A,** Sickle cell hemoglobin is produced by a recessive allele of the gene encoding the beta chain of the protein hemoglobin. It represents a single amino acid change from glutamic acid to valine at the sixth position of the chain. In the folded beta-chain molecule, the sixth position contacts the alpha chain and the amino acid change causes the hemoglobins to aggregate into long chains, altering the shape of the cell. **B,** Characteristic shape of sickled red blood cell (or cells). (**A** from Raven PH, Johnson GB: *Biology,* ed 3, Boston, 1993, Times Mirror Higher Education Group. **B** from Miale JB: *Laboratory medicine: hematology,* ed 6, St Louis, 1982, Mosby; courtesy Dr. M. Bessis.)

TABLE 21-2

Inheritance of Sickle Cell Disease

Hemoglobin Inherited From First Parent	Hemoglobin Inherited From Second Parent	Form of Sickle Cell Disease in Child
Hb S (an abnormal hemoglobin)	Hb S	Sickle cell anemia: homozygous inheritance in which the child's hemoglobin is mostly Hb S, with the remainder Hb F (fetal hemoglobin)
Hb S	Defective or insufficient alpha or beta chains of HbA (alpha- or beta-thalassemia)	Sickle cell–thalassemia disease (heterozygous inheritance of Hb S and alpha- or beta-thalassemia)
Hb S	Hb C or D (both abnormal hemoglobins)	Sickle cell–hemoglobin C (or D) disease (heterozygous inheritance of hemoglobin S and either C or D)
Hb S	Normal hemoglobins (mostly Hb A)	Sickle cell trait, the carrier state (heterozygous inheritance of Hb S and normal hemoglobin)

East, the Mediterranean area, and parts of India. In the United States, sickle cell disease is most common in blacks, with a reported incidence ranging from 1:400 to 1:500 live births. In the general population, the risk of two black parents having a child with sickle cell anemia is 0.7%. Sickle cell–hemoglobin C disease is less common (1 in 800 births), and sickle cell–thalassemia occurs in 1 in 1700 births.

Sickle cell trait occurs in 7% to 13% of African Americans, whereas its incidence among East Africans may be as high as 45%. The sickle cell trait may provide protection against lethal forms of malaria, a genetic advantage to carriers who reside in endemic regions for malaria (Mediterranean and African zones) but no advantage to carriers living in the United States.

PATHOPHYSIOLOGY Hemoglobin S is soluble and usually causes no problem when properly oxygenated. When oxygen tension decreases, the single amino acid substitution in the beta-globin chain of Hb S polymerizes, forming abnormal fluid polymers. As these polymers realign, they cause the red cell to deform into the sickle shape.[2] Sickling depends on the degree of oxygenation, pH, and dehydration of the individual. A decrease in oxygenation (hypoxemia) and pH, as well as dehydration, increases sickling. Deoxygenation is probably the most important variable in determining the occurrence of sickling.[3] Sickle-trait cells sickle at oxygen tensions of about 15 mm Hg, whereas those from an individual with sickle cell disease begin to sickle at about 40 mm Hg. Sickled erythrocytes tend to plug the blood vessels, increasing viscosity of the blood, which slows circulation and causes vascular occlusion, pain, and organ infarction. Viscosity increases the time of exposure to less oxygenation, promoting further sickling. Sickled cells undergo hemolysis in the spleen or become sequestered there, causing blood pooling and infarction of splenic vessels. The anemia that follows triggers erythropoiesis in the marrow and, in extreme cases, in the liver (Figure 21-3).

Sickling usually is not permanent; most sickled erythrocytes regain a normal shape after reoxygenation and rehydration. Irreversible sickling is caused by irreversible plasma membrane damage caused by sickling. In persons with sickle cell anemia, in which the erythrocytes contain a high percentage of Hb S (75% to 95%), up to 30% of the erythrocytes can become irreversibly sickled. Occasionally, irreversible sickling occurs in sickle cell disease but not in the carrier state (sickle cell trait). Sickling also can be triggered by increased plasma osmolality, decreased plasma volume, and low environmental temperature.

CLINICAL MANIFESTATIONS When sickling occurs, the general manifestations of hemolytic anemia—pallor, fatigue, jaundice, and irritability—sometimes are accompanied by acute manifestations called *crises*. Extensive sickling can precipitate the following four types of crises:

1. **Vasoocclusive crisis (thrombotic crisis).** This begins with sickling in the microcirculation. As blood flow is obstructed by sickled cells, vasospasm occurs and a "logjam" effect blocks all blood flow through the vessel. Unless the process is reversed, thrombosis and infarction (death caused by lack of oxygen) of local tissue follow. Vasoocclusive crisis is extremely painful and may last for days or even weeks, with an average duration of 4 to 6 days. The frequency of this type of crisis is variable and unpredictable.
2. **Sequestration crisis.** Large amounts of blood become acutely pooled in the liver and spleen. This type of crisis is seen only in the young child. Because the spleen can hold as much as one fifth of the body's blood supply at one time, up to 50% mortality has been reported, with death being caused by cardiovascular collapse.
3. **Aplastic crisis.** Profound anemia is caused by diminished erythropoiesis despite an increased need for new erythrocytes. In sickle cell anemia, erythrocyte survival is only 10 to 20 days. Normally a compensatory increase

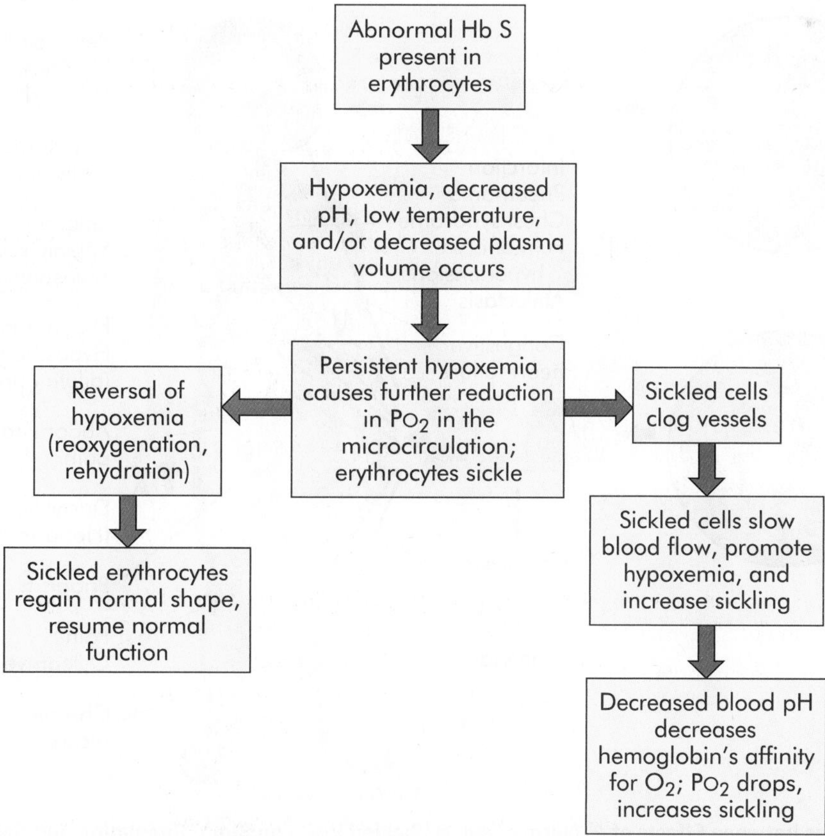

Figure 21-3 ■ **Sickling of Erythrocytes.**

in erythropoiesis (five to eight times normal) replaces the cells lost through premature hemolysis. If this compensatory response is compromised, aplastic crisis develops in a very short time.

4. **Hyperhemolytic crisis.** Although unusual, this may occur in association with certain drugs or infections.

The clinical manifestations of sickle cell disease usually do not appear until the infant is at least 6 months old, at which time the postnatal decrease in Hb F causes concentrations of Hb S to rise (Figure 21-4). Infection is the most common cause of death related to sickle cell disease. Sepsis and meningitis develop in as many as 10% of children with sickle cell anemia during the first 5 years of life, with a mortality rate of 25%. Survival time is unpredictable, but many individuals die in their 20s.

Sickle cell–Hb C disease is usually milder than sickle cell anemia. The main clinical problems are related to vasoocclusive crises and are believed to result from higher hematocrit values and viscosity. In older children, sickle cell retinopathy, renal necrosis, and aseptic necrosis of the femoral heads occur along with obstructive crises.

Sickle cell–thalassemia has the mildest clinical manifestations of all the sickle cell diseases. The normal hemoglobins, particularly Hb F, inhibit sickling. In addition, the erythrocytes tend to be small (microcytic) and to contain relatively little hemoglobin (hypochromic), making them less likely to occlude the microcirculation, even when in a sickled state.

EVALUATION AND TREATMENT The sickle cell trait does not affect life expectancy or interfere with daily activities. However, on rare occasions, severe hypoxia caused by shock, vigorous exercising at high altitudes, flying at high altitudes in unpressurized aircraft, or undergoing anesthesia is associated with vasoocclusive episodes in persons with sickle cell trait. These cells form an ivy shape instead of a sickle shape.

The parents' hematologic history and clinical manifestations may suggest that a child has sickle cell disease, but hematologic tests are necessary for diagnosis. If the sickle solubility test confirms the presence of Hb S in peripheral blood, hemoglobin electrophoresis provides information about the amount of Hb S in erythrocytes. Prenatal diagnosis can be made after chorionic villus sampling as early as 8 to 10 weeks' gestation or amniotic fluid analysis at 15 weeks' gestation. Newborn screening for sickle cell disease should be performed according to state law.

Treatment of sickle cell disease consists of supportive care aimed at preventing consequences of anemia and avoiding crises. Genetic counseling and psychologic support are important for the child and family.

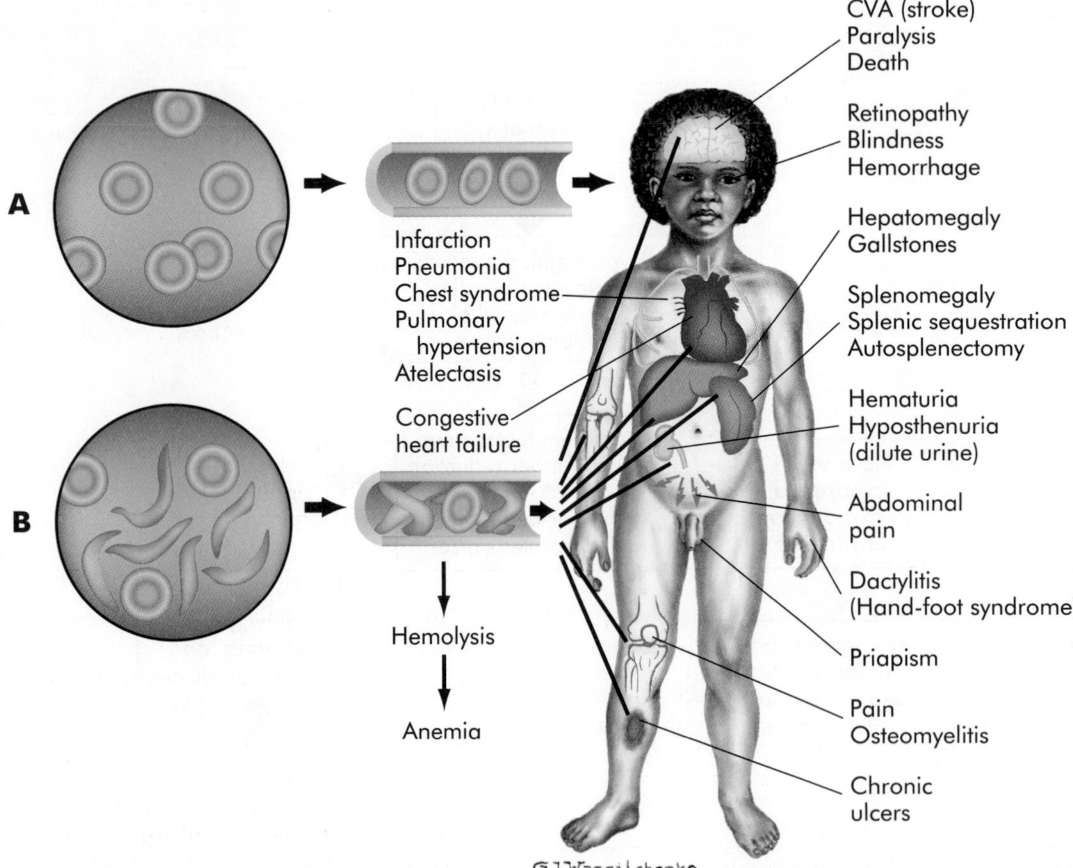

Figure 21-4 ■ **Differences between Effects of A, Normal, and B, Sickled RBCs on Blood Circulation and Selected Consequences in a Child.** (**A** and **B** adapted from Hockenberry MJ et al, editors: *Wong's nursing care of infants and children*, ed 8, St Louis, 2007, Mosby.)

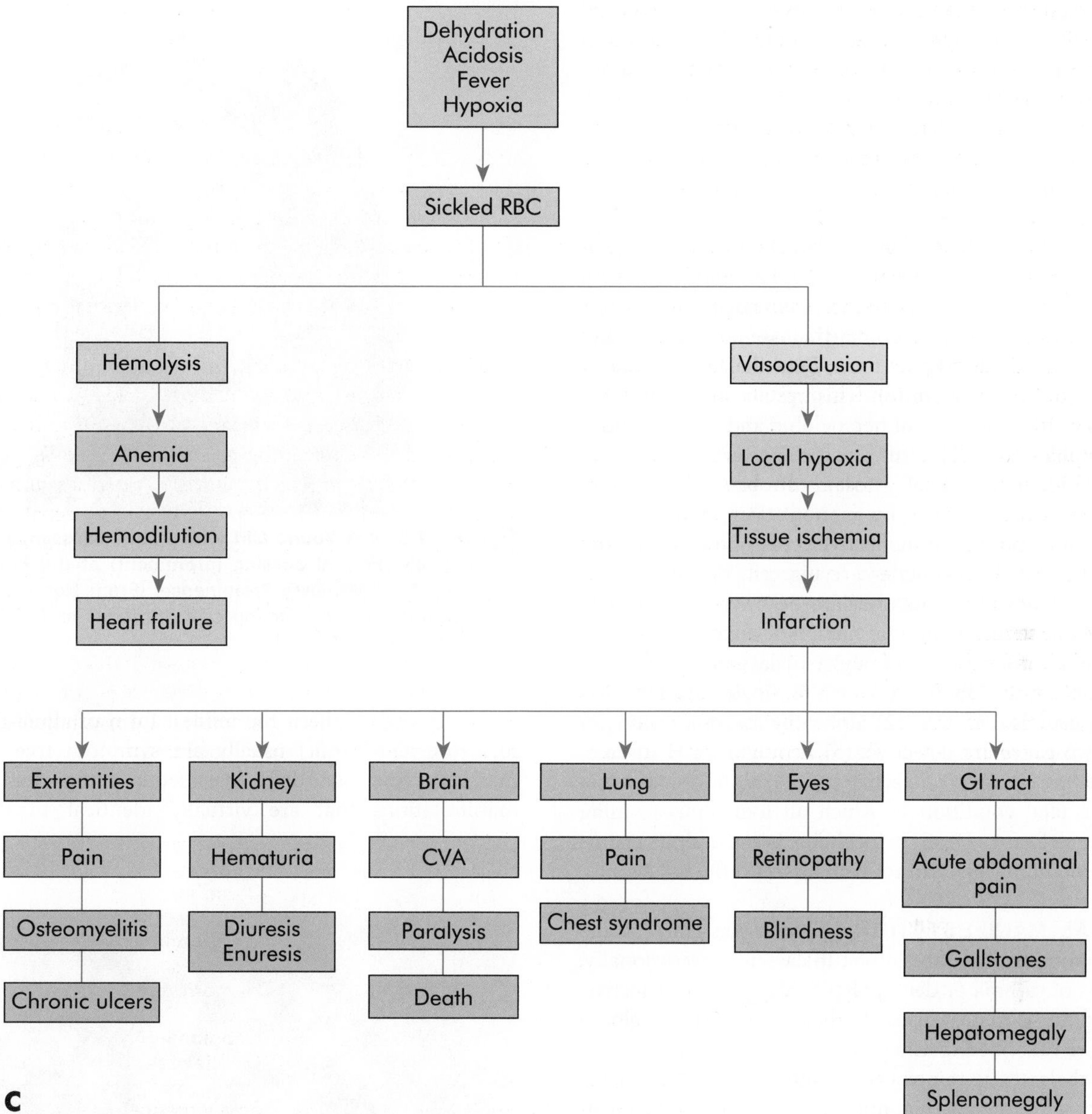

Figure 21-4 cont'd ■ **C, Tissue Effects of Sickle Cell Anemia.** *CVA,* Cerebrovascular accident; *RBC,* red blood cell; *GI,* gastrointestinal.

HEALTH ALERT

Hydroxyurea Treatment for Severe Sickle Cell Disease

Hydroxyurea is an antimetabolite that inhibits deoxyribonucleic acid (DNA) synthesis and causes an increase in the synthesis of hemoglobin F. According to one study, adults and children with severe sickle cell disease showed an increase in hemoglobin F and a significant reduction in vasoocclusive crises. Hospital admissions declined 30% as a result of hydroxyurea treatment, and the need for blood transfusion decreased by 58%. Hydroxyurea is well tolerated, with the most common side effect being myelosuppression.

Data from Ferguson RP et al: Hydroxyurea treatment of sickle cell anemia in hospital-based practices, *Am J Hematol* 70:326–328, 2002.

Thalassemias

The alpha- and beta-thalassemias are inherited autosomal recessive disorders that cause an impaired rate of synthesis of one of the two chains—alpha or beta—of adult hemoglobin (Hb A). The disorder was named **thalassemia,** which is derived from the Greek word for sea, because it was discovered initially in persons with origins near the Mediterranean Sea. Beta-thalassemia, in which synthesis of the beta-globin chain is slowed or defective, is prevalent among Greeks, Italians, and some Arabs and Sephardic Jews. Alpha-thalassemia, in which the alpha chain is affected, is most common among Chinese, Vietnamese, Cambodians, and Laotians. Both alpha- and beta-thalassemias are common among blacks.

Both alpha- and beta-thalassemias are referred to as major or minor, depending on how many of the genes that control alpha- or beta-chain synthesis are defective and whether the defects are inherited homozygously (thalassemia major) or heterozygously (thalassemia minor). Pathophysiologic effects range from mild microcytosis to death in utero, depending on the number of defective genes and mode of inheritance. The anemic manifestation of thalassemia is microcytic-hypochromic hemolytic anemia.

PATHOPHYSIOLOGY The fundamental defect in beta-thalassemia is the uncoupling of alpha- and beta-chain synthesis. Beta-chain production is depressed—moderately in the heterozygous form, **beta-thalassemia minor,** and severely in the homozygous form, **beta-thalassemia major** (also called **Cooley anemia**). This results in erythrocytes having a reduced amount of hemoglobin and accumulations of free alpha chains. The free alpha chains are unstable and easily precipitate in the cell. Most erythroblasts that contain precipitates are destroyed by mononuclear phagocytes in the marrow, resulting in ineffective erythropoiesis and anemia. Some of the precipitate-carrying cells do mature and enter the bloodstream, but they are destroyed prematurely in the spleen, resulting in mild hemolytic anemia.

There are four forms of alpha-thalassemia: (1) **alpha trait** (the carrier state), in which a single alpha chain–forming gene is defective, (2) **alpha-thalassemia minor,** in which two genes are defective, (3) **hemoglobin H disease,** in which three genes are defective, and (4) **alpha-thalassemia major,** a fatal condition in which all four alpha-forming genes are defective. Death is inevitable because alpha chains are absent and oxygen cannot be released to the tissues.

CLINICAL MANIFESTATIONS Beta-thalassemia occurs more commonly than does alpha-thalassemia. Occasionally, synthesis of gamma or delta polypeptide chains is defective, resulting in gamma- or delta-thalassemia. (Hemoglobin chains are described in Chapter 19.)

Beta-thalassemia minor causes mild to moderate microcytic-hypochromic anemia, mild splenomegaly, bronze coloring of the skin, and hyperplasia of the bone marrow. The degree of reticulocytosis depends on the severity of the anemia and results in skeletal changes (Figure 21-5). Hemolysis of immature (and therefore fragile) erythrocytes may cause a slight elevation in serum iron and indirect bilirubin levels. Persons with beta-thalassemia minor are usually asymptomatic.

Persons with beta-thalassemia major may become quite ill. Anemia is severe and results in a significant cardiovascular burden with high-output congestive heart failure. In the past, death resulted from cardiac failure. Today, blood transfusions can increase life span by 1 to 2 decades, and death usually is caused by hemochromatosis (from transfusions). Liver enlargement occurs as a result of progressive hemosiderosis, whereas enlargement of the spleen is caused by extramedullary hemopoiesis and increased destruction of red blood cells (Figure 21-6). Growth and maturation are retarded, and a characteristic chipmunk deformity develops on the face, caused by expansion of bones to accommodate hyperplastic marrow.

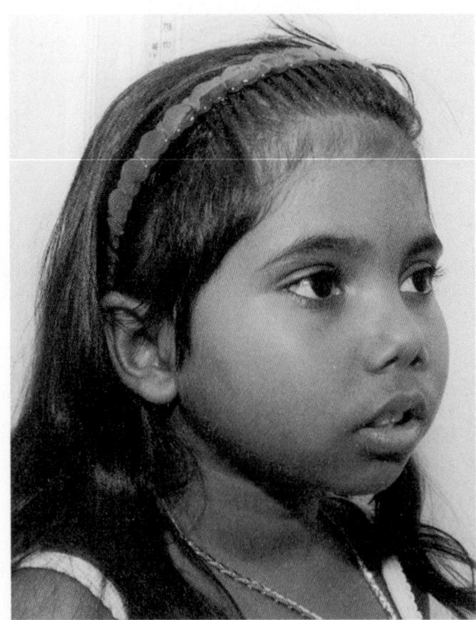

Figure 21-5 ■ A Young Girl with Beta-Thalassemia Demonstrating Mild Frontal Bossing (prominent) of the Right Forehead and Mild Maxillary Prominence. (From Hockenberry MJ et al, editors: *Wong's nursing care of infants and children,* ed 8, St Louis, 2007, Mosby.)

Persons who inherit the mildest form of alpha-thalassemia (the alpha trait) usually are symptom free or have mild microcytosis. Alpha-thalassemia minor has clinical manifestations that are virtually identical to those of

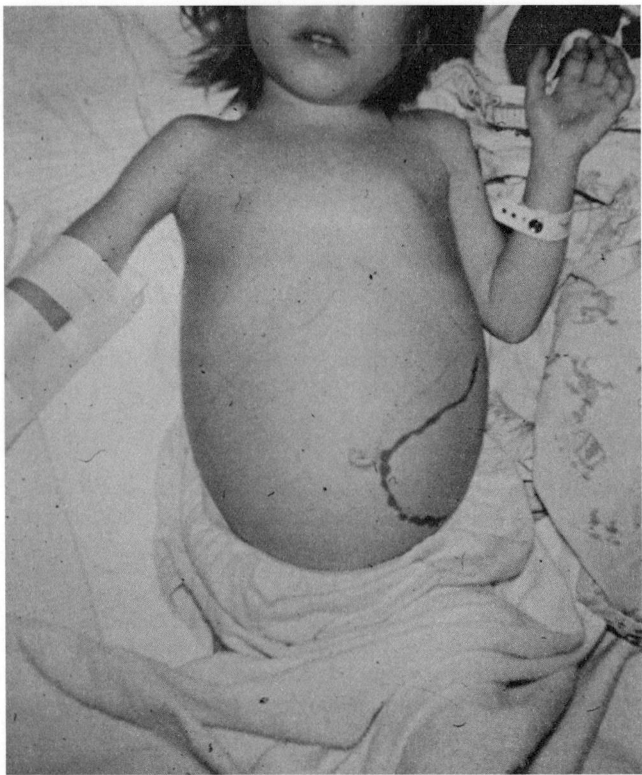

Figure 21-6 ■ A Child with Beta-Thalassemia Major Who Has Severe Splenomegaly. (From Jorde LB et al: *Medical genetics,* ed 3, updated, St Louis, 2006, Mosby.)

beta-thalassemia minor: mild microcytic-hypochromic reticulocytosis, bone marrow hyperplasia, increased serum iron concentrations, and moderate splenomegaly.

Signs and symptoms of alpha-thalassemia major are similar to those of beta-thalassemia major, but milder. Moderate microcytic-hypochromic anemia, enlargement of the liver and spleen, and bone marrow hyperplasia are evident.

Alpha-thalassemia major causes hydrops fetalis and fulminant intrauterine congestive heart failure. In addition to edema and massive ascites, the fetus has a grossly enlarged heart and liver. Diagnosis usually is made postmortem. Prenatal screening for this disorder can be performed by use of chorionic villus sampling. These cells can be analyzed, and a DNA genetic map can be constructed and evaluated for the abnormalities characteristic of hydrops fetalis.

Both alpha- and beta-thalassemia major are life threatening. Children with thalassemia major generally are weak, fail to thrive, show poor development, and experience cardiovascular compromise with high-output failure secondary to anemia. Untreated, they will die by 5 to 6 years of age.

EVALUATION AND TREATMENT Evaluation of thalassemia is based on familial disease history, clinical manifestations, and blood tests. Peripheral blood smears that show microcytosis and hemoglobin electrophoresis that demonstrates diminished amounts of alpha or beta chains are used to make the diagnosis. Analysis of fetal DNA from withdrawn amniotic fluid is used as a screening test to detect hydrops fetalis (alpha-thalassemia major). Newborn screening for thalassemia should be done according to state law.

Persons who are silent carriers or have thalassemia minor generally have few if any symptoms and require no specific treatment. Therapies to support and prolong life are necessary, however, for thalassemia major. There is no cure for either condition. For both symptom-free carriers and those with the disease, prenatal diagnosis and genetic counseling may be the most important therapeutic measures that can be offered.

QUICK CHECK 21-1

1. Why do clinical manifestations of sickle cell disease not appear until the infant is at least 6 months old?
2. Why is Rh incompatibility rare today?
3. Why do children with thalassemia major develop cardiovascular complications?

DISORDERS OF COAGULATION AND PLATELETS

Inherited Hemorrhagic Disease

Hemophilias

Awareness of a serious bleeding disorder in males was documented nearly 2000 years ago in the Babylonian Talmud, which exempted from the rite of circumcision those boys having male relatives prone to excessive bleeding. In 1803 the first description of this disorder appeared in the medical literature, where it was noted to be X-linked in nature and associated with joint bleeding and crippling.

Table 21-3 lists the coagulation factors that are associated with clinical bleeding. Until 1952, the term *hemophilia* was reserved for deficiency of factor VIII (antihemophilic factor). Since that time, two additional coagulation proteins, factor IX (plasma thromboplastin component [PTC]) and factor XI (plasma thromboplastin antecedent [PTA]), have been identified and their deficiency has been associated with similar clinical manifestations. Congenital deficiencies of these three plasma clotting factors—VIII, IX, and XI—account for 90% to 95% of the hemorrhagic bleeding disorders collectively called *hemophilia.* Table 21-3 lists coagulation factors and associated disorders, and the major types of hemophilia are summarized in Table 21-4.

PATHOPHYSIOLOGY Two types of defects dominate the hereditary defects of hemophilia to date: gene deletions and point mutations (base pair substitutions). Both types of genetic defects are associated with severe hemophilia A, in which no factor VIII circulates in the blood. Numerous gene mutations and deletions have been identified at the molecular level in factor VII and IX deficiency. The molecular defect that leads to hemophilia is identical among members of a given family; however, the deletion mutation has been unique in each family studied.[4,5]

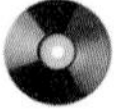

Point mutations, in which a single base in the DNA is mutated to another base, represent a second type of mutation that causes hemophilia. When a point mutation gives rise to a de novo stop codon (nonsense mutation), translation of the protein ceases and a shortened version of the protein is synthesized. Usually the protein is destroyed intracellularly and never reaches the plasma. This type of defect is associated with severe hemophilia—that is, with coagulant activity levels below 1%.[5] Point mutations in

TABLE 21-3
Coagulation Factors and Associated Disorders

Coagulation Factor	Associated Disorder
I	Fibrogen deficiency
II	Hypoprothrombinemia
V	Factor V deficiency, parahemophilia
VII	Factor VII deficiency
VIII	Factor VIII deficiency (hemophilia A); von Willebrand disease
IX	Factor IX deficiency (hemophilia B)
X	Factor X deficiency (Stuart-Prower deficiency)
XI	Factor XI deficiency (hemophilia C)
XII	Hageman trait
XIII	Factor XIII deficiency (fibrin stabilizing factor deficiency)

TABLE 21-4

The Hemophilias

Type	Description
Hemophilia A (classic hemophilia)	Caused by factor VIII deficiency; most common of hemophilias; inherited as X-linked recessive disorder; factor VIII gene has been mapped to the distal arm of X chromosome and clones; affects males and is transmitted by females; 1:5000–10,000 male births; occurs with varying degrees of severity
Hemophilia B (Christmas disease)	Caused by factor IX deficiency; transmitted as X-linked recessive trait; clinically indistinguishable from factor VIII deficiency, however, less severe than hemophilia A (the IX gene also has been cloned); 1:30,000 male births; occurs with varying degrees of severity
Hemophilia C	Caused by factor XI deficiency; inherited as an autosomal recessive disease; occurs equally in males and females; bleeding is usually less severe than with A or B
von Willebrand disease	Also caused by factor VIII deficiency; results from an inherited autosomal dominant trait encoded by a gene on chromosome 12; has variable clinical manifestations and hematologic findings; infusion of plasma causes factor VIII activity to increase

which one amino acid is substituted for another can cause phenotypes of varying severity. The mutation of an important amino acid can destroy protein function, activation, or folding; inhibit intracellular processing; or cause protein clearance. Unlike deletion mutations, point mutations at the same site have been recorded in different families with hemophilia.

Not all coagulation disorders are discussed in this chapter because some are extremely rare (e.g., congenital dysfibrinogenemias), whereas others have no clinical significance (e.g., Hageman factor deficiency, a condition in which profound laboratory deficiency of factor XII has absolutely no clinical effects on the child).

CLINICAL MANIFESTATIONS Children with severe hemophilia start to bleed at different ages. In one study, 44% of infants with hemophilia demonstrated their first bleeding episode before 1 year of age.[6] There is no transfer of maternal clotting factor to the fetus, yet many boys with hemophilia are circumcised without excessive bleeding. Normal hemostasis is achieved in these infants because clotting is activated through the extrinsic coagulation cascade.

During the first year, spontaneous bleeding often is minimal, but hematoma formation may result from injections and from firm holding (e.g., under the arms). Easy bruising, hemarthrosis (bleeding into joints), or both occur with ambulation. By age 3 to 4 years, 90% of children with hemophilia have had episodes of persistent bleeding from relatively minor traumatic lacerations (e.g., to the lip or tongue). This usually is the first clinical manifestation of hemophilia. Hemorrhage into the elbows, knees, and ankles causes pain, limits joint movement, and predisposes the child to degenerative joint changes. Spontaneous hematuria and epistaxis are troublesome but minor complications.

Recurrent bleeding, both spontaneous and after minor trauma, is a lifelong problem. Many affected persons experience phases or cycles of spontaneous bleeding episodes. Mechanisms that cause this phenomenon are unknown. Intracranial hemorrhage and bleeding into the tissues of the neck or abdomen constitute life-threatening emergencies.

EVALUATION AND TREATMENT Although laboratory tests are of primary value in the evaluation of hemorrhagic disorders, the history and physical assessment also are important. The phases of coagulation can be individually assessed by simple, reliable tests (Table 21-5).

The majority of children with hemophilia A (factor VIII deficiency) are treated with recombinant factor VIII, and children with hemophilia B (factor IX deficiency) are treated with recombinant factor IX. Plasma-derived factor is available and less expensive but carries with it the risk of viral infection (e.g., HIV, hepatitis).[7]

The prognosis for children with hemophilia is promising. Programs of comprehensive care and home treatment

TABLE 21-5

Laboratory Tests of Coagulation

Test	Significance
Thrombin time	Measures fibrinogen; usually elevated first because without fibrinogen, blood cannot clot
Prothrombin	A decrease indicates a deficiency of factors II, V, VII, or X; also used to monitor warfarin sodium (Coumadin) therapy
Activated partial thromboplastin time (PTT or APTT)	Assesses for factors XII, XI, IX, and VIII; also used to monitor heparin therapy
PT or APTT mixing study	Differentiates between factor deficiency and factor antibody activity
Specific factor assay	Measures specific factors; XIII, XII, XI, X, IX, VIII, VII, V II, fibrinogen (factor I)

have improved the quality of life for those with hemophilia and enhanced their general physical capabilities.

Antibody-Mediated Hemorrhagic Disease

The antibody-mediated hemorrhagic diseases are a group of disorders caused by the immune response. Antibody-mediated destruction of platelets or antibody-mediated inflammatory reactions to allergens damage blood vessels and cause seepage into tissues. The thrombocytopenic purpuras may be intrinsic or idiopathic, or they may be transient phenomena transmitted from mother to fetus. The inflammatory, or "allergic," purpuras, although rare, occur in response to allergens in the blood. All of these disorders first appear during infancy or childhood.

Idiopathic thrombocytopenic purpura

Acute **idiopathic thrombocytopenic purpura (ITP; autoimmune [primary] thrombocytopenic purpura)** is the most common disorder of platelet consumption. Antiplatelet antibodies bind to the plasma membranes of platelets, causing platelet sequestration and destruction by mononuclear phagocytes in the spleen and other lymphoid tissues at a rate that exceeds the ability of the bone marrow to produce them.

PATHOPHYSIOLOGY In approximately 70% of cases of ITP, there is an antecedent viral disease (e.g., cytomegalovirus [CMV], Epstein-Barr virus [EBV], parvovirus, or respiratory infection) that precedes the eruption of petechiae or purpura by 1 to 3 weeks. High levels of IgG have been found bound to platelets and may represent immune complexes on the platelet surface.

CLINICAL MANIFESTATIONS Bruising and a generalized petechial rash often occur with acute onset. Asymmetric bruising is typical and is found most often on the legs and trunk. Hemorrhagic bullae of the gums, lips, and other mucous membranes may be prominent, and epistaxis (nose bleeding) may be severe and difficult to control. Otherwise, the child appears well. The acute phase lasts 1 to 2 weeks, but thrombocytopenia often persists. Although the incidence is less than 1%, intracranial hemorrhage is the most serious complication of ITP. In some cases, the onset is more gradual, and clinical manifestations consist of moderate bruising and a few petechiae.

EVALUATION AND TREATMENT Laboratory examination reveals a low platelet count, and the few platelets observed on a smear are large, reflecting increased bone marrow production. The Ivy bleeding time is prolonged. Bone marrow aspiration reveals normal or increased megakaryocytes and normal erythrocytes and granulocytes.

Even without treatment, the prognosis for children with ITP is excellent. Seventy-five percent recover completely within 3 months. After the initial acute phase, spontaneous clinical manifestations subside. By 6 months after onset, 80% of affected children have regained normal platelet counts.[8]

QUICK CHECK 21-2

1. List the major disorders of coagulation and platelets found in children.
2. How do gene deletions differ from point mutations?
3. Why are persons with hemophilia at risk for developing degenerative joint changes?
4. What is the major abnormality in idiopathic thrombocytopenic purpura (ITP)?

NEOPLASTIC DISORDERS

Leukemia and Lymphoma

Leukemia, cancer of the blood-forming tissues, is the most common malignancy of childhood, representing approximately 33% of all childhood cancers. Childhood lymphoma, or cancer of the lymphoid system (primarily lymph nodes), is the third most common malignant neoplasm of children in the United States, representing approximately 11% of all childhood cancers. (See Chapter 20 for a discussion of leukemia in adults.) Table 21-6 defines the major classifications of leukemia.

Leukemia

Approximately 80% to 85% of leukemias in children are acute lymphoblastic leukemia (ALL). The remaining 15% to 20% are acute nonlymphocytic leukemias (ANLLs) (which include myeloblastic, promyelocytic, monocytic, and myelomonoblastic) and the rare red blood cell leukemia, erythroleukemia. Because the vast majority of ANLL cases involve the myeloblastic cell, many experts refer to the disease as acute myelogenous leukemia (AML). Both a juvenile form and an adult form of chronic myelocytic leukemia (CML) develop in children but are uncommon and account for only 2% of all leukemias in childhood. Chronic lymphocytic leukemia (CLL) is virtually nonexistent in children.

ALL is the most common malignancy in children, representing nearly one third of all pediatric cancers. Annual incidence of ALL is about 30 cases per million people, with a peak incidence in children 2 to 5 years of age, and affects almost twice as many white children as nonwhite children

TABLE 21-6
Major Classifications of Leukemia

Lympho	Leukemia involving the lymphoid tissue and the lymphatic system (e.g., lymphatic vessels, lymph nodes, spleen, thymus)
Myelo	Leukemias of bone marrow (myeloid) origin
Blastic and acute	Leukemias involving immature cells
Cytic and chronic	Leukemias involving mature cells

(4.2:100,000 versus 2.4:100,000, respectively). Childhood ALL also is more common in boys than in girls (1.3:1.0).

PATHOGENESIS Investigations into the causes of childhood leukemia have focused on genetic susceptibility, environmental factors, and viral infections. Observations of a familial tendency and links with a number of inherited disorders have implicated genetic factors in the origin of leukemia.

Inherited diseases that predispose a child to leukemia (both ALL and AML) include Down syndrome, Fanconi anemia, Bloom syndrome, and ataxia-telangiectasia. Leukemia also has been associated with known genetic diseases, such as congenital agammaglobulinemia. AML is attributable to prior chemotherapy, especially alkylating agents. AML can develop from preexisting myeloproliferative disorders that also are preleukemia syndromes. When these disorders progress to ANLL, an insidious pattern of leukemic dysfunction usually is revealed.

Many environmental factors (e.g., exposure to ionizing radiation and electromagnetic fields, parental use of alcohol and tobacco) have been investigated as potential risk factors, but none has been definitively shown to cause lymphoblastic leukemia in children.

There is no evidence that radon gas exposure causes cancer in children.[9] Likewise, electromagnetic field (EMF) exposure has not been demonstrated to be a causative factor in acute leukemias.[10] In addition, no evidence suggests a chemical or drug association either.

Leukemic clusters that represent a greater number of leukemia cases occurring in a particular geographic location have raised speculation about environmental factors and infectious patterns of transmission. Careful follow-up, however, has failed to document the abnormal clustering. Explanations for this phenomenon therefore are statistical artifact and coincidence.

Viruses clearly have been known to cause leukemia in a number of animals, including cats, fowl, and mice. Scientists have linked retroviruses with other types of cancer, but retroviruses have not been linked with childhood leukemia.

It appears that childhood leukemia is likely to be the result of a multiple interaction between hereditary or genetic predisposition and environmental influences.[11] This interaction is called *ecogenetics* and focuses on the genetic variations that occur in relation to environmental factors.

CLINICAL MANIFESTATIONS The onset of leukemia may be abrupt or insidious, but the most common symptoms reflect the consequence of bone marrow failure: decreased red blood cells and platelets and changes in white blood cells. Pallor, fatigue, petechiae, purpura, bleeding, and fever generally are present. Approximately 45% of children have a hemoglobin level below 7 g/dl. If acute blood loss occurs, characteristic symptoms of tachycardia, air hunger, restlessness, and thirst may be present. Epistaxis often occurs in children with severe thrombocytopenia.

Fever is usually present as a result of (1) infection associated with the decrease in functional neutrophils and (2) hypermetabolism associated with the ongoing rapid growth and destruction of leukemic cells. White blood cell counts greater than 200,000/mm^3 can cause leukostasis, an intravascular clumping of cells that results in infarction and hemorrhage, usually in the brain and lung.

Renal failure as a result of hyperuremia (high uric acid levels) can be associated with ALL, particularly at diagnosis or during active treatment. Extramedullary invasion with leukemic cells can occur in nearly all body tissue. The central nervous system (CNS) is a common site of infiltration of extramedullary leukemias, although fewer than 10% of children with ALL have CNS involvement at diagnosis. CNS infiltration manifests later in the course of the disease. The most common symptoms of CNS involvement relate to increased intracranial pressure, causing early morning headaches, nausea, vomiting, irritability, and lethargy.

Gonadal involvement can occur and leukemic infiltration into bones and joints is common. Reports of bone or joint pain actually lead to the diagnosis of leukemia in some children. In most children, bone pain is characterized as migratory, vague, and without areas of swelling or inflammation. If joint pain is the primary symptom and some swelling is associated with the pain, however, misdiagnoses of rheumatoid arthritis and rheumatic fever have occurred.

Other organs reported to be sites of leukemic invasion include the kidneys, heart, lungs, thymus, eyes, skin, and gastrointestinal tract. Children with leukemia usually have had symptoms for only 1 week before diagnosis.

EVALUATION AND TREATMENT Although blood test results can raise the clinician's suspicion of leukemia, a bone marrow aspiration is required to establish the diagnosis. The **blast cell** is the hallmark of acute leukemia (Figure 21-7). This relatively undifferentiated cell is characterized by diffusely distributed nuclear chromatin, with one or more nucleoli and basophilic cytoplasm. Healthy children have fewer than 5% blast cells in the bone marrow and none in the peripheral blood. In ALL, the bone marrow often is replaced by 80% to 100% blast cells, with a reduction in normal developing red blood cells and granulocytes. Occasionally, the marrow appears hypocellular, making the diagnosis difficult to differentiate from aplastic anemia. When this occurs, bone marrow biopsy or biopsy of extramedullary sites is necessary to confirm the diagnosis.

Combination chemotherapy, with or without radiation therapy to localized sites, such as the CNS, is the treatment of choice for acute leukemia. In ALL, identification of various risk groups has led to the development of different intensities of drug protocols. Thus, treatment is tailored specifically for a particular risk group. The 5-year relative survival rate for ALL is about 80%.

Lymphomas

Non-Hodgkin lymphoma (**NHL**) and Hodgkin lymphoma constitute approximately 11% of all childhood cancer. Approximately 750 cases of lymphoma occur in children between 0 and 14 years of age in the United States each year.[12] NHL occurs more often than Hodgkin lymphoma

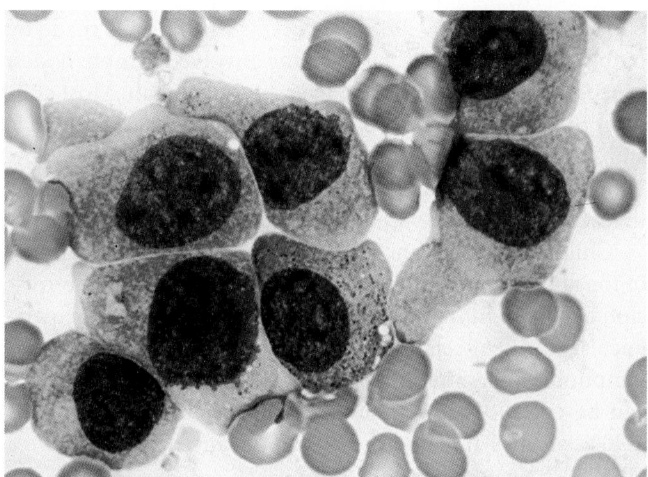

Figure 21-7 ■ Monoblasts from Acute Monoblastic Leukemia. Monoblasts in a marrow smear from a patient with acute monoblastic leukemia. The monoblasts are larger than myeloblasts and usually have abundant cytoplasm, often with delicate scattered azurophilic granules (an element that stains well with blue aniline dyes). (From Damjanov I, Linder J, editors: *Anderson's pathology,* ed 10, St Louis, 1996, Mosby.)

(4.5% versus 3.5% of all pediatric malignancies). Either group of diseases is rare before the age of 5 years, and the relative incidence increases throughout childhood. Boys are more likely to be diagnosed with a malignant lymphoma than are girls. At particular risk are children with inherited or acquired immunodeficiency syndromes, who have increased rates of lymphoreticular cancers that range between 100 and 10,000 times the rate of normal children.

HEALTH ALERT

Monoclonal Antibody Therapy to Treat Chronic Myeloid Leukemia

Cancer cells have specific and unique antigens on the cell surface. Monoclonal antibodies (MABs) seek out these antigens and bind to cancer cells. Once attached to cancer cells, MAB can alter activity of the targeted antigen and signal immune cells to destroy the cancer cells. The Food and Drug Administration approved the use of Gleevec (imatinib mesylate) in 2003 for the treatment of children with a rare, life-threatening form of cancer known as Philadelphia chromosome–positive (Ph+) chronic myeloid leukemia (CML), which accounts for about 2% of all leukemias in children. It was the first approval of a new agent to treat pediatric cancer in more than a decade. Approval of Gleevec for use in children with CML was granted under the accelerated drug approval program that makes treatments for serious or life-threatening diseases available earlier in the development process based on the evidence of a promising effect of the drug, such as tumor shrinkage. The most common side effects associated with Gleevec are nausea, vomiting, diarrhea, edema as a result of fluid retention, muscle cramps, and a reduction in white blood cells counts and platelets.

Data from Kaplow R: Innovations in antineoplastic therapy, *Nurs Clin North Am* 40:77–94, 2005.

Non-Hodgkin lymphoma

Generally, most classification systems divide NHL into two categories—nodular or diffuse—on the basis of cellular pattern. Whereas half of all adults with NHL have a nodular form of the disease, children rarely demonstrate this pattern. Nodular disease represents a less aggressive form of lymphoma. Almost without exception, childhood NHL becomes evident as a diffuse disease and can be further subdivided into three groups: (1) large cell (histiocytic), (2) lymphoblastic, and (3) small noncleaved cell (Burkitt or non-Burkitt lymphoma) (Figure 21-8). Large cell NHL often involves chromosomal translocations. Disease sites commonly involve extranodal sites, such as brain, lung, bone, and skin. Lymphoblastic NHL also shows chromosomal translocations, particularly chromosomes 7 and 14. Disease sites commonly include the mediastinum and peripheral lymph nodes. Small noncleaved cell NHL involves chromosome translocations of 8 and 14. Children with small noncleaved cell NHL commonly have intra-abdominal disease at diagnosis.

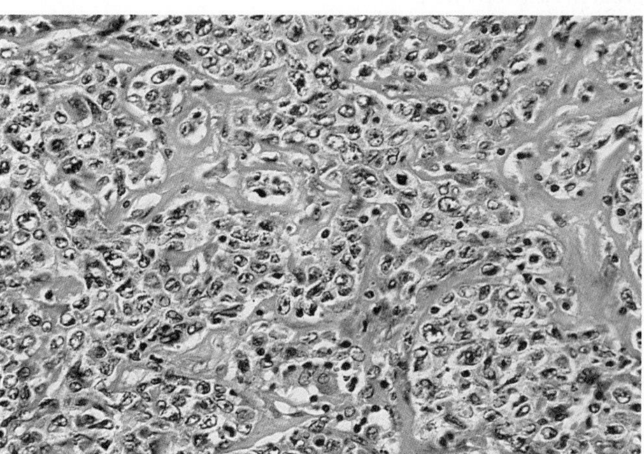

A

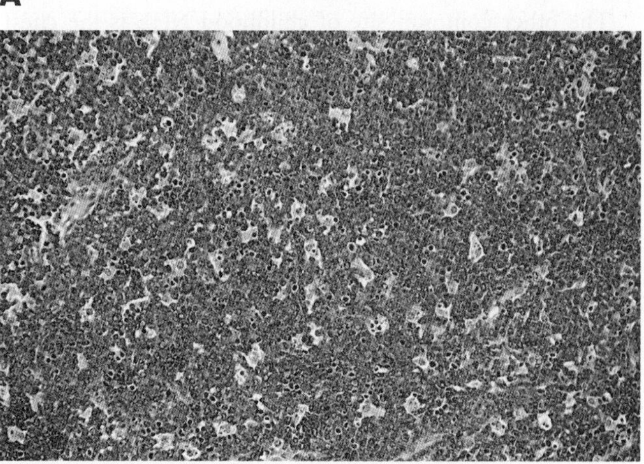

B

Figure 21-8 ■ Lymphomas. A, Large cell lymphoma. The tumor contains prominent areas of sclerosis. **B,** Burkitt lymphoma. A starry sky pattern is seen at low magnification. (From Damjanov I, Linder J: *Pathology: a color atlas,* St Louis, 2000, Mosby.)

As in ALL, immunophenotyping is an important part of the classification of childhood NHL. Almost 45% of cases of the disease in children originate from T cells; an equal number originate from B cells. The remaining group, which represents less than 10% of childhood NHLs, is classified as non-T, non-B.

PATHOGENESIS Viral etiology is suggested, with the strongest correlation between the Epstein-Barr virus and African Burkitt lymphoma. The relationship outside Africa is weak, however, even though the tumor is histopathologically and clinically indistinguishable. Chronic immunostimulation also has been suggested as a factor in the development of lymphomas, because these diseases are seen more often when chronic persistent antigenic stimulation occurs from infection, such as malaria or intestinal parasites. Genetic susceptibility also may play a role in the process of malignant transformation. There is increased evidence of NHL in children with congenital immunodeficiency syndromes, such as Wiskott-Aldrich syndrome, ataxia-telangiectasia, and Bloom syndrome. Children with acquired immunodeficiency syndrome (AIDS) also are at greater risk for NHL.[13]

CLINICAL MANIFESTATIONS NHL has been found to arise from any lymphoid tissue. Signs and symptoms therefore are specific for the site involved. Because childhood NHL is a rapidly progressive disease, symptoms generally are present only a few weeks before diagnosis is made. Rapidly enlarging lymphoid tissue and painless lymphadenopathy are common with abdominal sites of involvement, usually representing a gastrointestinal origin for the disease. Symptoms often include abdominal pain and vomiting, but a palpable mass is not always present. Most children with abdominal symptoms have diffuse, small noncleaved cell NHL (Burkitt or non-Burkitt) of B-cell origin. If the tumor recurs, it appears again in the abdomen before distant spread.

The other common site of childhood NHL is the chest region. An anterior mediastinal mass, with or without pleural effusion, often is present. If the mass is large enough, respiratory compromise, tracheal compression, and superior vena cava syndrome may arise, which constitute a medical emergency. Children with anterior mediastinal involvement often are male adolescents and usually have diffuse lymphoblastic lymphoma of T cell origin. This often evolves into extensive bone marrow involvement and is considered to be an overt leukemic phase, therefore referred to as *leukemic transformation.* CNS involvement and testicular infiltration often occur.

CNS involvement is common. A relatively small number (10% to 20%) of children with NHL have lymphoid tissue involvement of the head and neck (Waldeyer ring, nasopharynx, sinuses). Signs and symptoms include tonsillitis, sinusitis, and a painless nasopharynx mass. In African Burkitt lymphoma, involvement of facial bones, particularly the jaw, is common.

EVALUATION AND TREATMENT Diagnosis is made by biopsy of disease sites, usually the involved lymph nodes, tonsils, bone marrow, spleen, liver, bowel, or skin. Most children with NHL are cured of the disease. Optimal treatment is still being developed, but combination chemotherapy, with or without radiation therapy for prevention of CNS involvement, is being used successfully.

Children with advanced small noncleaved cell lymphoma of the abdomen have the poorest prognosis. Although remission occurs in more than 90% of these children, most experience subsequent relapses. Even in the presence of advanced lymphoblastic lymphoma, however, 60% to 80% of children can be cured. Overall, children with localized disease have a 90% survival rate and those with advanced disease have a 60% to 70% survival rate.[12]

Hodgkin lymphoma

Although the etiologic agent for **Hodgkin lymphoma,** a lymphoma, has not been identified in children, an infectious mode of transmission, particularly focused on viruses, has been implicated. Many persons with Hodgkin lymphoma have high Epstein-Barr virus titers. At this time, however, the evidence is not sufficient to link an Epstein-Barr virus infection to Hodgkin lymphoma.

Genetic susceptibility has been suggested, because observations show that siblings have a sevenfold increase in risk, particularly siblings of the same sex. In general, Hodgkin lymphoma is more common in males—in childhood, 60% of all cases occur in males.

Hodgkin lymphoma is rare in childhood. It occurs only infrequently in children younger than 2 years, and few cases are observed before the age of 5 years. A gradual rise in incidence occurs through the age of 11 years, with a marked increase through adolescence that continues into the 30s. The annual incidence of Hodgkin lymphoma in the United States is 4:1,000,000 in children younger than 15 years. Histologically, the tumor consists of neoplastic Reed-Sternberg cells that are typically found surrounded by small lymphocytes, macrophages, neutrophils, and plasma cells (Figure 21-9).

Painless adenopathy in the lower cervical chain, with or without fever, is the most common symptom in children. Other lymph nodes and organs also may be involved (Figure 21-10). Mediastinal involvement can cause pressure on the trachea or bronchi, leading to airway obstruction. Extranodal primary sites in Hodgkin lymphoma are rare. Initial symptoms consist of anorexia, malaise, and lassitude. Intermittent fever is present in 30% of children, and weight loss also may accompany these symptoms. Hodgkin lymphoma has a well-defined staging system that considers the extent and location of disease and the presence of fever, weight loss, or night sweats at diagnosis. Treatment for Hodgkin lymphoma includes chemotherapy and radiation therapy. For many years, the standard chemotherapy was a regimen of *m*echlorethamine, Oncovin (vincristine), *p*rocarbazine, and *p*rednisone (MOPP). However, these drugs

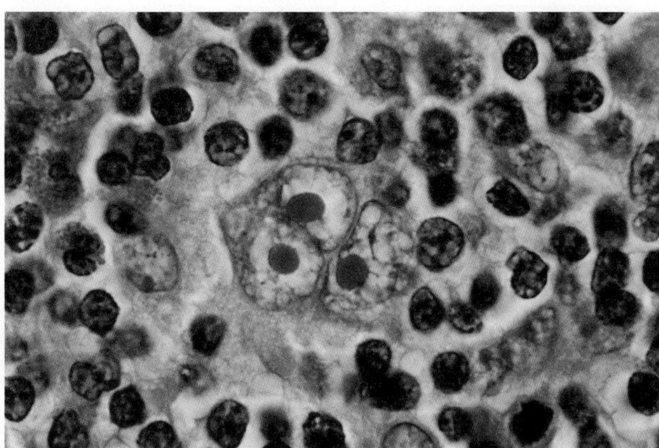

Figure 21-9 ■ **Diagnostic Reed-Sternberg Cell.** A large multinucleated or multilobated cell with inclusion body-like nucleoli surrounded by a halo of clear nucleoplasm. (From Damjanov I, Linder J: *Pathology: a color atlas,* St Louis, 2000, Mosby.)

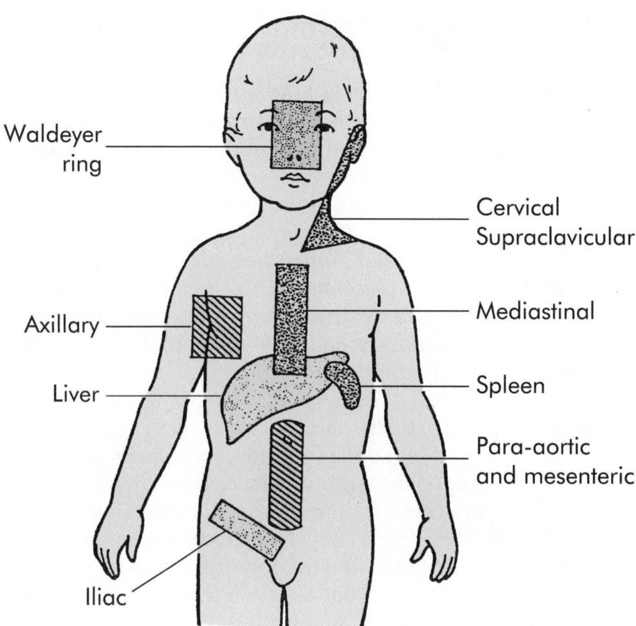

Figure 21-10 ■ **Main Areas of Lymphadenopathy and Organ Involvement in Hodgkin Lymphoma.** (From Hockenberry MJ et al, editors: *Wong's nursing care of infants and children,* ed 8, St Louis, 2007, Mosby.)

can cause permanent sterility. A new drug combination consisting of *A*driamycin (doxorubicin), *b*leomycin, *v*inblastine, and *d*acarbazine (ABVD) has been shown to be superior to MOPP; it is less toxic and requires 6 to 8 months of treatment rather than the traditional 12 months of MOPP treatment. The survival rate for children with Hodgkin lymphoma is high. Most children are seen initially with limited disease and have a 90% survival rate. Even children who are first seen with advanced disease have a 70% to 90% survival rate.[12]

QUICK CHECK 21-3

1. List the childhood leukemias in order of rate of incidence.
2. Why do children with leukemia experience bone or joint pain?
3. What are the common types of non-Hodgkin lymphoma (NHL) in children?

Did You Understand?

Disorders of Erythrocytes

1. Iron deficiency anemia is the most common blood disorder of infancy and childhood; the highest incidence occurs between 6 months and 2 years of age.
2. Hemolytic disease of the newborn (HDN) results from incompatibility between the maternal and the fetal blood, which may involve differences in Rh factors or blood type (ABO). Maternal antibodies enter the fetal circulation and cause hemolysis of fetal erythrocytes. Because the immature liver is unable to conjugate and excrete the excess bilirubin that results from the hemolysis, icterus neonatorum or kernicterus or both can develop. Kernicterus, which also may result from other causes, causes increased breakdown of red blood cells or decreased liver output of enzymes.
3. Infections of the newborn, often acquired by the mother and transmitted to the infant, may result in hemolytic anemia.
4. Sickle cell disease is a genetically determined defect of hemoglobin synthesis inherited by an autosomal recessive transmission; it causes a change in the shape of a red blood cell that results in decreased oxygen or hydration. It is most common among Africans and those of Mediterranean descent.
5. The thalassemias are a heterogeneous group of hereditary hypochromic anemias of varying severity. Basic genetic defects include abnormalities of messenger-RNA processing or deletion of genetic materials, resulting in a decrease in the chains for hemoglobin.

Disorders of Coagulation and Platelets

1. Hemophilia is a condition characterized by impairment of the coagulation of blood and a subsequent tendency to bleed. The classic disease is hereditary and limited to males, being transmitted through the female to the second generation. Many similar conditions attributable to the absence of various clotting factors are now recognized.

(Continued)

Did You Understand?—Cont'd

2. The acquired antibody-mediated hemorrhagic diseases include idiopathic thrombocytopenic purpura (ITP), transient neonatal thrombocytopenia, and autoimmune vascular purpura.
3. ITP, the most common of the childhood thrombocytopenic purpuras, is a disorder of platelet consumption in which antiplatelet antibodies bind to the plasma membranes of platelets. This results in platelet sequestration and destruction by mononuclear phagocytes at a rate that exceeds the ability of the bone marrow to produce them.

Neoplastic Disorders

1. The childhood leukemias include, in order of their rate of incidence, acute lymphoblastic, acute myeloblastic, and the very rare chronic myelocytic leukemia.
2. Although the cause of childhood leukemia is not known for certain, it is probably the result of multiple interactions between hereditary or genetic predisposition and environmental influences.
3. Acute lymphoblastic leukemia is a potentially curable disease, with about 80% of cases cured.
4. The lymphomas of childhood are Hodgkin lymphoma and non-Hodgkin lymphoma.
5. The origin of non-Hodgkin lymphoma is unknown. Factors that have been implicated include defective host immunity, a viral agent, chronic immunostimulation, and genetic predisposition.
6. Non-Hodgkin lymphoma has a favorable prognosis, with a 60% to 80% rate of cure.
7. Hodgkin lymphoma is thought to be caused by a yet unidentified etiologic agent.
8. Hodgkin lymphoma in children is a readily curable disease with survival statistics similar to those for adults.

Key Terms

Alpha trait, 558
Alpha-thalassemia major, 558
Alpha-thalassemia minor, 558
Aplastic crisis, 555
Beta-thalassemia major (Cooley anemia), 558
Beta-thalassemia minor, 558
Blast cell, 562
Erythroblastosis fetalis, 550
Glucose-6-phosphate dehydrogenase (G6PD) deficiency, 550
Hemoglobin H disease, 558
Hemoglobin S (Hb S), 553
Hemolytic anemia, 550
Hemolytic disease of the newborn (HDN) (erythroblastosis fetalis), 550
Hodgkin lymphoma, 564
Hydrops fetalis, 553
Hyperbilirubinemia, 553
Hyperhemolytic crisis, 556
Icterus gravis neonatorum, 553
Icterus neonatorum (neonatal jaundice), 553
Idiopathic thrombocytopenic purpura (ITP; autoimmune [primary] thrombocytopenic purpura), 561
Kernicterus, 553
Non-Hodgkin lymphoma (NHL), 562
Sequestration crisis, 555
Sickle cell anemia, 553
Sickle cell disease, 553
Sickle cell trait, 553
Sickle cell–Hb C disease, 553
Sickle cell–thalassemia, 553
Thalassemia, 557
Vasoocclusive crisis (thrombotic crisis), 555

References

1. Brotanek JM et al: Iron deficiency, prolonged bottle-feeding, and racial/ethnic disparities in young children, *Arch Pediatr Adolesc Med* 159(11):1038–1042, 2005.
2. Bain BJ: Diagnosis from the blood smear, *N Engl J Med* 353 (5):498–507, 2005.
3. Kyung P: Sickle cell disease and other hemoglobinopathies, *Int Anesthesiol Clin* 42(3):77–93, 2004.
4. Keeney S et al: The molecular analysis of haemophilia A: a guideline from the UK haemophilia centre doctors' organization haemophilia genetics laboratory network, *Haemophilia* 11(4):387–397, 2005.
5. Mitchell M et al: The molecular analysis of haemophilia B: a guideline from the UK haemophilia centre doctors' organization haemophilia genetics laboratory network, *Haemophilia* 11(4):398–404, 2005.
6. Pollman H et al: When are children diagnosed as having severe haemophilia and when do they bleed? A 10-year single center PUP study, *Eur J Pediatr* 158(suppl 3):166–170, 1999.
7. Sevier N: Inherited coagulation factor abnormalities: a pediatric review, *J Ped Onc Nurs* 22(3):137–144, 2005.
8. Sevier, N, Houston, M: Chronic refractory ITP in children: beyond splenectomy, *J Ped Onc Nurs* 22(3):145–151, 2005.
9. UK Childhood Cancer Study Investigators: The United Kingdom Childhood Cancer Study of exposure to domestic sources of ionizing radiation 1: radon gas, *Br J Cancer* 86(1): 1721–1726, 2002.
10. Ahlbom IC et al: Review of the epidemiologic literature on EMF and health, *Environ Health Perspect* 109(suppl 6): 911–933, 2001.
11. Davies SM, Ross JA: Childhood cancer etiology: recent reports, *Med Pediatr Oncol* 40:35–38, 2003.
12. American Cancer Society: *Cancer facts and figures 2006.* Atlanta, 2006, American Cancer Society.
13. Lim ST, Levine AM: Recent advances in acquired immunodeficiency syndrome (AIDS)-related lymphoma, *CA Can J Clin* 55:229–241, 2005.

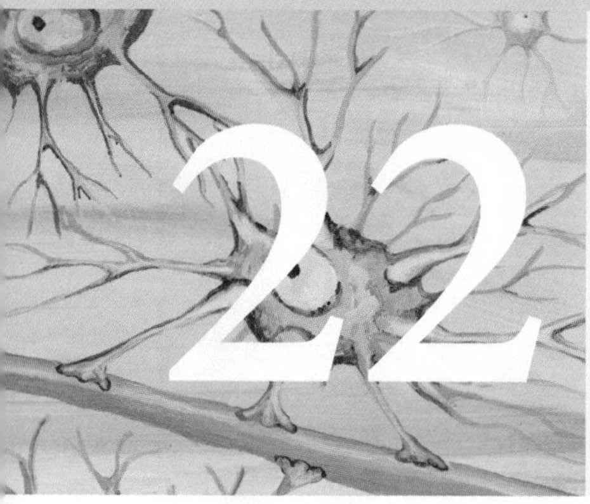

22 STRUCTURE AND FUNCTION OF THE CARDIOVASCULAR AND LYMPHATIC SYSTEMS

Kathryn L. McCance ▪ Valentina L. Brashers

CHAPTER OUTLINE

ELECTRONIC RESOURCES

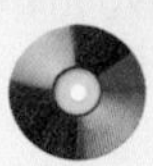

Companion CD
- Review Questions and Answers
- Animations

evolve Website
http://evolve.elsevier.com/Huether/
- Quick Check Answers
- Key Terms Exercises
- Critical Thinking Questions with Answers
- Algorithm Completion Exercises
- WebLinks

The function of the circulatory system is to deliver oxygen, nutrients, and other substances to all the body's cells and to remove the waste products of cellular metabolism. Delivery and removal are achieved by a complex array of tubing (the blood vessels) connected to a pump (the heart). The heart pumps blood continuously through the blood vessels with cooperation from other systems, particularly the nervous and endocrine systems, which are intrinsic regulators of the heart and blood vessels. Nutrients and oxygen are supplied by the digestive and respiratory systems; gaseous wastes of cellular metabolism are blown off by the lungs; and other wastes are removed by the kidneys. Of critical importance to cardiovascular function is the vascular endothelium. As a multifunctional organ, its health is essential to normal vascular physiology, and its dysfunction is a critical factor in the development of vascular disease.

THE CIRCULATORY SYSTEM

The heart pumps blood through two separate circulatory systems: one to the lungs and one to all other parts of the body. Structures on the right side of the heart, or **right heart,** pump blood through the lungs. This system is termed the **pulmonary circulation.** The left side of the heart, or **left heart,** sends blood throughout the **systemic circulation,** which supplies all of the body except the lungs (Figure 22-1). These two systems are serially connected; thus, the output of one becomes the input of the other.

Arteries carry blood flow from the heart to all parts of the body, where they branch into increasingly smaller vessels and ultimately become a fine meshwork of capillaries. Capillaries allow the closest contact and exchange between the blood and the interstitial space, or interstitium—the environment in which the cells live. Veins channel blood flow from capillaries in all parts of the body back to the heart. The plasma passes through the walls of the capillaries into the interstitial space. This fluid is eventually returned to the cardiovascular system by vessels of the lymphatic system.

THE HEART

The adult heart weighs less than 1 pound (2.2 kg) and is about the size of a fist. It lies obliquely (diagonally) in the **mediastinum,** an area above the diaphragm and between the lungs. Heart structures can be described with respect to three general categories of function:

1. *Structural support of heart tissues and circulation of pulmonary and systemic blood through the heart.* This includes the heart wall and fibrous skeleton, which enclose and support the heart and divide it into four chambers; the valves that direct flow through the chambers; and the great vessels that conduct blood to and from the heart.
2. *Maintenance of heart cells.* This comprises vessels of the coronary circulation—the arteries and veins that serve the

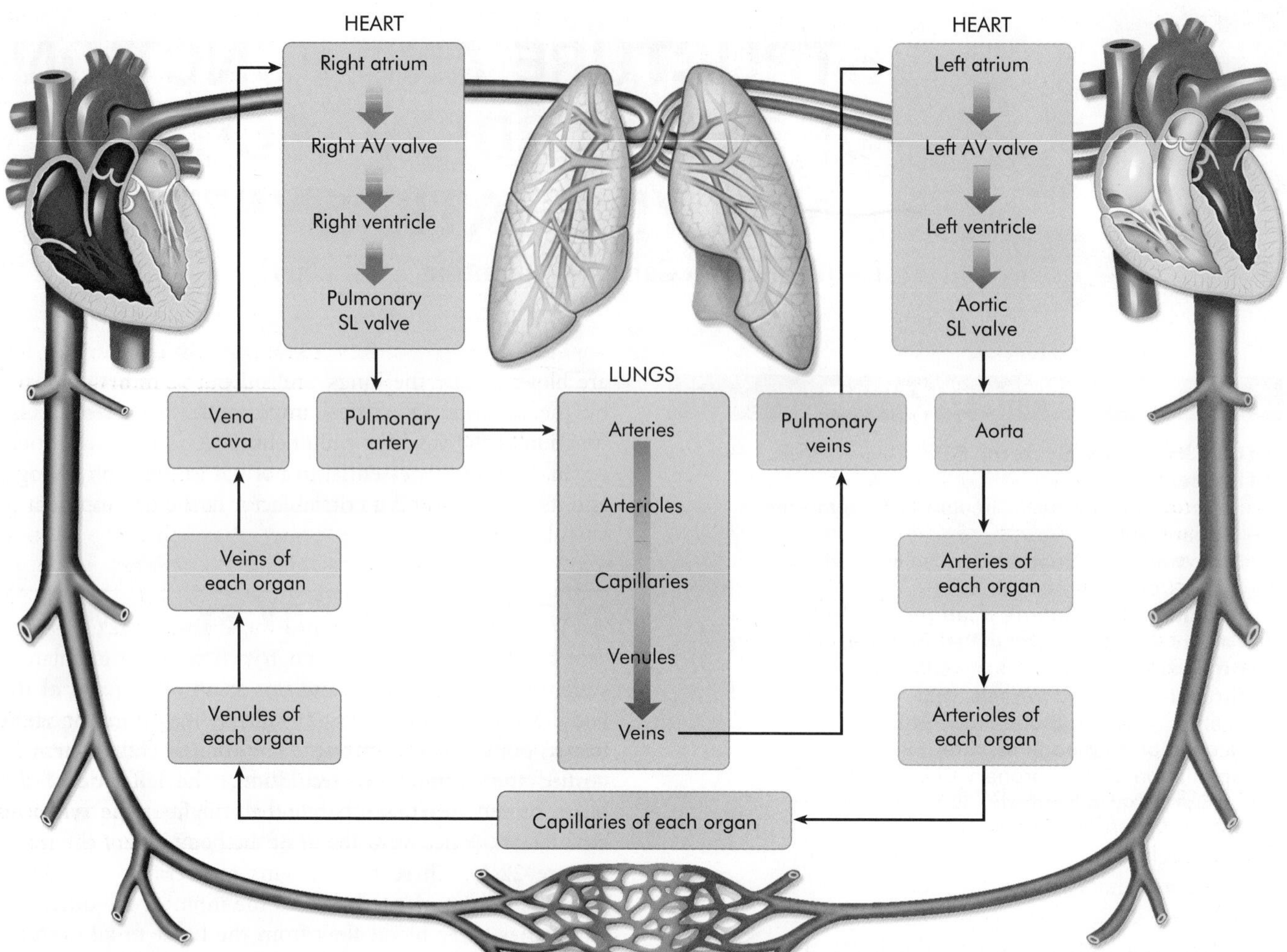

Figure 22-1 ■ Diagram Showing Serially Connected Pulmonary and Systemic Circulatory Systems and How to Trace the Flow of Blood. Right heart chambers propel unoxygenated blood through the pulmonary circulation, and the left heart propels oxygenated blood through the systemic circulation. (From Thibodeau GA, Patton KT: *Anatomy & Physiology,* ed 6, St Louis, 2007, Mosby.)

metabolic needs of all the heart cells—and the lymphatic vessels of the heart.

3. *Stimulation and control of heart action.* Among these structures are the nerves and specialized muscle cells that direct the rhythmic contraction and relaxation of the heart muscles, propelling blood throughout the pulmonary and systemic circulatory system.

Structures That Direct Circulation Through the Heart

The heart wall

The heart wall has three layers: the pericardium, myocardium, and endocardium (Figure 22-2). The **pericardium** is a double-walled membranous sac that encloses the heart and (1) prevents displacement of the heart during gravitational acceleration or deceleration, (2) serves as a physical barrier that protects the heart against infection and inflammation from the lungs and pleural space, and (3) contains pain receptors and mechanoreceptors to elicit reflex changes in blood pressure and heart rate. The two layers of the pericardium are the parietal and the visceral pericardia (see Figure 22-2). These are separated by a fluid-containing space called the **pericardial cavity.** The **pericardial fluid** (10 to 30 ml) is secreted by cells of the mesothelium and lubricates the membranes that line the pericardial cavity, enabling them to slide over one another with a minimum of friction as the heart beats. The amount and character of the pericardial fluid are altered if the pericardium is inflamed (see Chapter 23).

The thickest layer of the heart wall, the **myocardium,** is composed of cardiac muscle and is anchored to the heart's fibrous skeleton. The thickness of the myocardium varies tremendously in the various heart chambers and is related to the amount of resistance the muscle must overcome to pump blood from that chamber. The internal lining of the myocardium, the **endocardium,** comprises connective tissue and squamous cells (see Figure 22-2). This lining is continuous with the endothelium that lines all the arteries, veins, and capillaries of the body, creating a continuous, closed circulatory system.

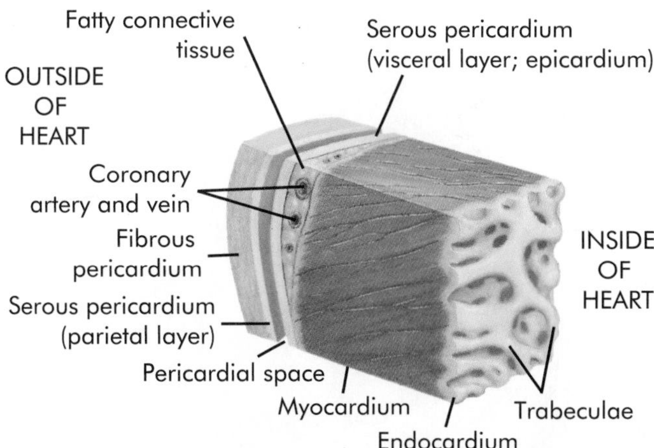

Figure 22-2 ■ **Wall of the Heart.** This section of the heart wall shows the fibrous pericardium, the parietal and visceral layers of the serous pericardium (with the pericardial space between them), the myocardium, and the endocardium. Note the fatty connective tissue between the visceral layer of the serous pericardium (epicardium) and the myocardium. Note also that the endocardium covers beamlike projections of myocardial muscle tissue called *trabeculae.* (From Thibodeau GA, Patton KT: *Anatomy & physiology,* ed 5, St Louis, 2003, Mosby.)

Chambers of the heart

The heart has four chambers: the **left atrium,** the **right atrium,** the **right ventricle,** and the **left ventricle.** (Blood flow through these chambers is illustrated in Figure 22-3.) The atria are smaller than the ventricles and have thinner walls. The ventricles have a thicker myocardial layer and constitute much of the bulk of the heart. The ventricles are formed by a continuum of muscle fibers originating from the fibrous skeleton at the base of the heart.

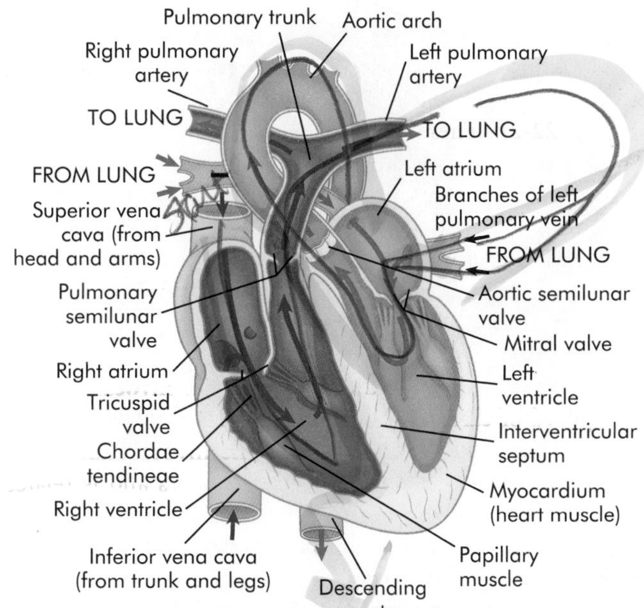

Figure 22-3 ■ **Structures That Direct Blood Flow Through the Heart.** Arrows indicate path of blood flow through chambers, valves, and major vessels.

The myocardial thickness of each cardiac chamber depends on the amount of pressure or resistance it must overcome to eject blood. The two atria have the thinnest walls because they are low-pressure chambers that serve as storage units and conduits for blood that is emptied into the ventricles. Normally, there is little resistance to flow from the atria to the ventricles. The ventricles, on the other hand, must propel blood all the way through the pulmonary or systemic circulation. The ventricular myocardium also must be strong enough to pump against pressures in the pulmonary or systemic vessels. The mean pulmonary capillary pressure is only 15 mmHg. By comparison, the mean systemic arterial pressure is about 92 mmHg. For this reason, the left ventricle's myocardium is several times thicker than that of the right ventricle.

The right ventricle is shaped like a crescent, or triangle, enabling a bellows-like action that efficiently ejects large volumes of blood through a very small valve into the low-pressure pulmonary system. The left ventricle is larger and bullet shaped, helping it to eject blood through a relatively large valve opening into the high-pressure systemic circulation.

The septal membrane separates the right and left sides of the heart and prevents blood from crossing over. The atria are separated by the interatrial septum, and the ventricles by the interventricular septum. Indentations of the endocardium form valves that separate the atria from the ventricles and the ventricles from the aorta and pulmonary arteries.

Fibrous skeleton of the heart

Four rings of dense fibrous connective tissue provide a firm anchorage for the attachments of the atrial and ventricular musculature, as well as the valvular tissue (Figure 22-4). The fibrous rings are adjacent and form a central, fibrous supporting structure collectively termed the *annuli fibrosi cordis.*

Valves of the heart

One-way blood flow through the heart is ensured by the four heart valves. During ventricular relaxation, the two **atrioventricular valves** open and blood flows from the atria to the relaxed ventricles. With increasing ventricular pressure, these valves close and prevent backflow into the atria as the ventricles contract. The **semilunar valves** of the heart open when intraventricular pressure exceeds aortic and pulmonary pressures and blood flows out of the ventricles and into the pulmonary and systemic circulations. After ventricular contraction and ejection, intraventricular pressure falls and the **pulmonic** and **aortic semilunar valves** close, preventing backflow into the right and left ventricles. The coordinated actions of the heart valves are shown in Figures 22-3 and 22-4.

The atrioventricular valve openings are guarded by flaps of tissue called *leaflets* or *cusps,* which are attached to the papillary muscles by the **chordae tendineae cordis** (see Figure 22-3). The **papillary muscles** are extensions of the myocardium that pull the cusps together and downward at the onset of ventricular contraction, thus preventing their backward expulsion into the atria.

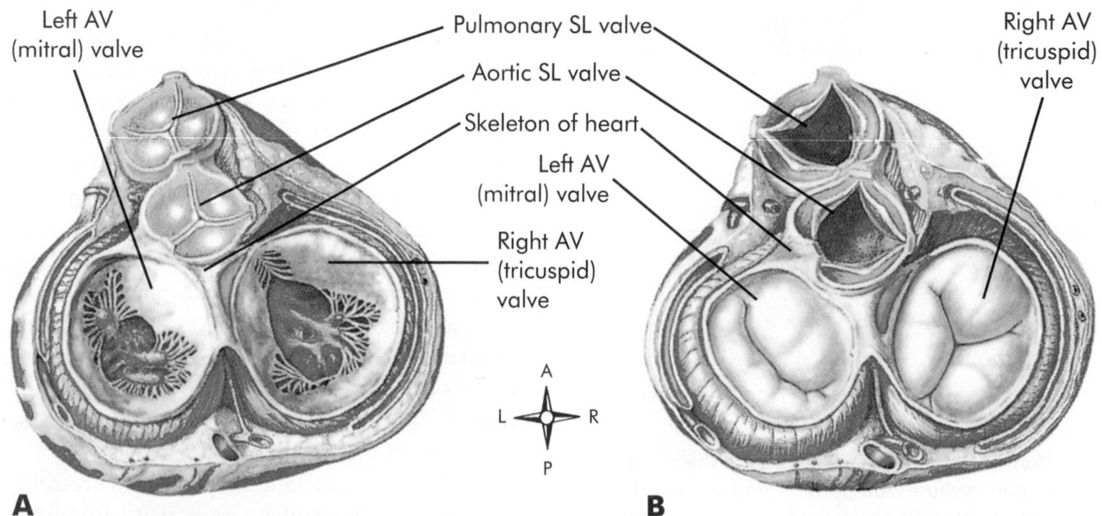

Figure 22-4 ■ **Structure of the Heart Valves. A,** The heart valves in this drawing are depicted as viewed from above (looking down into the heart). Note that the semilunar (SL) valves are closed and the atrioventricular (AV) valves are open, as when the atria are contracting. **B** is similar to **A** except that the semilunar valves are open and the atrioventricular valves are closed, as when the ventricles are contracting. (From Thibodeau GA, Patton KT: *Anatomy & physiology,* ed 6, St Louis, 2007, Mosby.)

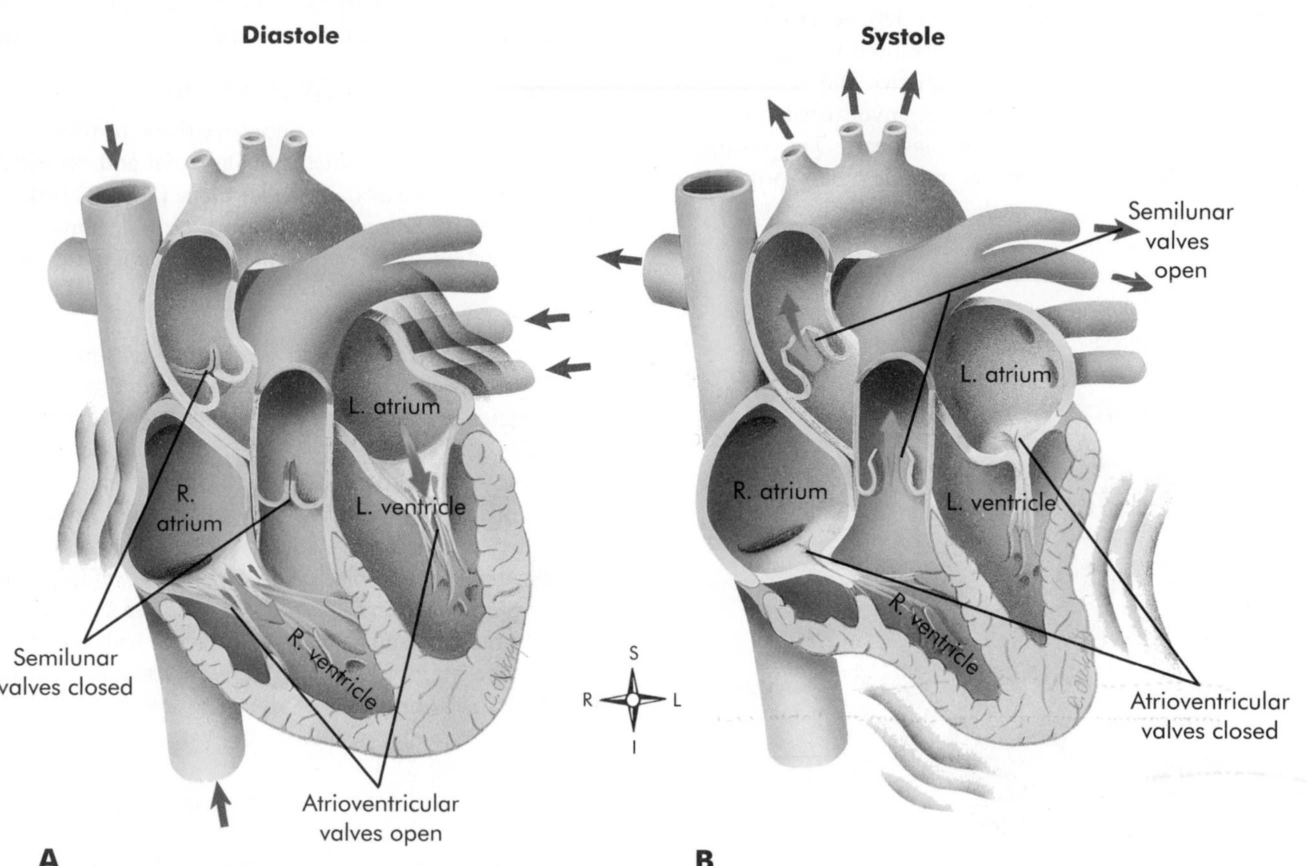

Figure 22-5 ■ **Blood Flow Through the Heart During a Single Cardiac Cycle. A,** During diastole, blood flows into atria, atrioventricular valves are pushed open, and blood begins to fill ventricles. Atrial systole squeezes any blood remaining in atria out into ventricles. **B,** During ventricular systole, ventricles contract, pushing blood out through semilunar valves into pulmonary artery (right ventricle) and aorta (left ventricle). (Modified from Thibodeau GA, Patton KT: *Anatomy & physiology,* ed 6, St Louis, 2007, Mosby.)

The right atrioventricular valve is called the **tricuspid valve** because it has three cusps. The left atrioventricular valve is a bicuspid (two-cusp) valve called the **mitral valve.** The tricuspid and mitral valves function as a unit because the atrium, fibrous rings, valvular tissue, chordae tendineae, papillary muscles, and ventricular walls are connected. Collectively, these six structures are known as the **mitral and tricuspid complex.** Damage to any one of the complex's six components can alter function significantly.

The great vessels

Blood moves in and out of the heart through several large vessels (see Figure 22-3). The right heart receives venous blood from the systemic circulation through the **superior** and **inferior venae cavae,** which enter the right atrium. Blood leaves the right ventricle and enters the pulmonary circulation through the **pulmonary artery.** This artery divides into right and left branches to transport unoxygenated blood from the right heart to the right and left lungs. The pulmonary arteries branch further into the pulmonary capillary bed, where oxygen and carbon dioxide exchange occurs.

The four **pulmonary veins,** two from the right lung and two from the left lung, carry oxygenated blood from the lungs to the left side of the heart. The oxygenated blood moves through the left atrium and ventricle and out into the **aorta,** which delivers it to systemic vessels that supply the body.

Blood flow during the cardiac cycle

The pumping action of the heart consists of contraction and relaxation of the myocardial layer of the heart wall. Each contraction and the relaxation that follows it constitute one **cardiac cycle.** (Blood flow through the heart during a single cardiac cycle is illustrated in Figure 22-5.) During relaxation, termed **diastole,** blood fills the ventricles. The ventricle fills rapidly in early diastole and again in late diastole when the atrium contracts. The ventricular contraction that follows, termed **systole,** propels the blood out of the ventricles and into the circulation. Contraction of the left ventricle is slightly earlier than contraction of the right ventricle.

The phases of the cardiac cycle can be identified on initiation of ventricular myocardial contraction (Figures 22-6 and 22-7). Expulsion of blood from the ventricles marks the end of one cardiac cycle.

Normal intracardiac pressures

Normal intracardiac pressures are shown in Table 22-1.

QUICK CHECK 22-1

1. Why are the two separate circulatory systems said to be "serially connected"?
2. Why does the thickness of the myocardium vary tremendously in the different heart chambers?
3. Trace blood flow through the heart during a single cardiac cycle.

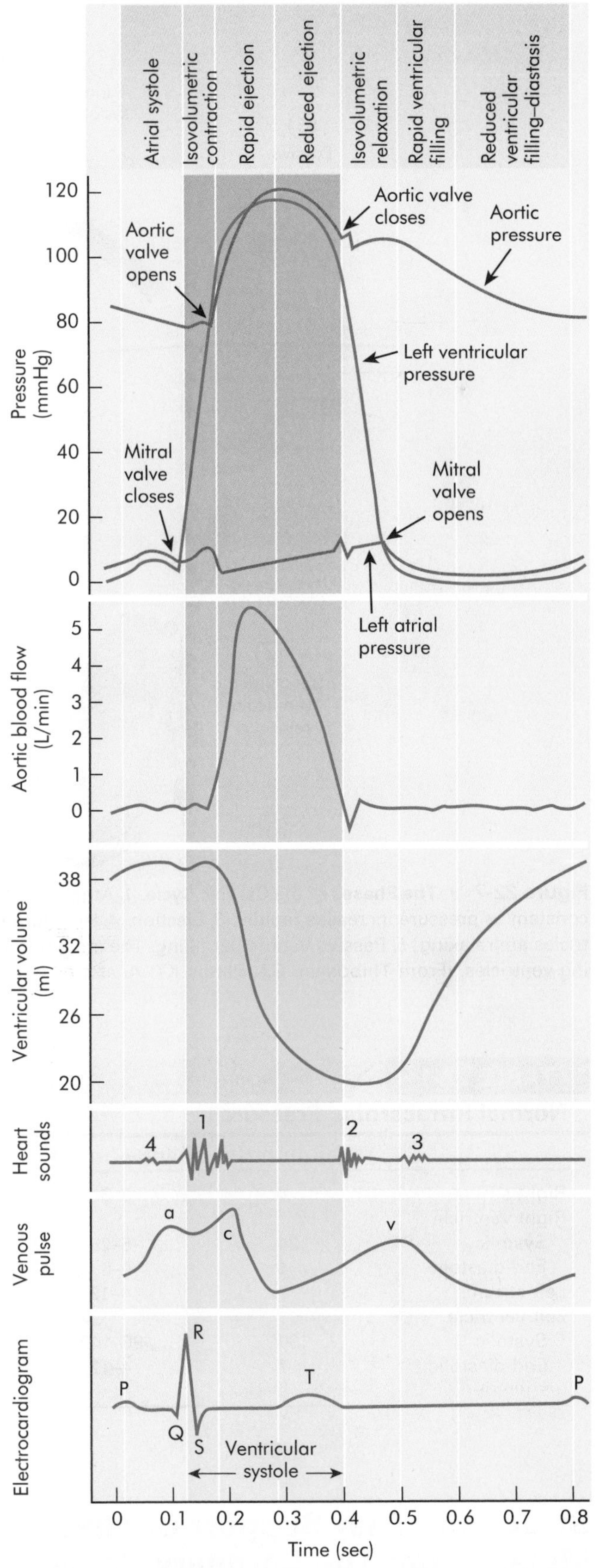

Figure 22-6 ■ **Composite Chart of heart function.** This chart is a composite of several diagrams of heart function (cardiac pumping cycle, blood pressure, blood flow, volume, heart sounds, venous pulse, and electrocardiogram [ECG]), all adjusted to the same timescale.

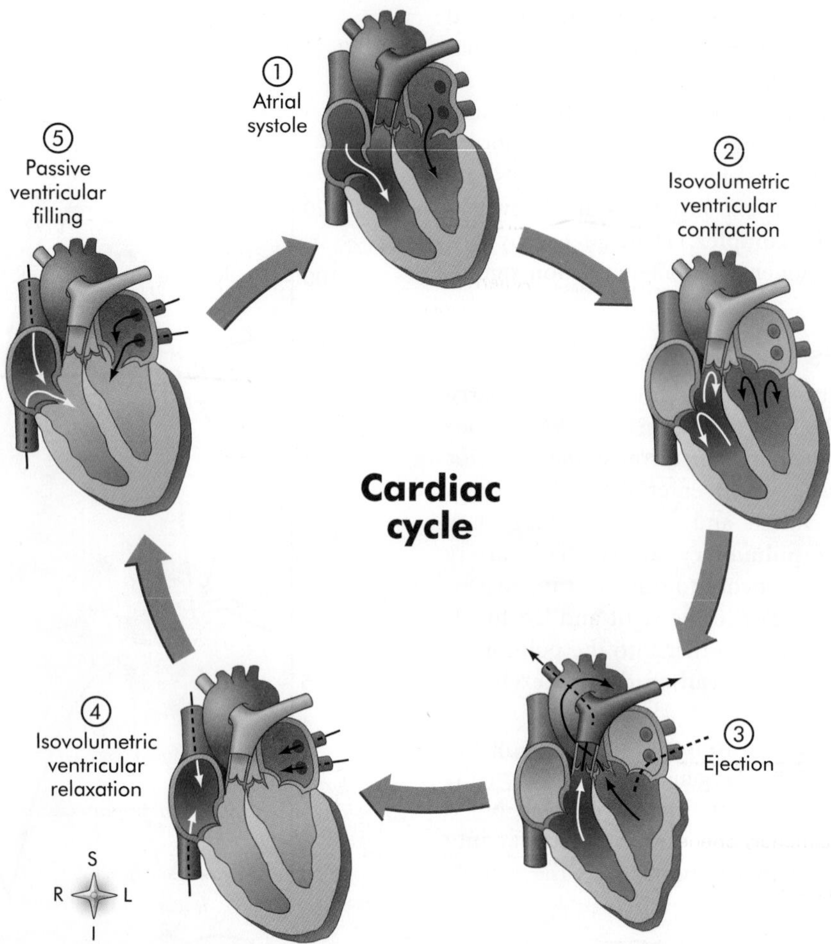

Figure 22-7 ■ **The Phases of the Cardiac Cycle.** *1,* Atrial systole. *2,* Isovolumetric ventricular contraction. Ventricular volume remains constant as pressure increases rapidly. *3,* Ejection. *4,* Isovolumetric ventricular relaxation. Both sets of valves are closed, and the ventricles are relaxing. *5,* Passive ventricular filling. The atrioventricular (AV) valves are forced open, and the blood rushes into the relaxing ventricles. (From Thibodeau GA, Patton KT: *Anatomy & physiology,* ed 6, St Louis, 2007, Mosby.)

TABLE 22-1

Normal Intracardiac Pressures

	Mean (mmHg)	Range (mmHg)
Right atrium	4	0–8
Right ventricle		
Systolic	24	15–28
End-diastolic	4	0–8
Left atrium	7	4–12
Left ventricle		
Systolic	130	90–140
End-diastolic	7	4–12

Structures That Support Cardiac Metabolism: The Coronary Vessels

The blood within the heart chambers does not supply oxygen and other nutrients to the cells of the heart. Like all other organs, including the lungs, heart structures are nourished by vessels of the systemic circulation. The branch of the systemic circulation that supplies the heart is termed the **coronary circulation** and consists of **coronary arteries,** which receive blood through openings in the aorta called the **coronary ostia,** and the **cardiac veins,** which empty into the right atrium through the opening of a large vein called the **coronary sinus** (Figure 22-8). (Regulation of the coronary circulation, which is similar to regulation of flow through systemic and pulmonary vessels, is described elsewhere.)

Coronary arteries

The **right coronary artery** and the **left coronary artery** (see Figure 22-8) traverse the epicardium, myocardium, and endocardium and branch to become arterioles and then capillaries.[1] Their main branches are outlined in Box 22-1.

Collateral arteries

The collateral arteries are really connections, or anastomoses, between two branches of the same or the opposite coronary artery. The epicardium contains more collateral vessels than the endocardium. Gradual coronary occlusion results in the growth of coronary collaterals. The collateral

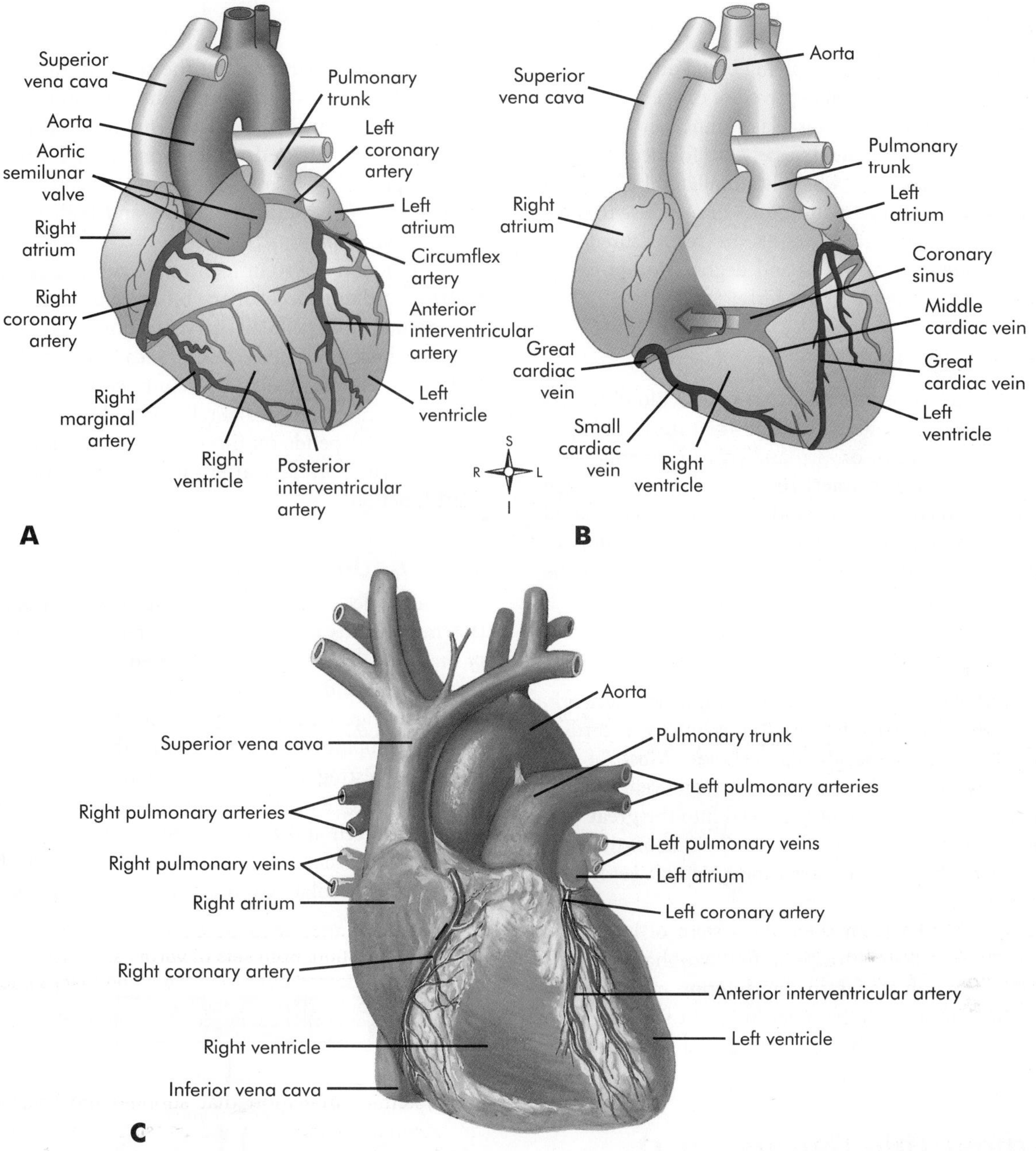

Figure 22-8 ■ **Coronary Circulation. A,** Arteries. **B,** Veins. Both **A** and **B** are anterior views of the heart. Vessels near the anterior surface are more darkly colored than vessels of the posterior surface seen through the heart. **C,** View of the anterior (sternocostal) surface. (**A** and **B** modified from Thibodeau GA, Patton KT: *Anatomy & physiology,* ed 6, St Louis, 2007, Mosby; **C** from Seeley RR, Stephens TD, Tate P: *Anatomy and physiology,* ed 3, St Louis, 1995, Mosby.)

BOX 22-1 Main Branches of the Coronary Arteries

Left coronary artery. Arises from single ostium behind left cusp of aortic semilunar valve; ranges from a few millimeters to a few centimeters long; passes between left arterial appendage and pulmonary artery and generally divides into two branches: the left anterior descending artery and the circumflex artery; other branches are distributed diagonally across the free wall of the left ventricle.

Left anterior descending artery (or anterior interventricular artery). Delivers blood to portions of left and right ventricles and much of interventricular septum; travels down the anterior surface of interventricular septum toward apex of the heart.

Circumflex artery. Travels in a groove *(coronary sulcus)* that separates left atrium from left ventricle and extends to left border of heart; supplies blood to left atrium and lateral wall of left ventricle; often branches to posterior surfaces of left atrium and left ventricle.

Right coronary artery. Originates from an ostium behind the right aortic cusp, travels from behind the pulmonary artery and extends around the right heart to the heart's posterior surface, where it branches to atrium and ventricle; three major branches are conus (supplies blood to upper right ventricle), right marginal branch (travels right ventricle to the apex), and posterior descending branch (lies in posterior interventricular sulcus and supplies smaller branches to both ventricles).

circulation is responsible for supplying blood and oxygen to the myocardium that has been deprived of oxygen following severe narrowing and reduced vasoelastic function of a major coronary artery. New collateral vessels are formed through the process of angiogenesis, which is stimulated by hypoxia and vascular endothelial growth factor.[2] In response to flow, stress, and pressure, collateral vessels are restructured and remodeled through the synthesis and degradation of extracellular matrix components in the vessel wall.

Coronary capillaries

The heart has an extensive capillary network. Blood travels from the arteries to the arterioles and then into the capillaries, where exchange of oxygen and other nutrients takes place. At rest, the heart extracts 70% to 80% of the oxygen delivered to it and coronary blood flow is directly correlated with myocardial oxygen consumption.[3] Any alteration of the cardiac muscles dramatically affects blood flow in the capillaries.

Coronary veins and lymphatic vessels

After passing through the extensive capillary network, blood from the coronary arteries drains into the cardiac veins, which travel alongside the arteries. Most of the venous drainage of the heart occurs through veins in the visceral pericardium. The veins then feed into the **great cardiac vein** (see Figure 22-8) and coronary sinus on the posterior surface of the heart, between the atria and ventricles, in the coronary sulcus.

The myocardium has an extensive system of lymphatic vessels. With cardiac contraction, the lymphatic vessels drain fluid to lymph nodes in the anterior mediastinum that eventually empty into the superior vena cava. The lymphatics are important for protecting the myocardium against injury.

Structures That Control Heart Action

The continuous, rhythmic repetition of the cardiac cycle (systole and diastole) depends on the transmission of electrical impulses, termed **cardiac action potentials,** through the myocardium. (Action potentials are described in Chapters 1 and 4.) The muscle fibers of the myocardium are uniquely joined so that action potentials pass from cell to cell rapidly and efficiently.

The myocardium also contains its own **conduction system**—specialized cells that enable it to generate and transmit action potentials without stimulation from the nervous system. These cells are concentrated at certain sites in the myocardium called **nodes.** The cardiac cycle is stimulated by these nodes of specialized cells and is fine-tuned as needed by the autonomic fibers. Although the heart is innervated by the autonomic nervous system (both sympathetic and parasympathetic fibers), neural impulses are not needed to maintain the cardiac cycle. Thus, the heart will beat in the absence of any nervous connection. The sympathetic and parasympathetic nerves affect the speed of the cardiac cycle (**heart rate,** or beats per minute) and the diameter of the coronary vessels (Figure 22-9). The sympathetic nervous system increases heart rate and conduction through the nodes, the parasympathetic nervous system slows heart rate and prolongs intranodal conduction time, and both systems cause coronary vasodilation.[4]

Heart action is also influenced by substances delivered to the myocardium in coronary blood. Nutrients and oxygen are needed for cellular survival and normal function, whereas hormones and biochemicals affect the strength and duration of myocardial contraction and the degree and duration of myocardial relaxation. Normal or appropriate function depends on the availability of these substances, which is why coronary artery disease can seriously disrupt heart function.

The conduction system

Normally, electrical impulses arise in the **sinoatrial node (SA node, sinus node),** which is often called the *pacemaker of the heart.* The SA node is located at the junction of the right atrium and superior vena cava, just above the tricuspid valve (Figure 22-10). The SA node is heavily innervated by both sympathetic and parasympathetic nerve fibers.[4]

In the resting adult the SA node generates about 75 action potentials per minute. Each one travels rapidly from cell to cell and through special pathways in the atrial myocardium, causing both atria to contract, beginning systole. Ventricular contraction is delayed because the

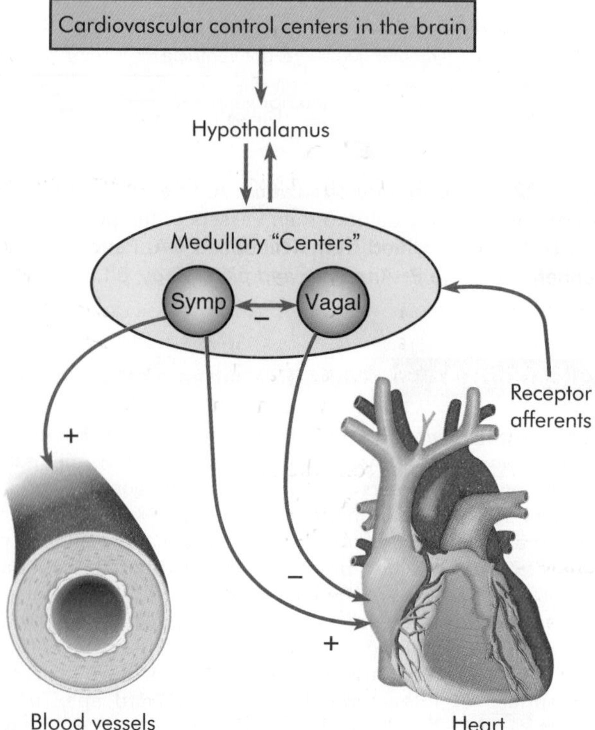

Figure 22-9 ■ **Autonomic innervation of cardiovascular system.** – = Inhibition; + = activation.

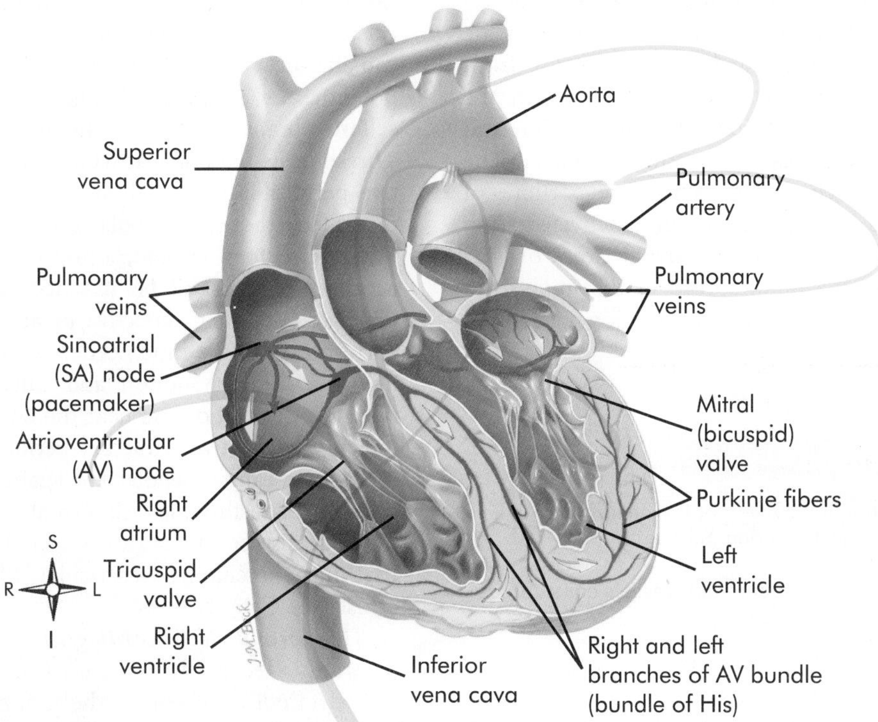

Figure 22-10 ■ **Conduction System of Heart.** Specialized cardiac muscle cells in the wall of the heart rapidly conduct an electrical impulse throughout the myocardium. The signal is initiated by the sinoatrial (SA) node (pacemaker) and spreads to the rest of the atrial myocardium and to the atrioventricular (AV) node. The AV node then initiates a signal that is conducted through the ventricular myocardium by way of the atrioventricular bundle (of His) and Purkinje fibers. (Modified from Thibodeau GA, Patton KT: *Anatomy & physiology,* ed 6, St Louis, 2007, Mosby.)

fibrous skeleton of the heart interrupts cell-to-cell transmission of the electrical impulses. The action potential is transmitted from the atrial to the ventricular myocardium through fibers of the conduction system, traveling first to the **atrioventricular node (AV node),** then to the **bundle of His (atrioventricular bundle, common bundle),** and finally through the **bundle branches** of the interventricular septum to Purkinje fibers in the heart wall (see Figure 22-10).

The AV node is well situated for mediating conduction between the atria and ventricles. It is located in the right atrial wall above the tricuspid valve and anterior to the ostium of the coronary sinus. Behind it are numerous autonomic parasympathetic ganglia. These ganglia serve as receptors for the vagus nerve and cause slowing of impulse conduction through the AV node.

Conducting fibers from the AV node converge to form the bundle of His, a triangle within the posterior border of the interventricular septum. The two lower ends of the triangle give rise to the right and left bundle branches. The **right bundle branch (RBB)** is thin and travels without much branching to the right ventricular apex. Because of its thinness and relative lack of branches, the RBB is susceptible to interruption by damage to the endocardium.

The **left bundle branch (LBB)** arises perpendicularly from the bundle of His and, in some hearts, divides into two branches, or fascicles. The left anterior bundle branch (LABB) passes the left anterior papillary muscle and the base of the left ventricle and crosses the aortic outflow tract. Damage to the aortic valve or the left ventricle can interrupt this branch. The left posterior bundle branch (LPBB) travels posteriorly, crossing the left ventricular inflow tract to the base of the left posterior papillary muscle. This branch spreads diffusely through the posterior inferior left ventricular wall. Blood flow through this portion of the left ventricle is relatively nonturbulent, so the LBB is somewhat protected from injury caused by wear and tear.

The **Purkinje fibers** are the terminal branches of the RBB and LBB. They extend from the ventricular apexes to the fibrous rings and penetrate the heart wall to the outer myocardium.

Because impulses from the SA node arrive at the AV node extremely quickly, investigators have proposed that these nodes are connected by internodal pathways called the **anterior, middle,** and **posterior internodal pathways.** These pathways consist of ordinary myocardial cells and specialized conducting fibers. The **anterior interatrial myocardial band** (or **Bachmann bundle**) conducts the impulse from the SA node to the left atrium. The posterior internodal pathway connects the right and left atria and the SA node and AV node for conduction from the SA to the AV node.[4,5]

From the SA node the impulse that begins contraction spreads throughout the right atrium at a conduction velocity of about 1 m/sec. The Bachmann bundle conducts the impulse from the SA node to the left atrium, and the posterior internodal pathway conducts the impulse from the SA node to the AV node. From the AV node, the impulse travels from the atrioventricular bundle and through the bundle branches to the Purkinje fibers. The first areas of the ventricles to be excited are portions of the interventricular septum. The septum is activated from both the RBB and the LBB. The extensive network of Purkinje fibers promotes the rapid spread of the impulse to the ventricular apices. The basal and posterior portions of the ventricles are the last to be activated.

QUICK CHECK 22-2

1. Outline the conduction system of the heart.
2. What happens ionically during depolarization; repolarization?
3. Why are the left and right coronary vessels considered the major coronary vessels?

Propagation of cardiac action potentials

Electrical activation of the muscle cells, termed **depolarization,** is caused by the movement of electrically charged solutes (ions) across cardiac cell membranes. Deactivation, called **repolarization,** occurs the same way. (Movement of ions across cell membranes is described in Chapter 1; electrical activation of muscle cells is described in Chapter 36.)

When ions move into and out of the cell, an electrical (voltage) difference across the cell membrane, called the *membrane potential,* is created. The resting membrane potential of myocardial cells is between −80 and −90 millivolts (mV), whereas that of the SA node is between −50 and −60 mV and the AV node is between −60 and −70 mV.[4] During depolarization, the inside of the cell becomes less negatively charged. In cardiac cells, the difference between resting membrane potential (in millivolts) and the decreased negative charge caused by depolarization is the cardiac action potential. Table 22-2 summarizes the intracellular and extracellular ionic concentrations of cardiac muscle. Hence, drugs that alter ion movement (e.g., calcium) have profound effects on the action potential and can alter heart rate. The various phases of the cardiac action potential are related to changes in the permeability of the cell membrane, primarily to sodium and potassium changes. Threshold is the point at which the cell membrane's selective permeability to sodium and potassium is temporarily disrupted, leading to depolarization.

A **refractory period,** during which no new cardiac action potential can be initiated by a stimulus, follows depolarization. This effective or absolute refractory period corresponds to the time needed for the reopening of channels that permit sodium and calcium influx. A relative refractory period occurs near the end of repolarization, following the effective refractory period. During this time, the membrane can be depolarized again but only by a greater-than-normal stimulus. Abnormal refractory periods as a result of disease can cause abnormal heart rhythms or dysrhythmias, including ventricular fibrillation and cardiac arrest (see Chapter 23).

The normal electrocardiogram. The normal electrocardiogram is recorded from electrical activity transmitted by skin electrodes and reflects the sum of all the cardiac action potentials (Figure 22-11). The **P wave** represents atrial depolarization. The **PR interval** is a measure of time from the onset of atrial activation to the onset of ventricular activation (normally 0.12 to 0.20 second). The PR interval represents the time necessary for electrical activity to travel from the sinus node through the atrium, AV node, and His-Purkinje system to activate ventricular myocardial cells. The **QRS complex** represents the sum of all ventricular muscle cell depolarizations. The configuration and amplitude of the QRS complex vary considerably among individuals. The duration is normally between 0.06 and 0.10 second. During the **ST interval,** the entire ventricular myocardium is depolarized. The **QT interval** is sometimes called the "electrical systole" of the ventricles. It lasts about 0.4 second but varies inversely with the heart rate.

Automaticity. **Automaticity,** or the property of generating spontaneous depolarization to threshold, enables the SA and AV nodes to generate cardiac action potentials without any stimulus. Cells capable of spontaneous depolarization are called **automatic cells.** Those of the cardiac conduction system can stimulate the heart to beat even when it is removed from the body. Spontaneous depolarization is possible in automatic cells because the membrane potential does not "rest" during return to the resting membrane potential. Instead, it slowly creeps toward threshold during the diastolic phase of the cardiac cycle. Because threshold is approached during diastole, return to the resting membrane potential in automatic cells is called **diastolic depolarization.** The electrical impulse normally begins in the SA node because its cells depolarize more rapidly than other automatic cells.

Rhythmicity. **Rhythmicity** is the regular generation of an action potential by the heart's conduction system. The SA node sets the pace because normally it has the fastest rate. The SA node depolarizes spontaneously 60 to 100

TABLE 22-2

Intercellular and Extracellular Ion Concentrations in the Myocardium

	Intracellular Concentration	Extracellular Concentration
Sodium (Na^+)	15 mM	145 mM
Potassium (K^+)	150 mM	4 mM
Chloride (Cl^-)	5 mM	120 mM
Calcium (Ca^{++})	10^{-7} mM	2 mM

mM, Millimoles per kilogram; *M,* moles per kilogram.

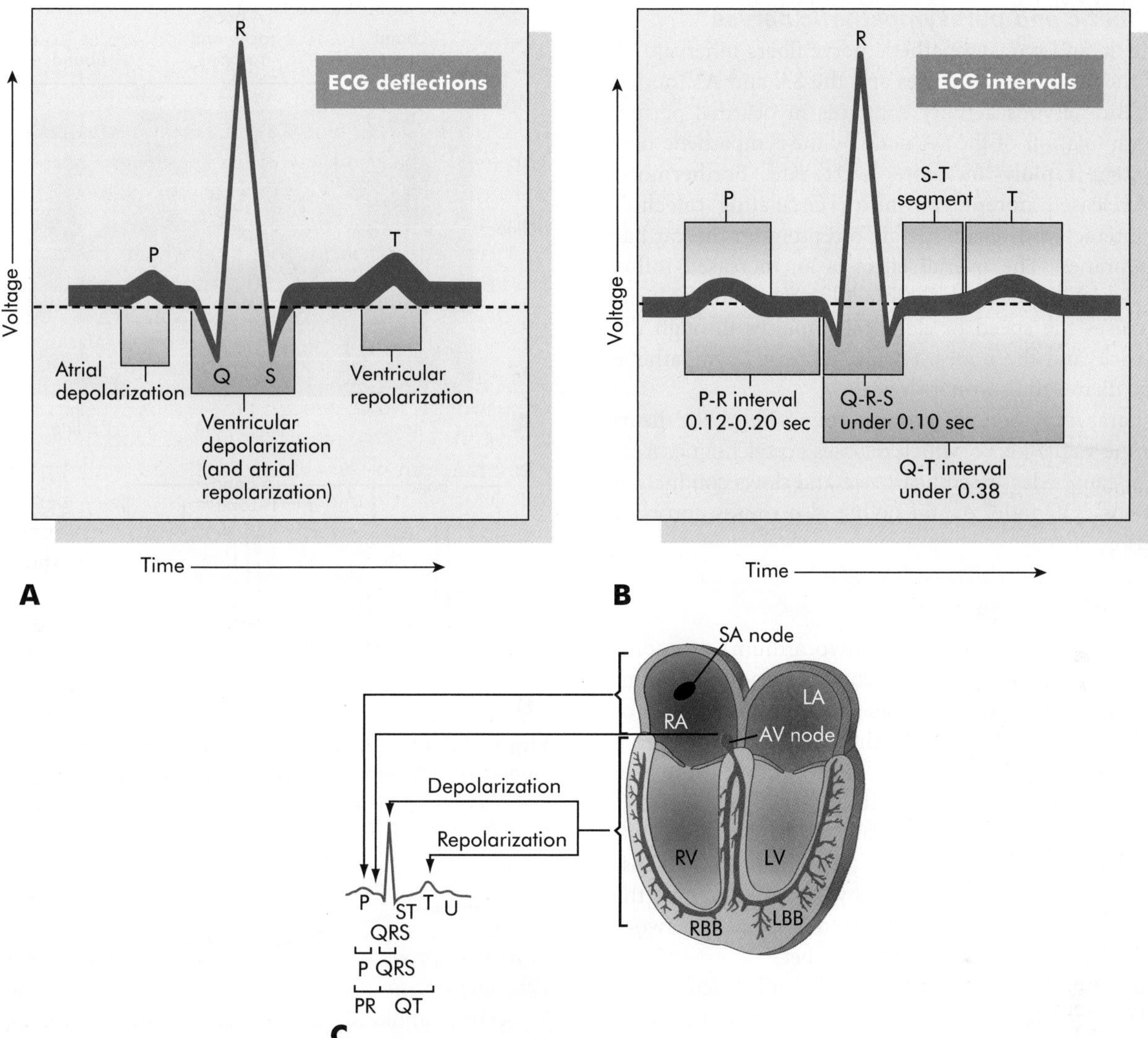

Figure 22-11 ■ **Electrocardiogram (ECG) and Cardiac Electrical Activity. A,** Normal ECG. Depolarization and repolarization. **B,** ECG intervals among P, QRS, and T waves. **C,** Schematic representation of ECG and its relationship to cardiac electrical activity. *RA,* Right atrium; *LA,* left atrium; *AV,* atrioventricular; *RV,* right ventricle; *LV,* left ventricle; *RBB,* right bundle branch; *LBB,* left bundle branch. (**A** and **B** from Thibodeau GA, Patton KT: *Anatomy & physiology,* ed 6, St Louis, 2007, Mosby.)

times per minute. If the SA node is damaged, the AV node will become the heart's pacemaker at a rate of about 40 to 60 spontaneous depolarizations per minute. Eventually, however, conduction cells in the atria usually take over from the AV node. Purkinje fibers are capable of spontaneous depolarization but at a rate of only 30 to 40 beats/min.[4]

QUICK CHECK 22-3

1. What does each of the electrocardiogram waves (P, Q, R, S, T) represent?
2. Define automaticity and rhythmicity.
3. What is the significance of autonomic neural transmission to the heart?

Cardiac innervation

Although the heart's nodes and conduction system generate cardiac action potentials independently, the autonomic nervous system influences the rate of impulse generation (firing), depolarization, and repolarization of the myocardium and the strength of atrial and ventricular contraction. Autonomic neural transmission produces changes in the heart and circulatory system faster than metabolic or humoral agents. Speed is important, for example, in stimulating the heart to increase its pumping action during times of stress or fear—the so-called fight-or-flight response. Although increased delivery of oxygen, glucose, hormones, and other blood-borne factors sustains increased cardiac activity, the rapid initiation of increased activity depends on the sympathetic and parasympathetic fibers of the autonomic nervous system.

Sympathetic and parasympathetic nerves

Sympathetic and parasympathetic nerve fibers innervate all parts of the atria and ventricles and the SA and AV nodes. Sympathetic nervous activity enhances myocardial performance. Stimulation of the SA node by the sympathetic nervous system rapidly increases heart rate. Furthermore, neurally released norepinephrine or circulating catecholamines interact with β-adrenergic receptors on the cardiac cell membranes. The overall effect is an increased influx of Ca^{++}, which increases the contractile strength of the heart and increases the speed of electrical impulses through the heart muscle and the nodes. Finally, increased sympathetic discharge dilates the coronary vessels.

The parasympathetic nervous system affects the heart through the vagus nerve, which releases acetylcholine. Acetylcholine causes decreased heart rate and slows conduction through the AV node. Acetylcholine also causes coronary vasodilation.

Myocardial cells

The cells of cardiac muscle (the myocardium) are composed of long, narrow fibers that contain bundles of longitudinally arranged myofibrils; a nucleus (cardiac muscle) or many nuclei (skeletal muscle); mitochondria; an internal membrane system (the sarcoplasmic reticulum); cytoplasm (sarcoplasm); and a plasma membrane (the sarcolemma), which encloses the cell. Cardiac and skeletal muscle cells also have an "external" membrane system made up of transverse tubules (T tubules) formed by invaginations of the sarcolemma. The sarcoplasmic reticulum forms a network of channels that surrounds the muscle fiber.

Because the myofibrils in both cardiac and skeletal fibers are made up of alternating light and dark bands of protein, the fibers appear striped, or striated. The dark and light bands of the myofibrils are called *sarcomeres* and are normally between 1.6 and 2.2 μm long (Figure 22-12). Length determines the limits of myocardial stretch at the end of diastole and subsequently the force of contraction during systole.

Differences between cardiac and skeletal muscle reflect heart function. Cardiac cells are arranged in branching networks throughout the myocardium, whereas skeletal muscle cells tend to be arranged in parallel units throughout the length of the muscle. Cardiac fibers have only one nucleus, whereas skeletal muscle cells have many nuclei. Other differences enable cardiac fibers to (1) transmit action potentials quickly from cell to cell, (2) maintain high levels of energy synthesis, and (3) gain access to more ions, particularly sodium and potassium, in the extracellular environment.

First, electrical impulses are transmitted rapidly from cardiac fiber to cardiac fiber because the network of fibers is connected at **intercalated disks,** which are thickened portions of the sarcolemma. The intercalated disks contain two junctions: desmosomes, which attach one cell to another, and gap junctions, which allow the electrical impulse to spread from cell to cell (see Chapter 1). Together, these junctions provide a low-resistance pathway for impulse propagation.

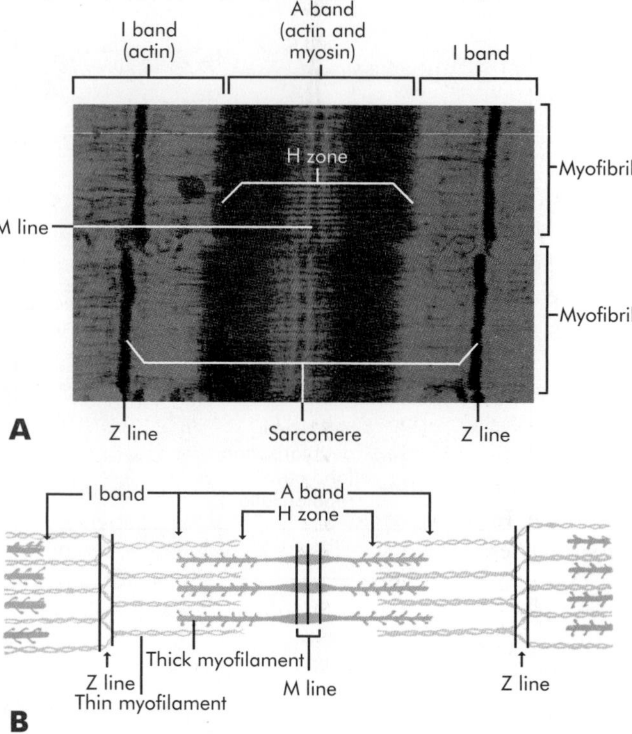

Figure 22-12 ■ **Sarcomere. A,** Electron photomicrograph of sarcomere. **B,** Schematic of location and interaction of actin and myosin. (Modified from Thibodeau GA, Patton KT: *Anatomy & physiology,* ed 3, St Louis, 1996, Mosby.)

Second, unlike skeletal muscle, the heart cannot rest and is in constant need of energy compounds such as adenosine triphosphate (ATP). Therefore, the cytoplasm surrounding the bundles of myofibrils in each cardiac muscle cell contains a superabundance of mitochondria (25% of the cellular volume). Cardiac muscle cells have more mitochondria than do skeletal muscle cells to provide the necessary respiratory enzymes for aerobic metabolism and supply quantities of ATP sufficient for the constant action of the myocardium.

Third, cardiac fibers contain more T tubules than do skeletal muscle fibers. This gives each myofibril in the myocardium ready access to molecules needed for the continuous transmission of action potentials, which involves transport of sodium and potassium through the walls of the T tubules. Because the T tubule system is continuous with the extracellular space and the interstitial fluid, it facilitates the rapid transmission of the electrical impulses from the surface of the sarcolemma to the myofibrils inside the fiber. This activates all the myofibrils of one fiber simultaneously. The sarcoplasmic reticulum is located around the myofibrils. When an action potential is transmitted through the T tubules, it induces the sarcoplasmic reticulum to release its stored calcium, which activates the contractile proteins actin and myosin.

Actin, myosin, and the troponin-tropomyosin complex

The thick filaments of **myosin** constitute the central dark band called the **anisotropic,** or **A, band** (see Figure 22-12). The myosin molecule resembles a golf club with two large bulbous heads protruding from one end of a straight shaft (see Figure 22-13, *A*). The bilobed heads contain an actin-binding site and a site of ATPase activity. A thick filament contains about 200 myosin molecules bundled together with the heads of the molecules (called *cross-bridges*) facing outward (Figure 22-14, *A*). The **actin** molecules are part of the thin filaments (Figure 22-14, *A*). The light bands are called **isotropic,** or **I, bands** (see Figure 22-12). The thin filaments of actin appear light and extend from the **Z line,** a dense fibrous line that crosses the center of each I band. The area from one dark Z line to an adjacent Z line is the sarcomere. In the center of the sarcomere is the H zone, a somewhat less dense region. A thin, dark **M line** travels the center of the H zone. A single **tropomyosin** molecule (a relaxing protein) lies alongside seven actin molecules. Troponin, another relaxing protein, associates with the tropomyosin molecule, forming the **troponin-tropomyosin complex** (see Figure 22-14). The troponin complex itself has three components. **Troponin T** aids in the binding of the troponin complex to actin and tropomyosin; **troponin I** inhibits the ATPase of actomyosin; and **troponin C** contains binding sites for the calcium ions involved in contraction. These troponin molecules are released into the bloodstream during myocardial infarction or injury, where they can be measured.

Myocardial metabolism

Cardiac muscle, like other muscle tissue, depends on the constant production of ATP for energy. ATP is produced within the mitochondria mainly from glucose, fatty acids, and lactate. If the myocardium is inadequately perfused because of coronary artery disease, anaerobic metabolism becomes an essential source of energy (see Chapter 1). The energy produced by metabolic processes is used for muscle contraction and relaxation, electrical excitation, membrane transport, and synthesis of large molecules. Normally, the amount of ATP produced supplies sufficient energy to pump blood throughout the system.

Cardiac work is often expressed in terms of **myocardial oxygen consumption ($M\dot{V}O_2$)**, which correlates closely with total cardiac energy requirements. $M\dot{V}O_2$ is determined by the following three major factors: (1) amount of wall stress during systole, which can be estimated by measuring the systolic blood pressure; (2) duration of systolic wall tension, which is measured indirectly by the heart rate; and (3) contractile state of the myocardium, for which no clinical measurement exists.

The oxygen supply to the myocardium is delivered exclusively by the coronary arteries. From 70% to 75% of the oxygen from the coronary arteries is used immediately by cardiac muscle, leaving little oxygen in reserve. Any increased energy needs can be met only by increasing coronary blood flow. When oxygen content decreases, the local concentration of metabolic factors increases. One of these, adenosine, dilates coronary arterioles, increasing coronary blood flow. Oxygen content of the blood cannot be increased under normal atmospheric conditions, nor can the amount of O_2 extracted from the blood be appreciably increased from the resting level. However, $M\dot{V}O_2$ can increase several-fold with exercise and decrease moderately under conditions such as hypotension and hypothermia.

Myocardial contraction and relaxation

Myocardial contractility is a change in developed tension at a given resting fiber length. In functional terms, contractility

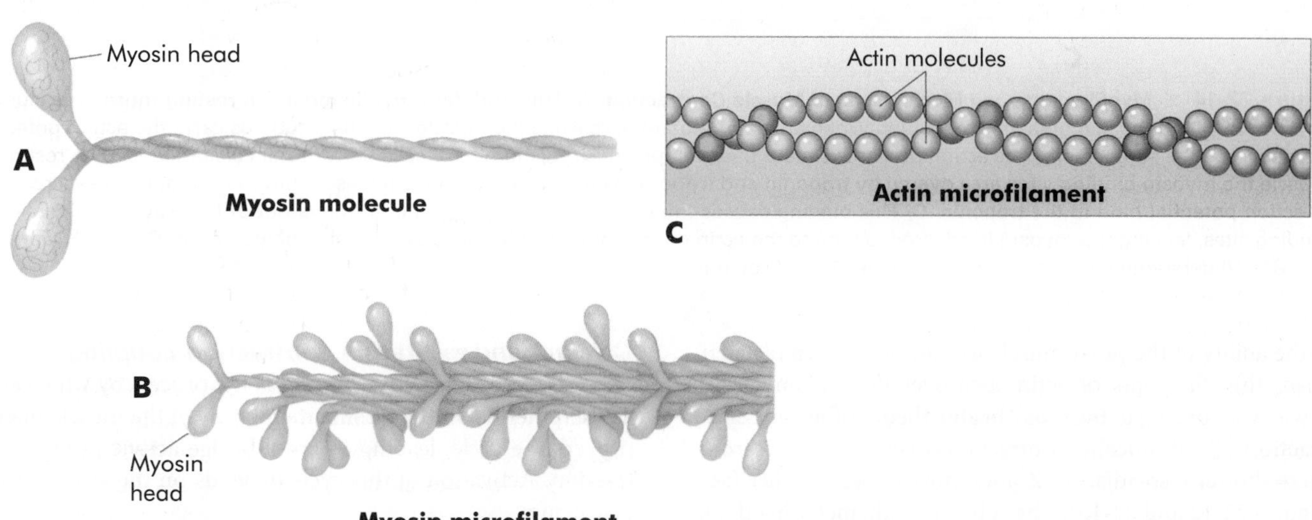

Figure 22-13 ■ **Structure of Myosin. A,** Each myosin molecule is a coil of two chains wrapped around one another. At the end of each chain is a globular region, much like a golf club, called the *head.* **B,** Myosin molecules usually are combined into filaments, which are stalks of myosin from which the heads protrude. **C,** Actin microfilament. (From Raven PH, Johnson GB: *Understanding biology,* ed 3, Dubuque, 1995, Brown.)

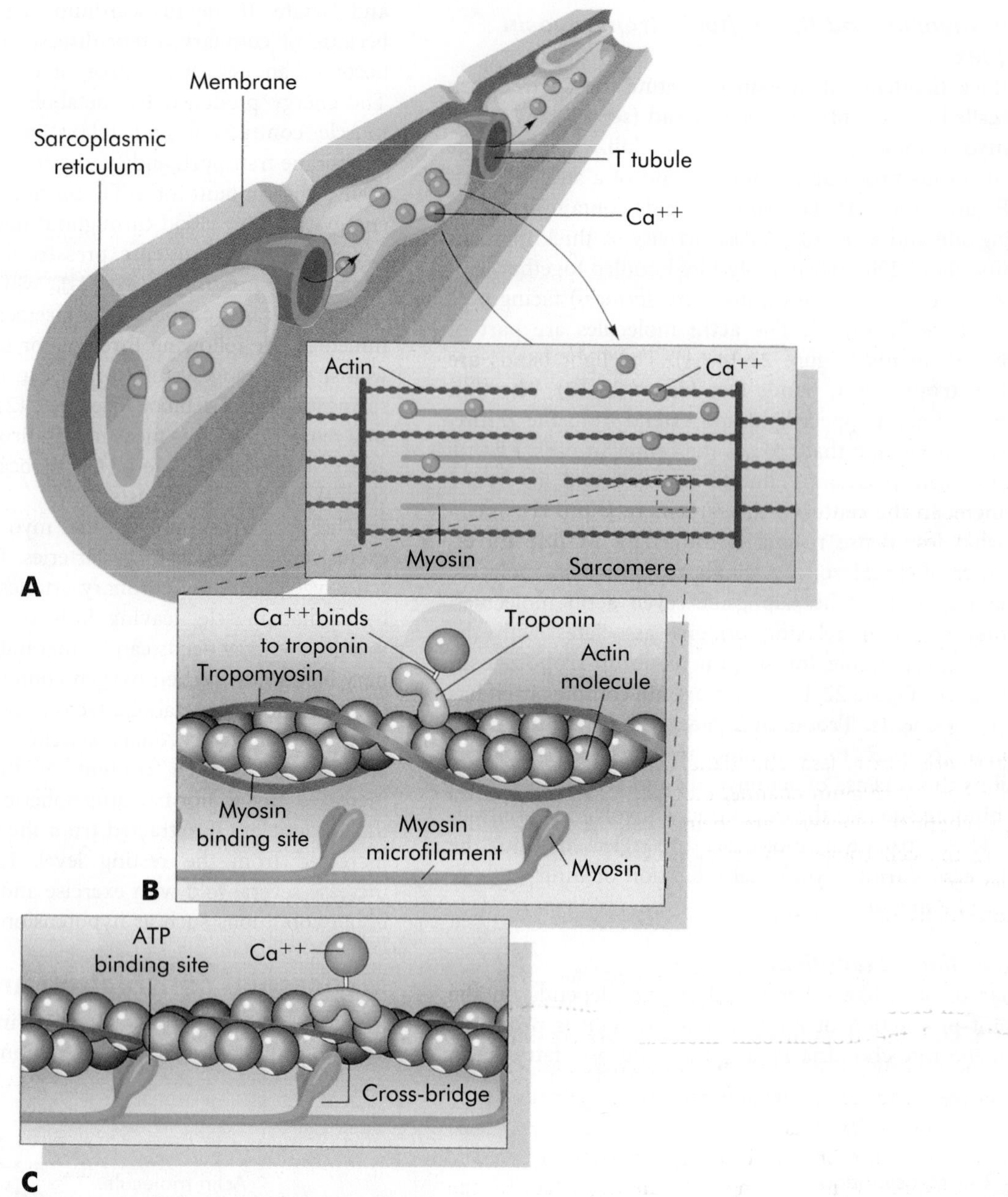

Figure 22-14 ■ **Myofilaments and Mechanisms of Muscle Contraction. A,** Thin and thick myofilaments. In resting muscle, calcium ions are stored in the sarcoplasmic reticulum. When an action potential reaches the muscle cell, the T tubules carry the action potential deep into the sarcoplasm. The action potential causes the sarcoplasmic reticulum to release the store of calcium ions. **B,** In resting muscle the myosin binding sites are covered by troponin and tropomyosin. The calcium ions released into the sarcoplasm as a result of action potential bind to the troponin. **C,** This binding causes the tropomyosin and troponin to move out of the way of the myosin binding sites, leaving the myosin heads free to bind to the actin microfilament. *ATP,* Adenosine triphosphate. (From Raven PH, Johnson GB: *Understanding biology,* ed 3, Dubuque, 1995, Brown.)

is the ability of the heart muscle to shorten. On a molecular basis, thin filaments of actin slide over thick filaments of myosin, according to the **cross-bridge theory of muscle contraction.**[4] Anatomically, contraction occurs when the sarcomere shortens, so adjacent Z lines move closer together (see Figures 22-12 and 22-15). The A band width, including thick myosin filaments, is unchanged, with the movement coming from the long sets of filaments. The degree of shortening depends on how much the thin filaments overlap the thick filaments.

Calcium and excitation-contraction coupling

Excitation-contraction coupling is the process by which an action potential in the plasma membrane of the muscle fiber triggers the cycle, leading to cross-bridge activity and contraction. Activation of this cycle depends on the availability of calcium.

Calcium is stored in the tubule system and the sarcoplasmic reticulum. It enters the myocardial cell from the interstitial fluid after electrical excitation, which increases membrane permeability to calcium. Two types of calcium

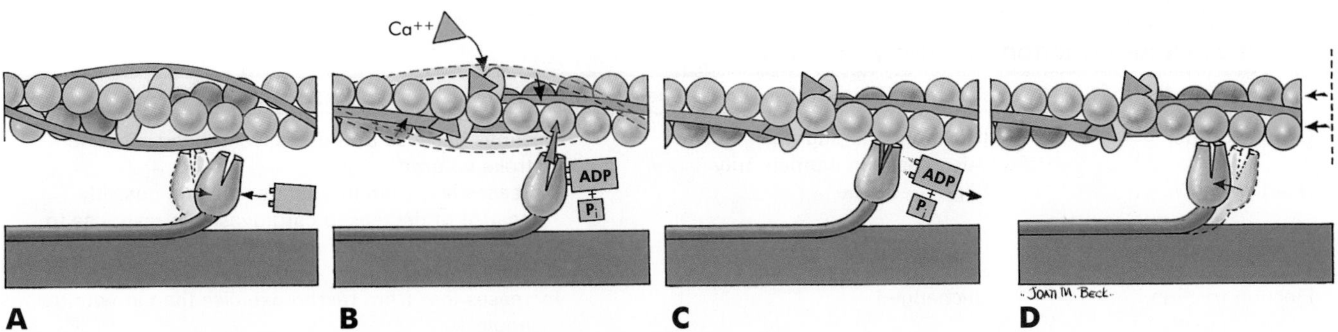

Figure 22-15 ■ **Cross-Bridge Theory of Muscle Contraction. A,** Each myosin cross-bridge in the thick filament moves into a resting position after an adenosine triphosphate (ATP) molecule binds and transfers its energy. **B,** Calcium ions released from the sarcoplasmic reticulum bind to troponin in the thin filament, allowing tropomyosin to shift from its position blocking the active sites of actin molecules. **C,** Each myosin cross-bridge then binds to an active site on a thin filament, displacing the remnants of ATP hydrolysis—adenosine diphosphate (ADP) and inorganic phosphate (P_i). **D,** The release of stored energy from step A provides the force needed for each cross-bridge to move back to its original position, pulling actin along with it. Each cross-bridge will remain bound to actin until another ATP molecule binds to it and pulls it back into its resting position, **A.** (From Thibodeau GA, Patton KT: *Anatomy & physiology,* ed 6, St Louis, 2007, Mosby.)

channels (L-type, T-type) are identified in cardiac tissues.[4,6] The L-type, or long-lasting, channels predominate and are the channels blocked by **calcium channel–blocking drugs** (verapamil, nifedipine, diltiazem).[6] The T-type, or transient, channels are much less abundant in the heart and are not blocked by calcium channel-blocking drugs, but novel T-type channel blockers are being explored.[7] Calcium entering the cell triggers the release of calcium from the storage sites, particularly the sarcoplasmic reticulum. Calcium then diffuses toward the myofibrils and binds with troponin.

The calcium-troponin complex interaction facilitates the contraction process. In the resting state, troponin I is bound to actin and the tropomyosin molecule covers the sites where the myosin heads bind to actin. Therefore, interaction between actin and myosin is prevented. Calcium binding to troponin inhibits troponin C (which enhances troponin I–actin binding) and causes tropomyosin to move away, consequently uncovering the binding sites on the myosin heads. Myosin and actin can now form cross-bridges, and ATP can be dephosphorylated to adenosine diphosphate (ADP). Under these circumstances, sliding of the thick and thin filaments can occur, and the muscle contracts.

Myocardial relaxation

Adequate relaxation is just as vital to optimal cardiac function as contraction; and calcium, troponin, and tropomyosin also facilitate relaxation. After contraction, free calcium ions are actively pumped out of the cell back into the interstitial fluid or reaccumulated in the sarcoplasmic reticulum and stored. Troponin releases its bound calcium. The tropomyosin complex blocks the active sites on the actin molecule, preventing cross-bridges with the myosin heads. A decreased ability by the myocardium to relax leads to increased diastolic filling pressures and eventually heart failure.[8]

✓ QUICK CHECK 22-4

1. What features distinguish myocardial cells from skeletal cells?
2. Describe the interactions of actin, myosin, and the troponin-tropomyosin complex in controlling heart function.
3. Define excitation-contraction coupling.

Factors Affecting Cardiac Performance

Cardiac performance can be quantified by measuring the **cardiac output.** Cardiac output is the volume of blood flowing through either the systemic or the pulmonary circuit per minute and is expressed in liters per minute. To determine cardiac output, heart rate is multiplied by stroke volume. Normal cardiac output is about 5 L/min for a resting adult.

The ventricle does not eject all the blood it contains, and the amount ejected is called the **ejection fraction,** which is the stroke volume divided by the end-diastolic volume. The end-diastolic volume of the normal ventricle is about 70 to 80 ml/m^2; the normal ejection fraction of the resting heart is about 60% to 75%. The ejection fraction is increased by factors that increase contractility (e.g., sympathetic nervous system activity). A decrease in ejection fraction is a hallmark of ventricular failure. The effects of aging on cardiovascular function are summarized in Table 22-3.

The factors that determine cardiac output are (1) preload, (2) afterload, (3) myocardial contractility, and (4) heart rate. Preload, afterload, and contractility affect stroke volume.

Preload

Preload is the volume and associated pressure generated in the ventricle at the end of diastole **(ventricular end-diastolic**

relaxation

TABLE 22-3

Cardiovascular Function in Elderly Persons

Determinant	Resting Cardiac Performance	Exercise Cardiac Performance
Cardiac output	Unchanged or slightly decreased in women only	Declines because of a decrease in heart rate and stroke volume
Heart rate	Slight decrease	Increases less than in younger people, possibly because of decreased cardiovascular response to catecholamines; overall slight decrease
Stroke volume	Slight increase	Slight increase
Ejection fraction	Unchanged	Increases less from rest to exercise than in younger people
Afterload	Increased	Uncertain
End-diastolic volume	Unchanged	Smaller for women
End-systolic volume	Unchanged	Lesser increase
Contraction	Increased because of prolonged relaxation	Decreases with vigorous exercise*
Cardiac dilation	No change	Increases at end-diastole and end-systole
$\dot{V}O_2$ max	Not applicable	Declines because of a decline in skeletal muscle mass

Data from Gerstenblith G, Lakatta EG: Aging and the cardiovascular system. In Willerson JT, Cohn JN, editors: *Cardiovascular medicine,* New York, 1995, Churchill Livingstone; Kaye D, Esler M: Sympathetic neuronal regulation of the heart in aging and heart failure, *Cardiovasc Res* 66(2):256–264, 2005; Kenny RA, Ceifer CM: Aging and geriatric heart disease. In Crawford MH, DiMarco JP: *Cardiology,* London, 2001, Mosby.
*As measured by end-systolic volume/systolic blood pressure (ESV/SBP), an index of contractility.

volume [VEDV] and **pressure** [VEDP]). Preload is determined by two primary factors: (1) the amount of venous return to the ventricle, and (2) the blood left in the ventricle after systole (end-systolic volume). End-systolic volume is dependent on the strength of ventricular contraction and the resistance to ventricular emptying.

The **Laplace law** describes the relationship by which the amount of tension generated in the wall of the ventricle (or any chamber or vessel) to produce a given intraventricular pressure depends on the size (radius and wall thickness) of the ventricle. **Ventricular end-diastolic volume,** which determines the size of the ventricle and the stretch of the cardiac muscle fibers, therefore affects the tension (or force) for contraction. Muscle fibers have an optimal resting length from which to generate the maximum amount of contractile strength. The **Frank-Starling law of the heart** describes the length-tension relationship of VEDV to myocardial contractility or stroke volume. Within a physiologic range of muscle stretching, increased preload increases cardiac output (Figure 22-16, *curve B*). Factors that increase contractility cause the heart to operate on a higher length-tension curve (Figure 22-16, *curve A*). Heart failure (Figure 22-16, *curve C*) is characterized by a lower length-tension curve (see Chapter 23). Excessive stretching causes actin and myosin to become completely disengaged and causes developed tension (force of contraction) to drop to zero. The relationship between stretch and contraction can be compared with that of a rubber band. To a certain point, the more the rubber band is stretched, the farther it will fly when one end is released. Beyond that point, however, the rubber band will break. Figure 22-17 illustrates the relationship between VEDV and cardiac output.

Heart failure occurs when it takes higher and higher filling pressures to accomplish normal contractile force. Increases in preload (VEDV) cause a decline in stroke volume and an increase in VEDP. Increased VEDP causes pressures to "back up" into the pulmonary or systemic venous circulation, where they force plasma out through vessel walls, causing fluid to accumulate in lung tissues (pulmonary edema; see Chapter 26) or in the peripheral tissues (peripheral edema).

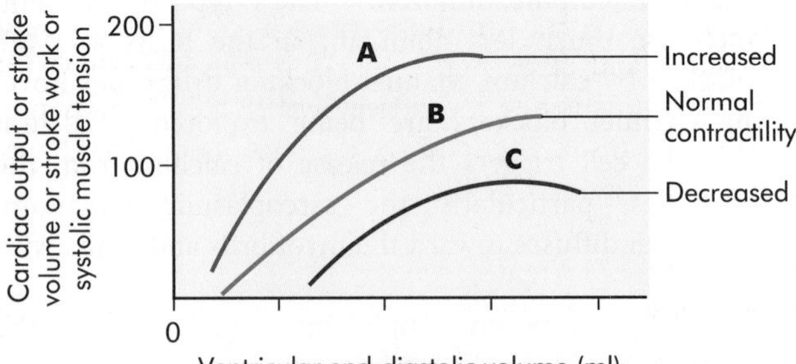

Figure 22-16 ■ **Frank-Starling Law of the Heart.** Relationship between length and tension in heart. End-diastolic volume determines end-diastolic length of ventricular muscle fibers and is proportional to tension generated during systole, as well as to cardiac output, stroke volume, and stroke work. A change in myocardial contractility causes the heart to perform on a different length-tension curve. *A,* Increased contractility, *B,* Normal contractility. *C,* Heart failure or decreased contractility. (See text for further explanation.)

Afterload

Left ventricular **afterload** is the resistance or impedance to ejection of blood from the left ventricle. It is the load the muscle must move after it starts to contract. Aortic systolic pressure is a good index of afterload. Pressure in the ventricle must exceed aortic pressure before blood can be pumped out during systole. Low aortic pressures (decreased

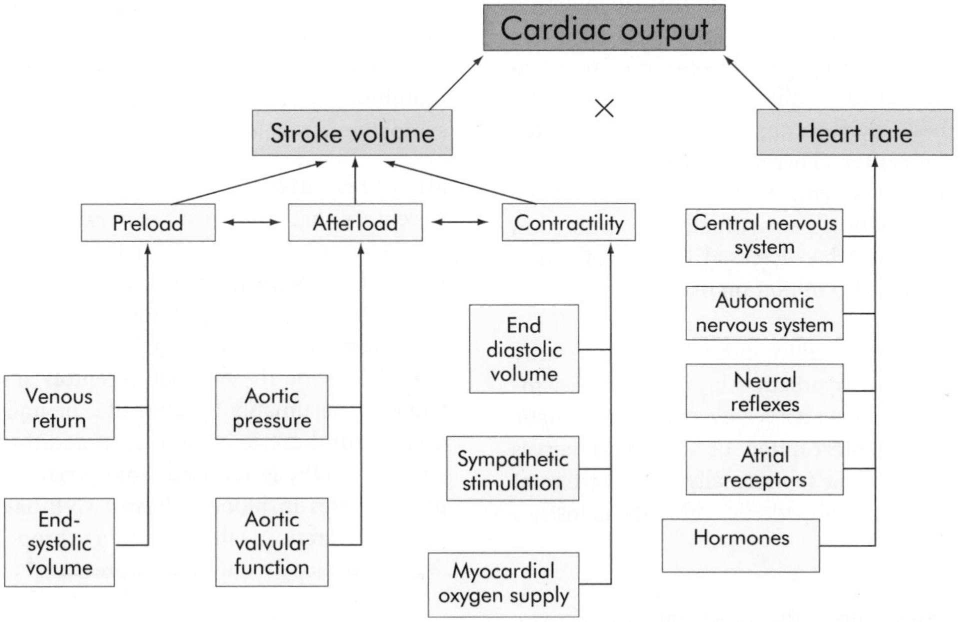

Figure 22-17 ■ **Factors Affecting Cardiac Performance.** Cardiac output, which is the amount of blood (in liters) ejected by the heart per minute, depends on heart rate (beats per minute) and stroke volume (milliliters of blood ejected during ventricular systole).

afterload) enable the heart to contract more rapidly, whereas high aortic pressures (increased afterload) slow contraction and cause higher workloads against which the heart must function so it can eject less blood. In some individuals, changes in afterload are the result of aortic valvular disease (see Figure 22-17).

Myocardial contractility

Stroke volume, or the volume of blood ejected per beat during systole, depends on the *force* of contraction, which depends on myocardial contractility or the degree of myocardial fiber shortening. Three major factors determine the force of contraction: (1) changes in the stretching of the ventricular myocardium caused by changes in ventricular volume (preload), (2) alterations in the sympathetic activation of the ventricles, and (3) adequacy of myocardial oxygen supply (see Figure 22-17). As discussed previously, increased blood flow from the veins into the heart distends the ventricle by increasing preload, which increases the stroke volume and, subsequently, cardiac output.

Chemicals affecting contractility are called **inotropic agents.** The most important positive inotropic agents are epinephrine and norepinephrine released from the sympathetic nervous system. Other positive inotropes include thyroid hormone and dopamine. The most important negative inotropic agent is acetylcholine released from the vagus nerve. Many drugs have positive or negative inotropic properties that can have profound effects on cardiac function.

Myocardial contractility is also affected by oxygen and carbon dioxide levels (tensions) in the coronary blood. With severe hypoxemia (arterial oxygen saturation less than 50%), contractility is decreased. With less severe hypoxemia (saturation more than 50%), contractility is stimulated. Moderate degrees of hypoxemia may increase contractility by enhancing the myocardial response to circulating catecholamines.[1] Preload, afterload, and contractility all interact with one another to determine stroke volume and cardiac output.

Heart rate

The average heart rate in normal adults is about 70 beats/min. This diminishes by 10 to 20 beats/min during sleep and can accelerate to more than 100 beats/min during muscular activity or emotional excitement. In well-conditioned athletes at rest, the heart rate is normally about 50 to 60 beats/min. In highly trained or elite athletes, the resting heart rate can be below 50 beats/min. Highly trained athletes have a lower resting heart rate, greater stroke volume, and lower peripheral resistance in active muscles than they had before training. The control of heart rate includes activity of the central nervous system, autonomic nervous system, neural reflexes, atrial receptors, and hormones (see Figure 22-17).

Cardiovascular control centers in the brain

The **cardiovascular control center** is in the brain stem in the medulla, with secondary areas in the hypothalamus, cerebral cortex, thalamus, and complex networks of exciting or inhibiting interneurons (connecting neurons) throughout the brain. The hypothalamic centers regulate cardiovascular responses to changes in temperature; the cerebral cortex centers adjust cardiac reaction to a variety of emotional states; and the medullary control center regulates heart rate and blood pressure (see Figure 22-9).

The nerve fibers from the cardiovascular control center synapse with autonomic neurons. When the parasympathetic nerves to the heart are stimulated, the sympathetic nerves to the heart, arterioles, and veins are usually inhibited. Because parasympathetic excitation and simultaneous sympathetic inhibition generally depress cardiac function (e.g., decrease the heart rate), these interneurons are often referred to as the **cardioinhibitory center.** Excitation occurs with parasympathetic inhibition and sympathetic stimulation, and these interneurons are collectively called the **cardioexcitatory center.** Therefore, heart rate can be slowed by (1) inhibition of sympathetic stimulation of the SA node and (2) activation of parasympathetic stimulation of the SA node; and it can be increased by (1) activation of sympathetic nerves and (2) inhibition of parasympathetic nerves.

The resting heart rate in healthy individuals is primarily under the control of parasympathetic stimulation. Parasympathetic effects from the vagus nerves override sympathetic effects in the SA node. Interruption of the vagus nerves causes significant tachycardia (abnormally fast heart rate) because the inhibitory parasympathetic influence is lost.

Neural reflexes

The **Bainbridge reflex** causes the heart rate to increase after intravenous infusions of blood or other fluid (Figure 22-18). The magnitude of the change in heart rate depends on the initial heart rate. If the initial rate is slow, intravenous infusion usually accelerates it, but if the initial rate is rapid, infusions will usually slow it down.[9]

The **baroreceptor reflex** facilitates blood pressure changes and heart rate changes. It is mediated by tissue pressure receptors (pressoreceptors) in the aortic arch and carotid arteries. The pressoreceptors increase their rate of discharge, sending neural impulses over the glossopharyngeal nerve (ninth cranial nerve) and through the vagus nerve to the cardiovascular control centers in the medulla. These centers increase parasympathetic activity and decrease sympathetic activity, causing blood vessels to dilate and heart rate to decrease. Responses to the baroreceptor reflex return the blood pressure to its previous level, which may or may not be normal. The higher the blood pressure, the greater the reflexive decrease in heart rate. If blood pressure is decreased, the baroreceptor reflex accelerates heart rate and causes vessels to constrict, raising blood pressure back toward normal (see Figure 22-18).[10] Baroreceptor function is discussed in more detail later in this chapter.

Neural receptors in the lungs cause heart rate to increase during inspiration and decrease during expiration. The vagal fibers are stretched in inspiration and inhibit the cardioinhibitory center of the medulla. This allows unopposed sympathetic acceleration of heart rate.

Atrial receptors

Receptors that influence heart rate exist in both atria (see Figure 22-18).[1,4] They are located in the right atrium at its junctions with the venae cava and in the left atrium at its junctions with the pulmonary veins. Distension of these atrial receptors sends impulses through C-fiber afferents. Stimulation of these atrial receptors also increases urine volume, presumably because of a neurally mediated reduction in antidiuretic hormone. In addition, atrial natriuretic peptide (ANP) is released from atrial tissue in response to the increases in blood volume. ANP has powerful diuretic and natriuretic (salt excretion) properties resulting in decreased blood volume and pressure.[4,11]

Hormones and biochemicals

Hormones and biochemicals affect the arteries, arterioles, venules, capillaries, and contractility of the myocardium. Norepinephrine increases heart rate, enhances myocardial contractility, and constricts blood vessels. Epinephrine dilates vessels of the liver and skeletal muscle and also causes an increase in myocardial contractility. Some adrenocortical hormones, such as hydrocortisone, potentiate the effects of these catecholamines.

Thyroid hormones enhance sympathetic activity, promoting increased cardiac output. A decrease in growth hormone, as well as in thyroid and adrenal hormones, results in bradycardia (heart rate below 60 beats/min), reduced cardiac output, and low blood pressure. (See other hormones in the Regulation of Blood Pressure section.)

QUICK CHECK 22-5

1. Why is the Frank-Starling law of the heart important to the understanding of heart failure?
2. Discuss the baroreceptor reflex and how it facilitates blood pressure and heart rate changes.
3. Summarize the cardiovascular changes with aging.

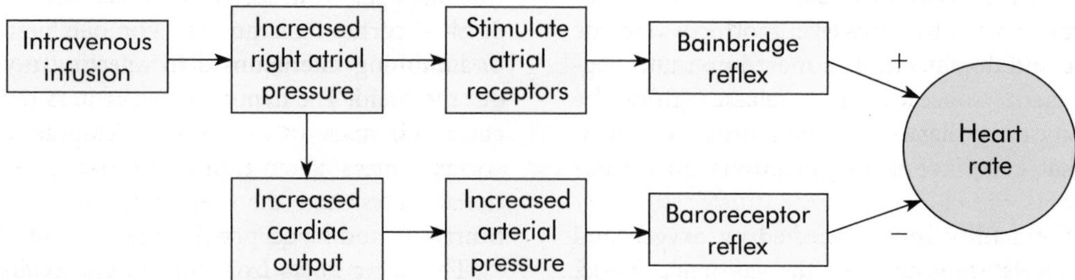

Figure 22-18 ■ Heart Rate and Intravenous Infusions. Intravenous infusions of blood or electrolyte solutions tend to increase heart rate through the Bainbridge reflex and to decrease heart rate through the baroreceptor reflex. The actual change in heart rate induced by such infusions is the result of these two opposing effects. (From Berne RM, Levy MN: *Cardiovascular physiology,* ed 8, St Louis, 2001, Mosby.)

THE SYSTEMIC CIRCULATION

The arteries and veins of the systemic circulation are illustrated in Figure 22-19. Blood from the left side of the heart flows through the aorta and into the systemic arteries. The **arteries** branch into small **arterioles,** which branch further into the smallest vessels, the **capillaries,** where nutrient exchange between the blood and tissues occurs. Blood from the capillaries then enters tiny **venules** that join to form the larger veins, which return venous blood to the right heart. **Peripheral vascular system** is an imprecise term used to describe the part of the systemic circulation that supplies the skin and the extremities, particularly the legs and feet.

Structure of Blood Vessels

Blood vessel walls are composed of three layers: (1) the **tunica intima** (innermost, or intimal, layer), (2) the **tunica media** (middle, or medial, layer), and (3) the **tunica externa** or **adventitia** (outermost, or external, layer). These structures are illustrated in Figure 22-20. Blood vessel walls vary in thickness depending on the thickness or absence of one or more of these three layers. Cells of the larger vessels are nourished by the **vasa vasorum,** small vessels located in the tunica externa.

Arterial vessels

Arterial walls are composed of elastic connective tissue, fibrous connective tissue, and smooth muscle. **Elastic arteries** have a thick tunica media with more elastic fibers than smooth muscle fibers. Examples include the aorta and its major branches and the pulmonary trunk. Elasticity allows the vessel to stretch as blood is ejected from the heart during systole. During diastole, elasticity promotes recoil of the arteries, maintaining blood pressure within the vessels.

Muscular arteries are medium-sized and small arteries and are farther from the heart than the elastic arteries. They contain more muscle fibers than the elastic arteries because they need less stretch and recoil. The muscular arteries distribute blood to arterioles throughout the body and help control blood flow because their smooth muscle can be stimulated to contract or relax. Contraction narrows the vessel **lumen** (the internal cavity of the vessel), which diminishes flow through the vessel **(vasoconstriction).** When the smooth muscle layer relaxes, more blood flows through the vessel lumen **(vasodilation).**

An artery becomes an arteriole where the diameter of its lumen narrows to less than 0.5 mm. The arterioles are composed almost exclusively of smooth muscle and regulate the flow of blood into the capillaries by vasoconstriction, which retards the flow of blood into the capillaries, and vasodilation, which permits blood to enter the capillaries freely (Figure 22-21). The thick smooth muscle layer of the arterioles is a major determinant of the resistance blood encounters as it flows through the systemic circulation.

The capillary network is composed of connective channels, or thoroughfares, called **metarterioles,** and "true" capillaries (Figure 22-22). The capillaries branch from the metarterioles, meeting at a ring of smooth muscle called the **precapillary sphincter.** As the sphincters contract and relax, they regulate blood flow through the capillaries. Appropriately stimulated, the precapillary sphincters help to maintain arterial pressure and regulate selective flow to vascular beds.

The capillary walls are very thin, making possible the rapid exchange of substrates, metabolites, and special products (e.g., hormones) between the blood and the interstitial fluid, from which they are taken up by the cells. A single endothelial cell may form the entire vessel wall if the capillary has no tunica media or tunica externa. In some capillaries, the endothelial cells contain oval windows or pores termed **fenestrations,** which are generally covered by a thin diaphragm.

Substances pass between the capillary lumen and the interstitial fluid (1) through junctions between endothelial cells, (2) through fenestrations in endothelial cells, (3) in vesicles moved by active transport across the endothelial cell membrane, or (4) by diffusion through the endothelial cell membrane. A single capillary may be only 0.5 to 1 mm in length and 0.01 mm in diameter, but the capillaries are so numerous that their total surface area may be more than 600 m^2, or larger than 100 football fields.

Endothelium

All tissues depend on a blood supply and the blood supply depends on **endothelial cells,** which form the lining, or **endothelium,** of the blood vessel (Figure 22-23). Endothelial cells are really quite remarkable in that they can adjust their number and arrangement to accommodate local requirements. Thus, they are a life-support tissue extending and remodeling the network of blood vessels to enable tissue growth, motion, and repair. Dysfunction of the endothelium has been implicated in virtually every type of vascular disorder, including atherosclerosis and hypertension (see Chapter 23).[4,12] Functions of the endothelium are summarized in Table 22-4.

Veins

The smallest venules closest to the capillaries have an inner lining, composed of the endothelium of the tunica intima and surrounded by fibrous tissue. The largest venules are surrounded by a few smooth muscle fibers constituting a thin tunica media.

Compared with arteries, **veins** are thin walled and fibrous and have a larger diameter (see Figure 22-20). Veins also are more numerous than arteries. In veins, the tunica externa has less elastic tissue than in arteries, so veins do not recoil after distention as quickly as do arteries. Like arteries, veins receive nourishment from the tiny vasa vasorum. Some veins, most commonly in the lower limbs, contain valves to regulate the one-way flow of blood toward the heart (Figure 22-24). These valves are folds of the tunica intima and resemble the semilunar valves of the heart. When a person stands up, contraction of the skeletal muscles of the legs compresses the deep veins of the legs and assists the flow of blood toward the heart. This important

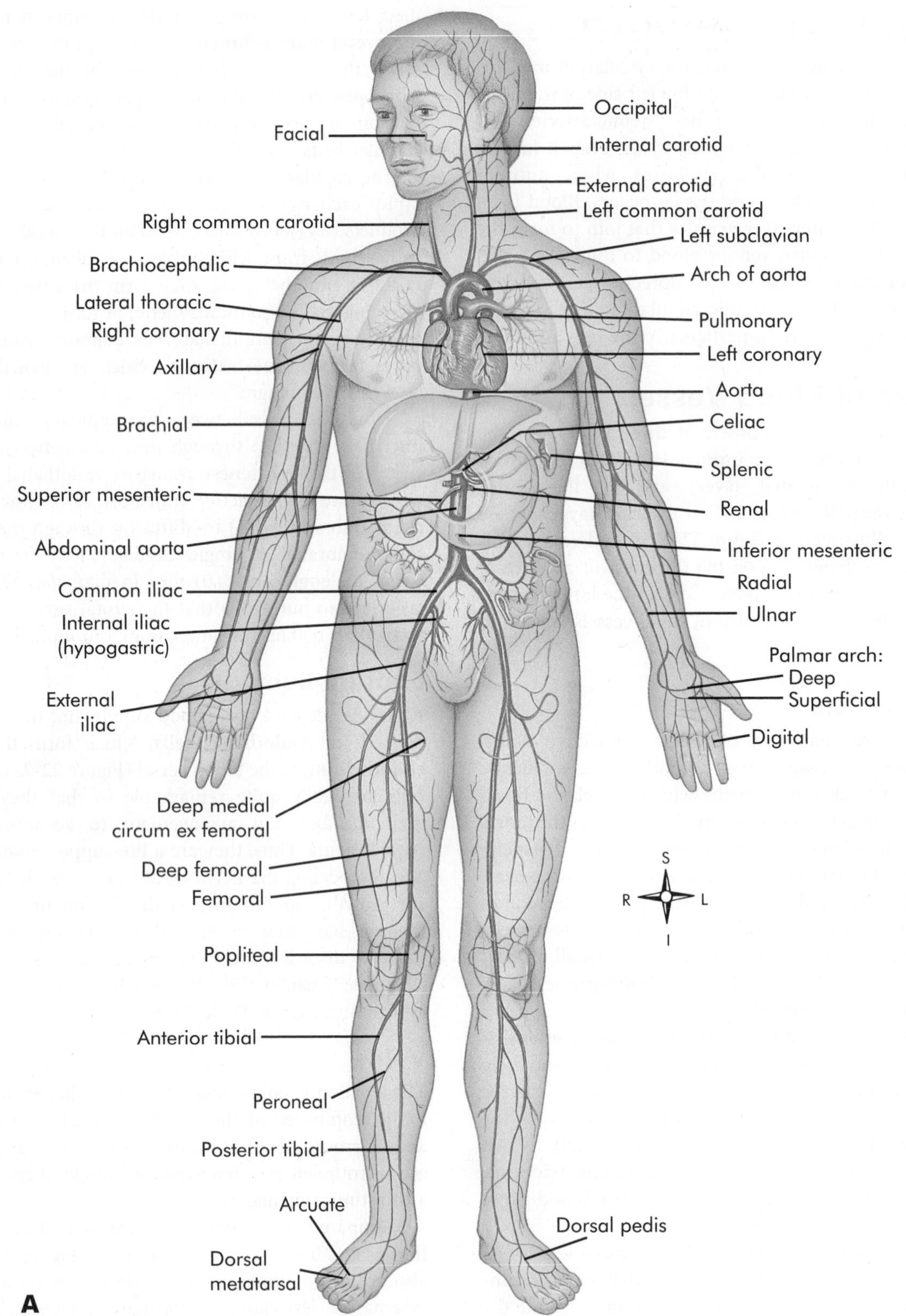

Figure 22-19 ■ **Circulatory System. A,** Principal arteries of body. (From Thibodeau GA, Patton KT: *Anatomy & physiology,* ed 6, St Louis, 2007, Mosby.)

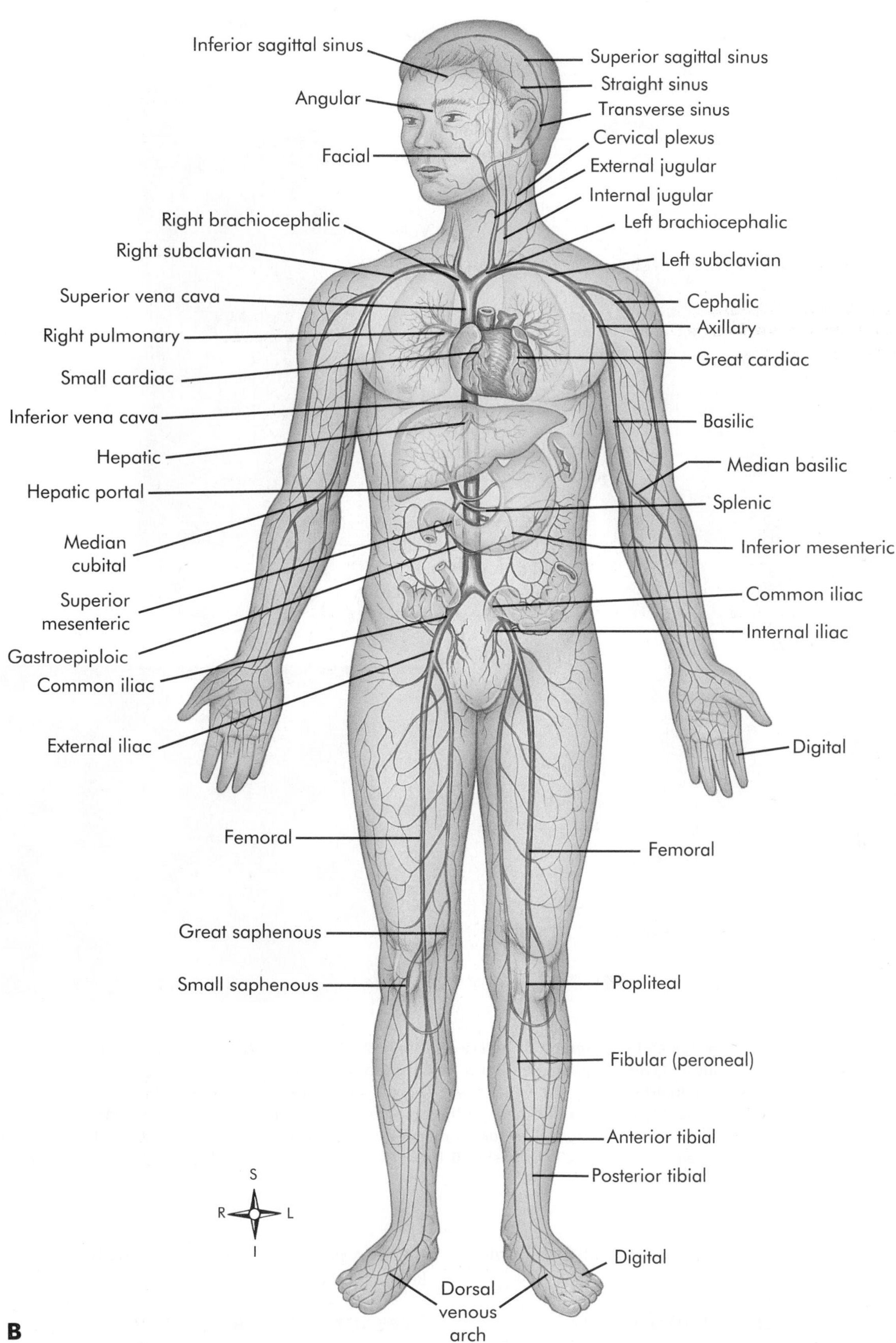

Figure 22-19 cont'd ■ **B,** Principal veins of body.

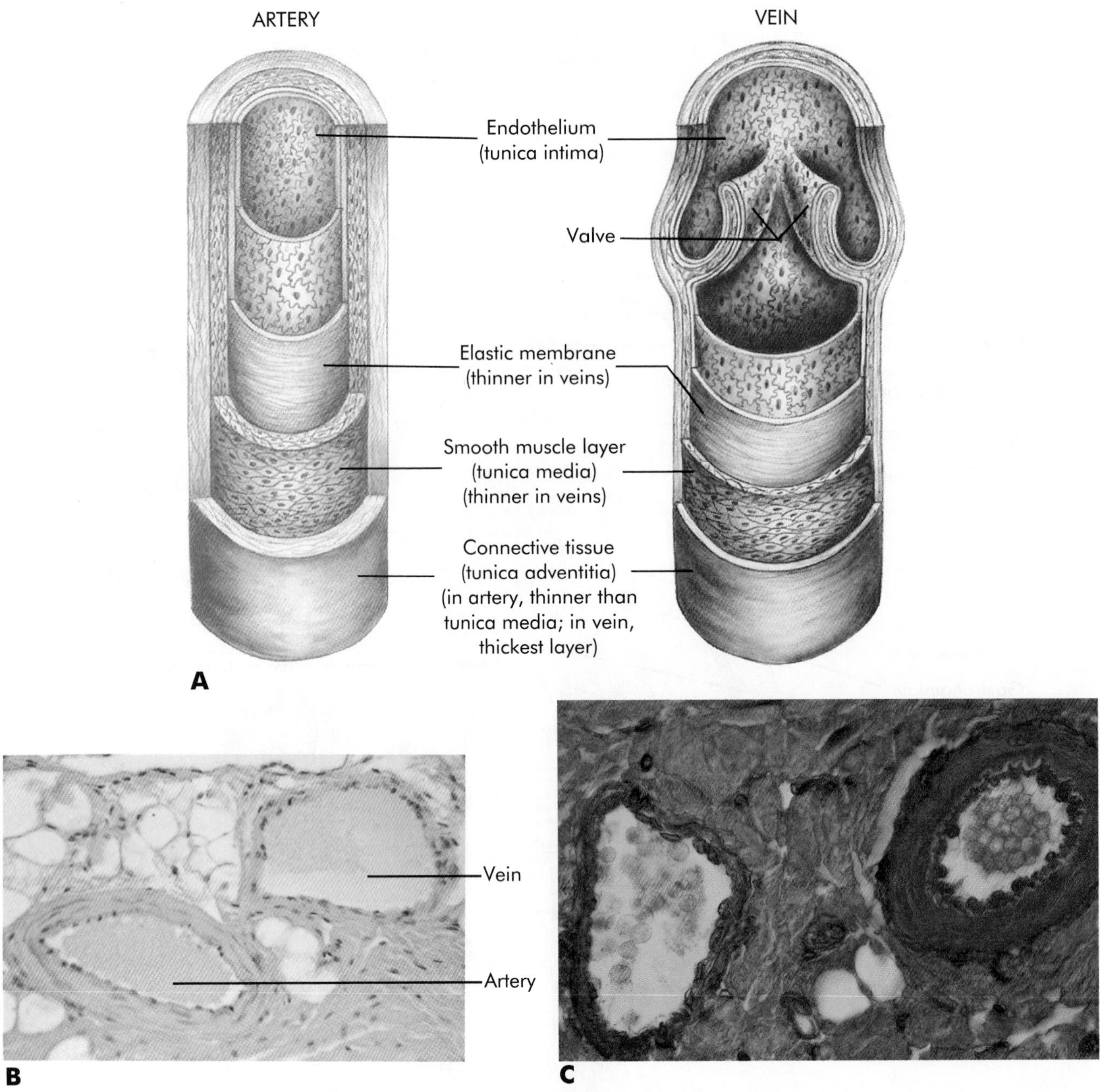

Figure 22-20 ■ **Schematic Drawings and Micrograph of Artery and Vein. A,** Shown are the comparative thickness of three layers: outer layer (tunica adventitia), muscle layer (tunica media), and lining of endothelium (tunica intima). Note that muscle and outer coats are much thinner in veins than in arteries and that veins have valves. **B,** Micrograph (× 250) of a cross section of tissue containing both an artery *(left)* and a vein *(right)*. Note the thickness of the smooth muscle (tunica media) in the artery compared with the vein. **C,** Micrograph showing both an artery and vein. The tunica media is much thicker in the artery. (**A** modified from Thompson JM et al: *Mosby's clinical nursing,* ed 5, St Louis, 2002, Mosby; **B** from Thibodeau GA, Patton KT: *Anatomy & physiology,* ed 6, St Louis, 2007, Mosby; **C,** Copyright Ed Reschke.)

mechanism of venous return is called the **muscle pump** (Figure 22-25).

Factors Affecting Blood Flow

Blood flow is the amount of fluid moved per unit of time and is usually expressed as liters or milliliters per minute (ml/min) or cubic centimeters per second (cm^3/sec). Flow is regulated by the same physical properties that govern the movement of simple fluids in a closed, rigid system—that is, pressure, resistance, velocity, turbulent versus laminar flow, and compliance.

Pressure and resistance

Pressure in a liquid system is the force exerted on the liquid per unit area and is expressed as dynes per square centimeter (dyn/cm^2), millimeters of mercury (mm Hg), or units of pressure (torr). Blood flow depends partly on the difference between pressures in the arterial and venous vessels

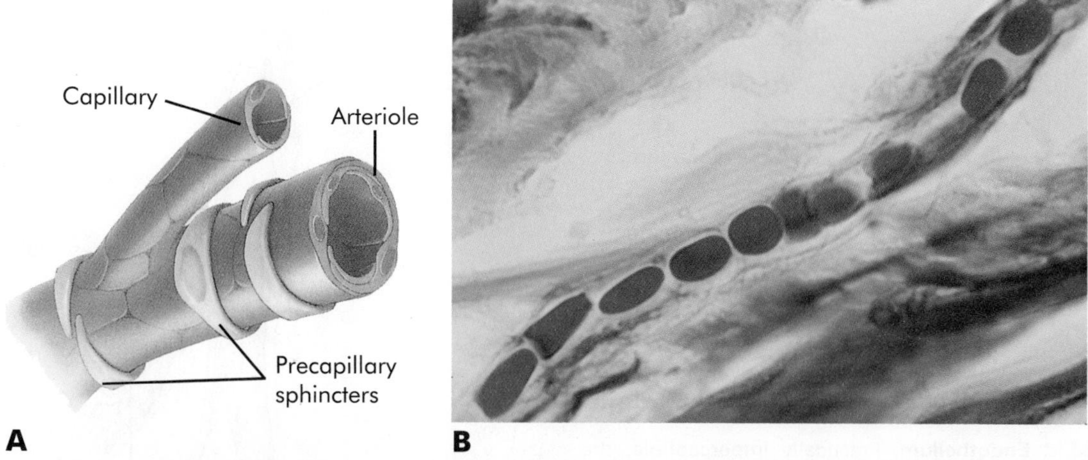

Figure 22-21 ■ **Capillary Wall. A,** Capillaries have a wall composed of only a single layer of flattened cells, whereas the walls of the larger vessels also have smooth muscle. **B,** Capillary with red blood cells in single file (× 500). (**A** from Thibodeau GA, Patton KT: *Anatomy & physiology,* ed 5, St Louis, 2003, Mosby; **B,** Copyright Ed Reschke.)

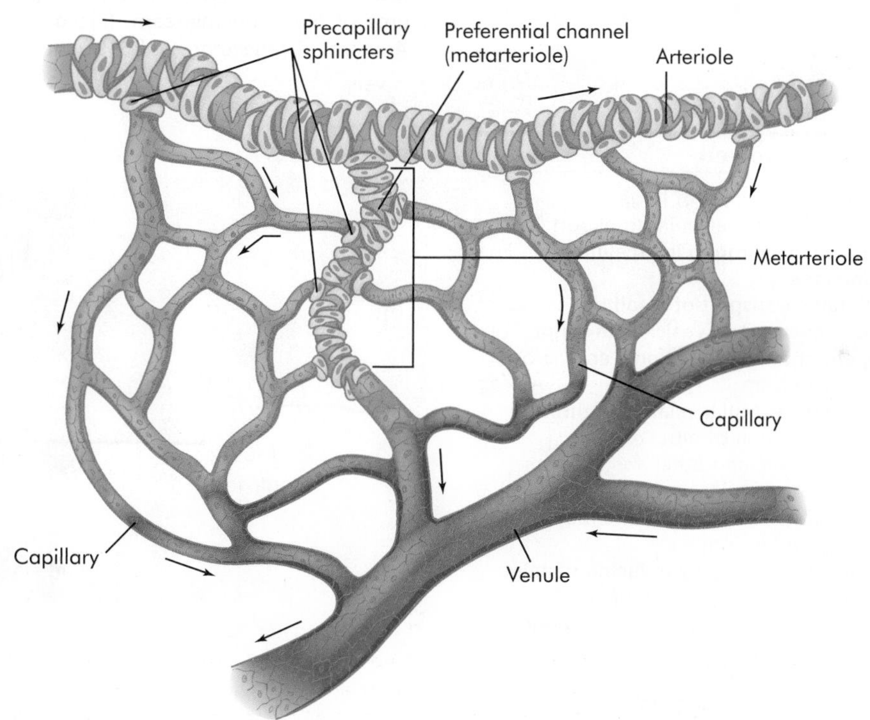

Figure 22-22 ■ **Capillary Network.** Blood enters network as arterial blood and exits as venous blood.

supplying the organ. Fluid moves from the arterial "side" of the capillaries, a region of greater pressure, to the venous side, a region of lesser pressure.

Resistance is the opposition to force. In the cardiovascular system, most opposition to blood flow is provided by the diameter and length of the blood vessels themselves. Therefore, changes in blood flow through an organ result from changes in the vascular resistance within the organ. Resistance in a vessel is inversely related to blood flow—that is, increased resistance leads to decreased blood flow. **Poiseuille law** shows the relationship among blood flow, pressure, and resistance:

$$Q = \frac{\delta P}{R}$$

where Q = blood flow, δP = the pressure difference ($P_1 - P_2$), and R = resistance. Resistance to flow cannot be measured directly, but it can be calculated if the pressure difference and flow volumes are known. Resistance to blood flow is influenced by (1) blood viscosity, (2) radius and length of the blood vessels, (3) whether vessels are arranged sequentially or in parallel, and (4) total cross sectional area.

1. Blood flow varies inversely with the **viscosity** of the fluid. Thick fluids move more slowly and experience greater resistance to flow than thin fluids. Blood that contains

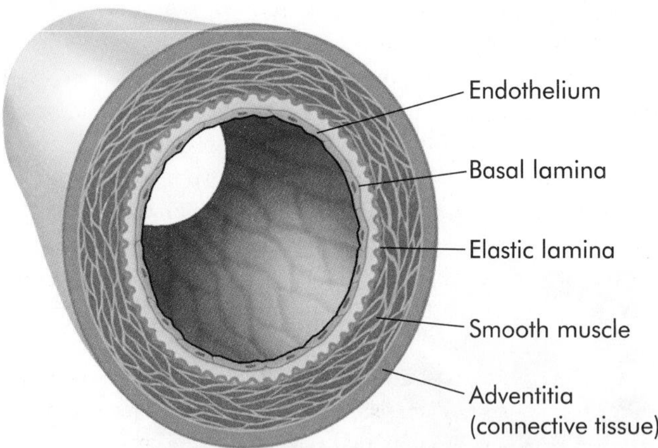

Figure 22-23 ■ **Endothelium.** Practically imperceptible, the endothelial cells arrange themselves as a fine lining that has numerous life-support functions (see Table 22-4).

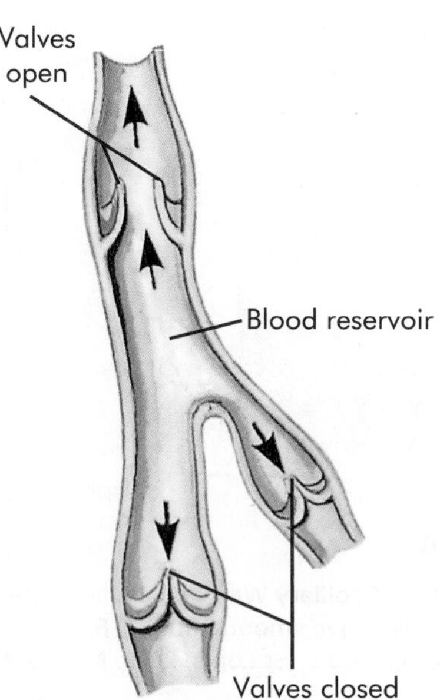

Figure 22-24 ■ **Valves of Vein.** Pooled blood is moved toward heart as valves are forced open by pressure from volume of blood downstream. (From Thibodeau GA, Patton KT: *Anatomy & physiology*, ed 5, St Louis, 2003, Mosby.)

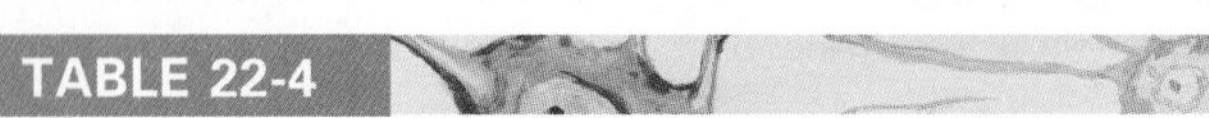

TABLE 22-4

Functions of the Endothelium

Function	Actions Involved
Filtration and permeability	Facilitates transport of large molecules via vesicular transport movement through intercellular junctions Facilitates transport of small molecules via movement of vesicles, through opening of tight junctions, and across the cytoplasm
Vasomotion	Stimulates vascular relaxation through the production of nitric oxide, prostacyclin, and other vasodilators Stimulates vascular constriction through the production of endothelin and angiotensin II
Clotting	Stimulates clotting by inducing platelet adhesion via production of von Willebrand factor, platelet-activating factor and others Prevents clotting through the production of endogenous anticoagulants such as heparin sulfate Promotes fibrinolysis via the production of tissue plasminogen activating factor (t-PH) and plasminogen activator inhibitor (PAI-A)
Inflammation	Expresses adhesion molecules that allow for monocyte and polymorphonucleocyte margination and diapedesis Expresses receptors for oxidized lipoproteins allowing them to enter the vascular intima

From Hansson GK, Nilsson J: Pathogenesis of atherosclerosis. In Crawford MH, DiMarco JP, editors: *Cardiology*, ed 2, London, 2004, Mosby.

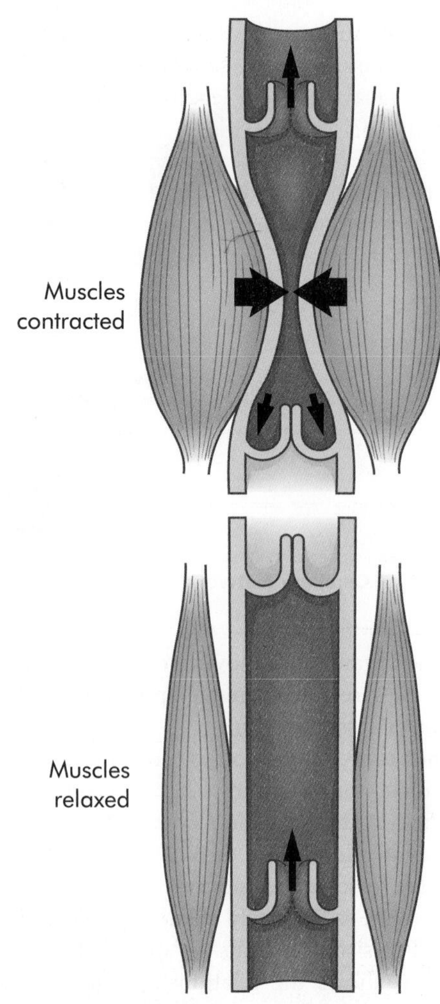

Figure 22-25 ■ **Muscle Pump.**

a high percentage of red cells is more viscous. This relationship is expressed as the hematocrit—the ratio of the volume of red blood cells to the volume of whole blood. A high hematocrit reduces flow through the blood vessels, particularly the **microcirculation** (arterioles, capillaries, venules). Conditions in which the hematocrit is elevated, for example, dehydration, cyanotic congenital heart disease, or polycythemia, can lead to increased cardiac work as a result of increased vascular resistance. The viscosity of blood also increases if blood flow becomes slow or stagnates **(anomalous viscosity).** This is generally not significant unless cardiac output is low as in shock. (Shock is described in Chapter 23.)

2. The most important factor determining resistance *in a single vessel* is the **radius** or diameter of the vessel's lumen, expressed in Poiseuille formula as its radius and in Figure 22-26 as its diameter. Small changes in the lumen's radius lead to large changes in vascular resistance. Another important factor is the **length** of the vessel. Generally, resistance to flow is greater in longer tubes because resistance increases with length. Blood flowing through the distributing arteries, beginning with branches off the aorta and ending at arterioles in the capillary bed, encounters more resistance than blood flowing through the capillary bed itself, where flow is distributed among many short, tiny branches arranged in parallel.

Poiseuille formula for resistance to fluid flow through a tube takes into account the viscosity of the fluid, the radius of the tube's lumen, and the length of the tube. Resistance *(R)* is proportional to a constant ($8/\pi$), the viscosity of the blood (η), and the length of the vessel *(l),* and it is inversely proportional to the fourth power of the lumen's radius (v_4).[1] Because this relationship was derived using straight, rigid tubes with steady, streamlined flow, it cannot be applied *directly* to the vascular system, but it is a useful model of vascular resistance.

3. Resistance to flow through a system of vessels, or **total resistance,** depends not only on characteristics of individual vessels but also on whether the vessels are arranged in series or in parallel (Figure 22-27). For vessels arranged in series, total resistance equals the sum obtained by adding all the individual resistances calculated using the Poiseuille formula. For vessels arranged in parallel, total resistance equals the sum of the reciprocals *(I/R)* of the individual resistances.

4. Total resistance is related to the total cross-sectional area of a system of vessels in parallel and to the number of vessels in parallel that make up the total cross-sectional area. The larger the total cross-sectional area, as in the capillary system, the lower the resistance. However, if a cross-sectional area is made up of a large number of parallel vessels, the overall resistance will be greater than it would be if the cross-sectional area were made up of only two or three parallel vessels. Therefore, resistance is greater in smaller vessels than in larger vessels. The total cross-sectional area of the arteriolar system is greater than that of the arterial system, yet the greater number of arterioles arranged in parallel leads to great resistance to flow in the arteriolar system. Although the capillary system has a larger number of vessels in parallel than the arteriolar system, the total cross-sectional area is greater, resulting in lower resistance overall through the capillary system. The relationship between flow and cross-sectional area has physiologic significance. Despite the narrow diameter of each vessel (which normally increases resistance), total resistance in any capillary bed is relatively low. This, plus the slow velocity of flow in each vessel, promotes optimal capillary-tissue exchange.

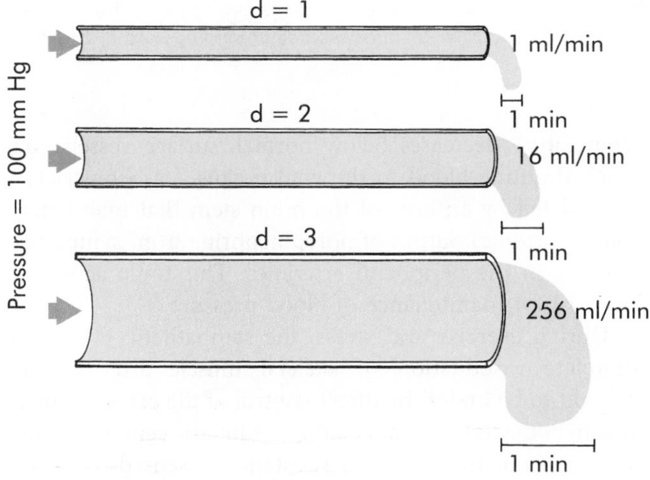

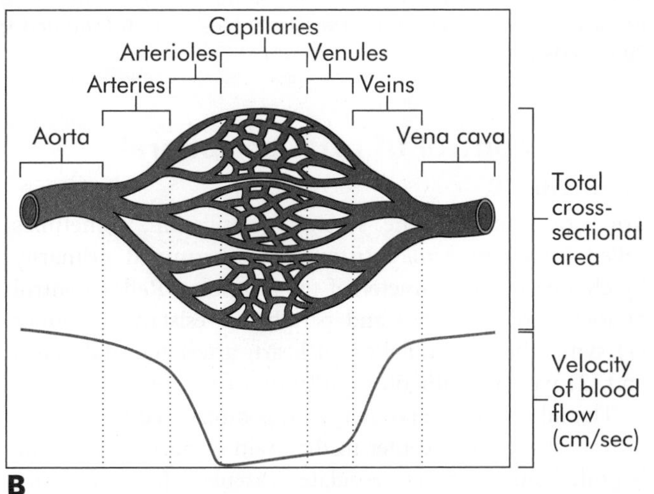

Figure 22-26 ■ **Lumen Diameter, Blood Flow, and Resistance. A,** Effect of lumen diameter on flow through vessel. *d,* Diameter. **B,** Blood flows with great speed in the large arteries. However, branching of arterial vessels increases the total cross-sectional area of the arterioles and capillaries, reducing the flow rate. When capillaries merge into venules and venules merge into veins, the total cross-sectional area decreases, causing the flow rate to increase. (**B** from Thibodeau GA, Patton KT: *Anatomy & physiology,* ed 5, St Louis, 2003, Mosby.)

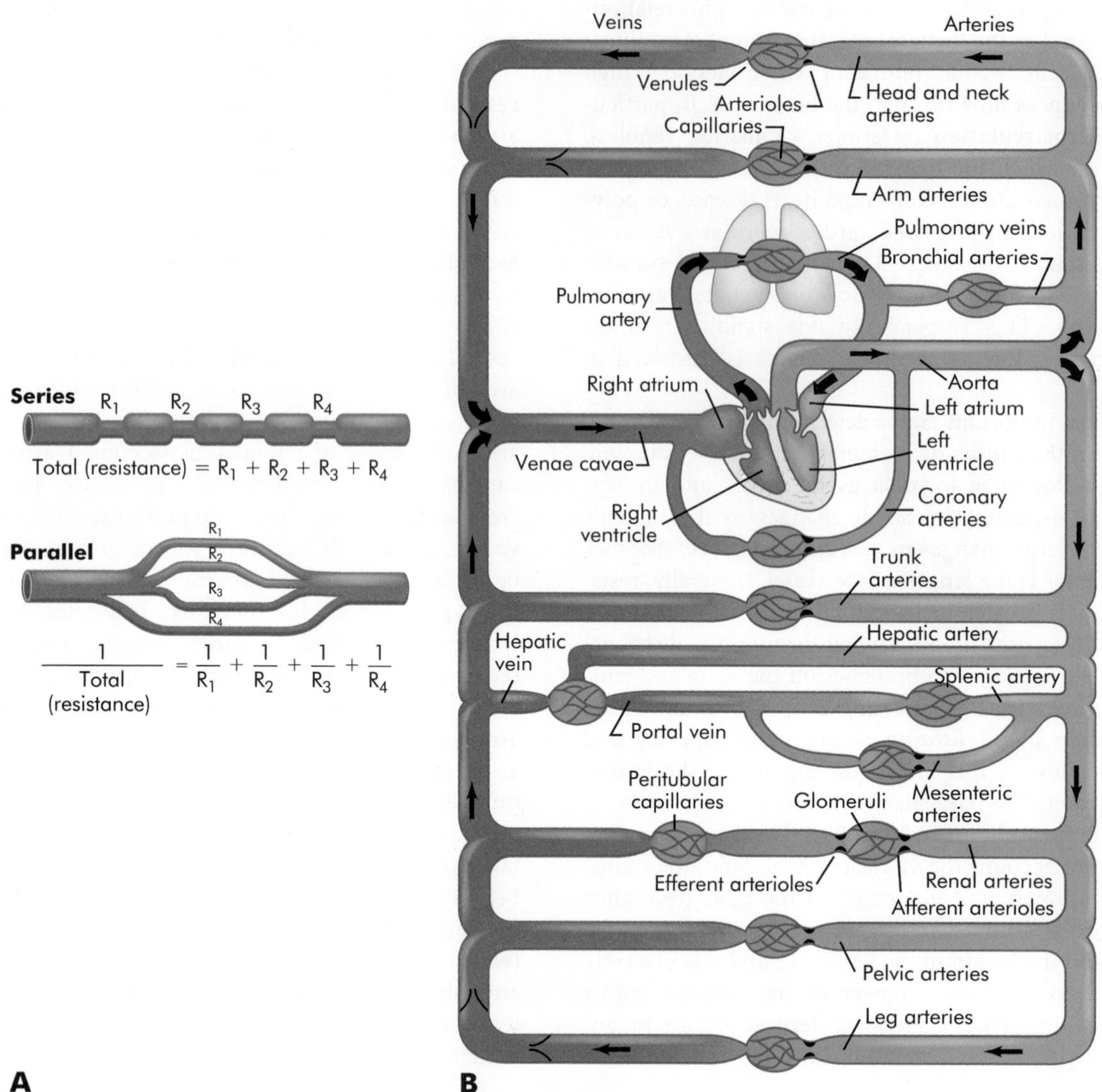

Figure 22-27 ■ **Schematic Diagram of the Parallel and Series Arrangement of the Vessels Composing the Circulatory System.** **A,** Resistance in blood vessels arranged in series or parallel. *R,* Resistance in an individual vessel. **B,** The capillary beds are represented by thin lines connecting the arterioles *(right)* and the veins *(left).* The crescent-shaped thickenings proximal to the capillary beds represent the arterioles (resistance vessels). (**B** modified from Berne RM, Levy MN: *Cardiovascular physiology,* ed 8, St Louis, 2001, Mosby.)

Neural control of total peripheral resistance

Total resistance in the systemic circulation, sometimes called *total peripheral resistance,* is determined primarily by change in the diameter of the arterioles. Reflex control of total cardiac output and peripheral resistance includes (1) sympathetic stimulation of heart, arterioles, and veins; and (2) parasympathetic stimulation of the heart.

The autonomic nervous system is monitored by the cardiovascular control center in the brain (Figure 22-28). The hypothalamic centers regulate vascular (and cardiac) responses to changes in temperature. When the body's core temperature exceeds normal, the hypothalamus reflex initiates dilation of arterioles and veins in the skin. This causes shunting of blood to the skin, where heat is lost from sweating, radiation, conduction, or convection. When body core temperature decreases below normal, surface vessels constrict, shunting blood to the vital organs. Vasoconstriction is regulated by an area of the brain stem that maintains a constant (tonic) output of norepinephrine from sympathetic fibers in the peripheral arterioles. This tonic activity is essential for maintenance of blood pressure.

During exercise and stress, the sympathetic fibers that stimulate vasodilation of skeletal muscle arterioles are thought to be under the direct control of the cerebral cortex and hypothalamus and *not* the medullary centers.[1] Information about pressure and resistance is sensed by neural receptors (baroreceptors, chemoreceptors) in arterial walls and delivered to the medullary centers.

Velocity

Blood velocity is the *distance* blood travels in a unit of time, usually centimeters per second (cm/sec). It is directly

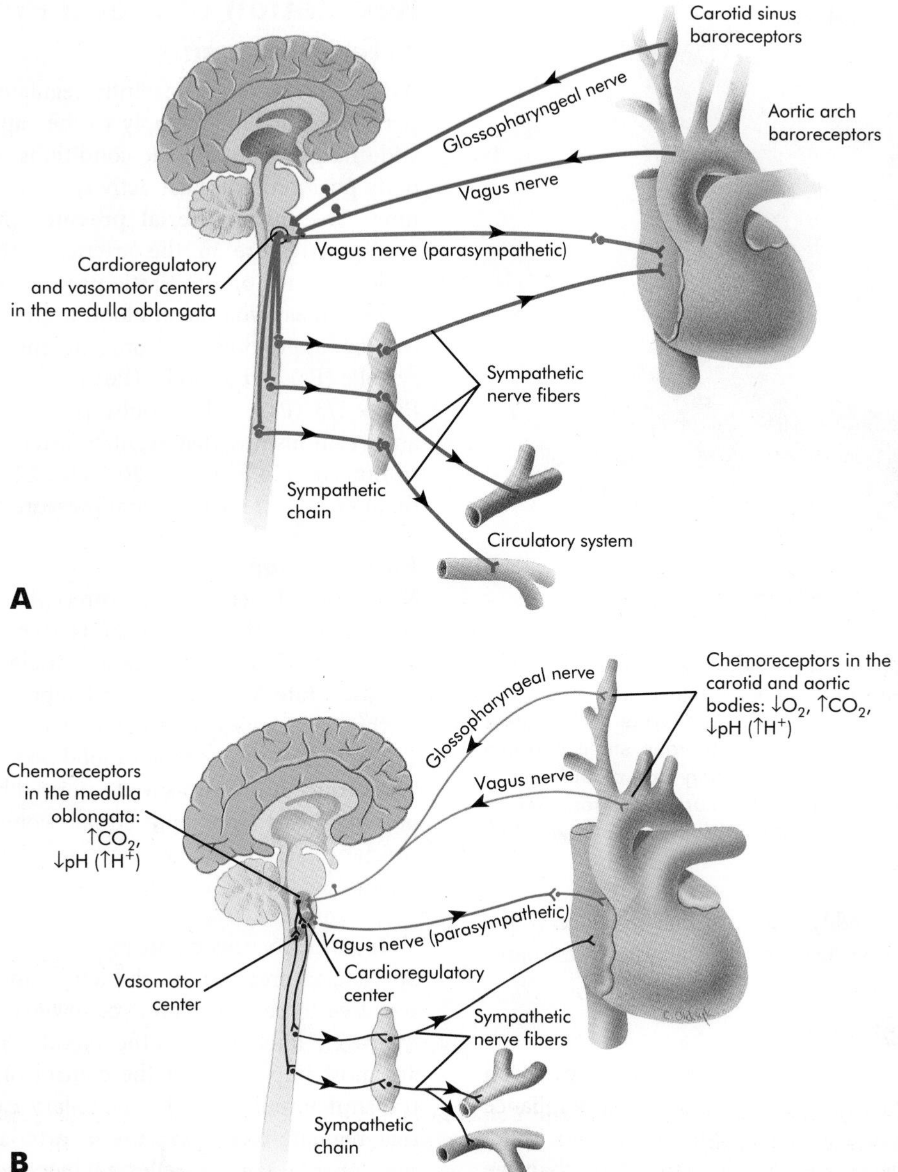

Figure 22-28 ■ **Baroreceptors and Chemoreceptor Reflex Control of Blood Pressure. A,** Baroreceptor reflexes. Baroreceptors located in the carotid sinuses and aortic arch detect changes in blood pressure. Action potentials are conducted to the cardioregulatory and vasomotor centers. The heart rate can be decreased by the parasympathetic system; the heart rate and stroke volume can be increased by the sympathetic system. The sympathetic system also can constrict or dilate blood vessels. **B,** Chemoreceptor reflexes. Chemoreceptors located in the medulla oblongata and in the carotid and aortic bodies detect changes in blood oxygen, carbon dioxide, or pH. Action potentials are conducted to the medulla oblongata. In response, the vasomotor center can cause vasoconstriction or dilation of blood vessels by the sympathetic system, and the cardioregulatory center can cause changes in the pumping activity of the heart through the parasympathetic and sympathetic systems. (From Seeley RR, Stephens TD, Tate P: *Anatomy and physiology,* ed 3, St Louis, 1995, Mosby.)

related to blood flow (*amount* of blood moved per unit of time) and inversely related to the cross-sectional area of the vessel in which the blood is flowing. As blood moves from the aorta to the capillaries, the total cross-sectional area of the vessels increases and velocity of flow decreases.

Laminar versus turbulent flow

Normally, blood flow through the vessels is *laminar* (**laminar flow),** meaning that concentric layers of molecules move "straight ahead." Each concentric layer flows at a different velocity (Figure 22-29). The cohesive attraction between the fluid and the vessel wall prevents the molecules of blood that are in contact with the wall from moving. The next thin layer of blood is able to slide slowly past the stationary layer and so on until, at the center, the blood velocity is greatest. Large vessels have room for a large center layer; therefore, they have less resistance to flow and greater flow and velocity than smaller vessels.

Where flow is obstructed, the vessel turns, or blood flows over rough surfaces, the flow becomes *turbulent* (**turbulent**

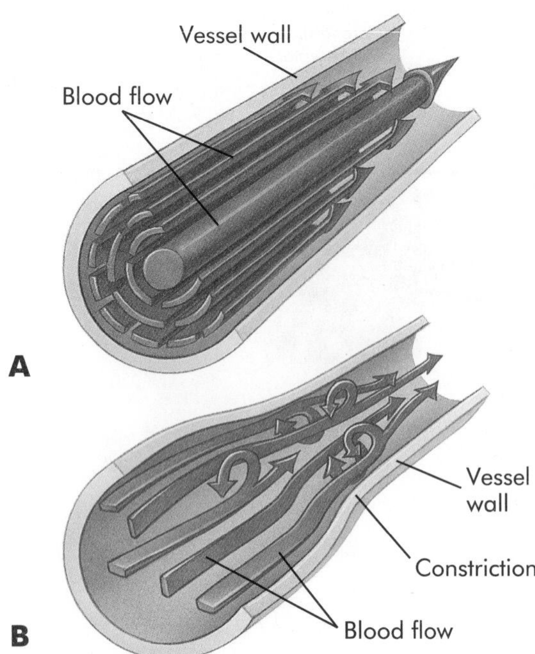

Figure 22-29 ■ **Laminar and Turbulent Blood Flow. A,** Laminar flow. Fluid flows in long, smooth-walled tubes as if it is composed of a large number of concentric layers. **B,** Turbulent flow. Turbulent flow is caused by numerous small currents flowing crosswise or oblique to the long axis of the vessel, resulting in flowing whorls and eddy currents. (From Seeley RR, Stephens TD, Tate P: *Anatomy and physiology,* ed 3, St Louis, 1995, Mosby.)

flow), with whorls or eddy currents that produce noise, causing a murmur to be heard on auscultation. Resistance increases with turbulence.

Vascular compliance

Vascular compliance is the increase in volume a vessel can accommodate for a given increase in pressure. Compliance depends on the ratio of elastic fibers to muscle fibers in the vessel wall. The elastic arteries are more compliant than the muscular arteries, and the veins are more compliant than either type of artery, and they can serve as storage areas for the circulatory system.

Compliance determines a vessel's response to pressure changes. For example, with a small increase in pressure, a large volume of blood can be accommodated by the venous system. In the less compliant arterial system, where smaller volumes and higher pressures are normal, small variations in pressure cause little or no change in the volume of blood within the arterial vessels.

Stiffness is the opposite of compliance. Several conditions and disorders can cause stiffness, with the most common being arteriosclerosis (see Chapter 23).

✔ QUICK CHECK 22-6

1. Define endothelial cells and endothelium.
2. Identify the functions of the endothelium.
3. Why does the total cross-sectional area in the capillary system lower the resistance to flow?

Regulation of Blood Pressure

Arterial pressure

Arterial pressure is constantly regulated to maintain tissue **perfusion,** or blood supply to the capillary beds, during a wide range of physiologic conditions, including changes in body position, muscular activity, and circulating blood volume. The **mean arterial pressure (MAP),** which is the average pressure in the arteries throughout the cardiac cycle, depends on the elastic properties of the arterial walls and the mean volume of blood in the arterial system. MAP can be approximated from the measured values of the systolic (Ps) and diastolic (Pd) pressures as follows: MAP = Pd + 1/3 (Ps − Pd, or pulse pressure). The major factors and relationships that regulate arterial blood pressure are summarized in Figure 22-30. Table 22-5 summarizes factors that affect both mean arterial pressure and capillary flow.

Baroreceptors

Major stretch receptors (baroreceptors) are located in the aorta and in the carotid sinus (see Figure 22-28). They respond to changes in smooth muscle fiber length by altering their rate of discharge and supply sensory information to the cardiovascular center that regulates blood pressure. The net effect of this major blood pressure–regulating reflex is to reduce blood pressure to normal by decreasing cardiac output (heart rate and stroke volume) and peripheral resistance. (Postural changes and the baroreceptor reflex are discussed in Chapter 23.)

Arterial chemoreceptors

Specialized areas within the aortic and carotid arteries are sensitive to concentrations of oxygen, carbon dioxide, and hydrogen ions (pH) in the blood. These chemoreceptors are most important for the control of respiration but also transmit impulses to the medullary cardiovascular centers that regulate blood pressure. If arterial oxygen concentration or pH falls, a reflexive increase in blood pressure occurs, whereas an increase in carbon dioxide causes a slight increase in blood pressure. The major chemoreceptive reflex is the result of alterations in arterial oxygen concentration, with only minor effects resulting from altered pH or carbon dioxide levels.

Antidiuretic hormone, renin-angiotensin system, natriuretic peptides, adrenomedullin, and insulin

Blood pressure can be influenced by factors that change the total volume of blood in the circulatory system. Recall that ADH (antidiuretic hormone) is released by the posterior pituitary and causes reabsorption of water by the kidney. With reabsorption, the blood plasma volume will increase, thereby increasing blood pressure (Figure 22-31) (see also Chapters 4 and 17).

Renin is an enzyme synthesized and secreted by the juxtaglomerular cells of the kidney. It also has been found in the adrenal cortex, salivary gland, prolactin-producing and luteinizing hormone–producing cells of the pituitary, arterial smooth muscle cells in the vascular endothelium, brain,

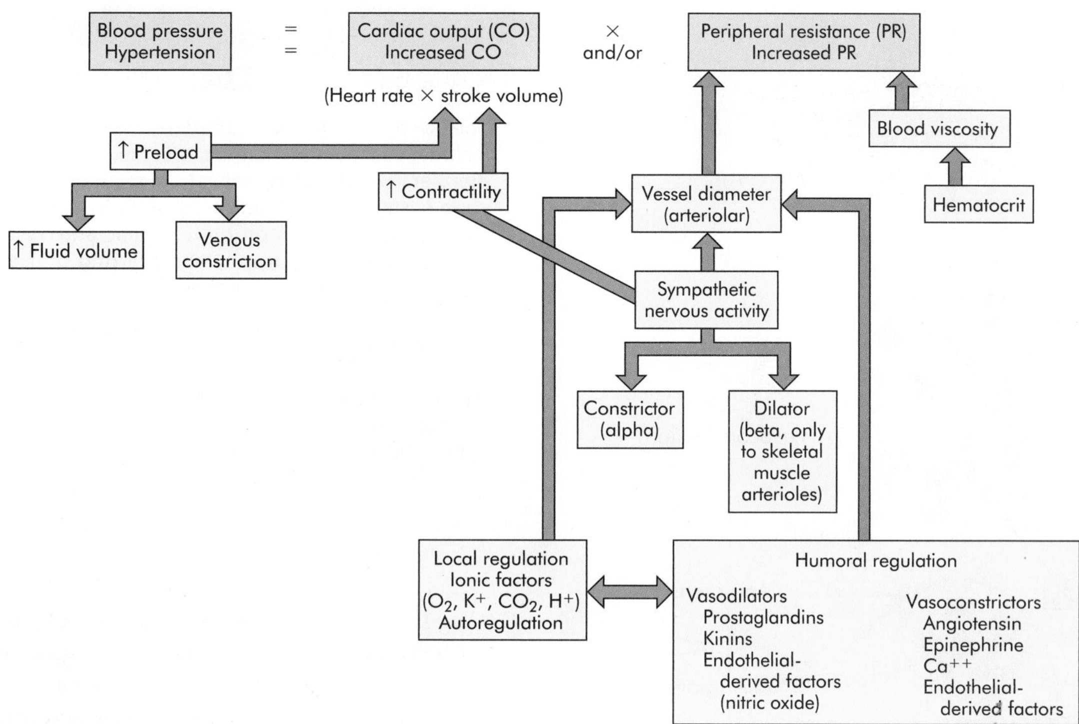

Figure 22-30 ■ **Factors Regulating Blood Pressure.**

TABLE 22-5

Factors That Affect Mean Arterial Pressure and Capillary Flow

	Mean Arterial Pressure	Capillary Flow
PERIPHERAL RESISTANCE*		
Increased	Increased	Decreased
Decreased	Decreased	Increased
HEART RATE†		
Increased	Increased	Increased
Decreased	Decreased	Decreased
STROKE VOLUME‡		
Increased	Increased	Increased
Decreased	Decreased	Decreased

From Little RC: *Physiology of the heart and circulation*, ed 3, St Louis, 1985, Mosby.
*Cardiac output constant.
†Peripheral resistance and stroke volume constant.
‡Peripheral resistance and heart rate constant.

myocardium, and possibly other tissues.[13] Factors that control renin release include the following:

1. A drop in blood pressure (detected as decreased flow in the renal artery)
2. A decrease in the amount of sodium chloride delivered to the kidney
3. β-adrenergic stimuli (increase renin release) and β-adrenergic inhibitors (decrease renin release)
4. Angiotensin II (reduces renin release)
5. Low potassium concentrations in plasma (increase renin release)

Once in the circulation, renin splits off a polypeptide from angiotensinogen to generate **angiotensin I (Ang I).** This is converted by an enzyme, angiotensin-converting enzyme (ACE), to **angiotensin II (Ang II),** a powerful vasoconstrictor that stimulates the secretion of **aldosterone** from the adrenal gland (see Figures 22-31 and 17-18). Ang II is now considered a growth promoter in cardiovascular tissues, resulting in myocyte and vascular hypertrophy and progression of hypertension.[14] The neural effects of Ang II include stimulation of thirst, release of antidiuretic hormone, and increases in sympathetic nervous system output (i.e., catecholamines). Aldosterone causes reabsorption of sodium in the kidneys and can have other direct deleterious effects on cardiovascular tissues.[15]

HEALTH ALERT

Aldosterone and Injury

Aldosterone has a number of deleterious effects, including myocardial necrosis and fibrosis, vascular stiffening and injury, reduced fibrinolysis, endothelial dysfunction, catecholamine release, and promotion of dysrhythmias. These effects are caused by aldosterone itself and are independent of aldosterone's stimulation of renal salt and water retention. Some mechanisms of aldosterone-induced cardiovascular dysfunction include activation of phospholipase C-mediated vasoconstriction, activation of the cyclooxygenase 2 pathway of inflammation, increased production of toxic oxygen radicals, and stimulation of smooth muscle cell proliferation.

Data from Schiffrin EL: Effects of aldosterone on the vasculature, *Hypertens* 47(3):312–318, 2006.

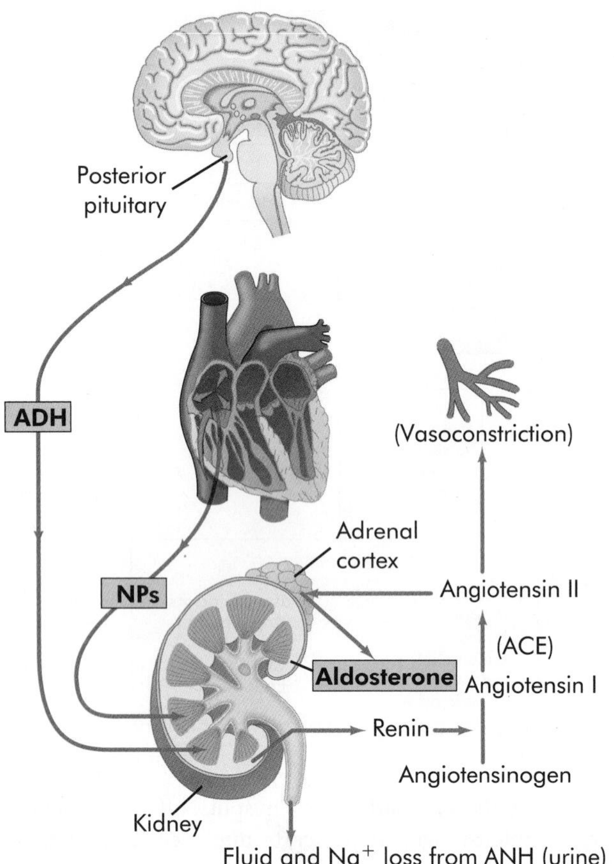

Figure 22-31 ■ **Three Mechanisms That Influence Total Plasma Volume.** The antidiuretic hormone (ADH) mechanism and renin-angiotensin and aldosterone mechanisms tend to increase water retention and thus increase total plasma volume. The natriuretic peptides antagonize these mechanisms by promoting water loss and sodium loss, thus promoting a decrease in total plasma volume. *NPs,* Natriuretic peptides; *ACE,* angiotensin converting enzyme. (Modified from Thibodeau GA, Patton KT: *Anatomy & physiology,* ed 5, St Louis, 2003, Mosby.)

This kidney-based renin-angiotensin system serves as an important regulatory loop. For example, decreases in blood pressure or sodium delivery to the kidneys (macula densa), as might occur after hemorrhage or extracellular volume deficits (dehydration), stimulate secretion of renin, which forms Ang I, which is converted to Ang II, and restores blood pressure. Sodium retention also results from increased secretion of aldosterone. Overall, the renin-angiotensin system is activated after volume depletion or hypotension, or both, and is suppressed after volume repletion. There also exists a tissue-based renin-angiotensin system that can be independently regulated from the circulation. The tissue renin-angiotensin system is activated in response to tissue injury.[14,16] This system is involved in maladaptive alterations, such as ventricular and vascular remodeling, alterations in renal function, and atherosclerosis[14,16,17] (see Chapter 23). Particularly significant is an increased recognition of the role of Ang II in these processes (Figure 22-32).

HEALTH ALERT
Angiotensin II

The systemic effects exerted by angiotensin II (Ang II) include vasoconstriction, increased blood pressure, glomerular hypertension, activation of the sympathetic nervous system, and retention of sodium and fluids. Ang II also has local effects on both cardiac and vascular tissue and can cause hypertrophy and scarring of tissues, a process that is called "remodeling."

Data from Daugherty A, Cassis L: Angiotensin II-mediated development of vascular diseases, *Trends Cardiovasc Med* 14 (3):117–120, 2004; Touyz RM: Molecular and cellular mechanisms in vascular injury in hypertension: role of angiotensin II, *Curr Opin Nephrol Hypertens* 14(2):125–131, 2005.

Ang II has two subtypes of receptors, AT_1 and AT_2 (Figure 22-33). Both subtypes, AT_1 and AT_2, are expressed in human hearts. AT_1 is also found on vascular smooth muscle and endothelial cells, nerve endings, and conduction tissues, adrenal cortex, liver, kidney and brain.[18] AT_2 has been found in fetal mesenchymal tissue, adrenal medulla, uterus and ovarian follicles, renal tubules, and vasculature.[18] The majority of Ang II actions occur through the **AT_1** receptor including vasoconstriction, stimulation of aldosterone release, inflammatory myocyte hypertrophy, fibroblast proliferation, collagen synthesis, smooth muscle cell growth, endothelial adhesion molecule expression, and catecholamine synthesis.[19,20] Ang II has been implicated in the progression of heart failure[21] (see Chapter 23). Therefore treatments such as angiotensin-converting enzyme (ACE) inhibitors and angiotensin receptor (ATR) antagonists that inhibit mostly AT_1 receptors are a main target in preventive and reparative strategies in cardiovascular diseases.

The role of **AT_2** receptors remains controversial. AT_2 stimulation results in NO-mediated vasodilation in many vascular beds and it is suggested that this receptor plays a modulating and protective role when AT_1 is activated.[22] However, other investigators suggest that AT_2 receptor stimulation may actually contribute to cardiovascular remodeling.[23] Numerous studies are under way to further elucidate the role of these important vascular receptors.

Another mechanism that can change blood plasma volume and, therefore, blood pressure is the **natriuretic peptides (NPs)** (see Figure 22-31). The natriuretic peptides include atrial natriuretic peptide (ANP), brain natriuretic peptide (BNP), C-type natriuretic peptide (CNP), and urodilatin. These peptides help regulate sodium excretion (natriuresis), diuresis, vasodilation, and antagonism of the renin-angiotensin system. All of these effects lead to the formation of a large volume of dilute urine that decreases blood volume and blood pressure.[24,25] **Atrial natriuretic peptide (ANP)** is a hormone secreted from cells in the right atrium when right atrial blood pressure increases. ANP inhibits antidiuretic hormone by increasing urine sodium

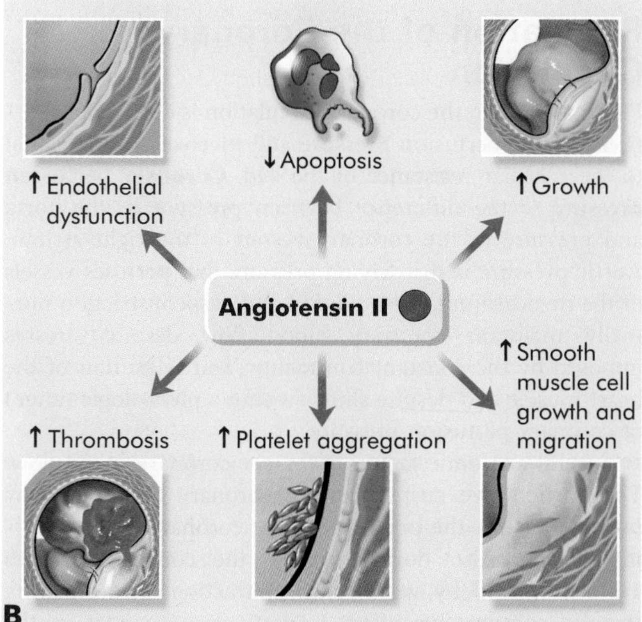

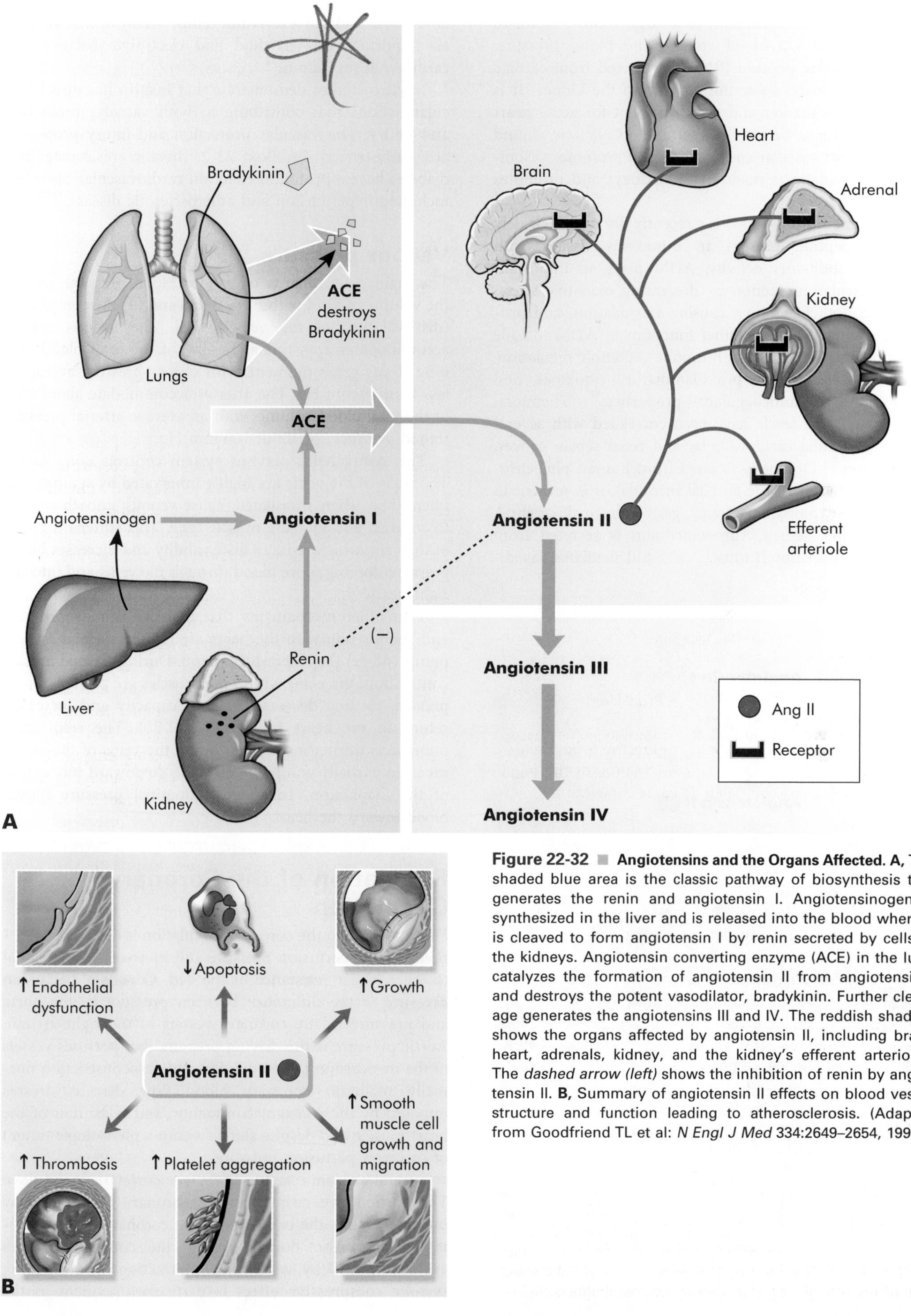

Figure 22-32 ■ **Angiotensins and the Organs Affected. A,** The shaded blue area is the classic pathway of biosynthesis that generates the renin and angiotensin I. Angiotensinogen is synthesized in the liver and is released into the blood where it is cleaved to form angiotensin I by renin secreted by cells in the kidneys. Angiotensin converting enzyme (ACE) in the lung catalyzes the formation of angiotensin II from angiotensin I and destroys the potent vasodilator, bradykinin. Further cleavage generates the angiotensins III and IV. The reddish shading shows the organs affected by angiotensin II, including brain, heart, adrenals, kidney, and the kidney's efferent arterioles. The *dashed arrow (left)* shows the inhibition of renin by angiotensin II. **B,** Summary of angiotensin II effects on blood vessel structure and function leading to atherosclerosis. (Adapted from Goodfriend TL et al: *N Engl J Med* 334:2649–2654, 1996.)

loss, leading to the formation of a large volume of dilute urine that decreases blood volume and blood pressure. **Brain natriuretic peptide (BNP)** is secreted from cardiac cells and also increases sodium loss from the kidney. It is used both as a marker and as a treatment for acute heart failure.[26] C-type natriuretic peptide (CNP) is found throughout the vascular endothelium and promotes vasodilation.[27] Urodilatin is made in the kidneys and promotes natriuresis.[28]

Adrenomedullin (ADM) is a recently discovered, widely dispersed peptide present in numerous tissues with powerful vasodilatory activity. ADM plays an important role in vascular protection by decreasing oxidative stress, limiting endothelial injury, causing vasodilation, and promoting angiogenesis.[29,30] Other functions of ADM include neurotransmission, growth, hormone secretion regulation, down-regulation of the proinflammatory cytokines, and modulation of anticoagulant properties.[31] Therefore, changes in ADM levels have been correlated with several diseases including cardiovascular and renal sepsis, cancer, and diabetes.[31] Originally isolated from human pheochromocytoma (tumor of the adrenal medulla), it is present in cardiovascular, pulmonary, renal, gastrointestinal, cerebral, and endocrine tissues. Adrenomedullin is secreted from endothelial and smooth muscle cells and mediates vasodilation and sodium excretion. Thus, ADM seems to play an important role in fluid and electrolyte balance and cardiorenal regulation.[32]

In vitro studies demonstrate that **insulin** has direct vascular actions that contribute to both vascular protection and injury. The vascular protection and injury properties are summarized in Box 22-2. Insulin resistance and diabetes have a profound effect on cardiovascular disorders including hypertension and atherosclerotic disease.[33,34]

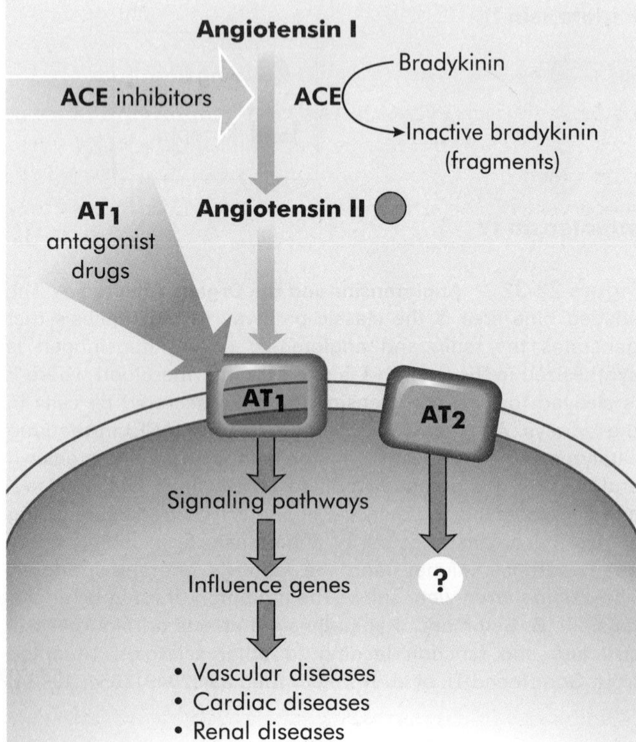

Figure 22-33 ■ Angiotensins and Their Receptors, AT_1 and AT_2. Blocking the angiotensin-converting enzyme (ACE) with ACE inhibitors decreases the amount of angiotensin II. Blocking the receptor AT_1 with drugs (AT_1 antagonists) blocks the attachment of angiotensin II to the cell preventing the cellular effects and decreasing the vascular, cardiac, and renal effects.

Venous pressure

The main determinants of venous blood pressure are (1) the volume of fluid within the veins and (2) the compliance (distensibility) of the vessel walls. The venous system accommodates approximately 60% of the total blood volume at any given moment, with venous pressure averaging less than 10 mm Hg. The arteries accommodate about 15% of the total blood volume, with an average arterial pressure (blood pressure) of about 100 mm Hg.

The sympathetic nervous system controls compliance. The walls of the veins are highly innervated by sympathetic fibers that, when stimulated, cause venous smooth muscle to contract and increase muscle tone. This stiffens the wall of the vein, which reduces distensibility and increases blood pressure, forcing more blood through the veins and into the right heart.

Two other mechanisms that increase venous pressure and venous return to the heart are (1) the skeletal muscle pump and (2) the respiratory pump. During skeletal muscle contraction, the veins within the muscles are partially compressed, causing decreased venous capacity and increased return to the heart (see Figure 22-25). The respiratory pump acts during inspiration, when the veins of the abdomen are partially compressed by the downward movement of the diaphragm. Increased abdominal pressure moves blood toward the heart.

Regulation of the Coronary Circulation

Flow of blood in the coronary circulation is directly proportional to the perfusion pressure and inversely proportional to the vascular resistance of the bed. **Coronary perfusion pressure** is the difference between pressure in the aorta and pressure in the coronary vessels of the right atrium. Aortic pressure is the driving pressure that perfuses vessels of the myocardium. Vasodilation and vasoconstriction normally maintain coronary blood flow despite stresses imposed by the constant contraction and relaxation of the heart muscle and despite shifts (within a physiologic range) of coronary perfusion pressure.

Several anatomic factors influence coronary blood flow. The aortic valve cusps obstruct coronary blood flow by pushing against the openings of the coronary arteries during systole. Also during systole, the coronary arteries are compressed by ventricular contraction. The resulting **systolic compressive effect** is particularly evident in the

BOX 22-2 Vascular Protection and Injury Properties of Insulin

Protection

Insulin has numerous protective actions on blood vessels:

1. Increases endothelial cell production of nitric oxide
   a. Nitric oxide (NO) (in vitro) inhibits growth of vascular smooth muscle cells
   b. NO decreases the inflammatory reaction by inhibiting the expression of adhesion molecules, inhibiting the activity of proinflammatory cytokines (e.g., TNF-α, monocyte chemoattractant protein-1 [MCP-1]). Thus NO decreases the binding of monocytes/macrophages to the vessel wall
2. Enhances acetylcholine-mediated vasodilation
3. Reduces platelet adherence and thus decreases thrombus formation
   a. Increased NO also inhibits the thrombotic process by preventing platelet adhesion and enhancing the effect of prostacyclin to inhibit platelet aggregation
   b. Insulin increases the endogenous anticoagulant plasminogen activator inhibitor
4. Is anti-inflammatory
   a. Reduces toxic oxygen radical production
   b. Decreases levels of C-reactive protein

Injury

Hyperinsulinemia has some deleterious effects on blood vessels:

1. Increases growth of vascular smooth muscle cells (VSMCs)
   a. Increases activity of insulin-like growth factor-1
   b. Increases angiotensin II–mediated vascular remodeling
2. Increases the effect of platelet-derived growth factor
3. Increases sympathetic nervous system activity and thus contributes to increased blood pressure

Insulin resistance is likely more important to the development of hypertension and the atherogenesis process than hyperinsulinemia:

1. Reduces NO production and increases vasoconstrictors such as angiotensin II and catecholamines
2. Promotes inflammation with increased production of toxic oxygen radicals and other inflammatory mediators
3. Increases clot formation
4. Contributes to endothelial damage
5. Contributes to deleterious lipid changes

Data from Bloomgarden ZT: Inflammation, atherosclerosis, and aspects of insulin action, *Diabetes Care* 28(9):2312–2319, 2005; Kuritzky L, Nelson SE: Beneficial effects of insulin on endothelial function, inflammation, and atherogenesis and their implications, *J Family Pract* 54(6):S7-S9, 2005; Sjoholm A, Nystrom T: Endothelial inflammation in insulin resistance, *Lancet* 365(9459):610–612, 2005; Sowers JR, Frohlich ED: Insulin and insulin resistance: impact on blood pressure and cardiovascular disease *Med Clin North Am* 88(1):63–82, 2004; Velloso LA et al: The multi-faceted cross-talk between the insulin and angiotensin II signaling systems, *Diabetes Metab Res Rev* 22(2):98–107, 2006; Zarich SW: Cardiovascular risk factors in the metabolic syndrome: impact of insulin resistance on lipids, hypertension, and the development of diabetes and cardiac events, *Rev Cardiovasc Med* 6(4):194–205, 2005.

subendocardial layers of the left ventricular wall and can greatly decrease coronary blood flow. Therefore, most coronary blood flow in the left ventricle occurs during diastole. During the period of systolic compression, when flow is slowed or stopped, oxygen is supplied by **myoglobin,** a protein present in heart muscle that binds oxygen during diastole and then releases it when blood levels of oxygen fall during systole.

Autoregulation

Autoregulation (automatic self-regulation) enables individual vessels to regulate blood flow by altering their own arteriolar resistances. Autoregulation in the coronary circulation maintains constant blood flow at perfusion pressures (mean arterial pressure) between 60 and 180 mm Hg, provided that other influencing factors are held constant. Thus, autoregulation ensures constant coronary blood flow despite shifts in the perfusion pressure within the stated range.

The mechanism of autoregulation is not known, but two explanations have been proposed. The **myogenic hypothesis** proposes that autoregulation originates in vascular smooth muscle, presumably of the arterioles, as a response to an increase in arterial pressure. Smooth muscle stretches in response to an increase in perfusion pressure. The stretching eventually stimulates contraction of the smooth muscles, which increases vascular resistance. Initially, coronary blood flow increases with the abrupt distention of the blood vessels. The return of more normal flow follows constriction of the arterioles. This mechanism also works in the opposite direction—that is, vasodilation is stimulated by decreased arterial pressure.

The **metabolic hypothesis** of autoregulation proposes that autoregulation of coronary vessels originates in the myocardium. The stimulus is a drop in coronary perfusion pressure or an increase in the metabolic needs of the myocardium (e.g., because of strenuous exercise). With an increased myocardial oxygen requirement, myocardial cells release substances that promote vasodilation. The best known of these substances is adenosine, a potent vasodilator released in response to a decrease in myocardial oxygenation. Low coronary blood flow, hypoxemia, or increased metabolic activity of the heart can all increase the heart muscle's need for oxygen.[1,35] An increased concentration of adenosine in the interstitial fluid decreases the resistance of the coronary arterioles and increases blood flow. Perfusion strongly correlates with the amount of adenosine released.[35] When coronary perfusion pressure is increased, the increased flow washes out the vasodilatory substances. As the dilators are washed out, vasoconstriction occurs and returns flow toward normal.

Autonomic regulation

Although the coronary vessels themselves contain sympathetic (α- and β-adrenergic) and parasympathetic neural receptors, coronary blood flow is regulated locally through metabolic autoregulation. Metabolic autoregulation overrides neurogenic influences.[4]

✓ QUICK CHECK 22-7

1. Why is capillary flow increased with increased mean arterial pressure?
2. Why is angiotensin significant in blood flow?
3. Identify the factors regulating blood pressure.
4. Define natriuretic peptides and adrenomedullin.

THE LYMPHATIC SYSTEM

The lymphatic system is a special vascular system that picks up excess tissue fluid and returns it to the bloodstream (Figure 22-34). Normally, fluid is forced out of the blood at the arterial end of the capillary bed and is reabsorbed into the bloodstream at the venous end. However, capillary outflow exceeds venous reabsorption by about 3 L/day, so some fluid lags behind in the interstitium. To maintain sufficient blood volume in the cardiovascular system, this fluid must eventually rejoin the bloodstream; this is the function of the lymphatic system.

The components of the lymphatic system are the lymphatic vessels and the lymph nodes (Figure 22-35). (Lymph nodes and lymphoid tissues are described in Chapters 5 and 7.) In this pumpless system, a series of valves ensures one-way flow of the excess interstitial fluid (now called lymph) toward the heart. The lymphatic capillaries are closed at the ends, as shown in Figure 22-36.

Lymph consists primarily of water and small amounts of dissolved proteins, mostly albumin, that are too large to be reabsorbed into the less permeable blood capillaries. Once

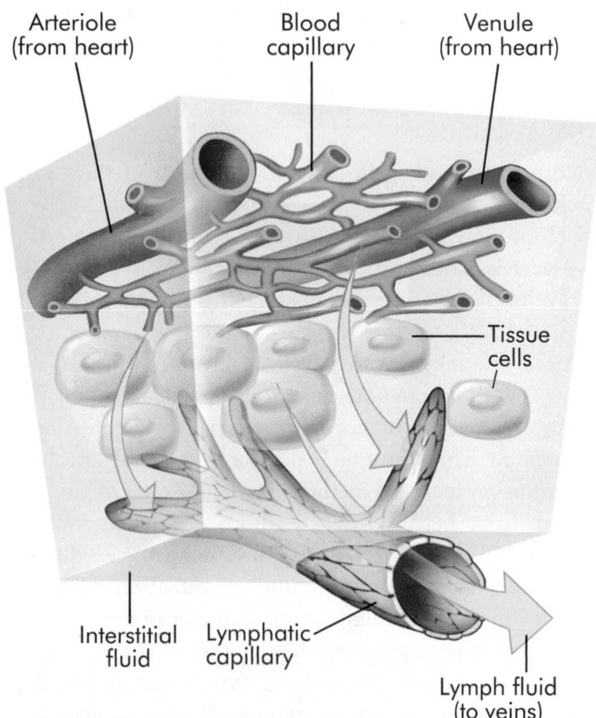

Figure 22-34 ■ Role of the Lymphatic System in Fluid Balance. Fluid from plasma flowing through the capillaries moves into interstitial spaces. Although much of this interstitial fluid is either absorbed by tissue cells or reabsorbed by capillaries, some of the fluid tends to accumulate in the interstitial spaces. As this fluid builds up, it tends to drain into lymphatic vessels that eventually return the fluid to the venous blood. (From Thibodeau GA, Patton KT: *Anatomy & physiology,* ed 6, St Louis, 2007, Mosby.)

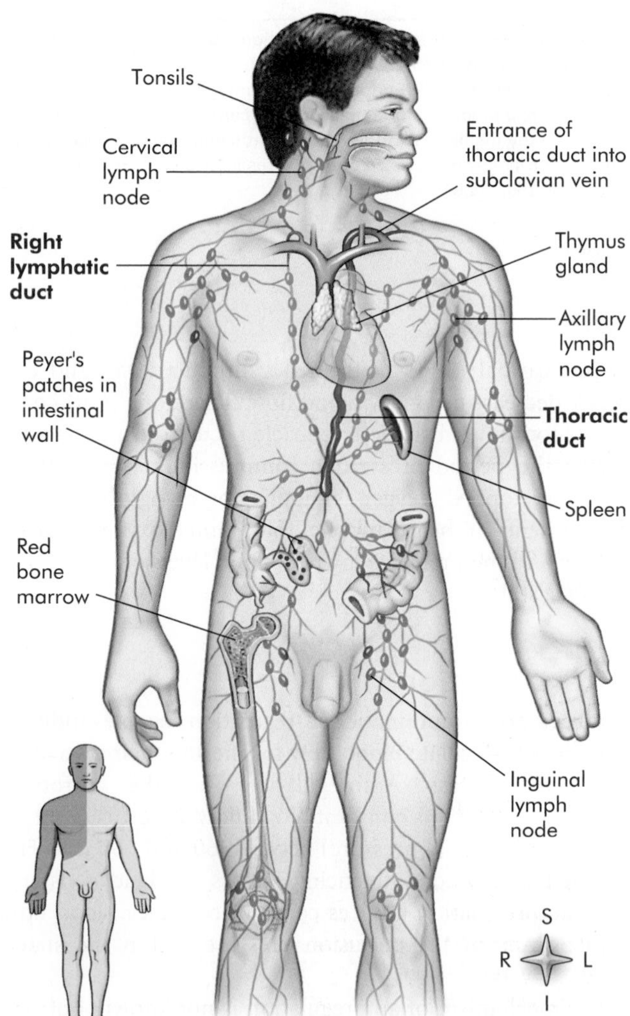

Figure 22-35 ■ Principle Organs of the Lymphatic System. The inset shows the areas drained by the right lymphatic duct *(green)* and the thoracic duct *(blue)*. (From Thibodeau GA, Patton KT: *Anatomy & physiology,* ed 6, St Louis, 2007, Mosby.)

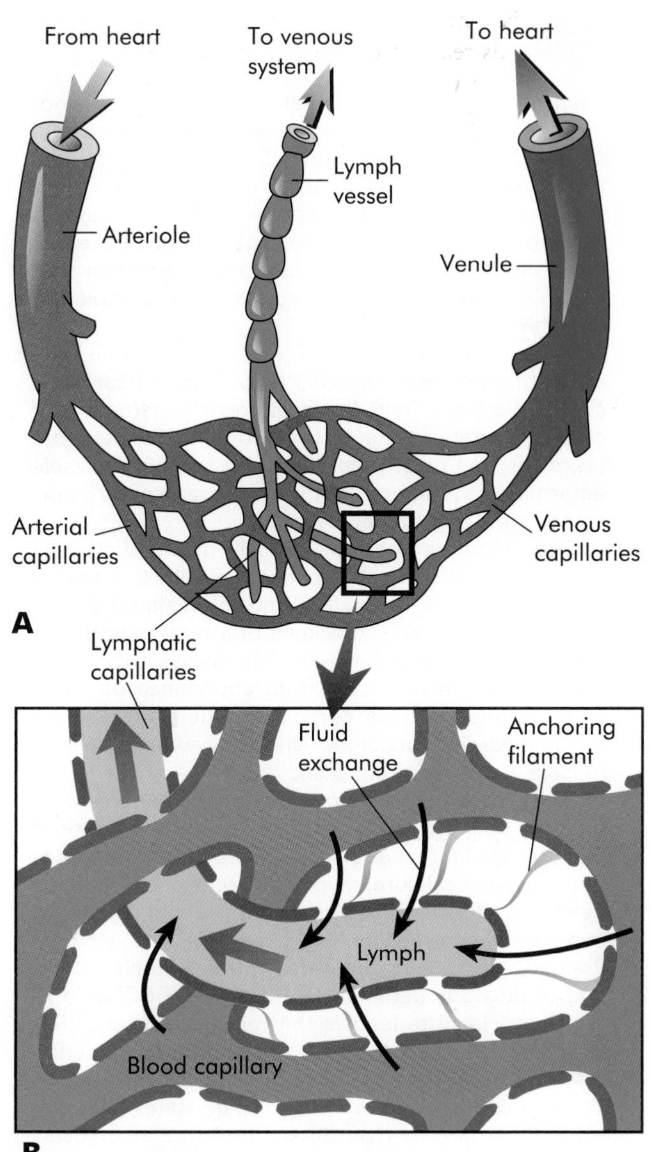

Figure 22-36 ■ **Lymphatic Capillaries. A,** Schematic representation of lymphatic capillaries. **B,** Anatomic components of microcirculation.

within the lymphatic system, lymph travels through larger vessels called **lymphatic venules** and **lymphatic veins.** The lymphatic vessels run alongside the arteries and veins and eventually drain into one of two large ducts in the thorax—the right lymphatic duct and the thoracic duct. The **right lymphatic duct** drains lymph from the right arm and the right side of the head and thorax, whereas the larger **thoracic duct** receives lymph from the rest of the body (see Figure 22-35). The right lymphatic duct and the thoracic duct drain lymph into the right and left subclavian veins, respectively.

The lymphatic veins are thin walled like the veins of the cardiovascular system. In the larger lymphatic veins, endothelial flaps form valves similar to those in the circulatory veins (see Figure 22-24). The valves permit lymph to flow in only one direction because lymphatic vessels are compressed intermittently by contraction of skeletal muscles, pulsatile expansion of an artery in the same sheath, and contraction of the smooth muscles in the walls of the lymphatic vessel.

As lymph is transported toward the heart, it is filtered through thousands of bean-shaped **lymph nodes** clustered along the lymphatic vessels (see Figure 22-35). Lymph enters the node through several **afferent lymphatic vessels,** filters through the sinuses in the node, and leaves by way of **efferent lymphatic vessels.** Lymph flows slowly through the node, which facilitates the phagocytosis of foreign substances within the node and prevents them from reentering the bloodstream. (Phagocytosis is described in Chapter 6.)

QUICK CHECK 22-8

1. Why is the lymphatic system considered a circulatory system?
2. What happens to lymph in lymph nodes?

Did You Understand?

The Circulatory System

1. The circulatory system is the body's transport system. It delivers oxygen, nutrients, metabolites, hormones, neurochemicals, proteins, and blood cells through the body and carries metabolic wastes to the kidneys and lungs for excretion.
2. The circulatory system consists of the heart and blood vessels and is made up of two separate, serially connected systems: the pulmonary circulation and the systemic circulation.
3. The pulmonary circulation is driven by the right side of the heart; its function is to deliver blood to the lungs for oxygenation.
4. The systemic circulation is driven by the left side of the heart, and its function is to move oxygenated blood throughout the body.
5. The lymphatic vessels collect fluids from the interstitium and return the fluids to the circulatory system.

The Heart

1. The heart consists of four chambers (two atria and two ventricles), four valves (two atrioventricular valves and two semilunar valves), a muscular wall, a fibrous skeleton, a conduction system, nerve fibers, systemic vessels (the coronary circulation), and openings where the great vessels enter the atria and ventricles.
2. The heart wall, which encloses the heart and divides it into chambers, is made up of three layers: the pericardium (outer layer), the myocardium (muscular layer), and the endocardium (inner lining).

(Continued)

Did You Understand?—Cont'd

3. The myocardial layer of the two atria, which receive blood entering the heart, is thinner than the myocardial layer of the ventricles, which have to be stronger to squeeze blood out of the heart.
4. The right and left sides of the heart are separated by portions of the heart wall called the *interatrial septum* and the *interventricular septum.*
5. Deoxygenated (venous) blood from the systemic circulation enters the right atrium through the superior and inferior venae cavae. From the atrium, the blood passes through the right atrioventricular (tricuspid) valve into the right ventricle. In the ventricle, the blood flows from the inflow tract to the outflow tract and then through the pulmonary semilunar valve (pulmonary valve) into the pulmonary artery, which delivers it to the lungs for oxygenation.
6. Oxygenated blood from the lungs enters the left atrium through the four pulmonary veins (two from the left lung and two from the right lung). From the left atrium, the blood passes through the left atrioventricular valve (mitral valve) into the left ventricle. In the ventricle, the blood flows from the inflow tract to the outflow tract and then through the aortic semilunar valve (aortic valve) into the aorta, which delivers it to systemic arteries of the entire body.
7. The heart valves ensure the one-way flow of blood from atrium to ventricle and from ventricle to artery.
8. Oxygenated blood enters the coronary arteries through an opening in the aorta, and unoxygenated blood from the coronary veins enters the right atrium through the coronary sinus.
9. The pumping action of the heart consists of two phases: diastole, during which the myocardium relaxes and the ventricles fill with blood, and systole, during which the myocardium contracts, forcing blood out of the ventricles. A cardiac cycle consists of one systolic contraction and the diastolic relaxation that follows it. Each cardiac cycle constitutes one "heartbeat."
10. The conduction system of the heart generates and transmits electrical impulses (cardiac action potentials) that stimulate systolic contractions. The autonomic nerves (sympathetic and parasympathetic fibers) can adjust heart rate and systolic force, but they do not stimulate the heart to beat.
11. The normal electrocardiogram is the sum of all action potentials. The P wave represents atrial depolarization; the QRS complex is the sum of all ventricular cell depolarizations. The ST interval occurs when the entire ventricular myocardium is depolarized.
12. Cardiac action potentials are generated by the sinoatrial node at the rate of about 75 impulses per minute. The impulses can travel through the conduction system of the heart, stimulating myocardial contraction as they go.
13. Cells of the cardiac conduction system possess the properties of automaticity and rhythmicity. Automatic cells return to threshold and depolarize rhythmically without outside stimulus. The cells of the sinoatrial node depolarize faster than other automatic cells, making it the natural pacemaker of the heart. If the sinoatrial node is disabled, the next fastest pacemaker, the atrioventricular node, takes over.
14. Each cardiac action potential travels from the sinoatrial node to the atrioventricular node to the bundle of His (atrioventricular bundle), through the bundle branches, and finally to the Purkinje fibers. There the impulse is stopped. It is prevented from reversing its path by the refractory period of cells that have just been polarized. The refractory period ensures that diastole (relaxation) will occur, thereby completing the cardiac cycle.
15. Adrenergic receptor number, type, and function govern autonomic (sympathetic) regulation of heart rate, contractile force, and the dilation or constriction of coronary arteries. The presence of specific receptors (α_1, α_2; β_1, β_2) on myocardium and coronary vessels determines the effects of the neurotransmitters norepinephrine and epinephrine.
16. Unique features that distinguish myocardial cells from skeletal cells enable myocardial cells to transmit action potentials faster (through intercalated disks), synthesize more ATP (because of a large number of mitochondria), and have readier access to ions in the interstitium (because of an abundance of transverse tubules). These combined differences enable the myocardium to work constantly, which skeletal muscle is not required to do.
17. Cross-bridges between actin and myosin enable contraction. Calcium and its interaction with the troponin complex facilitate the contraction process. With troponin release of calcium, myocardial relaxation begins.
18. Cardiac performance is affected by preload, afterload, myocardial contractility, and heart rate.
19. Preload, or pressure generated in the ventricles at the end of diastole, depends on the amount of blood in the ventricle. Afterload is the resistance to ejection of the blood from the ventricle. Afterload depends on pressure in the aorta.
20. The Frank-Starling law of the heart states that the myocardial stretch determines the force of myocardial contraction (the greater the stretch, the stronger the contraction).
21. Contractility is the potential for myocardial fiber shortening during systole. It is determined by the amount of stretch during diastole (i.e., preload) and by sympathetic stimulation of the ventricles.
22. Heart rate is determined by the sinoatrial node and by components of the autonomic nervous system, including cardiovascular control centers in the brain, neuroreceptors in the atria and aorta, hormones, and catecholamines (epinephrine, norepinephrine).

The Systemic Circulation

1. Blood flows from the left ventricle into the aorta and from the aorta into arteries that eventually branch into arterioles and capillaries, the smallest of the arterial vessels. Oxygen, nutrients, and other substances needed for cellular metabolism pass from the capillaries into the interstitium, where they are available for uptake by the cells. Capillaries also absorb products of cellular metabolism from the interstitium.
2. Venules, the smallest veins, receive capillary blood. From the venules, the venous blood flows into larger and larger veins until it reaches the venae cavae, through which it enters the right atrium.

Did You Understand?—Cont'd

3. Vessel walls consist of three layers: the tunica intima (inner layer), the tunica media (middle layer), and the tunica externa (the outer layer).
4. Layers of the vessel wall differ in thickness and composition from vessel to vessel, depending on the vessel's size and location within the circulatory system. In general, the tunica media of arteries close to the heart contains a greater proportion of elastic fibers because these arteries must be able to distend during systole and recoil during diastole. Distributing arteries farther from the heart contain a greater proportion of smooth muscle fibers because these arteries must be able to constrict and dilate to control blood pressure and volume within specific capillary beds.
5. Blood flow into the capillary beds is controlled by the contraction and relaxation of smooth muscle bands (precapillary sphincters) at junctions between metarterioles and capillaries.
6. Endothelial cells form the lining or endothelium of blood vessels. The endothelium is a life-support tissue and functions as a filter, altering permeability, changes in vasomotion (constriction and dilation), and is involved in clotting and inflammation.
7. Blood flow through the veins is assisted by the contraction of skeletal muscles (the muscle pump), and one-way valves prevent backflow in the lower body, particularly in the deep veins of the legs.
8. Blood flow is affected by blood pressure, resistance to flow within the vessels, blood consistency (which affects velocity), anatomic features that may cause turbulent or laminar flow, and compliance (distensibility) of the vessels.
9. Poiseuille law describes the relationship of blood flow, pressure, and resistance as the difference between pressure at the inflow end of the vessel and pressure at the outflow end divided by resistance within the vessel.
10. According to Poiseuille formula, resistance depends on the vessel's length and radius and on the viscosity of the blood. The greater the vessel's length and the blood's viscosity and the narrower the radius of the vessel's lumen, the greater the resistance within the vessel.
11. Total peripheral resistance, or the resistance to flow within the entire systemic circulatory system, depends on the combined lengths and radii of all the vessels within the system and on whether the vessels are arranged in series (greater resistance) or in parallel (lesser resistance).
12. Poiseuille law and Poiseuille formula are based on physical laws governing the behavior of fluids in a straight tube. In the body, blood flow is also influenced by neural stimulation (vasoconstriction or vasodilation) and by autonomic features that cause turbulence within the vascular lumen (e.g., protrusions from the vessel wall, twists and turns, bifurcations).
13. Arterial blood pressure is influenced and regulated by factors that affect cardiac output (heart rate, stroke volume), total resistance within the system, and blood volume.
14. Antidiuretic hormone, renin-angiotensin system, natriuretic peptides, adrenomedullin, and insulin can all alter blood volume and thus blood pressure.
15. The tissue renin-angiotensin system is activated in response to tissue injury. This system is gaining importance in the maladaptive alterations, such as ventricular and vascular remodeling, alterations in renal function, and atherosclerosis.
16. Particularly significant is an increased recognition of the role of angiotensin II for causing the systemic effects of vasoconstriction, hypertension, activation of the sympathetic nervous system, and retention of sodium and fluids.
17. Venous blood pressure is influenced by blood volume within the venous system and compliance of the venous walls.
18. Blood flow through the coronary circulation is governed not only by the same principles as flow through other vascular beds but also by adaptations dictated by cardiac dynamics. First, blood flows into the coronary arteries during diastole rather than systole, because during systole, the cusps of the aortic semilunar valve block the openings of the coronary arteries. Second, systolic contraction inhibits coronary artery flow by compressing the coronary arteries.
19. Autoregulation enables the coronary vessels to maintain optimal perfusion pressure despite systolic effects, and myoglobin in heart muscle stores oxygen for use during the systolic phase of the cardiac cycle.

The Lymphatic System

1. The vessels of the lymphatic system run in the same sheaths with the arteries and veins.
2. Lymph (interstitial fluid) is absorbed by lymphatic venules in the capillary beds and travels through ever larger lymphatic veins until it is emptied through the right or left thoracic duct into the right or left subclavian vein.
3. As lymph travels toward the thoracic ducts, it is filtered by thousands of lymph nodes clustered around the lymphatic veins. The lymph nodes are sites of immune function.

Key Terms

Actin, 579
Adrenomedullin (ADM), 598
Afferent lymphatic vessel, 601
Afterload, 582
Aldosterone, 595
Angiotensin I (Ang I), 595
Angiotensin II (Ang II), 595
Anisotropic band (A band), 579
Anomalous viscosity, 591
Anterior interatrial myocardial band (Bachmann bundle), 575
Anterior internodal pathway, 575
Aorta, 570
Aortic semilunar valve, 569
Arteriole, 585
Artery, 585
AT_1, 596
AT_2, 596
Atrial natriuretic peptide (ANP), 596
Atrioventricular node (AV node), 575
Atrioventricular valve, 569
Automatic cell, 576
Automaticity, 576
Autoregulation, 599
Bainbridge reflex, 584
Baroreceptor reflex, 584
Blood flow, 588
Blood velocity, 592
Brain natriuretic peptide (BNP), 598
Bundle branch, 575
Bundle of His (atrioventricular bundle common bundle), 575
Calcium channel–blocking drug, 581
Capillary, 585
Cardiac action potential, 574
Cardiac cycle, 571
Cardiac output, 581
Cardiac vein, 572
Cardioexcitatory center, 584
Cardioinhibitory center, 584
Cardiovascular control center, 583
Chordae tendineae cordis, 569
Conduction system, 574
Coronary artery, 572
Coronary circulation, 572
Coronary ostium (pl., ostia), 572
Coronary perfusion pressure, 598
Coronary sinus, 572
Cross-bridge theory of muscle contraction, 580
Depolarization, 576
Diastole, 571
Diastolic depolarization, 576
Efferent lymphatic vessel, 601
Ejection fraction, 581
Elastic artery, 585
Endocardium, 568
Endothelial cell, 585
Endothelium, 585
Excitation-contraction coupling, 580
Fenestration, 585
Frank-Starling law of the heart, 582
Great cardiac vein, 574
Heart rate, 574
Inferior vena cava, 571
Inotropic agent, 583
Insulin, 598
Intercalated disk, 578
Isotropic band (I band), 579
Laminar flow, 593
Laplace law, 582
Left atrium, 569
Left bundle branch (LBB), 575
Left coronary artery, 572
Left heart, 567
Left ventricle, 569
Length, 591
Lumen, 585
Lymph node, 601
Lymph, 600
Lymphatic vein, 601
Lymphatic venule, 601
M line, 579
Mean arterial pressure (MAP), 594
Mediastinum, 567
Metabolic hypothesis, 599
Metarteriole, 585
Microcirculation, 591
Middle internodal pathway, 575
Mitral and tricuspid complex, 571
Mitral valve (left atrioventricular valve, bicuspid valve), 571
Muscle pump, 588
Muscular artery, 585
Myocardial contractility, 579
Myocardial oxygen consumption ($M\dot{V}O_2$), 579
Myocardium, 568
Myogenic hypothesis, 599
Myoglobin, 599
Myosin, 579
Natriuretic peptide (NP), 596
Node, 574
P wave, 576
Papillary muscle, 569
Perfusion, 594
Pericardial cavity, 568
Pericardial fluid, 568
Pericardium, 568
Peripheral vascular system, 585
Poiseuille formula, 591
Poiseuille law, 589
Posterior internodal pathway, 575
PR interval, 576
Precapillary sphincter, 585
Preload, 581
Pressure, 588
Pulmonary artery, 571
Pulmonary circulation, 567
Pulmonary vein, 571
Pulmonic semilunar valve, 569
Purkinje fiber, 575
QRS complex, 576
QT interval, 576
Radius, 591
Refractory period, 576
Renin, 594
Repolarization, 576
Resistance, 589
Rhythmicity, 576
Right atrium, 569
Right bundle branch (RBB), 575
Right coronary artery, 572
Right heart, 567
Right lymphatic duct, 601
Right ventricle, 569
Semilunar valve, 569
Sinoatrial node (SA node, sinus node), 574
ST interval, 576
Stroke volume, 583
Superior vena cava, 571
Systemic circulation, 567
Systole, 571
Systolic compressive effect, 598
Thoracic duct, 601
Total resistance, 591
Tricuspid valve (right atrioventricular valve), 571
Tropomyosin, 579
Troponin C, 579
Troponin I, 579
Troponin T, 579
Troponin-tropomyosin complex, 579
Tunica externa (adventia; external layer), 585
Tunica intima (intimal layer), 585
Tunica media (medial layer), 585
Turbulent flow, 593
Vasa vasorum, 585
Vascular compliance, 594
Vasoconstriction, 585
Vasodilation, 585
Vein, 585
Ventricular end-diastolic pressure (VEDP), 582
Ventricular end-diastolic volume (VEDV), 581
Venule, 585
Viscosity, 589
Z line, 579

References

1. Berne RM, Levy MN: *Cardiovascular physiology*, ed 8, St Louis, 2001, Mosby.
2. Carmileit P: Angiogenesis in life, disease and medicine, *Nature* 483:932, 2005.
3. Ganong W: *Review of medical physiology*, ed 22, New York, 2005, McGraw-Hill.
4. Zipes D et al: *Braunwald's heart disease: a textbook of cardiovascular medicine*, ed 7, Philadelphia, 2005, Saunders.
5. Bailin SJ: Atrial lead implantation in the Bachmann bundle, *Heart Rhythm* 2(7):784–786, 2005.
6. Triggle DJ: L-type calcium channels, *Curr Pharmaceut Design* 12(4):443–457, 2006.
7. Tanaka H, Shigenobu K: Pathophysiological significance of T-type $Ca2^{+}$ channels: T-type $Ca2^{+}$ channels and drug development, *J Pharmacol Sci* 99(3):214–220, 2005.
8. Hay I et al: Role of impaired myocardial relaxation in the production of elevated left ventricular filling pressure, *Am J Physiol Heart Circ Physiol* 288(3):H1203–H1208, 2005.
9. Barbieri R, Triedman JK, Saul JP: Heart rate control and mechanical cardiopulmonary coupling to assess central volume: a systems analysis, *Am J Physiol Regul Integr Comp Physio* 283(5):R1210–R1220, 2002.
10. Parati G: Arterial baroreflex control of heart rate: determining factors and methods to assess its spontaneous modulation, *J Physiol* 565(Pt 3):706–707, 2005.
11. Potter LR, Abbey-Hosch S, Dickey DM: Natriuretic peptides, their receptors, and cyclic guanosine monophosphate-dependent signaling functions, *Endocr Rev* 27(1):47–72, 2006.
12. Felmeden DC, Lip GY: Endothelial function and its assessment, *Exp Opin Investig Drugs* 14(11):1319–1336, 2005.
13. Kim SD: Measurement of the renin-angiotensin system in heart failure, *Biol Res Nurs* 1(3):210, 2000.
14. Daugherty A, Cassis L: Angiotensin II-mediated development of vascular diseases, *Trends Cardiovasc Med* 14(3):117–120, 2004.
15. Schiffrin EL: Effects of aldosterone on the vasculature, *Hyperten* 47(3):312–318, 2006.
16. Touyz RM: Molecular and cellular mechanisms in vascular injury in hypertension: role of angiotensin II, *Curr Opin Nephrol Hypertens* 14(2):125–131, 2005.
17. Yasunari K et al: Left ventricular hypertrophy and angiotensin II receptor blocking agents, *Curr Med Chem Cardiovasc Hematol Agents* 3(1):61–67, 2005.
18. Smith GR, Missailidis S: Cancer, inflammation, and the AT_1 and AT_2 receptors, *J Inflamm* (Lond) 1(1):3, 2004.
19. Levy BI: How to explain the differences between renin angiotensin system modulators, *Am J Hypertens* 18(9 Pt 2): 134S–141S, 2005.
20. Suzuki H et al: Recent progress in signal transduction research of the angiotensin II type-1 receptor: protein kinases vascular dysfunction and structural requirement, *Curr Medicinal Chem Cardiovasc Hematol Agents* 3(4):305–322, 2005.
21. Schulz R, Heusch G: Angiotensin II in the failing heart, *Kidney Blood Press Res* 28(5–6):349–352, 2005.
22. Carey RM: Angiotensin type-2 receptors and cardiovascular function: are angiotensin type-2 receptors protective? *Curr Opin Cardiol* 20(4):264–269, 2005.
23. Booz GW: Cardiac angiotensin AT2 receptor: what exactly does it do? *Hypertens* 43:1162–1163, 2004.
24. Silver MA: The natriuretic peptide system: kidney and cardiovascular effects, *Curr Opin Nephrol Hypertens* 15(1):14–21, 2006.
25. Clerico A et al: M. Cardiac endocrine function is an essential component of the homeostatic regulation network: physiological and clinical implications, *Am J Physiol Heart Circ Physiol* 290(1):H17–29, 2006.
26. Wasywich CA, Whalley GA, Doughty RN: Brain natriuretic peptide in the contemporary management of congestive heart failure, *Exp Rev Cardiovas Ther* 3:71–84, 2005.
27. Scotland RS, Ahluwalia A, Hobbs AJ: C-type natriuretic peptide in vascular physiology and disease, *Pharmacol Ther* 105 (2):85–93, 2005.
28. Forssmann W, Meyer M, Forssmann K: The renal urodilatin system: clinical implications, *Cardiovas Res* 51(3):450–462, 2001.
29. Kato J et al: Adrenomedullin: a protective factor for blood vessels, *Arterioscler Thromb Vas Biol* 25(12):2480–2487, 2005.
30. Ribatti D et al: The role of adrenomedullin in angiogenesis, *Peptides* 26(9):1670–1675, 2005.
31. Bunton DC et al: The clinical relevance of adrenomedullin: a promising profile? *Pharmacol Therap* 103(3):179–201, 2004.
32. Hamid SA, Baxter GF: Adrenomedullin: regulator of systemic and cardiac homeostasis in acute myocardial infarction, *Pharmacol Therap* 105(2):95–112, 2005.
33. Sowers JR, Frohlich ED: Insulin and insulin resistance: impact on blood pressure and cardiovascular disease, *Med Clin North Am* 88(1):63–82, 2004.
34. Zarich SW: Cardiovascular risk factors in the metabolic syndrome: impact of insulin resistance on lipids, hypertension, and the development of diabetes and cardiac events, *Cardiovasc Med* 6(4):194–205, 2005.
35. Berne RM: The role of adenosine in the regulation of coronary blood flow, *Circ Res* 47(6):807–813, 1980.

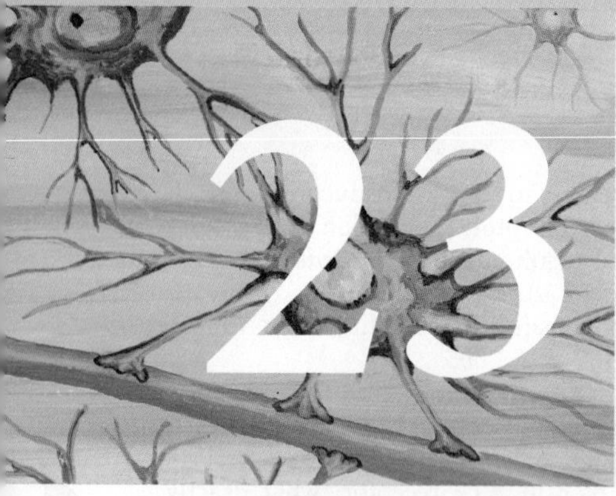

ALTERATIONS OF CARDIOVASCULAR FUNCTION

Valentina L. Brashers

CHAPTER OUTLINE

ELECTRONIC RESOURCES

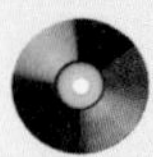

Companion CD
- Review Questions and Answers
- Animations

evolve Website
http://evolve.elsevier.com/Huether/
- Quick Check Answers
- Key Terms Exercises
- Critical Thinking Questions with Answers
- Algorithm Completion Exercises
- WebLinks

Our understanding of the pathophysiology of many cardiovascular diseases is evolving rapidly, especially atherosclerosis, hypertension, myocardial ischemia, and congestive heart failure. The role of genetics and its interaction with the environment in the etiology and progression of all forms of cardiovascular disease is just one example of new information that is leading to improvements in prevention and treatment.

DISEASES OF THE ARTERIES AND VEINS

Diseases of the Veins

Varicose veins and chronic venous insufficiency

A varicose vein is a vein in which blood has pooled, producing distended, tortuous, and palpable vessels. Veins are thin-walled, highly distensible vessels with valves to prevent backflow and pooling of blood. If a valve is damaged, a section of the vein is subjected to the pressure of a larger volume of blood under the influence of gravity. The vein becomes engorged with blood, which increases hydrostatic pressure and increases movement of plasma through the vessel wall, resulting in interstitial edema.

Venous distention can develop over time in individuals who habitually stand for long periods, wear constricting garments, or cross the legs at the knees, which diminishes the action of the muscle pump (see Figure 22-25). Risk factors also include age, female gender, a family history, obesity, pregnancy, phlebitis, and previous leg injury.[1] Eventually the pressure in the vein damages venous valves, rendering them incompetent and unable to maintain normal venous pressure. Hydrostatic pressure increases, further distending the vein and making it tortuous; edema then develops in the extremity.

Chronic venous insufficiency (CVI) is inadequate venous return over a long period. Venous hypertension, circulatory stasis, and tissue hypoxia lead to an inflammatory reaction in vessels and tissue leading to fibrosclerotic remodeling of the skin and then to ulceration.[2] Symptoms include chronic pooling of blood in the veins of the lower extremities and hyperpigmentation of the skin of the feet and ankles. Edema in these areas may extend to the knees.

Circulation to the extremities can become so sluggish that the metabolic demands of the cells for oxygen, nutrients, and waste removal are barely met. Any trauma or pressure can therefore lower the oxygen supply and cause cell death and necrosis **(venous stasis ulcers)** (Figure 23-1). Infection can occur because poor circulation impairs the delivery of the cells and biochemicals for the immune and inflammatory responses. This same sluggish circulation makes infection following reparative surgery a significant risk. Varicose veins and CVI may be associated with **deep venous thrombosis (DVT)** in up to 15% of affected individuals because of changes in collateral flow and shared risk factors; therefore, anyone with new-onset varicose veins should be evaluated for the possibility of underlying DVT.[3]

Treatment of varicose veins and CVI begins conservatively, and excellent wound healing results have followed noninvasive treatments, such as leg elevation, compression stockings, and physical exercise.[1] Invasive management includes sclerotherapy or surgical ligation and vein stripping.

Thrombus formation in veins

A **thrombus** is a blood clot that remains attached to a vessel wall (see Figures 23-2 and 20-16). A detached thrombus is a **thromboembolus.** Venous thrombi are more common than arterial thrombi because flow and pressure are lower in the veins than in the arteries. Deep venous thrombosis (DVT) occurs primarily in the lower extremity. Three factors (triad of Virchow) promote venous thrombosis: (1) venous stasis (e.g., immobility, age, congestive heart failure), (2) venous endothelial damage (e.g., trauma, medications), and (3) hypercoagulable states (e.g., inherited disorders, malignancy, pregnancy, oral contraceptives, hormone replacement). Orthopedic trauma or surgery, spinal cord injury, and obstetric/gynecologic conditions can be associated with up to a 100% likelihood of DVT. Numerous genetic abnormalities are associated with an increased risk for venous thrombosis primarily related to states of hypercoagulability. These inherited abnormalities include factor V Leiden mutation; prothrombin mutations; and deficiencies of protein C, protein S, and antithrombin and are commonly found in individuals who develop thrombi in the absence of the usual risk factors.[4]

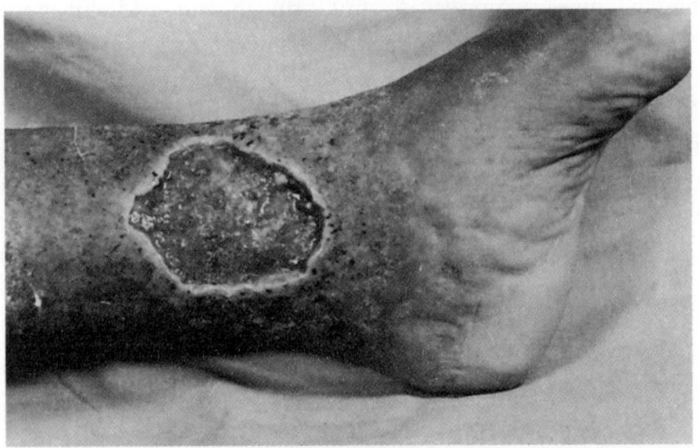

Figure 23-1 ■ **Venous Stasis Ulcer.** (From Rosai J: *Ackerman's surgical pathology,* ed 7, vol 2, St Louis, 1989, Mosby.)

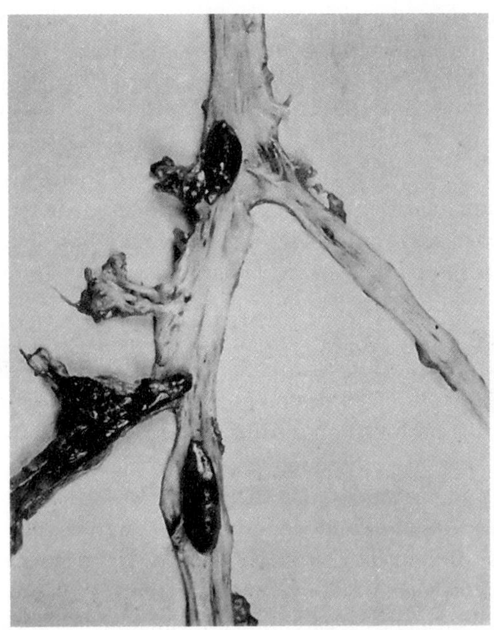

Figure 23-2 ■ **Multiple Venous Thrombi.** (From Rosai J: *Ackerman's surgical pathology,* ed 7, vol 2, St Louis, 1989, Mosby.)

Accumulation of clotting factors and platelets leads to thrombus formation in the vein, often near a venous valve. Inflammation around the thrombus promotes further platelet aggregation, and the thrombus propagates or grows proximally. This inflammation may cause pain and redness, but because the vein is deep in the leg, it is usually not accompanied by clinical symptoms or signs. If the thrombus creates significant obstruction to venous blood flow, increased pressure in the vein behind the clot may lead to edema of the extremity. Most thrombi will eventually dissolve without treatment, but untreated DVT is associated with a high risk of embolization of a part of the clot (pulmonary embolism) and may lead to persistent venous outflow obstruction and postthrombotic syndrome.

Prevention is important in at-risk individuals and includes early ambulation, pneumatic devices, and prophylactic anticoagulation. If thrombosis does occur, diagnosis is confirmed by a combination of serum D-dimer measurement and Doppler ultrasonography. Management consists of anticoagulation with heparin (low-molecular weight heparin) and warfarin. In selected individuals, thrombolytic therapy or placement of an inferior vena cava filter may be indicated.[5]

Superior vena cava syndrome

Superior vena cava syndrome (SVCS) is a progressive occlusion of the superior vena cava (SVC) that leads to venous distention in the upper extremities and head. Causes include bronchogenic cancer (75% of cases), followed by lymphomas (15%), and metastasis of other cancers (7%). The SVC is a relatively low-pressure vessel that lies in the closed thoracic compartment; therefore, tissue expansion can easily compress the SVC. The right main stem bronchus abuts the SVC so that cancers occurring in this bronchus may press on the SVC. Additionally, the SVC is surrounded by lymph nodes and lymph chains that commonly become involved in thoracic cancers and compress the SVC during tumor growth. Because onset of SVCS is slow, collateral venous drainage to the azygous vein usually has time to develop. Chronic cases of SVCS have also been attributed to arteriovenous shunt lesions, lymphadenopathy in cystic fibrosis, and goiter. Acute cases of SVCS have been attributed to pacemaker implantation, long-term indwelling central venous catheters, and pleural effusion.

Clinical manifestations of SVCS are edema and venous distention in the upper extremities and face, including the ocular beds. Affected persons complain of a feeling of fullness in the head or tightness of shirt collars, necklaces, and rings. Cerebral edema may cause headache, visual disturbance, and impaired consciousness. The skin of the face and arms may become purple and taut, and capillary refill time is prolonged. Respiratory distress may be present because of edema of bronchial structures or compression of the bronchus by a carcinoma. In infants, SVCS can lead to hydrocephalus.

Diagnosis is made by chest roentgenogram, Doppler studies, computed tomography (CT), magnetic resonance imaging (MRI), and ultrasound. Because of its slow onset and the development of collateral venous drainage, SVCS is generally not a vascular emergency, but it is an oncologic emergency. Treatment for malignant disorders can include radiation therapy; surgery; chemotherapy; and the administration of diuretics, steroids, and anticoagulants, as necessary. Treatment for nonmalignant causes may include bypass surgery using various grafts; thrombolysis, both locally and systemically; balloon angioplasty; and placement of intravascular stents.[6]

QUICK CHECK 23-1

1. What are the major risk factors for DVT?
2. What is chronic venous insufficiency, and how does it present clinically?
3. Name some causes of superior vena cava syndrome.

Hypertension

Hypertension is consistent elevation of systemic arterial blood pressure. Hypertension is the most common primary diagnosis in the United States. Approximately 65% of Americans older than the age of 60 have hypertension, and fewer than two thirds have their hypertension adequately controlled.[7] Hypertension is defined by the Seventh Joint National Committee Report[8] as a sustained systolic blood pressure of 140 mm Hg or greater systolic pressure or a diastolic pressure of 90 mm Hg or greater (Table 23-1). Normal blood pressure is associated with the lowest cardiovascular risk, whereas those who fall into the prehypertension category are at risk for developing hypertension unless lifestyle modification is instituted (over 90% will develop hypertension).[8] All stages of hypertension are associated with increased risk for target organ disease events, such as myocardial infarction, kidney disease, and stroke; thus both stage I and stage II hypertension need effective long-term therapy.[8] Systolic hypertension, even when not accompanied by an increase in diastolic pressure, is the most significant factor in causing target organ damage. The prevalence of hypertension increases with age and is higher for blacks than for whites.[9]

TABLE 23-1
Classification of Blood Pressure for Adults Age 18 Years or Older

	Systolic (mm Hg)	Diastolic Category (mm Hg)
Normal	<120	<80
Prehypertension	120–139	80–89
Stage 1 hypertension	140–159	90–99
Stage 2 hypertension	≥160	≥100

Data from Chobanian AV et al: The JNC 7 Report, *JAMA* 289 (19):2560–2572, 2003.

Individuals may have combined systolic and diastolic hypertension or isolated systolic hypertension. Most cases of combined systolic and diastolic hypertension are diagnosed as **primary hypertension** (also called **essential** or **idiopathic hypertension**). From 92% to 95% of hypertensive individuals have primary disease. **Secondary hypertension** is caused by an underlying disorder such as renal disease. This form of hypertension accounts for only 5% to 8% of cases.

Factors associated with primary hypertension

A specific cause for primary hypertension has not been identified, and a combination of genetic and environmental factors is thought to be responsible for its development. Genetic predisposition to hypertension is thought to be polygenic. The inherited defects are associated with renal sodium excretion, insulin and insulin sensitivity, activity of the renin-angiotensin-aldosterone system, cell membrane sodium or calcium transport, and sympathetic response to neurogenic hormones. A mutation in the adducin gene has been linked to changes in renal tubular sodium transport and hypertension (see Health Alert: Genes and the Risk for Hypertension). Factors associated with primary hypertension include (1) family history of hypertension; (2) advancing age; (3) gender (more common in men than women before age 55 years , more common in women after age 55); (4) black race; (5) high dietary sodium intake; (6) glucose intolerance (diabetes mellitus); (7) cigarette smoking; (8) obesity; (9) heavy alcohol consumption; and (10) low dietary intake of potassium, calcium, and magnesium (see *Risk Factors:* Primary Hypertension). Many of these factors are also risk factors for other cardiovascular disorders. In fact, hypertension, dyslipidemia, and glucose intolerance often are found together.

Although populations with high dietary sodium intake have long been shown to have an increased incidence of hypertension, studies indicate that low dietary potassium, calcium, and magnesium intakes are also risk factors because without their intake, sodium is retained.[10] The nicotine in cigarette smoke is a vasoconstrictor that can elevate both systolic and diastolic blood pressure acutely. In habitual smokers, an individual cigarette may not raise blood pressure, yet habitual smoking is associated with a high incidence of severe hypertension, myocardial hypertrophy, and death resulting from coronary artery disease (CAD). The incidence of hypertension is higher among heavy drinkers of alcohol (more than three drinks per day) than among abstainers, but moderate drinkers (two to four drinks per week) appear to have lower blood pressures, as well as lower cardiovascular mortality, than either abstainers or heavy drinkers. Obesity is recognized as an important risk factor for hypertension and contributes to many of the neurohumoral, metabolic, renal, and cardiovascular processes that cause hypertension, especially those factors that contribute to endothelial dysfunction and renal sodium retention.[11]

HEALTH ALERT

Genes and the Risk for Hypertension

Heritability accounts for an estimated 30% to 40% of primary hypertension. Gene polymorphisms that have been implicated include angiotensin II receptor genes, angiotensinogen, and renin genes; endothelial nitric oxide synthetase genes; G protein receptor kinase gene; aldosterone genes and adrenergic receptor genes; calcium transport and sodium-hydrogen antiporter genes (affect salt sensitivity); and genes that are associated with insulin resistance, obesity, hyperlipidemia, and hypertension as a cluster of traits. Adducin is a membrane-skeleton protein that plays an important role in the determination of cellular morphology and motility and in the regulation of membrane ion transport. It interacts with Na^+, K^+ ATPase and thus regulates the sodium-potassium pump. Mutations (e.g., *ADD1* Gly460Trp) of the gene that codes for adducin cause an increase in tubular renal reabsorption of sodium and are associated with an approximately 50% to 70% increase in risk for hypertension in whites. The presence of an adducin gene mutation indicates that the affected individual is more likely to be salt sensitive and to respond more effectively to diuretic treatment of his or her hypertension. These discoveries have led to potential new treatments for hypertension using gene therapy techniques.

Data from Bianchi G, Tripodi G: Genetics of hypertension: the adducin paradigm, *Ann NY Acad Sci* 986:660–668, 2003; Marteau JB et al: Genetic determinants of blood pressure regulation, *J Hypertens* 23(12):2127–2143, 2005; Phillips MI, Kimura B: Antisense therapeutics for hypertension: targeting the renin-angiotensin system, *Methods Molec Med* 106:51–68, 2005; Raizada MK, Der Sarkissian S: Potential of gene therapy strategy for the treatment of hypertension, *Hypertens* 47(1):6–9, 2006; Tanira MO, Al Balushi KA: Genetic variations related to hypertension: a review, *J Human Hypertens* 19:7–19, 2005.

RISK FACTORS Primary Hypertension

- Family history
- Advancing age
- Cigarette smoking
- Obesity
- Heavy alcohol consumption
- Gender (men > women before age 55, women > men after 55)
- Black race
- High dietary sodium intake
- Low dietary intake of potassium, calcium, magnesium
- Glucose intolerance

PATHOPHYSIOLOGY Hypertension results from a sustained increase in peripheral resistance (arteriolar vasoconstriction), an increase in circulating blood volume, or both.

Primary hypertension

Primary hypertension is the result of an extremely complicated interaction of genetics and the environment mediated by a host of neurohumoral effects. Multiple pathophysiologic mechanisms mediate these effects, including the sympathetic nervous system (SNS), the renin-angiotensin-aldosterone (RAA) system, and natriuretic peptides. Inflammation, endothelial dysfunction, and insulin resistance also contribute to both increased peripheral resistance and increased blood volume. Increased vascular volume is related to a decrease in renal excretion of salt, often referred to as a shift in the **pressure-natriuresis relationship** (Figure 23-3). This means that for a given blood pressure, individuals with hypertension tend to secrete less salt in their urine.[12]

The sympathetic nervous system has been implicated in both the development and the maintenance of elevated blood pressure and plays a role in hypertensive end-organ damage. Increased SNS activity causes increased heart rate and systemic vasoconstriction, thus raising the blood pressure. Additional mechanisms of SNS-induced hypertension include structural changes in blood vessels (vascular remodeling), renal sodium retention (shift in natriuresis curve), insulin resistance, increased renin and angiotensin levels, and procoagulant effects.[13]

The renin-angiotensin-aldosterone system plays an important role in blood pressure regulation by moderating vascular tone and influencing salt and water retention by the kidneys (see Figure 22-31). Further, angiotensin II mediates arteriolar remodeling, which is structural change in the vessel wall that results in permanent increases in peripheral resistance (see Figure 22-32). Angiotensin II is associated with end-organ effects of hypertension, including atherosclerosis, renal disease, and cardiac hypertrophy. Finally, aldosterone not only contributes to sodium retention by the kidney but also has other deleterious effects on the cardiovascular system.[14]

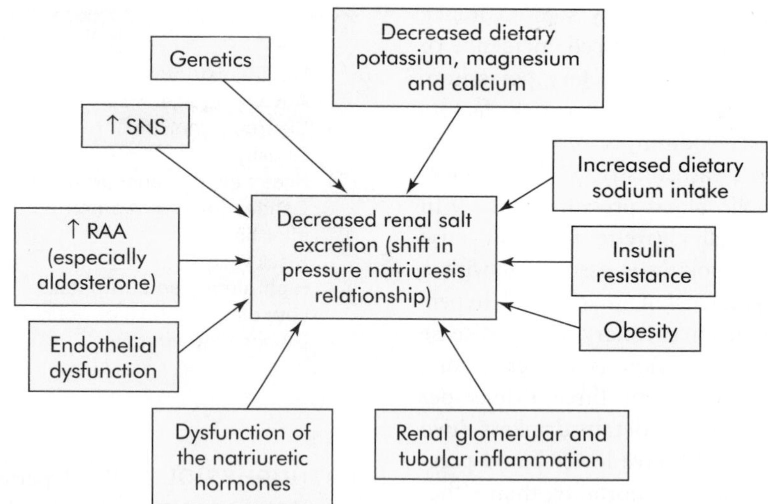

Figure 23-3 ■ **Factors that Cause a Shift in the Pressure-Natriuresis Relationship.** Numerous factors have been implicated in the pathogenesis of sodium retention in individuals with hypertension. These factors cause less renal excretion of salt than would normally occur with increased blood pressure. This is called a *shift in the pressure-natriuresis relationship* and is believed to be a central process in the pathogenesis of primary hypertension. *SNS,* Sympathetic nervous system; *RAA,* renin-angiotensin-aldosterone.

Natriuretic hormones modulate renal sodium (Na^+) excretion and include atrial natriuretic peptide (ANP), brain natriuretic peptide (BNP), C-type natriuretic peptide (CNP), and urodilatin. The function of these hormones can be affected by excessive sodium intake; inadequate dietary intake of potassium, magnesium, and calcium; and obesity.[10,15] Dysfunction of these hormones, along with alterations in the RAA system and the SNS, cause an increase in vascular tone and a shift in the pressure-natriuresis relationship. Salt retention leads to water retention and increased blood volume, which contributes to an increase in blood pressure. Subtle renal injury results, with renal vasoconstriction and tissue ischemia. Tissue ischemia causes inflammation of the kidney and contributes to dysfunction of the glomeruli and tubules and promotes additional sodium retention.

Inflammation plays a role in the pathogenesis of hypertension.[16] Endothelial injury and tissue ischemia result in the release of vasoactive inflammatory cytokines. Although many of these cytokines (e.g., histamine, prostaglandins) have vasodilatory actions in acute inflammatory injury, chronic inflammation contributes to vascular remodeling and smooth muscle contraction. Endothelial injury and dysfunction in primary hypertension is further characterized by a decreased production of vasodilators, such as nitric oxide, and increased production of vasoconstrictors, such as endothelin.

Obesity causes changes in systemic hemodynamics that may contribute to hypertension. It is also associated with increased activity of the sympathetic nervous system (perhaps because of high levels of leptin), and the RAA system. Obesity is linked to endothelial dysfunction (increased endogenous vasoconstrictors and insulin resistance) (see *Health Alert:* Obesity and Hypertension).[11]

HEALTH ALERT
Obesity and Hypertension

Several hemodynamic and metabolic abnormalities have been implicated in the development of hypertension in obesity. These include activation of the sympathetic nervous system and the renin-angiotensin-aldosterone system, insulin resistance, endothelial dysfunction, and renal functional abnormalities. One of the major mechanisms leading to the development of obesity-induced hypertension appears to be leptin-mediated effects on blood vessels and the kidney. Leptin is a circulating peptide hormone that is primarily secreted by adipocytes. Although obesity is generally associated with resistance to the weight-reducing actions of leptin, the resultant increased levels of this peptide cause an increase in sympathetic nervous system activity and adversely shift the renal pressure-natriuresis curve leading to sodium retention. Further studies aimed at achieving a better understanding of leptin signaling in the hypothalamus and in the renal and vascular systems may lead to new treatments for obesity-related hypertension.

Data from Correia ML, Haynes WG: Leptin, obesity and cardiovascular disease, *Curr Opin Nephrol Hypertens* 13(2): 215–223, 2004; Haynes WG: Role of leptin in obesity-related hypertension, *Experim Physiol* 90(5):683–688, 2005; Mukherjee R et al: Leptin as a common link to obesity and hypertension, *Drugs Today* 41(10):687–695, 2005; Rahmouni K et al: Obesity-associated hypertension: new insights into mechanisms, Hypertens 45(1):9–14, 2005.

Finally, insulin resistance is common in hypertension, even in individuals without clinical diabetes.[17] Insulin resistance is associated with decreased endothelial release of nitric oxide and other vasodilators. It also affects renal function and causes renal salt and water retention. Insulin resistance is associated with overactivity of the sympathetic nervous system and the renin-angiotensin-aldosterone system. It is interesting to note that in many individuals with diabetes treated with drugs that increase insulin sensitivity, blood pressure often declines, even in the absence of antihypertensive drugs.

It is likely that primary hypertension is an interaction between many of these factors leading to sustained increases in blood volume and peripheral resistance. The pathophysiology of primary hypertension is summarized in Figure 23-4.

Secondary hypertension

Secondary hypertension is caused by an underlying disease process or medication that raises peripheral vascular resistance or cardiac output. Examples include renal vascular or parenchymal disease, adrenocortical tumors, adrenomedullary tumors (pheochromocytoma), and drugs (oral contraceptives, corticosteroids, antihistamines). If the cause is identified and removed before permanent structural changes occur, blood pressure returns to normal.

Isolated systolic hypertension

Isolated systolic hypertension (ISH) is typically defined as a sustained systolic BP that is $\geq$140 mm Hg and diastolic BP that is below 90 mm Hg. ISH accounts for a substantial proportion of hypertension in individuals older than 65 years and is strongly associated with cardiovascular and cerebrovascular events.

An increased pulse pressure (PP) (systolic minus diastolic pressure) indicates reduced vascular compliance of large arteries. PP is always increased in isolated systolic hypertension. Mechanisms of aortic stiffening include gradual vascular calcification, changes in elastic fibers, and increases of a rigid component like collagen.

Complicated hypertension

Cardiovascular complications of sustained hypertension include left ventricular hypertrophy, angina pectoris, congestive heart failure (left heart failure), coronary artery disease, myocardial infarction, and sudden death. Myocardial hypertrophy in response to hypertension is mediated by several neurohormonal substances, including catecholamines from the SNS and angiotensin II.[18] This results in changes in the myocyte proteins, apoptosis of myocytes, and deposition of collagen in heart muscle. In addition, the increased size of the heart muscle increases demand for oxygen delivery over time, contractility of the heart is impaired and the individual is at increased risk for heart failure. Vascular complications include the formation, dissection, and rupture of aneurysms (outpouchings in vessel walls) and atherosclerosis leading to vessel occlusion. Possible renal complications are parenchymal damage, nephrosclerosis, renal arteriosclerosis, and renal insufficiency or failure.[18] Microalbuminuria (small amounts of protein in the urine) occurs in 10% to 25% of individuals with essential hypertension and is now recognized as an early sign of impending renal dysfunction and significantly increased risk for cardiovascular events, especially in those who also have diabetes.[19]

Changes in the vascular beds can be estimated by viewing the arterioles of the retina. Complications specific to the retina include retinal vascular sclerosis, exudation, and hemorrhage. Cerebrovascular complications are similar to those of other arterial beds and include transient ischemia, stroke, cerebral thrombosis, aneurysm, and hemorrhage. Chronic hypertension also has been linked to

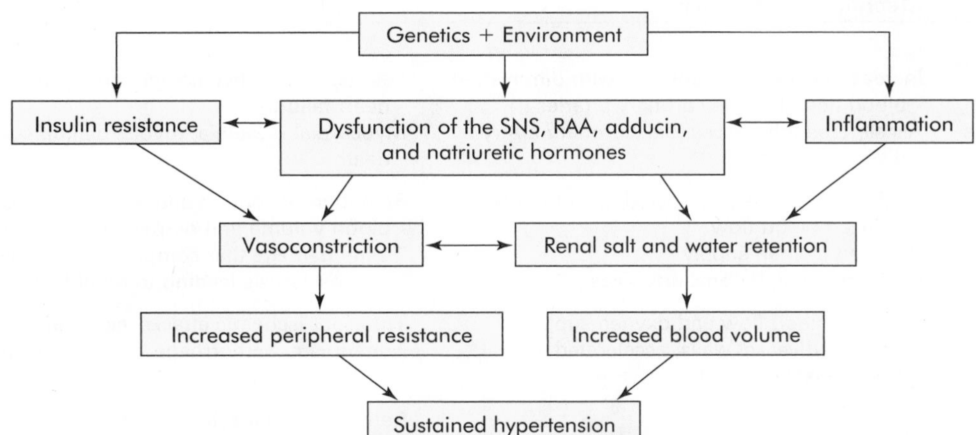

Figure 23-4 ■ **Pathophysiology of Hypertension.** Numerous genetic vulnerabilities have been linked to hypertension and these, in combination with environmental risks, cause neurohumoral dysfunction (sympathetic nervous system [SNS], renin-angiotensin-aldosterone [RAA] system, adducin, and natriuretic hormones) and promote inflammation and insulin resistance. Insulin resistance and neurohumoral dysfunction contribute to sustained systemic vasoconstriction and increased peripheral resistance. Inflammation contributes to renal dysfunction, which, in combination with the neurohumoral alterations, results in renal salt and water retention and increased blood volume. Increased peripheral resistance and increased blood volume are two primary causes of sustained hypertension.

cognitive decline in the elderly.[18] The pathologic effects of complicated hypertension are summarized in Table 23-2.

Malignant hypertension (rapidly progressive hypertension in which diastolic pressure is usually above 140 mm Hg) can cause encephalopathy, a profound cerebral edema that disrupts cerebral function and causes loss of consciousness. High arterial pressure renders the cerebral arterioles incapable of regulating blood flow to the cerebral capillary beds. High hydrostatic pressures in the capillaries cause vascular fluid to exude into the interstitial space. If blood pressure is not reduced, cerebral edema and cerebral dysfunction increase until death occurs. Organ damage resulting from malignant hypertension is life threatening. Besides encephalopathy, malignant hypertension can cause papilledema, cardiac failure, uremia, retinopathy, and cerebrovascular accident.

CLINICAL MANIFESTATIONS The early stages of hypertension have no clinical manifestations other than elevated blood pressure. Most important, there are no signs and symptoms to cause the individual to seek health care; thus, hypertension is called a silent disease. Some hypertensive individuals never have signs, symptoms, or complications, whereas others become very ill, and hypertension can be a cause of death. Still other individuals have anatomic and physiologic damage caused by past hypertensive disease, despite current blood pressures being within normal ranges.

The chance of developing primary hypertension increases with age. Although hypertension is usually thought to be an adult health problem, it is important to remember that hypertension does occur in children and is being diagnosed with increasing frequency (see Chapter 24). Usually, however, increased peripheral resistance and early hypertension develop in the second, third, and fourth decades of life. If elevated blood pressure is not detected and treated, it becomes established and may begin to accelerate its effects on tissues when the individual is 30 to 50 years of age. This sets the stage for the complications of hypertension that begin to appear during the fourth, fifth, and sixth decades of life.

Most clinical manifestations of hypertensive disease are caused by complications that damage organs and tissues outside the vascular system. Besides elevated blood pressure, the signs and symptoms therefore tend to be specific for the organs or tissues affected. Evidence of heart disease, renal insufficiency, central nervous system dysfunction, impaired vision, impaired mobility, vascular occlusion, or edema can all be caused by sustained hypertension.

EVALUATION AND TREATMENT A single elevated blood pressure reading does not mean that a person has hypertension. Diagnosis requires the measurement of blood pressure on at least two separate occasions averaging two readings at least 2 minutes apart, with the patient seated, the arm supported at heart level, after 5 minutes rest, with no smoking or caffeine intake in the previous 30 minutes.[8] Diagnostic tests for further evaluation of hypertension include 24-hour blood pressure monitoring in selected individuals, complete blood count, urinalysis, biochemical blood profile (plasma glucose, sodium, potassium, calcium, magnesium, creatinine, cholesterol, triglycerides), and an electrocardiogram. Individuals who have elevated blood

TABLE 23-2

Pathologic Effects of Sustained, Complicated Primary Hypertension

Site of Injury	Mechanism of Injury	Potential Pathologic Effect
HEART		
Myocardium	Increased workload combined with diminished blood flow through coronary arteries	Left ventricular hypertrophy, myocardial ischemia, left heart failure
Coronary arteries	Accelerated atherosclerosis (coronary artery disease)	Myocardial ischemia, myocardial infarction, sudden death
KIDNEYS	Renin and aldosterone secretion stimulated by reduced blood flow	Retention of sodium and water, leading to increased blood volume and perpetuation of hypertension
	Reduced oxygen supply	Tissue damage that compromises filtration
	High pressures in renal arterioles	Nephrosclerosis leading to renal failure
BRAIN	Reduced blood flow and oxygen supply; weakened vessel walls, accelerated atherosclerosis	Transient ischemic attacks, cerebral thrombosis, aneurysm, hemorrhage, acute brain infarction
EYES (RETINAS)	Reduced blood flow	Retinal vascular sclerosis
	High arteriolar pressure	Exudation, hemorrhage
AORTA	Weakened vessel wall	Dissecting aneurysm (see p. 614)
ARTERIES OF LOWER EXTREMITIES	Reduced blood flow and high pressures in arterioles, accelerated atherosclerosis	Intermittent claudication, gangrene

pressure are assumed to have primary hypertension unless their history, physical examination, or initial diagnostic screening indicates secondary hypertension. Once the diagnosis is made, a careful evaluation for other cardiovascular risk factors and for end-organ damage should be done.[8]

Treatment of primary hypertension depends on its severity. Lifestyle modification is important for preventing hypertension in those individuals who fall into the prehypertension category and for treating hypertension. Important lifestyle modifications include exercise, dietary modification, smoking cessation, and weight loss.[8] Figure 23-5 summarizes guidelines for the overall management of hypertension.

Orthostatic (Postural) Hypotension

The term **orthostatic (postural) hypotension** refers to a decrease in both systolic and diastolic arterial blood pressure on standing. Normally when an individual stands up, the gravitational changes on the circulation are compensated for by such mechanisms as reflex arteriolar and venous constriction, increased heart rate, and mechanical factors, such as the closure of valves in the venous system, pumping of the leg muscles, and a decrease in intrathoracic pressure. The normally increased sympathetic activity during upright posture is mediated through a stretch receptor (baroreceptor) reflex that responds to shifts in volume caused by postural changes. This reflex promptly increases heart rate and constricts the systemic arterioles. Thus, arterial blood pressure is maintained.

Orthostatic hypotension is often accompanied by dizziness, blurring or loss of vision, and syncope or fainting caused by insufficient vasomotor compensation and reduction of blood flow through the brain. This occurs because the normal or compensatory vasoconstrictor response to standing is absent so that there is blood pooling in the muscle vasculature, as well as in the splanchnic and renal beds.

Orthostatic hypotension may be acute and temporary or chronic. **Acute orthostatic hypotension** is caused when the normal regulatory mechanisms are sluggish as a result of (1) altered body chemistry, (2) drug action (e.g., antihypertensives, antidepressants), (3) prolonged immobility caused by illness, (4) starvation, (5) physical exhaustion, (6) any condition that produces volume depletion (e.g., dehydration, diuresis, potassium or sodium depletion), or (7) venous pooling (e.g., pregnancy, extensive varicosities of the lower extremities). Elderly persons are particularly susceptible to this type of orthostatic hypotension.

Chronic orthostatic hypotension may be (1) secondary to a specific disease or (2) idiopathic or primary. The

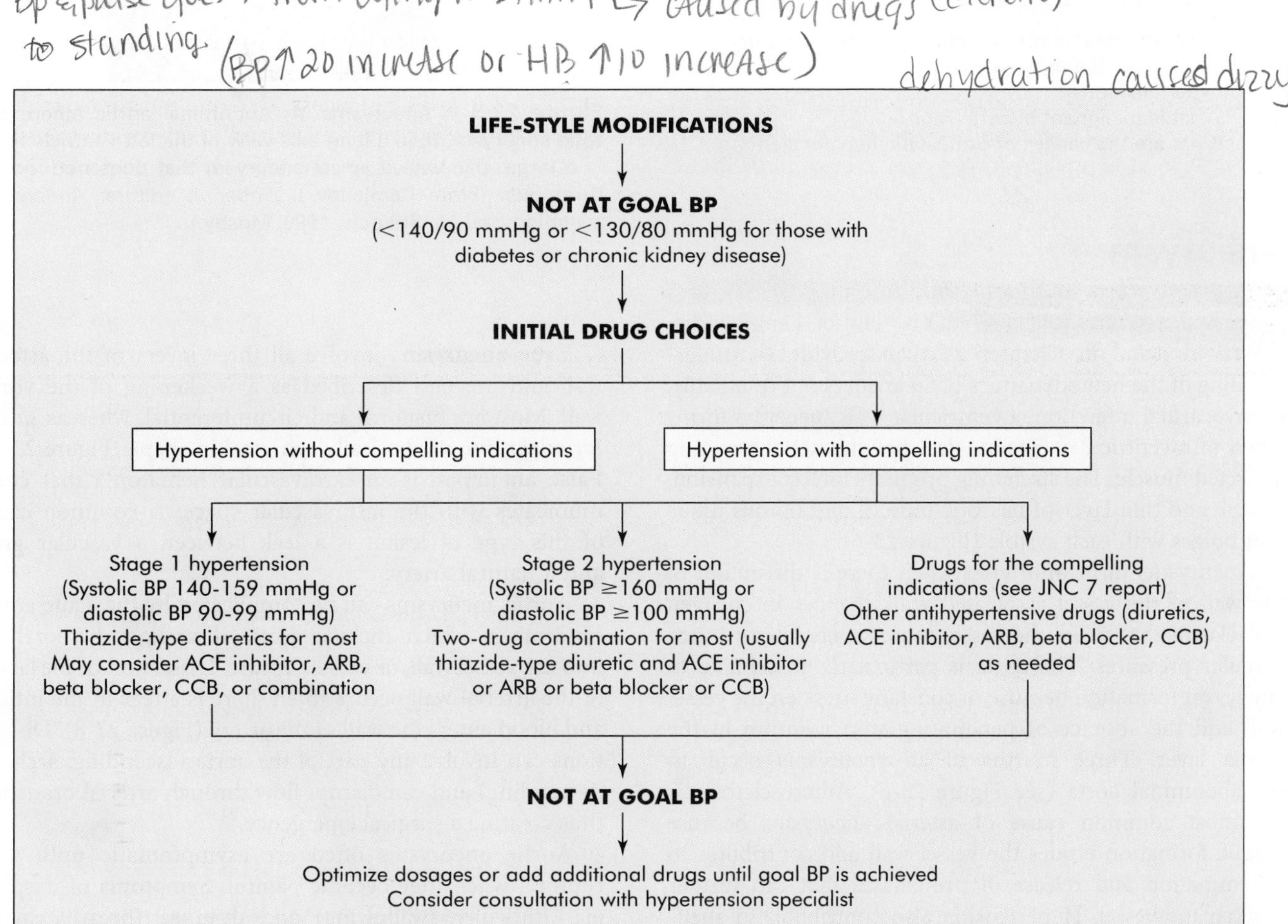

Figure 23-5 ■ **Summary of Treatment Recommendations for Hypertension.** *BP,* Blood pressure; *ACE,* angiotensin-converting enzyme; *ARB,* angiotensin-receptor blocker; *CCB,* calcium channel blocker. (Data from Chobanian AV et al: The JNC 7 Report, *JAMA* 289(19):2560–2572, 2003.)

diseases that cause secondary orthostatic hypotension are endocrine disorders (e.g., adrenal insufficiency, diabetes mellitus), metabolic disorders (e.g., porphyria), or diseases of the central or peripheral nervous systems (e.g., intracranial tumors, cerebral infarcts, Wernicke encephalopathy, peripheral neuropathies).

The term *idiopathic*, or *primary*, orthostatic hypotension implies no known initial cause. Some define the disorder as a separate entity, whereas others suggest it is a part of a generalized degenerative central nervous system disease. It affects men more often than women and usually occurs between the ages of 40 and 70 years. One third to half of the elderly population may be affected by primary orthostatic hypotension, and it is a significant risk factor for falls and associated injury.[20] In addition to cardiovascular symptoms, associated impotence and bowel and bladder dysfunction are common.

Although no curative treatment is available for idiopathic orthostatic hypotension, often it can be managed adequately with a combination of nondrug and drug therapies. For both acute and secondary forms, hypotension resolves when the underlying disorder is corrected.

QUICK CHECK 23-2

1. What are the major risk factors for hypertension?
2. Summarize the pathophysiology of primary hypertension.
3. What is malignant hypertension?
4. What are the causes of orthostatic hypotension?

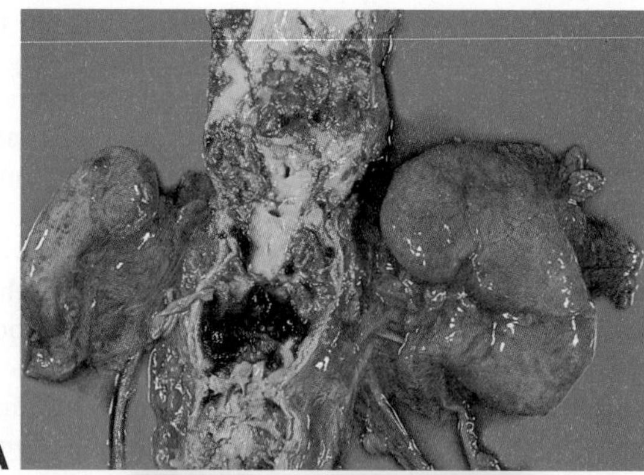

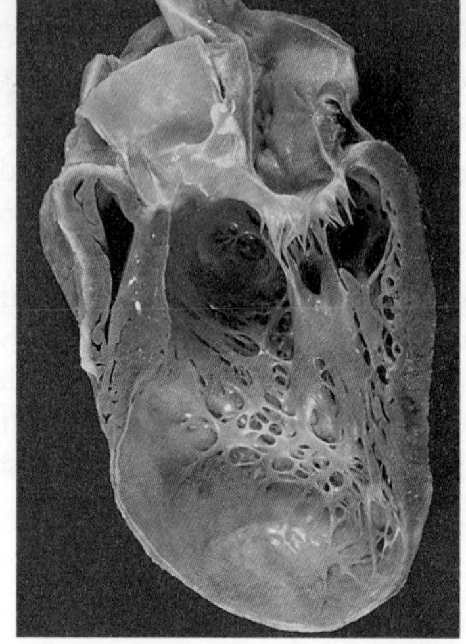

Figure 23-6 ■ **Aneurysms. A,** Abdominal aortic atherosclerotic aneurysm. **B,** In a long-axis view of the left ventricle there is a large, thin-walled apical aneurysm that does not contain thrombus. (From Damjanov I, Linder J, editors: *Anderson's pathology*, ed 10, St Louis, 1996, Mosby.)

Aneurysm

An **aneurysm** is a localized dilation or outpouching of a vessel wall or cardiac chamber. The law of Laplace (discussed in detail in Chapter 22) can provide an understanding of the hemodynamics of an aneurysm. Presumably, in myocardial infarction, a ventricular wall aneurysm forms when intraventricular tension stretches the noncontracting infarcted muscle. The stretching produces infarct expansion, a weak and thin layer of necrotic muscle, and fibrous tissue that bulges with each systole (Figure 23-6).

Aneurysms form in arteries when there is disruption of the wall of the vessel associated with changes in collagen and elastin that make the vessel more vulnerable to intravascular pressures. The aorta is particularly susceptible to aneurysm formation because of constant stress on the vessel wall and the absence of penetrating vasa vasorum in the media layer. Three fourths of all aneurysms occur in the abdominal aorta (see Figure 23-6). Atherosclerosis is the most common cause of arterial aneurysms because plaque formation erodes the vessel wall and contributes to inflammation and release of proteinases that can further weaken the vessel. Hypertension also contributes to aneurysm formation by increasing wall stress. Collagen-vascular disorders (e.g., Marfan syndrome), syphilis, and other infections that affect arterial walls also can cause aneurysms.

True aneurysms involve all three layers of the arterial wall and are best described as a weakening of the vessel wall. Most are fusiform and circumferential, whereas *saccular aneurysms* are basically spherical in shape (Figure 23-7). **False aneurysm** is an extravascular hematoma that communicates with the intravascular space. A common cause of this type of lesion is a leak between a vascular graft and a natural artery.

Aortic aneurysms can be complicated by the acute aortic syndromes, which include aortic dissection, hemorrhage into the vessel wall, or vessel rupture. Dissection of the layers of the arterial wall occurs when there is a tear in the intima and blood enters the wall of the artery (Figure 23-8). Dissections can involve any part of the aorta (ascending, arch, or descending) and can disrupt flow through arterial branches, thus creating a surgical emergency.[21]

Aortic aneurysms often are asymptomatic until they rupture, when they become painful. Symptoms of dysphagia (difficulty swallowing) and dyspnea (breathlessness) are caused by the pressure of a thoracic aneurysm on surrounding organs. An aneurysm that impairs flow to an extremity causes symptoms of ischemia. Cerebral aneurysms,

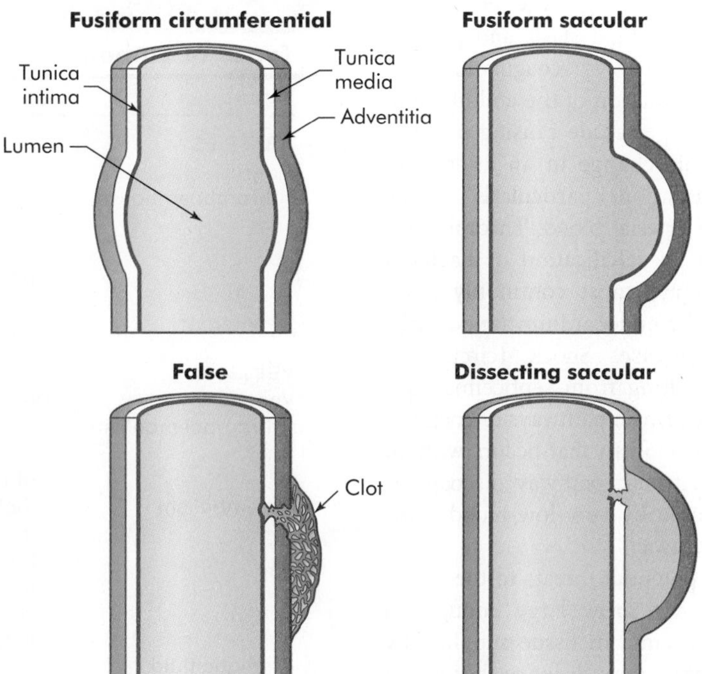

Figure 23-7 ■ **Longitudinal Sections Showing Types of Aneurysms.** The fusiform circumferential and fusiform saccular aneurysms are true aneurysms, caused by weakening of the vessel wall. False and saccular aneurysms involve a break in the vessel wall, usually caused by trauma.

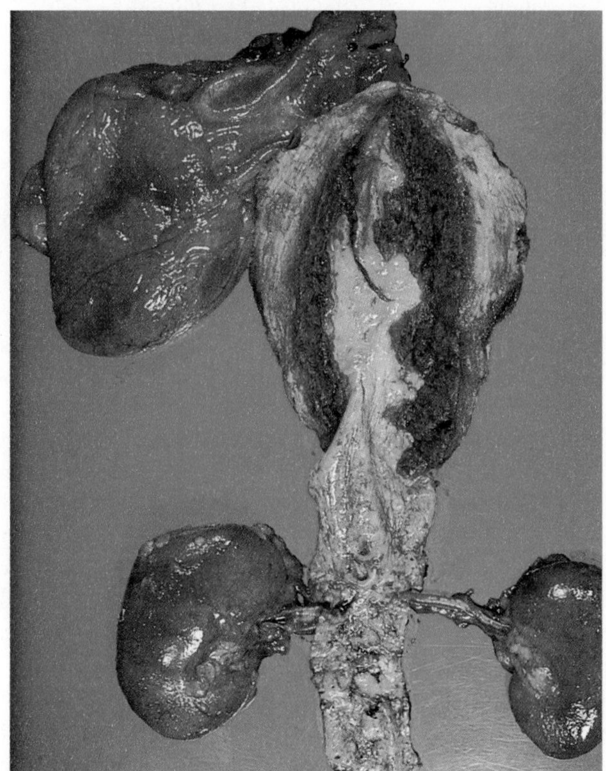

Figure 23-8 ■ **Dissecting Aneurysm of Thoracic Aorta.** (From Damjanov I, Linder J, editors: *Anderson's pathology,* ed 10, St Louis, 1996, Mosby.)

which often occur in the circle of Willis, are associated with signs and symptoms of increased intracranial pressure. Signs and symptoms of stroke occur when cerebral aneurysms leak. (Cerebral aneurysms are described in Chapter 15.)

The diagnosis of an aneurysm is usually confirmed by ultrasonography, computed tomography, magnetic resonance imaging, or angiography. The goals of medical treatment of aneurysms are to maintain a low blood volume and low blood pressure to decrease mechanical forces thought to contribute to vessel wall dilation. Medical treatment is indicated for slow-growing aortic aneurysms, particularly in early stages, and includes smoking cessation, reducing blood pressure (β-adrenergic blockage) and blood volume. For those aneurysms that are dilating rapidly, surgical treatment often is indicated. Surgery should be done when aortic aneurysms become large and usually includes replacement with a prosthetic graft. New endovascular surgical techniques make aneurysm repair possible for more individuals.[22]

Thrombus Formation

As in venous thrombosis, arterial thrombi tend to develop when intravascular conditions promote activation of coagulation, or when there is stasis of blood flow. These conditions include those in which there is intimal irritation or roughening (such as in surgical procedures), inflammation, traumatic injury, infection, low blood pressures, or obstructions that cause blood stasis and pooling within the vessels. (Mechanisms of coagulation are described in Chapter 19.) Inflammation of the endothelium leads to activation of the clotting cascade causing platelets to adhere readily. An anatomic change in an artery can contribute to thrombus formation, particularly if the change results in a pooling of arterial blood. Thrombi also form on heart valves altered by calcification or bacterial vegetation. Valvular thrombi are most commonly associated with inflammation of the endocardium (endocarditis) and rheumatic heart disease. Shock (circulatory failure), particularly shock resulting from septicemia, also can activate the intrinsic and extrinsic pathways of coagulation. The impaired cellular metabolism that occurs with all types of shock activates the extrinsic pathway of coagulation, whereas blood stasis caused by very low blood pressures activates the intrinsic pathway.

Arterial thrombi pose two potential threats to the circulation. First, the thrombus may grow large enough to occlude the artery, causing ischemia in tissue supplied by the artery. Second, the thrombus may dislodge, becoming a thromboembolus that travels through the vascular system until it occludes flow into a distal systemic vascular bed.

Diagnosis of arterial thrombi is usually accomplished through the use of Doppler ultrasonography and angiography. Pharmacologic treatment involves the administration of heparin, warfarin derivatives, thrombin inhibitors, or thrombolytics. A balloon-tipped catheter also can be used to remove or compress an arterial thrombus. Various combinations of drug and catheter therapies are sometimes used concurrently.

Embolism

Embolism is the obstruction of a vessel by an **embolus**—a bolus of matter circulating in the bloodstream. The embolus may consist of a dislodged thrombus; an air bubble; an aggregate of amniotic fluid; an aggregate of fat, bacteria, or cancer cells; or a foreign substance. An embolus travels in the bloodstream until it reaches a vessel through which it cannot fit. No matter how tiny it is, an embolus will eventually lodge in a systemic or pulmonary vessel determined by its source. Pulmonary emboli originate on the venous side (mostly from the deep veins of the legs) of the systemic circulation or in the right heart; systemic (or arterial) emboli most commonly originate in the left heart and are associated with thrombi after myocardial infarction, valvular disease, left heart failure, endocarditis, and dysrhythmias.

Embolism causes ischemia or infarction in tissues distal to the obstruction. Embolism of a central organ causes organ dysfunction and pain. Infarction and subsequent necrosis of a central organ are life threatening. Occlusion of a coronary artery will cause a myocardial infarction, whereas occlusion of a cerebral artery causes a stroke (see Chapter 15). The types of emboli are summarized in Table 23-3.

TABLE 23-3
Types of Emboli

Type	Characteristics
ARTERIES	
Arterial thromboembolism	Dislodged thrombus; source is usually from the heart; most common sites of obstruction are lower extremities (femoral and popliteal arteries), coronary arteries, and cerebral vasculature
VEINS	
Venous thromboembolism	Dislodged thrombus; source is usually from the lower extremities; obstructs branches of the pulmonary artery
Air embolism	A bolus of air displaces blood in the vasculature; source usually room air entering circulation through IV lines; trauma to the chest also may allow air from lungs to enter vascular space
Amniotic fluid embolism	A bolus of amniotic fluid; extensive intra-abdominal pressure attending labor and delivery can force amniotic fluid into bloodstream of mother; introduces antigens, cells, and protein aggregates that trigger inflammation, coagulation, and immune responses
Bacterial embolism	Aggregates of bacteria in bloodstream; source is subacute bacterial endocarditis or abscess
Fat embolism	Globules of fat floating in the bloodstream associated with trauma to long bones; the lungs in particular are affected
Foreign matter	Small particles or fibers introduced during trauma or through an IV or intra-arterial line; coagulation cascade is initiated and thromboemboli form around the particles

QUICK CHECK 23-3

1. How does the law of Laplace function in aneurysm?
2. What is a thrombus?
3. Why are emboli dangerous?

Peripheral Vascular Disease

Thromboangiitis obliterans (Buerger disease)

Thromboangiitis obliterans (Buerger disease), which tends to occur in young men who are heavy cigarette smokers, is an immune and inflammatory disease of the peripheral arteries. The pathogenesis of thromboangiitis obliterans is not known, although there is evidence of significant T cell activation and autoimmunity and inflammation.[23] The inflammation is accompanied by thrombi and vasospasm of arterial segments, which eventually occlude and obliterate portions of small and medium-sized arteries in the feet and sometimes in the hands. In addition, peripheral vessels are less responsive to acetylcholine, which normally causes vasodilation. Although collateral vessels develop in Buerger disease, they are inadequate to supply the extremities with blood. These collateral vessels have a characteristic corkscrew shape, believed to be a result of dilated vasa vasorum in the affected artery.

The chief symptom of thromboangiitis obliterans is pain and tenderness of the affected part. Clinical manifestations are caused by sluggish blood flow and include rubor (redness of the skin), which is caused by dilated capillaries under the skin. Cyanosis may also occur because of tissue ischemia and blood that remains in the capillaries after its oxygen has diffused into the interstitium. Chronic ischemia causes the skin to thin and become shiny, and it causes the nails to become thickened and malformed. In advanced disease, profound ischemia of the extremities resulting from vessel obliteration can cause gangrene necessitating amputation. Buerger disease has also been associated with cerebrovascular disease (stroke), mesenteric disease, and rheumatic symptoms (joint pain).[24]

The most important part of treatment is cessation of cigarette smoking. If smoking continues, the likelihood of recurrence of the disease and gangrene requiring amputation is high. Other measures are aimed at improving circulation to the foot or hand. Vasodilators are prescribed to alleviate vasospasm, and exercises are taught that use gravity to improve blood flow. If vasospasm persists, sympathectomy may be performed.

Raynaud phenomenon and disease

Raynaud phenomenon and **Raynaud disease** both are characterized by attacks of vasospasm in the small arteries and arterioles of the fingers and, less commonly, the toes. Although the clinical manifestations of the phenomenon and the disease are the same, their causes differ.

Raynaud phenomenon is secondary to systemic diseases, particularly collagen vascular disease (scleroderma), pulmonary hypertension, thoracic outlet syndrome, myxedema, trauma, serum sickness, or long-term exposure to environmental conditions, such as cold or vibrating machinery in the workplace. Raynaud disease is a primary vasospastic disorder of unknown origin; however, endothelial damage with an imbalance in endothelium-derived vasodilators (e.g., nitric oxide) and vasoconstrictors (e.g., endothelin-1) is implicated.[25] Platelet activation also may play a role. It tends to affect young women and to consist of vasospastic attacks triggered by brief exposure to cold or by emotional stress. Genetic predisposition may play a role in its development.

The clinical manifestations of the vasospastic attacks of either disorder are changes in skin color and sensation caused by ischemia. Vasospasm occurs with varying frequency and severity and causes pallor, numbness, and the sensation of cold in the digits. Attacks tend to be bilateral, and manifestations usually begin at the tips of the digits and progress to the proximal phalanges. Sluggish blood flow resulting from ischemia may cause the skin to appear cyanotic. Rubor, throbbing, and paresthesias follow as blood flow returns. Skin color returns to normal after the attack, but frequent, prolonged attacks interfere with cellular metabolism, causing the skin of the fingertips to thicken and the nails to become brittle. In severe, chronic Raynaud phenomenon or disease, ischemia can eventually cause ulceration and gangrene.

Treatment for Raynaud phenomenon consists of removing the stimulus or treating the primary disease process. Treatment of Raynaud disease begins with avoidance of stimuli that trigger attacks (e.g., cold, emotional stress), and cigarette smoking is stopped to eliminate the vasoconstricting effects of nicotine. If attacks of vasospasm become frequent or prolonged, vasodilators, such as calcium channel blockers or angiotensin II receptor blockers, are administered. Nitric oxide donors and endothelin antagonists are also being explored.[25] Sympathectomy may be indicated in severe cases, and if ischemia leads to ulceration and gangrene, amputation may be necessary.

✔ QUICK CHECK 23-4

1. What is Buerger disease and why does it occur?
2. Compare the physical manifestations of Buerger disease and Raynaud disease.

Arteriosclerosis

Arteriosclerosis is a chronic disease of the arterial system characterized by abnormal thickening and hardening of the vessel walls. Smooth muscle cells and collagen fibers migrate into the tunica intima, causing it to stiffen and thicken, gradually narrowing the arterial lumen (Figure 23-9). Changes in lipid, cholesterol, and phospholipid metabolism within the tunica intima also contribute to arteriosclerosis. Although these changes may be part of normal aging, pathophysiologic conditions such as hypertension, insufficient perfusion of tissues, or weakening and outpouching of arterial walls can be exacerbated.

Atherosclerosis

Atherosclerosis is the most common form of arteriosclerosis. It is characterized by soft deposits of intra-arterial fat and fibrin in the vessels walls that harden over time. Atherosclerosis is not a single disease entity but rather a pathologic process that can affect vascular systems throughout the body resulting in ischemic syndromes that can vary widely in their severity and clinical manifestations. It is the leading cause of coronary artery and cerebrovascular disease. (Atherosclerosis of the coronary arteries is described later in this chapter, and atherosclerosis of the cerebral arteries is described in Chapter 15.)

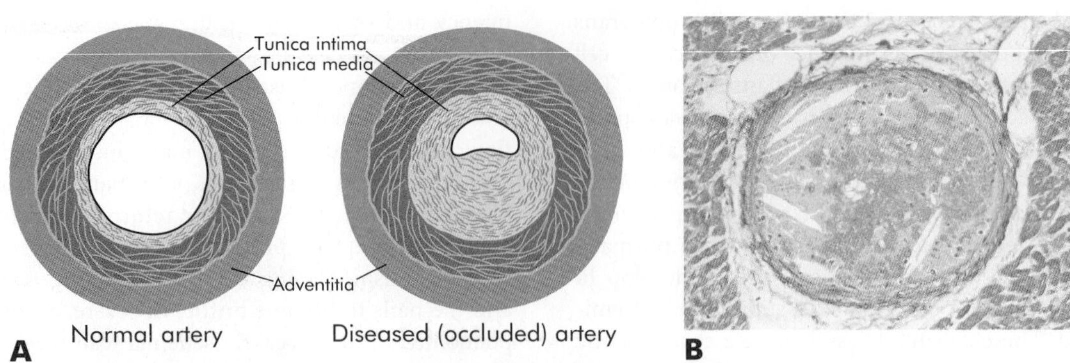

Figure 23-9 ■ **Arteriosclerosis. A,** Cross section of a normal artery and an artery altered by disease. **B,** A small artery in the myocardium is occluded by a mass of blue-staining platelets, yellow-staining red cells, and cholesterol bodies. (**B** from Damjanov I, Linder J, editors: *Anderson's pathology,* ed 10, St Louis, 1996, Mosby.)

PATHOPHYSIOLOGY Inflammation plays a fundamental role in mediating all of the steps in the initiation and progression of atherogenesis.[26–28] Atherosclerosis begins with injury to the endothelial cells that line artery walls. Possible causes of endothelial injury include the common risk factors for atherosclerosis, such as smoking, hypertension, diabetes, increased levels of low-density lipoprotein (LDL), decreased levels of high-density lipoprotein (HDL), and hyperhomocystinemia. Other causes of endothelial injury are called the "novel" risk factors, such as elevated C-reactive protein, increased serum fibrinogen, insulin resistance, oxidative stress, infection, and periodontal disease. These risk factors are discussed in more detail in the following section on coronary artery disease (see p. 622). There is recent evidence that individuals with a defect in the production of precursor endothelial cells in the bone marrow are at greater risk for atherosclerotic disease because these precursor cells are not available to repair injured endothelium.[29,30]

Injured endothelial cells become inflamed and cannot make normal amounts of antithrombic and vasodilating cytokines (Figures 23-10 and 23-11). The next step in

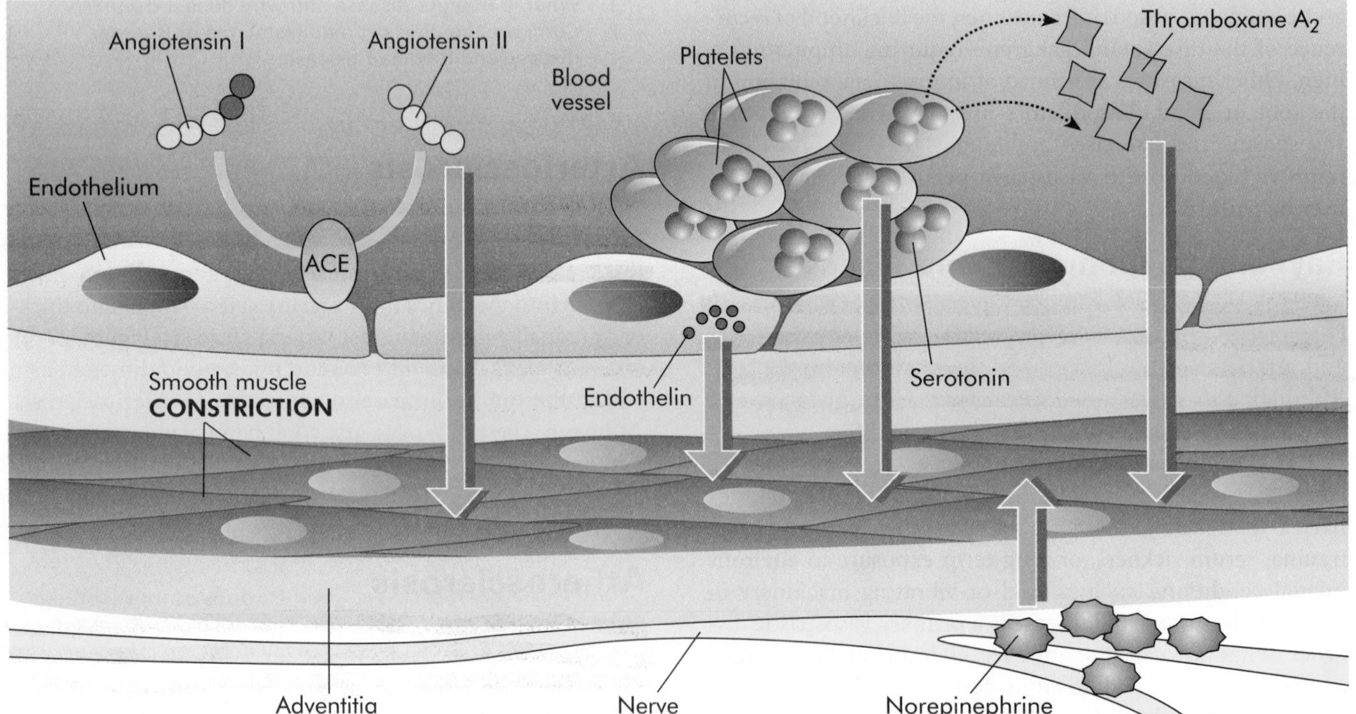

Figure 23-10 ■ **Endothelium Regulation of Vasomotion (Constriction and Dilation) and Platelet Aggregation.** With injury, the endothelium loses its normal ability to decrease clot formation (antithrombotic) and maintain vasodilation. Injury results in platelet aggregation with increases in thromboxane A_2 (which aspirin inhibits) and the release of serotonin and endothelin causing vasoconstriction, a decrease in blood flow, and ischemia. Sympathetic nerve activation causes vasoconstriction with the release of epinephrine. Endothelin is a potent amino acid peptide. The endothelium also converts angiotensin I into angiotensin II by the membrane-bound angiotensin-converting enzyme (ACE). Angiotensin II plays an important role in the pathophysiology of hypertension, atherosclerosis, myocardial infarction, and left heart failure (congestive heart failure) (see text under the heading for each). (Modified from Stern S, editor: *Silent myocardial ischemia,* St Louis, 1998, Mosby.)

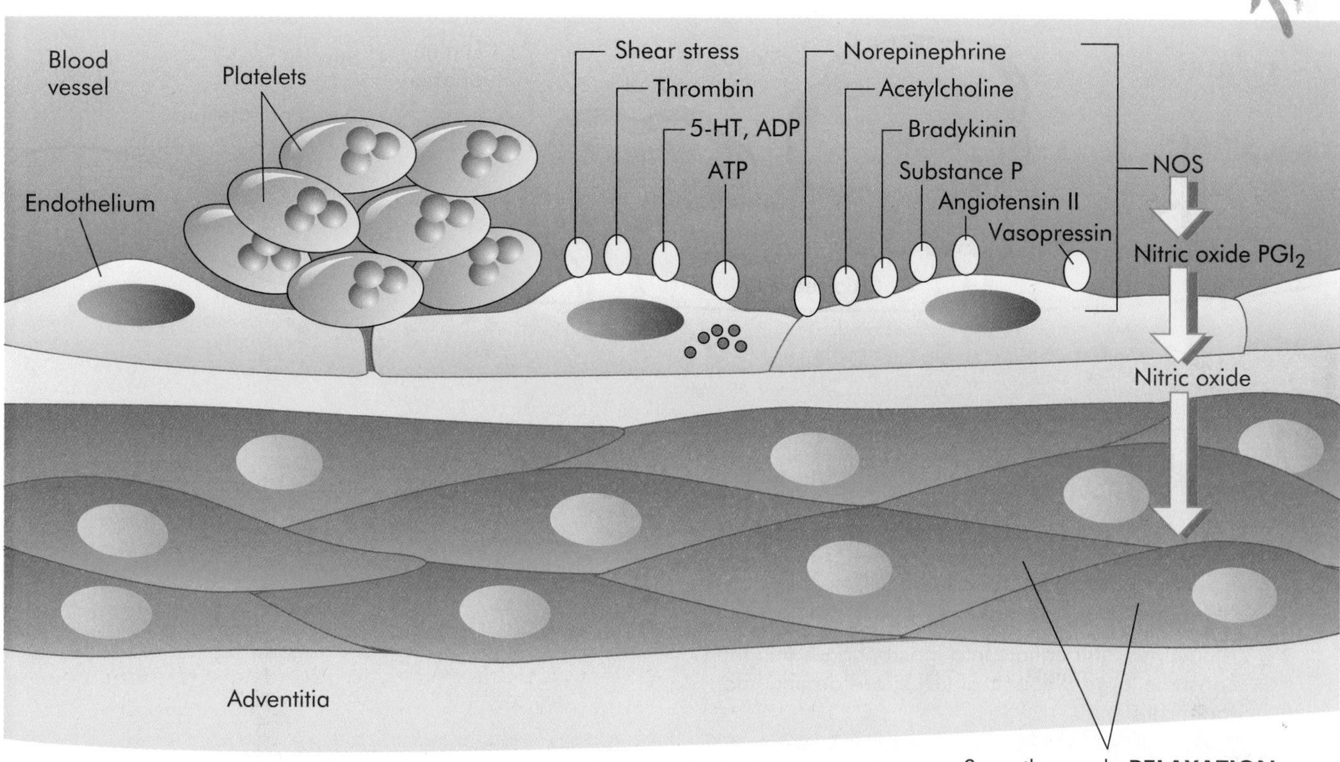

Figure 23-11 ■ Factors That Cause Endothelium-Dependent Vasodilation. Several pharmacologic and physiologic factors stimulate the release of nitric oxide synthase (NOS) that results in the release of nitric oxide (NO). These factors include norepinephrine, acetylcholine, bradykinin, substance P, angiotensin II, thrombin, vasopressin, ATP, 5-HT, and ADP. In addition, the continuous normal production of NO can be increased by physiologic events including shear stress (on the vessel walls) and movement of platelets. Nitric oxide leads to relaxation of the smooth muscle cells resulting in vasodilation. Prostacyclin (PGI2) also causes relaxation of the smooth muscle cells and inhibits platelet aggregation downstream. (Modified from Stern S, editor: *Silent myocardial ischemia,* St Louis, 1998, Mosby.)

atherogenesis occurs when inflamed endothelial cells express adhesion molecules that bind macrophages and other inflammatory and immune cells. Macrophages adhere to the injured endothelium and release numerous inflammatory cytokines (e.g., tumor necrosis factor alpha [TNF-α], interferons, interleukins, and C-reactive protein) and enzymes that further injure the vessel wall.[31] Toxic oxygen radicals generated by the inflammatory process cause oxidation (i.e. addition of oxygen) of LDL, which is the next important step in atherogenesis. Oxidized LDL is engulfed by macrophages, which then penetrate into the intima of the vessel. These lipid-laden macrophages are now called **foam cells,** and when they accumulate in significant amounts, they form a lesion called a **fatty streak** (Figures 23-12 and 23-13). These lesions can be found in the walls of arteries of most people, even young children. Once formed, fatty streaks produce more toxic oxygen radicals and cause immunologic and inflammatory changes resulting in progressive damage to the vessel wall. Treatment that lowers LDL may reverse this process.

Macrophages also release growth factors that stimulate smooth muscle cells proliferation. Smooth muscle cells in the region of endothelial injury proliferate, produce collagen, and migrate over the fatty streak forming a **fibrous plaque** (see Figure 23-12). The fibrous plaque may calcify, protrude into the vessel lumen, and obstruct blood flow to distal tissues (especially during exercise), which may cause symptoms (e.g., angina or intermittent claudication).

Many plaques, however, are "unstable," meaning they are prone to rupture even before they affect blood flow significantly and are clinically silent until they rupture. Plaque rupture occurs because of the inflammatory activation of proteinases, such as the matrix metalloproteinases and the cathepsins, and can be accelerated by bleeding within the lesion (plaque hemorrhage).[31] Plaques that have ruptured are called **complicated plaques** (see Figure 23-12). Once rupture occurs, exposure of underlying tissue results in platelet adhesion, initiation of the clotting cascade, and rapid thrombus formation. The thrombus may suddenly occlude the affected vessel resulting in ischemia and infarction. Aspirin or other antithrombotic agents are used to prevent this complication of atherosclerotic disease.

CLINICAL MANIFESTATIONS Atherosclerosis presents with symptoms and signs that result from inadequate perfusion of tissues because of obstruction of the vessels that supply them. Partial vessel obstruction may lead to transient ischemic events, often associated with exercise or stress. As the lesion becomes complicated, increasing obstruction with superimposed thrombosis may result in

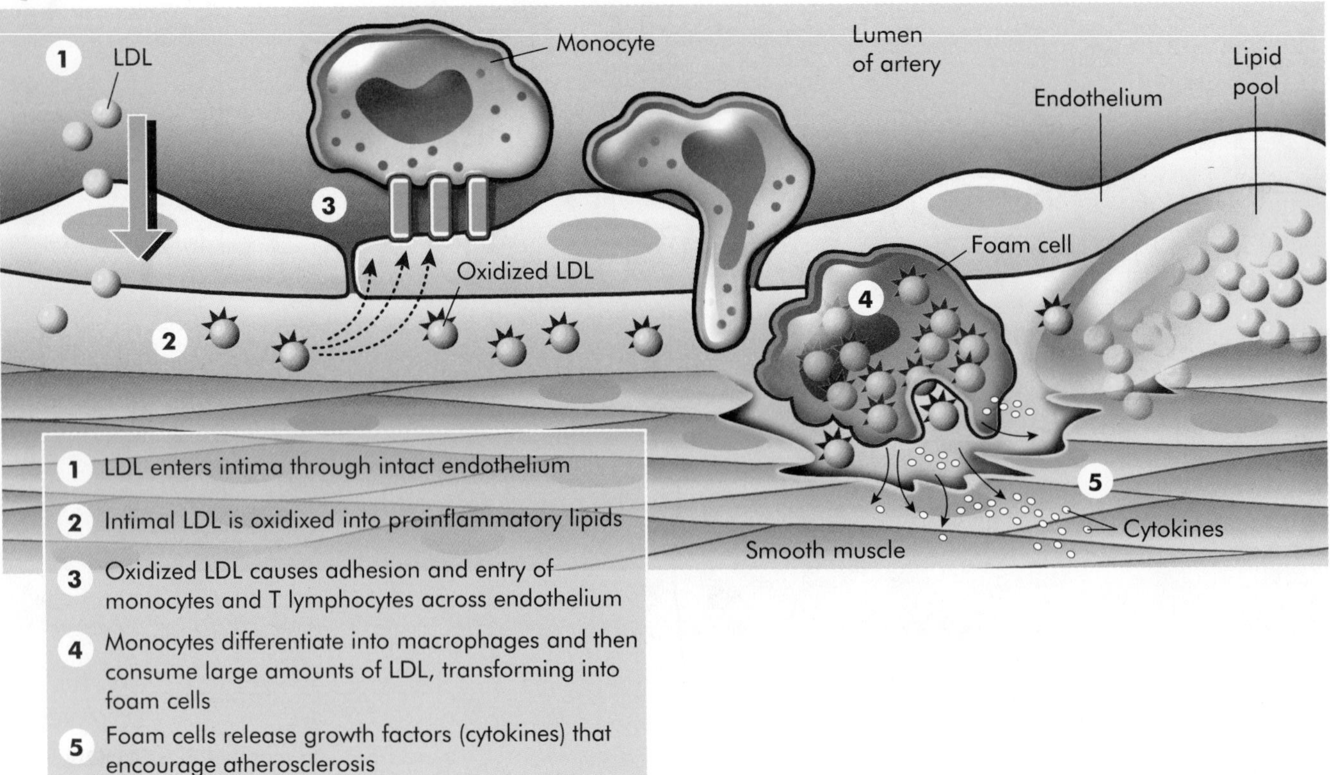

1
LDL
Monocyte
Lumen of artery
Lipid pool
Endothelium
3
Oxidized LDL
Foam cell
4
2
5
Cytokines
Smooth muscle
1 LDL enters intima through intact endothelium
2 Intimal LDL is oxidixed into proinflammatory lipids
3 Oxidized LDL causes adhesion and entry of monocytes and T lymphocytes across endothelium
4 Monocytes differentiate into macrophages and then consume large amounts of LDL, transforming into foam cells
5 Foam cells release growth factors (cytokines) that encourage atherosclerosis

Figure 23-12 ■ **Low-density Lipoprotein Oxidation.** Low-density lipoprotein (LDL) enters the arterial intima through an intact endothelium. In hypercholesterolemia, the influx of LDL exceeds the eliminating capacity and an extracellular pool of LDL is formed. This is enhanced by association of LDL with the extracellular matrix. Intimal LDL is oxidized through the actin of free oxygen radicals formed by enzymatic or nonenzymatic reactions. This generates proinflammatory lipids that induce endothelial expression of the adhesion molecule, vascular cell adhesion molecule-1 activate complement and stimulate chemokine secretion. All of these factors cause adhesion and entry of mononuclear leukocytes, particularly monocytes and T lymphocytes. Monocytes differentiate into macrophages. Macrophages up-regulate and internalize oxidized LDL and transform into foam cells. Macrophage uptake of oxidized LDL also leads to presentation of fragments of it to antigen-specific T cells. This induces an autoimmune reaction that leads to production of proinflammatory cytokines. Such cytokines include interferon-γ, tumor necrosis factor-α, and interleukin-1, which act on endothelial cells to stimulate expression of adhesion molecules and procoagulant activity; on macrophages to activate proteases, endocytosis, nitric oxide (NO), and cytokines; and on smooth muscle cells (SMCs) to include NO production and inhibit growth, collagen, and actin expression. *LDL,* low-density lipoprotein. (Modified from Crawford MH, DiMarco JP, editors: *Cardiology,* London, 2001, Mosby.)

tissue infarction. Obstruction of peripheral arteries can cause significant pain and disability. Coronary artery disease (CAD) caused by atherosclerosis is the major cause of myocardial ischemia and is one of the most important health issues in the United States. Atherosclerotic obstruction of the vessels supplying the brain is the major cause of stroke. Similarly, any part of the body may become ischemic when its blood supply is compromised by atherosclerotic lesions. Often, more than one vessel will become involved with this disease process such that an individual may present with symptoms from several ischemic tissues at the same time, and disease in one area may indicate that the individual is at risk for ischemic complications elsewhere.

EVALUATION AND TREATMENT In evaluating individuals for the presence of atherosclerosis, a complete health history (including risk factors), physical examination, and laboratory data, are considered. Judicious use of x-ray films, electrocardiography, ultrasonography, nuclear scanning, and angiography may be necessary to identify affected vessels, particularly coronary vessels.

The primary goal in the management of atherosclerosis is to restore adequate blood flow to the affected tissues. If an individual has presented with acute ischemia (e.g., myocardial infarction, stroke), interventions are specific to the diseased area and are discussed further under those topics. In situations where the disease process does not require

Figure 23-13 ■ **Progression of Atherosclerosis. A,** Damaged endothelium. **B,** Diagram of fatty streak and lipid core formation (see Figure 23-5 for a diagram of oxidized low-density lipoprotein [LDL]). **C,** Diagram of fibrous plaque. Raised plaques are visible: some are yellow; others are white. **D,** Diagram of complicated lesion; thrombus is red; collagen is blue. Plaque is complicated by red thrombus deposition.

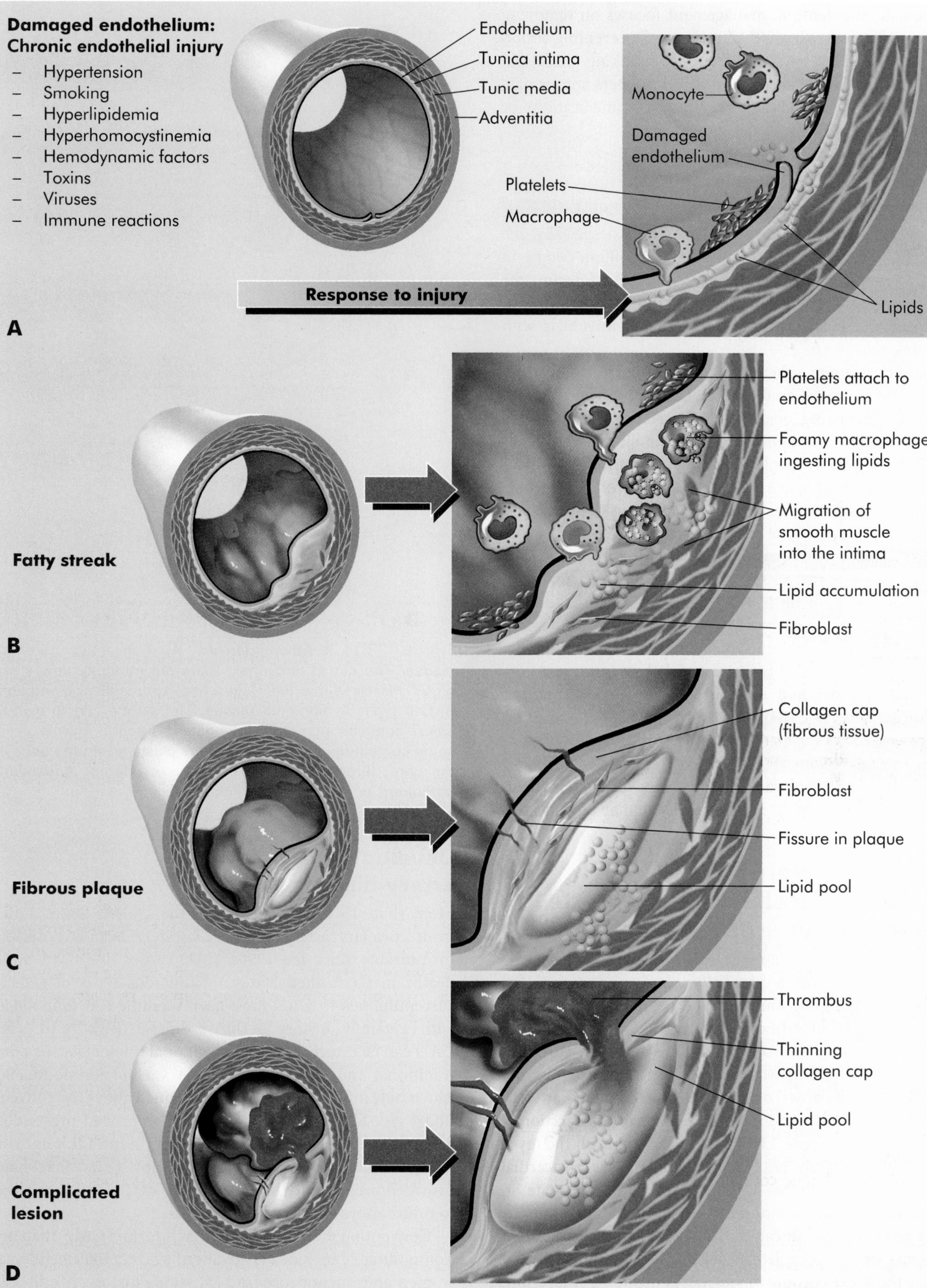
Damaged endothelium:
Chronic endothelial injury
– Hypertension
– Smoking
– Hyperlipidemia
– Hyperhomocystinemia
– Hemodynamic factors
– Toxins
– Viruses
– Immune reactions
Endothelium
Tunica intima
Tunic media
Adventitia
Monocyte
Damaged endothelium
Platelets
Macrophage
Lipids
Response to injury
A
Platelets attach to endothelium
Foamy macrophage ingesting lipids
Migration of smooth muscle into the intima
Lipid accumulation
Fibroblast
Fatty streak
B
Collagen cap (fibrous tissue)
Fibroblast
Fissure in plaque
Lipid pool
Fibrous plaque
C
Thrombus
Thinning collagen cap
Lipid pool
Complicated lesion
D

immediate intervention, management focuses on removing the initial causes of vessel damage and preventing lesion progression. This includes exercise, smoking cessation, and control of hypertension and diabetes where appropriate while reducing LDL cholesterol by diet or medications or both.

Peripheral Artery Disease

Peripheral artery disease (PAD) refers to atherosclerotic disease of arteries that perfuse the limbs, especially the lower extremities. It is estimated that 12 million people in the United States have significant PAD. The risk factors for PAD are the same as those previously described for atherosclerosis, and it is especially prevalent in individuals with diabetes.

Lower extremity ischemia resulting from arterial obstruction in PAD can be gradual or acute. In most individuals, gradually increasing obstruction to arterial blood flow to the legs caused by atherosclerosis in the iliofemoral vessels results in pain with ambulation called **intermittent claudication.** If a thrombus forms over the atherosclerotic lesion, perfusion can cease acutely with severe pain, loss of pulses, and skin color changes in the affected extremity.

PAD is often asymptomatic; therefore, evaluation for PAD requires a careful history and physical examination that focuses on looking for evidence of atherosclerotic disease (e.g., bruits) and noninvasive Doppler measurement of blood flow. Treatment includes risk factor reduction (smoking cessation and treatment of diabetes, hypertension, and dyslipidemia) and antiplatelet therapy. Symptomatic PAD should be managed with vasodilators in combination with antiplatelet or antithrombotic medications (aspirin, cilostazol, ticlopidine, or clopidogrel) and exercise rehabilitation.[32] If acute or refractory symptoms occur, emergent percutaneous or surgical revascularization may be indicated.

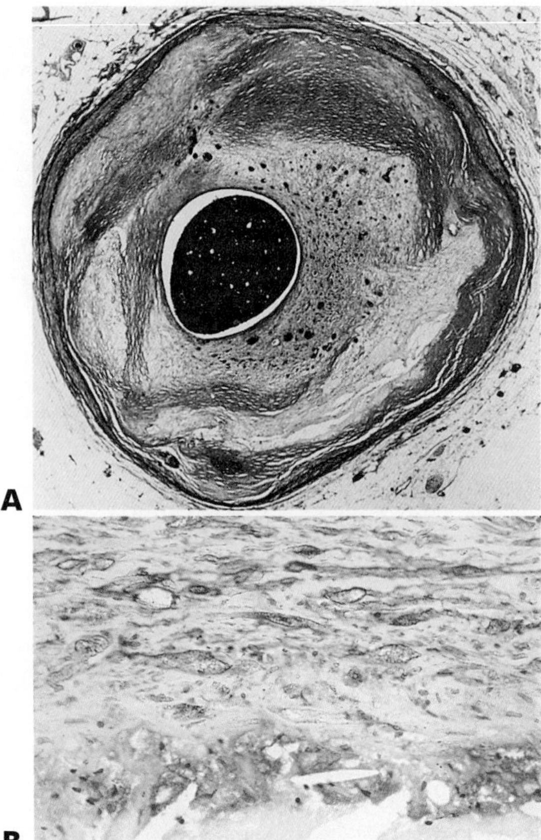

Figure 23-14 ■ **Atherosclerosis. A,** Concentric coronary plaque. The lumen is central. There are multiple, new small blood vessels within the plaque, the late result of disruption. **B,** Cell types in fibrolipid plaque. The plaque cap *(brownish color)* contains numerous elongated, smooth muscle cells; some contain lipid. Macrophages are clustered on the edge of the core. (From Damjanov I, Linder J, editors: *Anderson's pathology,* ed 10, St Louis, 1996, Mosby.)

Coronary Artery Disease, Myocardial Ischemia, and Acute Coronary Syndromes

Coronary artery disease, myocardial ischemia, and myocardial infarction form a pathophysiologic continuum that impairs the pumping ability of the heart by depriving the heart muscle of blood-borne oxygen and nutrients.[33] The earliest lesions of the continuum are those of **coronary artery disease (CAD),** which can result from any vascular disorder that narrows or occludes the coronary arteries. By far the most common cause of coronary obstruction is atherosclerosis (Figure 23-14). CAD can diminish the myocardial blood supply until deprivation impairs myocardial metabolism enough to cause **ischemia,** a local state in which the cells are temporarily deprived of blood supply. They remain alive but cannot function normally. Persistent ischemia or the complete occlusion of a coronary artery causes the **acute coronary syndromes** including **infarction,** or irreversible myocardial damage. Infarction constitutes the often-fatal event known as a *heart attack.*

Development of coronary artery disease

More than 13 million people in the United States suffer from coronary artery disease. Despite a dramatic decline in mortality since the 1990s, CAD causes one third of all deaths in the United States.[34] Numerous types of genetic susceptibilities to CAD have been identified in individuals with a family history of heart disease. Risk factors for CAD can be categorized as conventional (major) versus nontraditional (novel) and modifiable versus nonmodifiable. Much new information has been obtained about the conventional risk factors that has markedly improved prevention and management of CAD. In addition, nontraditional risk factors have been identified in recent years that have provided insight in to the pathogenesis of CAD and may lead to future more effective interventions.

Conventional or major risk factors for CAD that are nonmodifiable include (1) advanced age, (2) male gender or women after menopause, and (3) family history. Modifiable major risks include (1) dyslipidemia, (2) hypertension, (3) cigarette smoking, (4) diabetes and insulin resistance,

(5) obesity, (6) sedentary lifestyle, and (7) atherogenic diet (see *Health Alert:* The Basics on Fats). Fortunately, modification of these factors can dramatically reduce the risk for CAD.

HEALTH ALERT
The Basics on Fats

Saturated fats are found in animal fats (butter, cheese, beef, pork, lamb, chicken) and some tropical oils (e.g., palm kernel). All saturated fats are not the same; some are stickier than others. They consist of a long chain of atoms that take a longer time to burn than shorter-chained fats. The longer the fat takes to burn, the stickier it becomes. Those fats that become stickiest are more conducive to weight gain and heart disease.

Unsaturated fats consist of two types: monounsaturated and polyunsaturated. Both contain essential fatty acids (EFAs), but polyunsaturated fats have more.

Monounsaturated fats are liquid at room temperature but more solid when refrigerated. They are found in especially high concentration in olive and canola oils, which are high in oleic acid, a common monounsaturated fat. Monounsaturated fats are known to lower low-density lipoproteins (LDL) and raise high-density lipoproteins (HDL) levels. They are more stable in heat than other oils, thus they are often used for stir-frying and baking.

Polyunsaturated fats are liquid at any temperature and are found in vegetable oils, soy, fish, walnuts, pumpkin seeds, and flaxseed oil. They contain both omega-6 and omega-3 EFAs in varying ratios. Today people are eating many more omega-6 EFAs than omega-3. Too much omega-6 can contribute to clot formation; omega-3 fats have the opposite effect, so to reduce the risk of heart disease one needs more omega-3 and less omega-6. Omega-3 EFAs are found in fish oil, flaxseed (and flaxseed oil), canola oil, walnuts, pumpkins, and green leafy vegetables. Soy contains both omega-6 and omega-3. Populations that eat high amounts of omega-3 EFAs have a lower risk of heart disease. Omega-6 EFAs are found in vegetable oils such as corn, safflower, sunflower, cottonseed, peanut, sesame, grape seed, borage, primrose, and soy. Omega-6 EFAs have protective effects only when they are combined with omega-3 EFAs.

Trans-fats are primarily found in artificially solidified (hydrogenated) oils (e.g., margarine and vegetable shortening). By becoming more solid they lose EFAs. They can raise LDL and lower HDL levels. They also can raise lipoprotein-a levels, which increases risk of heart disease. Trans-fats raise blood-sugar levels and contribute to more weight gain than the same amount of other fats. "Partially hydrogenated" or "hydrogenated" on a food label means the food contains trans-fatty acids (e.g., cakes, cookies, crackers, processed cheese).

Dyslipidemia

The term **lipoprotein** refers to lipids, phospholipids, cholesterol, and triglycerides bound to carrier proteins. Lipids (cholesterol in particular) are required by most cells for the manufacture and repair of plasma membranes. Cholesterol is also a necessary component for the manufacture of such essential substances as bile acids and steroid hormones. Although cholesterol can easily be obtained from dietary fat intake, most body cells also can manufacture cholesterol. The cycle of lipid metabolism is complex. Dietary fat is packaged into particles known as **chylomicrons** in the small intestine. Chylomicrons are required for absorption of fat; they function by transporting exogenous lipid from the intestine to the liver and peripheral cells. Chylomicrons are the least dense of the lipoproteins and primarily contain triglyceride. Some of the triglyceride may be removed and either stored by adipose tissue or used by muscle as an energy source. The chylomicron remnants, composed mainly of cholesterol, are taken up by the liver. A series of chemical reactions in the liver results in the production of several lipoproteins that vary in density and function. These include **very-low-density lipoproteins (VLDLs),** primarily triglyceride and protein; **low-density lipoproteins (LDLs),** mostly cholesterol and protein; and **high-density lipoproteins (HDLs),** mainly phospholipids and protein.

Dyslipidemia (or **dyslipoproteinemia**) refers to abnormal concentrations of serum lipoproteins as defined by the Third Report of the National Cholesterol Education Program[35] (Table 23-4). It is estimated that nearly half of the U.S. population has some form of dyslipidemia. These abnormalities are the result of a combination of genetic and dietary factors. Primary or familial dyslipoproteinemias result from genetic defects that cause abnormalities in lipid-metabolizing enzymes and abnormal cellular lipid receptors. Secondary causes of dyslipidemia include several common systemic disorders, such as diabetes, hypothyroidism, pancreatitis, and renal nephrosis.

An increased serum concentration of LDL is a strong indicator of coronary risk.[35] Serum levels of LDL are normally controlled by hepatic receptors that bind LDL and limit liver synthesis of this lipoprotein. High dietary intake of cholesterol and fats, often in combination with a genetic predisposition to accumulations of LDL in the serum (e.g., dysfunction of the hepatic LDL receptor), results in high levels of LDL in the bloodstream. The term *LDL* actually describes several types of LDL molecules of which the

TABLE 23-4
Criteria for Dyslipidemia

	Optimal	Near Optimal	Desirable	Low	Borderline	High	Very High
Total cholesterol			<200		200–239	≥240	
LDL	<100	100–129			130–159	160–189	≥190
Triglycerides			<150		150–199	200–499	≥500
HDL				<40		≥60	

"small dense" LDL particles are the most atherogenic. LDL oxidation, migration into the vessel wall, and phagocytosis by macrophages are key steps in the pathogenesis of atherosclerosis (see Figure 23-12). LDL also plays a role in endothelial injury, inflammation, and immune responses that have been identified as being important in atherogenesis.[36] Aggressive reduction of LDL with diet and cholesterol-lowering drugs, such as the statins and ezetimibe, is associated with a dramatic decrease in risk for CAD.[37]

Low levels of HDL cholesterol also are a strong indicator of coronary risk, and high levels of HDL may be more protective for the development of atherosclerosis than low levels of LDL.[38] HDL is responsible for "reverse cholesterol transport," which returns excess cholesterol from the tissues to the liver for metabolism. HDL also participates in endothelial repair and decreases thrombosis.[39] It can be fractionated into several particle sizes that have different effects on vascular function. Exercise, weight loss, fish oil consumption, and moderate alcohol use can result in modest increases in HDL. Niacin, fibrates, and statins are drugs that can cause modest increases in HDL; however, new drugs are currently being studied to more directly increase HDL activity.[40]

Other lipoproteins associated with increased cardiovascular risk include elevated serum VLDL (triglycerides) and increased lipoprotein (a). Triglycerides are associated with an increased risk for CAD, especially in combination with other risk factors such as diabetes. **Lipoprotein (a) (Lp[a])** is a genetically determined molecular complex between LDL and a serum glycoprotein called *apolipoprotein A* and has been shown to be an important risk factor for atherosclerosis, especially in women.

Hypertension

Hypertension is responsible for a twofold to threefold increased risk of atherosclerotic cardiovascular disease. It contributes to endothelial injury, a key step in atherogenesis (see p. 617), and causes myocardial hypertrophy, which increases myocardial demand for coronary flow.

Cigarette smoking

Both direct and passive (environmental) smoking increase the risk of CAD. The mechanism by which smoking increases atherosclerosis is uncertain. Nicotine stimulates the release of catecholamines (epinephrine and norepinephrine), which increase heart rate and peripheral vascular constriction. As a result, blood pressure increases, as do cardiac workload and oxygen demand. Cigarette smoking is associated with an increase in LDL, a decrease in HDL, and contributes to vessel inflammation and thrombosis. The risk of CAD increases with heavy smoking and decreases when smoking is stopped.

Diabetes mellitus

Diabetes mellitus is an extremely important risk factor for CAD.[41] Insulin resistance and diabetes have multiple effects on the cardiovascular system including endothelial damage, thickening of the vessel wall, increased inflammation, increased thrombosis, glycation of vascular proteins, and decreased production of endothelial-derived vasodilators such as nitric oxide.[42] Diabetes is also associated with dyslipidemia.

Obesity/sedentary lifestyle

It is estimated that 65% of the adult population in the United States is overweight or obese, and an estimated 47 million U.S. residents have a combination of obesity, dyslipidemia, hypertension, and insulin resistance, called the **metabolic syndrome,** which is associated with an even higher risk for CAD events (see Health Alert: The Metabolic Syndrome in Chapter 18).[43,44] Abdominal obesity has the strongest link with increased CAD risk and is related to insulin resistance, decreased HDL, increased blood pressure, and decreased levels of a recently described cardioprotective protein called *adiponectin.*[45] Physical activity and weight loss offer substantial reductions in risk factors for CAD.[43]

Nontraditional risk factors

Nontraditional, or novel, risk factors for CAD include (1) increased serum markers for inflammation and thrombosis, (2) hyperhomocysteinemia, and (3) infection. The amount of risk conferred by these relatively newly identified factors is still being explored.

Markers of inflammation and thrombosis. Of the numerous markers of inflammation that have been linked to an increase in CAD risk (C-reactive protein, fibrinogen, protein C, plasminogen activator inhibitor), serum levels of C-reactive protein has been explored in the greatest depth. **C-reactive protein (C-rp)** is a protein mostly synthesized in the liver. C-rp is an indirect measure of atherosclerotic plaque-related inflammation and is an important indicator of CAD risk.[46] Other markers of inflammation associated with CAD include the erythrocyte sedimentation rate, von Willebrand factor concentration, interleukin-6, interleukin-18, tumor necrosis factor, fibrinogen, and CD 40 ligand (see *Health Alert:* Inflammatory Markers for Cardiovascular Risk).[46,47]

Hyperhomocysteinemia. **Hyperhomocysteinemia** occurs because of a genetic lack of the enzyme that breaks down homocysteine (an amino acid) or because of a nutritional deficiency of folate, cobalamin (vitamin B_{12}), or pyridoxine (vitamin B_6). It has been identified as a risk factor for CAD, although its significance in CAD and stroke continues to be explored. Routine serum measurement of homocysteine is not currently recommended, and prevention and management are focused on increasing the dietary intake of folate and B vitamins.

Infection. Emerging is evidence that infection may play a role in atherogenesis and CAD risk. Studies have found that several microorganisms, especially *Chlamydia pneumonae* and *Helicobacter pylori,* are often present in atherosclerotic lesions. Serum antibodies to microorganisms have been linked to an increased risk for CAD as has the presence of periodontal disease. Although a few early studies suggested that antibiotics used to treat these infections are associated with a decrease in CAD events, more recent studies have been less compelling.[48]

HEALTH ALERT

Inflammatory Markers for Cardiovascular Risk

Atherosclerosis is an inflammatory disease. A number of serum markers of inflammation have been found to be excellent predictors of cardiovascular risk, especially C-reactive protein (C-rp). Other inflammatory markers found to be predictive of cardiovascular risk include fibrinogen, erythrocyte sedimentation rate, von Willebrand factor, interleukin-6, interleukin-1, tumor necrosis factor-α, adhesion molecules (selectins, intercellular adhesion molecules [ICAMs]), and serum amyloid A. C-rp is made by the liver in response to inflammatory stimuli and has been demonstrated convincingly to be a good predictor of coronary artery disease. However, several problems remain in determining its use in clinical practice. C-rp must be measured by a high-sensitivity technique (hs-C-rp), and it is a nonspecific marker of inflammation. It can therefore be elevated in many other inflammatory states, and its use is limited to identifying high-risk individuals and for following individuals with known coronary disease. It should not be used to screen the general population.

Data from Danesh J et al: C reactive protein and other circulating markers of inflammation in the prediction of coronary heart disease, *N Engl J Med* 350:1387–1397, 2004; Fichtlscherer S, Heeschen C, Zeiher AM: Inflammatory markers and coronary artery disease, *Curr Opin Pharmacol* 4:124–131, 2004; Karaduman M et al: Leptin, soluble interleukin-6 receptor, C-reactive protein and soluble vascular cell adhesion molecule-1 levels in human coronary atherosclerotic plaque, *Clin Experim Immunol* 143(3):452–457, 2006; Tomai F et al: Elevated C-reactive protein levels and coronary microvascular dysfunction in patients with coronary artery disease, *Eur Heart J* 26(20):2099–2105, 2005.

Myocardial ischemia

PATHOPHYSIOLOGY The coronary arteries normally supply blood flow sufficient to meet the demands of the myocardium as it labors under varying workloads. Oxygen is extracted from these vessels with maximal efficiency. If demand inceases, healthy coronary arteries can dilate to increase the flow of oxygenated blood to the myocardium. Various pathologic mechanisms can interfere with blood flow through the coronary arteries, giving rise to myocardial ischemia. Narrowing of a major coronary artery by more than 50% impairs blood flow enough to hamper cellular metabolism when myocardial demand increases (Figure 23-15).

Myocardial ischemia develops if the flow or oxygen content of coronary blood is insufficient to meet the metabolic demands of myocardial cells. Imbalances between coronary blood supply and myocardial demand can result from a number of conditions. The most common cause of decreased coronary blood flow and resultant myocardial ischemia is the formation of atherosclerotic plaques in the coronary circulation.[33] As the plaque increases in size, it may partially occlude the vessel lumina, thus limiting coronary flow and causing ischemia especially during exercise. Some plaques are "unstable," meaning they are prone to ulceration or rupture.[31] When this occurs, underlying tissues of the vessel wall are exposed resulting in platelet adhesion and thrombus formation.[49] This can suddenly cut off blood supply to the heart muscle resulting in acute myocardial ischemia, and, if the vessel obstruction cannot be reversed rapidly, ischemia will progress to infarction. Myocardial ischemia also can result from other causes of decreased blood and oxygen delivery to the myocardium, such as coronary spasm, hypotension, arrhythmias, and decreased oxygen-carrying capacity of the blood (anemia, hypoxemia). Common causes of increased myocardial

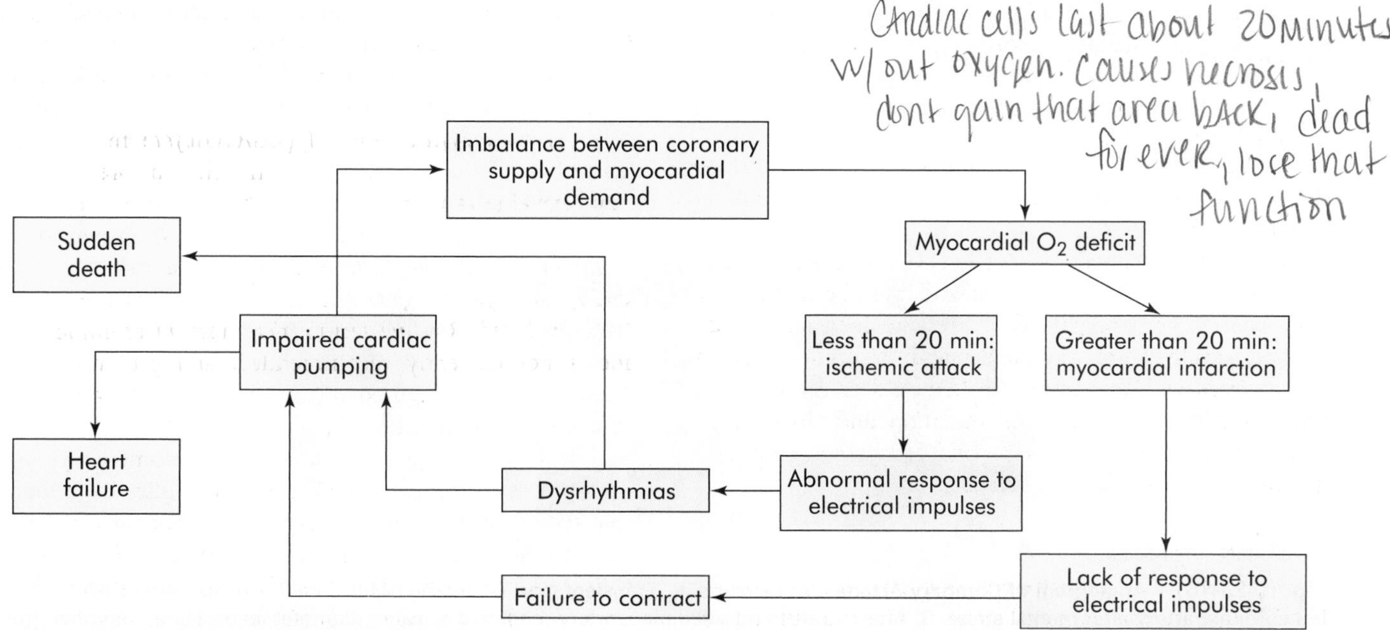

Figure 23-15 Cycle of Ischemic Events.

demand for blood include tachycardia, exercise, hypertension (hypertrophy), and valvular disease.

In CAD, ischemia develops within 10 seconds of coronary occlusion. After several minutes, the heart cells lose the ability to contract, thus hampering pump function and depriving the myocardium of a glucose source necessary for aerobic metabolism. Anaerobic processes take over, and lactic acid accumulates. Cardiac cells remain viable for approximately 20 minutes under ischemic conditions. If blood flow is restored, aerobic metabolism resumes, contractility is restored, and cellular repair begins. If perfusion is not restored, then myocardial infarction occurs (see Figure 23-15).

CLINICAL MANIFESTATIONS Individuals with reversible myocardial ischemia present clinically in several ways. Chronic coronary obstruction results in recurrent predictable chest pain called *stable angina.* Abnormal vasospasm of coronary vessels results in unpredictable chest pain called *Prinzmetal angina.* Myocardial ischemia that does not cause detectable symptoms is called *silent ischemia.*

1. **Stable angina pectoris.** Angina is chest pain caused by myocardial ischemia. The discomfort is usually transient, lasting approximately 3 to 5 minutes. If blood flow is restored, no permanent change or damage results. Angina pectoris is typically experienced as substernal chest discomfort, ranging from a sensation of heaviness or pressure to moderately severe pain. Individuals often describe the sensation by clenching a fist over the left sternal border. Discomfort may radiate to the neck, lower jaw, left arm, and left shoulder, or occasionally, to the back or down the right arm. Discomfort is commonly mistaken for indigestion. The pain is presumably caused by the buildup of lactic acid or abnormal stretching of the ischemic myocardium that irritates myocardial nerve fibers. These afferent sympathetic fibers enter the spinal cord from levels C3 to T4, accounting for the variety of locations and radiation patterns of anginal pain. Pallor, diaphoresis, and dyspnea may be associated with the pain. Stable angina is caused by gradual luminal narrowing and hardening of the arterial walls, so that affected vessels cannot dilate in response to increased myocardial demand associated with physical exertion or emotional stress. The pain is usually relieved by rest and nitrates; lack of relief indicates an individual may be developing infarction.
2. **Prinzmetal angina.** Prinzmetal angina is chest pain attributable to transient ischemia of the myocardium that occurs unpredictably and often at rest. Pain is caused by vasospasm of one or more major coronary arteries with or without associated atherosclerosis. The pain often occurs at night during rapid-eye-movement sleep and may have a cyclic pattern of occurrence. The angina may result from hyperactivity of the sympathetic nervous system, increased calcium flux in arterial smooth muscle, or endothelial dysfunction with impaired production or release of prostaglandin or thromboxane and abnormal responses to acetylcholine.[50]
3. **Silent ischemia.** Myocardial ischemia may not cause detectable symptoms such as angina. Ischemia can be totally asymptomatic and referred to as silent ischemia, and individuals may complain only of fatigue, dyspnea, or a feeling of unease. Silent ischemia and atypical symptoms are more common in women (see *Health Alert: Women and Coronary Artery Disease*). In addition, individuals who do experience angina often have additional silent episodes of myocardial ischemia. Studies have addressed the pathophysiologic differences between silent and symptomatic ischemia. One proposed mechanism for the absence of angina in silent myocardial ischemia is the presence of a global or regional abnormality in left ventricular sympathetic afferent innervation.[51] Such abnormality might occur as part of a metabolic dysfunction in diabetes mellitus, following surgical denervation during coronary artery bypass grafting (CABG) or cardiac transplantation, or following ischemic local nerve injury by myocardial infarction.
4. **Mental stress–induced ischemia.** Also of interest is the lack of angina, even though an artery is occluded, in some individuals during mental stress (Figures 23-16 through 23-18). Rozanski[52] documented myocardial ischemia by radionuclide angiography (RNA) during

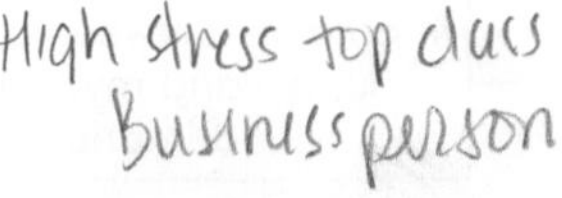

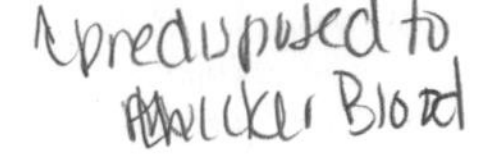

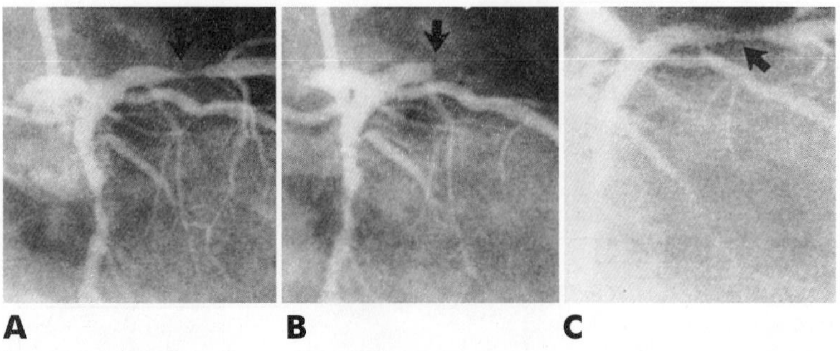

Figure 23-16 ■ **Angiogram of Coronary Arteries. A,** Baseline. **B,** Transient total occlusion of left anterior descending branch of the left coronary artery after mental stress. **C,** After nitrates and nifedipine, artery reopened to same diameter as baseline. (Modified from Stern S, editor: *Silent myocardial ischemia,* St Louis, 1998, Mosby.)

mental stress, and the majority of cases (83%) were silent. The researcher also noted a smaller increase in heart rate during mental stress than during exercise, although the systolic blood pressure response was comparable and the diastolic blood pressure response was even greater with mental stress. These observations, confirmed in similar studies, suggest that mental stress increases blood pressure and myocardial oxygen demand and thus results in mental stress–induced myocardial ischemia. Chronic stress has been linked to a hypercoagulable state that may contribute to acute ischemic events.[53] Stress management has been associated with a significant reduction in CAD events in men.[54]

HEALTH ALERT
Women and Coronary Artery Disease

Until recently, coronary artery disease (CAD) was the number one killer of women. Now, more women die from *CAD* and *stroke* than from all cancers combined. Women have a higher rate of mortality than men, in part because of underdiagnosis and treatment. Nearly two thirds of women who die from CAD had no prior warning symptoms, and symptoms that do occur are often different from those classically seen in men. One postulate is that women have more microvascular coronary disease than men, which can cause fewer and less recognizable symptoms. Women also have more avoidable risk factors than men, especially elevated cholesterol and physical inactivity, and women are less likely to receive counseling about nutrition, exercise, and weight control. In addition, CAD risk rises dramatically after menopause. Although many studies suggest that endogenous estrogen is protective of vascular function, several large prospective studies have determined that estrogen replacement regimens do not reduce the risk of CAD in postmenopausal women. In addition to lifestyle changes, the most effective interventions to reduce CAD risk in women have been found to be the HMG-CoA reductase drugs (statins) that lower cholesterol and exert both anti-inflammatory and plaque stabilizing effects. Research regarding the beneficial and adverse effects of statins is in progress.

Data from D'Antono B et al: Angina symptoms in men and women with stable coronary artery disease and evidence of exercise-induced myocardial perfusion defects, *Am Heart J* 151(4):813–819, 2006; Gauri AJ et al: Disparities in the use of primary prevention and defibrillator therapy among blacks and women, *Am J Med* 119 (2):167.e17–167.e21, 2006; Kuller LH, Women's Health Initiative: Hormone replacement therapy and risk of cardiovascular disease: implications of the results of the Women's Health Initiative, *Arterioscler Thromb Vasc Biol* 23(1):11–16, 2003; Morise AP: Assessment of estrogen status as a marker of prognosis in women with symptoms of suspected coronary artery disease presenting for stress testing, *Am J Cardiol* 97(3):367–371, 2006; Shaw LJ et al: Insights from the NHLBI-sponsored Women's Ischemia Syndrome Evaluation (WISE) study. Part I: Gender differences in traditional and novel risk factors, symptom evaluation, and gender-optimized diagnostic strategies, *J Am Coll Cardiol* 47(suppl)1s-71s, 2006; Vaccarino V et al: Sex and racial differences in the management of acute myocardial infarction, 1994 through 2002, *N Engl J Med* 353(7):671–682, 2005; Dale KM et al: Impact of gender on static efficacy, *Curr Med Res Opin* 23(3):565–574, 2007.

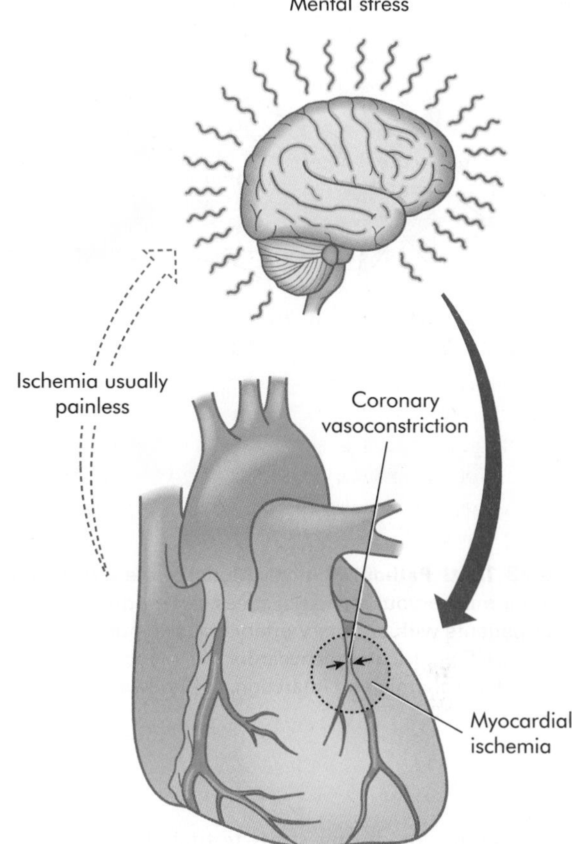

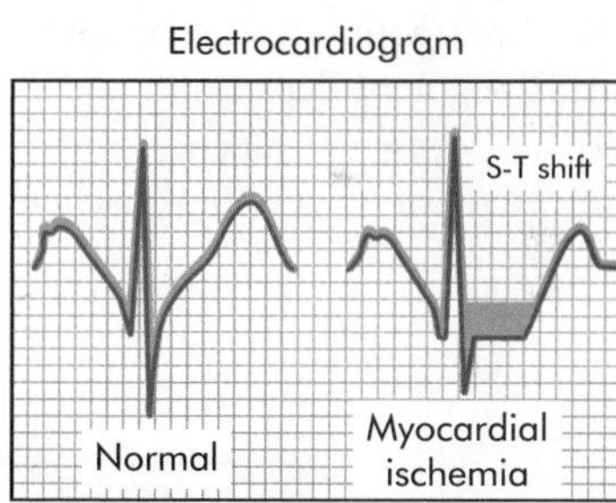

Figure 23-17 ■ **The Ischemic Cost of Aggravation.** Linkages among daily mental and emotional stimuli, brain activity, and coronary and myocardial physiology. (Modified from Papodemetrion V et al: *Am Heart J* 132:1299, 1996.)

EVALUATION AND TREATMENT Many individuals with reversible myocardial ischemia will have a normal physical examination between events. However, in those with chronic ischemia, the examination may disclose rapid pulse or extra heart sounds (left ventricular gallop or S_3), indicating impaired left ventricular function during ischemia. The presence of xanthelasmas (small fat deposits) around the eyelids or arcus senilis of the eyes (a yellow lipid ring around the cornea) suggests dyslipidemia and possible atherosclerosis.

Electrocardiography is a critical tool for the diagnosis of myocardial ischemia. Because many individuals have normal electrocardiograms when there is no pain, diagnosis requires that electrocardiography be performed during an

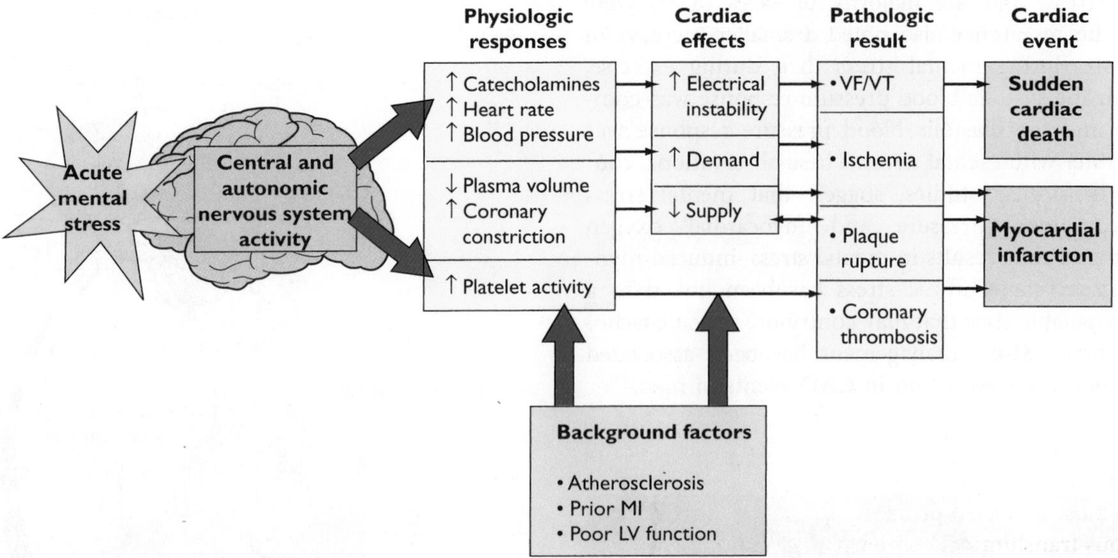

Figure 23-18 ■ **Pathophysiologic Model of the Effects of Acute Stress as a Trigger of Cardiac Clinical Events.** Acting via the central and autonomic nervous systems, stress can produce a cascade of physiologic responses that may lead to myocardial ischemia, especially in patients with coronary artery disease; potentially fatal dysrhythmia; plaque rupture; or coronary thrombosis. *VF,* Ventricular fibrillation; *VT,* ventricular tachycardia; *MI,* myocardial infarction; *LV,* left ventricular. (From Krantz DS et al: Mental stress as a trigger of myocardial ischemia and infarction. In Deedwania PC, Tofler GH, editors: *Triggers and timing of cardiac events,* ed 2, London, 1996, Saunders.)

attack of angina or during stress testing. The ST segment and the T wave segments of the electrocardiogram correlate with ventricular contraction and relaxation (see Figure 22-11). Transient ST segment depression and T wave inversion are characteristic signs of subendocardial ischemia. ST elevation, indicative of transmural ischemia, is seen in individuals with Prinzmetal angina and transmural myocardial infarction (Figure 23-19). The electrocardiogram also can indicate which coronary artery is involved. Exercise stress testing is useful in differentiating angina from other types of chest pain, as well as detecting ischemic changes that occur in the absence of anginal pain.

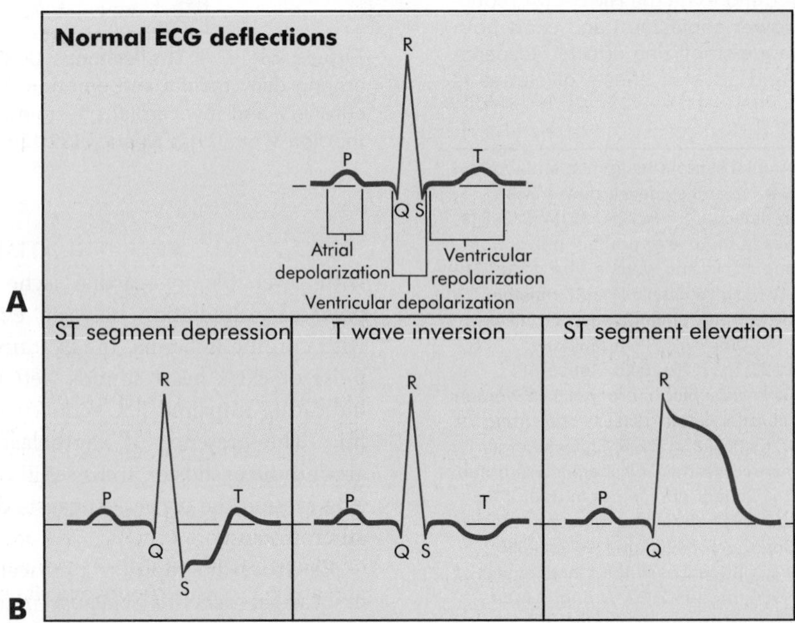

Figure 23-19 ■ **Electrocardiogram (ECG) and Ischemia. A,** Normal ECG. **B,** Electrocardiographic alterations associated with ischemia.

Stress testing is made more sensitive when radioisotope imaging is added to the ECG as an indicator of myocardial ischemia. Currently, the diagnostic modality of choice for the diagnosis of myocardial ischemia is single photon emission computerized tomography (SPECT), which is effective at identifying ischemia and estimating coronary risk. Radioisotope imaging with thallium-201 and stress echocardiography are other techniques used to diagnose CAD. Noninvasive tests for evaluating the presence of coronary atherosclerotic lesions include measurement of coronary artery calcium by computed tomography (CT), noninvasive coronary angiography using electron beam CT, protein-weighted magnetic resonance imaging, and intravascular ultrasound.[55]

Coronary angiography helps determine the anatomic extent of CAD. The procedure is expensive and carries some risk; thus, it is used primarily to evaluate for possible percutaneous transluminal coronary intervention (PTCI) or coronary artery bypass graft (CABG) surgery for individuals whose noninvasive studies suggest severe disease.

The primary aim of therapy for myocardial ischemia and angina is to reduce myocardial oxygen consumption by favorably altering its various determinants. The factors most amenable to pharmacologic manipulation are blood pressure, heart rate, contractility, and left ventricular volume. Medications that reduce vasospasm, lower cholesterol, and prevent clotting are also useful. These drugs include nitrates, β-adrenergic blocking agents, calcium channel blockers (verapamil, nifedipine, diltiazem), angiotensin-converting enzyme (ACE) inhibitors, lipid-lowering agents (statins), and antiplatelet agents (aspirin, clopidogrel, dipyridamole).[56] A new drug being tested is trimetazidine, which reduces myocardial fatty acid oxidation, thus reducing oxygen consumption by the myocardium.[57] There remain, however, controversies over how best to manage chronic stable angina.[58]

Percutaneous coronary intervention (PCI) is a procedure whereby stenotic (narrowed) coronary vessels are dilated with a catheter. Several different types of catheters can be used to open the blocked vessel. PCI is generally used to treat single-vessel disease, but it can be effective with multiple-vessel disease or restenosis of a coronary artery bypass graft. Restenosis of the artery is the major complication of the procedure; however, placement of a coronary stent can reduce this risk. Antithrombotic treatment with glycoprotein IIb/IIIa receptor antagonists after stenting also can greatly improve outcomes.[59]

Ischemic heart disease can be surgically treated by a coronary artery bypass graft (CABG), usually using the saphenous vein from the thigh. In selected individuals, a modified CABG procedure called *minimally invasive direct coronary artery bypass (MIDCAB)* can be used with much less surgical morbidity and more rapid recovery. In those individuals with refractory angina not amenable to standard bypass surgery, new techniques, such as transmyocardial laser revascularization, enhanced external counterpulsation, and myocardial gene therapy, are providing promising results.[60–62]

QUICK CHECK 23-5

1. Define atherosclerosis, and briefly describe how it forms.
2. Why do hypertension and increased cholesterol increase the development of coronary artery disease?
3. Discuss the relationships among myocardial ischemia, angina, and silent ischemia.

Acute coronary syndromes

The process of atherosclerotic plaque progression can be gradual. However, when there is sudden coronary obstruction caused by thrombus formation over a ruptured or ulcerated atherosclerotic plaque, the acute coronary syndromes result (Figure 23-20). **Unstable angina** is the result of reversible myocardial ischemia and is a harbinger of impending infarction. **Myocardial infarction (MI)** results when there is prolonged ischemia causing irreversible damage to the heart muscle. MI can be further subdivided into **non-ST elevation MI (non-STEMI)** and **ST elevation MI (STEMI).** Sudden cardiac death can occur as a result of any of the acute coronary syndromes.

The American Heart Association Committee on Vascular Lesions provided criteria for subdividing coronary

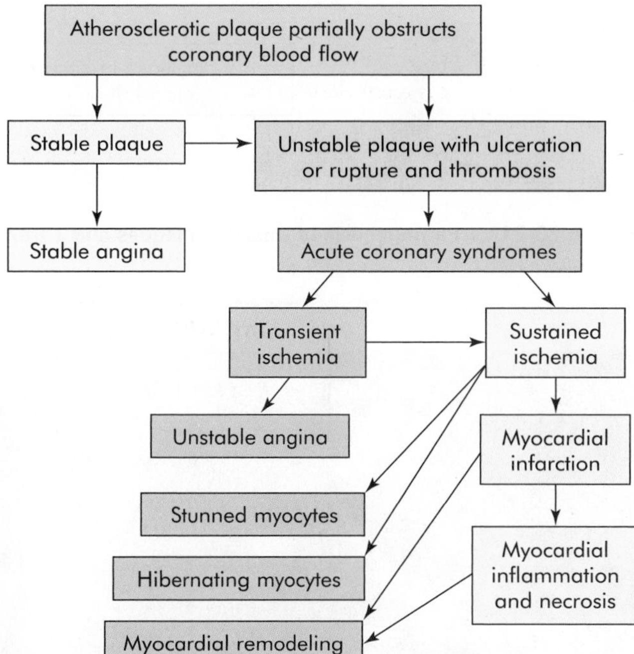

Figure 23-20 ■ Pathophysiology of Acute Coronary Syndromes. The atherosclerotic process can lead to stable plaque formation and stable angina or can result in unstable plaques that are prone to rupture and thrombus. Thrombus formation on a ruptured plaque that disperses in less than 20 minutes leads to transient ischemia and unstable angina. If the vessel obstruction is sustained, myocardial infarction with inflammation and necrosis of the myocardium results. In addition, myocardial infarction is associated with other structural and functional changes, including myocyte stunning and hibernation and myocardial remodeling.

atherosclerotic plaque progression into five phases with different lesion types corresponding to each phase.[63] The main point of this system is that some atherosclerotic lesions are "stable" and progress by gradually occluding the vessel lumen, whereas other lesions are "unstable" or complicated lesions and (even before there is any significant coronary occlusion) are prone to sudden plaque rupture and thrombus formation resulting in the acute coronary syndromes of unstable angina, myocardial infarction, and even sudden death. Figure 23-20 provides an overview of the steps in the development of the acute coronary syndromes. Plaque disruption (erosions, fissuring, or rupture) occurs because of shear forces, inflammation with release of multiple inflammatory mediators, secretion of macrophage-derived degradative enzymes, immune cell activation, and apoptosis of cells at the edges of the lesions (Figure 23-21).[31,33,64,65] Exposure of the plaque substrate activates the clotting cascade.[49] The resulting thrombus can form quickly (Figure 23-22, *A*). The thrombus may break up before permanent myocyte damage has occurred (unstable angina), or it may cause prolonged ischemia with infarction of the heart muscle (myocardial infarction) (Figure 23-22, *B*).[66]

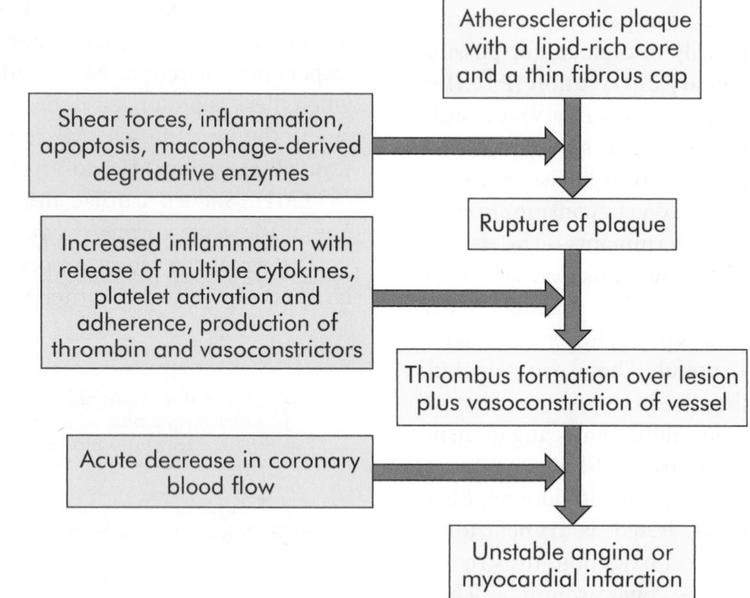

Figure 23-21 ■ Pathogenesis of Unstable Plaques and Thrombus Formation.

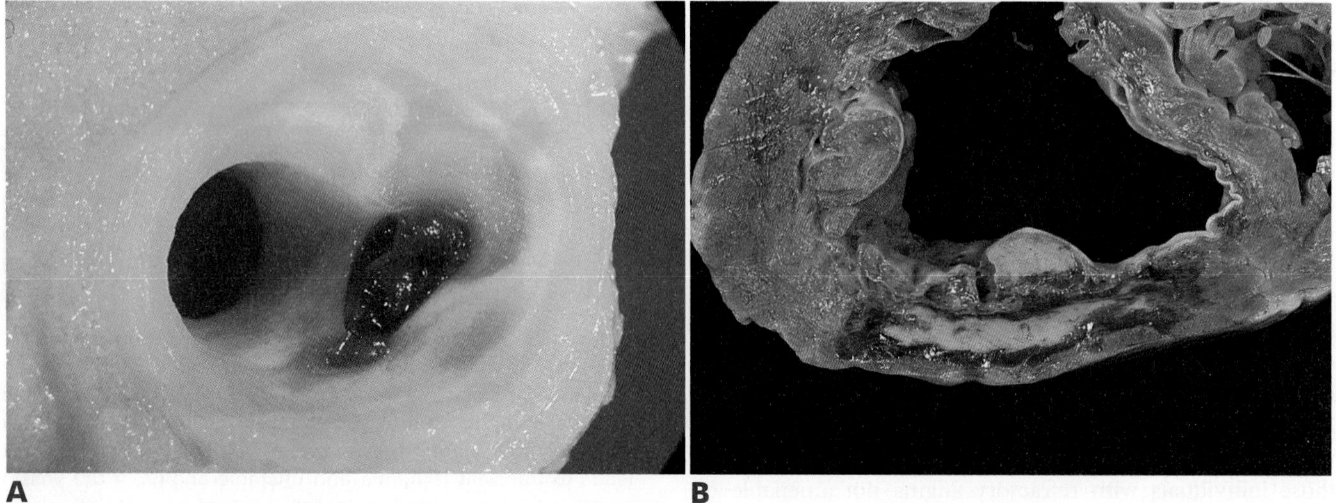

Figure 23-22 ■ Plaque Disruption and Myocardial Infarction. A, Plaque disruption. The cap of the lipid-rich plaque has become torn with the formation of a thrombus, mostly inside the plaque. **B,** Myocardial infarction. This infarct is 6 days old. The center is yellow and necrotic with a hemorrhagic red rim. The responsible artery occlusion is probably in the right coronary artery. The infarct is on the posterior wall. (From Damjanov I, Linder J, editors: *Anderson's pathology,* ed 10, St Louis, 1996, Mosby.)

Unstable angina

Unstable angina is a form of acute coronary syndrome that results from reversible myocardial ischemia. It is important to recognize this syndrome, because it signals that the atherosclerotic plaque has become complicated, and infarction may soon follow.[67] Unstable angina occurs when a fairly small fissuring or superficial erosion of the plaque leads to transient episodes of thrombotic vessel occlusion and vasoconstriction at the site of plaque damage. This thrombus is labile and occludes the vessel for no more than 10 to 20 minutes, with return of perfusion before significant myocardial necrosis occurs. Unstable angina presents as new-onset angina, angina that is occurring at rest, or angina that is increasing in severity or frequency. Individuals may experience increased dyspnea, diaphoresis, and anxiety as the angina worsens. Physical examination may reveal evidence of ischemic myocardial dysfunction such as tachycardia, or pulmonary congestion. The ECG most commonly reveals ST-segment depression and T wave inversion during pain that resolves as the pain is relieved. Approximately 20% of persons with unstable angina will progress to myocardial infarction or death. Management of unstable angina requires some form of antithrombotic therapy. In most cases, individuals are given aspirin and clopidogrel, or IIb/IIIa platelet receptor antagonists when emergent percutaneous coronary intervention (PCI) is anticipated. Anticoagulants such as low-molecular weight heparin or direct thrombin inhibitors also can be given.[68] Some individuals will require immediate intervention with PCI or coronary artery bypass grafting (CABG).

Myocardial infarction

When coronary blood flow is interrupted for an extended period of time, myocyte necrosis occurs.[69] This results in myocardial infarction (MI). Pathologically, there are two major types of myocardial infarction: subendocardial infarction and transmural infarction. Plaque progression, disruption, and subsequent clot formation are the same for myocardial infarction as they are for unstable angina (see Figures 23-20, 23-21, and 23-22).[70] In this case, however, the thrombus is less labile and occludes the vessel for a prolonged period, such that myocardial ischemia progresses to myocyte necrosis and death. If the thrombus breaks up before complete distal tissue necrosis has occurred, the infarction will involve only the myocardium directly beneath the endocardium (subendocardial MI). It is especially important to recognize this form of acute coronary syndrome because recurrent clot formation on the disrupted atherosclerotic plaque is likely unless some intervention is undertaken as soon as possible. If the thrombus lodges permanently in the vessel, the infarction will extend through the myocardium all the way from endocardium to epicardium, resulting in severe cardiac dysfunction (transmural MI). Clinically, it is important to identify those individuals with transmural infarction who are at highest risk for serious complications and who should receive definitive intervention without delay. Those individuals usually have marked elevations in the ST segments on ECG and are categorized as having ST-elevation MI, or STEMI. Those without T segment elevation are more likely to have subendocardial infarction and are said to have non-STEMI.

PATHOPHYSIOLOGY

Cellular injury. Cardiac cells can withstand ischemic conditions for about 20 minutes before cellular death takes place. After only 30 to 60 seconds of hypoxia, electrocardiographic changes are visible. Yet even if cells are metabolically altered and nonfunctional, they can remain viable if blood flow returns within 20 minutes.

After 8 to 10 seconds of decreased blood flow, the affected myocardium becomes cyanotic and cooler. Myocardial oxygen reserves are used quickly (within about 8 seconds) after complete cessation of coronary flow. Glycogen stores decrease as anaerobic metabolism begins. Unfortunately, glycolysis can supply only 65% to 70% of the total myocardial energy requirement and produces much less ATP than aerobic processes. Hydrogen ions and lactic acid accumulate. Because myocardial tissues have poor buffering capabilities and myocardial cells are sensitive to low cellular pH, accumulation of these products further compromises the myocardium. Acidosis may make the myocardium more vulnerable to the damaging effects of lysosomal enzymes and may suppress impulse conduction and contractile function, thereby leading to heart failure.

Oxygen deprivation also is accompanied by electrolyte disturbances, specifically the loss of potassium, calcium, and magnesium from cells. Myocardial cells deprived of necessary oxygen and nutrients lose contractility, thereby diminishing the pumping ability of the heart. Normally, the myocardium takes up varying quantities of catecholamines (epinephrine, norepinephrine). Significant arterial occlusion causes the myocardial cells to release catecholamines, predisposing the individual to serious imbalances of sympathetic and parasympathetic function, irregular heartbeats (dysrhythmia), and heart failure. Catecholamines mediate the release of glycogen, glucose, and stored fat from body cells. Therefore, plasma concentrations of free fatty acids and glycerol rise within 1 hour after the onset of acute myocardial infarction. Excessive levels of free fatty acids can have a harmful detergent effect on cell membranes. Norepinephrine elevates blood sugar levels through stimulation of liver and skeletal muscle cells and suppresses pancreatic β-cell activity, which reduces insulin secretion and elevates blood glucose further. Not surprisingly, hyperglycemia is noted approximately 72 hours after an acute myocardial infarction.[71]

Angiotensin II is released during myocardial ischemia and contributes to the pathogenesis of myocardial infarction in several ways. First, it results in the systemic effects of peripheral vasoconstriction and fluid retention. Second, it is a growth factor for vascular smooth muscle cells, myocytes, and cardiac fibroblasts resulting in structural changes in the myocardium called "remodeling."[72] Finally, angiotensin II promotes catecholamine release and causes coronary artery spasm.

Cellular death. After about 20 minutes of myocardial ischemia, irreversible hypoxic injury causes cellular death and tissue necrosis. This results in the release of intracellular enzymes such as creatinine phosphokinase MB (CPK-MB) and myocyte proteins such as the troponins, through the damaged cell membranes into the interstitial spaces. The lymphatics pick up the enzymes and transport them into the bloodstream, where they can be detected by serologic tests.

Structural and functional changes. With infarction, ventricular function is abnormal and ejection fraction falls which results in increases in ventricular end-diastolic volume (VEDV). If the coronary obstruction involves the perfusion to the left ventricle, pulmonary venous congestion ensues; if the right ventricle is ischemic, increases in systemic venous pressures occur.

Myocardial infarction results in both structural and functional changes of cardiac tissues (Figure 23-23). Gross tissue changes at the area of infarction may not become apparent for several hours, despite almost immediate onset (within 30 to 60 seconds) of electrocardiographic changes. Cardiac tissue surrounding the area of infarction also undergoes changes that can be categorized into (1) **myocardial stunning**—a temporary loss of contractile function that persists for hours to days after perfusion has been restored; (2) **hibernating myocardium**—tissue that is persistently ischemic and undergoes metabolic adaptation to prolong myocyte survival until perfusion can be restored; and (3) **myocardial remodeling**—a process mediated by angiotensin II, aldosterone, catecholamines, adenosine, and inflammatory cytokines that causes myocyte hypertrophy and loss of contractile function in the areas of the heart distant from the site of infarction.[72–75] All of these changes can be limited through rapid restoration of coronary flow and the use of angiotensin converting enzyme (ACE) inhibitors or angiotensin receptor blockers and beta-blockers after MI.

The severity of functional impairment depends on the size of the lesion and the site of infarction. Functional changes can include (1) decreased cardiac contractility with abnormal wall motion, (2) altered left ventricular compliance, (3) decreased stroke volume, (4) decreased ejection fraction, (5) increased left ventricular end-diastolic pressure, and (6) sinoatrial node malfunction. Life-threatening dysrhythmias and heart failure often follow myocardial infarction.

Repair. Myocardial infarction causes a severe inflammatory response that ends with wound repair (see Chapter 5). Damaged cells undergo degradation, fibroblasts proliferate, and scar tissue is synthesized. Many cell types, hormones, and nutrient substrates must be available for optimal healing to proceed. Within 24 hours, leukocytes infiltrate the necrotic area, and proteolytic enzymes from scavenger neutrophils degrade necrotic tissue. The collagen matrix that is deposited is initially weak, mushy, and vulnerable to reinjury. Unfortunately it is at this time in the recovery period (10 to 14 days after infarction) that individuals feel more like increasing activities and may stress the newly formed scar tissue. After 6 weeks, the necrotic area is completely replaced by scar tissue, which is strong but cannot contract and relax like healthy myocardial tissue.

CLINICAL MANIFESTATIONS The first symptom of acute myocardial infarction is usually sudden, severe chest pain. The pain is similar to angina pectoris but more severe and persistent and is not relieved by nitrates. It may be described as heavy and crushing, such as a "truck sitting on my chest." Radiation to the neck, jaw, back, shoulder, or left arm is common. Some individuals, especially those who are elderly or have diabetes, experience no pain, thereby having a "silent" infarction. Infarction often simulates a sensation of unrelenting indigestion. Nausea and vomiting may occur because of reflex stimulation of vomiting centers by pain fibers. Vasovagal reflexes from the area of the

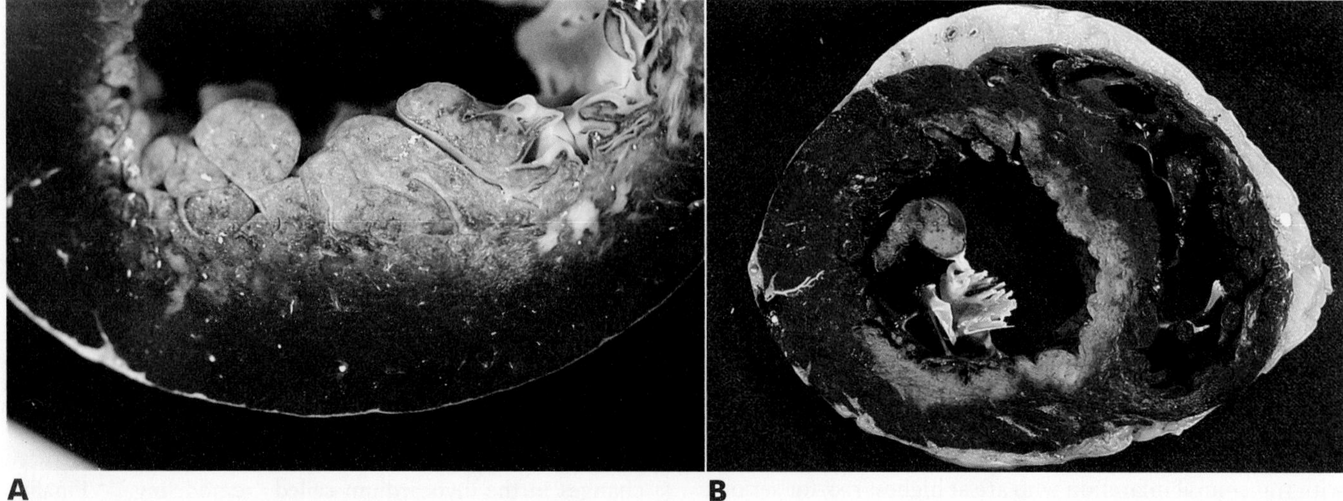

Figure 23-23 ■ **Myocardial Infarction. A,** Local infarct confined to one region. **B,** Massive large infarct caused by occlusion of three coronary arteries. (From Damjanov I, Linder J, editors: *Anderson's pathology,* ed 10, St Louis, 1996, Mosby.)

infarcted myocardium also may affect the gastrointestinal tract. Catecholamine release results in sympathetic stimulation, producing diaphoresis and peripheral vasoconstriction that cause the skin to become cool and clammy.

Various cardiovascular changes are found on physical examination:

1. Blood pressure initially decreases.
2. The sympathetic nervous system is reflexively activated to compensate, resulting in a temporary increase in heart rate and blood pressure.
3. Abnormal extra heart sounds reflect left ventricular dysfunction.
4. Pericardial friction rub (roughened membranes rubbing against each other) and cardiac murmurs may result from inflammation.
5. Pulmonary findings of congestion including dullness to percussion and inspiratory crackles at the lung bases can occur if the individual develops heart failure.

Complications. The number and severity of postinfarction complications depend on the location and extent of necrosis, the individual's physiologic condition before the infarction, and the availability of swift therapeutic intervention. Sudden cardiac death can occur in individuals with myocardial ischemia even if infarction is absent or minimal and is a multifactorial problem. Risk factors for sudden death are related to three factors: ischemia, left ventricular dysfunction, and electrical instability. These factors interact with each other (Figure 23-24). Table 23-5 lists the most common complications.

EVALUATION AND TREATMENT The diagnosis of acute myocardial infarction is made on the basis of history, physical examination, ECG, and serial enzyme alterations. The cardiac troponins (troponin I and troponin T) are the most specific indicators of MI. A transient rise in these plasma enzyme levels can confirm the occurrence of MI and indicate its severity. Other enzymes released by myocardial cells include creatine kinase (CK) and lactic dehydrogenase (LDH). These enzymes exist in several different active molecular forms called *isoenzymes,* which are present in different amounts within particular tissues. Blood is drawn for troponin and isoenzyme determinations as soon as possible after the onset of symptoms, and serial serum levels of these markers are assessed for several days. If serologic tests show abnormally high levels of troponin and isoenzymes associated with cardiac tissue (creatine kinase-myocardial bound [CK-MB], LDH_1), acute myocardial infarction probably has occurred. CK-MB is less specific

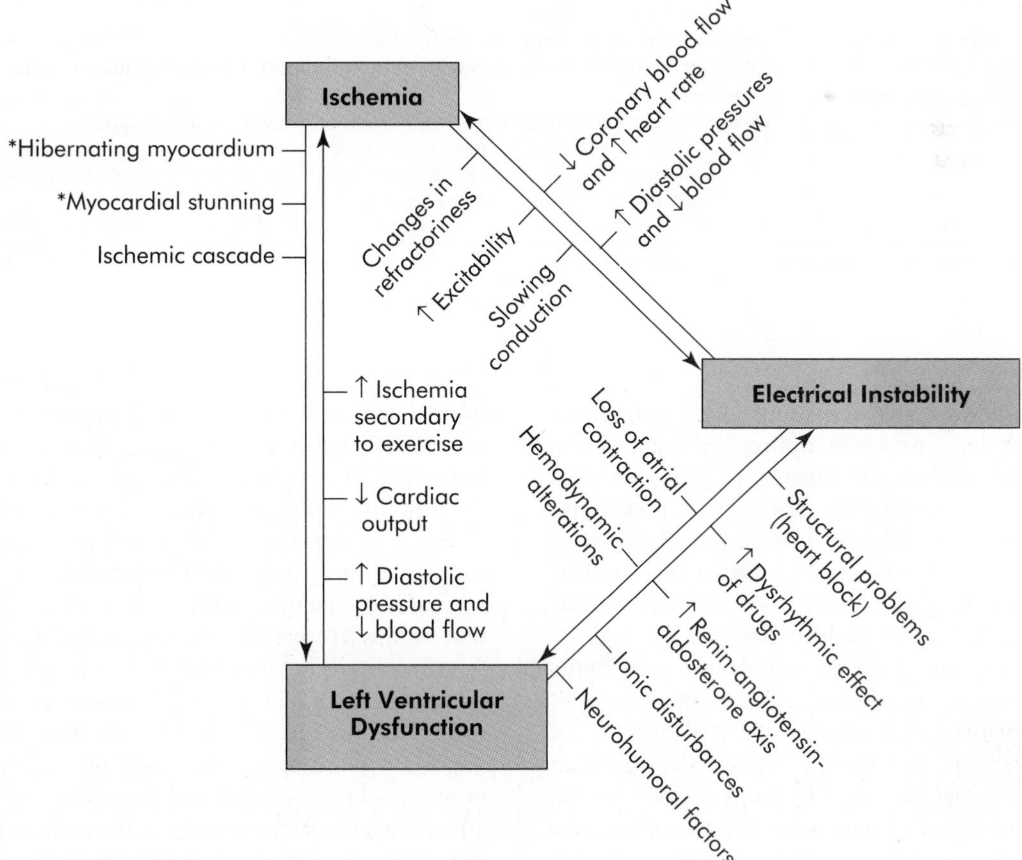

Figure 23-24 ■ **Three Interacting Factors Related to Sudden Cardiac Death.** The three factors are ischemia, left ventricular dysfunction, and electrical instability.

TABLE 23-5

Complications With Myocardial Infarctions

Type	Characteristics
Dysrhythmias	Disturbances of cardiac rhythm that affect 90% of cardiac infarction patients Caused by ischemia, hypoxia, autonomic nervous system imbalances, lactic acidosis, electrolyte abnormalities, alterations of impulse conduction pathways or conduction abnormalities, drug toxicity, or hemodynamic abnormalities
Left ventricular failure (congestive heart failure)	Characterized by pulmonary congestion, reduced myocardial contractility, and abnormal heart wall motion Cardiogenic shock can develop
Inflammation of the pericardium (pericarditis)	Includes pericardial friction rubs Often noted 2 to 3 days later and associated with anterior chest pain that worsens with respiratory effort
Dressler postinfarction syndrome	Essentially a delayed form of pericarditis that occurs 1 week to several months after acute MI syndrome Thought to be immunologic response to necrotic myocardium marked by pain, fever, friction rub, pleural effusion, and arthralgias
Organic brain syndrome	Occurs if blood flow to brain is impaired secondary to MI
Transient ischemic attacks or cerebrovascular accident	Occur if thromboemboli break loose from clots that form in the cardiac chambers or on cardiac valves
Rupture of heart structures	Caused by necrosis of tissue in or around papillary muscles Affects papillary muscles of chordae tendineae cordis Predisposing factors include thinning of wall, poor collateral flow, shearing effect of muscular contraction against stiffened necrotic area, marked necrosis at terminal end of blood supply and aging of myocardium with laceration of myocardial microstructure
Rupture of wall of infarcted ventricle	Can be caused by aneurysm formation when pressure becomes too great
Left ventricular aneurysm	Late (month to years) complication of MI that can contribute to heart failure and thromboemboli
Infarctions around septal structures	Occur in those structures that separate heart chambers and lead to septal rupture Associated with audible, harsh cardiac murmurs, increased left ventricular end-diastolic pressure, and decreased systemic blood pressure
Systemic thromboembolism	May disseminate from debris and clots that collect inside dilated aneurysmal sacs or from infarcted endocardium
Pulmonary thromboembolism	Usually from deep venous thrombi of legs Reduced incidence associated with early mobilization and prophylactic anticoagulation therapy
Sudden death	Dysrhythmias frequently causative, particularly ventricular fibrillation Risk of death increased by age more than 65 years, previous angina pectoris, hypotension or cardiogenic shock, acute systolic hypertension at time of admission, diabetes mellitus, dysrhythmias, and previous MI

MI, Myocardial infarction; *CPR*, cardiopulmonary resuscitation.

than troponins and may increase in individuals with certain other conditions (e.g., muscular dystrophy, hypothermia, chronic obstructive pulmonary disease [COPD] associated with left heart failure and pulmonary embolism, extensive third-degree burns, small bowel infarction). Elevation of troponin, CK-MB and LDH_1 may be noted at characteristic times, and laboratory confirmation that an infarction has occurred may be delayed up to 12 hours.

Myocardial infarction can occur in various regions of the heart wall and may be described as anterior, inferior, posterior, lateral, subendocardial, or transmural, depending on the anatomic location and extent of tissue damage from infarction. Twelve-lead electrocardiograms (ECGs) help to localize the affected area through identification of Q waves and changes in ST segments and T waves (Figure 23-25). The infarcted myocardium is surrounded by a zone of hypoxic injury, which may progress to necrosis or return to normal. Adjacent to this zone of hypoxic injury is a zone of reversible ischemia. Ischemic and injured myocardial tissue causes ST and T wave changes. As stated previously, if the thrombus breaks up before complete distal tissue necrosis has occurred, the infarction will involve only the myocardium directly beneath the endocardium. This type of myocardial infarction most often presents with no elevation of the ST segment on electrocardiogram (ECG) and therefore is termed non-STEMI.[76–78] In addition, this form of infarction will not be associated with the classic Q-wave tracing on the ECG (non-Q-wave MI). It is especially important to recognize this form of acute coronary syndrome because recurrent clot formation on the disrupted atherosclerotic plaque is likely, with resultant infarct expansion. If the thrombus lodges more permanently in the vessel, the infarction will extend through the myocardium from endocardium to epicardium, resulting in severe

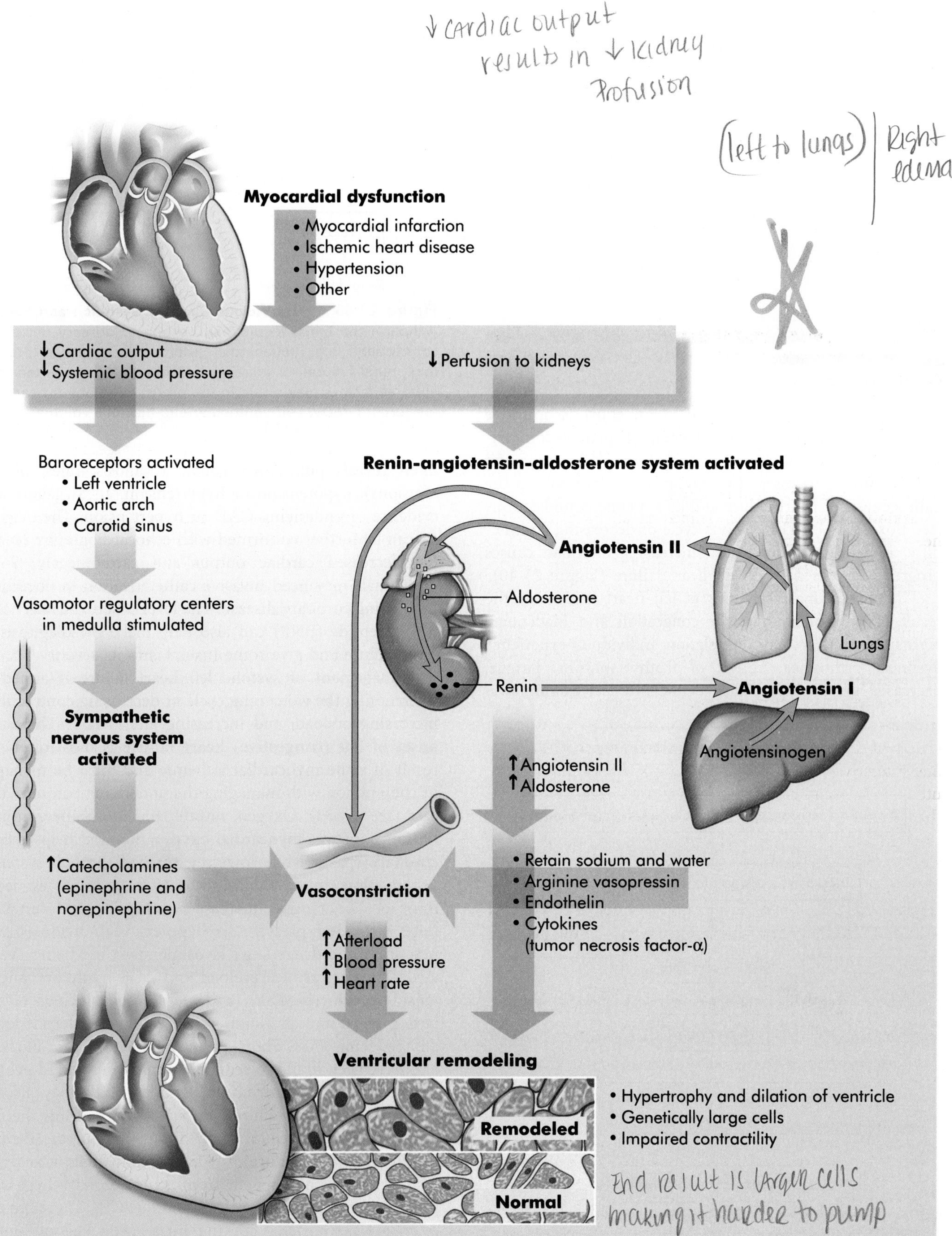

Figure 23-37 ■ **Pathophysiology of Ventricular Remodeling.** Myocardial dysfunction activates the renin-angiotensin-aldosterone and sympathetic nervous systems releasing neurohormones (angiotensin II, aldosterone, catecholamines, and cytokines). These neurohormones contribute to ventricular remodeling. (Redrawn from Carelock J, Clark AP: Heart failure: pathophysiologic mechanisms, *Am J Nurs* 101[12]:27, 2001.)

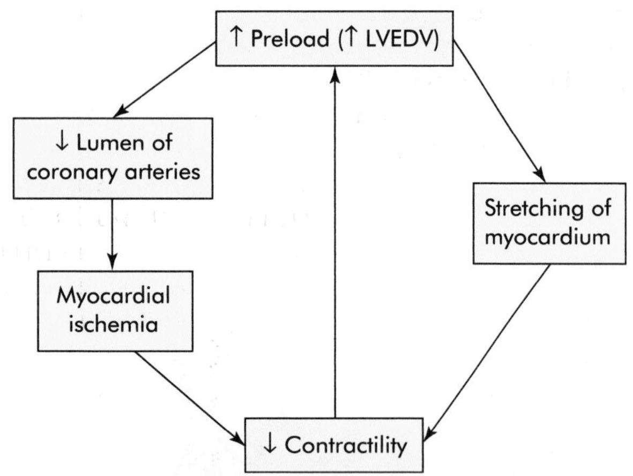

Figure 23-38 The Effect of Elevated Preload on Myocardial Oxygen Supply and Demand. *LVEDV,* Left ventricular end-diastolic volume.

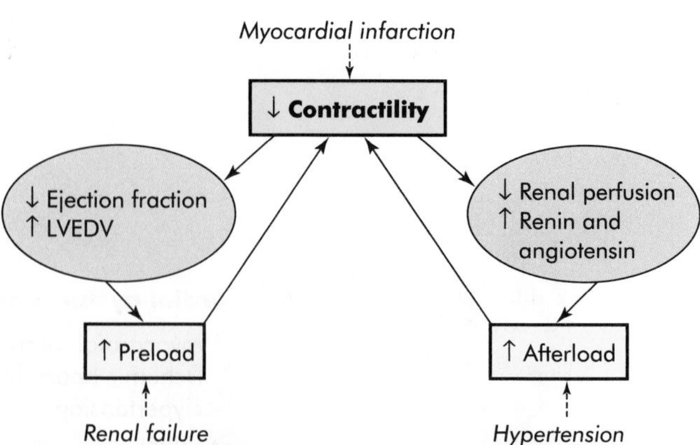

Figure 23-40 The Vicious Cycle of Systolic Heart Failure. Although the initial insult may be one of primary decreased contractility (e.g., myocardial infarction), increased preload (e.g., renal failure), or increased afterload (e.g., hypertension), all three factors play a role in the progression of left heart failure (LHF). *LVEDV,* Left ventricular end-diastolic volume.

natriuretic peptides are released in an effort to improve renal salt and water excretion but are inadequate to compensate for these neurohumoral perturbations.[102] Immune and inflammatory processes also play an important role in the pathogenesis of heart failure and its systemic complications (see Box 23-1).[103] This vicious cycle of decreasing contractility, increasing preload, and increasing afterload causes progressive worsening of left heart failure (Figure 23-40).

The clinical manifestations of left heart failure are the result of pulmonary vascular congestion and inadequate perfusion of the systemic circulation. Individuals experience dyspnea, orthopnea, cough of frothy sputum, fatigue, decreased urine output, and edema. Physical examination often reveals pulmonary edema (cyanosis, rales, pleural effusions), hypotension or hypertension, an S_3 gallop, and evidence of underlying CAD or hypertension. The diagnosis can be further confirmed with echocardiography revealing decreased cardiac output and cardiomegaly. Some individuals may need invasive catheterization to document underlying coronary disease. The level of serum brain natriuretic peptide (BNP) can also help make the diagnosis of heart failure and give some insight into its severity.[104]

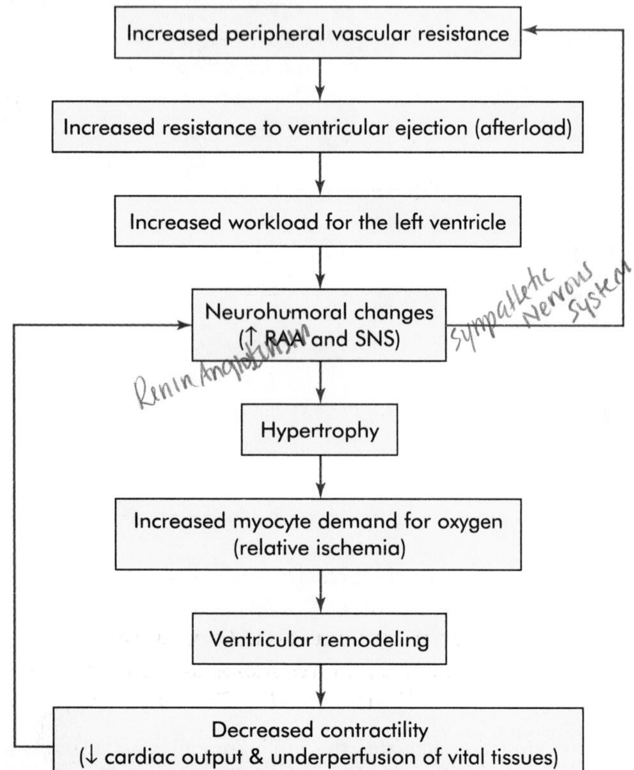

Figure 23-39 The Role of Increased Afterload in the Pathogenesis of Heart Failure.

Management of systolic left heart failure is aimed at interrupting the worsening cycle of decreasing contractility, increasing preload, and increasing afterload.[105] The **acute onset of left (congestive) heart failure** is most often the result of acute myocardial ischemia and must be managed in conjunction with managing the underlying coronary disease (see p. 633). Oxygen, nitrate, and morphine administration improves myocardial oxygenation and helps relieve coronary spasm while lowering preload through systemic venodilation. Intravenous inotropic drugs, such as dopamine or dobutamine, increase contractility and can help raise the blood pressure in hypotensive individuals, and new inotropic drugs (e.g., levosimendan) are being evaluated. Diuretics reduce preload and ACE inhibitors, angiotensin receptor blockers, and aldosterone blockers reduce both preload and afterload by decreasing aldosterone levels and reducing PVR. Short-acting intravenous beta-blockers also have been found to reduce mortality in selected people. Intravenous brain natriuretic peptide (BNP) may also be used in acute heart failure, although results of this therapy are mixed (see *Health Alert:* Brain Natriuretic Peptide [BNP] and Heart Failure).[104] Finally, individuals with severe systolic failure may benefit from acute coronary bypass or percutaneous coronary intervention (PCI). These people often are supported with the intra-aortic balloon pump (IABP) until they can be taken safely to the operating room. The IABP is positioned in the aorta just distal to the aortic valve and is inflated during diastole to improve coronary perfusion and deflated during systole to reduce afterload.

Management of **chronic left heart failure** also relies on increasing contractility and reducing preload and afterload. The current standard of care for chronic heart failure includes diuretics, ACE inhibitors, and beta-blockers for all clinical stages.[105] Salt restriction and diuretics (especially spironolactone) are effective in reducing preload. ACE inhibitors (or Ang II receptor blockers) reduce preload and afterload and have been shown to significantly reduce mortality in chronic left heart failure. Beta-blockers improve symptoms and increase survival but must be used carefully to avoid hypotension. The inotropic drug digoxin may be considered in some individuals, especially those with atrial fibrillation. Although many individuals with left heart failure die suddenly from dysrhythmias, prophylactic administration of antidysrhythmics has not been shown to improve survival. In individuals with sustained ventricular tachycardia, amiodarone or implantable cardioverter-defibrillators should be considered. Cardiac resynchronization therapy is proving to be an important modality in selected individuals.[105,106] Coronary bypass surgery or PTCI may improve perfusion to ischemic myocardium (hibernating myocardium) and improve cardiac output. Other types of surgical intervention that improve ventricular geometry may be considered. Finally, heart transplant may need to be considered. Experimental therapies including gene and stem cell therapies are being explored.[107,108]

HEALTH ALERT

Brain Natriuretic Peptide (BNP) and Heart Failure

Brain natriuretic peptide (BNP) is produced and released in response to pressure and volume overload of the cardiac chambers. This occurs in both systolic and diastolic heart failure. BNP causes arterial and venous dilation, natriuresis, and suppression of the renin-angiotensin-aldosterone system and the sympathetic nervous system. BNP inhibits myocardial fibrosis and hypertrophy and enhances diastolic function. Serum levels of BNP can be measured to help with determining the diagnosis, prognosis and response to treatment in heart failure. Recently, BNP levels have been found to be predictive of cardiovascular morbidity even in individuals without heart failure. Nesiritide, a human B-type natriuretic peptide (hBNP), is an effective agent for improving hemodynamic profiles and symptoms of disease in individuals with acute severe decompensated CHF.

Data from Bibbins-Domingo, K, et al: *N*-Terminal Fragment of the Prohormone Brain-Type Natriuretic Peptide (NT-proBNP), Cardiovascular Events, and Mortality in Patients With Stable Coronary Heart Disease, *JAMA* 297:169–176,2007; Fontana D: Nesiritide: the latest drug for treating heart failure, *Crit Care Nurs* 26(1):39–44, 46–47, 2006; Januzzi JL Jr: Natriuretic peptide testing: a window into the diagnosis and prognosis of heart failure, *Clev Clin J Med* 73(2):149–152:155–157, 2006; Jarai R, Wojta J, Huber K: Circulating B-type natriuretic peptides in patients with acute coronary syndromes: pathophysiological, prognostical and therapeutical considerations, *Thromb Haemost* 94(5):926–932, 2005; Sullivan DR, West M, Jeremy R: Utility of brain natriuretic peptide (BNP) measurement in cardiovascular disease, *Heart Lung Circ* 14(2):78–84, 2005.

Diastolic heart failure is also known as heart failure with preserved systolic function. Diastolic heart failure can occur singly or along with systolic heart failure. Isolated diastolic heart failure is defined as pulmonary congestion despite a normal stroke volume and cardiac output. It is the cause of 40% to 50% of all cases of left heart failure and is more common in women.[109] It results from decreased compliance of the left ventricle and abnormal diastolic relaxation such that a normal left ventricular end-diastolic volume (LVEDV) results in an increased left ventricular end-diastolic pressure (LVEDP). This pressure is reflected back into the pulmonary circulation and results in pulmonary edema. The major causes of diastolic dysfunction include hypertension-induced myocardial hypertrophy and myocardial ischemia with resultant ventricular remodeling. Like systolic heart failure, diastolic failure is characterized by sustained increases in the renin-angiotensin-aldosterone and sympathetic nervous systems.[109] Hypertrophy and ischemia cause a decreased ability of the myocytes to actively pump calcium from the cytosol, resulting in impaired relaxation. Other causes include aortic valvular disease, mitral valve disease, pericardial diseases, and cardiomyopathies. Diabetes also increases the risk for diastolic dysfunction.

Individuals with diastolic dysfunction present with dyspnea on exertion, fatigue, and evidence of pulmonary edema (crackles on auscultation, pleural effusions). There also may be evidence of underlying coronary disease, hypertension, or valvular disease. Diagnosis is made initially by echocardiography, which demonstrates poor ventricular filling with normal ejection fractions. Management is aimed at improving ventricular relaxation and prolonging diastolic filling times to reduce diastolic pressure. Calcium channel blockers, beta-blockers, ACE inhibitors, and angiotensin receptor blockers (ARBs) have been used with varying success. Inotropic drugs are not indicated in isolated diastolic heart failure because contractility and ejection fraction are not affected; however, digoxin may be used to slow the heart rate in individuals with atrial fibrillation. An innovative surgical technique that involves the transplantation of a portion of the latissimus dorsi muscle into the wall of the noncompliant left ventricle (dynamic cardiomyoplasty) is being tried, with some early success. Mortality is lower with diastolic failure than with systolic; however, risk of death is four times that of the population without heart failure.[105]

Right heart failure

Right heart failure can result from left heart failure when an increase in left ventricular filling pressure is reflected back into the pulmonary circulation. As pressure in the pulmonary circulation rises, the resistance to right ventricular emptying increases (Figure 23-41). The right ventricle is poorly prepared to compensate for this increased afterload and will dilate and fail. When this happens, pressure will rise in the systemic venous circulation, resulting in peripheral edema and hepatosplenomegaly. Treatment relies on

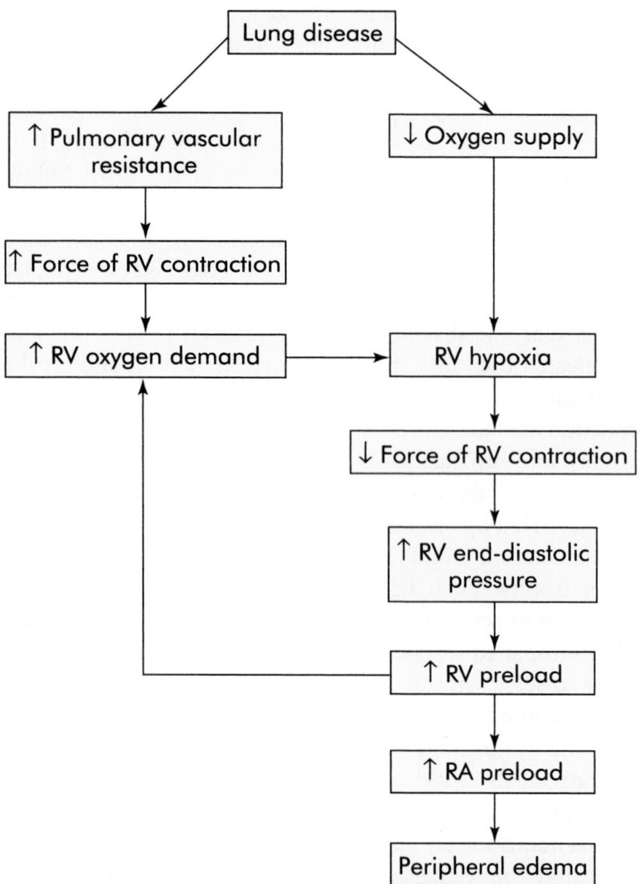

Figure 23-41 ■ **Right Heart Failure** *RV,* Right ventricular; *RA,* right atrial; *JVD,* jugular venous distension.

management of the left ventricular dysfunction as just outlined. When right heart failure occurs in the absence of left heart failure, it is caused most commonly by diffuse hypoxic pulmonary disease such as chronic obstructive pulmonary disease (COPD), cystic fibrosis, and adult respiratory distress syndrome (ARDS). These disorders result in an increase in right ventricular afterload. The mechanisms for this type of right ventricular dysfunction (cor pulmonale) are discussed in Chapter 26. Finally, myocardial infarction, cardiomyopathies, and pulmonic valvular disease interfere with right ventricular contractility and can lead to right heart failure.

High-output failure

High-output failure is the inability of the heart to adequately supply the body with blood-borne nutrients, despite adequate blood volume and normal or elevated myocardial contractility. In high-output failure, the heart increases its output but the body's metabolic needs are still not met. Common causes of high-output failure are anemia, septicemia, hyperthyroidism, and beriberi (Figure 23-42).

Anemia decreases the oxygen-carrying capacity of the blood. Metabolic acidosis occurs as the body's cells switch to anaerobic metabolism (see Chapter 4). In response to metabolic acidosis, heart rate and stroke volume increase in an attempt to improve tissue perfusion. If anemia is severe, however, even maximum cardiac output does not supply the cells with enough oxygen for metabolism.

In septicemia, disturbed metabolism, bacterial toxins, and the inflammatory process cause systemic vasodilation and fever. Faced with a lowered systemic vascular resistance (SVR) and an elevated metabolic rate, cardiac output increases to maintain blood pressure and prevent metabolic acidosis. In overwhelming septicemia, however, the heart may not be able to raise its output enough to compensate for vasodilation. Body tissues show signs of inadequate blood supply despite a high cardiac output.

Hyperthyroidism accelerates cellular metabolism through the actions of elevated levels of thyroxine from the thyroid gland. This may occur chronically (thyrotoxicosis) or acutely (thyroid storm). Because the body's demand for oxygen threatens to cause metabolic acidosis, cardiac output increases. If blood levels of thyroxine are high and the metabolic response to thyroxine is vigorous, even an abnormally elevated cardiac output may be inadequate.

In the United States, beriberi (thiamine deficiency) usually is caused by malnutrition secondary to chronic alcoholism. Beriberi actually causes a mixed type of heart failure. Thiamine deficiency impairs cellular metabolism in all tissues, including the myocardium. In the heart, impaired cardiac metabolism leads to insufficient contractile strength. In blood vessels, thiamine deficiency leads mainly to peripheral vasodilation, which decreases SVR. Heart failure ensues as decreased SVR triggers increased cardiac output, which the impaired myocardium is unable to deliver. The strain of demands for increased output in the face of impaired metabolism may deplete cardiac reserves until low-output failure begins.

✔ QUICK CHECK 23-10

1. Why are changes in LVEDV important for left heart failure?
2. What is ventricular remodeling?
3. What is the vicious cycle of systolic heart failure?

SHOCK

In **shock** the cardiovascular system fails to perfuse the tissues adequately, resulting in widespread impairment of cellular metabolism. Because tissue perfusion can be disrupted by any factor that alters heart function, blood volume, or blood pressure, shock has many causes and various clinical manifestations. Ultimately, however, shock progresses to organ failure and death, unless compensatory mechanisms reverse the process or clinical intervention succeeds. Untreated severe shock overwhelms the body's compensatory mechanisms through positive feedback loops that initiate and maintain a downward physiologic spiral.

The term **multiple organ dysfunction syndrome (MODS)** describes the failure two or more organ systems after severe illness and injury and is a frequent complication of severe shock. The disease process is initiated and

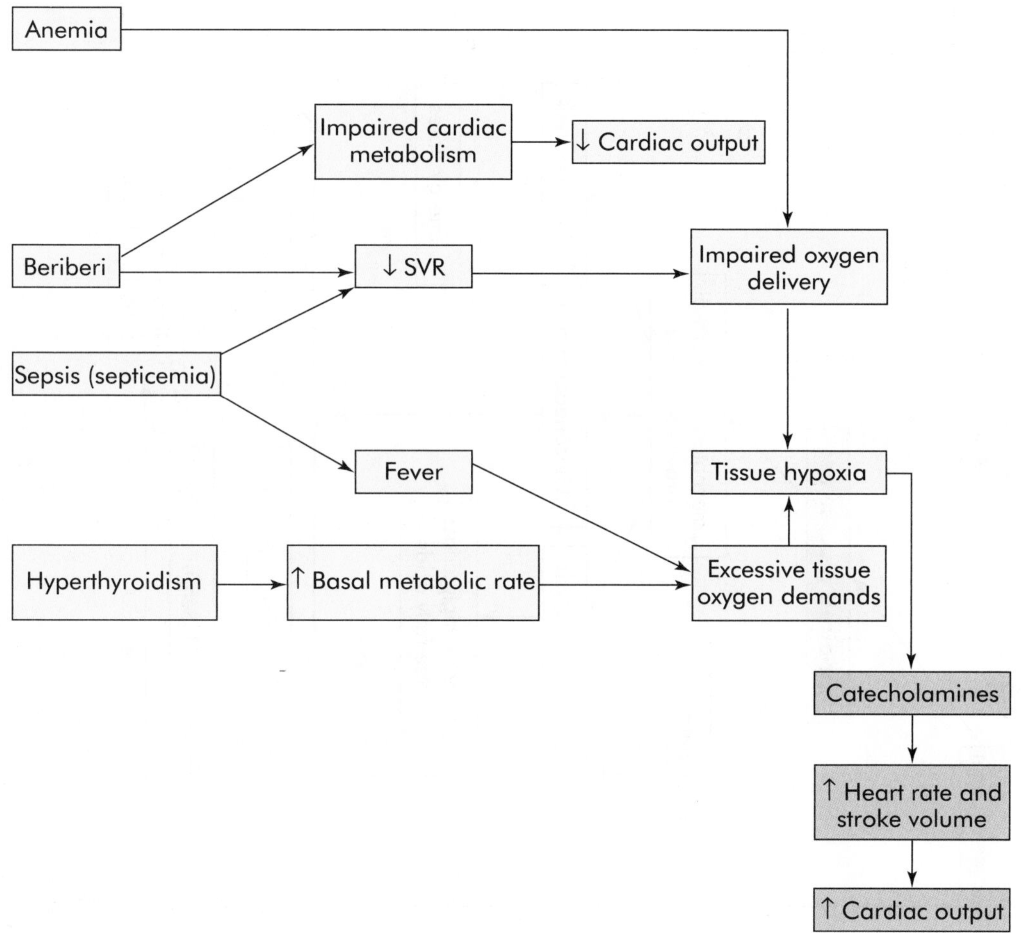

Figure 23-42 ■ **High-Output Failure.** *SVR,* Systemic vascular resistance.

perpetuated by uncontrolled inflammatory and stress responses. It is progressive and is associated with significant mortality.[110]

Impairment of Cellular Metabolism

The final common pathway in shock of any type is impairment of cellular metabolism. Figure 23-43 illustrates the pathophysiology of shock at the cellular level.

Impairment of oxygen use

In all types of shock, the cell either is not receiving an adequate amount of oxygen or is unable to use oxygen. Without oxygen, the cell shifts from aerobic to anaerobic metabolism. Anaerobic metabolism is a less efficient method of extracting energy from carbon bonds, and the cell begins to use its stores of adenosine triphosphate (ATP) faster than stores can be replaced. Without ATP, the cell cannot maintain an electrochemical gradient across its selectively permeable membrane. Specifically, the cell cannot operate the sodium-potassium pump. Sodium and chloride accumulate inside the cell, and potassium exits. Cells of the nervous system and myocardium are profoundly and immediately affected. The resting potentials of these cells are reduced, and action potentials decrease in amplitude. Various clinical manifestations of impaired central nervous system and myocardial function result.

As sodium moves into the cell, water follows. Throughout the body, the water drawn from the interstitium into the cells is "replaced" by water that is, in turn, drawn out of the vascular space. This decreases circulatory volume. Within the cells, water causes cellular edema that disrupts cellular membranes, releasing lysosomal enzymes that injure the cells internally and then leak into the interstitium.

Three positive feedback loops further impair oxygen use: (1) activation of the clotting cascade, (2) decreased circulatory volume, and (3) lysosomal enzyme release. The clotting cascade activates the inflammatory response and also accounts for common complications of shock, such as acute tubular necrosis (ATN), acute respiratory distress syndrome (ARDS), and disseminated intravascular coagulation (DIC). Decreased circulatory volume causes the second positive feedback loop and magnifies decreased tissue perfusion in all types of shock. Lysosomal enzymes, the third positive feedback loop, not only injure the cell that released them but also injure adjacent cells. By damaging the mechanisms of surrounding cells, lysosomal enzymes extend areas of impaired metabolism and cellular injury.

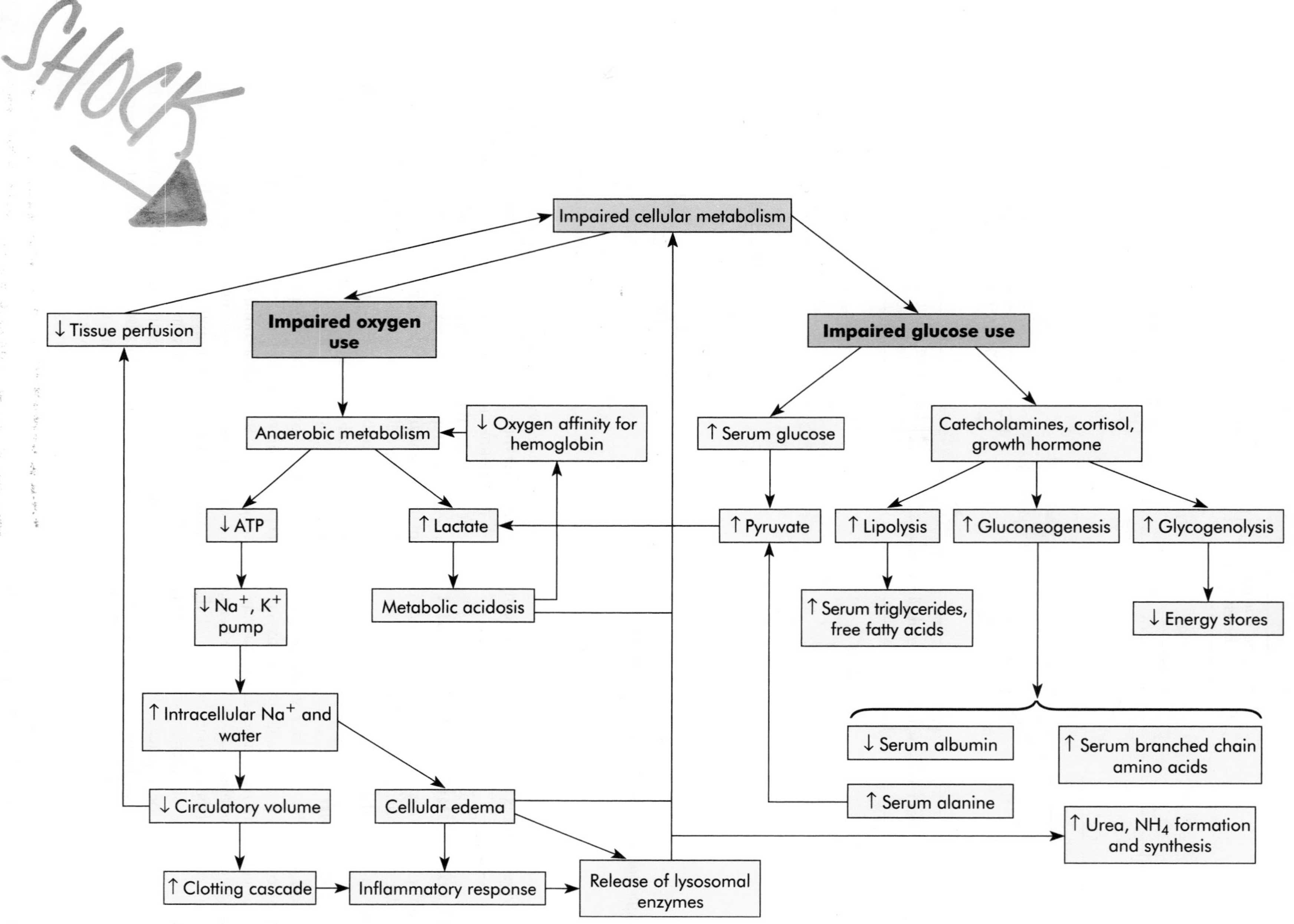

Figure 23-43 ■ **Impaired Cellular Metabolism in Shock.** *ATP,* Adenosine triphosphate.

In addition to decreasing ATP stores, anaerobic metabolism affects the pH of the cell, and metabolic acidosis develops. A compensatory mechanism enables cardiac and skeletal muscles to use lactic acid as a fuel source, but only for a limited time.

The decreasing pH of the cell that is functioning anaerobically has serious consequences. Enzymes necessary for cellular function dissociate under acid conditions. Enzyme dissociation stops cell function, repair, and division. As lactic acid is released systemically, blood pH drops, reducing the oxygen-carrying capacity of the blood (see Chapter 4). Therefore, less oxygen is delivered to the cells. Further acidosis triggers the release of more lysosomal enzymes because the low pH disrupts lysosomal membrane integrity.

Impairment of glucose use

Impaired glucose use can be caused by either impaired glucose delivery or impaired glucose uptake by the cells (see Figure 23-43). The reasons for inadequate glucose delivery are the same as those enumerated for inadequate oxygen delivery. In addition, in septic and anaphylactic shock, glucose metabolism may be increased or disrupted because of fever or bacteria, and glucose uptake can be prevented by the presence of vasoactive toxins, endotoxins, histamine, and kinins.

Some compensatory mechanisms activated by shock contribute to decreased glucose uptake by the cells. High serum levels of cortisol, thyroid hormone, and catecholamines account for hyperglycemia and insulin resistance, tachycardia, increased SVR, and increased cardiac contractility. Cells shift to glycogenolysis, gluconeogenesis, and lipolysis to generate fuel for survival (see Chapter 1). Except in the liver, kidneys, and muscles, the body's cells have extremely limited stores of glycogen. In fact, total body stores can fuel the metabolism for only about 10 hours. The depletion of fat and glycogen stores is not itself a cause of organ failure, but the energy costs of glycogenolysis and lipolysis are considerable and contribute to the cells' failure.

The depletion of protein also is a cause of organ failure. When gluconeogenesis causes proteins to be used for fuel, these proteins are no longer available to maintain cellular structure, function, repair, and replication. The breakdown of protein occurs in starvation states, hyperdynamic metabolic states, and septic shock. The breakdown of protein into amino acids that occurs with septicemia is called *septic autocannibalism*. During anaerobic metabolism, protein breakdown liberates alanine, which is converted to pyruvate. In sepsis, pyruvic acid is changed into lactic acid, and a positive feedback loop is formed.

As proteins are broken down anaerobically, ammonia and urea are produced. Ammonia is toxic to living cells. Uremia develops, and uric acid further disrupts cellular metabolism. Serum albumin and other plasma proteins are consumed for fuel first. Serum protein consumption decreases capillary osmotic pressure and contributes to the development of interstitial edema, creating another positive feedback loop that decreases circulatory volume. In septic shock, plasma protein breakdown includes breakdown of immunoglobulins, thereby impairing immune system function when it is most needed.

Muscle wasting caused by protein breakdown weakens skeletal and cardiac muscle. Skeletal muscle wasting impairs the muscles that facilitate breathing. Muscle wasting therefore alters the actions of both the heart and the lungs. The delivery of oxygen and glucose to the cells is directly reduced, as is the removal of waste products, forming another positive feedback loop.

A final outcome of impaired cellular metabolism is the buildup of metabolic end products in the cell and interstitial spaces. Waste products are toxic to the cells and further disrupt cellular function and membrane integrity. Once a sufficiently large number of cells from vital organs have damage to cellular membranes, leakage of lysosomal enzymes, and ATP depletion, shock can be irreversible.

Types of Shock

Shock is classified by cause as cardiogenic (caused by heart failure), hypovolemic (caused by insufficient intravascular fluid volume), neurogenic (caused by neural alterations of vascular smooth muscle tone), anaphylactic (caused by immunologic processes), or septic (caused by infection). As described previously, each of these share similar effects on tissues and cells but can vary in their clinical manifestations and severity.

Cardiogenic shock

Cardiogenic shock is defined as "decreased cardiac output and evidence of tissue hypoxia in the presence of adequate intravascular volume."[111] Most cases of cardiogenic shock follow myocardial infarction, but shock also can follow left heart failure, arrhythmias, acute valvular dysfunction, ventricular or septal rupture, myocardial or pericardial infections, and heart failure resulting from drug toxicity.[112] Cardiogenic shock is often unresponsive to treatment, with a mortality of more than 70% reported. Mortality improves with the use of percutaneous coronary angioplasty and thrombolytic/aspirin therapy.[112] The pathophysiology of cardiogenic shock is illustrated in Figure 23-44.

The clinical manifestations of cardiogenic shock are caused by widespread impairment of cellular metabolism. They include impaired mentation, elevated preload in the systemic and pulmonary vasculature, systemic and pulmonary edema, dusky skin color, marked hypotension, oliguria, ileus, and dyspnea.[111] Management of cardiogenic shock includes careful fluid and pressor administration followed by early angiography, intra-aortic balloon pump counterpulsation, and early revascularization (PCI or bypass surgery).[111,112] New therapies being explored include anti-inflammatory drugs and nitric oxide synthetase inhibitors.[112,113]

Hypovolemic shock

Hypovolemic shock is caused by loss of whole blood (hemorrhage), plasma (burns), or interstitial fluid (diaphoresis, diabetes mellitus, diabetes insipidus, emesis, diarrhea, or

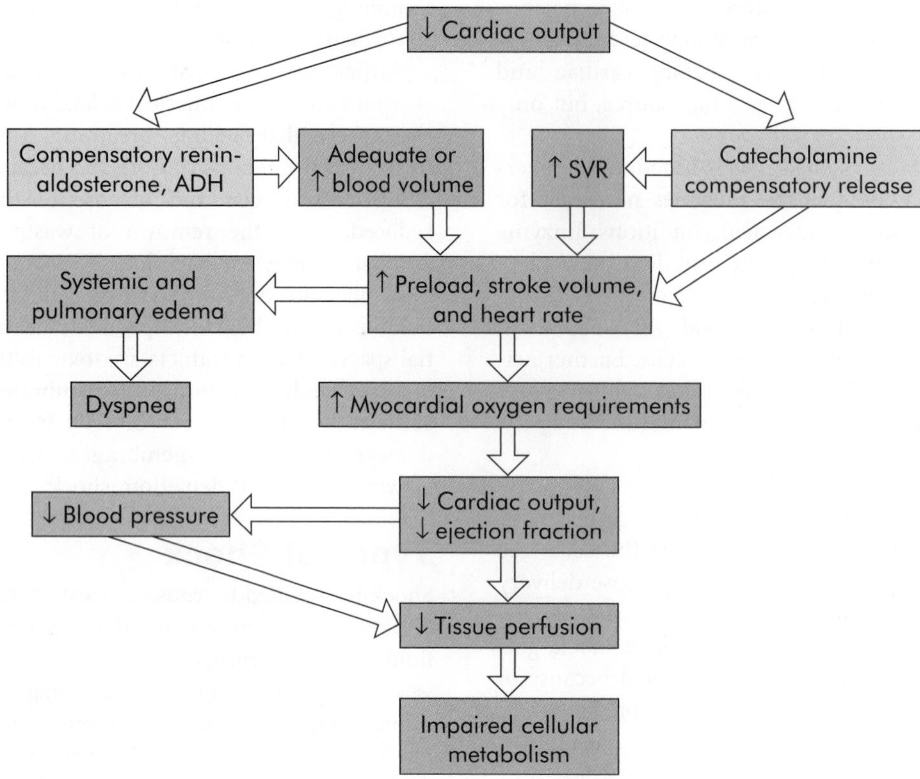

Figure 23-44 ■ **Cardiogenic Shock.** Shock becomes life threatening when compensatory mechanisms *(in blue)* cause increased myocardial oxygen requirements. Renal and hypothalamic adaptive responses (i.e., renin-angiotensin-aldosterone and antidiuretic hormone [ADH]) maintain or increase blood volume. The adrenal gland releases catecholamines (e.g., mostly epinephrine, some norepinephrine), causing vasoconstriction and increases in contractility and heart rate. These adaptive mechanisms, however, increase myocardial demands for oxygen and nutrients. These demands further strain the heart, which can no longer pump an adequate volume, resulting in shock and impaired metabolism. *SVR,* Systemic vascular resistance.

diuresis) in large amounts.[114] Hypovolemic shock begins to develop when intravascular volume has decreased by about 15%.

Hypovolemia is offset initially by compensatory mechanisms (Figure 23-45). Heart rate and SVR increase, boosting both cardiac output and tissue perfusion pressures. Interstitial fluid moves into the vascular compartment.[114] The liver and spleen add to blood volume by disgorging stored red blood cells and plasma. In the kidneys, renin stimulates aldosterone release and the retention of sodium (and hence water), whereas antidiuretic hormone (ADH) from the posterior pituitary gland increases water retention. However, if the initial fluid or blood loss is great or if loss continues, compensation fails, resulting in decreased tissue perfusion. As in cardiogenic shock, oxygen and nutrient delivery to the cells is impaired and cellular metabolism fails. Anaerobic metabolism and lactate production result in lactic acidosis and serum and cellular electrolyte abnormalities.

The clinical manifestations of hypovolemic shock include high SVR, poor skin turgor, thirst, oliguria, low systemic and pulmonary preloads, rapid heart rates, thready pulse, and mental status deterioration. The differences between the signs and symptoms of hypovolemic shock and those of cardiogenic shock are mainly caused by differences in fluid volume and cardiac muscle health. Management begins with rapid fluid replacement with crystalloids and blood products.[114] Hypothermia and coagulopathies frequently complicate treatment. If adequate tissue perfusion cannot be restored promptly, systemic inflammation and multiple organ dysfunction are likely.

Neurogenic shock

Neurogenic shock (sometimes called **vasogenic shock**) is the result of widespread and massive vasodilation that results from parasympathetic overstimulation and sympathetic understimulation (Figure 23-46) (see Chapter 22). This type of shock can be caused by any factor that stimulates parasympathetic or inhibits sympathetic stimulation of vascular smooth muscle. Trauma to the spinal cord or medulla and conditions that interrupt the supply of oxygen or glucose to the medulla can cause neurogenic shock by interrupting sympathetic activity. Depressive drugs, anesthetic agents, and severe emotional stress and pain are other causes. The loss of vascular tone results in "relative hypovolemia."[115] Blood volume has not changed, but the amount of space containing the blood has increased, so that SVR decreases drastically, meaning that pressure in the vessels is inadequate to drive nutrients across capillary membranes to the cells. In addition, bradycardia can occur with a decrease in cardiac output that further contributes to hypotension and underperfusion of tissues.[116] As with other

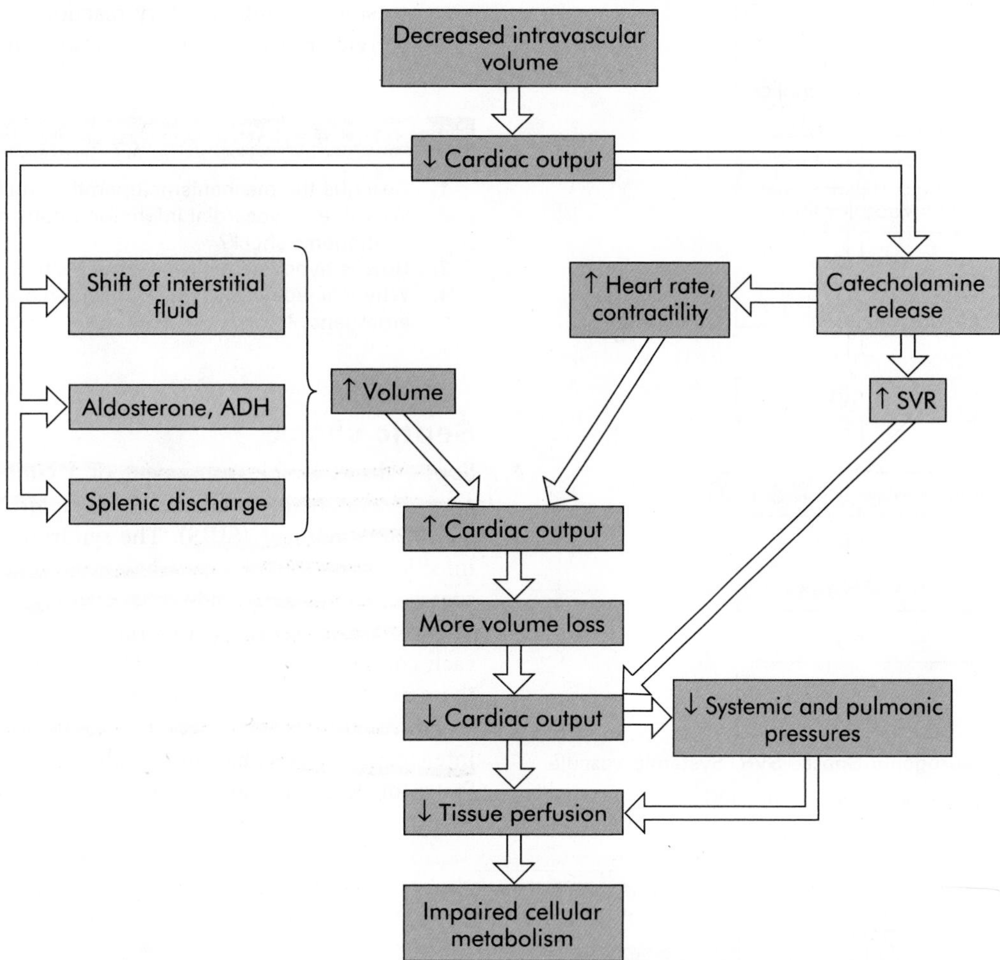

Figure 23-45 ■ **Hypovolemic Shock.** This type of shock becomes life threatening when compensatory mechanisms *(in purple)* are overwhelmed by continued loss of intravascular volume. *ADH,* Antidiuretic hormone; *SVR,* systemic vascular resistance.

types of shock, this leads to impaired cellular metabolism. Management includes the careful use of fluids and pressors until blood pressure stabilizes.[117]

Anaphylactic shock

Anaphylactic shock results from a widespread hypersensitivity reaction known as **anaphylaxis.** It is estimated that between 2% and 3% of people in the United States will develop anaphylaxis each year, most often as a result of penicillin, latex, and food allergies.[118–120] The basic physiologic alteration is the same as that of neurogenic shock: vasodilation, *peripheral pooling,* and relative hypovolemia, leading to decreased tissue perfusion and impaired cellular metabolism (Figure 23-47). Anaphylactic shock is often more severe than other types of normovolemic shock because the hypersensitivity reaction that triggers vasodilation has other pathophysiologic effects that rapidly involve the entire body.

Anaphylactic shock begins as an allergic reaction to an allergen. Common allergens known to cause these reactions are insect venoms, shellfish, peanuts, latex, and medications such as penicillin. In genetically predisposed individuals, these allergens initiate a vigorous humoral immune response (type I hypersensitivity) that results in the production of large quantities of immunoglobulin E (IgE) antibody (see Chapter 6). Allergen binds to IgE, initiating degranulation of mast cells. Mast cells release a large number of vasoactive and inflammatory cytokines. This provokes an extensive immune and inflammatory response, including vasodilation and increased vascular permeability, resulting in **peripheral pooling** and tissue edema.[118,121] Extravascular effects include constriction of extravascular smooth muscle, often causing respiratory difficulty because it affects smooth muscle layers in airway walls (e.g., the larynx and bronchioles; see Chapter 26).[118]

The onset of anaphylactic shock is usually sudden, and progression to death can occur within minutes unless emergency treatment is given. The first manifestations may be anxiety, difficulty breathing, gastrointestinal cramps, edema, hives (urticaria), and sensations of burning or itching of the skin.[118,120] A precipitous fall in blood pressure occurs, followed by impaired mentation. Other signs include decreased SVR, with high or normal cardiac output, and oliguria.[121] Treatment begins with removal of the antigen (if possible). Epinephrine is administered intramuscularly to cause vasoconstriction and reverse airway constriction.[120] Fluids are given intravenously to reverse the relative hypovolemia, and antihistamines and corticosteroids are

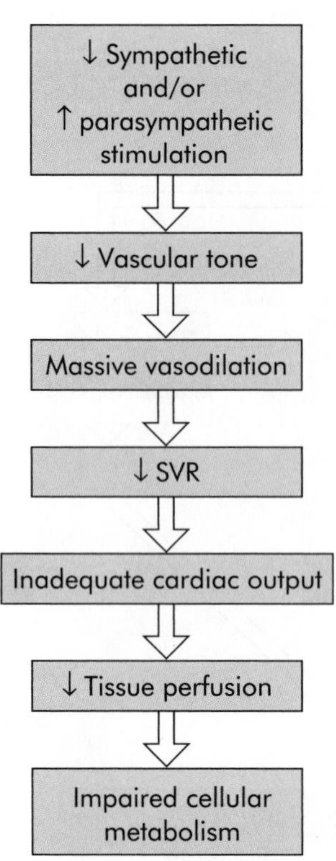

Figure 23-46 ■ **Neurogenic Shock.** *SVR,* Systemic vascular resistance.

given to stop the inflammatory reaction. Vasopressors and β-adrenergic bronchodilators may also be necessary.[120]

QUICK CHECK 23-11

1. Describe the mechanisms operative in shock.
2. Why does myocardial infarction often cause cardiogenic shock?
3. How is hypovolemic shock manifested?
4. Why is anaphylactic shock considered a medical emergency?

Septic shock

Septic shock is one component of a continuum of progressive dysfunction called the **systemic inflammatory response syndrome (SIRS).** The syndrome begins with an infection that progresses to bacteremia, then sepsis, then severe sepsis, then septic shock, and then multiple organ dysfunction syndrome (MODS). Consensus about definitions of each component was achieved in 1992 and revised in 2001; these definitions are presented in Table 23-11.[122, 123]

Septic shock, a common cause of death of individuals in intensive care units, has an overall mortality in the United States of 40% and can be caused by any class of micro-

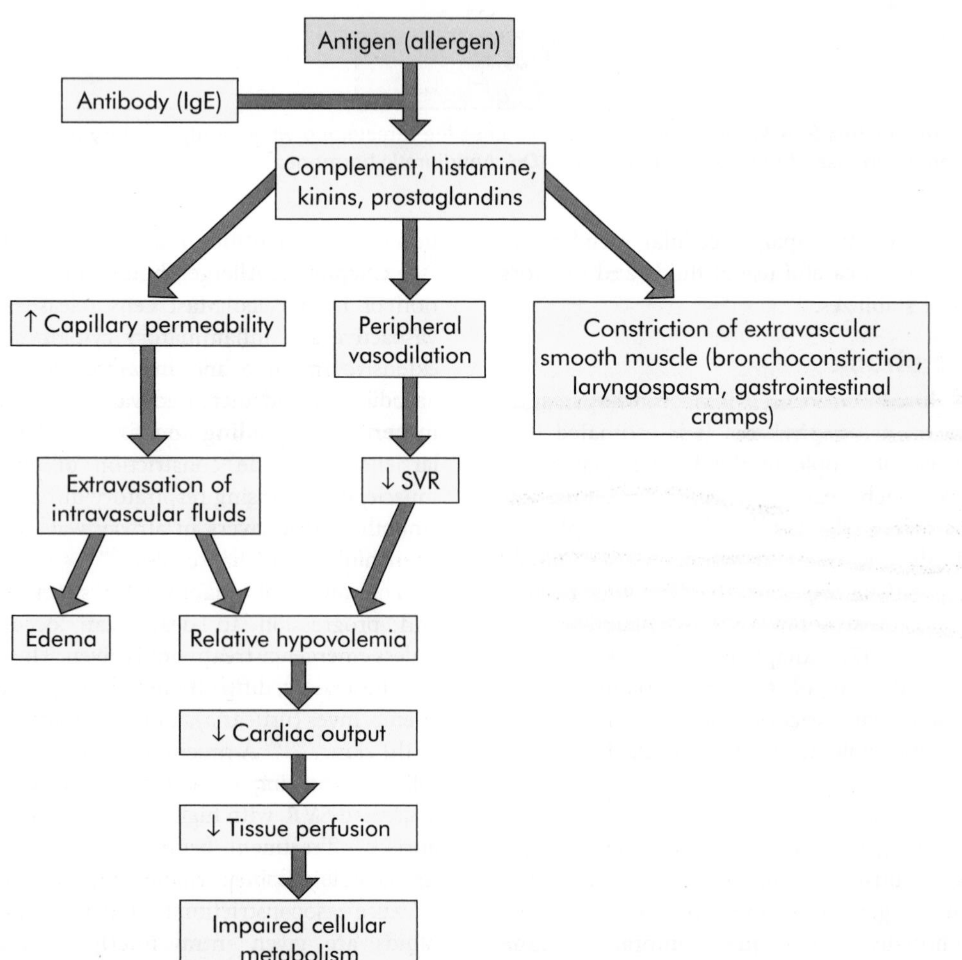

Figure 23-47 ■ **Anaphylactic Shock.** *IgE,* Immunoglobulin E; *SVR,* systemic vascular resistance.

TABLE 23-11

Causes and Definitions of Septic Shock

Cause	Definition
Infection	Microbial phenomenon characterized by an inflammatory response to the presence of microorganisms or the invasion of normally sterile host tissue by those microorganisms
Bacteremia	Presence of viable bacteria in the blood
Systemic inflammatory response syndrome (SIRS)	A systemic inflammatory response to a variety of severe clinical insults manifested by two or more of the following signs: Temperature >38° C or <36° C Heart rate >90 beats/min Respiratory rate >20 breaths/min or arterial blood carbon dioxide level <32 mm Hg White blood cell count >12,000 cells/mm^3, <4000 cells/mm^3, or containing <10% immature forms (bands)
Sepsis	SIRS caused by infection plus some of the following: Mental status changes Significant edema or positive fluid balance Hyperglycemia in the absence of diabetes Increased plasma C-reactive protein or proclacitonin Coagulation abnormalities Thrombocytopenia Hyperbilirubinemia Decreased capillary refill Hypoperfusion, or hypotension Hypoxemia Lactic acidosis Oliguria
Severe sepsis	Sepsis associated with organ dysfunction
Septic shock	Sepsis-induced hypotension or the requirement for vasopressors/inotropes (promote cardiac contractility) to maintain blood pressure despite adequate fluid resuscitation along with the presence of perfusion abnormalities that may include, but are not limited to, lactic acidosis, oliguria, or acute alteration in mental status
Multiple organ dysfunction syndrome	Presence of altered organ function in an acutely ill individual such that homeostasis cannot be maintained without intervention

Data adapted from American College of Chest Physicians/Society of Critical Care Medicine Consensus Conference: *Crit Care Med* 20(6):864–874, 1992; Levy MM et al: SCCM/ES/CM/ACCP/ATS/SIS International Sepsis Definitions Conference, *Crit Care Med* 31(4):1250–1256, 2003.

organism. Although 2 decades ago gram-negative bacteria were by far the microorganisms most often responsible for causing septic shock, gram-positive bacteria now have become the most common isolates.[124] Septic shock also can be caused by fungi and viruses, and in almost a third of cases, the infectious organism is never identified. The source and virulence of the infectious microorganism, as well as the underlying health of the affected individual, significantly affect prognosis.

Most septic shock begins when bacteria enter the bloodstream to produce bacteremia. These bacteria may directly stimulate an inflammatory response or they may release toxic substances into the bloodstream. Gram-negative microorganisms release endotoxins, and gram-positive microorganisms release exotoxins, lipoteichoic acids, and peptidoglycans. These substances trigger the septic syndrome by interacting with toll-like receptors on macrophages and activate complement, coagulation, kinins, and inflammatory cells (Figure 23-48).[124]

The release of inflammatory mediators triggers intense cellular responses and the subsequent release of secondary mediators, including cytokines, complement fragments, prostaglandins, platelet-activating factor, oxygen-free radicals, nitric oxide, and proteolytic enzymes. Chemotaxis, activation of granulocytes, and reactivation of the phagocytic cells and inflammatory cascades result. (Chapter 5 discusses the description and function of inflammatory cells and mediators.) This systemic inflammation, especially through the action of nitric oxide, leads to widespread vasodilation with compensatory tachycardia and increased cardiac output in the early stages of septic shock (hyperdynamic phase) (see *Health Alert:* The Role of Nitric Oxide in Severe Sepsis). Later in the course of disease, inflammatory mediators, such as complement and interleukins, depress myocardial contractility such that cardiac output falls and tissue perfusion decreases.[125] Tissue perfusion and cellular oxygen extraction also are affected by activation of the clotting cascade through the action of platelet-activating factor and depletion of the endogenous anticoagulant protein C. Furthermore, unresponsiveness to or depletion of vasoactive factors, such as vasopressin, contribute to hypotension and tissue hypoperfusion.[124,126] The inflammatory response can become overwhelming, leading to the systemic inflammatory response syndrome (SIRS), which can progress to widespread tissue hypoxia, necrosis, and apoptosis leading to MODS.[122] It has been determined that there is a parallel release of anti-inflammatory mediators and a depression in

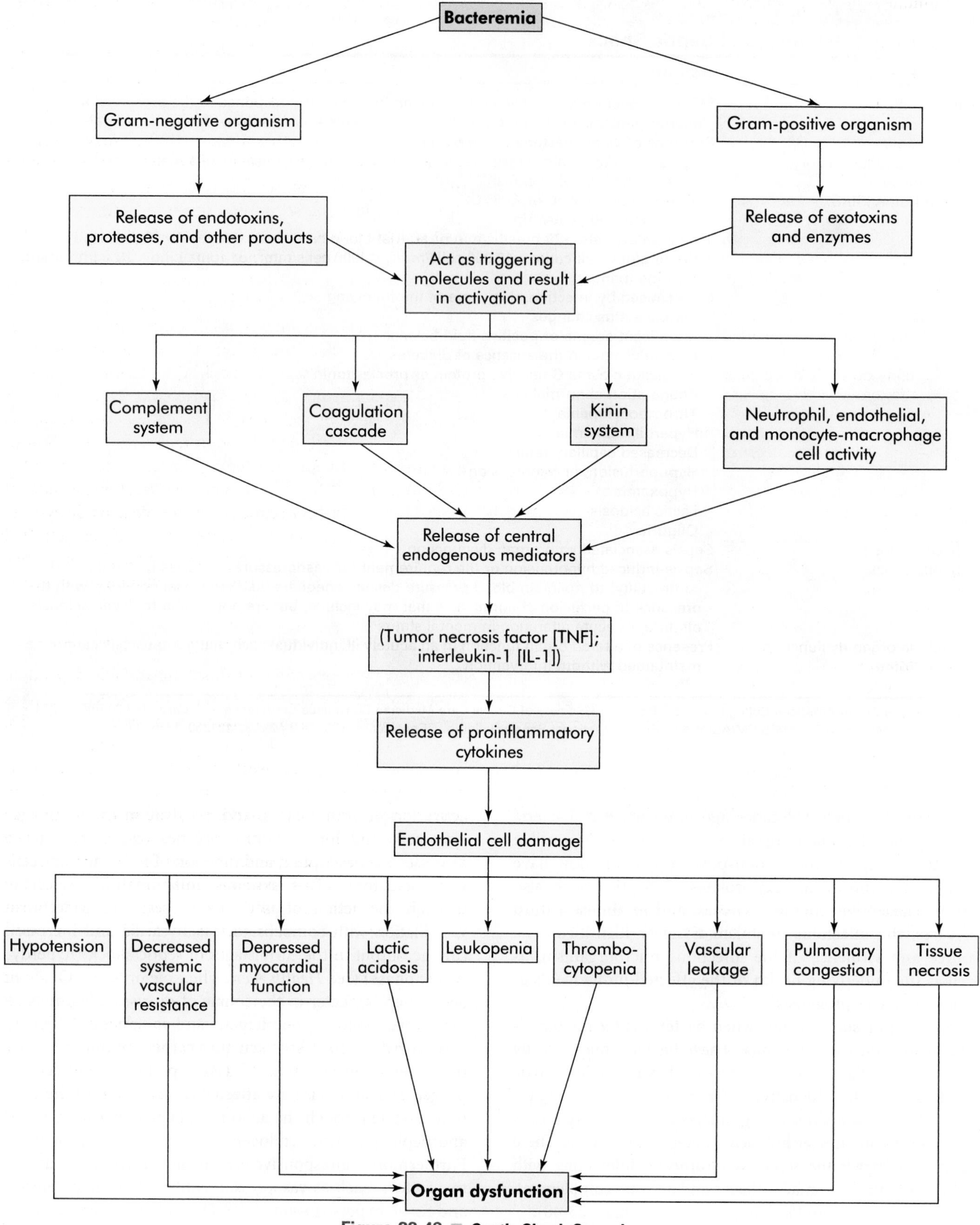

Figure 23-48 ■ **Septic Shock Cascade.**

the immune response that accompanies SIRS, which contributes to the overall shock syndrome (see *Risk Factors:* Inflammatory and Anti-inflammatory Mediators Contributing to Septic Shock).[126–128]

HEALTH ALERT

The Role of Nitric Oxide in Severe Sepsis

Nitric oxide (NO) is a free radical generated from L-arginine by a family of enzymes known as NO synthetases. The most important enzyme in sepsis is called *iNOS* (inducible NOS), which responds to immune/inflammatory insult and mediates tissue damage. In sepsis, iNOS is activated, and NO and $OONO^-$ (peroxynitrite) are produced in large quantities. In septic shock, nitric oxide has been shown to cause refractory peripheral vascular vasodilation, increase vascular permeability, and depress myocardial function. Nitric oxide contributes to the development of MODS because of its effects to decrease cellular protein synthesis, oxidize cell membranes, damage DNA, decrease glucose and glycogen production, and compete for cytochrome oxidase in the mitochondria thus decreasing tissue oxygen utilization. Studies are aimed at finding new treatments (such as antioxidants) to prevent the negative impact of this toxic free radical in sepsis.

Data from Dhillon SS et al: Neutrophils, nitric oxide, and microvascular permeability in severe sepsis, *Chest* 128(3):1706–1712, 2005; Kumar A, Kumar A: Nitric oxide and inflammatory cytokines in the heart: the presence of positive feedback loops, *Crit Care Med* 33(12):2851–2852, 2005; Levy RM, Prince JM, Billiar TR: Nitric oxide: a clinical primer, *Crit Care Med* 33(12 suppl):S492–S495, 2005; Victor VM et al: M. Role of free radicals in sepsis: antioxidant therapy, *Curr Pharm Des* 11(24):3141–3158, 2005.

RISK FACTORS **Inflammatory and Anti-inflammatory Mediators Contributing to Septic Shock**

The Interleukins

- Released by macrophages and lymphocytes in septic shock in response to bacterial toxins
- Net effect: produce fever, vasodilation and hypotension, edema, and elevated white blood count

Tumor Necrosis Factor

- Produced from macrophages, natural killer cells, and mast cells in response to endotoxin and interleukins
- Net effect: generates same symptoms of septic shock that interleukins do, thus is redundant

Platelet-Activating Factor

- Released from mononuclear phagocytes, platelets, and some endothelial cells in response to endotoxin
- Net effect: generates symptoms of shock as do interleukins and tumor necrosis factor but may also initiate multiple organ failure

Myocardial Depressant Factor

- Secreted from white blood cells in response to endotoxin
- Net effect: produces myocardial depression and ventricular dilation

Clinical manifestations of septic shock are low arterial pressure, low SVR from vasodilation, systemic edema, and an alteration in oxygen extraction by all cells. Tachycardia causes cardiac output to remain normal or become elevated, although myocardial contractility is reduced. Temperature instability is present, ranging from hyperthermia to hypothermia. Effects on other organ systems may result in deranged renal function, gastrointestinal mucosa changes that result in release of bacteria from the gut into the bloodstream, jaundice, clotting abnormalities, deterioration of mental status, and ARDS. Increased permeability of the gut not only allows bacteria to enter the bloodstream but also can lead to increased inflammation and immune reactions due to toxins carried by the intestinal lymphatics.[129] Present treatment includes multiple drug antibacterial therapy, removal of the source of infection if one is found, fluid resuscitation, and vasoactive medications to improve hemodynamic parameters. Many experimental treatments are under study, among them low- to moderate-dose corticosteroids, vasopressin, plasma filtration (apheresis), and immunomodulating therapy including monoclonal antibodies and vaccines.[124,128,130,131] Among the most promising of the new treatments for septic shock are nitric oxide synthetase inhibitors and novel anticoagulants such as activated protein C.[130,132] Because the septic syndrome is incompletely understood, recommended treatment continues to evolve.

Clinical Manifestations of Shock

The clinical manifestations of shock are variable depending on the type of shock, and observable and measurable signs and symptoms are often conflicting in nature. Subjective complaints in shock are usually nonspecific. The individual may report feeling sick, weak, cold, hot, nauseated, dizzy, confused, afraid, thirsty, and short of breath. Hypotension, characterized by a mean arterial pressure below 60 mm Hg is common to almost all shock states; however, it is a late sign of decreased tissue perfusion. Cardiac output and urinary output are usually variable early in shock states but generally become decreased as the shock syndrome progresses. Respiratory rate is usually increased, and a respiratory alkalosis may be an important early indicator of impending shock. Other variable indicators of shock include alterations of heart rate, core body temperature, skin temperature, systemic vascular resistance (SVR), and skin color. Altered sensorium may be another indicator of poor tissue perfusion. A decreased mixed venous oxygen saturation indicates poor tissue oxygenation and an alteration in cellular oxygen extraction and can be used to monitor response to therapy.

Treatment for Shock

The first treatment for shock is to discover and correct or remove the underlying cause. General supportive treatment includes intravenous fluid administered to expand intravascular volume, vasopressors, and supplemental oxygen. Further treatment depends on the cause and severity of the shock syndrome, which was discussed with each type of shock. Once positive feedback loops are established, intervention in shock is difficult. Prevention and very early treatment offer the best prognosis.

QUICK CHECK 23-12

1. What are some of the important causes of septic shock?
2. What is the systemic inflammatory response syndrome?
3. Why is correction of the underlying problem the most important treatment for all kinds of shock?

Multiple Organ Dysfunction Syndrome

Multiple organ dysfunction syndrome (MODS) is the progressive dysfunction of two or more organ systems resulting from an uncontrolled inflammatory response to a severe illness or injury. The organ dysfunction can progress to organ failure and death (Figure 23-49). Although sepsis and septic shock are the most common causes, any severe injury or disease process that activates a massive systemic inflammatory response in the host can initiate MODS. Clinical infection is not necessary for its development. Other common triggers are severe trauma, burns, acute pancreatitis, major surgery, circulatory shock, adult respiratory distress syndrome, and necrotic tissue.

MODS is a relatively new diagnosis, first recognized as a distinct clinical syndrome in the mid-1970s. Today MODS is the most common cause of mortality in intensive care units. Mortality for individuals with MODS is between 50% and 90%,[110] and it approaches 100% if there is failure of three or more organs. Moreover, mortality has not improved since the 1980s. People at greatest risk for developing MODS are elderly individuals and persons with significant tissue injury or preexisting disease (see *Risk Factors:* Development of Multiple Organ Dysfunction Syndrome).

RISK FACTORS Development of Multiple Organ Dysfunction Syndrome

- Age >65 years
- Baseline organ dysfunction (e.g., renal insufficiency)
- Bowel infarction
- Coma on admission
- Immunosuppression (e.g. corticosteroids)
- Inadequate, delayed resuscitation
- Malnutrition
- Multiple blood transfusions (>6 units/12 hr)
- Persistent infectious focus
- Preexisting chronic disease (e.g., cancer, diabetes)
- Significant tissue injury

PATHOPHYSIOLOGY As a result of the initiating insult (sepsis, injury, or disease), the neuroendocrine system is activated with the release of the stress hormones cortisol, epinephrine, and norepinephrine into the bloodstream (see Chapter 8). The sympathetic nervous system is stimulated to compensate for complications resulting from the injury, such as fluid loss and hypotension. Vascular endothelial damage occurs as a direct result of injury or from damage by bacterial toxins and inflammatory mediators released into the circulation. The vascular endothelium becomes permeable, allowing fluid and protein to leak into the interstitial spaces, contributing to hypotension and hypoperfusion. When the endothelium is damaged, platelets and tissue thromboplastin are activated, resulting in systemic microvascular coagulation that may lead to disseminated intravascular coagulation (DIC) (see Chapter 20).[133-135]

Because of the release of inflammatory mediators, three major plasma enzyme cascades are activated: complement, coagulation, and kallikrein/kinin. The overall effect of the activation of these cascades is a hyperinflammatory and hypercoagulant state that maintains the edema formation, cardiovascular instability, endothelial damage, and clotting abnormalities characteristic of MODS. A massive systemic immune/inflammatory response then develops involving neutrophils, macrophages, and mast cells (Table 23-12). The pathways by which neutrophils and macrophages are activated vary and involve multiple events rather than individual triggers. The inflammatory process initiated is the same as that described in septic shock and SIRS (see p. 662) and sets the stage for MODS.

The numerous inflammatory and clotting processes operating in MODS cause maldistribution of blood flow and hypermetabolism. Oxygen delivery to the tissues decreases despite the supranormal systemic blood flow for several reasons:

1. Shunting of blood past selected regional capillary beds, which is caused when inflammatory mediators override the normal vascular tone
2. Interstitial edema, resulting from microvascular changes in permeability, contributes to decreased oxygen delivery by creating a relative hypovolemia and by increasing the distance oxygen must travel to reach the cells
3. Capillary obstruction that occurs because of formation of microvascular thrombi and the aggregation of white blood cells

Hypermetabolism in MODS with accompanying alterations in carbohydrate, fat, and lipid metabolism is initially a compensatory measure to meet the body's increased demands for energy. The alterations in metabolism affect all aspects of substrate utilization. The net result of hypermetabolism is depletion of oxygen and fuel supplies.

Decreased oxygen delivery to the cells caused by the maldistribution of blood flow, coagulation, myocardial depression, and the hypermetabolic state combine to create an imbalance in oxygen supply and demand. This imbalance is critical in the pathogenesis of MODS because it

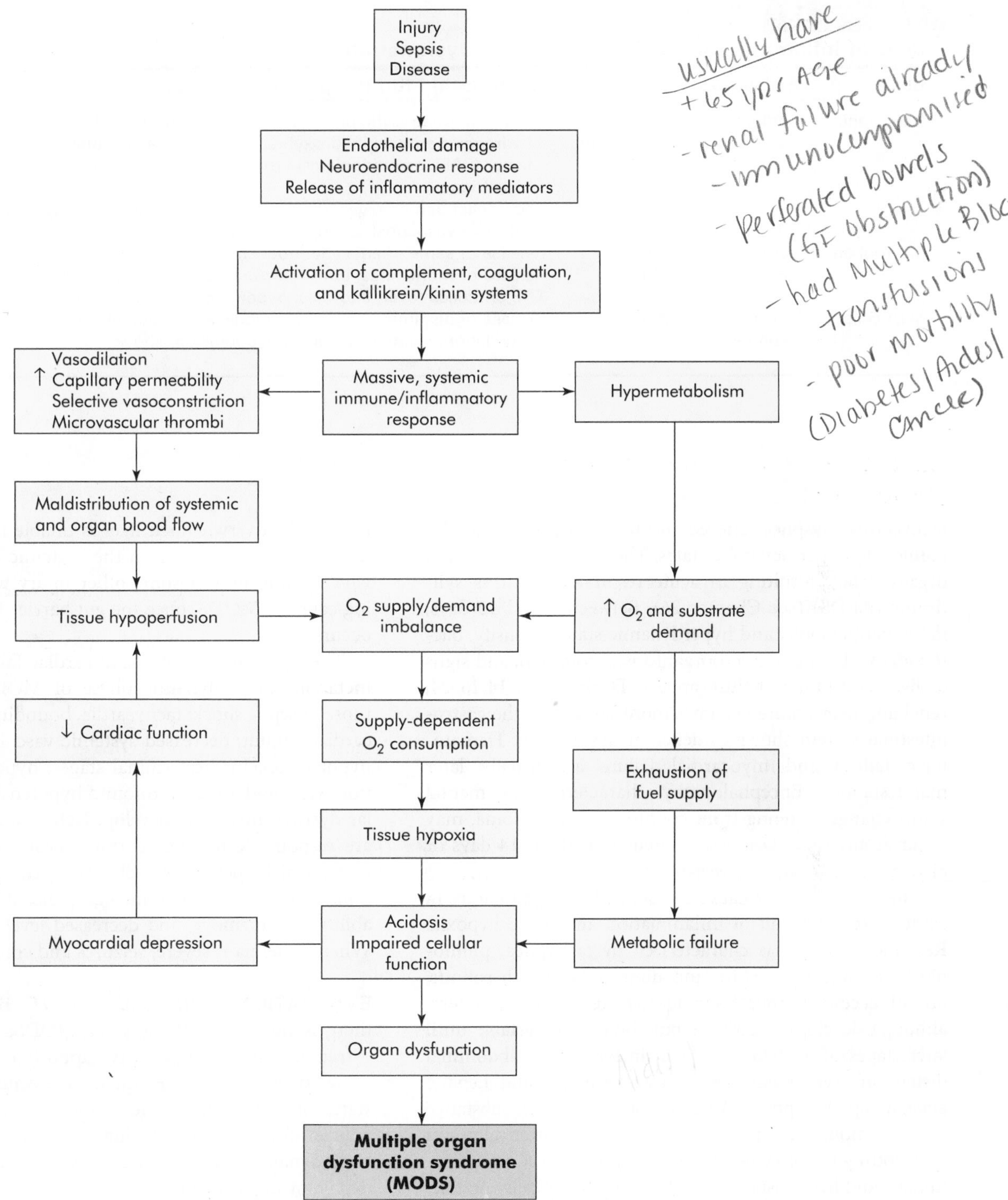

Figure 23-49 **Pathogenesis of Multiple Organ Dysfunction Syndrome.**

results in a pathologic condition known as **supply-dependent oxygen consumption.** Ordinarily, the amount of oxygen consumed by the cells depends only on the demands of the cells, because there is an adequate reserve of oxygen that can be delivered if needed. The reserve, however, has been exhausted in MODS, and the amount of oxygen consumed becomes dependent on the amount the circulation is able to deliver; this amount is inadequate in MODS. Therefore, tissue hypoxia with cellular acidosis and impaired cellular function ensue and result in the multiple organ failure.

CLINICAL MANIFESTATIONS There is often a predictable clinical pattern in the development of MODS,[110,136] although there is certainly some individual variation. After the inciting event and aggressive resuscitation for approximately 24 hours, the individual develops a low-grade fever,

TABLE 23-12

Cells of Inflammation and Multiple Organ Dysfunction

Cell	Activators	Contribution to Multiple Organ Dysfunction
Neutrophils	Complement, kinins, endotoxin, clotting factors	Release of phagocytic products: toxic oxygen-free radicals, superoxide ion, hydrogen peroxide, hydroxyl radicals, proteases, platelet-activating factor (PAF), arachidonic acid metabolites (prostaglandins, thromboxane, leukotrienes) Endothelial damage, vasodilation, vasopermeability, microvascular coagulation, selective vasoconstriction, hypotension, shock
Macrophages	Complement, endotoxin, chemotactic factors	Release of same phagocytic products as neutrophils Release of monokines: tumor necrosis factor (TNF), interleukin-1 (IL-1) TNF produces fever, anorexia, hyperglycemia, weight loss
Mast cells	Direct injury, endotoxin, complement	Release of histamine, PAF, arachidonic acid metabolites Vasodilation, vasopermeability, hypotension, shock

tachycardia, dyspnea, altered mental status, and hyperdynamic and hypermetabolic states. The lung is often the first organ to fail, resulting in acute respiratory distress syndrome (ARDS) (see Chapter 26). Between 7 and 10 days, the hypermetabolic and hyperdynamic states intensify, bacteremia with enteric microorganisms is common, and signs of liver and kidney failure appear. During days 14 to 24, renal and liver failure becomes more severe and the gastrointestinal system shows evidence of dysfunction. Hematologic failure and myocardial failure are usually later manifestations. Encephalopathy, characterized by mental status changes ranging from confusion to deep coma, may occur at any time. Death may occur as early as 14 days or after a period of several weeks.

The clinical manifestations of individual organ failure in MODS are the result of inflammation and tissue hypoxia. Respiratory failure is characterized by tachypnea, pulmonary edema with crackles and diminished breath sounds, use of accessory muscles, and hypoxemia. Liver failure, although developing early, is not clinically detectable until later stages of MODS, at which time jaundice, abdominal distention, liver tenderness, muscle wasting, and hepatic encephalopathy appear. All facets of metabolism, substance detoxification, and immune response are impaired, albumin and clotting factor synthesis decreases, protein wastes accumulate, and liver tissue macrophages (Kupffer cells) no longer function effectively.

Progressive oliguria, azotemia, and edema mark the development of renal failure. Anuria, hyperkalemia, and metabolic acidosis may occur if renal shutdown is severe. The gastrointestinal system is sensitive to ischemic and inflammatory injury. Clinical manifestations of bowel involvement are hemorrhage, ileus, malabsorption, diarrhea or constipation, vomiting, anorexia, and abdominal pain. Compounding the damage caused by injury to the bowel is the phenomenon of **bacterial translocation.** When mediators and severe ischemia injure the mucosal epithelium, bacteria and toxins pass from the gut into the portal circulation. The overwhelmed liver is unable to clear these products, and they move into the systemic circulation. Thus, whether infection or some other injury was the precipitating cause of MODS, once the gut barrier is damaged, sepsis occurs.

The signs and symptoms of cardiac failure in the hypermetabolic, hyperdynamic phase of MODS are similar to those of septic shock: tachycardia, bounding pulse, increased cardiac output, decreased systemic vascular resistance, and hypotension. In the terminal stages, hypodynamic circulation with bradycardia, profound hypotension, and ventricular dysrhythmias may develop. Ischemia and inflammation are responsible for the central nervous system manifestations, which include apprehension, confusion, disorientation, restlessness, agitation, headache, decreased cognitive ability and memory, and decreased level of consciousness. When ischemia is severe, seizures and coma can occur.

EVALUATION AND TREATMENT Because presently there is no specific therapy for MODS, early detection is extremely important so that supportive measures can be initiated immediately. Frequent assessment of the clinical status of individuals at known risk is essential. Once organ failure develops, monitoring of laboratory values and hemodynamic parameters also can be used to assess the degree of impairment.

Therapeutic management of MODS consists of prevention and support. First, if the initial insult is known, it is aggressively treated and sources of infection are removed. The second priority is restoration and maintenance of tissue oxygenation and cardiovascular function. Third, nutritional support must be provided (see *Health Alert:* Nutritional Support to Prevent and Treat MODS). Last, individual organs must be supported. Activated protein C (Drotrecogin alfa) has been shown to improve outcomes in those with DIC and may be useful for the general management of septic shock with multiple organ dysfunction syndrome.[132,137]

HEALTH ALERT
Nutritional Support to Prevent and Treat MODS

Maintaining the integrity of the gastrointestinal tract is an important step in preventing and managing sepsis and multiple organ dysfunction. Nutrition support not only prevents malnutrition but also helps maintain adequate functioning of the gut. Enteral nutrition (EN) has advantages over parenteral nutrition (PN) for postoperative/posttrauma individuals. Immediate and early EN improves mucosal blood flow, reduces intramucosal acidosis and permeability problems, and decreases the need for stress ulcer prophylaxis. EN also maintains the protective role of the gut by decreasing inflammatory cytokine production and improving mucosal IgA levels, which helps prevent infection. EN should be given as soon as is practical. Jejunal tube feedings have advantages over gastric tube feeding including faster metabolic recovery, less vomiting, and less risk of regurgitation and aspiration. Special attention should be given to the purity of water for the immunocompromised individual.

Data from Magnotti LJ, Deitch EA: Burns, bacterial translocation, gut barrier function, and failure, *J Burn Care Rehab* 26(5):383–391, 2005; Marla R, Dahn MS, Lange MP: Influence of enteral and parenteral nutrition on splanchnic hemodynamics in septic patients, *Surg Infect* 5(4):357–363, 2004; Sigalet DL, Mackenzie SL, Hameed SM: Enteral nutrition and mucosal immunity: implications for feeding strategies in surgery and trauma, *Can J Surg* 47(2):109–116, 2004.

QUICK CHECK 23-13

1. Why can MODS be initiated by either a septic or a nonseptic insult?
2. Why are inflammation and clotting triggered when the vascular endothelium is injured?
3. Describe the mechanisms that result in decreased oxygen delivery to the tissues in MODS.

Did You Understand?

Diseases of the Arteries and Veins

1. Varicosities are areas of veins in which blood has pooled, usually in the saphenous veins. Varicosities may be caused by damaged valves as a result of trauma to the valve or by chronic venous distention involving gravity and venous constriction.
2. Chronic venous insufficiency is inadequate venous return over a long period of time that causes pathologic ischemic changes in the vasculature, skin, and supporting tissues.
3. Venous stasis ulcers follow the development of chronic venous insufficiency and probably develop as a result of the borderline metabolic state of the cells in the affected extremities.
4. Deep venous thrombosis results from stasis of blood flow, endothelial damage or hypercoagulability. The most serious complication of deep venous thrombosis is pulmonary embolism.
5. Superior vena cava syndrome is a progressive occlusion of the superior vena cava that leads to venous distention in the upper extremities and head. Because this syndrome is usually caused by bronchogenic cancer, it is generally considered an oncologic emergency rather than a vascular emergency.
6. Hypertension is the elevation of systemic arterial blood pressure resulting from increases in cardiac output, total peripheral resistance, or both.
7. Hypertension can be primary, without a known cause, or secondary, caused by an underlying disease.
8. The risk factors for hypertension include a positive family history; male gender; advancing age; black race; obesity; high sodium intake; low magnesium, potassium or calcium intake; diabetes mellitus; cigarette smoking; and heavy alcohol consumption.
9. The exact cause of primary hypertension is unknown, although several hypotheses are proposed, including overactivity of the sympathetic nervous system; overactivity of the renin-angiotensin-aldosterone system; sodium and water retention by the kidneys; hormonal inhibition of sodium-potassium transport across cell walls; and complex interactions involving insulin resistance, inflammation, and endothelial function.
10. Clinical manifestations of hypertension result from damage of organs and tissues outside the vascular system. These include heart disease, renal disease, central nervous system problems, and musculoskeletal dysfunction.
11. Hypertension is managed with both pharmacologic and nonpharmacologic methods.
12. Orthostatic hypotension is a drop in blood pressure that occurs on standing. The compensatory vasoconstriction response to standing is replaced by a marked vasodilation and blood pooling in the muscle vasculature.
13. Orthostatic hypotension may be acute or chronic. The acute form is caused by a delay in the normal regulatory mechanisms. The chronic forms are secondary to a specific disease or are idiopathic in nature.
14. The clinical manifestations of orthostatic hypotension include fainting and may involve cardiovascular symptoms, as well as impotence and bowel and bladder dysfunction.

(Continued)

Did You Understand?—Cont'd

15. An aneurysm is a localized dilation of a vessel wall, to which the aorta is particularly susceptible.
16. A thrombus is a clot that remains attached to a vascular wall. Arteriosclerosis can generate thrombus formation through roughening of the intima that activates the clotting cascade. Thrombus formation may be discrete or diffuse.
17. An embolus is a mobile aggregate of a variety of substances that occludes the vasculature. Sources of emboli include clots, air, amniotic fluid, bacteria, fat, and foreign matter. These emboli cause ischemia and necrosis when a vessel is totally blocked.
18. The most common source of arterial thrombotic emboli is the heart as a result of mitral and aortic valvular disease and atrial fibrillation, followed by myxomas. Tissues affected include the lower extremities, the brain, and the heart.
19. Emboli to the central organs cause tissue death in lungs, kidneys, and mesentery.
20. The generation of air emboli requires a connection between the vascular compartment and a source of air.
21. Amniotic fluid may be forced into the bloodstream and generate an embolus during labor and childbirth.
22. Aggregates of bacteria in the vasculature may be large enough to form an embolus.
23. Fat emboli are caused mainly by trauma to the long bones, either through defective fat metabolism after trauma or through the release of fat globules from bone marrow exposed by fracture.
24. The introduction of foreign matter into the vasculature can occur with trauma and also can occur in a hospital setting in which intravenous and intra-arterial lines are being used.
25. Vasospastic disorders include Raynaud disease, involving arterioles of the extremities; Prinzmetal angina, involving coronary arteries; and Buerger disease, involving arteries of the hands and feet.
26. Arteriosclerosis is a thickening and hardening of the arteries, involving the intimal layer and leading to hypertension. It seems to be a part of the normal aging process, but it is a disease state when it occurs to the point of symptom development.
27. Arteriosclerosis raises the systolic pressure by decreasing arterial distensibility and lumen diameter.
28. Atherosclerosis is a form of arteriosclerosis and is the leading contributor to coronary artery disease (CAD) and cerebrovascular disease (CVD).
29. Atherosclerosis is an inflammatory disease that begins with endothelial injury (smoking, hypertension, diabetes [insulin resistance], hyperhomocystinemia, dyslipidemia, etc.) and progresses through several stages to become a fibrotic plaque.
30. Once a plaque has formed, it can rupture, resulting in clot formation and instability and vasoconstriction leading to obstruction of the lumen and inadequate oxygen delivery to tissues.
31. Peripheral artery disease is the result of atherosclerotic plaque formation in the arteries that supply the extremities, and it causes pain and ischemic changes in the nerves, muscles, and skin of the limb.
32. Coronary artery disease (CAD) is almost always the result of atherosclerosis that gradually narrows the coronary arteries or that ruptures and causes sudden thrombus formation and myocardial ischemia and even infarction. Many risk factors contribute to the onset and escalation of CAD, including dyslipidemia, smoking, hypertension, diabetes mellitus (insulin resistance), advancing age, obesity, sedentary lifestyle, psychosocial factors, hyperhomocysteinemia, and heavy consumption of alcohol.
33. The three risk factors most predictive of CAD are hypercholesterolemia, cigarette smoking, and hypertension.
34. Ischemic heart disease is most commonly the result of coronary artery disease and the resultant decrease in myocardial blood supply.
35. Angina pectoris is chest pain caused by myocardial ischemia.
36. Therapeutic interventions for CAD include use of vasodilators and medications to reduce cardiac workload (e.g., beta-blockers), as well as surgical procedures.
37. Atherosclerotic plaque progression can be gradual, but sudden coronary obstruction due to thrombus formation causes the acute coronary syndromes. These include unstable angina and myocardial infarction.
38. Unstable angina results in reversible myocardial ischemia.
39. Myocardial infarction is caused by prolonged, unrelieved ischemia that interrupts blood supply to the myocardium. After about 20 minutes of myocardial ischemia, irreversible hypoxic injury causes cellular death and tissue necrosis.
40. Myocardial infarction is clinically classified as non-STEMI or STEMI based on electrocardiographic findings which suggest the extent of myocardial damage (subendocardial versus transmural).
41. An increase in plasma enzyme levels is used to diagnose the occurrence of myocardial infarction and indicate its severity. Elevations of the isoenzymes creatine kinase (CK-MB), troponins, and lactic dehydrogenase (LDH-1) are most predictive of a myocardial infarction.
42. Treatment of a myocardial infarction includes revascularization (thrombolytics or PCI), antithrombotics, ACE inhibitors, and beta-blockers. Pain relief and fluid management also are key components of care. Dysrhythmias and cardiac failure are the most common complications of acute myocardial infarction.

Disorders of the Heart Wall

1. Inflammation of the pericardium, or pericarditis, may result from several sources (infection, drug therapy, tumors). Pericarditis presents with symptoms that are physically troublesome, but in and of themselves they are not life threatening.
2. Fluid may collect within the pericardial sac (pericardial effusion). Cardiac function may be severely impaired if the accumulation of fluid occurs rapidly and involves a large volume.
3. Cardiomyopathies are a diverse group of primary myocardial disorders that are usually the result of remodeling, neurohumoral responses, and hypertension. The cardiomyopathies are categorized as dilated (congestive), restrictive (rigid and noncompliant), and hypertrophic (asymmetric). The size of the cardiac muscle walls and chambers may increase or decrease depending on the type of cardiomyopathy, thereby altering contractile activity.

Did You Understand?—Cont'd

4. The hemodynamic integrity of the cardiovascular system depends to a great extent on properly functioning cardiac valves. Congenital or acquired disorders that result in stenosis, incompetence, or both can structurally alter the valves.
5. Characteristic heart sounds, cardiac murmurs, and systemic complaints assist in determining which valve is abnormal. If severely compromised function exists, a prosthetic heart valve may be surgically implanted to replace the faulty one.
6. Mitral valve prolapse (MVP) is a common finding, especially in young women. Although not grossly abnormal, the mitral valve leaflets do not position themselves properly during systole. Mitral valve prolapse may be a completely asymptomatic condition or can result in unpredictable symptoms. Afflicted valves are at greater risk for developing infective endocarditis.
7. Rheumatic fever is an inflammatory disease that results from a delayed immune response to a streptococcal infection in genetically predisposed individuals. The disorder usually resolves without sequelae if treated early.
8. Severe or untreated cases of rheumatic fever may progress to rheumatic heart disease, a potentially disabling cardiovascular disorder.
9. Infective endocarditis is a general term for infection and inflammation of the endocardium, especially the cardiac valves. The most common cause of infective endocarditis is staphylococcus aureus, followed by viridans streptococcus. In the mildest cases, valvular function may be slightly impaired by vegetations that collect on the valve leaflets. If left unchecked, severe valve abnormalities, chronic bacteremia, and systemic emboli may occur as vegetations break off the valve surface and travel through the bloodstream. Antibiotic therapy can limit the extension of this disease.
10. Human immunodeficiency virus (HIV) is associated with cardiac abnormalities, including myocarditis, endocarditis, pericarditis, and cardiomyopathy. Left heart failure is the most common clinical manifestation.

Manifestations of Heart Disease

1. A dysrhythmia (arrhythmia) is a disturbance of heart rhythm. Dysrhythmias range in severity from occasional missed beats or rapid beats to disturbances that impair myocardial contractility and are life threatening.
2. Dysrhythmias can occur because of an abnormal rate of impulse generation or the abnormal conduction of impulses.
3. Heart failure is an inability of the heart to supply the metabolism with adequate circulatory volume and pressure.
4. Right ventricular failure is usually the result of chronic pulmonary hypertension caused by left heart failure or chronic hypoxic lung disease.
5. Left heart failure (congestive heart failure) can be divided into systolic and diastolic heart failure.
6. The most common causes of left ventricular failure are myocardial infarction, fluid overload, hypertension, or valvular disease.
7. Systolic heart failure is caused by increased preload, decreased contractility, or increased afterload. These processes result in an increased left ventricular end-diastolic volume and an increase in left ventricular end-diastolic pressure that results in increased pulmonary venous pressures and pulmonary edema.
8. In addition to the hemodynamic changes of left ventricular failure, there is a neuroendocrine response that tends to exacerbate and perpetuate the condition.
9. The neuroendocrine mediators of congestive heart failure (CHF) include the sympathetic nervous system and the renin-angiotensin-aldosterone system; thus, diuretics, beta-blockers, and angiotensin-converting enzyme (ACE) inhibitors are important components of the pharmacologic therapy.
10. Diastolic heart failure is a clinical syndrome characterized by the symptoms and signs of heart failure, a preserved ejection fraction, and abnormal diastolic function.
11. Diastolic dysfunction means that the left ventricular end-diastolic pressure is increased, even if volume and cardiac output are normal.

Shock

1. Shock is a widespread impairment of cellular metabolism involving positive feedback loops that places the individual on a downward physiologic spiral leading to multiple organ dysfunction syndrome.
2. Types of shock are cardiogenic, hypovolemic, neurogenic, anaphylactic, and septic. Multiple organ dysfunction syndrome can develop from all types of shock.
3. The final common pathway in all types of shock is impaired cellular metabolism—cells switch from aerobic to anaerobic metabolism. Energy stores drop, and cellular mechanisms relative to membrane permeability, action potentials, and lysozyme release fail.
4. Anaerobic metabolism results in activation of the inflammatory response, decreased circulatory volume, and decreasing pH.
5. Impaired cellular metabolism results in cellular inability to use glucose because of impaired glucose delivery or impaired glucose intake, resulting in a shift to glycogenolysis, gluconeogenesis, and lipolysis for fuel generation.
6. Glycogenolysis is effective for about 10 hours. Gluconeogenesis results in the use of proteins necessary for structure, function, repair, and replication that leads to more impaired cellular metabolism.
7. Gluconeogenesis contributes to lactic acid, uric acid, and ammonia buildup, interstitial edema, and impairment of the immune system, as well as general muscle weakness leading to decreased respiratory function and cardiac output.
8. Cardiogenic shock is decreased cardiac output, tissue hypoxia, and the presence of adequate intravascular volume.

(Continued)

Did You Understand?—Cont'd

9. Hypovolemic shock is caused by loss of blood or fluid in large amounts. The use of compensatory mechanisms may be vigorous, but tissue perfusion ultimately decreases and results in impaired cellular metabolism.
10. Neurogenic shock results from massive vasodilation, causing a relative hypovolemia, even though cardiac output may be high, and results in impaired cellular metabolism.
11. Anaphylactic shock is caused by physiologic recognition of a foreign substance. The inflammatory response is triggered, and a massive vasodilation with fluid shift into the interstitium follows. The relative hypovolemia leads to impaired cellular metabolism.
12. Septic shock begins with impaired cellular metabolism caused by uncontrolled septicemia. The infecting agent triggers the inflammatory and immune responses. This inflammatory response is accompanied by widespread changes in tissue and cellular function.
13. Multiple organ dysfunction syndrome (MODS) is the progressive failure of two or more organ systems after a severe illness or injury. It can be triggered by chronic inflammation, necrotic tissue, severe trauma, burns, adult respiratory distress syndrome, acute pancreatitis, and other severe injuries.
14. MODS involves the stress response; changes in the vascular endothelium resulting in microvascular coagulation; release of complement, coagulation, and kinin proteins; and numerous inflammatory processes. Consequences of all these mediators are a maldistribution of blood flow, hypermetabolism, hypoxic injury, and myocardial depression.
15. Clinical manifestations of MODS include inflammation, tissue hypoxia, and hypermetabolism. All organs can be affected including the kidney, lung, liver, gastrointestinal tract and central nervous system.

Key Terms

Acute coronary syndromes, 622
Acute onset of left (congestive) heart failure, 654
Acute orthostatic hypotension, 613
Anaphylactic shock, 661
Anaphylaxis, 661
Aneurysm, 614
Aortic regurgitation, 639
Aortic sclerosis, 638
Aortic stenosis, 638
Arteriosclerosis, 617
Atherosclerosis, 617
Bacterial translocation, 668
Cardiogenic shock, 659
Cardiomyopathy, 637
Chronic left heart failure, 655
Chronic orthostatic hypotension, 613
Chronic venous insufficiency (CVI), 606
Chylomicron, 623
Complicated plaque, 619
Constrictive pericarditis (chronic pericarditis), 637
Coronary artery disease (CAD), 622
C-reactive protein (C-rp), 624
Deep venous thrombosis (DVT), 607
Diastolic heart failure, 655
Dyslipidemia (dyslipoproteinemia), 623
Dysrhythmia (arrhythmia), 647
Embolism, 616
Embolus, 616
False aneurysm, 614
Fatty streak, 619
Fibrous plaque, 619
Foam cell, 619
Heart failure, 652
Hibernating myocardium, 632
High-density lipoprotein (HDL), 623
High-output failure, 656
Hyperhomocysteinemia, 624
Hypertension, 608
Hypovolemic shock, 659
Infarction, 622
Infective endocarditis, 645
Intermittent claudication, 622
Ischemia, 622
Isolated systolic hypertension (ISH), 611
Left heart failure, 652
Lipoprotein (a) [Lp[a]), 624
Lipoprotein, 623
Low-density lipoprotein (LDL), 623
Malignant hypertension, 612
Mental stress–induced ischemia, 626
Metabolic syndrome, 624
Mitral regurgitation, 641
Mitral stenosis, 639
Mitral valve prolapse syndrome (MVPS), 642
Multiple organ dysfunction syndrome (MODS), 656
Myocardial infarction (MI), 629
Myocardial remodeling, 632
Myocardial stunning, 632
Myocarditis, 644
Neurogenic shock (vasogenic shock), 660
Nonbacterial thrombotic endocarditis, 646
Non-ST elevation MI (non-STEMI), 629
Orthostatic (postural) hypotension, 613
Percutaneous coronary intervention (PCI), 629
Pericardial effusion, 636
Peripheral artery disease (PAD), 622
Peripheral pooling, 661
Pressure-natriuresis relationship, 609
Primary hypertension (essential hypertension idiopathic hypertension), 608
Prinzmetal angina, 627
Raynaud disease, 617
Raynaud phenomenon, 617
Rheumatic fever, 643
Rheumatic heart disease (RHD), 643
Right heart failure, 655
Secondary hypertension, 608
Septic shock, 662
Shock, 656
Silent ischemia (induced ischemia), 626
Stable angina pectoris, 626
ST elevation MI (STEMI), 629
Superior vena cava syndrome (SVCS), 607
Supply-dependent oxygen consumption, 667
Systemic inflammatory response syndrome (SIRS), 662
Systolic heart failure, 652
Tamponade, 636
Thromboangiitis obliterans (Buerger disease), 616
Thromboembolus, 607
Thrombus, 607
Tricuspid regurgitation, 641
True aneurysm, 614
Unstable angina, 629
Valvular regurgitation (valvular insufficiency or valvular incompetence), 638
Valvular stenosis, 638
Varicose vein, 606
Venous stasis ulcer, 607
Ventricular remodeling, 652
Very-low-density lipoprotein (VLDL), 623

References

1. Eberhardt RT, Raffetto JD: Chronic venous insufficiency, *Circulation* 111(18):2398–2409, 2005.
2. Pascarella L, Schonbein GW, Bergan JJ: Microcirculation and venous ulcers: a review, *Ann Vasc Surg* 19(6):921–927, 2005.
3. Decousus H et al: Superficial vein thrombosis: risk factors, diagnosis, and treatment, *Curr Opin Pulm Med* 9(5): 393–397, 2003.
4. Caprini JA et al: Thrombophilia testing in patients with venous thrombosis, *Euro J VascEndovasc Surg* 30(5):550–555, 2005.
5. Kyrle PA, Eichinger S: Deep vein thrombosis, *Lancet* 365: 1163–1174, 2005.
6. Schifferdecker B et al: Nonmalignant superior vena cava syndrome: pathophysiology and management, *Catheter Cardiovas Interven* 65(3):416–423, 2005.
7. Wang TJ, Vasan RS: Epidemiology of uncontrolled hypertension in the United States, *Circulation* 112(11):1651–1662, 2005.
8. Chobanian AV: The Seventh Report of the Joint National Committee on prevention, detection, evaluation, and treatment of high blood pressure: the JNC Report, *JAMA* 289(19):2560–2572, 2003.
9. Mensah G et al: State of disparities in cardiovascular health in the United States, *Circulation* 111:1233–1241, 2005.
10. Townsend MS et al: Low mineral intake is associated with high systolic blood pressure in the Third and Fourth National Health and Nutrition Examination Surveys: could we all be right? *Am J Hyperten* 18(2 Pt 1):261–269, 2005.
11. Correia ML, Haynes WG: Leptin, obesity and cardiovascular disease, *Curr Opin Nephrol Hyperten* 13(2):215–223, 2004.
12. McDonough AA, Leong PK, Yang LE: Mechanisms of pressure natriuresis: how blood pressure regulates renal sodium transport, *Ann NY Acad Sci* 986:669–677, 2003.
13. Grisk O, Rettig R: Interactions between the sympathetic nervous system and the kidneys in arterial hypertension, *Cardiovasc Res* 61:238–246, 2004.
14. Mehta PK, Griendling KK: Angiotensin II cell signaling: physiological and pathological effects in the cardiovascular system, *Am J of Physiol—Cell Physiology* 292(1):C82–97, 2007.
15. Savoia C, Schiffrin EL: Significance of recently identified peptides in hypertension: endothelin, natriuretic peptides, adrenomedullin, leptin, *Med Clin North Am* 88:39–62, 2004.
16. Li JJ, Fang CH, Hui RT: Is hypertension an inflammatory disease, *Med Hypotheses* 64(2):236–240, 2005.
17. Sowers JR, Frohlich ED: Insulin and insulin resistance: impact on blood pressure and cardiovascular disease, *Med Clin North Am* 88:63–82, 2004.
18. Frohlich ED: Target organ involvement in hypertension: a promise of prevention and reversal, *Med Clin North Am* 88:209–221, 2004.
19. de Zeeuw D, Hillege HL, de Jong PE: The kidney, a cardiovascular risk marker, and a new target for therapy, *Kidney Int* (suppl 98):S25–S29, 2005.
20. Irvin DJ, White M: The importance of accurately assessing orthostatic hypotension, *Geriatric Nurs* 25(2):99–101, 2004.
21. Tsai TT, Nienaber CA, Eagle KA: Acute aortic syndromes, *Circulation* 112(24):3802–3813, 2005.
22. Katzen BT et al: Endovascular repair of abdominal and thoracic aortic aneurysms, *Circulation* 112(11):1663–1675, 2005.
23. Slavov ES et al: Cytokine production in thromboangiitis obliterans patients: new evidence for an immune-mediated inflammatory disorder, *Clin Experim Rheumatol* 23(2):219–226, 2005.
24. Calguneri M et al: Buerger's disease with multisystem involvement: a case report and a review of the literature, *Angiology* 55(3):325–328, 2004.
25. Boin F, Wigley FM: Understanding, assessing and treating Raynaud's phenomenon, *Curr Opin Rheumatol* 17(6): 752–760, 2005.
26. Hansson GK: Inflammation, atherosclerosis, and coronary artery disease, *N Engl J Med* 352:1685–1695, 2005.
27. Libby P: Inflammation and cardiovascular disease mechanisms, *Am J Clin Nutr* 83(2):456S–460S, 2006.
28. Libby P: Vascular biology of atherosclerosis: overview and state of the art, *Am J Cardiol* 91(3A):3A–6A, 2003.
29. Werner N, Nickenig G: Influence of cardiovascular risk factors on endothelial progenitor cells: limitations for therapy? *Arteriosc Thromb Vasc Biol* 26(2):257–266, 2006.
30. Goldschmidt-Clermont PJ et al: Atherosclerosis 2005: recent discoveries and novel hypotheses, *Circulation* 112(21): 3348–3353, 2005.
31. Boyle JJ: Macrophage activation in atherosclerosis: pathogenesis and pharmacology of plaque rupture, *Curr Vasc Pharmacol* 3:63–68, 2005.
32. Hankey GJ, Norman PE, Eikelboom JW: Medical treatment of peripheral arterial disease, *JAMA* 295(5):547–553, 2006.
33. Libby P, Theroux P: Pathophysiology of coronary artery disease, *Circulation* 111(25):3481–3488, 2005.
34. American Heart Association Writing Group: Heart disease and stroke statistics—2007 update, *Circulation* 115:e69–e171, 2007.
35. Expert Panel on Detection, Evaluation, and Treatment of High Blood Cholesterol in Adults: Executive summary of the third report of the National Cholesterol Education Program (NCEP) Expert Panel on Detection, Evaluation, and Treatment of High Blood Cholesterol in Adults (adult treatment panel III), *JAMA* 285:2486–2497, 2001.
36. Barter P: The inflammation: lipoprotein cycle, *Atheroscl* 6(suppl 2):15–20, 2005.
37. Grobbee DE, Bots ML: Statin treatment and progression of atherosclerotic plaque burden, *Drugs* 63:893–911, 2003.
38. Toth PP: High-density lipoprotein and cardiovascular risk, *Circulation* 109(15):1809–1812, 2004.
39. Ohashi R et al: Reverse cholesterol transport and cholesterol efflux in atherosclerosis, *QJM* 98(12):845–856, 2005.
40. Rader DJ: Mechanisms of disease: HDL metabolism as a target for novel therapies, *Nature Clinical Practice Cardiovascular Medicine* 4(2):102–109, 2007.
41. Schnell O: The links between diabetes and cardiovascular disease, *J Intervent Cardiol* 18(6):413–416, 2005.
42. Haffner SM: Insulin resistance, inflammation, and the prediabetic state, *Am J Cardiol* 92(suppl):18J–26J, 2003.
43. Poirier P et al: American Heart Association Obesity Committee of the Council on Nutrition, Physical Activity, and Metabolism. Obesity and cardiovascular disease: pathophysiology, evaluation, and effect of weight loss: an update of the 1997 American Heart Association Scientific Statement on Obesity and Heart Disease from the Obesity Committee of the Council on Nutrition, Physical Activity, and Metabolism, *Circulation* 113(6):898–918, 2006.
44. Koh KK, Han SH, Quon MJ: Inflammatory markers and the metabolic syndrome: insights from therapeutic interventions, *J Am Coll Cardiol* 46(11):1978–1985, 2005.
45. Skilton MR, Celermajer DS: The effects of obesity-related peptides on the vasculature, *Curr Vasc Pharmacol* 4(1):79–85, 2006.
46. Danesh J et al: C reactive protein and other circulating markers of inflammation in the prediction of coronary heart disease, *N Engl J Med* 350:1387–1397, 2004.
47. Ballantyne CM, Nambi V: Markers of inflammation and their clinical significance, *Atheroscler* 6(suppl 2):21–29, 2005.

References—Cont'd

48. Ieven MM, Hoymans VY: Involvement of *Chlamydia pneumoniae* in atherosclerosis: more evidence for lack of evidence, *J Clin Microbiol* 43:19–24, 2005.
49. Vorchheimer DA, Becker R: Platelets in atherothrombosis, *Mayo Clin Proc* 81(1):59–68, 2006.
50. Kawano H, Ogawa H: Endothelial function and coronary spastic angina, *Int Med* 44(2):91–99, 2005.
51. Almeda F et al: Silent myocardial ischemia: concepts and controversies, *Am J Med* 116:112–118, 2004.
52. Rozanski A: Mental stress and the induction of silent myocardial ischemia in patients with coronary artery disease, *N Engl J Med* 318(16):1005–1012, 1988.
53. von Kanel R et al: Effects of psychological stress and psychiatric disorders on blood coagulation and fibrinolysis: a biobehavioral pathway to coronary artery disease? *Psychosom Med* 63(4):531–544, 2001.
54. Blumenthal JA et al: Usefulness of psychosocial treatment of mental stress-induced myocardial ischemia in men, *Am J Cardiol* 89(2):164–168, 2002.
55. Raggi P et al: Atherosclerotic plaque imaging: contemporary role in preventive cardiology, *Arch Intern Med* 165(20): 2345–2353, 2005.
56. ACC/AHA: 2002 guideline update for the management of patients with chronic stable angina, *J Am Coll Cardiol* 41: 59–168, 2002.
57. McCullough PA: Chronic angina: new medical options for treatment, *Rev Cardiovas Med* 6(3):152–161, 2005.
58. Opie LH, Commerford PJ, Gersh BJ: Controversies in stable coronary artery disease, *Lancet* 367(9504):69–78, 2006.
59. Dery JP, Harrington RA, Tcheng JE: GP IIb/IIIa blockade in elective percutaneous coronary intervention, *Curr Pharm Design* 10(4):387–398, 2004.
60. Soran O et al: Two-year clinical outcomes after enhanced external counterpulsation (EECP) therapy in patients with refractory angina pectoris and left ventricular dysfunction (report from The International EECP Patient Registry), *Am J Cardiol* 97(1):17–20, 2006.
61. Goldberg RF, Fass AE, Frishman WH: Transmyocardial revascularization: defining its role, *Cardiol Rev* 13:52–55, 2005.
62. Isner JM: Myocardial gene therapy, *Nature* 415(6868): 234–239, 2002.
63. Stary HC et al: A definition of advanced types of atherosclerotic lesions and a histological classification of atherosclerosis: a report from the Committee on Vascular Lesions of the Council on Arteriosclerosis, American Heart Association, *Arterioscler Thromb Vasc Biol* 15(9):1512–1531, 1995.
64. Corti R, Fuster V, Badimon JJ: Pathogenetic concepts of acute coronary syndromes, *J Am Coll Cardiol* 41(4 suppl S):7S–14S, 2003.
65. Shah PK: Mechanisms of plaque vulnerability and rupture, *J Am Coll Cardiol* 41(4 suppl S):15S–22S, 2003.
66. Klein LW: Clinical implications and mechanisms of plaque rupture in the acute coronary syndromes, *Am Heart Hosp J* 3(4):249–255, 2005.
67. Wehrmacher WH, Bellows R: Unstable angina, *Compr Ther* 30:6–9, 2004.
68. ACC/AHA: 2002 guideline update for the management of patients with unstable angina and non-ST-segment elevation myocardial infarction, *J Am Coll Cardiol* 40:1366–1374, 2002.
69. Crossman DC: The pathophysiology of myocardial ischaemia, *Heart (Br Cardiac Soc)* 90:576–580, 2004.
70. Boersma E et al: Acute myocardial infarction, *Lancet* 361: 847–858, 2003.
71. Zarich SW: The role of intensive glycemic control in the management of patients who have acute myocardial infarction, *Cardol Clin* 23:109–117, 2005.
72. Maytin M, Colucci WS: Molecular and cellular mechanisms of myocardial remodeling, *J Nuclear Cardiol* 9(3):319–327, 2002.
73. Canty JM Jr, Fallavollita JA: Hibernating myocardium, *J Nuclear Cardiol* 12:104–119, 2005.
74. Depre C, Vatner SF: Mechanisms of cell survival in myocardial hibernation, *Trends Cardiovasc Med* 15(3):101–110, 2005.
75. Galinanes M, Fowler AG: Role of clinical pathologies in myocardial injury following ischaemia and reperfusion, *Cardiovas Res* 61:512–521, 2004.
76. Smith SW, Whitwam W: Acute coronary syndromes, *Emerg Med Clin North Am* 24(1):53–89, vi, 2006.
77. Cannon CP: Acute coronary syndromes: risk stratification and initial management, *Cardiol Clin* 23(4):401–409, v, 2005.
78. ACC/AHA: Guidelines for the management of patients with ST-elevation myocardial infarction, *J Am Coll Cardiol* 44(3): 671–719, 2004.
79. O'Keefe J et al: Optimal low-density lipoprotein is 50 to 70 mg/dl: better and physiologically normal, *J Am Coll Cardiol* 43:2142–2146, 2004.
80. Lange RA, Hillis LD: Clinical practice: acute pericarditis, *N Engl J Med* 351(21):2195–2202, 2004.
81. Imazio M et al: Colchicine in addition to conventional therapy for acute pericarditis: results of the Colchicine for acute PEricarditis (COPE) trial, *Circulation* 112(13): 2012–2016, 2005.
82. Mayosi BM, Burgess LJ, Doubell AF: Tuberculous pericarditis, *Circulation* 112(23):3608–3616, 2005.
83. Schofield RS et al: Left ventricular dysfunction after pericardiectomy for constrictive pericarditis, *Ann Thorac Surg* 77 (4):1449–1451, 2004.
84. Thiene G et al: Twenty years of progress and beckoning frontiers in cardiovascular pathology: cardiomyopathies, *Cardiovasc Pathol* 14(4):165–169, 2005.
85. Schoen FJ: Cardiac valves and valvular pathology: update on function, disease, repair, and replacement, *Cardiovasc Pathol* 14(4):189–194, 2005.
86. Freeman RV, Otto CM: Spectrum of calcific aortic valve disease: pathogenesis, disease progression, and treatment strategies, *Circulation* 111(24):3316–3326, 2005.
87. Carabello BA: Modern management of mitral stenosis, *Circulation* 112(3):432–437, 2005.
88. Tawn Z et al: Percutaneous valve procedures: present and future, *Int J Cardiovasc Interven* 7(1):14–20, 2005.
89. Bekeredjian R, Grayburn PA: Valvular heart disease: aortic regurgitation, *Circulation* 112(1):125–134, 2005.
90. Tanemoto K: Surgical treatment of ischemic mitral valve regurgitation, *Ann Thoracic Cardiovasc Surg* 11(4):228–231, 2005.
91. Hayek E, Gring CN, Griffin BP: Mitral valve prolapse, *Lancet* 365(9458):507–518, 2005.
92. Carapetis JR, McDonald M, Wilson NJ: Acute rheumatic fever, *Lancet* 366(9480):155–168, 2005.
93. Carapetis JR et al: The global burden of group A streptococcal diseases, *Lancet Infect Dis* 5(11):685–694, 2005.
94. Djani AS et al: Guidelines for the diagnosis of rheumatic fever: Jones criteria, updated 1993, *Circulation* 87:302, 1993.
95. WHO: *Rheumatic fever and rheumatic heart disease: report of a WHO Expert Consultation*, Geneva, Geneva, 2004, World Health Organization.
96. Hill EE et al: Evolving trends in infective endocarditis, *Clin Microbiol Infect* 12(1):5–12, 2006.
97. Durack DT, Lukes AS, Bright DK: New criteria for diagnosis of infective endocarditis: utilization of specific echocardiographic findings, *Am J Med* 96:200–209, 1994.
98. Habib G: Management of infective endocarditis, *Heart* 92(1): 124–130, 2006.

References—Cont'd

99. Zareba KM, Miller TL, Lipshultz SE: Cardiovascular disease and toxicities related to HIV infection and its therapies, *Exp Opin Drug Safety* 4(6):1017–1025, 2005.
100. McMurray JJ, Pfeffer MA: Heart failure, *Lancet* 365(9474): 1877–1889, 2005.
101. Jessup M, Brozena S: Heart failure, *N Engl J Med* 348: 2007–2018, 2003.
102. Stoupakis G, Klapholz M: Natriuretic peptides: biochemistry, physiology, and therapeutic role in heart failure, *Heart Dis* 5(3):215–223, 2003.
103. Aukrust P et al: Inflammatory and anti-inflammatory cytokines in chronic heart failure: potential therapeutic implications, *Ann Med* 37(2):74–85, 2005.
104. Prahash A, Lynch T: B-type natriuretic peptide: a diagnostic, prognostic, and therapeutic tool in heart failure, *Am J Crit Care* 13:46–53, 2004.
105. Hunt SA et al: ACC/AHA 2005 guideline update for the diagnosis and management of chronic heart failure in the adult: a report of the American College of Cardiology/American Heart Association Task Force on Practice Guidelines (Writing Committee to Update the 2001 Guidelines for the Evaluation and Management of Heart Failure): developed in collaboration with the American College of Chest Physicians and the International Society for Heart and Lung Transplantation: endorsed by the Heart Rhythm Society, *Circulation* 112(12):e154–235, 2005.
106. Ott P: Cardiac resynchronization therapy: a new therapy for advanced congestive heart failure, *Am J Geriatr Cardiol* 14: 31–34, 2005.
107. Bukhari F et al: Genetic maneuvers to ameliorate ventricular function in heart failure: therapeutic potential and future implications, *Exp Rev Cardiovasc Ther* 3:85–97, 2005.
108. Nanjundappa A et al: Cell transplantation for treatment of left-ventricular dysfunction due to ischemic heart failure: from bench to bedside, *Expert Review of Cardiovasc Ther* 5(1):125–131, 2007.
109. Sanderson JE: Heart failure with a normal ejection fraction, *Heart,* 93(2):155–158, 2007.
110. Cabre L et al: Multicenter study of the multiple organ dysfunction syndrome in intensive care units: the usefulness of Sequential Organ Failure Assessment scores in decision making, *Intens Care Med* 31(7):927–933, 2005.
111. Hollenberg SM: Cardiogenic shock, *Crit Care Clin* 17(2): 391–410, 2001.
112. Sanborn TA, Feldman T: Management strategies for cardiogenic shock, *Curr Opin Cardiol* 19(6):608–612, 2004.
113. Geppert A, Huber K: Inflammation and cardiovascular diseases: lessons that can be learned for the patient with cardiogenic shock in the intensive care unit, *Curr Opin Crit Care* 10(5):347–353, 2004.
114. Kelley DM: Hypovolemic shock: an overview, *Crit Care Nurs Q* 28(1):2–19, 2005.
115. Dumont RJ, et al: Acute spinal cord injury. Part I. Pathophysiologic mechanisms, *Clin Neuropharmacol* 24(5): 254–264, 2001.
116. Krassioukov A, Claydon VE: The clinical problems in cardiovascular control following spinal cord injury: an overview, *Progress Brain Res* 152:223–229, 2006.
117. Stevens RD et al: Critical care and perioperative management in traumatic spinal cord injury, *J Neurosurg Anesthesiol* 15(3): 215–229, 2003.
118. Lieberman P: Anaphylaxis, *Med Clin North Am* 90(1):77–95, viii, 2006.
119. Moneret-Vautrin DA et al: Epidemiology of life-threatening and lethal anaphylaxis: a review, *Allergy* 60(4):443–451, 2005.
120. Borchers A: The diagnosis and management of anaphylaxis, *Comp Therap* 30(2):111–120, 2004.
121. Brown SG: Cardiovascular aspects of anaphylaxis: implications for treatment and diagnosis, *Curr Opin Allerg Clin Immunol* 5(4):359–364, 2005.
122. Bone RC et al: Definitions for sepsis and organ failure and guidelines for the use of innovative therapies in sepsis, the ACCP/SCCM Consensus Conference Committee, American College of Chest Physicians/Society of Critical Care Medicine, *Chest* 101:1644–1655, 1992.
123. Levy MM et al: 2001 SCCM/ES/CM/ACCP/ATS/SIS International Sepsis Definitions Conference, *Crit Care Med* 31(4): 1250–1256, 2003.
124. Annane D et al: Septic shock *Lancet* 365(9453):63–78, 2005.
125. Hoesel LM et al: Complement-related molecular events in sepsis leading to heart failure, *Molecular Immunology* 44(1–3):95–102, 2007.
126. Landry DW, Oliver JA: Vasopressin and relativity: on the matter of deficiency and sensitivity, *Crit Care Med* 34(4): 1275–1277, 2006.
127. Asfar P et al: Catecholamines and vasopressin during critical illness, *Crit Care Clin* 22(1):131–149, 2006.
128. Monneret G et al: The anti-inflammatory response dominates after septic shock: association of low monocyte HLA-DR expression and high interleukin-10 concentration, *Immunol Letters* 95(2):193–198, 2004.
129. Fink MP, Delude RL: Epithelial barrier dysfunction: a unifying theme to explain the pathogenesis of multiple organ dysfunction at the cellular level, *Crit Care Clin* 21(2):177–196, 2005.
130. Rivers EP et al: Early and innovative interventions for severe sepsis and septic shock: taking advantage of a window of opportunity, *CMAJ* 25;173(9):1054–1065, 2005.
131. La Rosa SP: Use of corticosteroids in the sepsis syndrome: what do we know now? *Cleve Clin J Med* 72(12): 1121–1127, 2005.
132. Anonymous: Drotrecogin alfa (activated) for severe sepsis, *Drug Therap Bull* 44(1):5–8, 2006.
133. Wiel E et al: The endothelium in intensive care, *Crit Care Clin* 21(3):403–416, 2005.
134. Aird WC: Sepsis and coagulation, *Crit Care Clin* 21(3): 417–431, 2005.
135. Vincent JL, De Backer D: Does disseminated intravascular coagulation lead to multiple organ failure? *Crit Care Clin* 21(3):469–477, 2005.
136. Pettila V: Sequential assessment of multiple organ dysfunction as a predictor of outcome, *JAMA* 287(6):713–714, 2002.
137. Levi M: Disseminated intravascular coagulation: what's new? *Crit Care Clin* 21(3):449–467, 2005.

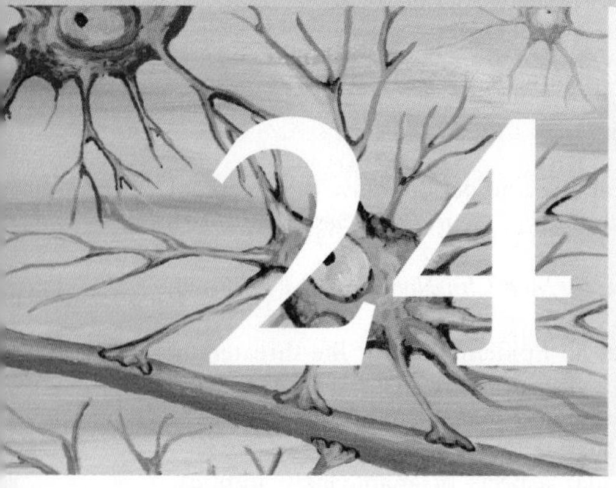

ALTERATIONS OF CARDIOVASCULAR FUNCTION IN CHILDREN

Nancy L. McDaniel ▪ Jean Anne Connor*

CHAPTER OUTLINE

ELECTRONIC RESOURCES

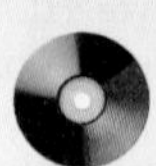

Companion CD
- Review Questions and Answers
- Animations

evolve Website
http://evolve.elsevier.com/Huether/
- Quick Check Answers
- Key Terms Exercises
- Critical Thinking Questions with Answers
- Algorithm Completion Exercises
- WebLinks

Cardiovascular disorders in children are classified as congenital or acquired. Congenital heart disease is the most common. The diagnosis and management of congenital heart defects continues to improve with the use of fetal echocardiography and early interventional catheterization or surgical repair. Acquired heart defects in children continue to present challenges to the practitioner. Although guidelines for diagnosing acquired defects are available, work is still needed in developing standards of treatment and long-term follow-up.

CONGENITAL HEART DISEASE

The incidence of **congenital heart disease (CHD)** varies from 4 to 8 per 1000 live births and is the major cause of death in the first year of life other than prematurity. Several environmental and genetic risk factors are associated with the incidence of different types of CHD. Among the environmental factors are (1) maternal conditions, such as intrauterine viral infections (especially rubella), diabetes mellitus, phenylketonuria, alcoholism, hypercalcemia, drugs (e.g., thalidomide, phenytoin), and complications of increased age; (2) antepartal bleeding; and (3) prematurity (Table 24-1).[1,2]

Genetic factors also have been implicated in the incidence of CHD, although the mechanism of causation is often unknown (Table 24-2). The incidence of CHD is three to four times higher in siblings of affected children, and chromosomal defects account for about 6% of all cases of CHD. Down syndrome, trisomies 13 and 18, Turner syndrome, and cri du chat syndrome have been associated with a relatively high incidence of heart defects. Only a small percentage of cases of CHD are clearly linked solely to genetic or environmental factors. The cause of most defects is multifactorial.[1,2]

Congenital heart defects can be described with respect to three principal areas:

1. *Anatomic defects* include valvular abnormalities; abnormal openings in the septa, including persistence of the foramen ovale; continued patency of the ductus arteriosus; and malformation or abnormal placement of the great vessels.
2. The *hemodynamic alterations* caused by these anatomic defects consist of (a) increases or decreases of blood flow through the pulmonary or systemic circulatory systems and (b) the mixing of pulmonary and systemic blood through an abnormal communication that permits flow between the two circulatory systems. The movement of blood between the normally separate pulmonary and systemic circulations is termed a **shunt.** Movement from the pulmonary to the systemic circulation (i.e., from the right heart to the left heart) is called a **right-to-left shunt.** Movement from the systemic to the pulmonary circulation (from the left heart to the right heart) is a **left-to-right shunt.** Shunt direction depends on relative pressures and resistances.
3. The *status of tissue oxygenation* is gauged by the presence or absence of cyanosis. **Cyanosis** is a bluish discoloration of the skin indicating that the tissues are not receiving normal amounts of oxygen, a condition known as *hypoxia.* (See Chapter 26 for more discussion about cyanosis and hypoxia. Acute hypoxic injury to cells is

*Jean Anne Connor, RN, MS, CPNP, contributed to this chapter in the previous edition.

TABLE 24-1

Maternal Conditions and Environmental Exposures and the Associated Congenital Heart Defects

Cause	Type of Congenital Heart Defect
INFECTION	
Intrauterine	Patent ductus arteriosus (PDA), pulmonary stenosis, coarctation of aorta
Systemic viral	PDA, pulmonary stenosis, coarctation of aorta
Rubella	PDA, pulmonary stenosis, coarctation of aorta
Coxsackie B5	Endocardial fibroelastosis
RADIATION	Specific cardiovascular effect not known
METABOLIC DISORDERS	
Diabetes	Ventricular septal defect (VSD), cardiomegaly, transposition of the great vessels
Phenylketonuria (PKU)	Coarctation of aorta, PDA
Hypercalcemia	Supravalvular aortic stenosis, pulmonic stenosis; aortic hyperplasia
DRUGS	
Thalidomide	No specific lesion
Dextroamphetamine	One case of reported transposition
Alcohol	Tetralogy of Fallot, atrial septal defect, VSD
PERIPHERAL CONDITIONS	
Increased maternal age	VSD, tetralogy of Fallot (relationship unclear)
Antepartal bleeding	Various defects (relationship unclear)
Prematurity	PDA, VSD
High altitude	PDA, atrial septal defect (increased incidence)

described in Chapter 3.) Hypoxia may result from any disorder that prevents oxygen from reaching the body's cells. Ischemia, for example, is hypoxia from lack of blood flow. Some congenital heart defects that cause hypoxia, and therefore cyanosis, involve a right-to-left shunt, which directs blood flow away from the lungs (Figure 24-1). These defects are commonly called **cyanotic defects.** Congenital defects that do not cause cyanosis, or **acyanotic defects,** may involve a left-to-right shunt, which directs blood toward the lungs, or no shunt at all. One way to categorize congenital heart defects is according to (a) whether they cause cyanosis, (b) whether they increase or decrease blood flow into the pulmonary circulation, and (c) whether they obstruct blood flow from the ventricles. Figure 24-2 categorizes the congenital heart defects based on these three characteristics. A description of the most common defects follows.

TABLE 24-2

Congenital Heart Disease in Selected Fetal Chromosomal Aberrations

Conditions	Incidence of CHD (%)	Common Defects (in Decreasing Order of Frequency)
5 p-(cri du chat syndrome)	25	VSD, PDA, ASD
Trisomy 13 syndrome	90	VSD, PDA, dextrocardia
Trisomy 18 syndrome	99	VSD, PDA, PS
Trisomy 21 (Down syndrome)	50	ECD, VSD
Turner syndrome (XO)	35	COA, AS, ASD
Klinefelter variant (XXXXY)	15	PDA, ASD

From Park MK: *Pediatric cardiology for practitioners,* ed 4, St Louis, 2002, Mosby.

VSD, Ventricular septal defect; *PDA,* patent ductus arteriosus; *ASD,* atrial septal defect; *PS,* pulmonary stenosis; *ECD,* endocardial cushion defect; *COA,* coarctation of the aorta; *AS,* aortic stenosis.

Obstructive Defects

Coarctation of the aorta

PATHOPHYSIOLOGY **Coarctation of the aorta (COA)** is a localized narrowing of the aorta near the insertion of the ductus arteriosus, resulting in increased blood pressure proximal to the defect (head and upper extremities) and decreased blood pressure distal to the obstruction (torso and lower extremities) (Figure 24-3). Prior to birth, the ductus arteriosis allows for blood to flow from the pulmonary artery into the distal aorta. However once the ductus closes after birth, blood flow to the lower extremities is limited by the coarctation of the aorta.

CLINICAL MANIFESTATIONS The location and severity of the COA determines whether an infant will become symptomatic after the ductus arteriosus closes. If the COA is severe, infants will present with low cardiac output, acidosis, and hypotension. Physical examination of the infant will reveal weak or absent femoral pulses with poor perfusion. Some infants with COA will remain asymptomatic after the closure of the ductus arteriosus. As they grow, older children with undiagnosed COA will present with unexplained hypertension. Children may complain of leg pain or cramping on exercise. They also may rarely experience dizziness, headaches, fainting, or epistaxis from hypertension.[1,2]

EVALUATION AND TREATMENT Physical examination and measurement of upper and lower extremity blood pressure will often suggest the diagnosis. Echocardiography, magnetic resonance imaging (MRI), and cardiac catheterization may be needed to confirm the diagnosis.

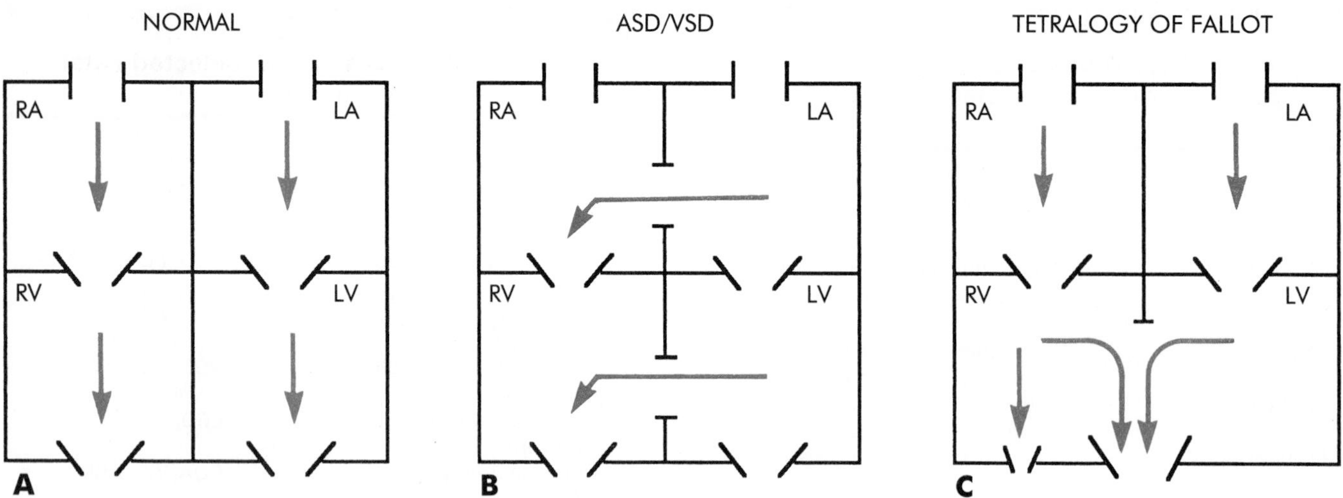

Figure 24-1 ■ **Shunting of Blood in Congenital Heart Disease. A,** Normal. **B,** Acyanotic defect. **C,** Cyanotic defect. *ASD,* Atrial septal defect; *VSD,* ventricular septal defect; *RA,* right atrium; *LA,* left atrium; *RV,* right ventricle; *LV,* left ventricle. (From Wong DL: *Whaley & Wong's essentials of pediatric nursing,* ed 4, St Louis, 1993, Mosby.)

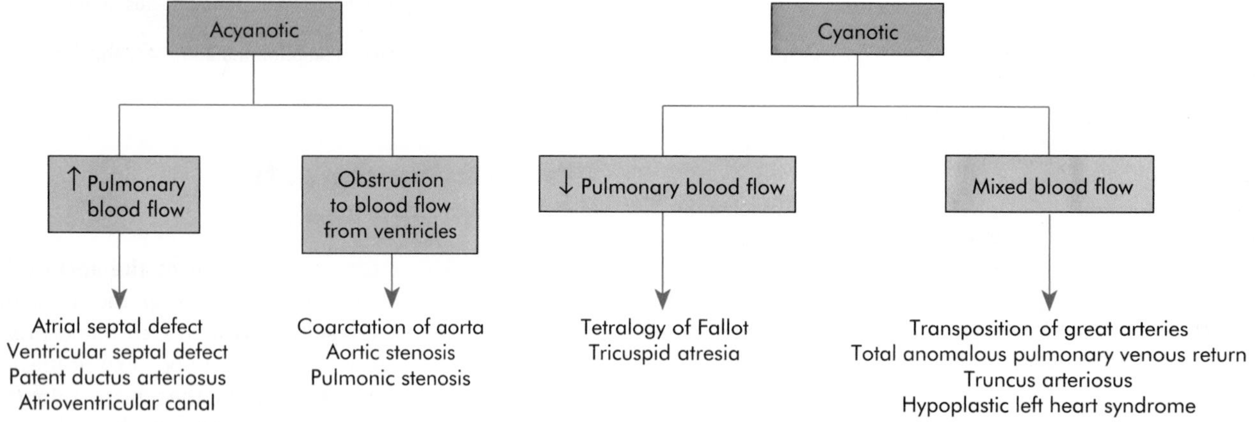

Figure 24-2 ■ **Comparison of Acyanotic-Cyanotic and Hemodynamic Classification Systems of Congenital Heart Disease.** (From Hockenberry MJ et al: *Wong's nursing care of infants and children,* ed 8, St Louis, 2007, Mosby.)

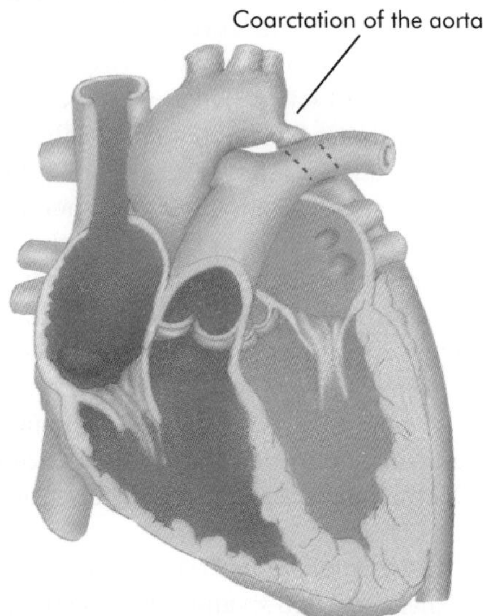

Figure 24-3 ■ **Coarctation of the Aorta (COA) (Postductal).** (From James SR, Ashwill JW: *Nursing care of children: principles and practice,* ed 3, St Louis, 2007, Saunders.)

Initial treatment in the symptomatic newborn consists of continuous intravenous infusion of prostaglandin E1 to reopen and maintain the ductus arteriosus. Once the symptomatic newborn is stabilized, surgical correction is indicated.[3,4]

Surgical correction consists of either resection of the narrowed portion of the aorta with an end-to-end anastomosis or enlargement of the constricted section using a graft taken from a portion of the left subclavian artery. Because this defect is outside the heart and pericardium, cardiopulmonary bypass usually is not required and a thoracotomy incision is used. However, coarctation repair may be part of a more complex operation, which might require a sternotomy incision and cardiopulmonary bypass. Postoperative hypertension is treated with intravenous medication, often a short-acting beta-blocker, followed by oral medications, such as an angiotensin enzyme converting inhibitor. Residual hypertension after repair of COA seems to be related to age and time of repair. Studies have shown that percutaneous balloon angioplasty has been effective in reducing residual postoperative coarctation in most children.[5–7]

Balloon angioplasty of COA as an initial intervention can also be considered. However, in infants younger than 7 months of age, most will experience recoarctation in only a short period of time after primary angioplasty. Other complications include aneurysm formation and blood vessel injury from arterial access. Data exist that support balloon angioplasty as an effective therapy in infants older than 7 months of age with discrete membranous or hourglass constrictions. Data also have revealed a decreased risk of aneurysm formation in the older age group.[3,5]

Aortic stenosis

PATHOPHYSIOLOGY **Aortic stenosis (AS)** is a narrowing or stricture of the aortic outlet, causing resistance of blood flow from the left ventricle into the aorta. If severe, there may be decreased cardiac output and pulmonary vascular congestion (Figure 24-4). The physiologic consequence of severe AS is hypertrophy of the left ventricular wall, which eventually leads to increased end-diastolic pressure, resulting in pulmonary venous and pulmonary arterial hypertension. Left ventricular hypertrophy also impedes coronary artery perfusion and may result in subendocardial ischemia and associated papillary muscle dysfunction causing mitral insufficiency.

Valvular AS occurs as a consequence of malformed or fused cusps resulting in a unicuspid or bicuspid valve. Valvular AS is a serious defect because (1) the obstruction tends to be progressive; (2) sudden episodes of myocardial ischemia, or low cardiac output, on rare occasions can result in sudden death in late childhood or adolescence; and (3) surgical repair will not result in a normal valve. This is one of the rare instances in which strenuous physical activity may be curtailed because of the cardiac condition.[3]

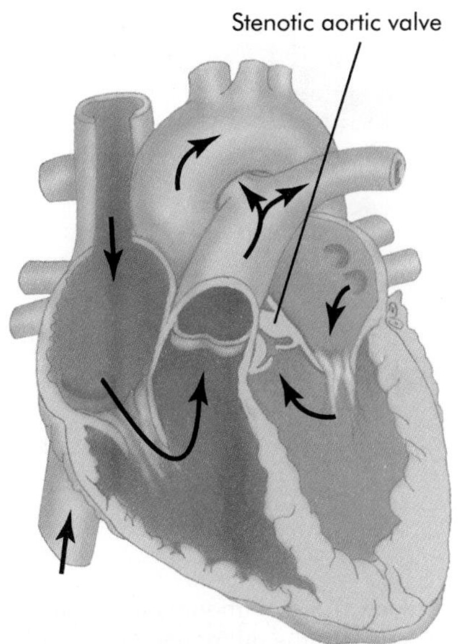

Figure 24-4 ■ **Aortic Stenosis (AS).** (From James SR, Ashwill JW: *Nursing care of children: principles and practice,* ed 3, St Louis, 2007, Saunders.)

Subvalvular AS is a stricture caused by a fibrous ring below a normal valve. It can also be caused by a narrowed left ventricular outflow tract in combination with a small aortic valve annulus. Supravalvular stenosis, a narrowing of the aorta just above the valve, occurs infrequently.

CLINICAL MANIFESTATIONS Infants with significant AS demonstrate signs of decreased cardiac output with faint pulses, hypotension, tachycardia, and poor feeding. A loud harsh systolic ejection murmur is expected. Children also may have complaints of exercise intolerance and chest pain. Children are at risk for bacterial endocarditis, coronary insufficiency, ventricular dysfunction, and, rarely, sudden death.

EVALUATION AND TREATMENT

Valvular aortic stenosis

Valvular AS is diagnosed by echocardiography. Mild to moderate valvular AS does not usually require intervention or restriction of activity. Treatment of severe valvular AS varies, with nonsurgical palliation the initial treatment of choice by many interventional cardiologists. Dilation of the stenotic valve with balloon angioplasty in the cardiac catheterization laboratory still carries a high morbidity and mortality in the critically ill neonate, but in older infants and children it compares favorably with surgical valvotomy.[4,5] Balloon angioplasty is, however, associated with the risk of aortic regurgitation (insufficiency). Children undergoing this procedure almost always require surgical intervention at some time to relieve recurrent narrowing or worsening regurgitation.[6,7]

Surgical treatment for valvular AS depends on the severity of the stenosis, previous interventions, and age of the child. Aortic valve commissurotomy or valvotomy may be used as an early intervention. Aortic valve replacement may be required if the valve is severely dysplastic. The Ross procedure, which involves moving the native pulmonary valve into the aortic position and replacing the pulmonary valve with a homograft (valvular tissue from a cadaver that has been cryopreserved), has become an option. The advantage of the Ross procedure over mechanical valve replacement, especially in a young child, is that there is no requirement for long-term anticoagulation. Mechanical valve replacement is usually deferred as long as possible. Data have shown that the pulmonary autograft has long-term durability and remains uncompromised by host reactions. Mortality for sick infants and young children is higher than for older children. Aortic stenosis requires lifelong evaluation and treatment. Multiple surgical or catheterization interventions are expected.[3]

Subvalvular aortic stenosis

Surgical correction for subvalvular AS involves incising the constricting fibromuscular ring. If the obstruction results from a narrow left ventricular outflow tract and a small aortic valve annulus, a patch may be required to enlarge the entire left ventricular outflow tract and annulus and replace the aortic valve, an approach known as the Konno procedure. An aortic homograft with a valve also may be used (extended aortic root replacement).

Pulmonic stenosis

PATHOPHYSIOLOGY **Pulmonic stenosis (PS)** is a narrowing or stricture of the pulmonary valve causing resistance to blood flow from the right ventricle to the pulmonary artery (Figure 24-5). Generally moderate to severe stenosis causes right ventricular hypertrophy. **Pulmonary atresia** is an extreme form of PS with total fusion of the valve leaflets (blood cannot flow to the lungs). The right ventricle may be hypoplastic. In some cases of obstruction, the narrowing is below the valve (infundibular or subvalve PS).

CLINICAL MANIFESTATIONS Most infants are asymptomatic if the PS is mild to moderate. Newborns with critical PS or pulmonary atresia will be cyanotic (from a right-to-left shunt through an atrial septal defect [ASD]) and may have signs of decreased cardiac output. A harsh systolic murmur is expected.

EVALUATION AND TREATMENT Echocardiography confirms the diagnosis and determines the severity of the PS. The treatment of choice for infants with moderate to severe pulmonary stenosis is balloon angioplasty (see Figure 24-5, *B*). A catheter with a special balloon device is used to dilate the area of narrowing.[6] The procedure has proved highly effective, with a 50% to 75% reduction in pressure gradient across the pulmonic valve and a low rate of complications.[7] Infrequently surgical valvotomy may be required. Pulmonary blood flood is supported with prostaglandin E1 infusion to open the ductus arteriosus in cases of pulmonary atresia until surgery is performed to supply pulmonary blood flow.

Both balloon dilation and surgical valvotomy leave the pulmonary valve incompetent (insufficient); however, children are usually able to tolerate pulmonary valve incompetence and are asymptomatic. Long-term problems with restenosis or clinically significant valve incompetence may occur, but reintervention for uncomplicated PS is rarely necessary.[6,8,9]

Defects With Increased Pulmonary Blood Flow

Patent ductus arteriosus

PATHOPHYSIOLOGY **Patent ductus arteriosus (PDA)** is failure of the fetal ductus arteriosus (artery connecting the aorta and pulmonary artery) to close within the first weeks of life (Figure 24-6). The continued patency of this vessel allows blood to flow from the higher-pressure aorta to the lower-pressure pulmonary artery, causing a left-to-right shunt.

CLINICAL MANIFESTATIONS Infants may be asymptomatic or show signs of pulmonary overcirculation, such as dyspnea, fatigue, and poor feeding. There is a characteristic machinery-like murmur. Aortic flow (run-off) into the lower pressure pulmonary circulation produces low

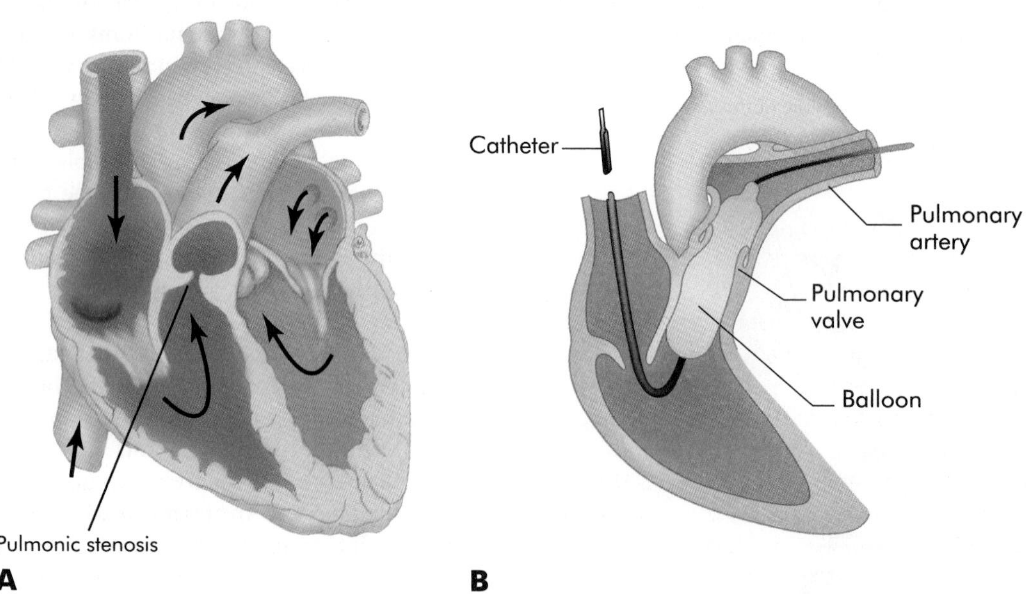

Figure 24-5 ■ **Pulmonic Stenosis (PS). A,** The pulmonary valve narrows at the entrance of the pulmonary artery. **B,** Balloon angioplasty is used to dilate the valve. A catheter is inserted across the stenotic pulmonic valve into the pulmonary artery, and a balloon at the end of the catheter is inflated while across the narrowed valve opening. (**A** from James SR, Ashwill JW: *Nursing care of children: principles and practice*, ed 3, St Louis, 2007, Saunders. **B** redrawn from Hockenberry MJ et al: *Wong's nursing care of infants and children*, ed 8, St Louis, 2007, Mosby.)

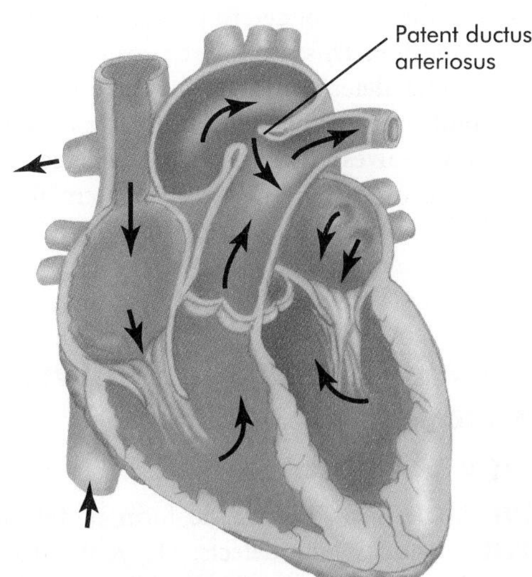

Figure 24-6 ■ **Patent Ductus Arteriosus (PDA).** (From James SR, Ashwill JW: *Nursing care of children: principles and practice*, ed 3, St Louis, 2007, Saunders.)

diastolic blood pressure, widened pulse pressure, and bounding pulses. Children are at risk for bacterial endocarditis and, rarely, may develop pulmonary hypertension in later life from chronic excessive pulmonary blood flow.

EVALUATION AND TREATMENT Diagnosis is confirmed with echocardiography. Administration of indomethacin (a prostaglandin inhibitor) has proved successful in closing a PDA in premature infants and some newborns. Surgical division of the PDA through a left thoracotomy also may be done; in some cases the procedure can be done with thoracoscopy. Closure with an occlusion device during cardiac catheterization is performed for most older children. Both surgical and nonsurgical procedures can be considered low risk.[3,8,9]

Atrial septal defect

PATHOPHYSIOLOGY An **atrial septal defect (ASD)** is an opening in the septal wall between the two atria. This opening allows blood to shunt from the higher pressure left atrium to the lower pressure right atrium. There are three types of ASDs. An **ostium primum ASD** is an opening low in the atrial septum and may be associated with abnormalities of the mitral valve. An **ostium secundum ASD** is an opening in the middle of the atrial septum and is the most common type. A **sinus venosus ASD** is an opening high up in the atrial wall and may be associated with partial anomalous pulmonary venous connection.[10]

CLINICAL MANIFESTATIONS Children with an ASD are usually asymptomatic. Infants with a large ASD may, in rare cases, develop pulmonary overcirculation and slow growth. Some older children and adults will experience shortness of breath with activity as the right ventricle becomes less compliant with age. Pulmonary hypertension and stroke are associated rare complications. A systolic ejection murmur and a widely split second heart sound are the expected findings on physical exam.

EVALUATION AND TREATMENT Diagnosis is confirmed by echocardiography. The ASD may be closed surgically with primary repair (sutured closed) or with a patch. Surgical repair involves open-heart surgery with cardiopulmonary bypass. Interventional catheterization closure involves placement of a closure device. Long-term follow-up finds atrial arrhythmias (10%) in both groups after closure.

Ventricular septal defect

PATHOPHYSIOLOGY A **ventricular septal defect (VSD)** is an opening of the septal wall between the ventricles. VSDs are the most common type of congenital heart defect. VSDs are classified by location. Perimembranous VSDs, are located high in the septal wall of the ventricle underneath the aortic valve. Muscular VSDs are located low in the septal wall. VSDs also can be located in the inlet or outlet portion of the ventricle. VSDs are similar to ASDs in that blood will shunt from left to right. Depending on the size and location, VSDs can spontaneously close, most often within the first 2 years of life.

CLINICAL MANIFESTATIONS Depending on the size, location, and degree of pulmonary vascular resistance, children may have no symptoms or have clinical effects from excessive pulmonary blood flow (commonly called congestive heart failure [CHF], although the heart muscle functions well in VSD). Clinically, large left-to-right shunts present with poor growth (failure to thrive) and tachypnea in infants. A holosystolic (pan-systolic) murmur is expected.

If the degree of shunting is significant and not corrected, the child is at risk for developing pulmonary hypertension. Irreversible pulmonary hypertension can result in **Eisenmenger syndrome,** a condition in which shunting of blood is reversed because of high pulmonary pressure and resistance (right-to-left shunt with cyanosis). Children with VSD are at risk for endocarditis.

EVALUATION AND TREATMENT Diagnosis is confirmed by echocardiogram. Cardiac catheterization may be needed to calculate the degree of right-to-left shunting. Depending on the size of the VSD and the degree of symptoms, management may be minimal. Smaller VSDs may close completely or to become small enough that surgical closure is not required. If the infant has severe CHF or failure to thrive that is unmanageable with medical therapy, early surgical repair is performed.

Surgical repair involves open-heart surgery with cardiopulmonary bypass. The opening is sutured closed primarily or with a patch. Nonsurgical intervention is available but only under restricted conditions.[8,9]

Atrioventricular canal defect

PATHOPHYSIOLOGY **Atrioventricular canal (AVC) defect,** also known as **atrioventricular septal defect (AVSD)** or by the traditional term of **endocardial cushion defect (ECD),** is the result of incomplete fusion of endocardial cushions (Figure 24-7). AVC defect consists of an ostium primum ASD and inlet VSD with associated abnormalities of the atrioventricular valve tissue. These valve abnormalities range from a cleft in the mitral valve to a common mitral and tricuspid valve. The directions and pathways of flow are determined by pulmonary and systemic resistance, left and right ventricular pressures, and the compliance of each chamber. Flow is generally from left to right. ACV is a common cardiac defect in children with Down syndrome. However, most children with this defect have normal chromosomes.

CLINICAL MANIFESTATIONS Infants with this defect often display moderate to severe heart failure due to left-to-right shunting. Infants with pulmonary hypertension and high pulmonary resistance have less shunting and therefore minimal signs of CHF. There may be mild cyanosis that increases with crying. Those with a large left-to-right shunt will have a murmur, and those with minimal shunt may not have a murmur. Children with AVC are at risk for developing irreversible pulmonary hypertension if left surgically untreated.

EVALUATION AND TREATMENT AVC is one of the most frequent diagnoses made with fetal echocardiography. Cardiac catheterization usually is not needed. Initial treatment goals include aggressive medical management of CHF. Infants are followed closely for signs or symptoms of failure to thrive. Complete surgical repair is performed between 3 and 6 months of age to prevent irreversible pulmonary hypertension. This procedure consists of patch closure of the septal defects and reconstruction of the AV valve tissue (either repair of the mitral valve cleft or fashioning of two AV valves). If the mitral valve defect is severe, a valve replacement may be needed. A potential problem following repair is mitral regurgitation, which may later require valve replacement.

Defects With Decreased Pulmonary Blood Flow

Tetralogy of fallot

PATHOPHYSIOLOGY The classic form of **tetralogy of Fallot (TOF)** includes four defects: (1) ventricular septal defect, (2) pulmonic stenosis, (3) overriding aorta, and (4) right ventricular hypertrophy (Figure 24-8). The pathophysiology varies widely, depending not only on the degree of pulmonary stenosis but also on the pulmonary and systemic vascular resistance to flow. If total resistance to pulmonary flow is higher than systemic resistance, the shunt is from right to left. If systemic resistance is higher than pulmonary resistance, the shunt is from left to right. Pulmonic stenosis decreases blood flow to the lungs and, consequently, the amount of oxygenated blood that returns to the left heart. Physiologic compensation to chronic hypoxia includes production of more red blood cells (polycythemia), development of collateral bronchial vessels, and enlargement of the nail beds (clubbing).

CLINICAL MANIFESTATIONS Some infants may be acutely cyanotic at birth. In others, progression of hypoxia and cyanosis may be more gradual over the first year of life

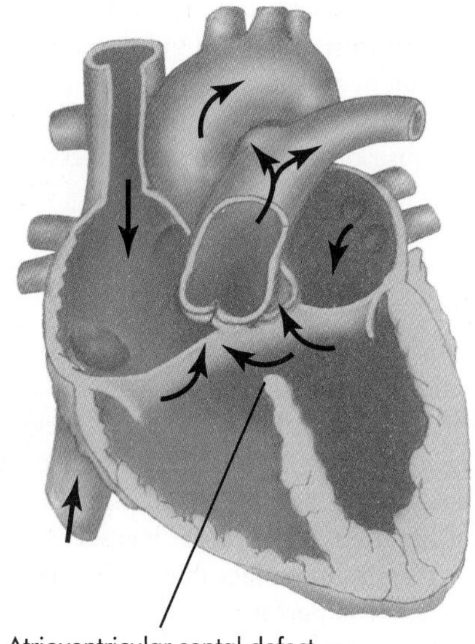

Figure 24-7 ■ **Atrioventricular Canal (AVC) Defect.** (From James SR, Ashwill JW: *Nursing care of children: principles and practice*, ed 3, St Louis, 2007, Saunders.)

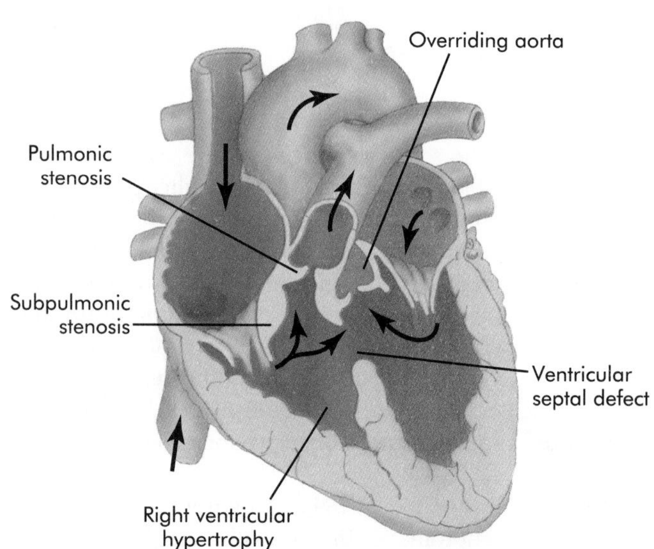

Figure 24-8 ■ **Tetralogy of Fallot (TOF).** (From James SR, Ashwill JW: *Nursing care of children: principles and practice*, ed 3, St Louis, 2007, Saunders.)

as the pulmonary stenosis worsens. Acute episodes of cyanosis and hypoxia can occur, called *hypercyanotic spells, blue spells,* or *"tet" spells.* These spells (increased right-to-left shunt) may occur during crying or after feeding. If prolonged or frequent, these spells are an indication for emergent evaluation and surgical treatment.

Chronic cyanosis may cause clubbing of the fingers, squatting, and poor growth in children. Children with unrepaired TOF are at risk for emboli, cerebrovascular disease, brain abscess, seizures, and loss of consciousness or sudden death following a tet spell.

EVALUATION AND TREATMENT Diagnosis is confirmed with echocardiography. Elective surgical repair is usually performed in the first year of life. Indications for earlier repair include increasing cyanosis or the development of hypercyanotic spells. Complete repair involves closure of the VSD, resection of the infundibular stenosis, and enlargement of the right ventricular outflow tract.

In very small infants who cannot undergo primary repair, a palliative procedure to increase pulmonary blood flow and increase oxygen saturation may be performed. This systemic artery to pulmonary artery procedure is the *Blalock-Taussig* or modified *Blalock-Taussig shunt,* which provides blood flow to the pulmonary arteries.

Tricuspid atresia

PATHOPHYSIOLOGY **Tricuspid atresia** is failure of the tricuspid valve to develop; consequently, there is no communication from right atrium to right ventricle (Figure 24-9). Blood flows through an atrial septal defect or a patent foramen ovale to the left atrium and through a ventricular septal defect to the right ventricle. This condition is often associated with pulmonic stenosis or transposition of the great arteries. There is complete mixing of unoxygenated and oxygenated blood in the left side of the heart, resulting in systemic desaturation and mild cyanosis. The physiology of the lesion is variable depending on the great vessel anatomy and amount of pulmonary stenosis.

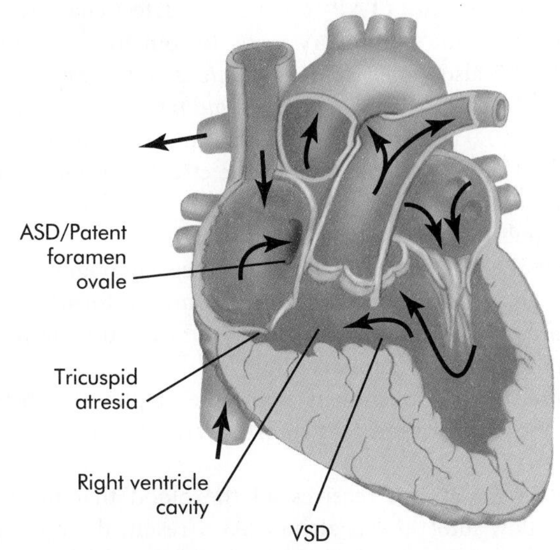

Figure 24-9 ■ **Tricuspid Atresia.** (From James SR, Ashwill JW: *Nursing care of children: principles and practice,* ed 3, St Louis, 2007, Saunders.)

CLINICAL MANIFESTATIONS A murmur is noted, and cyanosis is usually seen in the newborn period. Tachycardia, dyspnea, fatigue, and poor feeding may be noted with excessive pulmonary blood flow. Older children may have signs of chronic hypoxemia with clubbing. Children are at risk for bacterial endocarditis, brain abscess, and stroke.

EVALUATION AND TREATMENT After diagnosis is confirmed by echocardiography, the neonate with decreased pulmonary blood flow is treated with a continuous infusion of prostaglandin E1 until surgical intervention. If the ASD is restrictive, an atrial septostomy is done during cardiac catheterization. Treatment is accomplished in staged procedures. Once the infant is stabilized, a Blalock-Taussig shunt (systemic to pulmonary artery anastomosis) is placed to increase blood flow to the lungs. Some infants have increased pulmonary blood flow and require surgery to lessen the volume of blood to the lungs.

Further surgery is undertaken between 6 months and 2 years of age, depending on the child's growth and degree of pulmonary blood flow. The next step is usually a Glenn shunt in which the superior vena cava is anastomosed to the pulmonary artery. At that time, the pulmonary artery may be ligated or the Blalock-Taussig shunt may be taken down. The final separation of the pulmonary circulation from the systemic circulation is the *Fontan procedure.* In this stage, the inferior vena caval blood flow is routed to the pulmonary artery using a tube graft or baffle. The infant must have normal ventricular function and a low pulmonary vascular resistance for the procedure to be successful.

Postoperative complications that increase hospital stay include pleural and pericardial effusions, elevated pulmonary vascular resistance, and ventricular dysfunction. Exercise tolerance is limited in many children with the Fontan procedure, but general health is considered good.

Mixing Defects

Transposition of the great arteries or transposition of the great vessels

PATHOPHYSIOLOGY In **transposition of the great arteries (TGA)** or **transposition of the great vessels (TGV),** the pulmonary artery leaves the left ventricle and the aorta exits from the right ventricle (Figure 24-10). Associated defects, such as ASD, VSD or PDA, permit mixing of saturated and desaturated blood, which maintain adequate tissue oxygenation.

CLINICAL MANIFESTATIONS Clinical manifestations depend on the type and size of the associated defects. Children with limited communication between cardiac chambers are severely cyanotic, acidotic, and ill at birth. Those with large septal defects or a patent ductus arteriosus may

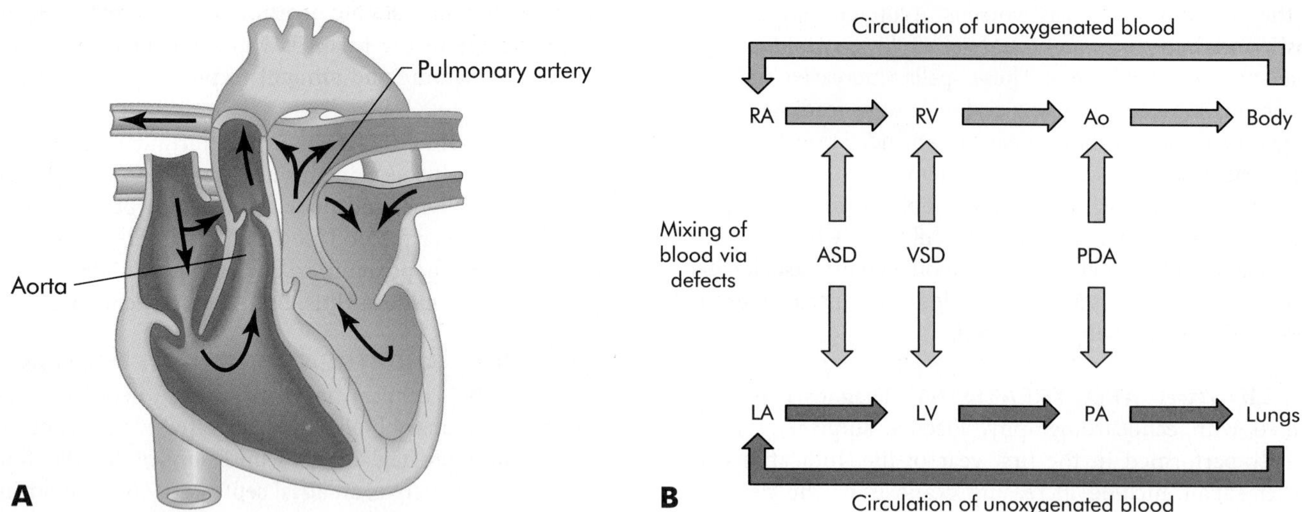

Figure 24-10 ■ **Hemodynamics in Transposition of the Great Vessels (TGV). A,** Complete transposition of the great vessels with an intact interventricular septum. The aorta arises from the right ventricle and the pulmonary artery from the left. **B,** Oxygen saturation in the two parallel circuits. *RA,* Right atrium; *RV,* right ventricle; *Ao,* aorta; *ASD,* atrial septal defect; *VSD,* ventricular septal defect; *PDA,* patent ductus arteriosus; *LA,* left atrium; *LV,* left ventricle; *PA,* pulmonary artery. (**A** redrawn from Hockenberry MJ et al: *Wong's nursing care of infants and children,* ed 8, St Louis, 2007, Mosby.)

be less severely cyanotic but may have symptoms of pulmonary overcirculation. No murmur is heard unless there is an associated VSD.

EVALUATION AND TREATMENT Diagnosis is suspected by physical examination and confirmed with echocardiography. Administration of intravenous prostaglandin E1 may be initiated to temporarily increase oxygen delivery. Enlargement of the patent foramen ovale by balloon atrial septostomy may also may be performed during cardiac catheterization to increase mixing and maintain cardiac output.

There are three types of corrective surgical repair for TGA or TGV. The most preferred type, performed in the first weeks of life, is the *arterial switch procedure.* It involves transecting the great arteries and anastomosing the main pulmonary artery to the native proximal aorta (just above the aortic valve) and anastomosing the ascending aorta to the native proximal pulmonary artery. The coronary arteries are moved with a "button" of tissue from the proximal aorta to the proximal pulmonary artery, creating a new aorta. Reimplantation of the coronary arteries is critical to the infant's survival, and the arteries must be reattached without torsion or kinking to provide the heart with its supply of oxygen. The advantage of the arterial switch procedure is the reestablishment of normal circulation with the left ventricle acting as the systemic pump. Potential complications of the arterial switch include narrowing at the great artery anastomosis or coronary artery insufficiency. Long-term results for the arterial switch operation are usually good.

A second type of surgical repair, now rarely performed, is the creation of an intraarterial baffle to divert venous blood to the mitral valve and pulmonary venous blood to the tricuspid valve using the individual's atrial septum *(Senning procedure)* or a prosthetic material *(Mustard procedure).* A disadvantage is the continuing role of the right ventricle as the systemic pump and the late development of right ventricular failure and rhythm disturbances.

A third type of surgical repair, for infants with TGA with VSD and severe PS, is the *Rastelli procedure.* It involves closure of the VSD with a baffle, directing left ventricular blood through the VSD into the aorta. The pulmonic valve is then closed, and a conduit is placed from the right ventricle to the pulmonary artery, creating a physiologically normal circulation.

Total anomalous pulmonary venous connection

PATHOPHYSIOLOGY **Total anomalous pulmonary venous connection (TAPVC)** is a rare defect characterized by failure of the pulmonary veins to join the left atrium. TAPVC is also called *total anomalous pulmonary venous return (TAPVR)* or *total anomalous pulmonary venous drainage (TAPVD)* (Figure 24-11). The pulmonary venous return is connected to the right side of the circulation rather than to the left atrium. The type of TAPVC is classified according to the pulmonary venous point of attachment:

- *Supracardiac.* Attachment above the diaphragm, usually to the superior vena cava (most common form)
- *Cardiac.* Direct attachment to the heart, usually to the right atrium or coronary sinus
- *Infracardiac.* Attachment below the diaphragm, such as to the inferior vena cava (most severe and least common form)

The right atrium receives all the blood that normally would flow into the left atrium. As a result, the right side of the heart is enlarged and the left side, especially the left atrium, is smaller than normal. An associated ASD or patent foramen ovale allows systemic venous blood to

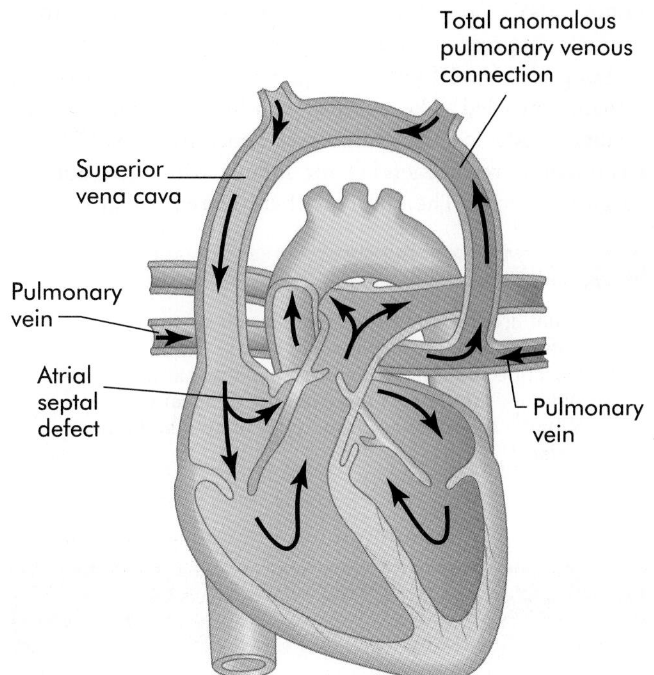

Figure 24-11 ■ **Total Anomalous Pulmonary Venous Connection (TAPVC).** (Redrawn from Hockenberry MJ et al: *Wong's nursing care of infants and children,* ed 8, St Louis, 2007, Mosby.)

shunt from the higher-pressure right atrium to the left atrium and into the left side of the heart. As a result, the oxygen saturation of the blood in both sides of the heart (and ultimately, in the systemic arterial circulation) is the same. If the pulmonary blood flow is large, pulmonary venous return is also large, and the amount of saturated blood is relatively high. However, if there is obstruction to pulmonary venous drainage, the infant has severe cyanosis and low cardiac output. Infracardiac TAPVC often is associated with obstruction of pulmonary venous drainage and is a surgical emergency.

CLINICAL MANIFESTATIONS Most infants develop cyanosis early in life. The degree of cyanosis is inversely related to the amount of pulmonary blood flow; the more pulmonary blood, the less cyanosis. Children with unobstructed TAPVC may be asymptomatic until pulmonary vascular resistance decreases during infancy, increasing pulmonary blood flow, with resulting signs of pulmonary overcirculation. Cyanosis becomes worse with pulmonary vein obstruction; once obstruction occurs, the infant's condition usually deteriorates rapidly. Without intervention, cardiac failure will progress to death. Murmur is not a common feature of TAPVC.

EVALUATION AND TREATMENT Diagnosis is suspected with echocardiography but may require confirmative angiography. Corrective repair is usually required in early infancy. The surgical approach varies with the anatomic defect. In general, however, the common pulmonary vein (venous confluence) is sewn to the left atrium, the ASD is closed, and the anomalous pulmonary venous connection may be ligated.

Truncus arteriosus

PATHOPHYSIOLOGY **Truncus arteriosus (TA)** is failure of normal septation and division of the embryonic outflow track into a pulmonary artery and an aorta, resulting in a single vessel that exits the heart. There is always an associated VSD with mixing of the systemic and arterial circulations (Figure 24-12) causing cyanosis. Blood ejected from the heart flows preferentially to the lower-pressure pulmonary arteries, causing increased pulmonary blood flow. The three types are as follows:

- *Type I:* A single pulmonary trunk arises near the base of the truncus and divides into the left and right pulmonary arteries.
- *Type II:* The left and right pulmonary arteries arise separately from the posterior aspect of the truncus.
- *Type III:* The pulmonary arteries arise independently and from the lateral aspect of the truncus.

CLINICAL MANIFESTATIONS Most infants are symptomatic with moderate heart failure and variable cyanosis, poor growth, and activity intolerance. Children are at risk for brain abscess and bacterial endocarditis.

EVALUATION AND TREATMENT Diagnosis is made by echocardiography. Corrective repair is a modification of the Rastelli procedure and is performed in the first few weeks or months of life. It involves closing the VSD so that the truncus arteriosus receives the outflow from the left ventricle, excising the pulmonary arteries from the aorta and attaching them to the right ventricle by means of a homograft. These children require additional procedures to replace the conduit as its size becomes inadequate in relation to growth.

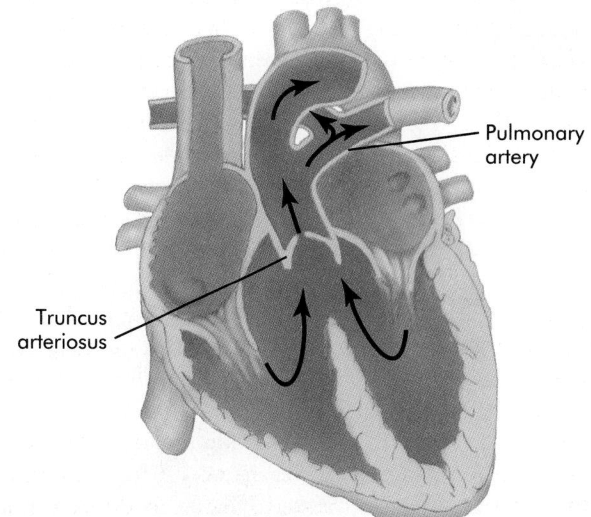

Figure 24-12 ■ **Truncus Arteriosus (TA).** (From James SR, Ashwill JW: *Nursing care of children: principles and practice,* ed 3, St Louis, 2007, Saunders.)

Hypoplastic left heart syndrome

PATHOPHYSIOLOGY **Hypoplastic left heart syndrome (HLHS)** is underdevelopment of the left side of the heart. Features include small left atrium, small or absent mitral valve, small or absent left ventricle, and a small or absent aortic valve. Coarctation also is expected (Figure 24-13). Most blood from the left atrium flows across the patent foramen ovale to the right atrium, to the right ventricle, and out the pulmonary artery. The descending aorta receives blood from the patent ductus arteriosus supplying systemic blood flow.

CLINICAL MANIFESTATIONS HLHS presents in the early newborn period if not already detected by fetal echocardiogram. Support of the systemic circulation is accomplished with prostaglandin E1 infusion. There is mild cyanosis with mild tachypnea. If HLHS is not suspected and the patent ductus arteriosus closes, there is progressive deterioration with cyanosis and decreased cardiac output, leading to cardiovascular collapse. If untreated, HLHS is usually fatal in the first months of life.

EVALUATION AND TREATMENT Echocardiography reveals all of the features of HLHS. Cardiac catheterization is rarely required. A several-stage repair approach is used. The first stage is the *Norwood procedure,* which is anastomosis of the main pulmonary artery to the aorta to create a new aorta, a shunt to provide pulmonary blood flow, creation of a large atrial septal defect, and coarctation repair. The second stage is a *bidirectional Glenn shunt* done at 6 to 9 months of age to relieve cyanosis and reduce the volume load on the right ventricle. The final repair is a *Fontan procedure.* Some centers perform heart transplantation in the newborn period rather than the staged procedure (Norwood, Glenn, Fontan). Problems of neonatal transplantation include the shortage of newborn organ donors, risk of rejection, long-term problems with chronic immunosuppression, and infection.

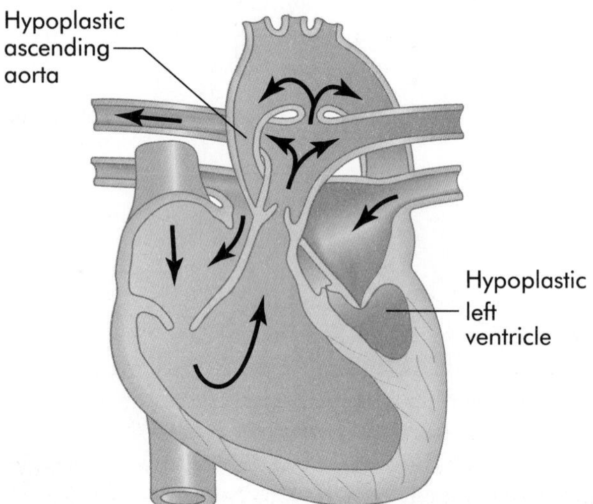

Figure 24-13 ■ **Hypoplastic Left Heart Syndrome (HLHS).** (Redrawn from Hockenberry MJ et al: *Wong's nursing care of infants and children,* ed 8, St Louis, 2007, Mosby.)

Long-term (>10 years) outcome from both procedures remains guarded. The survival continues to improve and quality of life for the children is generally good.[11–13] No treatment is recommended for infants with little hope of surgical survival. The family is then offered palliative care.

QUICK CHECK 24-1

1. What are the three principal classifications of congenital heart disease?
2. Describe the different characteristics that determine whether the defects are cyanotic or acyanotic.
3. What is the most common type of congenital heart defect?

HEALTH ALERT
Endocarditis Risk

Children with congenital heart disease are at risk for developing endocarditis. Although the risk is low, a transient bacteremia has been noted to follow dental and surgical procedures and instrumentation involving mucosal surfaces. A blood-borne pathogen can settle in areas of the heart where there is high turbulence, an abnormal valve or vessel, or an artificial material such as a valve or homograft. *Streptococcus viridans* (α-hemolytic streptococci) is the most commonly found pathogen following dental or oral procedures. *Enterococcus faecalis* (enterococci) is the most common bacterium found following genitourinary and gastrointestinal tract surgery or instrumentation. The American Heart Association has provided updated guidelines for the prevention of bacterial endocarditis. The type and dose of antibiotic prophylaxis recommended depend on the procedure and the cardiac classification of risk for endocarditis.

Data from the American Heart Association; www.americanheart.org.

Congestive Heart Failure

Congestive heart failure (CHF) is a common complication of many congenital heart defects. CHF occurs when the heart is unable to maintain sufficient cardiac output to meet the metabolic demands of the body. The most common causes congenital causes of CHF in infancy and childhood are listed in Table 24-3. CHF in children can also be acquired, usually resulting from cardiomyopathies. Pulmonary overcirculation from large left-to-right shunt is often called CHF but is not usually associated with decreased ventricular function and failure to meet metabolic demands. However, the clinical manifestations are similar, such as failure to thrive, tachypnea, tachycardia, and respiratory infections.[1]

In general, the pathophysiologic mechanisms of CHF in infants and children are similar to those in adults. It is most often a result of decreased left ventricular systolic function and the associated left atrial and pulmonary venous hyper-

TABLE 24-3

Causes of Congestive Heart Failure Resulting From Congenital Heart Disease

Age of Onset	Cause
At birth	HLHS Volume overload lesions Severe tricuspid or pulmonary insufficiency Large systemic AV fistula
First week	TGA PDA in small premature infants HLHS (with more favorable anatomy) TAPVR, particularly those with pulmonary venous obstruction Others Systemic AV fistula Critical AS or PS
1–4 wk	COA with associated anomalies Critical AS Large left-to-right shunt lesions (VSD, PDA) in premature infants All other lesions previously listed
4–6 wk	Some left-to-right shunt lesions, such as ECD
6 wk–4 months	Large VSD Large PDA Others, such as anomalous left coronary artery from the PA

From Park MK: *Pediatric cardiology for practitioners*, ed 4, St Louis, 2002, Mosby.

HLHS, Hypoplastic left heart syndrome; *AV*, atrioventricular; *TGA*, transposition of great arteries; *PDA*, patent ductus arteriosus; *TAPVR*, total anomalous pulmonary venous return; *AS*, aortic stenosis; *PS*, pulmonic stenosis; *COA*, coarctation of the aorta; *VSD*, ventricular septal defect; *ECD*, endocardial cushion defect; *PA*, pulmonary artery.

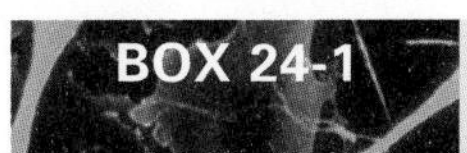

BOX 24-1 **Clinical Manifestations of Congestive Heart Failure**

Impaired Myocardial Function
Tachycardia
Sweating (inappropriate)
Decreased urinary output
Fatigue
Weakness
Restlessness
Anorexia
Pale, cool extremities
Weak peripheral pulses
Decreased blood pressure
Gallop rhythm
Cardiomegaly

Pulmonary Congestion
Tachypnea
Dyspnea
Retractions (infants)
Flaring nares
Exercise intolerance
Orthopnea
Cough, hoarseness
Cyanosis
Wheezing
Grunting

Excerpted from Hockenberry MJ et al: *Wong's nursing care of infants and children*, ed 8, St Louis, 2007, Mosby.

tension and pulmonary venous congestion. The same compensatory mechanisms are activated in the face of inadequate cardiac output (see Figure 23-40). Right ventricular failure is rare in childhood.

Left heart failure in infants is manifested as poor feeding and sucking, often leading to failure to thrive. In left heart failure, dyspnea, tachypnea, and diaphoresis may be accompanied by retractions, grunting, and nasal flaring. Wheezing, coughing, and rales are rare in childhood CHF.[2] Common skin changes, such as pallor or mottling, are often present (Box 24-1). Systemic venous congestion is rare in childhood. The presence of peripheral edema and weight gain suggests renal disease or nutritional disease much more often than cardiac dysfunction.

A thorough physical examination with emphasis on cardiac and pulmonary findings will often reveal the degree of CHF. Plotting the child's growth (height, weight, head circumference) is an important method of assessing a child's health. Infants with CHF or pulmonary overcirculation usually have low weight with normal length and head circumference. The failure to thrive is usually the result of increased metabolic expenditure relative to caloric intake. An electrocardiogram (ECG) also should be performed to determine the presence of dysrhythmia or hypertrophy. A chest x-ray is useful in assessing the presence of cardiomegaly and signs of increased pulmonary circulation.

Treatment is aimed at decreasing cardiac workload and increasing the efficiency of the heart function. Severe congenital heart disease is managed with surgical repair. Medical management initially consists of diuretics, such as furosemide. Depending on the degree of CHF, other diuretics can be used in combination with furosemide to counteract potassium losses. Agents that reduce afterload, such as captopril or enalapril and beta-blockers, have recently been employed to further manage severe CHF.[1,2]

ACQUIRED CARDIOVASCULAR DISORDERS

Acquired heart diseases refer to disease processes or abnormalities that occur after birth. They result from various causes, such as infection, genetic disorders, autoimmune processes in response to infection, environmental factors, or autoimmune diseases. Examples of acquired heart diseases include Kawasaki disease, myocarditis, rheumatic heart disease, cardiomyopathy, and systemic hypertension. This chapter discusses Kawasaki disease and systemic hypertension. Myocarditis, rheumatic heart disease, and cardiomyopathy are discussed in Chapter 23.

Kawasaki Disease

Kawasaki disease (KD), formerly known as mucocutaneous lymph node syndrome, is an acute, usually self-limiting systemic vasculitis that may result in cardiac sequelae. It was first identified in 1967. Although KD occurs throughout the world, the greatest number of cases are seen in Japan.[1,2] This reflects the genetic component of KD with the case rate being highest among Asians, less among Caucasian children, and rare in Black children.

Kawasaki disease is primarily a condition of young children. Eighty percent of cases are seen in children younger than 5 years of age, with the incidence peaking in the toddler age group. Males are affected slightly more than females. The peak incidence is in the winter and spring.[1,2]

The etiology of Kawasaki disease remains unknown. Current etiologic theories center on an immunologic response to an infectious, toxic, or antigenic substance (including superantigen).[14]

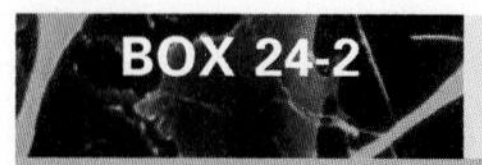

Diagnostic Criteria for Kawasaki Disease

The child must exhibit five of the following six criteria, including fever:

1. Fever for 5 or more days (often diagnosed with shorter duration of fever if other symptoms are present)
2. Bilateral conjunctival infection without exudation
3. Changes in the oral mucous membranes, such as erythema, dryness, and fissuring of the lips; oropharyngeal reddening; or "strawberry tongue"
4. Changes in the extremities, such as peripheral edema, peripheral erythema, and desquamation of palms and soles, particularly periungual peeling
5. Polymorphous rash, often accentuated in the perineal area
6. Cervical lymphadenopathy

Data from Hockenberry MJ et al: *Wong's nursing care of infants and children*, ed 8, St Louis, 2007, Mosby.

PATHOPHYSIOLOGY Kawasaki disease progresses pathologically and clinically in the following stages. In the early or acute phase, small capillaries, arterioles, and venules become inflamed, as does the heart itself. In the subacute state, inflammation spreads to larger vessels and aneurysms of the coronary arteries develop. In the convalescent stage, medium-sized arteries begin the granulation process, causing coronary artery thickening with increased risk for thrombosis. After the convalescent stage, inflammation wanes with scarring of the affected vessels, calcification, and stenosis.

CLINICAL MANIFESTATIONS The clinical course of the disease progresses in three stages: acute, subacute, and convalescent. In the acute phase, the child with classic of typical KD has fever, conjunctivitis, oral changes ("strawberry" tongue), rash, and lymphadenopathy and is often irritable. During this phase, myocarditis may develop. The subacute phase begins when the fever ends and continues until the clinical signs have resolved. It is at this time that the child is most at risk for coronary artery aneurysm development. Desquamation of the palms and soles occurs at this time, as well as marked thrombocytosis. The convalescent phase is marked by the continued elevation of the erythrocyte sedimentation rate and platelet count. Arthritis may be present. This phase continues until all laboratory values return to normal—usually about 6 to 8 weeks after onset.[2] Atypical KD is now described with the presentation of infants as young as 6 weeks who have fever and coronary aneurysms without the "classic" physical findings or typical time course. Recognition is difficult and may delay treatment.[2,14]

EVALUATION AND TREATMENT The diagnosis is based on the diagnostic criteria for Kawasaki disease, which state that the child must exhibit five of six criteria, including fever (Box 24-2). These children usually have leukocytosis, increased erythrocyte sedimentation rates, marked thrombocytosis, and elevated liver enzymes. An echocardiogram is obtained at the time of diagnosis as a baseline to assess for coronary aneurysms or inflammation. Serial echocardiograms are obtained after treatment to assess for development of coronary aneurysms or regression of those present early in the course. Treatment includes oral administration of aspirin and intravenous infusion of gamma globulin (most often only one dose). Aspirin is continued until the manifestations of inflammation are resolved.

Treatment with aspirin and intravenous immunoglobulin during the acute phase has decreased the morbidity of Kawasaki disease and has reduced the incidence of coronary abnormalities from approximately 20% to less than 10% at 6 to 8 weeks after initiation of therapy. Most children recover completely from Kawasaki disease, including regression of aneurysms. The most common cardiovascular sequela is coronary thrombosis.[14]

Systemic Hypertension

Systemic hypertension in children is defined as systolic and diastolic blood pressure levels greater than the ninety-fifth percentile for age and gender on at least three occasions (see Table 24-4). The Fourth Task Force on Blood Pressure Control in Children uses height as an additional criterion to the blood pressure guidelines.[2,15]

Hypertension is classified into two categories: primary, or essential hypertension, in which a specific cause cannot be identified, and secondary hypertension, in which a cause *can* be identified (see Box 24-3). Hypertension (HTN) in children differs from adult hypertension in etiology and presentation. Children, when diagnosed with HTN, are often found to have some underlying disease, such as renal disease or coarctation of the aorta (see Box 24-3). An increased prevalence of primary HTN in older children has been noted. Researchers are now focusing on primary HTN in older children in relation to morbidity and mortality and the presence of early atherosclerotic disease.[15–17] Certain factors influence blood pressure in children.

TABLE 24-4

Diagnosing Hypertension in Children (Selected Ages)

		NINETY-FIFTH PERCENTILE OF SYSTOLIC BP							NINETY-FIFTH PERCENTILE OF DIASTOLIC BP						
		Percentile of Height													
AGE	GENDER	5	10	25	50	75	90	95	5	10	25	50	75	90	95
1	Boys	98	99	103	104	104	106	106	54	54	55	56	57	58	58
	Girls	100	101	102	104	105	106	107	56	57	57	58	59	59	60
5	Boys	108	109	110	112	114	115	116	69	70	71	72	73	74	74
	Girls	107	107	108	110	111	112	113	70	71	71	72	73	73	74
10	Boys	115	116	117	119	121	122	123	77	78	79	80	81	81	82
	Girls	116	116	117	119	120	121	122	77	77	77	78	79	80	80
15	Boys	126	127	129	131	133	134	135	81	81	82	83	84	85	85
	Girls	124	125	126	127	129	130	131	82	82	82	83	84	85	85

Data from National High Blood Pressure Education Program Working Group on High Blood Pressure in Children and Adolescents: The fourth report on the diagnosis, evaluation, and treatment of high blood pressure in children and adolescents, *Pediatrics* 114:555–576, 2004.

Children who are overweight are often hypertensive.[17] Smoking is also associated with an increased risk for HTN. The gender or race of the child has not been an associated risk factor of primary HTN.[18]

PATHOPHYSIOLOGY In infants and children, a cause of HTN is almost always found. In general, the younger the child with significant hypertension, the more likely a correctable cause can be found. Therefore, a thorough evaluation needs to be done.[1,15]

The pathophysiology of primary HTN in children is not clearly understood but may result from a complex interaction of a strong predisposing genetic component with disturbances in sympathetic vascular smooth muscle tone, humoral agents (angiotensin, catecholamines), renal sodium excretion, and cardiac output. Ultimately these factors impair the ability of the peripheral vascular bed to relax.

CLINICAL MANIFESTATIONS Most children with systemic HTN are asymptomatic. It is necessary that a thorough history and physical examination be obtained. The examination should include an accurate blood pressure measurement on three separate occasions using an appropriate-size cuff.[16]

BOX 24-3 Conditions Associated With Secondary Hypertension in Children

Renal Disorders

Congenital defects
- Polycystic kidney, ectopic kidney, horseshoe kidney, etc.
- Obstructive anomalies
- Hydronephrosis

Renal tumor
- Wilms tumor
- Retrovascular

Abnormalities of renal arteries
Renal vein thrombosis
Acquired disorders
- Glomerulonephritis—acute or chronic
- Pyelonephritis
- Nephritis associated with collagen disease

Cardiovascular Disease

Coarctation of aorta
Arteriovenous fistulae
Patent ductus arteriosus
Aortic or mitral insufficiency

Metabolic and Endocrine Diseases

Adrenal tumors
- Adenoma
- Pheochromocytoma
- Neuroblastoma

Cushing syndrome
Adrenogenital syndrome
Hyperthyroidism
Aldosteronism
Hypercalcemia
Diabetes mellitus

Neurologic Disorders

Space-occupying lesions of cranium (increased intracranial pressure)
- Tumors, cysts, hematoma

Cerebral edema
Encephalitis (including Guillain-Barré and Reye syndromes)

Miscellaneous Causes

Drugs (corticosteroids, oral contraceptives, pressor agents, amphetamines)
Burns
Genitourinary surgery
Trauma (e.g., stretching of femoral nerve with leg traction)
Insect bites (e.g., scorpion)
Intravascular overload (blood, fluid)
Hypernatremia
Toxemia of pregnancy
Heavy metal poisoning

From Hockenberry MJ et al: *Wong's nursing care of infants and children*, ed 8, St Louis, 2007, Mosby.

HEALTH ALERT

U.S. Childhood Obesity and Its Association With Cardiovascular Disease

Childhood obesity is epidemic in the United States. The number of overweight children has doubled since the 1970s, and obesity has been called the most serious and prevalent nutritional disorder in the United States. Obesity is linked to insulin resistance and diabetes and increases cardiovascular risk, especially atherosclerosis, hypertension, and lipid abnormalities. The mechanisms by which insulin resistance and diabetes cause cardiovascular diseases include endothelial dysfunction, structural changes in arterial walls, abnormal vasoconstriction, and changes in renal function and salt transport. Research into genetics and insulin-regulated transcription factors suggest that obesity, insulin resistance, diabetes, and cardiovascular disease share important molecular etiologies and processes. These findings may lead investigators to important new treatments. For now, helping children develop good exercise and dietary habits has been shown to significantly improve arterial function and reduce cardiovascular risk.

Data from Arcaro G et al: Insulin causes endothelial dysfunction in humans: sites and mechanisms, *Circulation* 105(5):576–582, 2002; Chipkin SR, Klugh SA, Chasan-Taber L: Exercise and diabetes, *Cardiol Clin* 19(3):489–505, 2001; Rocchini AP: Childhood obesity and a diabetes epidemic, *N Engl J Med* 346(11):854–855, 2002; Sowers JR, Epstein M, Frohlich ED: Diabetes, hypertension, and cardiovascular disease: an update, *Hypertens* 37(4):1053–1059, 2001.

EVALUATION AND TREATMENT In children, the history and physical examination should be directed at determining the etiology of HTN, such as coarctation of the aorta or renal disease (Table 24-5). A complete blood count, serum chemistry levels, urinalysis, urine culture, lipid profile, and renal ultrasound are part of the routine evaluation for renal disease (Table 24-6). If coarctation of the aorta is found, surgical correction is initiated. If HTN is found to be essential, or primary, in nature, nonpharmacologic therapy is used initially. Moderate weight loss and exercise can decrease systolic and diastolic pressures in many children. Appropriate diet, regular physical activity, and avoidance of smoking have been shown to be effective in reducing blood pressure.[17] Ambulatory blood pressure monitoring (ABPM) has the potential to become an important tool in the evaluation and management of childhood hypertension.[19]

TABLE 24-5

Most Common Causes of Chronic Sustained Hypertension

Age-Group	Causes
Newborn	Renal artery thrombosis, renal artery stenosis, congenital renal malformation, COA, bronchopulmonary dysplasia
<6 yr	Renal parenchymal disease, COA, renal artery stenosis
6–10 yr	Renal artery stenosis, renal parenchymal disease, primary hypertension
>10 yr	Primary hypertension, renal parenchymal disease

From Park MK: *Pediatric cardiology for practitioners*, ed 4, St Louis, 2002, Mosby. See also National High Blood Pressure Education Program Working Group on High Blood Pressure in Children and Adolescents: The fourth report on the diagnosis, evaluation, and treatment of high blood pressure in children and adolescents, *Pediatrics* 114:555–576, 2004.

COA, Coarctation of the aorta.

TABLE 24-6

Routine and Special Laboratory Tests for Hypertension

Laboratory Tests	Significance of Abnormal Results
Urinalysis, urine culture, blood urea nitrogen, and creatinine levels	Renal parenchymal disease
Serum electrolyte levels (hypokalemia)	Hyperaldosteronism, primary or secondary Adrenogenital syndrome Renin-producing tumors
ECG, chest x-ray studies	Cardiac cause of hypertension, also baseline function
Intravenous pyelography (or ultrasonography, radionuclide studies, computed tomography of the kidneys)	Renal parenchymal diseases Renovascular hypertension Tumors (neuroblastoma, Wilms tumor)
Plasma renin activity, peripheral	High-renin hypertension Renovascular hypertension Renin-producing tumors Some caused by Cushing syndrome Some caused by essential hypertension Low-renin hypertension Adrenogenital syndrome Primary hyperaldosteronism
24-hr urine collection for 17-ketosteroids and 17-hydroxycorticosteroids	Cushing syndrome Adrenogenital syndrome
24-hr urine collection for catecholamine levels and vanillylmandelic acid	Pheochromocytoma Neuroblastoma
Aldosterone	Hyperaldosteronism, primary or secondary Renovascular hypertension Renin-producing tumors
Renal vein plasma renin activity	Unilateral renal parenchymal disease Renovascular hypertension
Abdominal aortogram	Renovascular hypertension Abdominal COA Unilateral renal parenchymal diseases Pheochromocytoma

From Park MK: *Pediatric cardiology for practitioners*, ed 4, St Louis, 2002, Mosby.

ECG, Electrocardiogram; *COA,* coarctation of the aorta.

Drug therapy is controversial in children with primary hypertension; however, when nonpharmacologic therapy fails, the approach is similar to the treatment of hypertension in adults with the use of angiotension-converting enzyme inhibitors or angiotension receptor blocker medications.[1] The current emphasis on preventive cardiology, especially for children, is significant because many investigators believe signs of atherosclerosis are present from childhood.[2,16]

QUICK CHECK 24-2

1. Why are the infant's height and weight important in the assessment of congestive heart failure?
2. Why is it of critical importance to recognize and treat children during the acute phase of Kawasaki disease?
3. Discuss the causes of the recent epidemic of obesity in children and the cardiovascular effects.

Did You Understand?

Congenital Heart Disease

1. Most congenital heart defects have begun to develop by the eighth week of gestation, and some have associated causes, both environmental and genetic.
2. Environmental risk factors associated with the incidence of congenital heart defects typically are maternal conditions. Maternal conditions include viral infections, diabetes, drug intake, and advanced maternal age.
3. Genetic factors associated with congenital heart defects include but are not limited to Down syndrome, trisomy 13, trisomy 18, cri du chat syndrome, and Turner syndrome.
4. Classification of congenital heart defects is based on (a) whether they cause blood flow to the lungs to increase, decrease, or remain normal; (b) whether they cause cyanosis; and (c) obstruction to flow.
5. Cyanosis, a bluish discoloration of the skin, indicates that the tissues are not receiving normal amounts of oxygenated blood. Cyanosis can be caused by defects that (a) restrict blood flow into the pulmonary circulation; (b) overload the pulmonary circulation, causing pulmonary hypertension, pulmonary edema, and respiratory difficulty; or (c) cause large amounts of unoxygenated blood to shunt from the pulmonary to the systemic circulation.
6. Congenital defects that maintain or create direct communication between the pulmonary and systemic circulatory systems cause blood to shunt from one system to another, mixing oxygenated and unoxygenated blood and increasing blood volume and, occasionally, pressure on the receiving side of the shunt.
7. The direction of shunting through an abnormal communication depends on differences in pressure and resistance between the two systems. Flow is always from an area of high pressure to an area of low pressure.
8. Obstruction of ventricular outflow is commonly caused by pulmonary stenosis (right ventricle) or aortic stenosis (left ventricle).
9. In less severe obstruction, ventricular outflow remains normal because of compensatory ventricular hypertrophy stimulated by increased afterload and, in postductal coarctation of the aorta, development of collateral circulation around the coarctation.
10. Acyanotic congenital defects that increase pulmonary blood flow consist of abnormal openings (atrial septal defect, ventricular septal defect, patent ductus arteriosus, or atrioventricular septal defect) that permit blood to shunt from left (systemic circulation) to right (pulmonary circulation). Cyanosis does not occur because the left-to-right shunt does not interfere with the flow of oxygenated blood through the systemic circulation.
11. If the abnormal communication between the left and right circuits is large, volume and pressure overload in the pulmonary circulation lead to left heart failure.
12. Cyanotic congenital defects in which saturated and desaturated blood mix within the heart or great arteries include truncus arteriosus, tricuspid atresia, tetralogy of Fallot, transposition of the great vessels, total anomalous pulmonary venous connection, and hypoplastic left heart syndrome.
13. In cyanotic heart defects that decrease pulmonary blood flow (tetralogy of Fallot), myocardial hypertrophy cannot compensate for restricted right ventricular outflow. Flow to the lungs decreases, and cyanosis is caused by an insufficient volume of oxygenated blood.
14. Initial treatment for congenital heart disease, depending on the defect, is aimed at controlling the level of congestive heart failure or cyanosis. Interventional procedures in the cardiac catheterization laboratory and surgical palliation or repair are performed to restore circulation to as normal as possible.
15. Congestive heart failure is usually the result of congenital heart defects that increase blood volume and pressure in the pulmonary circulation. A clinical manifestation of CHF unique to children is failure to thrive.

Acquired Cardiovascular Disorders in Children

1. Two examples of acquired heart disease in children are Kawasaki disease and systemic hypertension.
2. Kawasaki disease is an acute systemic vasculitis that also may result in the development of coronary artery aneurysms and thrombosis.
3. Systemic hypertension in children differs from adults in etiology and presentation. When significant hypertension is found in a child, the evaluation should rule out the presence of renal disease or coarctation.

Key Terms

Acyanotic defect, 677
Aortic stenosis (AS), 679
Atrial septal defect (ASD), 681
Atrioventricular canal (AVC) defect (also known as atrioventricular septal defect [AVSD] or endocardial cushion defect [ECD]), 682
Coarctation of the aorta (COA), 677
Congenital heart disease (CHD), 676
Congestive heart failure (CHF), 686
Cyanosis, 676
Cyanotic defect, 677
Eisenmenger syndrome, 681
Hypoplastic left heart syndrome (HLHS), 686
Kawasaki disease, 688
Left-to-right shunt, 676
Ostium primum ASD, 681
Ostium secundum ASD, 681
Patent ductus arteriosus (PDA), 680
Pulmonary atresia, 680
Pulmonic stenosis (PS), 680
Right-to-left shunt, 676
Shunt, 676
Sinus venosus ASD, 681
Subvalvular AS, 679
Systemic hypertension, 688
Tetralogy of Fallot (TOF), 682
Total anomalous pulmonary venous connection (TAPVC), 684
Transposition of the great arteries (TGA; transposition of the great vessels [TGV]), 683
Tricuspid atresia, 683
Truncus arteriosus (TA), 685
Valvular AS, 679
Ventricular septal defect (VSD), 681

References

1. Park MK: *Pediatric cardiology for practitioners,* ed 4, St Louis, 2002, Mosby.
2. Allen HD, editor: *Moss and Adams' heart disease in infants, children, and adolescents including the fetus and young adults,* ed 6, Philadelphia, 2001, Lippincott Williams & Wilkins.
3. Penny DJ et al: Management of the neonate with symptomatic congenital heart disease, *Arch Dis Child Fetal Neonatal Ed* 84:141–145, 2001.
4. McConnell ME et al: The neonate with suspected congenital heart disease, *Crit Care Nurs Q* 25(3):17–25, 2002.
5. Hornung TS et al: Intervention for aortic coarctation, *Cardiol Rev* 10:139–148, 2002.
6. Echigo S: Balloon valvuloplasty for congenital heart disease: immediate and long-term results of multi-institutional study, *Pediatr Int* 43(5):542–547, 2001.
7. Uzark K: Therapeutic cardiac catheterization for congenital heart disease—a new era in pediatric care, *J Pediatr Nurs* 16 (5):300–307, 2001.
8. Holzer R et al: Interventional approach to congenital heart disease, *Curr Opin in Cardiol* 19:84–90, 2004.
9. Andres RE et al: Interventional cardiac catheterization in congenital heart disease, *Arch Dis Child* 89:1168–1173, 2004.
10. Wong D et al: *Whaley & Wong's nursing care of infants and children,* ed 7, St Louis, 2002, Mosby.
11. Higgins S: Progress in congenital heart disease: decades added to fragile young lives, *J Pediatr Nurs* 16(5):297, 2001.
12. Kohl T: Congenital heart disease, Mending the tiniest hearts, *Lancet* 358(suppl):S17, 2001.
13. Ohye RG, Bove EL: Advances in congenital heart surgery, *Curr Opin Pediatr* 13(5):473–481, 2001.
14. Newberger JW et al: Diagnosis, treatment, and long-term management of Kawasaki disease: A statement for health professionals from the Committee on Rheumatic Fever, Endocarditis and Kawasaki Disease, Council on Cardiovascular Disease in the Young, American Heart Association, *Circulation* 110:2747–2771, 2004.
15. National High Blood Pressure Education Program Working Group on High Blood Pressure in Children and Adolescents: the fourth report on the diagnosis, evaluation, and treatment of high blood pressure in children and adolescents, *Pediatrics* 114:555–576, 2004.
16. Peters RM et al: Diagnosis and treatment of hypertension in children and adolescents, *J Am Acad Nurse Pract* 15(2): 56–63, 2003.
17. Couch SC et al: Diet and blood pressure in children, *Curr Opin Pediatr* 17(5):642–647, 2005.
18. Rosner B et al: Blood pressure difference between blacks and whites in relation to body size among US children and adolescents, *Am J of Epidemiol* 151(10):1007–1019, 2000.
19. Kennedy SE et al: Agreement on reporting of ambulatory blood pressure monitoring in children, *Pediatr Nephrol* 20: 1766–1768, 2005.

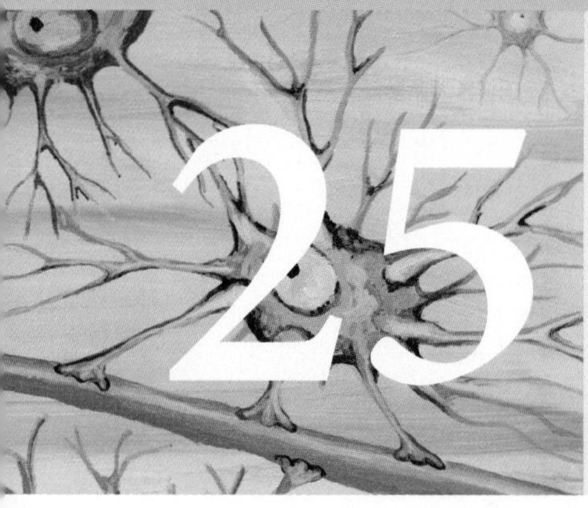

25 STRUCTURE AND FUNCTION OF THE PULMONARY SYSTEM

Valentina L. Brashers ▪ Sue E. Huether

CHAPTER OUTLINE

ELECTRONIC RESOURCES

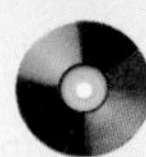

Companion CD
- Review Questions and Answers
- Animations

evolve Website
http://evolve.elsevier.com/Huether/
- Quick Check Answers
- Key Terms Exercises
- Critical Thinking Questions with Answers
- Algorithm Completion Exercises
- WebLinks

The pulmonary system consists of the lungs, airways, chest wall, and pulmonary circulation. Its primary function is the exchange of gases between the environmental air and the blood. The three steps in this process are (1) ventilation, the movement of air into and out of the lungs; (2) diffusion, the movement of gases between air spaces in the lungs and the bloodstream; and (3) perfusion, the movement of blood into and out of the capillary beds of the lungs to body organs and tissues. The first two functions are carried out by the pulmonary system and the third by the cardiovascular system (see Chapter 22). Normally the pulmonary system functions efficiently under a variety of conditions and with little energy expenditure.

STRUCTURES OF THE PULMONARY SYSTEM

The pulmonary system is made up of two lungs, their airways, the blood vessels that serve them (Figure 25-1), and the chest wall, or thoracic cage. The lungs are divided into lobes: three in the right lung (upper, middle, lower) and two in the left lung (upper, lower). Each lobe is further divided into segments and lobules. The space between the lungs, which contains the heart, great vessels, and esophagus, is called the *mediastinum.* A set of conducting airways, or bronchi, delivers air to each section of the lung. The lung tissue that surrounds the airways supports them, preventing their distortion or collapse as gas moves in and out during ventilation.

The lungs are protected from exogenous contaminants by a series of mechanical barriers (Table 25-1). These defense mechanisms are so effective that contamination of the lung tissue itself, particularly by infectious agents, is rare.

Conducting Airways

The conducting airways allow air into and out of the gas-exchange structures of the lung. The **nasopharynx, oropharynx,** and related structures are often called the *upper airway* (Figure 25-2). These structures are lined with a ciliated mucosa that warms and humidifies inspired air and removes foreign particles from it. The mouth and oropharynx are used for ventilation also when the nose is obstructed or when increased flow is required—for example, during e xercise. Filtering and humidifying are not, however, as efficient with mouth breathing.

The **larynx** connects the upper and lower airways and consists of the endolarynx and its surrounding triangular-shaped bony and cartilaginous structures. The endolarynx encompasses two pairs of folds: the false vocal cords (supraglottis) and the true vocal cords. The slit-shaped space between the true cords forms the glottis (see Figure 25-2). The vestibule is the space above the false vocal cords. The laryngeal box is formed of three large cartilages (epiglottis, thyroid, cricoid) and three smaller cartilages (arytenoid, corniculate, cuneiform) connected by ligaments. The supporting cartilages prevent collapse of the larynx during inspiration and swallowing. The internal laryngeal muscles control vocal cord length and tension, and the external

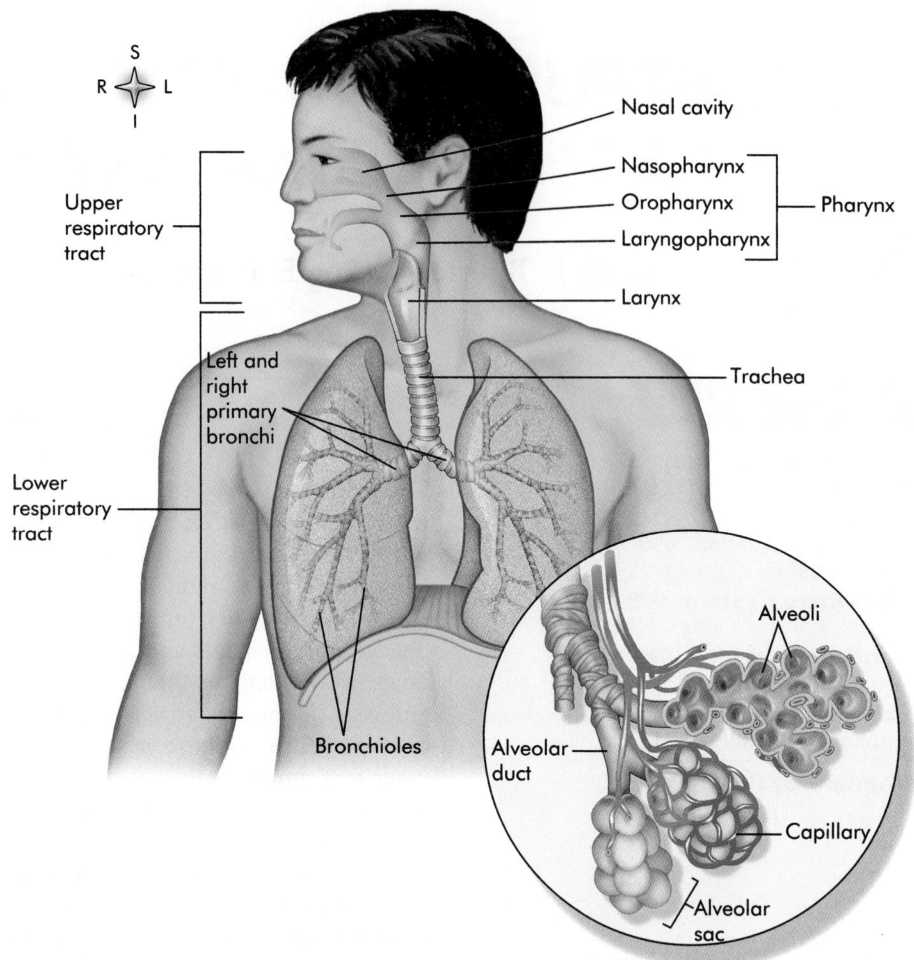

Figure 25-1 ■ **Structures of the Pulmonary System.** The enlargement in the circle depicts the acinus, where oxygen and carbon dioxide are exchanged. (From Thibodeau GA, Patton, KT: *Anatomy & physiology*, ed 6, St Louis, 2007, Mosby.)

laryngeal muscles move the larynx as a whole. Both sets of muscles are important to swallowing, ventilation, and vocalization.[1] The internal muscles contract during swallowing to prevent aspiration into the trachea. These muscles also contribute to voice pitch.

The **trachea,** which is supported by U-shaped cartilage, connects the larynx to the bronchi, the conducting airways of the lungs. The trachea branches into two main airways, or **bronchi** (sing., **bronchus**) at the **carina** (see Figure 25-1). The right and left main bronchi enter the

TABLE 25-1

Pulmonary Defense Mechanisms

Structure or Substance	Mechanism of Defense
Upper respiratory tract mucosa	Maintains constant temperature and humidification of gas entering the lungs; traps and removes foreign particles, some bacteria, and noxious gases from inspired air
Nasal hairs and turbinates	Trap and remove foreign particles, some bacteria, and noxious gases from inspired air
Mucus blanket	Protects trachea and bronchi from injury; traps most foreign particles and bacteria that reach the lower airways
Cilia	Propel mucus blanket and entrapped particles toward the oropharynx, where they can be swallowed or expectorated
Alveolar macrophages	Ingest and remove bacteria and other foreign material from alveoli by phagocytosis (see Chapters 5 and 6)
Irritant receptors in nares (nostrils)	Stimulation by chemical or mechanical irritants triggers sneeze reflex, which results in rapid removal of irritants from nasal passages
Irritant receptors in trachea and large airways	Stimulation by chemical or mechanical irritants triggers cough reflex, which results in removal of irritants from the lower airways

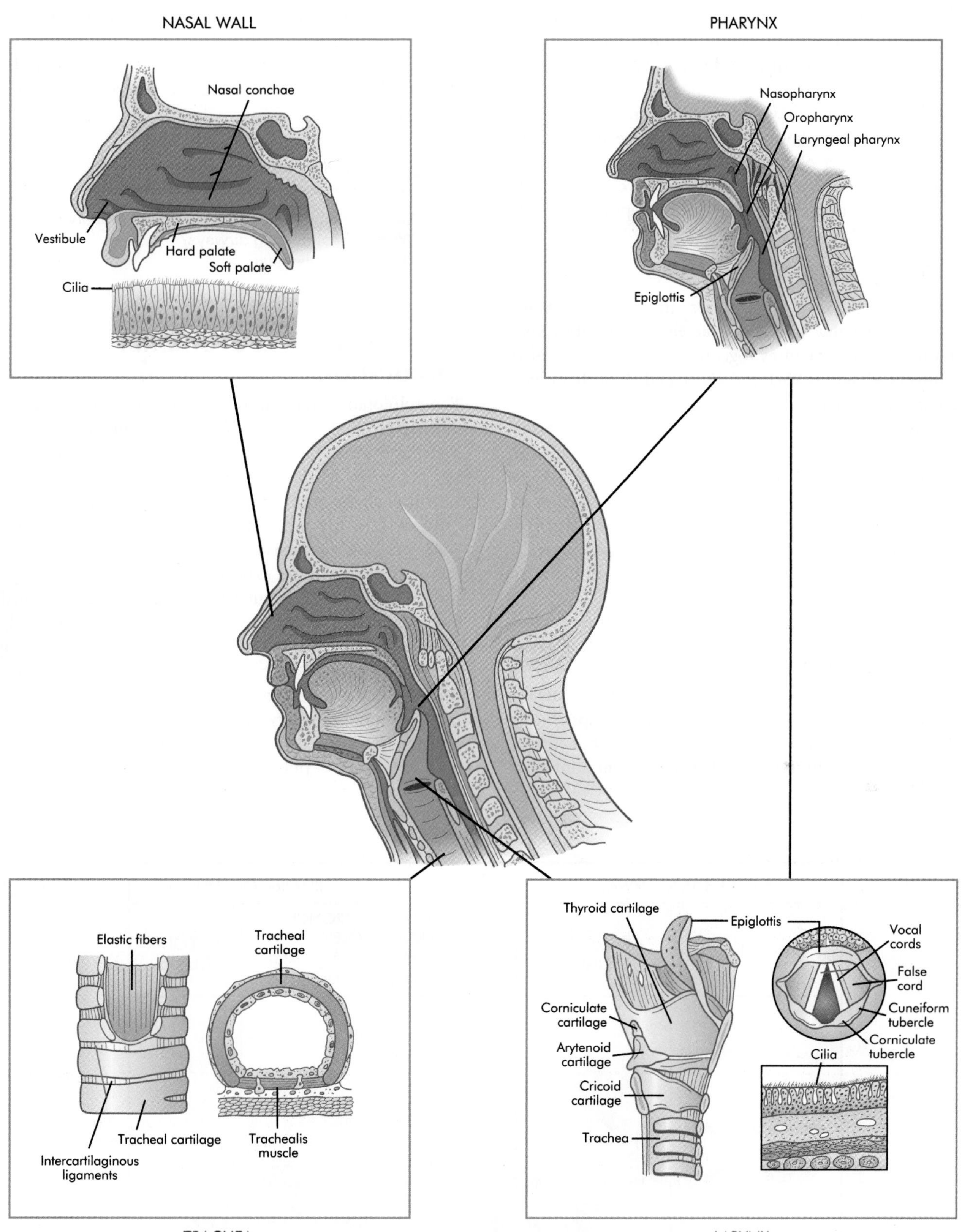

Figure 25-2 ■ **Structures of the Upper Airway.** (Redrawn from Thompson JM et al: *Mosby's clinical nursing*, ed 5, St Louis, 2002, Mosby.)

lungs at the **hila** (sing., **hilum**), or "roots" of the lungs, along with the pulmonary blood and lymphatic vessels. From the hila the main bronchi branch farther, as shown in Figure 25-3.

The bronchial walls have three layers: an epithelial lining, a smooth muscle layer, and a connective tissue layer. The epithelial lining of the bronchi contains single-celled exocrine glands—the mucus-secreting **goblet cells**—and ciliated cells. With branching, the layers of epithelium that line the bronchi become thinner (Figure 25-4).

Gas-Exchange Airways

The conducting airways terminate in the **respiratory bronchioles, alveolar ducts,** and **alveoli** (sing., **alveolus**). These thin-walled structures together are sometimes called the **acinus** (see Figures 25-1 and 25-3), and all of them participate in gas exchange.[2]

The alveoli are the primary gas-exchange units of the lung, where oxygen enters the blood and carbon dioxide is removed (Figure 25-5). Tiny passages called *pores of Kohn* permit some air to pass through the septa from alveolus to alveolus, promoting collateral ventilation and even distribution of air among the alveoli. The lungs contain approximately 25 million alveoli at birth and 300 million by adulthood.

Two major types of epithelial cells appear in the alveolus. Type I alveolar cells provide structure, and type II alveolar cells secrete **surfactant,** a lipoprotein that coats the inner surface of the alveolus and lowers alveolar surface tension at end-expiration and, thereby, prevents lung collapse.[1-4]

Like the bronchi, alveoli contain cellular components of inflammation and immunity, particularly the mononuclear phagocytes (called *alveolar macrophages*). These cells ingest foreign material that reaches the alveolus and prepare it for removal through the lymphatics. (Phagocytosis and the mononuclear phagocyte system are described in Chapters 5 and 6.)

QUICK CHECK 25-1

1. List the major components of the pulmonary system.
2. What are conducting airways?
3. Describe an alveolus.

Pulmonary and Bronchial Circulation

The pulmonary circulation facilitates gas exchange, delivers nutrients to lung tissues, acts as a reservoir for the left ventricle, and serves as a filtering system that removes clots, air, and other debris from the circulation.

Although the entire cardiac output from the right ventricle goes into the lungs, the pulmonary circulation has a lower pressure and resistance than the systemic circulation. Pulmonary arteries are exposed to about one-fifth the pressure of the systemic circulation. Usually about one third of the pulmonary vessels are filled with blood (perfused) at any given time. More vessels become perfused when right ventricular cardiac output increases. Therefore, increased delivery of blood to the lungs does not normally increase mean pulmonary artery pressure.

The arterioles divide at the terminal bronchioles to form a network of pulmonary capillaries around the acinus.

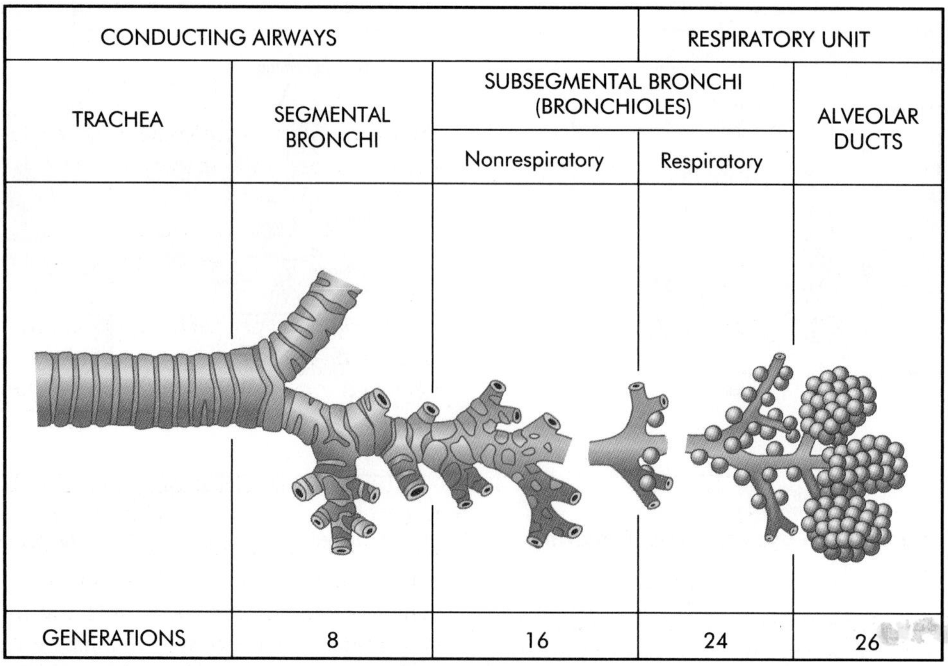

CONDUCTING AIRWAYS
RESPIRATORY UNIT
TRACHEA
SEGMENTAL BRONCHI
SUBSEGMENTAL BRONCHI (BRONCHIOLES)
Nonrespiratory
Respiratory
ALVEOLAR DUCTS
GENERATIONS
8
16
24
26

Figure 25-3 ■ **Structures of the Lower Airway.** (Redrawn from Thompson JM et al: *Mosby's clinical nursing,* ed 5, St Louis, 2002, Mosby.)

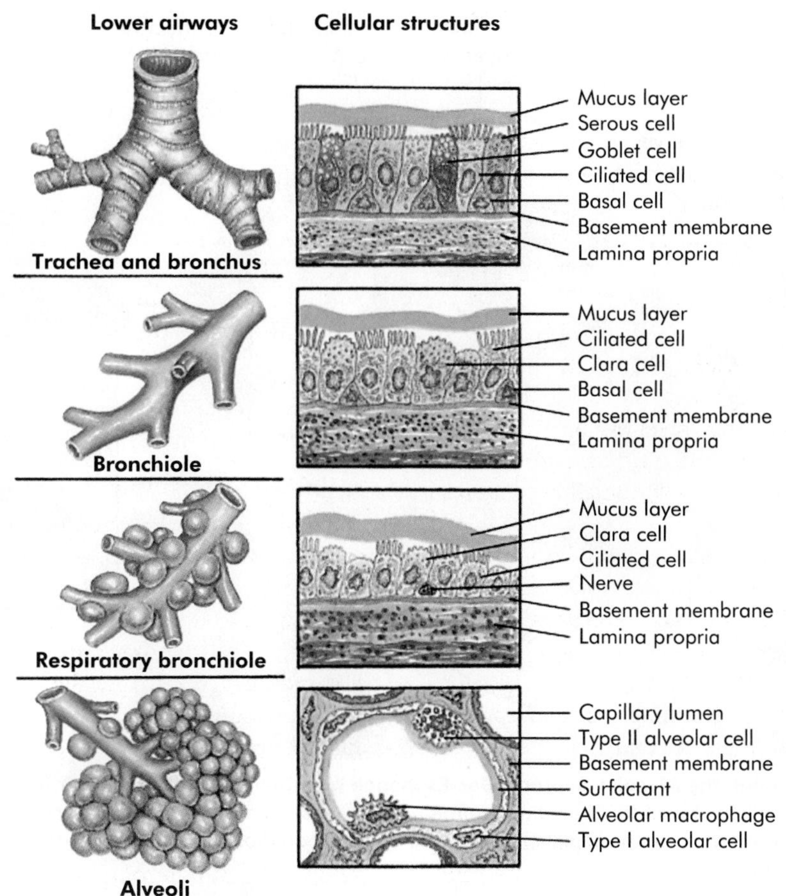

Figure 25-4 ■ **Changes in the Bronchial Wall With Progressive Branching.** (From Wilson SF, Thompson JM: *Respiratory disorders*, St Louis, 1990, Mosby.)

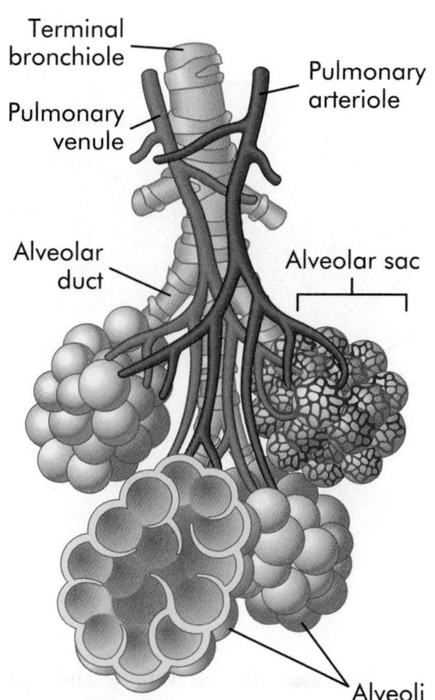

Figure 25-5 ■ **Alveoli.** Bronchioles subdivide to form tiny tubes called *alveolar ducts*, which end in clusters of alveoli called *alveolar sacs*. (From Thibodeau GA, Patton, KT: *Anatomy & physiology*, ed 6, St Louis, 2007, Mosby.)

Capillary walls consist of an endothelial layer and a thin basement membrane, which often fuses with the basement membrane of the alveolar septum. Therefore, very little separation exists between blood in the capillary and gas in the alveolus.

The shared alveolar and capillary walls compose the **alveolocapillary membrane** (Figure 25-6). Gas exchange occurs across this membrane. With normal perfusion, approximately 100 ml of blood in the pulmonary capillary bed is spread very thinly over 70 to 100 m^2 of alveolar surface area. Any disorder that thickens the membrane impairs gas exchange.

Each pulmonary vein drains several pulmonary capillaries. Unlike the pulmonary arteries, pulmonary veins are dispersed randomly throughout the lung and then leave the lung at the hila and enter the left atrium. They have no valves.

The bronchial circulation is part of the systemic circulation, and it supplies nutrients to the conducting airways, large pulmonary vessels, and membranes (pleurae) that surround the lungs. Not all of its capillaries drain into its own venous system. Some empty into the pulmonary vein and contribute to the normal venous mixture of oxygenated and deoxygenated blood or right-to-left shunt (right-to-left shunts are described in Chapter 26). The bronchial

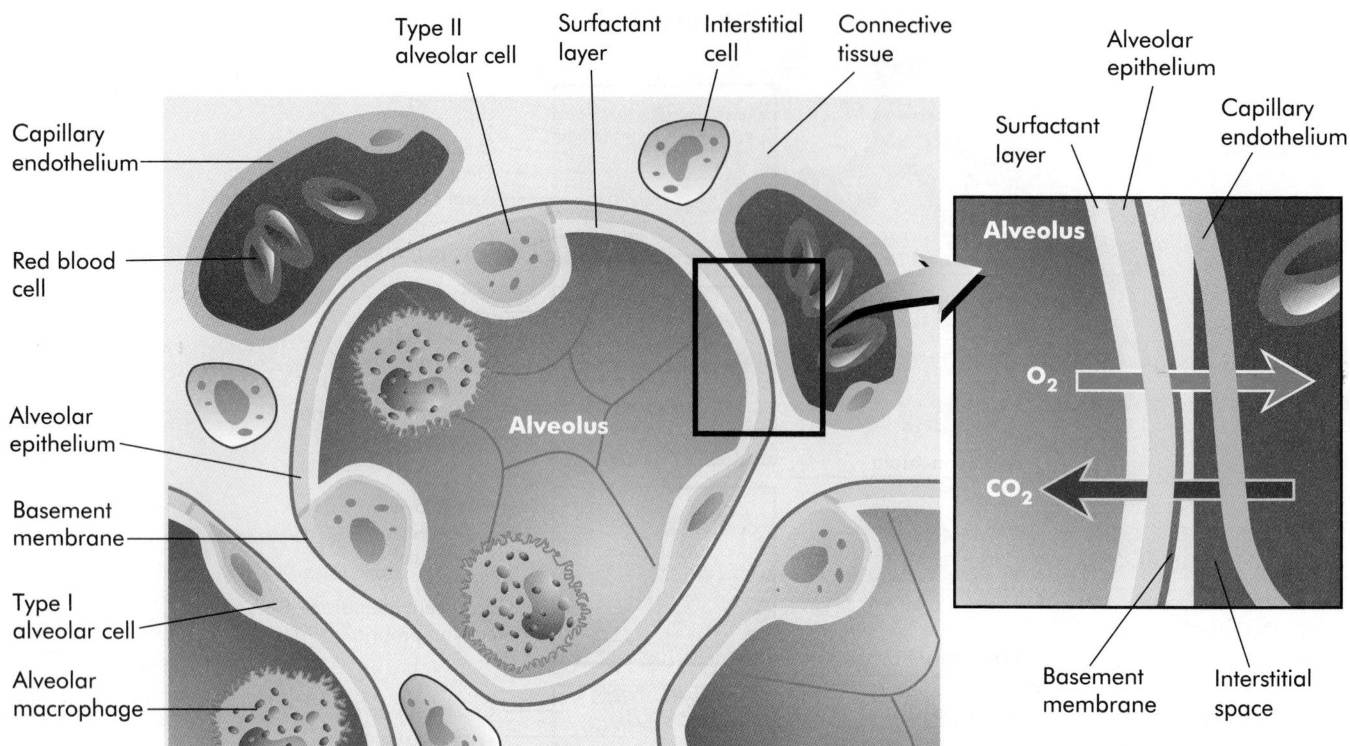

Figure 25-6 ■ **Section Through the Alveolar Septum (Gas-Exchange Membrane).** Inset shows a magnified view of the respiratory membrane composed of the alveolar wall (fluid coating, epithelial cells, basement membrane), interstitial fluid, and wall of a pulmonary capillary (basement membrane, endothelial cells). The gases CO_2 (carbon dioxide) and O_2 (oxygen) diffuse across the respiratory membrane.

circulation does not participate in gas exchange but warms and moistens inspired air and provides airway nourishment.[1]

Lung vasculature also includes deep and superficial lymphatic capillaries. Fluid and alveolar macrophages migrate from the alveoli to the terminal bronchioles, where they enter the lymphatic system. Both deep and superficial lymphatic vessels leave the lung at the hilum. The lymphatic system plays an important role in keeping the lung free of fluid. (The lymphatic system is described in Chapter 22.)

Chest Wall and Pleura

The chest wall (skin, ribs, intercostal muscles) protects the lungs from injury, and its muscles, along with the diaphragm, perform the muscular work of breathing. The **thoracic cavity** is contained by the chest wall and encases the lungs (Figure 25-7). A serous membrane called the **pleura** adheres firmly to the lungs and then folds over itself and attaches firmly to the chest wall. The membrane covering the lungs is the *visceral pleura;* that lining the thoracic cavity is the *parietal pleura.* The area between the two pleurae is called the **pleural space,** or **pleural cavity.** Normally, only a thin layer of fluid secreted by the pleura (pleural fluid) fills the pleural space, lubricating the pleural surfaces and allowing the two layers to slide over each other without separating. Pressure in the pleural space is usually negative or subatmospheric (−4 to −10 mm Hg).

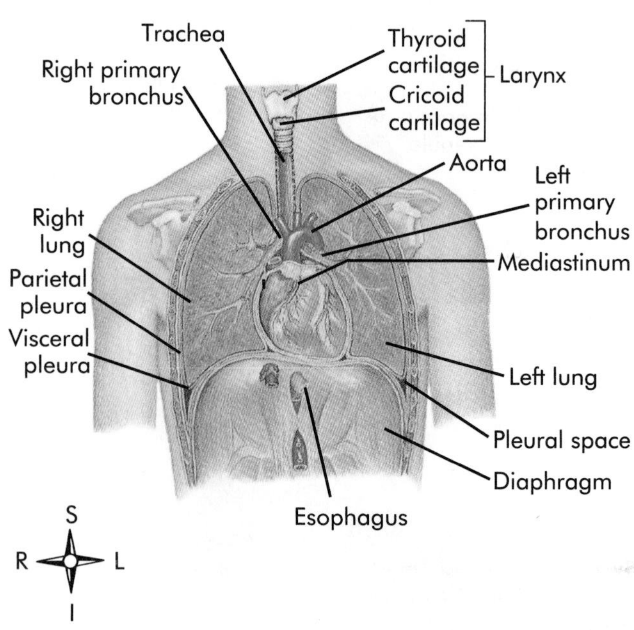

Figure 25-7 ■ **Thoracic (Chest) Cavity and Related Structures.** The thoracic (chest) cavity is divided into three subdivisions (left and right pleural divisions and mediastinum) by a partition formed by a serous membrane called the *pleura.* (From Thibodeau GA, Patton KT: *Anatomy & physiology,* ed 3, St Louis, 1996, Mosby.)

FUNCTION OF THE PULMONARY SYSTEM

The pulmonary system (1) ventilates the alveoli, (2) diffuses gases into and out of the blood, and (3) perfuses the lungs so that the organs and tissues of the body receive blood that is rich in oxygen and low in carbon dioxide. Each component of the pulmonary system contributes to one or more of these functions (Figure 25-8).

Ventilation

Ventilation is the mechanical movement of gas or air into and out of the lungs. It is often misnamed *respiration*, which is actually the exchange of oxygen and carbon dioxide during cellular metabolism. "Respiratory rate" is actually the ventilatory rate, or the number of times gas is inspired and expired per minute. The amount of effective ventilation is calculated by multiplying the ventilatory rate (breaths/minute) by the volume or amount of air per breath (liters/breath or tidal volume). This is called the **minute volume** and is expressed in liters/minute. Pulmonary function tests (PFTs) measure lung volumes and flow rates and can be used to diagnose lung disease (Figure 25-9).

Carbon dioxide (CO_2), the gaseous form of carbonic acid (H_2CO_3), is produced by cellular metabolism. The lung eliminates about 10,000 milliequivalents (mEq) of carbonic acid per day in the form of CO_2, which is produced at the rate of approximately 200 ml/min. Carbon dioxide is eliminated to maintain a normal arterial CO_2 ($PaCO_2$) of 40 mm Hg and normal acid-base balance. Adequate ventilation is necessary to maintain normal $PaCO_2$ levels. Diseases that limit ventilation result in CO_2 retention. The adequacy of alveolar ventilation *cannot* be accurately determined by observation of ventilatory rate, pattern, or effort. If a health care professional needs to determine the adequacy of ventilation, an arterial blood gas analysis must be performed to measure $PaCO_2$.

Neurochemical Control of Ventilation
(respiratory center, central and peripheral chemoreceptors)

↓

Mechanics of Breathing
(major and accessory muscles, lung elasticity, airway resistance, alveolar surface tension, work of breathing)

↓

Gas Transport
(distribution of ventilation and perfusion, oxygen transport, carbon dioxide transport)

↓

Control of the Pulmonary Circulation
(distribution of pulmonary blood flow)

Figure 25-8 ■ Functional Components of the Respiratory System. The central nervous system responds to neurochemical stimulation of ventilation and sends signals to the chest wall musculature. The response of the respiratory system to these impulses is influenced by several factors that impact the mechanisms of breathing and, therefore, affect the adequacy of ventilation. Gas transport between the alveoli and pulmonary capillary blood depends on a variety of physical and chemical activities. Finally, the control of the pulmonary circulation plays a role in the appropriate distribution of blood flow.

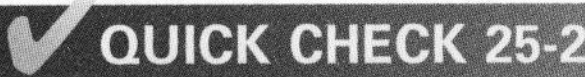
QUICK CHECK 25-2

1. List the major components of the pulmonary circulation.
2. What are the visceral and parietal pleurae?

Neurochemical Control of Ventilation

Breathing is usually involuntary, because homeostatic changes in ventilatory rate and volume are adjusted automatically by the nervous system to maintain normal gas exchange. Voluntary breathing is necessary for talking, singing, laughing, and deliberately holding one's breath. The mechanisms that control respiration are complex (Figure 25-10).

The **respiratory center** in the brain stem controls respiration by transmitting impulses to the respiratory muscles, causing them to contract and relax. The respiratory center is composed of several groups of neurons: the dorsal respiratory group (DRG), the ventral respiratory group (VRG), the pneumotaxic center, and the apneustic center.[1–4] The basic automatic rhythm of respiration is set by the DRG, which receives afferent input from **peripheral chemoreceptors** in the carotid and aortic bodies and from several different types of receptors in the lungs. The VRG contains both inspiratory and expiratory neurons and is almost inactive during normal, quiet respiration, becoming active when increased ventilatory effort is required. The pneumotaxic center and apneustic center, situated in the pons, do not generate primary rhythm but, rather, act as modifiers of the rhythm established by the medullary centers. The pattern of breathing can be influenced by emotion, pain, and disease.

Lung receptors

Three types of lung receptors send impulses from the lungs to the dorsal respiratory group:

1. **Irritant receptors** are found in the epithelium of all conducting airways. They are sensitive to noxious aerosols (vapors), gases, and particulate matter (e.g., inhaled dusts), which cause them to initiate the cough reflex. When stimulated, irritant receptors also cause bronchoconstriction and increased ventilatory rate.
2. **Stretch receptors** are located in the smooth muscles of airways and are sensitive to increases in the size or volume of the lungs. They decrease ventilatory rate and volume when stimulated, an occurrence sometimes referred to as the Hering-Breuer expiratory reflex. This reflex is active in newborns and assists with ventilation. In

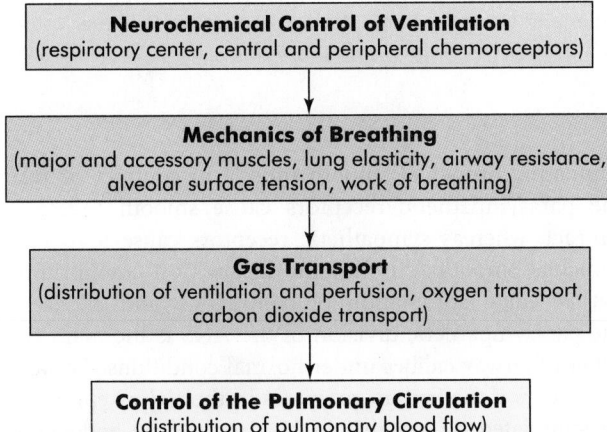

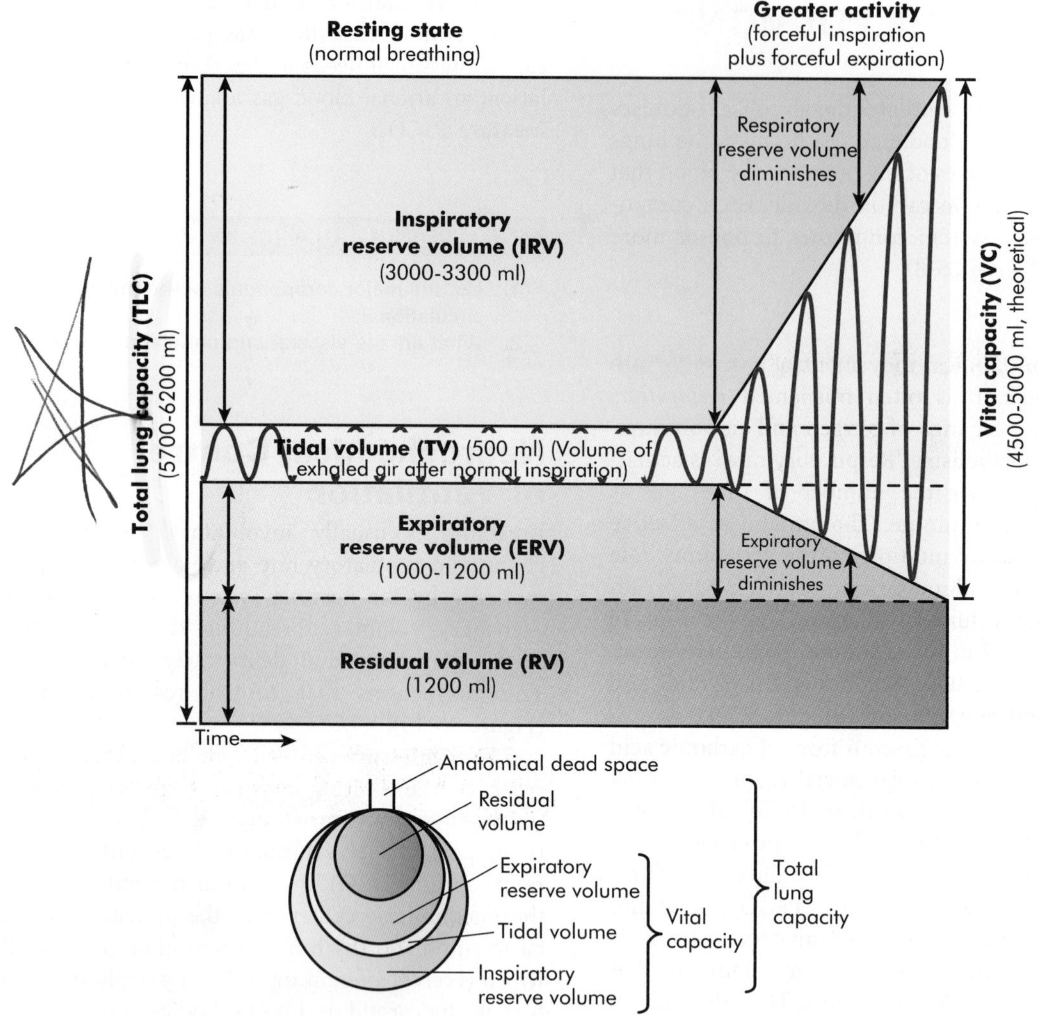

Figure 25-9 ■ **Spirogram.** During normal, quiet respirations, the atmosphere and lungs exchange about 500 ml of air (V_T). With a forcible inspiration, about 3300 ml more air can be inhaled (IRV). After a normal inspiration and normal expiration, approximately 1000 ml more air can be forcibly expired (ERV). Vital capacity (VC) is the amount of air that can be forcibly expired after a maximal inspiration and indicates, therefore, the largest amount of air that can enter and leave the lungs during respiration. Residual volume (RV) is the air that remains trapped in the alveoli. (From Thibodeau GA, Patton KT: *Anatomy & physiology*, ed 5, St Louis, 2003, Mosby.)

adults, this reflex is active only at high tidal volumes (such as with exercise) and may protect against excess lung inflation. Stretch receptors called rapidly adapting receptors (RARs) have been found to be an important mediator of cough.[5]

3. **J-receptors** (juxtapulmonary capillary receptors) are located near the capillaries in the alveolar septa. They are sensitive to increased pulmonary capillary pressure, which stimulates them to initiate rapid, shallow breathing, hypotension, and bradycardia.[4]

The lung is innervated by the autonomic nervous system (ANS). Fibers of the sympathetic division in the lung branch form the upper thoracic and cervical ganglia of the spinal cord. Fibers of the parasympathetic division of the ANS travel in the vagus nerve to the lung. (Structures and function of the ANS are covered in detail in Chapter 12.) The parasympathetic and sympathetic divisions control airway caliber (interior diameter of the airway lumen) by stimulating bronchial smooth muscle to contract or relax. The parasympathetic receptors cause smooth muscle to contract, whereas sympathetic receptors cause it to relax. Bronchial smooth muscle tone depends on equilibrium—that is, equal stimulation of contraction and relaxation. The parasympathetic division of the ANS is the main controller of airway caliber under normal conditions. Constriction occurs if the irritant receptors in the airway epithelium are stimulated by irritants in inspired air, by endogenous substances (e.g., histamine, serotonin, prostaglandins, leukotrienes), by many drugs, and by humoral substances.

Chemoreceptors

Chemoreceptors monitor the pH, $PaCO_2$, and PaO_2 of arterial blood. **Central chemoreceptors** monitor arterial blood indirectly by sensing changes in the pH of cerebrospinal fluid (CSF) (see Figure 25-10). They are located near the respiratory center and are sensitive to hydrogen ion

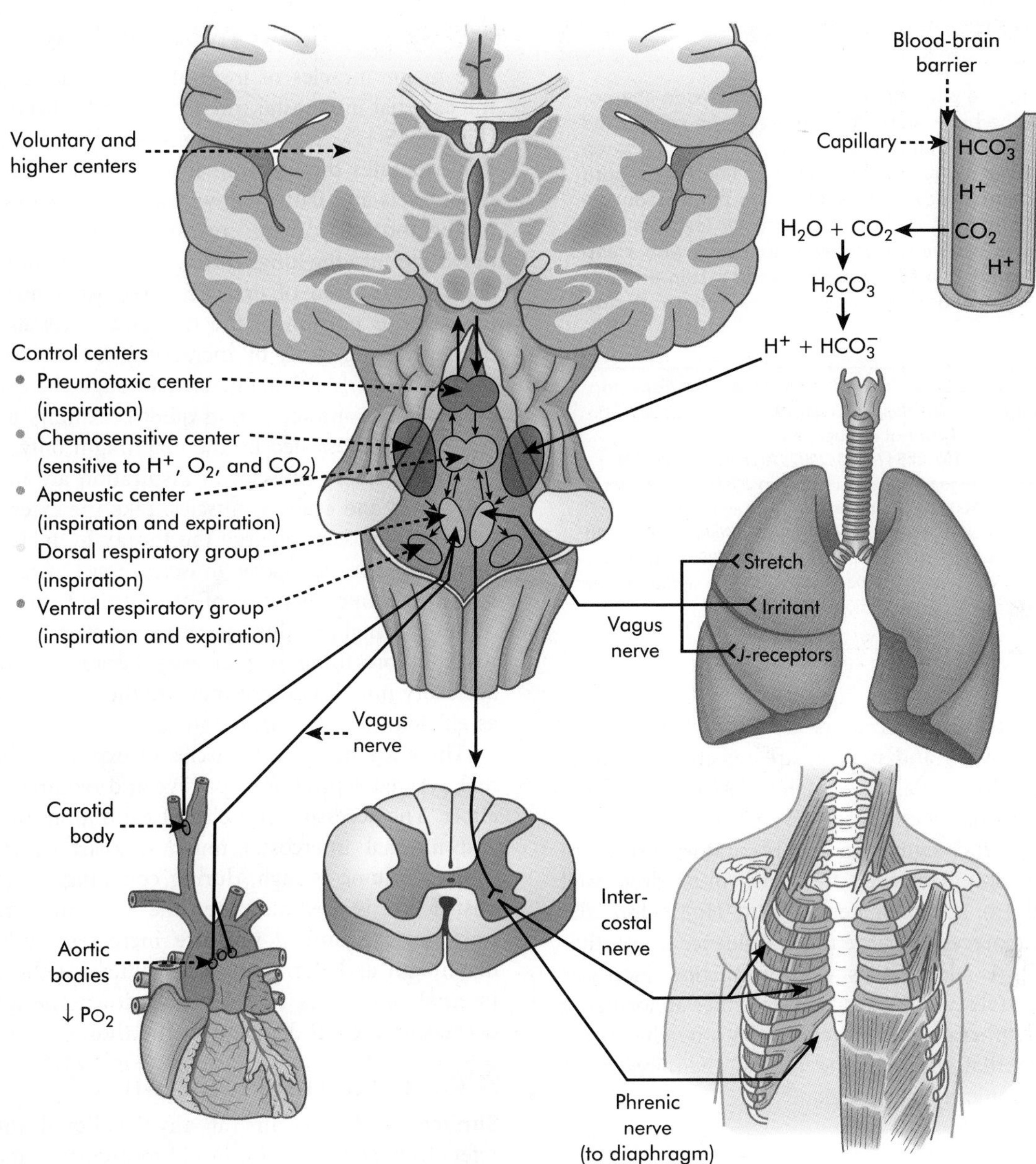

Figure 25-10 ■ **Neurochemical Respiratory Control System.**

concentration in the CSF. (Chapter 4 describes the relationship between ions and the pH, or acid-base status, of body fluids.) The pH of the CSF reflects arterial pH because carbon dioxide in arterial blood can diffuse across the blood-brain barrier (the capillary wall separating blood from cells of the central nervous system) into the CSF until the partial pressure of carbon dioxide (PCO_2) is equal on both sides. Carbon dioxide that has entered the CSF combines with H_2O to form carbonic acid, which subsequently dissociates into hydrogen ions that are capable of stimulating the central chemoreceptors. In this way, $PaCO_2$ regulates ventilation through its impact on the pH (hydrogen ion content) of the CSF.[1-4]

If alveolar ventilation is inadequate, $PaCO_2$ increases. Carbon dioxide diffuses across the blood-brain barrier until PCO_2 in blood and CSF reaches equilibrium. As the central chemoreceptors sense the resulting decrease in pH (increase in hydrogen ion concentration), they stimulate the respiratory center to increase the depth and rate of ventilation. Increased ventilation causes the PCO_2 of arterial blood to decrease below that of the CSF, and carbon dioxide diffuses back out of the CSF, returning its pH to normal.

The central chemoreceptors are sensitive to very small changes in the pH of CSF (equivalent to a 1 to 2 mm Hg change in PCO_2) and can maintain a normal $PaCO_2$ under many different conditions, including strenuous exercise. If inadequate ventilation, or hypoventilation, is long term (e.g., in chronic obstructive pulmonary disease), these receptors become insensitive to small changes in $PaCO_2$ ("reset") and regulate ventilation poorly.

HEALTH ALERT

Changes in the Chemical Control of Breathing During Sleep

There are multiple sites of central carbon dioxide chemosensitivity in the brain stem, and there may be specialized chemosensory sites that function only during certain sleep states. Chemical control of ventilation, related to both hypercapnia and hypoxia, appears to be blunted during sleep. This blunting increases with obesity (especially at altitude) and is severely disordered in those with sleep apnea. Congestive heart failure and hypertension are also associated with abnormal breathing responses during sleep.

Data from Parameswaran K, Todd DC, Soth M: Altered respiratory physiology in obesity, *Can Respir J* 13(4):203–210, 2006; Patil SP et al: Neuromechanical control of upper airway patency during sleep, *J Appl Physiol* 102(2):547–556, 2007; Arzt M, Bradley TD: Treatment of sleep apnea in heart failure, *Am J Respir Crit Care Med* 173(12):1300–1308, 2006; Shigemitsu M et al: Nocturnal oxygen therapy prevents progress of congestive heart failure with central sleep apnea, *Int J Cardiol* 115(3):354–360, 2007; Smith ML, Pacchia CF: Sleep apnoea and hypertension: role of chemoreflexes in humans, *Exp Physiol* 92(1):45–50, 2007.

The peripheral chemoreceptors are somewhat sensitive to changes in $PaCO_2$ and pH but are sensitive primarily to oxygen levels in arterial blood (PaO_2). As PaO_2 and pH decrease, peripheral chemoreceptors, particularly in the carotid bodies, send signals to the respiratory center to increase ventilation. However, the PaO_2 must drop well below normal (to approximately 60 mm Hg) before the peripheral chemoreceptors have much influence on ventilation. If $PaCO_2$ is elevated as well, ventilation increases much more than it would in response to either abnormality alone. The peripheral chemoreceptors become the major stimulus to ventilation when the central chemoreceptors are reset by chronic hypoventilation.[1]

QUICK CHECK 25-3

1. Describe three functions of the respiratory center in the brain stem.
2. What are the three types of lung receptors?
3. How do the functions of central and peripheral chemoreceptors differ?

Mechanics of Breathing

The mechanical aspects of inspiration and expiration are known collectively as the mechanics of breathing and involve (1) major and accessory muscles of inspiration and expiration, (2) elastic properties of the lungs and chest wall, and (3) resistance to airflow through the conducting airways. Alterations in any of these properties increase the work of breathing or the metabolic energy needed to achieve adequate ventilation and oxygenation of the blood.

Major and accessory muscles

The major muscles of inspiration are the diaphragm and the external intercostal muscles (muscles between the ribs) (Figure 25-11). The diaphragm is a dome-shaped muscle that separates the abdominal and thoracic cavities. When it contracts and flattens downward, it increases the volume of the thoracic cavity, creating a negative pressure that draws gas into the lungs through the upper airways and trachea. Contraction of external intercostal muscles elevates the anterior portion of the ribs and increases the volume of the thoracic cavity by increasing its front-to-back (anterior-posterior [AP]) diameter. Although the external intercostals may contract during quiet breathing, inspiration at rest is usually assisted by the diaphragm only.

The accessory muscles of inspiration are the sternocleidomastoid and scalene muscles. Like the external intercostals, these muscles enlarge the thorax by increasing its AP diameter. The accessory muscles assist inspiration when minute volume (volume of air inspired and expired per minute) is high, as during strenuous exercise, or when the work of breathing is increased because of disease. The accessory muscles do not increase the volume of the thorax as efficiently as the diaphragm does.

There are no major muscles of expiration because normal, relaxed expiration is passive and requires no muscular effort. The accessory muscles of expiration, the abdominal and internal intercostal muscles, assist expiration when minute volume is high, during coughing, or when airway obstruction is present. When the abdominal muscles contract, intraabdominal pressure increases, pushing up the diaphragm and decreasing the volume of the thorax. The internal intercostal muscles pull down the anterior ribs, decreasing the AP diameter of the thorax.

Alveolar surface tension

Surface tension occurs at any gas-liquid interface and refers to the tendency for liquid molecules that are exposed to air to adhere to one another. This phenomenon can be seen in the way liquids "bead" when splashed on a waterproof surface.

Within a sphere, such as an alveolus, surface tension tends to make expansion difficult. According to the law of Laplace, the pressure (P) required to inflate a sphere is equal to two times the surface tension $(2T)$ divided by the radius (r) of the sphere, or $P = (2T/r)$. As the radius of the sphere (or alveolus) becomes smaller, more and more pressure is required to inflate it. If the alveoli were lined only with a water-like fluid, taking breaths would be extremely difficult.

Alveolar ventilation, or distention, is made possible by surfactant, which lowers surface tension by coating the air-liquid interface in the alveoli. Surfactant, a lipoprotein produced by type II alveolar cells, has a detergent-like effect that separates the liquid molecules, thereby decreasing alveolar surface tension.

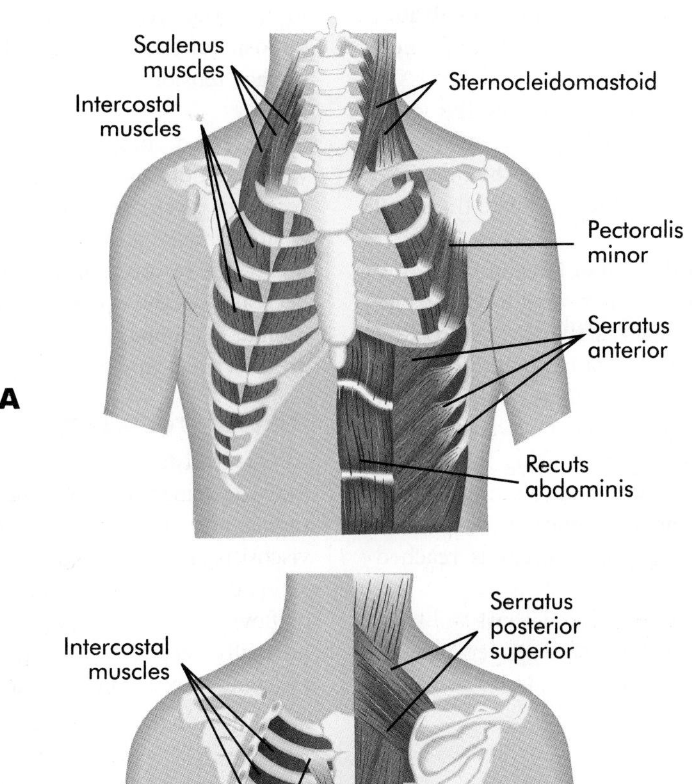

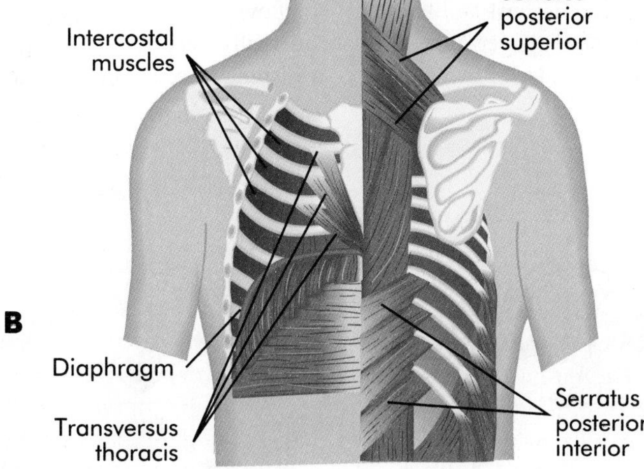

Figure 25-11 **Muscles of Ventilation. A,** Anterior view. **B,** Posterior view. (Modified from Thompson JM et al: *Mosby's clinical nursing*, ed 5, St Louis, 2002, Mosby.)

Surfactant lines the alveolar side of the alveolocapillary membrane and reverses the law of Laplace. As the radius of a surfactant-lined sphere (alveolus) grows smaller, the surface tension *decreases*, and as the radius grows larger, the surface tension *increases*. This occurs because the smaller radius causes surfactant molecules to crowd together and then repel one another strongly. A larger radius spreads them apart, decreasing their mutual repellence. Therefore, normal alveoli are much easier to inflate at low lung volumes (i.e., after expiration) than at high volumes (i.e., after inspiration). If surfactant is not produced in adequate quantities, alveolar surface tension increases and results in alveolar collapse, decreased lung expansion, increased work of breathing, and severe gas-exchange abnormalities.

The decrease in surface tension caused by surfactant is also responsible for keeping the alveoli free of fluid. In the absence of surfactant, water tends to move into the alveoli.

Elastic properties of the lung and chest wall

The lung and chest wall have elastic properties that permit expansion during inspiration and return to resting volume during expiration. Elastin fibers in the alveolar walls and surrounding the small airways and pulmonary capillaries, as well as surface tension at the alveolar air-liquid interface, produce this effect. The elasticity of the chest wall is the result of the configuration of its bones and musculature.

Elastic recoil is the tendency of the lungs to return to the resting state after inspiration. Normal elastic recoil permits passive expiration, eliminating the need for major muscles of expiration. Passive elastic recoil may be insufficient during labored breathing (high minute volume), when the accessory muscles of expiration may be needed. The accessory muscles are used also if disease compromises elastic recoil (e.g., in emphysema) or blocks the conducting airways.

Normal elastic recoil depends on an equilibrium between opposing forces of recoil in the lungs and chest wall. Under normal conditions, the chest wall tends to recoil by expanding outward. The tendency of the chest wall to recoil by expanding is balanced by the tendency of the lungs to recoil or inward collapse around the hila. The opposing forces of the chest wall and lungs create the small negative intrapleural pressure.

Balance between the outward recoil of the chest wall and inward recoil of the lungs occurs at the resting level, the end of expiration, where the functional residual capacity (FRC) is reached. During inspiration, the diaphragm and intercostal muscles contract, air flows into the lungs, and the chest wall expands. Muscular effort is needed to overcome the resistance of the lungs to expansion. During expiration, the muscles relax and the elastic recoil of the lungs causes the thorax to decrease in volume until, once again, balance between the chest wall and lung recoil forces is reached (Figure 25-12).

Compliance is the measure of lung and chest wall distensibility and is defined as volume change per unit of pressure change. It represents the relative ease with which these structures can be stretched and is, therefore, the opposite of elasticity. Compliance is determined by alveolar surface tension and the elastic recoil of the lung and chest wall.

Increased compliance indicates that the lungs or chest wall is abnormally easy to inflate and has lost some elastic recoil. A decrease indicates that the lungs or chest wall is abnormally stiff or difficult to inflate. Compliance is increased in normal aging and in emphysema and is decreased in the acute respiratory distress syndrome, pneumonia, pulmonary edema, and fibrosis. (These disorders are described in Chapter 26.)

Airway resistance

Airway resistance, which is similar to resistance to blood flow (described in Chapter 22), is determined by the length, radius, and cross-sectional area of the airways and density, viscosity, and velocity of the gas (Poiseuille law). Resistance (R) is computed by dividing change in pressure (P) by rate of flow (F), or $R = P/F$ (Ohm law). Airway resistance is normally very low. One half to two thirds of total airway resistance occurs in the nose. The next highest resistance

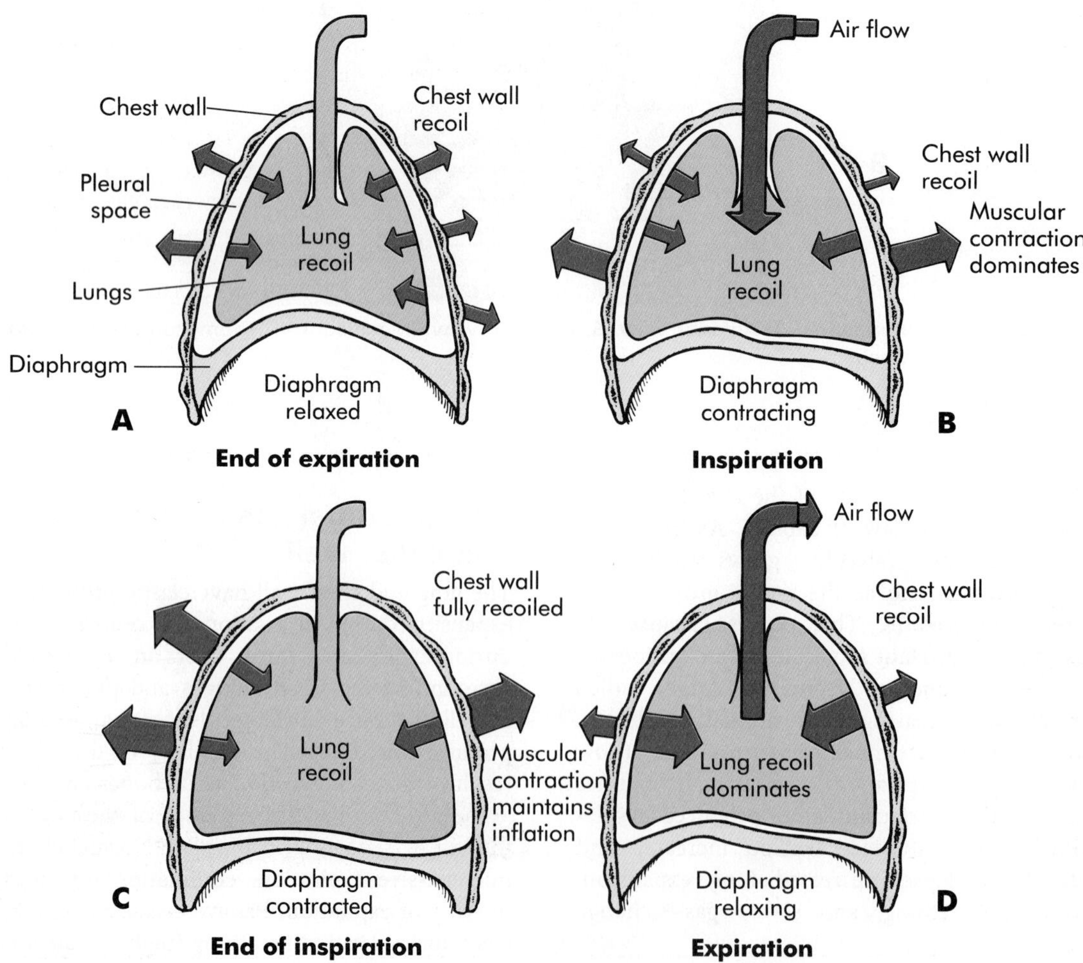

Figure 25-12 ■ **Interaction of Forces During Inspiration and Expiration. A,** Outward recoil of the chest wall equals inward recoil of the lungs at the end of expiration. **B,** During inspiration, contraction of respiratory muscles, assisted by chest wall recoil, overcomes the tendency of lungs to recoil. **C,** At the end of inspiration, respiratory muscle contraction maintains lung expansion. **D,** During expiration, respiratory muscles relax, allowing elastic recoil of the lungs to deflate the lungs.

is in the oropharynx and larynx. There is very little resistance in the conducting airways of the lungs because of their large cross-sectional area. Airway resistance increases when the diameter of the airways decreases. Bronchoconstriction, which increases airway resistance, can be caused by stimulation of parasympathetic receptors in the bronchial smooth muscle and by numerous irritants and inflammatory mediators.[2] Bronchodilation, which decreases resistance to airflow, is caused by β2-adrenergic receptor stimulation. Airway resistance can also be increased by edema of the bronchial mucosa and by airway obstructions such as mucus, tumors, or foreign bodies.

Work of breathing

The work of breathing is determined by the muscular effort (and therefore oxygen and energy) required for ventilation. Normally very low, the work of breathing may increase considerably in diseases that disrupt the equilibrium between forces exerted by the lung and chest wall. More muscular effort is required when lung compliance decreases (e.g., in pulmonary edema), chest wall compliance decreases (e.g., in spinal deformity or obesity), or airways are obstructed by bronchospasm or mucous plugging (e.g., in asthma or bronchitis).[6] An increase in the work of breathing can result in a marked increase in oxygen consumption and an inability to maintain adequate ventilation.

QUICK CHECK 25-4

1. Describe the work of the diaphragm in ventilation.
2. What is surfactant? What is its function?
3. How is elastic recoil related to compliance?
4. Where is airway resistance found?

Gas Transport

Gas transport, the delivery of oxygen to the cells of the body and the removal of carbon dioxide, has four steps: (1) ventilation of the lungs, (2) diffusion of oxygen from the alveoli into the capillary blood, (3) perfusion of systemic capillaries with oxygenated blood, and (4) diffusion of oxygen from systemic capillaries into the cells. Steps in the transport of carbon dioxide occur in reverse order: (1) diffusion of carbon dioxide from the cells into the systemic capillaries, (2) perfusion of the pulmonary capillary bed by venous blood, (3) diffusion of carbon dioxide into the alveoli, and (4) removal of carbon dioxide from the lung by ventilation. If any step in gas transport is impaired by a respiratory or cardiovascular disorder, gas exchange at the cellular level is compromised.

Measurement of gas pressure

A gas is made up of millions of molecules moving randomly and colliding with each other and with the wall of the space in which they are contained. These collisions exert pressure. If the same number of gas molecules is contained in a small and a large container, the pressure is greater in the small container because more collisions occur in the smaller space (Figure 25-13). Heat increases the speed of the molecules, which also increases the number of collisions and therefore the pressure.

Barometric pressure (P_B) (atmospheric pressure) is the pressure exerted by gas molecules in air at specific altitudes. At sea level, barometric pressure is 760 mm Hg and is the sum of the pressure exerted by each gas in the air at sea level. The portion of the total pressure exerted by any individual gas is its **partial pressure** (see Figure 25-13). At sea level the air is made up of oxygen (20.9%), nitrogen (78.1%), and

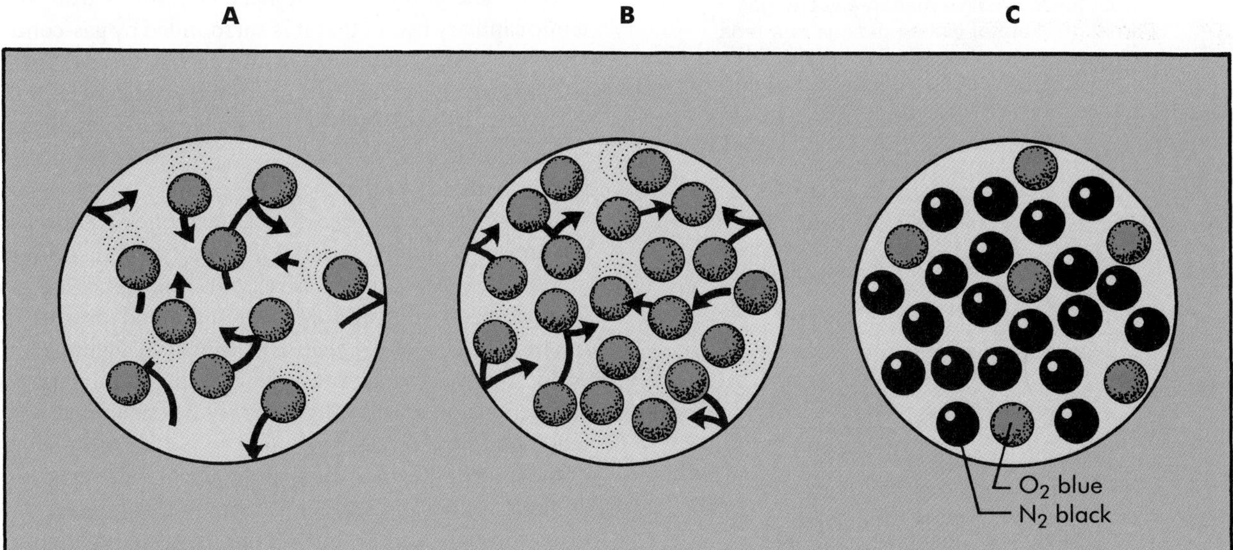

Figure 25-13 ■ **Relationship Between Number of Gas Molecules and Pressure Exerted by the Gas in an Enclosed Space. A,** Theoretically, 10 molecules of the same gas exert a total pressure of 10 within the space. **B,** If the number of molecules is increased to 20, total pressure is 20. **C,** If there are different gases in the space, each gas exerts a partial pressure: here the partial pressure of nitrogen (N_2) is 20, that of oxygen (O_2) is 6, and total pressure is 26.

a few other trace gases. The partial pressure of oxygen is equal to the percentage of oxygen in the air (20.9%) times the total pressure (760 mm Hg), or 159 mm Hg ($760 \times 0.209 = 158.84$). (Symbols used in the measurement of gas pressures and pulmonary ventilation are defined in Table 25-2.)

The amount of water vapor contained in a gas mixture is determined by the temperature of the gas and is unrelated to barometric pressure. Gas that enters the lungs becomes saturated with water vapor (humidified) as it passes through the upper airway. At body temperature (37° C), water vapor exerts a pressure of 47 mm Hg regardless of total (barometric) pressure. The partial pressure of water vapor must be subtracted from the barometric pressure before the partial pressure of other gases in the mixture can be determined. In saturated air at sea level, the partial pressure of oxygen is therefore $(760 - 47) \times 0.209 = 149$ mm Hg. All pressure and volume measurements made in pulmonary function laboratories specify the temperature and humidity of a gas at the time of measurement.

Many pressure measurements are stated as variations from barometric pressure, rather than percentages of it. On such scales, barometric pressure is considered zero, and pressure varies up or down from zero. Physiologic pressure measurements that involve fluids, rather than gases, are measured as variations from barometric pressure.

TABLE 25-2

Common Pulmonary Abbreviations

Symbol	Definition
V	Volume or amount of gas
Q	Perfusion or blood flow
P	Pressure (usually partial pressure) of a gas
PaO_2	Partial pressure of oxygen in arterial blood
P_AO_2	Partial pressure of oxygen in alveolar gas
$PaCO_2$	Partial pressure of carbon dioxide in arterial blood
PvO_2	Partial pressure of oxygen in mixed venous or pulmonary artery blood
$P(A–a)O_2$	Difference between alveolar and arterial partial pressure of oxygen (A–a gradient)
P_B	Barometric or atmospheric pressure
SaO_2	Saturation of hemoglobin (in arterial blood) with oxygen
SvO_2	Saturation of hemoglobin (in mixed venous blood) with
V_A	Alveolar ventilation
V_D	Dead-space ventilation
V_E	Minute capacity
V_T	Tidal volume or average breath
$\dot{V}/\dot{Q}$	Ratio of ventilation to perfusion
FiO_2	Fraction of inspired oxygen
FRC	Functional residual capacity
FVC	Forced vital capacity
FEV_1	Forced expiratory volume in 1 second

Subscripts identify the particular gas, volume, or pressure being discussed. A dot (·) means measurement over time, usually 1 minute.

For example, a systolic blood pressure of 120 mm Hg indicates that systolic pressure is 120 mm Hg above barometric pressure.

Distribution of ventilation and perfusion

Effective gas exchange depends on an approximately even distribution of gas (ventilation) and blood (perfusion) in all portions of the lungs. The lungs are suspended from the hila in the thoracic cavity. When an individual is in an upright position (sitting or standing), gravity pulls the lungs down toward the diaphragm and compresses their lower portions or bases. The alveoli in the upper portions, or apexes, of the lungs contain a greater residual volume of gas and are larger and less numerous than those in the lower portions. Because surface tension increases as the alveoli become larger, the larger alveoli in the upper portions of the lung are more difficult to inflate (less compliant) than the smaller alveoli in the lower portions of the lung. Therefore, during ventilation most of the tidal volume is distributed to the bases of the lungs, where compliance is greater.

The heart pumps against gravity to perfuse the pulmonary circulation. As blood is pumped into the lung apexes of a sitting or standing individual, some blood pressure is dissipated in overcoming gravity. As a result, blood pressure at the apexes is lower than that at the bases. Because greater pressure causes greater perfusion, the bases of the lungs are better perfused than the apexes (Figure 25-14). Thus, ventilation and perfusion are greatest in the same lung portions—the lower lobes—and depend on body position. If a standing individual assumes a supine or side-lying position, the areas of the lungs that are then most dependent become the best ventilated and perfused.

Distribution of perfusion in the pulmonary circulation also is affected by alveolar pressure (gas pressure in the alveoli). The pulmonary capillary bed differs from the systemic capillary bed in that it is surrounded by gas-containing alveoli. If the gas pressure in the alveoli exceeds the blood pressure in the capillary, the capillary collapses and flow ceases. This is most likely to occur in portions of the lung where blood pressure is lowest and alveolar gas pressure is greatest—that is, at the apex of the lung.

The lungs are divided into three zones on the basis of relationships among all the factors affecting pulmonary blood flow. Alveolar pressure plus the forces of gravity, arterial blood pressure, and venous blood pressure affect the distribution of perfusion, as shown in Figure 25-15.

In zone I, alveolar pressure exceeds pulmonary arterial and venous pressures. The capillary bed collapses, and normal blood flow ceases. Normally zone I is a very small part of the lung at the apex. In zone II, alveolar pressure is greater than venous pressure but not arterial pressure. Blood flows through zone II, but it is impeded to a certain extent by alveolar pressure. Zone II is normally above the level of the left atrium. In zone III, both arterial and venous pressures are greater than alveolar pressure and blood flow is not affected by alveolar pressure. Zone III is in the base of

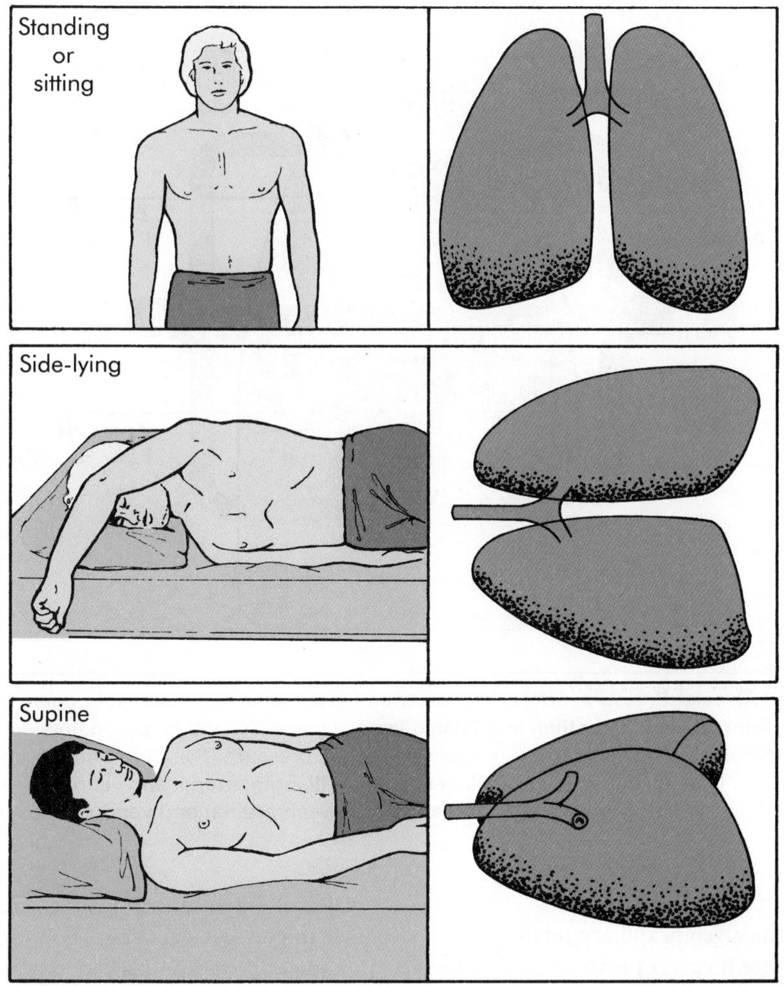

Figure 25-14 ■ **Pulmonary Blood Flow and Gravity.** The greatest volume of pulmonary blood flow normally will occur in the gravity-dependent areas of the lung. Body position has a significant effect on the distribution of pulmonary blood flow.

the lung. Blood flow through the pulmonary capillary bed increases in regular increments from the apex to the base.

Although both blood flow and ventilation are greater at the base of the lungs than at the apexes, they are not perfectly matched in any zone. Perfusion exceeds ventilation in the bases, and ventilation exceeds perfusion in the apexes of the lung. The relationship between ventilation and perfusion is expressed as a ratio called the **ventilation-perfusion ratio ($\dot{V}/\dot{Q}$)**. The normal $\dot{V}/\dot{Q}$ ratio is 0.8. This is the amount by which perfusion exceeds ventilation under normal conditions.

Oxygen transport

Approximately 1000 ml (1 L) of oxygen is transported to the cells of the body each minute. Oxygen is transported in the blood in two forms: a small amount dissolves in plasma, and the remainder binds to hemoglobin molecules. Without hemoglobin, oxygen would not reach the cells in amounts sufficient to maintain normal metabolic function. (Hemoglobin is discussed in detail in Chapter 19, and cellular metabolism is explored in Chapter 1.)

Diffusion across the alveolocapillary membrane

The alveolocapillary membrane is ideal for oxygen diffusion because it has a large total surface area (70 to 100 m^2) and is very thin (0.5 micrometer [μm]). In addition, the partial pressure of oxygen molecules in alveolar gas (P_AO_2) is much greater than in capillary blood, a condition that promotes rapid diffusion down the concentration gradient from the alveolus into the capillary. The partial pressure of oxygen (oxygen tension) in mixed venous or pulmonary artery blood ($P\bar{v}O_2$) is approximately 40 mm Hg as it enters the capillary, and alveolar oxygen tension (P_AO_2) is approximately 100 mm Hg at sea level. Therefore, a pressure gradient of 60 mm Hg facilitates the diffusion of oxygen from the alveolus into the capillary (Figure 25-16).

Blood remains in the pulmonary capillary for about 0.75 seconds, but only 0.25 seconds is required for oxygen concentration to equilibrate (equalize) across the alveolocapillary membrane. Therefore, oxygen has ample time to diffuse into the blood, even during increased cardiac output, which speeds blood flow, shortening the time the blood remains in the capillary.

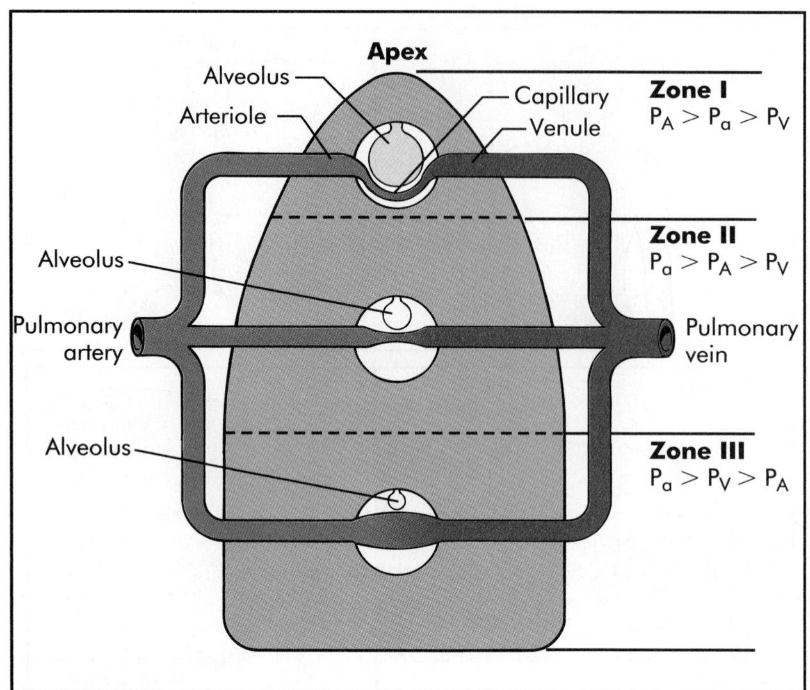

Figure 25-15 ■ Gravity and Alveolar Pressure. Effects of gravity and alveolar pressure on pulmonary blood flow in the three lung zones. In zone I, alveolar pressure (P_A) is greater than arterial and venous pressure, and no blood flow occurs. In zone II, arterial pressure (P_a) exceeds alveolar pressure, but alveolar pressure exceeds venous pressure (P_V). Blood flow occurs in this zone, but alveolar pressure compresses the venules (venous ends of the capillaries). In zone III, both arterial and venous pressures are greater than alveolar pressure and blood flow fluctuates depending on the difference between arterial and venous pressure.

Determinants of arterial oxygenation

As oxygen diffuses across the alveolocapillary membrane, it dissolves in the plasma, where it exerts pressure (the partial pressure of oxygen in arterial blood, or PaO_2). As the PaO_2 increases, oxygen moves from the plasma into the red blood cells (erythrocytes) and binds with hemoglobin molecules. Oxygen continues to bind with hemoglobin until the hemoglobin binding sites are filled or *saturated.* Oxygen then continues to diffuse across the alveolocapillary membrane until the PaO_2 (oxygen dissolved in plasma) and P_AO_2 (oxygen in the alveolus) equilibrate, eliminating the pressure gradient across the alveolocapillary membrane. At this point, diffusion ceases (see Figure 25-16).

The majority (97%) of the oxygen that enters the blood is bound to hemoglobin. The remaining 3% stays in the plasma and creates the partial pressure of oxygen (PaO_2). The PaO_2 can be measured in the blood by obtaining an arterial blood gas measurement. The **oxygen saturation (SaO_2)** is the percentage of the available hemoglobin that is bound to oxygen and can be measured using a device called an oximeter.

Because hemoglobin transports all but a small fraction of the oxygen carried in arterial blood, changes in hemoglobin concentration affect the oxygen content of the blood. Decreases in hemoglobin concentration below the normal value of 15 ml/dl of blood reduce oxygen content, and increases in hemoglobin concentration may increase oxygen content, minimizing the impact of impaired gas exchange. In fact, increased hemoglobin concentration is a major compensatory mechanism in pulmonary diseases that impair gas exchange. For this reason, measurement of hemoglobin concentration is important in assessing individuals with pulmonary disease. If cardiovascular function is normal, the body's initial response to low oxygen content is to speed up cardiac output. In individuals who also have cardiovascular disease, this compensatory mechanism does not work, making increased hemoglobin concentration an even more important compensatory mechanism. (Hemoglobin structure and function are described in Chapter 19.)

Oxyhemoglobin association and dissociation

When hemoglobin molecules bind with oxygen, **oxyhemoglobin (HbO_2)** forms. Binding occurs in the lungs and is called *oxyhemoglobin association* or *hemoglobin saturation with oxygen* (SaO_2). The reverse process, where oxygen is released from hemoglobin, occurs in the body tissues at the cellular level and is called *hemoglobin desaturation.* When hemoglobin saturation and desaturation are plotted on a graph, the result is a distinctive S-shaped curve known as the **oxyhemoglobin dissociation curve** (Figure 25-17).

Several factors can change the relationship between PaO_2 and SaO_2, causing the oxyhemoglobin dissociation curve to shift to the right or left (see Figure 25-17). A shift to the right depicts hemoglobin's decreased affinity for oxygen or an increase in the ease with which oxyhemoglobin dissociates and oxygen moves into the cells. A shift to the left depicts hemoglobin's increased affinity for oxygen,

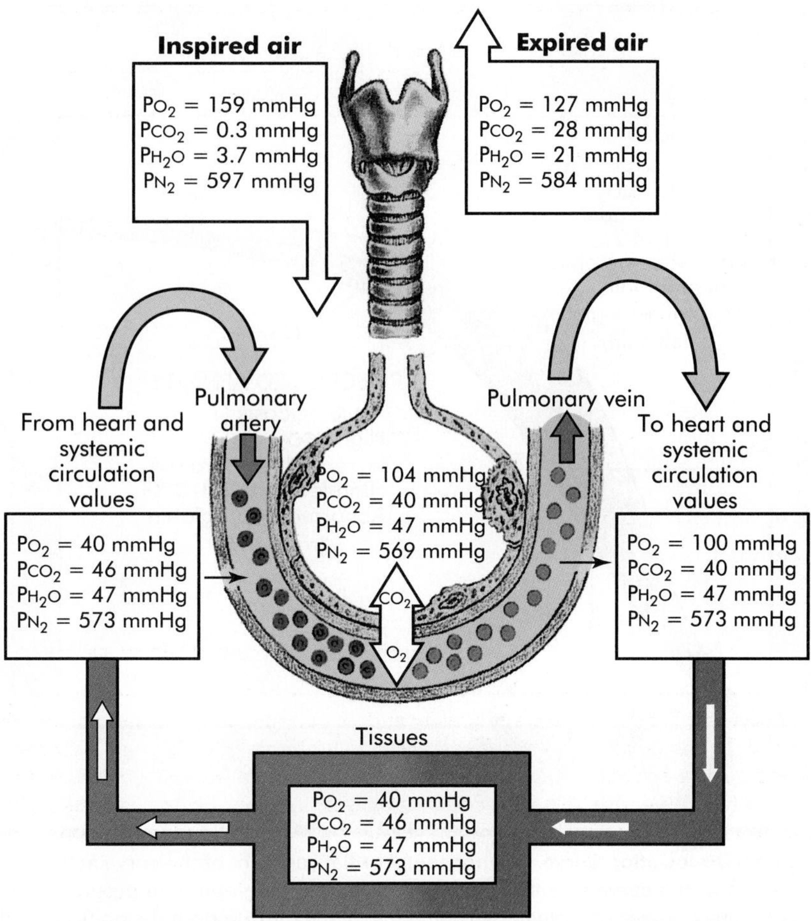

Figure 25-16 ■ **Partial Pressure of Respiratory Gases in Normal Respiration.** The numbers shown are average values near sea level. The values of PO_2, PCO_2, and PN_2 fluctuate from breath to breath. (Modified from Thompson JM et al: *Mosby's clinical nursing*, ed 5, St Louis, 2002, Mosby.)

which promotes association in the lungs and inhibits dissociation in the tissues.

The oxyhemoglobin dissociation curve is shifted to the right by acidosis (low pH) and hypercapnia (increased $PaCO_2$). In the tissues, the increased levels of carbon dioxide and hydrogen ions produced by metabolic activity decrease the affinity of hemoglobin for oxygen. The curve is shifted to the left by alkalosis (high pH) and hypocapnia (decreased $PaCO_2$). In the lungs, as carbon dioxide diffuses from the blood into the alveoli, the blood carbon dioxide level is reduced and the affinity of hemoglobin for oxygen is increased. The shift in the oxyhemoglobin dissociation curve caused by changes in carbon dioxide and hydrogen ion concentrations in the blood is called the **Bohr effect.**

The oxyhemoglobin curve is also shifted by changes in body temperature and increased or decreased levels of 2,3-diphosphoglycerate (2,3-DPG), a substance normally present in erythrocytes. Hyperthermia and increased 2,3-DPG levels shift the curve to the right. Hypothermia and decreased 2,3-DPG levels shift the curve to the left.

Carbon dioxide transport

Carbon dioxide is carried in the blood in three ways: (1) dissolved in plasma (PCO_2), (2) as bicarbonate, and (3) as carbamino compounds (including binding to hemoglobin).

As CO_2 diffuses out of the cells into the blood, it dissolves in the plasma. Approximately 10% of the total CO_2 in venous blood and 5% of the CO_2 in arterial blood are carried dissolved in the plasma ($PvCO_2$ and $PaCO_2$ respectively). As CO_2 moves into the blood, it diffuses into the red blood cells. Within the red blood cells, CO_2, with the help of the enzyme carbonic anhydrase, combines with water to form carbonic acid and then quickly dissociates into H^+ and HCO_3^-. As carbonic acid dissociates, the H^+ binds to hemoglobin, where it is buffered, and the HCO_3^- moves out of the red blood cell into the plasma. Approximately 60% of the CO_2 in venous blood and 90% of the CO_2 in arterial blood are carried in the form of bicarbonate. The remainder combines with blood proteins, hemoglobin in particular, to form carbamino compounds. Approximately 30% of the CO_2 in venous blood and 5% of the CO_2 in arterial blood are carried as carbamino compounds.

CO_2 is 20 times more soluble than O_2 and diffuses quickly from the tissue cells into the blood. The amount of CO_2 able to enter the blood is enhanced by diffusion of oxygen out of the blood and into the cells. Reduced hemoglobin (hemoglobin that is dissociated from oxygen) can carry more CO_2 than can hemoglobin that is saturated with O_2. Therefore, the drop in SO_2 at the tissue level increases the ability of hemoglobin to carry CO_2 back to the lung.

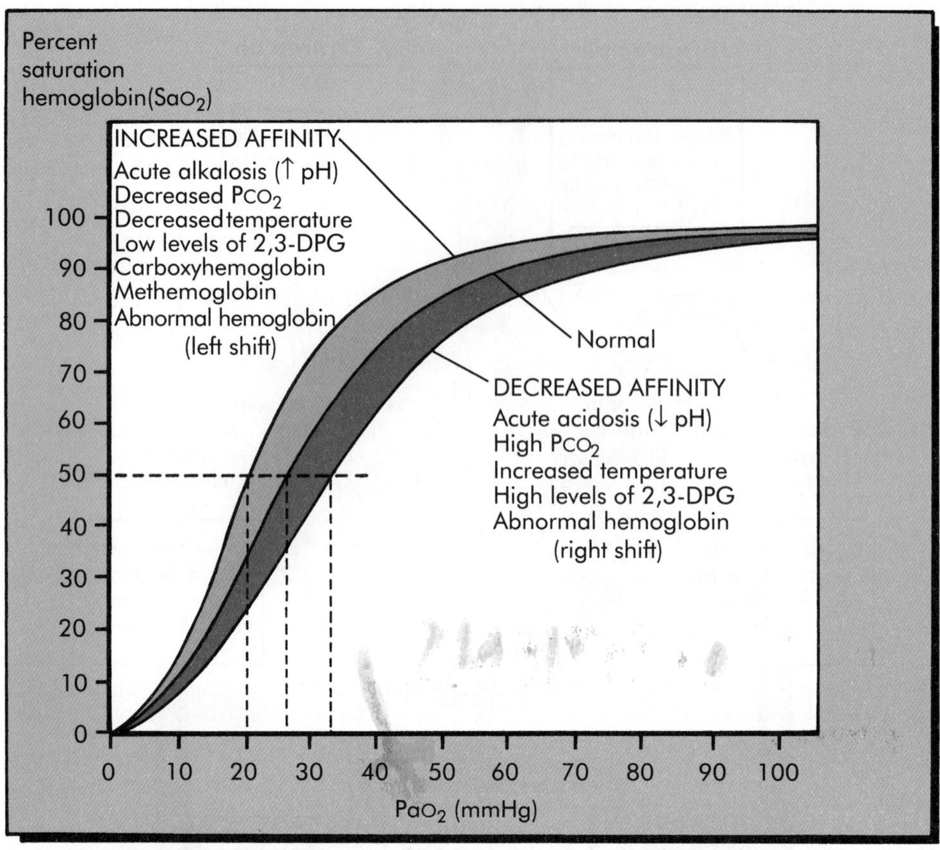

Figure 25-17 ■ Oxyhemoglobin Dissociation Curve. The horizontal or flat segment of the curve at the top of the graph is the arterial or association portion, or that part of the curve where oxygen is bound to hemoglobin and occurs in the lungs. This portion of the curve is flat because partial pressure changes of oxygen between 60 and 100 mm Hg do not significantly alter the percentage saturation of hemoglobin with oxygen and allow adequate hemoglobin saturation at a variety of altitudes. If the relationship between SaO_2 and PaO_2 were linear (in a downward sloping straight line) instead of flat between 60 and 100 mm Hg, there would be inadequate saturation of hemoglobin with oxygen. The steep part of the oxyhemoglobin dissociation curve represents the rapid dissociation of oxygen from hemoglobin that occurs in the tissues. During this phase there is rapid diffusion of oxygen from the blood into tissue cells. The P_{50} is the PaO_2 at which hemoglobin is 50% saturated, normally 26.6 mm Hg. A lower than normal P_{50} represents increased affinity of hemoglobin for O_2; a high P_{50} is seen with decreased affinity. Note that variation from the normal is associated with decreased (low P_{50}) or increased (high P_{50}) availability of O_2 to tissues *(dotted lines)*. The shaded area shows the entire oxyhemoglobin dissociation curve under the same circumstances. *2,3-DPG,* 2,3-Diphosphoglycerate. (From Lane EE, Walker JF: *Clinical arterial blood gas analysis,* St Louis, 1987, Mosby.)

The diffusion gradient for CO_2 in the lung is only approximately 6 mm Hg (venous $PCO_2 = 46$ mm Hg; alveolar $PCO_2 = 40$ mm Hg) (see Figure 25-16). Yet CO_2 is so soluble in the alveolocapillary membrane that the CO_2 in the blood quickly diffuses into the alveoli, where it is removed from the lung with each expiration. Diffusion of CO_2 in the lung is so efficient that diffusion defects that cause hypoxemia (low oxygen content of the blood) do not as readily cause hypercapnia (excessive carbon dioxide in the blood).

The diffusion of CO_2 out of the blood is also enhanced by oxygen binding with hemoglobin in the lung. As hemoglobin binds with O_2, the amount of CO_2 carried by the blood decreases. Thus, in the tissue capillaries, O_2 dissociation from hemoglobin facilitates the pickup of CO_2, and the binding of O_2 to hemoglobin in the lungs facilitates the release of CO_2 from the blood. This effect of oxygen on CO_2 transport is called the **Haldane effect.**[7]

QUICK CHECK 25-5

1. What are the eight steps of gas transport?
2. Describe the relationship between ventilation and pulmonary blood flow.
3. What is the alveolocapillary membrane? How does it function in ventilation and perfusion?
4. Describe the process of oxyhemoglobin association and dissociation.
5. What is barometric pressure? How is it related to physiologic pressure measurements?

Control of the Pulmonary Circulation

The caliber of pulmonary artery lumina decreases as smooth muscle in the arterial walls contracts. Contraction increases pulmonary artery pressure. Caliber increases as these muscles relax, decreasing blood pressure. Contraction (vasoconstriction) and relaxation (vasodilation) primarily occur in response to local humoral conditions, even though the pulmonary circulation is innervated by the ANS as is the systemic circulation.

The most important cause of pulmonary artery constriction is a low alveolar PO_2 (P_AO_2). Vasoconstriction caused by alveolar and pulmonary venous hypoxia, often termed **hypoxic pulmonary vasoconstriction,** can affect only one portion of the lung (i.e., one lobe that is obstructed, decreasing its P_AO_2) or the entire lung.[7] If only one segment of the lung is involved, the arterioles to that segment constrict, shunting blood to other, well-ventilated portions of the lung. This reflex improves the lung's efficiency by better matching ventilation and perfusion. If all segments of the lung are affected, however, vasoconstriction occurs throughout the pulmonary vasculature and pulmonary hypertension (elevated pulmonary artery pressure) can result. The pulmonary vasoconstriction caused by low alveolar PO_2 is reversible if the alveolar PO_2 is corrected. Chronic alveolar hypoxia can result in permanent pulmonary artery hypertension, which eventually leads to right heart failure (cor pulmonale).

Acidemia also causes pulmonary artery constriction. If the acidemia is corrected, the vasoconstriction is reversed. (Respiratory acidosis and metabolic acidosis are described in Chapter 4.) An elevated $PaCO_2$ without a drop in pH does not cause pulmonary artery constriction. Other biochemical factors that affect the caliber of vessels in pulmonary circulation are histamine, prostaglandins, serotonin, nitric oxide, and bradykinin.

QUICK CHECK 25-6

1. What is the most important factor causing pulmonary artery constriction? What other factors are involved?

AGING & The Pulmonary System

Elasticity/Chest Wall

Chest wall compliance decreases because ribs become ossified and joints grow stiffer, which results in increased work of breathing.

Kyphoscoliosis may curve the vertebral column.

Respiratory muscle strength decreases.

Elastic recoil diminishes, possibly the result of loss of elastic fibers.

Result: Lung compliance increases and ventilatory capacity (VC) declines, residual volume (RV) increases, total lung capacity (TLC) is unchanged, ventilatory reserves decline, ventilation-perfusion ratios fall.

Gas Exchange

Pulmonary capillary network decreases.

Alveoli dilate, and peripheral airways lose supporting tissues.

Surface area for gas exchange decreases.

pH and PCO_2 do not change much, but PO_2 declines.

Sensitivity of respiratory centers to hypoxia or hypercapnia decreases.

Ability to initiate an immune response against infection decreases.

NOTE: Maximum PaO_2 at sea level can be estimated by multiplying person's age by 0.3 and subtracting the product from 100.

Exercise

Decreased PaO_2 and diminished ventilatory reserve lead to decreased exercise tolerance.

Early airway closure inhibits expiratory flow.

Changes depend on activity and fitness levels earlier in life.

An active, physically fit individual has fewer changes in function at any age than does a sedentary individual.

Respiratory muscle strength and endurance decrease but can be enhanced by exercise.

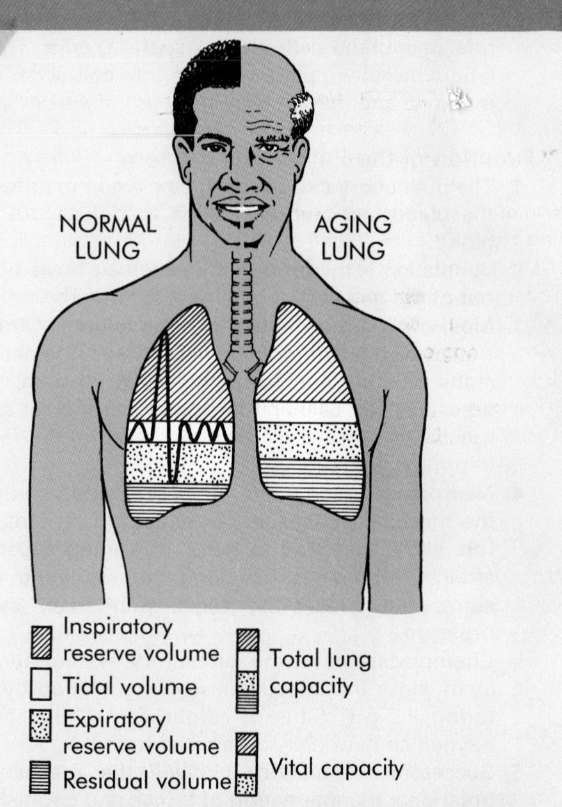

Changes in Lung Volumes With Aging. With aging, note particularly the dense vital capacity and the increase in residual volume. See also McClaran SR et al: Longitudinal effects of aging on lung function at rest and exercise in healthy active fit elderly adults, *J Appl Physiol* 78(5):1957–1968, 1995; Hardie JA et al: Reference values for arterial blood gases in the elderly, *Chest* 125(6):2053–2060, 2004; Zeleznik J: Normative aging of the respiratory system, *Clin Geriatr Med* 19(1):1–18, 2003; Meyer KC: The role of immunity in susceptibility to respiratory infection in the aging lung, *Respir Physiol* 128(1):23–31, 2001.

Did You Understand?

Structures of the Pulmonary System

1. The pulmonary system consists of the lungs, airways, chest wall, and pulmonary and bronchial circulation.
2. Air is inspired and expired through the conducting airways, which include the nasopharynx, oropharynx, trachea, bronchi, and bronchioles to the sixteenth division.
3. Gas exchange occurs in structures beyond the sixteenth division: the respiratory bronchioles, alveolar ducts, and the alveoli. Together these structures compose the acinus.
4. The chief gas-exchange units of the lungs are the alveoli. The membrane that surrounds each alveolus and contains the pulmonary capillaries is called the *alveolocapillary membrane.*
5. The gas-exchange airways are served by the pulmonary circulation, a separate division of the circulatory system. The bronchi and other lung structures are served by a branch of the systemic circulation called the *bronchial circulation.*
6. The chest wall, which contains and protects the contents of the thoracic cavity, consists of the skin, ribs, and intercostal muscles, which lie between the ribs.
7. The chest wall is lined by a serous membrane called the *parietal pleura*; the lungs are encased in a separate membrane called the *visceral pleura.* The area where these two pleurae come into contact and slide over one another is called the *pleural space.*
8. The alveoli produce surfactant, a lipoprotein that lines the alveoli. Surfactant reduces alveolar surface tension and permits the alveoli to expand as air flows in.
9. Compliance is the ease with which the lungs and chest wall expand during inspiration. Lung compliance is ensured by an adequate production of surfactant, whereas chest wall expansion depends on elasticity.
10. Elastic recoil is the tendency of the lungs and chest wall to return to their resting state after inspiration. The elastic recoil forces of the lungs and chest wall are in opposition and pull on each other, creating the normally negative pressure of the pleural space.
11. Gas transport depends on ventilation of the alveoli, diffusion across the alveolocapillary membrane, perfusion of the pulmonary and systemic capillaries, and diffusion between systemic capillaries and tissue cells.
12. Efficient gas exchange depends on an even distribution of ventilation and perfusion within the lungs. Both ventilation and perfusion are greatest in the bases of the lungs because the alveoli in the bases are more compliant (their resting volume is low) and perfusion is greater in the bases as a result of gravity.
13. Almost all the oxygen that diffuses into pulmonary capillary blood is transported by hemoglobin, a protein contained within red blood cells. The remainder of the oxygen is transported dissolved in plasma.
14. Oxygen enters the body by diffusing down the concentration gradient, from high concentrations in the alveoli to lower concentrations in the capillaries. Diffusion ceases when alveolar and capillary oxygen pressures equilibrate.
15. Oxygen is loaded onto hemoglobin by the driving pressure exerted by PaO_2 in the plasma. As pressure decreases at the tissue level, oxygen dissociates from hemoglobin and enters tissue cells by diffusion, again down the concentration gradient.
16. Carbon dioxide is more soluble in plasma than oxygen is. Therefore, carbon dioxide diffuses readily from tissue cells into plasma. Carbon dioxide returns to the lungs dissolved in plasma, as bicarbonate, or in carbamino compounds (e.g., bound to hemoglobin).
17. The pulmonary circulation is innervated by the autonomic nervous system (ANS), but vasodilation and vasoconstriction are controlled mainly by local and humoral factors, particularly arterial oxygenation and acid-base status.

Function of the Pulmonary System

1. The pulmonary system enables oxygen to diffuse into the blood and carbon dioxide to diffuse out of the blood.
2. Ventilation is the process by which air flows into and out of the gas-exchange airways.
3. Most of the time, ventilation is involuntary. It is controlled by the sympathetic and parasympathetic divisions of the autonomic nervous system, which adjust airway caliber (by causing bronchial smooth muscle to contract or relax) and control the rate and depth of ventilation.
4. Neuroreceptors in the lungs (lung receptors) monitor the mechanical aspects of ventilation. Irritant receptors sense the need to expel unwanted substances, stretch receptors sense lung volume (lung expansion), and J-receptors sense pulmonary capillary pressure.
5. Chemoreceptors in the circulatory system and brain stem sense the effectiveness of ventilation by monitoring the pH status of cerebrospinal fluid and the oxygen content (PO_2) of arterial blood.
6. Successful ventilation involves the mechanics of breathing: the interaction of forces and counterforces involving the muscles of inspiration and expiration, alveolar surface tension, elastic properties of the lungs and chest wall, and resistance to airflow.
7. The major muscle of inspiration is the diaphragm. When the diaphragm contracts, it moves downward in the thoracic cavity, creating a vacuum that causes air to flow into the lungs.

AGING & the Pulmonary System

1. Aging affects the mechanical aspects of ventilation by decreasing chest wall compliance and elastic recoil of the lungs. Changes in these elastic properties reduce ventilatory reserve.
2. Aging causes the PaO_2 to decrease.

Key Terms

Acinus, 696
Alveolar duct, 696
Alveolar ventilation, 699
Alveolocapillary membrane, 697
Alveolus (pl. alveoli), 696
Bohr effect, 709
Bronchus (pl. bronchi), 694
Carina, 694
Central chemoreceptor, 700
Compliance, 704
Elastic recoil, 703
Goblet cell, 696
Haldane effect, 710
Hilus (pl. hila), 696
Hypoxic vasoconstriction, 711
Irritant receptor, 699
J-receptor, 700
Larynx, 693
Minute volume, 699
Nasopharynx, 693
Oropharynx, 693
Oxygen saturation (SaO_2), 708
Oxyhemoglobin (HbO_2), 708
Oxyhemoglobin dissociation curve, 708
Partial pressure (of a gas), 705
Peripheral chemoreceptor, 699
Pleura (pl. pleurae), 698
Pleural space (pleural cavity), 698
Respiratory bronchiole, 696
Respiratory center, 699
Stretch receptor, 699
Surface tension, 702
Surfactant, 696
Thoracic cavity, 698
Trachea, 694
Ventilation, 699
Ventilation-perfusion ratio $\dot{V}/\dot{Q}$, 707

References

1. Lumb AB: *Nunn's applied respiratory physiology*, ed 6, Elsevier, 2005.
2. Ganong W: *Review of medical physiology*, ed 22, New York, 2005, McGraw-Hill.
3. Clouter M, Thrall R: The respiratory system. In Berne R et al, editors: *Physiology*, ed 5, St Louis, 2004, Mosby.
4. West JB: *Respiratory physiology: the essentials*, ed 7, Philadelphia, 2005, Lippincott Williams & Wilkins.
5. Canning BJ: Anatomy and neurophysiology of the cough reflex, *Chest* 129:33s–47s, 2006.
6. Des Jardins T, Burton GC: *Clinical manifestations and assessment of respiratory disease*, ed 5, St Louis, 2006, Mosby.
7. Aaronson PI et al: Hypoxic pulmonary vasoconstriction: mechanisms and controversies, *J Physiol* 570(pt 1):53–58, 2006.

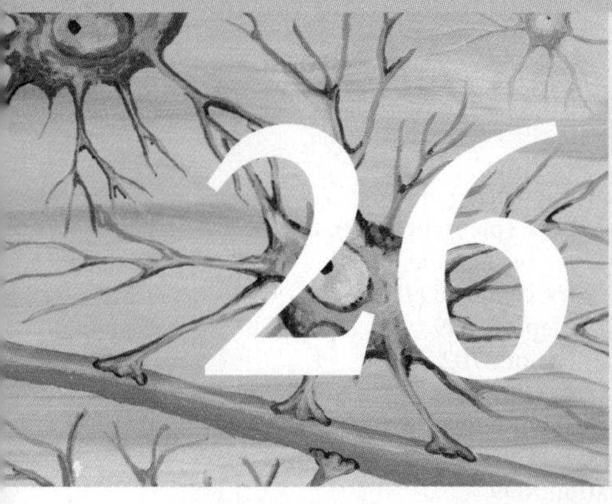

26 ALTERATIONS OF PULMONARY FUNCTION

Valentina L. Brashers

CHAPTER OUTLINE

ELECTRONIC RESOURCES

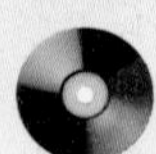

Companion CD
- Review Questions and Answers
- Animations

evolve Website
http://evolve.elsevier.com/Huether/
- Quick Check Answers
- Key Terms Exercises
- Critical Thinking Questions with Answers
- Algorithm Completion Exercises
- WebLinks

Pulmonary disease is often classified as acute or chronic, obstructive or restrictive, or infectious or noninfectious and is caused by alteration in the lung or heart. Because skillful and knowledgeable clinical care plays a major role in decreasing respiratory mortality and morbidity, the clinician who has a clear understanding of the pathophysiology of common respiratory problems can greatly affect the outcome for each individual.

The lungs, with their large surface area, are constantly exposed to the external environment. Therefore, lung disease is greatly influenced by conditions of the environment, occupation, and personal and social habits. Symptoms of lung disease are common and associated not only with primary lung disorders but also with diseases of other organ systems.

CLINICAL MANIFESTATIONS OF PULMONARY ALTERATIONS

Signs and Symptoms of Pulmonary Disease

Pulmonary disease is associated with many signs and symptoms, the most common of which are cough and dyspnea. Others include chest pain, abnormal sputum, hemoptysis, altered breathing patterns, cyanosis, and fever.

Dyspnea

Dyspnea is the subjective sensation of uncomfortable breathing, the feeling of being unable to get enough air. It is often described as breathlessness, air hunger, shortness of breath, labored breathing, and preoccupation with breathing.

Dyspnea can be caused by diffuse or focal pulmonary disease. Disturbances of ventilation, gas exchange, or ventilation-perfusion relationships can cause dyspnea, as can increased work of breathing or any disease that damages lung tissue (lung parenchyma). One proposed mechanism for dyspnea is a mismatch between sensory and motor input from the respiratory center such that there is more urge to breathe than there is response by the respiratory muscles. Other causes of dyspnea include stimulation of central and peripheral chemoreceptors, and stimulation of afferent receptors in the lung and chest wall.[1,2]

The signs of dyspnea include flaring of the nostrils, use of accessory muscles of respiration, and retraction (pulling back) of the intercostal spaces. In dyspnea caused by parenchymal disease (e.g., pneumonia), retractions of tissue between the ribs (subcostal and intercostal retractions) may be observed, although retractions are more common in children than in adults. In upper airway obstruction, supercostal retractions (retractions of tissues above the ribs) predominate. Dyspnea can be quantified by the use of both ordinal rating scales and visual analog scales and is frequently associated with significant anxiety.[3]

Dyspnea can occur transiently or can become chronic. Often the first episode occurs with exercise and is called *dyspnea on exertion*. This type of dyspnea is common to many pulmonary disorders. One cause of dyspnea is pulmonary congestion usually resulting from heart disease. Pulmonary congestion tends to cause dyspnea when the individual is lying down **(orthopnea).** The horizontal position redistributes body water, causes the abdominal contents to exert pressure on the diaphragm, and decreases the efficiency of the respiratory muscles. Sitting up in a forward-leaning posture or supporting the upper body on several pillows generally relieves orthopnea. Some individuals with pulmonary or cardiac disease wake up at night gasping for air and have to sit up or stand to relieve the dyspnea **(paroxysmal nocturnal dyspnea [PND])**.

Abnormal breathing patterns

Normal breathing (eupnea) is rhythmic and effortless. The resting ventilatory rate is 8 to 16 breaths per minute, and tidal volume ranges from 400 to 800 ml. A short expiratory pause occurs with each breath, and the individual takes an occasional deeper breath, or sighs. Sigh breaths, which help to maintain normal lung function, are usually 1 ½ to 2 times the normal tidal volume and occur approximately 10 to 12 times per hour.

The rate, depth, regularity, and effort of breathing undergo characteristic alterations in response to physiologic and pathophysiologic conditions. Patterns of breathing automatically adjust to minimize the work of respiratory muscles. Strenuous exercise or metabolic acidosis induces **Kussmaul respiration (hyperpnea),** which is characterized by a slightly increased ventilatory rate, very large tidal volumes, and no expiratory pause.

Labored breathing occurs whenever there is an increased work of breathing, especially if the airways are obstructed. If the large airways are obstructed, a slow ventilatory rate, large tidal volume, increased effort, prolonged inspiration and expiration and stridor or audible wheezing (depending on the site of obstruction) are typical. In small airway obstruction like that seen in asthma and chronic obstructive pulmonary disease, a rapid ventilatory rate, small tidal volume, increased effort, and prolonged expiration are often present.

Restricted breathing is commonly caused by disorders such as pulmonary fibrosis that stiffen the lungs or chest wall and decrease compliance. Small tidal volumes, rapid ventilatory rate (tachypnea), and rapid expiration are characteristic.

Shock and severe cerebral hypoxia (insufficient oxygen in the brain) contribute to gasping respirations that consist of irregular, quick inspirations with an expiratory pause. Anxiety can cause sighing respirations, which consist of irregular breathing characterized by frequent, deep sighing inspirations.

Cheyne-Stokes respirations are characterized by alternating periods of deep and shallow breathing. Apnea lasting from 15 to 60 seconds is followed by ventilations that increase in volume until a peak is reached; then ventilation (tidal volume) decreases again to apnea. Cheyne-Stokes respirations result from any condition that slows the blood flow to the brain stem, which in turn slows impulses sending information to the respiratory centers of the brain stem. Neurologic impairment above the brain stem is also a contributing factor.

Hypoventilation/hyperventilation

Hypoventilation is inadequate alveolar ventilation in relation to metabolic demands. Hypoventilation occurs when minute volume (tidal volume times respiratory rate) is reduced. It is caused by alterations in pulmonary mechanics or in the neurologic control of breathing. When alveolar ventilation is normal, carbon dioxide (CO_2) is removed from the lungs at the same rate as that produced by cellular metabolism; therefore, arterial and alveolar PCO_2 values remain at normal levels (40 mm Hg). With hypoventilation, CO_2 removal does not keep up with CO_2 production and the level of CO_2 in the arterial blood ($PaCO_2$) increases, causing **hypercapnia** ($PaCO_2$ more than 44 mm Hg) (see Table 25-2 for a definition of gas partial pressures and other pulmonary abbreviations). This results in respiratory acidosis that can affect the function of many tissues throughout the body. Hypoventilation is often overlooked until it is severe because breathing pattern and ventilatory rate may appear to be normal and changes in tidal volume can be difficult to detect clinically. Blood gas analysis (i.e., measurement of the $PaCO_2$ of arterial blood) reveals the hypoventilation. Pronounced hypoventilation can cause somnolence or disorientation.

Hyperventilation is alveolar ventilation exceeding metabolic demands. The lungs remove CO_2 faster than it is produced by cellular metabolism, resulting in decreased $PaCO_2$, or **hypocapnia** ($PaCO_2$ less than 36 mm Hg). Hypocapnia results in a respiratory alkalosis that also can interfere with tissue function. Like hypoventilation, hyperventilation can be determined by arterial blood gas analysis. Increased respiratory rate or tidal volume can occur with severe anxiety, acute head injury, pain, and in response to conditions that cause insufficient oxygenation of the blood.

Cyanosis

Cyanosis is a bluish discoloration of the skin and mucous membranes caused by increasing amounts of desaturated or reduced hemoglobin (which is bluish) in the blood. It generally develops when 5 g of hemoglobin is desaturated, regardless of hemoglobin concentration.

Cyanosis can be caused by decreased arterial oxygenation (low PaO_2), pulmonary or cardiac right-to-left shunts, decreased cardiac output, cold environment, or anxiety. Lack of cyanosis does not necessarily indicate that oxygenation is normal. In adults, cyanosis is not evident until severe hypoxemia is present and, therefore, is an insensitive indication of respiratory failure. Severe anemia (inadequate hemoglobin concentration) and carbon monoxide poisoning (in which hemoglobin binds to carbon monoxide instead of to oxygen) can cause inadequate oxygenation of tissues without causing cyanosis. Individuals with polycythemia (an abnormal increase in numbers of red blood cells), however, may have cyanosis when oxygenation is adequate. Therefore, cyanosis must be interpreted in relation to the underlying pathophysiology. If cyanosis is suggested, the PaO_2 should be measured. Central cyanosis (decreased oxygen saturation of hemoglobin in arterial blood) is best seen in buccal mucous membranes and lips. Peripheral cyanosis (slow blood circulation in fingers and toes) is best seen in nail beds.

Clubbing

Clubbing is the selective bulbous enlargement of the end (distal segment) of a digit (finger or toe) (Figure 26-1). Usually it is painless. Clubbing is commonly associated with diseases that cause chronic hypoxemia, such as lung cancer, bronchiectasis, cystic fibrosis, pulmonary fibrosis, lung abscess, and congenital heart disease. It can sometimes be seen in individuals with lung cancer even without hypoxemia.

Cough

A **cough** is a protective reflex that cleanses the lower airways by an explosive expiration. Inhaled particles, accumulated mucus, inflammation, or the presence of a foreign body initiates the cough reflex by stimulating the irritant receptors in the airway. There are few such receptors in the most distal bronchi and the alveoli, thus it is possible for significant amounts of secretions to accumulate in the distal respiratory tree without cough being initiated. The cough consists of inspiration, closure of the glottis and vocal cords, contraction of the expiratory muscles, and reopening of the glottis, causing a sudden, forceful expiration that removes the offending matter. The effectiveness of the cough depends on the depth of the inspiration and the degree to which the airways narrow, increasing the velocity of expiratory gas flow. Cough occurs frequently in healthy individuals.

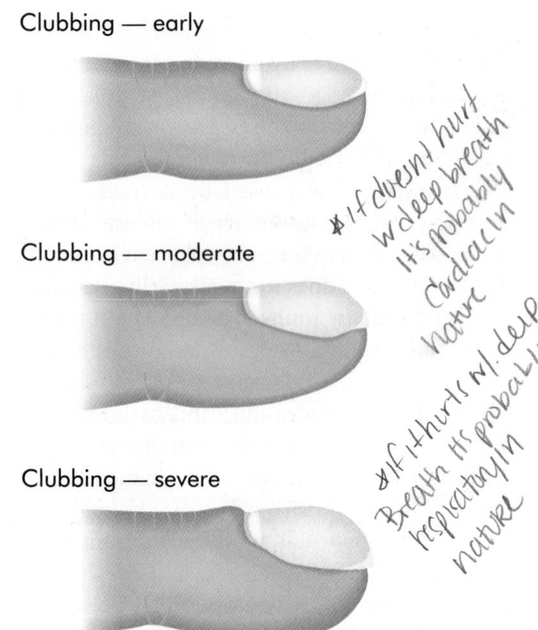

Figure 26-1 ■ Clubbing of Fingers Caused by Chronic Hypoxemia. (Modified from Seidel HM et al: *Mosby's guide to physical examination,* ed 5, St Louis, 2003, Mosby.)

Acute cough is cough that resolves within 2 to 3 weeks of the onset of illness or resolves with treatment of the underlying condition. It is most commonly the result of upper respiratory infections, allergic rhinitis, acute bronchitis, pneumonia, congestive heart failure, pulmonary embolus, or aspiration. *Chronic cough* is defined as cough that has persisted for more than 3 weeks. In nonsmokers, chronic cough is almost always the result of postnasal drainage syndrome, asthma, or gastroesophageal reflux disease. In smokers, chronic bronchitis is the most common cause of chronic cough, although lung cancer must always be considered.[4] Chronic cough can result in a significantly decreased quality of life.[5]

Hemoptysis

Hemoptysis is the coughing up of blood or bloody secretions. This is sometimes confused with hematemesis, which is the vomiting of blood. Blood that is coughed up is usually bright red, has an alkaline pH, and is mixed with frothy sputum, whereas blood that is vomited is dark, has an acidic pH, and is mixed with food particles.

Hemoptysis indicates a localized abnormality, usually infection or inflammation that damages the bronchi (bronchitis, bronchiectasis) or the lung parenchyma (tuberculosis, lung abscess). Other causes include cancer and pulmonary infarction. The amount and duration of bleeding provide important clues about its source. Bronchoscopy, combined with chest computed tomography (CT) is used to confirm the site of bleeding.

Abnormal sputum

Changes in the amount and consistency of sputum provide information about progression of disease and effectiveness of therapy. The gross and microscopic appearances of sputum enable the clinician to identify cellular debris or microorganisms, which aids in diagnosis and choice of therapy.

Pain

Pain caused by pulmonary disorders originates in the pleurae, airways, or chest wall. Infection and inflammation of the parietal pleura (pleurodynia) cause sharp or stabbing pain when the pleura stretches during inspiration. The pain is usually localized to a portion of the chest wall, where a unique breath sound called a *pleural friction rub* may be heard over the painful area. Laughing or coughing makes pleural pain worse. Pleural pain is common with pulmonary infarction (tissue death) caused by pulmonary embolism and emanates from the area around the infarction.

Pulmonary pain is central chest pain that is pronounced after coughing and occurs in individuals with infection and inflammation of the trachea or bronchi (tracheitis or tracheobronchitis). It can be difficult to differentiate from cardiac pain. High blood pressure in the pulmonary circulation (pulmonary hypertension) can cause pain during exercise that is often mistaken for cardiac pain (angina pectoris).

Pain in the chest wall is muscle pain or rib pain. Excessive coughing (which makes the muscles sore) and rib fractures produce such pain. Inflammation of the costochondral junction (costochondritis) also can cause chest wall pain. Chest wall pain can often be reproduced by pressing on the sternum or ribs.

Conditions Caused by Pulmonary Disease or Injury

Hypercapnia

Hypercapnia, or increased carbon dioxide in the arterial blood (increased $PaCO_2$), is caused by hypoventilation of the alveoli. As discussed in Chapter 25, carbon dioxide is easily diffused from the blood into the alveolar space; thus, minute volume (respiratory rate times tidal volume) determines not only alveolar ventilation but also $PaCO_2$. Hypoventilation is often overlooked because the breathing pattern and ventilatory rate may appear to be normal; therefore, it is important to obtain blood gas analysis to determine the severity of hypercapnia and resultant respiratory acidosis (acid-base balance is described in Chapter 4).

There are many causes of hypercapnia. Most are a result of decreased drive to breathe or an inadequate ability to respond to ventilatory stimulation. Some of these causes include (1) depression of the respiratory center by drugs; (2) diseases of the medulla, including infections of the central nervous system or trauma; (3) abnormalities of the spinal conducting pathways, as in spinal cord disruption or poliomyelitis; (4) diseases of the neuromuscular junction or of the respiratory muscles themselves, as in myasthenia gravis or muscular dystrophy; (5) thoracic cage abnormalities, as in chest injury or congenital deformity; (6) large airway obstruction, as in tumors or sleep apnea; and (7) increased work of breathing or physiologic dead space, as in emphysema.

Hypercapnia and the associated respiratory acidosis result in electrolyte abnormalities that may cause dysrhythmias. Individuals also may present with somnolence and even coma because of changes in intracranial pressure associated with high levels of arterial carbon dioxide, which causes cerebral vasodilation. Alveolar hypoventilation with increased alveolar CO_2 limits the amount of oxygen available for diffusion into the blood, thereby leading to secondary hypoxemia.

Hypoxemia

Hypoxemia, or reduced oxygenation of arterial blood (reduced PaO_2), is caused by respiratory alterations, whereas **hypoxia,** or reduced oxygenation of cells in tissues, may be caused by alterations of other systems as well. Although hypoxemia can lead to tissue hypoxia, tissue hypoxia can result from other abnormalities unrelated to alterations of pulmonary function, such as low cardiac output or cyanide poisoning.

Hypoxemia results from problems with one or more of the major mechanisms of oxygenation:

1. Oxygen delivery to the alveoli
   a. Oxygen content of the inspired air (FiO_2)
   b. Ventilation of the alveoli
2. Diffusion of oxygen from the alveoli into the blood
   a. Balance between alveolar ventilation and perfusion ($\dot{V}/\dot{Q}$ match)
   b. Diffusion of oxygen across the alveolar capillary barrier
3. Perfusion of pulmonary capillaries.

The amount of oxygen in the alveoli is called the PAO_2 and is dependent on two factors. The first factor is the presence of adequate oxygen content of the inspired air. The amount of oxygen in inspired air is expressed as the percentage or fraction of air that is composed of oxygen called the FiO_2. The FiO_2 of air at sea level is approximately 21% or 0.21. Anything that decreases the FiO_2 (such as high altitude) decreases the PAO_2. The second factor is the amount of alveolar minute volume (tidal volume times respiratory rate). Hypoventilation results in an increase in $PACO_2$ and a decrease in PAO_2 such that there is less oxygen available in the alveoli for diffusion into the blood. This type of hypoxemia can be completely corrected if alveolar ventilation is improved by increases in the rate and depth of breathing. Hypoventilation causes hypoxemia in unconscious persons; in persons with neurologic, muscular, or bone diseases that restrict chest expansion; and in individuals who have chronic obstructive pulmonary disease.

Diffusion of oxygen from the alveoli into the blood is also dependent on two factors. The first is the balance between the amount of air getting into alveoli ($\dot{V}$) and the amount of blood perfusing the capillaries around the alveoli ($\dot{Q}$) An abnormal ventilation-perfusion ratio ($\dot{V}/\dot{Q}$) is the most common cause of hypoxemia (Figure 26-2). Normally, alveolocapillary lung units receive almost equal amounts of ventilation and perfusion. The normal $\dot{V}/\dot{Q}$ is 0.8 to 0.9 because perfusion is somewhat greater than ventilation in the lung bases and because some blood is normally shunted to the bronchial circulation. $\dot{V}/\dot{Q}$ mismatch refers to an

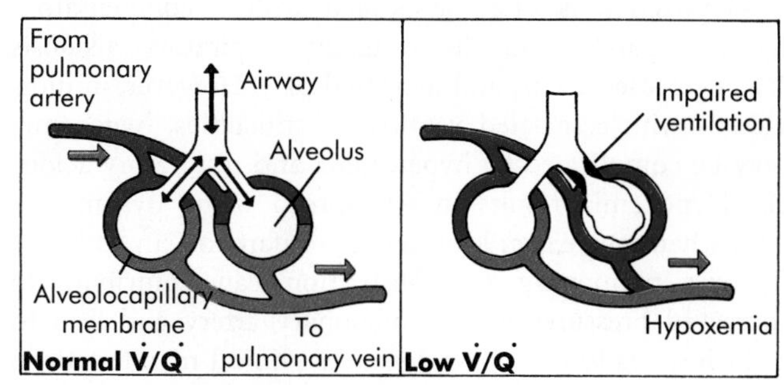

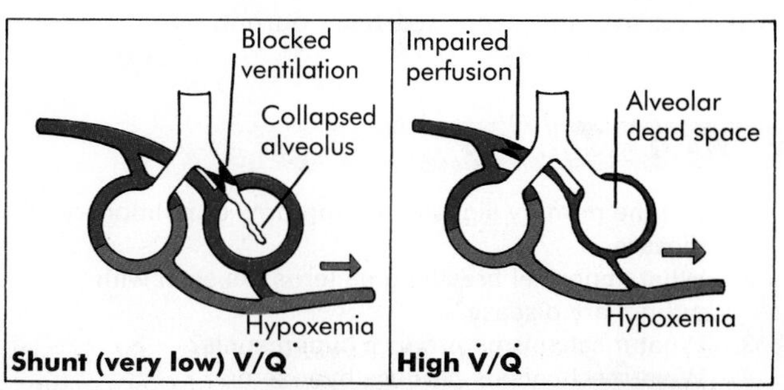

Figure 26-2 ■ **Ventilation-Perfusion ($\dot{V}/\dot{Q}$) Abnormalities.**

abnormal distribution of ventilation and perfusion. Hypoxemia can be caused by inadequate ventilation of well-perfused areas of the lung (low $\dot{V}/\dot{Q}$). Mismatching of this type, called **shunting,** occurs in atelectasis, in asthma as a result of bronchoconstriction, and in pulmonary edema and pneumonia when alveoli are filled with fluid. When blood passes through portions of the pulmonary capillary bed that receive no ventilation, right-to-left shunt occurs, resulting in decreased systemic PaO_2 and hypoxemia. Hypoxemia also can be caused by poor perfusion of well-ventilated portions of the lung (high $\dot{V}/\dot{Q}$), resulting in wasted ventilation. The most common cause of high $\dot{V}/\dot{Q}$ is a pulmonary embolus that impairs blood flow to a segment of the lung. An area where alveoli are ventilated but not perfused is termed **alveolar dead space.**

The second factor affecting diffusion of oxygen from the alveoli into the blood is the alveolocapillary barrier. Diffusion of oxygen through the alveolocapillary membrane is impaired if the membrane is thickened or the surface area available for diffusion is decreased. Thickened alveolocapillary membranes, as occur with edema (tissue swelling) and fibrosis (formation of fibrous lesions), increase the time required for oxygen to diffuse from the alveoli into the capillaries. If diffusion is slowed enough, the PO_2 of alveolar gas and capillary blood do not have time to equilibrate during the fraction of a second that blood remains in the capillary. Destruction of alveoli, as in emphysema, decreases the surface area available for diffusion. Hypercapnia is seldom produced by impaired diffusion because carbon dioxide diffuses so easily from capillary to alveolus that the individual with impaired diffusion would die from hypoxemia before hypercapnia could occur.

Finally, hypoxemia can result from blood flow bypassing the lungs. This can occur because of intracardiac defects that cause right to left shunting or because of intrapulmonary arteriovenous malformations.

Hypoxemia is often associated with a compensatory hyperventilation and the resultant respiratory alkalosis (i.e., decreased $Paco_2$ and increased pH). However, in individuals with associated ventilatory difficulties, hypoxemia may be complicated by hypercapnia and respiratory acidosis. Hypoxemia results in widespread tissue dysfunction and, when severe, can lead to organ infarction. In addition, hypoxic pulmonary vasoconstriction can contribute to increased pressures in the pulmonary artery and lead to right heart failure or *cor pulmonale.* Clinical manifestations of acute hypoxemia may include cyanosis, confusion, tachycardia, edema, and decreased renal output.

QUICK CHECK 26-1

1. List the primary signs and symptoms of pulmonary disease.
2. What abnormal breathing patterns are seen with pulmonary disease?
3. What mechanisms produce hypercapnia?
4. What mechanisms produce hypoxemia?

Acute respiratory failure

Respiratory failure is defined as inadequate gas exchange such that $PaO_2 \leq 50$ mm Hg or $PaCO_2 \geq 50$ mm Hg with pH ≤ 7.25. Respiratory failure can result from direct injury to the lungs, airways, or chest wall or indirectly because of injury to another body system, such as the brain or spinal cord. It can occur in individuals who have an otherwise normal respiratory system or in those with underlying chronic pulmonary disease. Most pulmonary diseases can cause episodes of acute respiratory failure. If the respiratory failure is primarily hypercapnic, it is the result of inadequate alveolar ventilation and the individual must receive ventilatory support, such as with a bag-valve mask or mechanical ventilator. If the respiratory failure is primarily hypoxemic, it is the result of inadequate exchange of oxygen between the alveoli and the capillaries and the individual must receive supplemental oxygen therapy. Many people will have combined hypercapnic and hypoxemic respiratory failure and will require both kinds of support.

Respiratory failure is an important potential complication of any major surgical procedure, especially those that involve the central nervous system, thorax, or upper abdomen. The most common postoperative pulmonary problems are atelectasis, pneumonia, pulmonary edema, and pulmonary emboli. Smokers are at risk, particularly if they have preexisting lung disease. Limited cardiac reserve, chronic renal failure, chronic hepatic disease, and infection also increase the tendency to develop postoperative respiratory failure.

Prevention of postoperative respiratory failure includes frequent turning, deep breathing, and early ambulation to prevent atelectasis and accumulation of secretions. Humidification of inspired air can help loosen secretions. Incentive spirometry gives individuals immediate feedback about tidal volumes, which encourages them to breathe deeply. Supplemental oxygen is given for hypoxemia, and antibiotics are given as appropriate to treat infection. If respiratory failure develops, the individual may require mechanical ventilation for a time.

Pulmonary edema

Pulmonary edema is excess water in the lung. The normal lung is kept dry by lymphatic drainage and a balance among capillary hydrostatic pressure, capillary oncotic pressure, and capillary permeability. In addition, surfactant lining the alveoli repels water, keeping fluid from entering the alveoli. Predisposing factors for pulmonary edema include heart disease, acute respiratory distress syndrome, and inhalation of toxic gases. The pathogenesis of pulmonary edema is shown in Figure 26-3.

The most common cause of pulmonary edema is heart disease. When the left ventricle fails, filling pressures on the left side of the heart increase and vascular volume redistributes into the lungs, subsequently causing an increase in pulmonary capillary hydrostatic pressure.[6] When the hydrostatic pressure exceeds oncotic pressure (which holds fluid in the capillary), fluid moves out into the interstitium,

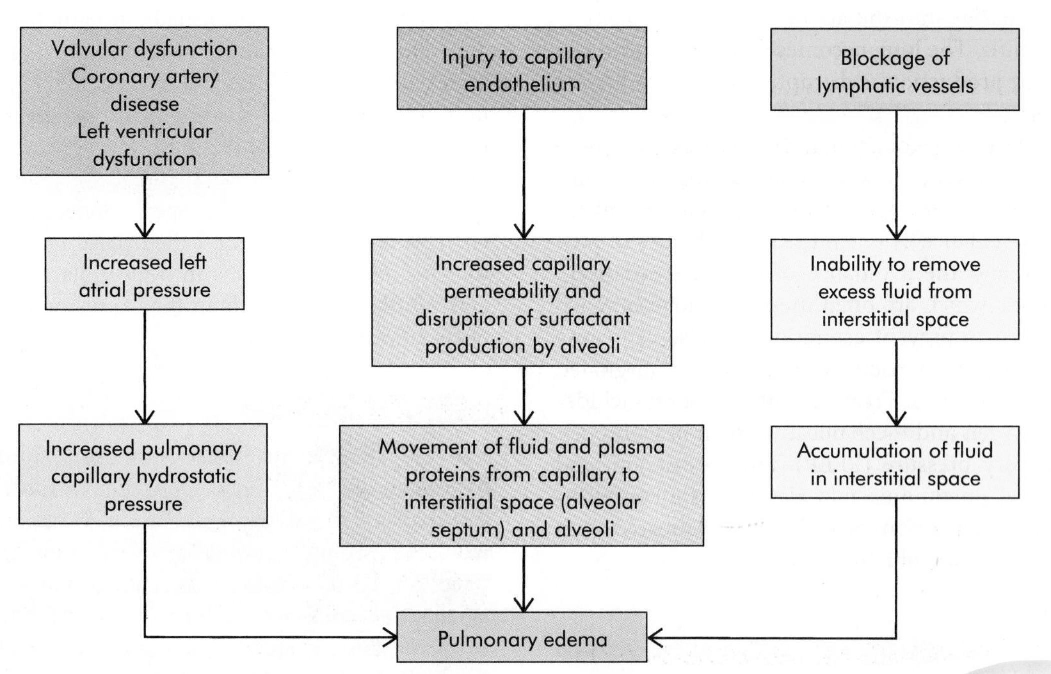

Figure 26-3 ■ **Pathogenesis of Pulmonary Edema.**

or interstitial space (the space within the alveolar septum between alveolus and capillary). When the flow of fluid out of the capillaries exceeds the lymphatic system's ability to remove it, pulmonary edema develops.

Another cause of pulmonary edema is capillary injury that increases capillary permeability, as in cases of acute respiratory distress syndrome or inhalation of toxic gases, such as ammonia. Capillary injury causes water and plasma proteins to leak out of the capillary and move into the interstitium, increasing the interstitial oncotic pressure, which is usually very low. As the interstitial oncotic pressure begins to equal capillary oncotic pressure, water moves out of the capillary and into the lung. (This phenomenon is discussed in Chapter 4, Figures 4-1 and 4-2.)

Pulmonary edema also can result from obstruction of the lymphatic system. Drainage can be blocked by compression of lymphatic vessels by edema, tumors, and fibrotic tissue and by increased systemic venous pressure.

Clinical manifestations of pulmonary edema include dyspnea, hypoxemia, and increased work of breathing. Physical examination may reveal inspiratory crackles (rales) and dullness to percussion over the lung bases. In severe edema, pink frothy sputum is expectorated and $PaCO_2$ increases.

The treatment of pulmonary edema depends on its cause. If the edema is caused by increased hydrostatic pressure that results from heart failure, therapy is geared toward improving cardiac output with diuretics, vasodilators, and drugs that improve the contraction of the heart muscle. If edema is the result of increased capillary permeability resulting from injury, the treatment is focused on removing the offending agent and supportive therapy to maintain adequate ventilation and circulation. Individuals with either type of pulmonary edema require supplemental oxygen. Positive-pressure mechanical ventilation may be needed if edema significantly impairs ventilation and oxygenation.

Aspiration

Aspiration is the passage of fluid and solid particles into the lung. It tends to occur in individuals whose normal swallowing mechanism and cough reflex are impaired by central or peripheral nervous system abnormalities. Predisposing factors include an altered level of consciousness caused by substance abuse, sedation, or anesthesia; seizure disorders; cerebrovascular accident; and neuromuscular disorders that cause dysphagia. The right lung, particularly the right lower lobe, is more susceptible to aspiration than the left lung because the branching angle of the right main stem bronchus is straighter than the branching angle of the left main stem bronchus.

The aspiration of large food particles or foreign bodies can obstruct a bronchus, resulting in bronchial inflammation and collapse of airways distal to the obstruction. Clinical manifestations include the sudden onset of choking, cough, vomiting, dyspnea, and wheezing. If the aspirated solid is not identified and removed by bronchoscopy, a chronic, local inflammation develops that may lead to recurrent infection and bronchiectasis (permanent dilation of the bronchus). Once the pathologic process has progressed to bronchiectasis, surgical resection of the affected area is usually required.

Aspiration of acidic gastric fluid (pH <2.5) may cause severe pneumonitis (lung inflammation). Bronchial damage includes inflammation, loss of ciliary function, and bronchospasm. In the alveoli, acidic fluid damages the alveolocapillary membrane, allowing plasma and blood cells to move from capillaries into the alveoli, resulting in hemorrhagic pneumonitis. The lung becomes stiff and noncompliant as surfactant production is disrupted, leading to further edema and collapse.

Preventive measures for individuals at risk are more effective than treatment of known aspiration. The most important preventive measures include the semirecumbent position, the surveillance of enteral feeding, the use of promotility agents, and the avoidance of excessive sedation.[7] Nasogastric tubes, which are often used to remove stomach contents, are used to prevent aspiration but also can cause aspiration if fluid and particulate matter are regurgitated as the tube is being placed. Treatment of aspiration includes supplemental oxygen and mechanical ventilation with positive end-expiratory pressure (PEEP), fluid restriction, and steroids. Bacterial pneumonia may develop as a complication of aspiration pneumonitis and must be treated with broad-spectrum antimicrobials.

Atelectasis

Atelectasis is the collapse of lung tissue. There are two types of atelectasis:

1. **Compression atelectasis** is caused by external pressure exerted by tumor, fluid, or air in pleural space or by abdominal distention pressing on a portion of lung, causing alveoli to collapse.
2. **Absorption atelectasis** results from removal of air from obstructed or hypoventilated alveoli or from inhalation of concentrated oxygen or anesthetic agents.

Clinical manifestations of atelectasis are similar to those of pulmonary infection including dyspnea, cough, fever, and leukocytosis.

Atelectasis tends to occur after surgery.[8] Postoperative patients may have received supplemental oxygen or inhaled anesthetics, and they are usually in pain, breathe shallowly, are reluctant to change position, and produce viscous secretions that tend to pool in dependent portions of the lung. Prevention and treatment of postoperative atelectasis usually include deep breathing, frequent position changes, and early ambulation. Deep breathing and the use of an incentive spirometer helps open connections between patent and collapsed alveoli, called *pores of Kohn* (Figure 26-4). This allows air to flow into the collapsed alveoli (collateral ventilation) and aids in the expulsion of intrabronchial obstructions.

Bronchiectasis

Bronchiectasis is persistent abnormal dilation of the bronchi. It usually occurs in conjunction with other respiratory conditions and can be caused by obstruction of an airway with mucus plugs, atelectasis, aspiration of a foreign body, infection, cystic fibrosis, tuberculosis, congenital weakness of the bronchial wall, or impaired defense mechanisms. Bronchiectasis is often associated with inflammation of the bronchi (bronchitis) and has similar symptoms (see p. 735).

The symptoms of bronchiectasis may date back to a childhood illness or infection. The disease is commonly associated with recurrent lower respiratory tract infections and expectoration of voluminous amounts of purulent sputum (measured in cupfuls). If the individual is not receiving antibiotics, the sputum has a foul odor. Hemoptysis and clubbing of the fingers are common. Pulmonary function studies show decreased vital capacity (VC) and expiratory flow rates. Bronchiectasis is often associated with bronchitis and atelectasis. Hypoxemia eventually leads to cor pulmonale (see p. 738).

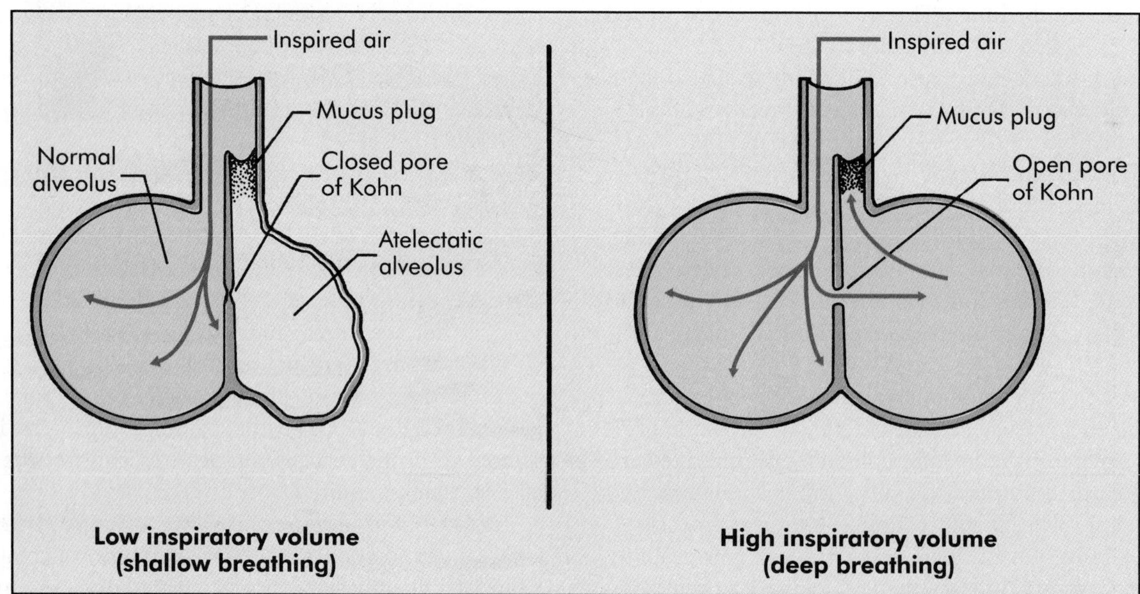

Figure 26-4 ■ **Pores of Kohn. A,** Absorption atelectasis caused by lack of collateral ventilation through pores of Kohn. **B,** Restoration of collateral ventilation during deep breathing.

Bronchiolitis

Bronchiolitis is an inflammatory obstruction of the small airways or bronchioles, occurring most commonly in children. In adults, it usually accompanies chronic bronchitis but can occur in otherwise healthy individuals in association with an upper or lower respiratory infection or inhalation of toxic gases. Bronchiolitis is also a serious complication of lung transplantation. Atelectasis or emphysematous destruction of the alveoli may develop distal to the inflammatory lesion. Bronchiolitis is usually diffuse. **Bronchiolitis obliterans** is a fibrotic process that occludes airways and causes permanent scarring of the lungs. This process can occur in all causes of bronchiolitis but is most common after lung transplantation. Bronchiolitis obliterans can be further complicated by the development of organizing pneumonia (BOOP). Bronchiolitis frequently presents with a rapid ventilatory rate; marked use of accessory muscles; low-grade fever; dry, nonproductive cough; and hyperinflated chest. A decrease in the ventilation-perfusion ratio results in hypoxemia. Bronchiolitis is treated with appropriate antibiotics, steroids, and chest physical therapy (humidified air, coughing and deep breathing, postural drainage) as indicated by the underlying cause.

Pleural abnormalities

Pneumothorax

Pneumothorax is the presence of air or gas in the pleural space caused by a rupture in the visceral pleura (which surrounds the lungs) or the parietal pleura and chest wall. As air separates the visceral and parietal pleurae, it destroys the negative pressure of the pleural space and disrupts the equilibrium between elastic recoil forces of the lung and chest wall. The lung then tends to recoil by collapsing toward the hilum (Figure 26-5).

Spontaneous pneumothorax, which occurs unexpectedly in healthy individuals (usually men) between 20 and 40 years of age, is caused by the spontaneous rupture of blebs (blister-like formations) on the visceral pleura. Bleb rupture can occur during sleep, rest, or exercise. The ruptured bleb or blebs are usually located in the apexes of the lungs. The cause of bleb formation is not known.

A secondary or traumatic pneumothorax can be caused by chest trauma (such as a rib fracture or stab and bullet wounds that tear the pleura; rupture of a bleb or bulla [larger vesicle], as occurs in chronic obstructive pulmonary disease; or mechanical ventilation, particularly if it includes positive end-expiratory pressure [PEEP]).

Both spontaneous and secondary pneumothorax can present as either open or tension. In **open pneumothorax (communicating pneumothorax),** air pressure in the pleural space equals barometric pressure because air that is drawn into the pleural space during inspiration (through the damaged chest wall and parietal pleura or through the lungs and damaged visceral pleura) is forced back out during expiration. In **tension pneumothorax,** however, the site of pleural rupture acts as a one-way valve, permitting air to enter on inspiration but preventing its escape by closing up during expiration. As more and more air enters the pleural space, air pressure in the pneumothorax begins to exceed barometric pressure. The pathophysiologic effects of tension pneumothorax are life threatening. Air pressure in

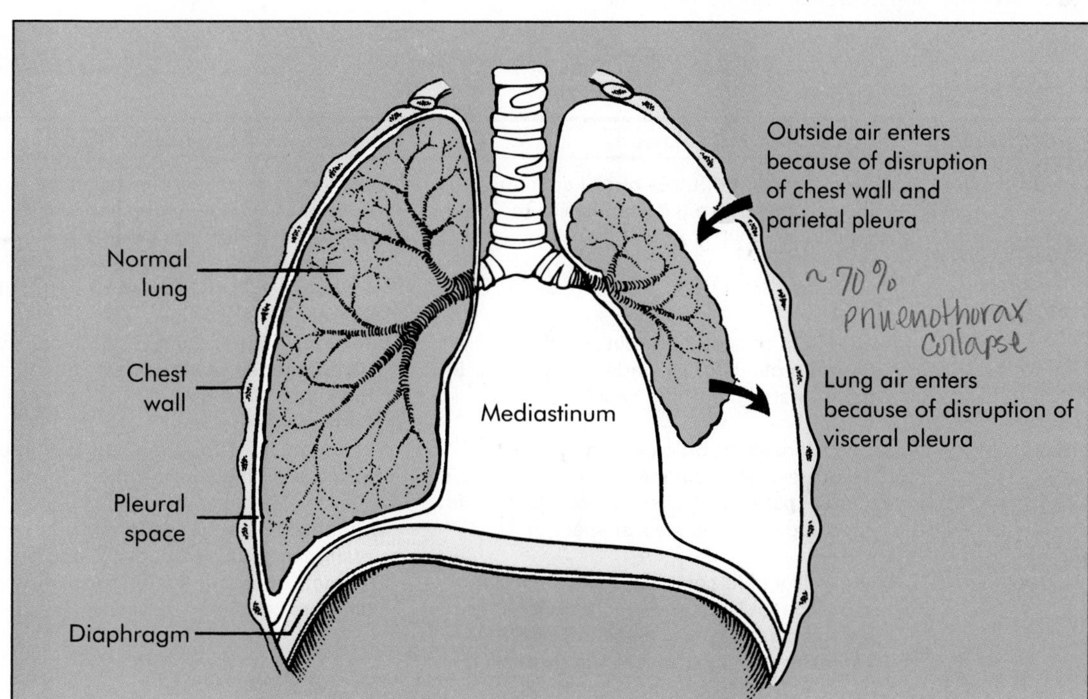

Figure 26-5 ■ **Pneumothorax.** Air in the pleural space causes the lung to collapse around the hilus and may push mediastinal contents (heart and great vessels) toward the other lung.

the pleural space pushes against the already recoiled lung, causing compression atelectasis, and against the mediastinum, compressing and displacing the heart and great vessels.

Clinical manifestations of spontaneous or secondary pneumothorax begin with sudden pleural pain, tachypnea, and dyspnea. The manifestations depend on the size of the pneumothorax. Physical examination may reveal absent or decreased breath sounds and hyperresonance to percussion on the affected side. Tension pneumothorax may be complicated by severe hypoxemia, tracheal deviation away from the affected lung, and hypotension (low blood pressure). Deterioration occurs rapidly and immediate treatment is required. Diagnosis of pneumothorax is made with chest radiographs and computed tomography (CT). Pneumothorax is treated with insertion of a chest tube that is attached to a water-seal drainage system with suction. After the pneumothorax is evacuated and the pleural rupture is healed, the chest tube is removed.

Pleural effusion

Pleural effusion is the presence of fluid in the pleural space. The most common mechanism of pleural effusion is migration of fluids and other blood components through the walls of intact capillaries bordering the pleura. Pleural effusions that enter the pleural space from the intact blood vessels can be **transudative** (watery) or **exudative** (high concentrations of white blood cells and plasma proteins). Other types of pleural effusion characterized by the presence of pus (empyema), blood (hemothorax), or chyle (chylothorax). Mechanisms of pleural effusion are summarized in Table 26-1. Milky looking

Small collections of fluid normally can be drained away by the lymphatics. Dyspnea, compression atelectasis with impaired ventilation, and mediastinal shift occur with large effusions. Pleural pain is present if the pleura is inflamed, and cardiovascular manifestations occur in a large, rapidly developing effusion. Physical exam reveals decreased breath sounds and dullness to percussion on the affected side. A pleural friction rub can be heard over areas of extensive effusion.

Diagnosis is confirmed by chest x-ray and thoracentesis (needle aspiration), which can determine the type of effusion and provide symptomatic relief. If the effusion is large, drainage usually requires the placement of a chest tube.

Empyema

Empyema (infected pleural effusion) is the presence of pus in the pleural space. It is thought to develop when the pulmonary lymphatics become blocked, leading to an outpouring of contaminated lymphatic fluid into the pleural space. Empyema occurs most commonly in older adults and children and usually develops as a complication of pneumonia, surgery, trauma, or bronchial obstruction from a tumor.[9] Commonly documented infectious organisms include *Staphylococcus aureus, Escherichia coli,* anaerobic bacteria, and *Klebsiella pneumoniae.*

Individuals with empyema present clinically with cyanosis, fever, tachycardia (rapid heart rate), cough, and pleural pain. Breath sounds are decreased directly over the empyema. Diagnosis is made by chest radiographs, thoracentesis, and sputum culture.

The treatment for empyema includes the administration of appropriate antimicrobials and drainage of the pleural

TABLE 26-1

Mechanism of Pleural Effusion

Type of Fluid/Effusion	Source of Accumulation	Primary or Associated Disorder
Transudate (hydrothorax)	Watery fluid that diffuses out of capillaries beneath the pleura (i.e., capillaries in lung or chest wall)	Cardiovascular disease that causes high pulmonary capillary pressures; liver or kidney disease that disrupts plasma protein production, causing hypoproteinemia (decreased oncotic pressure in the blood vessels)
Exudate	Fluid rich in cells and proteins (leukocytes, plasma proteins of all kinds; see Chapter 5) that migrates out of the capillaries	Infection, inflammation, or malignancy of the pleura that stimulates mast cells to release biochemical mediators that increase capillary permeability
Pus (empyema)	Debris of infection (microorganisms, leukocytes, cellular debris) dumped into the pleural space by blocked lymphatic vessels	Pulmonary infections, such as pneumonia; lung abscesses; infected wounds
Blood (hemothorax)	Hemorrhage into the pleural space	Traumatic injury, surgery, rupture, or malignancy that damages blood vessels
Chyle (chylothorax)	Chyle (milky fluid containing lymph and fat droplets) that is dumped by lymphatic vessels into the pleural space instead of passing from the gastrointestinal tract to the thoracic duct	Traumatic injury, infection, or disorder that disrupts lymphatic transport

The principles of diffusion are described in Chapter 1; mechanisms that increase capillary permeability and cause exudation of cells and proteins are discussed in Chapter 5

space with a chest tube. In severe cases, instillation of fibrinolytic agents or deoxyribonuclease (DNase) into the pleural space is needed for adequate drainage.

Chest wall restriction

If the chest wall is deformed, traumatized, immobilized, or made heavy by fat, the work of breathing increases and ventilation may be compromised because of a decrease in tidal volume. The degree of ventilatory impairment depends on the severity of the chest wall abnormality. Grossly obese individuals are often dyspneic on exertion or when recumbent. Individuals with severe kyphoscoliosis (lateral bending and rotation of the spinal column, with distortion of the thoracic cage) often present with dyspnea on exertion that can progress to respiratory failure. Such individuals are also susceptible to lower respiratory tract infections. Both obesity and kyphoscoliosis are risk factors for respiratory disease in hospital patients admitted for other problems, particularly those who require surgery. Other musculoskeletal abnormalities that can impair ventilation are ankylosing spondylitis (rheumatoid arthritis of the spine; see Chapter 37) and pectus excavatum, or funnel chest (a deformity characterized by depression of the sternum).

Impairment of respiratory muscle function caused by neuromuscular disease also can restrict the chest wall and impair pulmonary function. Muscle weakness can result in hypoventilation, inability to remove secretions, and hypoxemia. Respiratory difficulty is the most common cause of hospital admission for individuals with neuromuscular diseases such as poliomyelitis, muscular dystrophy, myasthenia gravis, and Guillain-Barré syndrome. (See Unit 4 for a more complete discussion of these disorders.)

Chest wall restriction results in a decrease in tidal volume. An increase in respiratory rate can compensate for small decreases in tidal volume, but many patients will progress to hypercapnic respiratory failure. Diagnosis of chest restriction is made by pulmonary function testing (reduction in forced vital capacity [FVC]), arterial blood gas measurement (hypercapnia), and radiographs. Treatment is aimed at any reversible underlying cause but is otherwise supportive. In severe cases, mechanical ventilation may be indicated.

Flail chest

Flail chest results from the fracture of several consecutive ribs in more than one place or the fracture of the sternum plus several consecutive ribs. These multiple fractures result in instability of a portion of the chest wall, causing paradoxic movement of the chest with breathing. During inspiration the unstable portion of the chest wall moves inward, and during expiration it moves outward, impairing movement of gas in and out of the lungs (Figure 26-6).

The clinical manifestations of flail chest are pain, dyspnea, unequal chest expansion, hypoventilation, and hypoxemia. Treatment is internal fixation by controlled mechanical ventilation until the chest wall can be stabilized surgically.

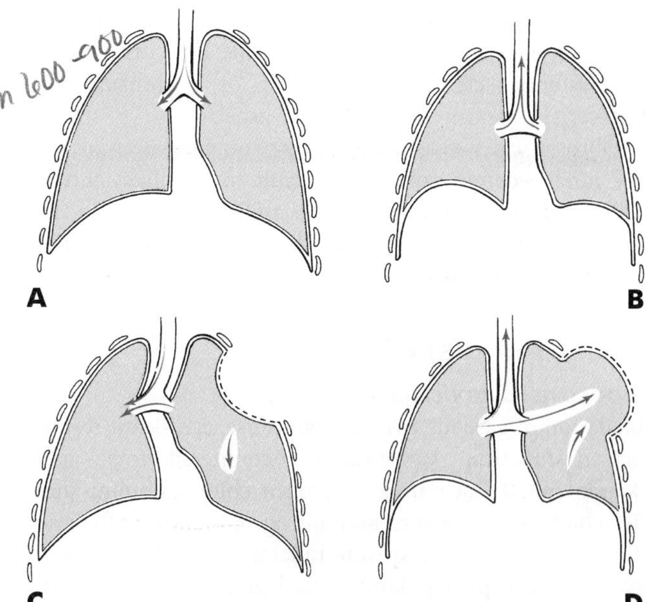

Figure 26-6 ■ **Flail Chest.** Normal respiration: **A,** inspiration; **B,** expiration. Paradoxical motion: **C,** inspiration, area of lung underlying unstable chest wall sucks in on inspiration; **D,** expiration, unstable area balloons out. Note movement of mediastinum toward opposite lung during inspiration.

QUICK CHECK 26-2

1. Describe pulmonary edema, and list two causes.
2. Contrast atelectasis and bronchiectasis.
3. How does pneumothorax differ from pleural effusion?
4. What causes empyema?
5. How does chest wall restriction affect ventilation?

PULMONARY DISORDERS

Restrictive Lung Diseases

Restrictive lung diseases are characterized by decreased compliance of the lung tissue and resultant increased work of breathing. Individuals with lung restriction complain of dyspnea and have an increased respiratory rate and decreased tidal volume. Pulmonary function testing reveals a decrease in forced vital capacity (FVC). Restrictive lung diseases commonly affect the alveolocapillary membrane and cause decreased diffusion of oxygen from the alveoli into the blood resulting in hypoxemia. Some of the most common restrictive lung diseases in adults are pulmonary fibrosis, inhalational disorders, pneumoconiosis, allergic alveolitis, and the acute respiratory distress syndrome.

Pulmonary fibrosis

Pulmonary fibrosis is an excessive amount of fibrous or connective tissue in the lung. The most common form of pulmonary fibrosis has no known cause and therefore is called idiopathic pulmonary fibrosis. Pulmonary fibrosis also can be caused by formation of scar tissue after active pulmonary disease (e.g., acute respiratory distress syndrome, tuberculosis), in association with a variety of autoimmune disorders (e.g., rheumatoid arthritis, progressive systemic sclerosis, sarcoidosis), or by inhalation of harmful substances (e.g., coal dust, asbestos).

Fibrosis causes a marked loss of lung compliance. The lung becomes stiff and difficult to ventilate, and the diffusing capacity of the alveolocapillary membrane may decrease, causing hypoxemia. Diffuse pulmonary fibrosis has a poor prognosis.

Inhalation disorders

Exposure to toxic gases

Inhalation of gaseous irritants can cause significant respiratory dysfunction. Commonly encountered toxic gases include smoke, ammonia, hydrogen chloride, sulfur dioxide, chlorine, phosgene, and nitrogen dioxide. Inhalation of a toxic gas results in severe inflammation of the airways, alveolar and capillary damage, and pulmonary edema. Initial symptoms include burning of the eyes, nose, and throat; coughing; chest tightness; and dyspnea. Hypoxemia is common. Treatment includes supplemental oxygen, mechanical ventilation with PEEP, and support of the cardiovascular system. Steroids are sometimes used, although their effectiveness has not been well documented. Most individuals respond quickly to therapy. Some, however, may improve initially and then deteriorate as a result of bronchiectasis or bronchiolitis (inflammation of the bronchioles).

Prolonged exposure to high concentrations of supplemental oxygen can result in a relatively rare condition known as **oxygen toxicity.** The basic underlying mechanism of injury is a severe inflammatory response mediated primarily by oxygen radicals. Toxicity is often undetected because it occurs in individuals who are already in acute respiratory failure. Treatment involves ventilatory support and a reduction of inspired oxygen concentration to less than 60% as soon as the individual can tolerate this change.

Pneumoconiosis

Pneumoconiosis represents any change in the lung caused by inhalation of inorganic dust particles, usually in the workplace. As in all cases of environmentally acquired lung disease, the individual's history of exposure is important in determining the diagnosis. Pneumoconiosis often occurs after years of exposure to the offending dust, with progressive fibrosis of lung tissue.

The dusts of silica, asbestos, and coal are the most common causes of pneumoconiosis. Others include talc, fiberglass, clays, mica, slate, cement, cadmium, beryllium, tungsten, cobalt, aluminum, and iron. Deposition of these materials in the lungs leads to chronic inflammation with scarring of the alveolar capillary membrane leading to pulmonary fibrosis (see p. 723).[10] These dust deposits are permanent and lead to progressive pulmonary deterioration. Clinical manifestations with advancement of disease include cough, chronic sputum production, dyspnea, decreased lung volumes, and hypoxemia. Diagnosis is confirmed by chest x-ray and computed tomography (CT).[11] Treatment is usually palliative and focuses on preventing further exposure, particularly in the workplace.

Allergic alveolitis

Inhalation of organic dusts can result in an allergic inflammatory response called **extrinsic allergic alveolitis,** or **hypersensitivity pneumonitis.** Many allergens can cause this disorder, including grains, silage, bird droppings or feathers, wood dust (particularly redwood and maple), cork dust, animal pelts, coffee beans, fish meal, mushroom compost, and molds that grow on sugarcane, barley, and straw. The lung inflammation, or pneumonitis, occurs after repeated, prolonged exposure to the allergen.

Allergic alveolitis can be acute, subacute, or chronic. The acute form causes a fever, cough, and chills a few hours after exposure. In the subacute form, coughing and dyspnea are common and sometimes necessitate hospital care. Recovery is complete if the offending agent can be avoided in the future. With continued exposure, the disease becomes chronic and pulmonary fibrosis develops.

Acute respiratory distress syndrome

Acute respiratory distress syndrome (ARDS) is characterized by acute lung inflammation and diffuse alveolocapillary injury. In the United States, over 30% of ICU admissions are complicated by this syndrome. Advances in therapy have decreased overall mortality in people younger than 60 years to approximately 40%, although mortality in older adults and those with severe infections remains much higher.[12] The most common predisposing factors are sepsis and multiple trauma; however, there are many other causes, including pneumonia, burns, aspiration, cardiopulmonary bypass surgery, pancreatitis, blood transfusions, drug overdose, inhalation of smoke or noxious gases, fat emboli, high concentrations of supplemental oxygen, radiation therapy, and disseminated intravascular coagulation.

PATHOPHYSIOLOGY All disorders causing ARDS cause massive pulmonary inflammation that injures the alveolocapillary membrane and produces severe pulmonary edema, shunting, and hypoxemia (Figure 26-7). The damage can occur directly, as with the aspiration of highly acidic gastric contents or the inhalation of toxic gases, or indirectly from chemical mediators released in response to systemic disorders such as sepsis. Injury to the pulmonary capillary endothelium stimulates platelet aggregation and intravascular thrombus formation. Endothelial damage also initiates the complement cascade, stimulating neutrophil and macrophage activity and the inflammatory response.[13]

Once activated, macrophages produce toxic mediators such as tumor necrosis factor (TNF) and interleukin 1 (IL-1). The role of neutrophils is central to the development of ARDS. Activated neutrophils release a battery of inflammatory mediators, including proteolytic enzymes, toxic oxygen products, arachidonic acid metabolites (prostaglandins, thromboxanes, leukotrienes), and platelet-activating factor.[13] These mediators extensively damage

Acute insult
(e.g., pneumonia, aspiration, smoke inhalation)
↓
Release of cytokines
(e.g., IL-1β, TNF)
↓
Influx of inflammatory cells to lung
(i.e., neutrophils, macrophages, activated platelets)
↓
Release of ROS and cytokines
Activation of complement system
↓

- Damage to type II pneumocytes → Atelectasis and decreased lung compliance
- Disruption of alveolar-capillary membrane → Noncardiogenic pulmonary edema and intrapulmonary shunting
- Microthrombi in pulmonary circulation → Pulmonary hypertension
- Release of fibroblast growth factors (e.g., TGF-β, PDGF) → Pulmonary fibrosis

Figure 26-7 ■ **Proposed Mechanisms for the Pathogenesis of Acute Respiratory Distress Syndrome (ARDS).** IL-1-*β*, Interleukin-1-β; *TNF,* tumor necrosis factor; *ROS,* reactive oxygen species; *TGF-β,* transforming growth factor-β; *PDGF,* platelet derived growth factor. (From Soubani AO, Pieroni R: Acute respiratory distress syndrome: a clinical update, *South Med J* 92[5]:452, 1999.)

the alveolocapillary membrane and greatly increase capillary membrane permeability. This allows fluids, proteins, and blood cells to leak from the capillary bed into the pulmonary interstitium and alveoli. The resulting pulmonary edema severely reduces lung compliance and impairs alveolar ventilation. Mediators released by neutrophils and macrophages also cause pulmonary vasoconstriction, which leads to worsening $\dot{V}/\dot{Q}$ mismatching and hypoxemia.

The initial lung injury also damages the alveolar epithelium. This type II alveolar cell injury increases alveolocapillary permeability, increases susceptibility to bacterial infection and pneumonia, and decreases surfactant production.[13] Alveoli and respiratory bronchioles fill with fluid or collapse. The lungs become less compliant, ventilation of alveoli decreases, and pulmonary blood flow is shunted right to left. The work of breathing increases. The end result is acute respiratory failure.

Twenty-four to 48 hours after the acute phase of ARDS, hyaline membranes form, and after approximately 7 days, fibrosis progressively obliterates the alveoli, respiratory bronchioles, and interstitium (fibrosing alveolitis). Functional residual capacity declines, and more severe right-to-left shunting is evident.

The chemical mediators responsible for the alveolocapillary damage of ARDS often cause widespread inflammation, endothelial damage, and capillary permeability throughout the body resulting in the systemic inflammatory response syndrome (SIRS), which then leads to multiple organ dysfunction syndrome (MODS). In fact, death may not be caused by respiratory failure alone but by MODS associated with ARDS. (MODS is discussed in Chapter 23.)

CLINICAL MANIFESTATIONS The classic signs and symptoms of ARDS are marked dyspnea; rapid, shallow breathing; inspiratory crackles; respiratory alkalosis; decreased lung compliance; hypoxemia unresponsive to oxygen therapy (refractory hypoxemia); and diffuse alveolar infiltrates seen on chest radiographs, without evidence of cardiac disease. Symptoms develop progressively, as follows:

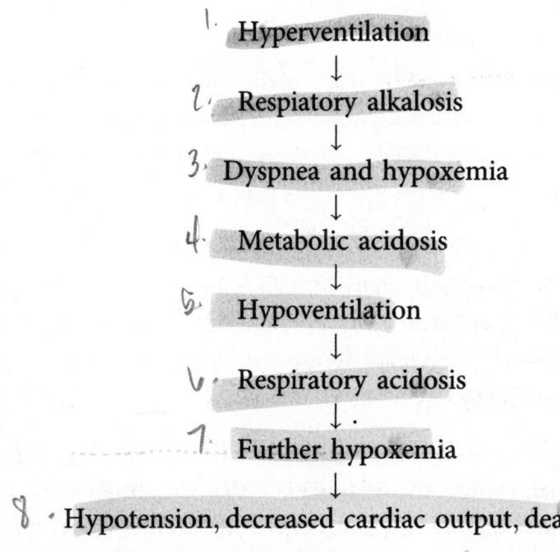

Hyperventilation
↓
Respiratory alkalosis
↓
Dyspnea and hypoxemia
↓
Metabolic acidosis
↓
Hypoventilation
↓
Respiratory acidosis
↓
Further hypoxemia
↓
Hypotension, decreased cardiac output, death

EVALUATION AND TREATMENT Diagnosis is based on physical examination, analysis of blood gases, and radiologic examination. Treatment is based on early detection, supportive therapy, and prevention of complications. Supportive therapy is focused on maintaining adequate oxygenation and ventilation while preventing infection. This often requires alternative modes of mechanical ventilation.[13,14] Surfactant can be given to improve lung compliance. Many studies are under way that investigate new ways to prevent or treat ARDS. Anticoagulant therapy with recombinant human-activated protein C improves outcomes in sepsis associated with ARDS and continues to be evaluated.[14,15]

QUICK CHECK 26-3

1. What are some of the causes of pulmonary fibrosis?
2. What symptoms are produced by inhalation of toxic gases?
3. Describe pneumoconiosis, and give two examples.
4. Briefly describe the role of neutrophils in the acute respiratory distress syndrome (ARDS).

Obstructive Lung Diseases

Obstructive lung disease is characterized by airway obstruction that is worse with expiration. More force (i.e., use of accessory muscles of expiration) is required to expire a given volume of air, or emptying of the lungs is slowed, or both. In adults, the major obstructive lung diseases are asthma, chronic bronchitis, and emphysema. **Asthma** is one of the most common lung disorders in the U.S. and is one of the few that is increasing in prevalence. Because many individuals have both chronic bronchitis and emphysema, these diseases together are often called *chronic obstructive pulmonary disease (COPD)*. Asthma is more acute and intermittent than COPD, even though it can be chronic (Figure 26-8). The unifying symptom of obstructive lung diseases is dyspnea, and the unifying sign is wheezing. Individuals have an increased work of breathing, ventilation/perfusion mismatching, and a decreased forced expiratory volume in one second (FEV_1).

Asthma

Asthma is defined as follows:

> A chronic inflammatory disorder of the airways in which many cells and cellular elements play a role, in particular, mast cells, eosinophils, T lymphocytes, macrophages, neutrophils, and epithelial cells. In susceptible individuals, this inflammation causes recurrent episodes of wheezing, breathlessness, chest tightness, and coughing, particularly at night or in the early morning. These episodes are usually associated with widespread but variable airflow obstruction that is often reversible, either spontaneously or with treatment. The inflammation also causes an associated increase in the existing bronchial hyperresponsiveness to a variety of stimuli. Subbasement membrane fibrosis may occur in some patients with asthma, and these changes contribute to persistent abnormalities of lung function.[16]

Asthma occurs at all ages, with approximately half of all cases developing during childhood and another third before age 40. In the United States, more than 5% of children under the age of 18 report having asthma attacks.[16] Mortality rates have declined since 1995, but the incidence of asthma has increased since the 1980s, especially in urban areas.[16]

Asthma is a familial disorder, and over 20 genes have been identified that may play a role in the susceptibility and pathogenesis of asthma, including those that influence the production of interleukins 4 and 5, IgE, eosinophils, mast cells, beta adrenergic receptors, and bronchial hyperresponsiveness.[17,18] Risk factors for asthma, in addition to family history, include allergen exposure, urban residence, exposure to air pollution and cigarette smoke, recurrent respiratory viral infections, and other allergic diseases, such as allergic rhinitis.[17,19] There is considerable evidence that exposure to high levels of certain allergens during childhood increases the risk for asthma. Furthermore, decreased exposure to certain infectious organisms appears to create an immunologic imbalance that favors the development of allergy and asthma. This complex relationship has been called the *hygiene hypothesis*.[20,21] Urban exposure to pollution and cockroaches and decreased exercise by young people also play a role in the increasing prevalence of asthma.[19,21]

PATHOPHYSIOLOGY Inflammation resulting in hyperresponsiveness of the airways is the major pathologic feature of asthma. It is initiated by a Type I hypersensitivity reaction (see Chapter 7). Exposure to allergens (with subsequent immunologic activation in the atopic individual with production IL-4 and IgE) or irritants results in a cascade of events beginning with mast cell degranulation and the release of multiple inflammatory mediators (Figure 26-9). Some of the most important mediators that are released during an asthma attack are histamine, interleukins, prostaglandins, leukotrienes, and nitric oxide. Vasoactive effects of these cytokines include vasodilation and increased capillary permeability. Chemotactic factors are produced that result in bronchial infiltration by neutrophils, eosinophils, and lymphocytes. Eosinophils release a variety of toxic chemicals that contribute to inflammation and tissue damage. The resulting inflammatory process produces bronchial smooth muscle spasm, vascular congestion, edema formation, production of thick mucus, impaired mucociliary function (see Figure 26-8), thickening of airway walls, and increased bronchial hyperresponsiveness. In addition, the autonomic control of bronchial smooth muscle is dysregulated because of production of toxic neuropeptides leading to acetylcholine-mediated bronchospasm. These changes, combined with epithelial cell damage caused by eosinophil infiltration, produce airway hyperresponsiveness and obstruction and, untreated, can lead to long-term airway damage that is irreversible.[22,23]

Airway obstruction increases resistance to airflow and decreases flow rates, primarily expiratory flow. Impaired expiration causes air trapping and hyperinflation distal to

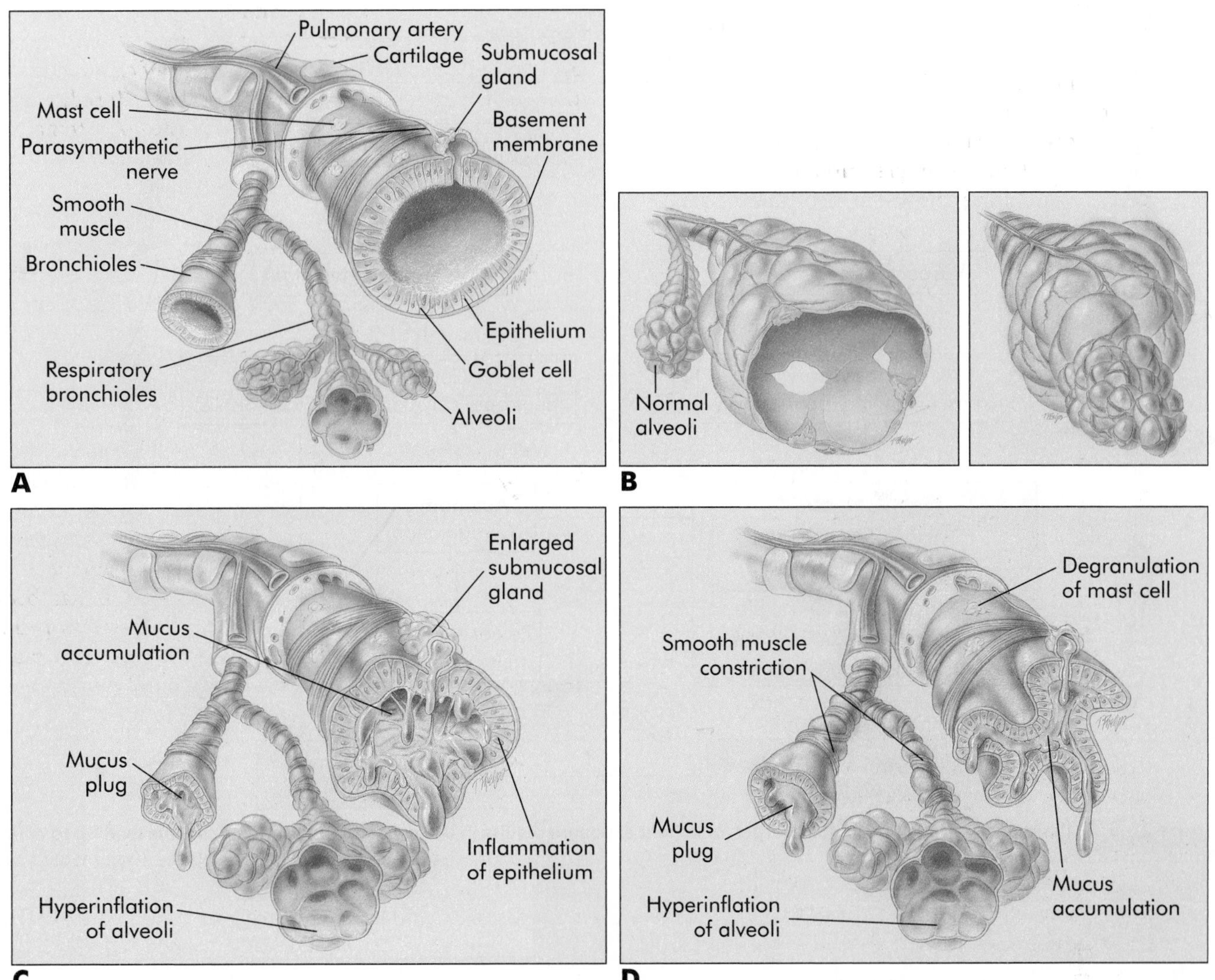

Figure 26-8 **Airway Obstruction Caused by Emphysema, Chronic Bronchitis, and Asthma. A,** The normal lung. **B,** Emphysema: enlargement and destruction of alveolar walls with loss of elasticity and trapping of air; *(left)* panlobular emphysema showing abnormal weakening and enlargement of all air spaces distal to the terminal bronchioles (normal alveoli shown for comparison only); *(right)* centrilobular emphysema showing abnormal weakening and enlargement of the respiratory bronchioles in the proximal portion of the acinus. **C,** Chronic bronchitis: inflammation and thickening of mucous membrane with accumulation of mucus and pus leading to obstruction; characterized by cough. **D,** Bronchial asthma: thick mucus, mucosal edema, and smooth muscle spasm causing obstruction of small airways; breathing becomes labored, and expiration is difficult. (Modified from Des Jardins T, Burton GG: *Clinical manifestations and assessment of respiratory disease,* ed 5, St Louis, 2006, Mosby.)

obstructions and increases the work of breathing. Intrapleural and alveolar gas pressures rise and cause decreased perfusion of the alveoli. These changes lead to uneven ventilation-perfusion relationships causing hypoxemia. Hyperventilation is triggered by lung receptors responding to hyperinflation and causes decreased $PaCO_2$ and increased pH (respiratory alkalosis). As the obstruction becomes more severe, however, the number of alveoli being adequately ventilated and perfused decreases. Air trapping continues to worsen and the work of breathing increases further, leading to hypoventilation (decreased tidal volume), CO_2 retention, and respiratory acidosis. Respiratory acidosis signals respiratory failure.

CLINICAL MANIFESTATIONS Between attacks, individuals are asymptomatic and pulmonary function tests are normal. At the beginning of an attack, the individual experiences chest constriction, expiratory wheezing, dyspnea, nonproductive coughing, prolonged expiration, tachycardia, and tachypnea. Severe attacks involve the accessory muscles of respiration and wheezing is heard during inspiration and expiration. A **pulsus paradoxus** (decrease in systolic blood pressure during inspiration of more than 10 mm Hg) may be noted. Peak flow measurements should be obtained. Because the severity of blood gas alterations is difficult to evaluate by clinical signs alone, arterial blood gas tensions should be measured if oxygen

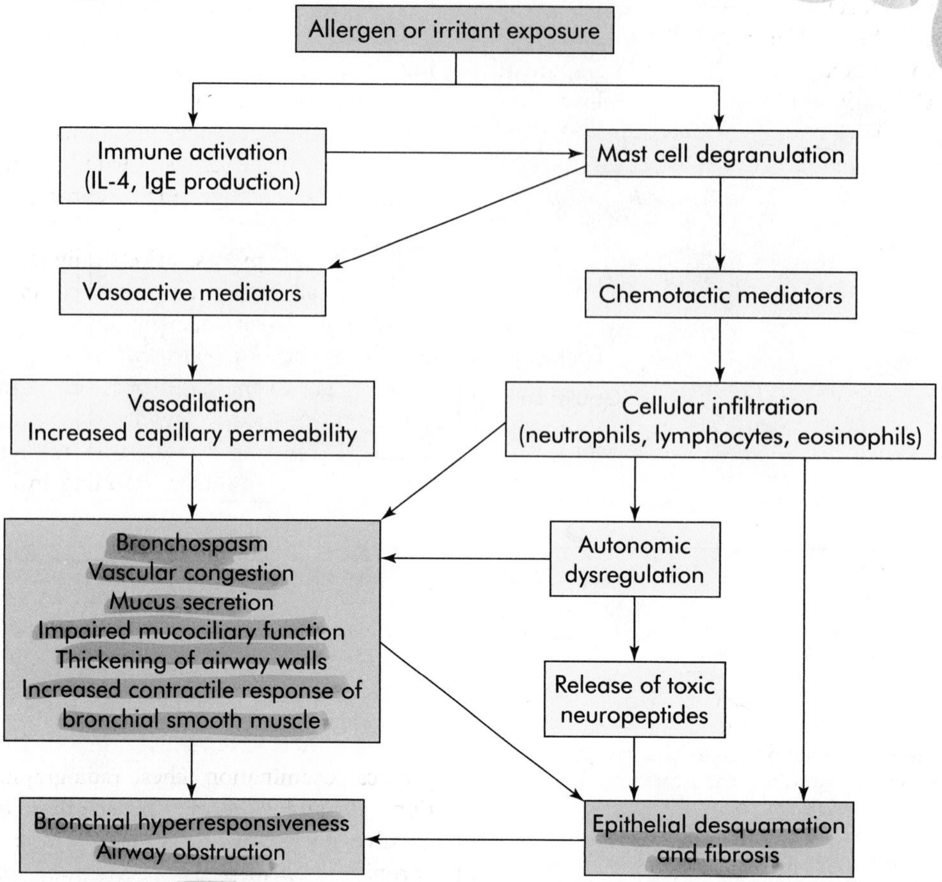

Allergen or irritant exposure

Immune activation (IL-4, IgE production)

Mast cell degranulation

Vasoactive mediators

Chemotactic mediators

Vasodilation
Increased capillary permeability

Cellular infiltration (neutrophils, lymphocytes, eosinophils)

Bronchospasm
Vascular congestion
Mucus secretion
Impaired mucociliary function
Thickening of airway walls
Increased contractile response of bronchial smooth muscle

Autonomic dysregulation

Release of toxic neuropeptides

Bronchial hyperresponsiveness
Airway obstruction

Epithelial desquamation and fibrosis

Figure 26-9 ■ **Pathophysiology of Asthma.** Allergen or irritant exposure results in a cascade of inflammatory events leading to acute and chronic airway dysfunction.

saturation falls below 90%. Usual findings are hypoxemia with an associated respiratory alkalosis.

If bronchospasm is not reversed by usual measures, the individual is considered to have severe bronchospasm or **status asthmaticus.** If status asthmaticus continues, hypoxemia worsens, expiratory flows and volumes decrease further, and effective ventilation decreases. Acidosis develops as $PaCO_2$ begins to rise. Asthma becomes life threatening at this point if treatment does not reverse this process quickly. A silent chest (no audible air movement) and a $PaCO_2$ over 70 mm Hg are ominous signs of impending death.

EVALUATION AND TREATMENT Between attacks, the diagnosis of asthma is supported by a history of allergies and recurrent episodes of breathlessness or exercise intolerance. Further evaluation includes spirometry, which may document reversible decreases in FEV_1 during an induced attack. Gastroesophageal reflux disease may contribute to asthma severity and should be investigated.

Management of asthma begins with avoidance of allergens and irritants and patient education. Individuals with asthma tend to underestimate the severity of their illness and should be taught the use of a home peak-flowmeter. Acute attacks are treated with oral corticosteroids and inhaled beta-agonists. Staging of asthma (mild intermittent, mild persistent, moderate persistent, severe persistent) is based on the frequency and severity of symptoms as well as pulmonary function tests (decreases in FEV_1).[16,17] Chronic management is based on the stage of asthma and includes the regular use of anti-inflammatory medications such as inhaled corticosteroids, cromolyn sodium, or leukotriene inhibitors.[16,17,24] Inhaled bronchodilators such as β_2-agonists and ipratropium are added to supplement symptom control. Immune therapies such as allergy shots and monoclonal antibodies to IgE have been found to be extremely helpful in allergic individuals.[16,17,24–26]

Chronic obstructive pulmonary disease

Chronic obstructive pulmonary disease (COPD) is a syndrome that includes the pathologic lung changes consistent with emphysema or chronic bronchitis. It is characterized by abnormal tests of expiratory airflow that do not change markedly over time nor exhibit major reversibility in response to pharmacologic agents. A 2006 update of the Global Strategy for the Diagnosis, Management, and Prevention of COPD consensus report (GOLD) defines COPD as "a preventable and treatable disease with some significant extrapulmonary effects that may contribute to the severity in individual patients. Its pulmonary component is characterized by airflow limitation that is not fully reversible. The airflow limitation is usually progressive and associated with an abnormal inflammatory response of the lung to noxious particles or gases."[27] It is currently the fourth leading cause of death in the United States and is one of the few causes of death that have increased in incidence since the 1970s.[28] COPD is primarily caused by cigarette smoke, and both active and passive smoking have been implicated. Other risks include occupational exposures and air pollution. Genetic susceptibilities also have been identified.[29]

HEALTH ALERT
Monoclonal Antibodies to IgE for Treatment of Asthma

In genetically predisposed individuals, exposure to inhaled allergens can lead to an allergic response that is manifested clinically as asthma. This immunologic response is a type I hypersensitivity reaction (see Chapter 7) and results from a complex interaction of macrophages, T lymphocytes, antibodies, mast cells, and eosinophils. The immune response leads to a profound inflammatory response, with resultant bronchospasm, mucus formation, and mucosal edema in the airways. Allergen avoidance and immunotherapy (allergy shots) can be effective in preventing this type I hypersensitivity reaction. Omalizumab (Xolair) is humanized monoclonal anti-immunoglobulin E (IgE) antibody that is indicated for individuals with moderate or severe asthma who do not respond to standard therapy. Omalizumab can improve symptoms, reduce hospitalizations, and limit the need for systemic corticosteroid therapy.

Data from Mathur SK, Busse WW: Asthma: diagnosis and management, *Med Clin North Am* 90(1):39–60, 2006; Davydov L: Omalizumab (Xolair) for treatment of asthma, *Am Family Phys* 71:341–342, 2005; Marcus P, Practice Management Committee, American College of Chest Physicians: Incorporating anti-IgE (omalizumab) therapy into pulmonary medicine practice: practice management implications, *Chest* 129(2):466–474, 2006.

Chronic bronchitis

Chronic bronchitis is defined as hypersecretion of mucus and chronic productive cough for at least 3 months of the year (usually the winter months) for at least 2 consecutive years. It is almost always caused by cigarette smoking and by exposure to air pollution.

PATHOPHYSIOLOGY Inspired irritants result in airway inflammation with infiltration of neutrophils, macrophages, and lymphocytes into the bronchial wall. Continual bronchial inflammation causes bronchial edema and increases the size and number of mucous glands and goblet cells in the airway epithelium.[30] Thick, tenacious mucus is produced and cannot be cleared because of impaired ciliary function. The lung's defense mechanisms are, therefore, compromised, increasing susceptibility to pulmonary infection and injury. Frequent infectious exacerbations are complicated by bronchospasm with dyspnea and productive cough.[31] The pathogenesis of chronic bronchitis is shown in Figure 26-10.[28,30]

Initially this process affects only the larger bronchi, but eventually all airways are involved. As the airways become increasingly narrowed, expiratory airway obstruction results (Figure 26-11). The airways collapse early in expiration, trapping gas in the distal portions of the lung. Eventually ventilation-perfusion mismatch and hypoxemia occurs. Extensive air trapping puts the respiratory muscles at a mechanical disadvantage, resulting in hypoventilation and hypercapnia.

CLINICAL MANIFESTATIONS Table 26-2 lists the common clinical manifestations of chronic obstructive lung disease including chronic bronchitis.

EVALUATION AND TREATMENT Diagnosis is based on physical examination, chest radiograph, pulmonary function tests, and blood gas analyses; these tests reflect the progressive nature of the disease. The best "treatment" for chronic bronchitis is prevention, because pathologic changes are not reversible. By the time an individual seeks medical care for symptoms, considerable airway damage is present. If the individual stops smoking, disease progression can be halted. If smoking is stopped before symptoms occur, the risk of chronic bronchitis decreases considerably.

Bronchodilators, expectorants, and chest physical therapy are employed as needed to control cough and reduce dyspnea.[32] Teaching of individuals includes nutritional counseling, respiratory hygiene, recognition of the

TABLE 26-2
Clinical Manifestations of Chronic Obstructive Lung Disease

Clinical Manifestations	Bronchitis	Emphysema
Productive cough	Classic sign	Late in course with infection
Dyspnea	Late in course	Common
Wheezing	Intermittent	Common
History of smoking	Common	Common
Barrel chest	Occasionally	Classic
Prolonged expiration	Always present	Always present
Cyanosis	Common	Uncommon
Chronic hypoventilation	Common	Late in course
Polycythemia	Common	Late in course
Cor pulmonale	Common	Late in course

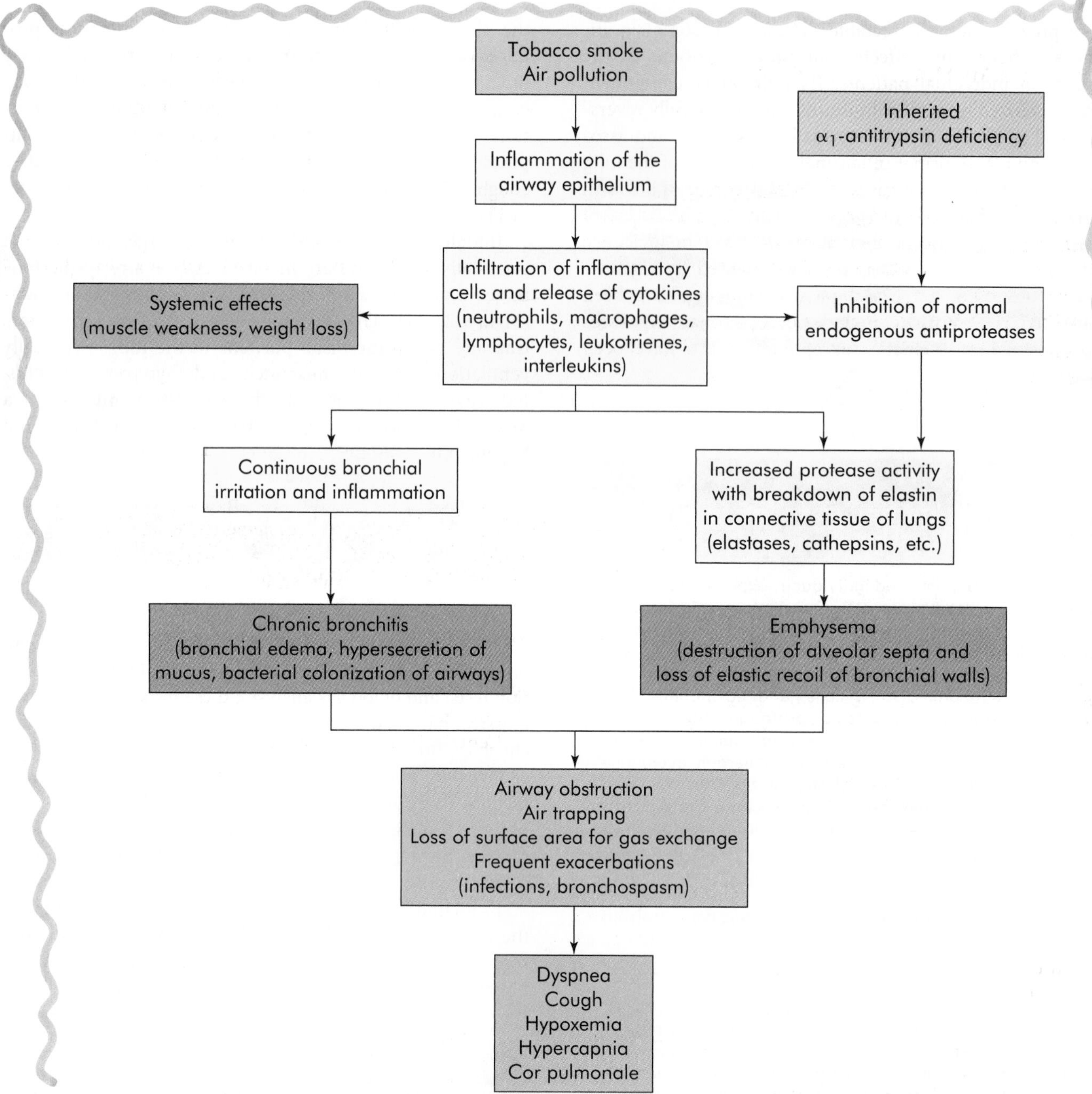

Figure 26-10 ■ **Pathogenesis of Chronic Bronchitis and Emphysema (Chronic Obstructive Pulmonary Disease [COPD]).**

HEALTH ALERT

Nutrition and Chronic Obstructive Pulmonary Disease

Malnutrition is a major concern for individuals with chronic obstructive pulmonary disease (COPD) because they have increased energy expenditure, decreased energy intake, and impaired oxygenation. The disproportionate muscle wasting is similar to what occurs with other chronic diseases, such as cancer, heart failure, and AIDS. Systemic inflammatory mediators may impair appetite and contribute to hypermetabolism. Malnutrition (1) adversely affects exercise tolerance by limiting skeletal and respiratory muscle strength and aerobic capacity, (2) limits surfactant production, (3) reduces cell-mediated immune responses, (4) reduces protein synthesis, and (5) increases morbidity and mortality. The medical nutrition therapy goal is to maintain an acceptable and stable weight for the person. This can be accomplished by including foods of high energy density, frequent snacking, soft foods and beverages, assistance with shopping, and meal preparation. Increasing omega-3 fatty acids and antioxidant intake may modulate the effects of systemic inflammation. Protein intake should be maintained at 1.0 to 1.5 g/kg of body weight, and a daily vitamin C supplement should be added to the diet if the individual is still smoking.

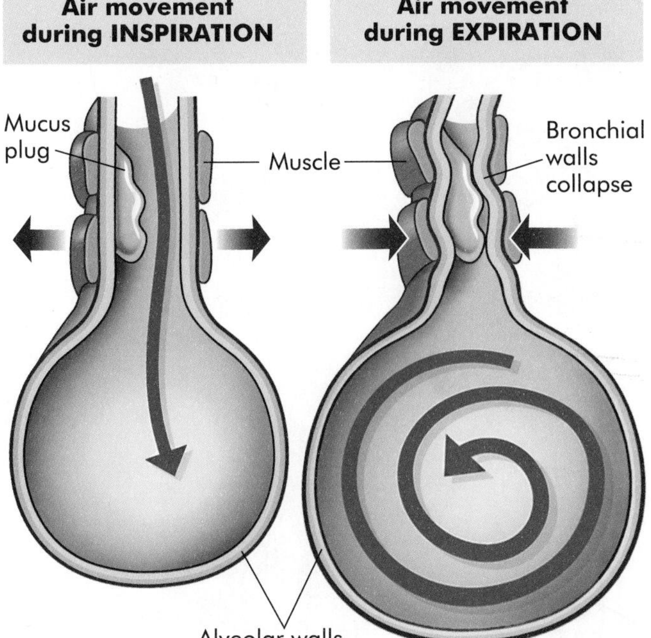

Figure 26-11 ■ **Mechanisms of Air Trapping in COPD.** Mucus plugs and narrowed airways cause air trapping and hyperinflation on expiration. During inspiration, the airways are pulled open allowing gas to flow past the obstruction. During expiration, decreased elastic recoil of the bronchial walls results in collapse of the airways and prevents normal expiratory airflow.

early signs of infection, and techniques that relieve dyspnea, such as pursed-lip breathing. During acute exacerbations (infection and bronchospasm), individuals require treatment with antibiotics and steroids and may need mechanical ventilation.[33] Chronic oral steroids may be needed late in the course of the disease but should be considered a last resort. Individuals with severe hypoxemia will require home oxygen therapy.

Emphysema

Emphysema is abnormal permanent enlargement of gas-exchange airways (acini) accompanied by destruction of alveolar walls without obvious fibrosis. Obstruction results from changes in lung tissues, rather than mucus production and inflammation as in chronic bronchitis. The major mechanism of airflow limitation is loss of elastic recoil (see Figure 26-11).[30] The major cause of emphysema by far is cigarette smoking, although air pollution and childhood respiratory infections are known to be contributing factors.

Primary emphysema, which accounts for 1% to 3% of all cases of emphysema, is commonly linked to an inherited deficiency of the enzyme α_1-antitrypsin, a major component of α_1-globulin, a plasma protein.[34] Normally α_1-antitrypsin inhibits the action of many proteolytic enzymes, therefore α_1-antitrypsin deficiency (an autosomal recessive trait) produces an increased likelihood of developing emphysema because proteolysis in lung tissues is not inhibited. α_1-Antitrypsin deficiency is suggested in individuals who develop emphysema before 40 years of age and in nonsmokers who develop the disease.

PATHOPHYSIOLOGY Emphysema begins with destruction of alveolar septa, which eliminates portions of the pulmonary capillary bed and increases the volume of air in the acinus. It is postulated that inhaled oxidants in tobacco smoke and air pollution inhibit the activity of endogenous antiproteases and stimulate inflammation with increased activity of the proteases (e.g., elastase). Thus, the balance is tipped toward alveolar destruction and loss of the normal elastic recoil of the bronchi (see Figure 26-10). Alveolar destruction produces large air spaces within the lung parenchyma (bullae) and air spaces adjacent to pleurae (blebs). Bullae and blebs are not effective in gas exchange and result in significant ventilation-perfusion ($\dot{V}/\dot{Q}$) mismatching and hypoxemia. Expiration becomes difficult because loss of elastic recoil reduces the volume of air that can be expired passively and air is trapped in the lungs (see Figure 26-11). Air trapping causes hyperexpansion of the chest, which puts the muscles of respiration at a mechanical disadvantage. This results in increased workload of breathing, so that late in the course of disease, many individuals will develop hypoventilation and hypercapnia.

Emphysema can be centriacinar (centrilobular) or panacinar (panlobular), depending on the site of involvement (Figure 26-12).[30]

1. **Centriacinar emphysema.** Septal destruction occurs in the respiratory bronchioles and alveolar ducts, causing inflammation in bronchioles. Alveolar sac is intact. Tends to occur in persons who smoke and persons with chronic bronchitis.
2. **Panacinar emphysema.** Involves entire acinus, with damage more randomly distributed and involving lower lobes of lung. Tends to occur in elderly persons and persons with α_1-antitrypsin deficiency.

CLINICAL MANIFESTATIONS The clinical manifestations of emphysema are listed in Table 26-2.

EVALUATION AND TREATMENT Pulmonary function testing, chest x-ray, high-resolution computed tomograph (CT), and arterial blood gas measurement are used to diagnose emphysema.[27,35] Pulmonary function measurements, especially FEV_1 values, also are helpful in determining the stage of disease, appropriate treatment, and prognosis.[27] Treatment for emphysema is similar to that for chronic bronchitis and includes smoking cessation, bronchodilating drugs, nutrition, breathing retraining, relaxation exercises, anti-inflammatory medications, and antibiotics for acute infections. The most recent recommendations for the management of chronic symptoms of COPD are based on the four stages of severity of airflow limitation and include bronchodilators, such as ipratropium and β_2-agonists.[27,36] Treatment of severe COPD may require the use of methylxanthines, inhaled or oral steroids, and home oxygen.[27,36,37] A new class of drugs called *phosphodiesterase E4 (PDE4)* inhibitors are proving to be effective in selected patients

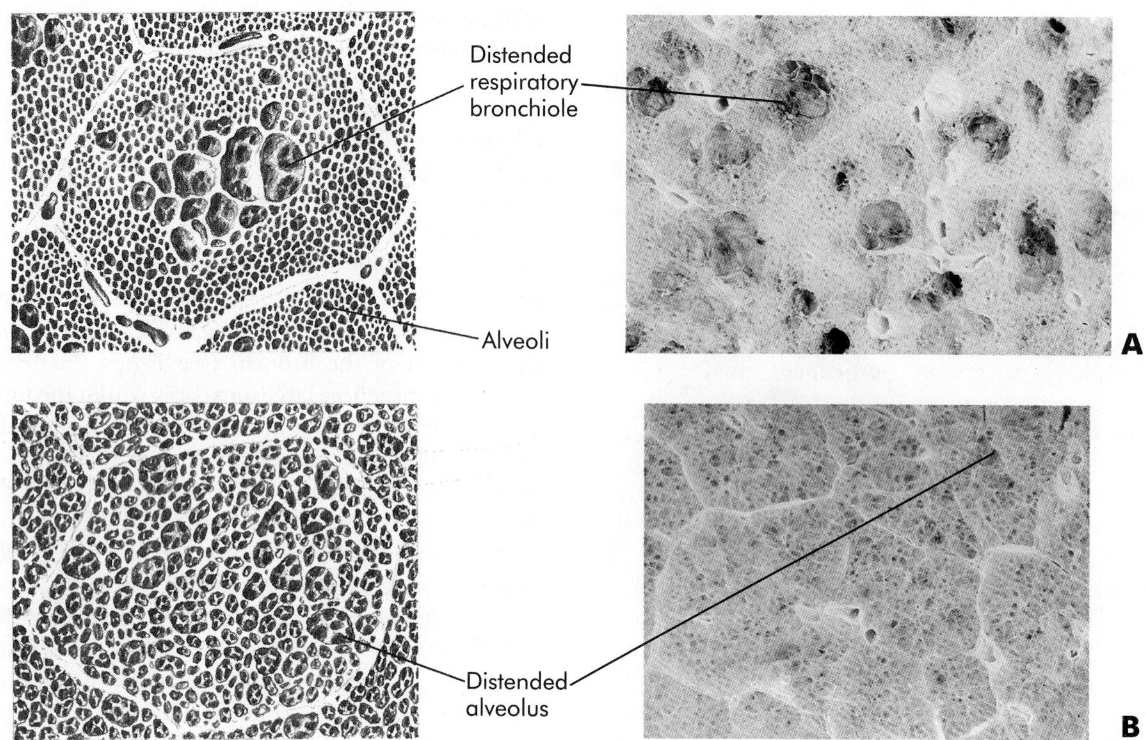

Figure 26-12 ■ **Types of Emphysema. A,** Centriacinar emphysema. **B,** Panacinar emphysema. (Micrographs from Damjanov I, Linder J, editors: *Anderson's pathology,* ed 10, St Louis, 1996, Mosby.)

with severe COPD.[38] Selected individuals with severe emphysema can benefit from lung reduction surgery or lung transplantation.

QUICK CHECK 26-4

1. What mechanisms cause obstruction in asthma?
2. How does emphysema affect oxygenation and ventilation?
3. Define chronic bronchitis.

Respiratory Tract Infections

Respiratory tract infections are the most common cause of short-term disability in the United States. Most of these infections—the common cold, pharyngitis (sore throat), and laryngitis—involve only the upper airways. Although the lungs have direct contact with the atmosphere, they usually remain sterile. Infections of the lower respiratory tract occur most often in individuals whose normal defense mechanisms are impaired.

Pneumonia

Pneumonia is infection of the lower respiratory tract caused by bacteria, viruses, fungi, protozoa, or parasites. It is the sixth leading cause of death in the United States. The incidence and mortality of pneumonia are highest in the elderly. Risk factors for pneumonia include advanced age, immunocompromise, underlying lung disease, alcoholism, altered consciousness, smoking, endotracheal intubation, malnutrition, and immobilization. The causative microorganism influences how the individual presents clinically, how the pneumonia should be treated, and the prognosis. Community-acquired pneumonia (CAP) tends to be caused by different microorganisms as compared with those infections acquired in the hospital (nosocomial). In addition, the characteristics of the individual are important in determining which etiologic microorganism is likely; for example, immunocompromised individuals tend to be susceptible to opportunistic infections that are uncommon in normal adults. In general, nosocomial infections and those affecting immunocompromised individuals have a higher mortality than CAPs. Some of the most common causal microorganisms include the following[39-41]:

Community-Acquired Pneumonia (CAP)	Nosocomial Pneumonia	Immunocompromised Individuals
Streptococcus pneumoniae	*Pseudomonas aeruginosa*	*Pneumocystis jiroveci*
Mycoplasma pneumoniae	*Staphylococcus aureus*	*Mycobacterium tuberculosis*
Haemophilus influenza	*Klebsiella pneumoniae*	Atypical mycobacteria
Oral anaerobic bacteria	*Escherichia coli*	Fungi
Influenza virus		Respiratory viruses
Legionella pneumophila		Protozoa
Chlamydia pneumoniae		Parasites
Moraxella catarrhalis		

The most common community-acquired pneumonia is caused by *Streptococcus pneumoniae* (also known as the *pneumococcus*), which has a relatively high mortality in the elderly.[42] *Mycoplasma pneumoniae* is a common cause of pneumonia in young people, especially those living in group housing such as dormitories and army barracks.[43] Influenza is the most common viral community-acquired pneumonia in adults; in children, respiratory syncytial virus and parainfluenza virus are common etiologic microorganisms.[44] *Legionella* species is an important cause of community-acquired pneumonia, and Legionnaire's disease has increased in incidence since it was first described in the 1976 incident at the American Legion Convention in Philadelphia.[45] *Pseudomonas aeruginosa,* other gram-negative microorganisms, and *Staphylococcus aureus* are the most common etiologic agents in nosocomial pneumonia.[40] Immunocompromised patients (HIV, transplant) are especially susceptible to *Pneumocystis jiroveci* (formerly called *P. carinii*), mycobacterial infections, and fungal infections of the respiratory tract.[41,46] These infections can be difficult to treat and have a high mortality.

PATHOPHYSIOLOGY Aspiration of oropharyngeal secretions is the most common route of lower respiratory tract infection; thus, the nasopharynx and oropharynx constitute the first line of defense for most infectious agents. Another route of infection is through the inhalation of microorganisms that have been released into the air when an infected individual coughs, sneezes, or talks, or from aerosolized water such as that from contaminated respiratory therapy equipment. This route of infection is most important in viral and mycobacterial pneumonias and in *Legionella* outbreaks. Pneumonia also can occur when bacteria are spread to the lung in the blood from bacteremia that can result from infection elsewhere in the body or from IV drug abuse.

In healthy individuals, pathogens that reach the lungs are expelled or held in check by mechanisms of self-defense (see Chapters 5, 6, and 7). If a microorganism gets past the upper airway defense mechanisms, such as the cough reflex and mucociliary clearance, the next line of defense is the alveolar macrophage. This phagocyte is capable of removing most infectious agents without setting off significant inflammatory or immune responses. However, if the microorganism is virulent or present in large enough numbers, it can overwhelm the alveolar macrophage. This results in a full-scale activation of the body's defense mechanisms, including the release of multiple inflammatory mediators, cellular infiltration, and immune activation.[47,48] These inflammatory mediators and immune complexes can damage bronchial mucous membranes and alveolocapillary membranes causing the acini and terminal bronchioles to fill with infectious debris and exudate. In addition, some microorganisms release toxins from their cell walls that can cause further lung damage. The accumulation of exudate in the acinus leads to dyspnea and to $\dot{V}/\dot{Q}$ mismatching and hypoxemia.

Pneumococcal pneumonia

In pneumococcal pneumonia, *S. pneumoniae* microorganisms initiate the inflammatory response, and inflammatory exudate causes alveolar edema, which leads to the other changes shown in Figure 26-13.[48]

Viral pneumonia

Although viral pneumonia can be severe (see Health Alert: Avian Influenza), it is usually mild and self-limiting but can set the stage for a secondary bacterial infection by providing an ideal environment for bacterial growth and by damaging ciliated epithelial cells, which normally prevent pathogens from reaching the lower airways. Viral pneumonia can be a primary infection or a complication of another viral illness, such as chickenpox or measles (spread from the blood). The virus not only destroys the ciliated epithelial cells but also invades the goblet cells and bronchial mucous glands. Sloughing of destroyed bronchial epithelium occurs throughout the respiratory tract, preventing mucociliary clearance. Bronchial walls become edematous and infiltrated with leukocytes. In severe cases, the alveoli are involved with decreased compliance and increased work of breathing.

HEALTH ALERT

Avian Influenza

A highly pathogenic virus called H5N1 influenza virus has been causing massive infections in poultry in Asia and was first found to infect humans in 1997. So far, most human infections have occurred only in those individuals who have been in close contact with infected birds. However, there has been at least one instance in which several cases of flu were documented within an extended family. This raises concerns that the virus is mutating to a form that can be passed from human to human. The H5N1 virus can be carried by migratory birds and is expected to spread to the United States and throughout the world. Human infection with avian influenza results in symptoms of fever, cough, sore throat, and muscle aches, eye infections (conjunctivitis), pneumonia, acute respiratory distress, and other severe and life-threatening complications. As of March 2007, a total of 279 cases and 169 deaths have been attibuted to avian influenza worldwide, most were reported in Indonesia and Vietnam. In preparation for possible viral mutation and potential human pandemic, stockpiles of two effective antivirals (oseltamivir and zanamivir) are being created. In February 2007, the WHO announced that several new vaccines have been developed that are demonstrating significant immune effectiveness and appear to be safe even in the elderly and in children. Extensive research on vaccine development is continuing.

Data from the Centers for Disease Control and Prevention, available at www.cdc.gov/flu/avian/gen-info/avian-flu-humans.htm; and the World Health Organization, available at www.who.int/csr/disease/avian_influenza/en/index.html

CLINICAL MANIFESTATIONS Many cases of pneumonia are preceded by an upper respiratory infection, which is often viral. Individuals then develop fever, chills, productive

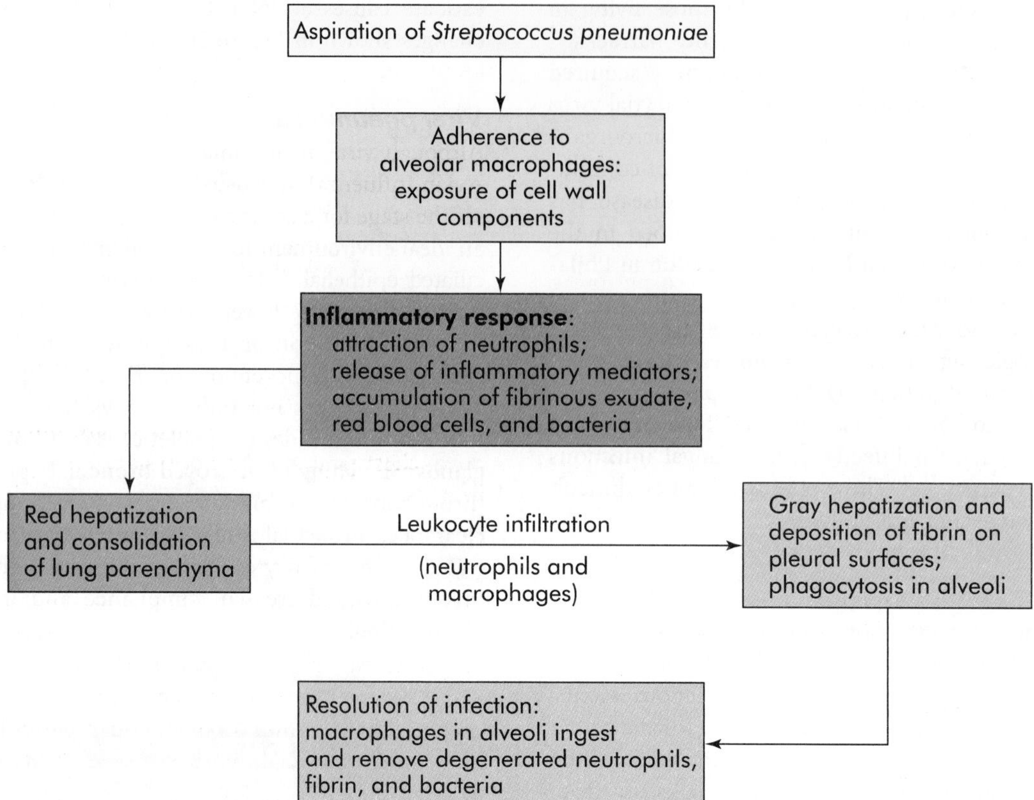

Figure 26-13 ■ **Pathophysiologic Course of Pneumococcal Pneumonia.**

or dry cough, malaise, pleural pain, and sometimes dyspnea and hemoptysis. Physical examination may reveal signs of pulmonary consolidation, such as dullness to percussion, inspiratory crackles, increased tactile fremitus, egophony, and whispered pectoriloquy. Individuals also may demonstrate symptoms and signs of underlying systemic disease or sepsis.

EVALUATION AND TREATMENT Diagnosis is made on the basis of physical examination, white blood cell count, chest x-ray, stains and cultures of respiratory secretions, and blood cultures.[49] The white blood cell count is usually elevated, although it may be low if the individual is debilitated or immunocompromised. Chest radiographs show infiltrates that may involve a single lobe of the lung or may be more diffuse. Once the diagnosis of pneumonia has been made, the pathogen is identified by means of sputum characteristics (gram stain, color, odor) and cultures or, if sputum is absent, blood cultures. Because many pathogens exist in the normal oropharyngeal flora, the specimen may be contaminated with pathogens from oral secretions. If sputum studies fail to identify the pathogen, the individual is immunocompromised, or the individual's condition worsens, further diagnostic studies may include bronchoscopy or lung biopsy. Positive identification of viruses can be difficult. Blood cultures often help to identify the virus if systemic disease is present.

Antibiotics are used to treat bacterial pneumonia; however, resistant strains of pneumococcus are on the rise.[50] Empiric antibiotics are chosen based on the likely causative microorganism.[49] Viral pneumonia is usually treated with supportive therapy alone; however, antivirals may be needed in severe cases. Infections with opportunistic microorganisms may be polymicrobial and require multiple drugs, including antifungals. Adequate hydration and good pulmonary hygiene (e.g., deep breathing, coughing, chest physical therapy) are important aspects of treatment for all types of pneumonia.

Tuberculosis

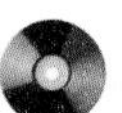

Tuberculosis (TB) is an infection caused by *Mycobacterium tuberculosis,* an acid-fast bacillus that usually affects the lungs but may invade other body systems. Tuberculosis is the leading cause of death from a curable infectious disease in the world. TB cases increased greatly during the mid-1990s as a result of the acquired immunodeficiency syndrome (AIDS).[51] In 2005, a total of 14,093 TB cases were reported in the United States, representing a 3.8% decline in the rate from 2004. This decline was the result of more effective treatment of HIV-infected individuals. Even so, individuals with AIDS are highly susceptible to infection with multidrug resistant tuberculosis that is difficult to manage.[52,53] Emigration of infected individuals from high-prevalence countries, transmission in crowded institutional settings, homelessness, substance abuse, and lack of access to medical care also have contributed to the spread of TB.

HEALTH ALERT

Multidrug Resistant Tuberculosis in HIV Infection

Tuberculosis is the leading cause of death from a curable infectious disease in the world, with 8.8 million new cases of tuberculosis documented in 2005. Although the total number of cases continues to increase, the rate of new TB cases appears to be leveling off for the first time. Africa continues to have the highest estimated incidence rate, but the majority of patients with tuberculosis live in the most populous countries of Asia including Bangladesh, China, India, Indonesia, and Pakistan. The incidence rate in these countries is highest among young adults, and most cases are the result of recent infection or reinfection. Much of the increase in global tuberculosis incidence seen since 1980 is attributable to the spread of HIV, especially in Africa. HIV infection is the most common identifiable risk factor for progression from latent TB to active disease (reactivation). Treatment of TB in HIV-infected persons is characterized by relatively good short-term responses (especially if rifampicin [rifampin] is used as a primary drug) but becomes more difficult as both diseases progress and is associated with more adverse reactions to the antituberculous medications. This scenario is made even more challenging by the increasing prevalence of multidrug resistant TB microorganisms.

Data from de Jong BC et al: Clinical management of tuberculosis in the context of HIV infection, *Annu Rev Med* 55:283–301, 2004; Nunn P et al: Tuberculosis control in the era of HIV, *Nat Rev Immunol* 5(10):819–826, 2005; and the World Health Organization at http://www.who.int/tb/en/.

PATHOPHYSIOLOGY Tuberculosis is transmitted from person to person in airborne droplets. Microorganisms lodge in the lung periphery, usually in the upper lobe. Once the bacilli are inspired into the lung, they multiply and cause nonspecific pneumonitis (lung inflammation). Some bacilli migrate through the lymphatics and become lodged in the lymph nodes, where they encounter lymphocytes and initiate the immune response.

Inflammation in the lung causes activation of alveolar macrophages and neutrophils. These cells are phagocytes that engulf the bacilli and begin the process by which the body's defense mechanisms isolate the bacilli, preventing their spread. The neutrophils and macrophages seal off the colonies of bacilli, forming a granulomatous lesion called a *tubercle* (see Chapter 5). Infected tissues within the tubercle die, forming cheeselike material called *caseation necrosis.*[54,55] Collagenous scar tissue then grows around the tubercle, completing isolation of the bacilli. The immune response is complete after about 10 days, preventing further multiplication of the bacilli.

Once the bacilli are isolated in tubercles and immunity develops, tuberculosis may remain dormant for life.[54,55] If the immune system is impaired, however, or if live bacilli escape into the bronchi, active disease occurs and may spread through the blood and lymphatics to other organs. Endogenous reactivation of dormant bacilli may be caused by poor nutritional status, insulin-dependent diabetes, long-term corticosteroid therapy, the use of antirejection drugs, HIV infection, and other debilitating diseases.

CLINICAL MANIFESTATIONS In many infected individuals, tuberculosis is asymptomatic. In others, symptoms develop so gradually that they are not noticed until the disease is advanced. Common clinical manifestations include fatigue, weight loss, lethargy, anorexia (loss of appetite), and a low-grade fever that usually occurs in the afternoon. A cough that produces purulent sputum develops slowly and becomes more frequent over several weeks or months. Night sweats and general anxiety are often present. Dyspnea, chest pain, and hemoptysis may occur as the disease progresses. Extrapulmonary TB disease is common in HIV infected individuals and may cause neurologic deficits, meningitis symptoms, bone pain, and urinary symptoms.[56]

EVALUATION AND TREATMENT Tuberculosis is usually diagnosed by a positive tuberculin skin test, sputum culture, and chest radiographs. Newer diagnostic tests include the enzyme-linked immunospot and quantitative blood interferon-gamma assay that improve the sensitivity and specificity of skin testing.[57,58]

Treatment consists of antibiotic therapy to control active or dormant tuberculosis and prevent transmission. Today, with the increased numbers of immunosuppressed individuals and drug-resistant bacilli, the recommended treatment includes a combination of drugs to which the organism is susceptible, including use of isoniazid, rifampin, pyrazinamide, ethambutol, and streptomycin. Treatment usually is continued for a minimum of 3 months.[58,59] Infection in immunocompromised individuals often require the use of newer drugs for longer periods of time.[52,53,58,59]

In the past, individuals with active tuberculosis were isolated from the community and their families in sanitariums. Today, individuals remain at home or, rarely, in the hospital, until sputum cultures show that the active bacilli have been eliminated. This usually takes a few weeks to 2 months if antibiotics are taken conscientiously. Long-acting antituberculous medications have improved adherence in outpatient clinical settings. If the individual's cooperation is in question, it is advisable for the administration of the drugs to be supervised by health care workers.

Acute bronchitis

Acute bronchitis is acute infection or inflammation of the airways or bronchi and is usually self-limiting. In the vast majority of cases, acute bronchitis is caused by viruses.[60] Many clinical manifestations are similar to those of pneumonia (i.e., fever, cough, chills, malaise), but chest radiographs show no infiltrates. Individuals with viral bronchitis present with a nonproductive cough that often occurs in paroxysms and is aggravated by cold, dry, or dusty air. In some cases, purulent sputum is produced. Chest pain often develops from the effort of coughing. Treatment consists of rest, aspirin, humidity, and a cough suppressant, such as codeine.[60]

Bacterial bronchitis is rare in previously healthy adults except after viral infection but is common in patients with COPD. Although individuals with bronchitis do not have signs of pulmonary consolidation on physical examination (e.g., crackles, egophony), many will require chest x-ray evaluation to exclude the diagnosis of pneumonia. Bacterial bronchitis is treated with rest, antipyretics, humidity, and antibiotics.

Abscess formation and cavitation

An **abscess** is a circumscribed area of suppuration and destruction of lung parenchyma. Abscess formation follows **consolidation** of lung tissue, in which inflammation causes alveoli to fill with fluid, pus, and microorganisms. Necrosis (death and decay) of consolidated tissue may progress proximally until it communicates with a bronchus. **Cavitation** is the process of the abscess emptying into a bronchus and cavity formation. The diagnosis is made by chest radiography.

Pneumonia caused by aspiration, *Klebsiella,* or *Staphylococcus* is the most common cause of abscess formation. Aspiration abscess is usually associated with alcohol abuse, seizure disorders, general anesthesia, and swallowing disorders. The clinical manifestations of abscess formation are similar to those of pneumonitis: fever, cough, chills, sputum production, and pleural pain. Abscess communication with a bronchus causes a severe cough, copious amounts of often foul-smelling sputum, and occasionally hemoptysis.

Treatment includes the administration of appropriate antibiotics and chest physical therapy, including chest percussion and postural drainage. Sometimes bronchoscopy is performed to drain the abscess.

✔ QUICK CHECK 26-5

1. Compare pneumococcal and viral pneumonia as to severity of disease.
2. Describe the pathophysiologic features of tuberculosis.
3. How does lung abscess present clinically?

Pulmonary Vascular Disease

Blood flow through the lungs can be disrupted by disorders that occlude the vessels, increase pulmonary vascular resistance, or destroy the vascular bed. Effects of altered pulmonary blood flow may range from insignificant dysfunction to severe and life-threatening changes in ventilation-perfusion ratios. Major disorders include pulmonary embolism, pulmonary hypertension, and cor pulmonale.

Pulmonary embolism

Pulmonary embolism is occlusion of a portion of the pulmonary vascular bed by an embolus, which can be a thrombus (blood clot), tissue fragment, lipids (fats), foreign body, or an air bubble. More than 90% of pulmonary emboli result from clots formed in the veins of the legs and pelvis.

Risk factors for **pulmonary thromboembolism,** or the obstruction of a pulmonary vessel by a thrombus, include conditions and disorders that promote blood clotting as a result of venous stasis (slowing or stagnation of blood flow through the veins), hypercoagulability (increased tendency of the blood to form clots), and injuries to the endothelial cells that line the vessels. Genetic risks include factor V Leiden, antithrombin II, protein S, protein C, and prothrombin gene mutations.[49] No matter its source, a blood clot becomes an embolus when all or part of it breaks away from the site of formation and begins to travel in the bloodstream. (Thromboembolism is described further in Chapter 20.)

Although the overall incidence of pulmonary embolism has declined, it remains an important cause of death, especially in elderly and hospitalized persons.[50] Trauma, especially head injuries and fractures of the lower extremities, spine, or pelvis, confers a high risk for venous thromboembolism.[51]

PATHOPHYSIOLOGY The impact or effect of the embolus depends on the extent of pulmonary blood flow obstruction, the size of the affected vessels, the nature of the embolus, and the secondary effects. Pulmonary emboli can occur as any of the following:

1. Massive occlusion: an embolus that occludes a major portion of the pulmonary circulation (i.e., main pulmonary artery embolus)
2. Embolus with infarction: an embolus that is large enough to cause infarction (death) of a portion of lung tissue
3. Embolus without infarction: an embolus that is not severe enough to cause permanent lung injury
4. Multiple pulmonary emboli: may be chronic or recurrent

The pathogenesis of pulmonary embolism caused by a thrombus is summarized in Figure 26-14.

If the embolus does not cause infarction, the clot is dissolved by the fibrinolytic system and pulmonary function returns to normal. If pulmonary infarction occurs, shrinking and scarring develop in the affected area of the lung.

CLINICAL MANIFESTATIONS In most cases, the clinical manifestations of pulmonary embolism are nonspecific, so evaluation of risk factors and predisposing factors is an important aspect of diagnosis. Although most emboli originate from clots in the lower extremities, deep vein thrombosis is often asymptomatic, and clinical examination has low sensitivity for the presence of clot, especially in the thigh.

An individual with pulmonary embolism usually presents with the sudden onset of pleuritic chest pain, dyspnea, tachypnea, tachycardia, and unexplained anxiety. Occasionally syncope (fainting) or hemoptysis occurs. With large emboli, a pleural friction rub, pleural effusion, fever, and leukocytosis may be noted. Recurrent small emboli may

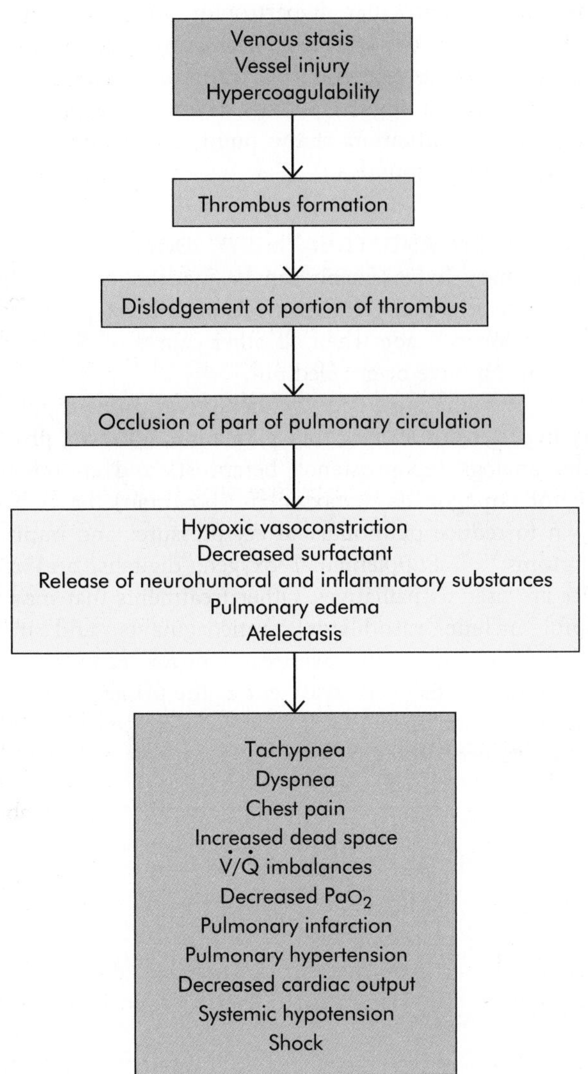

Figure 26-14 ■ Pathogenesis of Massive Pulmonary Embolism Caused by a Thrombus (Pulmonary Thromboembolism).

not be detected until progressive incapacitation, precordial pain, anxiety, dyspnea, and right ventricular enlargement are exhibited. Massive occlusion causes severe pulmonary hypertension and shock.

EVALUATION AND TREATMENT Routine chest radiographs and pulmonary function tests are not definitive for pulmonary embolism. On chest radiographs, the infarcted portion of the lung appears as a nonspecific infiltrate in a classic wedge shape bordering the pleura. Arterial blood gas analyses usually demonstrate hypoxemia and hyperventilation (respiratory alkalosis). A ventilation/perfusion scan ($\dot{V}/\dot{Q}$ scan), in which lungs are scanned after injection and inhalation of a radioactive substances, may indicate embolism; however, this test is rarely definitive. Today, the diagnosis is made by measuring elevated levels of D-dimer in the blood in combination with spiral computed tomography (CT).[61–63]

The ideal treatment for pulmonary embolism is prevention through elimination of predisposing factors for individuals at risk. Venous stasis in hospital patients is minimized by leg elevation, bed exercises, position changes, early postoperative ambulation, and pneumatic calf compression. Clot formation is also prevented by prophylactic low-dose anticoagulant therapy usually with low-molecular-weight heparin or warfarin. Newer medications such as the antithrombotics fondaparinux, idraparinux, and ximelagatran are superior to standard prevention in high-risk individuals undergoing orthopedic surgery.[64]

Anticoagulant therapy is the primary treatment for pulmonary embolism. Intravenous administration of heparin is begun immediately and is followed by oral doses of coumarin. Studies suggest that low-molecular-weight heparins (e.g., enoxaparin) are as safe and effective as standard heparin but are easier to administer.[63,64] If a massive life-threatening embolism occurs, a fibrinolytic agent, such as streptokinase, is sometimes used, and some individuals will require surgical thrombectomy.

Pulmonary hypertension

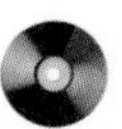

Pulmonary hypertension is defined as a mean pulmonary artery pressure 5 to 10 mm Hg above normal or above 20 mm Hg. Pulmonary hypertension is classified as primary or secondary.

Primary pulmonary hypertension (PPH) is an idiopathic form of pulmonary artery hypertension and is characterized by pathologic changes in precapillary pulmonary arteries.[65,66] Primary pulmonary hypertension is rare, has no known cause, usually occurs in women between the ages of 20 and 40 years, and may be hereditary, although only 10% to 20% of those with a genetic predisposition actually develop the disease. Risk factors for PPH include HIV infection, collagen vascular diseases, and the use of appetite suppressants.

Most pulmonary hypertension is called *secondary pulmonary hypertension* and results from diseases of the respiratory system that cause hypoxemia and are characterized by pulmonary arteriolar vasoconstriction and arterial remodeling.[65] In some cases, pulmonary hypertension is the result of recurrent pulmonary emboli; however, this is relatively uncommon. Pulmonary venous hypertension is caused by congestive heart failure and is discussed in Chapters 20 and 23.

PATHOPHYSIOLOGY PPH is considered an idiopathic disorder characterized by endothelial dysfunction with overproduction of vasoconstrictors, such as thromboxane and endothelin, and decreased production of vasodilators, such as prostacyclin.[66] Vascular growth factors are released that cause changes in the vascular smooth wall called *remodeling.* Angiotensin II, serotonin, electrolyte transporter mechanisms, and nitric oxide also play a role in the pathogenesis of this disorder. Together, this results in pathologic changes in the pulmonary vasculature characterized by fibrosis and thickening of the vessel wall with luminal narrowing and abnormal vasoconstriction. These changes cause resistance to pulmonary artery blood flow, thus increasing the pressure in the pulmonary arteries. As resistance and pressure increase, the workload of the right ventricle increases and subsequent right ventricular hypertrophy, followed by failure, may occur *(cor pulmonale)*. This eventually results in the death of most individuals with PPH.

Secondary pulmonary hypertension can often be reversed if the primary disorder is resolved quickly. If hypertension persists, hypertrophy occurs in the medial smooth muscle layer of the arterioles. The larger arteries stiffen, and hypertension progresses until pulmonary artery pressure equals systemic blood pressure, causing right ventricular hypertrophy and eventually cor pulmonale. The pathogenesis of pulmonary hypertension and cor pulmonale resulting from disease of the respiratory system is shown in Figure 26-15.

CLINICAL MANIFESTATIONS Pulmonary hypertension may not be detected until it is quite severe. The symptoms are often masked by primary pulmonary or cardiovascular disease. The first indication of pulmonary hypertension may be an abnormality seen on a chest radiograph (enlarged right heart border) or an electrocardiogram that shows right ventricular hypertrophy. Manifestations of fatigue, chest discomfort, tachypnea, and dyspnea, particularly with exercise, are common. Examination may reveal peripheral edema, jugular venous distension, a precordial heave, and accentuation of the pulmonary component of the second heart sound.

COPD
Interstitial fibrosis
Obesity-hypoventilation syndrome
↓
Chronic hypoxemia
Chronic acidosis
↓
Pulmonary artery vasoconstriction
↓
Increased pulmonary artery pressure
↓
Intimal fibrosis and hypertrophy of medial smooth muscle layer of pulmonary arteries
↓
Chronic pulmonary hypertension
↓
Cor pulmonale (hypertrophy and dilation of right ventricle)
↓
Right heart failure

Progression of pulmonary hypertension can be reversed at this point with effective treatment of primary or underlying disease

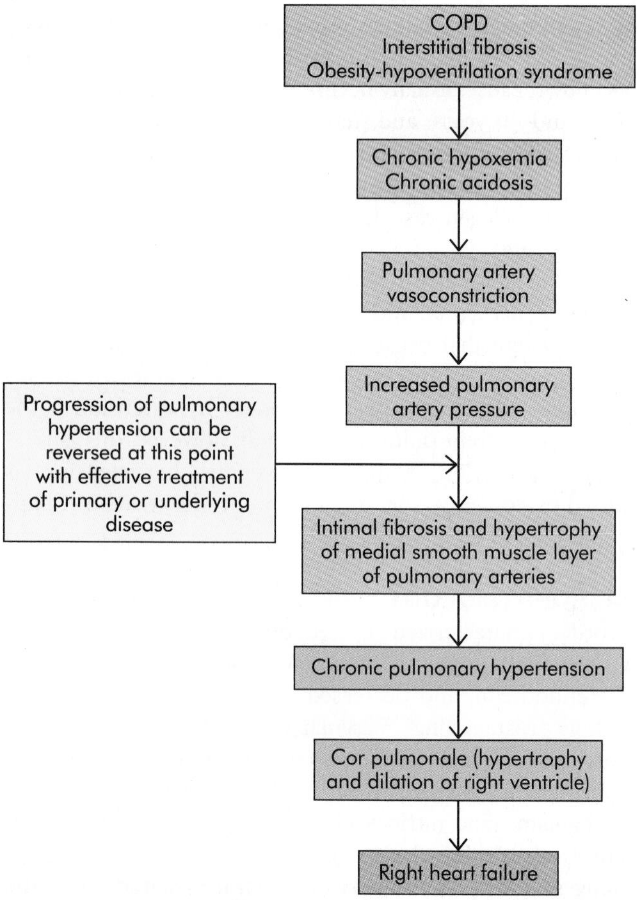

Figure 26-15 ■ Pathogenesis of Pulmonary Hypertension and Cor Pulmonale.

EVALUATION AND TREATMENT Definitive diagnosis of pulmonary hypertension can be made only with right heart catheterization. The diagnosis of primary pulmonary hypertension is made when all other causes of pulmonary hypertension have been ruled out.

Currently, the most effective therapy for primary pulmonary hypertension is lung transplantation; however, prostacyclin analogs (epoprostenol, beraprost) and endothelin-receptor antagonists (sitaxsentan, bosentan) have been shown to reduce pulmonary artery pressures and improve symptoms.[67-69] Supplemental oxygen, digitalis, and diuretics are used as palliatives. Other treatments that may be helpful include vasodilators, anticoagulants, and nitric oxide.[67,68] The most effective treatment for secondary pulmonary hypertension is treatment of the primary disorder. Treatment often includes supplemental oxygen to reverse hypoxic vasoconstriction.

Cor pulmonale

Cor pulmonale, also called *pulmonary heart disease,* consists of right ventricular enlargement (hypertrophy, dilation, or both) and failure. It is caused by primary or secondary pulmonary hypertension (see Figure 26-15).

PATHOPHYSIOLOGY Cor pulmonale develops as pulmonary hypertension creates chronic pressure overload in the right ventricle, similar to that created in the left ventricle by systemic hypertension. (Systemic hypertension is discussed in Chapter 23.) Pressure overload increases the work of the right ventricle and first causes hypertrophy of the normally thin-walled heart muscle, but eventually leads to dilation and failure of the ventricle. Acute hypoxemia, as with pneumonia, can exaggerate pulmonary hypertension and dilate the ventricle as well. The right ventricle usually fails when pulmonary artery pressure equals systemic blood pressure.

CLINICAL MANIFESTATIONS The clinical manifestations of cor pulmonale may be obscured by primary respiratory disease and appear only during exercise testing. The heart may appear normal at rest, but with exercise, cardiac output falls. The electrocardiogram may show right ventricular hypertrophy. The pulmonary component of the second heart sound, which represents closure of the pulmonic valve, may be accentuated, and a pulmonic valve murmur also may be present. Tricuspid valve murmur may accompany the development of right ventricular failure. Increased pressures in the systemic venous circulation cause jugular venous distension, hepatosplenomegaly, and peripheral edema.

EVALUATION AND TREATMENT Diagnosis is based on physical examination, radiologic examination, electrocardiogram, and echocardiography. The goal of treatment for cor pulmonale is to decrease the workload of the right ventricle by lowering pulmonary artery pressure. Treatment is the same as for pulmonary hypertension, and its success depends on reversal of the underlying lung disease.

QUICK CHECK 26-6

1. What factors influence the impact of an embolus?
2. List three causes of pulmonary hypertension.
3. What is cor pulmonale?

Respiratory Tract Malignancies

Lip cancer

Cancer of the lip is more prevalent in men, with 2000 new cases per year.[70] Long-term exposure to sun, wind, and cold over a period of years results in dryness, chapping, hyperkeratosis, and predisposition to malignancy. In addition, immunosuppression, such as that seen in individuals with renal transplants, increases the risk for lip cancer. The lower lip is the most common site.

PATHOPHYSIOLOGY The most common form of lower lip cancer is termed *exophytic.* The lesion usually develops in the outer part of the lip along the vermilion border. The lip becomes thickened and evolves to an ulcerated center with a raised border (Figure 26-16). Verrucous-type lesions are less common. They have an irregular surface, follow cracks in the lip, and tend to extend toward the inner surface. Squamous cell carcinoma is the most common cell type. Basal cell carcinoma does not develop unless there is extension from the mucous membrane or vermilion border of the lip.

CLINICAL MANIFESTATIONS Malignant lesions are often preceded by the development of a blister that evolves into a superficial ulceration. There may be a history of recurrent scales that precede development of a bleeding ulceration. Metastases to the cervical lymph nodes have a low rate of occurrence (2% to 8%) and are more likely when the primary lesion is larger and exists for a longer period.

EVALUATION AND TREATMENT Diagnosis is commonly made by clinical history and presentation of the lesion. Biopsy confirms the presence of malignant cells. The staging for lip cancer is summarized in Box 26-1. Surgical excision is effective for smaller lesions. A relatively new surgical technique, called the *Mohs micrographic surgery,* has been found to be highly effective and is associated with a low risk of local recurrence (8%). Larger lesions that require extensive resection may be followed by cosmetic surgeries. The prognosis for recovery is excellent, and deaths are usually the result of inadequate treatment.

Laryngeal cancer

Cancer of the larynx represents approximately 2% to 3% of all cancers in the United States, and 11,300 new cases are estimated for 2007.[70] The risk of laryngeal cancer is increased by the amount of tobacco smoked; risk is further heightened with the combination of smoking and alcohol consumption. More recently, the human papillomavirus (HPV) has been implicated as a cause of laryngeal cancer.[71] The highest incidence is in men between 50 and 75 years of age.

PATHOPHYSIOLOGY Carcinoma of the true vocal cords (glottis) is more common than that of the supraglottic structures (epiglottis, aryepiglottic folds, arytenoids, false cords). Tumors of the subglottic area are rare. Squamous cell carcinoma is the most common cell type, although small cell carcinomas also occur (Figure 26-17). Metastasis develops by spread to the draining lymph nodes, and distant metastasis, usually to the lung, is rare.

CLINICAL MANIFESTATIONS The presenting symptoms of laryngeal cancer include hoarseness, dyspnea, and cough. Progressive hoarseness is the most significant symptom and can result in voice loss. Dyspnea is rare with

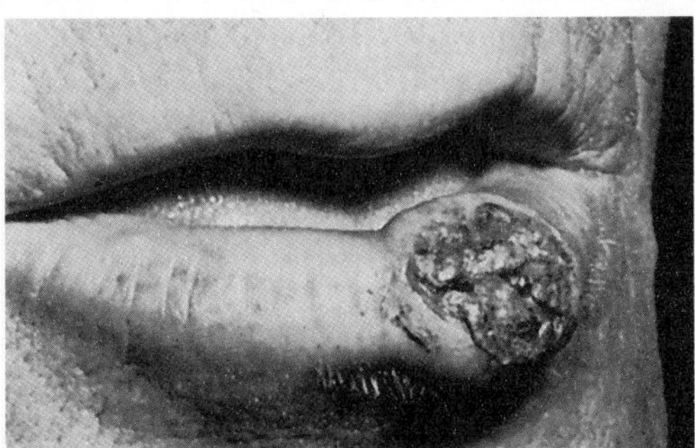

Figure 26-16 ■ **Lip Cancer.** Carcinoma of lower lip with central ulceration and raised, rolled borders. (From del Regato JA, Spjut HJ, Cox JD: *Ackerman and del Regato's cancer,* ed 2, St Louis, 1985, Mosby.)

BOX 26-1 Staging of Lip Cancer

Stage I
Primary tumor less than 2 cm; no palpable nodes

Stage II
Primary tumor 2 to 4 cm; no palpable nodes

Stage III
Primary tumor over 4 cm; metastasis to lymph nodes

Stage IV
Large primary tumors; nodes fixed to mandible or distant metastases

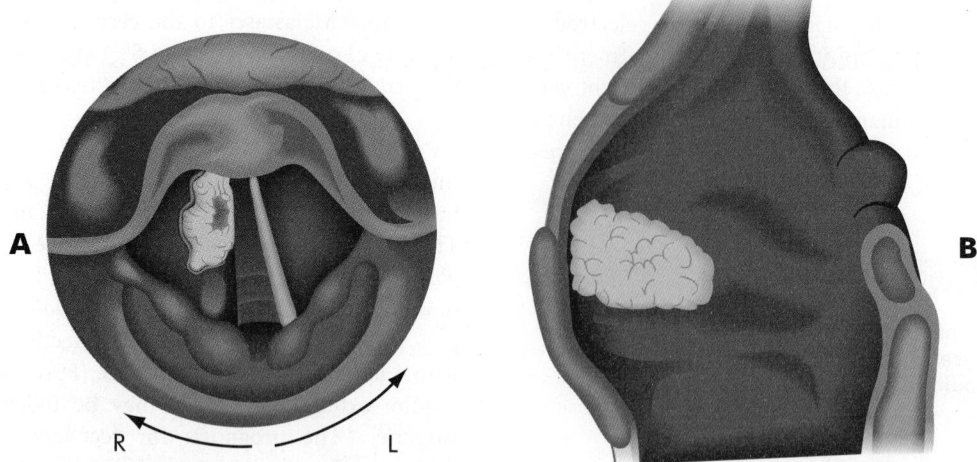

Figure 26-17 ■ **Laryngeal Cancer. A,** Mirror view of carcinoma of the right false cord partially hiding the true cord. **B,** Lateral view. (Redrawn from del Regato JA, Spjut HJ, Cox JD: *Ackerman and del Regato's cancer,* ed 2, St Louis, 1985, Mosby.)

supraglottic tumors but can be severe in subglottic tumors. Cough occurs less commonly and may follow swallowing. Laryngeal pain or a sore throat is likely with supraglottic lesions.

EVALUATION AND TREATMENT Evaluation of the larynx includes external inspection and palpation of the larynx and the lymph nodes of the neck. Indirect laryngoscopy provides a stereoscopic view of the structure and movement of the larynx. A biopsy also can be obtained during this procedure. Direct laryngoscopy provides specific visualization of the tumor. Plain films of the larynx and computed tomography facilitate the identification of tumor boundaries and the degree of extension to surrounding tissue.

Radiation therapy has shown good results for early carcinoma of the vocal cords and is used as an adjunct to surgery in more advanced disease. Endoscopic laser for partial laryngectomies is emerging as the preferred treatment for small supraglottic and subglottic malignancies. Total laryngectomy is required when lesions are extensive and involve the cartilage. Efforts to preserve voice function and improve quality of life continue to be evaluated.[72]

Lung cancer

Lung cancers (bronchogenic carcinomas) arise from the epithelium of the respiratory tract. Therefore, the term *lung cancer* excludes other pulmonary tumors, including sarcomas, lymphomas, blastomas, hematomas, and mesotheliomas. Lung cancer is an epidemic in the United States, with an estimated 213,380 new cases in 2007 (15% of all cancer sites).[70] It is the most common cause of cancer death and is responsible for 29% of all deaths in the United States.

Deaths caused by lung cancer in men have declined, and the death rate in women is approaching a plateau after a long period of increase. One-year survival in individuals with lung cancer increased from 37% to 42% since the early 1980s, but overall 5-year survival remains low at 16%.[70]

The most common cause of lung cancer is cigarette smoking. Secondhand (environmental) smoke exposure has also been identified as a risk for lung cancer. Smokers with obstructive lung disease (low FEV_1) are at even greater risk. Genetic predisposition to developing lung cancer, which is evident in analysis of pedigrees, also plays a role in its pathophysiology. Other risk factors for lung cancer include occupational exposures to certain workplace toxins, radiation, air pollution, and tuberculosis.

Types of lung cancer

Primary lung cancers arise from the bronchi within the lungs and are therefore called *bronchogenic carcinomas.* Although there are many types of lung cancer, lung cancer is divided into two major categories, non–small cell lung carcinoma (NSCLC, 75% to 85% of all lung cancers) and small cell lung carcinoma (SCLC, 15% to 20% of all lung cancers). The category of non–small cell carcinoma can be subdivided into three common types of lung cancer: squamous cell carcinoma, adenocarcinoma, and large cell undifferentiated carcinoma. Characteristics of these tumors, including clinical manifestations, are listed in Table 26-3. Many cancers that arise in other organs of the body metastasize to the lungs; however, these are not considered lung cancers and are categorized by their primary site of origin.

Non-small cell lung cancer. **Squamous cell carcinoma** accounts for about 30% of bronchogenic carcinomas, representing a sharp decline in incidence since the mid-1980s. These tumors are typically located near the hilum and project into bronchi (Figure 26-18, *A*). Because of the location in the central bronchi, obstructive manifestations are nonspecific and include nonproductive cough or hemoptysis. Pneumonia and atelectasis are often associated with

TABLE 26-3

Characteristics of Lung Cancers

Tumor Type	Growth Rate	Metastasis	Means of Diagnosis	Clinical Manifestations and Treatment
NON–SMALL CELL CARCINOMA				
Squamous cell carcinoma	Slow	Late; mostly to hilar lymph nodes	Biopsy, sputum analysis, bronchoscopy, electron microscopy, immunohistochemistry	Cough, hemoptysis, sputum production, airway obstruction, hypercalcemia; treated surgically, chemotherapy and radiation as adjunctive therapy
Adenocarcinoma	Moderate	Early; to lymph nodes, pleura, bone, adrenal glands and brain	Radiography, fiber-optic bronchoscopy, electron microscopy	Pleural effusion; treated surgically, chemotherapy as adjunctive therapy
Large cell carcinoma	Rapid	Early and widespread	Sputum analysis, bronchoscopy, electron microscopy (by exclusion of other cell types)	Chest wall pain, pleural effusion, cough, sputum production, hemoptysis, airway obstruction resulting in pneumonia; treated surgically
SMALL CELL CARCINOMA				
	Very rapid	Very early; to mediastinum, lymph nodes, brain, bone marrow	Radiography, sputum analysis, bronchoscopy, electron microscopy, immunohistochemistry	Cough, chest pain, dyspnea, hemoptysis, localized wheezing, airway obstruction, signs and symptoms of excessive hormone secretion; treated by chemotherapy and ionizing radiation to thorax and central nervous system

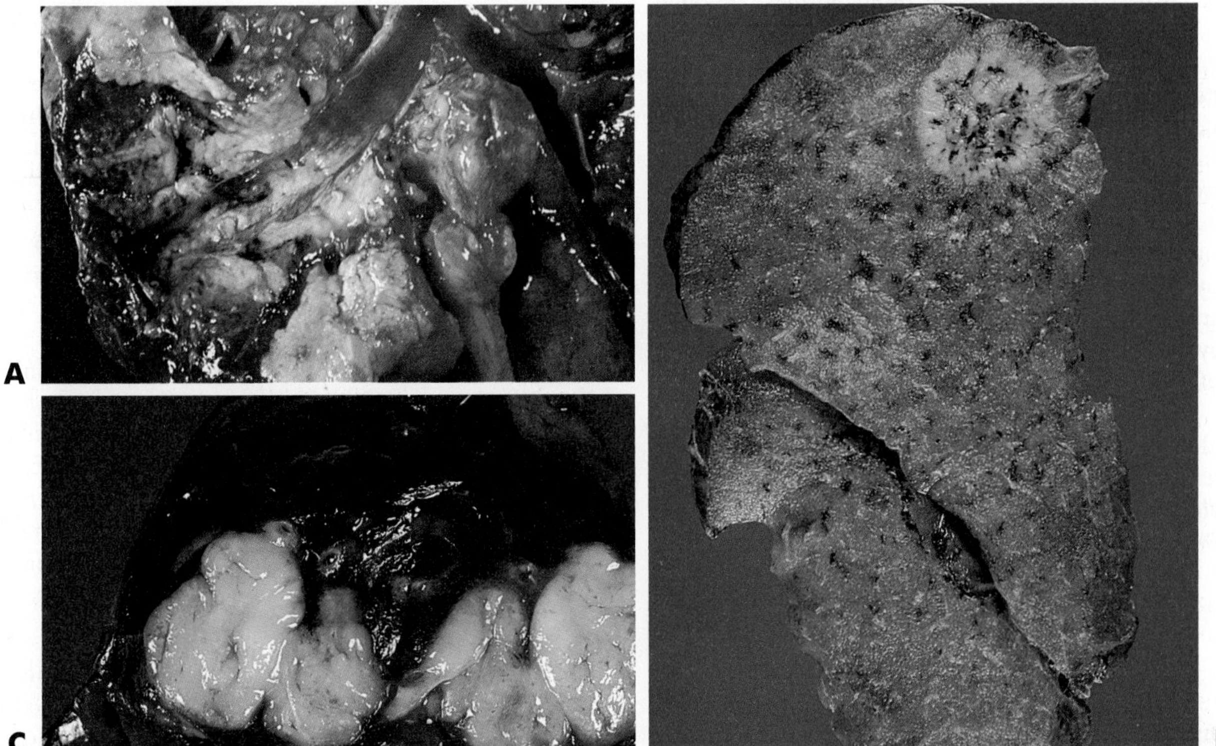

Figure 26-18 ■ **Lung Cancer. A,** Squamous cell carcinoma. This hilar tumor originates from the main bronchus. **B,** Peripheral adenocarcinoma. The tumor shows prominent black pigmentation, suggestive of having evolved in an anthracotic scar. **C,** Small cell carcinoma. The tumor forms confluent nodules. On cross section, the nodules have an encephaloid appearance. (From Damjanov I, Linder J, editors: *Anderson's pathology,* ed 10, St Louis, 1996, Mosby.)

squamous cell carcinoma (see Figure 26-18, *A*). Chest pain is a late symptom associated with large tumors. These tumors can remain fairly well localized and tend not to metastasize until late in the course of the disease. The preferred treatment is surgical resection, although once metastasis has taken place, total surgical resection is more difficult and survival rates dramatically decrease.[73,74] Adjunctive radiation and chemotherapy improve outcomes in many individuals.[75]

Adenocarcinoma (tumor arising from glands) of the lung constitutes 35% to 40% of all bronchogenic carcinomas (Figure 26-18, *B*). The increase in incidence of adenocarcinoma has been ascribed to the increasing occurrence of lung cancer in women, environmental and occupational carcinogens, and changes in the histologic criteria for diagnosis. These tumors, which are usually smaller than 4 cm, more commonly arise in the peripheral regions of the pulmonary parenchyma. They may be asymptomatic and discovered by routine chest roentgenogram in the early stages, or the individual may present with pleuritic chest pain and shortness of breath from pleural involvement by the tumor.

Included in the category of adenocarcinoma is bronchioloalveolar cell carcinoma. These tumors tend to arise from the terminal bronchioles and alveoli. They are slow-growing tumors with an unpredictable pattern of metastasis. Metastasis occurs through the pulmonary arterial system and mediastinal lymph nodes. This cell type has the weakest association with smoking.

Surgical resection is possible in a high proportion of cases, but because metastasis occurs early, the 5-year survival rate is less than 15%. Newer chemotherapy agents are resulting in increased survival rates in recent studies, although benefits must be balanced with the considerable toxicities of these drugs.[75]

Large cell carcinomas constitute 10% to15% of bronchogenic carcinomas. This cell type has lost all evidence of differentiation and is therefore sometimes referred to as undifferentiated large cell anaplastic cancer. Because large cell carcinomas show none of the histologic findings of squamous cell carcinoma or adenocarcinoma, they are diagnosed by a process of exclusion. The cells are large and contain darkly stained nuclei. These tumors commonly arise centrally and can grow to distort the trachea and cause widening of the carina. Once metastasis has occurred, surgical therapy is limited to palliative procedures (comfort measures) designed to relieve obstructive pneumonitis or prevent recurrence of pleural effusion.

Small cell lung cancer. **Small cell carcinomas** constitute 15% to 20% of bronchogenic carcinomas. Most of these tumors are central in origin (Figure 26-18, *C*). Cell sizes range from 6 to 8 µm. This cell type has the strongest correlation with cigarette smoking. Because these tumors show a rapid rate of growth and tend to metastasize early and widely, small cell carcinomas have the worst prognosis. Survival time for untreated small cell carcinoma is usually 1 to 3 months. Approximately 14% of treated individuals are alive 2 years after diagnosis.

Small cell carcinoma is most often associated with ectopic hormone production. Neuroendocrine cells (NE cells) containing neurosecretory granules exist throughout the tracheobronchial tree and may be associated with small cell carcinoma.[76] Ectopic hormone production is important to the clinician because resulting signs and symptoms (called *paraneoplastic syndromes*) may be the first manifestation of the underlying cancer. Small cell carcinomas most commonly produce antidiuretic hormone from associated neuroendocrine cells (the syndrome of inappropriate antidiuretic hormone secretion [SIADH]). They also can produce gastrin-releasing peptide, calcitonin, arginine vasopressin, and adrenocorticotropic hormone (ACTH). As a result of ACTH secretion, individuals with lung cancer secrete large quantities of 17-hydroxysteroids and 17-ketosteroids, leading to the development of an atypical Cushing syndrome. Signs and symptoms related to this condition include muscular weakness, facial edema, hypokalemia, alkalosis, hyperglycemia, hypertension, and increased pigmentation. Treatment of small cell carcinoma is usually palliative. More than 85% of tumors will have metastasized by the time of diagnosis. Chemotherapy and radiation can significantly prolong life and relieve symptoms, but relapse is inevitable in most individuals.[77]

PATHOPHYSIOLOGY Tobacco smoke contains more than 30 carcinogens and is responsible for causing 80% to 90% of lung cancers. These carcinogens, along with probable inherited genetic predisposition to cancers, result in multiple genetic abnormalities in bronchial cells including deletions of chromosomes, activation of oncogenes, and inactivation of tumor suppressor genes.[78] The most common genetic abnormality associated with lung cancer is loss of the tumor suppressor gene *p53;* mutations in this gene have been found in 50% to 60% of non–small cell lung cancers and 90% of small cell cancers.[79] Once lung cancer is initiated by these carcinogen-induced mutations, further tumor development is promoted by growth factors such as epidermal growth factor. Further cellular toxicity is enhanced through smoke-induced toxic oxygen radical production.

The bronchial mucosa suffers multiple carcinogenic "hits" due to repetitive exposure to cigarette smoke, and eventually epithelial cell changes begin to be visible on biopsy. These changes progress from metaplasia to carcinoma in situ, and finally to invasive carcinoma. Further tumor progression includes invasion of surrounding tissues and finally metastasis to distant sites including the brain, bone marrow, and liver.

CLINICAL MANIFESTATIONS Table 26-3 summarizes the characteristic clinical manifestations according to tumor type. By the time there are manifestations severe enough to motivate the individual to seek medical advice, the disease is usually advanced.

EVALUATION AND TREATMENT Diagnostic tests for the evaluation of lung cancer include chest x-ray, sputum cytology, chest-computed tomography, fiberoptic bronchoscopy, and biopsy. Low-dose helical computed tomography is emerging as a sensitive and specific diagnostic test. Biopsy determines the cell type, and the evaluation of lymph nodes and other organ systems is used to determine the stage of the cancer. The histologic cell type and the stage of the disease are the major factors that influence choice of therapy. The current accepted system for the staging of non–small cell cancer is the **TNM classification.** This system is a code in which *T* denotes the extent of the primary tumor, *N* indicates the nodal involvement, and *M* describes the extent of metastasis. Small cell carcinoma is so rapidly progressive that its staging system consists of only two stages: limited versus extensive disease.

The only proven way of reducing the risk for lung cancer is the cessation of smoking, although chemopreventative measures are being explored. To date, trials evaluating the use of various early screening modalities such as chest x-ray and computed tomography have not resulted in a decrease in lung cancer mortality.[80] The management of lung cancer has been outlined here under each cell type, but it generally is chosen on the basis of tumor stage and patient functional status. Current modalities include combinations of surgical resection, chemotherapy, and radiation; however, new genetic and immunologic therapies are being explored[81-85] (see *Health Alert:* Genetic and Immunologic Breakthroughs in Lung Cancer Treatment).

HEALTH ALERT

Genetic and Immunologic Breakthroughs in Lung Cancer Treatment

Although new chemotherapeutic agents have improved outcomes slightly in the management of lung cancer, overall survival rates remain poor and toxicities of these regimens limit their use. New understandings of the genetic and immunologic features of lung cancer cells have led to new treatments. Gene therapy is emerging as a way of restoring normal tumor suppressor gene function (e.g., *p53*) and increasing tumor responsiveness to chemoradiation. Immunologic therapies include antibodies to growth factor receptors (e.g., epidermoid growth factor receptors [EGFR]) and antiangiogenesis drugs. The effectiveness of these strategies is still being evaluated, but new knowledge is leading to new opportunities for treatment.

Data from González G et al: Therapeutic vaccination with epidermal growth factor (EGF) in advanced lung cancer: analysis of pooled data from three clinical trials, *Hum Vaccin* 3(1):8–13, 2007; Ruttinger D et al: Immunotherapy of lung cancer: an update, *Onkologie* 29(1–2):33–38, 2006; Sandler AB: Targeting angiogenesis in lung cancer, *Sem Oncol* 32(6 suppl 10):S16–S22, 2005; Toloza EM: Gene therapy for lung cancer, *Thorac Surg Clin* 16(4):397–419, 2006.

QUICK CHECK 26-7

1. What are the principal features of lip cancer?
2. Describe squamous cell carcinoma of the vocal cords.
3. Compare three types of lung cancer as to cause and survival.

Did You Understand?

Clinical Manifestations of Pulmonary Alterations

1. Dyspnea is the feeling of breathlessness and increased respiratory effort.
2. Abnormal breathing patterns are adjustments made by the body to minimize the work of respiratory muscles. They include Kussmaul, obstructed, restricted, gasping, Cheyne-Stokes respirations, and sighing.
3. Hypoventilation is decreased alveolar ventilation caused by airway obstruction, chest wall restriction, or altered neurologic control of breathing. Hypoventilation causes increased $PaCO_2$.
4. Hyperventilation is increased alveolar ventilation produced by anxiety, head injury, or severe hypoxemia. Hyperventilation causes decreased $PaCO_2$.
5. Coughing is a protective reflex that expels secretions and irritants from the lower airways.
6. Hemoptysis is expectoration of bloody mucus, which can be caused by bronchitis, tuberculosis, abscess, neoplasms, and other conditions that cause hemorrhage from damaged vessels.
7. Cyanosis is a bluish discoloration of the skin caused by desaturation of hemoglobin, polycythemia, or peripheral vasoconstriction.
8. Chest pain can result from inflamed pleurae, trachea, bronchi, or respiratory muscles.
9. Clubbing of the fingertips is associated with diseases that interfere with oxygenation of the tissues.
10. Hypercapnia is an increased $PaCO_2$ caused by hypoventilation.
11. Hypoxemia is a reduced PaO_2 caused by (a) decreased oxygen content of inspired gas, (b) hypoventilation, (c) diffusion abnormality, (d) ventilation-perfusion mismatch, or (e) shunting.
12. Pulmonary edema is excess water in the lung caused by disturbances of capillary hydrostatic pressure, capillary oncotic pressure, or capillary permeability. A common cause is left heart failure that increases the hydrostatic pressure in the pulmonary circulation.
13. Atelectasis is the collapse of alveoli resulting from compression of lung tissue or absorption of gas from obstructed alveoli.
14. Bronchiectasis is abnormal dilation of the bronchi secondary to another pulmonary disorder, usually infection or inflammation.
15. Pneumothorax is the accumulation of air in the pleural space. It can be caused by spontaneous rupture of weakened areas of a pleura, or it can be secondary to pleural damage caused by disease, trauma, or mechanical ventilation.

(Continued)

Did You Understand?—Cont'd

16. Pneumothorax can be open, which means that the lung will only partially collapse, or tension, which means that pressure builds up in the pleural space and can compress both the affected lung and the mediastinum.
17. Pleural effusion is the accumulation of fluid in the pleural space, usually resulting from disorders that promote transudation or exudation from capillaries underlying the pleura but occasionally resulting from blockage or injury that causes lymphatic vessels to drain into the pleural space.
18. Empyema is the presence of pus in the pleural space (infected pleural effusion).
19. Chest wall compliance is diminished by obesity and kyphoscoliosis, which compress the lungs, and by neuromuscular diseases that impair chest wall muscle function.
20. Flail chest results from rib or sternal fractures that disrupt the mechanics of breathing.

Pulmonary Disorders

1. Pulmonary fibrosis is an excessive amount of connective tissue in the lung. It diminishes lung compliance and may be idiopathic or caused by disease.
2. Inhalation of noxious gases or prolonged exposure to high concentrations of oxygen can damage the bronchial mucosa or alveolocapillary membrane and cause inflammation or acute respiratory failure.
3. Pneumoconiosis, which is caused by inhalation of dust particles in the workplace, can cause pulmonary fibrosis, susceptibility to lower airway infection, and tumor formation.
4. Allergic alveolitis is an allergic or hypersensitivity reaction to many allergens.
5. Bronchiolitis is the inflammatory obstruction of small airways. It is most common in children.
6. Acute respiratory distress syndrome (ARDS) results from an acute, diffuse injury to the alveolocapillary membrane and decreased surfactant production, which increases membrane permeability and causes edema and atelectasis.
7. Obstructive lung disease is characterized by airway obstruction that causes difficult expiration. Obstructive disease can be acute or chronic in nature and includes asthma, chronic bronchitis, and emphysema.
8. Asthma is the result of a type 1 hypersensitivity immune response involving the activity lymphocytes, IgE, mast cells, and eosinophils.
9. In asthma, obstruction is caused by episodic attacks of bronchospasm, bronchial inflammation, mucosal edema, and increased mucus production.
10. Dysregulation of the parasympathetic division of the autonomic nervous system is thought to facilitate bronchospasm in individuals with asthma.
11. Asthma staging is based on clinical severity from mild intermittent to severe persistent and is used to determine therapy.
12. Chronic bronchitis causes airway obstruction resulting from bronchial smooth muscle hypertrophy and production of thick, tenacious mucus.
13. In emphysema, destruction of the alveolar septa and loss of passive elastic recoil lead to airway collapse and obstruct gas flow during expiration.
14. Chronic obstructive pulmonary disease (COPD) is the coexistence of chronic bronchitis and emphysema.
15. COPD is an important cause of hypoxemic and hypercapnic respiratory failure.
16. Upper respiratory tract infections, which are the most common cause of short-term disability in the United States, include rhinitis (the common cold), pharyngitis, and laryngitis.
17. Serious lower respiratory tract infections occur most often in the elderly and in individuals with impaired immunity or underlying disease.
18. *Pneumococcal* pneumonia is an acute lung infection resulting in an inflammatory response with four phases: (a) consolidation, (b) red hepatization, (c) gray hepatization, and (d) resolution.
19. Viral pneumonia can be severe, but is more often an acute, self-limiting lung infection usually caused by the influenza virus.
20. Tuberculosis is a lung infection caused by *Mycobacterium tuberculosis* (tubercle bacillus).
21. In tuberculosis, the inflammatory response proceeds to isolate colonies of bacilli by enclosing them in tubercles and surrounding the tubercles with scar tissue.
22. Bacilli may remain dormant within the tubercles for life or, if the immune system breaks down, cause recurrence of active disease.
23. Pulmonary vascular diseases are caused by embolism or hypertension in the pulmonary circulation.
24. Pulmonary embolism is occlusion of a portion of the pulmonary vascular bed by a thrombus (most common), tissue fragment, or air bubble. Depending on its size and location, the embolus can cause hypoxic vasoconstriction, pulmonary edema, atelectasis, pulmonary hypertension, shock, and even death.
25. Pulmonary hypertension (pulmonary artery pressure 5 to 10 mm Hg above normal) is caused by (a) elevated left ventricular pressure, (b) increased blood flow through the pulmonary circulation, (c) obliteration or obstruction of the vascular bed, or (d) active constriction of the vascular bed produced by hypoxemia or acidosis.
26. Cor pulmonale is right ventricular enlargement caused by chronic pulmonary hypertension. Cor pulmonale progresses to right ventricular failure if the pulmonary hypertension is not reversed.
27. Lip cancer is most common in men. In the most common cell type, squamous cell, metastasis is rare when lesions are diagnosed and treated early.
28. Laryngeal cancer occurs primarily in men and represents 2% to 3% of all cancers. Squamous cell carcinoma of the true vocal cords is most common and presents with a clinical symptom of progressive hoarseness.
29. Lung cancer, the most common cause of cancer death in the United States, is commonly caused by cigarette smoking.
30. Cancer cell types include non–small cell carcinoma (squamous cell, adenocarcinoma, and large cell) and small cell carcinoma. Each type arises in a characteristic site or type of tissue, causes distinctive clinical manifestations, and differs in likelihood of metastasis and prognosis.

Key Terms

References

1. Lumb AB: *Nunn's applied respiratory physiology*, ed 6, St Louis, 2005, Elsevier.
2. Scano G, Stendardi L: Dyspnea and asthma, *Curr Opin Pulmon Med* 12(1):18–22, 2006.
3. Lansing RW, Moosavi SH, Banzett RB: Measurement of dyspnea: word labeled visual analog scale vs. verbal ordinal scale, *Respir Physiol Neurobiol* 134(2):77–83, 2003.
4. Brashers VL, Haden K: Differential diagnosis of cough: focus on lung malignancy, *Lippincott's Prim Care Pract*, 4(4): 374–389, 2000.
5. Irwin RS: Complications of cough, *Chest* 129:54s–58s, 2006.
6. Ganter BG, Jakob SM, Takala J: Pulmonary capillary pressure: a review, *Minerva Anestesiologica*, 72(1–2):21–36, 2006.
7. d'Escrivan T, Guery B: Prevention and treatment of aspiration pneumonia in intensive care units, *Treat Resp Med* 4 (5):317–324, 2005.
8. Duggan M, Kavanagh BP: Pulmonary atelectasis: a pathogenic perioperative entity, *Anesthesiol* 102(4):838–854, 2005.
9. Chapman SJ, Davies RJ: Recent advances in parapneumonic effusion and empyema, *Curr Opin Pulmon Med* 10(4): 299–304, 2004.
10. Rimal B, Greenberg AK, Rom WN: Basic pathogenetic mechanisms in silicosis: current understanding, *Curr Opin Pulmon Med* 11(2):169–173, 2005.
11. Chong S et al: Pneumoconiosis: comparison of imaging and pathologic findings, *Radiographics* 26(1):59–77, 2006.
12. Rubenfeld GD: Epidemiology of acute lung injury, *Crit Care Med* 31(4 suppl):S276–S284, 2003.
13. Ware LB, Matthay MA: The acute respiratory distress syndrome, *N Engl J Med* 342(18):1334–1349, 2000.
14. Santacruz JF, Zavala ED, Arroliga AC: Update in ARDS management: recent randomized controlled trials that changed our practice, *Clev Clin J Med* 73(3):217–219, 223–225, 229 passim, 2006.
15. Esper AM, Martin GS: Evolution of treatments for patients with acute lung injury, *Exp Opin Investig Drugs* 14(5): 633–645, 2005.
16. Second Expert Panel on the Management of Asthma, National Heart, Lung, and Blood Institute: *Highlights of the expert panel report 2: guidelines for the diagnosis and management of asthma*, Bethesda, Md, 1997, National Institutes of Health (pub no NIH 97-4051A).
17. NAEPP Expert Panel Report Guidelines for the Diagnosis and Management of Asthma: *Update on selected topics*, Bethesda, Md, 2002, National Institutes of Health.
18. Contopoulos-Ioannidis DG et al: Genetic predisposition to asthma and atopy, *Respiration*. 74(1):8–12, 2007.
19. Lemanske RF Jr, Busse RF: Asthma: Factors underlying inception, exacerbation, and disease progression, *J Allergy Clin Immunol* 117(2 suppl mini-primer):S456–S461, 2006.
20. Renz H et al: The immunological basis of the hygiene hypothesis, *Chem Immunol Allergy*, 91:30–48, 2006.
21. Platts-Mills TA et al: Is the hygiene hypothesis still a viable explanation for the increased prevalence of asthma? *Allergy* 60(suppl 79):25–231, 2005.
22. Busse WW, Rosenwasser LJ: Mechanisms of asthma, *J Allergy Clin Immunol* 11(3 suppl):S799–S804, 2003.
23. Effros RM, Nagaraj H: Asthma: new developments concerning immune mechanisms, diagnosis and treatment, *Current Opinion in Pulmonary Medicine*, 13(1):37–43, 2007.
24. Mathur SK, Busse WW: Asthma: diagnosis and management, *Med Clin North Am* 90(1):39–60, 2006.
25. Davydov L: Omalizumab (Xolair) for treatment of asthma, *Am Family Phys* 71:341–342, 2005.
26. Marcus P, Practice Management Committee, American College of Chest Physicians: Incorporating anti-IgE (omalizumab) therapy into pulmonary medicine practice: practice management implications, *Chest* 129(2):466–474, 2006.

References—Cont'd

27. Executive Summary 2006 Global Strategy for the Diagnosis, Management and Prevention of COPD. December, http://www.goldcopd.org/Guidelineitem.asp?l1=2&l2=1&intId=996 Page 1.
28. Barnes PJ: Chronic obstructive pulmonary disease, *N Engl J Med* 343(4):269–280, 2000.
29. Molfino NA: Genetics of COPD, *Chest* 125:1929–1940, 2004.
30. Hogg JC: Pathophysiology of airflow limitation in chronic obstructive pulmonary disease, *Lancet* 364:709–721, 2004.
31. O'Donnell DE, Parker CM: COPD exacerbations. 3: pathophysiology, *Thorax* 61(4):354–361, 2006.
32. Braman SS: Chronic cough due to chronic bronchitis: ACCP evidence-based clinical practice guidelines, *Chest* 129 (1 suppl):104S–115S, 2006.
33. Martinez FJ, Anzueto A: Appropriate outpatient treatment of acute bacterial exacerbations of chronic bronchitis, *Am J Med* 118(suppl 7A):39S–44S, 2005.
34. Stoller JK, Aboussouan LS: Alpha 1-antitrypsin deficiency, *Lancet* 365(9478):2225–2236, 2005.
35. Dewar M, Curry RW Jr: Chronic obstructive pulmonary disease: diagnostic considerations, *Am Family Phys* 73(4): 669–676, 2006.
36. Sutherland ER, Cherniack RM: Current concepts: management of chronic obstructive pulmonary disease, *N Engl J Med* 350(26):2689–2697, 2004.
37. Meinke L et al: Advances in the management of chronic obstructive pulmonary disease, *Expert Opinion on Pharmacotherapy,* 8(1):23–37, 2007.
38. Kroegel C, Foerster M: Phosphodiesterase-4 inhibitors as a novel approach for the treatment of respiratory disease: cilomilast. *Expert Opinion on Investigational Drugs,* 16(1): 109–124, 2007.
39. Andrews J et al: Community-acquired pneumonia., *Curr Opin Pulmon Med* 9(3):175–180, 2003.
40. Flanders SA, Collard HR, Saint S: Nosocomial pneumonia: state of the science, *Am J Infect Control* 34(2):84–93, 2006.
41. Waite S, Jeudy J, White CS: Acute lung infections in normal and immunocompromised hosts, *Radiol Clin North Am* 44 (2):295–315, ix, 2006.
42. Ortqvist A, Hedlund J, Kalin M: *Streptococcus pneumoniae*: epidemiology, risk factors, and clinical features, *Sem Respir-Crit Care Med* 26(6):563–574, 2005.
43. Blasi F, Allegra L et al: *Chlamydia pneumoniae* and *Mycoplasma pneumoniae, Sem Respir Crit Care Med* 26(6):617–624, 2005.
44. Lahti E et al: Influenza pneumonia, *Pediat Infect Dis J* 25 (2):160–164, 2006.
45. Pedro-Botet ML, Sabria M: Legionellosis, *Sem Respir Crit Care Med* 26(6):625–634, 2005.
46. Pop SM, Kolls JK, Steele C: Pneumocystis: immune recognition and evasion, *Int J Biochem Cell Biol* 38(1):17–22, 2006.
47. Delclaux C, Azoulay E: Inflammatory response to infectious pulmonary injury, *Eur Respir J Suppl* 42:10s–14s, 2003.
48. Kadioglu A, Andrew PW: The innate immune response to pneumococcal lung infection: the untold story, *Trends Immunol* 25(3):143–149, 2004.
49. Hoare Z, Lim WS: Pneumonia: update on diagnosis and management, *Br Med J* 332(7549):1077–1079, 2006.
50. Lynch JP 3rd, Zhanel GG: Escalation of antimicrobial resistance among Streptococcus pneumoniae: implications for therapy, *Sem Respir Crit Care Med* 26(6):575–616, 2005.
51. Dye C: Global epidemiology of tuberculosis, *The Lancet* 367 (9514):938–940, 2006.
52. de Jong BC et al: Clinical management of tuberculosis in the context of HIV infection, *Annu Rev Med* 55:283–301, 2004.
53. Nunn P et al: Tuberculosis control in the era of HIV, *Nat Rev Immunol* 5(10):819–826, 2005.
54. Yew WW, Leung CC: Update in tuberculosis 2005, *Am J Respir Crit Care Med* 173(5):491–498, 2006.
55. Russell DG: Who puts the tubercle in tuberculosis? *Nature Reviews Microbiology,* 5(1):39–47, 2007.
56. Golden MP, Vikram HR: Extrapulmonary tuberculosis: an overview, *Am Fam Phys* 72(9):1761–1768, 2005.
57. Giovanni Ferrara et al: Use in routine clinical practice of two commercial blood tests for diagnosis of infection with *Mycobacterium tuberculosis*: a prospective study, *The Lancet* 367 (9519):1328–1334, 2006.
58. Campbell IA, Bah-Sow O: Pulmonary tuberculosis: diagnosis and treatment, *Br Med J* 332(7551):1194–1197, 2006.
59. Potter B, Rindfleisch K, Kraus CK: Management of active tuberculosis, *Am Fam Phys* 72(11):2225–2232, 2005.
60. Braman SS: Chronic cough due to acute bronchitis: ACCP evidence-based clinical practice guidelines, *Chest* 129(1 suppl): 95S–103S, 2006.
61. Blann AD, Lip GY: Venous thromboembolism, *Br Med J* 332 (7535):215–219, 2006.
62. McRae SJ, Ginsberg JS: Update in the diagnosis of deep-vein thrombosis and pulmonary embolism, *Curr Opin Anaesthesiology* 19(1):44–51, 2006.
63. Langan CJ, Weingart S: New diagnostic and treatment modalities for pulmonary embolism: one path through the confusion, *Mt Sinai J Med* 73(2):528–541, 2006.
64. Segal JB et al: Management of venous thromboembolism: a systematic review for a practice guideline, *Annals of Internal Medicine,* 146(3):211–222, 2007.
65. Carbone R et al: Secondary pulmonary hypertension—diagnosis and management, *Eur Rev Med Pharmacol Sci* 9(6): 331–342, 2005.
66. Hoeper MM, Rubin LJ: Update in pulmonary hypertension 2005, *Am J Resp Crit Care Med* 173(5):499–505, 2006.
67. Dandel M, Lehmkuhl HB, Hetzer R: Advances in the medical treatment of pulmonary hypertension, *Kidney Blood Press Res* 28(5–6):311–324, 2005.
68. Haj RM, Cinco JE, Mazer CD: Treatment of pulmonary hypertension with selective pulmonary vasodilators, *Curr Opin Anaesthesiol* 19(1):88–95, 2006.
69. Barst RJ: Sitaxsentan: a selective endothelin-A receptor antagonist, for the treatment of pulmonary arterial hypertension, *Expert Opinion on Pharmacotherapy* 8(1):95–109, 2007.
70. American Cancer Society: Cancer facts and figures 2007, www;cancer.org/downloads/STT/CAFF2007PWSecured.pdf.
71. Syrjanen S: Human papillomavirus (HPV) in head and neck cancer, *J Clin Virol* 32(suppl 1):S59–S66, 2005.
72. Back G, Sood S: The management of early laryngeal cancer: options for patients and therapists, *Curr Opin Otolaryngol Head Neck Surg* 13(2):85–91, 2005.
73. Collins LG et al: Lung cancer: diagnosis and management, *American Family Physician,* 75(1):56–63, 2007.
74. Posther KE, Harpole DH Jr: The surgical management of lung cancer, *Can Invest* 24(1):56–67, 2006.
75. Huang CL et al: Tailor-made chemotherapy for non-small cell lung cancer patients, *Future Oncol* 2(2):289–299, 2006.
76. Onganer PU, Seckl MJ, Djamgoz MB: Neuronal characteristics of small-cell lung cancer, *Br J Can* 93(11):1197–1201, 2005.
77. Rocha Ciombor KK, Lima CM: Management of small cell lung cancer, *Curr Treat Options Oncol* 7(1):59–68, 2006.
78. Vincenzi B et al: Cell cycle alterations and lung cancer, *Histol Histopathol* 21(4):423–435, 2006.

References—Cont'd

79. Liu G, Zhou W, Christiani DC: Molecular epidemiology of non-small cell lung cancer, *Sem Respir Crit Care Med* 26 (3):2652–2672, 2005.
80. Black C et al: Population screening for lung cancer using computed tomography, is there evidence of clinical effectiveness? A systematic review of the literature, *Thorax* 62(2):131–138, 2007.
81. Byrne BJ, Garst J: Epidermal growth factor receptor inhibitors and their role in non-small-cell lung cancer, *Curr Oncol Rep* 7(4):241–247, 2005.
82. Nemunaitis J, Nemunaitis J: A review of vaccine clinical trials for non-small cell lung cancer, *Expert Opinion on Biological Therapy,* 7(1):89–102, 2007.
83. Ruttinger D et al: Immunotherapy of lung cancer: an update, *Onkologie* 29(1–2):33–38, 2006.
84. Sandler AB: Targeting angiogenesis in lung cancer, *Sem Oncol* 32(6 suppl 10):S16–S22, 2005.
85. Toloza EM: Gene therapy for lung cancer, *Sem Thorac Cardiovasc Surg* 17(3):205–212, 2005.

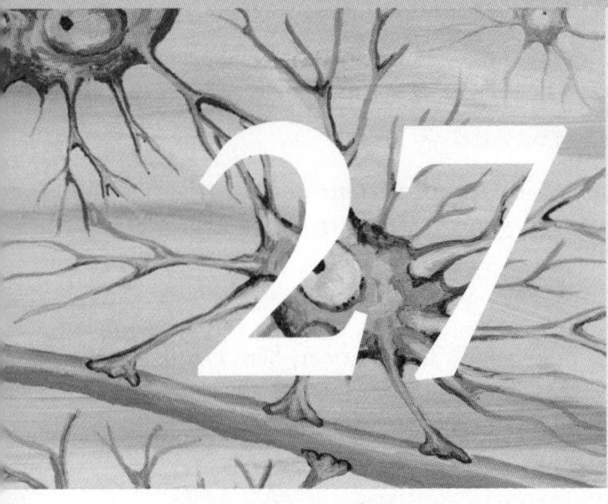

27 ALTERATIONS OF PULMONARY FUNCTION IN CHILDREN

Deborah K. Froh ▪ Sue E. Huether

CHAPTER OUTLINE

ELECTRONIC RESOURCES

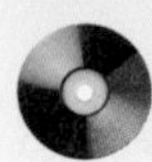

Companion CD
- Review Questions and Answers
- Animations

evolve Website
http://evolve.elsevier.com/Huether/
- Quick Check Answers
- Key Terms Exercises
- Critical Thinking Questions with Answers
- Algorithm Completion Exercises
- WebLinks

Alterations of respiratory function in children are influenced by physiologic maturation as a function of age, genetics, and environmental conditions. A variety of upper and lower airway infections can cause respiratory compromise or play a role in the pathogenesis of more chronic pulmonary disease. Infants, especially premature infants, may present special problems because of immaturity of lung, airway, and chest wall structures, as well as immaturity of pulmonary homeostasis (e.g., surfactant production) and immunologic immaturity. Immunization and attentive medical care can greatly reduce the incidence and severity of pulmonary disorders in children.

PULMONARY DISORDERS

Pulmonary dysfunction can be categorized into disorders of either the upper or lower airways.

Disorders of the Upper Airways

Table 27-1 compares different upper airway infections.

Croup

Classic croup is an acute laryngotracheobronchitis and almost always occurs in children between 6 months and 5 years of age.[1] In 85% of cases, croup is caused by a virus, most commonly parainfluenza and in other instances by influenza A or respiratory syncytial virus. The incidence of croup is higher in males and is most common during the winter months. Approximately 15% of affected children have a strong family history of croup, with laryngitis tending to recur in the same child.

PATHOPHYSIOLOGY Airway obstruction occurs in the subglottic region of the trachea, just below the vocal cords. Contributory factors include mucosal edema and secretions related to the viral infection. Anatomically, the subglottic region is slightly narrower than the rest of the trachea, and in children the subglottic mucous membrane is more loosely attached and more vascular than in adults. These factors make the airway susceptible to compromise in children. If there is significant narrowing of the airway in this area, the child will have to breathe hard to move air, and the excessive negative pressure generated may even cause the airway structures higher up to collapse with inspiration (Figure 27-1). The turbulent flow across this obstruction will cause stridor on inspiration and sometimes also on expiration (Figure 27-2). Croup tends to affect younger children more prominently because they have smaller airways that are therefore compromised more easily (see Figures 27-1 and 27-3).

CLINICAL MANIFESTATIONS Typically, the child experiences rhinorrhea, sore throat, and low-grade fever for a few days, then develops a seal-like barking cough. Most cases resolve spontaneously within 24 to 48 hours and do not warrant hospital admission. The presence of inspiratory stridor or respiratory distress suggests a more severe situation.

Spasmodic croup is characterized by similar hoarseness, barking cough, and stridor but usually occurs in older children. It is of sudden onset and usually occurs at night and without prodromal symptoms. It usually resolves quickly. The etiology is unknown.

The clinical manifestations of croup are produced primarily by inflammatory edema of the upper trachea. A child with severe croup usually displays deep retractions (Figure 27-4), stridor, agitation, tachycardia, and sometimes pallor or cyanosis.

EVALUATION AND TREATMENT The degree of symptoms determines the level of treatment. Most children with

TABLE 27-1

Comparison of Upper Airway Infections

Condition	Age	Onset	Etiology	Pathophysiology	Symptoms
Acute laryngotracheobronchitis	6 mo-3 yr	Usually gradual	Viral	Inflammation from larynx to bronchi	Harsh cough; stridor; low-grade fever; may have nasal discharge, conjunctivitis
Acute tracheitis	1–12 yr	Abrupt or following viral illness	*Staphylococcus aureus*	Inflammation of upper trachea	High fever; toxic appearance; harsh cough; purulent secretions
Acute epiglottitis	2–6 yr	Abrupt	*Haemophilus influenzae* group A streptococcus	Inflammation of supraglottic structures	Severe sore throat; dysphasia; high fever; toxic appearance; muffled voice; may drool; dyspnea; sits erect and quietly

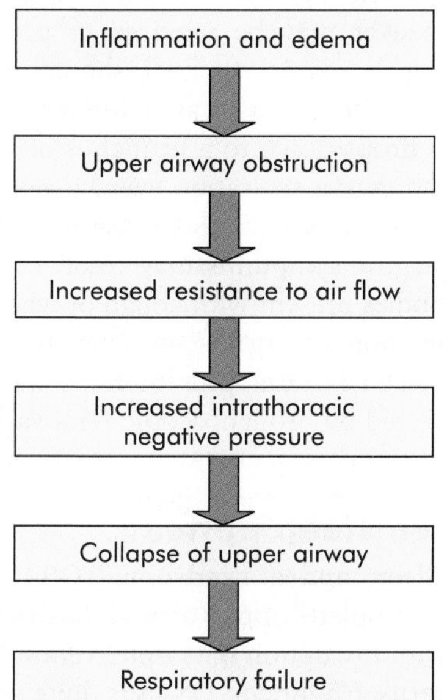

Figure 27-1 ■ Upper Airway Obstruction With Croup.

croup require no treatment. Some cases are treated, but appear mild enough to do so as outpatients. These patients usually have only mild stridor or retractions and appear alert, playful, and able to eat. Glucocorticoids, either injected or oral (dexamethasone) or nebulized (budesonide) appear to be helpful in managing the patient through the illness. The presence of stridor at rest, moderate or severe retractions of the chest, or agitation suggests more severe disease and does require in-hospital observation and treatment. For acute respiratory distress, nebulized racemic epinephrine stimulates α- and β-adrenergic receptors and decreases mucosal edema. The racemic epinephrine effects last only for 2 to 3 hours; either systemic or nebulized steroids are used concomitantly to control and reduce inflammation after the effects of epinephrine have waned.[2] In rare and extreme situations, placement of an endotracheal tube becomes necessary to secure the airway.

Acute epiglottitis

Historically, **acute epiglottitis** was caused by *Haemophilus influenzae* type B. However, since the advent of *H. influenzae* vaccine, the overall incidence of acute epiglottis has been reduced by 80% to 90%. Current cases in children usually are caused by other pathogens, such as group A *Streptococcus.*

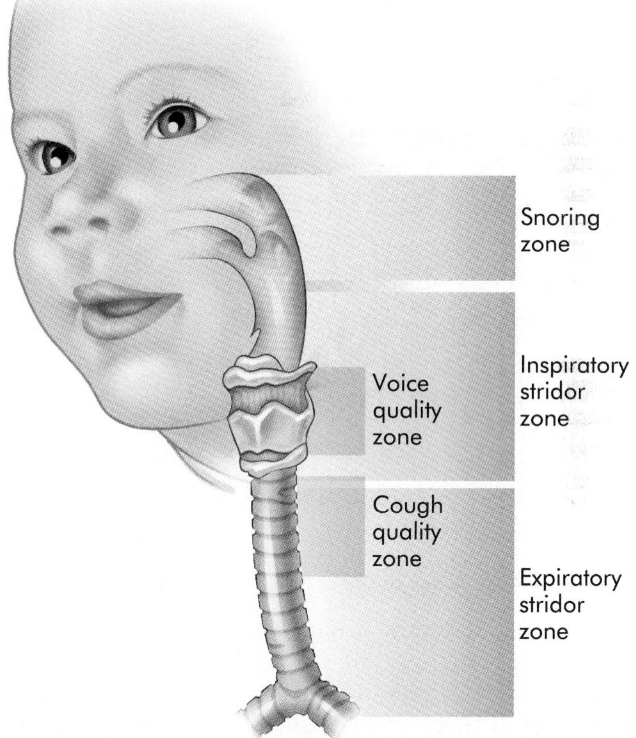

Figure 27-2 ■ Listening Can Help Locate the Site of Airway Obstruction. A loud, gasping snore suggests enlarged tonsils or adenoids. In inspiratory stridor, the airway is compromised at the level of the supraglottic larynx, vocal cords, subglottic region, or upper trachea. Expiratory stridor results from a narrowing or collapse in the trachea or bronchi. Airway noise during both inspiration and expiration often represents a fixed obstruction of the vocal cords or subglottic space. Hoarseness or a weak cry is a by-product of obstruction at the vocal cords. If a cough is croupy, suspect constriction below the vocal cords (Redrawn from Eavey RD: *Contemp Ped* 3(6):79, 1986; original illustration by Paul Singh-Roy.)

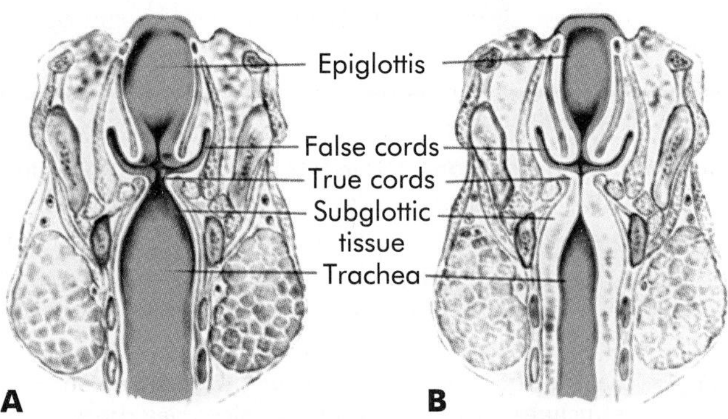

Figure 27-3 ■ **The Larynx and Subglottic Trachea. A,** Normal. **B,** Narrowing and obstruction from edema caused by croup. (From Hockenberry MJ et al: *Wong's nursing care of infants and children,* ed 8, St Louis, 2007, Mosby.)

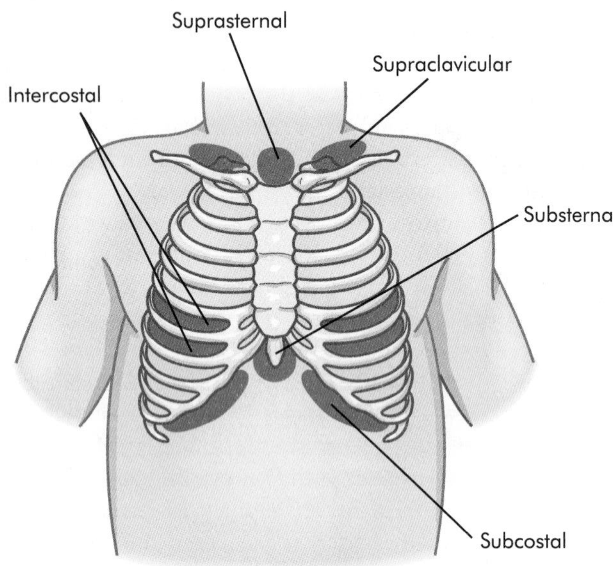

Figure 27-4 ■ **Areas of Chest Muscle Retraction.**

CLINICAL MANIFESTATIONS In the classic form of the disease, a child between 2 and 7 years of age suddenly develops fever, inspiratory stridor, and severe respiratory distress.[3] The child appears anxious and has a voice that sounds muffled. Drooling and dysphagia (inability to swallow) are common. Death can occur in a few hours. Nasotracheal intubation or tracheotomy is mandatory in instances of rapidly increasing obstruction. Pneumonia, cervical lymph node inflammation, otitis, and, rarely, meningitis or septic arthritis may occur concomitantly because of bacterial sepsis.

EVALUATION AND TREATMENT Acute epiglottitis is a life-threatening emergency. Efforts should be made to keep the child calm and undisturbed. Examination of the throat should not be attempted as it may trigger laryngospasm and cause respiratory collapse. With severe airway obstruction, the airway may be secured with intubation, and the disease may be treated with antibiotics. Resolution with treatment is usually rapid.

Aspiration of foreign bodies

Aspiration of foreign bodies into the airways usually occurs in children 1 to 3 years of age. Most objects are expelled by the cough reflex, but some objects may lodge in the larynx, trachea, or bronchi. Large objects (e.g., a bite of hot dog, peanuts, popcorn, grapes, beans, toy pieces, fragments of popped balloons, or coins) may occlude the airway and become life threatening. Foreign bodies lodged in the larynx or upper trachea cause cough, stridor, hoarseness or inability to speak, respiratory distress, and agitation or panic; the presentation is often dramatic and frightening. If the child is acutely hypoxic and unable to move air, immediate action such as sweeping the oral airway or performing the Heimlich maneuver may be required to prevent tragedy. Otherwise, bronchoscopic removal should be performed urgently. Most often, an aspirated foreign body is small enough that it drops down to a bronchus before becoming lodged. Commonly the aspiration event is not witnessed or is not recognized when it happens, because the coughing, choking, or gagging symptoms may resolve quickly. Bronchial foreign bodies present with cough or wheezing or with atelectasis, pneumonia, lung abscess, or blood-streaked sputum if the object has been present for some time. These patients are treated by bronchoscopic removal of the object and antibiotics as necessary.

Obstructive sleep apnea

Obstructive sleep apnea syndrome (OSAS) is defined by partial or complete upper airway obstruction (UAO) during sleep with disruption of normal ventilation and normal sleep patterns. Childhood OSAS is quite common, with an estimated prevalence of 1% to 10%.[4] In children, unlike adults, OSAS occurs equally among girls and boys.

PATHOPHYSIOLOGY By far the most common predisposing factor to OSAS in children is adenotonsillar hypertrophy, which causes physical impingement on the nasopharyngeal airway. OSAS also may occur in children with obesity, craniofacial anomalies (with structurally small nasopharyngeal airways), or reduced motor tone of the upper airways (as may be seen in neurologic disorders, cerebral palsy, and Down syndrome).

CLINICAL MANIFESTATIONS There usually is a history of snoring and labored breathing during sleep, which may be continuous or intermittent. There may be episodes of increased respiratory effort but no audible airflow, often terminated by snorting, gasping, repositioning, or arousal. Sleep is often described as restless. Daytime sleepiness is occasionally reported. Often the child is a chronic mouth breather and has large tonsils.

EVALUATION AND TREATMENT All parents should be asked if their child exhibits snoring, a symptom that is often not spontaneously reported to the healthcare provider.[4] The most definitive evaluation is the polysomnographic sleep study, which documents obstructed breathing and physiologic impairment. If obstructive sleep apnea is documented or strongly suspected clinically, children are most often referred for tonsillectomy and adenoidectomy (T & A) on the basis of described symptoms and physical findings, such as enlarged tonsils, adenoidal facies, and mouth breathing. For severely affected children who do not respond to T & A or who have different problems, such as obesity, that cannot be remedied rapidly, continuous positive airway pressure (CPAP) may be delivered through a tight-fitting nasal mask used during sleep.

QUICK CHECK 27-1

1. Compare and contrast pathology, clinical presentations, and severity of croup and epiglottis.
2. What symptoms indicate aspiration of a foreign body?
3. What signs and symptoms suggest obstructive sleep apnea?

Disorders of the Lower Airways

A number of disorders of the lower respiratory tract are specific to children, such as newborn respiratory distress syndrome, bronchopulmonary dysplasia, and congenital malformations, Lower airway infections, such as viral bronchiolitis and bacterial pneumonia, occur fairly often in children. Chronic pulmonary conditions, such as asthma and cystic fibrosis, frequently first present clinically in childhood.

Respiratory distress syndrome of the newborn

The name **respiratory distress syndrome (RDS) of the newborn** (previously also called *hyaline membrane disease [HMD])* refers to the lung disorder that remains a significant cause of neonatal morbidity and mortality.[5] It occurs almost exclusively in premature infants. RDS occurs in 60% born at less than 28 weeks gestation, 30% of those born at 28 to 34 weeks, and fewer than 5% of those born after 34 weeks. The incidence and death rates have declined significantly since the introduction of antenatal steroid therapy and postnatal surfactant therapy.[6] Risk factors are summarized in *Risk Factors:* Respiratory Distress Syndrome of the Newborn.

RISK FACTORS Respiratory Distress Syndrome of the Newborn

- Premature birth
- Male gender
- Cesarean delivery without labor
- Diabetic mother
- Perinatal asphyxia

PATHOPHYSIOLOGY RDS is caused by surfactant deficiency and also a deficiency in alveolar surface area for gas exchange. Surfactant is the material that lines the alveoli and is required for maintaining their inflation. Without surfactant, which lowers surface tension, alveoli would tend to collapse at the end of each exhalation. Surfactant is normally not secreted by the alveolar cells until approximately 30 weeks gestation. In addition to the functional surfactant deficiency of the premature lung, structural immaturity is a problem. Premature infants are born with many underdeveloped and small alveoli that are difficult to inflate. In the most extreme premature infants, the "alveoli" have thick walls and inadequate capillary blood supply such that gas exchange is significantly impaired. Furthermore, the infant's chest wall is weak and highly compliant and, thus, the rib cage tends to collapse inward with respiratory effort. The net effect of all these adverse factors is *atelectasis* (collapsed alveoli), which is difficult for the neonate to overcome because it requires a significant negative inspiratory pressure to open the alveoli with each breath. The infant uses more oxygen to sustain the work of breathing and becomes hypoxemic and hypercapnic. Hypoxia and atelectasis cause pulmonary vasoconstriction and increase intrapulmonary resistance and shunting (Figure 27-5). This results in hypoperfusion of the lung and a decrease in effective pulmonary blood flow. Increased pulmonary vascular resistance may even cause a partial return to fetal circulation, with right-to-left shunting of blood through the ductus arteriosus and foramen ovale.

Pulmonary capillary permeability increases and the alveolar epithelium may be damaged because of ventilation-induced injury, and together these conditions result in the leakage of plasma proteins into the alveoli. Fibrin deposits in the airspaces create the appearance of "*hyaline membranes,*" for which the disorder was named. The plasma proteins leaked into the airspace have the additional adverse effect of interfering with the function of surfactant that may be present. The pathogenesis of RDS is summarized in Figure 27-5.

CLINICAL MANIFESTATIONS Signs of RDS appear within minutes of birth. Some neonates require immediate resuscitation because of asphyxia or severe respiratory distress. Characteristic signs are tachypnea (respiratory rate over 60 breaths/min), expiratory grunting, intercostal and subcostal retractions, nasal flaring, and poor color. The natural course is characterized by progressive hypoxemia and dyspnea. Apnea and irregular respirations occur as the infant tires. The typical chest radiograph shows diffuse, fine granular densities within the first 6 hours of life. Ventilatory support is often required. In most cases the clinical manifestations reach a peak within 3 days, after which there is gradual improvement.

EVALUATION AND TREATMENT Diagnosis is made on the basis of prematurity or other risk factors, chest radiographs, and, occasionally, confirmatory analysis (for example,

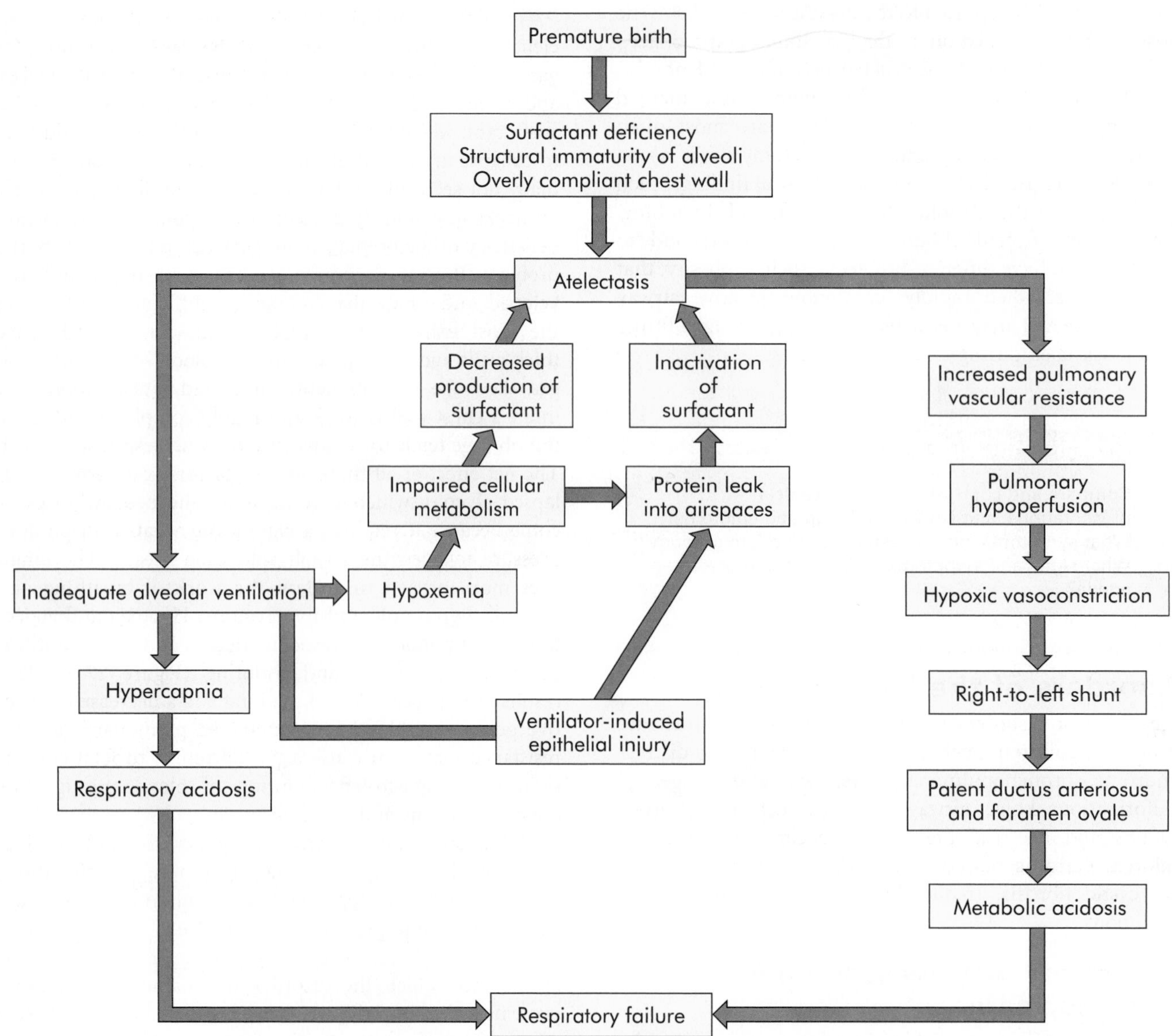

Figure 27-5 ■ **Pathogenesis of Respiratory Distress Syndrome (RDS) of the Newborn.**

lecithin/sphingomyelin ratio [L/S ratio]) of amniotic fluid or tracheal aspirates. The ultimate treatment for RDS would be prevention of premature birth.

Antenatal treatment with glucocorticoids is given to women at 24 to 34 weeks gestation and in preterm labor, unless delivery is imminent. Glucocorticoids induce a significant and rapid acceleration of lung maturation, and there is extensive evidence that maternal steroid therapy significantly reduces the incidence of RDS and death.[7]

Current protocols recommend prophylactic administration of exogenous surfactant to infants weighing less than 1000 g, beginning within 15 to 30 minutes of birth, after the infant is stabilized.[8] There is usually a dramatic improvement in oxygenation. For infants weighing more than 1000 g, surfactant replacement is based on clinical need. Surfactant therapy should be considered complementary to antenatal glucocorticoids.

Supportive care includes oxygen and often such measures as continuous positive airway pressure (CPAP) or mechanical ventilation. Tidal volume must be carefully monitored to minimize ventilation injury; the extremely preterm infant is particularly vulnerable.[9] Ventilation may interfere with alveolarization and surfactant metabolism and may aggravate the proinflammatory state that is believed to accompany premature birth and RDS, as reflected by abnormal cytokine profiles in the lung. A combination of factors may lead to subsequent development of chronic lung disease or bronchopulmonary dysplasia.

Most infants survive RDS with treatment. In many cases, recovery may be complete within 10 to 14 days. However, the incidence of subsequent chronic lung disease is significant among very-low-birth-weight infants.

Bronchopulmonary dysplasia

Bronchopulmonary dysplasia (BPD), also known as *chronic lung disease of infancy,* is the term used for persisting lung disease following neonatal lung injury, usually associated with premature birth and perinatal respiratory

RISK FACTORS Bronchopulmonary Dysplasia (BPD)

- Prematurity (especially ≤28 weeks)
- Positive-pressure ventilation
- Supplemental oxygen administration
- Antenatal chorioamnionitis
- Postnatal sepsis or pneumonia
- Patent ductus arteriosus
- Nutritional deficiencies
- Early adrenal insufficiency

support.[10] Risk factors for BPD are summarized in the *Risk Factors:* Bronchopulmonary Dysplasia (BPD) box.

In the current era of neonatology, the widespread use of antenatal glucocorticoids and postnatal surfactant has lessened the incidence and severity of RDS, and BPD is occurring primarily in the smallest premature infants (24 to 28 weeks gestation) who have received mechanical ventilation. Surprisingly, some of these tiny infants who develop BPD have had few or no clinical signs of RDS at birth or have initially received only low levels of supplemental oxygen or ventilatory support, sometimes for other reasons such as apnea.[11] Nevertheless, a highly significant predictor of subsequent BPD seems to be ventilation on the day of birth.[12]

The reported incidence of BPD varies because diagnostic criteria are not uniform. Criteria are based on persistent oxygen requirement, abnormalities visible on chest x-rays, and clinical criteria. It is estimated that 30% to 50% of infants with birthweights under 1000 g develop BPD.[13]

PATHOPHYSIOLOGY *Classic BPD* evolves over several weeks, with an early exudative inflammatory phase followed by a fibroproliferative phase. However, this severe form, resulting in evidence of marked airway injury and cyst formation, is no longer common. Instead, the predominant histopathologic findings in the *"new BPD"* are those of disrupted lung development with poor formation of the alveolar architecture.[14] Alveoli are large and fewer in number, thereby presenting decreased surface area for gas exchange. Furthermore, there is evidence of reduced ingrowth of the pulmonary capillaries to the formative alveolar units, which leads to impaired gas exchange, ventilation perfusion mismatch, and poor capacity to exercise. In more severe cases of BPD, pulmonary hypertension may develop because of abnormal muscularization of the primary vasculature in response to recurrent hypoxemia or inflammatory stimuli. Figure 27-6 illustrates the pathophysiology of BPD.

CLINICAL MANIFESTATIONS Clinically, the infant exhibits hypoxemia and hypercapnia caused by ventilation-perfusion mismatch and diffusion defects. The work of breathing increases, and the ability to feed may be impaired. Intermittent bronchospasm, mucus plugging, and pulmonary hypertension characterize the clinical course. Of the most severely affected infants, dusky spells may occur with agitations, feeding, or gastroesophageal reflux. Infants with mild BPD may demonstrate only mild tachypnea and difficulty handling respiratory infections.

EVALUATION AND TREATMENT Infants with severe BPD require prolonged assisted ventilation. Home oxygen therapy by nasal canula is commonly used for BPD. Diuretics are used to control pulmonary edema. Bronchodilators reduce airway resistance. Early antiinflammatory therapies, such as steroids, may facilitate weaning from mechanical ventilation and may or may not cause risks, such as abnormal neurologic development.[15] Nutritional needs are high and must be met to promote growth and healing.

Death from BPD is usually caused by infection, cor pulmonale, or respiratory failure. However, most infants with BPD improve substantially during the first year or two of life. Nevertheless, there is an increased incidence of asthma during childhood and pulmonary function abnormalities may persist for many years.[13,16]

QUICK CHECK 27-2

1. Why do premature infants get RDS?
2. Describe the pathologic findings of "new BPD."

Respiratory infections

Respiratory infections are common in children and are a frequent cause for emergency room visits and hospitalizations. Clinical presentation, age of the child, and season of the year can often provide clues to the etiologic agent, even when the agent cannot be proven.

Bronchiolitis

Bronchiolitis is a rather common, viral-induced lower respiratory tract infection that occurs almost exclusively in infants and young toddlers. It has a seasonal, yearly incidence, from approximately November to April, and is the leading cause of hospitalization for infants during the winter season. The most common associated pathogen is respiratory syncytial virus (RSV), which accounts for 50% to 75% of cases,[17,18] but also may be associated with adenoviruses, influenza, parainfluenza, and mycoplasma. Rhinovirus and human metapneumovirus have been linked to infant bronchilitis.[19] Healthy infants usually make a full recovery from RSV bronchiolitis, but infants who were premature (birthweight <2500 g) or who have underlying BPD or heart disease may have a much higher risk for a more severe or even deadly course.

PATHOPHYSIOLOGY Viral infection causes necrosis of the bronchial epithelium and destruction of ciliated epithelial cells. There is infiltration with lymphocytes around the bronchioles and a cell-mediated hypersensitivity to viral

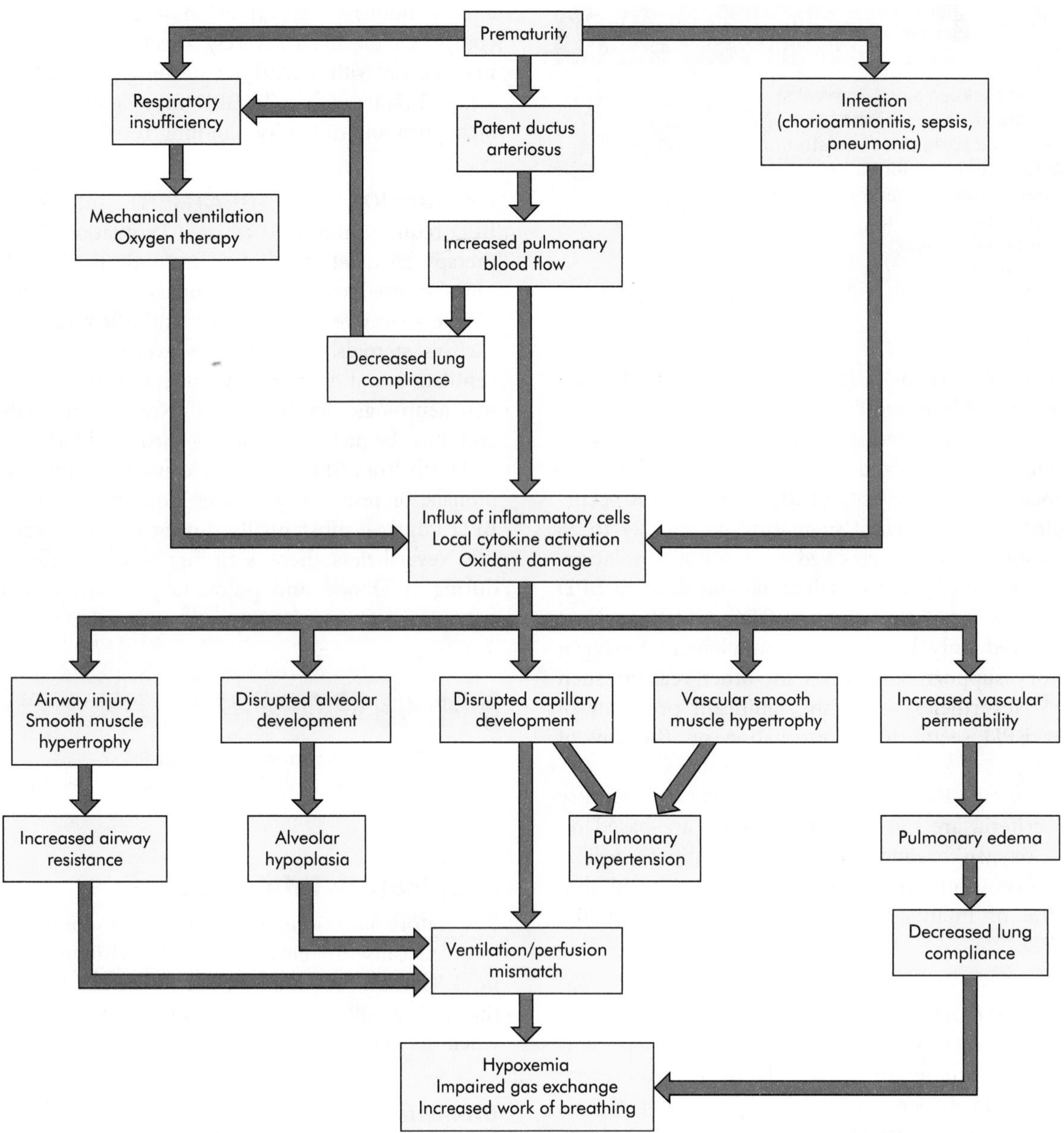

Figure 27-6 ■ Pathophysiology of Bronchopulmonary Dysplasia (BPD).

antigens with release of lymphokines causing inflammation, as well as activation of eosinophils, neutrophils, and monocytes.[20] The submucosa becomes edematous and cellular debris and fibrin form plugs within the bronchioles.

Edema of the bronchiolar wall, accumulation of mucus and cellular debris, and, perhaps, bronchospasm narrow many peripheral airways. Other airways become partially or completely occluded. Atelectasis occurs in some areas of the lung and hyperinflation in others.

The mechanics of breathing are disrupted by bronchiolitis. There is air trapping, and functional residual capacity (FRC) is greatly increased. Compliance is decreased because the lungs are already highly inflated and because airway resistance within the lung is uneven and increased. The decrease in compliance and the increase in airway resistance result in a substantial increase in the work of breathing. Serious alterations in gas exchange occur because of airway obstruction and patchy atelectasis. Hypoxemia develops because of ventilation-perfusion mismatch (see Chapter 26), and hypercapnia may occur in severe cases.

CLINICAL MANIFESTATIONS Symptoms usually begin with significant rhinorrhea followed with a tight cough over the next several days, along with systemic signs of poor feedings, lethargy, and, often, fever. Infants typically have tachypnea, variable degrees of respiratory distress, and abnormal auscultatory findings of the chest. Wheezing is most common, but rales or rhonchi also may be present. Chest radiographs often reveal hyperexpanded lungs, patchy or peribronchial infiltrates, and, sometimes, atelectasis of the right upper lobe. Very young infants may present with severe apneas before lower respiratory tract symptoms appear, and these apneas frequently require mechanical ventilation.

EVALUATION AND TREATMENT Diagnosis of bronchiolitis is made by review of signs and symptoms (e.g., rhinitis, cough, wheezing, chest retractions, tachypnea) and radiologic examination. Nasal washings may be tested for specific viral agents, such as RSV. Treatment is determined by the severity of the disease and the age of the child. Most cases are mild and require no specific treatment and may be monitored as outpatients. Inhaled bronchodilators and steroids remain controversial.[17,21,22] They have not been validated as effective therapies but are widely tried on a case-by-case basis. Babies with underlying lung disease usually do benefit from inhaled therapies, and those with BPD often need increased diuretic therapy during the acute illness. Mechanical ventilation is occasionally necessary. Preventive treatment with RSV-specific monoclonal antibody, provided as a monthly injection through the RSV season, is recommended for high-risk infants under 2 years old who meet specific criteria.[17]

Pneumonia

Pneumonia involves inflammation and infection in the terminal airways and alveoli. It is a major cause of morbidity and mortality, particularly in developing countries. The most common agents are viruses, followed by bacteria and mycoplasma (Table 27-2). Widespread childhood vaccination has decreased the incidence of *Haemophilus influenzae (H. influenzae)* type b and *Streptococcus pneumoniae* infections.[23]

Viral pneumonia is acquired by direct contact, droplet transmission, or aerosol. There is initial destruction of ciliated epithelium of the distal airway with sloughing of cellular material. A mononuclear-predominant inflammatory response occurs, in the interstitium initially, and later may involve the alveoli as well.

The most common cause of viral pneumonia in infants is respiratory syncytial virus (RSV),[24] usually occurring in the winter to early spring. A number of other viruses are important, including parainfluenza, influenza, and adenoviruses. Certain serotypes of adenovirus can cause necrotizing disease, sometimes leading to bronchiolitis obliterans and significant lung disability.

Bacterial pneumonia usually results from inhalation of microbes dispersed in ambient air or in secretion droplets (person-to-person spread) or by aspiration of one's own nasopharyngeal bacteria. Once in the alveolar region, bacteria will encounter local host defenses, such as opsonins and IgG, which prepare bacteria for ingestion by alveolar macrophages. If these mechanisms fail, neutrophils will be recruited and an intense, cytokine-mediated inflammation will ensue. Vascular engorgement, edema, and a fibrinopurulent exudate occur. Alveolar filling precludes gas exchange and, if extensive, can lead to respiratory failure.[25] If sepsis occurs at the same time, shock and end-organ hypoperfusion will cause metabolic acidosis. A spreading viral infection of the lower respiratory tract sometimes sets the stage for bacterial infection by causing epithelial damage and reduced mucociliary clearance. One study showed that among childhood pneumonias requiring hospitalization, one-fourth were associated with mixed viral and bacterial pathogens.[26]

Pneumococcal pneumonia is the most common cause of community-acquired bacterial pneumonia and presents acutely and with variable severity. In 2000, a polyvariant pneumococcal vaccine was incorporated into routine childhood immunizations and appears to have lessened the

TABLE 27-2

Common Types of Pneumonia in Children

Type	Causal Agent	Age	Onset	Signs/Symptoms
Viral pneumonia	Respiratory syncytial virus (RSV), influenza, adenovirus, others	Infants for RSV, all ages for others	Acute or gradual, winter and early spring	Mild to high fever, cough, rhinorrhea, malaise, rales, rhonchi, or wheezing, apnea, variable radiographic pattern
Pneumococcal pneumonia	Pneumococci *(Streptococcus pneumoniae)*	Usually 1–4 yr	Acute, follows an upper respiratory infection, winter and early spring	High fever, productive cough, pleuritic pain, increased respiration rate, decreased breath sounds in area of consolidation; lobar infiltrate or "round pneumonia" on radiograph
Staphylococcal pneumonia	*Staphylococcus aureus* (including methicillin-resistant strains)	1 wk–2 yr	Acute, winter	High fever, cough, respiratory distress, empyema or pneumatoceles common
Streptococcal pneumonia	Group A β-hemolytic streptococci	All ages	Acute, any season	High fever, chills, respiratory distress, sepsis, or shock
Mycoplasma and chlamydia pneumonia	*Mycoplasma pneumoniae, Chlamydia pneumoniae*	School-age and adolescents	Gradual	Low-grade fever, cough

incidence of pneumococcal pneumonia in children under 2 years of age.[27] Staphylococcal and group A streptococcal pneumonia can be particularly fulminant (sudden, severe) and necrotizing (causing cell death) with a high incidence of accompanying empyema, pneumatocele, and sepsis. *H. influenzae* pneumonia has become rare because of widespread immunization.

Atypical pneumonia *(Mycoplasma pneumoniae, Chlamydia pneumoniae)* is the most common cause of community-acquired pneumonia for school-age children and young adults. *Chlamydia* pneumonia is clinically indistinguishable from and is typically grouped with *Mycoplasma* as "atypical pneumonia."[28,29] Transmission is from person to person with a 2- to 3-week incubation period.

Mycoplasmic microorganisms lack cell walls but have a limiting membrane and a specialized receptor for attaching to ciliated respiratory epithelial cells. Local sloughing of cells occurs. Peribronchial lymphocytic infiltration develops, along with neutrophil recruitment to the airway lumen. The pattern resembles bronchitis or bronchopneumonia.

Onset is usually gradual, resembling a typical upper respiratory infection but with low-grade fever and prominent cough. Cases are not usually clinically severe, and full recovery should be expected.

EVALUATION AND TREATMENT Diagnosis of pneumonia is based on clinical findings and chest radiograph confirmation; the etiologic agent can sometimes be inferred from the age of the child and clinical scenario.[23] A bacterial pneumonia will initially produce a patchy infiltration and later cause a segmental or lobar disease. A unilateral lobar consolidation on a chest x-ray film is often associated with *Streptococcus pneumoniae.* The formation of small areas of airway dilatation (called pneumatoceles) most commonly suggest a *Staphylococcal pneumoniae.* Pleural effusions are rarely seen with viral pneumonias or atypical pneumonias.

Some pneumonias may be treated on an outpatient basis; however, many children require oxygen supplementation and, occasionally, assisted ventilation. This is particularly true with infants who have a viral interstitial pneumonia, such as RSV. In addition, adequate hydration, nutrition, and supportive pulmonary therapy are required to reduce the duration and severity of illness. Many infants are markedly tachypneic and unable to coordinate their breathing with swallowing; they may require enteral feeding. Aspiration is always a risk with infants in respiratory distress.

Appropriate antibiotic administration for bacterial pneumonias should be instituted for a minimum of 10 days, and longer for *Staphylococcus aureus* or group A streptococcus.[23,30]

✓ QUICK CHECK 27-3

1. Describe the typical presentation of RSV bronchiolitis.
2. What clinical features distinguish bacterial pneumonia from atypical pneumonia?

Aspiration pneumonitis

Aspiration pneumonitis is caused by a foreign substance, such as food, secretions, or environmental compounds, entering the lung and resulting in inflammation. The aspiration of meconium from amniotic fluid can occur at birth. Meconium contains bile salts from the fetal intestinal tract that cause inflammation. Neurologically compromised children or children undergoing sedation or anesthesia may aspirate oral secretions and their anaerobic bacteria or stomach contents. The severity of lung injury after an aspiration incident is determined by pH of the aspirated material and presence of pathogenic bacteria. Very low pH or extremely high pH will cause a significant inflammatory response. With hydrocarbon ingestions, lung injury is determined by the volatility and viscosity of the aspirated substance. A low-viscosity substance, such as gasoline or lighter fluid, is the most toxic, and high-viscosity hydrocarbons, such as petroleum jelly or mineral oil, are much less likely to cause a pneumonitis. Treatment for aspiration pneumonitis depends on the material aspirated.

Bronchiolitis obliterans

Bronchiolitis obliterans is fibrotic obstruction of the respiratory bronchioles and alveolar ducts secondary to intense inflammation. Cases of bronchiolitis obliterans in children are rare but are most often sequelae of a severe viral pulmonary infection (e.g., influenza, adenovirus, pertussis [whooping cough], or measles). It also may occur after lung transplantation. While the child initially improves after the acute insult, the progression of disease is then reflected by increasing dyspnea, cough, sputum production, and wheezing and is related to airway obstruction.[31]

There is no specific treatment for bronchiolitis obliterans. Some children deteriorate rapidly and die within weeks, whereas others follow a more chronic course.

Asthma

Asthma is an inflammatory, obstructive airway disease characterized by reversible airflow obstruction and bronchial hyperreactivity, usually in response to an allergen or viral infection. It is the most prevalent chronic disease in childhood, affecting 5% to 10% of all children, and has become more prevalent in the past 2 decades. The economic burden on society is huge, including both medical and indirect costs, such as parental time lost from work.[32] In the prepubertal years, more boys than girls are affected. It is noteworthy that inner-city black and Hispanic children have higher morbidity and mortality than white children.[33] Mortality rates associated with childhood asthma seem to have leveled off after many years of rising.[34] Asthma-related deaths almost always occur outside the hospital setting.

There are currently many theories regarding the mechanisms of disease in childhood asthma. The wide spectrum of clinical disease probably reflects a complex interaction between *genetic* susceptibility and *environmental* factors, including early exposure to allergens and infections, particularly viral respiratory infections.[35–38]

HEALTH ALERT
Asthma Genes and Tailored Therapies

Genomic screening of populations suggests that there is no single "asthma gene" but rather numerous genes that may be associated with asthma. It may ultimately be possible to associate certain gene variants with specific clinical patterns of asthma and with responsiveness to specific asthma treatments. For example, one variant (or polymorphism) is the gene for the β-2-adrenergic receptor that has been shown to be associated with a poor or even adverse response to albuterol in one study. If findings such as these can be corroborated and expanded in larger studies, it ultimately may be possible to develop individual profiles to optimize asthma therapy.

Data from Steinke JW, Borish L: Genetics of allergic disease, *Med Clin N Am* 90(1):1–15, 2006; Meurer JR, Lustig JV, Jacob HJ: Genetic aspects of the etiology and treatment of asthma, *Pediatr Clin North Am* 53(4):715-25, 2006.

PATHOPHYSIOLOGY Examination of postmortem lung specimens of individuals who died from asthma reveals abnormalities consistent with both acute and chronic changes in the airways. These include extensive mucous plugging, mucosal edema, and denudation of bronchial and bronchiolar epithelium. Eosinophilia is present in the submucosa, and a multicellular inflammatory infiltrate accumulates in the airways. Thickening of the basement membrane, airway smooth muscle hypertrophy, and mucous gland hypertrophy are often noted, sometimes even in pathology specimens from mild asthmatics, providing evidence that there may be long-term airway structural changes associated with asthma. In chronic asthma, increased numbers of inflammatory cells may lead to long-term changes, such as goblet cell hyperplasia and airway wall remodeling (subepithelial fibrosis, smooth muscle hypertrophy). The pathophysiology of asthma in children is the same as in adults (see Chapter 26, p. 726 and Figure 26-9).

In a full-blown asthma attack **(status asthmaticus),** there is bronchospasm and acute airway inflammation. Mucus plugging, edema, and cellular infiltration lead to further airway narrowing. Partial obstruction creates a "ball-valve" effect leading to segmental hyperinflation, which may become extreme and compromise effective tidal volume. Expiratory flow rates, such as FEV_1, and peak flow are markedly reduced.

For acute allergen-induced asthma, the paradigm of the *early asthmatic response* remains useful (Figure 27-7, *A*). This begins immediately after exposure and lasts up to 2 hours. The allergen binds to preformed IgE on the surface of mucosal mast cells, and cross-linking of these IgE molecules triggers degranulation of the mast cell, releasing mediators such as histamine, leukotrienes, prostaglandin D_2, platelet activating factor, and certain cytokines. These mediators cause airway smooth muscle constriction (bronchospasm), increased vascular permeability (mucosal edema), and mucus secretion. The *late asthmatic response* starts at 4 to 8 hours postexposure and may persist up to 24 hours (Figure 27-7, *B*). The response is characterized by inflammatory cell recruitment (neutrophils, eosinophils, basophils, lymphocytes) that was triggered earlier by chemotactic factors and up-regulation of endothelial adhesion molecules. Another wave of mediator release occurs, again inciting bronchospasm, edema, and mucus secretion. Epithelial damage and impaired mucociliary function may be seen because of direct toxic effects of products such as major basic protein from eosinophils. This local injury stimulates local nerve endings, which may aggravate bronchoconstriction and mucus secretion through autonomic pathways. In *chronic asthma,* some of these mechanisms may be operational on an ongoing basis. Chronically increased numbers of inflammatory cells may lead to long-term changes, such as goblet cell hyperplasia and airway wall remodeling (subepithelial fibrosis, smooth muscle hypertrophy).

The typical arterial blood gas abnormalities in acute asthma are hypoxemia, hypocarbia, and respiratory alkalosis. As bronchial obstruction is nonuniform, ventilation is likewise uneven, causing ventilation-perfusion mismatch and hypoxemia. The degree of hypoxemia is usually mild, however, and arterial saturations of less than 90% indicate severe airway obstruction. Pulmonary circulation may be altered by regional hypoxic vasoconstriction, as well as the effect of increased intra-alveolar pressure (caused by hyperinflation) to decrease perfusion of alveolar capillaries. Typically, respiratory rate is elevated to compensate for hypoxemia with reduced minute ventilation because of increased airway resistance and lung hyperinflation. Thus, arterial pCO_2 is low (30 to 35 mm Hg) and even a normal value should be of concern. Retention of CO_2 is a late finding, usually only occurring if FEV_1 falls to around 15% to 20% of predicted values, and reflects inadequate alveolar ventilation and increased functional dead space as little air is being moved. Alterations of pH homeostasis usually start with respiratory alkalosis caused by hyperventilation. With severe airway obstruction, the end result of the pathophysiologic processes may be respiratory failure with acute CO_2 retention and respiratory acidosis. Metabolic acidosis may accompany life-threatening asthma, especially when left ventricular filling and thus cardiac output becomes compromised because of severe hyperinflation.

CLINICAL MANIFESTATIONS In a typical acute asthma attack, the major complaints are cough, wheeze, and shortness of breath. There may or may not have been signs of a preceding upper respiratory infection, such as rhinorrhea or low-grade fever. In children, about 70% to 80% of acute wheezing episodes are associated with viral respiratory infections. In infants and toddlers under 2 years old, the most common of these is respiratory syncytial virus (RSV). In older children and adults, the major viral trigger is rhinovirus (the "common cold" virus).[39]

On physical examination, there is expiratory wheezing that is often described as high pitched and musical, and there is prolongation of the expiratory phase of the respiratory cycle. Breath sound may become faint when air movement is poor. The child may speak in clipped sentences or not at all because of dyspnea. Sometimes hyperinflation (barrel chest) is visible. Respiratory rate and heart rate are elevated. Nasal flaring and use of accessory muscles with retractions in the substernal, subcostal, intercostal, suprasternal, or sternocleidomastoid areas are evident. Infants may appear to be "head bobbing" because of

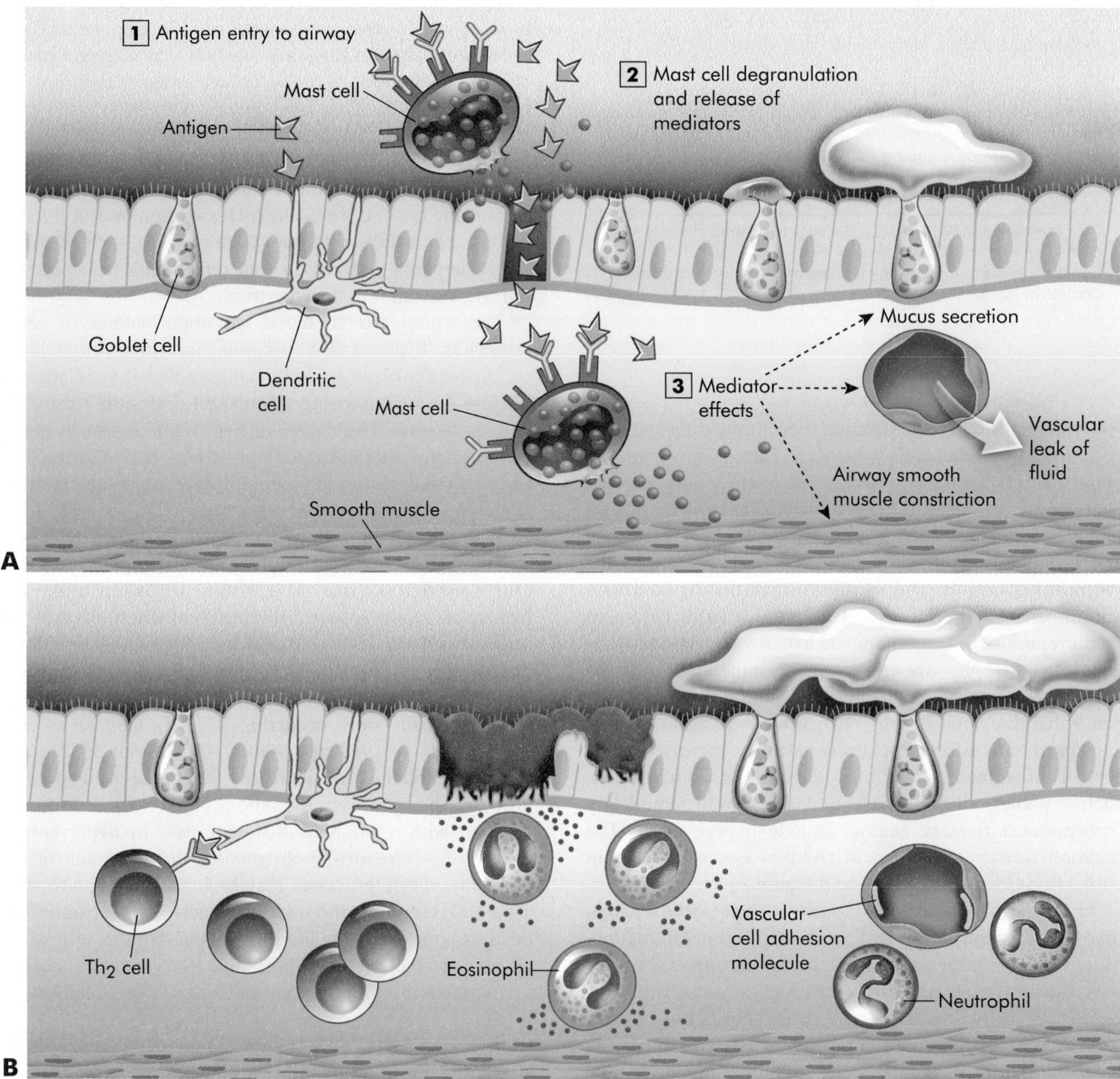

Figure 27-7 ■ **Asthmatic Responses. A,** In the early asthmatic response, inhaled antigen *(1)* binds to preformed IgE on mast cells. Mast cells degranulate *(2)* and release mediators such as histamine, leukotrienes, prostaglandin D_2, platelet activating factor, and others. Acute inflammation opens intercellular tight junctions, allowing allergen to penetrate and activate submucosal mast cells. Secreted mediators *(3)* induce active bronchospasm, edema, and mucus secretion. Inflammatory responses are set in motion by chemotactic factors and up-regulation of adhesion molecules *(not shown)*. At the same time, as shown on the left, antigen may be received by dendritic cells and later present it, either in regional lymph nodes to naïve (Th_o) T-lymphocytes or locally to memory Th_2 cells in the airway mucosa (see **B**). **B,** In the late asthmatic response, there are areas of epithelial damage caused at least in part by toxicity of eosinophil products (major basic protein, eosinophilic cationic protein, eosinophil-derived neurotoxin, and eosinophil peroxidase). Many inflammatory cells are recruited by chemokines and up-regulation of vascular cell adhesion molecules. Local T-lymphocytes display a predominant Th_2 cytokine profile. They produce IL-4 and IL-13, which promote switching of B cells to favor IgE production, and IL-3, IL-5, and granulocyte-macrophage colony-stimulating factor, which encourage eosinophil differentiation and survival.

sternocleidomastoid muscle use. Pulsus paradoxus may be present. The child may appear anxious or diaphoretic, important signs of respiratory compromise.

Findings in chronic asthma may include hyperinflation of the thorax or pectus excavatum. Clubbing should not be seen with asthma and, if present, should trigger evaluation for other conditions such as cystic fibrosis.

EVALUATION AND TREATMENT For objective evaluation of asthma, the best indicators are measures of pulmonary function using spirometry. For home management of asthma, peak flow meters are often used to help guide treatment in the face of increased symptoms or intercurrent illness.

Rapid-acting bronchodilators, such as albuterol or levalbuterol (β_2 agonist), are typically used for management of acute asthma, as well as systemic steroids for moderate to severe attacks to decrease inflammatory responses in the lung.[40] Inhaled ipratropium bromide is an anticholinergic agent that contributes to bronchodilation by inhibiting vagal tone; it is sometimes used additive effect or sometimes as an alternative for those who cannot tolerate β_2 agonists because of side effects.

There is a growing number of options for management of chronic asthma depending on chronicity and severity of symptoms, as well as individual compliance issues. Guidelines have been outlined and widely distributed by a National Institutes of Health (NIH) expert panel.[41] The most important element of chronic asthma management seems to be reduction of inflammation. For individuals with persistent symptoms, daily "controller" medication is recommended. The most widely preferred controller therapy remains inhaled corticosteroids. However, montelukast (an oral leukotriene receptor antagonist) is frequently used as supplemental therapy or, for milder or exercise-induced asthma, as monotherapy.[42,43] Inhaled cromolyn and nedocromil remain available anti-inflammatory therapies, but their use has declined in favor of other therapies, at least in the United States. Long-acting β_2-adrenergic agonists, such as salmeterol, also may be applied to pediatric asthma except in the youngest children. For allergic asthma, anti-IgE therapy has become available for select individuals (see *Health Alert:* Monoclonal Antibodies to IgE for Treatment of Asthma in Chapter 26, p. 729).

QUICK CHECK 27-4

1. What are the key features of the early and late asthmatic responses?
2. Explain the full progression of blood gas abnormalities in a severe asthma attack.

Acute respiratory distress syndrome

Acute respiratory distress syndrome (ARDS) is a dramatic, life-threatening condition resulting from a direct pulmonary insult (such as pneumonia, aspiration, near drowning, or smoke inhalation) or a systemic insult (such as sepsis or multiple trauma), either of which activates an inflammatory response that causes alveolocapillary injury. Clinically, ARDS is characterized by severe hypoxemia, decreased pulmonary compliance, and diffuse densities on chest radio-. graph. ARDS accounts for approximately 10% of total patient days and one third of all deaths in pediatric intensive care units.[44] Mortality in pediatric ARDS remains high, at approximately 50%.[45]

PATHOPHYSIOLOGY The hallmark of ARDS is lung inflammation. There is activation of the inflammatory response (see Figure 26-7), including complement, cytokines, arachidonic acid metabolites, platelet-activating factor, reactive oxygen species, and others. Sources of these mediators include neutrophils, activated platelets, macrophages, and injured endothelium. In early ARDS, there is pulmonary neutrophil influx along with intraluminal fibrin and platelet aggregation. Injury to pulmonary capillary endothelium results in capillary leak and noncardiogenic pulmonary edema. Edema fluid contains plasma proteins that can inactivate surfactant, contributing further to alveolar collapse. This fluid also has procoagulant activity, leading to fibrin clotting within airspaces. During the acute phase, the pulmonary microcirculation is compromised by the formation of thrombi composed of fibrin, platelets, and leukocytes.

The early accumulation of edema fluid in the airspaces results in decreased lung compliance, decreased functional residual volume, and increased dead space. There is ventilation/perfusion mismatching, intrapulmonary shunting, and hypoxemia. Diffuse pulmonary thrombosis contributes further to the formation of pulmonary edema by increasing capillary hydrostatic pressure and may lead to pulmonary hypertension.

In the fibroproliferative phase, type II alveolar cells proliferate, and alveolar septal thickening and collagen deposition occur. Interstitial fibrosis can be evident as early as 10 days from the initial insult. Similarly, vascular changes may occur including obliteration of the microcirculation and thickening of the walls of pulmonary arterioles and arteries, which can then lead to chronic pulmonary hypertension in survivors.

CLINICAL MANIFESTATIONS ARDS develops acutely after the initial insult, usually within 24 hours, though occasionally it is delayed up to a few days. There is progressive respiratory distress and severe hypoxemia with poor response to oxygen supplementation. Chest radiograph shows diffuse bilateral opacities. Initially, hyperventilation occurs, but CO_2 retention may ultimately occur as well because of inadequate functional airspace and respiratory muscle fatigue. Severity of the overall picture is modified by comorbid factors, such as the presence of sepsis or multiorgan failure, and whether or not there are complications, such as nosocomial pneumonia. Some children who recover have residual pulmonary abnormalities.

EVALUATION AND TREATMENT Treatment for ARDS remains supportive in nature, and the goals are to maintain adequate tissue oxygenation, minimize acute lung injury, and avoid iatrogenic pulmonary complications. Most individuals with ARDS require mechanical ventilation and often relatively high levels of positive end-expiratory pressure (PEEP) to promote alveolar ventilation and stabilization, and redistribution of alveolar edema fluid into the interstitium. Ventilation strategies may include low tidal volume, permissive hypercapnia, prone positioning, and high-frequency oscillation.[46]

Cystic fibrosis

Cystic fibrosis (CF) is an autosomal recessive inherited disease that results from defective epithelial chloride ion transport. The CF gene has been located on chromosome 7. Its mutation results in the abnormal expression of the protein, **cystic fibrosis transmembrane conductance regulator (CFTR),** which is a chloride channel present on the surface of many types of epithelial cells including airways, bile ducts, pancreas, sweat ducts, and vas deferens.[47] CF affects primarily whites (approximately 1 in 3200) but is occasionally seen in other groups as well. The estimated carrier frequency is high, 1 in 28 whites in the United States. Carriers are not affected by the mutation.

PATHOPHYSIOLOGY Although CF is a multiorgan disease, its most important effects are on the lungs, and respiratory failure is almost always the cause of death. The typical features of CF lung disease are mucus plugging, chronic inflammation, and chronic infection. The mucus plugging seen in CF probably results from both increased production of mucus and altered physicochemical properties of the mucus. Mucus-secreting airway cells (goblet cells and submucosal glands) are increased in number and size. CF mucus is dehydrated and viscous because of defective chloride secretion and excess sodium absorption. The periciliary fluid layer is depleted in volume, impairing the mobility of the cilia and thereby allowing mucus to adhere to the airway epithelium, along with bacteria and injurious by-products from neutrophils.[48,49]

Chronic inflammation is believed to contribute to long-term lung damage, and there is evidence that this process may even begin in infancy. Abnormal cytokine profiles promote a proinflammatory state.[50]

Neutrophils are present in great excess in the airways and release damaging oxidants and proteases.[51] One such protease in particular, neutrophil elastase, causes (1) direct damage to lung structural proteins, such as elastin; (2) induction of airway cells to produce interleukin-8 (IL-8), a potent attractant for neutrophils and thus a means for augmenting a local "vicious cycle" of inflammation; (3) cleavage of IgG and complement components important for opsonization and phagocytosis of pathogens; and (4) stimulation of mucus secretion, a strong effect of IL-8.

Children with CF have a propensity for chronic endobronchial infection that remains poorly understood. It is likely that local factors in the CF airway microenvironment favor bacterial colonization, because there is no systemic immune defect. *Staphylococcus aureus* is common, and *Pseudomonas aeruginosa* ultimately colonizes airways in at least 75% of children with CF. *Pseudomonas* acquisition has been linked with more rapid decline in pulmonary function.[49,52] Persistence of this microorganism incites chronic local inflammation and airway damage. Combined with chronic bacterial infection, these lead to microabscess formation, bronchiectasis, patchy consolidation and pneumonia, peribronchial fibrosis, and cyst formation (Figure 27-8). There is a progressive decrease in the amount of available and functional lung tissue. The pathophysiology for these changes is outlined in Figure 27-9. Peripheral bullae may develop because of obstruction and airway wall weakening and pneumothorax may occur. Hemoptysis, sometimes life threatening, may occur because of the erosion of enlarged bronchial arteries that develop in response to the inflammation associated with bronchiectasis. Over a long period of time, pulmonary vascular remodeling occurs because of localized hypoxia and arteriolar vasoconstriction,

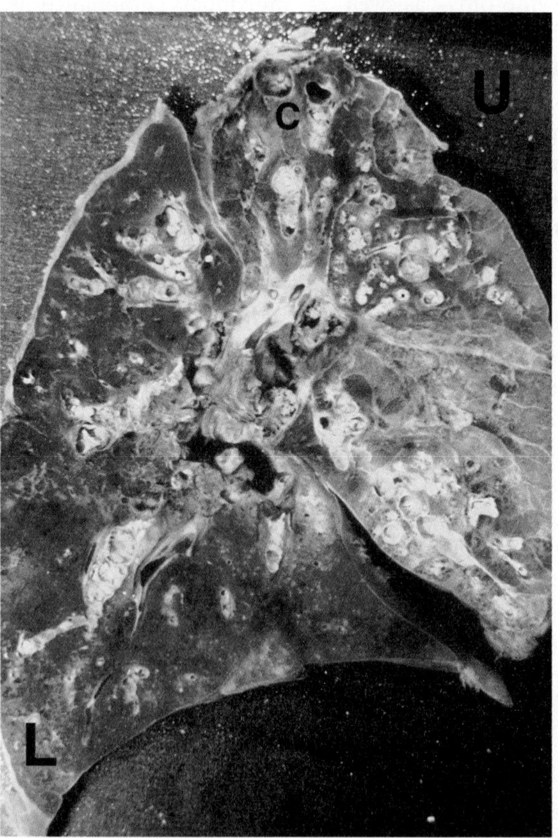

Figure 27-8 ■ Pathology of the Lung in End-Stage Cystic Fibrosis. Key features are widespread mucus impaction of airways and bronchiectasis (especially from upper lobe *[U]*), with hemorrhagic pneumonia in the lower lobe *(L)*. Small cysts *(C)* are present at the apex of the lung. (From Kleinerman J, Vauthy P: *Pathology of the lung in cystic fibrosis,* Atlanta, 1976, Cystic Fibrosis Foundation.)

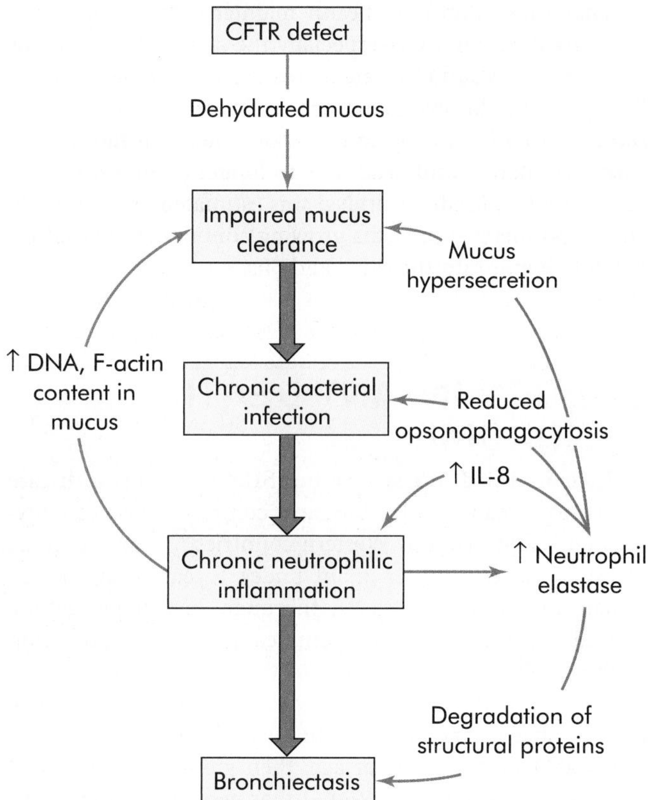

Figure 27-9 ■ **Pathogenesis of Cystic Fibrosis Lung Disease.** *CFTR,* Cystic fibrosis transmembrane conductance regulator.

and pulmonary hypertension and cor pulmonale may develop in the late stages of disease.

CLINICAL MANIFESTATIONS The median age at diagnosis is 6 months and nearly 75% of cases are diagnosed by 1 year. Approximately 10% of cases are not diagnosed until after age 10, however, and these children or even adults usually have milder symptoms. The most common presentations are respiratory or gastrointestinal. Respiratory symptoms include persistent cough or wheeze and recurrent or severe pneumonia. Physical signs that develop over time include barrel chest and digital clubbing. Classic gastrointestinal presentations include meconium ileus at birth, which is pathognomic for CF and prompts the diagnosis in 20% of all children with CF. Approximately half of all children present with failure-to-thrive and malabsorptive symptoms, such as frequent, loose, and oily stools. More subtle presentations include chronic sinusitis, nasal polyps, and rectal prolapse. Newborn screening for CF is expanding rapidly throughout the United States and will increase the numbers of early, presymptomatic diagnosis[53] (see *Health Alert:* Newborn Screening for Cystic Fibrosis). Complications of CF may include liver disease (approximately 5%) and diabetes mellitus (10% to 25%). Overall severity of CF is variable and is not generally predictable on the basis of genotype.

HEALTH ALERT

Newborn Screening for Cystic Fibrosis

Unfortunately, the diagnosis of cystic fibrosis (CF) is still frequently missed or significantly delayed, after perplexing and frustrating struggles for the child and family. Often there have been hospitalizations, unexplained recurrent respiratory symptoms, and failure to thrive. Several states piloted newborn screening for CF starting in the 1980s (Colorado, Wisconsin, and Wyoming), and many others have recently added programs. Long-term data show that patients with CF identified by newborn screening have better nutritional status and growth than those identified by symptomatic presentation, not only at diagnosis but persisting for at least 7 years. This has important implications because poor nutritional status has been linked to poor clinical outcome over the long term. Several studies support the presence of an advantage in pulmonary function and, possibly, delayed colonization with *Pseudomonas aeruginosa.* Based on available evidence, the Centers for Disease Control and Prevention issued a recommendation in 2004 supporting neonatal screening for CF. It is anticipated that most states will implement this screening by 2010. However, the methodologies involved in screening are rather cumbersome. An initial screen is performed on the routine newborn bloodspot based on a biochemical marker, immunoreactive trypsinogen (IRT). Positive screens are followed up by either repeat blood test for IRT or CF mutation screen. Screening programs require a high level of support from CF centers and genetic counseling professionals, as well as education of primary physicians and the community. Difficult problems include handling initial false positive IRT results, appropriate information for those with select "mild" mutations that are not well understood, and making sure that the many CF gene carriers that will be identified do not misunderstand their status. States choosing to adopt screening will have to tailor the details of their programs to match available resources statewide.

Data from Castellani C: Evidence for newborn screening for cystic fibrosis, *Paediatric Resp Rev* 4(4):278–284, 2003; Centers for Disease Control and Prevention: *MMWR* 53(RR-13), 2004; Lai HJ et al: Association between initial disease presentation, lung disease outcomes, and survival in patients with cystic fibrosis, *Am J Epidemiol* 159(6):537–546, 2004; Lai HJ et al: Evidence on improved outcomes with early diagnosis of cystic fibrosis through neonatal screening: enough is enough. *J Pediatr* 147(3 suppl):S57–S63, 2005; Grosse SD, Rosenfeld M, Devine OJ, Lai HJ, Farrell PM: Potential impact of newborn screening for cystic fibrosis on child survival: a systematic review and analysis, *J Pediatr* 149(3):362–6, 2006.

EVALUATION AND TREATMENT The standard method of diagnosis is the sweat test, which reveals sweat chloride concentration in excess of 60 mEq/L. Genotyping for CFTR mutations is available as an alternative or supplemental method but may fail to confirm up to 10% of cases because of a lack of ability to screen for every described CF-associated mutation (there are over 1000 CF-associated mutations).

Treatment is primarily focused on pulmonary health and nutrition. Common pulmonary therapies include techniques to promote mucus clearance, such as chest physical therapy and related mechanical devices, bronchodilators, and aerosolized DNase, which liquefies mucus. Inhaled maintenance antibiotics (i.e., tobramycin) can be used to suppress *Pseudomonas aeruginosa* when it is present, and this has a beneficial clinical impact.[49] Oral antibiotics are used fairly liberally for minor pulmonary exacerbations. Intravenous antibiotics are used to treat major flareups of pulmonary infection, which may be either subacute or acute in presentation. Individuals with end-stage lung disease may consider lung transplantation.

Approximately 90% of children with CF have pancreatic insufficiency and therefore need to take pancreatic enzymes (for absorption of nutrients) before meals and snacks for their entire lifetime. Fat-soluble vitamins must be supplemented. Caloric needs are high, especially with advancing lung disease, and high-calorie supplements or even gastrostomy feeding may be warranted. Nutritional care for children with CF has become increasingly aggressive because of the documented link to better long-term outcomes.

HEALTH ALERT
A Cure for Cystic Fibrosis?

After sequencing the cystic fibrosis (CF) gene in 1989, hopes were voiced for a gene therapy "cure" within 5 years. Ideally, the normal cystic fibrosis transmembrane conductance regulator (CFTR) gene could be inhaled or sprayed into the lungs and thereby halt disease progression. The task has proven more formidable than expected. Different methods, such as viral vectors or lipid-DNA complexes, have demonstrated problems of low efficiency of gene transfer, lack of persistence of gene transfer, or significant host immune responses. Since 1993, a number of limited gene transfer experiments have been completed in individuals with CF. Some of these have provided "proof of concept" in that normal CFTR mRNA (transcribed from the transferred DNA) was seen in at least a small portion of epithelial cells, and local chloride transport could be at least partially corrected. It is hoped that continued development of strategies may one day make the process efficient, practical, and safe.

Lung transplantation is an option for selected individuals with end-stage lung disease from CF. Complications are usually related to infection or rejection, and survival at 5 years posttransplant is approximately 50%. Unfortunately, the demand exceeds the supply of available transplantable lungs. Usual guidelines suggest consideration of listing when FEV_1 has deteriorated to approximately 30% of predicted, or somewhat higher if the clinical course is rapidly declining.

Data from Liou TG, Woo MS, Cahill BC: Lung transplantation for cystic fibrosis, *Curr Opin Pulm Med* 12(6):459–463, 2006; Griesenbach U, Geddes DM, Alton EWFW: Advances in cystic fibrosis gene therapy, *Curr Opin Pulmon Med* 10:542–546, 2004; Lee TW, Matthews DA, Blair GE: Novel molecular approaches to cystic fibrosis gene therapy, *Biochem J* 387(Pt 1):1–15, 2005; Rosenecker J, Huth S, Rudolph C: Gene therapy for cystic fibrosis lung disease: current status and future perspectives, *Curr Opin Mol Ther* 8(5): 439–445, 2006; Nathan SD: Lung transplantation: disease-specific considerations for referral, *Chest* 127:1006–1016, 2005.

There are often high health maintenance requirements for individuals with CF (especially the demanding schedule of medications and respiratory treatments), yet most should be expected to be able to participate in normal activities and function well for a long time. Frequent hospitalizations and early debilitation and death are no longer common in children with CF. Median survival was estimated at 37 years in 2006, and there is, in fact, a growing contingent of adult CF patients living into their 40s and 50s.

SUDDEN INFANT DEATH SYNDROME

Sudden infant death syndrome (SIDS) remains a disease of unknown cause and is the most common cause of unexplained infant death in Western countries.[54,55] It is defined as "sudden death of an infant under 1 year of age which remains unexplained after a thorough case investigation, including performance of a complete autopsy, examination of the death scene, and review of the clinical history."[54]

The incidence of SIDS is low during the first month of life but sharply increases in the second month of life and peaks at 3 to 4 months of age, then gradually declines. It is more common in male (60%) than female (40%) infants. It almost always seems to occur during nighttime sleep, when infants are least likely to be observed. A seasonal variation has been noted, with higher frequencies during the winter months. This has been related to a higher rate of respiratory tract infection during those months and, in fact, such infections are often reported to have preceded the death.

Clinical risk groups include babies who were preterm or low birth weight, who were one of simultaneous multiple births, and who were siblings of prior SIDS victims. Nevertheless, about three quarters of all SIDS victims have no known predisposing clinical risk factor.

Additional risk factors fall into the categories of socioeconomic or maternal factors, and factors in the baby's sleeping situation. Maternal factors that predict increased SIDS risk are maternal smoking, young maternal age (under 20 years), less prenatal care, poverty, and illicit drug use. Risk factors that relate to the baby's sleeping situation are prone positioning, sleeping on a soft surface, and overheating.[56–58] Prone sleeping was concluded to be a major and modifiable risk factor. Epidemiologic studies have now shown lowering of SIDS rates by 40% to 70% in countries, including the United States, where massive public campaigns warned against prone sleeping for infants. Infants should sleep on their backs, even in preference over side sleeping. Other avoidable risk factors include sleeping on top of any soft surface (such as sheepskins, quilts, comforters, pillows, porous mattresses, waterbeds) and loose bedding. Overwrapping the infant or overheating the room also appear to increase risk, particularly if the infant is sleeping prone.

RISK FACTORS Sudden Infant Death Syndrome (SIDS)

- Prone sleeping position
- Soft sleep surfaces and/or loose bedding
- Overheated sleeping environment
- Lower socioeconomic status
- Mothers younger than 20
- Low birth weight
- Preterm delivery
- Multiple birth
- Sibling who died of SIDS
- Smoking during pregnancy
- Exposure to tobacco smoke
- Lack of prenatal care

Data from Kohlendorfer U, Kiechl S, Sperl W: Sudden infant death syndrome: risk factor profiles for distinct subgroups. *Am J Epidemiol* 147(10):960–968, 1998; Ponsonby AL, Dwyer T, Cochrane J: Population trends in sudden infant death syndrome, *Semin Perinatol* 26(4):296–305, 2002; Centers for Disease Control and Prevention: Sudden infant death syndrome (SIDS): risk factors. Last reviewed 5/24/2006 at http://www.cdc.gov/SIDS/riskfactors.htm

The etiology of SIDS remains unknown but probably involves a combination of predisposing factors and external stressors.[54,55] A leading hypothesis is that there may be developmental immaturity of ventilatory and arousal responses to hypoxemia or hypercarbia. Alternative theories involve airway obstruction events; increased vagal tone; sudden intrapulmonary shunting because of abnormalities of surfactant or pulmonary vessels; or exaggerated inflammation, eosinophil degranulation, and massive cytokine release causing pulmonary edema in response to either bacterial pathogens from the nasopharynx or viral respiratory tract infections. Even genetic factors may be linked including those for congenital cardiac conduction abnormalities (e.g., long-QT syndrome).[59,60]

Currently, the best strategies for reducing SIDS seem to be avoidance of all the controllable risk factors. Parents of infants with clinical risk should be taught cardiopulmonary resuscitation (CPR) as a precaution. Although home monitoring has not been proven to decrease the incidence of SIDS, some at-risk infants may warrant cardiorespiratory monitoring after careful consideration of the individual situation.[61]

QUICK CHECK 27-5

1. How are the alveoli and capillaries affected by the inflammation of acute respiratory distress syndrome (ARDS)?
2. What aspects of lung disease in cystic fibrosis are the focus of current therapies?
3. What are the risk factors for SIDS?

Did You Understand?

Pulmonary Disorders in Children

1. Croup is an acute respiratory illness of young children, usually caused by parainfluenza virus. This infection causes swelling of the upper trachea. The typical sign is a seal-like barking cough, which appears after a few days of rhinorrhea, sore throat, and low-grade fever.
2. Spasmodic croup is characterized by a similar barking cough but occurs in older children, is of sudden onset at night, without fever, and has unknown etiology.
3. Acute epiglottitis is a potentially life-threatening airway infection, whose incidence has decreased dramatically since the advent of *H. influenzae* vaccine. Now other pathogens, such as group A *Streptococcus,* are usually the causative agents.
4. Aspiration of foreign bodies that lodge in the airways may cause cough, hoarseness, stridor or wheezing, and dyspnea. The severity of the situation depends on the location of the foreign body within the airway and the degree of obstruction. Blockage of the larynx or trachea can be fatal, whereas bronchial obstruction may not even be diagnosed immediately.
5. Obstructive sleep apnea syndrome (OSAS) is defined by partial or complete upper airway obstruction during sleep with disruption of normal ventilation and normal sleep patterns. The most common cause in children is adenotonsillar hypertrophy.
6. Respiratory distress syndrome (RDS) of the newborn usually occurs in premature infants who are born before surfactant production and alveolocapillary development are complete. Atelectasis and hypoventilation cause shunting, hypoxemia, and hypercapnia. Prenatal steroids and postnatal surfactant are beneficial therapies.
7. Bronchopulmonary dysplasia (BPD) is the result of tissue injury and repair and disrupted alveolar development in the lungs of infants who required ventilatory support during a time when their lungs were underdeveloped because of their prematurity. Infants with BPD may require oxygen and additional therapies for many months.
8. Bronchiolitis presents with runny nose, wheezing, cough, and tachypnea in infants and is usually caused by infection with respiratory syncytial virus (RSV). Babies with risk factors of prematurity or underlying lung or heart disease may receive immunizations to prevent RSV disease, which can be extremely serious in these patients.
9. Viral pneumonia and bacterial pneumonia cause varying degrees of illness in children, most often mild.

(Continued)

Did You Understand?—Cont'd

10. Aspiration pneumonitis is caused by inhalation of a foreign substance, such as food, milk, secretions, or environmental compounds, into the lung, and results in inflammation.
11. Bronchiolitis obliterans is an uncommon postinflammatory condition in which the bronchioles and some small bronchi are partially or completely obliterated by fibrous tissue, causing pulmonary impairment and disability.
12. Asthma is a prevalent and important pediatric problem. Its origins are probably multifactorial, including genetic, allergic, and viral-triggered mechanisms. Effective management is aimed at decreasing chronic inflammation in the lungs, eliminating known triggers from the environment, and early recognition and treatment of acute symptoms.
13. Acute respiratory distress syndrome (ARDS) can occur when there is an insult to the lung that activates an inflammatory response causing alveolar capillary injury, usually within 24 hours. There is progressive respiratory distress with severe hypoxemia and respiratory failure.
14. Cystic fibrosis is an autosomal recessive genetic disease that affects many organ systems, especially the lungs and digestive system. Airway secretions are particularly thick and tenacious, and the airways develop chronic bacterial infection with pathogens such as *Pseudomonas aeruginosa* and *Staphylococcus aureus*. Chronic infection, plugged airways, and severe inflammation cause long-term lung damage and ultimately death. However, the prognosis is improving, and most patients with CF now survive to adulthood.

Sudden Infant Death Syndrome (SIDS)

1. Sudden infant death syndrome is the leading cause of postnatal death for infants outside of the hospital setting and is associated with low birth weight, prone sleeping position, and other environmental factors. Some risk factors are modifiable; the prime example is the profound reduction in SIDS since widespread adoption of recommendations for supine positioning of infants during sleep.

Key Terms

References

1. Wright RB, Pomerantz WJ, Luria JW: New approaches to respiratory infections in children: bronchiolitis and croup, *Emerg Med Clin North Am* 20(1):93–114, 2002.
2. Wright RB et al: Current pharmacological options in the treatment of croup, *Exp Opin Pharmacother* 6(2):255–261, 2005.
3. Raferi K, Lichenstein R: Airway infectious disease emergencies, *Pediatr Clin N Am* 53:215–242, 2006.
4. Chan J, Edman JC, Kattai PJ: Obstructive sleep apnea in children, *Am Fam Physician* 69(5):1147–1154, 1159–1160, 2004.
5. Fraser M, Walls M, McGuire W: Respiratory complications of preterm birth, *Br Med J* 329:962–965, 2004.
6. Malloy MH, Freeman DH: Respiratory distress syndrome mortality in the United States, 1987 to 1995, *J Perinatol* 20 (7):414–420, 2000.
7. Roberts D, Dalziel S: Antenatal corticosteroids for accelerating fetal lung maturation for women at risk of preterm birth, *Cochrane Database Syst Rev*, Jul 19; 3:CD004454, 2006.
8. Lacaze-Masmonteil T: Exogenous surfactant therapy: newer developments, *Semin Neonatol* 8(6):433–440, 2003.
9. Ambalavanan N, Carlo WA: Ventilatory strategies in the prevention and management of bronchopulmonary dysplasia, *Semin Perinatol* 30(4):192–199, 2006.
10. Van Marter LJ et al: Chorioamnionitis, mechanical ventilation, and postnatal sepsis as modulators of chronic lung disease in preterm infants, *J Pediatr* 140(2):171–176, 2002.
11. Bancalari E, Claure N, Sosenko IRS: Bronchopulmonary dysplasia: changes in pathogenesis, epidemiology, and definition, *Semin Neonatol* 8(1):63–71, 2003.
12. Van Marter LJ et al: Do clinical markers of barotrauma and oxygen toxicity explain interhospital variation in rates of chronic lung disease? *Pediatrics* 105(6):1194–1201, 2000.
13. Bhandari A, Bhandari V: Pathogenesis, pathology, and pathophysiology of pulmonary sequelae of bronchoppulmonary dysplasia in premature infants, *Front Biosci* 8:e370–e380, 2003.
14. Coalson JJ: Pathology of new bronchopulmonary dysplasia, *Semin Neonatol* 8(1):73–81, 2003.
15a. Rademaker KJ et al: Neonatal hydrocortisone treatment: neurodevelopmental outcome and MRI at school age in preterm-born children, *J Pediatr* 150(4):351–357, 2007.

References—Cont'd

15b. Parikh et al: Postnatal dexamethasone therapy and cerebral tissue volumes in extremely low birth weight infants, *Pediatrics* 119(2):265–272, 2007.

16. Mai XM et al: Asthma, lung function and allergy in 12-year-old children with very low birth weight: a prospective study, *Ped Allergy Immunol* 14(3):184–192, 2003.
17. Coffin SE: Bronchiolitis: in-patient focus, *Pediatr Clin N Am* 52:1047–1057, 2005.
18. Holman RC et al: Risk factors for bronchiolitis-associated deaths among infants in the United States, *Pediatr Infect Dis* 22:483–489, 2003.
19. Williams JV et al: Human metapneumovirus and lower respiratory tract disease in otherwise healthy infants and children, *N Engl J Med* 350:443–450, 2004.
20. Ogra PL: Respiratory syncytial virus, the disease and the immune response, *Paediatr Respir Rev* 5(Suppl A): S119–S126, 2004.
21. Patel H et al: Glucocorticoids for acute viral bronchiolitis in infants and young children, *Cochrane Database Syst Rev* (3): CD004878, 2004.
22. American Academy of Pediatrics Subcommittee on Diagnosis and Management of Bronchiolitis. Diagnosis and management of bronchiolitis, *Pediatr* 118(4):1774–1793, 2006.
23. Ostapchuk M, Roberts DM, Haddy R: Community-acquired pneumonia in infants and children, *Am Fam Physician* 70 (5):899–908, 2004.
24. van Drunen Little et al: Immunopathology of RSV infection: prospects for developing vaccines without this complication, *Rev Med Virol* 17(1):5–34, 2007.
25. Light RB: Pulmonary pathophysiology of pneumococcal pneumonia, *Semin Respir Infect* 14(3):218–226, 1999.
26. Michelow IC et al: Epidemiology and clinical characteristics of community-acquired pneumonia in hospitalized children, *Pediatr* 113:701–707, 2004.
27. Toltzis P, Jacobs MR: The epidemiology of childhood pneumococcal disease in the United States in the era of conjugate vaccine use, *Infect Dis Clin N Am* 19(3):629–645, 2005.
28. Waites KB: New concepts of *Mycoplasma pneumoniae* infections in children, *Pediatr Pulmonol* 36(4):267–278, 2003.
29. Hammerschlag MR: Pneumonia due to *Chlamydia pneumoniae* in children: epidemiology, diagnosis, and treatment, *Pediatr Pulmonol* 36(5):384–390, 2003.
30. Low DE, Pichichero ME, Schaad UB: Optimizing antibacterial therapy for community-acquired respiratory tract infections in children in an era of bacterial resistance, *Clin Pediatr (Phil)* 43(2):135–151, 2004.
31. Chan PW, Muridan R, Debruyne JA: Bronchiolitis obliterans in children: clinical profile and diagnosis, *Respirology* 5 (4):369–375, 2000.
32. Bousquet J et al: The public health implications of asthma, *Bull World Health Org* 83(7):548–554, 2005.
33. Gupta RS, Carrion-Carire V, Weiss KB: The widening black/white gap in asthma hospitalizations and modality, *J All Clin Immunol* 117(2):351–358, 2006.
34. Guill MF: Asthma update: epidemiology and pathophysiology, *Pediatr Rev* 25(9):299–305, 2004.
35. Friedlarden SL et al: Viral infections, cytokine dysregulation and the origins of childhood asthma and allergic diseases, *Pediatr Infect Dis J* 24(11 suppl):5170–5176, 2005.
36. Platts-Mills TA, Rakes G, Heymann PW: The relevance of allergen exposure to the development of asthma in childhood, *J Allergy Clin Immunol* 105(2 Pt 2):S503–S508, 2000.
37. Steinke JW, Borish L: Genetics of allergic disease, *Med Clin N Am* 90(1):1–15, 2006.
38. Weschler ME, Israel E: How pharmacogenetics will play a role in the management of asthma, *Am J Resp Care* 172:12–18, 2005.
39. Heymann PW et al: Viral infections in relation to age, atopy, and season of admission among children hospitalized for wheezing, *J Allergy Clin Immunol* 114(2):239–247, 2004.
40. Szefler SJ: Advances in pediatric asthma 2006, *J Allergy Clin Immunol* 119(3):558–562, 2007.
41. Guill MF: Asthma update: clinical aspects and management, *Pediatr Rev* 25(10):335–344, 2004.
42. Capristo C, Rigotti E, Boner AL: Update on the use of montelukast in pediatric asthma, *Allergy Asthma Proc* 27(4):312–318, 2006.
43. Szefler SJ: Current concepts in asthma treatment for children, *Curr Opin Pediatrics* 16(3):299–304, 2004.
44. Schears GJ, Costarino AT: Complexity of inflammatory mediators in acute respiratory distress syndrome (ARDS), *J Pediatr* 135(2 Pt 1):144–146, 1999.
45. Moloney-Harmon PA: When the lung fails: acute respiratory distress syndrome in children, *Crit Care Nurs Clin North Am* 11(4):519–528, 1999.
46. Mehta NM, Arnold JH: Mechanical ventilation in children with acute respiratory failure, *Curr Opin Crit Care* 10(1): 7–12, 2004.
47. Ameen N et al: Endocytic trafficking of CFTR in health and disease, *J Cyst Fibros* 6(1):1–14, 2007.
48. Boucher RC: New concepts of the pathogenesis of cystic fibrosis lung disease, *Eur Respir J* 23(1):156–158, 2004.
49. Gibson RL, Burns JL, Ramsey BW: Pathophysiology and management of pulmonary infections in cystic fibrosis, *Am J Respir Crit Care Med* 168(8):918–951, 2003.
50. Rao S, Grigg J: New insights into pulmonary inflammation in cystic fibrosis, *Arch Dis Child* 91(9):786–788, 2006.
51. Conese M et al: Neutrophil recruitment and airway epithelial cell involvement in chronic cystic fibrosis lung disease, *J Cyst Fibros* 2(3):129–135, 2003.
52. Emerson J et al: *Pseudomonas aeruginosa* and other predictors of mortality and morbidity in young children with cystic fibrosis, *Pediatr Pulmonol* 34(23):91–100, 2002.
53. Grosse SD et al: Newborn screening for cystic fibrosis: evaluation of benefits and risks and recommendations for state newborn screening programs, *MMWR* 53(RR-13):1–36, 2004.
54. Daley KC: Update on sudden infant death syndrome, *Curr Opin Pediatr* 16(2):227–232, p. 227, 2004.
55. Byard RW, Krous HF: Sudden infant death syndrome: overview and update, *Perspect Pediatr Pathol* 6:112–127, 2003.
56. American Academy of Pediatrics Task Force on Infant Sleep Position and Sudden Infant Death Syndrome: Changing concepts of sudden infant death syndrome: implications for infant sleeping environment and sleep position, *Pediatrics* 105(3 Pt 1):650–656, 2000.
57. Kemp JS et al: Unsafe sleep practices and an analysis of bed-sharing among infants dying suddenly and unexpectedly: results of a four-year, population-based, Death-Scene Investigation Study of Sudden Infant Death Syndrome and Related Deaths, *Pediatrics* 106(3):E41, 2000.
58. Hauck FR et al: Sleep environment and the risk of sudden infant death in an urban population: the Chicago Infant Mortality Study, *Pediatrics* 111(5 Pt 2):1207–1214, 2003.
59. Hunt CE: Gene-environment interactions: implications for sudden unexpected deaths in infancy, *Arch Dis Child* 90 (1):48–53, 2005.
60. Berul CI, Perry JC: Contribution of long-QT syndrome genes to sudden infant death syndrome: is it time to consider newborn electrocardiographic screening? *Circulation,* 115(3): 294–296, 2007.
61. Committee on Fetus and Newborn, American Academy of Pediatrics: Apnea, sudden infant death syndrome, and home monitoring, *Pediatrics* 111(4 Pt 1):914–917, 2003.

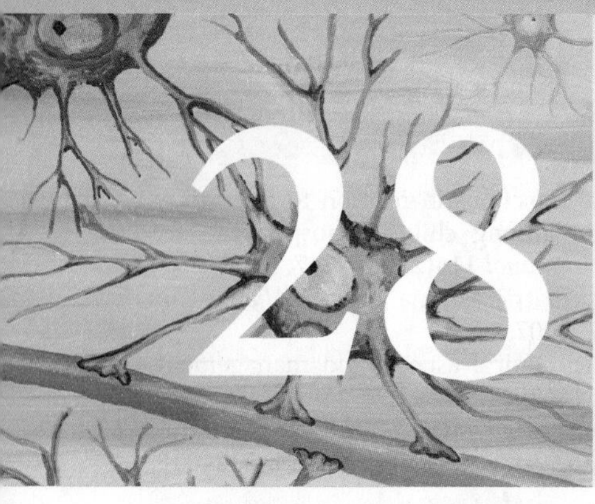

28 STRUCTURE AND FUNCTION OF THE RENAL AND UROLOGIC SYSTEMS

Sue E. Huether

CHAPTER OUTLINE

ELECTRONIC RESOURCES

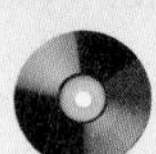

Companion CD
- Review Questions and Answers
- Animations

evolve Website
http://evolve.elsevier.com/Huether/
- Quick Check Answers
- Key Terms Exercises
- Critical Thinking Questions with Answers
- Algorithm Completion Exercises
- WebLinks

The primary function of the kidney is to maintain a stable internal environment for optimal cell and tissue metabolism. The kidneys accomplish these life-sustaining tasks by balancing solute and water transport, excreting metabolic waste products, conserving nutrients, and regulating acids and bases. The kidney also has an endocrine function and secretes the hormones renin, erythropoietin, and 1,25-dihydroxyvitamin D_3 for regulation of blood pressure, erythrocyte production, and calcium metabolism, respectively. In times of severe fasting, the kidney also can synthesize glucose from amino acids, performing the process of gluconeogenesis. The formation of urine is achieved through the processes of glomerular filtration, and tubular reabsorption, and secretion within the kidney. The bladder stores the urine that it receives from the kidney by way of the ureters. Urine is then released from the bladder through the urethra.

STRUCTURES OF THE RENAL SYSTEM

Structures of the Kidney

The **kidneys** are paired organs located on the posterior abdominal wall outside the peritoneal cavity. They lie on either side of the vertebral column with their upper and lower poles extending from the twelfth thoracic vertebra to the third lumbar vertebra (Figure 28-1). Each kidney is approximately 11 cm long, 5 to 6 cm wide, and 3 to 4 cm thick. A tightly adhering capsule (the **renal capsule**) surrounds each kidney, and the kidney then is embedded in a mass of fat. The capsule and fatty layer are covered with a double layer of **renal fascia,** fibrous tissue that attaches the kidney to the posterior abdominal wall. The cushion of fat and the position of the kidney between the abdominal organs and muscles of the back protect it from trauma.

The right kidney is slightly lower than the left; it is displaced downward by the overlying liver. A medial indentation (the **hilum**) in the kidney is the location of the entry and exit for the renal blood vessels, nerves, lymphatic vessels, and ureter.

The outer layer of the kidney is called the **cortex** and it contains all of the glomeruli, most of the proximal tubules, and some segments of the distal tubule. The **medulla** forms the inner part of the kidney and consists of regions call **pyramids.** The pyramids extend into the renal pelvis and contain the loops of Henle and collecting ducts. The **calyces** are chambers that receive urine from the collecting ducts and form the entry into the renal pelvis.

The structural unit of the kidney is the lobe. Each **lobe** is composed of a pyramid and the overlying cortex. There are about 14 lobes in each kidney. The gross structure of the kidney can be reviewed in Figure 28-2.

Nephron

The **nephron** is the functional unit of the kidney. Each kidney contains approximately 1.2 million nephrons. The nephron is a tubular structure with subunits that include the renal corpuscle, proximal convoluted tubule, loop of Henle, distal convoluted tubule, and collecting duct, all of which contribute to the formation of final urine (Figure 28-3).

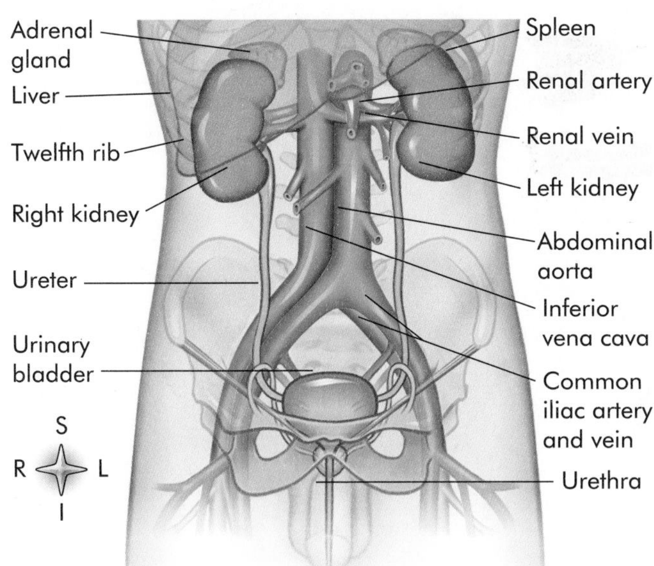

Figure 28-1 ■ **Organs of the Urinary System.** (From Thibodeau GA, Patton KT: *Anatomy & physiology,* ed 6, St Louis, 2007, Mosby.)

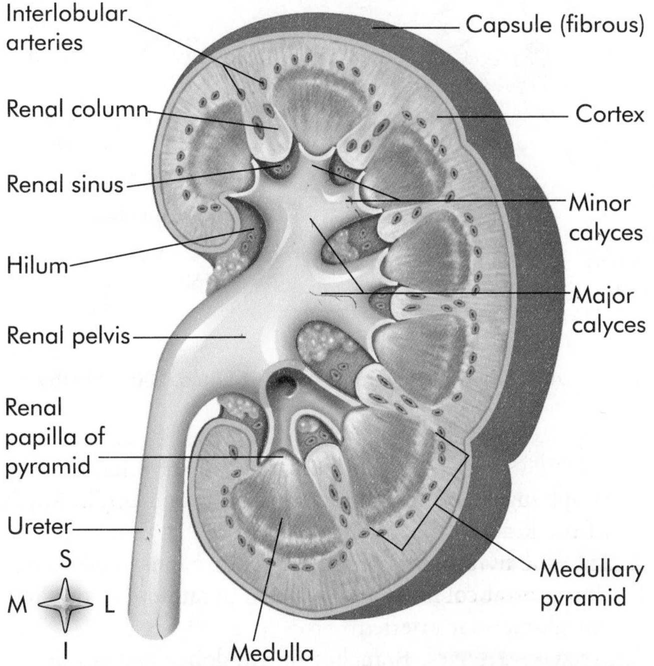

Figure 28-2 ■ **Kidney Structure.** (From Thibodeau GA, Patton KT: *Anatomy & physiology,* ed 6, St Louis, 2007, Mosby.)

The different structures of the epithelial cells lining various segments of the tubule facilitate the special functions of secretion and reabsorption (Figure 28-4).

The kidney has (1) **cortical nephrons** (85% of all nephrons), which extend only partially into the medulla, and (2) **juxtamedullary nephrons,** which lie close to and extend deep into the medulla and are important for the concentration of urine (Figure 28-5). The **glomerulus** is a tuft of capillaries that loop into **Bowman capsule,** like fingers pushed into bread dough. Together, the glomerulus and Bowman capsule are called the *renal corpuscle.* **Mesangial cells** (similar to monocytes) and the mesangial matrix lie between and support the capillaries (Figure 28-6). Mesangial cells have phagocytic ability similar to monocytes and can contract to regulate glomerular capillary blood flow.[1,2] The space inside Bowman capsule is called **Bowman space.**

The **glomerular filtration membrane** filters blood components through its three layers: (1) an inner capillary endothelium, (2) a middle basement membrane, and (3) an outer layer of capillary epithelium. The capillary endothelium is composed of cells in continuous contact with the basement membrane and contains pores. The middle basement membrane is a selectively permeable network of glycoproteins and mucopolysaccharides. The epithelium has specialized cells called **podocytes** from which pedicles radiate and adhere to the basement membrane. The pedicles interlock with the pedicles of adjacent podocytes, forming an elaborate network of intercellular clefts (**filtration slits,** or slit membranes).[3,4] The endothelium, basement membrane, and podocytes are covered with protein molecules bearing anionic (negative) charges that retard the filtration of anionic proteins and prevent proteinuria. The glomerular filtration membrane separates the blood of the glomerular capillaries from the fluid in Bowman space. The glomerular filtrate passes through the three layers of the glomerular membrane and forms the primary urine.

The glomerulus is supplied by the afferent arteriole and drained by the efferent arteriole. A group of specialized cells known as **juxtaglomerular cells** (renin-releasing cells) are located around the afferent arteriole where it enters the renal corpuscle (see Figure 28-3). Between the afferent and efferent arterioles is the **macula densa** (sodium-sensing cells) of the distal tubule (see Figure 28-6). Together the juxtaglomerular cells and macula densa cells form the **juxtaglomerular apparatus** (see Figure 28-3). Control of renal blood flow, glomerular filtration, and renin secretion occurs at this site.[5,6]

The **proximal tubule** continues from Bowman space and has an initial convoluted segment (pars convoluta) and then a straight segment (pars recta) that descends toward the medulla (see Figure 28-3). The proximal tubular lumen consists of one layer of cuboidal cells. This is the only surface inside the nephron where the cells are covered with microvilli (a brush border). This greatly expands the surface area of the tubule and enhances its reabsorptive function (see Figure 28-4). The proximal tubule joins the **loop of Henle,** which extends into the medulla. The tube then loops and becomes a thickening ascending segment that extends toward the cortex. A thin segment is composed of thin squamous cells with no active transport function. The cells of the thick segment are cuboidal and actively transport several solutes.

The major structural difference between the glomeruli in the two types of nephrons is the length of the loop of Henle. In cortical nephrons, the loop is short and may not extend

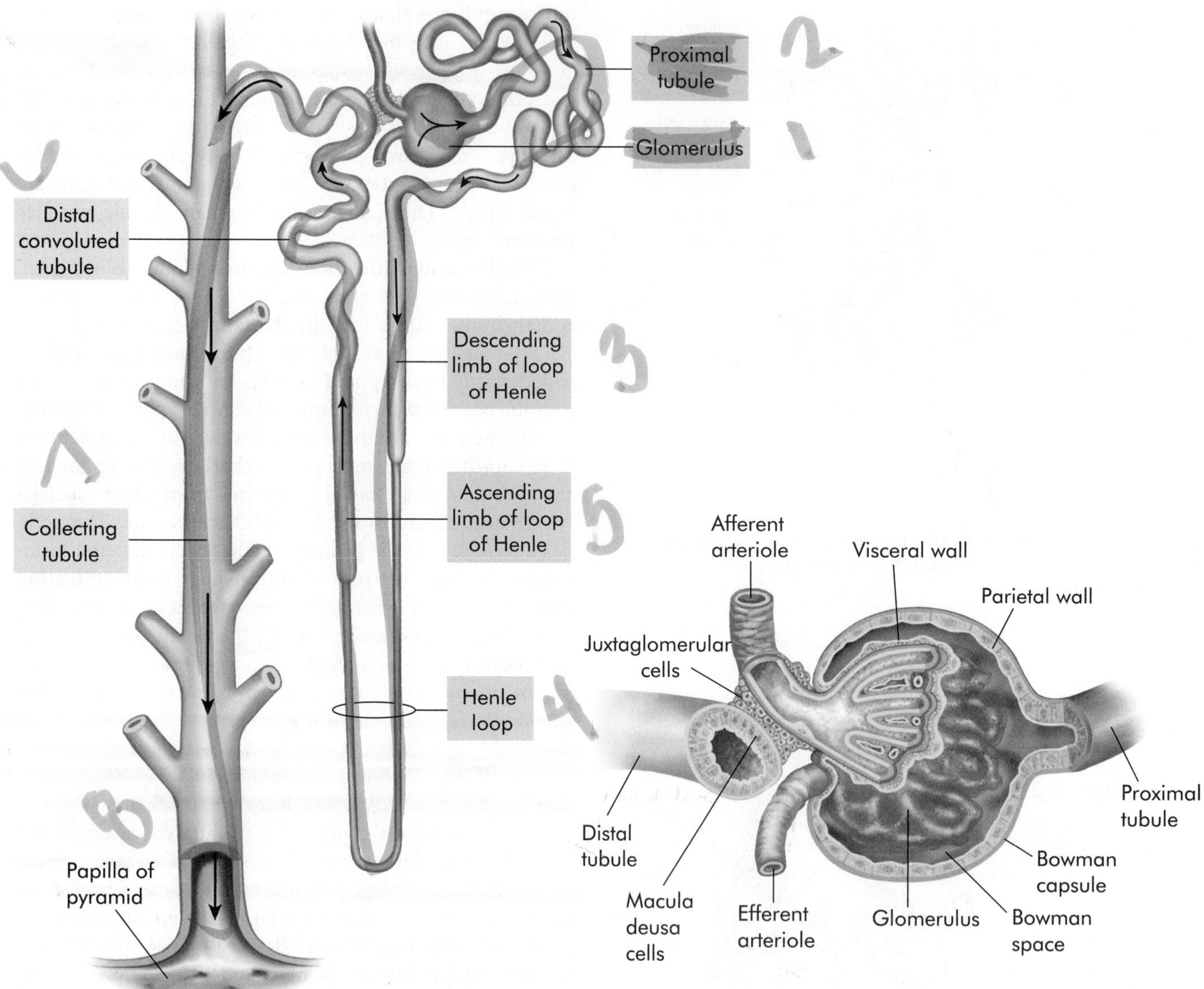

Figure 28-3 ■ **Components of Nephron.** (From Thibodeau GA, Patton KT: *Anatomy & physiology,* ed 6, St Louis, 2007, Mosby.)

into the medulla. The loops of Henle for the juxtamedullary nephrons, however, may extend the whole length of the medulla (40 mm). Juxtamedullary nephrons represent about 12% of the total number of nephrons.

The **distal tubule** has straight and convoluted segments. It extends from the macula densa to the **collecting duct,** a large tubule that descends down the cortex, through the renal pyramids of the inner and outer medullae, and into the minor calyx. In the distal tubule, **principal cells** reabsorb sodium and secrete potassium and **intercalated cells** reabsorb potassium and bicarbonate and secrete hydrogen.

Blood vessels of the kidney

The blood vessels of the kidney closely parallel nephron structure. The major vessels are as follows:

1. **Renal arteries.** Arise as the fifth branches of the abdominal aorta, divide into anterior and posterior branches at the renal hilum, then subdivide into lobar arteries supplying blood to the lower, middle, and upper thirds of the kidney.
2. **Interlobar arteries.** Further subdivisions that travel down renal columns and between pyramids; form afferent glomerular arteries.
3. **Arcuate arteries.** Branches of interlobar arteries at the cortical medullary junction; arch over the base of the pyramids and run parallel to the surface.
4. **Glomerular capillaries.** Four to eight vessels in a fistlike structure; arise from the afferent arteriole and empty into the efferent arteriole, which carries blood to the peritubular capillaries.
5. **Peritubular capillaries.** Surround convoluted portions of the proximal and distal tubules and the loop of Henle; adapted for cortical and juxtamedullary nephrons.
6. **Vasa recta.** Network of capillaries that forms loops and closely follows the loops of Henle; only blood supply to the medulla.

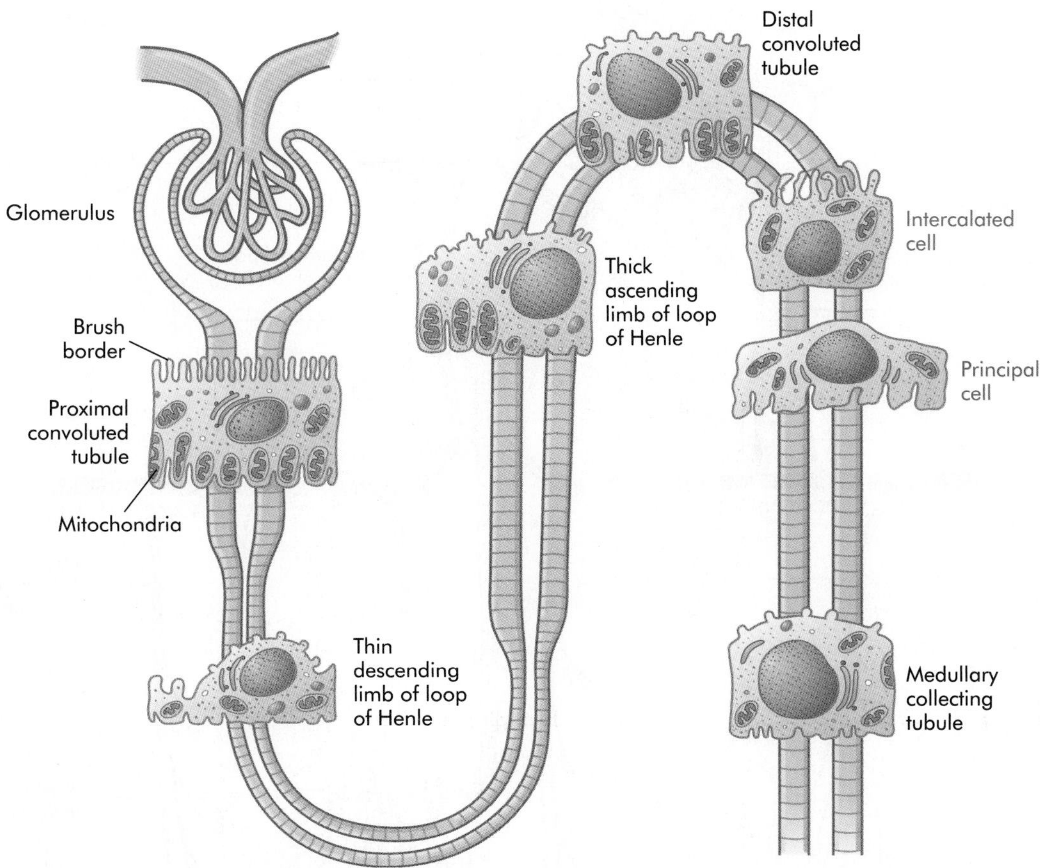

Figure 28-4 ■ **Epithelial Cells of the Various Segments of Nephron Tubules.** The brush border and high number of mitochondria in cells of the proximal tubule promote reabsorption of 50% of the glomerular filtrate. Intercalated cells *(blue type)* secrete either H^+ (resorb HCO_3^-) or HCO_3^- and reabsorb K^+. Principal cells *(magenta type)* reabsorb Na^+ and water and secrete K^+.

7. **Renal veins.** Follow arterial path and have same names as the arteries; eventually empty into the inferior vena cava.

Note that the lymphatic vessels tend also to follow the distribution of the blood vessels.

QUICK CHECK 28-1

1. Describe the physical characteristics of the kidneys.
2. What does the nephron do?
3. Why are proteins not filtered at the glomerulus?

Urinary Structures

Ureters

The urine formed by the nephrons flows from the distal tubules and collecting ducts through the duct of Bellini and the **renal papillae** (projections of the ducts) and into the calyces and is collected in the renal pelvis (see Figure 28-2). From the renal pelvis, urine is funneled into the **ureters.** Each adult ureter is approximately 30 cm long and is composed of long, intertwining muscle bundles. The lower ends pass obliquely through the posterior aspect of the bladder wall. The close approximation of muscle cells permits the direct transmission of electrical stimulation, and the resulting peristaltic activity propels urine into the bladder. Peristaltic activity is affected by urine volume. When urine flow is slow, the contraction is segmented, with downward propulsion of urine. Increasing flow rates increase peristalsis. Peristalsis is maintained even when the ureter is denervated, so ureters can be transplanted. The upper part of the ureter is innervated by the tenth thoracic nerve roots, with referred pain to the umbilicus. The innervation of lower segments arises from the sacral nerves with referred pain to the vulva or penis. Contraction of the bladder during **micturition** (urination) compresses the lower end of the ureter, preventing reflux. The ureters have a rich blood supply from the kidney with contributions by the lumbar and superior vesical arteries.

Bladder and urethra

The **bladder** is a bag of smooth muscle fibers that forms the detrusor muscle and its smooth lining of transitional epithelium. As the bladder fills with urine, it distends and the layers of transitional epithelium slide past each other and become thinner. The uroepithelium maintains an important barrier function to prevent movement of water and solutes between the urine and the blood.[7] The **detrusor** is the smooth muscle coat of the bladder, and the **trigone** is

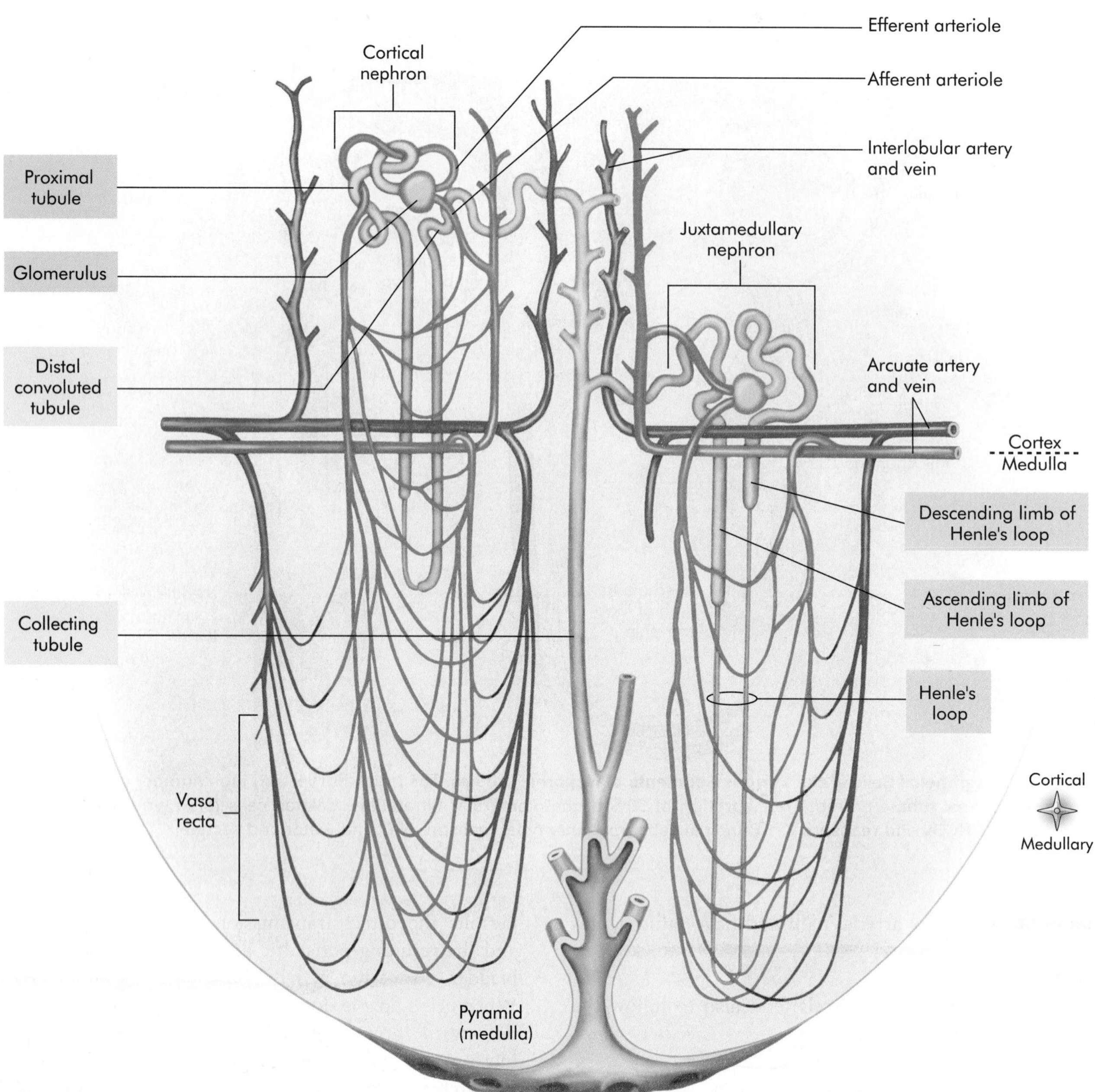

Figure 28-5 ■ **The Nephron Unit With Its Blood Vessels.** Blood flows through nephron vessels as follows: interlobular artery, afferent arteriole, glomerulus, efferent arteriole, peritubular capillaries (around the tubules), venules, interlobular vein. The vasa recta capillaries distribute along the long loops of Henle of the juxtamedullary nephrons. (From Thibodeau GA, Patton KT: *Anatomy & physiology,* ed 6, St Louis, 2007, Mosby.)

a smooth triangular area between the openings of the two ureters and the urethra (Figure 28-7). The position of the bladder varies with age and gender. The bladder has a profuse blood supply, accounting for the bleeding that readily occurs with trauma, surgery, or inflammation.

The **urethra** extends from the inferior side of the bladder to the outside of the body. A ring of smooth muscle forms the **internal urethral sphincter** at the junction of the urethra and bladder. The **external urethral sphincter** is composed of striated muscles and is under voluntary control. The entire urethra is lined with mucus-secreting glands. The female urethra is short (3 to 4 cm). The male urethra is long (18 to 20 cm) and has three segments: prostatic, membranous, and cavernous. The prostatic urethra is closest to the bladder. It passes through the prostate gland and contains the openings of the ejaculatory ducts. The membranous urethra passes through the floor of the pelvis. The cavernous segment forms the remainder of the tube. It is surrounded by erectile tissue and contains the openings of the bulbourethral mucous glands.

The innervation of the bladder and internal urethral sphincter is supplied by parasympathetic fibers of the autonomic nervous system. The reflex arc required for micturition is stimulated by mechanoreceptors that respond

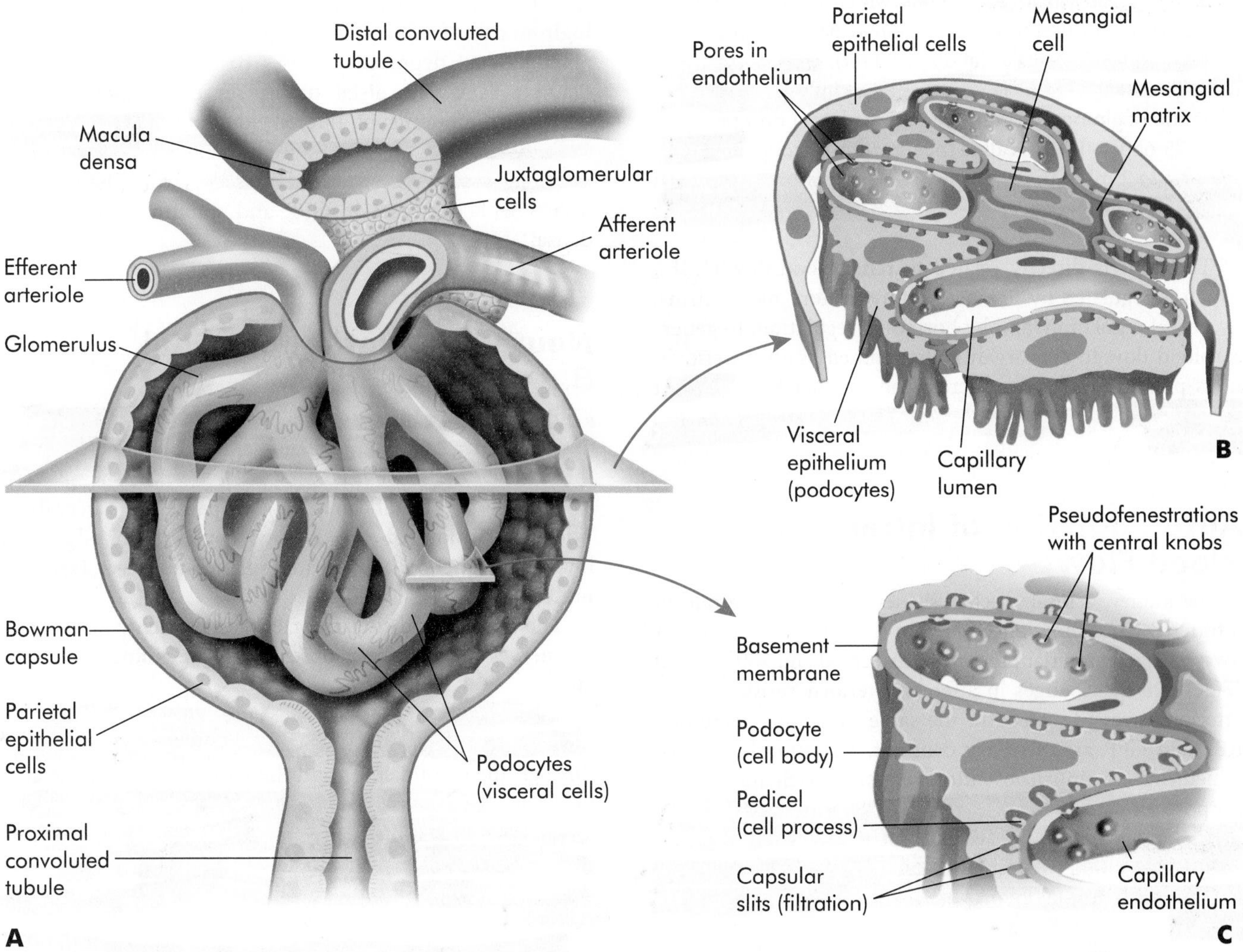

Figure 28-6 ■ **Anatomy of the Glomerulus and Juxtaglomerular Apparatus. A,** Longitudinal cross section of glomerulus and juxtaglomerular apparatus. **B,** Horizontal cross section of glomerulus. **C,** Enlargement of glomerular capillary filtration membrane.

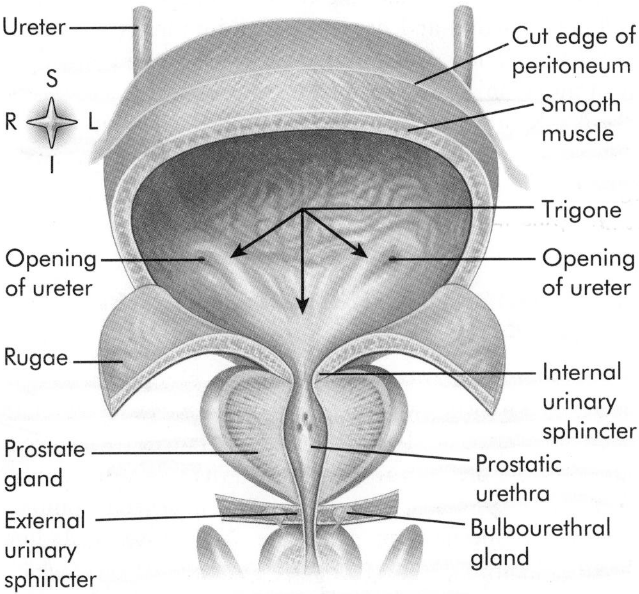

Figure 28-7 ■ **Structure of the Urinary Bladder.** Frontal view of a dissected urinary bladder (male) in a fully distended position. (From Thibodeau GA, Patton KT: *Anatomy & physiology,* ed 6, St Louis, 2007, Mosby.)

to stretching of tissue, sensing bladder fullness and sending impulses to the sacral level of the cord. When the bladder accumulates 250 to 300 ml of urine, the bladder contracts and the internal urethral sphincter relaxes through activation of the spinal reflex arc (known as the *micturition reflex*). At this time, a person feels the urge to void. In older children and adults, the reflex can be inhibited or facilitated by impulses coming from the brain, resulting in voluntary control of micturition by the relaxation or contraction of the external sphincter.

RENAL BLOOD FLOW

The kidneys are highly vascular organs and usually receive 1000 to 1200 ml of blood per minute, or about 20% to 25% of the cardiac output. With a normal hematocrit of 45%, about 600 to 700 ml of blood flowing through the kidney per minute is plasma. From the renal plasma flow (RPF), 20% (approximately 120 to 140 ml/min) is filtered at the glomerulus and passes into Bowman capsule. The filtration of the plasma per unit of time is known as the

glomerular filtration rate (GFR), which is directly related to the perfusion pressure of the glomerular capillaries.

The remaining 80% (about 480 ml) of plasma flows through the efferent arterioles to the peritubular capillaries. The ratio of glomerular filtrate to renal plasma flow per minute (125/600 = 0.20) is called the *filtration fraction.* Normally all but 1 to 2 ml of the glomerular filtrate is reabsorbed from nephron tubules and returned to the circulation by the peritubular capillaries.

The GFR is directly related to renal blood flow (RBF), which is regulated by intrinsic autoregulatory mechanisms, by neural regulation, and by hormonal regulation. In general, blood flow to any organ is determined by the arteriovenous pressure differences across the vascular bed. If mean arterial pressure decreases or vascular resistance increases, RBF falls.

Autoregulation of Intrarenal Blood Flow

In the kidney, a local mechanism tends to keep the rate of intrarenal blood flow and therefore the GFR fairly constant over a range of arterial pressures between 80 and 180 mm Hg (Figure 28-8). Changes in afferent arteriolar resistance and arteriolar pressure occur in the same direction. Therefore, RBF and GFR are relatively constant, a relationship maintained by an intrinsic autoregulatory mechanism. The purpose of **autoregulation of blood flow** is to prevent large changes in GFR when there are increases or decreases in systemic blood pressure. Solute and water excretion and thus blood volume are regulated when arterial pressure changes.[8]

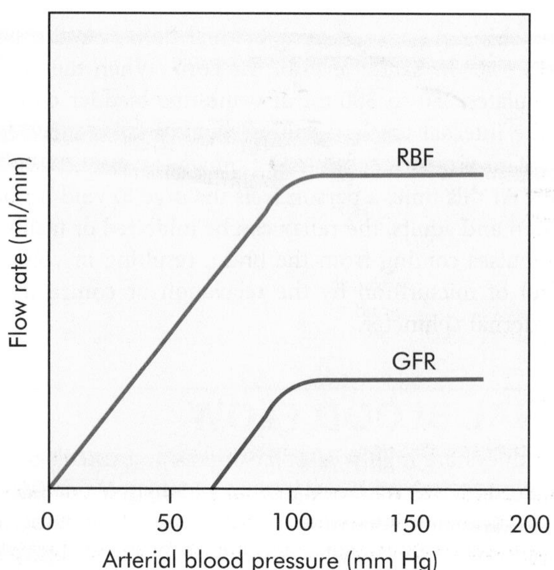

Figure 28-8 ■ **Renal Autoregulation.** Blood flow and glomerular filtration rate are stabilized in the face of changes in perfusion pressure. (From Levy MN, editors: *Berne & Levy Principles of physiology,* ed 4, Philadelphia, 2006, Mosby.)

A mechanism that keeps RBF and GFR constant is **tubuloglomerular feedback.** As the glomerular filtration rate in an individual nephron increases or decreases, the macula densa cells in the distal tubule sense the increasing or decreasing amounts of filtered sodium. When GFR and sodium increase, the macula densa cells stimulate afferent arteriolar vasoconstriction and decrease GFR. The opposite occurs with decreases in GFR and sodium at the macula densa.

Neural Regulation of Renal Blood Flow

The blood vessels of the kidney are innervated by the autonomic nervous system through sympathetic fibers that cause vasoconstriction and decrease renal blood flow. There is no significant parasympathetic innervation. The innervation of the kidney comes primarily from the celiac ganglion and greater splanchnic nerve (see Figure 12-24).

The afferent and efferent arterioles are richly innervated, but nerves have not been observed in the glomerular capillaries.

When systemic arterial pressure decreases, increased renal sympathetic nerve activity is mediated reflexively through the carotid sinus and the baroreceptors of the aortic arch. This stimulates renal arteriolar vasoconstriction and decreases both RBF and GFR. The decreased RBF also diminishes excretion of sodium and water, promoting an increase in blood volume and thus an increase in systemic pressure.

Exercise, body position, and hypoxia also influence RBF. Exercise and change of body position activate renal sympathetic neurons and cause mild vasoconstriction. Severe hypoxia stimulates the chemoreceptors of the carotid and aortic bodies and decreases RBF by means of sympathetic stimulation. Hemorrhage induces intense sympathetic stimulation and vasoconstriction, and both GFR and blood flow are reduced. The sympathetic nervous system also participates in hormonal regulation of renal blood flow.

Hormonal Regulation of Renal Blood Flow

A major hormonal regulator of renal blood flow is the **renin-angiotensin system,** which can increase systemic arterial pressure and change RBF. Renin is an enzyme formed and stored in the cells of the arterioles of the juxtaglomerular apparatus (see Figure 28-3). Several complex physiologic mechanisms stimulate its release, including decreased blood pressure in the afferent arterioles, which reduces the stretch of the juxtaglomerular cells, decreased sodium chloride concentration in the distal convoluted tubule, and sympathetic nerve stimulation of β-adrenergic receptors on the juxtaglomerular cells.[9] Numerous physiologic effects of the renin-angiotensin system stabilize systemic blood pressure and preserve the extracellular fluid volume during hypotension or hypovolemia, including sodium reabsorption, systemic vasoconstriction, sympathetic nerve stimulation, thirst stimulation, and drinking. The effects of aldosterone combine with antidiuretic hormone in regulating blood volume. The effects are summarized in Figure 28-9.

QUICK CHECK 28-2

1. Where is pain from the ureters referred?
2. How do the bladder and urethra function in urine formation?
3. What is autoregulation in the kidney? What other regulatory mechanisms are at work in renal function?

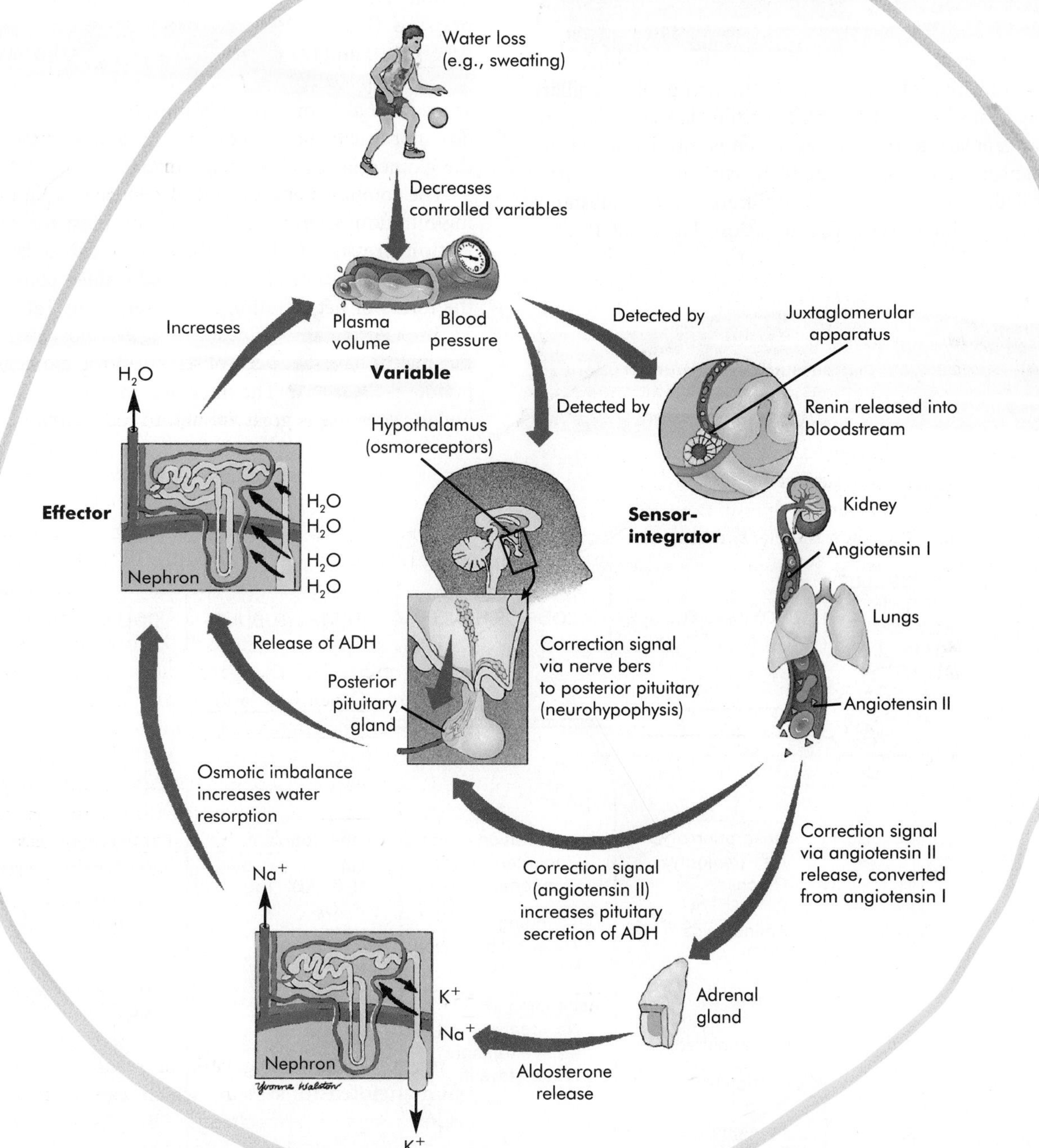

Figure 28-9 ■ **Cooperative Roles of Antidiuretic Hormone (ADH) and Aldosterone in Regulating Urine and Plasma Volume.** The drop in blood pressure that accompanies loss of fluid from the internal environment triggers the hypothalamus to rapidly release ADH from the posterior pituitary gland. ADH increases water reabsorption by the kidney by increasing water permeability of the distal tubules and collecting ducts. The drop in blood pressure is also detected by each nephron's juxtaglomerular apparatus, which responds by secreting renin. Renin triggers the formation of angiotensin II, which stimulates release of aldosterone from the adrenal cortex. Aldosterone then slowly boosts water reabsorption by the kidneys by increasing reabsorption of Na^+. Because angiotensin II also stimulates secretion of ADH, it serves as an additional link between the ADH and aldosterone mechanisms. (From Thibodeau GA, Patton KT: *Anatomy & physiology,* ed 6, St Louis, 2007, Mosby.)

KIDNEY FUNCTION

Nephron Function

The nephron can perform many functions simultaneously, as follows:

1. Filters plasma at glomerulus
2. Reabsorbs and secretes different substances along tubular structures
3. Forms a filtrate of protein-free fluid (**ultrafiltration**)
4. Regulates the filtrate to maintain body fluid volume, electrolyte composition, and pH within narrow limits

Tubular reabsorption is the movement of fluids and solutes from the tubular lumen to the peritubular capillary plasma. Transfer of substances from the plasma of the peritubular capillary to the tubular lumen is **tubular secretion.** The transport mechanisms are both active and passive (processes defined in Chapter 1). The elimination of a substance in the final urine is known as **excretion** (Figure 28-10).

Glomerular filtration

The fluid filtered by the glomerular capillary filtration membrane is protein free but contains electrolytes, such as sodium, chloride, and potassium, and organic molecules, such as creatinine, urea, and glucose, in the same concentrations as in plasma. Like other capillary membranes, the glomerulus is freely permeable to water and relatively impermeable to large colloids, such as plasma proteins. The molecule's size and electrical charge affect the permeability of substances crossing the glomerulus.

Capillary pressure also affects glomerular filtration. The hydrostatic pressure within the capillary is the major force for moving water and solutes across the filtration membrane and into Bowman capsule. Two forces oppose the filtration effects of the glomerular capillary hydrostatic pressure (P_{GC}): (1) the hydrostatic pressure in Bowman space (P_{BC}) and (2) the effective oncotic pressure of the glomerular capillary blood (π_{GC}). Because the fluid in Bowman space normally contains only minute amounts of protein, it does not usually have an oncotic influence on the plasma of the glomerular capillary (Figure 28-11).

The combined effect of forces favoring and forces opposing filtration determines the filtration pressure. The **net filtration pressure (NFP)** is the sum of forces favoring and opposing filtration. The estimated values contributing to the forces of net filtration are presented in Table 28-1.

As the protein-free fluid is filtered into Bowman capsule, the plasma oncotic pressure increases and the hydrostatic pressure decreases. The increase in glomerular capillary oncotic pressure is great enough to reduce the net filtration

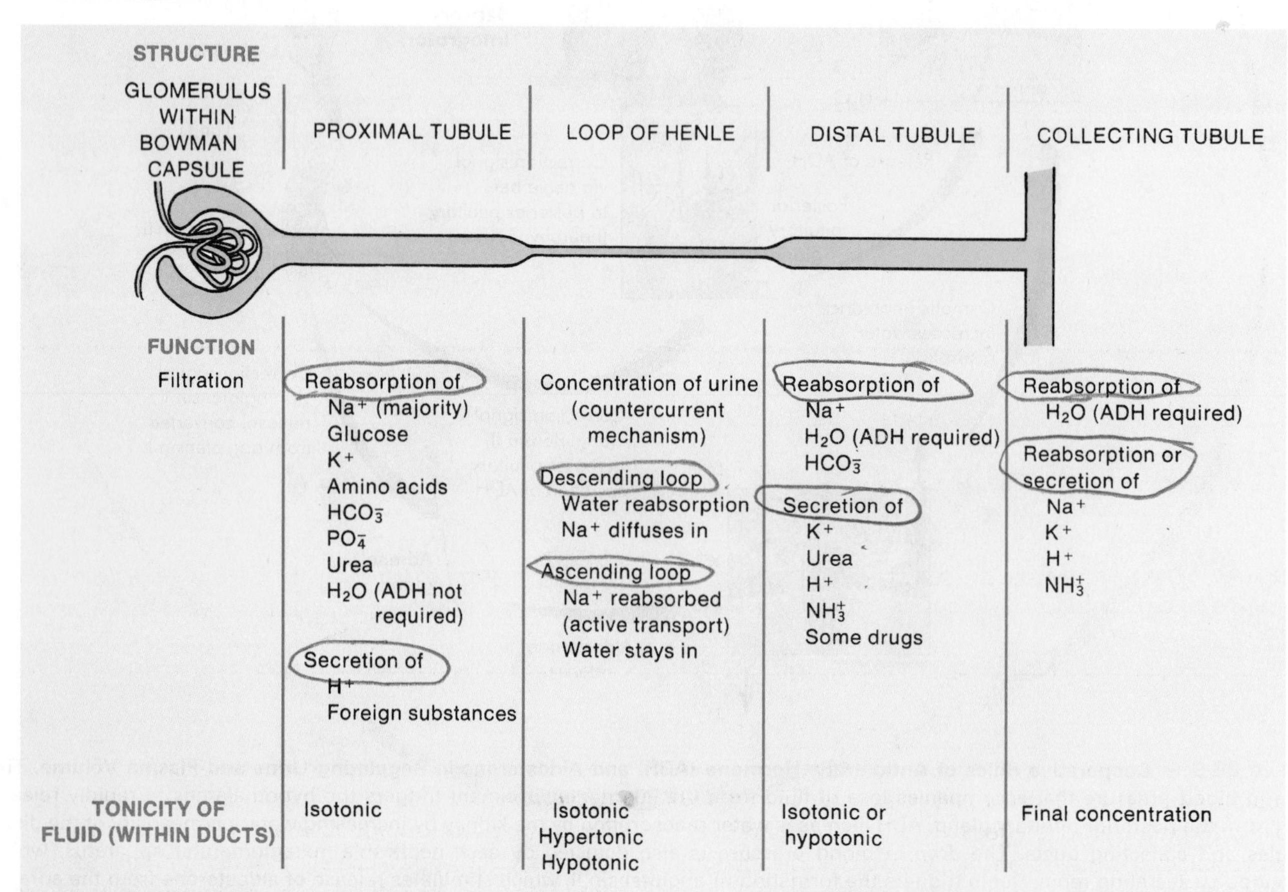

STRUCTURE
GLOMERULUS WITHIN BOWMAN CAPSULE
PROXIMAL TUBULE
LOOP OF HENLE
DISTAL TUBULE
COLLECTING TUBULE
FUNCTION
Filtration
Reabsorption of
Na+ (majority)
Glucose
K+
Amino acids
HCO3-
PO4-
Urea
H2O (ADH not required)
Secretion of
H+
Foreign substances
Concentration of urine (countercurrent mechanism)
Descending loop
Water reabsorption
Na+ diffuses in
Ascending loop
Na+ reabsorbed (active transport)
Water stays in
Reabsorption of
Na+
H2O (ADH required)
HCO3-
Secretion of
K+
Urea
H+
NH3+
Some drugs
Reabsorption of
H2O (ADH required)
Reabsorption or secretion of
Na+
K+
H+
NH3+
TONICITY OF FLUID (WITHIN DUCTS)
Isotonic
Isotonic
Hypertonic
Hypotonic
Isotonic or hypotonic
Final concentration

Figure 28-10 **Major Functions of Nephron Segments.** *ADH,* Antidiuretic hormone. (Modified from Hockenberry MJ et al: *Wong's nursing care of infants and children,* ed 8, St Louis, 2007, Mosby.)

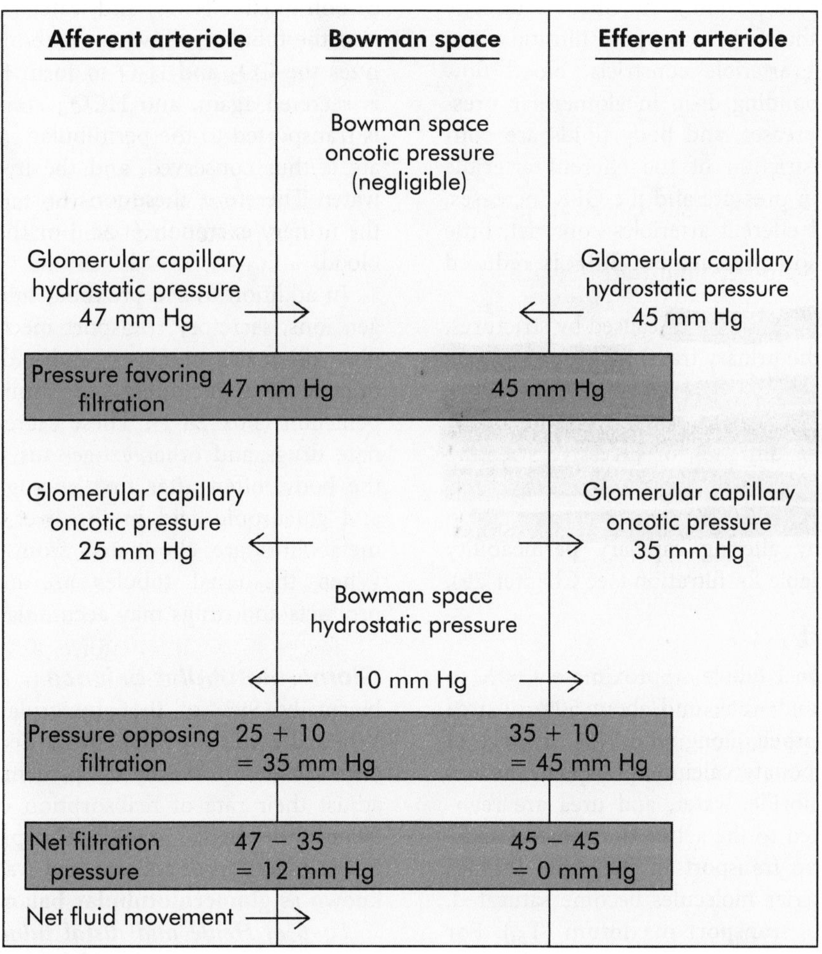

Figure 28-11 ■ **Glomerular Filtration Pressures.**

TABLE 28-1

Glomerular Filtration Pressures

		PRESSURES (mm Hg)	
Forces	**Pressures**	**Beginning of Capillary**	**End of Capillary**
PROMOTING FILTRATION			
Glomerular capillary hydrostatic pressure	P_{GC}	47	45
Bowman capsule oncotic pressure	π_{BC}	Negligible effect	Negligible effect
OPPOSING FILTRATION			
Bowman capsule hydrostatic pressure	P_{BC}	10	10
Glomerular capillary oncotic pressure	π_{GC}	25	35
Net filtration pressure		12	0

pressure to zero at the efferent end of the capillary and to stop the filtration process effectively. The low hydrostatic pressure and the increased oncotic pressure in the efferent arteriole then are transferred to the peritubular capillaries and facilitate reabsorption of fluid from the proximal tubules.

Filtration rate

The total volume of fluid filtered by the glomeruli averages 180 L/day, or approximately 120 ml/min, a phenomenal amount considering the size of the kidneys. Because only 1 to 2 L of urine is excreted per day, 99% of the filtrate is reabsorbed into the peritubular capillaries and returned to the blood. The factors determining the GFR are directly related to the pressures that favor or oppose filtration. For example, if the afferent arteriole constricts, blood flow decreases with a corresponding drop in glomerular pressure. The GFR then decreases, and body fluids are conserved. Conversely, constriction of the efferent arteriole increases the net filtration pressure and the GFR increases. When both afferent and efferent arterioles constrict, little change occurs in filtration pressure but RBF is reduced and so is the GFR.

Obstruction to the outflow of urine (caused by strictures, stones, or tumors along the urinary tract) can cause a retrograde increase in pressure at Bowman capsule and a decrease in GFR. Excessive loss of protein-free fluid from vomiting, diarrhea, use of diuretics, or excessive sweating can increase glomerular capillary oncotic pressure and decrease the GFR. Renal disease also can cause changes in pressure relationships by altering capillary permeability and the surface area available for filtration (see Chapter 29).

Tubular transport

By the end of the proximal tubule, approximately 60% to 70% of filtered sodium and water and about 50% of urea have been actively reabsorbed, along with 90% or more of potassium, glucose, bicarbonate, calcium, phosphate, amino acids, and uric acid. Chloride, water, and urea are reabsorbed passively but linked to the active transport of sodium (co-transport). Active transport in the renal tubules can be limited as the carrier molecules become saturated, a phenomenon known as **transport maximum (T_m)**. For example, when the carrier molecules for glucose become saturated (i.e., with the development of hyperglycemia) the excess will be excreted in the urine.

Proximal tubule

Active reabsorption of sodium is the primary function of the proximal tubule. Water, most electrolytes, and organic substances are co-transported with sodium. The osmotic force generated by active sodium transport promotes the passive diffusion of water out of the tubular lumen and into the peritubular capillaries. Passive transport of water is further enhanced by the elevated oncotic pressure of the blood in the peritubular capillaries, which is created by the previous filtration of water at the glomerulus. The reabsorption of water leaves an increased concentration of urea within the tubular lumen, creating a gradient for its passive diffusion to the peritubular plasma.

As the positively charged sodium ions leave the tubular lumen, negatively charged chloride ions passively follow to maintain electroneutrality. Because the proximal tubular cell has a limited permeability to chloride, chloride reabsorption lags behind sodium. Hydrogen ions are actively exchanged for sodium ions. The hydrogen ions (H^+) then combine with bicarbonate (HCO_3^-). Bicarbonate is completely filtered at the glomerulus, and approximately 90% is reabsorbed in the proximal tubule. In the tubular lumen, hydrogen and bicarbonate ions form carbonic acid (H_2CO_3), which rapidly breaks down, or dissociates, to carbon dioxide (CO_2) and water (H_2O). These then diffuse into the tubular cell, where carbonic anhydrase again catalyzes the CO_2 and H_2O to form HCO_3^- and H^+. The H^+ is secreted again, and HCO_3^- combines with sodium and is transported to the peritubular capillary blood. Bicarbonate is thus conserved, and the hydrogen is reabsorbed as water. Therefore, these ions normally do not contribute to the urinary excretion of acid or the addition of acid to the blood.

In addition to the proximal tubular secretion of hydrogen ions, secretory transport mechanisms exist for creatinine, other organic bases, and endogenous and exogenous organic acids including para-aminohippurate (PAH) and penicillin (Box 28-1). These secretory mechanisms eliminate drugs and other exogenous chemical products from the body, often after first conjugating them with sulfate and glucuronic acid in the liver. Many drugs and their metabolites are eliminated from the body in this way. When the renal tubules are damaged, metabolic by-products and drugs may accumulate, causing toxic levels.

Glomerulotubular balance

Normally, 99% of the glomerular filtrate is reabsorbed. When the GFR spontaneously decreases or increases, the renal tubules, primarily the proximal tubules, automatically adjust their rate of reabsorption of sodium and water to balance the change in GFR. This prevents wide fluctuations in the excretion of sodium and water into the urine and is known as **glomerulotubular balance.**

Loop of Henle and distal tubule. Urine can be hypotonic, isotonic, or hypertonic. The **concentration** or **dilution of urine** occurs principally in the loop of Henle, distal tubules, and collecting ducts. The structural features of the medullary hairpin loops allow the kidney to concentrate urine and conserve water for the body. The transition of the filtrate into the final urine reflects the concentrating ability of the loops. Final adjustments in urine composition are made by the distal tubule and collecting duct according to body needs.

Producing a concentrated urine involves a **countercurrent exchange system,** in which fluid flows in opposite directions through the parallel tubes of the loop of Henle. A concentration gradient causes fluid to be exchanged

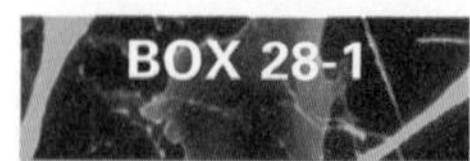

Substances Transported by Renal Tubules

Reabsorption	Secretion
Albumin	Choline
Ascorbate	Creatinine
Fructose	Histamine
Galactose	Methyl guanidine
Glutamate	Para-aminohippurate
Glucose	Penicillin
Phosphate	Steroid glucuronides
Sulfate	Thiamine
Xylose	

across the parallel pathways. The longer the loop, the greater the concentration gradient and the concentration gradient increases from the cortex to the tip of the medulla. The loops of Henle multiply the concentration gradient, and the vasa recta act as a countercurrent exchanger for maintaining the gradient.[9,10]

The process is initiated in the thick ascending limb of the loop of Henle with the active transport of chloride and sodium out of the tubular lumen and into the medullary interstitium (Figure 28-12). Because the lumen of the ascending limb is impermeable to water, water cannot follow the sodium-chloride transport. This causes the ascending tubular fluid to become hypoosmotic and the medullary interstitium to become hyperosmotic. The descending limb of the loop, which receives fluid from the proximal tubule, is highly permeable to water but it is the only place in the nephron that does not actively transport either sodium or chloride. Sodium and chloride may, however, diffuse into the descending tubule from the interstitium. The hyperosmotic medullary interstitium causes water to move out of the descending limb, and the remaining fluid in the descending tubule becomes increasingly concentrated as it flows toward the tip of the medulla. As the tubular fluid rounds the loop and enters the ascending limb, sodium and chloride are removed and water is retained. The fluid then becomes more and more dilute as it encounters the distal tubule.

The slow rate of blood flow and the hairpin structure of the vasa recta allow blood to flow through the medullary tissue without disturbing the osmotic gradient. As blood flows into the descending limb of the vasa recta, it encounters the increasing osmotic concentration gradient of the medullary interstitium. Water moves out and sodium and chloride diffuse into the descending vasa recta. The plasma becomes increasingly concentrated as it flows toward the tip of the medulla.

As the blood flow passes into the ascending limb and back toward the cortex, the surrounding interstitial fluid becomes comparatively more dilute. Water then moves back into the vasa recta, and sodium and chloride diffuse out. The net result is a preservation of the medullary osmotic gradient. If blood were to flow rapidly through the vasa recta, as occurs in some renal diseases, the medullary concentration gradient would be washed away and the ability to concentrate urine and conserve water would be lost. The efficiency of water conservation is related to the length of the loops: the longer the loops, the greater the ability to concentrate the urine.

Another important function of the loop of Henle is the production of Tamm-Horsfall protein, the most abundant protein in human urine. This protein binds to uropathogens to prevent urinary tract infection, protects the uroepithelium from injury, and may also activate cell-mediated immunity.[11]

The convoluted portion of the distal tubule is poorly permeable to water but readily reabsorbs ions and contributes to the dilution of the tubular fluid. The later, straight segment of the distal tubule and the collecting duct are permeable to water as controlled by antidiuretic hormone (ADH). Sodium is readily reabsorbed by the later segment of the distal tubule and collecting duct under the regulation of the hormone aldosterone (see Chapter 17). Potassium is actively secreted in these segments and is also controlled by aldosterone and other factors related to the concentration of potassium in body fluids.

Acidification of urine. Hydrogen is also secreted by the distal tubule and combines with nonbicarbonate buffers (i.e., ammonium and phosphate) for the elimination of acids in the urine. The distal tubule thus contributes to the regulation of acid-base balance by excreting hydrogen ions into the urine and by adding new bicarbonate to the plasma. The mechanism is similar to the conservation of

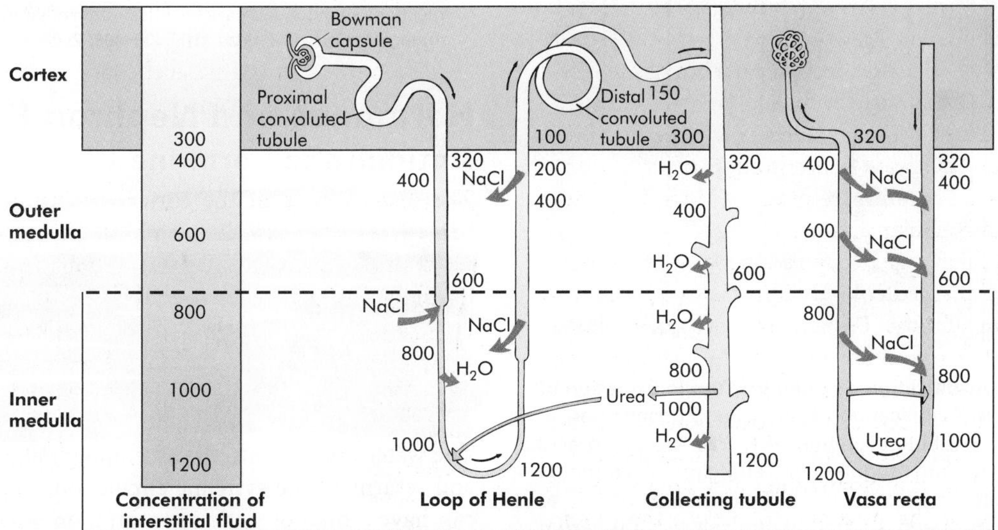

Figure 28-12 ■ **Countercurrent Mechanism for Concentrating and Diluting Urine.** (NOTE: Numbers on illustration represent milliosmoles [mOsm].)

bicarbonate by the proximal tubule, except that the hydrogen ion is excreted in the urine and influences acid-base balance (Figure 28-13). (The specific mechanisms of acid-base balance and acid excretion are described in Chapter 4.)

Urea is the major constituent of urine along with water. The glomerulus freely filters urea, and tubular reabsorption depends on urine flow rate, with less reabsorption at higher flow rates. Approximately 50% of urea is excreted in the urine, and 50% is recycled within the kidney. This recycling contributes to the osmotic gradient within the medulla and is necessary for the concentration and dilution of urine (see Figure 28-12). Because urea is an end product of protein metabolism, individuals with protein deprivation cannot maximally concentrate their urine.

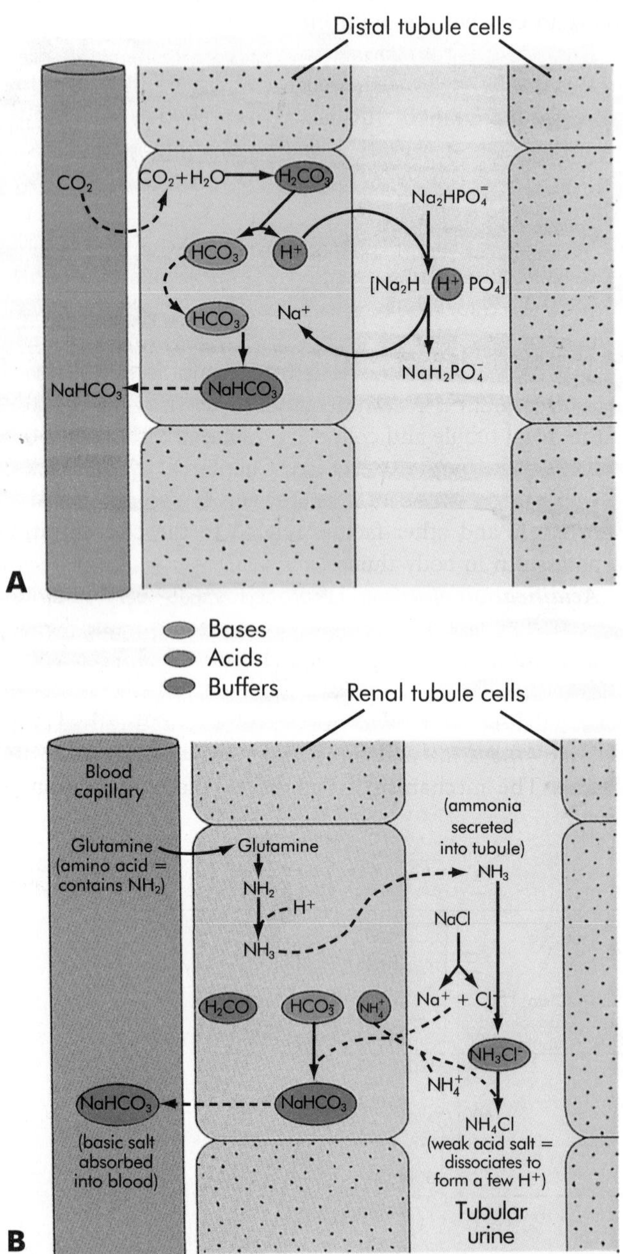

Figure 28-13 **Acidification of Urine by Tubule Excretion of Ammonia (NH_3). A,** Acidification of urine and conservation of base by distal renal tubule excretion of H^+. **B,** An amino acid (glutamine) moves into tubule cell and forms ammonia (NH_3) which is secreted into the urine. To combine with H^+ to form ammonia (NH_4^+) and an ammonium salt (NH_4Cl). (From Thibodeau, GA, Patton KT: *Anatomy & physiology,* ed 4, St Louis, 1999, Mosby.)

Urine

Urine is normally clear yellow or amber in color. Cloudiness may indicate the presence of bacteria, cells, or high solute concentration. The pH ranges from 4.6 to 8.0, but it is normally acidic, providing protection against bacteria. Specific gravity ranges from 1.001 to 1.035. Normal urine does not contain glucose or blood cells and only occasionally contains traces of protein, usually in association with rigorous exercise.

HEALTH ALERT
Cranberry Juice and Urinary Tract Infection

Cranberry juice (CBJ) has long been used to prevent and treat uncomplicated urinary tract infections (UTIs). Although CBJ is not bacteriostatic nor does it acidify the urine, it does inhibit bacterial adhesion to uroepithelial cells by the action of epicatechin, a proanthocyanidin. Randomized trials of cranberry juice ingestion show a significant effect in preventing *E. coli* uropathogenic adherence and UTI, particularly in women. Randomized controlled trials are needed to determine the effectiveness of CBJ for treatment of recurrent UTI in children. The cost of CBJ for prophylaxis also may be more expensive than antibiotic prophylaxis and other preventive measures.

Data from Di Martino P et al: Reduction of *Escherichia coli* adherence to uroepithelial bladder cells after consumption of cranberry juice: a double-blind randomized placebo-controlled cross-over trial, *World J Urol* 24(1):21–27, 2006; Liu Y et al: Role of cranberry juice on molecular-scale surface characteristics and adhesion behavior of *Escherichia coli, Biotechnol Bioeng* 93(2): 297–305, 2006; Regal RE, Pham CQ, Bostwick TR: Urinary tract infections in extended care facilities: preventive management strategies, *Consult Pharm* 21(5):400–409, 2006.

Hormones and Nephron Function

Antidiuretic hormone

The distal tubule in the cortex receives the hypoosmotic urine from the ascending limb of the loop of Henle. The concentration of the final urine is controlled by antidiuretic hormone (ADH), which is secreted from the posterior pituitary or neurohypophysis. ADH increases water permeability and reabsorption in the last segment of the distal tubule and along the entire length of the collecting ducts, which pass through the inner and outer zones of the medulla. The water diffuses into the ascending limb of the vasa recta and returns to the systemic circulation. The excreted urine can have a high osmotic concentration, up to 1400 mOsm. The volume is normally reduced to about 1% of what was filtered at the glomerulus.

ADH secretion is therefore one cause of **oliguria,** or diminished excretion of urine that is less than 400 ml/day or 30 ml/hr. Fluid imbalance may be related to the syndrome of inappropriate secretion of ADH, which is a cause of water excess (see Chapter 4). Inadequate secretion of ADH results in diabetes insipidus, the excretion of a large volume of dilute urine (see Chapter 18).

In the absence of ADH, **water diuresis,** an increase in excretion of a highly dilute urine, takes place. The distal tubules and collecting ducts become impermeable to water. Water remains in the tubular lumen and is excreted as a dilute and large volume of urine. Because ADH has no effect on sodium reabsorption, it continues to be actively transported from the distal tubule. (The mechanism for the regulation of ADH and plasma osmolality is described in Chapters 4 and 17).

Aldosterone

Aldosterone is synthesized and secreted by the adrenal cortex under the regulation of the renin-angiotensin system (see Chapter 17, p. 441). Aldosterone stimulates the epithelial cell of the distal tubule and collecting duct to reabsorb sodium (promoting water reabsorption) and increases the excretion of potassium and hydrogen ion.

Atrial natriuretic peptide

Atrial natriuretic peptide (ANP) is secreted from cells in the right atrium of the heart. When right atrial pressure rises, ANP inhibits secretion of renin, inhibits angiotensin-induced secretion of aldosterone, relaxes vascular smooth muscle, and inhibits sodium and water absorption by kidney tubules. The result is decreased blood volume and blood pressure. Natriuretic hormones are also produced by other tissues including the brain and vascular system and have effects on heart tissue, vasodilation and bone growth.[12]

Diuretics as a factor in urine flow

A **diuretic** is any agent that enhances the flow of urine. Clinically, diuretics interfere with renal sodium reabsorption and reduce extracellular fluid volume. Diuretics are commonly used to treat hypertension and edema caused by heart failure, cirrhosis, and nephrotic syndrome.

Diuretics are divided into four general categories: (1) osmotic diuretics, (2) carbonic anhydrase inhibitors (inhibitors of urinary acidification), (3) inhibitors of loop sodium or chloride transport, and (4) aldosterone antagonists. (The physiologic mechanism related to each category is summarized in Table 28-2.)

Renal Hormones

Certain hormones are either activated or synthesized by the kidney. These hormones have significant systemic effects and include urodilatin, the active form of vitamin D, and erythropoietin.

Urodilatin

Urodilatin, a natriuretic peptide, is produced by the distal tubule and collecting ducts when there is increased circulating volume and increased blood pressure. It inhibits sodium

TABLE 28-2

Action of Diuretics

Diuretic	Site of Action	Action	Side Effects
OSMOTIC DIURETIC			
Mannitol Glycerol Urea	Proximal tubule	Freely filtered but not reabsorbed; osmotically attracts water and diminishes sodium reabsorption	Hypokalemia, dehydration
CARBONIC ANHYDRASE INHIBITORS			
Acetazolamide	Proximal tubule	Inhibits carbonic anhydrase; blocks hydrogen ion secretion and reabsorption of sodium and bicarbonate	Hypokalemia, systemic acidosis, alkaline urine
INHIBITORS OF SODIUM/CHLORIDE REABSORPTION			
Thiazides	Between end of ascending loop and beginning of distal tubule	Blocks sodium and chloride reabsorption; mildly suppresses carbonic anhydrase	Hypokalemia, metabolic alkalosis
Furosemide Ethacrynic acid	Thick ascending limb of Henle's loop	Block active transport of chloride, sodium, and potassium	Hypokalemia, uric acid retention
Torsemide Bumetanide	Cortical vasodilation	Increased rate of urine formation	Hypokalemia, uric acid retention
POTASSIUM SPARING			
Spironolactone	Distal tubule/collecting duct	Inhibits aldosterone, blocks sodium reabsorption, and results in potassium retention	Hyperkalemia, nausea, confusion, gynecomastia
Triamterene and amiloride	Distal tubule/collecting duct	Block sodium reabsorption and inhibit potassium excretion	Nausea, vomiting, headache, granulocytopenia, skin rash

and water resorption from the medullary part of the collective duct producing diuresis.

Vitamin D

in intestines

Vitamin D is a hormone that can be obtained in the diet or synthesized by the action of ultraviolet radiation on cholesterol in the skin. These forms of vitamin D_3 (cholecalciferol) are inactive and require two hydroxylations to establish a metabolically active form. The first step occurs in the liver and the second in the kidneys.

Vitamin D is necessary for the absorption of calcium and phosphate by the small intestine. The renal hydroxylation step is stimulated by parathyroid hormone. A decreased plasma calcium level (less than 10 mg/dl) stimulates the secretion of parathyroid hormone. Parathyroid hormone then stimulates a sequence of events that help restore plasma calcium back toward normal:

1. Calcium mobilization from bone
2. Synthesis of 1,25-dihydroxyvitamin D_3
3. Absorption of calcium from the intestine
4. Increased renal calcium reabsorption
5. Decreased renal phosphate reabsorption

Serum phosphate fluctuations also influence the renal hydroxylation of vitamin D. Decreased levels stimulate active 1,25-dihydroxyvitamin D_3 formation, and increased levels inhibit formation. This results in compensatory changes in phosphate absorption from bone and intestine. Individuals with renal disease have a deficiency of 1,25-dihydroxyvitamin D_3 (1,25-OH_2D_3) and manifest symptoms of disturbed calcium and phosphate balance (see Chapters 4 and 29).

Erythropoietin

in kidneys

Erythropoietin stimulates the bone marrow to produce red blood cells in response to tissue hypoxia. (Erythrocyte production is discussed in Chapter 19.) The stimulus for erythropoietin release is decreased oxygen delivery in the kidneys. The anemia of chronic renal failure, in which kidney cells have become nonfunctional, can be related to the lack of this hormone.[13]

QUICK CHECK 28-3

1. Outline the process of glomerular filtration.
2. What types of absorption/reabsorption take place in the proximal tubule, the loops of Henle, and the distal tubule?
3. What is the countercurrent exchange system? What substances are involved?
4. What hormones are activated or synthesized by the kidney?

The Concept of Clearance

A number of specific renal functions can be measured by renal clearance. Renal clearance techniques determine how much of a substance can be cleared from the blood by the kidneys per given unit of time. The application of this principle permits an indirect measure of GFR, tubular secretion, tubular reabsorption, and RBF.

Clearance and glomerular filtration rate

The GFR provides the best estimate of functioning renal tissue. Loss or damage to nephrons leads to a corresponding decrease in GFR. The measurement of GFR requires the use of a substance that has a stable plasma concentration, is freely filtered at the glomerulus, and is not secreted, reabsorbed, or metabolized by the tubules. Inulin (a fructose polysaccharide) is one substance that meets the criteria for measurement of GFR.

The accurate determination of inulin clearance requires constant infusion to maintain a stable plasma level. This is time consuming and inconvenient. Therefore, the clearance of creatinine, a natural substance produced by muscle and released into the blood at a relatively constant rate, is commonly used clinically. It is freely filtered at the glomerulus, but a small amount is secreted by the renal tubules. Therefore, creatinine clearance overestimates the GFR but within tolerable limits. Creatinine clearance provides a good measure of GFR because only one blood sample is required in addition to a 24-hour volume of urine. Cystatin C, a stable protein in serum, is also a marker for estimating GFR particularly for mild to moderate impaired renal function.[14]

The GFR can also be estimated using formulas. The Cockcroft and Gault formula is one that is commonly used and considers age, body weight, and plasma creatinine (P_{cr}) values:[15]

$$\text{GFR (ml/min)} = \frac{(140 - \text{age}) \times \text{Weight (kg)} \times 0.85\ \text{(women)}}{P_{cr} \times 72}$$

The National Kidney Foundation recommends the Modification of Diet in Renal Disease (MDRD) equation.[16]

An abbreviated version is as follows:

$$\text{GFR (ml/min)} = 186 \times P_{cr}^{-1.154} \times \text{Age}^{-0.203} \times (0.742 \text{ if female; } 1.210 \text{ if black})$$

Calculators for the MDRD are readily available on the Internet.

Substances freely filtered at the glomerulus but with a clearance less than inulin or creatinine have been reabsorbed along the tubules. For example, glucose is completely reabsorbed and has a clearance rate of nearly zero. Conversely, substances secreted by the tubules have a clearance rate greater than inulin or creatinine (i.e., greater than 1.0).

Plasma creatinine concentration

A chronic decline in the GFR over weeks or months is reflected in the **plasma creatinine (P_{cr}) concentration** (normal value = 0.7 to 1.2 mg/dl). The P_{cr} concentration has a stable value when the GFR is stable, because creatinine has a constant rate of production as a product of muscle metabolism. The amount filtered is approximately equal

important to know persons baseline ↗ normal (P_{cr})

to the amount excreted. When the GFR declines, the P_{cr} increases proportionately. Thus, the GFR and P_{cr} are inversely related. If the GFR were to decrease by 50%, the filtration and excretion of creatinine would be reduced by 50% and creatinine would accumulate in plasma to twice the normal value. Therefore, elevated P_{cr} values represent decreasing GFR. In the new steady state, however, the total amount of creatinine excreted in the urine would remain the same because of the proportionate decrease in GFR and increase in P_{cr}.

The application of this principle is simple and useful for monitoring progressive changes in renal function. The test is most valuable for monitoring the progress of chronic rather than acute renal disease because it takes 7 to 10 days for the plasma creatinine level to stabilize when GFR declines. Serial measures can be obtained over a long time and plotted as a curve of glomerular function. The P_{cr} also becomes elevated during trauma or the breakdown of muscle tissue. In such instances, the value is then not useful for estimating GFR.

Blood urea nitrogen

The concentration of urea nitrogen in the blood reflects glomerular filtration and urine-concentrating capacity. Because urea is filtered at the glomerulus, blood urea nitrogen (BUN) levels increase as glomerular filtration drops. Because urea is reabsorbed by the blood through the permeable tubules, the BUN rises in states of dehydration and acute and chronic renal failure when passage of fluid through the tubules slows. BUN also changes as a result of altered protein intake and protein catabolism. The normal range for BUN in the adult is 10 to 20 mg/dl of blood. Urine tests are listed in Table 28-3. Bladder function tests are listed in Table 28-4.

TABLE 28-3

Normal Renal Function Tests

Test	Normal Value	Interpretation
URINE		
Color	Amber-yellow	Drugs and foods may change color
Turbidity	Clear	Purulent matter will make cloudy
pH	4.6–8.0	Bacteria create an alkaline urine
Specific gravity (density of water =1.000)		Represents concentrating ability or density of urine in relation to density of water (i.e., higher when contains glucose or protein; lower with dilute urine)
Adults	1.010–1.025	
Infants	1.010–1.018	
Blood	Negative	Bleeding along urinary tract
MICROSCOPIC URINE		
Bacteria	None	Infection
Red blood cells	Negative	Bleeding along urinary tract
White blood cells	Negative	Urinary tract infection
Crystals	Negative	May have potential for stones
Fat	Negative	Can be associated with nephrosis
Casts	Occasional	A few are normal, may represent renal disease
URINARY CHEMISTRY		
Bilirubin	Negative	Increases may cause dark orange color
Urobilinogen	Less than 4 mg/24 hr	Increases may indicate red blood cell hemolysis
Ketones	Negative	Represents an increase in fat metabolism
Glucose	Negative	Usually signifies hyperglycemia
Sodium	100–260 mEq/24 hr	Can increase or decrease with renal disease
Potassium	25–100 mEq/24 hr	Can increase or decrease with renal disease, potassium intake, aldosteronism or use of diuretics
Protein	Negative-trace	Dysfunction of the glomerulus
NORMAL SERUM VALUES		
BUN	7–18 mg/dl	Elevated with diseased kidneys
Creatinine		Elevated with decreased GFR
Male	0.6–1.5 mg/dl	
Female	0.6–1.1 mg/dl	
Cystatin C	0.8–2.1 mg/L	Early detection of decreased GFR
Potassium		Elevated in renal failure

TABLE 28-4

Bladder Function Tests

Procedure	Description
URODYNAMIC TESTS	
Cystometry (cystometrogram)	Measurement of bladder pressure determined using a pressure measuring catheter; fluid volume and pressures are measured as the bladder is filled with fluid; simultaneous pressures may be measured in the rectum; sensations of bladder fullness are also recorded; coughing or straining can lead to involuntary bladder contractions Bladder capacity: male: 350–750 ml; female 350–550 ml Intrabladder pressure with empty bladder: 40 cm H_2O Detrusor pressure: <10 cm H_2O Residual urine: <30 ml
Uroflowmetry	Measures the time it takes to empty a full bladder of urine; flow rates may be faster with urge incontinence or slower with prostatic obstruction
Postvoid residual urine	Measures residual urine in the bladder after voiding; urine can be removed with a catheter or by use of ultrasound imaging; postvoid residual of more than 200 mL is abnormal and requires further evaluation
Measurement of leak point pressure	Pressure at which bladder fluid will leak from the bladder without warning
Pressure flow study	Measures the pressure required to empty the bladder; a pressure flow study identifies bladder outlet obstruction as may be experienced with prostate enlargement
Electromyography	Measures nerve impulses and muscle activity in the urethral sphincter by placing sensors on the skin near the urethra and rectum or by placing sensors on a catheter placed in the urethra or rectum
Video urodynamics	Imaging of x-rays or ultrasound waves during fluid filling of the bladder; shows size and shape of the urinary tract
DIRECT VISUALIZATION DIAGNOSTIC PROCEDURE	
Cystoscopy	A cystoscope (a type of endoscope) is inserted through the urethra and is used to visualize the inside of the bladder
Ureteroscopy	A ureteroscope is inserted through the urethra, bladder, and directly into the ureter and upper urinary tract to visualize the upper urinary tract

PEDIATRICS & Renal Function

Glomerular filtration in infants does not reach adult values until 1 to 2 years of age, and newborns have a decreased ability to efficiently remove excess water and solutes. Their shorter loops of Henle also decrease concentrating ability and produce a more dilute urine than that produced by adults. Risks for metabolic acidosis are increased during the first few months of life as the mechanisms for excreting acid and retaining bicarbonate are maturing. These normal developmental processes result in a narrow safety margin for fluid and electrolyte balance when there is any disturbance such as diarrhea, infection, fasting for diagnostic tests, improper feeding, or fluid replacement. An increased risk of toxicity accompanies drug administration.

Data from Brandt JR et al: Estimating absolute glomerular filtration rate in children, *Pediatr Nephrol* 21(12):1865–1872, 2006; Miller M: Fluid and electrolyte homeostasis in the elderly: physiological changes of ageing and clinical consequences. *Baillieres Clin Endocrinol Metab* 11(2):367–387, 1997.

✔ QUICK CHECK 28-4

1. Why is creatinine clearance a good estimate of glomerular filtration rate?
2. What is the relationship between plasma creatinine concentration and glomerular filtration rate?

AGING & Renal Function

- There is a slow decline in GFR in most individuals, but generally it is not significant enough to lead to severe loss of renal function. The number of nephrons decreases and degenerative changes can occur, so nephrons are less able to concentrate urine with decreases in ability to tolerate dehydration or excessive water loads.
- Response to acid-base changes and reabsorption of glucose may be delayed.
- Drugs eliminated by the kidney can accumulate in the plasma, causing toxic reactions; drug dosage should be carefully evaluated.
- Alterations in thirst and water intake may alter water balance.
- Impairment in renal blood flow, hormonal regulatory systems, and use of medications may alter sodium and water balance.

Data from Long DA, Mu W, Price KL, Johnson RJ: Blood vessels and the aging kidney. *Nephron Exp Nephrol* 101(3), 2005; Buemi M, Nostro L, Aloisi C, Cosentini V, Criseo M, Frisina N: Kidney aging: from phenotype to genetics. *Rejuvenation Res* 8(2):101–109, 2005; Merle L, Laroche ML, Dantoine T, Charmes JP: Predicting and preventing adverse drug reactions in the very old. *Drugs Aging* 22(5):375–379, 2005.

Did You Understand?

Structures of the Renal System

1. The kidneys are paired structures lying bilaterally between the twelfth thoracic and third lumbar vertebrae.
2. The kidney is composed of an outer cortex and an inner medulla.
3. The calyces join to form the renal pelvis, which is continuous with the upper end of the ureter.
4. The nephron is the urine-forming unit of the kidney and is composed of the glomerulus, proximal tubule, hairpin loops of Henle, distal tubule, and collecting duct.
5. The glomerulus contains loops of capillaries. The capillary walls serve as a filtration membrane for the formation of the primary urine.
6. The proximal tubule is lined with microvilli to increase surface area and enhance reabsorption.
7. The hairpin loops of Henle transport solutes and water, contributing to the hypertonic state of the medulla.
8. The distal tubule adjusts acid-base balance by excreting acid into the urine and forming new bicarbonate ions.
9. The ureters extend from the renal pelvis to the posterior wall of the bladder. Urine flows through the ureters by means of peristaltic contraction of the ureteral muscles.
10. The bladder is a bag composed of the detrusor and trigone muscles and innervated by parasympathetic fibers. When accumulation of urine reaches 250 to 300 ml, mechanoreceptors, which respond to stretching of tissue, stimulate the micturition reflex.

Renal Blood Flow

1. Renal blood flows at about 1000 to 1200 ml/min, or 20% to 25% of the cardiac output.
2. Blood flow through the glomerular capillaries is maintained at a constant rate in spite of a wide range of arterial pressures.
3. The glomerular filtration rate (GFR) is the filtration of plasma per unit of time and is directly related to the perfusion pressure of renal blood flow.
4. Autoregulation of renal blood flow and neural regulation of vasoconstriction maintain a constant GFR.
5. Renin is an enzyme secreted from the juxtaglomerular apparatus and causes the generation of angiotensin, a potent vasoconstrictor. The renin-angiotensin system is thus a regulator of renal blood flow.

Kidney Function

1. The major function of the nephron is urine formation, which involves the processes of glomerular filtration, tubular reabsorption, and tubular secretion and excretion.
2. Glomerular filtration is favored by capillary hydrostatic pressure and opposed by oncotic pressure in the capillary and hydrostatic pressure in Bowman capsule. The balance of favoring and opposing filtration forces is known as net filtration pressure (NFP).
3. The GFR is approximately 120 ml/min, and 99% of the filtrate is reabsorbed.
4. The proximal tubule reabsorbs about 60% to 70% of the filtered sodium and water and 90% of other electrolytes.
5. Because most molecules are reabsorbed by active transport, the carrier mechanism can become saturated at a point known as the transport maximum (T_m). Molecules not reabsorbed are excreted with the urine.
6. The distal tubules actively reabsorb sodium and secrete potassium and hydrogen for the regulation of electrolyte and acid-base balance.
7. The concentration of the final urine is a function of the level of antidiuretic hormone (ADH) that stimulates the distal tubules and collecting ducts to reabsorb water. The countercurrent exchange system of the long loops of Henle and their accompanying capillaries establishes a concentration gradient within the renal medulla to facilitate the reabsorption of water from the collecting duct.
8. The distal nephron regulates acid-base balance by excreting hydrogen ions and forming new bicarbonate.
9. The kidney secretes or activates a number of hormones that have systemic effects, including 1,25-dihydroxyvitamin D_3, erythropoietin, and natriuretic hormone.
10. Creatinine, a substance produced by muscle, is measured in both plasma and urine to calculate a commonly used clinical measurement of GFR.
11. Both the plasma creatinine concentration and the blood urea nitrogen (BUN) levels indicate glomerular function. Plasma creatinine is measured to monitor progressive renal dysfunction; BUN is an indicator of hydration status.

PEDIATRICS & Renal Function

1. Infants and children have more dilute urine than do adults because of higher blood flow and shorter loops of Henle.
2. Children are more affected than adults by fluid imbalances resulting from diarrhea, infection, or improper feeding because of their limited ability to quickly regulate changes in pH or osmotic pressure.

AGING & Renal Function

1. Older adults have a decreased ability to concentrate urine and are less able to tolerate dehydration or water loads because they have fewer nephrons.
2. Response to acid-base changes and reabsorption of glucose are delayed in older adults.
3. In older adults, drugs eliminated by the kidney can accumulate in the plasma, causing toxic reactions.

Key Terms

Aldosterone, 779
Arcuate artery, 768
Atrial natriuretic peptide (ANP), 779
Autoregulation of blood flow, 772
Bladder, 769
Bowman capsule, 767
Bowman space, 767
Calyx (calyces), 766
Collecting duct, 768
Concentration of urine, 776
Cortex, 766
Cortical nephron, 767
Countercurrent exchange system, 776
Detrusor, 769
Dilution of urine, 776
Distal tubule, 768
Diuretic, 779
Excretion, 774
External urethral sphincter, 770
Filtration slit, 767
Glomerular capillary, 768
Glomerular filtration membrane, 767
Glomerular filtration rate (GFR), 772
Glomerulotubular balance, 776
Glomerulus, 767
Hilum, 766
Intercalated cell, 768
Interlobar artery, 768
Internal urethral sphincter, 770
Juxtaglomerular apparatus, 767
Juxtaglomerular cell, 767
Juxtamedullary nephron, 767
Kidney, 766
Lobe, 766
Loop of Henle, 767
Macula densa, 767
Medulla, 766
Mesangial cell, 767
Micturition, 769
Nephron, 766
Net filtration pressure (NFP), 774
Oliguria, 779
Peritubular capillary, 768
Plasma creatinine (P_{cr}) concentration, 780
Podocyte, 767
Principal cell, 768
Proximal tubule, 767
Pyramid, 766
Renal artery, 768
Renal capsule, 766
Renal fascia, 766
Renal papilla, 769
Renal vein, 769
Renin-angiotensin system, 772
Transport maximum (T_m), 776
Trigone, 769
Tubular reabsorption, 774
Tubular secretion, 774
Tubuloglomerular feedback, 772
Ultrafiltration, 774
Urea, 778
Ureter, 769
Urethra, 770
Urodilatin, 779
Vasa recta, 768
Water diuresis, 779

References

1. Gomez-Guerrero C et al: Mesangial cells and glomerular inflammation: from the pathogenesis to novel therapeutic approaches, *Curr Drug Targets Inflamm Allergy* 4(3):341–351, 2005.
2. Herrera GA: Plasticity of mesangial cells: a basis for understanding pathological alterations, *Ultrastruct Pathol* 30(6): 471–479, 2006.
3. de Zoysa JR, Topham PS: Podocyte biology in human disease, *Nephrology (Carlton)* 10(4):362–367, 2005.
4. Pavenstadt H: Roles of the podocyte in glomerular function, *Am J Physiol Renal Physiol* 278(2):F173–F179, 2000.
5. Ollerstam A, Persson AE: Macula densa neuronal nitric oxide synthase, *Cardiovasc Res* 56(2):189–196, 2002.
6. Schweda F, Kurtz A: Cellular mechanism of renin release, *Acta Physiol Scand* 181(4):383–390, 2004.
7. Apodaca G: The uroepithelium: not just a passive barrier, *Traffic* 5(3):117–128, 2004.
8. Mattson DL: Importance of the renal medullary circulation in the control of sodium excretion and blood pressure, *Am J Physiol Regul Integr Comp Physiol* 284(1):R13–R27, 2003.
9. Field M, Pollock C, Harris D: *The renal system,* Churchill Livingstone, Edinburgh, 2001, 37–40.
10. Guthrie D, Yucha C: Urinary concentration and dilution, *Nephrol Nurs J* 31(3):297–301, 2004.
11. Saemann MD et al: Tamm-Horsfall protein: a multilayered defence molecule against urinary tract infection, *Eur J Clin Invest* 35(4):227–235, 2005.
12. Maack T: The broad homeostatic role of natriuretic peptides, *Arq Bras Endocrinol Metabol* 50(2):198–207, 2006.
13. Buemi M, Nostro L, Romeo A, Giacobbe MS, Aloisi C, Sturiale A, Bolignano D, Allegra A, Grasso G, Frisina N: From the oxygen to the organ protection: erythropoietin as protagonist in internal medicine, *Cardiovasc Hematol Agents Med Chem* 4(4):299–311, 2006.
14. Hojs R, Bevc S, Ekart R, Gorenjak M, Puklavec L: Serum cystatin C as an endogenous marker of renal function in patients with mild to moderate impairment of kidney function, *Nephrol Dial Transplant* 21(7):1855–1862, 2006.
15. Stevens LA, Levey AS: Measurement of kidney function, *Med Clin North Am* 89(3):457–473, 2005.
16. Rigalleau V et al: Estimation of glomerular filtration rate in diabetic subjects: Cockcroft formula or modification of Diet in Renal Disease Study equation? *Diabetes Care* 28(4): 838–843, 2005.

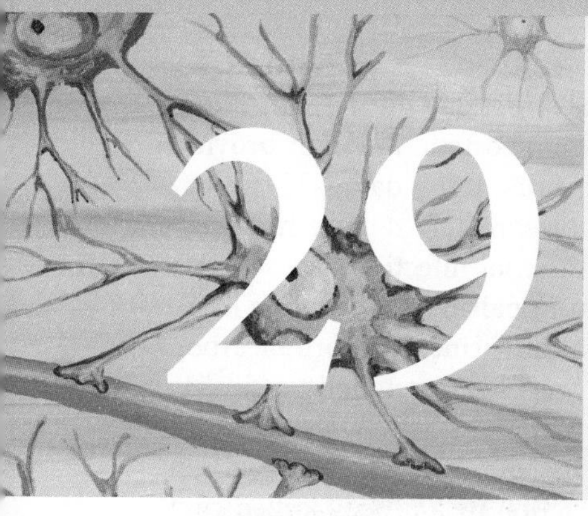

29 ALTERATIONS OF RENAL AND URINARY TRACT FUNCTION

Sue E. Huether ▪ Mikel Gray

CHAPTER OUTLINE

ELECTRONIC RESOURCES

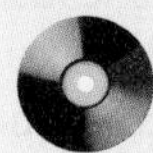

Companion CD
- Review Questions and Answers
- Animations

evolve Website
http://evolve.elsevier.com/Huether/
- Quick Check Answers
- Key Terms Exercises
- Critical Thinking Questions with Answers
- Algorithm Completion Exercises
- WebLinks

Renal and urinary function can be affected by a variety of disorders. The most common type of urinary dysfunction is infection of the bladder. Stones or tumors also can obstruct the urinary tract. Renal function can be impaired by disorders of the kidney itself or by many other systemic diseases. Because the kidney filters the blood, it is directly linked to every other organ system. Renal failure, whether acute or chronic, is therefore a life-threatening condition.

URINARY TRACT OBSTRUCTION

Urinary tract obstruction is an interference with the flow of urine at any site along the urinary tract (Figure 29-1). An obstruction may be anatomic or functional; it impedes flow proximal to the blockage, dilates the urinary system, increases the risk for infection, and compromises renal function. Anatomic changes in the urinary system caused by obstruction are referred to as **obstructive uropathy.** The severity of an obstructive uropathy is determined by (1) the location of the obstructive lesion, (2) whether one or both upper urinary tracts are involved, (3) the severity (completeness) of the blockage, (4) its duration, and (5) the nature of the obstructive lesion.[1,2] Obstructions may be relieved or partially alleviated by correction of the obstruction, although permanent impairments occur if a complete or partial obstruction persists over a period of weeks to months or longer.

Upper Urinary Tract Obstruction

Common causes of upper urinary tract obstruction include stricture or congenital compression of a calyx or the ureteropelvic or ureterovesical junction (i.e., stones [calculi]); compression from an aberrant vessel, tumor, or abdominal inflammation and scarring (retroperitoneal fibrosis); or ureteral blockage from stones or a malignancy of the renal pelvis, ureter, bladder, or prostate.

Obstruction of the upper urinary tract causes dilation of the ureter, renal pelvis, calyces, and renal parenchyma proximal to the site of urinary blockage. Dilation of the ureter is referred to as **hydroureter** (accumulation of urine in the ureter), and dilation of the renal pelvis and calyces proximal to a blockage leads to **hydronephrosis** (enlargement of the renal pelvis and calyces) or **ureterohydronephrosis** (dilation of both the ureter and pelvicaliceal system) (Figure 29-2). Dilation of the upper urinary tract is an early response to obstruction. It reflects smooth muscle hypertrophy and accumulation of urine above the level of blockage (urinary stasis). Unless the obstruction is relieved, this dilation leads to enlargement and fibrosis affecting the distal nephron within approximately 7 days. By 14 days, obstruction has adversely affected both distal and proximal aspects of the nephron. Within 28 days, the glomeruli of the kidney have been damaged and the renal cortex and medulla are reduced in size (thinned). Tubular damage initially decreases the kidney's ability to concentrate urine, causing an increase in urine volume despite a decrease in glomerular filtration rate (GFR). The affected kidney is unable to conserve sodium, bicarbonate, and water or to excrete hydrogen or potassium, leading to metabolic acidosis and dehydration. The magnitude of this damage, and the kidney's ability to recover normal

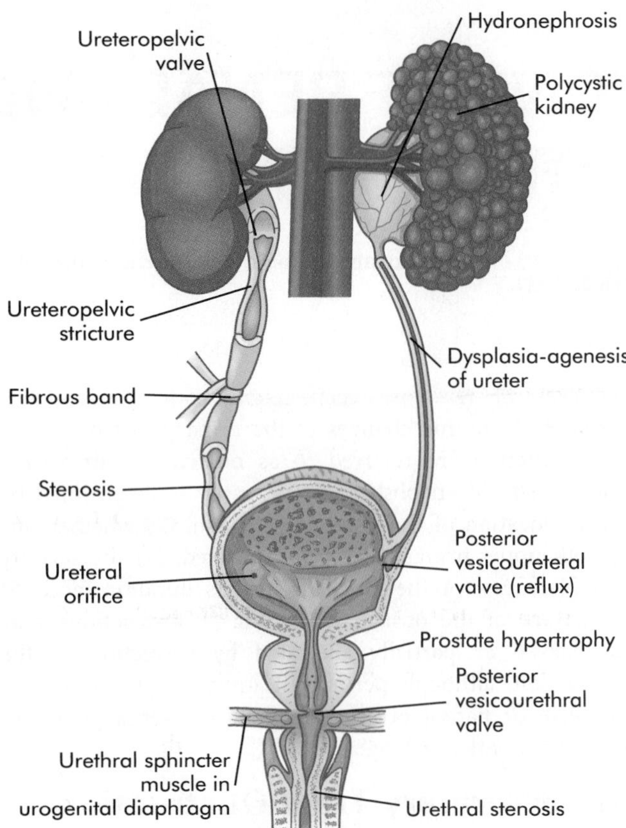

Figure 29-1 ■ **Major Sites of Urinary Tract Obstruction.**

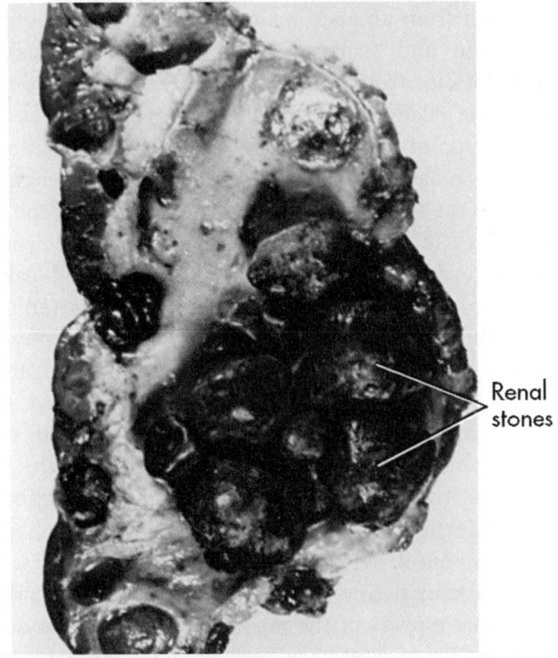

Figure 29-2 ■ **Hydronephrosis.** Hydronephrosis with renal stones in renal pelvis and calyces. (From Kissane JM, editor: *Anderson's pathology,* ed 9, St Louis, 1990, Mosby.)

homeostatic function, is affected by the severity and duration of the obstruction. With complete obstruction, damage to the renal tubules occurs in a matter of hours, and irreversible damage occurs within 4 weeks. Nevertheless, even in the face of a complete obstruction, the human kidney may recover at least partial homeostatic function provided the blockage is removed within 56 to 69 days.[1] This recovery requires a period of approximately 4 months. Partial obstruction, in the absence of renal infection, leads to subtler but ultimately permanent impairments including loss of the kidney's ability to concentrate urine, reabsorb bicarbonate, excrete ammonia, or regulate metabolic acid-base balance.

The body is able to partially counteract the negative consequences of unilateral obstruction by a process called **compensatory hypertrophy.**[1] Compensatory hypertrophy is the result of two growth processes: obligatory growth occurs under the influence of growth hormone, and compensatory growth occurs under the influence of a yet-to-be-identified hormone or hormones. These processes cause the contralateral (unobstructed) kidney to increase the size of individual glomeruli and tubules but not the total number of functioning nephrons. The ability of the body to engage in compensatory hypertrophy diminishes with age, and the process is reversible when relief of obstruction results in recovery of function by the obstructed kidney.

Relief of bilateral, partial urinary tract obstruction, or complete obstruction of one kidney is usually followed by diuresis (commonly called **postobstructive diuresis**).[1,2] It is a physiologic response and is typically mild, representing a restoration of fluid and electrolyte imbalance caused by the obstructive uropathy. Occasionally, relief of obstruction will cause rapid excretion of large volumes of water, sodium, or other electrolytes, resulting in a urine output of 10 L/day or more. Rapid postobstructive diuresis causes dehydration and fluid and electrolyte imbalances that must be promptly corrected. Risk factors for severe postobstructive diuresis include chronic, bilateral obstruction, impairment of one or both kidneys' ability to concentrate urine or reabsorb sodium *(nephrogenic diabetes insipidus),* hypertension, edema and weight gain, congestive heart failure, and uremic encephalopathy.

Kidney stones

Calculi, or **urinary stones,** are masses of crystals, protein, or other substances that are a common cause of urinary tract obstruction in adults. The prevalence of stones in the United States is approximately 5% in women and 12% in men.[3] The recurrence rate is approximately 30% to 50% within 5 years.[4] The risk of urinary calculi formation is influenced by a number of factors, including age, gender, race, geographic location, seasonal factors, fluid intake, diet, and occupation. Most persons develop their first stone before age 50 years. Geographic location influences the risk of stone formation because of indirect factors, including average temperature, humidity, and rain fall, and its influence on fluid and dietary patterns. Persons who regularly consume an adequate volume of water and those who are physically active are at reduced risk when compared to persons who are inactive or consume lower volumes of fluid.

Urinary calculi can be described according to the primary minerals (salts) that make up the stones. The most common stone types include calcium oxalate or phosphate (70% to 80%), struvite (magnesium, ammonium, and phosphate) (15%), and uric acid (7%). Cystine stones are rare, less than 1%.

PATHOPHYSIOLOGY Calculus formation is based on (1) supersaturation of one or more salts in the urine, (2) precipitation of the salts from a liquid to a solid state, (3) growth through crystallization or agglomeration (sometimes called *aggregation*), and (4) the presence or absence of stone inhibitors.[5] *Supersaturation* is the presence of a higher concentration of a salt within a fluid (in this case, the urine) than the volume is able to dissolve to maintain equilibrium.

Human urine contains many ions capable of *precipitating* from solution and forming a variety of salts. The salts form crystals that can grow into stones. *Crystallization* is the process by which crystals grow from a small *nidus* (nucleus) to larger stones in the presence of supersaturated urine. Although supersaturation is essential for stone formation, the urine need not remain continuously supersaturated for a calculus to grow once its nidus has precipitated from solution. Intermittent periods of supersaturation after the ingestion of a meal or during times of dehydration are sufficient for stone growth in many individuals. In addition, the renal tubules and papillae have many surfaces that may attract a crystalline nidus and add biologic material (matrix) to the forming stone. *Matrix* is an organic material that is formed in the presence of urea-splitting pathogens.

Temperature and pH of the urine also influence the risk of precipitation and calculus formation, and pH is most important. An alkaline urinary pH significantly increases the risk of a calcium phosphate stone formation, whereas acidic urine increases the risk of a uric acid stone. Cystine and xanthine precipitates more readily in acidic urine.

Stone or *crystal growth inhibiting substances*, such as potassium citrate, pyrophosphate, and magnesium, are capable of crystal growth inhibition, thereby reducing the risk of calcium phosphate or calcium oxalate precipitation in the urine and preventing subsequent stone formation.

The size of a stone determines the likelihood that it will pass through the urinary tract and be excreted through micturition.[6] A stone that is smaller than 5 mm in size has about a 50% chance of spontaneous passage, whereas a stone that is 1 cm has almost no chance of spontaneous passage. Nevertheless, the person with ureteral dilation from the previous passage of a stone may be able to excrete larger stones when compared with the person experiencing an initial obstructing calculus.

Retention of *crystal particles* occurs primarily at the papillary collecting ducts. Although most crystals are flushed from the tract through antegrade urine flow, urinary stasis, anatomic abnormalities, or inflamed epithelium within the urinary tract may prevent prompt flushing of crystals from the system, thus increasing the risk of calculus formation.

Calcium stones (calcium phosphate or calcium oxalate) account for 70% to 80% of all stones requiring treatment. Most of these individuals have *idiopathic calcium urolithiasis (ICU)*, a condition whose exact etiology has not yet been defined. However, hypercalciuria, hyperoxaluria, hyperuricosuria, hypocitraturia, mild renal tubular acidosis, or crystal growth inhibitor deficiencies are associated with calcium stones. Hypercalciuria is usually attributable to intestinal hyperabsorption of dietary calcium. Hyperthyroidism and bone demineralization associated with prolonged immobilization are also known to cause hypercalciuria. Although oxalate in the diet influences the risk of calcium stones, primary hyperoxaluria is a rare, inherited disorder.

Struvite stones primarily contain magnesium-ammonium-phosphate as well as varying levels of matrix. Matrix forms in an alkaline urine and during infection with a urease-producing bacterial pathogen, such as a *Proteus*, *Klebsiella*, or *Pseudomonas*. Struvite calculi may grow quite large and branch into a staghorn configuration that approximates the pelvicaliceal collecting system.

Uric acid is primarily a product of biosynthesis of endogenous purines and is secondarily affected by consumption of purines in the diet. Persons who excrete excessive uric acid in the urine, such as those with gouty arthritis, are at particular risk for **uric acid stones.** A consistently acidic urine greatly increases this risk. Cystine and xanthine are amino acids that precipitate more readily in acidic urine. *Cystinuria* and *xanthinuria* are both genetic disorders of amino acid metabolism, and their excess in urine can cause stone formation in the presence of a low urine pH of 5.5 or less.

CLINICAL MANIFESTATIONS **Renal colic,** described as moderate to severe pain often originating in the flank and radiating to the groin, usually indicates obstruction of the renal pelvis or proximal ureter.[7] Colic that radiates to the lateral flank or lower abdomen typically indicates obstruction in the midureter, and bothersome lower urinary tract symptoms (urgency, frequent voiding, urge incontinence) indicate obstruction of the lower ureter or ureterovesical junction. The pain can be severe and incapacitating and may be accompanied by nausea and vomiting. Gross or microscopic hematuria may be present.

EVALUATION AND TREATMENT The evaluation and diagnosis of urinary calculi is based on presenting symptoms and history combined with a focused physical assessment, imaging studies, and possibly a functional study of renal pelvic and ureteral pressures.[8] The history also queries the age of the first stone episode, stone analysis, and presence of complicating factors including hyperparathyroidism or recent gastrointestinal or genitourinary surgery. Urinalysis (including pH) is obtained and a 24-hour urine is completed to identify calcium oxalate, citrate, and other significant constituents. In addition, every effort is made to retrieve and analyze calculi that are passed spontaneously or retrieved through aggressive intervention. Additional tests are obtained in selected individuals, such as those with suspected hyperparathyroidism or cystine or uric acid stones, in order to diagnose and manage underlying metabolic disorders. A KUB radiograph (x-ray film of the kidneys, ureters, and bladder) is obtained to evaluate radiopaque stones (comprising more than 90% of all stones) and an ultrasound, intravenous pyelogram (IVP), or computerized tomographic (CT) scan or ultrasonography are obtained to determine the location of the calculi, the severity of obstruction, and associated obstructive uropathy.[9]

The goals of treatment are to reduce the size of stones already formed and prevent new stone formation. The components of treatment include (1) reducing the concentration of stone-forming substances by increasing urine flow rate with high fluid intake, (2) decreasing the amount of stone-forming substances in the urine by decreasing dietary intake or endogenous production or by altering urine pH,[10] and (3) removing stones using endoscopy or ultrasonic or laser lithotripsy to fragment stones for excretion in the urine.[11]

Lower Urinary Tract Obstruction

Obstructive disorders of the lower urinary tract (LUT) are primarily related to storage of urine in the bladder or emptying of urine through the bladder outlet. The causes of the obstruction include both neurogenic and anatomic alterations or, in some instances, a combination of both. Incontinence is a common symptom and types of incontinence are reviewed in Table 29-1.

Neurogenic bladder

Neurogenic bladder is a general term for bladder dysfunction caused by neurologic disorders (Table 29-2). The types of dysfunction are related to the sites in the nervous system that control sensory and motor bladder function. Lesions that develop in upper motor neurons of the brain and spinal cord result in **dyssynergia** (loss of coordinated neuromuscular contraction) and overactive or hyperreflexive bladder function. Lesions in the sacral area of the spinal cord or peripheral nerves result in underactive, hypotonic, or atonic (flaccid) bladder function, often with loss of bladder sensation.

Neurologic disorders that develop above the pontine micturition center result in **detrusor hyperreflexia,** also known as an uninhibited or reflex bladder. This is an upper motor neuron disorder in which the bladder empties automatically when it becomes full and the external sphincter functions normally. Because the pontine micturition center remains intact, there is coordination between detrusor

TABLE 29-1

Types of Incontinence

Type	Description
Urge incontinence (most common in older adults)	Involuntary loss of urine associated with an abrupt and strong desire to void (urgency); often associated with involuntary contractions of the detrusor; when associated with a neurologic disorder, this is called detrusor hyperreflexia; when no neurologic disorder exists, this is called detrusor instability; may be associated with decreased bladder wall compliance.
Stress incontinence (most common in women under 60 years and men who have had prostate surgery)	Involuntary loss of urine during coughing, sneezing, laughing or other physical activity associated with increased abdominal pressure.
Overflow incontinence	Involuntary loss of urine with overdistention of the bladder; associated with neurologic lesions below S1, polyneuropathies and urethral obstruction (i.e., an enlarged prostate in men).
Mixed incontinence (most common in older women)	A combination of both stress and urge incontinence.
Functional incontinence	Involuntary loss of urine due to dementia or immobility.

Data from Agency for Health Care Policy and Research: *Overview: urinary incontinence in adults, clinical practice guideline update*, Rockville, MD, 1996; www.ahrq.gov/clinic/uiovervw.htm.

TABLE 29-2

Neurogenic Bladder

Site of Lesion	Cause (Symptoms)	Diseases
Lesions above C2 Involve pontine micturition center	Detrusor hyperreflexia (urgency and urine leakage)	Stoke, traumatic brain injury, multiple sclerosis (MS), hydrocephalus, cerebral palsy, Alzheimer disease, brain tumors
Lesions between C2 and S1	Detrusor sphincter dyssynergia with detrusor hyperreflexia (functional bladder outlet obstruction)	Spinal cord injury C2-T12, MS, transverse myelitis, "Guillain-Barré" syndrome, disk problems
Lesions below S1 (cauda equina syndrome)	Acontractile detrusor, with or without urethral sphincter incompetence (stress urinary incontinence)	Myelodysplasia, peripheral polyneuropathies, MS, tabes dorsalis, spinal injury T12-S1, cauda equina syndrome, herpes simplex/zoster

muscle contraction and the relaxation of the urethral sphincter. Stroke, traumatic brain injury, dementia, and brain tumors are examples of disorders that result in detrusor hyperreflexia. Symptoms include urine leakage and incontinence.

Neurologic lesions that occur below the pontine micturition center but above the sacral micturition center (between C2 and S1) are also upper motor neuron lesions and result in **detrusor sphincter dyssynergia with detrusor hyperreflexia.** There is loss of pontine coordination of detrusor muscle contraction and external sphincter relaxation, so both the bladder and the sphincter are contracting at the same time causing a functional obstruction of the bladder outlet.[12] Spinal cord injury, multiple sclerosis, Guillain Barré syndrome, and disk problems are causes of this disorder. There is diminished bladder relaxation during storage with small urine volumes and high intravesicular (inside the bladder) pressures. This results in an overactive bladder syndrome with symptoms of frequency, urgency, and urge incontinence and increased risk for urethral turbulence and urinary tract infection.

Lesions that involve the sacral micturition center (below S1; may also be termed *cauda equina syndrome*) or peripheral nerve lesions result in **detrusor areflexia** (acontractile detrusor), a lower motor neuron disorder. The result is an acontractile detrusor or atonic bladder with retention of urine and distention. This is an *underactive bladder syndrome* and may have symptoms of stress and overflow incontinence. Myelodysplasia, multiple sclerosis, tabes dorsalis, and peripheral polyneuropathies are associated with this disorder.

Overactive bladder syndrome

Overactive bladder syndrome is a syndrome of detrusor overactivity characterized by involuntary detrusor contractions during the bladder filling phase that may be spontaneous or provoked.[13] There is coordination between the contracting bladder and the external sphincter, but the detrusor is too weak to empty the bladder, resulting in urinary retention with overflow or stress incontinence. Overactive bladder as defined by the International Continence Society as a *symptom syndrome* of urgency, with or without urge incontinence and usually associated with frequency and nocturia.[14] Overactive bladder syndrome affects millions of men and women who are often reluctant to discuss this syndrome with their health care provider. Diagnosis is usually made by evaluation of symptoms. Urodynamic evaluation confirms the diagnosis. Antimuscarinics are the most common treatment and in intractable cases, surgery is recommended.[15] When left untreated, overactive bladder syndrome impairs health and quality of life, causes depression, and leads to social isolation; in the elderly it may cause risk for falls and urinary tract infection.[16]

Obstructions to urine flow

Anatomic causes of resistance to urine flow include urethral stricture, prostatic enlargement in men, and pelvic organ prolapse in women. Symptoms of obstruction are more common in men and include (1) frequent daytime voiding (urination more than every 2 hours while awake); (2) nocturia (awakening more than once each night to urinate for adults less than 65 years of age or more than twice for older adults); (3) poor force of stream; (4) intermittency of urinary stream; (5) bothersome urinary urgency, often combined with hesitancy; and (6) feelings of incomplete bladder emptying despite micturition.

A **urethral stricture** is a narrowing of its lumen. It occurs when infection, injury, or surgical manipulation produces a scar that reduces the caliber of the urethra.[17] The vast majority of urethral strictures occur in men; they are rare in women.[18] The severity of obstruction is influenced by its location within the urethra, its length, and the minimum caliber of urethral lumen within the stricture. Specifically, proximal urethral strictures cause more severe obstruction than do strictures of the distal urethra, longer strictures tend to be more obstructive, and the magnitude of blockage is in *reverse* proportion to the urethral caliber.

Prostate enlargement is caused by acute inflammation, benign prostatic hyperplasia, or prostate cancer (see Chapter 32). Each of these disorders can cause encroachment on the urethra with obstruction to urine flow and the symptoms summarized previously.

Severe **pelvic organ prolapse** (see Chapter 32) in a woman causes bladder outlet obstruction when a cystocele (the downward protrusion of the bladder into the vagina) descends below the level of the urethral outlet. Cystoceles that reach or protrude beyond the vaginal introitus create the greatest risk for obstruction, particularly if the bladder neck has been surgically repaired without simultaneous repair of the cystocele. In men the bladder may rarely herniate into the scrotum causing a similar type of obstruction.

Partial obstruction of the bladder outlet or urethra initially causes an increase in the force of detrusor contraction. If the blockage persists, afferent nerves within the bladder wall are adversely affected, leading to urinary urgency and, in some cases, overactive detrusor contractions (a myogenic cause of overactive bladder). When obstruction persists, there is an increased deposition of collagen within the smooth muscle bundles of the detrusor muscle *(trabeculation)*, possibly in an attempt to increase the force of its contraction strength. Ultimately, the bladder wall loses its ability to stretch and accommodate urine, a condition called **low bladder wall compliance,** and the detrusor loses its ability to contract efficiently. Low bladder wall compliance chronically elevates intravesicular pressure, greatly increasing the problems of hydroureter, hydronephrosis, and impaired renal function.

EVALUATION AND TREATMENT Although the history and physical examination are critical to the evaluation of lower urinary tract disorders, it must be remembered that no symptom or cluster of symptoms has been identified that accurately differentiates the various causes of these disorders. For example, symptoms such as urgency, urge incontinence, frequent urination, and nocturia may develop because of overactive bladder or either increased or decreased bladder outlet resistance. Reduced resistance is associated with the symptom of stress incontinence (incontinence with coughing or sneezing) and symptoms of increased resistance are similar to bladder outlet obstruction, including poor force of urinary stream, hesitancy, and feelings of incomplete bladder emptying.

Various diagnostic tests assist with evaluation. The *post-void urine* is measured by catheterization within 5 to 15 minutes of urination or through a bladder ultrasound machine that measures bladder height and width to provide an approximation of urine within the vesicle. This measurement may be combined with *uroflowmetry*, a graphic representation of the force of the urinary stream expressed as milliliters voided per second. Each of these measurements assesses the lower urinary tract's efficiency in evacuating urine through micturition but neither differentiates poor detrusor contraction strength from obstruction as a cause of urinary retention. Instead, *multichannel urodynamic testing* is used to identify obstruction, quantify its severity, and measure detrusor contraction strength (Figure 29-3). *Video-urodynamic recordings* can also demonstrate overactive bladder and detrusor sphincter dyssynergia. An evaluation of renal function, including functional imaging studies and serum creatinine, is completed particularly when obstruction is severe and associated with elevated residuals or urinary tract infection.

Because the bladder neck consists of circular smooth muscle with adrenergic innervation, detrusor sphincter dyssynergia may be managed by alpha-adrenergic blocking (antimuscarinic) medications. Obstruction that is not adequately managed by pharmacotherapy may require bladder neck incision. Detrusor sphincter dyssynergia may be managed by intermittent catheterization in combination with higher dose antimuscarinic drugs to prevent overactive detrusor contractions and associated dyssynergia while ensuring regular, complete bladder evacuation via catheterization. Alternatively, men with dyssynergia may be managed by condom catheter containment, supplemented by an alpha-adrenergic-blocking drug or transurethral sphincterotomy (surgical incision of the striated sphincter) in order to relieve obstruction. Low bladder wall compliance may be managed by antimuscarinic drugs and intermittent catheterization; however, more severe cases may require augmentation enterocystoplasty (enlargement of the low compliant bladder wall using a detubularized piece of small bowel), urinary diversion, or long-term indwelling catheterization.

Prostate enlargement is managed by treating the underlying cause of the prostate enlargement with medication or surgery. Acute prostatitis is initially managed by broad-spectrum antibiotics until the results of a urine culture are obtained. Urinary retention may require transient

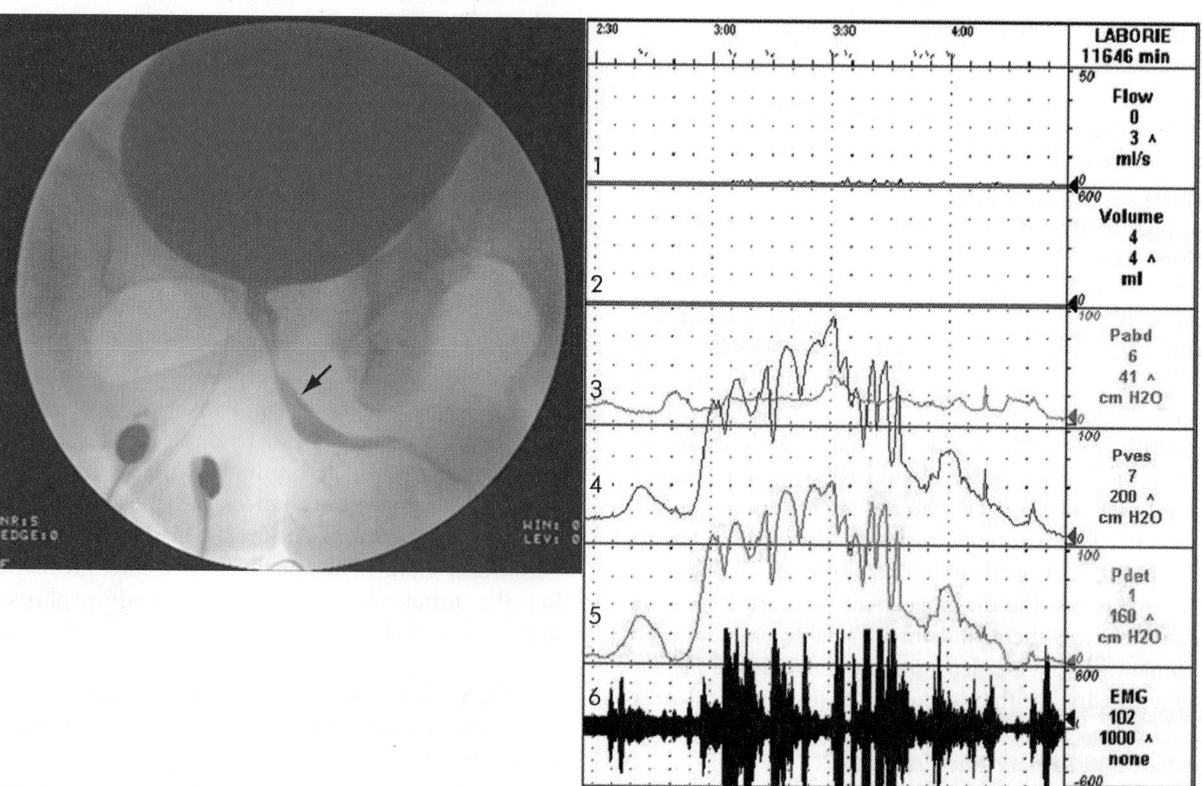

Figure 29-3 ■ **Neurogenic Detrusor Overactivity With Vesico-Sphincter.** The *arrow* indicates narrowing of the striated sphincter consistent with electromyographic activity *(line 6)* noted on the urodynamic tracing. Note the characteristic poor flow pattern *(line 1)* with elevated voiding pressures *(lines 4 and 5)* indicating obstruction. *Line 1,* Urine flow rate; *line 2,* urine volume; *line 3,* abdominal pressure (Pabd); *line 4,* intravesicular (inside bladder) pressure (Pues); *line 5,* detrusor muscle pressure (Pdet); *line 6,* bladder electromyelogram (EMG).

placement of a suprapubic catheter. The management of benign prostatic hyperplasia and treatment options for prostate cancer are presented in Chapter 32.

Urethral stricture is treated with urethral dilation accomplished by using a steel instrument shaped like a catheter (urethral sound) or a series of incrementally increasing catheter-like tubes (filiforms and followers). Long, dense strictures typically require surgical repair to prevent recurrence.

A pessary (rubber or silicone device designed to compensate for vaginal wall prolapse) may be inserted to mechanically reverse severe pelvic organ (bladder, uterus, or rectum) prolapse. Depending on the device, the woman may be able to remove, cleanse, and replace the pessary, or it may be changed during a clinic visit. Intravaginal hormone replacement therapy and regular follow-up are critical to the long-term success of a pessary. Alternatively, pelvic organ prolapse may be repaired surgically; the procedure may be combined with a urethral suspension to correct stress urinary incontinence or rectocele repair.

Tumors

Renal tumors

Renal tumors account for about 51,190 (3.5%) of new cancer cases and 12,890 deaths each year,[19] and there are a number of different types of kidney tumors. **Renal adenomas** (benign tumors) are uncommon but are increasing in number. The tumors are encapsulated and are usually located near the cortex of the kidney. Because they can become malignant, they are usually surgically removed. **Renal cell carcinoma (RCC)** is the most common renal neoplasm (85% of all renal neoplasms) and represents about 2% of cancer deaths. Renal cell carcinoma usually occurs in men (two times more often than in women) between 50 and 60 years of age. Black races, cigarette smokers, and those who are obese have a higher incidence.[20] Five-year survival is less than 50% and less than 2% with metastasis.[21]

PATHOGENESIS A moderate association has been identified between tobacco use, obesity, hypertension, and the incidence of RCC.[22] Estrogen administration is linked to renal cell carcinoma in animals.[23] The actual etiology is unknown.

Renal cell carcinomas are adenocarcinomas that usually arise from tubular epithelium commonly in the renal cortex. They are classified according to cell type and extent of metastasis. *Clear cell tumors,* the most common, present a better prognosis than granular cell or spindle tumors. Confinement within the renal capsule, together with treatment, is associated with a better survival rate. The tumors usually occur unilaterally (Figure 29-4). About 25% of individuals with RCC present with metastasis.[24]

CLINICAL MANIFESTATIONS The classic clinical manifestations of renal tumors are hematuria, flank pain, palpable flank mass, and weight loss, but all of these symptoms occur in fewer than 10% of cases. Further, they represent an advanced stage of disease, whereas earlier stages are often silent. The most common sites of distant metastasis are the lung, lymph nodes, liver, bone, thyroid, and central nervous system.[25]

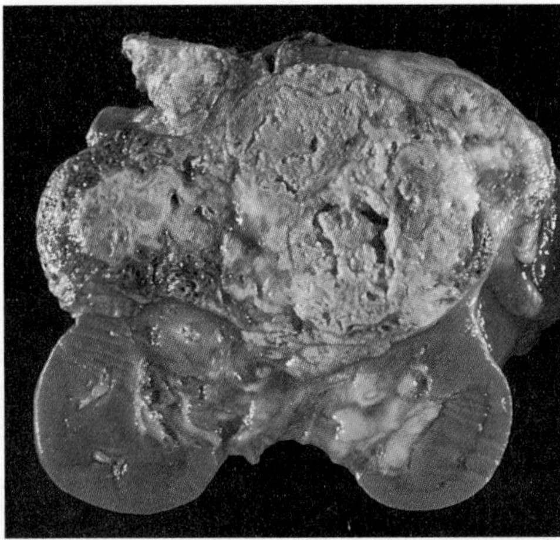

Figure 29-4 ■ Renal Cell Carcinoma. Renal cell carcinomas usually are spheroidal masses composed of yellow tissue mottled with hemorrhage, necrosis, and fibrosis. (From Damjanov I, Linder J, editors: *Anderson's pathology,* ed 10, St Louis, 1996, Mosby.)

EVALUATION AND TREATMENT Diagnosis is based on the clinical symptoms, plain x-ray films of the abdomen, intravenous pyelography, renal angiography, and computed tomography. (Staging of renal cell carcinoma is presented in Table 29-3.) Staging systems using molecular tumor markers are rapidly advancing.[26] Treatment for localized disease is surgical removal of the affected kidney (radical nephrectomy) with combined use of chemotherapeutic agents. Radiation therapy also may be used. Immunotherapy (i.e., interferon-alpha and interleukin-2) is promising in selected cases and new targeted therapies are being developed.[27]

Bladder tumors

Bladder tumors represent about 1% of all malignant tumors and are the fifth most common malignancy.[19,28] Approximately 67,160 people develop bladder cancer each year, and 13,750 die of it.[19,28] The development of bladder cancer

TABLE 29-3

Staging of Renal Cell Carcinoma

Stage	Metastasis
I	Tumor confined within kidney capsule ≤7 cm in size
II	Invasion through renal capsule and renal vein but within surrounding fascia >7 cm in size
III	Involvement of one lymph node, or vena cava, or adrenal glands
IV	Distant metastases (e.g., liver and lung) and more than one lymph node

Adapted from American Cancer Society: *Detailed guide: kidney cancer. How is kidney cancer (renal cell carcinoma) staged?* www.cancer.org/docroot/CRI/content/CRI_2_4_3X_How_is_kidney_cancer_staged_22.asp?rnav=cri (accessed April, 2007).

is most common in men older than 60 years. *Transitional cell carcinoma* is the most common bladder malignancy.

PATHOGENESIS The risk of primary bladder cancer is greater among people who smoke or are exposed to metabolites of aniline dyes or other aromatic amines.[29] Bladder cancer results from a genetic alteration in normal bladder epithelium.[30] Metastasis is usually to lymph nodes, liver, bones, or lungs. Staging for bladder carcinoma is presented in Table 29-4. Secondary bladder cancer develops by invasion of cancer from bordering organs, such as cervical carcinoma in women or prostatic carcinoma in men.

CLINICAL MANIFESTATIONS Gross painless hematuria is the archetypal clinical manifestation of bladder cancer. Episodes of hematuria tend to recur, and they are often accompanied by bothersome lower urinary tract symptoms including daytime voiding frequency, nocturia, urgency, and urge urinary incontinence. Flank pain may occur if tumor growth obstructs one or both ureterovesical junctions. Bothersome lower urinary tract symptoms are particularly intense in individuals with carcinoma in situ.

EVALUATION AND TREATMENT Urinalysis for evidence of hematuria in the absence of infection provides a useful screening tool for high-risk patients. Several bladder tumor antigen-testing systems have been developed for screening, but they have proved more useful in monitoring patients with known cancer as compared to being used for primary screening. Urine cytology (pathologic analysis of sloughed cells within the urine) is completed in individuals with evidence of hematuria from unknown causes; cystoscopy with tissue biopsy confirms the diagnosis. Transurethral resection or laser ablation, combined with intravesical chemotherapy or immunotherapy, is effective for superficial tumors, but radical cystectomy with urinary diversion and adjuvant chemotherapy is required for locally invasive tumors.

TABLE 29-4

Staging of Bladder Carcinoma (TNM* System)

Stage	Description
PRIMARY TUMOR	
T0	No primary tumor identified
Ta	Noninvasive papillary carcinoma—not in bladder muscle
Tis	Carcinoma in situ (CIS)
T1	Tumor invades connective tissue
T2	Tumor invades detrusor muscle
T3	Invasion of fatty tissue around bladder
T4	Tumor has invaded adjacent structures
REGION OF LYMPH NODES	
N0	No lymph node involvement
N1 to N3	Lymph node metastasis to pelvic or adjacent region
DISTANT METASTASIS	
M0	No metastasis
M1	Distant metastasis

**T,* Tumor; *N,* node; *M,* metastasis.

Adapted from American Cancer Society: *Detailed guide: bladder cancer. How is bladder cancer staged?* www.cancer.org/docroot/CRI/content/CRI_2_4_3X_How_is_bladder_cancer_staged_44.asp?sitearea= (accessed April, 2007).

QUICK CHECK 29-1

1. List two common complications of urinary tract obstruction, and briefly describe them.
2. How do kidney stones form?
3. Who are at greatest risk of bladder tumors?

URINARY TRACT INFECTION

Causes of Urinary Tract Infection

A **urinary tract infection (UTI)** is an inflammation of the urinary epithelium usually caused by bacteria from gut flora. A UTI can occur anywhere along the urinary tract including the urethra, prostate, bladder, ureter, or kidney. At risk are premature newborns; prepubertal children; sexually active and pregnant women; women treated with antibiotics that disrupt vaginal flora; spermicide users; estrogen-deficient postmenopausal women; individuals with indwelling catheters; and persons with diabetes mellitus, neurogenic bladder, or urinary tract obstruction. Cystitis is more common in women because of the shorter urethra and the closeness of the urethra to the anus (increasing the possibility of bacterial contamination). Up to 50% of women may have a lower UTI at some time in their life.[31]

Several factors normally combine to protect against UTIs. Most bacteria are washed out of the urethra during micturition. The low pH and high osmolality of urea, the presence of Tamm-Horsfall protein, and secretions from the uroepithelium provide a bactericidal effect. The ureterovesical junction closes during bladder contraction, preventing reflux of urine to the ureters and kidneys. Both the longer urethra and prostatic secretions decrease the risk of infection in men.

Types of Urinary Tract Infection

Acute cystitis

Acute cystitis is an inflammation of the bladder and is the most common site of UTI. The morphologic appearance of the bladder through cystoscopy describes different types of cystitis. With mild inflammation, the mucosa is hyperemic (red). More advanced cases may show diffuse hemorrhage (termed *hemorrhagic cystitis*), pus formation, or suppurative exudates (termed *suppurative cystitis*) on the epithelial surface of the bladder. Prolonged infection may lead to sloughing of the bladder mucosa with ulcer formation (termed *ulcerative cystitis*). The most severe infections may cause necrosis of the bladder wall (termed *gangrenous cystitis*).

Generally, infections are mild, without complications, and occur in individuals with a normal urinary tract; these infections are termed *uncomplicated UTI.* A *complicated UTI* develops when there is an abnormality in the urinary system or there is a health problem that compromises host defenses or response to treatment. UTI may occur alone or in association with pyelonephritis or prostatitis.

PATHOPHYSIOLOGY The most common infecting microorganisms are *Escherichia coli* and less commonly *Klebsiella, Proteus, Pseudomonas, Staphylococcus,* fungi, viruses, parasites, or tubercular bacilli. Bacterial contamination of the normally sterile urine usually occurs by retrograde movement of gram-negative bacilli into the urethra and bladder and then to the ureter and kidney. Expression of type 1 fibriae by *E. coli* with attachment to the uroepithelium is thought to be the initial step of infection. Some women may be genetically susceptible to certain strains of *E. coli* attachment.[32] Hematogenous infections are uncommon and often preceded by septicemia. Infection initiates an inflammatory response and the symptoms of cystitis. The inflammatory edema in the bladder wall stimulates discharge of stretch receptors initiating symptoms of bladder fullness with small volumes of urine and producing the urgency and frequency of urination associated with cystitis.

CLINICAL MANIFESTATIONS Many individuals with bacteriuria are asymptomatic and the elderly have the highest risk. Clinical manifestations of cystitis, however, usually include frequency, urgency, dysuria (painful urination), and suprapubic and low back pain. Hematuria, cloudy urine, and flank pain are more serious symptoms. Approximately 10% of individuals with bacteriuria have no symptoms, and 30% of individuals with symptoms are abacteriuric. Elderly persons with cystitis may be asymptomatic or demonstrate confusion or vague abdominal discomfort. The elderly with recurrent UTI and other concurrent illness have a higher risk of mortality.[33]

EVALUATION AND TREATMENT Infections are diagnosed by urine culture of specific microorganisms with counts of 10,000/ml or more from freshly voided urine. Risk factors, such as urinary tract obstruction, should be identified and treated. Evidence of bacteria from urine culture and antibiotic sensitivity warrants treatment with a microorganism-specific antibiotic. A single large dose of antibiotic or a 3-day course may be effective when symptoms are of short duration and there are no complications. Three to 7 days of treatment is most common; elderly people with obstructive disorders may require 7 to 14 days of treatment. From 20% to 25% of women have relapsing infection within 7 to 10 days requiring prolonged antibiotic treatment.[34] Follow-up urine cultures should be obtained 1 week after initiation of treatment and at monthly intervals for 3 months. Clinical symptoms are frequently relieved, but bacteriuria may still be present. Repeat cultures should be obtained every 3 to 4 months until 1 year after treatment for evaluation of recurrent infection.[35]

HEALTH ALERT

Urinary Tract Infection and Antibiotic Resistance

Uncomplicated urinary tract infection (UTI) occurs primarily in sexually active women with fewer cases among older and pregnant women and older men. The leading cause of UTI is *Escherichia coli (E. coli),* and antibiotics are the mainstay of treatment. Of major concern is the worldwide emergence of bacterial strains resistant to specific antibiotics in both hospital- and community-acquired infections. The resistance is caused in part by high human use of antibiotics and antibiotics in animal feed. Rates of resistance are highest in regions with the highest rates of prescription; ampicillin and trimethoprim-sulfamethoxazole (TMP-SMX) have a high rate of resistance. Risks for resistance include TMP-SMX treatment within last 3 months, diabetes mellitus, recent hospitalization, and specific antibiotic resistance rates in a community of greater than 20%. However, reliable data regarding the true prevalence of resistance in a community are often lacking. Other factors to consider in choice of antibiotic treatment include infection severity, complicated or uncomplicated UTI, accuracy of diagnosis, broad-spectrum (i.e., trimethoprim-sulfamethoxazole, ampicillin, and cephalothin) versus narrow-spectrum (i.e., nitrofurantoin and ciprofloxacin) antibiotic sensitivity, cost-effectiveness, and instructing consumers about the correct use of antibiotics.

Data from Nicolle L, Anderson PA, Conly J, Mainprize TC, Meuser J, Nickel JC, Senikas VM, Zhanel GG: Uncomplicated urinary tract infection in women. Current practice and the effect of antibiotic resistance on empiric treatment; *Can Fam Physician* 52:612–618, 2006; Chulain MN et al: Antimicrobial resistance in *E. coli* associated with urinary tract infection in the west of Ireland, *Ir J Med Sci* 174(4):6–9, 2005; Mehnert-Kay SA: Diagnosis and management of uncomplicated urinary tract infections, *Am Fam Physician* 72(3):451–456, 2005.

Painful bladder syndrome/interstitial cystitis

Painful bladder syndrome/interstitial cystitis (PBS/IC) is a condition that includes nonbacterial infectious cystitis (viral, mycobacterial, chlamydial, fungal), noninfectious cystitis (radiation, chemical, autoimmune, hypersensitivity), and interstitial cystitis. It occurs most commonly in women ages 20 to 30 years who have symptoms of cystitis, such as frequency, urgency, dysuria and, nocturia, but with negative urine cultures and no other known etiology. Nonbacterial infectious cystitis is most common among those who are immunocompromised. Noninfectious cystitis is associated with radiation or chemotherapy treatment for pelvic and urogenital cancers.

Interstitial cystitis (IC) is a persistent and chronic form of "nonbacterial" cystitis. The cause is not known, but an autoimmune reaction may be responsible for the inflammatory response, which includes mast cell activation, altered epithelial permeability, and increased sensory nerve sensitivity. The inflammation is associated with a derangement of the bladder mucosa that makes it more susceptible to penetration by bacteria. Inflammation and fibrosis of the bladder wall are accompanied by the presence of hemorrhagic ulcers (Hunner ulcers), and bladder volume may decrease as a result of fibrosis. More recently, the identification of antiproliferative factor (APF), a protein expressed by the bladder uroepithelium in those with IC, is important. APF appears to block the normal growth of cells that line the inside wall of the bladder and indirectly increases bladder sensation.[36] Characteristic symptoms of IC include bladder fullness, frequency (including nocturia), small urine volume, and chronic pelvic pain with symptoms lasting longer than 9 months. Diagnosis of IC requires the exclusion of other diagnoses, and extensive evaluations are completed.[37] No single treatment is effective, and different approaches are used for symptom relief.[38]

Acute pyelonephritis

Pyelonephritis is an infection of the renal pelvis and interstitium. Common causes are summarized in Table 29-5. Urinary obstruction and reflux of urine from the bladder (vesicoureteral reflux) are the most common underlying risk factors. One or both kidneys may be involved. Most cases occur in women. The responsible microorganism is usually *E. coli, Proteus,* or *Pseudomonas.* The latter two microorganisms are more commonly associated with infections after urethral instrumentation or urinary tract surgery. These microorganisms also split urea into ammonia, making alkaline urine that increases the risk of stone formation.

PATHOPHYSIOLOGY The infection is probably spread by ascending microorganisms along the ureters, but spread also may occur by way of the bloodstream. The inflammatory process is usually focal and irregular, primarily affecting the pelvis, calyces, and medulla. The infection causes medullary infiltration of white blood cells with renal inflammation, renal edema, and purulent urine. In severe infections, localized abscesses may form in the medulla and extend to the cortex. Primarily affected are the tubules; the glomeruli usually are spared. Necrosis of renal papillae can develop. After the acute phase, healing occurs with deposition of scar tissue and atrophy of affected tubules (Figure 29-5). The number of bacteria decreases until the urine again becomes sterile. Acute pyelonephritis rarely causes renal failure.[39]

CLINICAL MANIFESTATIONS The onset of symptoms is usually acute, with fever, chills, and flank or groin pain. Symptoms characteristic of a UTI, including frequency, dysuria, and costovertebral tenderness, may precede systemic signs and symptoms. Children and older adults may have nonspecific symptoms, such as fever and malaise.

EVALUATION AND TREATMENT Differentiating symptoms of cystitis from those of pyelonephritis by clinical assessment alone is difficult. The specific diagnosis is established by urine culture, urinalysis, and clinical signs and symptoms. White blood cell casts indicate pyelonephritis, but they are not always present in the urine. Complicated pyelonephritis requires blood cultures and urinary tract imaging.[40]

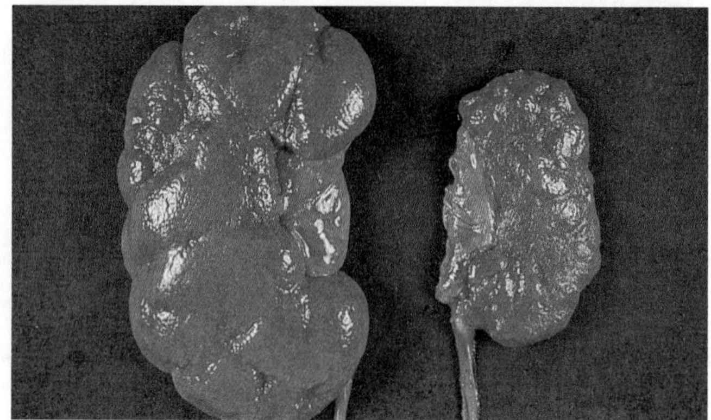

Figure 29-5 ■ **Pyelonephritis.** *Right:* Small, shrunken, irregularly scarred kidney of an individual with chronic pyelonephritis. *Left:* Kidney is of normal size but also shows scarring on the upper pole. (From Damjanov I: *Pathology for the health professions,* ed 3, St Louis, 2006, Saunders.)

TABLE 29-5
Common Causes of Pyelonephritis

Predisposing Factor	Pathologic Mechanisms
Kidney stones	Obstruction and stasis of urine contributing to bacteriuria and hydronephrosis; irritation of epithelial lining with entrapment of bacteria
Vesicoureteral reflux	Chronic reflux of urine up the ureter and into kidney during micturition, contributing to bacterial infection
Pregnancy	Dilation and relaxation of ureter with hydroureter and hydronephrosis; partly caused by obstruction from enlarged uterus and partly from ureteral relaxation caused by higher progesterone levels
Neurogenic bladder	Neurologic impairment interfering with normal bladder contraction with residual urine and ascending infection
Instrumentation	Introduction of organisms into urethra and bladder by catheters and endoscopes introduced into the urinary tract for diagnostic purposes
Female sexual trauma	Movement of organisms from the urethra into the bladder with infection and retrograde spread to kidney

Uncomplicated acute pyelonephritis responds well to 2 to 3 weeks of microorganism-specific antibiotic therapy. Follow-up urine cultures are obtained at 1 and 4 weeks after treatment if symptoms recur. Antibiotic-resistant microorganisms or reinfection may occur in cases of urinary tract obstruction or reflux. Intravenous pyelography and voiding cystourethrography identify surgically correctable lesions.

Chronic pyelonephritis

Chronic pyelonephritis is a persistent or recurrent infection of the kidney leading to scarring of the kidney. One or both kidneys may be involved. The specific cause of chronic pyelonephritis is difficult to determine. Recurrent infections from acute pyelonephritis may be associated with chronic pyelonephritis. Generally, chronic pyelonephritis is more likely to occur in patients who have renal infections associated with some type of obstructive pathologic condition, such as renal stones and vesicoureteral reflux.

PATHOPHYSIOLOGY Chronic urinary tract obstruction starts a process of progressive inflammation, altered renal pelvis and calyces, destruction of the tubules, atrophy or dilation and diffuse scarring, and finally impaired urine-concentrating ability, leading to chronic renal failure.

The lesions of chronic pyelonephritis are sometimes termed *chronic interstitial nephritis* because the inflammation and fibrosis are located in the interstitial spaces between the tubules (see Figure 29-5). Causes other than chronic pyelonephritis include drug toxicity from analgesics such as phenacetin, aspirin, and acetaminophen; ischemia; irradiation; and immune-complex diseases.

CLINICAL MANIFESTATIONS The early symptoms of chronic pyelonephritis are often minimal and may include hypertension, frequency, dysuria, and flank pain. Progression leads to renal failure.

EVALUATION AND TREATMENT Urinalysis, intravenous pyelography, and ultrasound are used diagnostically. Treatment is related to the underlying cause. Obstruction must be relieved. Antibiotics may be given, with prolonged antibiotic therapy for recurrent infection.

QUICK CHECK 29-2

1. Why is cystitis more common in women?
2. What is interstitial cystitis?
3. How does pyelonephritis differ from cystitis?

GLOMERULAR DISORDERS

The onset of glomerular disease may be sudden or insidious. Damage to the glomerulus is the result of inflammatory processes initiated by immune responses, metabolic disorders, or circulatory disturbances. Most glomerular diseases are the result of immune dysregulation mediated by type II (cell lysis) or type III (immune complex deposition) hypersensitivity reactions (see Chapter 7). Damage to the glomerulus results in changes in GFR and capillary wall structure, with proteinuria and hematuria.[41] Severe glomerular disease is usually associated with diffuse lesions and may cause oliguria, hypertension, and renal failure. Focal lesions tend to produce less severe clinical symptoms.

Different types of glomerular disease may be associated with patterns of urinary sediment. Urine in diseases associated with **nephrotic sediment** contains massive amounts of protein and lipids and either a microscopic amount of blood or no blood. Urine in diseases associated with **nephritic sediment** is characterized by the presence of blood in the urine with red cell casts, white cell casts, and varying degrees of protein, which usually is not severe. The sediment of chronic glomerular disease has waxy casts, granular casts, and less protein and blood than does nephrotic or nephritic sediment.

Glomerular damage reduces glomerular membrane surface area, glomerular capillary blood flow, and driving hydrostatic pressure. Injury to the glomeruli causes various signs and symptoms as a result of changes in capillary wall structure and GFR. Proteinuria is caused by increased permeability of glomerular capillaries and loss of electrical negative charge. The loss of negative charge allows the escape of plasma proteins, which are normally repelled because they also have a negative charge. Hematuria results from increased glomerular permeability or bleeding along the nephron.

Reduced GFR during glomerular disease is evidenced by elevated plasma urea, cystatin C and creatinine concentration or reduced creatinine clearance (see Chapter 28). Edema, caused by excessive sodium and water retention, may require the use of diuretics or dialysis. The volume expansion that accompanies salt and water retention leads to hypertension. During the first few weeks, the major life-threatening problems are acute renal insufficiency with fluid, electrolyte, and acid-base imbalances; acute hypertension that may cause hypertensive encephalopathy; circulatory failure; and pulmonary edema.

Glomerulonephritis

Glomerulonephritis is an inflammation of the glomerulus caused by numerous factors, including immunologic abnormalities, ischemia, free radicals, drugs, toxins, vascular disorders, and systemic diseases, including diabetes mellitus and lupus erythematosus. Glomerular disease is the most common cause of chronic and end-stage renal failure.[42]

Types of glomerulonephritis

The classification of glomerulonephritis can be described according to cause, pathologic lesions (Table 29-6), disease progression (acute, rapidly progressive, chronic), or clinical presentation (nephrotic syndrome, nephritic syndrome, acute or chronic renal failure). Features of types of glomerulonephritis are summarized in Table 29-7. In nearly all types of glomerulonephritis, the epithelial or podocyte layer

TABLE 29-6

Types of Glomerular Lesions

Lesion	Characteristics
GLOMERULAR LESIONS	
Diffuse	Relatively uniform involvement of most or all glomeruli; most common form of glomerulonephritis
Focal	Changes in only some glomeruli, whereas others are normal
Segmental-local	Changes in one part of the glomerulus with other parts unaffected
LESION CHARACTERISTICS	
Mesangial	Deposits of immunoglobulins in the mesangial matrix, mesangial cell proliferation
Membranous	Thickening of the glomerular capillary wall with immune deposits
Proliferative	Increase in the number of glomerular cells
Sclerotic	Glomerular scarring from previous glomerular injury
Crescentic	Accumulation of proliferating cells within Bowman space, making the appearance of a crescent

TABLE 29-7

Features of the Common Types of Glomerulonephritis

Type and Cause	Pathophysiology
Acute glomerulonephritis Group A β-hemolytic streptococcus	Diffuse deposits of immune complexes in glomerular capillary wall and infiltration of inflammatory cells with decreased capillary blood flow and GFR
Rapidly progressive or crescentic Nonspecific response to glomerular injury; can occur in any severe glomerular disease	Accumulation of immune deposits and inflammatory cells and debris that proliferate into Bowman space and form crescent-shaped lesions that decrease capillary blood flow and glomerular filtration Formation of antiglomerular membrane antibodies, which can damage the glomerulus, leading to renal failure
Membranoproliferative Usually idiopathic; associated with low complement levels	Activation of inflammatory processes that cause thickening of glomerular basement membrane, reduce glomerular blood flow and GFR
Mesangial proliferative Usually associated with IgA nephropathy	Deposits of immune complexes in the mesangium with mesangial proliferation; results in decreased glomerular blood flow
IgA nephropathy (Berger disease) Usually idiopathic; elevated IgA plasma levels	Deposits of IgA and proliferation of inflammatory cells into Bowman space with sclerosis and fibrosis of glomerulus and decreased GFR
Minimal change disease (lipoid nephrosis) Usually idiopathic No immune deposits	Disruption of capillary filtration membrane and loss of negative charge, which cause increased permeability, loss of protein, and nephrotic syndrome
Focal segmented glomerulosclerosis Usually idiopathic	Similar to minimal change disease
Membranous nephropathy Usually idiopathic; can be associated with systemic diseases, (i.e., hepatitis B virus, systemic lupus erythematous, solid malignant tumors)	Thickening of glomerular capillary wall caused by inflammatory process with increased permeability, proteinuria, and nephrotic syndrome IgG depository on epithelium of glomerular basement membrane

of the glomerular capillary membrane is disturbed with loss of negative charges and changes in membrane permeability; the mesangial matrix may be expanded or the basement membrane thickened.

Acute glomerulonephritis

Acute glomerulonephritis often is associated with a streptococcal infection (acute poststreptococcal glomerulonephritis). The disease begins abruptly and usually occurs 7 to 10 days after a streptococcal infection of the skin (impetigo) or of the throat (pharyngitis) and commonly affects children (see Chapter 30). Sporadic occurrences have been observed after bacterial endocarditis, which may be associated with streptococcal or staphylococcal microorganisms, or after viral diseases such as varicella and hepatitis B and C. Glomerular injury is immune mediated with streptococcal antigen-antibody complexes depositing in the glomerular basement membrane (GBM). The antigen-antibody complex activates complement and the release of inflammatory mediators that damage endothelial and epithelial cells lying on the basement membrane.[43]

Symptoms usually occur 10 to 21 days after infection and include hematuria, red blood cell casts, proteinuria, decreased GFR, oliguria, hypertension, edema around the eyes or feet and ankles, and, occasionally, ascites or pleural effusions. Immunofluorescent findings from renal biopsy indicate immune complex deposits in the glomerulus, with diffuse mesangial cell and capillary endothelial cell proliferation. The thickened glomerular membrane contributes to the decreased GFR. More severe renal disease is observed after a prolonged infection and before antibiotic therapy. Most individuals, especially children, recover without significant loss of renal function or recurrence of the disease.

Rapidly progressive glomerulonephritis

Rapidly progressive glomerulonephritis (RPGN) is also known as subacute, crescentic, or extracapillary glomerulonephritis. The disease develops over a period of days to weeks. The disease affects primarily adults in their 50s and 60s and may be idiopathic or associated with a proliferative glomerular disease (with diffuse proliferation of extracapillary cells), such as poststreptococcal glomerulonephritis and antineutrophil cytoplasmic antibodies.[44] By the time RPGN is diagnosed, renal insufficiency is apparent. There is extensive proliferation of cells into the Bowman space with crescent formation. Typically, the glomerular injury is accompanied by a rapid decline in glomerular function, progressing to renal failure in a few weeks or months.[45] Hematuria is common and may or may not be accompanied by proteinuria, edema, or hypertension.

Antiglomerular basement membrane disease (Goodpasture syndrome) is a type of RPGN. The disease is rare and associated with antibody formation against both pulmonary capillary and glomerular basement membranes, with activation of complement and neutrophils that damage the GBM. The disease occurs most often in men 20 to 30 years of age, often accompanied by pulmonary hemorrhage and renal failure.

RPGN has a relatively poor prognosis if not diagnosed and treated early. Anticoagulants may be of some benefit in reducing the fibrin component of crescent formation. Plasmapheresis is usually combined with steroids and immunosuppression therapy, including plasma exchange. Dialysis or transplantation is required when failure is irreversible.[46]

Chronic glomerulonephritis

Chronic glomerulonephritis encompasses several glomerular diseases with a progressive course leading to chronic renal failure. There may be no history of renal disease before the diagnosis. Hypercholesterolemia and proteinuria have been associated with progressive glomerular and tubular injury. The proposed mechanism is related to glomerulosclerosis and interstitial injury.[47] The primary cause may be difficult to establish because advanced pathologic changes may obscure specific disease characteristics (Figure 29-6). Diabetes mellitus and lupus erythematosus are secondary causes of chronic glomerular injury.[48]

PATHOPHYSIOLOGY Two types of immune mechanisms commonly contribute to glomerular injury: (1) deposition of circulating soluble antigen-antibody complexes, often with complement components, and (2) formation of antibodies specific for the glomerular basement membrane (anti-GBM antibodies). The severity of glomerular damage and renal insufficiency is related to the size, number, location (focal or diffuse), duration of exposure, and type of antigen-antibody complexes.

Activation of biochemical mediators of inflammation (complement, leukocytes, fibrin) begins after the antibody or antigen-antibody complexes have localized in the glomerular capillary wall. Complement is deposited with the antibodies, and its activation can cause cell lysis or serve as a chemotactic stimulus for attraction of leukocytes.[49] The phagocytes further the inflammatory reaction by releasing lysosomal enzymes, reactive oxygen species, and cytokines, which damage glomerular cell walls and contribute to proliferation of the extracellular matrix causing a decrease in glomerular blood flow and GFR.[50]

The inflammatory processes also alter membrane permeability and may cause loss of the negative electrical charge across the glomerular filtration membrane, enhancing filtration of proteins. Membrane damage can lead to platelet aggregation and degranulation, whereby platelets release substances that increase glomerular permeability, permitting the passage of protein molecules or red blood cells into the urine and causing proteinuria or hematuria. The coagulation system also may be activated and lead to fibrin deposition in Bowman space, contributing to crescent formation (deposition of substances in the Bowman space forming the shape of a crescent moon). Renal blood flow decreases, and glomerular filtration is reduced.

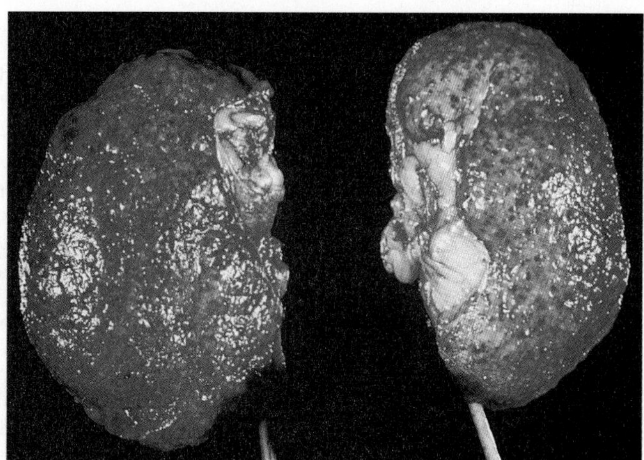

Figure 29-6 ■ **Chronic Glomerulonephritis.** The kidneys appear small, are uniformly shrunken, and have a finely granular external surface (From Damjanov I: *Pathology for the health professions*, ed 3, St Louis, 2006, Saunders.)

CLINICAL MANIFESTATIONS Injury to the glomeruli causes various signs and symptoms consequent to changes in glomerular capillary wall structure and GFR. Two major changes distinctive of more severe glomerulonephritis are (1) hematuria with red blood cell casts and (2) proteinuria exceeding 3 to 5 g/day with albumin as the major protein. Gross proteinuria is associated with nephrotic syndrome; a decrease in urine output accompanies a decreased GFR (see Chapter 28).

Several disorders may produce hematuria, because bleeding can occur anywhere along the urinary tract. The characteristics of hematuria from red blood cells escaping through the glomerular membrane include a smoky brown–tinged urine, red blood cell casts, and an accompanying proteinuria. Bleeding from sites lower in the urinary tract may produce a pink- or red-colored urine. Glomerular bleeding provides prolonged contact with the acidic urine and transforms hemoglobin to methemoglobin, which has a brownish color and no blood clots. The history and physical examination may disclose findings that differentiate glomerular disease from another source of urinary tract bleeding.

The immune-mediated inflammatory response with cellular infiltration decreases GFR, which leads to fluid retention. Salt and water are also reabsorbed, contributing to fluid volume expansion, edema, and hypertension.

After 10 to 20 years, renal insufficiency usually begins to develop, followed by nephrotic syndrome and an accelerated progression to end-stage renal failure. Symptom patterns vary depending on the underlying cause. Steroids usually do not change the course of chronic glomerular disease, and dialysis or kidney transplantation ultimately may be needed.

EVALUATION AND TREATMENT The diagnosis of glomerular disease is confirmed by the progressive development of clinical manifestations and laboratory findings of abnormal urinalysis with proteinuria, red blood cells, white blood cells, and casts. Microscopic evaluation from renal biopsy provides a specific determination of renal injury and type of pathologic condition.

Patterns of antigen-antibody complex deposition within the glomerular capillary filtration membrane have been established using light, electron, and immunofluorescent microscopy for different disease processes. The findings on light microscopy provide information about the distribution and extent of immune response injury (Table 29-8). Electron microscopy differentiates morphologic changes within the glomerular capillary wall. Staining with fluorescein identifies different antibodies (i.e., immunoglobulin G [IgG] or immunoglobulin A [IgA]) and their configurations when viewed under ultraviolet (black) light with a microscope.

Management principles for treating glomerulonephritis are related to treating the primary disease, preventing or minimizing immune responses, and correcting accompanying problems, such as edema, hypertension, and hyperlipidemia. Specific treatment regimens are necessary for particular types of glomerulonephritis. Antibiotic therapy is essential for the management of underlying infections that may be contributing to ongoing antigen-antibody responses. Corticosteroids decrease antibody synthesis and suppress inflammatory responses. Cytotoxic agents (i.e., cyclophosphamide) may be used to suppress the immune response. Anticoagulants may be useful for controlling fibrin crescent formation in RPGN.

Nephrotic Syndrome

Nephrotic syndrome is the excretion of 3.5 g or more of protein in the urine per day and is characteristic of glomerular injury. Lipoid nephrosis (minimal change disease), membranous glomerulonephritis, and focal glomerulosclerosis are directly related to nephrotic syndrome, although these

TABLE 29-8

Immunologic Pathogenesis of Glomerulonephritis

Glomerular Injury	Mechanism
Soluble immune-complex glomerulonephritis (90%)	Formation of antibodies stimulated by the presence of endogenous or exogenous antigens results in circulating soluble antigen-antibody complexes, which are deposited in glomerular capillaries; glomerular injury occurring with complement activation and release of immunologic substances that lyse cells and increase membrane permeability; severity of glomerular injury related to the number of complexes formed; a type III hypersensitivity
Antiglomerular basement membrane glomerulonephritis (5%)	Antibodies are formed and act directly against the glomerular basement membrane; immune response causes accumulation of inflammatory cells in the Bowman space (in the shape of a crescent moon) surrounding and compressing the glomerular capillaries; generally associated with rapidly progressive renal failure, such as Goodpasture syndrome; a type II hypersensitivity
Alternative complement pathway	A relatively obscure mechanism associated with low levels of complement and membranoproliferative glomerulonephritis; a type III hypersensitivity
Cell-mediated immunity	A delayed hypersensitivity response that damages the glomerulus; actual cellular mechanism not clearly understood; a type IV hypersensitivity

conditions can occur with other types of glomerular disease.[51] Nephrotic syndrome is more common in children than adults (see Chapter 30).

Secondary forms of nephrotic syndrome occur in systemic diseases, including diabetes mellitus, amyloidosis, systemic lupus erythematosus, and Henoch-Schönlein purpura. Nephrotic syndrome is also seen with certain drugs, infections, malignancies, and vascular disorders. When present as a secondary complication with renal diseases, nephrotic syndrome often signifies a more serious prognosis.

PATHOPHYSIOLOGY Disturbances in the glomerular basement membrane leads to increased permeability to protein and loss of electrical negative charge. Loss of plasma proteins, particularly albumin and some immunoglobulins, occurs across the injured glomerular filtration membrane.[51] Hypoalbuminemia results from urinary loss of albumin combined with a diminished synthesis of replacement albumin by the liver. Albumin is lost in the greatest quantity because of its high plasma concentration and low molecular weight. Decreased dietary intake of protein from anorexia or malnutrition or accompanying liver disease may also contribute to lower levels of plasma albumin. Loss of albumin stimulates lipoprotein synthesis by the liver and hyperlipidemia. Loss of immunoglobulins may increase susceptibility to infections.

CLINICAL MANIFESTATIONS Many clinical manifestations of nephrotic syndrome are related to loss of serum proteins (see Table 29-9). They include edema, hyperlipidemia, lipiduria, and vitamin D deficiency.[51,52] Vitamin D deficiency is related to loss of serum transport proteins and decreased vitamin D activation by the kidney. Alterations in coagulation factors cause hypercoagulability and may lead to thromboembolic events.[53]

EVALUATION AND TREATMENT Nephrotic syndrome is diagnosed when the protein level in a 24-hour urine collection is greater than 3.5 g. Serum albumin decreases (to less than 3 g/dl), and serum cholesterol, phospholipids, and triglycerides increase. Fat bodies may be present in the urine. The specific pathologic condition is identified by renal biopsy.

Nephrotic syndrome is commonly treated with a normal-protein (i.e., 1 g/kg body weight/day), low-fat diet, salt restriction, diuretics, immunosuppression, and heparinoids. When diuretics are used, care must be taken to observe for hypovolemia and hypokalemia or potassium toxicity in the presence of renal insufficiency. Aldactone may be combined with loop diuretics to suppress aldosterone activity to conserve potassium. Steroids may be particularly effective for the initial treatment of nephrotic syndrome in children.[54]

QUICK CHECK 29-3

1. What is glomerulonephritis? List two types.
2. What immune mechanisms are operative in glomerulonephritis?
3. What causes nephrotic syndrome?

RENAL FAILURE

Types of Renal Failure

Acute renal failure

Acute renal failure (ARF) occurs rapidly over a period of days or weeks with a reduction in glomerular filtration rate (GFR) and elevation of blood urea nitrogen (BUN), plasma creatinine and cystatin C levels. It is usually associated with oliguria (urine output of less than 30 ml/hr or less than 400 ml/day), although urine output may be normal or increased. Fluid is still filtered at the glomerulus but there is an alteration in tubular secretion or reabsorption. Most types of acute renal failure are reversible if diagnosed and treated early. Acute renal failure can be classified as prerenal, intrarenal, or postrenal (obstructive) (Table 29-10).[55]

TABLE 29-9
Clinical Manifestations of Nephrotic Syndrome

Manifestation	Contributing Factors	Result
Proteinuria	Increased glomerular permeability, decreased proximal tubule reabsorption	Edema, increased susceptibility to infection from loss of immunoglobulins
Hypoalbuminemia	Increased urinary losses of protein	Edema
Edema	Hypoalbuminemia (decreased plasma oncotic pressure, sodium and water retention, increased aldosterone and antidiuretic hormone [ADH] secretion), unresponsiveness to atrial natriuretic peptides	Soft, pitting, generalized edema
Hyperlipidemia	Decreased serum albumin; increased hepatic synthesis of very low-density lipoproteins; increased cholesterol, phospholipids, triglycerides	Increased atherogenesis
Lipiduria	Sloughing of tubular cells containing fat (oval fat bodies); free fat from hyperlipidemia	Fat droplets that may float in urine

TABLE 29-10

Classification of Acute Renal Failure

Area of Dysfunction	Possible Causes
Prerenal	Hypovolemia Hemorrhagic blood loss (trauma, gastrointestinal bleeding, complications of childbirth) Loss of plasma volume (burns, peritonitis) Water and electrolyte losses (severe vomiting or diarrhea, intestinal obstruction, uncontrolled diabetes mellitus, inappropriate use of diuretics) Hypotension or hypoperfusion Septic shock Cardiac failure or shock Massive pulmonary embolism Stenosis or clamping of renal artery
Intrarenal	Acute tubular necrosis (postischemic or nephrotoxic) Glomerulopathies Acute interstitial necrosis (tumors or toxins) Vascular damage Malignant hypertension, vasculitis Coagulation defects Renal artery/vein occlusion Bilateral acute pyelonephritis
Postrenal	Obstructive uropathies (usually bilateral) Ureteral destruction (edema, tumors, stones, clots) Bladder neck obstruction (enlarged prostate) Neurogenic bladder

PATHOPHYSIOLOGY **Prerenal acute renal failure** is the most common cause of ARF and is caused by impaired renal blood flow. The GFR declines because of the decrease in filtration pressure. Poor perfusion can result from renal vasoconstriction, hypotension, hypovolemia, hemorrhage, or inadequate cardiac output. Acute prerenal failure may occur when chronic renal failure exists if a sudden stress is imposed on already marginally functioning kidneys. Failure to restore blood volume or blood pressure and oxygen delivery cause cell injury and acute tubular necrosis or acute interstitial necrosis.

Intrarenal acute renal failure usually results from **acute tubular necrosis (ATN).** ATN caused by ischemia occurs most often after surgery (40% to 50% of cases) but is also associated with sepsis, obstetric complications, severe trauma, including severe burns, and nephrotoxins (radiocontrast media and some antimicrobials). Hypotension associated with hypovolemia produces ischemia, generating toxic oxygen-free radicals that cause cell swelling, injury, and necrosis.[56] Dehydration, advanced age, concurrent renal insufficiency, and diabetes mellitus tend to enhance nephrotoxicity from either antibiotics or radiocontrast media. Aminoglycosides (neomycin, gentamicin, tobramycin) and other antibiotics tend to accumulate in the renal cortex and may not cause renal failure until after treatment is complete. Other substances, such as excessive myoglobin (oxygen-transporting substance from muscles), carbon tetrachloride, heavy metals (mercury, arsenic), or methoxyflurane anesthetic, and bacterial toxins may promote renal failure. Necrosis caused by nephrotoxins is usually uniform and limited to the proximal tubules. Ischemic necrosis tends to be patchy and may be distributed along any part of the nephron.

Three pathophysiologic explanations have been proposed to account for the oliguria of ATN.[55,57] All three mechanisms probably contribute to oliguria in varying combinations and degrees throughout the course of the disease (Figure 29-7). These theories[58] are as follows:

1. *Tubular obstruction theory.* Necrosis of the tubules causes sloughing of cells, cast formation, or ischemic edema that results in tubular obstruction, which in turn causes a retrograde increase in pressure and reduces the GFR. Renal failure can occur within 24 hours.
2. *Back leak theory.* Glomerular filtration remains normal, but tubular reabsorption of filtrate is accelerated as a result of permeability caused by ischemia.
3. *Alterations in renal blood flow.* Afferent arteriolar vasoconstriction may be produced by intrarenal release of angiotensin II or by redistribution of blood flow from the cortex to the medulla. Autoregulation of blood flow may be impaired, resulting in decreased GFR. Changes in glomerular permeability and decreased GFR may also result from the ischemia.

Postrenal acute renal failure usually occurs with urinary tract obstruction that affects the kidneys bilaterally (e.g., bladder outlet obstruction, prostatic hypertrophy, bilateral ureteral obstruction) or neurogenic bladder. A pattern of several hours of anuria with flank pain followed by polyuria is a characteristic finding. This type of renal failure can occur after diagnostic catheterization of the ureters, a procedure that may cause edema of the tubular lumen.

CLINICAL MANIFESTATIONS The clinical progression of acute renal failure with recovery of renal function occurs in three phases: oliguria, diuresis, and recovery. *Oliguria* begins within 1 day after a hypotensive event and lasts 1 to 3 weeks, but it may regress in several hours or extend for several weeks, depending on the duration of ischemia or severity of injury or obstruction. Renal failure can present with nonoliguria, particularly with intrinsic renal failure associated with nephrotoxins. The urine output may vary in volume, but the BUN and plasma creatinine concentrations increase (plasma creatinine is inversely proportional to the GFR). Other early manifestations depend on the underlying cause of renal failure.

As renal function improves, increase in urine volume (diuresis) is progressive. During the early *diuretic phase*, the tubules are still damaged and recovering their function. Fluid and electrolyte balance must be carefully monitored and excessive urinary losses replaced.

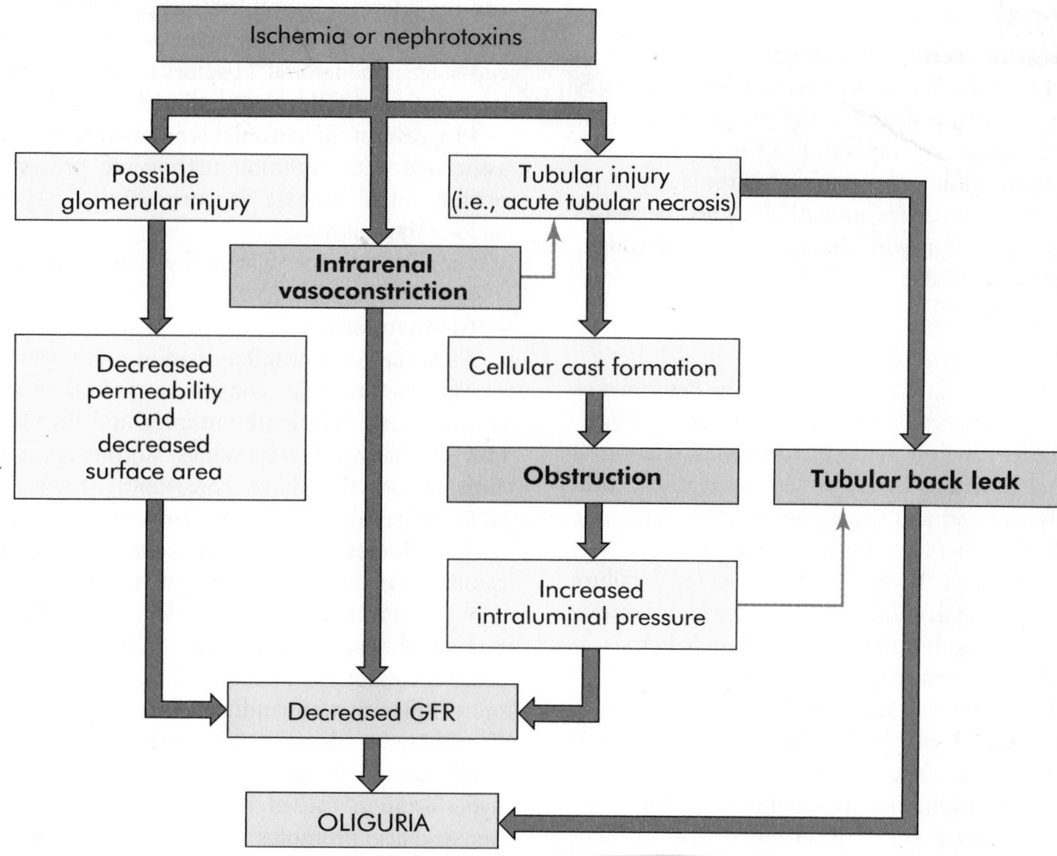

Figure 29-7 ■ **Mechanisms of Oliguria in Acute Renal Failure.** *GFR,* Glomerular filtration rate.

Serial measurements of plasma creatinine provide an index of renal function during the *recovery phase.* Return to normal status may take from 3 to 12 months, and some individuals do not have full recovery of a normal GFR or tubular function.

EVALUATION AND TREATMENT The diagnosis of acute renal failure is related to the cause of the disease. A history of surgery, trauma, or cardiovascular disorders is common, and exposure to nephrotoxins must be considered. Obstructive uropathies (i.e., an enlarged prostate) also need consideration. The diagnostic challenge is to differentiate prerenal acute renal failure from intrarenal acute renal failure, and some evidence is available from urinalysis, plasma creatinine, and BUN (Table 29-11). Prevention of acute renal failure is a major treatment factor and involves maintenance of fluid volume before and after surgery or diagnostic procedures and use of vasoactive drugs or diuretics.[59]

The primary goal of therapy is to maintain the individual's life until renal function has been recovered. Management principles directly related to physiologic alterations generally include (1) correcting fluid and electrolyte disturbances, (2) treating infections, (3) maintaining nutrition, and (4) remembering that drugs or their metabolites are not excreted. Renal replacement therapy may be indicated. The mortality rate is greater than 30%[60] and is associated with the underlying cause of renal failure.

TABLE 29-11
Differentiation of Acute Oliguric Renal Failure

	Urine Volume	Urine Specific Gravity	Urine Osmolality	Urine Sodium	BUN/Plasma Creatinine	FE_{Na}*
Prerenal failure	<400 ml	1.016–1.020	>500 mOsm	<10 mEq/L	>15:1	<1% (also seen in acute glomerulonephritis)
Intrarenal failure (i.e., acute tubular necrosis)	<400 ml	1.010–1.012	<400 mOsm	>30 mEq/L	<15:1	>1% (also seen in acute urinary tract obstruction and renal parenchymal disease)

$$*FE_{Na} = \frac{\text{Urine Na/plasma Na}}{\text{Urine creatinine/plasma creatinine}} = \times 100$$

Chronic renal failure

Chronic renal failure (CRF) is the progressive loss of renal function over a period of months or years. CRF develops as a complication of systemic diseases, such as hypertension or diabetes mellitus, or as a complication of many renal diseases (i.e., chronic glomerulonephritis, chronic pyelonephritis, or chronic obstructive uropathies). CRF decreases GFR and tubular functions with changes manifest throughout all organ systems (Table 29-12).[61]

Stages of chronic renal failure

Stages of chronic renal failure can generally be described as chronic renal insufficiency, chronic renal failure, and end-stage renal failure. **Chronic renal insufficiency** refers to a decline in renal function. Levels of serum creatinine and urea are mildly elevated and usually there are no systemic symptoms. CRF is a significant loss of renal function with systemic manifestations. Progressive chronic renal failure leads to **end-stage renal failure (ESRF)** in which there is less than 10% of remaining renal function and dialysis or kidney transplant is required to sustain life. Table 29-13 summarizes the progressive stages of CRF as a measure of declining glomerular filtration rate. **Azotemia** is increased serum urea levels and, often, increased creatinine levels as well. Chronic renal insufficiency or renal failure causes azotemia. Uremia is a *syndrome* of renal failure and includes elevated blood urea and creatinine levels accompanied by fatigue, anorexia, nausea, vomiting, pruritus, and neurologic changes. Uremia represents the numerous consequences related to renal failure, including retention of toxic wastes, deficiency states, and electrolyte disorders. Both azotemia and uremia indicate an accumulation of nitrogenous waste products in the blood.

PATHOPHYSIOLOGY The kidneys have a remarkable ability to adapt to loss of nephron mass.[62] Symptomatic changes resulting from increased creatinine, urea, potassium, and alterations in salt and water balance usually do not become apparent until renal function declines to less than 25% of normal when adaptive renal reserves have been exhausted.

The *intact nephron hypothesis* proposes that loss of nephron mass with progressive kidney damage causes the surviving nephrons to sustain normal kidney function. These nephrons are capable of a compensatory hypertrophy and expansion or hyperfunction in their rates of filtration, reabsorption, and secretion and can maintain a constant rate of excretion in the presence of overall declining GFR. The intact nephron hypothesis explains adaptive changes in solute and water regulation that occur with advancing renal failure. Although the urine of an individual with chronic renal failure may contain abnormal amounts of protein and red and white blood cells or casts, the major end products of excretion are similar to those of normally functioning kidneys until the advanced stages of renal failure when there is a significant reduction of functioning nephrons.[63,64] The continued loss of functioning nephrons and the adaptive hyperfiltration probably results in further nephron injury and ultimately results in uremia and end-stage renal failure.[64] Factors involved in the pathophysiology of renal failure are outlined in Table 29-14.

Progression of chronic renal failure is thought to be associated with common pathogenic processes regardless of the initial disease (Figure 29-8).[65] These processes include the following:

- Glomerular hypertension, hyperfiltration, and hypertrophy
- Glomerulosclerosis
- Tubulointerstitial inflammation and fibrosis

The factors that contribute to the pathogenesis of chronic renal failure are complex and involve the interaction of many cells, cytokines, and structural alterations. Two factors that have consistently been recognized to advance renal disease are proteinuria and angiotensin II.[66–69] Glomerular hyperfiltraion and increased glomerular capillary permeability lead to proteinuria. **Proteinuria** contributes to tubulointerstitial injury by accumulating in the interstitial space and activating complement proteins and other mediators and cells, such as macrophages, that promote inflammation and progressive fibrosis. Angiotensin II activity is elevated with progressive nephron injury. **Angiotensin II** promotes glomerular hypertension and hyperfiltration caused by efferent arteriolar vasoconstriction and also promotes systemic hypertension. The chronically high intraglomerular pressure increases glomerular capillary permeability contributing to proteinuria. Angiotensin II also may promote the activity of inflammatory cells and growth factors that participate in tubulointerstitial fibrosis and scarring.

CLINICAL MANIFESTATIONS The clinical manifestations of chronic renal failure are often described using the term *uremia.* **Uremia** refers to the accumulation of nitrogenous wastes from protein metabolism as well as the systemic symptoms caused by decline in renal function with the accumulation of toxins in the plasma. Sources of toxins include end products of protein metabolism, alterations in electrolytes, metabolic acidosis, and intestinal absorption of toxins produced by gut bacteria. Uremia represents a proinflammatory state with many systemic effects.[70] Generally, the symptoms include hypertension, anorexia, nausea, vomiting, diarrhea, weight loss, pruritus, edema, anemia, and neurologic and skeletal changes. The many systemic manifestations associated with chronic renal failure are summarized in Table 29-12 and discussed next.

Creatinine and urea clearance

Creatinine is constantly released from muscle and excreted primarily by glomerular filtration. In chronic renal failure (CRF), as glomerular filtration rate (GFR) declines, the plasma creatinine level increases by a reciprocal amount to maintain a constant rate of excretion. As GFR continues to decline, plasma creatinine concentration increases. The clearance of *urea* follows a similar pattern, but urea is both filtered and reabsorbed and varies with the state of hydration.

TABLE 29-12
Systemic Effects of Uremia

System	Manifestations	Mechanisms	Treatment
Skeletal	Spontaneous fractures and bone pain Deformities of long bones	Osteitis fibrosa: bone inflammation with fibrous degeneration related to hyperparathyroidism Osteomalacia: bone resorption associated with vitamin D and calcium deficiency	Control of hyperphosphatemia to reduce hyperparathyroidism; administration of calcium and aluminum hydroxide antacids, which bind phosphate in the gut, together with a phosphate-restricted diet; vitamin D replacement; avoidance of magnesium antacids because of impaired magnesium excretion
Cardiopulmonary	Pulmonary edema, Kussmaul respirations	Fluid overload associated with pulmonary edema and metabolic acidosis leading to Kussmaul respirations	ACE inhibitors; combination of propranolol, hydralazine, and minoxidil for those with high levels of renin; bilateral nephrectomy with dialysis or transplantation
Cardiovascular	Left ventricular hypertrophy, cardiomyopathy, and ischemic heart disease; hypertension, arrhythmias, accelerated atherosclerosis; pericarditis with fever, chest pain, and pericardial friction rub	Extracellular volume expansion and hypersecretion of renin associated with hypertension; anemia increases cardiac workload; hyperlipidemia promotes atherosclerosis; toxins precipitate into pericardium	Volume reduction with diuretics that are not potassium sparing (to avoid hyperkalemia); dialysis
Neurologic	Encephalopathy (fatigue, loss of attention, difficulty with problem solving); peripheral neuropathy (pain and burning in the legs and feet, loss of vibration sense and deep tendon reflexes); loss of motor coordination, twitching, fasciculations, stupor, and coma with advanced uremia	Progressive accumulation of uremic toxins associated with end-stage renal disease Stroke or intracerebral hemorrhage associated with chronic dialysis	Dialysis or successful kidney transplantation
Hematologic	Anemia, usually normochromic normocytic; platelet disorders with prolonged bleeding times	Reduced erythropoietin secretion and reduced red cell production; uremic toxins shorten red blood cell survival and alter platelet function	Dialysis; recombinant human erythropoietin and iron supplementation; conjugated estrogens; DDAVP (1-desamino-8-$_D$-arginine vasopressin); transfusion
Gastrointestinal	Anorexia, nausea, vomiting; mouth ulcers, stomatitis, urinous breath (uremic factor), hiccups, peptic ulcers, gastrointestinal bleeding, and pancreatitis associated with end-stage renal failure	Retention of metabolic acids and other metabolic waste products	Protein-restricted diet for relief of nausea and vomiting
Integumentary	Abnormal pigmentation and pruritus	Retention of urochromes, contributing to sallow, yellow color; high plasma calcium levels and neuropathy associated with pruritus	Dialysis with control of serum calcium levels
Immunologic	Increased risk of infection that can cause death; increased risk of carcinoma	Suppression of cell-mediated immunity; reduction in number and function of lymphocytes, diminished phagocytosis	Routine dialysis
Reproductive	Sexual dysfunction: menorrhagia, amenorrhea, infertility, and decreased libido in women; decreased testosterone levels, infertility, and decreased libido in men	Dysfunction of ovaries and testes; presence of neuropathies	No specific treatment

With data from Keane WF: *Kidney Int Suppl* 75:S27-S31, 2000; Uribarri J: *Semin Dial* 13(4):232–234, 2000.

TABLE 29-13

Stages of Chronic Kidney Disease

Stage	Severity	GFR ml/min	Progression	Symptoms
—	At increased risk	≥60	(Chronic kidney disease risk factors present)	None
1	Kidney damage: normal or increased GFR	≥90	None apparent	None
2	Kidney damage: mild ↓GFR	60–89	Increasing PTH Early bone disease	Subtle
3	Moderate: ↓GFR	30–59	Erythropoietin deficiency, anemia	Mild
4	Severe: ↓GFR	15–29	Increased triglycerides Metabolic acidosis Hyperkalemia Salt/water retention	Moderate
5	End-stage kidney disease; kidney failure	<15	Uremia	Severe

GFR, Glomerular filtration rate; *PTH,* parathyroid hormone.

Adapted from National Kidney Foundation, Clinical Practice Guidelines for Chronic Kidney Disease: *Evaluation, classification, stratification: definition and classification of stages of chronic kidney disease,* 2002; Available at http://www.kidney.org/professionals/kdoqi/guidelines_ckd/p4_class_g1.htm (accessed April, 2007).

TABLE 29-14

Factors Representing Progression of Chronic Renal Failure

Factor	Characteristics
Proteinuria	Glomerular hyperfiltration of protein contributes to tubular interstitial injury by accumulating in the interstitial space and promoting inflammation and progressive fibrosis.
Creatinine and urea clearance	In chronic renal failure, the GFR falls and the plasma creatinine concentration increases by a reciprocal amount; because there is no regulatory adjustment for creatinine, plasma levels continue to rise and serve as an index of changing glomerular function. As GFR declines, urea clearance increases. (NOTE: Urea is both filtered and reabsorbed and varies with the state of hydration.)
Sodium and water balance	In chronic renal failure, sodium load delivered to nephrons exceeds normal, so excretion must increase, thus less is reabsorbed. Obligatory loss occurs, leading to sodium deficits and volume depletion. As GFR is reduced, ability to concentrate and dilute urine diminishes.
Phosphate and calcium balance	Changes in acid-base balance affect phosphate and calcium balance. The major disorders associated with chronic renal failure are reduced renal phosphate excretion, decreased renal synthesis of 1,25-$(OH)_2$ vitamin D_3, and hypocalcemia. Hypocalcemia leads to secondary hyperparathyroidism, GFR falls, and progressive hyperphosphatemia, hypocalcemia, and dissolution of bone result.
Hematocrit	Because of anemia that accompanies chronic renal failure, lethargy, dizziness, and low hematocrit are common.
Potassium balance	In chronic renal failure, tubular secretion of potassium increases until oliguria develops. Use of potassium-sparing diuretics also may precipitate elevated serum potassium levels. As disease progresses, total body potassium levels can rise to life-threatening levels and dialysis is required.
Acid-base balance	In early renal insufficiency, acid excretion and bicarbonate reabsorption are increased to maintain normal pH. Metabolic acidosis begins when GFR reaches 30% to 40%. Metabolic acidosis and hyperkalemia may be severe enough to require dialysis when end-stage renal failure develops.
Dyslipidemia	Chronic hyperlipidemia may induce glomerular and tubulointerstitial injury, contributing to the progression of chronic renal disease.

GFR, Glomerular filtration rate.

However, as the GFR decreases, plasma urea concentration increases.

Fluid and electrolyte balance

Fluid and electrolyte balance is significantly disturbed with chronic renal failure. When the GFR decreases to 25%, there is an obligatory loss of 20 mEq to 40 mEq of *sodium* per day with osmotic loss of water. Dietary intake must be maintained to prevent sodium deficits and volume depletion. As GFR continues to decline, there also is loss of tubular function to dilute and concentrate the urine and urine-specific gravity becomes fixed at about 1.010.

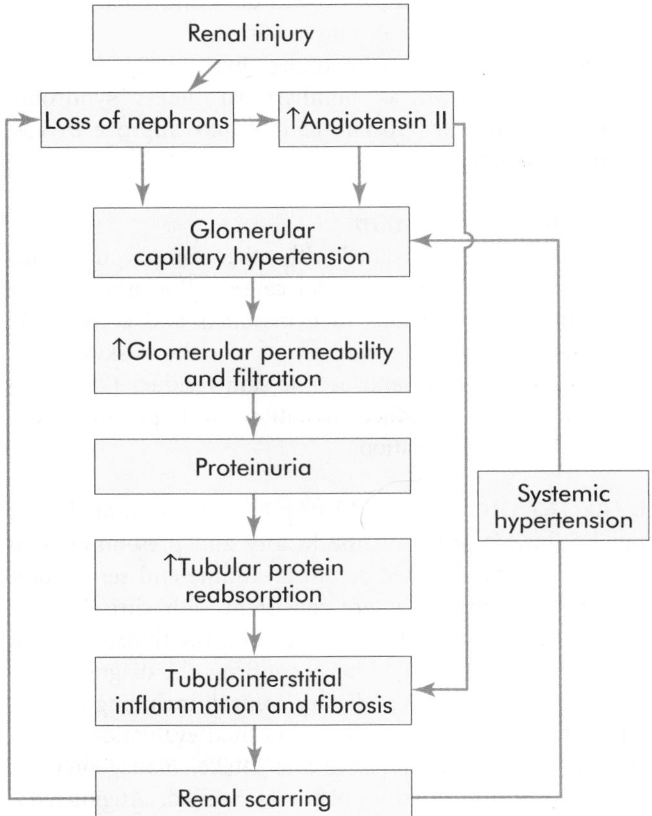

Figure 29-8 ■ Mechanisms Related to the Progression of Chronic Renal Failure.

Ultimately the kidney loses its ability to regulate sodium and water balance. Both sodium and water are retained, contributing to edema and hypertension.

In early renal failure, tubular secretion of *potassium* is maintained and larger amounts of potassium are lost through the bowel. With the onset of oliguria, total body potassium can increase to life-threatening levels and must be controlled by dialysis.

Metabolic acidosis develops when GFR decreases to less than 20% to 25% of normal. The causes of acidosis are primarily related to decreased hydrogen ion elimination and decreased bicarbonate reabsorption. With end-stage renal failure, metabolic acidosis may be severe enough to require dialysis.[71]

Musculoskeletal system

Bone and skeletal changes develop with alterations in calcium and phosphate metabolism. These changes begin when GFR decreases to 25% or less. *Hypocalcemia* is accelerated by impaired renal synthesis of 1,25-vitamin D with decreased intestinal absorption of calcium. Renal phosphate excretion also decreases and the increased serum phosphate binds calcium, further contributing to hypocalcemia. Acidosis also contributes to a negative calcium balance. Decreased serum calcium stimulates parathyroid hormone secretion with mobilization of calcium from bone. The combined effect of *hyperparathyroidism* and *vitamin D deficiency* can result in renal osteodystrophies (i.e., *osteomalacia* and *osteitis fibrosis*) with increased risk for fractures.[72]

Protein, carbohydrate, and fat metabolism

Protein, carbohydrate, and fat metabolism are altered in CRF. Proteinuria and a catabolic state contribute to a negative nitrogen balance. Serum proteins diminish, including albumin, complement, and transferrin, and there is loss of muscle mass. Glucose intolerance related to insulin resistance is common and may be related to alterations in adipokines (high leptin and low adiponectin) that interfere with insulin action. Hyperparathyroidism also decreases insulin sensitivity and impairs glucose tolerance.[73]

Hyperlipidemia is common among individuals with CRF. There is a high ratio of low-density lipoprotein (LDL) to high-density lipoprotein (HDL) with accelerated atherosclerosis and vascular calcification. Uremia causes a deficiency in lipoprotein lipase and decreased hepatic triglyceride lipase. Decreased lipolytic activity results in a reduction in HDL. Apolipoprotein B is also elevated, thereby accelerating atherogenesis.[74]

Cardiovascular system

Cardiovascular disease is a major cause of morbidity and mortality in CRF. Proinflammatory mediators, oxidative stress, and metabolic derangements are significant contributors.[75] *Hypertension* is the result of excess sodium and fluid volume. Elevated renin also stimulates the secretion of aldosterone, increasing sodium reabsorption. Hyperlipidemia promotes atheromatous plaque formation. Endothelial cell dysfunction and calcium deposits lead to a loss of vessel elasticity and vascular calcification. The resulting vascular disease increases the risk for *ischemic heart disease, left ventricular hypertrophy, congestive heart failure, stroke,* and *peripheral vascular disease* in individuals with uremia. Declining erythropoietin production causes anemia, thereby increasing demands for cardiac output and adding to cardiac workload. *Pericarditis* can develop from inflammation caused by the presence of uremic toxins. Accumulation of fluid in the pericardial space can compromise ventricular filling and cardiac output.

Pulmonary system

Pulmonary complications are associated with fluid overload and congestive heart failure. Pulmonary edema develops and metabolic acidosis can cause Kussmaul respirations.

Hematologic system

Hematologic alterations include *normochromic-normocytic anemia, impaired platelet adhesiveness,* and *hypercoagulability.* Inadequate production of erythropoietin decreases red blood cell production and requires treatment with recombinant erythropoietin. Uremia also decreases the red blood cell life span. Lethargy, dizziness, and low hematocrit are common findings. Defective platelet aggregation and altered vascular endothelium promotes an increased bleeding tendency with uremia and an increased risk for bruising, epistaxis, gastrointestinal bleeding, or cerebrovascular hemorrhage. Alterations in thrombin and other clotting factors contribute to hypercoagulability, thus control of coagulation is essential during dialysis.

Immune system

Immune system dysregulation with immune suppression, deficient response to vaccination, and increased risk for infection develops with CRF. Chemotaxis, phagocytosis, antibody production, and cell-mediated immune responses are suppressed. Malnutrition, metabolic acidosis, and hyperglycemia may amplify immunosuppression. Dialysis usually improves immune responses.

Neurologic system

Neurologic symptoms are common and progressive with CRF. Symptoms may include headache, drowsiness, sleep disorders, impaired concentration, memory loss, and impaired judgment. Neuromuscular irritation can cause hiccups, muscle cramps, and muscle twitching. In advanced stages of renal failure, symptoms may progress to seizures and coma. Peripheral neuropathies can also develop with impaired sensations particularly in the lower limbs.

Gastrointestinal system

Gastrointestinal complications are common in individuals with CRF. Uremic gastroenteritis can cause bleeding. Nonspecific symptoms include anorexia, nausea, and vomiting. Uremic fetor is a form of bad breath caused by the breakdown of urea by salivary enzymes. Malnutrition is common.

Endocrine and reproductive systems

Endocrine and reproductive alterations develop with progression of CRF. Both males and females have a decrease in circulating sex steroids. Males often experience a reduction in testosterone levels and may be impotent. Oligospermia and germinal cell dysplasia can rèsult in infertility. Females have reduced estrogen levels, amenorrhea, and difficulty maintaining a pregnancy to term. A decrease in libido occurs in both genders.

Insulin resistance is common in uremia, and as CRF progresses the ability of the kidney to degrade insulin is reduced and the half-life of insulin is prolonged. Individuals with diabetes mellitus and CRF need to carefully manage their insulin dosages. Low-protein diets and renal replacement therapy improve insulin sensitivity.[76]

CRF also causes alterations in thyroid hormone metabolism, known as nonthyroidal illness syndrome. A low-protein, low-phosphorus diet may improve thyroid hormone function.[77]

Integumentary system

Skin changes are associated with other complications that develop with CRF. Anemia can cause pallor and bleeding into the skin and results in hematomas and ecchymosis. Retained urochromes manifest as a sallow skin color. Hyperparathyroidism and uremic skin residues (known as "uremic frost") produce irritation and pruritus with scratching and excoriation.

EVALUATION AND TREATMENT Evaluation of chronic renal failure is based on the history and presenting signs and symptoms. Elevated serum creatinine and serum urea nitrogen concentrations are consistent with chronic renal failure. Ultrasound, CT scan, or plain x-ray films will show small kidney size. Renal biopsy confirms the diagnosis.

Management involves dietary control, including moderate protein restriction, sodium, and fluid evaluation, potassium restriction, adequate caloric intake, management of dylipidemias and erythropoietin as needed. Angiotensin-converting enzyme (ACE) inhibitors or receptor blockers are often used to provide renoprotection and control systemic hypertension.[78] End-stage renal failure related to diabetic nephropathy can be significantly reduced with control of hyperglycemia by intense insulin therapy.[79] End-stage renal failure is treated with dialysis, supportive therapy, and renal transplantation.[80]

✔ QUICK CHECK 29-4

1. What mechanisms cause prerenal acute renal failure?
2. How does intrarenal acute failure differ from postrenal failure?
3. Briefly describe the causes of anemia, cardiovascular disease, and bone and neurologic changes associated with chronic renal failure.

Did You Understand?

Urinary Tract Obstruction

1. Obstruction can occur anywhere in the urinary tract, and it may be anatomic or functional, including renal stones, an enlarged prostate gland, or urethral strictures. The most serious complications are hydronephrosis, hydroureter, ureterohydronephrosis, and infection caused by the accumulation of urine behind the obstruction.
2. Hypertrophy of the opposite kidney compensates for loss of function of the kidney with obstructive disease.
3. Relief of obstruction is usually followed by postobstructive diuresis and may cause fluid and electrolyte imbalance.
4. Persistent obstruction of the bladder outlet leads to residual urine volumes, low bladder wall compliance, and risk for vesicoureteral reflux and infection.
5. Kidney stones are caused by supersaturation of the urine with precipitation of stone-forming substances, changes in urine pH, or urinary tract infection.
6. The most common kidney stone is formed from calcium oxylate and most often causes obstruction by lodging in the ureter.
7. Obstructions of the bladder are a consequence of neurogenic or anatomic alteration bladder or both.
8. A neurogenic bladder is caused by a neural lesion that interrupts innervation of the bladder.
9. Upper motor neuron lesions result in overactive or hyperreflexive bladder function and dyssynergia (lack of coordinated neuromuscular contraction).
10. Lower motor neuron lesions result in underactive, hypotonic, or atonic bladder function.
11. Overactive bladder (OAB) syndrome is an uncontrollable or premature contraction of the bladder that results in urgency with or without incontinence, frequency, and nocturia.
12. Underactive bladder (UAB) is a condition in which the duration or strength of contraction is inadequate to empty the bladder resulting in distention and overflow incontinence.
13. Detrusor sphincter dyssynergia is failure of the urethrovesical junction smooth muscle to release urine during micturition and causes a functional obstruction.
14. Other causes of lower urinary tract obstruction include prostatic enlargement, urethral stricture, and pelvic organ prolapse in women.
15. Partial obstruction of the bladder can result in overactive bladder contractions with urgency. There is deposition of collagen in the bladder wall over time, resulting in decreased bladder wall compliance and ineffective detrusor muscle contraction.
16. Renal cell carcinoma is the most common renal neoplasm. The larger neoplasms tend to metastasize to the lung, liver, and bone.
17. Bladder tumors are commonly composed of transitional cells with a papillary appearance and a high rate of recurrence.

Urinary Tract Infection

1. Urinary tract infections (UTIs) are commonly caused by the retrograde movement of bacteria into the urethra and bladder. UTIs are uncomplicated when the urinary system is normal or complicated when there is an abnormality.
2. Cystitis is an inflammation of the bladder commonly caused by bacteria and may be acute or chronic.
3. Painful bladder syndrome/interstitial cystitis includes nonbacterial infectious cystitis (viral, mycobacterial, chlamydial, fungal), noninfectious cystitis (i.e., radiation injury), and interstitial cystitis, which is related to autoimmune injury.
4. Pyelonephritis is an acute or chronic inflammation of the renal pelvis often related to obstructive uropathies and may cause abscess formation and scarring with an alteration in renal function.

Glomerular Disorders

1. Glomerular disorders are a group of related diseases of the glomerulus that can be caused by immune responses, toxins or drugs, vascular disorders, and other systemic diseases.
2. Acute glomerulonephritis commonly results from inflammatory damage to the glomerulus as a consequence of immune reactions after a streptococcal infection.
3. The urine sediment may contain large amounts of protein (nephrotic sediment) or have red and white blood cells and protein (nephritic sediment).
4. Rapidly progressive glomerulonephritis (RPGN) is associated with injury that results in the proliferation of glomerular capillary endothelial cells and a rapid loss of renal function.
5. Chronic glomerulonephritis is related to a variety of diseases that cause deterioration of the glomerulus and a progressive loss of renal function.
6. Immune mechanisms in glomerulonephritis are the deposition of antigen-antibody complexes often with complement components and the formation of antibodies specific for the glomerular basement membrane.
7. Nephrotic syndrome is the excretion of at least 3.5 g protein (primarily albumin) in the urine per day because of glomerular injury with increased capillary permeability and loss of membrane negative charge. Its principal signs are hypoproteinuria, hyperlipidemia, and edema. The liver cannot produce enough protein to adequately compensate for urinary loss.

Renal Failure

1. Acute renal failure is classified as prerenal, intrarenal, or postrenal and is usually accompanied by oliguria with an elevated plasma BUN and plasma creatinine levels.
2. Prerenal acute renal failure is caused by decreased renal perfusion with a decreased GFR, ischemia, and tubular necrosis.
3. Intrarenal acute renal failure is associated with several systemic diseases but is commonly related to acute tubular necrosis (ATN).
4. Postrenal failure is associated with diseases that obstruct the flow of urine from the kidneys.
5. Chronic renal failure represents a progressive loss of renal function. Plasma creatinine levels gradually become elevated as GFR declines; sodium is lost in the urine; potassium is retained; acidosis develops; calcium metabolism and phosphate metabolism are altered and erythropoietin production is diminished. All organs systems are affected by CRF.

Key Terms

References

1. Gillenwater JY: Hydronephrosis, In Gillenwater JY et al, editors: *Adult and pediatric urology*, ed 4, Philadelphia, 2002, Lippincott Williams & Wilkins.
2. Gulmi FA, Felsen D, Vauchan ED: Pathophysiology of urinary tract obstruction, In Walsh PC et al, editors: *Campbell's urology*, ed 8, Philadelphia, 2002, Saunders.
3. Coe FL, Evan A, Worcester E: Kidney stone disease, *J Clin Invest* 115(10):2598–2608, 2004.
4. Menon M, Resnick MI: Urinary lithiasis: etiology, diagnosis, and medical management, In Walsh PC et al, editors: *Campbell's urology*, ed 8, Philadelphia, 2002, Saunders.
5. Moe OW: Kidney stones: pathophysiology and medical management, *Lancet* 367(9507):333–344, 2006.
6. Lingeman JE, Lifshitz DA, Evan AP: Surgical management of urinary lithiasis, In Walsh PC et al, editors: *Campbell's urology*, ed 8, Philadelphia, 2002, Saunders.
7. Teichman JMH: Acute renal colic from ureteral calculus, *N Engl J Med* 350:684–693, 2004.
8. Pietrow PK, Karellas ME: Medical management of common urinary calculi, *Am Fam Physician* 74(1):86–94, 2006.
9. Park S, Pearle MS: Imaging for percutaneous renal access and management of renal calculi, *Urol Clin North Am* 33(3): 353–364, 2006.
10. Borghi L, Meschi T, Maggiore U, Prati B: Dietary therapy in idiopathic nephrolithiasis, *Nutr Rev* 64(7 Pt 1):301–312, 2006.
11. Tiselius HG: Removal of ureteral stones with extracorporeal shock wave lithotripsy and ureteroscopic procedures: what can we learn from the literature in terms of results and treatment efforts? *Urol Res* 33(3):185–190, 2005.
12. Karsenty G et al: Understanding detrusor sphincter dyssynergia—significance of chronology, *Urology* 66(4):763–768, 2005.
13. Chu FM, Dmochowski R: Pathophysiology of overactive bladder, *Am J Med* 119(3 suppl 1):3–8, 2006.
14. Abrams P et al: The standardisation of terminology of lower urinary tract function: report from the Standardisation Subcommittee of the International Continence Society, *Am J Obstet Gynecol* 187(1):116–126, 2002.
15. Staskin DR, MacDiarmid SA: Using anticholinergics to treat overactive bladder: the issue of treatment tolerability, *Am J Med* 119(3 suppl 1):9–15, 2006.
16. Staskin DR, MacDiarmid SA: Pharmacologic management of overactive bladder: practical options for the primary care physician, *Am J Med* 119(3 suppl 1):24–28, 2006.
17. Fenton AS et al: Anterior urethral strictures: etiology and characteristics, *Urology* 65(6):1055–1058, 2005.
18. Valchanov K et al: An unusual cause of acute renal failure: urethral stricture in a female, *Nephron* 87(1):89–90, 2001.
19. American Cancer Society: *Cancer facts & figures—2007*, Atlanta, 2007, Author.
20. Lipworth L, Tarone RE, McLaughlin JK: The epidemiology of renal cell carcinoma, *J Urol* 176(6 Pt 1):2353–2358, 2006.
21. Meloni-Ehrig AM: Renal cancer: cytogenetic and molecular genetic aspects, *Am J Med Genet* 115(3):164–172, 2002.
22. Lipworth L, Tarone RE, McLaughlin JK: The epidemiology of renal cell carcinoma, *J Urol* 176(6 Pt 1):2353–2358, 2006.
23. Ogushi T et al: Estrogen receptor-binding fragment-associated antigen 9 is a tumor-promoting and prognostic factor for renal cell carcinoma, *Cancer Res* 65(9):3700–3706, 2005.
24. Lane BR, Kattan MW: Predicting outcomes in renal cell carcinoma, *Curr Opin Urol* 15(5):289–297, 2005.
25. Tigrani VS et al: Potential role of nephrectomy in the treatment of metastatic renal cell carcinoma: a retrospective analysis, *Urology* 55(1):36–40, 2000.
26. Lam JS et al: Renal cell carcinoma 2005: new frontiers in staging, prognostication, and targeted molecular therapy, *J Urol* 173(6):1853–1862, 2005.
27. Gore ME, Harrison ML, Montes A: New drug therapies for advanced renal cell carcinoma, *Expert Rev Anticancer Ther* 7(1):57–71, 2007.
28. Pelucchi C, Bosetti C, Negri E, Malvezzi M, La Vecchia C: Mechanisms of disease: The epidemiology of bladder cancer, *Nat Clin Pract Urol* 3(6):327–340, 2006.
29. Sonpavde G: Bladder cancer update. Current evaluation methods and standard of care, *Postgrad Med* 19(3):30–37, 2006.
30. Lokeshwar VB, Selzer MG: Urinary bladder tumor markers, *Urol Oncol* 24(6):528–537, 2006.
31. Griebling TL: Urologic diseases in America project: trends in resource use for urinary tract infections in women, *J Urol* 173(4):1281–1287, 2005.
32. Bouckaert J et al: Receptor binding studies disclose a novel class of high-affinity inhibitors of the *Escherichia coli* FimH adhesion, *Mol Microbiol* 55(2):441–455, 2005.
33. Ginde AA, Rhee SH, Katz ED: Predictors of outcome in geriatric patients with urinary tract infections, *J Emerg Med* 27(2): 101–108, 2004.
34. Mehnert-Kay SA: Diagnosis and management of uncomplicated urinary tract infections, *Am Fam Physician* 72(3):451–456 review, 2005.

References—Cont'd

35. Czaja CA, Hooton TM: Update on acute uncomplicated urinary tract infection in women, *Postgrad Med* 119(1):39–45, 2006.
36. Graham E, Chai TC: Dysfunction of bladder urothelium and bladder urothelial cells in interstitial cystitis, *Curr Urol Rep* 7 (6):440–446, 2006.
37. National Kidney and Urologic Diseases Information Clearinghouse: *Interstitial cystitis/painful bladder syndrome, June 2005;* http://kidney.niddk.nih.gov/kudiseases/pubs/interstitialcystitis.
38. Phatak S, Foster HE Jr: The management of interstitial cystitis: an update, *Nat Clin Pract Urol* 3(1):45–53, 2006.
39. Funfstuck R, Ott U, Naber KG: The interaction of urinary tract infection and renal insufficiency, *Int J Antimicrob Agents* 28(suppl 1):S72–77, 2006.
40. Ramakrishnan K, Scheid DC: Diagnosis and management of acute pyelonephritis in adults, *Am Fam Physician* 71(5): 933–942, 2005.
41. Cunard R, Kelly CJ: Immune-mediated renal disease, *J Allergy Clin Immunol* 111(2 suppl):S637–S644, 2003.
42. Cattran DC: Outcomes research in glomerulonephritis, *Semin Nephrol* 23(4):340–354, 2003.
43. Garcia GE et al: Mononuclear cell-infiltrate inhibition by blocking macrophage-derived chemokine results in attenuation of developing crescentic glomerulonephritis, *Am J Pathol* 162(4):1061–1073, 2003.
44. Hotta O, Ishida A, Kimura T, Taguma Y: Improvements in treatment strategies for patients with antineutrophil cytoplasmic antibody-associated rapidly progressive glomerulonephritis, *Ther Apher Dial* 10(5):390–395, 2006.
45. Little MA, Pusey CD: Rapidly progressive glomerulonephritis: current and evolving treatment strategies, *J Nephrol* 17(suppl 8):S10–S19, 2004.
46. Levy JB et al: Long-term outcome of anti-glomerular basement membrane antibody disease treated with plasma exchange and immunosuppression, *Ann Intern Med* 134(11): 1033–1042, 2001.
47. Liu Y: Renal fibrosis: new insights into the pathogenesis and therapeutics, *Kidney Int* 69(2):213–217, 2006.
48. Johnson DW: Evidence-based guide to slowing the progression of early renal insufficiency, *Intern Med J* 34(1–2):50–57, 2004.
49. Turnberg D, Cook HT: Complement and glomerulonephritis: new insights, *Curr Opin Nephrol Hypertens* 14(3):223–228, 2005.
50. Gomez-Guerrero C et al: Mesangial cells and glomerular inflammation: from the pathogenesis to novel therapeutic approaches, *Curr Drug Targets Inflamm Allergy* 4(3):341–351, 2005.
51. Crew RJ, Radhakrishnan J, Appel G: Complications of the nephrotic syndrome and their treatment, *Clin Nephrol* 62(4): 245–259, 2004.
52. Fehally J, Floege J, Johnson R: *Comprehensive clinical nephrology*, St Louis, 2007, Mosby Elsevier.
53. Nickolas TL, Radhakrishnan J, Appel GB: Hyperlipidemia and thrombotic complications in patients with membranous nephropathy, *Semin Nephrol* 23(4):406–411, 2003.
54. Anochie I, Eke F, Okpere A: Childhood nephrotic syndrome: change in pattern and response to steroids, *J Natl Med Assoc* 98(12):1977–1981, 2006.
55. Agrawal M, Swartz R: Acute renal failure, *Am Fam Physician* 61(7):2077–2088, 2000. Erratum in *Am Fam Physician* 63(3): 445, 2001.
56. Devarajan P: Cellular and molecular derangements in acute tubular necrosis, *Curr Opin Pediatr* 17(2):193–199, 2005.
57. Hladunewich M, Rosenthal MH: Pathophysiology and management of renal insufficiency in the perioperative and critically ill patient, *Anesthesiol Clin North America* 18(4): 773–789, 2000.
58. Safirstein RL: Pathophysiology of acute renal failure. In Greenberg A, editor: *National Kidney Foundation primer on kidney disease*, p 283, Elsevier Saunders, 2005, Philadelphia.
59. Venkataraman R: Prevention of acute renal failure, *Crit Care Clin* 21(2):281–289, 2005.
60. Ympa YP et al: Has mortality from acute renal failure decreased? A systematic review of the literature, *Am J Med* 118(8):827–832, 2005.
61. Snyder S, Pendergraph B: Detection and evaluation of chronic kidney disease, *Am Fam Physician* 72(9):1723–1732, 2005.
62. Mene P, Polci R, Festuccia F: Mechanisms of repair after kidney injury, *J Nephrol* 16(2):186–195, 2003.
63. Bricker NS, Morrin PA, Kime SW Jr: The pathologic physiology of chronic Bright's disease: an exposition of the "intact nephron hypothesis," *J Am Soc Nephrol* 8(9):1470–1476, 1997.
64. Tall MW, Luychx VA, Brenner BM: Adaptation to nephron loss. In Brenner BM, editor: *Brenner and Rector's the kidney*, ed 7, p. 1954, Philadelphia, 2004, Saunders.
65. Schieppati A, Pisoni R, Remuzzi G: Pathophysiology and management of chronic kidney disease. In Greenberg A, editor: *Primer on kidney diseases*, ed 4, pp 445–447, St Louis, 2005, Elsevier Saunders.
66. Hirschberg R, Wang S: Proteinuria and growth factors in the development of tubulointerstitial injury and scarring in kidney disease, *Curr Opin Nephrol Hypertens* 14(1):43–52, 2005.
67. Sean Eardley K, Cockwell P: Macrophages and progressive tubulointerstitial disease, *Kidney Int* 68(2):437–455, 2005.
68. Durvasula RV, Shankland SJ: The renin-angiotensin system in glomerular podocytes: mediator of glomerulosclerosis and link to hypertensive nephropathy, *Curr Hypertens Rep* 8(2): 132–138, 2006.
69. Zandi-Nejad K et al: Why is proteinuria an ominous biomarker of progressive kidney disease? *Kidney Int Suppl* (92): S76–S89, review, 2004.
70. Guarnieri G et al: Chronic systemic inflammation in uremia: potential therapeutic approaches, *Semin Nephrol* 24(5): 441–445, 2004.
71. Kraut JA, Kurtz I: Metabolic acidosis of CKD: diagnosis, clinical characteristics, and treatment, *Am J Kidney Dis* 45 (6):978–993, 2005.
72. Mondry A, Wang Z, Dhar PK: Bone and the kidney: a systems biology approach to the molecular mechanisms of renal osteodystrophy, *Curr Mol Med* 5(5):489–496, 2005.
73. Procopio M, Borretta G: Derangement of glucose metabolism in hyperparathyroidism, *J Endocrinol Invest* 26(11):1136–1142, 2003.
74. Qunibi WY: Dyslipidemia and progression of cardiovascular calcification (CVC) in patients with end-stage renal disease (ESRD), *Kidney Int Suppl* (95):S43–S50, 2005.
75. Axelsson J, Heimburger O, Stenvinkel P: Adipose tissue and inflammation in chronic kidney disease, *Contrib Nephrol* 151:165–174, 2006.
76. Rigalleau V, Gin H: Carbohydrate metabolism in uraemia, *Curr Opin Clin Nutr Metab Care* 8(4):463–469, 2005.
77. Rosolowska-Huszcz D, Kozlowska L, Rydzewski A: Influence of low protein diet on nonthyroidal illness syndrome in chronic renal failure, *Endocrine* 27(3):283–288, 2005.
78. Ferrari P: Prescribing angiotensin-converting enzyme inhibitors and angiotensin receptor blockers in chronic kidney disease, *Nephrology* (Carlton) 12(1):81–89, 2007.
79. Schena FP, Gesualdo L: Pathogenetic mechanisms of diabetic nephropathy, *J Am Soc Nephrol* 16(suppl 1):S30–S33, 2005.
80. Nolan CR: Strategies for improving long-term survival in patients with ESRD, *J Am Soc Nephrol* 16(suppl 2):S120–S127, 2005.

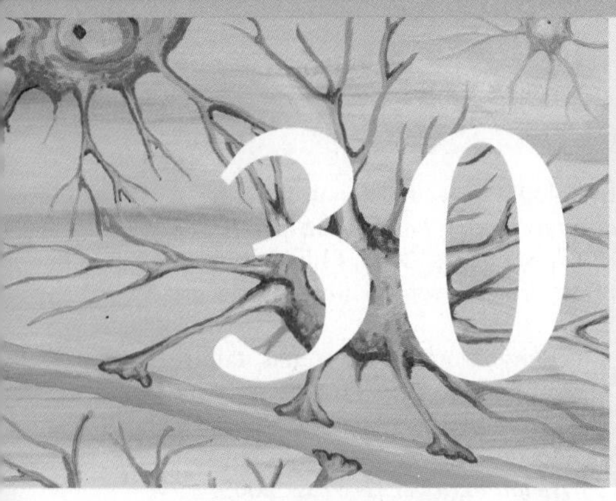

30 ALTERATIONS OF RENAL AND URINARY TRACT FUNCTION IN CHILDREN

Sue E. Huether

CHAPTER OUTLINE

ELECTRONIC RESOURCES

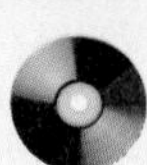

Companion CD
- Review Questions and Answers
- Animations

evolve Website
http://evolve.elsevier.com/Huether/
- Quick Check Answers
- Key Terms Exercises
- Critical Thinking Questions with Answers
- Algorithm Completion Exercises
- WebLinks

The incidence and type of renal and urinary tract disorders experienced by children varies with age and maturation, and newborn disorders may involve congenital malformations. During childhood, the kidney and genitourinary structures continue to develop, so renal dysfunction may be associated with mechanisms and manifestations that differ from those found in adults.

STRUCTURAL ABNORMALITIES

Variations from the normal anatomic structure of the urinary tract occur in 10% to 15% of the total population. These abnormalities range from minor, nonpathologic, or easily correctable anomalies to those that are incompatible with life. For example, the kidneys may fail to ascend from the pelvis to the abdomen, causing ectopic kidneys—which usually function normally. The kidneys also may fuse as they ascend, causing a single, U-shaped **horseshoe kidney.** Approximately one third of individuals with horseshoe kidneys are asymptomatic, and the most common problems are hydronephrosis, infection, stone formation, and, rarely, renal malignancies.[1,2] Collectively, structural anomalies of the renal system account for approximately 45% of cases of renal failure in children, and many are linked to gene defects.[3,4]

Certain structural anomalies are commonly associated with urinary tract malformations,[5] including the following:

Low-set, malformed ears
Chromosomal disorders, especially trisomy 13 (Patau syndrome) and trisomy 18
Absent abdominal muscles (prune-belly syndrome)
Anomalies of the spinal cord and lower extremities
Imperforate anus or genital deviation
Neuroblastoma (Wilms tumor)
Congenital ascites
Cystic disease of the liver
Positive family history of renal disease (hereditary nephritis or cystic disease)

Hypospadias

Hypospadias is a congenital condition in which the urethral meatus is located on the ventral side or undersurface of the penis. The meatus can be located anywhere on the glans, the penile shaft, at the base of the penis, the penoscrotal junction, or the perineum (Figure 30-1). This is the most common anomaly of the penis; it occurs in about 100 in 300 infant boys, and the incidence appears to be increasing.[6] The cause of this condition is multifactorial and includes maternal intake of progestin, androgen synthesis, advanced maternal age, 5α-reductase mutations, and environmental factors.[6] **Chordee** or penile torsion may accompany cases of hypospadias. In chordee, skin tethering and shortening of subcutaneous tissue cause the penis to bend or "bow" ventrally (Figure 30-2). Penile

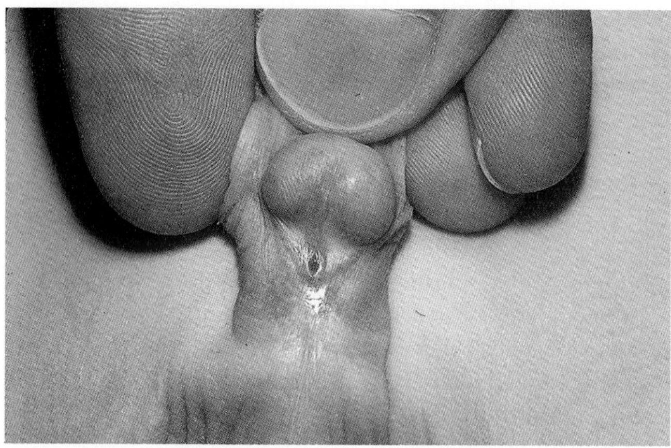

Figure 30-1 ■ **Hypospadias.** (Courtesy H. Gil Rushton, MD, Children's National Medical Center, Washington, DC; from Hockenberry MJ, Wilson D: *Wong's nursing care of infants and children*, ed 8, St Louis, 2007, Mosby.)

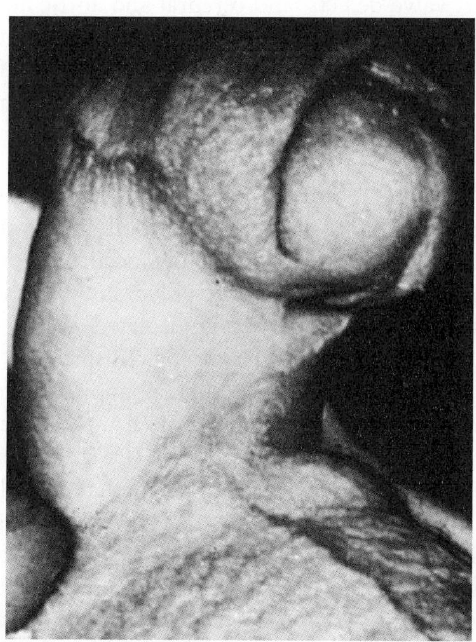

Figure 30-2 ■ **Hypospadias with Significant Chordee.** (From Shirkey HC, editor: *Pediatric therapy*, ed 6, St Louis, 1980, Mosby.)

torsion is rotation of the penile shaft to either the right or the left. Partial absence of the foreskin and cryptorchidism (undescended testes; see Chapter 32) are associated with the anomaly.[7]

The goals for corrective surgery on the child with hypospadias are (1) a straight penis when erect to facilitate intercourse as an adult, (2) a uniform urethra of adequate caliber to prevent spraying during urination, (3) a cosmetic appearance satisfactory to the individual, and (4) repair completed in as few procedures as possible. Surgery is most effective, psychologically as well as physically, when performed between 4 and 8 months of age.[8]

Epispadias and Exstrophy of the Bladder

Epispadias and exstrophy of the bladder are the same congenital defect expressed to differing degrees. In male epispadias, the urethral opening is on the dorsal surface of the penis. In females, a cleft along the ventral urethra usually extends to the bladder neck. The incidence of epispadias is 1 in 40,000 to 118,000 births. Twice as many boys as girls present with this defect.[9]

In boys, the urethral opening may be small and situated behind the glans (anterior epispadias), or a fissure may extend the entire length of the penis and into the bladder neck (posterior epispadias). Children with anterior epispadias can be continent with perhaps only stress incontinence, but those with posterior epispadias will experience constant dribbling of urine.[10]

Exstrophy of the bladder is a rare extensive congenital anomaly in which the bladder opens directly onto the abdominal wall. The bony part of the pelvis remains open (Figure 30-3), and the posterior portion of the bladder mucosa is exposed through the abdominal opening and appears bright red. The incidence of exstrophy of the bladder is about 1 in 40,000 live births and occurs equally in males and females.[11]

Exstrophy of the bladder is caused by intrauterine failure of the abdominal wall and the mesoderm of the anterior bladder to fuse. The rectus muscles below the umbilicus are separated, and the pubic rami (bony projections of the pubic bone) are not joined. This causes a waddling gait when the child first learns to walk, but most children quickly learn to compensate. The clitoris in girls is divided into two halves with the urethra between them. The penis in boys is epispadiac. Urine seeps onto the abdominal wall from the ureters, causing a constant odor of urine and excoriation of the surrounding skin. Because the exposed bladder mucosa becomes hyperemic and edematous, it bleeds easily and is painful.

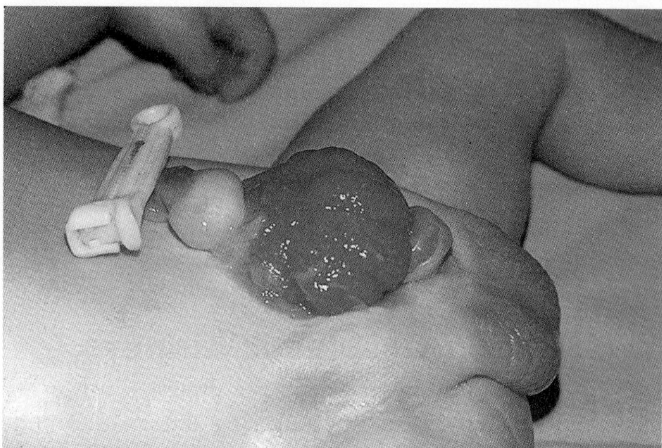

Figure 30-3 ■ **Exstrophy of Bladder.** (Courtesy H. Gil Rushton, MD, Children's National Medical Center, Washington, DC; from Hockenberry MJ, Wilson D: *Wong's nursing care of infants and children*, ed 8, St Louis, 2007, Mosby.)

The unrepaired exstrophic bladder is prone to cancerous changes as soon as 1 year after birth. Surgical reconstruction is performed usually within the first year as either a complete primary repair or as staged procedures. Staged procedures include bladder augmentation, bladder neck closure, or reconstruction, or both bladder neck closures and reconstruction.[12] Ideally, the bladder and pubic defect should be closed before the infant is 48 hours old. Objectives of management include preservation of renal function, attainment of urinary control, prevention of infection, and improvement of sexual function.[13] Diagnosis is often made by prenatal ultrasound.

Cloacal exstrophy is the most rare and severe form of bladder exstrophy. The intestine and spine may be involved, and reconstruction with restored urine and fecal control is difficult.

Bladder Outlet Obstruction

Congenital causes of bladder outlet obstruction are rare and include urethral valves and polyps. A **urethral valve** is a thin membrane of tissue that occludes the urethral lumen and obstructs urinary outflow in males. Most valves occur in the posterior urethra, although a few arise from the embryologically distinct anterior urethra. Urethral polyps rarely arise from the prostatic urethra. They often cause relatively severe obstruction and may impair renal embryogenesis and lead to renal failure.[14] Urethral valves or polyps are resected during the first days of life using a small cystoscope.[15]

Ureteropelvic Junction Obstruction

Ureteropelvic junction (UPJ) obstruction is a blockage of the tapered point where the renal pelvis transitions into the ureter.[16] It is the most common cause of hydronephrosis in neonates. An intrinsic malformation of smooth muscle or urothelial development produces obstruction in 90% of cases, and approximately 10% are caused by extrinsic compression.[16,17] During infancy or childhood, **secondary ureteropelvic junction (UPJ) obstruction** is caused by kinking or secondary scarring in the presence of high-grade vesicoureteral reflux (see p. 815). An increased risk of vesicoureteral reflux in children with UPJ obstruction affects both the obstructed and contralateral kidneys; whether this represents a sequela of the embryonic defect leading to the UPJ defect is not known. Diagnosis can be made by ultrasound, and surgical or endoscopic pyeloplasty relieves the obstruction.[18] Obstruction of the distal ureter causes dilation of the entire ureter, renal pelvis, and caliceal system.[19] *Ureterocele* occurs when a short acontractile segment of ureter develops just above the ureterovesical junction. UPJ obstructions are usually corrected surgically.

Hypoplastic/Dysplastic Kidneys

During embryologic development, the ureteric duct grows into the metanephric tissue, triggering the formation of the kidneys. If this growth does not occur, the kidney is absent—a condition called **renal aplasia.** Occasionally, a **hypoplastic kidney,** a very small normal kidney, may develop. These aberrations may be unilateral or bilateral; the occurrence may be incidental or familial. Bilateral hypoplastic kidneys are a common cause of chronic renal failure in children. Segmental hypoplasia, the Ask-Upmark kidney, is a deformity acquired secondary to intrarenal reflux and can be associated with arterial hypertension.[20]

Renal dysplasia usually results from abnormal differentiation of the renal tissues; for example, primitive glomeruli and tubules, cysts, and nonrenal tissue, such as cartilage, are found in the dysplastic kidney. Dysplasia is usually also associated with obstruction of the collecting system. The obstruction may begin before birth, as in prune-belly syndrome (congenital absence of abdominal muscles), posterior urethral valves, or ureteroceles.

Polycystic Kidneys

Polycystic kidney disease is an autosomal dominant (PDK1 or PDK2 gene) and autosomal recessive inherited disorder. It occurs in about 1 in 1000 live births.[21] The affected kidney has large fluid-filled cysts that include the tubules and collecting ducts. Other organs also may have cysts, including the liver, pancreas, and ovaries. Hypertension, heart valve defects, and cerebral and aortic aneurysms may develop. Symptoms may not develop until adulthood. Cyst formation is related to tubular cell proliferation, basement membrane remodeling, and fluid accumulation with obstruction.

Renal Agenesis

Renal agenesis (the absence of one or both kidneys) may be unilateral or bilateral and randomly occurring or clearly hereditary. The kidney is usually polycystic and dysplastic. The condition may occur as an isolated entity or as a problem associated with other urologic disorders.[22]

Unilateral renal agenesis occurs in approximately 1 of 1000 live births. Males are more often affected, and it is usually the left kidney that is absent. The single remaining kidney is often completely normal so that the child can expect a normal, healthy life. By the time the child is several years old, the volume of this kidney may approach twice the normal size. In some instances, however, the single kidney is abnormally formed and associated with abnormalities of its collecting system. Extrarenal congenital abnormalities are relatively more common with unilateral renal agenesis.

Bilateral renal agenesis (also called *Potter syndrome*) occurs in about 1 to 4 in 10,000 live births, 75% being male.[23] The term **Potter syndrome** refers to the association with a specific group of facial anomalies (wide-set eyes, parrot-beak nose, low-set ears, and receding chin). Affected infants rarely live more than a few hours. Approximately 40% of affected infants are stillborn. Renal agenesis can be detected prenatally by ultrasound.

QUICK CHECK 30-1

1. Describe hypospadias.
2. Why does bladder exstrophy occur?
3. Contrast dysplastic kidney and hypoplastic kidney.

GLOMERULAR DISORDERS

Glomerular disorders in children can present in different ways including glomerulonephritis, immunoglobin A (IgA) nephropathy, nephrotic syndrome, and hemolytic uremic syndrome. The disease can be acute or chronic and rarely leads to renal failure.

Glomerulonephritis

Glomerulonephritis includes a number of renal disorders in which proliferation and inflammation of the glomeruli are secondary to an immune mechanism (Box 30-1). Chronic glomerulonephritis accounts for about 53% of renal failure in children and is the causative factor for most school-age and teenage children that require dialysis and kidney transplantation.

Poststreptococcal glomerulonephritis

Acute poststreptococcal glomerulonephritis is one of the most common immune complex-mediated renal diseases in children. The sudden onset of gross hematuria, edema, hypertension, and renal insufficiency occurs after a throat or skin infection with certain strains of group A β-hemolytic streptococci.

Pharyngeal infections are most common during cold weather. Skin infections from impetigo, infected insect bites, or varicella sores usually occur during warm weather.

Glomerulonephritis develops with the deposition of antigen-antibody complexes in the glomerulus. The immune injury results in activation of complement and inflammation, which increases glomerular capillary permeability and loss of the negative charge. These changes lead to hematuria and proteinuria.

Symptoms of varying severity develop about 1 to 3 weeks after the streptococcal infection. As many as half the children affected are asymptomatic and show only microscopic hematuria with otherwise normal renal function. The most severely affected develop acute renal failure with oliguria.

The onset of symptoms in the child is abrupt and consists of flank or midabdominal pain, irritability, general malaise, and fever. Acute hypertension may cause headache, vomiting, somnolence, and other central nervous system (CNS) manifestations, including seizures. Cardiovascular symptoms are related to circulatory overload and are compounded by hypertension. These include dyspnea, tachypnea, and an enlarged, tender liver.

The disease usually runs its course in 1 month, but urine abnormalities may be found for up to 1 year after the onset. Children become oliguric less commonly and develop rapidly progressive glomerulonephritis, whereas others slowly progress to chronic glomerulonephritis. Prolonged proteinuria and abnormal glomerular filtration rate (GFR) indicate an unfavorable prognosis. More than 95% recover completely. Treatment is symptom specific.

Immunoglobulin A Nephropathy

Immunoglobulin A (IgA) nephropathy is the most common form of glomerulonephritis worldwide and occurs more often in males. It is characterized by deposition mainly of immunoglobulin IgA and some IgM and complement proteins in glomerular capillaries and the mesangium. No systemic immunologic disease is evident.[24] Deposits of IgA cause immune injury to the glomerulus that is usually reversible. **Henoch-Schönlein purpura nephritis** is a particular form of IgA nephropathy that involves a systemic vasculitis. The pathogenesis is unknown.

Children with the disease have recurrent gross hematuria, often after a respiratory infection. Most continue to have microscopic hematuria between the attacks of gross hematuria and have a mild proteinuria as well. Treatment is supportive because kidney damage is generally insignificant. Approximately 20% of affected children develop the progressive form of the disease, however, with hypertension and decreasing renal function. These children eventually require dialysis and transplantation.

Nephrotic Syndrome

Nephrotic syndrome is a symptom complex related to loss of protein in the urine. In children with nephrotic syndrome, the kidney is usually the only organ involved, termed **primary nephrotic syndrome,** and the cause is usually unknown (idiopathic). If it is caused by a systemic disease or other causes (e.g., drugs, toxins), it is called **secondary nephrotic syndrome.** Primary nephrotic syndrome is found predominantly in the preschool child, with

BOX 30-1 Primary Glomerulonephritis in Children

Cause
Poststreptococcal infection related to other bacterial or viral infection; unknown; idiopathic; minimal change nephropathy; idiopathic IgA nephropathy

Immunologic Mechanism
Antigen-antibody complex deposition and formation in situ; complement activation; anti-glomerular basement membrane (GBM) disease; no specific immunologic cause established

Glomerular Histopathology
No lesion; diffuse, focal, or segmented; membranous, proliferative, or combination of types; lobular, exudative, necrotizing, and other types; chronic with glomerular proliferation

Manifestations of Glomerulonephritis
Hematuria, proteinuria, lipiduria, with or without oliguria; edema, hypertension, hyperlipidemia

a peak incidence of onset between 2 and 3 years of age. It is rare after 8 years of age. Boys are affected more often than girls. No prevalent racial or geographic distributions are evident. The incidence is approximately 3 per 100,000 children per year.

PATHOPHYSIOLOGY The most common causes of primary or idiopathic nephrotic syndrome in children are minimal change nephropathy and focal segmental glomerulosclerosis. **Minimal change nephropathy (MCN) (lipoid nephrosis)** is characterized by fusion of the glomerular podocyte foot processes. The glomeruli often appear normal, and there are few other renal structural abnormalities. A systemic immune mechanism is a likely cause of the disease, and an unidentified circulating permeability factor, released by T lymphocytes, has been proposed.[25] In idiopathic **focal segmental glomerulosclerosis (FSGS)** there is segmental loss of glomerular capillaries with proliferation of the mesangial matrix and adhesion of the capillaries to Bowman's capsule. In both MCN and FSGS there is loss of the glomerular basement membrane negative charge and an increase in glomerular capillary permeability, which leads to proteinuria and the symptoms of nephrotic syndrome: hypoproteinemia, hyperlipidemia, lipiduria, and edema (see Chapter 29). Sodium retention also contributes to the edema.[26]

CLINICAL MANIFESTATIONS Parents become alerted to nephrotic syndrome when they notice diminished, frothy, or foamy urine output and when edema becomes pronounced with periorbital swelling, ascites, respiratory difficulty from pleural effusion, and labial or scrotal swelling. Edema of the intestinal mucosa may cause anorexia, poor absorption, and diarrhea. Edema often masks the malnutrition caused by malabsorption and protein loss. Because of protein deficiency, changes in the quality of hair indicate a malnourished state. Pallor, with shiny skin and prominent veins, is also common. Blood pressure is usually normal or slightly decreased. The child has an increased susceptibility to infection, especially pneumonia, peritonitis, cellulitis, and septicemia. Irritability, fatigue, and lethargy are common. **Congenital nephrotic syndrome (Finnish type)** is caused by the NPHS1 gene that encodes an immunoglobulin-like protein, nephrin, at the podocyte slit membrane, which causes heavy proteinuria.[27] Babies born with congenital nephrotic syndrome have large fontanelles and separated cranial sutures and may show gingival hyperplasia.[28]

EVALUATION AND TREATMENT The diagnosis of nephrotic syndrome is evident from the finding of proteinuria, hyperlipidemia, and lipiduria. Several different diagnostic tests, including kidney biopsy, may be required to determine whether the cause is an intrinsic renal disease or a consequence of systemic disease. Basic management of nephrotic syndrome includes activity as tolerated; a low-sodium, well-balanced diet; glucocorticosteroids (prednisone), diuretics (furosemide, metolazone), and skin care. Immunosuppressive agents (i.e., cyclophosphamide and levamisole) may be given to children who have relapses, are resistant to steroid therapy, or both.[29,30]

Hemolytic Uremic Syndrome

Hemolytic uremic syndrome (HUS) is an acute disorder characterized by hemolytic anemia, thrombocytopenia, and acute renal failure. HUS is the most common cause of acute renal failure in children. The disease occurs most often in infants and children younger than 4 years of age but has been known to occur in adolescents and adults. The prognosis has improved dramatically, with more than 90% of children surviving and most regaining normal renal function.[31]

PATHOPHYSIOLOGY HUS has been associated with bacterial and viral agents, as well as endotoxins, especially that from *Escherichia coli* 0157:H7.[32] In HUS, the endothelial lining of the glomerular arterioles becomes swollen and occluded with platelets and fibrin clots. Narrowed vessels damage erythrocytes as they pass through. These damaged red blood cells are removed by the spleen, causing acute hemolytic anemia. Fibrinolysis, the process of dissolution of a clot, acts on precipitated fibrin, causing the fibrin split products to appear in serum and urine. Platelet thrombi develop within damaged vessels, and platelet removal produces thrombocytopenia. Varying degrees of vascular occlusion cause altered renal perfusion and renal insufficiency or failure.[32]

CLINICAL MANIFESTATIONS A prodromal gastrointestinal illness (fever, vomiting, diarrhea) or, less frequently, an upper respiratory infection often precedes the onset of HUS by 1 to 2 weeks. After a symptom-free 1- to 5-day period, the sudden onset of pallor, bruising or purpura, irritability, and oliguria heralds the onset of the disease. Slight fever, anorexia, vomiting, diarrhea (with the stool characteristically watery and blood stained), abdominal pain, mild jaundice, and circulatory overload are accompanying symptoms. Seizures and lethargy indicate CNS involvement. Renal failure is apparent within the first days of onset. The renal failure causes metabolic acidosis, azotemia, hyperkalemia, and often hypertension.

EVALUATION AND TREATMENT Clinical evaluation includes history of preexisting illness, presenting symptoms, and urine and blood analysis. Management is supportive. When renal failure occurs, early and frequent dialysis is indicated. Blood transfusions with packed red cells are needed to maintain reasonable hemoglobin levels. Kidney transplant may be required.[33]

Other Renal Disorders

Other disorders of the kidney occurring in children include renal tubular acidosis and acute and chronic renal failure. The pathophysiology for these conditions is similar to that in adults and is described in Chapter 29.

BLADDER DISORDERS

Urinary Tract Infections

Urinary tract infections (UTIs) are rare in newborns, and when they do occur they are usually caused by bacteria from the bloodstream that have settled in the urinary tract. Urinary tract infections in children are most common in 7- to 11-year-old girls (8.1%) as a result of perineal bacteria, especially *E. coli*, ascending the urethra.[34,35] Individual susceptibility, bacterial virulence, and the host's anatomy (presence of reflux, obstruction, stasis, or stones) affect the severity of the disease. An abnormal urinary tract is particularly susceptible to infection.[36] Sexually active female adolescents are more likely to have a UTI.

Cystitis, or infection of the bladder, results in mucosal inflammation and congestion. This causes detrusor muscle hyperactivity and a resulting decrease in bladder capacity. It may also cause distortion of the ureterovesical (UV) junction leading to transient reflux of infected urine up the ureters, causing acute or chronic pyelonephritis.[37]

Differentiating whether an infection is in the bladder or the kidneys is difficult based on symptoms alone. Infants may be asymptomatic or develop fever, lethargy, vomiting, diarrhea, or jaundice. Children may present with fever of undetermined origin, frequency, urgency, dysuria, enuresis or incontinence in a previously dry child, abdominal pain, and sometimes hematuria. **Acute pyelonephritis** usually causes chills, fever, and flank or abdominal pain, along with enlarged kidney(s) caused by inflammatory edema. **Chronic pyelonephritis** may be asymptomatic.

Diagnosis of UTIs is by urine culture and urinalysis. Dipstick analyses for nitrite or leukocyte esterase are also sensitive, particularly for children with a low likelihood of UTI. A positive result requires urine culture. Diagnostic imaging may be necessary to rule out obstructions, renal scarring, or functional abnormalities.[38]

With treatment, UTI symptoms are usually relieved in 1 to 2 days, and the urine becomes sterile. Sulfonamides are the drug of choice, with the usual empiric treatment given in four doses. More potent medications may be required if the child has been previously treated for a UTI or has congenital abnormalities of the urinary tract, such as urethral valves. If there is no improvement in 2 days, the child should be reevaluated.

HEALTH ALERT
Childhood Urinary Tract Infections

Childhood urinary tract infections are often seen in primary care settings and can cause significant longer-term morbidity if not treated. Children younger than 2 years often have few, nonspecific signs of infection, including fever, irritability, poor feeding, failure to thrive, and diarrhea. Circumcision status is controversial; however, more recent studies have shown an increased risk in uncircumcised boys. The American Academy of Pediatrics position is that scientific evidence shows medical benefits of neonatal circumcision, but data are insufficient to support routine neonatal circumcision. Obtaining a proper urine sample and culture is vital because true infections require radiographic studies. Antibiotic prophylaxis is promoted because of the link between vesicoureteral reflux, recurrent UTIs, and renal scarring and hypertension. Prophylactic antibiotics may be required until children are 3 or 4 years old, especially when there is risk of damage from reflux. Surgical management is sought only when medical management has failed and there are recurrent infections and pyelonephritis or poor renal growth.

Data from American Academy of Pediatrics: Circumcision policy statement Task Force on Circumcision, *Pediatrics* 103(3):686–693, 1999; Chang SL, Shortliffe LD: Pediatric urinary tract infections, *Pediatr Clin North Am* 53(3):379–400, 2006; Zorc JJ, Kiddoo DA, Shaw KN: Diagnosis and management of pediatric urinary tract infections, *Clin Microbial Rev* 18(2):417–422, 2005; Zorc JJ et al: Clinical and demographic factors associated with urinary tract infection in young febrile infants, *Pediatrics* 116(3):644–648, 2005.

Vesicoureteral Reflux

Vesicoureteral reflux (VUR) is the retrograde flow of urine from the bladder into the ureters. Reflux allows infected urine from the bladder to be repeatedly swept up into the

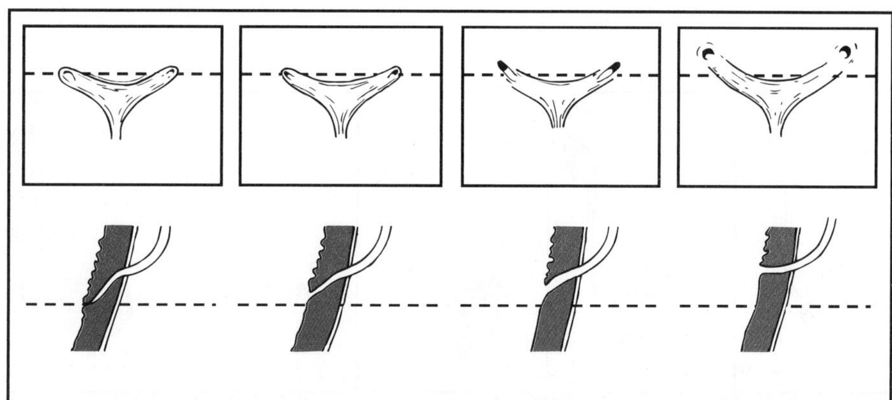

Figure 30-4 ■ Normal and Abnormal Configuration of the Ureterovesical Junction. Shown from left to right, progressive lateral displacement of the ureteral orifices and shortening of the intramural tunnels. *(Top)* Endoscopic appearance. *(Bottom)* Sagittal view through the intramural ureter. (From Behrman R et al, editors: *Nelson textbook of pediatrics,* ed 16, Philadelphia, 2000, Saunders.)

kidneys. The reflux perpetuates infection by preventing complete emptying of the bladder and allows the maximal intravesical pressure to be transmitted to the renal calyces and pyramids. The combination of reflux and infection is an important cause of pyelonephritis, especially in children younger than 5 years.

Vesicoureteral reflux occurs more often in girls by a ratio of 10:1 and is uncommon in blacks. Its incidence is approximately 1 in 1000 children. Siblings of those affected have a 50% chance of having reflux, but children with parents who had childhood reflux have almost a 70% chance of reflux.[39] Although reflux is considered abnormal at any age, the shortness of the submucosal segment of the ureter during infancy and childhood renders the antireflux mechanism relatively inefficient and delicate. Thus reflux is seen commonly in association with infections during early childhood but rarely in older children and adults.

PATHOPHYSIOLOGY Primary reflux results from a congenitally abnormal or ectopic insertion of the ureter into the bladder. Secondary reflux is more serious and may be transient or persistent. It develops in association with infection, malformations of the ureterovesical (UV) junction (Figure 30-4), increased intravesical pressures, and surgery on the UV junction.

Reflux may be unilateral or bilateral, and it can be classified or graded using the International Classification for comparative purposes[40] (Figure 30-5):

Grade I: reflux into a nondilated distal ureter
Grade II: reflux into the upper collecting system without dilation
Grade III: reflux into dilated ureter or blunting of calyceal fornices
Grade IV: reflux into a grossly dilated ureter and calyces
Grade V: massive reflux with urethral dilation and tortuosity and effacement of the calyceal details

CLINICAL MANIFESTATIONS Children with reflux have recurrent urinary tract infection or unexplained fever, poor growth and development, irritability, and feeding problems. The family history reveals reflux or urinary tract infection, pain with voiding, and signs of urinary obstruction or nephropathy.

EVALUATION AND TREATMENT In addition to the history of recurrent urinary tract infection and other symptoms, a voiding cystourethrogram is the primary diagnostic procedure. Most children with vesicoureteral reflux respond to nonoperative management aimed at prevention and treatment of infection. Spontaneous remission of grades I and II reflux may occur in 30% to 60% of children younger than 5 years. Children with grades III and IV reflux need careful monitoring. Recurrent infection requires surgical intervention or endoscopic injection. In cases of grade V reflux, early surgical intervention may be indicated to prevent renal scarring.[41]

QUICK CHECK 30-2

1. What is the cause of proteinuria?
2. How does the cause of urinary tract infections (UTIs) in newborns differ from that in older children?
3. Why does vesicoureteral reflux occur?

NEPHROBLASTOMA

Nephroblastoma (Wilms tumor) is a rare embryonal tumor of the kidney arising from undifferentiated mesoderm and represents 5% to 6% of childhood cancers in the United States.[42] Its incidence remains constant in the United States, with 7.8 cases per 1 million population ages 1 to 14 years. Approximately 500 children are diagnosed each year in the United States, most between 1 and 5 years of age. The peak incidence occurs between 2 and 3 years of age. Nephroblastoma is the most common solid tumor occurring in children. Paternal preconception toxin exposure (hydrocarbons and heavy metals) may be associated with increased risk in offspring.[43] Nephroblastoma is slightly more common in black children than in white children.

PATHOGENESIS Nephroblastoma has both sporadic and inherited origins. The sporadic form occurs in children with no known genetic predisposition. Inherited cases,

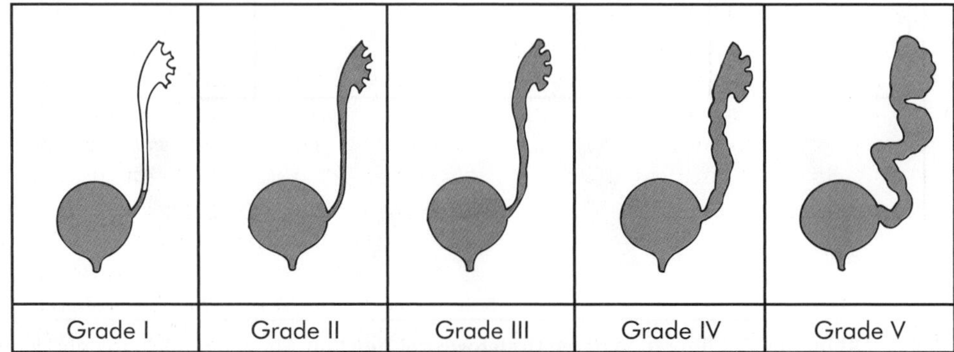

Figure 30-5 ■ Grades of Visicoureteral Reflux.

which are relatively rare, are transmitted in an autosomal dominant fashion. Nephroblastoma has been linked to mutation of several tumor suppressor genes (i.e., WT1 mutations).[44]

Eighteen percent of children who have nephroblastoma also have a number of congenital anomalies. The anomalies associated with nephroblastoma are aniridia (lack of an iris in the eye), hemihypertrophy (an asymmetry of the body), and genitourinary malformations (i.e., horseshoe kidneys, hypospadias, ureteral duplication, polycystic kidneys).[45] Children with both congenital anomalies and nephroblastoma are more likely to have the inherited bilateral form of the disease.

CLINICAL MANIFESTATIONS Most nephroblastoma usually present as enlarging asymptomatic abdominal masses before the age of 5 years. Many tumors are actually discovered by the child's parent, who feels or notices an abdominal swelling, usually while dressing or bathing the child. The child appears healthy and thriving. Other presenting complaints include vague abdominal pain (37%), hematuria (18%), and fever (22%).[46] Hypertension also may be present. In 25% to 63% of cases, there may be excess renin secretion.

Nephroblastoma may occur in any part of the kidney and varies greatly in size at the time of diagnosis. The tumor generally appears as a solitary mass surrounded by a smooth, fibrous external capsule and also may contain cystic or hemorrhagic areas. A pseudocapsule generally separates the tumor from the renal parenchyma.

EVALUATION AND TREATMENT On physical examination, the tumor feels firm, nontender, smooth, and is generally confined to one side of the abdomen. If the tumor is palpable past the midline of the abdomen, it may be large or may be arising from a horseshoe or ectopic kidney. Once an abdominal mass is detected, an abdominal ultrasound may be the initial means of study. Abdominal computed tomography (CT) scan or MRI also may be obtained before biopsy and surgical removal of the tumor.

Diagnosis is based on surgical biopsy. Additional laboratory and radiologic studies are used to evaluate the presence or absence of metastasis. The most common sites of metastasis are regional lymph nodes and the lungs. Metastases also occur in the liver, brain, and bone.

Several staging systems for nephroblastoma have been developed. The most widely accepted system was developed by the National Wilms Tumor Study Group (Table 30-1). Primary treatment is usually surgical exploration and resection or chemotherapy and then surgical resection. Survival approaches 90% for localized disease and 70% for metastatic disease.[47]

TABLE 30-1
Staging of Nephroblastoma Tumor*

Stage	Tumor Characteristics
I	Tumor limited to the kidney; can be completely resected
II	Tumor ascending beyond the kidney but is totally resected
III	Residual nonhematogenous tumor confined to the abdomen
IV	Hematogenous metastases to organs such as lungs, liver, bone, or brain
V	Bilateral disease either at diagnosis or later, then staged for each kidney

*Staging system of the National Wilms Tumor Study Group.

ENURESIS

Enuresis refers to the involuntary passage of urine by a child who is beyond the age when voluntary bladder control should have been acquired. Bladder control is accomplished by most children before the age of 4 years. Five years of age is more accurate and widely accepted, however, being largely determined by cultural beliefs and practices of parents regarding toilet training. In 80% of children, enuresis occurs at night only, in which case it is called **nocturnal enuresis.** Wetness during the day is called **diurnal enuresis.**

Types of Enuresis

In **primary enuresis,** the child has never been continent. In **secondary enuresis,** or acquired enuresis, the child has experienced a period of dryness of at least 3 to 6 months after toilet training and then becomes incontinent. Secondary enuresis may be diurnal, nocturnal, or a combination of both. (Types of incontinence are defined in Table 30-2.)

The incidence of enuresis is difficult to determine because it is not a problem that parents readily share with others and because definitions vary according to cultural norms and family practices. Some families start toilet training before 1 year of age and expect continence by the age of 1 to 1½ years, whereas other families do not expect dryness earlier than 5 years. The incidence of enuresis in children older than 5 years ranges from 10% to 20%. Boys represent more cases of enuresis than girls by a ratio of 3:2. Teenage and adult enuresis is rare and usually is a continuation of childhood bed-wetting.

PATHOGENESIS A combination of factors is likely to be responsible for enuresis.[48] Organic causes account for 2% to 10% of cases and include UTIs; neurologic disturbances; congenital defects of the meatus, urethra, and bladder neck; and allergies. Disorders that increase the normal output of urine, such as diabetes mellitus and diabetes insipidus, or disorders that impair the concentrating ability of the kidney, such as chronic renal failure or sickle cell disease, must be considered in the evaluation of enuresis.

Genetic factors as a cause of enuresis are likely, and the condition shows a familial tendency. Bed-wetting occurs with high frequency among parents, siblings, and other

TABLE 30-2
Classification of Incontinence

Type	Definition
Total incontinence	Inability to store any urine; indicates an anatomic or functional absence of urinary sphincters (e.g., epispadias or myelomeningocele) or a bypassing of urinary sphincters (e.g., vesicovaginal fistula)
Overflow incontinence	Frequent dribbling that relieves a constantly full bladder; occurs when urinary outlet is obstructed
Urge incontinence	Sudden and uncontrollable need to void that cannot be suppressed; suggests bladder irritation
Precipitate voiding	Voiding without a preceding urge to void; suggests neurologic origin
Stress incontinence	Uncontrollable voiding that occurs when intravesical pressure momentarily exceeds intravesical resistance, as in "giggle incontinence"; suggests alteration in intrinsic sphincter integrity
Paradoxic incontinence	Incontinence in spite of normal voiding; suggests an ectopic ureteral orifice outside the urinary sphincter mechanism (e.g., as when a girl is constantly wet, yet voids normally)

near relatives of symptomatic children. These observations are further supported by a high concordance rate in monozygotic twins with enuresis.

Other problems may be associated with enuresis, such as perinatal anoxia, CNS trauma, seizures, developmental delay, UTI, radiation therapy, imperforate anus, bladder trauma or surgery, and occult spinal dysraphism. Difficult sleep arousal, prolonged rapid eye movement (REM) sleep intervals, and the presence of obstructive sleep apnea syndrome are also associated with nocturnal enuresis.[49] Stressful psychologic situations, such as a new sibling, may cause enuresis to develop.

Therapeutic management of enuresis includes enuresis alarms, fluid management, diet therapy, drugs (desmopressin, an antidiuretic), treatment of obstructive sleep apnea, and behavioral therapy.[50,51] The main goals of therapy should be to have the child awaken and get up to use the toilet during the night to preserve self-esteem in moving toward the goal and to relieve psychologic stress.[50,51]

QUICK CHECK 30-3

1. What is Wilms tumor, and what cellular components are involved?
2. What organic causes are operative in enuresis?

Did You Understand?

Structural Abnormalities

1. Congenital renal disorders affect 10% to 15% of the population. These disorders range in severity from minor, easily correctable anomalies to those incompatible with life.
2. Hypospadias is a congenital condition in which the urethral meatus can be located anywhere on the ventral surface of the glans, the penile shaft, the midline of the scrotum, or the perineum.
3. Epispadias is a congenital condition in which the urethral opening is located on the dorsal surface of the penis. Epispadias is a mild form of exstrophy, a congenital condition that affects the urethra and bladder neck.
4. Exstrophy of the bladder is a congenital malformation in which the pubic bones are separated, the lower portion of the abdominal wall and anterior wall of the bladder are missing, and the back wall of the bladder is everted through the opening.
5. Urethral valves and polyps are congenital formations of tissue that block the urethra.
6. Ureteropelvic junction obstruction causes urethral obstruction by a malformation of junctional smooth muscle.
7. A dysplastic kidney is the result of abnormal differentiation of renal tissues. The hypoplastic kidney is a small but otherwise normal kidney.
8. Polycystic kidneys are an inherited disorder that results in large, fluid-filled cysts within the kidneys.
9. Renal agenesis is the failure of a kidney to grow or develop. The condition may be unilateral or bilateral and may occur as an isolated entity or in association with other disorders.

Glomerular Disorders

1. Glomerulonephritis is an inflammation of the glomeruli characterized by hematuria, edema, and hypertension. The cause is unknown but is often immune mediated. Glomerulonephritis may follow infections, especially those of the upper respiratory tract caused by strains of group A β-hemolytic streptococcus. Increases in glomerular capillary permeability lead to hematuria and proteinuria.
2. IgA nephropathy occurs with deposition of IgA in the glomerulus causing glomerular injury with gross hematuria.
3. *Nephrotic syndrome* is a term used to describe a symptom complex characterized by proteinuria, hypoproteinemia, hyperlipidemia, and edema. Metabolic, biochemical, or physiochemical disturbances in the glomerular basement membrane may lead to increased permeability to protein.

Did You Understand?—Cont'd

4. Hemolytic uremic syndrome is an acute disorder characterized by hemolytic anemia, acute renal failure, and thrombocytopenia.

Obstructive Disorders

1. Urinary tract infections can result from general sepsis in the newborn but are caused by bacteria ascending the urethra in older children. The bladder alone is infected in cystitis. The infection ascends to one or both kidneys in pyelonephritis. Urinary tract anomalies must be surgically corrected to prevent frequent recurrent infections.
2. Vesicoureteral reflux is the retrograde flow of bladder urine into the ureters providing a mechanism for pyelonephritis in children, whose ureters are shorter than those of adults.

Nephroblastoma

1. Nephroblastoma (Wilms tumor) is an embryonal tumor of the kidney that usually presents between birth and 5 years of age. The tumor can be successfully treated by surgery, a combination of drugs, and, sometimes, radiation therapy.

Enuresis

1. Enuresis refers to the involuntary passage of urine. Enuresis may occur during the day (diurnally) or during the night (nocturnally). The disorder tends to occur during non-REM sleep and can have a variety of organic and psychologic causes.

Key Terms

Acute pyelonephritis, 815
Chordee, 810
Chronic pyelonephritis, 815
Congenital nephrotic syndrome (Finnish type), 814
Cystitis, 815
Diurnal enuresis, 817
Enuresis, 817
Epispadias, 811
Exstrophy of the bladder, 811
Focal segmental glomerulosclerosis (FSGS), 814
Glomerulonephritis, 813
Hemolytic uremic syndrome (HUS), 814
Henoch-Schönlein purpura nephritis, 813
Horseshoe kidney, 810
Hypoplastic kidney, 812
Hypospadias, 810
Immunoglobulin A (IgA) nephropathy, 813
Minimal change nephropathy (MCN; lipoid nephrosis), 814
Nephroblastoma (Wilms tumor), 816
Nocturnal enuresis, 817
Polycystic kidney disease, 812
Potter syndrome, 812
Primary enuresis, 817
Primary nephrotic syndrome, 813
Renal agenesis, 812
Renal aplasia, 812
Renal dysplasia, 812
Secondary enuresis, 817
Secondary nephrotic syndrome, 813
Secondary ureteropelvic junction (UPJ) obstruction, 812
Ureteropelvic junction (UPJ) obstruction, 812
Urethral valve, 812
Urinary tract infection (UTI), 815
Vesicoureteral reflux (VUR), 815

References

1. Sawicz-Birkowska K et al: Malignant tumours in a horseshoe kidney in children: a diagnostic dilemma, *Eur J Pediatr Surg* 15(1):48–52, 2005.
2. Weizer AZ et al: Determining the incidence of horseshoe kidney from radiographic data at a single institution, *J Urol* 170(5):1722–1726, 2003.
3. Glassberg KI: Normal and abnormal development of the kidney: a clinician's interpretation of current knowledge, *J Urol* 167(6):2339–2350, discussion 2350–2351, 2002.
4. Kemper MJ, Mueller-Wiefel DE: Renal function in congenital anomalies of the kidney and urinary tract, *Curr Opin Urol* 11(6):571–575, 2001.
5. Belman AB, Lowell RK, Kramer SR: *Clinical pediatric urology*, ed 4, London, 2002, Martin Dunitz.
6. Nelson CP et al: The increasing incidence of congenital penile anomalies in the United States, *J Urol* 174(4 Pt 2):1573–1576, 2005.
7. Baskin LS, Himes K, Colborn T: Hypospadias and endocrine disruption: is there a connection? *Environ Health Perspect* 109(11):1175–1183, 2001.
8. Stokowski LA: Hypospadias in the neonate, *Adv Neonatal Care* 4(4):206–215, 2004.
9. Surer I et al: Continent urinary diversion and the exstrophy-epispadias complex, *J Urol* 169(3):1102–1105, 2003.
10. Grady RW, Mithcell ME: Management of epispadias, *Urol Clin North Am* 29(2):349–360, 2002.
11. Nelson CP, Dunn RL, Wei JT: Contemporary epidemiology of bladder exstrophy in the United States, *J Urol* 173(5): 1728–1731, 2005.
12. Borer et al: Bladder growth and development after complete primary repair of bladder exstrophy in the newborn with comparison to staged approach, *J Urol* 174(4 Pt 2): 1553–1557, 2005.
13. Kiddoo DA et al: Initial management of complex urological disorders: bladder exstrophy, *Urol Clin North Am* 31(3): 417–426, 2004.
14. Lopez Pereira P, Martinez Urrutia MJ, Jaureguizar E: Initial and long-term management of posterior urethral valves, *World J Urol* 22(6):418–424, 2004.
15. Narasimhan KL et al: Does mode of treatment affect outcome of neonatal posterior urethral valves? *J Urol* 171(6 Pt 1): 2423–2426, 2004.
16. Zhang PL, Peters CA, Rosen S: Ureteropelvic junction obstruction: morphological and clinical studies, *Pediatr Nephrol* 14(8–9):820–826, 2000.
17. Rooks VJ, Lebowitz RL: Extrinsic ureteropelvic obstruction from a crossing renal vessel: demography and imaging, *Pediatr Radiol* 31(2):120–124, 2001.

References—Cont'd

18. Capello SA et al: Prenatal ultrasound has led to earlier detection and repair of ureteropelvic junction obstruction, *J Urol* 174(4 Pt 1):1425–1428, 2005.
19. Tsai JD et al: Intermittent hydronephrosis secondary to ureteropelvic junction obstruction: clinical and imaging features, *Pediatrics* 117(1):139–146, 2006.
20. Babin J et al: The Ask-Upmark kidney: a curable cause of hypertension in young patients, *J Hum Hypertens* 19(4): 315–316, 2005.
21. Ong AC, Harris PC: Molecular pathogenesis of ADPKD: the polycystin complex gets complex, *Kidney Int* 67(4): 1234–1247, 2005.
22. Damen-Elias HA et al: Concomitant anomalies in 100 children with unilateral multicystic kidney, *Ultrasound Obstet Gynecol* 25(4):384–388, 2005.
23. Parikh CR et al: Congenital renal agenesis: case-control analysis of birth characteristics, *Am J Kidney Dis* 39:680–694, 2002.
24. Yoshikawa N, Tanaka R, Iijima K: Pathophysiology and treatment of IgA nephropathy in children, *Pediatr Nephrol* 16(5): 446–457, 2001.
25. Saha TC, Singh H: Minimal change disease: a review, *South Med J* 99(11):1264–70, 2006.
26. Vande Walle JG, Donckerwolcke RA: Pathogenesis of edema formation in the nephrotic syndrome, *Pediatr Nephrol* 16(3): 283–293, 2001.
27. Papez KE, Smoyer WE: Recent advances in congenital nephrotic syndrome, *Curr Opin Pediatr* 16(2):165–170, 2004.
28. Mattoo TK: Gingival hyperplasia in congenital and infantile nephrotic syndrome [letter to the editor], *Pediatr Nephrol* 11(3):388, 1997.
29. Durkan A et al: Non-corticosteroid treatment for nephrotic syndrome in children, *Cochrane Database Syst Rev* Apr 18(2): CD002290, 2005.
30. Hodson EM et al: Corticosteroid therapy for nephrotic syndrome in children, *Cochrane Database Syst Rev* Jan 25(1): CD001533, 2005.
31. Siegler R, Oakes R: Hemolytic uremic syndrome; pathogenesis, treatment, and outcome, *Curr Opin Pediatr* 17(2): 200–2004, 2005.
32. Razzaq S: Hemolytic uremic syndrome: an emerging health risk, *Am Fam Physician* 74(6):991–996, 2006.
33. Reppetto HA: Long-term course and mechanisms of progression of renal disease in hemolytic uremic syndrome, *Kidney Int* Suppl(97):S102–S106, 2005.
34. American Academy of Pediatrics, Committee on Quality Improvement, Subcommittee on Urinary Tract Infection: Practice parameter: the diagnosis, treatment, and evaluation of the initial urinary tract infection in febrile infants and young children, *Pediatrics* 103(4 pt 1):843–852, 1999.
35. Chang SL, Shortliffe LD: Pediatric urinary tract infections, *Pediatr Clin North Am* 53(3):379–400, 2006.
36. Yeung CK et al: The characteristics of primary vesico-ureteric reflux in male and female infants with prenatal hydronephrosis, *Br J Urol* 80:319–327, 1997.
37. Brandt J et al: Invasive pneumococcal disease and hemolytic uremic syndrome, *Pediatrics* 110(2 Pt 1):371–376, 2002.
38. Alper BS, Curry SH: Urinary tract infection in children, *Am Fam Physician* 72(12):2483–2488, 2005.
39. Mak RH, Kuo HJ: Primary ureteral reflux: emerging insights from molecular and genetic studies, *Curr Opin Pediatr* 15(2): 181–185, 2003.
40. Lebowitz RL et al: International system of radiographic grading of vesicoureteric reflux. International Reflux Study in Children, *Pediatr Radiol* 15(2):105–109, 1985.
41. Greenbaum LA, Mesrobian HG: Vesicoureteral reflux, *Pediatr Clin North Am* 53(3):413–27, 2006.
42. American Cancer Society: Detailed Guide: Wilms' Tumor: What Are the Key Statistics for Wilms Tumor? http://www.cancer.org/docroot/CRI/content/CRI_2_4_1X_What_are_the_key_statistics_for_Wilms_tumor_46.asp?rnav=cri (accessed April, 2007).
43. Pritchard-Jones K: Controversies and advances in the management of Wilms' tumour, *Arch Dis Child* 87(3):241–244, 2002.
44. Scott RH, Stiller CA, Walker L, Rahman N: Syndromes and constitutional chromosomal abnormalities associated with Wilms tumour, *J Med Genet* 43(9):705–15, 2006.
45. Sakamoto J et al: A novel WT1 gene mutation associated with Wilms' tumor and congenital male genitourinary malformation, *Pediatr Res* 50(3):337–344, 2001.
46. Amar AM et al: Clinical presentation of rhabdoid tumors of the kidney, *J Pediatr Hematol Oncol* 23(2):105–108, 2001.
47. Metzger ML, Dome JS: Current therapy for Wilms' tumor, *Oncologist* 10(10):815–826, 2005.
48. Butler RJ: Childhood nocturnal enuresis: developing a conceptual framework, *Clin Psychol Rev* 24(8):909–931, 2004.
49. Brooks LJ, Topol HI: Enuresis in children with sleep apnea, *J Pediatr* 142(5):515–518, 2003.
50. Berry AK: Helping children with nocturnal enuresis: the wait-and-see approach may not be in anyone's best interest, *Am J Nurs* 106(8):56–63, 2006.
51. Lyon C, Schnall J: What is the best treatment for nocturnal enuresis in children? *J Fam Pract* 54(1):905–906, 909, 2005.

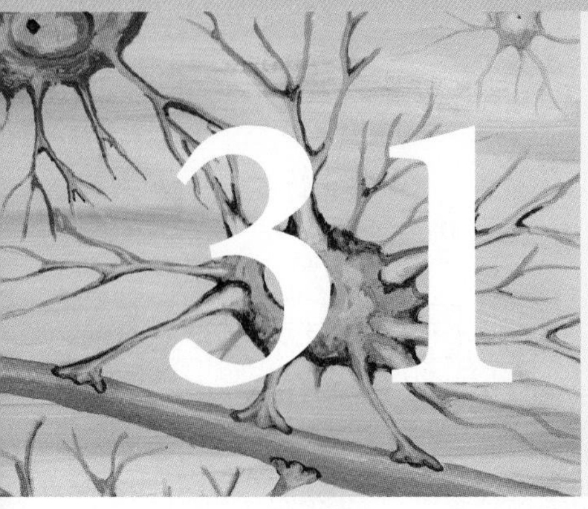

STRUCTURE AND FUNCTION OF THE REPRODUCTIVE SYSTEMS

Angela Deneris ▪ Sue E. Huether

CHAPTER OUTLINE

ELECTRONIC RESOURCES

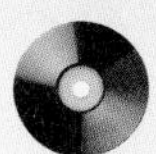

Companion CD

- Review Questions and Answers
- Animations

evolve Website
http://evolve.elsevier.com/Huether/

- Quick Check Answers
- Key Terms Exercises
- Critical Thinking Questions with Answers
- Algorithm Completion Exercises
- WebLinks

The male and female reproductive systems have several anatomic and physiologic features in common. Most obvious is their major function—reproduction—through which a 23-chromosome female gamete, the ovum, and a 23-chromosome male gamete, the **spermatozoon (sperm cell),** unite to form a 46-chromosome zygote that is capable of developing into a new individual. The male reproductive system produces sperm and delivers them to the female reproductive tract. The female reproductive system produces the **ovum** (*pl.,* ova) and, if the ovum is fertilized (then called the embryo and developing fetus), can nurture and protect it and expel it at birth. These functions are determined not only by anatomic structures but also by complex hormonal, neurologic, and psychogenic factors.[1]

DEVELOPMENT OF THE REPRODUCTIVE SYSTEMS

The structure and function of both male and female reproductive systems depend on steroid hormones called **sex hormones**. Hormonal effects on the reproductive systems begin during embryonic development and continue in varying degrees throughout life.

Sexual Differentiation in Utero

Until the eighth week of gestation, the initial reproductive structures of male and female embryos are homologous (the same), consisting of one pair of primary sex organs, or **gonads,** and two pairs of ducts: the mesonephric ducts (wolffian ducts) and the paramesonephric ducts (müllerian ducts) (Figure 31-1). Both pairs of ducts empty into the urogenital sinus.

At about 7 to 8 weeks of gestation, the gonads of genetically male embryos begin to produce **testosterone.** Under its influence, the male gonads develop into the two testes, which produce sperm after puberty. The paramesonephric ducts degenerate, and the mesonephric ducts develop into the vas deferens—the two tubes that carry sperm from the testes to the urethra.

The presence of *estrogen* and the absence of testosterone cause the two female gonads to develop into ovaries, which will produce ova. In females, the mesonephric ducts deteriorate, and the lower ends of the paramesonephric ducts join to become the uterus. The upper portions of the paramesonephric ducts develop into the fallopian (uterine) tubes. These two ducts will carry ova from the ovaries to the uterus during a woman's reproductive years.

Like the internal reproductive structures, the external structures develop from homologous embryonic tissues. During the first 7 to 8 weeks of gestation, both male and female embryos develop an elevated structure called the *genital tubercle* (Figure 31-2). Testosterone is necessary for the genital tubercle to differentiate into male genitalia;

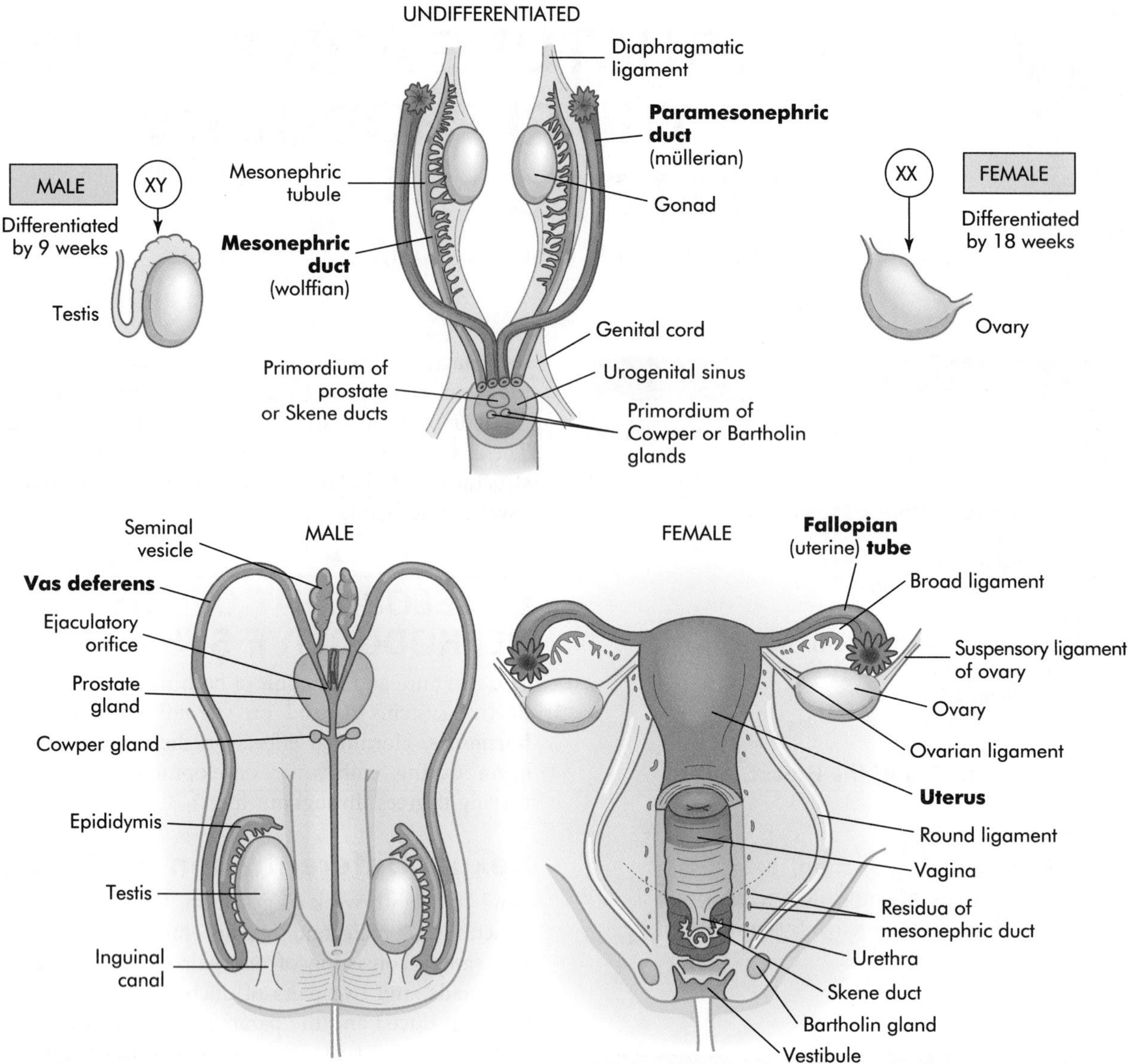

Figure 31-1 ■ **Internal Genitalia Development.** Embryonic and fetal development of the internal genitalia.

otherwise, female genitalia develop, which may occur even in the absence of ovaries, possibly because of the presence of placental estrogens.[1] By 9 months of gestation, the internal and external genital structures are all present and the male gonads (the testes) have descended into the scrotum.

At a term pregnancy, a sensitive negative-feedback system, which includes the **gonadostat** (also known as the **gonadotropin-releasing hormone pulse generator**), is operative in the human fetus. The gonadostat responds to high placental estrogens by releasing low levels of **gonadotropin-releasing hormone (GnRH).** Soon after birth, sex hormones (estrogen and testosterone) drop precipitously; negative feedback action of the sex hormones on the hypothalamus and pituitary is removed, and gonadotropin is released. Gonadostat is remarkably sensitive (6 to 15 times more sensitive than in the adult) to negative feedback,[1] and GnRH secretion is restrained by extraordinarily low levels of sex hormones.

Puberty

Between the ages of 8 and 12 years, the gonads begin to produce more of the sex hormones. This triggers sexual maturation, or puberty. Puberty is the process that involves a complex series of interrelated physiologic changes leading to reproductive maturation.[1] In girls, puberty begins at about age 8 to 9 years with thelarche (breast development). In boys, it begins later—at about age 11 years. Puberty lasts 2 or 3 years and is complete when the individual is capable of reproduction.

Although the exact trigger for puberty is unknown, it has been linked to obesity and, more recently, to the presence of **leptin,** a hormone secreted from adipose tissue.[2,3] Leptin may have an independent and direct effect on the hypothalamic-pituitary-gonadal axis or may affect it indirectly through an unidentified intermediary factor.[1]

Reproductive maturation involves the central nervous system (hypothalamus), the endocrine system (anterior

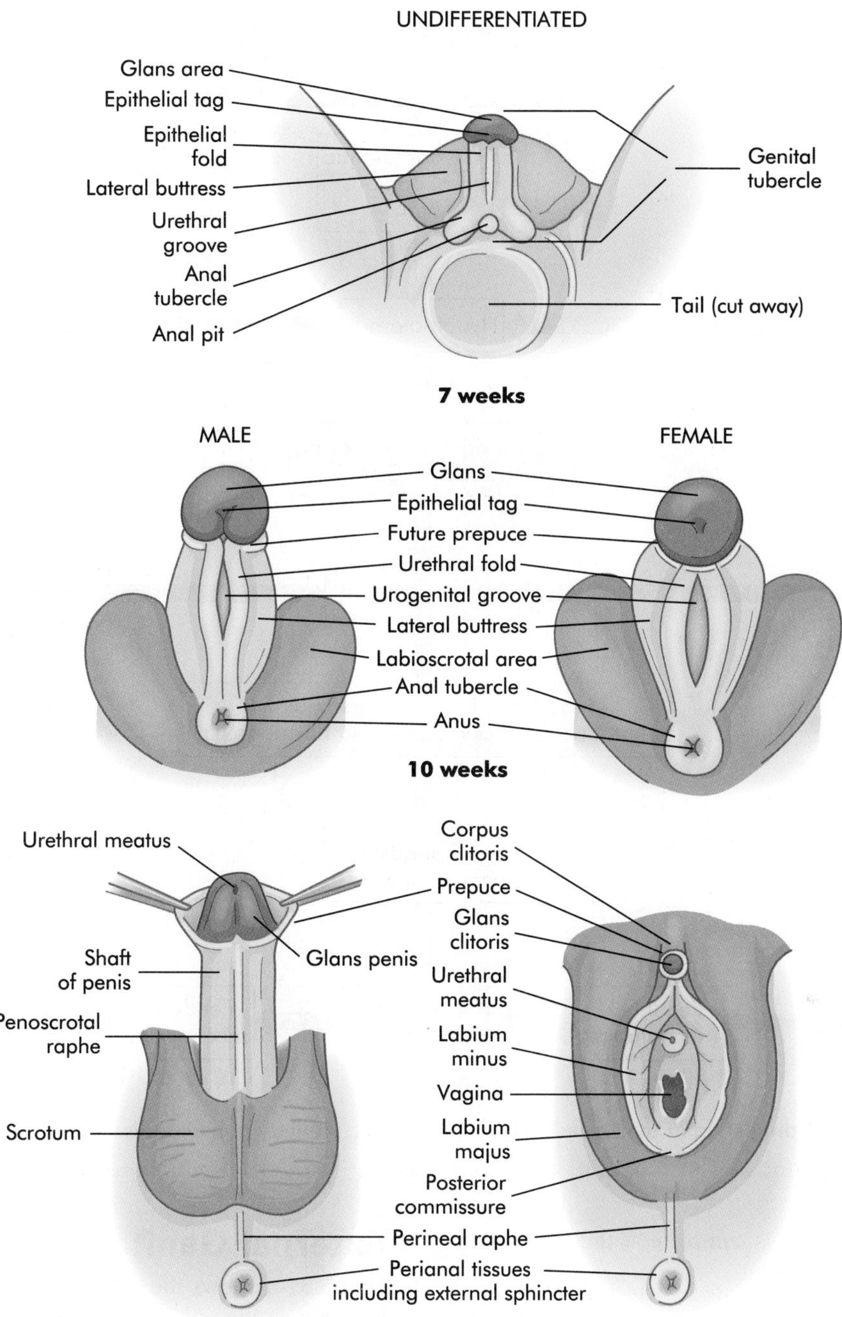

Figure 31-2 ■ **External Genitalia Development.** Embryonic and fetal development of the external genitalia.

pituitary), and the gonads themselves (ovaries and testes) (Figure 31-3). As puberty approaches, three critical endocrine changes occur: (1) **adrenarche,** which is the increase in production of adrenal androgens; (2) decreased gonadostat sensitivity, which establishes a pulsatile pattern of GnRH; and (3) development of a positive feedback system between the gonadotropins **luteinizing hormone (LH), follicle-stimulating hormone (FSH),** and GnRH. The hypothalamus produces greater amounts of GnRH, which stimulate the anterior pituitary to increase its production of LH and FSH. These gonadotropins then stimulate the gonads to produce more of the sex hormones, estrogen or testosterone, through a positive feedback loop.

Increased sex hormone production causes the genitalia to grow into their adult proportions and stimulates the development of male and female secondary sex characteristics (beard, voice changes, breast development, and pubic and axillary hair). The most important hormonal effects occur in the gonads, however. In males, the testes begin to produce mature sperm capable of fertilizing an ovum. Male puberty is complete with the first ejaculation that contains mature sperm. In females, the ovaries begin to release

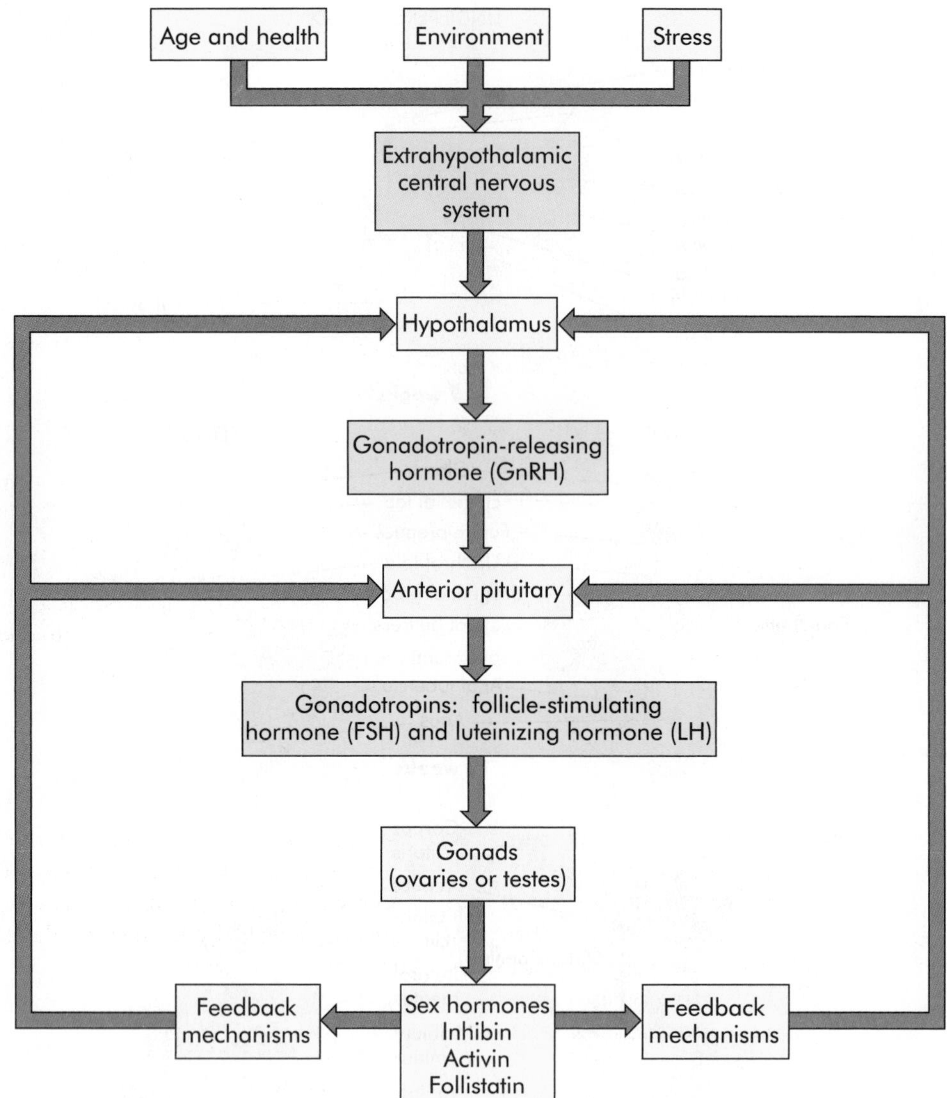

Figure 31-3 ■ **Hormonal Stimulation of the Gonads.** The hypothalamic-pituitary-gonadal axis.

mature ova. Female puberty is complete at the time of the first ovulatory menstrual period.

QUICK CHECK 31-1

1. When do sex hormones first exhibit an effect on sexual development?
2. Why are sex hormones necessary for reproduction?

THE FEMALE REPRODUCTIVE SYSTEM

In females, the most important reproductive organs, or genitalia, are internal. These organs are essential to reproduction and include ovaries, fallopian tubes, uterus, and vagina. The external genitalia protect body openings and play an important role in sexual functioning.[1,4,5]

External Genitalia

Figure 31-4 shows the external female genitalia, known collectively as the **vulva,** or pudendum. The major structures are as follows:

Mons pubis. Fatty layer of tissue over pubic symphysis (joint of the pubic bones); during puberty it becomes covered with pubic hair, and sebaceous and sweat glands become more active. Estrogen causes fat to be deposited under the skin, gives the mons pubis a moundlike shape, and protects the pubic symphysis during sexual intercourse.

Labia majora (*sing., labium majus*). Two folds of skin arising at mons pubis and extending back to fourchette, forming a cleft; during puberty the amount of fatty tissue increases, pubic hair grows on lateral surfaces, and sebaceous glands on hairless medial surfaces secrete lubricants. Highly sensitive to temperature, touch, pressure, and pain; homologous to the male scrotum; and protects the inner structures of the vulva.

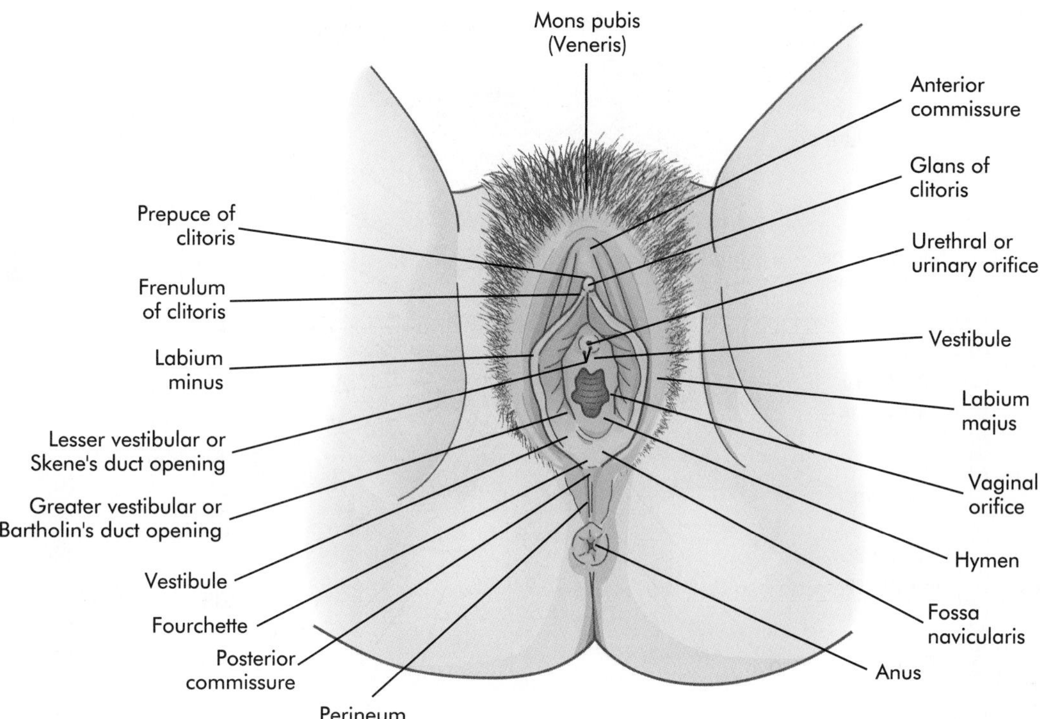

Figure 31-4 ■ **External Female Genitalia.**

Labia minora (sing., labium minus). Two smaller, thinner, asymmetrical folds of skin within the labia majora that form the clitoral hood (prepuce) and frenulum, then split to enclose vestibule, and converge near anus to form fourchette. Hairless, pink, moist, well supplied with nerves, blood vessels, and sebaceous glands that secrete bactericidal fluid with distinctive odor that lubricates and waterproofs vulvar skin. They swell with blood during sexual arousal.

Clitoris. Richly innervated erectile organ between labia minora; has a visible glans and a shaft that lies beneath the skin, homologous to the penis. Secretes smegma with a unique odor that may be sexually arousing to male. With sexual arousal, erectile tissue fills with blood causing it to enlarge slightly. Major site of sexual stimulation and orgasm.

Vestibule. Area protected by labia minora that contains openings to vagina and urethra or urinary meatus (orifice).

Introitus. Vaginal orifice covered by thin, perforated membrane (hymen).

Skene glands. Lesser vestibular or paraurethral glands that secrete fluids that help to lubricate the urinary meatus and vestibule and facilitate coitus.

Bartholin glands. Greater vestibular or vulvovaginal glands that secrete mucus to lubricate the inner labial surfaces and enhance the viability and motility of sperm. Also facilitate coitus.

Perineum. Area with less hair, skin, and subcutaneous tissue lying between vaginal orifice and anus; contains very little subcutaneous fat, so skin lies just above underlying muscles; stretches remarkably.

Perineal body. Fibrous structure composed of highly elastic fiber, connective tissue, and common attachment of bulbocavernosus, external anal sphincter, and levator ani muscles; covered by perineum. Varies in length from 2 to 5 cm.

Internal Genitalia

Vagina

The **vagina** is an elastic, fibromuscular canal that is 9 to 10 cm in length. It extends up and back from the introitus to the lower portion of the uterus. As Figure 31-5 shows, the vagina lies between the urethra (and part of the bladder) and the rectum. Mucosal secretions from the upper genital organs, menstrual fluids, and products of conception leave the body through the vagina, which also receives the penis during coitus. During sexual excitement, the vagina lengthens and widens and the anterior third becomes congested with blood.

The vaginal wall is composed of four layers:

1. Mucous membranous lining of squamous epithelial cells that thickens and thins in response to hormones, particularly estrogen. The squamous epithelial membrane is continuous with the membrane that covers the lower part of the uterus. In women of reproductive age, the mucosal layer is arranged in transverse wrinkles, or folds, called **rugae** (*sing.,* ruga) that permit stretching during coitus and childbirth.
2. Fibrous connective tissue containing numerous blood and lymphatic vessels.
3. Smooth muscle.
4. Connective tissue and a rich network of blood vessels.

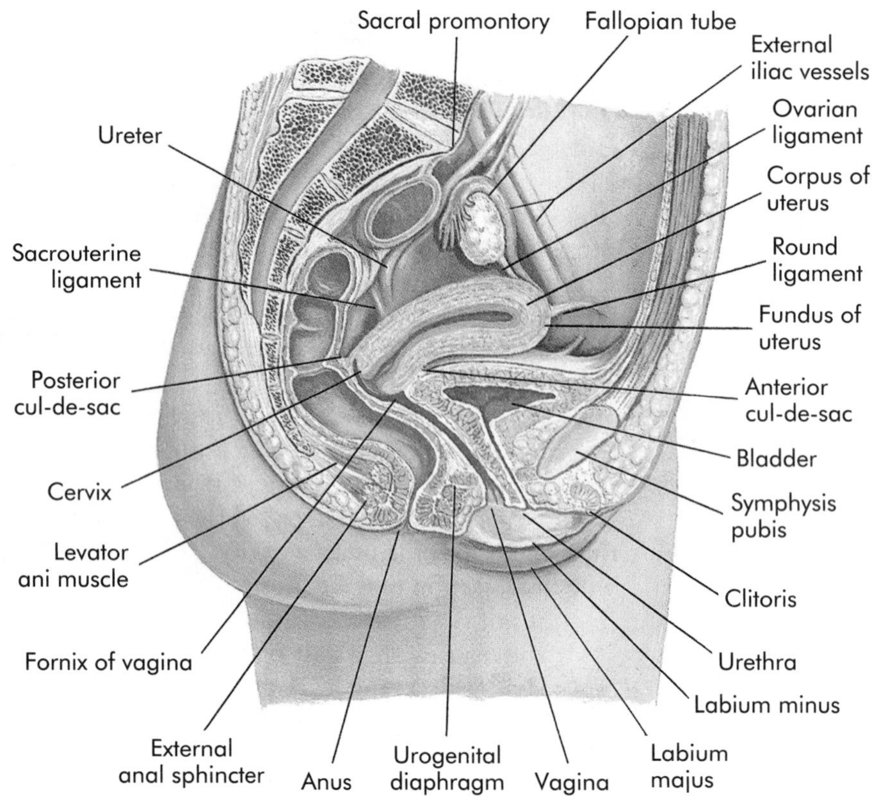

Figure 31-5 ■ Internal Female Genitalia and Other Pelvic Organs. (From Seidel HM et al: *Mosby's guide to physical examination,* ed 6, St Louis, 2006, Mosby.)

The upper part of the vagina surrounds the cervix, the lower end of the uterus (see Figure 31-5). The recessed space around the cervix is called the **fornix** of the vagina. The posterior fornix is "deeper" than the anterior fornix because of the angle at which the cervix meets the vaginal canal. In most women this angle is about 90 degrees. A pouch called the **cul-de-sac** separates the posterior fornix and the rectum.

Its elasticity and relatively sparse nerve supply enhance the vagina's function as the birth canal. During sexual arousal, the vaginal wall becomes engorged with blood, like the labia minora and clitoris. Engorgement pushes some fluid to the surface of the mucosa, enhancing lubrication. The vaginal wall does not contain mucus-secreting glands; rather, secretions drain into the vagina from the endocervical glands or enter from the vestibule from the Bartholin glands.

Two factors help to maintain the self-cleansing action of the vagina and to defend it from infection, particularly during the reproductive years. They are (1) an acid-base balance that discourages the proliferation of most pathogenic bacteria and (2) the thickness of the vaginal epithelium. Before puberty, vaginal pH is about 7.0 (neutral) and the vaginal epithelium is thin. At puberty, the pH becomes more acidic (4.0 to 5.0) and the squamous epithelial lining thickens. These changes are maintained until menopause (cessation of menstruation), when the pH rises again to more alkaline levels and the epithelium thins out. Therefore, protection from infection is greatest during the years when a woman is most likely to be sexually active. Both defenses are greatest when estrogen levels are high and the vagina contains a normal population of *Lactobacillus acidophilus,* a harmless resident bacterium that helps to maintain pH at acidic levels. Any condition that causes vaginal pH to rise, such as douching or use of vaginal sprays or deodorants, low estrogen levels, or destruction of *L. acidophilus* by antibiotics, lowers vaginal defenses against infection.

Uterus

The **uterus** is a hollow, pear-shaped organ whose lower end opens into the vagina. It anchors and protects a fertilized ovum, provides an optimal environment while the ovum develops, and pushes the fetus out at birth. In addition, the uterus plays an important role in sexual response and conception. During sexual excitement, the opening of the lower uterus (the cervix) dilates slightly. At the same time, the uterus increases in size and moves upward and backward, creating a tenting effect in the midvagina that results in the cervix "sitting" in a pool of semen. During orgasm, rhythmic contractions facilitate movement of sperm through the cervical os while also enhancing physical pleasure.

At puberty, the uterus attains its adult size and proportions and descends from the abdomen to the lower pelvis, between the bladder and the rectum (see Figure 31-5). The uterus of a mature, nonpregnant female is approximately 7 to 9 cm long and 6.5 cm wide, with muscular

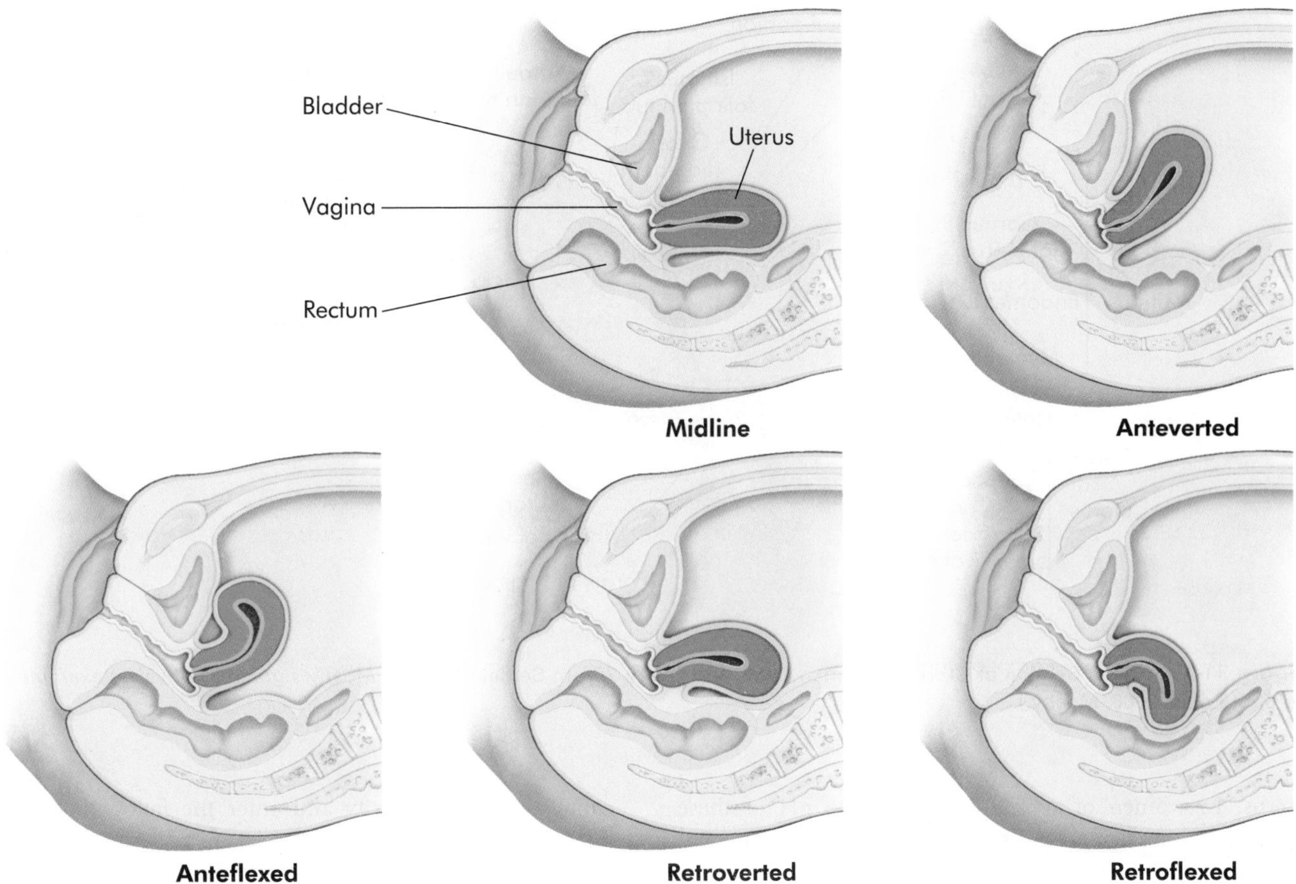

Figure 31-6 ■ **Uterine Positions.**

walls 3.5 cm thick.[1] It is held loosely in position by ligaments, peritoneal tissue folds, and pressure of adjacent organs, especially the urinary bladder, sigmoid colon, and rectum. In most women, the uterus is tipped forward (anteverted) so that it rests on the urinary bladder, but it may be tipped backward (retroverted). Various degrees of flexion are normal (Figure 31-6).

The uterus has two major parts: the body, or **corpus,** and the cervix (Figure 31-7). The top of the corpus, above the insertion of the fallopian tubes, is called the **fundus.** The diameter of the uterine cavity is widest at the fundus and narrowest at the **isthmus,** just above the **cervix** (see Figure 31-5). The cervix, or "neck of the uterus," extends from the isthmus to the vagina. The passageway between the cervix's upper opening (the internal os) and its lower opening (the external os) is called the **endocervical canal** (see Figure 31-7). The entire uterus, like the upper vagina, is innervated exclusively by motor and sensory fibers of the autonomic nervous system.

The uterine wall is composed of three layers (see Figure 31-7). The **perimetrium (parietal peritoneum)** is the outer serous membrane that covers the uterus. The **myometrium** is the thick, muscular middle layer. It is thickest at the fundus, apparently to facilitate birth. The **endometrium,** or uterine lining, is composed of a functional layer (superficial compact layer and spongy middle layer) and a basal layer. The functional layer of the endometrium responds to sex hormones, estrogen and progesterone. Between puberty and menopause, this layer proliferates and sloughs off monthly. The basal layer, which is attached to the myometrium, regenerates the functional layer after sloughing (menstruation).

The endocervical canal does not have an endometrial layer but is lined with columnar epithelial cells (see Box 1-1). It is continuous with the lining of the outer cervix and vagina, which are lined with squamous epithelial cells. The point where the two types of cells meet is called the *transformation zone,* or **squamous-columnar junction.** The transformation zone is the usual site of cervical dysplasia or carcinoma in situ and are the cells sampled during a Papanicolaou (Pap) smear.[1]

The cervix acts as a mechanical barrier to infectious microorganisms from the vagina. The external cervical os is a very small opening that contains thick, sticky mucus (the mucus "plug") during most of the menstrual cycle and all of pregnancy. During ovulation, the mucus changes under the influence of estrogen and forms watery strands, or **spinnbarkeit mucus,** to facilitate the transport of sperm into the uterus. In addition, the downward flow of cervical secretions moves microorganisms away from the cervix and

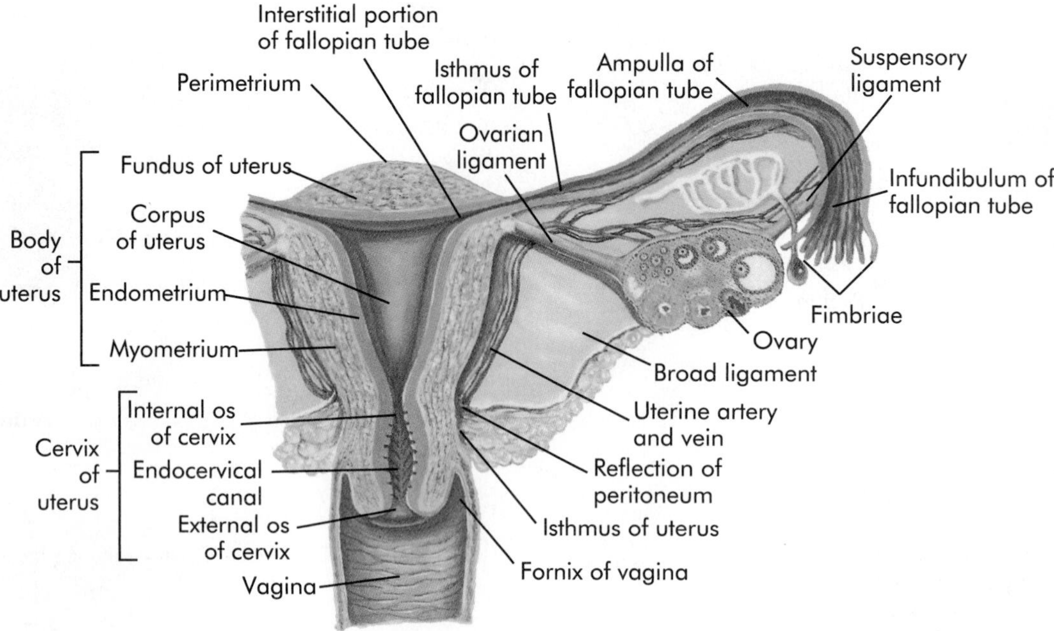

Figure 31-7 ■ Cross Section of Uterus, Fallopian Tube, and Ovary. (From Seidel HM et al: *Mosby's guide to physical examination,* ed 6, St Louis, 2006, Mosby.)

uterus. In women of reproductive age, the pH of these secretions is inhospitable to most bacteria. Further, mucosal secretions contain enzymes and antibodies (mostly immunoglobulin A [IgA]) of the secretory immune system. Uterine pathophysiology includes infection, displacement of the uterus within the pelvis, benign growths of the uterine wall, and cancer.

✓ QUICK CHECK 31-2

1. Name three functions of the uterus.
2. Where are the Bartholin glands located? What is their function?
3. What is the name of the cells in which cervical cancer is most likely to grow?

Fallopian tubes

The two **fallopian tubes** (oviducts, **uterine tubes**) enter the uterus bilaterally just beneath the fundus (see Figure 31-7). They conduct the ova from the spaces around the ovaries to the uterus. From the uterus, the fallopian tubes curve up and over the two ovaries. Each tube is 8 to 12 cm long and about 1 cm in diameter, except at its ovarian end, which flares out like the bell of a trumpet and is fringed or fimbriated **(infundibulum).** The **fimbriae** (fringes) move, creating a current that draws the ovum into the infundibulum. Once the ovum enters the fallopian tube, cilia and peristalsis (muscle contractions) keep it moving toward the uterus.

The ampulla, or distal third, of the fallopian tube is the usual site of fertilization (see Figure 31-7). Sperm released into the vagina travel upward through the endocervical canal and uterine cavity and enter the fallopian tubes. If an ovum is present in either tube, fertilization can occur. Whether or not the ovum encounters sperm, it continues to travel through the fallopian tube to the uterus. If fertilized, the ovum (then called a *blastocyst*) implants itself in the endometrial layer of the uterine wall. If not fertilized, the ovum breaks down and leaves the uterus with menstrual fluids. Disorders that affect the fallopian tubes (e.g., congenital malformations, infection, inflammation) block the path of both sperm and ovum and may cause infertility or ectopic (tubal) pregnancy.

Ovaries

The **ovaries,** the female gonads, are the primary female reproductive organs. Their two main functions are secretion of female sex hormones and development and release of female gametes, or ova.

The almond-shaped ovaries are located on both sides of the uterus and are suspended and supported by the mesovarian portions of the broad ligament, ovarian ligaments, and suspensory ligaments (see Figure 31-7). The ovaries are smaller than their male homologs, the testes. In women of reproductive age, each ovary is 3 to 5 cm long, 2.5 cm wide, and 2 cm thick and weighs 4 to 8 g. Size and weight vary somewhat from phase to phase of the menstrual cycle (see p. 831).

Figure 31-8 shows a cross section of an ovary. At birth, the cortex of each ovary contains approximately 1 million ova within immature **ovarian follicles.** By puberty, the number ranges between 200,000 and 400,000, and some of the follicles and the ova within them begin to mature. Between puberty and menopause, the ovarian cortex always contains follicles and ova in various stages of development.

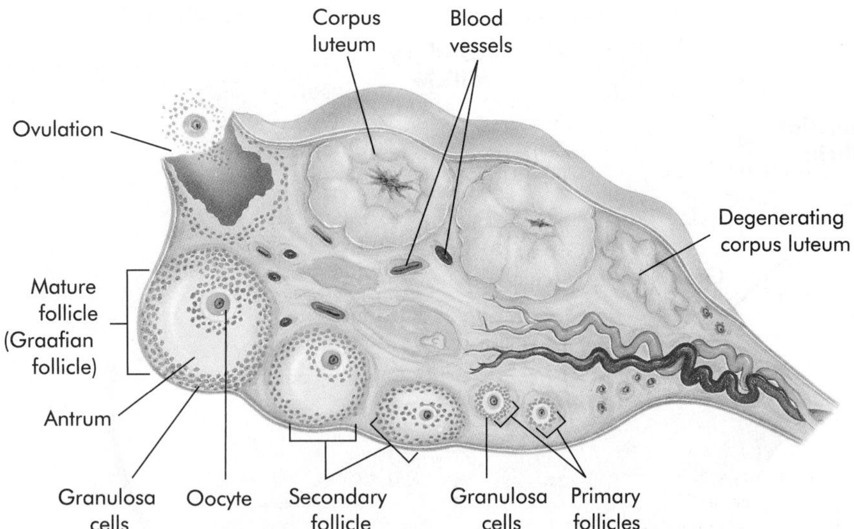

Figure 31-8 ■ **Cross Section of Ovary During Reproductive Years.** (From Thibodeau GA, Patton KT: *Anatomy & physiology,* ed 6, St Louis, 2007, Mosby.)

Once every menstrual cycle (about every 28 days), one of the follicles reaches maturation and discharges its ovum through the ovary's outer covering, the germinal epithelium. During the reproductive years, 300 to 500 ovarian follicles mature completely and release an ovum **(ovulation).** The rest either fail to develop at all or degenerate without maturing completely.[1]

Having ejected a mature ovum, the follicle develops into another structure, the **corpus luteum** (see Figure 31-8). If fertilization occurs, the corpus luteum enlarges and begins to secrete hormones that maintain and support pregnancy. If fertilization does not occur, the corpus luteum secretes these hormones for approximately 14 days and then degenerates, which triggers the maturation of another follicle. The **ovarian cycle**—the process of follicular maturation, ovulation, corpus luteum development, and corpus luteum degeneration—is continuous from puberty to menopause, except during pregnancy or hormonal contraceptive use. At menopause, this process ceases and the ovaries atrophy to the point that they cannot be felt during a pelvic examination.

Sex hormones are secreted by four types of cells present within the ovarian cortex: cells of the stroma, or tissue matrix; two types of cells in the ovarian follicle, **granulosa cells** and **theca cells;** and cells of the corpus luteum (Figure 31-9). These cells all contain receptors for the gonadotropins (LH, FSH) or for the sex hormones, which are discussed in the next section.

Because ovarian function is regulated by hormones, any disorder, such as abnormal pituitary or thyroid function, that disrupts hormone secretion or reception by target cells can cause ovarian dysfunction and infertility. Benign or malignant growths, cysts, infection, or inflammation also can cause ovarian pathologic conditions.

Female Sex Hormones

The sex hormones are all steroid hormones—that is, they are synthesized from cholesterol (see Chapter 17). Most of them, both male and female, are present in adults of both genders all the time. The female body contains low levels of testosterone, for example, and the male body contains low levels of estrogen. The effects of the sex hormones depend on their amount and concentration in the blood.

Steroid hormones produced by the ovaries maintain female characteristics throughout life. During fetal development, infancy, and childhood, sex hormone production is low. At puberty, hormone production surges, causing sexual maturation and development of secondary sex characteristics. From puberty to menopause, the sex hormones control the ovarian-menstrual cycle, pregnancy, and lactation. The dominant female sex hormones are estrogen and progesterone.[1,5] These two hormones are not produced steadily. Rather, their production surges and diminishes monthly, creating the ovarian-menstrual cycle.

Estrogens

Estrogen is a generic term for any of three similar hormones: estradiol, estrone, and estriol. **Estradiol (E2)** is the most potent and plentiful of the three and is principally produced (95%) by the ovaries (ovarian follicle and corpus luteum). Limited amounts are secreted by the cortices of the adrenal glands and the placenta during pregnancy. Androgens are converted to estrone in ovarian and peripheral adipose tissue; estriol is the peripheral metabolite of estrone and estradiol.

Estrogen is needed for maturation of reproductive organs, development of secondary sex characteristics, closure of long bones after the pubertal growth spurt, regulation of the ovarian-menstrual cycle, endometrial regeneration after menstruation, endometrial maintenance during pregnancy, and it promotes growth of the breast ductile system in preparation for lactation.[6] Estrogen also has metabolic effects on the bones, liver, blood vessels, blood, central nervous system, kidneys, and skin. During the reproductive years, estrogen helps to maintain the density

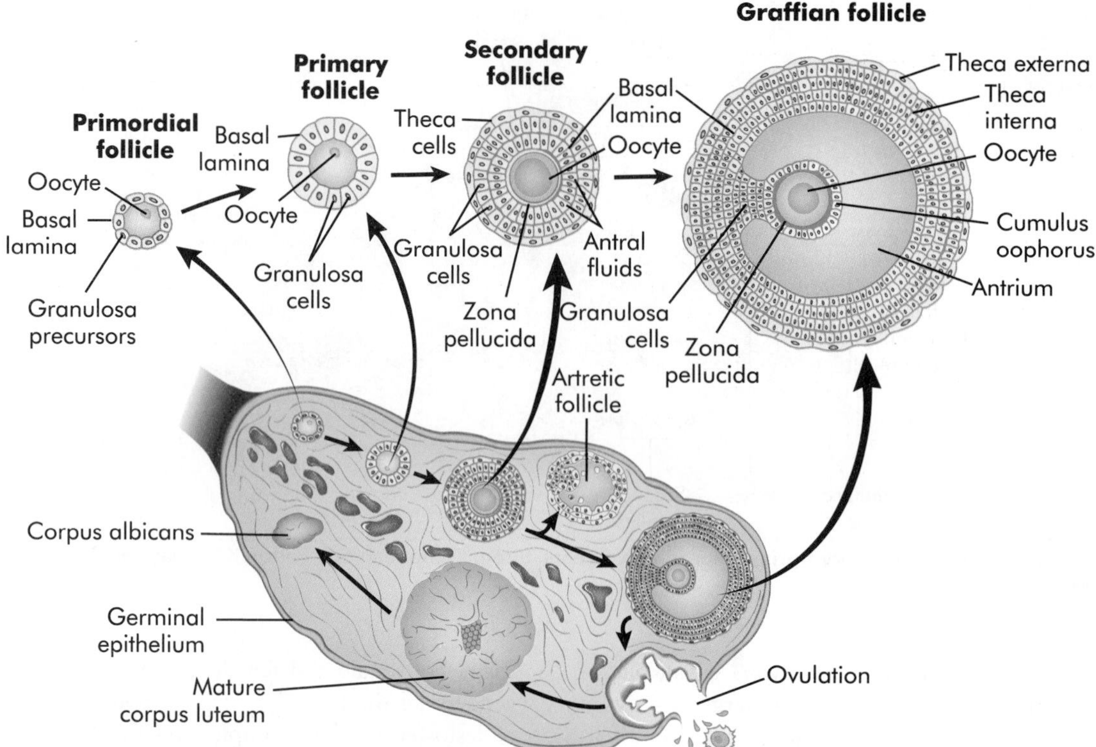

Figure 31-9 ■ **Development of an Ovarian Follicle.** Schematic representation (not to scale) of the structure of the ovary, showing the various stages in the development of the follicle and its successor structure, the corpus luteum. (Adapted from Berne RM, Levy MN, editors: *Physiology,* ed 5, St Louis, 2003, Mosby.)

of bone. After menopause, the ovaries dramatically reduce production of estradiol and secretion of estrone is also markedly diminished. For this reason, postmenopausal women are susceptible to osteoporosis, a condition in which bone density is reduced.

Disturbances of estrogen production can be caused by abnormalities that affect (1) secretion of GnRH by the hypothalamus, (2) secretion of LH or FSH by the anterior pituitary, (3) hormonal feedback mechanisms, or (4) structural integrity of the ovaries. Estrogen's role in the menstrual cycle is described on pages 832-833.

Progesterone

Luteinizing hormone (LH) from the anterior pituitary stimulates the corpus luteum to secrete **progesterone,** the second major female sex hormone. With estrogen, progesterone controls the ovarian-menstrual cycle. Large amounts of progesterone are secreted while the corpus luteum is active, about 9 to 13 days after ovulation. Small amounts of progesterone are secreted steadily by the adrenal cortices.

Progesterone secreted by the corpus luteum stimulates the thickened endometrium to become more complex in preparation for implantation of a blastocyte. If conception and implantation do occur, the corpus luteum persists and secretes progesterone (and estrogen) throughout pregnancy.

Progesterone is sometimes called the *hormone of pregnancy.* During pregnancy, it is produced not only by the corpus luteum but also by the placenta. During pregnancy, it (1) maintains the thickened endometrium; (2) relaxes smooth muscle in the myometrium, which prevents premature contractions and helps the uterus to expand; (3) thickens the myometrium, which prepares it for the muscular work of labor; (4) promotes growth of lobules and alveoli in the breast in preparation for lactation[6] but prevents lactation until the fetus is born; and (5) prevents additional maturation of ova by suppressing FSH and LH, thereby stopping the menstrual cycle. Progesterone and estrogen have some opposing and complementary effects, which are summarized in Table 31-1.

Androgens

Although **androgens** are primarily male sex hormones, small amounts of them are produced in the ovaries and adrenal cortices of females. Some androgens are precursors of female sex hormones, notably estrogen and androstenedione. At puberty, androgens contribute to the skeletal growth spurt and cause growth of pubic and axillary hair. The androgens also activate sebaceous glands, accounting for some cases of acne during puberty; they also play a role in libido function.

TABLE 31-1

Complementary and Opposing Effects of Estrogen and Progesterone

Structure	Effect of Estrogen	Effect of Progesterone
Vaginal mucosa	Proliferation of squamous epithelium; increase in glycogen content of cells; layering (cornification) of cells	Thinning of squamous epithelium; decornification
Cervical mucosa	Production of abundant fluid secretions that favor survival and enhance motility of sperm	Production of thick, sticky secretions that tend to plug the cervical os
Fallopian tube	Increase of motility and ciliary action	Decrease of motility and ciliary action
Uterine muscle	Increase of blood flow; increase of contractile proteins and uterine muscle and myometrial excitability and action potential; increase of sensitization to oxytocin	Relaxation of myometrium; decrease of sensitization to oxytocin
Endometrium	Stimulation of growth; increase in number of progesterone receptors	Activation of glands and blood vessels; decrease in number of estrogen receptors
Breasts	Growth of ducts; promotion of prolactin effects	Growth of lobules and alveoli; inhibition of prolactin effects

QUICK CHECK 31-3

1. What hormones does the ovary produce?
2. Why is the ovary the most essential female reproductive organ?

Menstrual Cycle

Besides pregnancy, the obvious manifestation of female reproductive functioning is menstrual bleeding (the menses), which starts with **menarche** (first menstruation) and ends with **menopause** (cessation of menstrual flow). In the United States, the average age of first menstruation is 12.5 years, with a range from 9 to 17 years. Menarche appears to be related to body weight, especially percentage of body fat (ratio of fat to lean tissue), which may trigger a change in the metabolic rate and lead to hormonal changes associated with ovulation. The presence of leptin, a hormone secreted from adipose tissue, is thought to inhibit the gonadostat and trigger puberty.[2] At first, cycles are anovulatory and may vary in length from 10 to 60 days or more. As adolescence proceeds, regular patterns of menstruation and ovulation are established at intervals ranging between 30 and 35 days.[7] During adulthood, menstruation continues to recur in a recognizable and characteristic pattern, with the length of the menstrual cycle varying considerably among women. The commonly accepted cycle average is 28 (25 to 30) days, with rhythmic intervals of 21 to 45 days considered normal. Approximately 2 to 8 years before menopause, cycles begin to lengthen again. Menstrual cyclicity and regular ovulation are dependent on (1) the activity of the gonadostat (GnRH pulse generator); (2) the pituitary secretion of gonadotropins; and (3) estrogen (estradiol) positive feedback for the preovulatory LH surge, oocyte maturation, and corpus luteum formation.[2]

Phases of the menstrual cycle

The menstrual cycle consists of one event and three phases. The event is ovulation: the release of an ovum from a mature ovarian follicle. The three phases are the follicular (ovarian)/proliferative (endometrium) phase, the luteal (ovarian)/secretory (endometrium) phase, and the ischemic (endometrium)/menstrual (endometrium) phase (Figure 31-10).

During **menstruation (menses),** the functional layer of the endometrium disintegrates and is discharged through the vagina. Menstruation is followed by the **follicular/proliferative phase.** This phase is named for two simultaneous processes: maturation of an ovarian follicle and proliferation of the endometrium (see Figure 31-10). During this phase, the anterior pituitary gland secretes FSH, which causes an ovarian follicle to develop. While the follicle is developing, its granulosa cells secrete estrogen and the estrogen causes cells of the endometrium to proliferate. By the time the ovarian follicle is mature, the endometrial lining is restored and ovulation occurs.

Ovulation marks the beginning of the **luteal/secretory phase** of the menstrual cycle. The ovarian follicle begins its transformation into a corpus luteum (see Figure 31-8). LH from the anterior pituitary stimulates the corpus luteum to secrete progesterone, which in turn initiates the secretory phase of endometrial development. Glands and blood vessels in the endometrium branch and curl throughout the functional layer, and the glands begin to secrete a thin, glycogen-containing fluid. If conception occurs, the nutrient-laden endometrium is ready for implantation. If conception and implantation do not occur, the corpus luteum degenerates and ceases its production of progesterone and estrogen. Without progesterone or estrogen to maintain it, the endometrium enters the ischemic ("blood-starved") phase and disintegrates, the **ischemic/menstrual phase.** Then menstruation occurs, marking the beginning of another cycle.

Ovulatory cycles appear to have a minimum length of 24 to 26.5 days: the ovarian follicle requires 10 to 12.5 days to develop, and the luteal phase appears fixed at 14 days (±3 days). Menstrual blood flow usually lasts 3 to 7 days but may last as long as 8 days or stop after 2 days and still be considered within normal limits. Bleeding is consistently scant to heavy and varies from 30 ml to 80 ml, with most blood loss occurring during the first 3 days of menses. Menstrual discharge consists of blood, mucus, and desquamated endometrial tissue and fails to clot under normal

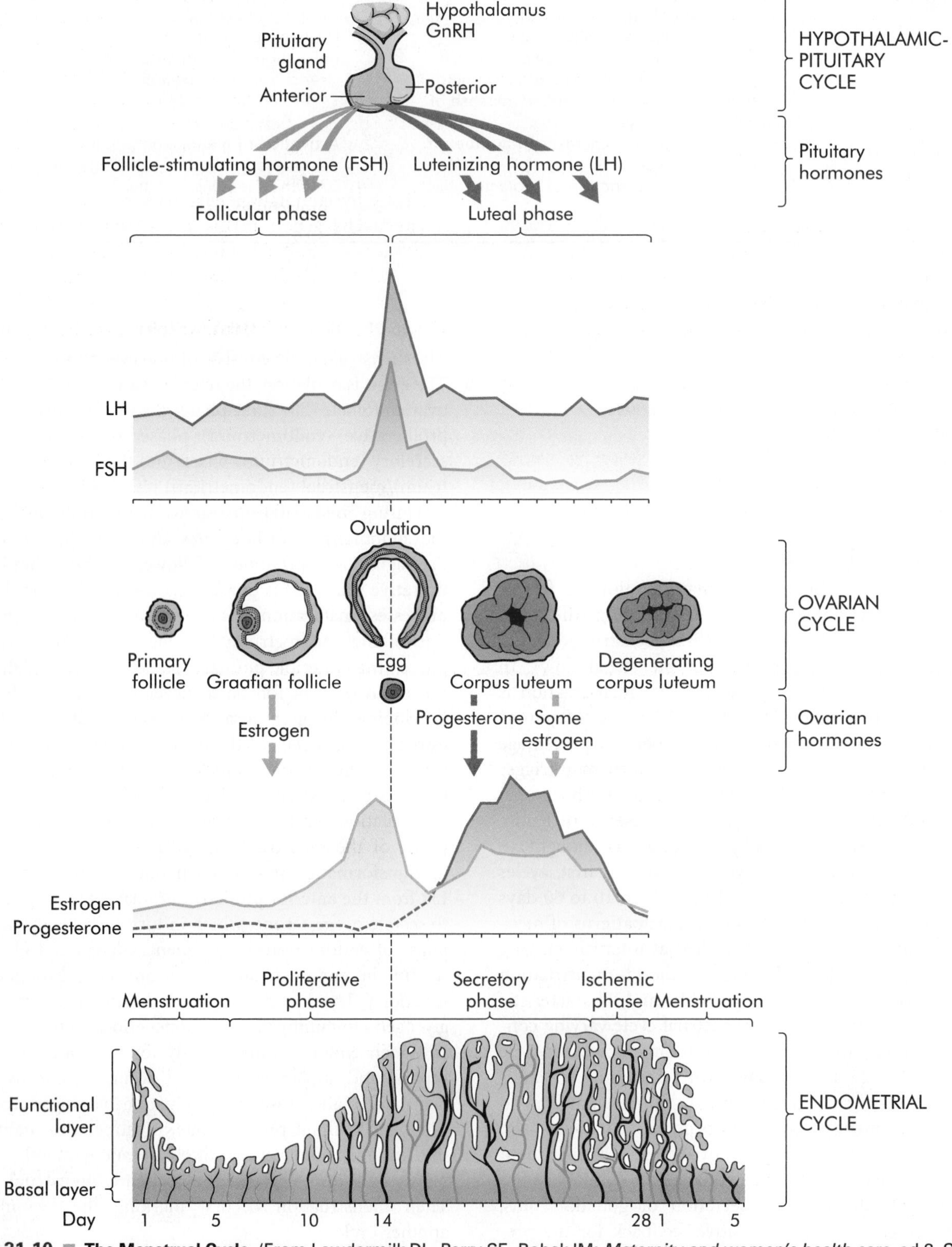

Figure 31-10 ■ **The Menstrual Cycle.** (From Lowdermilk DL, Perry SE, Bobak IM: *Maternity and women's health care*, ed 8, St Louis, 2004, Mosby.)

circumstances. It is usually dark and produces a characteristic musty odor on oxidation. Environmental factors (e.g., severe emotional stress, illness, malnutrition, seasonal variation) may affect the length of the menstrual cycle.[1,8]

Hormonal controls

Hormonal control of the menstrual cycle depends on complex interactions among the hypothalamus, the anterior pituitary, and the ovaries (or hypothalamic-pituitary-ovarian [H-P-O] axis)[9] (Table 31-2). GnRH is secreted by the hypothalamus into the hypophyseal portal system and travels to the anterior pituitary, where it stimulates the secretion of FSH and LH. FSH and LH are released from the anterior pituitary in pulses that correspond to the secretion of GnRH.

Blood levels of estrogen and progesterone exert a feedback effect on the hypothalamus and the anterior pituitary, thereby determining how much and when FSH and LH are secreted (see Table 31-2). FSH and LH secretion are not completely parallel—that is, FSH and LH are not secreted simultaneously in equal amounts throughout the menstrual cycle. Nonparallel secretion is caused by cyclic changes in feedback mechanisms. During the early follicular phase, low levels of estrogen inhibit the FSH-secreting cells of the anterior pituitary. In addition, the developing ovarian follicle secretes **inhibin,** a protein hormone that inhibits both GnRH and FSH secretion. As the ovarian follicle grows, it produces more and more estrogen. During the late follicular phase, a rise in progesterone facilitates a positive feedback loop whereby estrogen levels begin to increase, stimulating a surge of FSH and LH secretion from the anterior pituitary. The midcycle surge of LH causes ovulation. Rising estrogen and progesterone levels during the luteal phase may inhibit the anterior pituitary and thus LH and FSH secretion. Just before menstruation, FSH and LH levels begin to increase slightly, probably because of declining estrogen and progesterone levels (Figure 31-11).

A variety of growth factors and autocrine/paracrine peptides influence hormonal control and follicular response.[1] During the early follicular stage, FSH stimulates FSH and LH receptors, insulin-like growth factor-I, and production of inhibin and activin in the ovary. **Activin** has a positive feedback by stimulating FSH release in the pituitary and augments its action in the ovary and possibly increases FSH receptors but does not increase LH release. Inhibin inhibits FSH synthesis and secretion, inhibits prolactin and growth hormone release, interferes with GnRH receptors, and promotes breakdown of intracellular gonadotropins.[1,8,10] To a lesser degree, **follistatin,** a polypeptide produced by the pituitary but found primarily in the follicles, suppresses FSH activity, probably by binding to activin. In summary, the balance between activin and inhibin regulates FSH secretion and follistatin inhibits activin and boosts inhibin activity. Inhibin and activin also regulate LH stimulation of androgen synthesis in theca cells.

TABLE 31-2

Hormonal Feedback Mechanism in the Menstrual Cycle

Phase of Cycle and Ovarian Hormone Levels	Feedback to Hypothalamus and Anterior Pituitary	Resultant GnRH, FSH, and LH Levels	Ovarian and Menstrual Events
Early follicular phase: estrogen levels low; minute amount of progesterone secreted	Negative and inhibitory	All low	Ovarian follicle develops; endometrium proliferates
Late follicular (preovulatory) phase: estrogen levels high; progesterone increases with small surge before ovulation	Positive and stimulatory	All surge; LH dominates	Process of ovulation begins; endometrial proliferation complete
Ovulatory phase: estrogen levels dip; progesterone levels begin to rise	Negative and inhibitory	All fall sharply	Corpus luteum begins to develop; endometrium enters secretory phase
Early luteal phase: estrogen and progesterone levels high; progesterone dominates	Negative and inhibitory	All continue to decline, but gradually	Corpus luteum fully developed; endometrium ready for implantation
Late luteal phase: estrogen and progesterone levels fall sharply	Negative and inhibitory; feedback lessens slightly	All rise slightly	Corpus luteum regresses; endometrium breaks down; menstruation begins
Menstrual phase: estrogens levels low; minute amount of progesterone secreted	Negative and inhibitory	All low	More ovarian follicles begin to develop; functional layer of endometrium is shed

GnRH, Gonadotropin-releasing hormone; *FSH,* follicle-stimulating hormone; *LH,* luteinizing hormone.

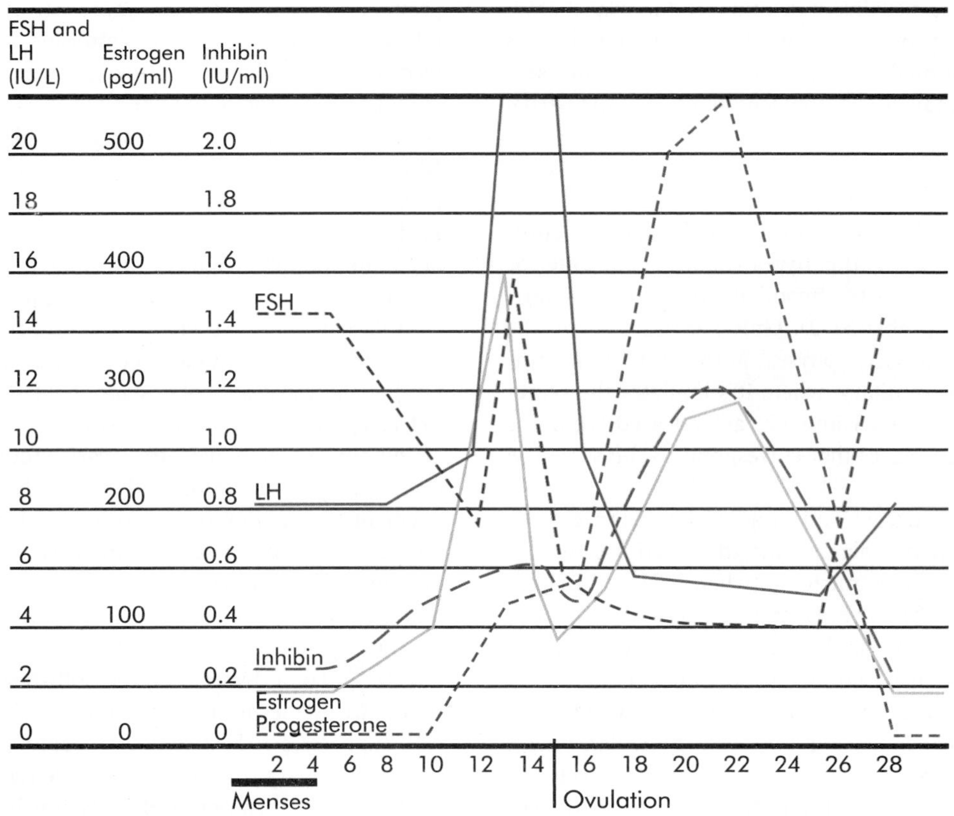

Figure 31-11 ■ **Estrogen, Progesterone, Gonadotropin, and Inhibin Fluctuations Over the Menstrual Cycle.** Inhibin rises slowly but steadily throughout the follicular phase, peaking at midcycle and again during the midluteal phase. The midcycle peak coincides with surges of luteinizing hormone (LH) and follicle-stimulating hormone (FSH).

Figure 31-11 depicts fluctuating estrogen, progesterone, gonadotropin, and inhibin levels.

Ovarian cycle

By stimulating follicles, gonadotropins initiate their growth and maturation. The most important hormonal event is a rise in FSH. The decline in luteal phase estrogen, progesterone, and inhibin secretion allows FSH to rise; concurrently there is a slight increase in LH levels (see Figure 31-11). FSH stimulates granulosa cell growth and initiates estrogen production in these cells. At this time, a group of ovarian follicles is recruited and begins to mature; the exact number depends on the remaining pool of inactive follicles. As the follicles mature, granulosa cells multiply, increasing estradiol secretion. Within a few days of the cycle, one follicle becomes dominant and the others atrophy. The dominant follicle begins to secrete progressively larger amounts of estradiol, which exerts a positive-feedback effect causing the LH surge. Ovulation occurs about 12 to 36 hours after the onset of the LH surge. Progesterone, proteolytic enzymes, and prostaglandins trigger follicular rupture and the release of ovum.[1]

The LH surge also transforms the granulosa cells of the ovulatory follicle into the corpus luteum. This secretes both estrogen and progesterone in amounts that depend, in part, on adequate development of the follicle before ovulation. Progesterone suppresses new follicular growth during the early to midluteal phases. If pregnancy does not occur, the corpus luteum persists for 14 days and then regresses and eventually disappears.[7]

Uterine phases

Uterine phases of the menstrual cycle—the proliferative phase, the secretory phase, and menstruation—involve the cyclic changes that occur in the endometrium. During the midfollicular phase, increasing levels of estrogen contribute to endometrial repair and proliferation, thus increasing endometrial thickness. Once ovulation occurs and serum progesterone levels increase, the endometrial tissue develops secretory characteristics. If implantation of a fertilized ovum does not take place, endometrial tissue begins to break down approximately 11 days after ovulation (ischemic phase of menstruation; see Figure 31-10). Sloughing of tissue (menstrual bleeding) begins about 14 days after ovulation.

Cervical mucus also undergoes cyclic changes. During the proliferative phase, the cervical mucus is thin and watery. With the preovulatory surge of LH and estradiol, it becomes more elastic and abundant (spinnbarkeit). Increasing estrogen levels apparently contribute to the development of tiny channels in cervical mucus, providing access for sperm. Changes in the consistency of cervical mucus can be used to identify fertile intervals.[7]

Vaginal response

The vaginal endothelium also responds to the cyclic hormonal changes of the menstrual cycle. Under the influence of estrogen, cells of the vaginal epithelium grow maximally during the follicular/proliferative phase. After ovulation, layers of keratinized cells overgrow the basal epithelium, a process known as **cornification.** Near the end of the luteal phase, leukocytes invade vaginal epithelium, removing the outer layers in a process termed **decornification.**

Body temperature

Basal body temperature (BBT) undergoes characteristic biphasic changes during menstrual cycles in which ovulation occurs. During the follicular phase, the BBT fluctuates around 98° F (37° C). During the luteal phase, the average temperature increases by 0.4° to 1.0° F (0.2° to 0.5° C). At the end of the luteal phase, 1 to 3 days before the onset of menstruation, BBT declines to follicular-phase levels. The shift in temperature is related to ovulation, corpus luteum formation, and increased serum progesterone levels. Progesterone probably acts on the thermoregulatory center of the hypothalamus to increase body temperature. Changes in BBT are used to document ovulatory cycles but are not useful to predict the exact timing of ovulation.

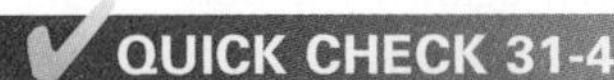

1. Why does menstruation occur?
2. What event is associated with the luteal/secretory phase of the menstrual cycle?

THE MALE REPRODUCTIVE SYSTEM

In men, the external genitalia perform the major functions of reproduction. Sperm are produced in the male gonads, the testes, and delivered by the penis. The internal male genitalia have a more accessory function. They consist of conducting tubes and fluid-producing glands, all of which aid in the transport of sperm from the testes to the urethral opening of the penis. The male reproductive and urinary structures are shown in Figure 31-12.

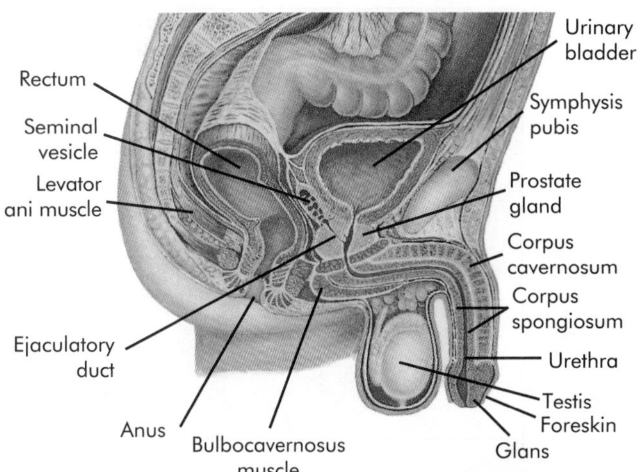

Figure 31-12 ■ **Structure of the Male Reproductive Organs.** (From Seidel HM et al: *Mosby's guide to physical examination,* ed 6, St Louis, 2006, Mosby.)

External Genitalia

Testes

In men, the testes are the essential organs of reproduction.[11] Like the ovaries, the testes have two functions: (1) production of gametes (i.e., sperm) and (2) production of sex hormones (i.e., androgens and testosterone). The testes are suspended outside the pelvic cavity.

During embryonic and fetal life, the testes develop within the abdomen (see Figure 31-1). About 3 months before birth, the testes start to descend toward the developing scrotum. About 1 month before birth, they enter twin passageways called **inguinal canals.** The inguinal canals are vaginal processes created by outpouchings of the peritoneum (lining of the abdominal cavity). The descent of a testis is shown in Figure 31-13. When descent is complete, the abdominal end of each vaginal process closes up, and the inguinal canal disappears. Failure of the testes to descend through the inguinal canal is known as cryptorchidism. The scrotal end of each vaginal process becomes the outer covering of the testis, the **tunica vaginalis.**

Figure 31-14 shows a sagittal section of a mature testis. The adult **testis** is oval and varies considerably in length (3 to 6 cm), width (2 to 3.5 cm), depth (3 to 4 cm), and weight (10 to 40 g). The testis is almost entirely surrounded by the tunica vaginalis, which separates the testis from the scrotal wall, and the **tunica albuginea.** Inward extensions of the tunica albuginea separate the testis into about 250 compartments, or lobules, each of which contains several tortuously coiled ducts called **seminiferous tubules.** Sperm are produced in these tubules. (Sperm production, termed *spermatogenesis,* is described on pp. 838-839.) Tissue surrounding these ducts contains **Leydig cells,** which occur in clusters and produce androgens, chiefly testosterone.

The two ends of each seminiferous tubule join and leave the lobule through the **tubulus rectus,** which lead to the central portion of the testis, the **rete testis.** The sperm then move through the **efferent tubules,** or vasa efferentia, to the epididymis, where they mature.

The testes are innervated by adrenergic fibers whose sole function apparently is to regulate blood flow to the Leydig cells. Arterial blood from the internal spermatic and differential arteries flows over the surface of the testes before entering the parenchyma (functional tissues). Surface flow cools the blood to temperatures that promote spermatogenesis, approximately 1° to 2° C below body core temperature.

Epididymis

The **epididymis** (*pl.,* epididymides) is a comma-shaped structure that curves over the posterior portion of each testis (see Figure 31-14). It consists of a single, 60- to 70-cm, densely packed and markedly coiled duct measuring 5 cm

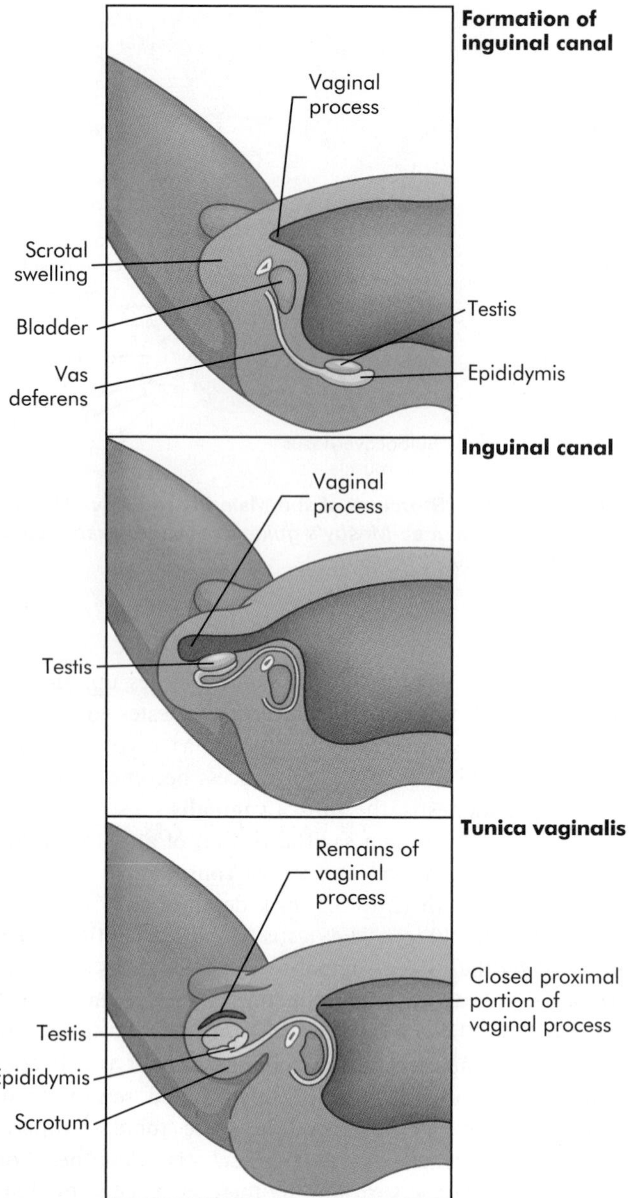

Figure 31-13 ■ **Descent of a Testis.** The testes descend from the abdominal cavity to the scrotum during the last 3 months of fetal development.

in length. The epididymis has structural and physiologic functions. Its structural function is to conduct sperm from the efferent tubules to the vas deferens, while physiologic functions include maturation, mobility, and fertility. When sperm enter the head of the epididymis, they are not fully mature or motile, nor can they fertilize an ovum. During the 12 days (or more) sperm take to travel the length of the epididymis, they receive nutrients and testosterone and their capacity for fertilization is enhanced.

After traveling the length of the epididymis, sperm are stored in the epididymal tail and vas deferens. The **vas deferens** is a duct with muscular layers capable of powerful peristalsis that transports sperm toward the urethra. The vas deferens enters the pelvic cavity through the spermatic cord (see Figure 31-14).

Scrotum

The testes, epididymides, and spermatic cord are enclosed and protected by the **scrotum,** a skin-covered, fibromuscular sac homologous to the female labia majora (see Figure 31-2). The skin of the scrotum is thin and has rugae (wrinkles or folds), which enable it to enlarge or relax away from the body. At puberty the scrotal skin darkens, develops active sebaceous glands, and becomes sparsely covered with hair. Just under the skin lies a layer of connective tissue (fascia) and smooth muscle, the **tunica dartos** (see Figure 31-13). The tunica dartos also forms a septum that separates the two testes. Exposure to cold temperatures causes the tunica dartos to contract, pulling the testes close to the warm body. In warm temperatures, the tunica dartos relaxes, suspending the testes away from body heat. These mechanisms promote optimal temperatures for spermatogenesis. In addition, scrotal sensitivity to touch, pressure, temperature, and pain protects the testes from potential harm. During sexual excitement, the scrotal skin and tunica thicken, the scrotum tightens and lifts, and the spermatic cords shorten, partially elevating the testes toward the body. As excitement plateaus, the engorged testes increase 50% in size, rotate anteriorly, and flatten against the body, signaling impending ejaculation.

Penis

The **penis** has two main functions: delivery of sperm and elimination of urine. (Urine formation and excretion are discussed in Chapter 28.) Embryonically, the penis is homologous to the female clitoris (see Figure 31-2).

Figure 31-12 shows a sagittal section of the adult penis and its anatomic relation to other urogenital structures. Externally, the penis consists of a shaft with a tip, the **glans,** which contains the opening of the urethra (Figure 31-15). The skin of the glans folds over the tip of the penis, forming the **prepuce,** or **foreskin.** The skin of the penis is continuous with that of the groin, scrotum, and inner thighs. It is hairless, movable, and darker than surrounding skin.

Internally, the penis consists of the urethra and three compartments: two **corpora cavernosa** and the **corpus spongiosum** (Figure 31-15) separated by Buck fascia; like the testes, the compartments are enclosed by a tunica albuginea. The **urethra** passes through the corpus spongiosum and ends at a sagittal slit in the glans. If the urethra is not completely surrounded by the corpus spongiosum, the meatus may open on the ventral surface of the penile shaft (hypospadias) or on the dorsal surface (epispadias).

Penetration of the female vagina is made possible by the **erectile reflex,** a process in which erectile tissues within the corpora cavernosa and corpus spongiosum become engorged with blood. The erectile tissues consist of vascular spaces, or chambers, supplied with blood by arterioles (small arteries). Usually, the arterioles are constricted, so that not much blood flows through the erectile tissues. Sexual stimulation, however, causes the arterioles to dilate and fill with blood, expanding the erectile tissues and causing an erection. Erection apparently is maintained by compression

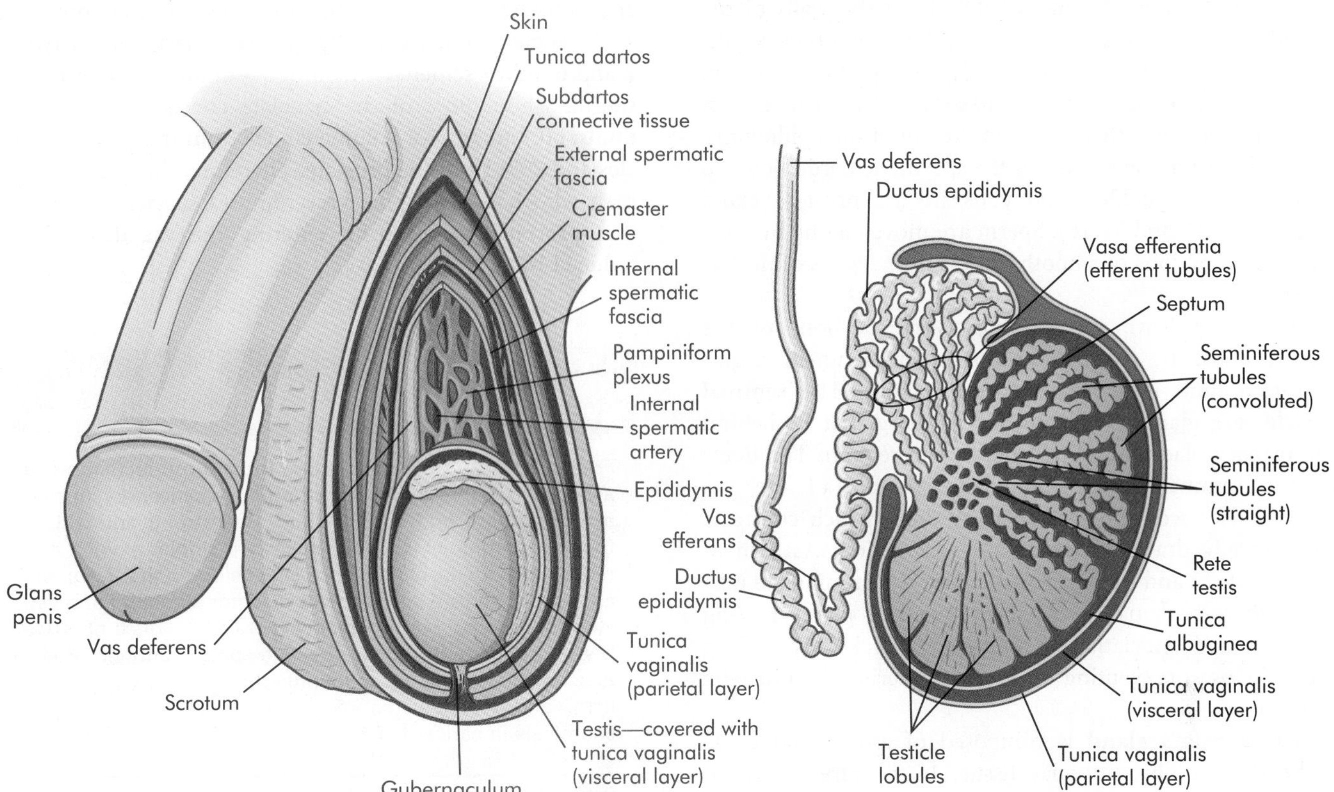

Figure 31-14 ■ **The Testes.** External and sagittal views showing interior anatomy. (Redrawn from Seidel HM et al: *Mosby's guide to physical examination*, ed 5, St Louis, 2003, Mosby.)

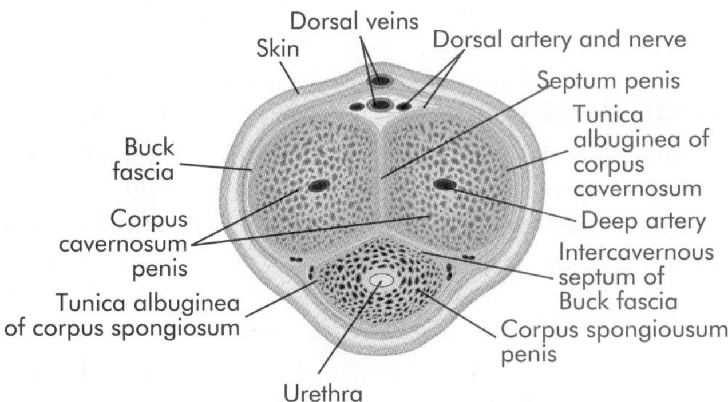

Figure 31-15 ■ **Cross Section of the Penis.** (From Thompson JM et al, editors: *Mosby's clinical nursing*, ed 5, St Louis, 2002, Mosby.)

or constriction of veins that drain the corpora cavernosa and corpus spongiosum. When sexual stimulation ceases or orgasm and ejaculation occur, these veins open, blood flows out of the arterioles, and the penis becomes flaccid (soft and pendulous).[11] Erection is under the control of the autonomic nervous system but can be stimulated or inhibited by central nervous system input, such as stress, medications, and pictures.

Erections begin in utero and continue throughout life, but ejaculation does not occur until sperm production begins at puberty. Growth of the penis and scrotal contents continues well past puberty, however, and may not be complete until the late teens or early 20s. Penis size, when flaccid, varies considerably; with an erection, difference in penis size diminishes. Sexual excitement causes the corpora cavernosa to increase in length and width and become rigid; the penis becomes erect. Stimulation of the glans, which is endowed with copious sensitive nerve endings, provides maximum erotic sensation. With sexual arousal, skin color deepens, the glans doubles in size, and the urethral meatus dilates. Ejaculation occurs with frequent, strong contractions of the vas deferens, epididymis, seminal vesicles, prostate, urethra, and penis.

Internal Genitalia

Figure 31-12 shows the anatomy of the internal genitalia and their relation to other pelvic organs. The internal genitalia consist of ducts and glands, as follows:

Ducts. Consist of two vasa deferentia, ejaculatory duct, urethra; conduct sperm and glandular secretions from testes to urethral opening of the penis

Glands. Consist of prostate gland, two seminal vesicles, two Cowper (bulbourethral) glands; secrete fluids that serve as a vehicle for sperm transport and create nutritious alkaline medium that promotes sperm motility and survival

Together the sperm and the glandular fluids compose **semen.**

Sperm leave the epididymides and travel rapidly through the internal ducts **(emission).** Emission occurs just seconds before ejaculation, at the moment when sexual arousal peaks. It always leads to ejaculation.

Emission occurs as smooth muscle in the walls of the epididymides and vasa deferentia begins to contract rhythmically, pushing sperm and epididymal secretions through the vasa deferentia. Each vas deferens is a firm, elastic, fibromuscular tube that begins at the tail of the epididymis, enters the pelvic cavity within the spermatic cord, loops up and over the bladder, and ends in the prostate gland (Figures 31-12 and 31-16). Sperm are moved along by peristaltic contractions of smooth muscle in the walls of the vas deferens.

As sperm leave the ampulla (wide portion) of the vas deferens, the seminal vesicles secrete a nutritive, glucose-rich fluid into the ejaculate (semen). The **seminal vesicles** are glands about 4 to 6 cm long that lie behind the urinary bladder and in front of the rectum. The ducts of the seminal vesicles join the ampulla of the vas deferens to become the **ejaculatory duct,** which contracts rhythmically during emission and ejaculation. As seen in Figures 31-12 and 31-16, the ejaculatory duct joins the urethra, where both pass through the prostate gland. During emission and ejaculation, a sphincter (muscle surrounding a duct) closes, preventing urine from entering the prostatic urethra.

The **prostate gland** is composed of alveoli and ducts embedded in fibromuscular tissue. It measures 4 cm in diameter and weighs approximately 20 g. While semen moves through the prostatic portion of the urethra, the prostate gland contracts rhythmically and secretes prostatic fluid (a thin, milky substance with an alkaline pH that helps sperm to survive in the acid environment of the female reproductive tract) into the mixture. In addition, substances in seminal and prostatic fluids help to mobilize sperm after ejaculation.

The last pair of glands to add fluid to the ejaculate are **Cowper glands (bulbourethral glands),** whose ducts secrete mucus into the urethra near the base of the penis. Ejaculation occurs as semen reaches the base of the penis and muscles there begin the rhythmic contractions that push semen out. Normally a man ejaculates between 2 and 6 ml of semen, containing 75 million to 400 million sperm. About 98% of the ejaculate consists of glandular fluids; 60% to 70% of volume comes from the seminal vesicles and 20% from the prostate. Therefore, the ejaculate of a man who has undergone vasectomy (a surgical procedure that prevents sperm from entering the vas deferens) is reduced by only about 2%.

HEALTH ALERT
Lycopene and Prostate Cancer

Frequent intake of tomatoes and tomato products may be associated with a lower risk of prostate cancer. Lycopene, a red pigment and a carotenoid, is a strong antioxidant found in tomatoes. Lycopene can trap singlet oxygen and reduce mutagenesis. Evidence is developing that lycopene also may interfere with growth receptor signaling and cell cycle progression in prostate cancer cells, reduce prostate DNA damage, and reduce prostate specific antigen (PSA). Research is continuing to identify the absorption, metabolism, and mechanisms of lycopene and other tomato chemicals in cancer risk reduction.

Data from Edinger MS, Koff WJ: Effect of the consumption of tomato paste on plasma prostate-specific antigen levels in patients with benign prostate hyperplasia, *Braz J Med Biol Res* 39(8):1115–1119, 2006; Kirsh VA et al: A prospective study of lycopene and tomato product intake and risk of prostate cancer, *Cancer Epidemiol Biomarkers Prev* 15(1):92–98, 2006.

Spermatogenesis

Spermatogenesis begins at puberty and continues for life. In this respect, spermatogenesis differs markedly from oogenesis (production of primordial ova), which occurs during fetal life only.

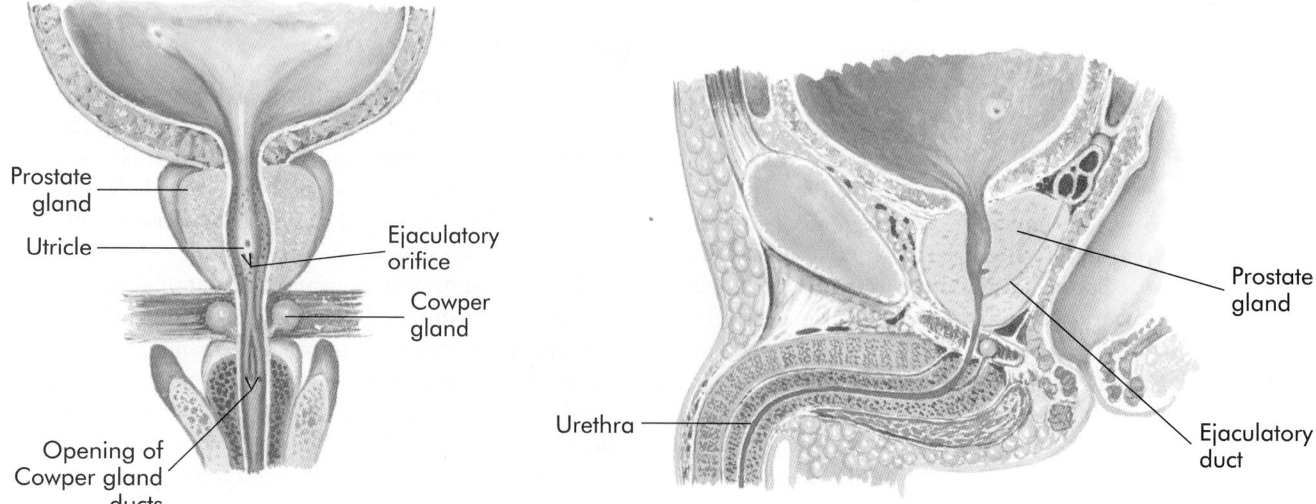

Figure 31-16 ■ **Anatomy of the Prostate Gland and Seminal Vesicles.** (From Seidel HM et al: *Mosby's guide to physical examination,* ed 6, St Louis, 2006, Mosby.)

Spermatogenesis takes place within the seminiferous tubules of the testes (see Figure 31-14). The basement membrane of each seminiferous tubule is lined with diploid (46-chromosome) germ cells called **spermatogonia** (*sing.,* spermatogonium). These cells undergo continuous mitotic division. (Mitotic division, in which a cell divides into two identical cells, is described in Chapter 1.) Some spermatogonia move away from the basement membrane and mature, becoming **primary spermatocytes** (Figure 31-17). These undergo meiosis, a type of cell division that results in two haploid (23-chromosome) cells called **secondary spermatocytes.** (Meiosis is described and illustrated in Chapter 2.) The secondary spermatocytes then undergo meiosis, resulting in four **spermatids.** The spermatids differentiate into spermatozoa, or sperm, each of which contains 23 chromosomes (Figure 31-18).

The development of spermatids into sperm depends on the presence of **Sertoli cells (nondividing support cells)** within the seminiferous tubules. Spermatids attach themselves to the Sertoli cells where they receive nutrients and hormonal signals necessary to develop into sperm.

The process of spermatogenesis, from mitotic division of a spermatogonium to maturation of the spermatids, takes about 70 to 80 days. Mature sperm migrate from

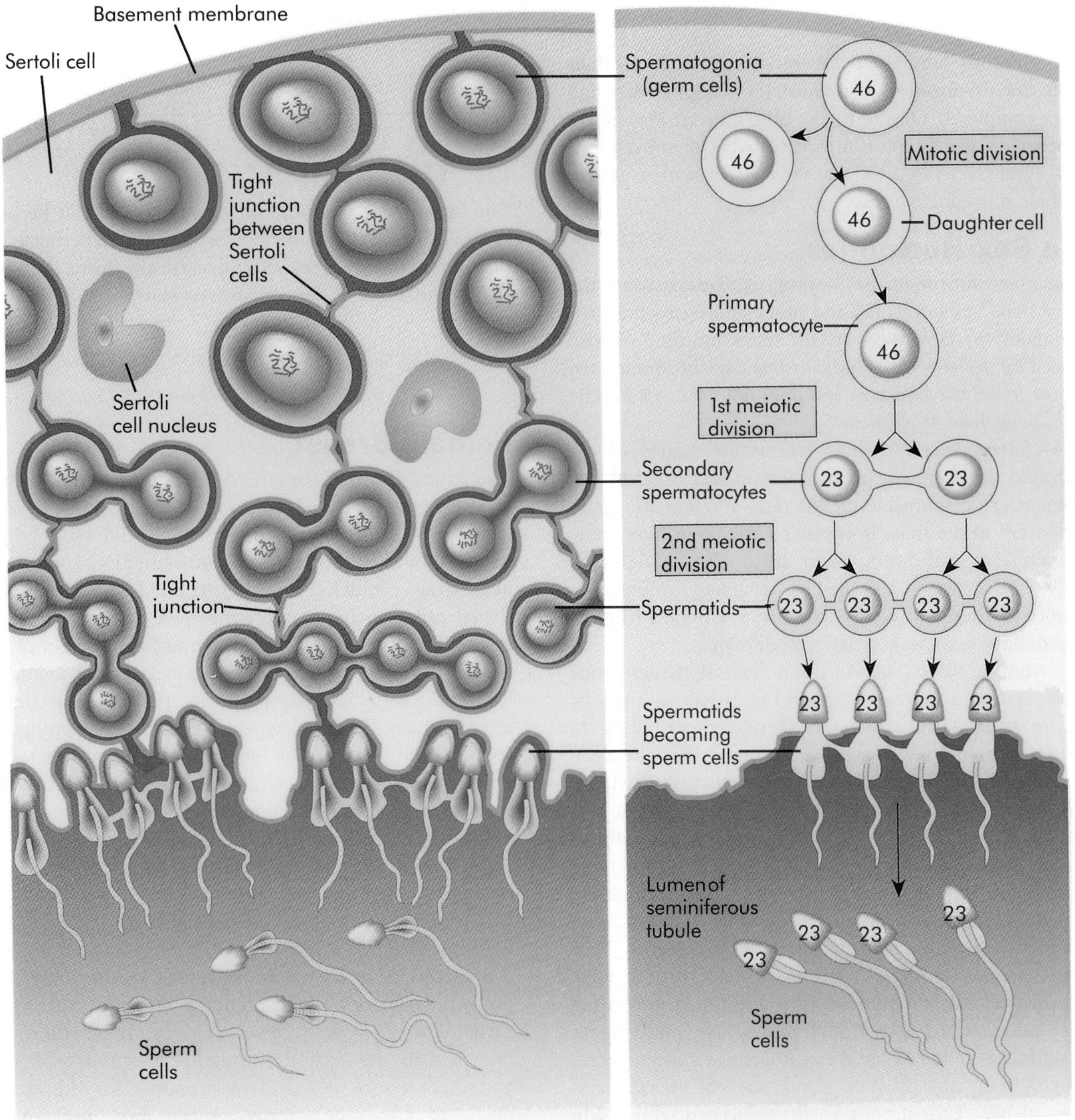

Figure 31-17 ■ **Seminiferous Tubule.** Section shows process of meiosis and sperm cell formation. (From Thibodeau GA, Patton KT: *Anatomy & physiology,* ed 6, St Louis, 2007, Mosby.)

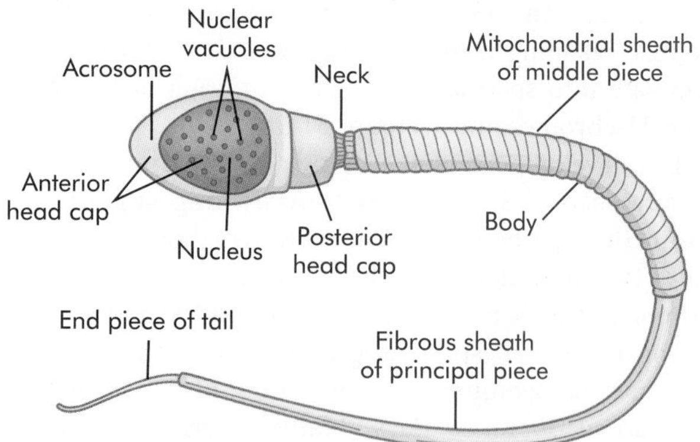

Figure 31-18 ■ **Mature Sperm Cell (Spermatozoon).** Anatomy of mature sperm cell.

the seminiferous tubules to the epididymides, where their capacity for fertilization continues to develop. Although they are completely mature by the time they are ejaculated, the sperm do not become motile (capable of movement) until they are activated by biochemicals in semen and in the female reproductive tract.

Male Sex Hormones

The male sex hormones are androgens. Testosterone, the primary male sex hormone, and other androgens are produced mainly by Leydig cells of the testes, but they are also produced by the adrenal glands. In men, sex hormone production is relatively constant and does not occur in a cyclic pattern, as it does in women.

The androgens' physiologic actions are related to the growth and development of male tissues and organs.[1,11,12] Androgens are responsible for the fetal differentiation and development of the male urogenital system and have some effects on the fetal brain. After birth, the Leydig cells become quiescent until activated by the gonadotropins during puberty. Then androgens cause the sex organs to grow and secondary sex characteristics to develop.

Testosterone affects nervous and skeletal tissues, bone marrow, skin and hair, and sex organs. It has an anabolic effect on skeletal muscle tissue, thereby contributing to the difference in body weight and composition between men and women. Testosterone also stimulates growth of the musculature and cartilage of the larynx, causing a permanent deepening of the voice. Testosterone directly stimulates the bone marrow and indirectly stimulates renal erythropoietin production to achieve increased hemoglobin and hematocrit levels. Because sebaceous gland activity is stimulated by testosterone, acne may develop. Hair becomes coarser in texture, and facial, axillary, and pubic hair grows in male patterns. Later in life, testosterone causes baldness in genetically susceptible individuals. Testosterone is required for spermatogenesis and for secretion of fluid by the prostate gland, seminal vesicles, and Cowper glands. Testosterone is also associated with **libido** (sex drive). Other, less-understood effects of testosterone include alterations in fatty acid and cholesterol metabolism.

The regulation of androgen production and spermatogenesis is achieved by a complex feedback system involving the extrahypothalamic central nervous system, the hypothalamus, the anterior pituitary, the testes, and the androgen-sensitive end organs. These relationships, which are essentially the same in women, are summarized in Figure 31-3. Extrahypothalamic influences include such variables as physiologic and psychologic stress. These factors may inhibit or augment hypothalamic activity.

✓ QUICK CHECK 31-5

1. Which cells produce testosterone?
2. Why do sperm take 12 days to travel the length of the epididymis?
3. What is the purpose of prostatic secretion?

STRUCTURE AND FUNCTION OF THE BREAST

The **breasts** are modified sebaceous glands that lie on the ventral surface of the thorax, within the superficial fascia of the chest wall. They extend vertically from the second rib to the sixth or seventh intercostal space and laterally from the side of the sternum to the midaxillary line. Breast tissue also may extend into the axilla; this tissue is known as the *tail of Spence.*

Female Breast

The female breast is composed of 15 to 20 pyramid-shaped lobes that are separated and supported by Cooper ligaments (Figure 31-19). Each lobe contains 20 to 40 lobules (alveoli), which subdivide further into many functional units called **acini** (*sing.*, acinus). Each acinus is lined with a layer of epithelial cells capable of secreting milk and a layer of subepithelial cells capable of contracting to squeeze milk from the acinus. The acini empty into a network of lobular collecting ducts, which empty into interlobular collecting and ejecting ducts. These ducts reach the skin through openings (pores) in the nipple. The lobes and lobules are surrounded and separated by muscle strands and fatty connective tissue. The amount of fatty connective tissue varies from individual to individual, depending on weight, genetic, and endocrine factors and contributes to the diversity of breast size and shape.[6]

An extensive capillary network surrounds the acini and is supplied by the internal and lateral thoracic arteries and the intercostal arteries. Venous return follows arterial supply, with relatively rapid emptying into the superior vena cava. The breasts receive sensory innervation from branches of the second through sixth intercostal nerves and the cervical plexus. This accounts for the fact that breast pain may be referred to the chest, back, scapula, medial arm, and neck. Lymphatic drainage of the breast occurs largely through axillary nodes, but approximately

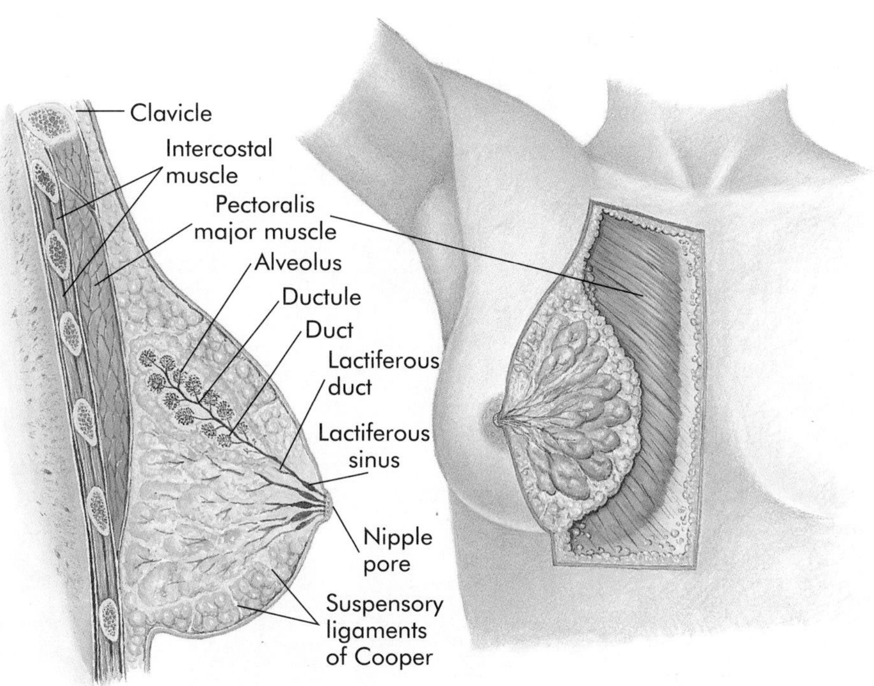

Figure 31-19 ■ **The Female Breast.** (From Seidel HM et al: *Mosby's guide to physical examination,* ed 6, St Louis, 2006, Mosby.)

25% occurs through transpectoral and internal mammary routes[6] (Figure 31-20).

The **nipple** is a pigmented, cylindrical structure usually located at the fourth or fifth intercostal space. On its surface lie multiple openings, one from each lobe. It measures 0.5 to 1.3 cm in diameter and is approximately 10 to 12 mm in height when erect. The **areola** is the pigmented, circular area around the nipple. It may be 15 to 60 mm in diameter. A number of sebaceous glands, the **glands of Montgomery,** are located within the areola and aid in lubrication of the nipple during lactation. The nipple and areola contain smooth muscles, which receive motor innervation from the sympathetic nervous system. Sexual stimulation, breast-feeding, and exposure to cold cause the nipple to become erect.

The fetal and early postnatal development of breast tissue does not depend on hormones, although fetal breast tissue does become progressively responsive to hormonal stimulation. During childhood, breast growth is latent and growth of the nipple and areola keeps pace with body surface growth. At the onset of puberty in the female, estrogen secretion stimulates mammary growth. Breast development, or **thelarche,** is usually the first sign of puberty in the female. Full differentiation and development of breast tissue are mediated by several hormones, including estrogen, progesterone, prolactin, growth hormone, thyroid and parathyroid hormones, insulin, and cortisol.

During the reproductive years, the breast undergoes cyclic changes in response to changes in the levels of estrogen and progesterone associated with the menstrual cycle. Estrogen promotes development of the lobular ducts; progesterone stimulates development of cells lining the acini. Lactation (milk production) occurs after childbirth in response to increased levels of prolactin. Prolactin secretion, in turn, increases by continued breast-feeding. **Oxytocin,** another hormone released after delivery, controls milk ejection (let down) from acini cells. During the follicular/proliferative phase of the menstrual cycle, high estradiol levels increase the vascularity of breast tissue and stimulate proliferation of ductal and acinar tissue. This effect is sustained into the luteal/secretory phase of the cycle. During this phase, progesterone levels increase and contribute to the breast changes induced by estradiol. Specific effects of progesterone include dilation of the ducts and conversion of the acinar cells into secretory cells. Most women experience some degree of premenstrual breast fullness, tenderness, and increased breast nodularity. Breast volume may increase as much as 10 to 30 ml. Because the length of the menstrual cycle does not allow for complete regression of new cell growth, breast growth continues at a slow rate until approximately 35 years of age. Because of the cyclic changes that occur in breast tissue, breast examination should be conducted at the conclusion of or a few days after the menstrual cycle, when hormonal effects are minimal and breasts are at their smallest.

The function of the female breast is primarily to provide a source of nourishment for the newborn. Physiologically, breast milk is the most appropriate nourishment for newborns. Not only does its composition change over time to meet the changing digestive capabilities and nutritional requirements of the infant, but also breast milk contains specific immunoglobulins, especially IgA, and nonspecific antimicrobial factors, such as lysosomes and lactoferrin, that protect the infant against infection. During lactation,

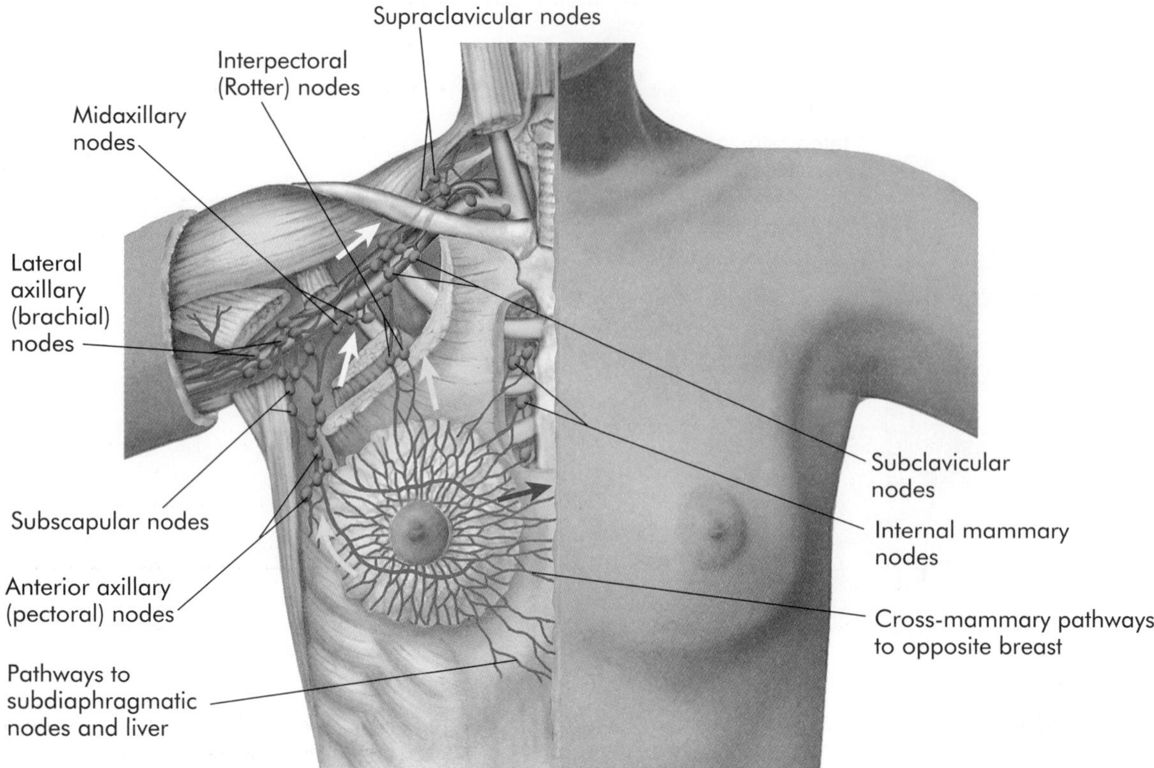

Figure 31-20 ■ **Lymphatic Drainage of the Female Breast.** (From Seidel HM et al: *Mosby's guide to physical examination,* ed 6, St Louis, 2006, Mosby.)

high prolactin levels interfere with hypothalamic-pituitary hormones that stimulate ovulation. This mechanism suppresses the menstrual cycle and prevents ovulation.[6] In many parts of the world (underdeveloped or Third World countries), breast-feeding is the major means of contraception. Breasts are also a source of pleasurable sexual sensation and in Western cultures have become a sexual symbol.

Male Breast

Until puberty, development of the male breast is similar to that of the female breast. In the absence of sufficiently high levels of estrogen and progesterone, the male breast does not develop any further. The normal male breast consists of a small, underdeveloped nipple; some fatty and fibrous tissue; and a few ductlike structures in the subareolar area. The male breast may appear enlarged in obese men because of accumulation of fatty tissue. During puberty, some males experience gynecomastia, a condition in which the breasts enlarge temporarily as a result of hormonal fluctuations.

AGING & Reproductive Function

Aging and the Female Reproductive System

Menopause is a normal developmental event that is universally experienced by the average age of 48 to 55 years, and a median age of 51.4 years.[1] It is not affected by age at menarche, childbearing, weight, socioeconomic factors, oral contraception, or race. However, it is genetically predetermined, which has been documented by family history. It can occur 2 years sooner on average for smokers, and thinner women also tend to experience menopause at a slightly younger age.

Changes are caused primarily by declining ovarian function and a resulting decrease in ovarian hormone secretion. The primary changes of menopause are as follows:

Perimenopause: This is the transitional period between reproductive and nonreproductive years and can last 1 to 8 years. Five to 10 years before menopause, approximately 90% of women note mild to extreme variability in frequency and quality of menstrual flow. Symptoms usually begin with a shortening of the menstrual cycle, which correlates with a shorter follicular phase, followed by unpredictable or irregular ovulation and a lengthening of the menstrual cycle. The perimenopause varies between women and from cycle to cycle in the same woman.

Ovarian changes: Around 37 to 38 years of age, women experience accelerated follicular loss, which ends when the supply of follicles is depleted at menopause. This accelerated loss is correlated with increased FSH stimulation, a declining inhibin production, and slightly elevated estradiol levels (Figure 31-21). The ovarian response to high FSH recruits increasing numbers of follicles; these follicles only partially develop, with a net effect of irregular ovulation, lower progesterone levels,

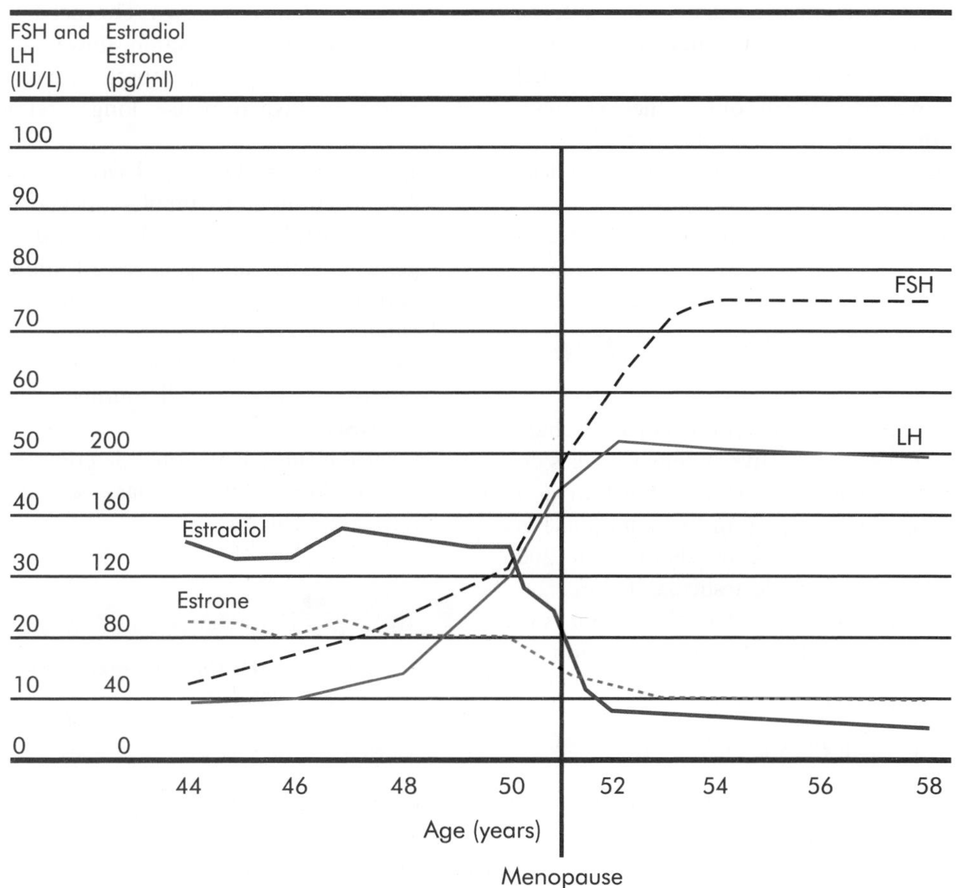

Figure 31-21 ■ **The Perimenopausal Transition.** Mean circulating hormone levels. (From Speroff L et al: *Clinical gynecologic endocrinology and infertility,* ed 7, Baltimore, 2005, Lippincott.)

and depleted follicle reserve. The ovaries begin to decrease in size around age 30; this decrease accelerates after age 60.

Uterine changes: The increase in anovulatory cycles allows for proliferative growth of the endometrium. With this longer exposure to unopposed estrogen and greater thickness of the endometrium, 50% of perimenopausal women will experience dysfunctional uterine bleeding that is heavy and unpredictable. In the past, this has put women at high risk for hysterectomy. Newer treatment includes progesterone administration or endometrial ablation by laser or electrocautery. New methods of decreasing the function of the endometrial tissue are being developed.

Systemic changes: **Vasomotor flushes** are characterized by a rise in skin temperature, dilation of peripheral blood vessels, increased blood flow in the hands, increased skin conductance, and transient increase in heart rate followed by a temperature drop and profuse perspiration over the area of flush distribution. This usually occurs in the face and neck and may radiate into the chest and other parts of the body. Dizziness, nausea, headaches, or palpitations may accompany the flush. These flushes can vary in frequency, intensity, and duration and are experienced by up to 85% of perimenopausal to postmenopausal women from 1 to 15 years (mean 1 to 5 years). It is thought to be caused by rapid change in estrogen levels, and estrogen replacement therapy can ameliorate these symptoms. Rapid changes in estrogen levels also can increase emotional stress with unpredictable mood swings, weight gain, migraine headaches, and insomnia. Lower estrogen levels will decrease skin thickness and diminish skin elasticity, thereby causing increased skin dryness and wrinkling.

Menopause: Menopause is defined by the point that marks 12 consecutive months of amenorrhea. This means that it is determined retrospectively after a woman has not had a menstrual period for 1 year. It is characterized by loss of ovarian function, low estrogen and progesterone levels, and high FSH and LH levels (see Figure 31-21).[13]

Breast tissue changes: Breast tissue becomes involuted; fat deposits and connective tissue increase; and breasts are reduced in size and firmness.

Urogenital tract changes: The ovaries shrink; the uterus atrophies; and the vagina shortens, narrows, and loses some elasticity. Lubrication of the vagina diminishes and vaginal pH increases, creating higher incidence of vaginitis. The cervix atrophies, cervical os shrinks; vaginal epithelium atrophies; labia major and minora become less prominent; some pubic hair is lost; urethral tone declines along with muscle tone throughout the pelvic area; urinary frequency or urgency, urinary tract infections, and incontinence may occur. Regular sexual activity and orgasm may diminish some of these changes. Sexually active women have less vaginal atrophy.

Skeletal changes: Bone mass is lost, leading to increased brittleness and porosity and possibly osteoporosis.

Cardiac change: The risk of coronary heart disease increases significantly.

Aging and the Male Reproductive System

No known discrete event, comparable to menopause, characterizes aging of the male reproductive system. Changes do occur, however, in testicular structure and function and sexual behavior. Androgen deficiency in the aging male is known as **andropause** and occurs in about 1 in 200 men.[14] Contributing factors include testicular failure and changes in the hypothalamus and pituitary gland.[15] Obesity also contributes to decreased testosterone production in aging men.[16] Primary changes are summarized as follows[17,18]:

Sexual drive (libido). Influenced by changes in health status with aging.

Erectile/ejaculatory capacity. The need for longer stimulation to achieve full erection, slower and less forceful ejaculation, less pelvic muscle involvement; decreased vasocongestive response; longer refractory time, up to 24 hours.

Testicular changes. Decreased weight, atrophy, softening of testes; seminiferous tubules thicken in basement membrane area, have germ cell arrest, decrease in spermatogenic activity, and collapse of tubules; then sclerosis and fibrosis cause complete obstruction.

Hormonal changes. Hormone synthesis decreases and target tissues decline in responsiveness; testosterone levels reduce as Leydig cell numbers fall; gonadotropins increase.

Associated change. Functional deterioration of accessory sex organs; loss of muscle mass, strength, and endurance; decrease in libido.

QUICK CHECK 31-6

1. How does breast development differ between adult men and women?
2. What happens to estradiol levels in perimenopausal women?

Did You Understand?

Development of the Reproductive Systems

1. Differentiation of female and male genitalia begins around 7 to 8 weeks of embryonic development, when the gonads of genetically male embryos begin to secrete male sex hormones, primarily testosterone. Until that time, the primitive reproductive organs of males and females are homologous (the same).
2. The structure and function of both male and female reproductive systems depend on interactions among the central nervous system (hypothalamus), the endocrine system (anterior pituitary), the gonads (ovaries, testes), and the hypothalamic-pituitary-gonadal (H-P-G) axis. A set of complex neurologic and hormonal interactions accelerate at puberty and lead to sexual maturation and reproductive capability
3. Extrahypothalamic factors cause the hypothalamus to secrete gonadotropin-releasing hormone (GnRH), which stimulates the anterior pituitary to secrete gonadotropin follicle-stimulating hormone (FSH) and luteinizing hormone (LH) that stimulate the gonads (ovaries and testes) to secrete female or male sex hormones. Paracrine hormones (inhibin, activin, and follistatin) influence the positive and negative feedback loops that occur along the H-P-G axis.
4. Production of primitive female gametes (ova) occurs solely during fetal life. From puberty to menopause, one female gamete matures per menstrual cycle. Production of the male gametes (sperm) begins at puberty; after that, millions are produced daily, usually for life.

The Female Reproductive System

1. The function of the reproductive system is to produce mature ova and, when they are fertilized, to protect and nourish them through embryonic and fetal life and expel them at birth.
2. The external female genitalia are the mons pubis, labia majora, labia minora, clitoris, vestibule (urinary and vaginal openings), Bartholin glands, and Skene glands. They protect body openings and may play a role in sexual functioning.
3. The internal female genitalia are the vagina, uterus, fallopian tubes, and ovaries. Although all these organs are needed for reproduction, the ovaries are the most essential because they produce the female gametes and female sex hormones.
4. The vagina is a fibromuscular canal that receives the penis during sexual intercourse and is the exit route for menstrual fluids and products of conception. The vagina leads from the introitus (its external opening) to the cervical portion of the uterus.
5. The uterus is the hollow, muscular organ in which a fertilized ovum develops until birth. The uterine walls have three layers: the endometrium (lining), myometrium (muscular layer), and perimetrium (outer covering, which is continuous with the pelvic peritoneum). The endometrium proliferates (thickens) and sloughs off in response to cyclic changes in levels of female sex hormones. The cervix is the narrow, lower portion of the uterus that opens into the vagina.

Did You Understand?—Cont'd

6. The two fallopian tubes extend from the uterus to the ovaries. Their function is to conduct ova from the spaces around the ovaries to the uterus. Fertilization normally occurs in the distal third of the fallopian tubes.
7. From puberty to menopause, the ovaries are the site of (a) ovum maturation and release and (b) production of female sex hormones (estrogen, progesterone) and androgens. The female sex hormones are involved in sexual differentiation and development, the menstrual cycle, pregnancy, and lactation. Although they are primarily male sex hormones, androgens in women are precursors of female sex hormones and contribute to the prepubertal growth spurt, pubic and axillary hair growth, and activation of sebaceous glands.
8. Estrogen (primarily estradiol) is produced by cells in the developing ovarian follicle (structure that encloses the ovum). Progesterone is produced by cells of the corpus luteum, the structure that develops from the ruptured ovarian follicle after ovulation (ovum release). Androgens are produced within the ovarian follicle, adrenal glands, and adipose tissue.
9. The average menstrual cycle lasts 27 to 30 days and consists of three phases, which are named for ovarian and endometrial changes: the follicular/proliferative phase, the luteal/secretory phase, and menstruation.
10. Ovarian events of the menstrual cycle are controlled by gonadotropins and follicular secretion of inhibin. High follicle-stimulating hormone (FSH) levels stimulate follicle and ovum maturation (follicular phase); then a surge of luteinizing hormone (LH) causes ovulation, which is followed by development of the corpus luteum (luteal phase).
11. Uterine (endometrial) events of the menstrual cycle are caused by ovarian hormones. During the follicular phase of the ovarian cycle, estrogen produced by the follicle causes the endometrium to proliferate (proliferative phase). During the luteal phase, estrogen maintains the thickened endometrium, while progesterone causes it to develop blood vessels and secretory glands (secretory phase). As the corpus luteum degenerates, production of both hormones drops sharply and the "starved" endometrium degenerates and sloughs off, causing menstruation.
12. Cyclic changes in hormone levels also cause thinning and thickening of the vaginal epithelium, thinning and thickening of cervical secretions, and changes in basal body temperature.

The Male Reproductive System

1. The function of the male reproductive system is to produce male gametes (sperm) and deliver them to the female reproductive tract.
2. The external male genitalia are the testes, epididymides, scrotum, and penis. The internal genitalia are the vas deferens, ejaculatory duct, prostatic and membranous sections of the urethra, seminal vesicles, prostate gland, and Cowper glands.
3. The testes (male gonads) are paired glands suspended within the scrotum. The testes have two functions: spermatogenesis (sperm production) and production of male sex hormones (androgens, chiefly testosterone).
4. The epididymis is a long, coiled tube arranged in a comma-shaped compartment that curves over the top and rear of the testis. The epididymis receives sperm from the testis and stores them while they develop further. Sperm travel the length of the epididymis and then are ejaculated into the vas deferens, which transports sperm to the urethra.
5. The scrotum is a skin-covered, fibromuscular sac that encloses the testes and epididymides, which are suspended within the scrotum by the spermatic cord. The scrotum keeps these organs at optimal temperatures for sperm survival (about 1° to 2° C lower than body temperature) by contracting in cold environments and relaxing in warm environments.
6. The penis is a cylindrical organ consisting of three longitudinal compartments (two corpora cavernosa and one corpus spongiosum) and the urethra. The urethra runs through the corpus spongiosum. The corpora cavernosa and corpus spongiosum consist of erectile tissue. Externally the penis consists of a shaft and a tip, which is called the *glans*.
7. The penis has two functions: delivery of sperm and elimination of urine.
8. Sexual intercourse is made possible by the erectile reflex, in which tactile or psychogenic stimulation of the parasympathetic nerves causes arterioles in the corpora cavernosa and corpus spongiosum to dilate and fill with blood, causing the penis to enlarge and become firm.
9. Emission, which occurs at the peak of sexual arousal, is the movement of semen from the epididymides to the penis. Ejaculation, which is a continuation of emission, is the pulsatile ejection of semen from the penis.
10. Spermatogenesis is a continuous process because spermatogonia, the primitive male gametes, undergo continuous mitosis within the seminiferous tubules of the testes. Some spermatogonia develop into primary spermatocytes, which divide meiotically into secondary spermatocytes and then spermatids. The spermatids develop into sperm with the help of nutrients and hormonal signals from Sertoli cells.
11. Production of the male sex hormones (like production of the female sex hormones) is controlled by interactions among the hypothalamus, anterior pituitary, and gonads. The male hormones are produced steadily rather than cyclically, however.

Structure and Function of the Breast

1. Until puberty, the female and male breasts are similar, consisting of a small, underdeveloped nipple, some fatty and fibrous tissue, and a few ductlike structures under the areola. At puberty, however, a variety of hormones (estrogen, progesterone, prolactin, growth hormone, insulin, cortisol) cause the female breast to develop into a system of glands and ducts that is capable of producing and ejecting milk.

(Continued)

Did You Understand?—Cont'd

2. The basic functional unit of the female breast is the lobe, a system of ducts that branches from the nipple to milk-producing units called *lobules.* The lobules contain *acini cells,* which are convoluted spaces lined with epithelial cells, that contract moving milk into the system of ducts that leads to the nipple.
3. Each breast contains 15 to 20 lobes, which are separated and supported by Cooper ligaments.
4. Milk production occurs in response to prolactin, a hormone that is secreted in larger amounts after childbirth. Milk ejection is under the control of oxytocin, another hormone of pregnancy and lactation.
5. During the reproductive years, breast tissue undergoes cyclic changes in response to hormonal changes of the menstrual cycle. At menopause, the tissue involutes, fat deposits and connective tissue increase, and the breasts reduce in size and firmness.
6. Perimenopause is the transitional period between reproductive and nonreproductive years in women.
7. Menopause the point that marks 12 consecutive months of amenorrhea.
8. Andropause is androgen deficiency in the aging male.

Key Terms

Acinus (*pl.*, acini) of breast, 840
Activin, 833
Adrenarche, 823
Androgen, 830
Andropause, 844
Areola, 841
Breast, 840
Cervix, 827
Cornification, 835
Corpus (body of uterus), 827
Corpus cavernosum (*pl.*, corpora cavernosa), 836
Corpus luteum, 829
Corpus spongiosum, 836
Cowper gland (bulbourethral gland), 838
Cul-de-sac, 826
Decornification, 835
Efferent tubule, 835
Ejaculatory duct, 838
Emission, 837
Endocervical canal, 827
Endometrium, 827
Epididymis (*pl.*, epididymides), 835
Erectile reflex, 836
Estradiol (E2), 829
Estrogen, 829
Fallopian tube (uterine tube), 828
Fimbriae, 828
Follicle-stimulating hormone (FSH), 823
Follicular/proliferative phase, 831
Follistatin, 833
Fornix, 826
Fundus, 827
Glands of Montgomery, 841
Glans, 836
Gonad, 821
Gonadostat (gonadotropin-releasing hormone pulse generator), 822
Gonadotropin-releasing hormone (GnRH), 822
Granulosa cell, 829
Infundibulum, 828
Inguinal canal, 835
Inhibin, 833
Ischemic/menstrual phase, 831
Isthmus, 827
Leptin, 822
Leydig cell, 835
Libido, 840
Luteal/secretory phase, 831
Luteinizing hormone (LH), 823
Menarche, 831
Menopause, 831
Menstruation (menses), 831
Myometrium, 827
Nipple, 841
Ovarian cycle, 829
Ovarian follicle, 828
Ovary, 828
Ovulation, 829
Ovum (*pl.*, ova), 821
Oxytocin, 841
Penis, 836
Perimetrium (parietal peritoneum), 827
Prepuce (foreskin), 836
Primary spermatocyte, 839
Progesterone, 830
Prostate gland, 838
Rete testis, 835
Ruga (*pl.*, rugae; pertains to vagina and testes), 825
Scrotum, 836
Secondary spermatocyte, 839
Semen, 837
Seminal vesicle, 838
Seminiferous tubule, 835
Sertoli cell (nondividing support cell), 839
Sex hormone, 821
Spermatid, 839
Spermatogenesis, 839
Spermatogonium (*pl.*, spermatogonia), 839
Spermatozoon (sperm cell), 821
Spinnbarkeit mucus, 827
Squamous-columnar junction, 827
Testis, 835
Testosterone, 821
Theca cell, 829
Thelarche, 841
Tubulus rectus, 835
Tunica albuginea, 835
Tunica dartos, 836
Tunica vaginalis, 835
Urethra, 836
Uterus, 826
Vagina, 825
Vas deferens, 836
Vasomotor flush, 843
Vulva, 824

References

1. Speroff L et al: *Clinical gynecologic endocrinology and infertility*, ed 7, Baltimore, 2005, Lippincott.
2. Gordan K, Oehninger S: Reproductive physiology, In Copeland LJ, Ferrell JF, editors: *Textbook of gynecology*, ed 2, Philadelphia, 2000, Saunders.
3. Klein KO et al: Effect of obesity on estradiol level, and its relationship to leptin, bone maturation, and bone mineral density in children, *J Clin Endocrinol Metab* 83(10):3469–3475, 1998.
4. Berne RM, Levy MN, editors: *Physiology*, ed 5, St Louis, 2003, Mosby.
5. Lowdermilk DL, Perry SE, Bobak IM: *Maternity and women's health care*, ed 8, St Louis, 2004, Mosby.
6. Riordan J: *Breastfeeding and human lactation*, ed 3, Sudsberry, MA, 2005, Jones & Barrlett.
7. Schuiling KD, Likis FE: Women's gynecologic health, Sudsberry, MA, 2005, Jones & Bartlett.
8. Stenchevor MA et al: *Comprehensive gynecology*, ed 4, St Louis, 2001, Mosby.
9. Golub S: *Periods: from menarche to menopause*, Newbury Park, NJ, 1992, Sage.
10. de Kretser DM et al: Inhibins, activans and follistatin in reproduction, *Hum Reprod Update* 8(6):529–541, 2002.
11. McAninch DW, Tanagho EA, editors: *Smith's general urology*, ed 15, Norwalk, Conn, 2002, McGraw-Hill/Appleton & Lange.
12. Blackburn ST: *Maternal, fetal, and neonatal physiology: a clinical perspective*, ed 2, St Louis, 2003, WB Saunders.
13. Zacur H et al: *Menopause health and hormones: enhancing patient management*, Baltimore, 2002, Johns Hopkins.
14. Morales A, Tenover JL: Androgen deficiency in the aging male: when, who, and how to investigate and treat, *Urol Clin North Am* 29(4):975–982, 2002.
15. Wespes E, Schulman CC: Male andropause: myth, reality, and treatment, *Int J Impot Res* 14(suppl 1):S93–S98, 2002.
16. Tan RS, Pu SJ: Impact of obesity on hypogonadism in the andropause, *Int J Androl* 25(4):195–201, 2002.
17. Handelsman DJ, Liu PY: Andropause: invention, prevention, rejuvenation, *Trends Endocrinol Metab* 16(2):39–45, 2005.
18. Kevorkian R: Andropause, *Mo Med* 104(1):68–71, 2007.

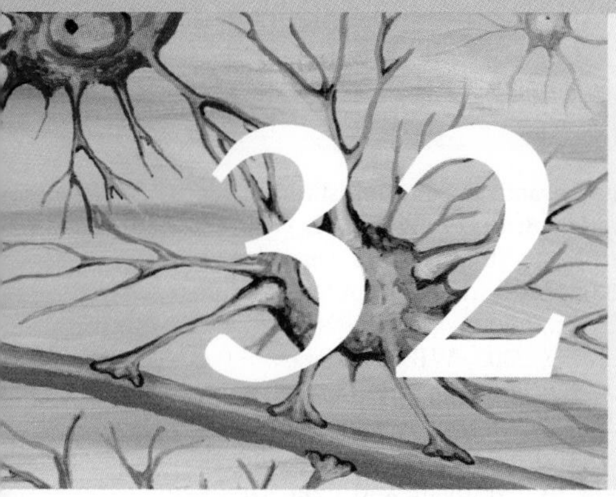

ALTERATIONS OF THE REPRODUCTIVE SYSTEMS, INCLUDING SEXUALLY TRANSMITTED INFECTIONS

Katherine Morgan ▪ Kathryn L. McCance

CHAPTER OUTLINE

ELECTRONIC RESOURCES

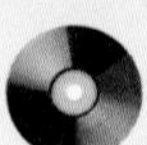

Companion CD
- Review Questions and Answers
- Animations

evolve Website
http://evolve.elsevier.com/Huether/
- Quick Check Answers
- Key Terms Exercises
- Critical Thinking Questions with Answers
- Algorithm Completion Exercises
- WebLinks

Alterations of the reproductive system span a wide range of concerns from delayed sexual development and suboptimal sexual performance to structural and functional abnormalities. Many common reproductive disorders carry potentially serious physiologic or psychologic consequences. For example, sexual or reproductive dysfunction, such as impotence or infertility, can dramatically affect self-concept, relationships, and overall quality of life. Conversely, organic and psychosocial problems, such as alcoholism, depression, situational stressors, chronic illness, and medications, can affect ovulation and menstruation, sexual performance, and fertility and may be risk factors for the development of some types of reproductive tract cancers. Prostate cancer is the second leading cause of cancer deaths in men, and breast cancer is the second leading cause of cancer deaths in women.[1] Diagnosis and treatment of reproductive system disorders, however, are often complicated by the stigma and symbolism associated with the reproductive organs and emotion-laden beliefs and behaviors related to reproductive health. Treatment or diagnosis for any problem may be delayed because of embarrassment, guilt, fear, or denial.

ALTERATIONS OF SEXUAL MATURATION

The process of sexual maturation, or puberty, is marked by the development of secondary sex characteristics, rapid growth, and, ultimately, the ability to reproduce. The average age of puberty has been occurring earlier than previously defined. A variety of congenital and endocrine disorders can disrupt the timing of puberty. Puberty that occurs too late (delayed puberty) or too early (precocious puberty) is caused by the inappropriate onset of sex hormone production.

Delayed Puberty

About 3% of children living in North America experience delayed development of secondary sex characteristics.[2] The first sign of puberty in girls is thelarche, or breast development; it should begin by 13 years of age. Normally, boys tend to mature later than girls, around 14 to 14.5 years of age. In boys, the first sign of maturity is enlargement of testes and thinning of the scrotal skin. In **delayed puberty,** these secondary sex characteristics develop later.

In about 95% of cases, hormonal levels are normal, the hypothalamic-pituitary-gonadal (ovarian or testicular) axis is intact but maturation is slow. This is much more common in boys than in girls. Treatment is seldom needed unless the delayed puberty is causing psychosocial problems.

The other 5% of cases are caused by disruption of the hypothalamic-pituitary-gonadal axis or a systemic disease. Treatment depends on the cause (Box 32-1), and referral to a pediatric endocrinologist is necessary.

BOX 32-1 Causes of Delayed Puberty

Hypergonadotropic Hypogonadism (Increased Follicle-Stimulating Hormone [FSH] and Luteinizing Hormone [LH])

1. Gonadal dysgenesis, most commonly Turner syndrome (45,X/46,XX; structural X or Y abnormalities; or mosaicism)
2. Klinefelter syndrome (47,XXY)
3. Bilateral gonadal failure
   a. Traumatic or infectious
   b. Postsurgical, postirradiation, or postchemotherapy
   c. Autoimmune
   d. Idiopathic empty-scrotum or vanishing-testes syndrome (congenital anorchia) or resistant-ovary syndrome

Hypogonadotropic Hypogonadism (Decreased LH, Depressed FSH)

1. Reversible
   a. Physiologic delay
   b. Weight loss/anorexia
   c. Strenuous exercise
   d. Severe obesity
   e. Illegal drug use, especially marijuana
   f. Primary hypothyroidism
   g. Congenital adrenal hyperplasia
   h. Cushing syndrome
   i. Prolactinomas
2. Irreversible
   a. Gonadotropin-releasing hormone (GnRH) deficiency (Kallmann syndrome) or idiopathic hypogonadotropic hypogonadism (IHH)
   b. Hypopituitarism
   c. Congenital central nervous system (CNS) defects
   d. Other pituitary adenomas
   e. Craniopharyngioma
   f. Malignant pituitary tumors

Eugonadism

These conditions are associated with amenorrhea but may have otherwise normal pubertal development

1. Congenital anomalies
   a. Müllerian agenesis
   b. Vaginal septum or imperforate hymen
2. Androgen insensitivity syndrome
3. Inappropriate positive feedback

Precocious Puberty

Precocious puberty is a rare event, affecting about 1 in 10,000 girls and fewer than 1 in 50,000 boys. Precocious puberty has been defined as sexual maturation occurring before age 6 in black girls or age 7 in white girls and before age 9 in boys.[3] Precocious puberty may be caused by many conditions (Box 32-2), including lethal central nervous system tumors. With 75% of precocity in girls being idiopathic,[4] all cases of precocious puberty require thorough evaluation.

All forms of precocious puberty are treated by identifying and removing the underlying cause or administering appropriate hormones. In many cases, precocious puberty can be reversed. However, **idiopathic isosexual precocity** (development consistent with the sex of the individual) is difficult to treat and can cause long bones to stop growing before the child has reached normal height.

QUICK CHECK 32-1

1. Why does puberty occur too late or too early in some individuals?

BOX 32-2 The Three Forms of Precocious Puberty

Isosexual Precocious Puberty

Premature development of sex characteristics appropriate for the child's gender

Normal but premature functioning of hypothalamic-pituitary-ovarian axis

Lethal central nervous system tumor may be the cause in about 10% of cases

Heterosexual Precocious Puberty

Development of some secondary sex characteristics not appropriate for the child's gender (e.g., breast enlargement in males)

Common causes are adrenal hyperplasia or androgen-secreting tumors

Incomplete Precocious Puberty

Partial development of appropriate secondary sex characteristics

Premature thelarche (breast budding) seen in girls between 6 months and 2 years of age

Progression to complete puberty (ovulation and menstruation) is arrested

Premature adrenarche (growth of axillary and pubic hair); tends to occur between 5 and 8 years of age

Progression to complete precocious puberty may occur; estrogen-secreting neoplasms may be the cause or it may be a variant of normal pubertal development

See also Ritzen EM: Early puberty: what is normal and when is treatment indicated? *Horm Res* 60(suppl 3):31–34, 2003.

DISORDERS OF THE FEMALE REPRODUCTIVE SYSTEM

Hormonal and Menstrual Alterations

Dysmenorrhea

Primary dysmenorrhea is painful menstruation associated with the release of prostaglandins in ovulatory cycles but not with pelvic disease. Between 50% and 75% of women ages 15 to 25 years are affected—some (up to 15%)[5] are affected severely enough to cause missed work or school. Primary dysmenorrhea begins with the onset of ovulatory cycles. The incidence steadily rises, peaks in women in their mid-20s, and decreases slowly thereafter.

Secondary dysmenorrhea is related to pelvic pathology, manifests later in the reproductive years, and may occur any time in the menstrual cycle.

PATHOPHYSIOLOGY Primary dysmenorrhea results from excessive prostaglandin F ($PGF_{2\alpha}\alpha$) found in secretory endometrium. These lipid hormones increase myometrial contractions and constrict endometrial blood vessels, causing ischemia and endometrial shedding. In addition, prostaglandins and prostaglandin metabolites can cause gastrointestinal complaints, headache, and syncope.

Secondary dysmenorrhea results from disorders such as endometriosis, pelvic adhesions, inflammatory disease, uterine fibroids, or adenomyosis.

CLINICAL MANIFESTATIONS The chief symptom of dysmenorrhea is pelvic pain associated with the onset of menses. The severity is directly related to length and amount of menstrual flow. The pain often radiates into the groin and may be accompanied by backache, anorexia, vomiting, diarrhea, syncope, and headache. Usually, the discomfort begins shortly before the onset of menstruation and rarely persists beyond the second day.

EVALUATION AND TREATMENT Primary dysmenorrhea can be differentiated from secondary dysmenorrhea by a thorough medical history and pelvic examination. In women who desire contraception, dysmenorrhea may be relieved with hormonal contraceptives. Hormonal contraception stops ovulation and creates an atrophic endometrium, thereby decreasing prostaglandin synthesis and myometrial contractility. Prostaglandin inhibitors work in a majority of women with primary dysmenorrhea and should be taken before or at the onset of bleeding or cramping. Regular exercise seems to prevent or reduce symptoms. Other comfort measures include local application of heat, massage, or relaxation techniques. Orgasm may relieve or worsen symptoms.

Primary amenorrhea

Amenorrhea means lack of menstruation. **Primary amenorrhea** is defined as the failure of menarche and the absence of menstruation by age 14 years with no development of secondary sex characteristics or the absence of menstruation by age 16 years regardless of the presence of secondary sex characteristics. Causes include a diverse group of abnormalities, such as congenital defects of gonadotropin production; genetic disorders (Turner syndrome); congenital central nervous system (CNS) defects (e.g., hydrocephalus); congenital anatomic malformations of the reproductive system (e.g., absence of vagina or uterus); and acquired CNS lesions, including trauma, infection, and tumors.

PATHOPHYSIOLOGY In some congenital or acquired syndromes, the hypothalamic-pituitary-ovarian (H-P-O) axis is dysfunctional. Because of anatomic defects of the CNS, the ovary does not receive the hormonal signals that normally initiate the development of secondary sex characteristics and menarche (beginning of menstruation). In other cases, CNS lesions develop between the onset and conclusion of puberty. Therefore, skeletal growth may occur and secondary sex characteristics may develop, but sexual maturation is interrupted before menarche.

Primary amenorrhea also has been associated with congenital absence or hypoplasia of the uterus and some genetic disorders, including gonadal dysgenesis (Turner syndrome), androgen insensitivity syndrome (AIS) (formerly known as testicular feminization), and poly-X (superfemale) syndrome. In Turner syndrome (XO), the ovaries lack gametes and ovarian failure is complete. In AIS, the individual is male genetically but female morphologically. The gonads are found either in the abdomen or in the inguinal canal and produce both androgens and estrogens. Because target tissues lack androgen receptors but have estrogen receptors, most individuals with AIS acquire female secondary sex characteristics and female external genitalia but, except for a small vagina, lack internal female genitalia. Removal of the gonads prevents malignancy but should be delayed until puberty is complete.

CLINICAL MANIFESTATIONS The major clinical manifestation of primary amenorrhea is the absence of menarche. The cause of the amenorrhea determines whether secondary sex characteristics and height are affected.

EVALUATION AND TREATMENT Diagnosis of primary amenorrhea is based on history and physical examination. Laboratory studies may be required to document abnormal levels of gonadotropins and ovarian hormones. Diagnostic imaging is used to document structural abnormalities.

Treatment involves correction of any underlying disorders and hormone replacement therapy to induce the development of secondary sex characteristics. Although surgical alteration of the genitalia may be undertaken to correct abnormalities, it should be postponed until the individual can make a truly informed decision.

Secondary amenorrhea

Secondary amenorrhea is the absence of menstruation for a time equivalent to three or more cycles or 6 months in

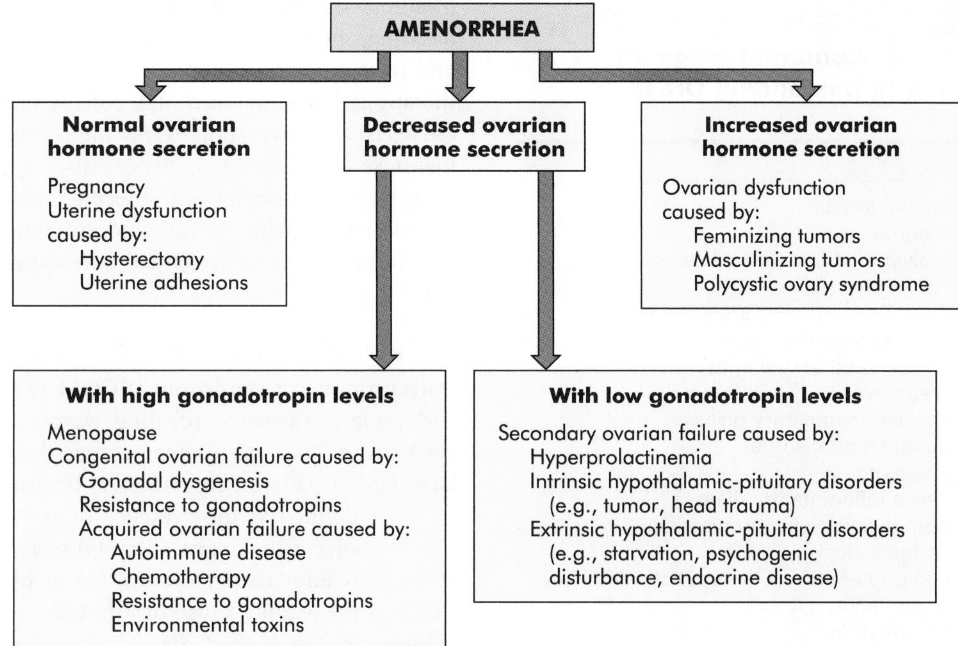

Figure 32-1 ■ **Causes of Secondary Amenorrhea.**

women who have previously menstruated. Many disorders and physiologic conditions are associated with secondary amenorrhea. Secondary amenorrhea is normal during early adolescence, pregnancy, lactation, and the perimenopausal period.

PATHOPHYSIOLOGY The pathophysiology of secondary amenorrhea is summarized in Figure 32-1.

CLINICAL MANIFESTATIONS The major manifestation of secondary amenorrhea is the absence of menses. Depending on the underlying cause of the amenorrhea, infertility, vasomotor flushes, vaginal atrophy, acne, and hirsutism (abnormal hairiness) also may be present.

EVALUATION AND TREATMENT Pregnancy is the most common cause of secondary amenorrhea and must be ruled out before any further evaluation. Diagnosis of secondary amenorrhea involves identifying underlying hormonal or anatomic alterations. A complete history and physical examination are done. Evaluation may include a progesterone challenge to induce withdrawal bleeding. Evaluation of thyroid-stimulating hormone (TSH) or prolactin levels may be indicated. Depending on the cause of the amenorrhea, treatment may involve hormone replacement therapy or a corrective procedure, such as surgical removal of pituitary tumors.

Abnormal uterine bleeding

Menstrual irregularity or abnormal bleeding patterns (Table 32-1) account for 20% of all gynecologic visits and 25% of all gynecologic surgeries. The most common cause of cycle irregularity is failure to ovulate related to age or endocrinopathy. Common causes of abnormal bleeding based on age group and frequency are presented in Table 32-2.

PATHOPHYSIOLOGY **Dysfunctional uterine bleeding (DUB)** is abnormal uterine bleeding resulting from a disturbance of the menstrual cycle, usually anovulation. DUB is a diagnosis of exclusion made only after other causes have been ruled out. Although DUB may occur at any time during the reproductive years, it is most likely to affect women at the extremes of the reproductive years.

In anovulatory cycles, progesterone secretion is absent while variable amounts of estrogen continue to be secreted by the ovary. Estrogen stimulates proliferation and hyperplasia of the endometrial glands. Without the usual stromal

TABLE 32-1

Definitions of Abnormal Menstrual Bleeding

Term	Definition
Polymenorrhea	Cycles shorter than 3 wk; may indicate disturbance in endocrine control of ovulation
Oligomenorrhea	Cycles longer than 6–7 wk; may indicate disturbance in endocrine control of ovulation
Metrorrhagia	Intermenstrual bleeding or bleeding of light character occurring irregularly between cycles; may be a sign of organic disease
Menorrhagia	Increased amount and duration of flow
Menometrorrhagia	Prolonged flow associated with irregular and intermittent spotting between bleeding episodes

TABLE 32-2

Common Causes of Abnormal (Vaginal/Genital) Bleeding in Descending Order of Frequency

Age Group	Cause
Prepubescence	Sexual assault Trauma Presence of foreign bodies Precocious puberty
Adolescence	Anovulation (immature hypothalamic-pituitary-ovarian axis) Trauma and sexual abuse Pregnancy Pelvic inflammatory disease Coagulation disorder
Reproductive years	Pregnancy Pelvic inflammatory disease Complication of contraceptives Endometriosis Benign neoplasms (submucosal fibroids) Anovulation
Premenopause	Anovulation Malignancy Pregnancy Endometriosis Benign neoplasms (myomas, adenomyosis)
Postmenopause	Malignancy

support induced by progesterone and periodic menstruation, the endometrium attains an abnormal height with increasing hypervascularity and back-to-back glandularity. Random breakdown of endometrial tissue occurs, and exposure of vascular channels leads to irregular, prolonged, and excessive bleeding. In addition, unopposed estrogen induces a progression of endometrial responses that may end with atypia (atypical hyperplasia) and carcinoma.

Abnormal bleeding in ovulatory cycles is less common, and mechanisms underlying the bleeding are unclear. Excessive fibrinolytic activity and changes in prostaglandin production may be implicated. Infection or structural abnormalities also may be present.

CLINICAL MANIFESTATIONS DUB is characterized by unpredictable and variable bleeding in terms of amount and duration. Especially during perimenopause, dysfunctional bleeding also may involve flooding and the passing of large clots.[6] Although large clots often indicate excessive blood loss, it is difficult to estimate the severity of blood loss; healthy women usually do not become anemic until blood loss exceeds 1.6 L over a short time or with chronic heavy flow. Heavy bleeding may be preceded by episodes of amenorrhea and be perceived by individuals as a miscarriage.

EVALUATION AND TREATMENT DUB is diagnosed after other organic conditions that could cause abnormal bleeding are eliminated. Goals of therapy are to control bleeding, prevent hyperplasia, prevent or treat anemia, and treat concurrent endocrine problems if present. Usual therapy is hormonal and may consist of intense progestin-estrogen therapy, short-term high-dose estrogen, cyclic low-dose contraceptives, progestins, progesterone, or the progesterone-releasing intrauterine system (IUS). Treatment for DUB with dilation and curettage (D & C) or hysterectomy is not recommended unless medical management fails.[6]

Polycystic ovary syndrome

Polycystic ovary syndrome (PCOS) is the most common endocrine disturbance affecting women. The name "polycystic ovary" is a misnomer because there is an absence of large cysts (>20 mm in diameter) because of anovulation.[7] PCOS is defined as the presence of any two of the following: (1) polycystic (i.e., small cysts) ovary, (2) oligo-anovulation (few anovulatory cycles), (3) or hyperandrogenism.[8] PCOS is the leading cause of infertility, especially in young women, in the United States.[8] Prevalence rates are estimated at between 6% and 10% in the United States. Although common, PCOS remains poorly understood with no clear etiology. Confusing the issue is the frequency, expression, and timing of PCOS. Eighty percent of women with normal ovaries also experience one or more PCOS symptoms. Signs and symptoms of women with PCOS may change over time. The differential diagnosis of PCOS includes (1) Cushing syndrome, (2) congenital adrenal hyperplasia, (3) thyroid disease, (4) androgen-producing adrenal tumors or ovarian tumors, and (5) syndromes with hyperprolactinemia.[9,10] In addition, PCOS may be associated with other endocrine disorders.

PATHOPHYSIOLOGY The direct cause of PCOS is unknown. Hyperinsulinemia plays a key role in androgen excess, anovulation, and pathogenesis of PCOS.[11] For years, PCOS has been deemed an ovarian disease. PCOS is associated with other long-term health issues, including hypertension, dyslipidemia, and hyperinsulinemia (Figure 32-2).[12] Insulin stimulates androgen secretion by the ovarian stroma and reduces serum sex hormone-binding globulin (SHBG) directly and independently. The net effect is an increase in free testosterone levels. Excessive androgens affect follicular growth, and insulin affects follicular decline by suppressing apoptosis and enabling follicles, which would normally disintegrate, to survive (Figure 32-3) Further, there seems to be a genetic ovarian defect in PCOS that makes the ovary either more susceptible to or at least sensitive to insulin's stimulation of androgen production in the ovary.[12]

Inappropriate gonadotropin secretion triggers the beginning of a vicious cycle that perpetuates anovulation. Typically, levels of follicle-stimulating hormone (FSH) are low or below normal, and the luteinizing hormone (LH) level is elevated. Persistent LH elevation causes an increase in androgens (dehydroepiandrosterone sulfate [DHEAS] from the adrenal glands and testosterone, androstenedione, and

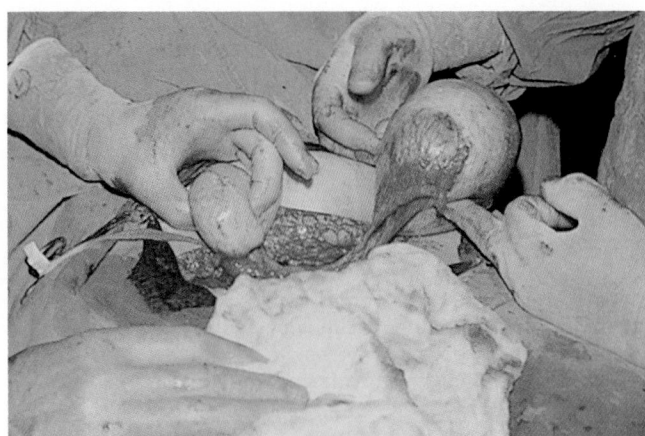

Figure 32-2 ■ **Polycystic Ovary.** Both ovaries shown are enlarged with multiple cysts. (From Symonds EM, Macpherson, MBA: *Diagnosis in color: obstetrics and gynecology,* London, 1997, Mosby.)

dehydroepiandrosterone [DHEA] from the ovary). Androgens are converted to estrogen in peripheral tissues, and increased testosterone levels cause a significant reduction (approximately 50%) in SHBG, which, in turn, causes increased levels of free estradiol. Elevated estrogen levels trigger a positive-feedback response in LH and a negative-feedback response in FSH. Because FSH levels are not totally depressed, new follicular growth is continuously stimulated, but not to full maturation and ovulation (see Figure 32-3).[12]

CLINICAL MANIFESTATIONS Clinical manifestations of PCOS are related to anovulation and elevated testosterone levels and include dysfunctional bleeding or amenorrhea, hirsutism, and infertility (Box 32-3). Approximately 38% of women with PCOS are obese, and 20% are asymptomatic. In addition, 30% of women with PCOS will develop diabetes by the age of 30.

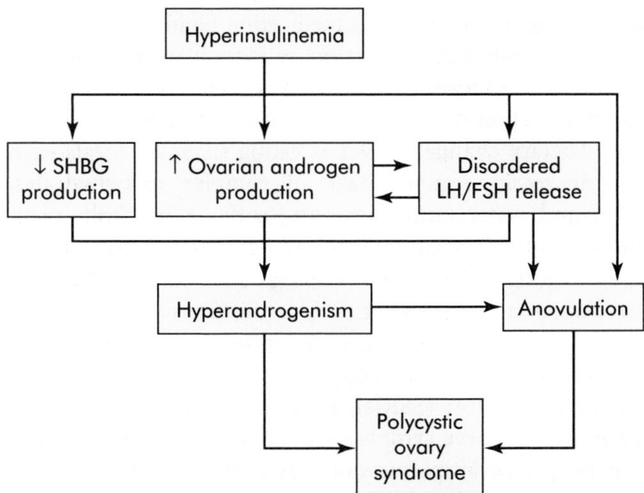

Figure 32-3 ■ **Insulin Resistance and Hyperinsulinemia in PCOS.** See text for explanation. *SHBG,* Sex hormone-binding globulin; *LH,* luteinizing hormone; *FSH,* follicle-stimulating hormone.

Sequelae include type 2 diabetes mellitus, cardiovascular disease, and endometrial carcinoma (caused by unopposed estrogen). Pregnant women with PCOS may be at increased risk for glucose intolerance.[5]

EVALUATION AND TREATMENT Diagnosis of PCOS is based on evidence of androgen excess, chronic anovulation, and inappropriate gonadotropin secretion. Treatment of PCOS with insulin sensitizers seems to increase fertility while decreasing predisposition to type 2 diabetes. Adding an antiandrogen agent may enhance results. For women who do not desire pregnancy, hormonal contraception may be used to suppress androgen production and reduce endometrial hyperplasia.

Premenstrual syndrome

Premenstrual syndrome (PMS) is the cyclic recurrence (in the luteal phase of the menstrual cycle) of distressing physical, psychologic, or behavioral changes that impair interpersonal relationships or interfere with usual activities.[13] An estimated 5% to 10% of menstruating women have severe to disabling symptoms; 3% to 8% of these women have cyclic dysphoria (exaggerated feeling of depression), known as **premenstrual dysphoric disorder (PMDD),** warranting treatment. Making study of this syndrome difficult, it seems that (1) symptoms are experienced to some degree by all ovulating adolescent and adult women and they may occur throughout all menstrual phases, (2) the presence and severity of symptoms in any one woman may be inconsistent from month to month, and (3) the menstrual phase for peak symptom severity may differ depending on the population studied.[14,15]

PATHOPHYSIOLOGY The exact etiology of PMS is unknown. The cause of PMS is considered to be multifactorial. Fluctuating estrogen and progesterone levels may trigger this biologic response but are not sufficient alone to cause PMS. Research suggests that serotonin levels play a role in type and severity of symptoms. Low-dose fluoxetine, a selective serotonin reuptake inhibitor, significantly reduces premenstrual mood-related symptoms, whereas higher doses also decrease breast tenderness, bloating, and joint/muscle pain.

A predisposition for PMS runs in families, perhaps because of genetics or shared environment. A woman's menstrual experience tends to be similar to her mother's or her sister's experience. Further evidence supports a relationship between the severity and frequency of premenstrual symptoms and reports of major affective disorder, personality characteristics, and family conflict. In turn, when premenstrual symptoms are perceived as distressing, the quality of interpersonal relationships and self-image are negatively affected.

CLINICAL MANIFESTATIONS The pattern of symptom frequency and severity is more important than specific

BOX 32-3 Clinical Manifestations of Polycystic Ovary Syndrome (PCOS)

Presenting Signs and Symptoms (Percentage of Women Affected)

Obesity (38%)
Menstrual disturbance (66%)
Oligomenorrhea (47%)
Amenorrhea (19%)
Regular menstruation (48%)
Hyperandrogenism (48%)
Infertility (73% of anovulatory infertility)
Asymptomatic (20% of those with PCOS)

Hormonal Disturbances

Increased insulin (independent of obesity)
Decreased SHBG
Increased androgens (testosterone, androstenedione)
Increased LH (genetic variant subunit)
Increased prolactin
Increased leptin, especially in obesity (independent of insulin)
Suggested decreased insulin-like growth factor (IGF-I) receptors on theca cells
Possible decreased estrogen receptors (intraovarian and along hypothalamic-pituitary axis)

Possible Late Sequelae

Dyslipidemia: increased low-density lipoproteins, decreased high-density lipoproteins, increased triglycerides
Diabetes mellitus (30% of women with or without obesity will develop type 2 diabetes mellitus by age 30)
Cardiovascular disease; hypertension
Endometrial carcinoma (anovulatory women are hyperestrogenic)

Other

It is controversial if women with PCOS are at increased risk of glucose intolerance and preeclampsia during pregnancy

See also Haakova L et al: Pregnancy outcome in women with PCOS and in controls matched by age and weight, *Hum Reprod* 18(7):1438–1441, 2003.
PCOS, Polycystic ovary syndrome; *SHBG*, sex hormone-binding globulin; *LH*, luteinizing hormone.

complaints. More than 200 physical, emotional, and behavioral symptoms have been attributed to PMS. Emotional symptoms, particularly depression, anger, irritability, and fatigue, have been reported as the most prominent and the most distressing, whereas physical symptoms seem to be the least prevalent and problematic. Approximately 6% of women have classic PMS (distressing luteal symptoms), and 7% report premenstrual magnification of symptoms that are present during the entire cycle. A typical premenstrual symptom pattern may appear after the treatment of a systemic disease. Likewise, underlying physical or psychologic disease may be aggravated premenstrually.

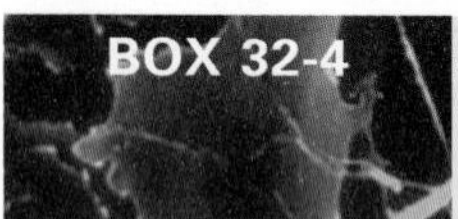

BOX 32-4 General Criteria for Premenstrual Dysphoric Disorder

Premenstrual dysphoria is the predominant feature of premenstrual dysphoric disorder (PMDD) and is triggered (not caused) by the endocrine changes that occur in the late luteal phase of the menstrual cycle. Although PMDD is not an accepted diagnostic entity in the *Diagnostic and Statistical Manual of Mental Disorders* (DSM-IV-TR, 2000) text, recognition is given to the severe and incapacitating dysphoria that characterizes the disorder by listing PMDD as an example under "Mood Disorders, Depression, Not Otherwise Specified" in the main text. To encourage further research, PMDD remains in the appendix of DSM-IV. Criteria for PMDD include a rigorous prospective assessment confirming a regular premenstrual pattern of severe depressive symptoms.

Data from American Psychiatric Association: *DSM-IV-TR diagnostic and statistical manual of mental disorders*, ed 4, Washington, DC, 2000, American Psychiatric Association.

EVALUATION AND TREATMENT Diagnosis of PMS is based on health history and symptoms. Research and diagnostic criteria for premenstrual dysphoric disorder (PMDD) are presented in Box 32-4. Current treatment for PMS is symptomatic because the cause is complex and cannot be reduced to a single biologic explanation and because the occurrence and severity are mediated by lifestyle, social, and psychologic factors. Nonpharmacologic therapies, with or without medication, tend to be more effective in controlling symptoms than medication alone.

Initial treatment focuses on validation of premenstrual experience, education about PMS, self-help techniques, and elimination of contributing factors or coexisting disorders. Dietary changes—such as eating six small meals each day; increasing one's intake of complex carbohydrates, fiber, and water; and decreasing caffeine, alcohol, sugar, and animal fat consumption—are beneficial.

After a trial of nonpharmacologic therapies, or if criteria for diagnosis of PMDD is met, medications may be added to the treatment regimen. Drugs often prescribed include vitamin and mineral supplements, selective serotonin reuptake inhibitors (SSRIs), antiprostaglandins, and alprazolam. SSRIs relieve symptoms in about 60% of women and may be given continuously or only during the premenstrual period. Long-acting SSRIs, such as fluoxetine, should be tapered to prevent withdrawal symptoms. Edema associated with PMS is a result of local fluid shifts rather than fluid retention, therefore diuretics are not recommended.

Women tend to respond immediately to SSRIs whether prescribed intermittently or consistently, suggesting that premenstrual depression is mediated differently than major mood disorders.[16] Although controversial because evidence demonstrating efficacy is lacking, the most widely prescribed treatment in Great Britain is progestogens, including progesterone.[17]

In severe cases, menses is abolished, which eliminates cyclic ovarian hormones and thus the biologic trigger for PMS. This is accomplished by the use of oral contraceptives, depomedroxyprogesterone acetate, or GnRh agonists.

QUICK CHECK 32-2

1. Why do prostaglandin inhibitors decrease symptoms associated with primary dysmenorrhea?
2. Why does amenorrhea occur?
3. Why do anovulatory cycles lead to dysfunctional uterine bleeding?
4. What other conditions are associated with PCOS?

Infection and Inflammation

Infections of the genital tract may result from exogenous or endogenous microorganisms. Exogenous pathogens are most often sexually transmitted. Endogenous causes of infection include microorganisms that are normally resident in the vagina, bowel, or vulva. Infection occurs if these microorganisms migrate to a new location or overproliferate when the immune system and other defense mechanisms are impaired.

Skin disorders that can affect the vulva include reactive dermatitis, contact dermatitis, psoriasis, and impetigo. (For a discussion of skin disorders, see Chapter 39.) Most infectious disorders that affect the vulva and vagina are sexually transmitted, however. These disorders are described in Table 32-15 (on pp. 900-901).

Pelvic inflammatory disease

Pelvic inflammatory disease (PID) is an acute inflammatory process caused by infection (Figure 32-4). PID may involve any organ, or combination of organs, of the upper genital tract—the uterus, fallopian tubes, or ovaries—and, in its most severe form, the entire peritoneal cavity. Inflammation of the fallopian tubes is termed **salpingitis** (Figure 32-5); inflammation of the ovaries is called **oophoritis.** Most cases of PID are caused by sexually transmitted microorganisms that migrate from the vagina to the uterus, fallopian tubes, and ovaries.[18]

PATHOPHYSIOLOGY The development of upper genital tract infections is mediated by a number of defense mechanisms. Virulence of the organism, size of the inoculum, and immune status of the individual may overwhelm defenses. PID usually is considered a polymicrobial infection, and although mostly initiated by gonorrhea or chlamydia, mixed bacteria also contribute, including anaerobes (*Bacteroides* species and peptostreptococci) and facultative organisms (*Gardnerella vaginalis, Haemophilus influenzae,* and streptococci). Recovery of *Neisseria gonorrhoeae, Chlamydia trachomatis,* or both, have been reported in 50% to 60% of women with acute PID. These microorganisms induce necrosis with repeated infections and predispose an individual to PID. In addition, *Mycoplasma hominis* and *Ureaplasma urealyticum* might be etiologic agents of PID. After one episode of pelvic infection, 15% to 25% of women develop long-term sequelae, such as infertility, ectopic pregnancy, chronic pelvic pain, dyspareunia (painful intercourse), pelvic adhesions, perihepatitis, and tubo-ovarian (fallopian tube and ovary) abscess. The incidence of complications increases markedly with repeated infections. Mortality associated with PID is 0.29 deaths per

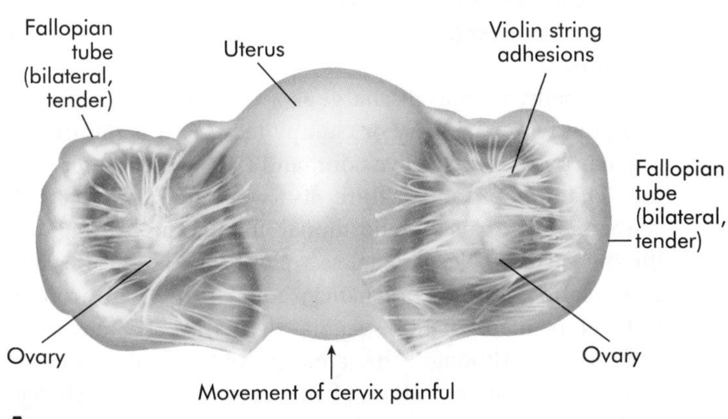

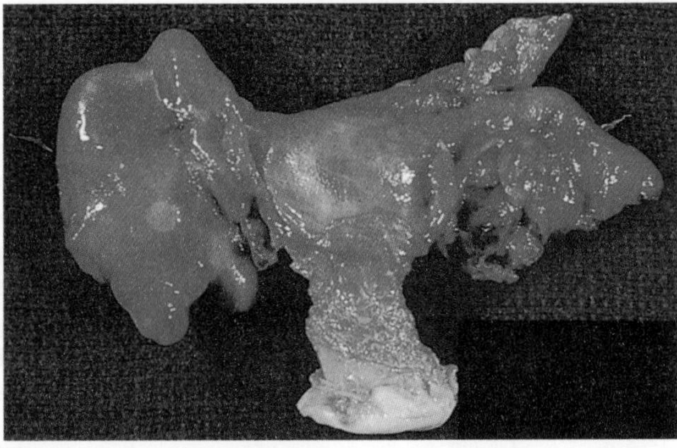

Figure 32-4 ■ **Pelvic Inflammatory Disease. A,** Drawing depicting involvement of both ovaries and fallopian tubes. **B,** Total abdominal hysterectomy and bilateral salpingo-oophorectomy specimen showing unilateral pyosalpinx. (**A** from Seidel HM et al: *Mosby's guide to physical examination,* ed 6, St Louis, 2006, Mosby; **B** from Morse SA, Ballard RC, Holmes KK, Moreland AA: *Atlas of sexually transmitted diseases and AIDS,* ed 3, Edinburgh, 2003, Mosby.)

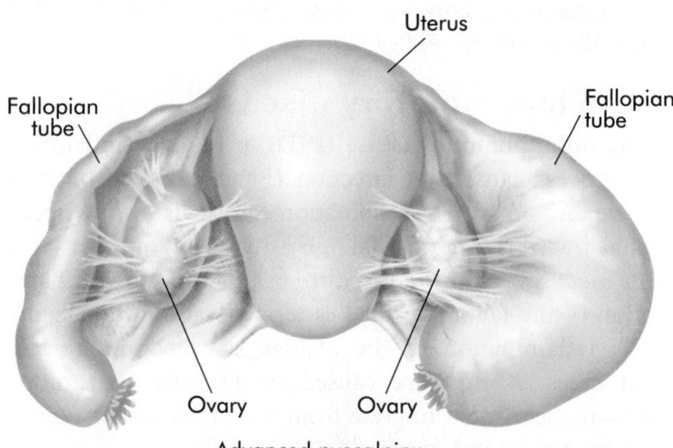

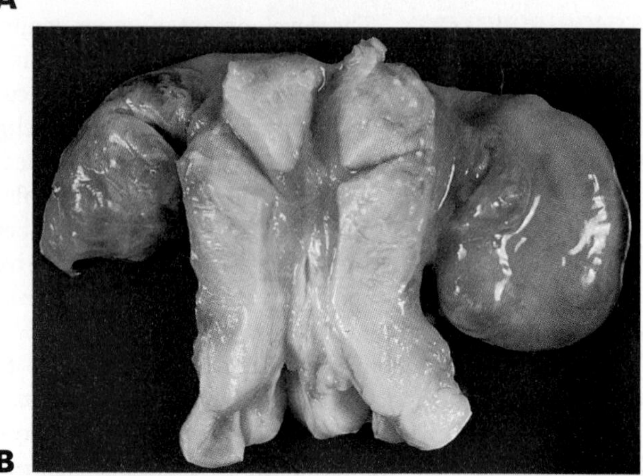

Figure 32-5 ■ **Salpingitis. A,** Note the swollen fallopian tubes. **B,** Bilateral, retort-shaped, swollen sealed tubes and adhesions of ovaries are typical of salpingitis. (**A** from Seidel HM et al: *Mosby's guide to physical examination,* ed 6, St Louis, 2006, Mosby; **B** from Damjanov I, Linder J, editors: *Anderson's pathology,* ed 10, St Louis, 1996, Mosby.)

100,000 women age 15 to 44.[19] Most deaths resulting from PID are caused by septic shock (see Chapter 23).

CLINICAL MANIFESTATIONS The clinical manifestations of PID vary from sudden, severe abdominal pain with fever to no symptoms at all. An asymptomatic cervicitis may be present for some time before PID develops. Of women with salpingitis, 67% to 75% may have a subclinical infection. The first sign of the ascending infection may be the onset of low bilateral abdominal pain, often characterized as dull and steady with a gradual onset. Symptoms are more likely to develop during or immediately after menstruation. The pain of PID may worsen with walking, jumping, or intercourse. Other manifestations of PID include dysuria (difficult or painful urination) and irregular bleeding.

EVALUATION AND TREATMENT The diagnosis of PID is based on history, abdominal tenderness, presence of uterine and cervical movement tenderness on bimanual pelvic examination, mucopurulent discharge at the cervical os, white blood cells on Gram stain or wet mount of cervical discharge, leukocytosis, and increased erythrocyte sedimentation rate. To support the diagnosis, tests for chlamydia and gonorrhea are done; sonography, laparoscopy, and culdocentesis are indicated when a woman has recurrent symptoms or symptoms unresponsive to outpatient treatment regimen, fever greater than 38° C, or an adnexal mass. Other conditions that cause pelvic pain must be excluded, including ectopic pregnancy, threatened abortion, or appendicitis.

Because of the significance of the complications of PID, aggressive treatment is recommended. Treatment involves bed rest, avoidance of intercourse, and combined antibiotic therapy. From 25% to 40% of women require hospitalization for intravenous administration of antibiotics and treatment of peritonitis or a tuboovarian abscess. To prevent recurrence, sexual partners are also treated with antibiotic combinations.

Vaginitis

Vaginitis is infection of the vagina. The major causes are sexually transmitted pathogens, bacterial vaginosis, and *Candida albicans.* The incidence of sexually transmitted vaginitis remains highest in women 10 to 24 years of age.[18]

The development of vaginitis is related to local defense mechanisms, such as skin integrity and, particularly, vaginal pH. The pH of the vagina depends on cervical secretions and the presence of normal flora that help maintain an acidic environment. Variables that alter the vaginal pH, and therefore the bactericidal nature of secretions (see Chapter 31) and the predisposition to infection, include douching; use of soaps, spermicides, feminine hygiene sprays, deodorant menstrual pads or tampons; and conditions associated with increased glycogen content of vaginal secretions, such as pregnancy, diabetes, and conditions that compromise the immune system.

The use of antibiotics may destroy *Lactobacillus acidophilus,* an anaerobic, gram-positive rod normally found in the vagina that helps maintain an acidic pH. In its absence, alkalinity increases and the vagina is more susceptible to trichomoniasis and bacterial vaginosis; moreover, there may be an overgrowth of *C. albicans,* causing a yeast vaginitis.

Normally, vaginal discharge is a clear, milky, or cloudy secretion with a slippery or clumpy texture. It is nonirritating, has a mild inoffensive odor, and turns yellow after drying. The amount and texture of a woman's discharge will change in response to hormonal fluctuation throughout the menstrual cycle. Vaginal secretions increase at the time of ovulation, during pregnancy, and with sexual arousal; just before menstruation, vaginal discharge becomes thick and sticky. Although the amount of vaginal discharge alone is not an indication of infection, any other change in discharge may indicate a problem. Infection is suggested with a marked change in color or if the discharge becomes copious, malodorous, or irritating.

Diagnosis is based on history, physical examination, and examination of the discharge by wet mount. Treatment involves developing and maintaining an acidic environment, relieving symptoms (usually pruritus), and administering antimicrobial or antifungal medications to eradicate the infectious organism. If the infection can be sexually transmitted, a woman's partner will also be treated.

Cervicitis

Cervicitis is a nonspecific term used to describe inflammation of the cervix before the identification of pathogens. **Mucopurulent cervicitis (MPC)** is usually caused by one or more sexually transmitted pathogens, such as *Trichomonas,* gonorrhea, *Chlamydia, Mycoplasma,* or *Ureaplasma.* Infection causes the cervix to become red and edematous. A mucopurulent (mucus- and pus-containing) exudate drains from the external cervical os, and the individual may report vague pelvic pain, bleeding, or dysuria. The infectious organisms are cultured or identified by immunoassay. Definitive diagnosis is followed by oral antibiotic therapy. Sexual partners are usually treated to prevent reinfection.[18]

Vulvitis

Inflammation of the vulva is termed **vulvitis.** Acute vulvitis is an inflammation of the skin (dermatitis) of the vulva and often of the perianal area. Vulvitis can be caused by contact with soaps, detergents, lotions, hygienic sprays, shaving, menstrual pads, or perfumed toilet paper and can be aggravated by nonabsorbent or tight-fitting clothes. Vulvitis may increase susceptibility to vaginal infection. Likewise vulvitis is also caused by vaginal infections (e.g., candidiasis, trichomoniasis) that spread to the labia, where they cause inflammation and edema. The vulva also can be affected by other skin diseases, such as tinea cruris, lichen sclerosis, psoriasis, and inflammation of the apocrine (sweat) glands (see Chapter 39).

Avoidance of irritants; wearing loose, cotton clothing; and appropriate antimicrobial/antifungal treatment for recurrent vaginitis are usually effective cures for acute vulvitis. Chronic vulvitis is usually treated with fluorinated hydrocortisone. Biopsy specimens of persistent lesions are examined for the presence of malignancy.

Bartholinitis

Bartholinitis (Bartholin cyst) is an inflammation of one or both of the ducts that lead from the introitus (vaginal opening) to the Bartholin glands (Figure 32-6). The usual causes are microorganisms that infect the lower female reproductive tract, such as streptococci, staphylococci, and sexually transmitted pathogens. Acute bartholinitis may be preceded by an infection, such as cervicitis, vaginitis, or urethritis. Cultures for gonorrhea and chlamydia are recommended.

Infection or trauma causes inflammatory changes that narrow the distal portion of the duct, leading to obstruction and stasis of glandular secretions. The obstruction, or cyst, varies from 1 to 8 cm in diameter and is located in the posterolateral portion of the vulva. The affected area is usually red and painful, and pus may be visible at the opening of the duct. This exudate should be cultured. The individual may have fever and malaise.

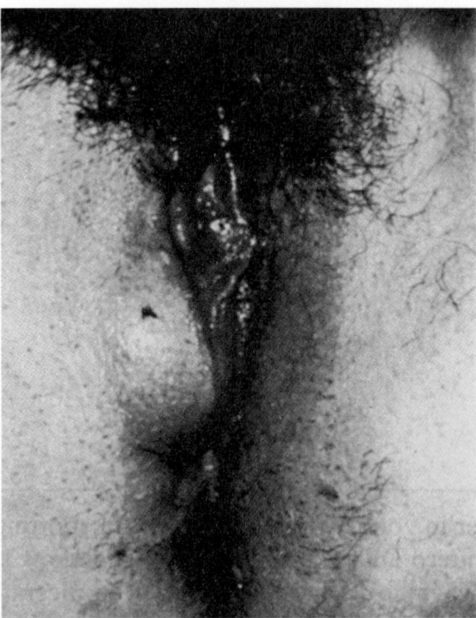

Figure 32-6 ■ **Inflammation of Bartholin Glands.** (From Gardner HL, Kaufman RH: *Benign diseases of the vulva and vagina,* St Louis, 1969, Mosby.)

Chronic bartholinitis is characterized by the presence of a small cyst that is slightly tender but otherwise is asymptomatic. Most Bartholin cysts require no treatment. Symptoms only occur if an exacerbation of infection causes an abscess to form in the gland itself.

Diagnosis is based on the clinical manifestations and the identification of infectious microorganisms. Infection is treated with antibiotics, and pain is relieved with analgesics and warm sitz baths. If an abscess forms, it may be surgically drained.

Pelvic Relaxation Disorders

The bladder, urethra, and rectum are supported by the endopelvic fascia and perineal muscles. This muscular and fascial tissue loses tone and strength with aging and may fail to maintain the pelvic organs in the proper position. Uterine displacement can be caused by progressive relaxation of the pelvic support structures or trauma, such as childbirth or pelvic surgery, that damages or weakens the supporting structures. Pelvic relaxation is progressive and is related to the inherent strength or weakness of the woman's musculofascial tissue. Malpositioning of the bladder, urethra, or rectum (and hence the uterus) may occur many years after an initial injury to the supporting structure. A strong familial tendency and, possibly, a multifactorial genetic component place some women at risk for the development of prolapse.

Figure 32-7 shows vaginal prolapse caused by cystocele, rectocele, and enterocele. **Cystocele** is descent of the bladder and the anterior vaginal wall into the vaginal canal. In severe cases, the bladder and anterior vaginal wall bulge outside the introitus (vaginal opening). A cystocele may cause the woman to lose urine when she laughs, sneezes,

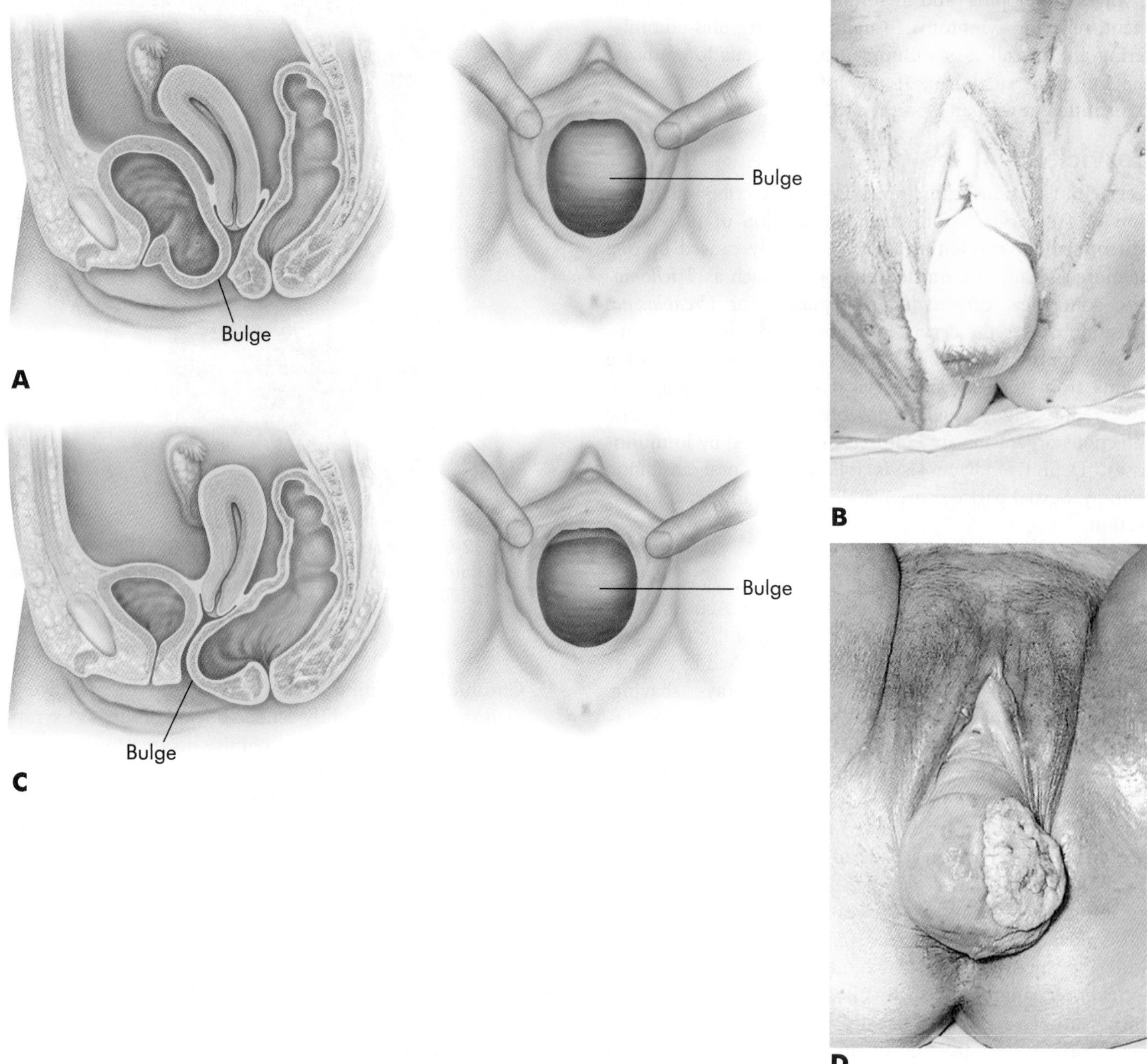

Figure 32-7 ■ **Vaginal Prolapse. A,** Anatomic positioning involving cystocele. **B,** Large cystocele. **C,** Anatomic positioning involving rectocele. **D,** Rectocele associated with ulceration of vaginal wall. (**A** and **C** from Seidel HM et al: *Mosby's guide to physical examination,* ed 4, St Louis, 1999, Mosby; **B** and **D** from Symonds EM, Macpherson MBA: *Color atlas of obstetrics and gynecology,* London, 1994, Mosby.)

coughs, or does anything that strains the abdominal muscles, a condition called **stress incontinence.** Cystocele is usually accompanied by **urethrocele,** or sagging of the urethra. Urethrocele is usually caused by the shearing effect of the fetal head on the urethra during childbirth. A **rectocele** is the bulging of the rectum and posterior vaginal wall into the vaginal canal. If this condition is severe, defecation is difficult and can be accomplished only by applying manual pressure to the posterior vaginal wall. An **enterocele** is herniation of the rectouterine pouch into the rectovaginal septum (between the rectum and posterior vaginal wall). It is usually associated with other pelvic relaxation disorders, such as uterine prolapse, cystocele, and rectocele. Table 32-3 summarizes the causes, symptoms, and treatment of cystocele, urethrocele, and rectocele.

Uterine prolapse is descent of the cervix or entire uterus into the vaginal canal (Figure 32-8). In severe cases, the uterus falls completely through the vagina and protrudes from the introitus. First-degree uterine prolapse is not treated unless it causes discomfort. Second- and third-degree prolapses cause feelings of fullness, heaviness, and collapse through the vagina. Symptoms of other pelvic relaxation disorders also may be present. Treatment in these cases is the insertion of a **pessary,** which is a removable mechanical device that holds the uterus in position.[20] The pelvic fascia may be strengthened through Kegel exercises—a repetitive,

TABLE 32-3

Cystocele, Urethrocele, and Rectocele

Condition	Etiology	Symptoms	Treatment
Cystocele	Laceration, stretching, or weakening of supporting fascial tissue; usually caused by prolonged labor, multiple births, or birth of a large baby	Urinary frequency, urgency, incontinence Difficulty in complete emptying of the bladder Low backache Symptoms become problematic premenopausally or postmenopausally	Depending on age of woman and severity of the condition, includes the following: Isometric exercise to strengthen the pubococcygeal muscle Oral or topical estrogen to improve tone and vascularity of fascial support Pessary, a removable device that holds the bladder in position Surgical correction
Urethrocele	Pressure of fetal head on urethra and attachments beneath the symphysis pubis Familial or genetic predisposition	Asymptomatic unless it occurs in conjunction with cystocele Stress incontinence	Isometric exercises (see cystocele)
Rectocele	Trauma to the fascia and levator muscles; usually caused by childbirth	Constipation or feeling of rectal fullness Difficult defecation Pressure and sensation of fullness in the vagina	Isometric exercises Diet counseling to prevent constipation Stool softeners or laxatives Surgery

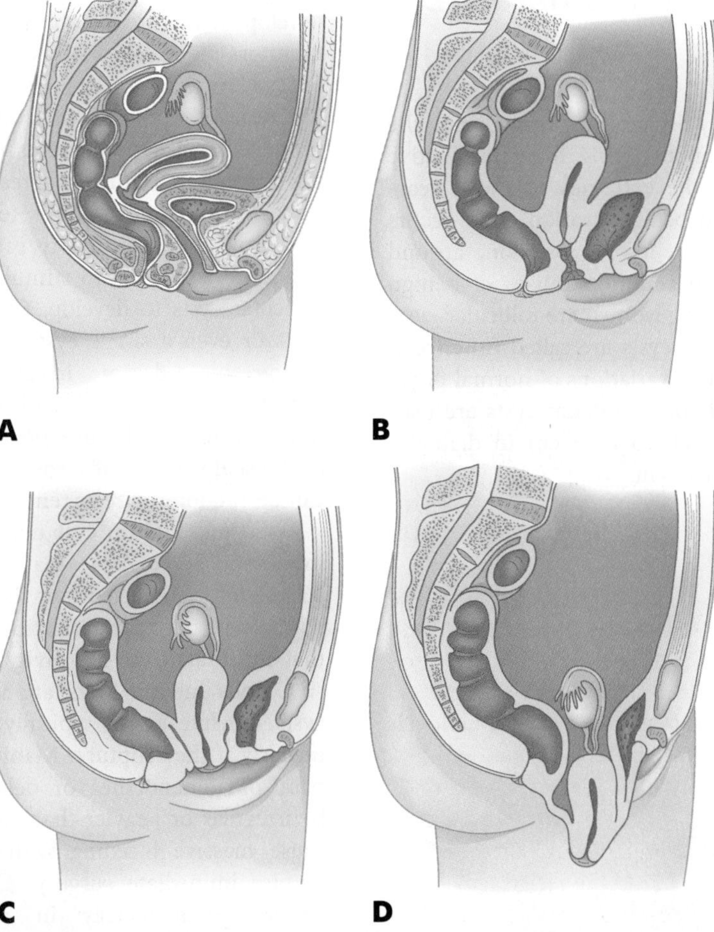

Figure 32-8 ■ Degrees of Uterine Prolapse. A, Normal positioning of uterus. **B,** First-degree prolapse: descent within the vagina. **C,** Second-degree prolapse: the cervix protrudes through the introitus. **D,** Third-degree prolapse: the vagina is completely everted.

isometric tightening and relaxing of the pubococcygeal muscles—or by a course of estrogen therapy, particularly if the woman is past menopause. Surgical repair with or without hysterectomy may be necessary. Prevention of constipation, maintaining a healthy body mass index, and early treatment of respiratory ailments that cause coughing may help (see *Health Alert:* Dietary Interventions and Lifestyle Changes).[21]

HEALTH ALERT

Dietary Interventions and Lifestyle Changes for Pelvic Prolapse

Constipation contributes to chronic straining and pelvic prolapse. Increasing fiber to 25 to 35 mg/day and water intake to 8 to 10 glasses per day will prevent constipation and consequently straining and prolapse. Other lifestyle changes may help also. These include achieving and maintaining ideal weight, doing pelvic floor exercises, avoiding or reducing heavy lifting, avoiding high-impact aerobics or jogging, and quitting smoking.

Data from Jelovsek JE, Maher C, Barber MD: Pelvic organ prolapse, *Lancet* 369(9566):1027–1038, 2007; Forrest DE: Common gynecologic pelvic disorders. In Youngkin EQ, Davis MS, editors: *Women's health: a primary care clinical guide,* ed 3, Upper Saddle River, NJ, 2004, Prentice Hall.

Benign Growths and Proliferative Conditions

Benign ovarian cysts

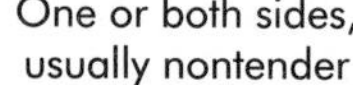

Benign cysts of the ovary may occur at any time during the life span but are most common during the reproductive years and, in particular, at the extremes of those years (Figure 32-9). An increase in benign ovarian cysts occurs when hormonal imbalances are more common, around puberty and menopause. Two common causes of benign ovarian enlargement in ovulating women are follicular cysts and corpus luteum cysts. These cysts are called **functional cysts** because they are caused by variations of normal physiologic events. Follicular and corpus luteum cysts are usually unilateral. They are typically 5 to 6 cm in diameter but can grow as large as 8 to 10 cm.

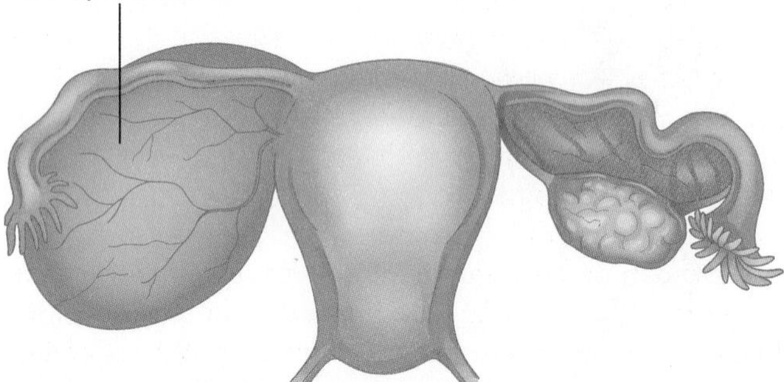

Figure 32-9 ■ **Depiction of Ovarian Cyst.**

Benign cysts of the ovary are produced when a follicle or a number of follicles are stimulated but no dominant follicle develops and completes the maturity process. Every month about 3 to 12 follicles are stimulated, but normally only one succeeds in ovulation of a mature ova.

Normally, in the early follicular phase of the menstrual cycle, follicles of the ovary respond to hormonal signals from the brain. The pituitary produces FSH to mature follicles in the ovary. As the follicles enlarge, granulosa cells in the follicle multiply and secrete estradiol. As a dominant follicle develops, it secretes higher levels of estradiol, which stimulates the LH surge that comes from the pituitary. The LH surge stimulates the follicle to rupture, releasing the ova and transforming the granulosa cells of the dominant follicle into the corpus luteum. If the dominant follicle develops properly before ovulation, the corpus luteum becomes vascularized and secretes progesterone. Progesterone arrests development of other follicles in both ovaries in that cycle. Progesterone, proteolytic enzymes, and prostaglandins trigger follicular rupture and release of the ovum.

Follicular cysts can be caused by a transient condition in which the dominant follicle fails to rupture or one or more of the nondominant follicles fail to regress. This disturbance is not well understood. It may be that the hypothalamus does not receive or send a message strong enough to increase FSH levels to the degree necessary to develop or mature a dominant follicle. The hypothalamus monitors blood levels of estradiol and progesterone; when FSH is low, estradiol does not increase enough to stimulate LH. Research indicates that when progesterone is not being produced, the hypothalamus releases gonadotropin-releasing hormone (GnRh) to increase the FSH level.[22] FSH continues to stimulate follicles to mature, and the granulosa cells grow and, presumably, estradiol increases. This abnormal cycle continues to stimulate follicular size and causes follicular cysts to develop. Clinical symptoms of follicular cysts or even a single cyst are pelvic pain, a sensation of feeling bloated, or irregular menses. After several subsequent cycles in which hormone levels once again follow a regular cycle and progesterone levels are restored, cysts usually will be absorbed or will regress. Follicular cysts can be random or recurrent events.

A **corpus luteum cyst** may develop because there is an intracystic hemorrhage that occurs in the vascularization stage, and the effected cyst then consists of blood. In normal cycles, the vascularization is replaced by a clear fluid that accumulates in the cavity of the corpus luteum.

Corpus luteum cysts are less common than follicular cysts, but luteal cysts typically cause more symptoms, particularly if they rupture. Manifestations include dull pelvic pain and amenorrhea or delayed menstruation, followed by irregular or heavier-than-normal bleeding. Rupture can cause massive bleeding with excruciating pain and can require immediate surgery. Corpus luteum cysts usually regress spontaneously in nonpregnant women. Oral contraceptives may be used to prevent cysts from forming in the future.

Dermoid cysts are ovarian teratomas that contain elements of all three germ layers; they are common ovarian neoplasms. These growths may contain mature tissue including skin, hair, sebaceous and sweat glands, muscle fibers, cartilage, and bone. Dermoid cysts are usually asymptomatic and are found incidentally on pelvic examination. Dermoid cysts have malignant potential and should be removed.

Torsion of the ovary may occur as a complication of ovarian cysts or tumors or enlargement of the ovary associated with infertility treatments. **Ovarian torsion** is rare but is a gynecologic emergency when present. Individuals present with acute, severe unilateral abdominal or pelvic pain related to a change of position.

QUICK CHECK 32-3

1. Why is prompt treatment of pelvic inflammatory disease (PID) critical to reproductive health?
2. Why do benign ovarian cysts develop in women who ovulate?
3. What is the difference between a follicular cyst and a corpus luteum cyst?

Endometrial polyps

An **endometrial polyp** is a mass of endometrial tissue and contains a variable amount of glands, stroma, and blood vessels. Endometrial polyps are usually solitary and originate at the fundus but also may be multiple (20% of the time) or originate from the lower uterine segment or upper endocervix and contain mixed epithelium. Polyps are morphologically diverse and are usually classified as hyperplastic, atrophic (or inactive), or functional. In the latter case, the surface epithelium may be "out of phase" with other endometrial tissue. Hyperplastic polyps are often pedunculated and may be mistaken for endometrial hyperplasia or, if large, adenosarcoma (Figure 32-10). Although polyps most often develop in women between ages 40 and 60 years, they can occur at all ages.[23]

Most polyps are asymptomatic; however, some endometrial polyps often cause intermenstrual bleeding or even excessive menstrual bleeding. Diagnosis is made by hysteroscopy or direct examination of tissue obtained by curettage. The lesions are removed with small, curved forceps. Coexistence of a separate endometrial atypical hyperplasia or adenocarcinoma is possible.

Leiomyomas

Leiomyomas, commonly called *uterine fibroids,* are benign tumors that develop from smooth muscle cells in the myometrium. Leiomyomas are the most common benign tumors of the uterus, and most remain small and asymptomatic. Prevalence increases in women ages 30 to 50 years but decreases with menopause. In the United States, it is estimated that myomas develop in 30% of white and 50% of black women by the age of 50 years. The incidence of leiomyomas in black and Asian women is two to five times higher than that in white women.

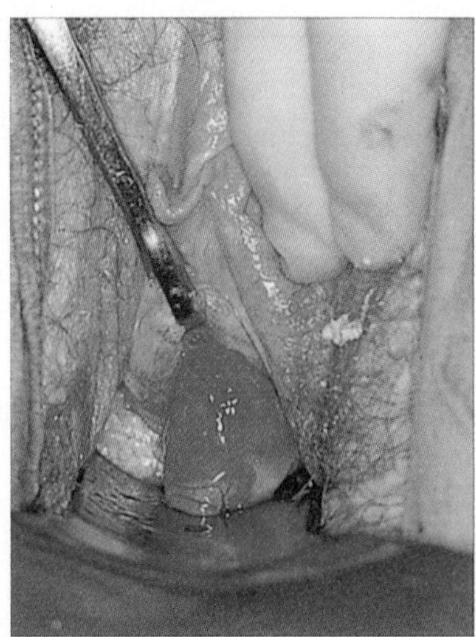

Figure 32-10 ■ **Endometrial Polyp.** Polyp is protruding through the cervical os. (From Symonds EM, Macpherson MBA: *Color atlas of obstetrics and gynecology,* London, 1994, Mosby.)

The cause of uterine leiomyomas is unknown, although their size appears to be related to hormonal fluctuations (particularly estrogen). Uterine leiomyomas are not seen before menarche, and those that develop during the reproductive years generally shrink after menopause. Tumors in pregnant women enlarge rapidly but often decrease in size after termination of the pregnancy.

PATHOPHYSIOLOGY Most leiomyomas occur in multiples in the fundus of the uterus, although they may occur singly and throughout the uterus. Leiomyomas are classified as subserous, submucous, or intramural, according to their location within the various layers of the uterine wall (Figure 32-11). Uterine leiomyomas are usually firm and surrounded by a pseudocapsule composed of compressed but otherwise normal uterine myometrium. Degenerative changes, such as ulceration and necrosis, may occur when the leiomyoma outgrows its blood supply and therefore are more common in larger tumors.

CLINICAL MANIFESTATIONS Although fibroids rarely present problems, they occasionally cause cramping, excessive bleeding, and symptoms related to pressure on nearby structures. The leiomyoma can make the uterine cavity larger, thereby increasing the endometrial surface area. This increase may account for the increased menstrual bleeding, particularly with submucosal leiomyomas. Pain or cramping occurs with the devascularization of larger leiomyomas and is associated with blood vessel compression that limits blood supply to adjacent structures. Because the tumor is relatively slow growing, enabling adjacent structures to adapt to pressure, symptoms of abdominal pressure develop slowly. Pressure on the bladder may contribute to urinary frequency, urgency, and dysuria. Pressure on the ureter

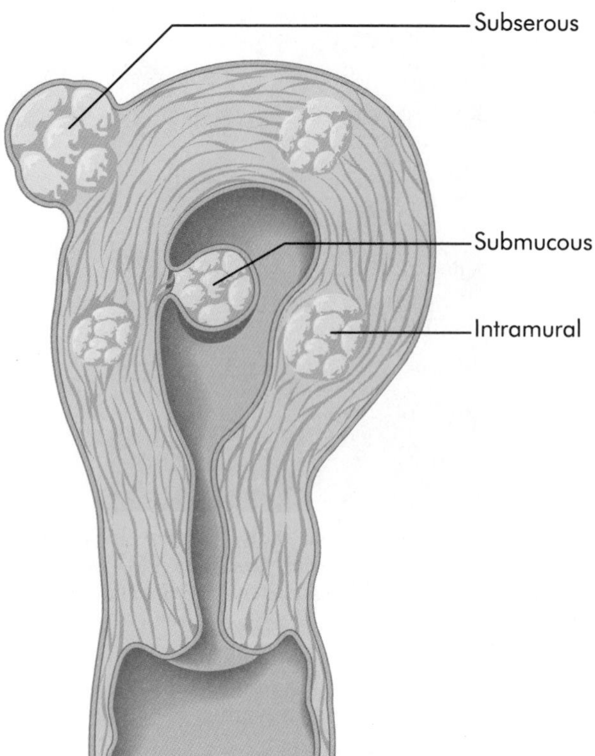

Figure 32-11 ■ **Leiomyomas.** Depiction of uterine section showing whorl-like appearance and locations of leiomyomas, also called *uterine fibroids.*

may cause it to become distended "upstream" from the pressure point; rectosigmoid pressure may lead to constipation. Larger tumors may cause a sensation of abdominal or genital heaviness.

EVALUATION AND TREATMENT Uterine leiomyomas are suspected when bimanual examination discloses irregular, nontender nodularity of the uterus. Pelvic sonography or MRI confirms the diagnosis. Treatment depends on symptoms, tumor size, age, reproductive status, and the overall health of the individual. Most myomas can be treated conservatively. Conservative treatment is aimed at shrinking the myoma using a GnRH agonist (GnRHa), progesterone, or oral contraceptives. Mifepristone (formerly RU486), an antiprogesterone, also may be useful as a conservative treatment. Aromatase inhibitors also show promise as medical therapy.[24,25] Myomectomy may be undertaken and has been the surgical treatment of choice. Newer surgical alternatives are being designed, such as therapeutic embolization of uterine arteries under guided magnetic resonance imagery (MRI). As with any treatment, risks accompany these newer treatments, especially arterial embolization.[26]

Adenomyosis

Adenomyosis is the presence of islands of endometrial glands surrounded by benign endometrial stroma within the uterine myometrium. It commonly develops during the late reproductive years, with the highest incidence among women in their 40s and women taking tamoxifen. Adenomyosis has been found in 18% of hysterectomy specimens and 53% of specimens from women taking tamoxifen.[27] Adenomyosis may be asymptomatic or may be associated with abnormal menstrual bleeding, dysmenorrhea, uterine enlargement, and uterine tenderness during menstruation. Secondary dysmenorrhea becomes increasingly severe as disease progresses. On examination, the uterus is enlarged, globular, and most tender just before or after menstruation. Diagnosis is confirmed with ultrasonography or MRI. Treatment, when necessary, includes surgical resection of localized areas of adenomyosis or, if severe, hysterectomy. Adenomyosis is typically unresponsive to hormone treatment.

Endometriosis

Endometriosis is the presence of functioning endometrial tissue or implants outside the uterus. Like normal endometrial tissue, the ectopic (out-of-place) endometrium responds to the hormonal fluctuations of the menstrual cycle. Endometriosis affects 10% to 15% of reproductive-age women and 50% of infertile women.[28] Theories of the cause of endometriosis are shown in Box 32-5.

PATHOPHYSIOLOGY Endometrial implants can occur throughout the body but occur primarily in the abdominal and pelvic cavities. The most common sites of implantation are the ovaries, uterine ligaments, rectovaginal septum, and pelvic peritoneum (Figure 32-12). Less common sites include the sigmoid colon, small intestine, rectum, appendix, bladder, uterus, vulva, vagina, cervix, lymph nodes, extremities, pleural cavity, lungs, laparotomy scars, and hernial sacs.

If the blood supply is sufficient, the ectopic endometrium proliferates, breaks down, and bleeds in conjunction with the normal menstrual cycle. The bleeding causes inflammation and pain in surrounding tissues. The inflammation may lead to fibrosis, scarring, and adhesions.

CLINICAL MANIFESTATIONS The clinical manifestations of endometriosis vary in frequency and severity and

BOX 32-5 Theories of Endometriosis

- Implantation of endometrial cells during retrograde menstruation, in which menstrual fluids move through the fallopian tubes and empty into the pelvic cavity; occurs in most women, but few develop endometriosis as a result.
- Spread of endometrial cells through the vascular or lymphatic systems—helps explain the rare sites
- Immunologic factors that may include depressed cytotoxic T cell response to endometrial cells
- Stimulation of multipotential epithelial cells covering the reproductive organs that develop into endometrial cells
- Genetic predisposition based on familial tendencies

Data from Speroff L, Fritz MA: *Clinical gynecologic endocrinology and infertility,* ed 7, Philadelphia, 2005, Lippincott Williams & Wilkins.

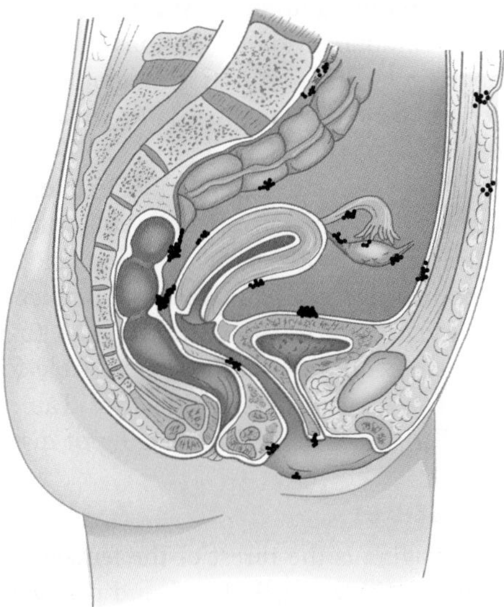

Figure 32-12 ■ Pelvic Sites of Endometrial Implantation. Endometrial cells may enter the pelvic cavity during retrograde menstruation.

include primarily infertility and pain, dysmenorrhea, dyschezia (pain on defecation), dyspareunia (pain on intercourse), and, less commonly, constipation and abnormal vaginal bleeding. If implants are located within the pelvis, an asymptomatic pelvic mass having irregular, movable nodules and a fixed, retroverted uterus is found on examination. Most symptoms can be explained by the proliferation, breakdown, and bleeding of the ectopic endometrial tissue with subsequent formation of adhesions. In many instances, however, the degree of endometriosis is not related to the frequency or severity of symptoms. Dysmenorrhea, for example, does not appear to be related to the degree of endometriosis. With involvement of the rectovaginal septum or the uterosacral ligaments, dyspareunia develops. Dyschezia, a hallmark symptom of endometriosis, occurs with bleeding of ectopic endometrium in the rectosigmoid musculature and subsequent fibrosis.

Up to one third of individuals with endometriosis are infertile, presumably because of (1) mechanical interference with ovulation or ovum transport through the fallopian tube, (2) phagocytosis of sperm by macrophages in the reproductive tract, (3) changes in prostaglandin secretion, (4) luteal phase defect, (5) unruptured luteinizing follicle syndrome, (6) hyperprolactinemia, and (7) autoimmune and genetic factors.

EVALUATION AND TREATMENT A presumptive diagnosis is based on the previously described symptoms, but pelvic laparoscopy is required for a definitive diagnosis.[21] The American Fertility Society has proposed that endometriosis be classified by the extent of the disease as stage I, mild; stage II, moderate; stage III, severe; and stage IV, extensive. All treatment is based on the stage of the disease and aimed toward preventing progression of the disease, alleviating pain, and establishing or restoring fertility. Medical therapies include suppression of ovulation with various medications. Conservative surgical treatment includes laparoscopic removal of endometrial implants with conventional or laser techniques and presacral neurectomy for severe dysmenorrhea. All treatments have risks or side effects, and recurrent symptoms will develop in as many as 45% of women within 5 years.

Cancer

Malignant tumors of the female reproductive system are common. Endometrial carcinoma accounts for approximately 6% of all cancers in women; ovarian tumors, 3.6%; and cervical tumors, 2%.[1] Malignant neoplasms of the female reproductive tract account for about 1 of 8 diagnosed cancers and 1 of 10 cancer deaths in women in the United States.[1]

Cervical cancer

Invasive cancer of the cervix accounts for approximately 12% of all gynecologic cancers and less than 2% of all cancers in women in the United States. Because of the increased prevalence of Papanicolaou (cytologic) screening (Pap smear), rates of invasive cancer have declined steadily (greater than 55% since the early 1970s). Although mortality for blacks declined more rapidly than for whites, mortality risks for black women continue to be more than two times those of white women.

Precancerous dysplasia, also called **cervical intraepithelial neoplasia (CIN),** is more common than invasive cancer and occurs more often in younger women.[1] CIN has genetic abnormalities, loss of cellular functions, and some phenotypic characteristics of cancer that predict risk of developing invasive cancer.[29] An estimated one in eight young women will have cervical dysplasia by age 20. Human papillomavirus (HPV) is a necessary precursor to the development of cervical cancer (see *Health Alert:* Vaccine Offers Promise of Cervical Cancer Prevention).[18,30] Intercourse before 16 years of age and multiple sexual partners or a male partner with multiple partners also place a woman at risk. Smoking is considered a cofactor. Poor nutrition also increases risks, perhaps by depressing the immune system. Likewise, human immunodeficiency virus (HIV)–positive women are at greater risk for developing cervical cancer.[31,32] The role of other sexually transmitted infections is not clear; however, coinfections with HPV and *Chlamydia trachomatis* may increase risk.[33]

HEALTH ALERT

Vaccine Offers Promise of Cervical Cancer Prevention

In 2006 the Food and Drug Administration approved a vaccine (Gardisil) produced by the pharmaceutical maker Merck & Company against human papillomavirus (HPV) types 6, 11, 16, and 18. HPV types 16 and 18 are responsible for 70% of all cervical cancers, and HPV types 6 and 11 are associated with benign genital warts. The vaccine is given in a series of three shots to girls and young women ages 9 to 26. In clinical trials, the vaccine was 90% effective in preventing these types of HPV.[205–207] However, it does not replace screening with a Pap test.

PATHOGENESIS Cervical cancer is a progressive disease—that is, it moves from normal cervical epithelial cells to dysplasia to CIS to invasive cancer (Table 32-4). Figure 32-13 summarizes the progressive degrees of CIN. Premalignant lesions usually occur 10 to 12 years before the development of invasive carcinoma. There is extensive evidence that chromosomes *3p*, *4q*, and *11q* contain tumor suppressor genes and loss of heterozygosity (LOH) (whereby a large segment of a chromosome is lost, consequently a loss of heterozygosity [see Chapter 9]). LOH is associated with the development of invasive cervical cancers.

CLINICAL MANIFESTATIONS Because cervical neoplasms are often asymptomatic, regular cytologic screening (Pap smear) is necessary. About 90% of cervical cancers can be detected early through the use of Pap and HPV testing. If symptoms are present, they may include a change in vaginal discharge or bleeding. Bleeding varies and may occur after intercourse or between menstrual periods. At times, women will complain of abnormal menses or postmenopausal bleeding. A less common symptom may be a serosanguineous or yellowish vaginal discharge. A new or foul odor also may be present. Severe bleeding may cause anemia. Pelvic or epigastric pain is experienced only with large lesions. Advanced disease may cause urinary or rectal symptoms and pelvic or back pain.

EVALUATION AND TREATMENT When dysplasia is detected, cervical biopsy and endocervical curettage are required. Colposcopy is used to suggest sites for biopsy. If invasive carcinoma is found, lymphangiography, computed tomography (CT) scan, ultrasonography, or radioimmunodetection methods are used to assess lymphatic involvement.

The treatment depends on the degree of neoplastic change, the size and location of the lesion, and the extent of metastatic spread. With early detection and treatment, prognosis for invasive cervical cancer is excellent. Overall, the 5-year survival rate is 70% and increases to 92% with early diagnosis. A cure rate of 100% is possible for women with dysplasia or carcinoma in situ.[1] See Table 32-5 for recommended treatment based on staging of disease.

Vaginal cancer

Cancer of the vagina is the rarest of the female genital cancers. It can occur at any age but is found predominantly in women 60 years of age and older. More than 90% of women with vaginal cancer have squamous cell carcinoma, although rare melanomas, sarcomas, and adenocarcinomas are also found. (Types of tumors are described in Chapter 9.) Metastatic cancers are more common than primary lesions in older women.

Vaginal and cervical cancers are thought to have similar epidemiology. Both start as intraepithelial lesions and occur in sexually active women. HPV infection and prior carcinoma of the cervix place a woman at higher risk for developing vaginal cancer.[34] In addition, exposure in utero to nonsteroidal estrogens (diethylstilbestrol [DES]) also has been identified as a risk factor. DES was given to millions

TABLE 32-4

Clinical Staging for Cancer of the Cervix

Stage		Characteristics
0		Cancer in situ, intraepithelial carcinoma; earliest stage of cancer; cancer confined to its original site
I		Carcinoma confined to cervix (extension to corpus disregarded)
	IA	Earliest form of stage I; there is very small amount of cancer, which is visible only under a microscope
	IA1	Area of invasion is <3 mm (about $^1/_8$ inch) deep and <7 mm (about $^1/_3$ inch) wide
	IA2	Area of invasion is between 3 mm and 5 mm (about $^1/_5$ inch) deep, and <7 mm (about $^1/_3$ inch) wide
IB		Includes cancers that can be seen without a microscope; also includes cancers seen only with a microscope that have spread deeper than 5 mm (about $^1/_5$ inch) into connective tissue of the cervix or are wider than 7 mm
	IB1	A IB cancer that is no longer than 4 cm (about $1^3/_5$ inches)
	IB2	A IB cancer that is >4 cm
II		Cancer has spread beyond the cervix to the upper part of the vagina; cancer does not involve the lower third of the vagina
	IIA	Cancer has spread beyond the cervix to the upper part of the vagina; cancer does not involve the lower third of the vagina
	IIB	Cancer has spread to the tissue next to the cervix, called the *parametrial tissue*
III		Cancer has spread to the lower part of the vagina or the pelvic wall; cancer may be blocking the ureters (tubes that carry urine from the kidneys to the bladder)
	IIIA	Cancer has spread to the lower third of the vagina but not to the pelvic wall
	IIIB	Cancer extends to the pelvic wall or blocks urine flow to the bladder
IV		Most advanced stage of cervical cancer; cancer has spread to other parts of the body
	IVA	Cancer has spread to the bladder or rectum, which are organs close to the cervix
	IVB	Cancer has spread to distant organs beyond the pelvic area, such as the lungs

Excerpted from the American Cancer Society: *Detailed guide: Cervical cancer: How is cervical cancer staged?*

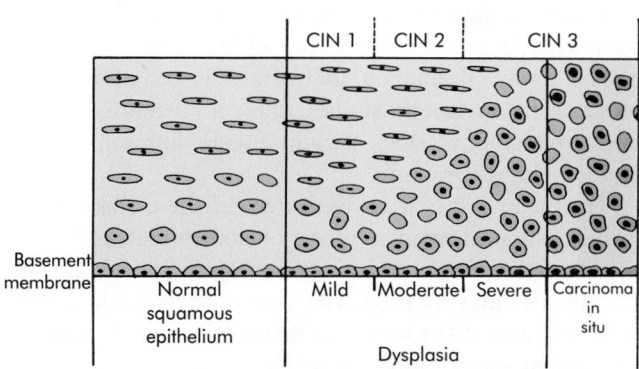

CIN 1 | CIN 2 | CIN 3

Basement membrane | Normal squamous epithelium | Mild | Moderate | Severe | Carcinoma in situ

Dysplasia

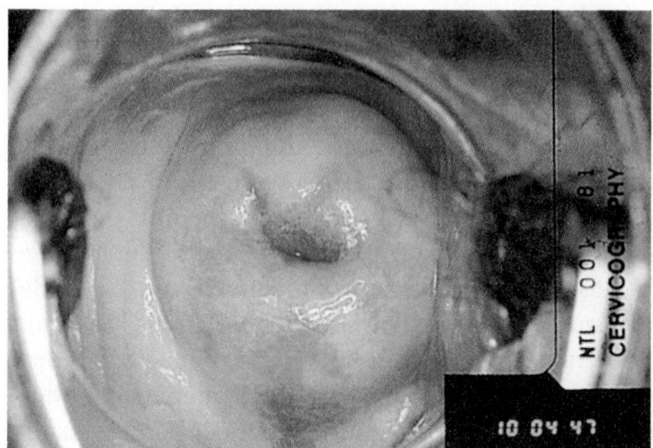

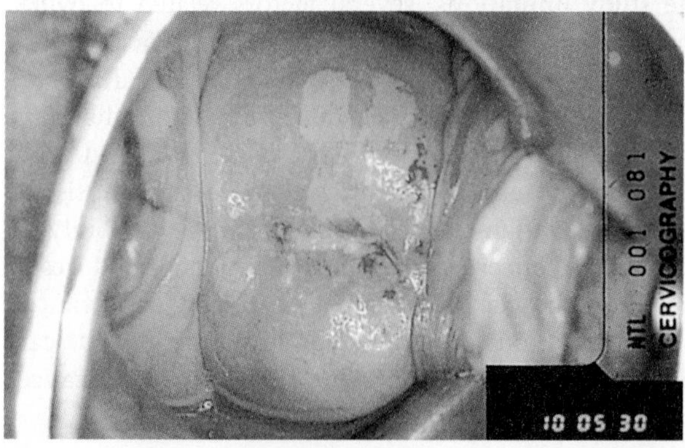

C

Figure 32-13 ■ Cervical Intraepithelial Neoplasia (CIN). **A,** Diagram of cervical endothelium showing progressive degrees of CIN. **B,** Normal multiparous cervix. **C,** CIN stage 1. Note the white appearance of part of the anterior lip of the cervix associated with neoplastic changes. (**A** from Herbst AL et al: *Comprehensive gynecology,* ed 2, St Louis, 1992, Mosby; **B** and **C** from Symonds EM, Macpherson MBA: *Color atlas of obstetrics and gynecology,* London, 1994, Mosby.)

of women between 1938 and 1971 to prevent miscarriage. Between 0.14 and 1.4 cases of vaginal cancer develop per 1000 women at risk. The average age at which clear cell carcinoma develops as a result of DES exposure is 19 years.

Like cervical neoplasms, vaginal cancers are classified as intraepithelial neoplasia (dysplasia), carcinoma in situ, or invasive carcinoma. The lesion usually is not invasive, and it most often occurs in the upper third of the vagina.

TABLE 32-5

Recommended Treatment Based on Clinical Staging for Cancer of the Cervix

Stage	Treatment
0	Cryosurgery, laser surgery, loop electrosurgical excision procedure (LEEP), electrocautery
I	Loop electrosurgical excision procedure (LEEP), laser surgery, conization, cryosurgery, radiation without surgery, total hysterectomy with or without bilateral pelvic lymphadenectomy
II	Radiation, radical hysterectomy and pelvic lymphadenectomy often followed by radiation
III	Radiation with external beam or implant(s) with or without hydroxyurea
IV	Radiation with external beam of implant(s) with or without hydroxyurea, chemotherapy (cisplatin or ifosfamide with distant site involvement)

Vaginal cancer is generally asymptomatic. Therefore, regular pelvic examinations, particularly for women with a history of intrauterine DES exposure, are extremely important. Clinical manifestations that occur include abnormal vaginal bleeding or discharge and urinary symptoms. Pain is a symptom of advanced disease or an infected lesion.

Biopsy techniques confirm the tumor type and determine its size, location, and extent. Treatment depends on these findings and on the age of the individual. Surgery may be followed by radiation and chemotherapy.

Vulvar cancer

Cancer of the vulva was responsible for approximately 3490 new cases of cancer reported in 2007.[1] Cancers arising in younger women are likely to be squamous cell carcinoma caused by HPV, whereas in older women, epithelial disorders, such as chronic inflammation, may be involved. Melanoma and sarcoma may occur on the vulva, and it is possible, although rare, to develop cancer of the Bartholin gland. Early detection is critical, and all suspicious lesions should be biopsied. Treatment includes surgery, radiation, and chemotherapy. Prognosis depends on lesion size, location, histology, and lymph involvement.[35]

Endometrial cancer

Carcinoma of the endometrium is the most prevalent gynecologic malignancy (Figure 32-14). It accounts for about 6% of cancers affecting women and more than 51% of gynecologic cancers. Estimates include 39,080 reported new cases in 2007, with approximately 7400 deaths.[1] Although the cause of endometrial cancer is not clear, a number of risk

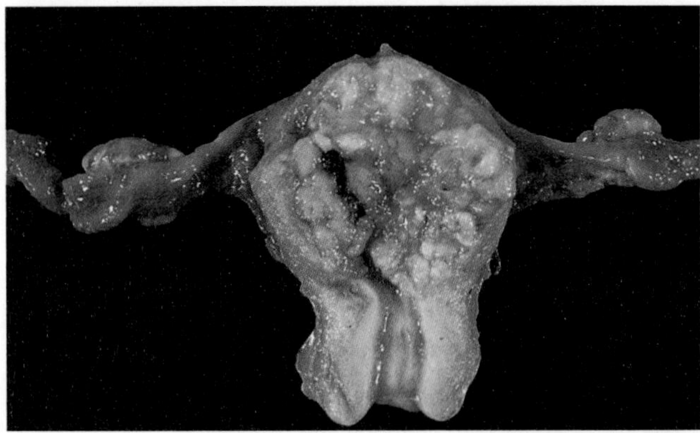

Figure 32-14 ■ **Endometrial Cancer.** Tumor fills the endometrial cavity. Obvious myometrial invasion is shown. (From Damjanov I, Linder J, editors: *Anderson's pathology,* ed 10, St Louis. 1996, Mosby.)

factors have been identified (see *Risk Factors:* Endometrial Cancer). Ninety-five percent of endometrial cancers occur in women age 40 years or older, with an average age of 60 years at diagnosis. Whites are about 70% more likely than blacks to develop this kind of cancer, but survival rates for whites are higher than for blacks.[1]

RISK FACTORS Endometrial Cancer

- History of obesity (>30 pounds overweight)
- High-fat diet (animal fat)
- Higher socioeconomic status (may be caused by diet)
- Infertility or no pregnancies
- Early menarche (<12 years)
- Late menopause (>52 years)
- Family history of endometrial cancer
- Personal history of breast or ovarian cancer
- Prior pelvic radiotherapy
- Age ≥40 years
- White race
- Prolonged estrogen use or tamoxifen therapy after menopause
- Diabetes
- Hereditary nonpolyposis colon cancer
- Gallbladder disease

Data from American Cancer Society: *Cancer facts and figures—2006,* New York, 2006, American Cancer Society.

Delayed menarche, pregnancy, and the use of hormonal contraception have a protective effect. After 12 months use of oral contraception, a 50% reduction in risk continues for at least 10 years.

All postmenopausal women with unscheduled bleeding or obese women with persistent irregular bleeding are evaluated for endometrial cancer. Diagnosis is made by direct cytologic sampling of the endometrium. This may be accomplished by endometrial biopsy or fractional curettage that includes biopsies of all sectors of the uterus. Transvaginal ultrasound is used to measure endometrial thickness. An endometrial depth of less than 5 mm suggests atrophy. Evaluation for metastasis includes routine blood work, metabolic studies, chest x-ray films, intravenous pyelography (IVP), barium enema, ultrasonography, and lymphangiography.

Treatment is based on the extent of the disease, and it includes surgical removal of the obvious tumor and radiation for control of residual microscopic disease. Chemotherapy also may be used. The 5-year survival rate is 95%, 60%, and 26% if the cancer is diagnosed at local, regional, and distant stages, respectively.[1,36]

Ovarian cancer

The American Cancer Society (ACS) estimated 22,430 new cases and 15,280 cancer deaths in 2007 (Figure 32-15).[1] In other words, ovarian cancer accounts for over 5% of all female cancer deaths and causes more deaths than any other cancer of the female reproductive system.[37] Incidence rates increase with age and peak in the eighth decade.[38]

The cause of ovarian cancer is unknown, and the epidemiologic studies, because of several limitations, has confused interpretations. Multiple epidemiologic studies, however, do agree that an increased risk of epithelial ovarian cancer has been linked to advancing age, family history of breast or ovarian cancer, and frequency of ovulation.[37] Despite study limitations, several factors related to ovulation have been consistently associated with increased or decreased risk of developing ovarian cancer (see *Risk Factors:* Ovarian Cancer). Risk is reduced by factors that suppress ovulation (pregnancy, breast-feeding, and oral contraceptive pill use).[37] The dismal overall prognosis for women with ovarian cancer results from an inability to detect ovarian cancer early when treatment might result in cure, from the lack of effective treatment for advanced disease, and from our incomplete understanding of the early changes in the ovary before the development of cancer and the initiators of these changes.[37]

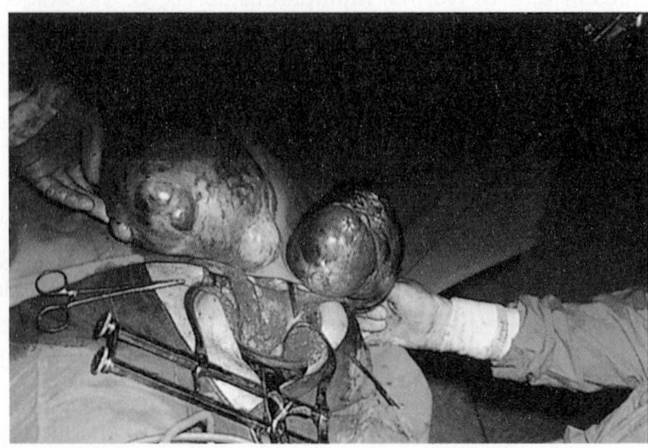

Figure 32-15 ■ **Ovarian Tumors.** Bilateral multicystic ovarian tumors. (From Symonds EM, Macpherson MBA: *Color atlas of obstetrics and gynecology,* London, 1994, Mosby.)

RISK FACTORS Ovarian Cancer

- Family history of ovarian, breast, uterine, pancreatic, or colon cancer
- Personal history of breast cancer
- Age: postmenopausal
- Infertility or prolonged use of fertility drugs without achieving pregnancy
- Early menarche, late menopause, or no children or first child after age 30 years (uninterrupted ovulation)
- Genetic predisposition

Data from American Cancer Society: *Cancer facts and figures—2006*, New York, 2006, American Cancer Society; American Cancer Society: *Overview: ovarian* cancer, New York, 2006, American Cancer Society.

PATHOGENESIS More than 90% of ovarian cancers arise from epithelial cells, ovarian surface epithelium.[39] Cancers also can arise from germ cells or theca cells of the ovarian stroma. Germ cell tumors occur in younger women, whereas those from epithelial tissue occur in women over 40 years of age. Ovarian cancers exhibit a distinctive pattern of progression spreading intra-abdominally over the surface of the peritoneum. As a clonal disease, ovarian cancer arises from a single cell in more than 90% of individuals. Amplification or deletion of several chromosomes is observed. Loss of tumor-suppressor genes and activation of oncogenes have both been described. Most ovarian cancers are sporadic and not associated with any pattern of inheritance. Germline mutations of *p53* are rarely the cause. Of the 5% to 10% that are inherited, the majority are associated with mutations of the breast cancer susceptibility gene (*BRCA1* and *BRCA2*).[40,41] Endometrial ovarian cancers may arise from endometriosis because they can share common genetic changes; this link, however, has yet to be proven.[42]

CLINICAL MANIFESTATIONS Ovarian cancer is generally considered a silent disease, meaning that by the time the individual experiences symptoms and seeks treatment, the disease has spread beyond the primary site. The most obvious symptoms are pain and abdominal swelling (ascites) that arise from the primary ovarian mass. Gastrointestinal manifestations may include dyspepsia, vomiting, and alterations in bowel habits caused by the mechanical obstruction by the tumor. Abnormal vaginal bleeding may occur if the postmenopausal endometrium is stimulated by a hormone-secreting tumor. The tumor also may cause ulcerations through the vaginal wall that result in bleeding. There also can be a feeling of pressure in the pelvis and leg pain.[38]

Systemic manifestations of nonmetastatic malignant disease include connective tissue inflammation (dermatomyositis), abnormal pigmentation (acanthosis nigricans), and subacute cerebellar degeneration. Tumor obstruction of vascular channels can cause venous and, occasionally, arterial thrombosis. Alterations in coagulability also occur, contributing to clot formation. Metastasis often causes pleural effusion (Figure 32-16).

EVALUATION AND TREATMENT Because ovarian cancer has no early symptoms and there are no effective screening techniques to detect it, the disease is usually advanced by the time treatment is sought. Transvaginal ultrasound and a tumor marker (CA-125) may assist diagnosis but are not recommended for routine screening. Research is ongoing to develop more effective screening in high-risk women. Diagnosis is made after ultrasound, CT scan, magnetic resonance imaging (MRI), or other imaging techniques that enable clinicians to localize the tumor mass. The International Federation of Gynecologists and Obstetricians (FIGO) staging system is described in Table 32-6. Other preoperative studies used to determine the extent of metastasis include an upper gastrointestinal series, barium enema, intravenous pyelogram, mammography, and lymphography.

The initial approach to treatment is surgery, which is performed to determine the stage of disease and to remove as much of the tumor as possible. Radiation therapy may follow if the tumor is smaller than 2 cm in size and is confined to the abdominopelvic area without involvement of the kidneys or liver. The success of chemotherapy depends on the extent of disease, whether the tumor is a discrete mass, and whether there has been prior exposure to chemotherapeutic agents. Research into prevention and treatment of ovarian cancer is ongoing and expanding.

The mortality associated with ovarian cancer has not changed significantly since the 1980s, mainly because the disease is already advanced at the time of diagnosis. Five-year mortality for women for all stages is 53%.[1] If ovarian cancer is diagnosed and treated early, the rate is 95%; however, less than one in four cases are detected at the localized stage[1] (see *Health Alert:* Recovery After Cancer Treatment).

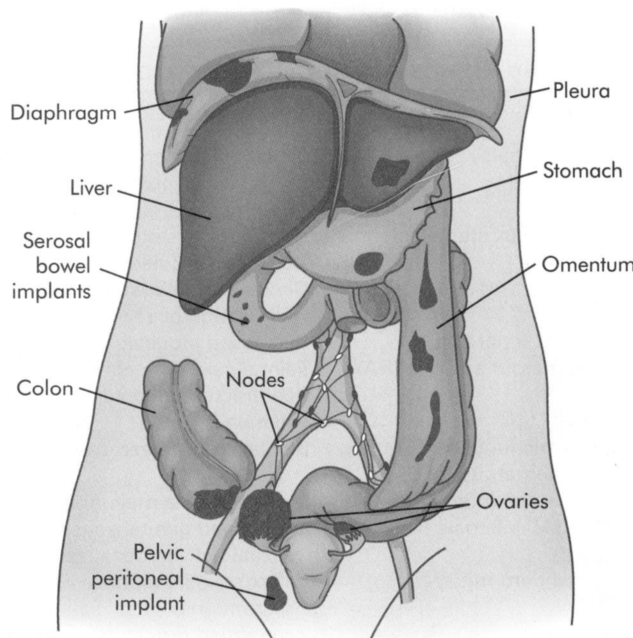

Figure 32-16 ■ **Metastasis of Ovarian Cancer.** Pattern of spread for epithelial cancer of the ovary.

TABLE 32-6

FIGO* Staging of Carcinoma of the Ovary

Stage	Characteristics
I	Growth limited to the ovaries
II	Growth involving one or both ovaries with pelvic extension
III	Cancer involves one or both ovaries, and one or both of the following are present: (1) cancer has spread beyond the pelvis to the lining of the abdomen, (2) cancer has spread to lymph nodes
IV	Growth involving one or both ovaries with distant metastases; if pleural effusion is present, there must be positive cytology to allow designating a case as stage IV; parenchymal liver metastases indicate stage IV
Recurrent	Cancer recurred after completion of treatment

*The International Federation of Gynecologists and Obstetricians.

HEALTH ALERT

Recovery After Cancer Treatment

Recovery after cancer treatment can be enhanced through lifestyle changes:

- Stop tobacco use
- Limit alcohol to less than 1 drink per day
- Improve nutrition—increase intake of fruits, vegetables, whole grains, and high-fiber foods; limit fat, especially animal fats
- Exercise daily
- Rest frequently
- Join a support group and attend meetings (family members should attend support groups also)
- Communicate openly, honestly, and frequently with members of the cancer care team

See American Cancer Society: *What happens after treatment?* at www.cancer.org/docroot/CRI/content/CRI_2-4-5X_What_happens_after_treatment_8.asp

Sexual Dysfunction

Increased awareness of female sexual dysfunction is relatively new; most of what is known comes from clinical observations and anecdotal reports from women, and adequate research is lacking. Both organic and psychosocial disorders can be implicated in sexual dysfunction. Organic problems may be the underlying cause in 10% to 20% of cases and may contribute to another 15%. Chronic illness can affect sexual functioning and response. Table 32-7 outlines possible effects of specified chronic diseases on female sexual functioning.

Disorders of desire (inhibited sexual desire, decreased libido) may be a biologic manifestation of depression, alcohol or other substance abuse, prolactin-secreting pituitary tumors, or testosterone deficiency. β-Adrenergic blockers used for heart disease also may inhibit sexual desire.

Vaginismus is an involuntary muscle spasm of the pubococcygeal muscle in response to attempted penetration.

TABLE 32-7

Possible Effects of Chronic Disease on Sexual Functioning in Women

Disease	Sexual Function
Cerebral palsy	Intact genital sensations, decreased lubrication; difficulty with sexual activity/positioning be cause of muscle spasticity, rigidity, or weakness; pain with positioning caused by contracture of knees and hips or because of increased spasms with arousal
Cerebrovascular accident (CVA)	Difficulties in sexual positioning and sensitivity because of impaired motor strength, coordination, or paralysis; decreased sex drive with stroke on the dominant side of the brain
Diabetes	Diminished intensity of orgasm and gradual decline in ability to achieve orgasm; decreased lubrication or recurrent vaginal infections with resultant dyspareunia
Chronic renal failure	Decreased arousal; increasingly rare and less intense orgasms; decreased lubrication
Rheumatoid arthritis (RA)	Painful sexual activity/positions because of swollen, painful joints, muscular atrophy, and joint contracture; decreased sex drive because of pain, fatigue, or medication; genital sensations remain intact
Systemic lupus erythematous (SLE)	Similar to RA; decreased lubrication and vaginal lesions result in painful penetration
Myocardial infarction (MI)	Most literature male-oriented; problems related to medications
Multiple sclerosis (MS)	Diminished genital sensitivity; decreased lubrication; declining orgasmic ability; difficulty with sexual activity because of muscle weakness, pain, or incontinence
Spinal cord injury	Reflex sexual response with injury above sacral area; disrupted response with lesion at or below sacrum; loss of sensation, decreased lubrication; spasticity, incontinence, or pain with arousal; continued orgasmic sensations or sensations diffused in general or to specific body parts, such as breast or lips

Common psychologic causes include prior sexual trauma and fear of sex. Organic causes are similar to those that cause dyspareunia. Even after the underlying organic problem is detected and successfully treated, vaginismus may persist.

Anorgasmia (orgasmic dysfunction) is the inability of a woman to reach or achieve orgasm. Specific disorders that may block orgasm are diabetes, alcoholism, neurologic disturbances, hormonal deficiencies, and pelvic disorders, such as infections, trauma, and surgical scarring. Other inhibitors include drugs, such as narcotics, tranquilizers, antidepressants, and antihypertensive medications.

Dyspareunia (painful intercourse) is common. Women may experience pain at any time from the beginning of arousal to after intercourse. The pain may have a burning, sharp, searing, or cramping quality and may be described as external, vaginal, deep abdominal, or pelvic. A variety of psychosocial and organic causes have been identified. Inadequate lubrication may make penetration or intercourse difficult or painful. Drugs with a drying effect, such as antihistamines, certain tranquilizers, and marijuana, and disorders such as diabetes, vaginal infections, and estrogen deficiency can decrease lubrication. Other causes include skin problems around the introitus or affecting the vulva; irritation or infection of the clitoris; disorders of the vaginal opening, such as scarring from episiotomy or chronically infected hymenal remnants; intact hymen; bartholinitis; disorders of the urethra or anus; disorders of the vagina, such as infections, thinning of the walls caused by aging or decreased estrogen, or irritation caused by spermicides or douches; and pelvic disorders, such as infection, tumors, cervical or uterine abnormalities, or torn uterine ligaments.

Sexual dysfunction may develop as a coping mechanism. Women with a history of sexual trauma—rape, incest, or molestation—often have problems with desire, arousal, or orgasm or experience pain with sexual activity. In extreme cases, total sexual aversion may develop. At other times, sexual dysfunction may be a symptom of marital or relationship problems. Often, unresolved anger manifests as inhibited desire or diminished arousal.

Impaired Fertility

Infertility affects approximately 15% of all couples and is defined as the inability to conceive after 1 year of unprotected intercourse. Fertility can be impaired by factors in the man or in the woman or in both partners. Male factors include diminished quality and production of sperm. Causes include infections or inflammation, endocrine or hormonal disorders, immunologic problems in which men produce antibodies to their own sperm, and environmental or lifestyle factors.[43] Female infertility factors are associated with malfunctions of the fallopian tubes, the ovaries, or the reproductive hormones. Adhesions from pelvic infection may cause blockage of one or both fallopian tubes, preventing access of the sperm to the ovum. Hormonal or local factors may disrupt ovulation or prevent a fertilized egg from implantation. Endometriosis also may contribute to infertility. A number of diagnostic procedures are required in the routine investigation of the infertile couple. Initial workup includes semen analysis and determination of ovulation. In many instances, no cause may be identified.

Treatment of infertility is aimed toward correcting problems identified during the diagnostic workup. The best treatment for infertility is prevention of sexually transmitted infection that can result in scarring and adhesion formation in the reproductive tract of either the man or the woman.

QUICK CHECK 32-4

1. Why is cervical cancer considered a sexually transmitted infection?
2. Why does the American Cancer Society recommend screening for cervical cancer?
3. What are the risk factors for endometrial cancer?
4. What factors reduce the risk of ovarian cancer?

DISORDERS OF THE MALE REPRODUCTIVE SYSTEM

Disorders of the Urethra

Urethritis and urethral strictures are common disorders of the male urethra. Urethral carcinoma, an extremely rare form of cancer, can occur in men older than 60 years.

Urethritis

Urethritis is an inflammatory process that is usually, but not always, caused by a sexually transmitted microorganism. Infectious urethritis caused by *N. gonorrhoeae* is often called *gonococcal urethritis (GU);* urethritis caused by other microorganisms is called *nongonococcal urethritis (NGU).* Nonsexual origins of urethritis include inflammation or infection as a result of urologic procedures, insertion of foreign bodies into the urethra, anatomic abnormalities, or trauma.

Noninfectious urethritis is rare and is associated with the ingestion of wood or ethyl alcohol or turpentine. It is also seen with Reiter syndrome.[44]

Symptoms of urethritis include urethral tingling or itching or a burning sensation, and frequency and urgency with urination. The individual may note a purulent or clear mucus-like discharge from the urethra. Nucleic acid detection amplification tests allow early detection of *N. gonorrhoeae* and *C. trachomatis* in urine tests. Treatment consists of appropriate antibiotic therapy for infectious urethritis and avoidance of future exposure or mechanical irritation.

Urethral strictures

A **urethral stricture** is a narrowing of the urethra caused by scarring. The scars may be congenital but are more likely to result from trauma (e.g., injury or urologic instrumentation) or untreated or severe urethral infections. Prostatitis and infection secondary to urinary stasis are common complications. Severe and prolonged obstruction can result in hydronephrosis and renal failure.

Clinical manifestations include urinary frequency and hesitancy, diminished force and caliber of the urinary stream, dribbling after voiding, and nocturia. Urethral stricture is diagnosed on the basis of history, physical examination, and cystoscopy. Treatment is usually surgical and may involve urethral dilation, urethrotomy, or a variety of open surgical techniques. The choice of surgical intervention depends on the age of the individual and the severity of the problem.

Disorders of the Penis

Phimosis and paraphimosis

Phimosis and paraphimosis are both disorders in which the foreskin (prepuce) is "too tight" to move easily over the glans penis. **Phimosis** is a condition in which the foreskin cannot be retracted back over the glans, whereas **paraphimosis** is the opposite: the foreskin is retracted and cannot be moved forward (reduced) to cover the glans (Figure 32-17). Both conditions can cause penile pathologic conditions.

The inability to retract the foreskin is normal in infancy and is caused by congenital adhesions. During the first 3 years of life, congenital adhesions (between the foreskin and glans) separate naturally with penile erections and are not an indication for circumcision. Phimosis can occur at any age and is most commonly caused by poor hygiene and chronic infection. It rarely occurs with normal foreskin.

Reasons for seeking treatment include edema, erythema, and tenderness of the prepuce and purulent discharge; inability to retract the foreskin is a less common complaint. Circumcision, if needed, is performed after infection has

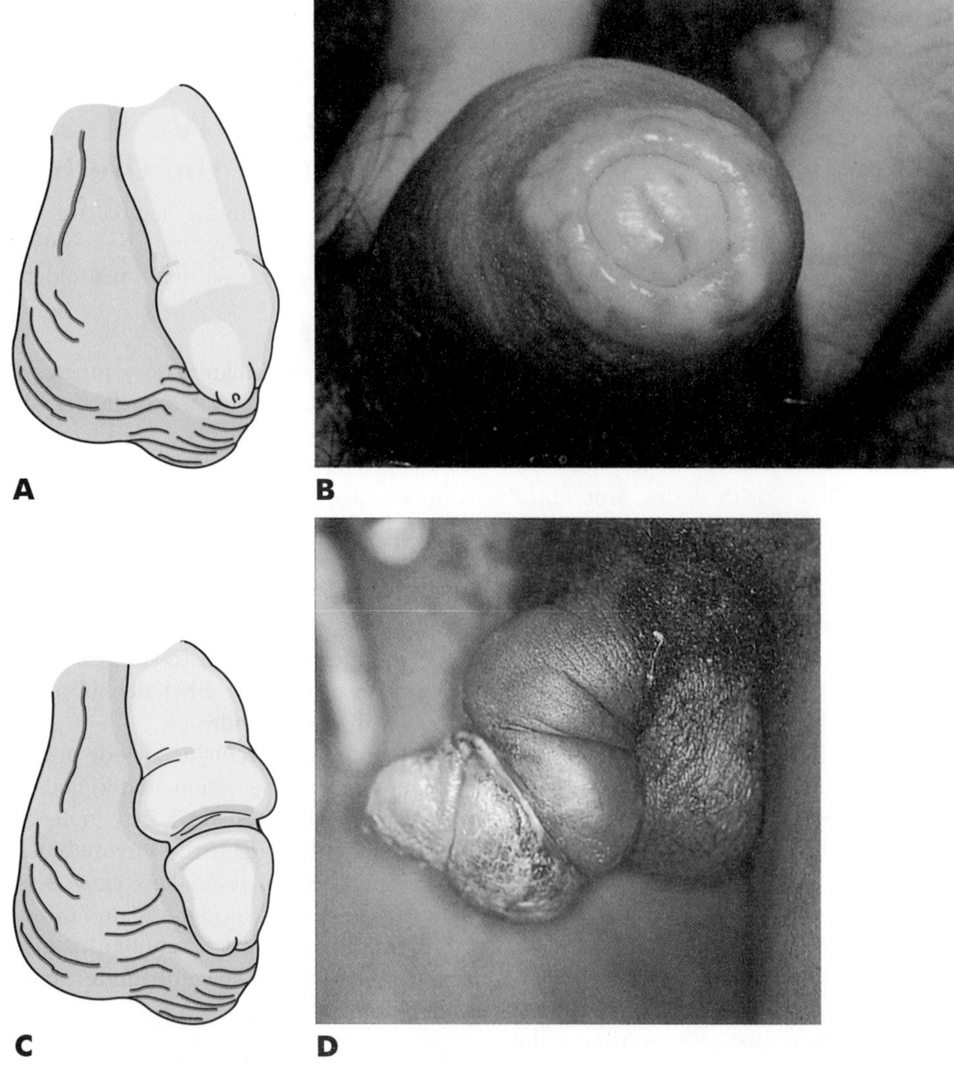

Figure 32-17 ■ **Phimosis and Paraphimosis. A,** Phimosis: the foreskin has a narrow opening that is not large enough to permit retraction over the glans. **B,** Lesions on the prepuce secondary to infection cause swelling, and retraction of foreskin may be impossible. Circumcision is usually required. **C,** Paraphimosis: the foreskin is retracted over the glans but cannot be reduced to its normal position. Here it has formed a constricting band around the penis. **D,** Ulcer on the retracted prepuce with edema. (**A** and **C** from Monahan FD et al: *Phipps' Medical-surgical nursing: health and illness perspectives,* ed 8, St Louis, 2007, Mosby; **B** from Taylor PK: *Diagnostic picture tests in sexually transmitted diseases,* St Louis, 1995, Mosby; **D** from Morse SA, Ballard RC, Holmes KK, Moreland AA: *Atlas of sexually transmitted diseases and AIDS,* ed 3, Edinburgh, 2003, Mosby.)

been eradicated. Complications of phimosis include inflammation of the glans (balanitis) or prepuce (posthitis) and paraphimosis. There is a higher incidence of penile carcinoma in uncircumcised males, but chronic infection and poor hygiene are usually the underlying factors in such cases.

Paraphimosis, in which the foreskin is retracted, can constrict the penis, causing edema of the glans. If the foreskin cannot be reduced manually, surgery must be performed to prevent necrosis of the glans caused by constricted blood vessels. Severe paraphimosis is a surgical emergency.

Peyronie disease

Peyronie disease ("bent nail syndrome") is a fibrotic condition that causes lateral curvature of the penis during erection (Figure 32-18). Peyronie disease develops slowly and is characterized by tough fibrous thickening of the fascia in the erectile tissue of the corpora cavernosa. A dense, fibrous plaque is usually palpable on the dorsum of the penile shaft. The problem usually affects middle-aged men and is associated with painful erection, painful intercourse (for both partners), and poor erection distal to the involved area. In some cases, impotence or unsatisfactory penetration occurs. When the penis is flaccid, there is no pain.

A local vasculitis-like inflammatory reaction occurs, and decreased tissue oxygenation results in fibrosis and calcification. The exact cause is unknown. Peyronie disease is associated with Dupuytren contracture (a flexion deformity of the fingers or toes caused by shortening or fibrosis of the palmar or plantar fascia), diabetes, predisposition to keloids, and, in rare cases, use of beta-blocker medications.[45]

Surgical treatments include intracavernosal plaque excision, including newer minimally invasive repair strategies.[46] Plication and surgical resection of the fibrous plaque followed by grafting have been successful.

Priapism

Priapism is an uncommon condition of prolonged penile erection. It is usually painful and is not associated with sexual arousal (Figure 32-19). Priapism is idiopathic in 60% of cases; the remaining 40% of cases can be associated with spinal cord trauma, sickle cell disease, leukemia, pelvic tumors, or intracavernous injection therapy for impotence.

Priapism must be considered a urologic emergency. Treatment within hours is effective and prevents impotence. Conservative approaches include iced saline enemas, ketamine administration, and spinal anesthesia. Newer drug therapy for recurrent ischemic priapism includes phosphodiesterase 5 inhibitors.[47] Needle aspiration of blood from the corpus through the dorsal glans is often effective and is followed by catheterization and pressure dressings to maintain decompression. More aggressive surgical treatments include the creation of vascular shunts to maintain blood flow. Erectile dysfunction results in up to 50% of cases.

Balanitis

Balanitis is an inflammation of the glans penis (Figure 32-20) and usually occurs in conjunction with posthitis, an inflammation of the prepuce. (Inflammation of the glans and the prepuce is called *balanoposthitis.*) It is associated with poor hygiene and phimosis. The accumulation under the foreskin of glandular secretions (smegma), sloughed epithelial cells, and *Mycobacterium smegmatis* can irritate the glans directly or lead to infection. Skin disorders (e.g., psoriasis, lichen planus, eczema) and candidiasis must be differentiated from inflammation resulting from poor hygienic practices. Balanitis is most commonly seen in men with poorly controlled diabetes mellitus and candidiasis. The infection is treated with antimicrobials. After the inflammation has subsided, circumcision can be considered to prevent recurrences.

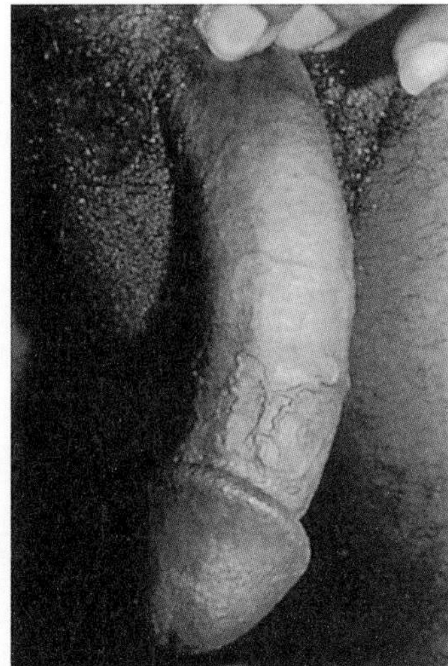

Figure 32-18 ■ **Peyronie Disease.** This person complained of pain and deviation of his penis to one side on erection. (From Taylor PK: *Diagnostic picture tests in sexually transmitted diseases,* London, 1995, Mosby.)

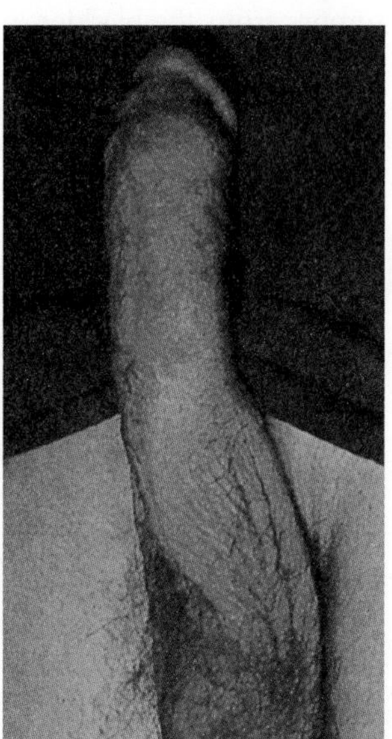

Figure 32-19 ■ **Priapism.** (From Lloyd-Davies RW et al: *Color atlas of urology,* ed 2, London, 1994, Wolfe Medical.)

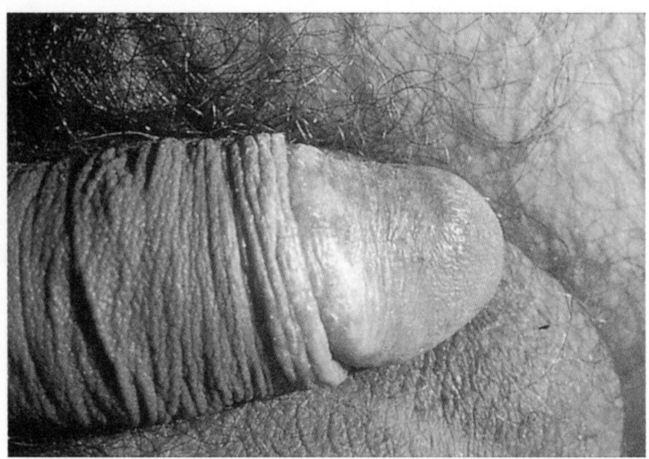

Figure 32-20 ■ **Balanitis.** (From Taylor PK: *Diagnostic picture tests in sexually transmitted diseases,* London, 1995, Mosby.)

Penile cancer

Carcinoma of the penis is rare in the United States, constituting less than 0.16%[1] of all malignancies in men. It does account, however, for about 10% of cancers in African and South American men. It can affect men 50 to 70 years of age, with 40% of diagnosed men being younger than 60 years. The disease occurs almost twice as often in blacks as in whites in the United States and tends to be more common in lower socioeconomic groups. Although the exact cause is unknown, major risks factors include HPV infection, smoking, and psoriasis.

Squamous cell carcinoma accounts for 95% of invasive penile cancers. Other premalignant lesions, or in situ forms of epidermal carcinoma, that occur on the penis include leukoplakia (white plaque), Paget disease (red, inflamed areas), erythroplasia of Queyrat (raised red areas), and Buschke-Löwenstein patches (large venous areas). Condylomata (genital warts) caused by HPV may be involved in the development of precancerous lesions and squamous cell cancers.[35] At times, the penis might be the site of metastatic spread of solid tumors from the bladder, prostate, rectum, or kidney. Early squamous cell carcinoma and premalignant epidermal lesions are easily treated, but delays in seeking treatment are attributed to denial, embarrassment, failure to detect lesions under a phimotic foreskin, fear, guilt, and ignorance.

Squamous cell carcinoma usually begins as a small, fat, ulcerative or papillary lesion on the glans or foreskin that grows to involve the entire penile shaft. Extensive lesions are associated with metastases and a poor prognosis. These lesions are not as painful as the amount of tissue involvement would seem to indicate. The regional femoral and iliac nodes are common metastatic sites; the urethra and bladder are rarely involved. Weight loss, fatigue, and malaise accompany chronic suppurative lesions. Untreated, progressive disease causes death within 2 years.

The specific diagnosis is made by biopsy after examination to document the location, size, and fixation of the lesion. After a positive biopsy, the extent of cancer spread is determined by imaging studies, such as ultrasound, computed tomography, or magnetic resonance. Distant metastases are uncommon. Stages of carcinoma of the penis are presented in Box 32-6.

Penile carcinoma requires surgery. Palliative treatment with radiation or chemotherapy may be used when the disease is inoperable and bulky inguinal metastases have occurred. Options for individuals with carcinoma in situ include local excision, radiation, laser surgery, cryosurgery, chemosurgery, or chemotherapy with topical (5%) 5-fluorouracil. The 5-year survival rate for stage I disease is more than 80%, the average 5-year survival rate for all stages is 50%.[48]

QUICK CHECK 32-5

1. Why are priapism and severe paraphimosis considered urologic emergencies?
2. What are the risk factors for cancer of the penis?

Disorders of the Scrotum, Testis, and Epididymis

Disorders of the scrotum

Varicocele, hydrocele, and spermatocele are common intrascrotal disorders. A **varicocele** is an abnormal dilation

BOX 32-6 Tumor, Node, Metastasis (TNM)* Staging for Penile Cancer

Stage 0	Stage I	Stage II
T_{is}, N_0, M_0 T_a, N_0, M_0	T_1, N_0, M_0	T_1, N_1, M_0 T_2, N_0, M_0 T_2, N_1, M_0
Stage III	**Stage IV**	**Recurrent**
T_1, N_2, M_0 T_2, N_2, M_0 T_3, N_0, M_0 T_3, N_1, M_0 T_3, N_2, M_0 T_2, N_1, M_0	T_4, any N, M_0 Any T, N_3, M_0 Any T, any N, M_1	Any local or distant penile cancer that returns after treatment

*See Figure 9-3 on p. 226 for T, N, and M definitions.

of a vein within the spermatic cord and is classically described as a "bag of worms" (Figure 32-21). Varicoceles are the most common abnormal finding among infertile men. Advancements in diagnostic techniques indicate that the incidence of varicoceles is significantly greater than previously reported.[49] Most (95%) occur on the left side and may be painful or tender. Varicocele occurs in 10% to 15% of males and is seen most often after puberty.[50] Unilateral right-sided varicoceles are rare and result from compression or obstruction of the inferior vena cava by a tumor or thrombus. Varicoceles may be less likely to be diagnosed among obese men.[51]

The cause of varicocele is incompetent or congenitally absent valves in the spermatic veins. Blood pools in the veins rather than flowing into the venous system. Varicocele decreases blood flow through the testis, interfering with spermatogenesis and causing infertility. If infertility is a problem, treatment consists of ligation of the spermatic vein. If varicocele is mild and fertility is not an issue, a scrotal support is usually sufficient to relieve symptoms of scrotal heaviness or "dragging." Color Doppler ultrasonography is used to confirm diagnosis.

A **hydrocele** is a collection of fluid within the tunica vaginalis (Figure 32-22). It is the most common cause of scrotal swelling. Hydroceles occur in 6% of male newborns and are congenital malformations that often resolve spontaneously in the first year of life. Surgical ligation is recommended if hydrocele persists after age 1 year.[52] Hydroceles in adults may be caused by an imbalance between the secreting and absorptive capacities of scrotal tissues. Hydroceles range in size from slightly larger than the normal testes to a grapefruit size or larger and may be flaccid or tense. Compression of testicular blood supply may lead to atrophy.

The exact mechanism of idiopathic hydrocele is unknown. Secondary hydrocele may result from trauma or infection of the testis or epididymis or from a testicular tumor. Rapid accumulation of fluid occurs after local injury, radiotherapy, or infection, or it may accompany testicular neoplasm. Chronic hydrocele is more common and occurs in men over 40 years of age because of an imbalance between fluid secretion and resorption in the tunica vaginalis. Treatment for uncomplicated hydrocele is aspiration of the fluid and injection of a sclerosing agent into the scrotal sac (cystic dilation) to excise the tunica vaginalis.[53]

A **spermatocele** is a painless diverticulum of the epididymis located between the head of the epididymis and the testis. Spermatoceles are filled with a milky fluid containing sperm (Figure 32-23). Spermatoceles that cause pain or discomfort are excised. Both spermatoceles and epididymal cysts present clinically as discrete, firm, freely mobile masses distinct from the testis that may be transilluminated. Usually, however, spermatoceles are asymptomatic or produce mild discomfort that is relieved by scrotal support. Neither hydroceles nor spermatoceles are associated with infertility.

Cryptorchidism

In **cryptorchidism,** one or both testes fail to descend into the scrotum. It is the most common congenital condition involving the testes. About 3% to 6% of all full-term males and 20% to 30% of all premature males have undescended testes at birth. The testes may remain in the abdomen, or descent may be arrested in the inguinal canal or the

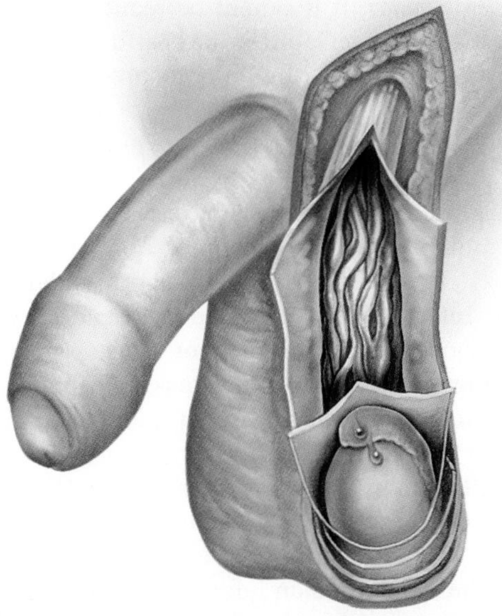

Figure 32-21 ■ **Depiction of a Varicocele.** Dilation of veins within the spermatic cord. (From Seidel HM et al: *Mosby's guide to physical examination,* ed 6, St Louis, 2006, Mosby.)

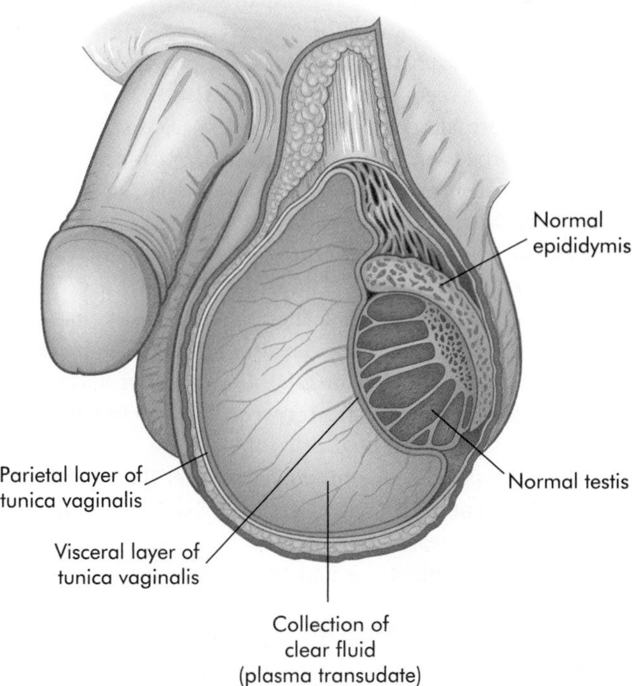

Figure 32-22 ■ **Depiction of a Hydrocele.** Accumulation of clear fluid between the visceral (inner) and parietal (outer) layers of the tunica vaginalis.

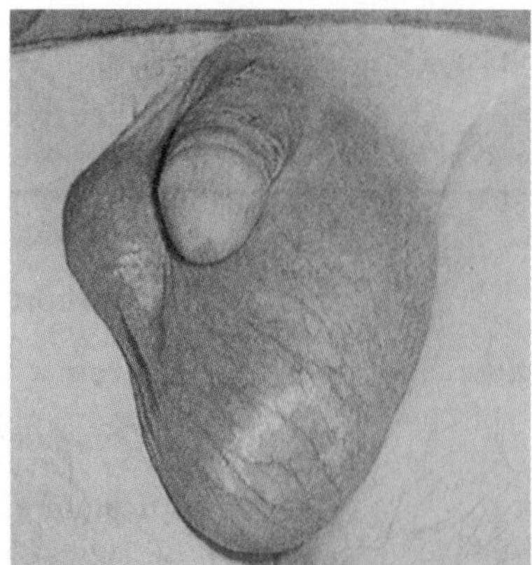

Figure 32-23 ■ **Spermatocele.** Retention cyst of the head of the epididymis or of an aberrant tubule or tubules of the rete testis. The spermatocele lies outside the tunica vaginalis; therefore, on palpation it can be readily distinguished and separated from the testis. (From Lloyd-Davies RW et al: *Color atlas of urology,* ed 2, London, 1994, Wolfe Medical.)

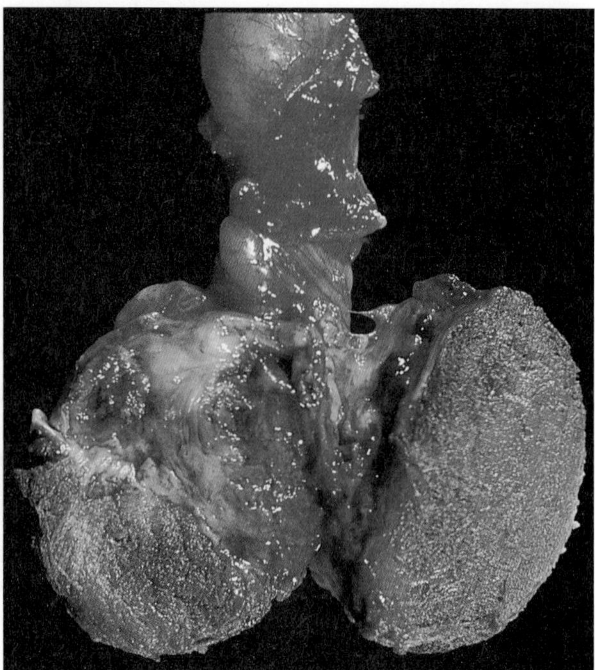

Figure 32-24 ■ **Torsion of the Testis.** The testes appear dark red and partially necrotic owing to hemorrhagic infarction. (From Damjanov I, Linder J, editors: *Anderson's pathology,* ed 10, St Louis, 1996, Mosby.)

puboscrotal junction. In approximately 75% to 90% of infants with cryptorchidism, the testes descend into the scrotum by 1 year of age, leaving a true incidence of 0.8% of the male population.

Cryptorchidism may result from a developmental delay, a defect of the testis, deficient maternal gonadotropin stimulation, or some mechanical factor that prevents descent through the inguinal canal. Mechanical possibilities include a short spermatic cord, fibrous bands or adhesions in the normal path of the testes, or a narrowed inguinal canal. Chromosomal studies do not support a genetic component.

Untreated cryptorchidism is associated with a lowered sperm count and, therefore, impaired fertility. Impaired spermatogenesis is caused by higher temperatures within the abdomen. Cryptorchidism does not prevent puberty or maintenance of secondary sex characteristics if the testis is otherwise normal. Undescended testes are susceptible to neoplastic processes: the risk of testicular cancer is 35 to 50 times greater for men with cryptorchidism or a history of cryptorchidism than for the general male population.

Physical examination discloses the absence of one or both testes in the scrotum. Ultrasonography or a CT scan can help clinicians locate a nonpalpable testis that has migrated intra-abdominally. Treatment often begins with hormonal therapy. If hormonal therapy is not successful, to preserve fertility, surgical correction (orchiopexy) of cryptorchidism is attempted when the child is about 2 years of age. Orchiopexy is recommended no later than age 5 or 6 years. Placement of the cryptorchid testis into the scrotal sac does not decrease the potential for malignancy, but it does facilitate examination and tumor detection.

Torsion of the testis

In **torsion of the testis,** the testis rotates on its vascular pedicle, interrupting its blood supply (Figure 32-24). Torsion of the testis is one of several conditions that cause an acute scrotum, which is testicular pain and swelling. It is responsible for 16% to 42% of cases of boys with acute scrotum.[52] This event can occur at any age but is most common among neonates and adolescents, particularly at puberty.[52] Onset may be spontaneous or follow physical exertion or trauma. Torsion twists the arteries and veins in the spermatic cord, reducing or stopping circulation to the testis. Vascular engorgement and ischemia develop, causing scrotal swelling and pain not relieved by rest or scrotal support. Diagnostic testing includes urinalysis (for infection) and color Doppler ultrasonography.[53-55] Torsion of the testis is a surgical emergency. If it cannot be reduced manually (scrotal elevation), surgery must be performed within 6 hours after the onset of symptoms to preserve normal testicular function.

Orchitis

Orchitis is an acute inflammation of the testes (Figure 32-25) and is uncommon except as a complication of systemic infection or as an extension of an associated epididymitis (see p. 876). Infectious organisms may reach the testes through the blood or the lymphatics or, most commonly, by ascent through the urethra, vas deferens, and epididymis. Most cases of orchitis are actually cases of epididymoorchitis. Occasionally in middle-aged men, a nonspecific, apparently noninfectious, inflammatory process (called *granulomatous orchitis*) can occur, apparently a granulomatous response to spermatozoa.

Mumps is the most common infectious cause of orchitis and usually affects postpubertal males. The onset is sudden, occurring 3 to 4 days after the onset of parotitis. Signs and symptoms include high fever, reaching 40° C (104° F),

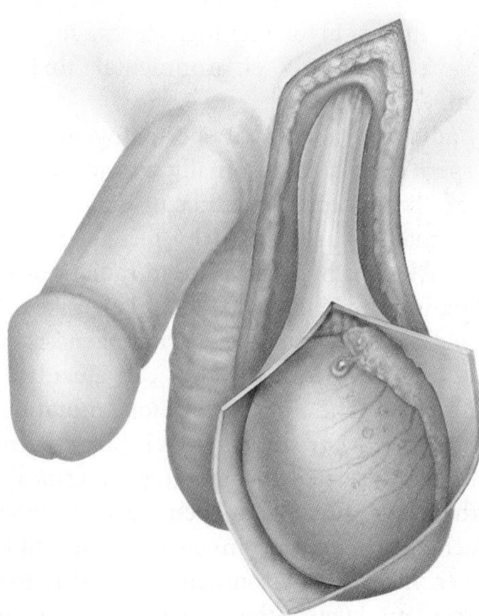

Figure 32-25 ■ **Depiction of Orchitis.** (From Seidel HM et al: *Mosby's guide to physical examination,* ed 6, St Louis, 2006, Mosby.)

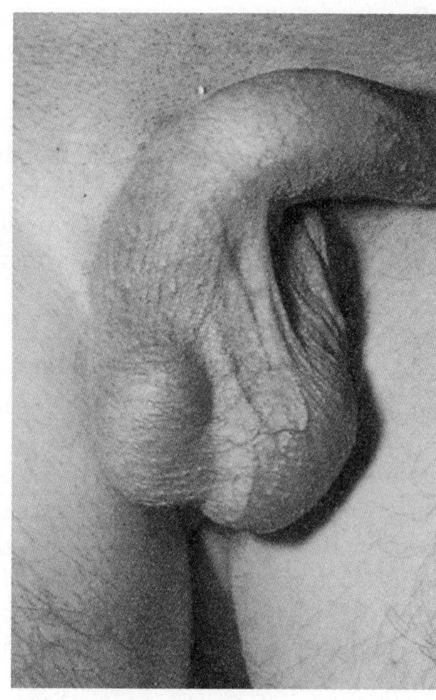

Figure 32-26 ■ **Testicular Tumor.** (From *400 Self-assessment picture tests in clinical medicine,* London, 1984, Wolfe Medical.)

marked prostration, bilateral or unilateral erythema, edema and tenderness of the scrotum, and leukocytosis. An acute hydrocele may develop. Urinary signs and symptoms, which accompany epididymitis, are absent. Atrophy with irreversible damage to spermatogenesis may result in 30% of affected testes. Bilateral orchitis does not affect androgenic function but may cause permanent sterility.

Treatment is supportive and includes bed rest, scrotal support, elevation of the scrotum, hot or cold compresses, and analgesic agents for relief of pain. If an acute hydrocele develops, it is aspirated. Testicular abscess usually requires orchiectomy (removal of the testis). Appropriate antimicrobial drugs should be used for bacterial orchitis, and corticosteroids are indicated in proved cases of nonspecific granulomatous orchitis.

Cancer of the testis

Testicular cancer is among the most curable of cancers, with cure rates greater than 95%. Overall, testicular cancers are uncommon, accounting for approximately 1% of all male cancers and 0.13% of cancer deaths in men; yet they are the most common solid tumor of young adult men.[1] Cancer of the testis occurs most commonly in men between the ages of 15 and 35 years.[1] In the United States, the lifetime probability of developing testicular cancer is 0.3% for white men, an incidence that is 4.5 times higher than in blacks. Testicular tumors are slightly more common on the right side than on the left, a pattern that parallels the occurrence of cryptorchidism, and they are bilateral in 1% to 3% of cases (Figure 32-26).

PATHOPHYSIOLOGY Ninety percent of testicular cancers are germ cell tumors, arising from the male gametes. Germ cell tumors include seminomas, embryonal carcinomas, teratomas, and choriosarcomas. Testicular tumors also can arise from specialized cells of the gonadal stroma. These tumors, which are named for their cellular origins, are the Leydig cell, Sertoli cell, granulosa cell, and theca cell tumors.

The cause of testicular neoplasms is unknown (see *Risk Factors:* Cancer of the Testis). A genetic predisposition is suggested by the fact that the incidence is higher among brothers, identical twins, and other close male relatives. Genetic predisposition is supported statistically showing that the disease is relatively rare among black Africans, black Americans, Asians, and native New Zealanders. A history of trauma or infection also is associated with the development of testicular neoplasms, but it may be that coexisting testicular tumors are discovered by accident in men who undergo examination because of trauma or infections.

RISK FACTORS Cancer of the Testis

- History of cryptorchidism
- Abnormal testicular development
- Klinefelter syndrome
- History of testicular cancer

CLINICAL MANIFESTATIONS Painless testicular enlargement commonly is the first sign of testicular cancer. Occurring gradually, it may be accompanied by a sensation of testicular heaviness or a dull ache in the lower abdomen. Occasionally acute pain occurs because of rapid growth resulting in hemorrhage and necrosis. Ten percent of affected men have epididymitis, 10% have hydroceles, and 5% have breast enlargement (gynecomastia). The testicular mass is usually discovered by the individual or by his sexual partner. At the time of initial diagnosis, approximately 10% of individuals already have symptoms related to metastases. Lumbar pain also may be present and usually is caused by retroperitoneal node metastasis. Signs of metastasis to the lungs include cough, dyspnea, and bloody sputum (hemoptysis). Supraclavicular node involvement may cause difficulty swallowing (dysphagia) and neck swelling. With metastasis to the CNS, alterations in vision or mental status, papilledema, and seizures may be experienced.

EVALUATION AND TREATMENT Evaluation begins with careful physical examination, including palpation of the scrotal contents with the individual in the erect and supine positions. Signs of testicular cancer include abnormal consistency, induration, nodularity, or irregularity of the testis. The abdomen and lymph nodes are palpated to seek evidence of metastasis, and tumor type is identified after orchiectomy. Testicular biopsy is not recommended because it may cause dissemination of the tumor and increase the risk of local recurrence. Primary testicular cancer can be assessed rapidly and accurately by scrotal ultrasonography. Tumor markers, α-fetoprotein and β-subunit gonadotropin, and lactate dehydrogenase (LDH) are usually elevated. Chest x-ray films, lymphangiograms, intravenous pyelograms, abdominal ultrasound or CT scan, and measurement of serum markers are used in clinical staging of the disease. Besides surgery, treatment involves radiation and chemotherapy singly or in combination. Factors influencing the prognosis include histology of the tumor stage of the disease and selection of appropriate treatment. Most patients treated for cancer of the testis can expect a normal life span; some have persistent paresthesias, Raynaud phenomenon, or infertility. Almost 90% of disease-related deaths occur in the first 2 years after cessation of therapy; a person who is disease-free after 3 years is considered to be cured. Orchiectomy does not affect sexual function.

Impairment of sperm production and quality

Spermatogenesis requires adequate secretion of follicle-stimulating hormone (FSH) and luteinizing hormone (LH) by the pituitary and sufficient secretion of testosterone by the testes. Inadequate secretion of gonadotropins may be caused by hypothyroidism, hyperadrenocortisolism, hyperprolactinemia, or hypogonadotropic hypogonadism. In the absence of adequate gonadotropin levels, the Leydig cells are not stimulated to secrete testosterone, and sperm maturation is not promoted in the Sertoli cells. Spermatogenesis also depends on an appropriate response by the testes. Defects in testicular response to the gonadotropins result in decreased secretion of testosterone and inhibin B and occur as a result of normal feedback mechanisms and high levels of circulating gonadotropins. In the absence of adequate testosterone levels, spermatogenesis is impaired. Newer studies demonstrate the importance of inhibin B as an important marker of the competence of Sertoli cells and spermatogenesis.[56] Impaired spermatogenesis also can be caused by testicular trauma, infection, atrophy of the testes, systemic illness involving high fever, ingestion of various drugs, exposure to environmental toxins, and cryptorchidism.

Fertility is adversely affected if spermatogenesis is normal but the sperm are chromosomally or morphologically abnormal or are produced in insufficient quantities. Chromosomal abnormalities are caused by genetic factors and by external variables, such as exposure to radiation or toxic substances. Because the Y chromosome plays a key role in testis determination and control of spermatogenesis, understanding how the genes work together can elucidate exact causes of infertility. The most common mutations are microdeletion of the Y chromosome (AZ [azoospermia] a, b, and c).[57] Research related to mapping the critical genes and gene pathways is the current focus of male infertility. Common mechanisms may be involved in infertility and testicular cancer. In utero environmental exposure to endocrine disruptors modulates the genetic makeup of the gonad and may result in both infertility and testicular cancer.[57–62]

Sperm motility also may affect fertility. Motility appears to be affected by characteristics of semen. Prostatic dysfunction, excessive semen viscosity, presence of drugs or toxins in the semen, and presence of antisperm antibodies are associated with impaired sperm motility. However, new data show that motile density may not be a good indicator of infertility.[63] Approximately 17% of infertile males have antisperm antibodies in their semen. These antibodies may be (1) cytotoxic antibodies, which attack sperm and reduce their number in the semen, or (2) sperm-immobilizing antibodies, which impair sperm motility and reduce their ability to traverse the endocervical canal.

Treatment for impaired spermatogenesis involves correcting any underlying disorders, avoiding radiation and toxins, and using hormones to enhance spermatogenesis. In addition, semen can be modified to improve sperm motility; modifications are followed by artificial insemination.

Epididymitis

Epididymitis, or inflammation of the epididymis, generally occurs in sexually active young males (younger than 35 years) and is rare before puberty (Figure 32-27). In young men, the usual cause is a sexually transmitted microorganism, such as *N. gonorrhoeae* or *C. trachomatis.* Men who practice unprotected anal intercourse may acquire sexually transmitted epididymis that results from infection with *E. coli, H. influenza,* tuberculosis, or *Cryptococcus* or *Brucella* species.[64] In men older than 35 years, *Enterobacteriaceae* (intestinal bacteria) and *Pseudomonas aeruginosa* associated with urinary tract infections and prostatitis also may cause epididymitis. Epididymitis also may result from a chemical inflammation caused by the reflux of sterile urine into the ejaculatory ducts and is then called **chemical epididymitis.**[64,65] It is associated with urethral strictures, congenital posterior valves, and excessive physical straining in which increased abdominal pressure is transmitted to the bladder. Chemical epididymitis is usually self-limiting and

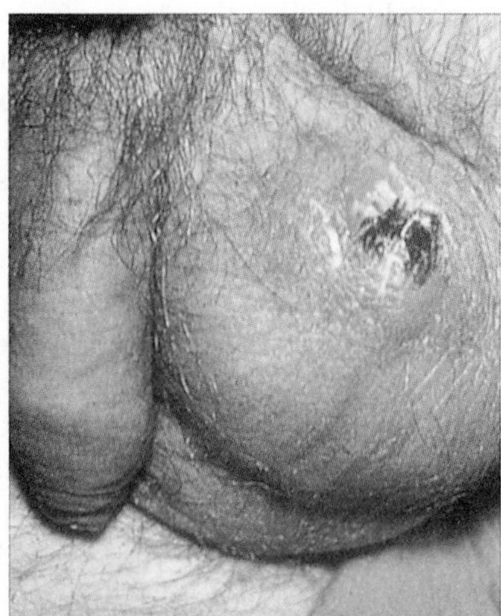

Figure 32-27 ■ Epididymitis Secondary to Gonorrhea or Nongonococcal Urethritis. This infection spread to the testes, and rupture through the scrotal wall is threatened. (From Taylor PK: *Diagnostic picture tests in sexually transmitted disease,* London, 1995, Mosby.)

does not require evaluation or intervention unless it persists.

PATHOPHYSIOLOGY The pathogenic microorganism usually reaches the epididymis by ascending the vasa deferentia from an already infected urethra or bladder. The resulting inflammatory response causes symptoms of bacterial epididymitis. Epididymitis caused by heavy lifting or straining results from reflux of urine from the bladder into the vas deferens and epididymis. Urine is extremely irritating to the epididymis and initiates the inflammatory response called *chemical epididymitis.*

CLINICAL MANIFESTATIONS The main symptom of epididymitis is scrotal or inguinal pain caused by inflammation of the epididymis and surrounding tissues. The pain is usually acute and severe. Flank pain may occur if, as the urethra passes over the spermatic cord, edematous swelling of the cord obstructs the urethra. The individual may have pyuria, bacteriuria, and a history of urinary symptoms, including urethral discharge. The scrotum on the involved side is red and edematous. The tail of the epididymis near the lower pole of the testis usually swells first; then swelling ascends to the head of the epididymis. The spermatic cord also may be swollen and tender.

Complications include abscess formation, infarction of the testis, recurrent infection, and infertility. Infarction is probably caused by thrombosis (obstruction by blood clots) of the prostatic vessels secondary to severe inflammation. Recurrent epididymitis may result from inadequate initial treatment or failure to identify or treat predisposing factors. Chronic epididymitis can cause scarring of the epididymal endothelium and infertility. Once scarring has occurred, treatment with antibiotics is ineffective because adequate antibiotic levels cannot be achieved within the epididymis.

EVALUATION AND TREATMENT A history of recent urinary tract infection or urethral discharge suggests the diagnosis of epididymitis. The relief of pain when the inflamed testis and epididymis are elevated (Phren sign) is also diagnostic. Definitive diagnosis is based on culture or Gram stain of a urethral swab. Epididymal aspiration may be necessary to obtain a specimen, especially if the individual has been taking antibiotics and has sterile urine.

Treatment includes antibiotic therapy for the infection itself and various measures to provide symptomatic relief. Complete resolution of swelling and pain may take several weeks to months. The individual's sexual partner should be treated with antibiotics if the causative microorganism is a sexually transmitted pathogen.

QUICK CHECK 32-6

1. Why is a genetic predisposition suggested for testicular cancer?
2. Why is epididymitis rare in prepubescent males?
3. Why is testicular torsion considered a urologic emergency?

Disorders of the Prostate Gland

Benign prostatic hyperplasia

Benign prostatic hyperplasia (BPH), also called **benign prostatic hypertrophy,** is the enlargement of the prostate gland (Figure 32-28). Because the major prostatic changes are caused by hyperplasia, not hypertrophy, benign prostatic hyperplasia is the preferred term. This condition becomes problematic as prostatic tissue compresses the urethra, where it passes through the prostate, resulting in frequency of lower urinary tract symptoms. About 80% of men will have prostatic enlargement before age 80 years, and there is a 25% to 30% lifetime chance of needing prostatectomy for BPH once a man reaches 50 years of age.[50] At birth, the prostate is pea sized, and growth of the gland is gradual until puberty. At that time, there is a period of rapid development that continues until the third decade of life when the prostate reaches adult size (see Chapter 31). When the man reaches about 40 to 45 years of age, benign hyperplasia begins and continues slowly until death. Although androgens, such as dihydrotestosterone (DHT), are necessary for normal prostatic development, their role in BPH remains unclear. Among all the androgen-metabolizing enzymes within the prostate, 5-α-reductase is the most powerful one. This reductase corresponds to an age-dependent DHT level. Therefore, although 5-α-reductase and DHT decrease with age in the epithelium, they remain constant in the stroma (microenvironment) of the prostate gland. Current causative theories of BPH focus on levels and ratios of endocrine factors such as androgens, estrogens (androgen/estrogen ratio), gonadotropins, and prolactin and on changes in the balance between autocrine/paracrine growth-stimulating and growth-inhibiting factors. These

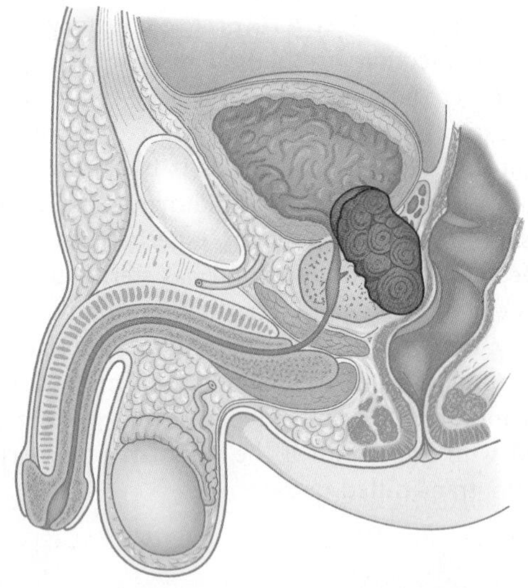

A

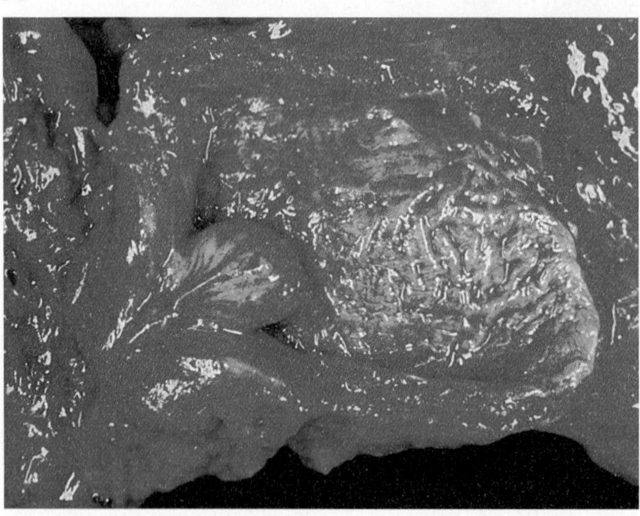

B

Figure 32-28 ■ **Benign Prostatic Hyperplasia (BPH). A,** Condition becomes a problem as prostatic tissue compresses the urethra. **B,** Gross appearance of BPH showing transition zone resulting from bulging nodules of varying size. (**B** from Damjanov I, Linder J, editors: *Anderson's pathology,* ed 10, St Louis, 1996, Mosby.)

factors include insulin-like growth factors (IGFs) as well as several others. Investigators are also studying whether abnormal blood flow patterns in the aging prostate gland might lead to hypoxia-stimulated prostate growth.[67] This hypothesis seems important with the new understanding that in most men symptoms result from a combination of BPH *and* age-related bladder dysfunction.[68,69] Conflicting data relate BPH to anthropometric measures (height, weight, waist, hip) or metabolic syndrome, or both.[70,71]

BPH begins in the periurethral glands, which are the inner glands or layers of the prostate. The prostate enlarges as nodules form and grow (nodular hyperplasia) and glandular cells enlarge (hypertrophy). As nodular hyperplasia and cellular hypertrophy progress, tissues that surround the prostatic urethra compress it, usually but not always causing **bladder outflow obstruction.**

Symptoms include the urge to urinate often, some delay in starting urination, and decreased force of the urinary stream. As the obstruction progresses, often over several years, the bladder cannot empty all the urine, and the increasing volume leads to long-term urine retention. The volume of urine retained may be great enough to produce uncontrolled "overflow incontinence" with any increase in intraabdominal pressure. At this stage, the force of the urinary stream is significantly reduced, and much more time is required to initiate and complete voiding.

Progressive bladder distention causes diverticular outpouchings of the bladder wall. The ureters may be obstructed where they pass through the hypertrophied detrusor muscle, potentially causing hydroureter, hydronephrosis, and bladder or kidney infection.

Digital rectal examination (DRE) and **prostate-specific antigen (PSA)** are conducted to determine hyperplasia. **Prostate-specific antigen density (PSAD)** is helpful in differentiating BPH from prostatic cancer. PSAD is calculated by dividing prostate-specific antigen (PSA) serum levels by the volume of prostate tissue, which is determined by transrectal ultrasound (TRUS). Treatment depends on the severity of symptoms, including postvoid residual urine (PVR), pressure-flow study, creatinine and BUN, and subjective symptoms score. Thirty percent of men with mild to moderate symptoms improve with watchful waiting. Those with moderately elevated symptom scores or severe symptom scores without large PVR levels can be treated with medications, such as 5-α-reductase inhibitors (e.g., finasteride) or selective α_1-blocking agents (e.g., Prazosin, Tamsulosin).[72,73] Candidates for surgical intervention include those with severe symptoms, large PVR, or complications, or those who fail to improve with medical therapy. Treatment from holmium laser enucleation (HoLEP) is emerging.[66] With improved medical treatments available, the number of men undergoing surgery is declining.[68]

Prostatitis

Prostatitis is an inflammation of the prostate. Some degree of prostatic inflammation is present in 4% to 36% of the male population, increasing to 50% in older men. Inflammation is usually limited to a few of the gland's excretory ducts.

Prostatitis is characterized as (1) acute bacterial prostatitis, (2) chronic bacterial prostatitis, or (3) nonbacterial prostatitis. Prostatitis can be in the form of **prostatodynia** (pain in the prostate). Men with prostatodynia have the same clinical manifestations as those with nonbacterial prostatitis, but physical and laboratory examinations do not show prostatic pathologic findings. Prostatodynia may be caused by spasms in the genitourinary tract or tension in the muscles of the pelvic floor.

Defense mechanisms protecting the lower urogenital tract from infection include urethral length, micturition (urination), ejaculation, and antimicrobial substances in the prostatic fluid. The most important of these is the zinc-containing polypeptide known as **prostatic antibacterial factor (PAF).** Coliform bacteria, particularly *Enterobacter, E. coli, Enterococcus, Klebsiella,* and *Pseudomonas* are common pathogens causing bacterial prostatitis. *Ureaplasma* and *C. trachomatis* also may be causative agents of infectious prostatitis.[55]

Bacterial prostatitis

Acute bacterial prostatitis is an ascending infection of the urinary tract that tends to occur in men between the ages of 30 and 50 years but is also associated with BPH in older men. Infection stimulates an inflammatory response in which the prostate becomes enlarged, tender, firm, or boggy. The onset of prostatitis may be acute and unrelated to previous illnesses, or it may follow catheterization or cystoscopy.

Clinical manifestations of acute bacterial prostatitis are those of urinary tract infection or pyelonephritis. Sudden onset of malaise, low back and perineal pain, high fever (up to 40° C [104° F]) and chills is common, as are dysuria, inability to empty the bladder, nocturia, and urinary retention. The individual also may have symptoms of lower urinary tract obstruction, such as slow, small, "narrowed" urinary stream, which may be a medical emergency. Acute inflammatory prostatic edema can compress the urethra, causing urinary obstruction. Systemic signs of infection include sudden onset of a high fever, fatigue, arthralgia, and myalgia. Prostatic pain may occur, especially when the individual is in an upright position, because the pelvic floor muscles tighten with standing and compression of the prostate gland occurs. Some individuals experience low back pain, painful ejaculation, and rectal or perineal pain. Palpation discloses an enlarged, extremely tender and swollen prostate that is firm, indurated, and warm to the touch.

Because acute bacterial prostatitis is usually associated with a bladder infection caused by the same microorganism, urine cultures disclose its identity. Prostatic massage may express enough secretions from the urethra for direct bacterial examination, but massage may be painful and increases the risk that the infection will ascend to adjacent structures or enter the bloodstream and cause septicemia.

To resolve the infection and control its spread, long-term, broad-spectrum antibiotic therapy (up to 6 weeks) may be required. In severe cases, the individual is hospitalized and treated with intravenous aminoglycoside and ampicillin for 7 days, followed by 4 to 6 weeks of oral antibiotics. Analgesics, antipyretics, bed rest, and adequate hydration are also therapeutic. Complications include urinary retention that resolves with antibiotic therapy; prostatic abscess that may rupture into the urethra, rectum, or perineum; epididymitis; bacteremia; and septic shock. Urinary retention requiring drainage is best managed with a suprapubic catheter; Foley catheterization is contraindicated during acute infection.

Chronic bacterial prostatitis is characterized by recurrent urinary tract symptoms and persistence of pathogenic bacteria (usually gram negative) in urine or prostatic fluid. This form of prostatitis is the most common recurrent urinary tract infection in men. Symptoms may be similar to those of an acute bladder infection: frequency, urgency, dysuria, perineal discomfort, low back pain, myalgia, arthralgia, and sexual dysfunction. The prostate may be only slightly enlarged or boggy, but it may be fibrotic because repeated infections can cause it to be firm and irregular in shape.

When the initial urine sample is bacteria-free, prostatic massage is used to express secretions. Subsequently, the first 10 ml of voided urine is collected and examined microscopically. Prostatic secretions showing more than 10 white blood cells (WBCs) per high-power field (hpf) and macrophages containing fat are indicative of bacterial infection; diagnosis is confirmed by culture. A pelvic x-ray or transurethral ultrasound (TRUS) may show prostatic calculi.

Treatment of chronic bacterial prostatitis is difficult because it is often caused by prostatic calculi. Calculi are silent and are found in up to 50% of men with prostatitis, and infected calculi can serve as a source of bacterial persistence and relapsing urinary tract infection.[55] Calculi harbor pathogens within the stone and, consequently, pathogens cannot be eradicated from the urinary tract. Permanent cure is achieved by surgical removal of the stones through transurethral prostatectomy, which may not be a viable option for young men. More common symptoms are tempered with chronic suppressive therapy. Comfort measures include nonsteroidal anti-inflammatory drug (NSAID) therapy and the liberal use of sitz baths.

Nonbacterial prostatitis

Nonbacterial prostatitis is the most common prostatitis syndrome. It consists of prostatic inflammation without evidence of bacterial infection. Symptoms tend to be milder but are persistent and annoying. Presumably, noninfectious prostatitis or prostatodynia is caused by reflux of sterile urine into the ejaculatory ducts because of high-pressure voiding.[55] Reflux may be triggered by spasms of the external or internal sphincters. Quinolones, because of their bioavailability and penetration into prostatic tissue, are the treatment of choice; drug therapy lasts for a minimum of 3 to 4 weeks. If symptoms do not subside, other infectious microorganisms are considered and treated accordingly.[55]

Men with nonbacterial prostatitis may complain of pain or a dull ache that is continuous or spasmodic in the suprapubic, infrapubic, scrotal, penile, or inguinal area. Other symptoms are pain on ejaculation and urinary symptoms, such as frequency of urination. The prostate gland generally feels normal on palpation.

Nonbacterial prostatitis is a diagnosis by exclusion. Digital examination of the prostate, bacterial cultures of the urogenital tract, microscopic examination of expressed prostatic fluid, urethroscopy, and urodynamic studies are used to verify the diagnosis of nonbacterial prostatitis.

There is no generally accepted treatment for nonbacterial prostatitis. Hot sitz baths, bed rest, alpha-blockers, anticholinergics, and anti-inflammatory drugs can relieve symptoms.

Cancer of the prostate

Prostate cancer is among the most common male cancers, but the incidence varies greatly worldwide. It is the most common cancer in American males but the third most common cancer worldwide. Figure 32-29 shows the remarkable worldwide variation. Prostate cancer accounts for more than 29% of all cancers in men in the United States and more than 14% of all cancer deaths; only lung cancer accounts for more deaths. Among countries with reliable cancer statistics, prostate cancer rates are highest in Westernized countries such as the United States and Western Europe and lowest in Asian countries. More than any other cancer, prostate cancer incidence warrants interpretation in the context of diagnostic intensity and screening behavior. Screening with PSA can amplify the incidence of prostate cancer by allowing the detection of prostatic lesions that, while meeting the pathologic criteria for malignancy, many believe to have low potential for growth and metastasis; this is, however, controversial. Thus screening can amplify the incidence of prostate cancer by allowing the detection of these localized lesions. Therefore, incidence rates in some countries, such as the United States, reflect both clinical and latent (or preclinical) disease compared to other countries with only clinical disease. Comparing data in the pre-PSA era, however, reflects less extreme incidence rates but country ranking reveals the United States as still being in the lead. Data from the Surveillance, Epidemiology, and End Results (SEER) program show that U.S. incidence rates for white men increased 80% from 1983–1987 to 1988–1992, and they about doubled between 1983–1987 and 1993–1995.[74]

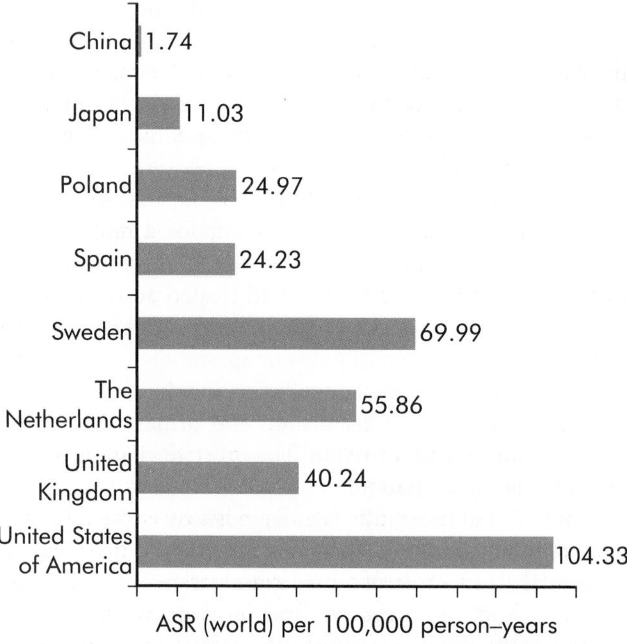

Figure 32-29 ■ Selected World Population Age-Standardized (to the World Population) Incidence Rates of Prostate Cancer. ASR, Age-standardized rate. (Data from Ferlay J et al: *GLOBOCAN 2000: cancer incidence, mortality, and prevalence worldwide,* Lyon, 2001, International Agency for Research on Cancer.)

Prostate cancer death rates in the United States declined after 1991 in white men and after 1992 in black men.[75] The decline may reflect increased screening using PSA.[75] The overall mortality rates are predominantly in men over the age of 65; within younger age groups, mortality has been stable across decades. Incidence increases with advancing age, with more than 75% of all prostate cancers diagnosed in men older than 65 years. By age 85 years, about one in six American men will develop prostate cancer in their lifetime, and approximately 3% will die from it. Most of the androgen-metabolizing enzymes undergo significant alteration with aging. Although worldwide the incidence is low in black African men, black African-American men have the highest rate of prostate cancer in the world and in the United States. Age is the strongest risk factor with few other established factors including family history of prostate cancer, a Western lifestyle, and an African-American heritage. Expanding literature suggests a possible link between chronic inflammation and prostate cancer. The molecular pathogenesis of prostate cancer has shown several alterations of genes involved in defenses against inflammatory damage and tissue recovery (see the Pathogenesis section presented later in the chapter).[76]

Dietary factors

The worldwide distribution of prostate cancer suggests that diet may play a role in the development of prostate cancer, especially if the diet affects hormone levels. Consistency across studies indicates that a high intake of fat (total and especially saturated fat) is a risk factor for prostate cancer, but the strength of the associations is modest and may be greater for African Americans than for European Americans.[77–79] Several hypotheses exist concerning the enhancing effect of fat on prostate carcinogenesis, including hormonal mediation and the generation of free radicals. Fat intake from dairy products increases calcium, itself a proposed risk factor. Calcium can suppress circulating levels of dihydroxyvitamin D, a possible protective factor for prostate cancer.[80] In addition, a low intake of dietary fiber and complex carbohydrates and a high intake of protein are associated with an increased risk of prostate cancer.[79] Controversial is whether obesity or an increased body mass index is a risk factor for prostate cancer. Unclear is if high-energy intake (consumption of excess calories) increases insulin levels and insulin-like growth factor-1 (IGF-1). High levels of IGF-1 and low levels of IGF-binding protein-3 (IGFBP-3) have been implicated in experimental studies related to prostate cancer growth, survival, and progression. Yet data suggest a much weaker association of IGF-1 with prostate cancer development but a stronger protective effect of IGFBP-3.[81] Interestingly, data showed lycopene increased the levels of IGFBP-3 and decreased in vitro prostate cancer cell proliferation.[82]

Individual nutrients or foods and their associations with prostate cancer risk are not strong, yet migration of individuals from low-risk geographic areas of the world, such as Japan, to high-risk countries, such as the United States, increases risk considerably. These changes in risk probably reflect differences in lifestyle and dietary habits. Geographically, individuals who reside in regions with less sunlight have a higher risk of prostate cancer. The highest rates of mortality from prostate cancer in the world are in Scandinavian countries, where exposure to ultraviolet light is low; the possible link is less vitamin D induced by less sun exposure. The Cure of Cancer of the Prostate (CaP CURE) Report states that of all the risk factors for prostate cancer, only nutrition seems to explain the differences in global distribution of prostate cancer.[83]

Animal studies suggest a protective effect of retinoids (vitamin A) and prostate carcinogenesis; however, consistency is lacking among epidemiologic studies. Vegetarian men have a lower incidence of prostate cancer than omnivorous males.[84,85] Low levels of dietary selenium are associated with increased prostate cancer risk.[86] Vitamin D (1,25-[OH]2D3) inhibited the growth of certain human prostate cancer cell lines by function of an androgen-dependent mechanism.[87] Lycopene, a carotenoid that gives vegetables their red color and is found in large amounts in tomatoes, has been associated with a lower risk of prostate cancer. Many chemopreventive agents, including silibinin, inositol hexaphosphate, decursin, apigenin, acacetin, grape seed extract, curcumin, and epigallocatechin-3 gallate, have been identified in laboratory studies, which might be useful in altering or preventing prostate cancer progression (see *Health Alert:* Nutritional and Chemopreventive Agents for Risk Reduction of Prostate Cancer).[82,88–90]

HEALTH ALERT

Nutritional and Chemopreventive Agents for Risk Reduction of Prostate Cancer

Several areas of investigation are identifying prospective therapies for prostate cancer prevention. Several studies found antioxidants to be potential chemopreventive agents. Individuals with the highest quartile of antioxidant levels (vitamin E, selenium, and lycopene) have a 42% reduction in prostate cancer risk. The effect was higher (59% reduction) in those with high-grade or high-stage cancer risk. Many chemopreventive agents that have been identified in laboratory studies—including silibinin (from milk thistle), inositol hexaphosphate (IP6, a form of carbohydrate in cereals, legumes, oil seeds, and nuts), decursin (from the roots of Angelica giga), apigenin and acacetin (fruits and vegetables), grape seed extract, curcumin, and epigallocatechin-3 (green tea)—could be useful against prostate cancer. Molecular mechanisms include cell signaling, cell-cycle regulators, and survival/apoptosis.

Data from Kantoff P: Prevention, complementary therapies, and new scientific developments in the field of prostate cancer, *Rev Urol* 8(suppl 1):S9-S14, 2006; Singh RP, Agarwal R: Mechanisms of action of novel agents for prostate cancer chemoprevention, *Endocr Relat Cancer* 13(3):751–778, review, 2006.

Hormones

Prostate cancer develops in an androgen-dependent epithelium and is usually androgen sensitive. In addition, a few case reports of prostate cancer in men who used androgenic steroids as anabolic agents or for medical purposes suggest a causal relationship.[78,91–93] Population studies have not, however, provided clear and convincing patterns involving associations between circulating (e.g., not tissue concentrations) hormone concentrations and prostate cancer risk.[77,94] Only a few associations with prostate cancer risk have been observed consistently (in at least three studies), and those associations are weak: (1) slightly higher circulating testosterone and estrogen levels and lower DHEA (sulfate) levels in high-risk African-American men as compared with lower-risk European-American men and (2) a cytosine-adenine-guanine (CAG) repeat-length polymorphism in the androgen-receptor gene associated with increased risk and increased receptor activity (androgen receptor). Evidence for involvement of activity of the enzyme 5-α-reductase, which is critical in androgen activity in the prostate, is contradictory and inconsistent.[77,94] A prevention study has provided some of the strongest hormonal data with the drug finasteride which inhibits 5-α reductase. The 7-year intervention study reduced prostate cancer risk in healthy men by about 25%.[95] Important, however, was that more high-grade tumors were found in those men who developed prostate cancer while on the drug. In men younger than 50 years, circulating levels of androgens and estrogens appear to be higher in men of African descent than in European-American men.

Investigations directed at understanding the hormonal basis of prostate (as well as breast) carcinogenesis have numerous problems. The complexities of interacting hormones and separating out the effects of a single hormone are profound. In addition, only single *blood* samples are generally available, *tissue* hormone samples important for paracrine signaling are not consistently measured, and within-subject variations over time and differences in circadian rhythms cannot be adequately measured. The results of several animal studies do support elevation of bioavailable and bioactive androgens in the circulation and in target tissue as an important risk factor. Animal studies also indicate that increased biologic activity of the androgen receptor may be associated with prostate cancer. A more thorough discussion of the role of hormones in the pathogenesis of prostate cancer is in the Pathogenesis section.

Vasectomy

Vasectomy has been identified as a possible risk factor for prostate cancer in both case-controlled studies and cohort studies.[81,96] Three mechanisms by which vasectomy could increase risk are (1) elevation of circulating androgens; (2) immunologic mechanisms involving antisperm antibodies; and (3) reduction of seminal fluid levels of 5α-dihydrotestosterone, the active metabolite of testosterone in the prostate, in vasectomized men. Other investigators reported a decrease in sex hormone–binding globulin (SHBG) and an increase in the ratio of testosterone to SHBG.[97] These results suggest an elevation of circulating free testosterone after vasectomy.[94] The epidemiologic literature is consistent with no appreciable association of vasectomy and prostate cancer or a weak positive association.[89]

Chronic inflammation

The results of a 5-year, longitudinal study of the influence of chronic inflammation and prostate cancer have been reported.[98] The study included 144 men, 33 of whom presented with chronic inflammation in their initial biopsy. Biopsies revealed prostatic hyperplasia and proliferative inflammatory atrophy in those with chronic inflammation. Upon repeat biopsy, 29 new cancers were diagnosed representing a new cancer incidence of 20%.[98] In contrast, of the 33 men initially showing no inflammation, 2 (6%) were found to have adenocarcinoma. Thus, chronic inflammation may be an important risk factor for prostatic adenocarcinoma. An inflammatory process could possibly account for the evidence that antioxidants (e.g., lycopene, vitamin E, selenium) and nonsteroidal anti-inflammatory drugs, such as aspirin, may be protective.[80,89,98]

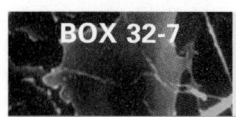

Determining the Grade of Prostate Cancer With the Gleason Score

Grade 1. The cancer cells closely resemble normal cells. They are small, uniform in shape, evenly spaced, and well differentiated (i.e., they remain separate from one another).

Grade 2. The cancer cells are still well differentiated, but they are arranged more loosely and are irregular in shape and size. Some of the cancer cells have invaded the neighboring prostate tissue.

Grade 3. This is the most common grade. The cells are less well differentiated (some have fused into clumps) and are more variable in shape.

Grade 4. The cells are poorly differentiated and highly irregular in shape. Invasion of the neighboring prostate tissue has progressed further.

Grade 5. The cells are undifferentiated. They have merged into large masses that no longer resemble normal prostate cells. Invasion of the surrounding tissue is extensive.

Familial factors

Other possible causes are those of genetic predisposition (familial and hereditary forms). Genetic studies suggest that strong familial predisposition may be responsible for 5% to 10% of prostate cancers.[65] Hereditary cancer is an autosomal dominant disease caused by a rare but highly penetrant gene—that is, 88% of gene carriers develop prostate cancer by age 85 years. Hereditary cancer differs from the familial form, which occurs in individuals with a positive family history but who do not exhibit early age of onset.[99] The hereditary form constitutes about 9% of all prostate cancers and approximately 43% of cancers in men younger than 55 years of age.[100] There is no clear evidence of a causal link between BPH and prostate cancer, even though they may often occur together. Data substantiate that tobacco use has a significant impact on the occurrence of fatal prostate cancer.[101]

PATHOGENESIS More than 95% of prostatic neoplasms are adenocarcinomas,[102] and most occur in the periphery of the prostate. The biologic aggressiveness of the neoplasm appears to be related to the degree of differentiation rather than the size of the tumor (Box 32-7).

Although steroid hormonal factors are strongly implicated in prostate carcinogenesis, little is known about their involvement. Just as the testicles are the male equivalent of the female ovaries, the prostate is the male equivalent of the female uterus; in both cases, they originate from the same embryonic cells. This may be important in understanding the role of the associated hormones testosterone (T), dihydrotestosterone (DHT), and estradiol in prostate carcinogenesis.

Testosterone is the major *circulating* androgen, whereas DHT predominates in prostate tissue and binds to the androgen receptor (AR) with greater affinity than does T.[103] Testosterone is the major androgen that comes from the interstitial cells of the testis (Leydig cells). Its production in men is almost 5 mg/day. The adrenal cortex contributes the far less potent androstenedione as its major androgen, at about 3 mg/day. In the target tissues and, to a lesser extent, in the testes themselves, testosterone is converted to dihydrotestosterone (DHT) by the enzyme 5-α-reductase (Figure 32-30). Thus, DHT is the most potent intraprostatic androgen.

Normally, a small amount of estrogen is produced per day—65 μg of estrone and 45 μg of estradiol—by the aromatization of androstenedione and testosterone, respectively. This reaction is catalyzed by the enzyme system aromatase. A small quantity of estradiol is released by the testes (see Figure 32-30); the rest of the estrogens in males are produced by adipose tissue, liver, skin, brain, and other nonendocrine tissue. Thus, testosterone is a precursor of the two hormones, DHT and estradiol.

Most of the androgen-metabolizing enzymes undergo a significant age-dependent alteration. In epithelium, both the blood levels of 5-α-reductase activity and the DHT level decrease with age; whereas in stroma (prostate), not only the 5-α-reductase activity but also the stromal DHT level

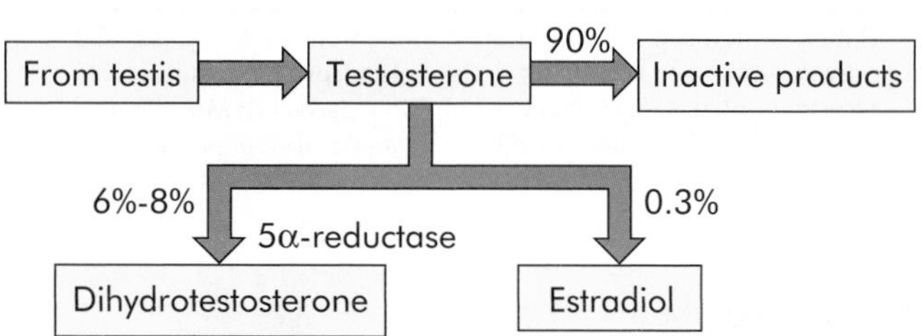

Figure 32-30 ■ Testosterone and Conversion to Dihydrotestosterone (DHT).

is rather constant over the whole range. In contrast to the relatively unaltered DHT level over time, the estrogen content follows an age-dependent increase. Thus the age-dependent decrease of the DHT accumulation in epithelium and the concomitant increase of the estrogen accumulation in stroma lead to a tremendous increase with age of the estrogen/androgen ratio in the human prostate. In animal studies, chronic exposure to testosterone plus estradiol is strongly carcinogenic, whereas testosterone alone is weakly carcinogenic.[77] The mechanism is not clearly understood and may involve estrogen-generated oxidative stress and DNA toxicity, and it requires androgen and estrogen receptor–mediated processes, such as changes in sex steroid metabolism and receptor status.[77] In addition, there are changes in the balance between autocrine/paracrine growth-stimulatory and growth-inhibitory factors, such as the insulin growth factors (IGFs). One promising advance in our understanding of the etiology of prostate cancer is the action of IGF-1. IGF-1 is known to be a potent mitogen that can increase cell proliferation and decrease cell death, or apoptosis—thus allowing a mutated cell to live and proliferate. Both normal and malignant prostate cells produce IGF-1 and several of its binding proteins. Some studies have provided compelling evidence that IGF-1 may be a key risk factor for prostate cancer.[104–106]

From all of these observations, the following multifactorial general hypothesis of prostate carcinogenesis emerges: (1) androgens act as strong tumor promoters through androgen receptor–mediated mechanisms to (2) enhance the weak but continuously present genotoxic carcinogen, estradiol-17 beta, and (3) possibly unknown environmental carcinogens. All of these factors are modulated by diet and genetic determinants, such as hereditary susceptibility genes and polymorphic genes, which encode receptors and enzymes involved in the metabolism and action of steroid hormones.[77]

The microenvironment (stroma) surrounding the prostatic tumor actively fuels the progression of prostate cancer from localized growth, to invasion, to development of distant metastases.[107] The most common sites of distant metastasis are the lymph nodes, bones, lungs, liver, and adrenals. The pelvis, lumbar spine, femur, thoracic spine, and ribs are the most common sites of bone metastasis. Local extension is usually posterior, although late in the disease the tumor may invade the rectum or encroach on the prostatic urethra and cause bladder outlet obstruction (Figure 32-31). The spread of cancer through blood vessels is illustrated in Figure 32-32.

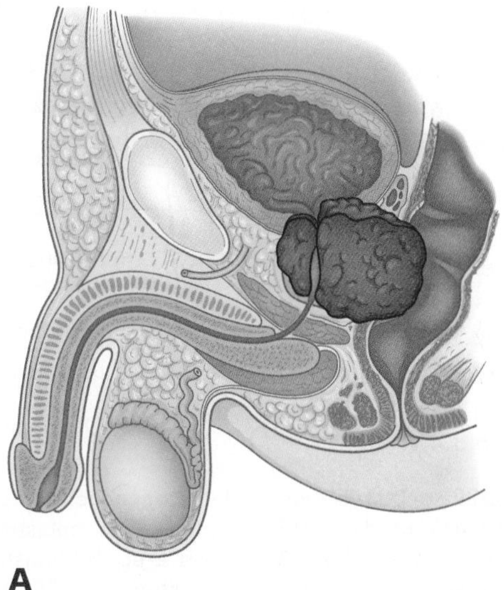

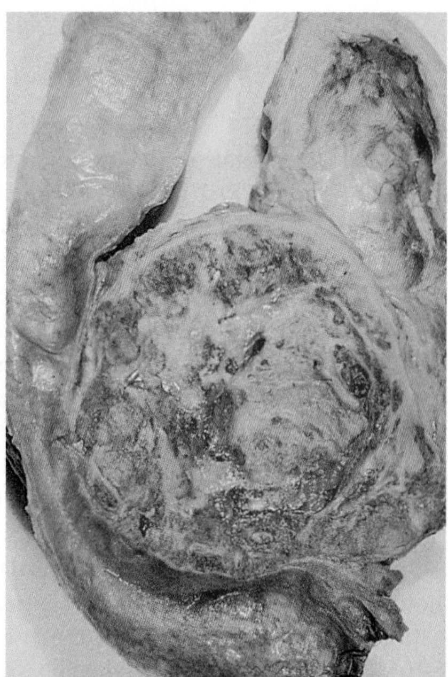

Figure 32-31 ■ Carcinoma of Prostate. A, Schematic of carcinoma of the prostate. **B,** Carcinoma of the prostate extending into the rectum and urinary bladder. (**B** from Damjanov I, Linder J, editors: *Pathology: a color atlas,* St Louis, 2000, Mosby.)

CLINICAL MANIFESTATIONS Prostatic cancer often causes no symptoms until it is far advanced. Therefore, routine screening is recommended for asymptomatic men beginning at age 50 years or at age 45 years if they are considered at high risk. The first manifestations of disease are those of bladder outlet obstruction: slow urinary stream, hesitancy, incomplete emptying, frequency, nocturia, and dysuria. Unlike the symptoms of obstruction caused by BPH, the symptoms of obstruction caused by prostatic cancer are progressive and do not remit. Local extension of prostatic cancer can obstruct the upper urinary tract ureters as well. Rectal obstruction also may occur, causing the individual to experience large bowel obstruction or difficulty in defecation. Symptoms of late disease include bone pain at sites of bone metastasis, edema of the lower extremities, enlargement of lymph nodes, liver enlargement, pathologic bone fractures, and mental confusion associated with brain metastases. Prostatic cancer and its treatment can affect sexual functioning.

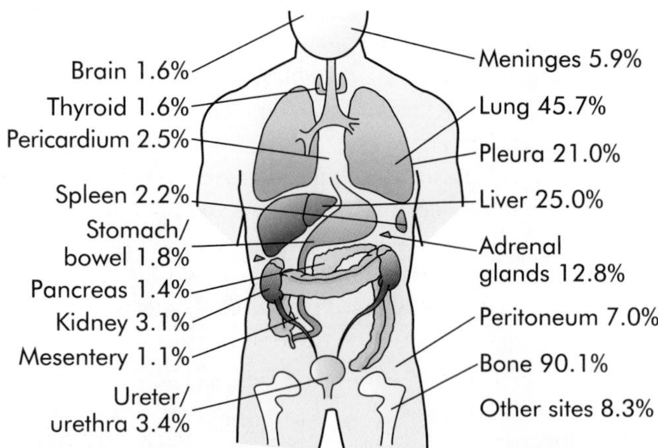

Figure 32-32 ■ Distribution of Hematogenous Metastases in Prostate Cancer. Study of 556 individuals with metastatic prostate cancer. (Adapted from Budendorf L et al: Metastatic patterns of prostate cancer: an autopsy study of 1,589 patients, *Hum Pathol* 31:578, 2000.)

EVALUATION AND TREATMENT Screening for prostatic cancer includes digital rectal examination (DRE), prostate-specific antigen (PSA) blood tests, and transrectal ultrasound (TRUS). Cancer diagnosis is confirmed through tissue biopsy and microscopic examination of tissue. Lymphography, bone scans, MRI, and CT scans also may be used to determine metastasis to lymph, bone, or other adjacent tissue. Important for treatment is to accurately measure the size of the index (longest) tumor and its percentage Gleason grade of differentiation.[108]

Treatment of prostatic cancer depends on the stage of the disease (see Box 32-7), the anticipated effects of treatment, and the age, general health, and life expectancy of the individual. Options range from hormonal or radiation therapy or chemotherapy to surgery (contemporary nerve sparing or robotic surgery), any combination of these, or no treatment. Palliative treatment is aimed at relieving urinary, bladder outlet, or colon obstruction, spinal cord compression, and pain.

Prognosis and survival rates have improved steadily since the 1950s. Currently, 85% of all prostate cancers are discovered in the local and regional stages; in these stages, the 5-year survival rate is 100%.[109] For those men whose cancer has spread to distant tissue when it is found, the 5-year survival is 34%.[109]

Treatment for prostate cancer may lead to loss of urinary control, which can return to normal after several weeks or months. Mild stress incontinence can occur after surgery and mild urge incontinence after radiation therapy. Prostate cancer and its treatment can affect sexual functioning. Most men will need assistance (medication) with obtaining an erection for 3 to 12 months after surgery. Sensation of orgasm is not usually affected, but smaller amounts of ejaculate will be produced or men may experience a "dry" ejaculate because of retrograde ejaculation.

Sexual Dysfunction

In males, the normal sexual response involves erection, emission, and ejaculation. **Sexual dysfunction** is the impairment of any or all of these processes and can be caused by various physiologic, psychologic, and emotional factors.

Until the late 1970s, most cases of male sexual dysfunction were considered psychogenic. Now there is evidence that 89% to 90% of cases involve organic factors and include (1) vascular, endocrine, and neurologic disorders; (2) chronic disease, including renal failure and diabetes mellitus; (3) penile diseases and penile trauma; and (4) iatrogenic factors, such as surgery and pharmacologic therapies. Most of these disorders cause erectile dysfunction.[110]

PATHOPHYSIOLOGY Sexual dysfunction can have a specific physiologic cause, can be associated with many chronic diseases and their treatment, or may be related to low energy levels, stress, or depression. For example, vascular disease may cause impotence, and endocrine disorders or conditions that cause decreased testosterone levels or testicular atrophy can diminish sexual functioning or libido. In addition, neurologic disorders and spinal cord injuries can interfere with sympathetic, parasympathetic, and CNS mechanisms required for erection, emission, and ejaculation.

Drug-induced sexual dysfunction consists of decreased desire, decreased erectile ability, or decreased ejaculatory ability. Alcohol and other CNS depressants, antihypertensives, antidepressants, antihistamines, and hormonal preparations are commonly used drugs that affect sexual functioning. Other pharmacologic agents may diminish the quality or quantity of sperm or cause priapism.

CLINICAL MANIFESTATIONS AND TREATMENT Evaluation of sexual dysfunction includes a thorough history and physical examination. Particular attention is given to drug history and examination of the genitalia, prostate, and nervous system. Basic laboratory tests are used to identify the presence of endocrinopathies or other underlying disorders that can cause dysfunction. Psychologic evaluation is indicated for younger men with a sudden onset of sexual dysfunction or men of any age who can achieve but not maintain an erection. If no physiologic cause is found and the condition does not improve with psychotherapy, the man is referred for further investigation of organic causes.

Treatments for organic sexual dysfunction include both medical and surgical approaches. The drug Viagra (sildenafil) has created much enthusiasm over its ability to help a man maintain an erection. For a small percentage of men (1%), however, this improvement in sexual function is accompanied by heart attacks and death. Whether these effects are the result of sexual performance or Viagra has been controversial. Research has shown that Viagra increases blood concentrations of an enzyme, cGMP-dependent protein kinase (PKG), which increases blood flow to the penis. PKG, however, plays a dual role: first it increases platelet aggregation and then, minutes later, it decreases clot size. The initial clot could cause some men with heart disease to experience cardiac arrest.[111] Nonsurgical approaches include correction of underlying disorders, particularly drug-induced dysfunction and endocrinopathy-related (e.g., reduced testosterone associated with chronic renal failure) dysfunction. Vasodilators and cessation of smoking can benefit individuals with vasculogenic erectile dysfunction. Surgical approaches include penile implants, penile revascularization, and correction of other anatomic defects contributing to sexual dysfunction.

QUICK CHECK 32-7

1. What is the current understanding of hormones in the pathophysiology of prostate cancer?

DISORDERS OF THE BREAST

Disorders of the Female Breast

Galactorrhea

Galactorrhea (inappropriate lactation) is the persistent and sometimes excessive secretion of a milky fluid from the breasts of a woman who is not pregnant or nursing an infant. Galactorrhea, which also can occur in men, may involve one or both breasts and is not associated with breast cancer.[112]

The incidence of galactorrhea is difficult to estimate because of differences among definitions of the condition, examination techniques, and populations of women who have been studied. Prevalence has been documented as 0.1% to 32% of all women.

PATHOPHYSIOLOGY Galactorrhea is not a breast disorder but, rather, a manifestation of pathophysiologic processes elsewhere in the body. These processes are chiefly hormone imbalances caused by hypothalamic-pituitary disturbances, pituitary tumors, or neurologic damage. Exogenous causes include drugs, estrogen (e.g., in oral contraceptives), and manipulation of the nipples.

The most common cause of galactorrhea is **nonpuerperal hyperprolactinemia,** or excessive amounts of prolactin in the blood not related to pregnancy or childbirth. Nonpuerperal hyperprolactinemia can be caused by any factor that (1) stimulates or overstimulates the prolactin-secreting units of the pituitary gland; (2) interferes with production of **prolactin-inhibiting factor (PIF),** a neurotransmitter (probably dopamine) that inhibits prolactin secretion; or (3) interferes with pituitary receptors for PIF.

Certain drugs can cause nonpuerperal hyperprolactinemia. They include the phenothiazines, reserpine, and methyldopa; exogenous estrogens, particularly in oral contraceptives; morphine; and the tricyclic antidepressants.

Hypothyroidism causes increased secretion of hypothalamic thyroid-releasing hormone (TRH), which stimulates prolactin release from the pituitary. Hypothyroidism also is associated with reduced metabolic clearance of prolactin, which prolongs its effects.

Many types of pituitary tumors cause hyperprolactinemia, particularly prolactinoma. Prolactinomas cause hyperprolactinemia by secreting prolactin, decreasing production of PIF, or putting pressure on the pituitary stalk, thus preventing delivery of PIF to the anterior pituitary. Growth hormone–secreting pituitary tumors may cause galactorrhea through the intrinsic lactogenic effect that growth hormone appears to have on mammary tissue. Prolactin-secreting lung and kidney tumors also cause hyperprolactinemia.

Galactorrhea can be induced by persistent and repeated sucking or squeezing of the nipples and has been documented in women who manipulate their breasts and nipples daily. Monthly examination of the breasts for nipple discharge usually is not associated with the development of galactorrhea.

CLINICAL MANIFESTATIONS Inappropriate lactation is manifested by the appearance of a milky breast secretion from one or both breasts of nonpregnant, nonlactating women. Most women with galactorrhea experience menstrual abnormality. If a pituitary process is involved, the woman usually experiences hirsutism and infertility; if a hypothalamic lesion is present, she may report CNS symptoms, such as intractable headache, visual field disturbances, sleep disturbances, and abnormal temperature, thirst, or appetite.[113]

EVALUATION AND TREATMENT Galactorrhea in nulliparous women (women who have never been pregnant) or in parous women who have not breast-fed for 12 months must be thoroughly evaluated. Serum prolactin levels are measured, and at least two positive results are needed to diagnose hyperprolactinemia. Prolactin levels higher than 25 to 30 ng/ml (measured by radioimmunoassay) are considered elevated. Those in the range of 75 to 100 ng/ml are considered to be caused by a pituitary tumor until proven otherwise. Serum T_4 and TSH levels are measured to rule out hypothyroidism, and LH and FSH levels are obtained if the individual is menorrheic. CT, MRI, and carotid angiography may assist in the localization of adenomas.

Treatment for galactorrhea consists of identification and treatment of the cause. Medical and surgical therapies may be involved.

Benign breast conditions

Numerous benign alterations in ducts and lobules occur in the breast. The most common symptoms reported by women are pain, palpable mass, or nipple discharge; the majority of these prove to have a benign cause. Benign epithelial lesions can be broadly classified according to their future risk of developing breast cancer as (1) nonproliferative breast lesions, (2) proliferative breast disease, and (3) atypical (atypia) hyperplasia.

Nonproliferative breast lesions

The term *nonproliferative* is used to discriminate from the "proliferative" changes associated with increased risk for development of breast cancer. This nonproliferative group includes **fibrocystic changes (FCC)**—the most widely accepted term—for physiologic nodularity and breast tenderness that waxes and wanes with the menstrual cycle. On palpation, breasts are lumpy or bumpy and, from radiology studies, breast tissue appears dense with cysts. These lesions mimic carcinoma and women seek medical attention because they produce palpable lumps or nipple discharge. **Cysts**, fluid-filled sacs, are a specific type of lump that commonly occurs in women in their 30s, 40s, and early 50s. Cysts feel squishy when they occur close to the surface of the breast but when deeply embedded they can feel hard. It has become increasingly clear that FCC is a heterogeneous group of lesions that should be diagnosed separately. An estimated 50% to 80% of women normally experience some of these changes. The prevalence of fibrocystic lesions is probably related to hormonal changes, which in turn are affected by genetic background, age, parity, history of lactation, caffeine, and use of exogenous hormones.[114] Cystic change can be induced in experimental animals by altering ratios of estrogens and progesterone. It is assumed, therefore, that breast cysts are the result of ovarian alterations, but the exact mechanism is unknown. Calcifications, found in cysts and adenosis or an increase in the number of acini per lobule, can form mammographically suspicious alterations.[115] Cysts also can be associated with unilateral nipple discharge. Cystic changes by themselves do not appear to be premalignant alterations. Cysts often rupture with release of secretory material into the adjacent tissue. The resulting chronic inflammation and scarring fibrosis contribute to the palpable firmness of the breast.[115] Fibrous tissue increases progressively until menopause and regresses thereafter.

The College of American Pathologists has classified biopsy tissue according to breast cancer risk. These classifications are listed in Box 32-8. In addition to FCC, many women experience several other types of benign breast tumors (Table 32-8). In general, the frequency of chromosome abnormalities is lower in benign lesions than in breast cancer. Genetic aberrations are more common in proliferative than in nonproliferative lesions.[115]

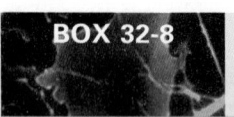

Classification of Breast Biopsy Tissue According to Risk for Breast Cancer

No Increased Risk
Adenosis (sclerosing or florid)
Apocrine metaplasia
Macrocysts or microcysts
Fibroadenoma
Fibrosis
Mild hyperplasia (3–4 cells deep)
Mastitis or periductal mastitis
Squamous metaplasia

Slightly Increased Risk (One and One-Half to Two Times)
Moderate or florid hyperplasia
Papilloma

Moderately Increased Risk (Three to Five Times)
Atypical hyperplasia (ductal or lobular)

Proliferative breast lesions without atypia

These disorders are characterized by proliferation of ductal epithelium or stroma without cellular signs of malignancy. The following structurally diverse lesions are included: (1) moderate or florid epithelial hyperplasia, (2) sclerosing adenosis, (3) complex sclerosing lesions (radial scar), (4) papillomas, and (5) fibroadenoma with complex features.[115] **Epithelial hyperplasia** is defined by the presence of *more* than two cell layers above the basement membrane. In the normal breast, only myoepithelial cells and a single layer of luminal cells are present above the basement membrane.[115] Moderate to **florid hyperplasia** is more than four cell layers above the basement membrane. The proliferating epithelium fills and distends the ducts and lobules by both luminal and myoepithelial cells.

Sclerosing adenosis is present when the number of acini per terminal duct is greater than twice the number found in uninvolved lobules.[115] Calcification is commonly present within the lumens; however, the normal lobular arrangement is maintained. The acini are structurally altered, and myoepithelial cells are prominent. Occasionally, stromal fibrosis may mimic the appearance of invasive carcinoma.[115]

Complex sclerosing lesion (radial scar) refers to an irregular, radial proliferation of ductlike small tubules entrapped in a dense central fibrosis. The term *scar* refers to the structural appearance only because these lesions are not associated with prior injury or surgery. Radial scar also has been called *radial sclerosing lesions* and *sclerosing papillary proliferation.* Among women with atypical hyperplasia, as compared to women with nonproliferative disease, the relative risk of breast cancer was 5.8 for those with radial scars and 3.8 for those without radial scars. Radial scars are now considered an independent histologic risk factor for breast cancer.[116] The appearance in mammograms, as well as the gross and microscopic appearance, can cause it to be confused with infiltrating ductal carcinoma.[117]

Papillomas consist of multiple, finger-like projections or branching axis lined by myoepithelial cells and luminal cells. Hyperplasia and metaplasia are often present within the ducts. Small duct papillomas increase the risk of subsequent carcinoma; it is unknown whether large duct papillomas do as well.

TABLE 32-8

Examples of Benign Breast Disorders

Benign Breast Disease	Period of Greatest Risk	Pathophysiology	Clinical Manifestations of Lesion	Treatment
Fibroadenoma	Puberty, early adulthood, rare after menopause	Unknown but thought to be associated with exposure to increased estrogen levels	Painless, firm, solitary, well-circumscribed mobile mass; usually in upper outer quadrant of breast	Surgical excision of mass or careful observation
Mammary duct ectasia (comedomastitis)	Menopause, postmenopause, during pregnancy and lactation	Subareolar ducts become dilated and fill with cellular debris, initiating inflammatory reaction; rupture of ducts may occur	Blood-stained, sticky, thick, spontaneous, multiple-duct discharge; ductal rupture creates palpable mass; burning pain, swelling of areolar area may occur	Condition usually resolves 7–10 days after onset with or without antibiotic therapy
Solitary intraductal papilloma	Age 40–50 yr	Unknown	Lesion is slow-growing and cauliflower-like and extends length of involved duct; nipple discharge from one or two ductal openings may be watery, serous, serosanguineous, or sanguineous	Surgical excision of involved duct
Multiple papillomas	Age 35–40 yr	Unknown	Similar to solitary intraductal papilloma, except that discharge is from multiple ductal openings	Depends on extent of involvement; if lesion is small, excision of that breast segment; total mastectomy if disease is widespread
Fat necrosis	Age 14–80 yr, average age 50 yr	Breast trauma, including silicone injections and breast biopsy, cause hemorrhage and induration, leading to formation of a palpable mass	Unilateral, fairly immobile breast mass, located close to the surface; mass is usually tender and painful	Mass may be reabsorbed spontaneously or local excision

Proliferative breast lesions with atypia

Proliferative breast lesions with some abnormal structure or *atypia* include atypical ductal hyperplasia (ADH) and atypical lobular hyperplasia (ALH).[115] Overall, proliferative disease, unlike nonproliferative changes, is correlated with increases in breast cancer risk.

Atypical hyperplasia is an increase in the number of cells, and the cells have some variation in structure. **Ductal hyperplasia** is an increased number of cells mostly within the lumen of the terminal ducts. It includes a continuum of changes—cell structure and placement—ranging from an increase in cellularity to features of ductal carcinoma in situ (DCIS; see p. 896). In ADH, the cells fail to completely fill ductal spaces as compared to DCIS. **Lobular hyperplasia** refers to proliferation of small, uniform cells in the lumen of lobular units. The abnormal cells of ALH and lobular carcinoma in situ (LCIS) are identical, but the cells in ALH do not distend more than 50% of the acini within a lobule.[115] ALH can extend into ducts, and this is associated with an increased risk of invasive carcinomas.[115]

Breast cancer

Breast cancer, the most common cancer in American women, is the leading cause of death in women 40 to 44 years of age and the second most common killer of women of all ages after lung cancer. Incidence of invasive breast cancer has increased since the 1990s in Asian Americans/Pacific Islanders; decreased in American Indian/Alaska Natives; and did not change significantly among whites, African Americans, and Hispanics/Latinos.[118] Incidence rates of ductal carcinoma in situ (DCIS) has increased in all age groups since the 1980s, presumably as a direct result of detection by mammography.[118] A sharp decline in incidence of estrogen receptor positive tumors occurred in 2003 continuing in 2004 possibly related to a decline in HRT usage (see hormones, p. 889). Age-specific incidence

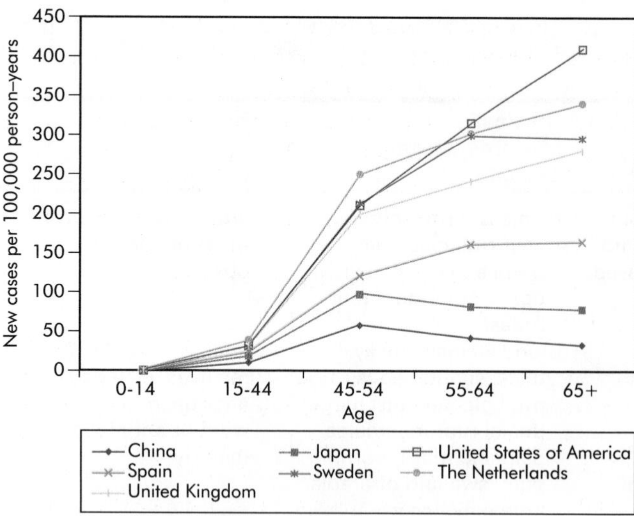

Figure 32-33 ■ Age-Specific Incidence Rates of Breast Cancer Among Women. (Data from Ferlay J et al: *GLOBOCAN 2000: cancer incidence, mortality, and prevalence worldwide,* Lyon, 2001, International Agency for Research on Cancer.)

and mortality rates vary internationally (Figure 32-33). Data reveal that death rates declined 1.4% per year from 1989 to 1995 and 3.2% thereafter, with the largest decreases in younger women—both whites and African Americans. The causes for the decline are unknown. For all ages combined, white women are more likely to develop breast cancer than black women; yet the incidence of breast cancer is higher in blacks among women younger than 45 years. In addition, for all ages, black women are more likely to die of breast cancer (29.3/100,000) compared with white women (26/100,000).[118] Breast cancers account for about 30% of all cancer cases found in women and 16% of cancer deaths. The highest rates of breast cancer are in North America and Europe, and the lowest rates are in Asia.

Risk factors and possible causes of breast cancer can be classified as reproductive, hormonal, environmental, and familial (Table 32-9). Although high-risk populations can be identified, and it is unknown what percentage of breast cancers are due to endogenous levels of hormones (because of measurement challenges) the majority (75%) of breast cancers occur in women whose only known risk factors are gender and age.[118]

Reproductive factors

A woman's age when her first child is born affects her risk for developing breast cancer. The younger she is, the lower the risk. The main mechanism for the protective effect of pregnancy is controversial. The most widely accepted explanation proposes that the development and differentiation of the breast are completed *only* by the end of the first term of pregnancy. The protection seems to be the *interval of time* between menarche and the first pregnancy, because a greater risk is noted with an interval of more than 14 years. The protection conveyed early persists into old age, possibly because of lasting genetic change through differentiation.[119]

TABLE 32-9

Factors Associated With Increased Risk of Breast Cancer*

Category	Risk Factor	Relative Risk†
Race	Blacks have higher incidence up to age 40 yr; whites have higher incidence over age 40 yr	1.1–1.9
Family history	Breast cancer in first-degree relative before age 60 yr	2.0–3.0
	Premenopausal or bilateral breast cancer	>4.0
	Postmenopausal in first-degree relative	≤2.0
	Breast cancer in two first-degree relatives	4.0–6.0
	BRCA1 or BRCA2	≥4.0
	p53 (Li Fraumeni syndrome)	>4.0
Previous medical history	Moderate or florid mammary hyperplasia	1.5–2.0
	Mammary papilloma	1.5–2.0
	Atypical mammary hyperplasia	4.0–5.0
	DCIS, LCIS‡	8.0–10.0
Estrogen exposure	Early menarche (before age 12 yr)	1.1–1.9
	Late menopause (after age 55 yr)	1.1–1.9
	Postmenopausal estrogen therapy	1.4§
	Oral contraceptive use	1.5
Pregnancy	Nulliparous or late first pregnancy (after age 35 yr)	1.1–1.9
Radiation	Atomic bomb	3.0
	Repeated fluoroscopy	1.5–2.0§
Obesity and stature	Postmenopausal	1.2
Dietary/alcohol	Tallness	≤2.0
	High alcohol consumption	1.4–2.0
	High energy intake	≤2.0
	Advanced age	2.0–4.0
	Xenobiotics	≤2.0
Social	Smoking	2.0–4.0
	Higher socioeconomic status	≤2.0
	Low physical activity	≤2.0
Environmental	Excess radiation to breasts	?§
	Chemical carcinogens	≤2.0-?
	Infectious agents	≤2.0-?

*Normal lifetime risk in white non-Hispanic women: 1 in 8.
†Relative risk is defined and discussed in Chapter 2.
‡Data from Lester SC: The breast. In Kumar V, Abbas AK, Fausto N, editors: *Robbins and Cotran pathologic basis of disease,* ed 7, Philadelphia, 2005, Saunders.
§Currently being debated.
DCIS, Ductal carcinoma in situ; *LCIS,* lobular carcinoma in situ.

These findings have, however, been challenged.[120] Investigators using animal models abolished the pregnancy-associated protection against breast cancer by altering the hormonal environment of the animal.[120] Important is their findings that both pregnancy or hormone treatment with pregnancy levels of bioidentical estrogen and progesterone significantly decreased the animals' risk of chemically induced breast tumor development. The activity of growth hormone and IGF-1 also was fundamental in determining the level of breast carcinogenesis. In addition, there are several other hormones, besides estrogen and progesterone, including prolactin, chorionic gonadotropin, growth hormone, and insulin growth factor-1 (IGF-1), that have a heightened effect during pregnancy that involves promoting mammary tissue differentiation, and these hormones may offer additional clues. Unknown are the hormones that may be involved because of weight gain (see Diet, p. 892).

The duration of a woman's reproductive life also affects her risk of developing breast cancer. Late menarche and early menopause (i.e., a short reproductive life) reduce risk (see Pathogenesis). Menarche marks the onset of the mature hormonal milieu—that is, cyclic hormonal changes that result in ovulation, menstruation, and cellular proliferation in the breast. Thus, the younger the age at menarche, the earlier a young woman experiences steroid hormone levels and ovulatory cycles. Although data are limited, women with earlier menarche may have higher levels of endogenous estrogen.[121,122] Age of menarche is a relatively weak risk factor overall; however, it may be important in understanding the international variation, for example, mean age of menarche in China of 16 to 17 years versus 12 to 13 years in the United States.[123]

Hormonal factors

Endogenous hormones have long been implicated in the development of breast cancer. Most significant are the findings of (1) the protective effect of an early first pregnancy; (2) the protective effect of bilateral ovariectomy before age 45 years; (3) the increased risk associated with early menarche, late menopause, and nulliparity; and (4) the hormone-dependent development and differentiation of mammary gland structures (see the Pathogenesis section). A vast majority of breast cancers are *initially* hormone-dependent (estrogen receptor [ER] positive or progesterone receptor [PR] positive or both) with estrogen playing a crucial role in their development.[124]

Epidemiologic prospective cohort studies have shown that *postmenopausal* women who have elevated *plasma* levels of either androgens (i.e., dehydroepiandrosterone [DHEA] or its sulfate (DHEAS)], androstenedione, and testosterone) of adrenal or ovarian origin or estrogens (i.e., estrone and estradiol) have an increased risk of breast cancer.[125] Epidemiologic studies among *premenopausal* women and plasma levels of hormones have produced conflicting results. These studies are more difficult because circulating levels of hormones vary greatly during the menstrual cycle and the low numbers of women with breast cancer among premenopausal women.

It is possible to consider four major hormonal hypotheses for breast cancer: (1) ovarian androgen excess, (2) estrogens and progesterone levels, (ovarian), (3) estrogens alone (ovarian)), and (4) local biosynthesis of estrogens in breast tissue. These hypotheses, however, may not be mutually exclusive. In addition, the percent contribution from exogenous hormones (HRT) has been estimated between 2%-10% and delays or hinders breast cancer diagnosis because of increased breast density.[125a]

The first hypothesis that breast cancer risk is increased among women who have an ovarian androgen excess also includes chronic anovulation and reduction of luteal-phase (menstrual cycle) progesterone production. Therefore, it is also called the "ovarian hyperandrogenism/luteal inadequacy hypothesis." This hypothesis, actually proposed by Grattarola in the 1960s, was based on the observation that women with breast cancer also reveal hyperplasia of the endometrium—a common symptom of ovarian, androgen excess chronic anovulation, and progesterone deficiency.[125] Some initial studies confirmed that women with breast cancer had higher plasma or urinary levels of testosterone or its urinary metabolites than those without cancer. A prospective Italian study showed a significant increase in breast cancer risk for premenopausal women who had elevated levels of testosterone and lower levels of progesterone.[126] Experimental (in vitro) studies, however, showed conflicting results of androgens and breast tissue. Elevated serum androgens may indirectly lead to increased estrogenic exposure of breast tissue because of enzymes (i.e., aromatase) that promote the formation of estrogen from androgenic precursors (Figure 32-34).

The second hypothesis is breast cancer risk is increased among women with elevations of both estrogens and progesterone. These observations revealed increased proliferation rates of breast epithelium during the luteal phase of the menstrual cycle when the ovaries produce both estradiol and progesterone. Data supporting the "estrogen-plus-progesterone hypothesis" suggest hormone replacement therapy (HRT) with estrogen plus progestin increases breast cancer risk to a greater degree than estrogen alone.[127,128] In addition, incidence of breast cancer in the United States declined 7% between 2002 and 2003, and the number of women aged 50 to 69 diagnosed with ER+ breast cancer declined 12% over the same period. Although it is not really known why these changes occurred, millions of women stopped taking HRT after the Women's Initiative Study published in 2002.[129] Another study also found a greater incidence of breast abnormalities in women taking HRT.[130] In the most recent European Perspective Investigation into Cancer (EPIC) study, no correlations were found between plasma progesterone (natural) levels and breast cancer risk.[125]

The third hypothesis is often called the "estrogen-alone hypothesis." This hypothesis is gaining support because of consistent prospective cohort studies and the EPIC cohort that *postmenopausal* women who have elevated plasma concentrations of estrone (E_1) and estradiol (E_2) have an increased breast cancer risk. Experimental studies (in vitro)

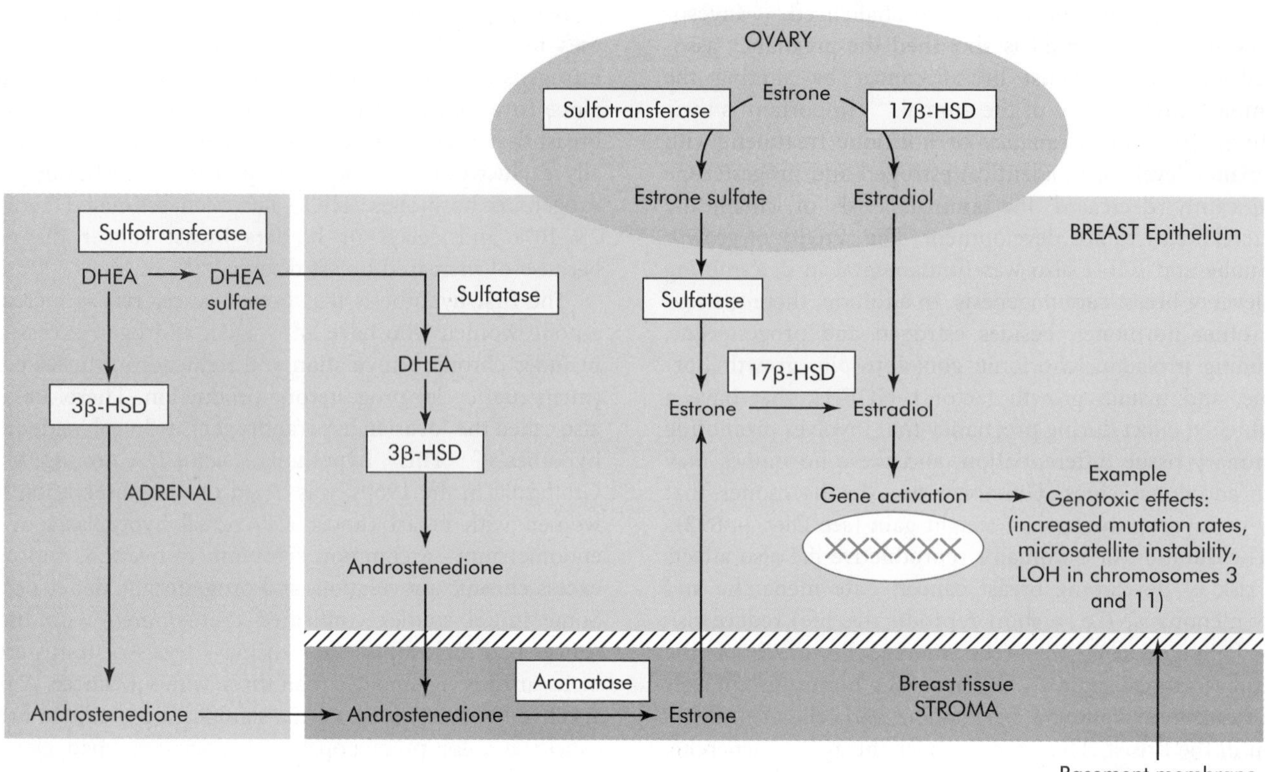

Figure 32-34 ■ **Local Biosynthesis of Estrogens.** Three main enzyme complexes *(yellow)* involved in estrogen formation in breast tissue, including aromatase, sulfatase, and 17β-estradiol hydroxysteroid dehydrogenase (HSD). Thus, despite low levels of circulating estrogens in postmenopausal women with breast cancer, the tissue levels are several-fold higher than these in plasma, suggesting tumor accumulation of these estrogens. Data suggest that most abundant is sulfatase in both premenopausal and postmenopausal women with breast cancer. Numerous agents can block the aromatase action, exploration of progesterone, and various progestins to inhibit sulfatase and 17β-HSD or stimulate sulfotransferase (i.e., breast cancer cells cannot inactivate estrogens because they lack sulfotransferase) may provide new possibilities for treatment. *LOH,* Loss of heterozygosity (see Chapter 9). (Adapted from Russo J, Russo I: *Molecular basis of breast cancer: prevention and treatment,* Germany, 2004, Springer.)

have also provided strong and consistent evidence that estrogens can promote and possibly *initiate* breast tumor development and growth (see the Pathogenesis section).[125]

EPIC and other studies, however, observed no clear relationship between plasma estrogen levels and breast cancer risk in *premenopausal* women.[125] From these data it is possible that a clear direct relationship with estrogen levels exists only within the lower (plasma not breast tissue) levels of the postmenopausal range of estrogen levels and not at higher premenopausal estrogen concentrations. These relationships may also affect estrogen receptor concentrations—that is, with lower endogenous levels of estrogen this may increase (up-regulate) estrogen receptors. Studies have reported higher concentrations of estrogen receptors in older women.[131]

The fourth hypothesis suggests that *local* (in situ; paracrine) formation of estrogens in breast tumors is more important than circulating estrogens in *plasma* for the growth and survival of estrogen-dependent breast cancer in postmenopausal women.[132] The rationale is based on the following evidence: (1) estradiol (E_2) levels in breast tumors are equivalent to those of premenopausal women, despite plasma E_2 levels being lower after menopause; (2) E_2 concentrations in breast tumors of postmenopausal women are 10 to 40 times higher than serum levels; and (3) biosynthesis of estrogens in breast tumors occurs through two different routes, one is the aromatase pathway and the other is the steroid sulfate (STS) pathway (see Figure 32-34).[132]

Breast tissue (endogenous) metabolism of estrogens through the aromatase-mediated pathway is correlated with the risk of breast carcinogenesis. Breast tissue, however, may contain higher sulfatase activity than aromatase activity and produce estrone through the hydrolysis of estrone sulfate (see Figure 32-34).[132] Thus, quantitatively estrone sulfate may be the most important circulating estrogen in women; it increases the reservoir for the production of estrone and, ultimately, estradiol. It was found that E_2, itself, has anti-sulfatase action.[133] This paradoxical effect of estradiol could be related to some studies that have found estrogen replacement therapy (ERT) to have either no effect or to decrease breast cancer mortality in postmenopausal women.[133] In summary, the blockage of estradiol through both the aromatase and sulfatase pathways, as well as the stimulation of sulfotransferase activity (i.e., sulfation is important to estrogens because the addition of the charged sulfonate group protects the hormones [estrogens] from binding to their receptors and, consequently, inhibiting cell growth) can provide new and potentially powerful applications in breast cancer.

Two main mechanisms of carcinogenicity of estrogens involve (1) a receptor-mediated hormonal activity shown to stimulate cellular proliferation resulting in increased opportunities for accumulation of genetic damage and (2) oxidative catabolism of estrogens mediated by various cytochromes complexes (e.g., p450) that eventually activate and generate reactive oxygen species (ROS) (Box 32-9). Oxidative metabolites of estrogens, if found, can develop ultimate carcinogens that react with DNA to cause mutations leading to carcinogenesis. For example, the gonadal estrogen 17β-estradiol (E_2) is metabolized into various compounds that activate pathways that either induce or block cancer (Figure 32-35). The 4- and 16α-hydroxy catechols pathways are tumor promoting; conversely, the 2-hydroxy catechol pathway has been demonstrated to be less tumor promoting and, possibly, inhibiting.[134] Thus, imbalances in estrogen metabolites in breast tissue correlate with the development of tumors and suggest possible biomarkers related to the risk of developing breast cancer.

BOX 32-9 Estrogen Carcinogenesis

Standard Theory

Estrogen and perhaps progesterone affect the rate of cell division and thus affect the risk of breast cancer by causing proliferation of breast epithelial cells. Proliferating cells are susceptible to genetic errors during DNA replication; if uncorrected, these errors can ultimately lead to a malignant phenotype.

Updated Theory

Although estrogen-induced proliferation undoubtedly has an important role in the carcinogenic process, mounting evidence supports a complementary pathway involving direct and indirect genotoxiciy originating from estrogen metabolites (for example, 4-hydroxy catechol):

- *Indirect.* Oxidative DNA damage through redox cycling leads to reactive oxygen species
- *Direct.* Estrogen-quinone DNA adducts (see Figure 32-35)

Perhaps less carcinogenic effects: through 2-methoxy catechol (see Figure 32-35)

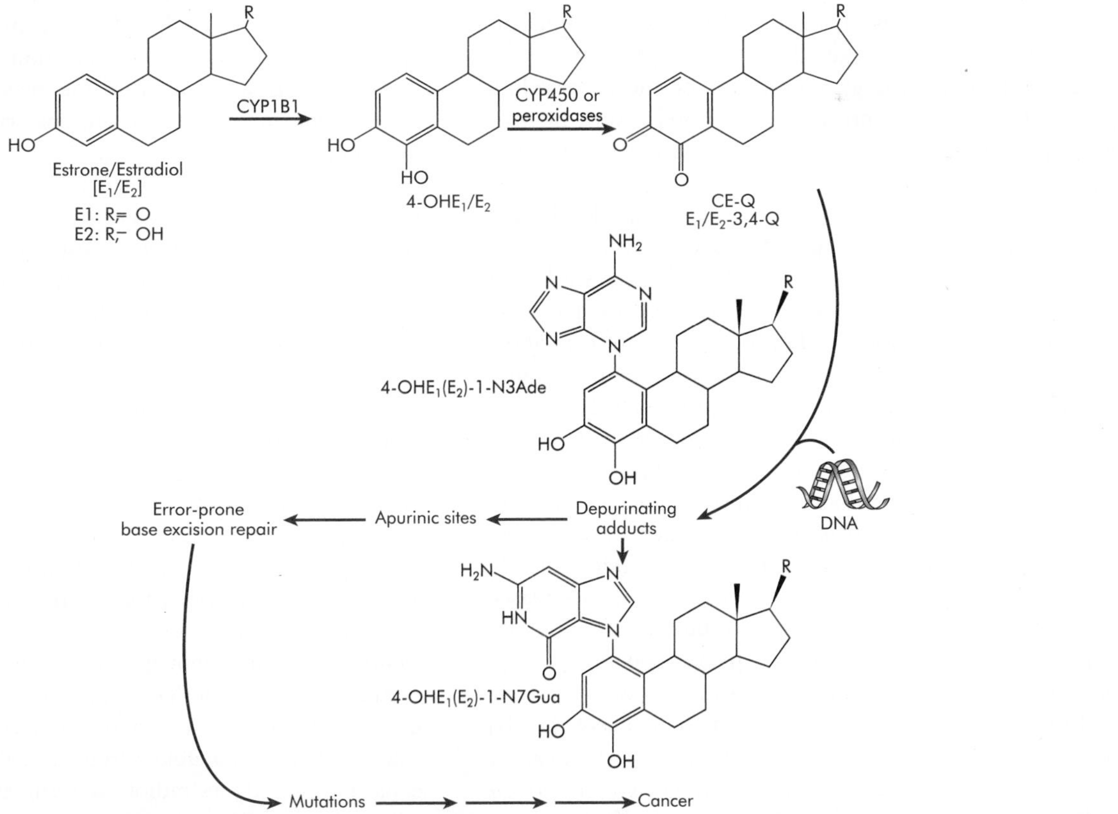

Insulin-like growth factors (IGFs) regulate cellular functions involving cell proliferation, differentiation, and apoptosis. Insulin-like growth factor-1 (IGF-1) is a protein hormone with a structure similar to insulin. The growth hormone-IGF-1 axis can stimulate proliferation of both breast cancer and normal breast epithelial cells.[135] IGF-1 levels seem to be more of a risk factor for premenopausal women. In addition, premenopausal mammographic breast density (a risk factor for breast cancer) was positively correlated with IGF-1 levels; this relationship was not found in postmenopausal women.[136] Estradiol increases IGF-1 activity in the breast.[137] Hormones are discussed further in the pathogenesis section.

Human chorionic gonadotropin (hCG) increases during the first trimester of pregnancy and then rapidly declines to a steady state throughout pregnancy. Data indicate that

Figure 32-35 ■ **Formation, Metabolism, and DNA Adducts of Estrogen.** Catechol estrogens are the major metabolites of E_1 and E_2. If these metabolites are oxidized to the electrophilic (CE-Q), they may react with DNA. The carcinogenic 4-OHE$_1$ (E_2) are oxidized to E_1 (E_2-3,4-Q), which reacts with DNA to form depurinating adducts. These adducts are complexes that form when a chemical (e.g., estrogen metabolites) binds to DNA and damages DNA. These adducts generate the damaged sites—known as apurinic sites—that may lead to misrepair and cancer-initiating pathways. Activating enzymes and depurinating adducts are in *purple*.

hCG may be useful in developing new therapies because it has antiproliferative and anti-invasive effects.[138]

Depending on the tissue, progesterone is classified as either a proliferative or differentiative hormone. Studies reveal progesterone is capable of stimulating or inhibiting cell growth depending on whether treatment is transient or continuous.[139,140] Investigators have reported that different signal transduction pathways are used by natural versus synthetic progestins for the induction of vascular endothelial growth factor (VEGF), which promotes angiogenesis. However, the safe use of progesterone/progestins, in terms of breast cancer, is not now established.

Controversy remains about the relationship between oral contraceptive (OC) use and breast cancer risk; however, the efficacy of OCs in protecting against ovarian cancer and endometrial cancer is well established.

Environmental factors

The environmental causes of breast cancer probably affect the glandular epithelial cells of the breast during the early differential stages from undifferentiated cells to alveolar buds and lobules (see Pathogenesis). During these early phases, mitotic activity and cell division are greater than later in life.[141]

Radiation. High doses of ionizing radiation are associated with an increased risk of breast cancer, especially if exposure occurs during adolescence or pregnancy, when breast cells are proliferating rapidly. Radiologic exposure of the upper spine, heart, ribs, lungs, shoulders, and esophagus also exposes breast tissue to radiation. A hot topic currently is the effect of low-dose ionizing radiation. The debate is that low-energy x-rays may be more hazardous per unit dose than previously reported. New biologic understandings of low doses of radiation are presented in Chapter 10.

Diet. The association between individual foods and breast cancer is inconsistent, and new data on *dietary patterns* are emerging. The prudent pattern includes a higher intake of fruits, vegetables, whole grains, low-fat dairy products, fish, and poultry. The Western pattern includes higher intake of red and processed meats, refined grains, sweets and desserts, and high-fat dairy products. In general, however, neither of the patterns was associated with overall risk of postmenopausal breast cancer. A positive association, however, was found among smokers and the Western pattern.[142] In addition, lower risk of estrogen receptor-negative cancer was observed with those on a prudent diet.[142] Observations with diets high in flavonols found a decreased risk with intake of beans or lentils but not tea, onions, apples, string beans, broccoli, green pepper, or blueberries.[143] All of these findings need further study.

Prospective studies do not support the concept that fat intake in middle life has a major relation to breast cancer risk.[144] Moreover, there is limited evidence that modest reductions in fat intake (less than 20% of caloric intake) reduces breast cancer risk.[145] Even so, because breast cancer incidence varies widely around the world, and offspring that migrate from countries with low incidence to countries with high incidence have the same rates as those in the new country, nutrition remains an important area of study. The dominant hypothesis has been that high-fat intake increases risk.[144] Studies in animal models, and observations in humans, however, have provided evidence that a high intake of omega-6–polyunsaturated fatty acids (omega-6 PUFAs) stimulates several stages in the development of mammary and colon cancer and possibly prostate cancer—from an increase in oxidative DNA damage that effects cell proliferation and increased free estrogen levels that effect hormonal catabolic products.[146–149] Conversely, fish oil–derived omega-3 fatty acids may *prevent* cancer by influencing the activity of enzymes and proteins related to intracellular signaling and, eventually, cell proliferation.[150,151] Fish oil, rich in iodine, may protect against oxidative stress.[152] Studies that show protective effects of fish oil and decreased cancer risk have been confined to countries with high fish intake. Fat tissue in the breast may be a source of high concentrations of fat-soluble chemicals (including estrogens), some of which may be carcinogens.[153]

Obesity has been associated with a *reduced* risk of *premenopausal* breast cancer. One mechanism suggested is the direct relationship between irregular menstrual cycling, especially anovulatory cycling and obesity. The anovulatory cycling would result in a decrease in both estrogens and progesterone and thus a decreased risk of breast cancer. Some obese women have polycystic ovaries. With this condition they may have anovulatory cycling, abnormal menstrual periods, elevated androgens, hyperinsulinemia, and alterations in gonadotropic secretions. It is possible that higher insulin levels increase the enzymatic conversion of testosterone to dihydrotestosterone, rather than estradiol, lowering their estrogen levels.[153]

Obesity, however, is *weakly* related to increasing the risk of breast cancer in *postmenopausal* women.[144] Despite strong links with endogenous estrogen levels, body fat has been consistently but *weakly* related to increased postmenopausal risk.[154] This observation has been surprising because obese postmenopausal women have endogenous estrogen levels (estrone and estradiol) nearly double those of lean women.[154,155] This weak association is possibly related to two factors. First, the premenopausal reduction in breast cancer risk related to being overweight possibly persists, opposing the adverse effect of elevated estrogens after menopause. Thus, *weight gain* should be more strongly related to postmenopausal breast cancer risk than attained weight. In two case-control studies and prospective studies, this was indeed true.[156-159] Premenopausal and postmenopausal weight gain is also associated with higher estradiol and estrone levels and lower sex-hormone–binding globulin (SHBG) as a transporter protein; low levels cause higher bioavailable estrogen.[160] The increase in estrogens, particularly estradiol, is from aromatization in the adipose tissue. Second, use of exogenous hormones postmenopausally obscures the variation in endogenous estrogens caused by adiposity and elevates breast cancer risk regardless of body weight.[154] Among newer users of postmenopausal hormones, those gaining at least 55 pounds after age 18 years had double the breast cancer risk of women who maintained their weight.

Obesity is associated with poor survival among women with breast cancer and the association of obesity with mortality from breast cancer appears to be stronger than its association with incidence.[154,158] The increase in breast cancer risk with increasing BMI among postmenopausal women is possibly the result of increases in estrogen, especially with estradiol.[144,161] However, studies of hormones secreted by adipose tissue, *leptin*, and *adiponectin* may underlie the association between obesity and breast cancer risk. Because increasing BMI and central fat are associated with increased risk for breast cancer in prospective studies, increased leptin exposure associated with obesity and central adiposity could explain the greater incidence of breast cancer in overweight or obese postmenopausal women. In vitro studies have shown leptin stimulated breast carcinogenesis.[162,163] Adiponectin has been shown to exert antiproliferative effects in vitro of human breast cancer cells.[162,164]

Age at menarche also indicates childhood energy balance. Prospective studies document weight, height, and body fat as predictors of age at menarche.[165,166] Age at menarche is 12 to 13 years in Western countries; in rural China (where the risk of breast cancer is low) the typical age of menarche has been 17 to 18.[167]

Most prospective studies have not supported a link between fiber intake and breast cancer.[168,169] Carbohydrate quality, however, rather than absolute amount may be important for breast cancer risk, especially for premenopausal women.

Substantial evidence exists that alcohol consumption increases breast cancer risk. In a pooled analysis of the six largest cohort studies, the risk of breast cancer increased incrementally with increasing intake of alcohol.[141] Beer, wine, and liquor all contribute to the positive association. Differences in alcohol intake, however, explain only a small fraction of breast cancer rates.[170,171] In large prospective studies, high intake of folic acid appeared to decrease completely the excess risk for breast cancer caused by alcohol.[172–174] The mechanisms by which alcohol intake increases the risk of breast cancer are unknown. It is not known whether decreasing or stopping alcohol consumption in midlife decreases the risk of breast cancer.

Data from observational studies suggest a possible protection effect of vitamin A intake, particularly carotenoids, on breast cancer risk. This effect is only noted for premenopausal women.[144] Vitamin E has inhibited breast tumors in some animal studies.[175] None of the prospective studies, however, have reported a significant association.[144] Yet epidemiologic evidence indicates a higher risk of breast cancer development with a combination of low vitamin E and low selenium levels.[132,176,177] No significant overall association between vitamin C and breast cancer was observed in prospective studies.[178,179]

Soy products are a hot topic because of their consumption in Asian countries that have low rates of cancer. These isoflavone compounds, including diadzen and genistein, can bind estrogen receptors but are far less potent than estradiol. Soy may act like other antiestrogens, tamoxifen for example, by blocking the action of endogenous estrogens to reduce breast cancer risk. Thus, depending on the estradiol concentration, soy exhibits weak estrogenic or antiestrogenic activity. Isoflavones can influence transcription and cell proliferation. They modulate enzyme activities, as well as signal transduction, and have antioxidant properties.[180] Results of clinical studies on the effects of soy products or isolated isoflavones on vasomotor symptoms are contradictory. Concerns, however, are that soy or isoflavones may increase proliferating cells. A study of nipple aspirate fluid from women who had ingested high soy diets and were either premenopausal or took estrogen replacement therapy showed an increase in proliferating cells.[181] Controversy has ensued on whether breast stimulation can equal breast cancer growth. Soy may cause breast cells to grow; however, in vitro properties of soy for blocking invasion and antiangiogenesis may be more important in preventing breast cancer. In vitro and animal studies show soy to inhibit breast cancer growth, and additional work showed this effect on cancer cells that are both ER+ and ER−.[182] In addition, soy may optimize extrarenal 1,25 (OH)2 cholecalciferol or vitamin D_3 (a prodifferentiating vitamin D metabolite), which could result in growth control and, conceivably, inhibition of tumor progression.[183]

Iodine deficiency is hypothesized as contributing to the development of breast pathology and cancer.[152,184] Evidence reveals that iodine is an antioxidant and antiproliferative agent contributing to the integrity of normal mammary tissue.[184] Seaweed, which is iodine-rich, is an important dietary item in Asian communities and has been associated with the *low* evidence of benign and breast cancer disease in Japanese women.[185] Molecular iodine (I[2]) supplementation exerts an inhibitory effect on the development and size of benign and cancerous tissue.[186]

Environmental Chemicals. Evidence for linking chemicals to the cause of breast cancer is difficult. It is challenging because it is a life history of exposure that is important—not just a single chemical but complex mixtures of chemicals and their interaction with endogenous hormones. In addition, newer investigative models with epigenetic alterations may increase understanding. The highest rates of breast cancer are found in superindustrialized countries—North America and Europe—and the lowest rates in Central Africa and Asia. With development, breast cancer rates increase. An estimated 85,000 synthetic chemicals are registered for use in the United States, and toxicologic screening for these chemicals is minimal. Chemicals persist in the environment, accumulate in adipose tissue, interact with local adipose tissue physiology in an endocrine/paracrine manner, and remain in breast tissue for decades. Some of these chemicals have been linked to breast tumors in animals. Women who immigrate to the United States from Asian countries experience an enormous percent increase in risk within one generation. A generation later, the rate of their daughter's risk approaches that of women born in the United States. This change in risk suggests that utero exposures affect subsequent disease risk. It is difficult to know whether these changes in risk come from nutritional content, pollutants, food additives, or other factors.

Xenoestrogens are synthetic chemicals that mimic the actions of estrogens and are found in many pesticides, fuels, plastics, detergents, and drugs.[117] Because many factors correlated with breast cancer (early menarche, delayed pregnancy and breastfeeding, late menopause, etc.) are associated with lifetime exposure to estrogens, investigators reasoned that environmental chemicals affect estrogen metabolism and contribute to breast cancer. The most significant chemicals may be polychlorinated biphenyls (PCBs), such as dichlorodiphenyltrichloroethane (DDT). Such chemicals are fat soluble, and the estrogenic effect would require that they bind to either the nuclear estrogen receptor and then cause cell division or gene transcription or that they activate ROS through exudative catabolism of estrogens (see p. 891.)

Physical Activity. Regular physical activity may reduce overall risk of breast cancer, especially in premenopausal or young postmenopausal women.[187–189] Activity also may reduce invasive breast cancer.[190] Mechanisms for this protective effect are not known but include alterations in endogenous free radical formation and oxidative damage, effects on DNA repair capacity, alteration in carcinogen-metabolizing enzymes, increased intestinal transit times (i.e., reduced exposures to carcinogens), weight loss, and changes in endogenous sex hormone levels.[188,189]

Familial factors

Genetically, breast cancer can be divided into three main groups: (1) sporadic, the majority or 40% of women with breast cancer have no known family history; (2) inherited autosomal dominant cancer gene syndromes; and (3) probably polygenic, where there is family history but it is not passed on to future generations as a dominant gene. Unknown are the genes in the polygenic model that could be involved, the nature of the interactions among these genes, and their interaction with environmental factors. One study has, however, identified a large number of previously uncharacterized *CAN*-genes (e.g., CANdidate CANcer). These data suggest that the number of mutational events occurring during the progression from a benign to metastatic state is *much* larger than previously thought. These investigators estimate there are 81 to 105 mutant genes in the typical colorectal or breast cancer, respectively. Of these, 14 and 20, respectively, would be possible *CAN*-genes.[191] These findings have large implications for future research including the possibility that a subset of *CAN*-genes can also be dysregulated epigenetically through changes in chromatin or DNA methylation rather than from mutation.

A history of breast cancer in first-degree relatives (mother or sister) increases a woman's risk two to three times. Risk increases even more if two first-degree relatives are involved, especially if the disease occurred before menopause and was bilateral. A small total proportion of breast cancers (5% to 10%, although the prevalence is significant) are the result of highly penetrant dominant genes (i.e., hereditary breast cancers). The most important of the dominant genes are the breast cancer susceptibility genes *(BRCA1, BRCA2). BRCA1* is located on chromosome 17 and *BRCA2* is located on chromosome 13. A family history of both breast and ovarian cancer increases the risk that an individual with breast cancer carries a *BRCA1* mutation. Up to age 40, a woman with *BRCA1* mutation is estimated to have a 20-times greater risk of breast cancer compared to the general population and a lifetime risk of 60% to 85%.[189] Race is also an important distinction for genetic risk. A population-based study showed that whereas 3.3% of white women with breast cancer had *BRCA1* mutations, none of the 88 black women with breast cancer had a *BRCA1* mutation.[192] Carriers of the *BRCA1* gene are also at higher risk for ovarian cancer. *BRCA1* is a tumor suppressor gene; therefore, any mutation in the gene may inhibit or retard its suppressor function, leading to uncontrolled cell proliferation.[193] Men who develop breast cancer are more likely to have a *BRCA2* mutation than a *BRCA1* mutation. Another suppressor gene, *p53,* is mutated in approximately 20% to 40% of individuals with breast cancer.[194] *p53* is a regulatory gene (i.e., a policeman) that increases DNA repair and, if damage is great, cell death (i.e., apoptosis) occurs in mutated cells. Thus, it helps to get rid of cancer proliferating cells. When *p53* is mutated, its regulatory properties are radically altered, conferring a loss of tumor-suppressor activity and, possibly, even a gain of tumor-promotion function.

PATHOGENESIS Most breast cancers arise from the ductal epithelium. Tumors of the infiltrating ductal type do not grow to a large size, but they metastasize early. This type accounts for 70% of breast cancers. Table 32-10 lists the different types of breast carcinomas and summarizes their major characteristics.

Breast cancer is a disease of the glandular epithelium, and pathogenesis probably involves several main steps. First, modifications of the deoxyribonucleic acid (DNA) of the breast epithelial ductal cells are caused by genetic alterations, environmental agents, or their interactions. The initiated changes in DNA may occur early in a woman's life—before full differentiation of the breast tissue.[141] Second, alterations involve chromosomal alterations, gene mutations, and suppression of apoptosis. Breast cells produce other growth factors as well as the surrounding stroma (Figure 32-36). The production of these factors is to some degree regulated by estrogen.[170] Third is the progressive modification of specific oncogenes or the loss of specific suppressor genes leading to advanced metastatic disease. Changes in malignant cells are accompanied by or preceded by alterations in the supporting tissue and stromal cells because of genetic and epigenetic events and disruption of normal signaling pathways. Studies on tissue from both breast and colon carcinomas indicate that genetic changes occur in the stroma during the earliest stages of pathogenesis suggesting that a genetically unstable stroma may increase genetic instability in the overlying epithelium.[195]

TABLE 32-10

Types of Breast Carcinomas and Major Distinguishing Features

Histologic Type	Distinguishing Features
CARCINOMA OF MAMMARY DUCTS	
Papillary	Well-delineated cystic masses in multiple areas; hemorrhage often present; majority appear in 40- to 60-yr age group; often involves skin
Intraductal (comedo)	Often accompanied by evidence of inflammation; well-circumscribed tumors within the duct; rarely ulcerates the skin
INFILTRATING CARCINOMA	
Ductal	Fibrous, firm, glistening, gray-tan mass with chalky streaks, mixture of patterns; may cause discharge from the nipple; represents about 70% of all breast cancer
Mucinous	Usually large, >3 cm in diameter, circumscribed and encapsulated, glistening appearance, varies in color; two types: pure and mixed; pure tumor is surrounded by mucin; infrequent; found in the lateral half of the breast; tends to occur in women over 70 yr
Medullary	Encapsulated and grows to be very large (7–8 cm in diameter); can be surrounded by lymphocytic inflammatory infiltrate; occurs after age 50 yr
Tubular	Well-differentiated with orderly tubules in center (stroma) of mass; can be associated with noninfiltrating ductal carcinoma; occurs in women about 50 yr of age; nodal metastasis infrequent; occurrence rare
Adenoid cystic	Very rare; well-circumscribed, painless mass arising from the nipple and areola
Metaplastic	Involves cartilage or bone, mixed tumors or osteogenic sarcomas
Squamous cell	Frequent in blacks; originates in ductal epithelium
CARCINOMA OF MAMMARY LOBULES	
Lobular carcinoma in situ	Found in individuals with fibrocystic disease; localized to upper breast quadrants; risk of 10%-35% becoming invasive; occurs frequently in mid-40s; infiltrating variety occurs in early 50s
Infiltrating lobular	Infiltrates from duct; firm mass with chalky streaks
Inflammatory carcinoma	Not a histologic type; fairly diffuse within the breast tissue, diffuse edema of the overlying skin; extremely undifferentiated, very rare, most metastasize to axilla
SARCOMA OF THE BREAST	
Cystosarcoma phyllodes	Usually large (>17 cm in diameter); mostly localized but can rupture through the skin; rarely metastasizes to lymph nodes; history of painless nodule present for years before it forms a large mass; ulceration and bleeding of skin often present; occurs in wide age range (13–77 yr)
Fibrosarcoma	Well-circumscribed, firm, and usually does not involve the skin or nipple; well-differentiated to extremely undifferentiated; arises from connective tissue; extremely rare (e.g., liposarcoma, angiosarcoma)

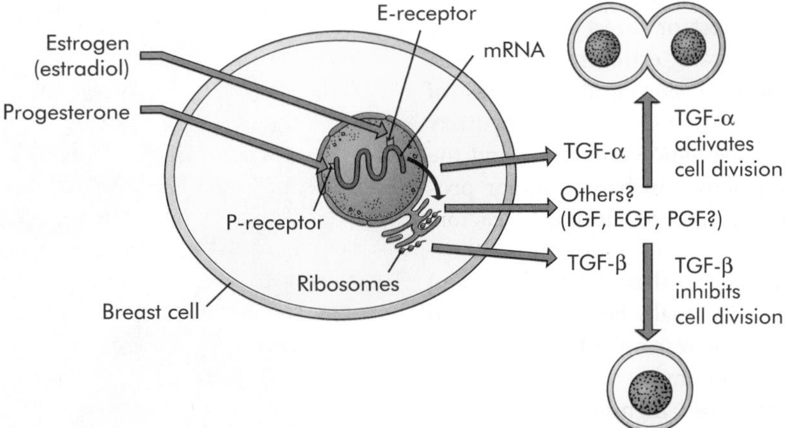

Figure 32-36 ■ **Control of Breast Cell Growth.** Two levels of control of breast cell growth: (1) paracrine signaling by estrogen (E-receptor) and progesterone (P-receptor) steroids and (2) autocrine signaling by locally secreted growth factors, such as transforming growth factor (TGF-α and -β) and others, including insulin-like growth factor (IGF), epidermal growth factor (EGF), and platelet-derived growth factor (PGF). *mRNA,* Messenger ribonucleic acid.

Unlike most human organs that are differentiated at the end of fetal life, the mammary gland develops and differentiates after puberty. Factors that affect full differentiation of the breast may be essential for countering the development of breast cancer (see p. 888).

Mammary epithelial cells achieve rapid renewal by a small number of mitotic divisions of immortal stem cells. (Cell renewal is discussed in Chapters 1 and 9.) Because the number of mutations is proportional to the rate and number of stem cell divisions, factors that accelerate cell division can have a carcinogenic effect. Hormones may act as accelerators, as well as initiators, and influence the susceptibility of the breast epithelium to environmental carcinogens, because hormones control the differentiation of the mammary gland epithelium and thereby regulate the rate of stem cell division.

The highest proliferative activity of mammary epithelium stem cells is during each ovulatory cycle between puberty and either the first full-term pregnancy or menopause among nulliparous women. The greatest increase in mitotic activity in the breast is during the luteal phase. During the estrogen follicular phase, terminal ductules are few and there is no mitotic activity. During the luteal phase, because of increased progesterone levels perhaps resulting from the estrogen priming or as a result of cooperation between the two hormones, there is increased mitotic activity.[196,197] Investigators have determined that 17 β-estradiol (E_2), the predominant circulating ovarian steroid, initiated complete cancerous transformation (in vitro) in human breast epithelial cells. The study model demonstrated a sequence of chromosomal changes that correlated with stages of neoplastic progression. E_2 treatment induced the expression of anchorage-independent growth, loss of breast duct anatomic structure, invasiveness, and loss of chromosome 9p11–13.[198] These data supported the concept that E2 acted as a carcinogenic agent without the need of the estrogen receptor-alpha (ER-α). Thus prolonged exposure to high levels of estrogens gives relevance to this study model of estrogen induced carcinogenesis.[198]

Although estrogen-induced cell alterations have an important if not essential role in estrogen carcinogenesis, other pathways involving indirect or direct DNA toxicity (i.e., genotoxicity) originate from estrogen metabolites. Among the metabolites formed during the process of metabolism and elimination are the 4- and 16-α hydroxy catechols pathways shown to be tumor promoting and the 2-hydroxy catechol pathway shown to be less tumor promoting and possibly inhibiting (see the Hormonal Factors section and Figure 32-35).

Emerging is the understanding that the biologic and structural features of carcinomas usually begin at the in situ stage.[199] The in situ lesion closely resembles the developing invasive carcinoma.[199] For example, low-grade DCIS with well-differentiated carcinomas, high-grade DCIS with high-grade carcinomas, and lobular carcinomas are associated with lobular carcinoma in situ (LCIS). DCIS is a clonal proliferation usually confined to a single ductal system. LCIS, unlike DCIS, has a uniform appearance in which the cells occur in noncohesive clusters in ducts and lobules. Several lines of evidence, however, support the concept that different types of DCIS show different genetic alterations suggesting there may be multiple pathways for the evolution of DCIS.[200–202]

The majority of carcinomas of the breast occur in the upper outer quadrant, where most of the glandular tissue of the breast is located. The lymphatic spread of cancer to the opposite breast, to lymph nodes in the base of the neck, and to the abdominal cavity is caused by obstruction of the normal lymphatic pathways or destruction of lymphatic vessels by surgery or radiotherapy (see Figure 31-20). The less common inner quadrant tumors may spread to mediastinal nodes or Rotter nodes, which are located between the pectoral muscles (see Figure 31-20).

Internal mammary chain nodes are also common sites of metastasis. Metastases from the vertebral veins can involve the vertebrae, pelvic bones, ribs, and skull. The lungs, kidneys, liver, adrenal glands, ovaries, and pituitary gland are also sites of metastasis.

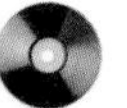

CLINICAL MANIFESTATIONS The first sign of breast cancer is usually a painless lump. Lumps caused by breast tumors do not have any classic characteristics. Other presenting signs include palpable nodes in the axilla, retraction of tissue (dimpling) (Figure 32-37), or bone pain caused by metastasis to the vertebrae. Table 32-11 summarizes the clinical manifestations of breast cancers. Manifestations vary according to the type of tumor and stage of disease.

EVALUATION AND TREATMENT Mammography, ultrasound, percutaneous needle aspiration, biopsy or minimally invasive biopsy called **Mammotome,** palpation, and hormone receptor assays are generally used in evaluating breast alterations and cancer. Biopsy is the definitive diagnostic test.

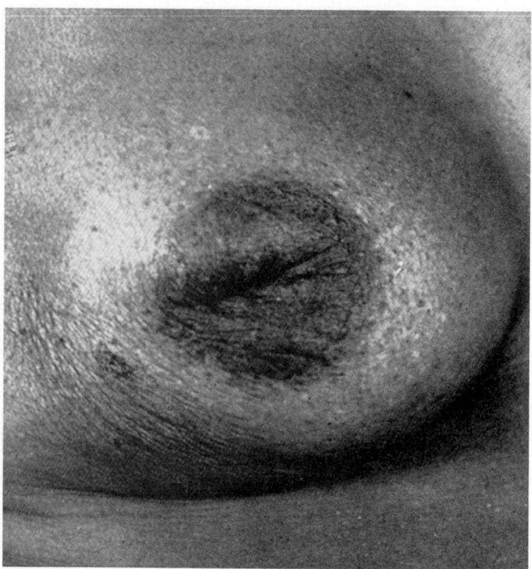

Figure 32-37 ■ Retraction of Nipple Caused by Carcinoma. (From del Regato JA, Spjut HJ, Cox JD: *Ackerman and del Regato's cancer: diagnosis, treatment, and prognosis,* ed 6, St Louis, 1985, Mosby.)

Treatment is based on the extent or stage of the cancer (Table 32-12). The extent of the tumor at the primary site, the presence and extent of lymph node metastasis, and the presence of distant metastases are all evaluated to determine the stage of disease. Surgery, radiation, chemotherapy, hormone therapy, biologic therapy, and bone marrow transplantation may be used to treat breast cancer.

QUICK CHECK 32-8

1. What types of fibrocystic breast changes increase the risk of breast cancer?
2. What is the role of hormones and growth factors in the pathophysiology of breast cancer?
3. Why are reproductive factors, such as early menarche and late menopause, important for the pathogenesis of breast cancer?

TABLE 32-11

Clinical Manifestations of Breast Cancer

Clinical Manifestation	Pathophysiology
Local pain	Local obstruction caused by the tumor
Dimpling of the skin	Can occur with invasion of the dermal lymphatics because of retraction of Cooper ligament or involvement of the pectoralis fascia
Nipple retraction	Shortening of the mammary ducts
Skin retraction	Involvement of the suspensory ligament
Edema	Local inflammation or lymphatic obstruction
Nipple/areolar eczema	Paget disease
Pitting of the skin (similar to the surface of an orange *[peau d'orange]*)	Obstruction of the subcutaneous lymphatics, resulting in the accumulation of fluid
Reddened skin, local tenderness, and warmth	Inflammation
Dilated blood vessels	Obstruction of venous return by a fast-growing tumor; obstruction dilates superficial veins
Nipple discharge in a nonlactating woman	Spontaneous and intermittent discharge caused by tumor obstruction
Ulceration	Tumor necrosis
Hemorrhage	Erosion of blood vessels
Edema of the arm	Obstruction of lymphatic drainage in the axilla
Chest pain	Metastasis to the lung

Modified from Griffiths MJ, Murray KH, Russo PC: *Oncology nursing: pathophysiology, assessment, and intervention*, Macmillan, New York, 1984.

Disorders of the Male Breast

Gynecomastia

Gynecomastia is the overdevelopment of breast tissue in a male. Gynecomastia accounts for approximately 85% of all masses that develop in the male breast and affects 32% to 40% of the male population. If only one breast is involved, it is typically the left. Incidence is greatest among adolescents and men older than 50 years.

Gynecomastia results from hormonal alterations, which may be idiopathic or caused by systemic disorders, drugs, or neoplasms. Gynecomastia usually involves an imbalance of the estrogen/testosterone ratio. The normal estrogen/testosterone ratio can be altered in one of two ways. First, estrogen levels may be excessively high, although testosterone levels are normal. This is the case in drug-induced and tumor-induced hyperestrogenism. Second, testosterone levels may be extremely low, although estrogen levels are normal, as is the case in hypergonadism. Gynecomastia also can be caused by alterations in breast tissue responsiveness to hormonal stimulation. Breast tissue may have increased responsiveness to estrogen or decreased responsiveness to androgen. Alterations of responsiveness may cause many cases of idiopathic gynecomastia.

Besides puberty and aging, estrogen/testosterone imbalances are associated with hypogonadism, Klinefelter syndrome, and testicular neoplasms. Hormone-induced gynecomastia is usually bilateral. Pubertal gynecomastia is a self-limiting phenomenon that usually disappears within 4 to 6 months. Senescent gynecomastia usually regresses spontaneously within 6 to 12 months.

Systemic disorders associated with gynecomastia include cirrhosis of the liver, infectious hepatitis, chronic renal failure, chronic obstructive lung disease, hyperthyroidism, tuberculosis, and chronic malnutrition. It may be that these disorders ultimately alter the estrogen/testosterone ratio, initiating the gynecomastia.

Gynecomastia is often seen in males receiving estrogen therapy, either in preparation for a sex-change operation or in the treatment of prostatic carcinoma. Other drugs that can cause gynecomastia include digitalis, cimetidine, spironolactone, reserpine, thiazide, isoniazid, ergotamine, tricyclic antidepressants, amphetamines, vincristine, and busulfan. Gynecomastia is usually unilateral in these instances.

Malignancies of the testes, adrenals, or liver can cause gynecomastia if they alter the estrogen/testosterone ratio. Pituitary adenomas and lung cancer also are associated with gynecomastia.

PATHOPHYSIOLOGY The enlargement of the breast consists of hyperplastic stroma and ductal tissue. Hyperplasia results in a firm, palpable mass that is at least 2 cm in diameter and located beneath the areola.

EVALUATION AND TREATMENT The diagnosis of gynecomastia is based on physical examination. Identification and treatment of the cause are likely to be followed by resolution of the gynecomastia. The man should be

TABLE 32-12

Staging of Breast Cancer

T—Primary Tumor Size		N—Regional Lymph Nodes		M—Distant Metastasis	
TX	Primary tumor cannot be assessed	NX	Regional lymph nodes cannot be assessed (e.g., previously removed)	MX	Presence of distant metastasis cannot be assessed
T0	No evidence of primary tumor	N0	No regional lymph node metastasis	M0	No distant metastasis
Tis	Carcinoma in situ: intraductal carcinoma, lobular carcinoma in situ, or Paget disease of the nipple with node	N1	Metastasis to movable ipsilateral axillary lymph nodes(s)	M1	Distant metastasis (includes metastasis to ipsilateral supraclavicular lymph node[s])
T1	Tumor 2 cm or less in greatest dimension	N2	Metastasis to ipsilateral axillary lymph nodes(s) fixed to one another or to other structures		
T2	Tumor more than 2 cm but not more than 5 cm in greatest dimension	N3	Metastasis to ipsilateral internal mammary lymph node(s)		
T3	Tumor more than 5 cm in greatest dimension				

NOTE: Paget disease associated with a tumor is classified according to the size of the tumor.

STAGE GROUPING			
Stage	Tis	N0	M0
Stage I	T1	N0	M0
Stage IIa	T0	N0	M0
	T1	N1	M0
	T2	N0	M0
Stage IIB	T2	N1	M0
	T3	N0	M0
Stage IIIA	T0	N2	M0
	T1	N2	M0
	T2	N2	M0
	T3	N1	M0
	T3	N2	M0
Stage IIIB	T4	Any N	M0
	Any T	N3	M0
Stage IV	Any T	Any N	M1

From Beahrs OH, Hutter RV, Kennedy BJ, editors: *Breast manual for staging of cancer*, ed 45, Philadelphia, 1992, Lippincott.

taught to perform breast self-examination and is reexamined at 6- and 12-month intervals if the gynecomastia persists.

Carcinoma

Breast cancer in males accounts for 0.26% of all male cancers and 1.1% of all breast cancers. About 2030 new cases of breast cancer in men are estimated in 2007.[1] It is seen most commonly after the age of 60 years, with the peak incidence between 60 and 69 years. It has, however, been reported in males as young as 6 years old and in adolescents. Possible risk factors include gynecomastia, radiation of the chest wall, and family history of breast cancer. The effects of inheritance of the breast cancer susceptibility gene (*BRCA1*) in men are unclear. Although the risk of developing breast cancer is almost nonexistent, they may have a slight increase in prostate cancer; this is still under investigation. Male carriers of the *BRCA1* gene, however, can pass the gene on to their daughters.[1] In terms of breast cancer susceptibility genes, men who develop breast cancer are more likely to have a *BRCA2* mutation than a *BRCA1* mutation.[203]

Male breast tumors often resemble carcinoma of the breast in women. Estrogen receptors have been found in 77% to 87% of biopsy specimens from men. The malignant male breast lesion is usually a unilateral solid mass located near the nipple. Because the nipple is commonly involved, crusting and nipple discharge are typical clinical manifestations. Other findings include skin retraction, ulceration of the skin over the tumor, and axillary node involvement. Patterns of metastasis are similar to those in females.

The diagnosis of cancer is confirmed by biopsy. Because of delays in seeking treatment, male breast cancer tends to be advanced at the time of diagnosis and therefore has a poor prognosis. Treatment protocols are similar to those for female breast cancer, but endocrine therapy is used more often for males because a higher percentage of male tumors are hormone dependent. Orchiectomy is performed to treat metastatic disease.

SEXUALLY TRANSMITTED INFECTIONS

Sexually contracted infections affect more than 19 million Americans per year[18] and account for about one third of the reproductive mortality in the United States (Table 32-13).[204] Untreated or undertreated chlamydial infections are the primary cause of preventable infertility and ectopic pregnancy. Reportable infections do not include some of the most prevalent sexually transmitted infections (STIs), including human papillomavirus (HPV) or herpes (HSV). Complications of STIs include pelvic inflammatory disease (PID), infertility, ectopic pregnancy, chronic pelvic pain, neonatal morbidity and mortality, genital cancer, and epidemiologic synergy with HIV transmission. Long-term sequelae of untreated or undertreated STIs may be disastrous and can impact a person's physical, emotional, and financial well-being. (STIs are shown following Table 32-15.)

Sexually transmitted diseases are infections contracted by intimate as well as sexual contact and include systemic infections, such as tuberculosis and hepatitis, that can spread to a sexual partner. Etiology of an STI may be bacterial, viral, protozoan, parasitic, or fungal (Table 32-14). Although the majority of STIs can be treated, viral-induced STIs are considered incurable.

The current increase in severity and incidence of STIs can be attributed to demographic, lifestyle, and behavioral factors.[18] First, indulgence in high-risk sexual behaviors and poor health habits, such as failure to use a condom or nonmonogamous or new relationships, drug use, and douching, increases an individual's risk of exposure or the severity of infection if exposed. Second, many infected individuals do not seek treatment because symptoms are absent, minor, or transient. Last, a rise in the number of single or never-married individuals, involvement in premarital or extramarital sexual affairs, and bisexuality contribute to an increase in the number of lifetime sexual partners and the increased exposure to STIs. Perhaps partly as a result of risk-taking behavior, adolescents tend to be at highest risk for STI exposure and infection. Table 32-15 summarizes the major STIs.

TABLE 32-13

Estimated New Cases of STIs Each Year

Infection	Number of Cases
Chlamydia	976,445
Gonorrhea	339,593
Syphilis	35,878
Herpes	1 million
Human papillomavirus	5.5 million
Hepatitis B	120,000
Trichomonas	5 million

Data from Centers for Disease Control and Prevention: Tracking the hidden epidemics: trends in STDs in the United States, 2000; www.cdc.gov/nchstp/dstd/Stats_Trends2000.pdf

TABLE 32-14

Currently Recognized Sexually Transmitted Infections

Causal Microorganism	Disease
BACTERIA	
Campylobacter	Campylobacter enteritis
Calymmatobacterium granulomatis	Granuloma inguinale
Chlamydia trachomatis	Urogenital infections; lymphogranuloma venereum
POLYMICROBIAL ORGANISMS	
Gardnerella vaginalis plus Mycoplasma hominis and various anaerobic bacteria	Bacterial vaginosis
Haemophilus ducreyi	Chancroid
Mycoplasma	Mycoplasmosis
Neisseria gonorrhoeae	Gonorrhea
Shigella	Shigellosis
Treponema pallidum	Syphilis
VIRUSES	
Cytomegalovirus	Cytomegalic inclusion disease
Hepatitis A, B and C virus	Hepatitis
Herpes simplex virus (HSV)	Genital herpes
Human immunodeficiency virus (HIV)	Acquired immunodeficiency syndrome (AIDS)
Human papillomavirus (HPV)	Condylomata acuminata
Molluscum contagiosum virus	Molluscum contagiosum
PROTOZOA	
Entamoeba histolytica	Amebiasis; amebic dysentery
Giardia lamblia	Giardiasis
Trichomonas vaginalis	Trichomoniasis
ECTOPARASITES	
Phthirus pubis	Pediculosis pubis
Sarcoptes scabiei	Scabies
FUNGUS	
Candida albicans	Candidiasis

HEALTH ALERT

Anti-Infective Treatment for Victims of Sexual Assault

Victims of sexual assault are given prophylaxis against gonorrhea, trichomonas, bacterial vaginosis, and chlamydia using the current recommended treatment based on Centers for Disease Control (CDC) guidelines. Hepatitis B vaccination is highly recommended, and emergency contraception is also available.

TABLE 32-15

Major Sexually Transmitted Infections

Source of Infection	Epidemiology/Clinical Manifestations	Evaluation and Treatment
BACTERIA		
Bacterial vaginosis *(Haemophilus, Corynebacterium, Gardnerella vaginalis/Mycoplasma hominis)*	Occurs almost exclusively in sexually active women, but does not infect men Risk factors include multiple or new male partners Manifestations include discharge (sometimes "fishy" odor); males generally asymptomatic; may predispose women to other STIs or preterm labor	Diagnosed from specimen of vaginal secretions (wet mount) Weeklong treatment with oral or vaginal antibiotics Treatment of sex partner is not recommended
Chancroid *(Haemophilus ducreyi)*	Incidence is low in United States; women are generally asymptomatic, whereas men develop inflamed, painful genital ulcer Secondary infections can occur	Definitive diagnosis is from cultured specimens Treat with antibiotics
Chlamydial infections *(Chlamydia trachomatis)*	Most common bacterial STI in United States; leading cause of infertility for both men and women; cause of ectopic pregnancy; leading cause of blindness worldwide; often asymptomatic Acute course is fairly self-limited followed by chronic, low-grade, persistent infections over years; infections in men can cause urethritis and epididymitis; *C. trachomatis* causes acute urethral syndrome (dysuria, polyuria, pus in urine) in young women; newborns can be infected; perinatal exposure involves the eye, oropharynx, urogenital tract and rectum	Diagnosed by amplified DNA or fluorescent monoclonal antibody screening of discharge; urine assay Treatment of both sexual partners with antibiotics
Gonorrhea *(Neisseria gonorrhoeae)*	Adolescents 15–19 yr at high risk; transmitted by oral, anal, or vaginal intercourse; mother-to-child transmission during vaginal delivery Manifestations include urethral or anorectal infections; vaginal discharge; bleeding or spotting and heavy menses; women may be asymptomatic	Gram-stained slides; DNA screening or culture of endocervical, pharyngeal, and anal secretions; concomitant screening for chlamydia Treat both sexual partners with antibiotics
Lymphogranuloma venereum (LGV) *(C. trachomatis)*	Often confused with syphilis, herpes, or chancroid Begins as skin lesion, spreads to lymphatic tissue; appears as multivesicular ulcer on penis or scrotum in men and appears on vaginal wall, cervix, or labia in women; anorectal lesions, from anal intercourse, can appear in both men and women	Diagnosed through LGV complement-fixation tests, tissue culture, and monoclonal antibody tests Treated with antibiotics
Syphilis *(Treponema pallidum)*	Incidence is decreasing; higher incidence in low-income, minority, heterosexual couples; transmitted during first few years of infection; can be transmitted to fetus during pregnancy to fetus Hard chancre develops in primary stage; systemic symptoms include low-grade fever, malaise, sore throat, hoarseness, anorexia, headache, joint pain, skin rashes; latent (tertiary) stages usually asymptomatic Neurosyphilis and life-threatening hypersensitivities can develop without treatment	Dark-field or fluorescent antibody examination of fluid from syphilitic chancre; VDRL or RPR Treatment includes penicillin injections for primary or secondary infections

TABLE 32-15

Major Sexually Transmitted Infections—Cont'd

Source of Infection	Epidemiology/Clinical Manifestations	Evaluation and Treatment
VIRUSES		
Condylomata acuminata (human papillomavirus [HPV])	Most common viral STI in United States Risk factors include multiple sexual partners, early onset of sexual activity (16–25 yr of age); HPV is associated with cervical and vulvar cancer in females and anorectal and squamous cell carcinoma of the penis in men; genital warts contagious; infants can be infected during delivery HPV can be asymptomatic Warts are soft, skin-colored, whitish pink to reddish brown; may occur singly or in clusters	Diagnosis based in clinical manifestations; Pap smears and HPV DNA tests Treated with topical acids, cryosurgery or immune system modifiers; cervical and extensive vaginal lesions treated with 5-FU or surgical excision Treatment is not curative
Genital herpes (type 1 [HSV-1] or type 2 [HSV-2])	Most common cause of genital ulceration in United States; reaching epidemic status Neonatal infections can occur in utero, intrapartum, and postpartum; virus undergoes local replication in dermis and epidermis leading to vesicles; can remain in latent stage until reactivated; cause of reactivation unknown but may be related to stress, sun exposure, hormonal fluctuations, or illness	Diagnosis based on clinical manifestations, tissue culture or serologic antibody testing No curative treatment; oral acyclovir, famciclovir, or valacyclovir may be used; IV acyclovir reserved for severely immunocompromised persons
PARASITES		
Pediculosis pubis (*Phthirus pubis* [crab louse])	Commonly transmitted sexually, causes "crabs"; most common in single persons ages 15–25 yr Ranges from mild itching to severe, intolerable itching	Definitive diagnosis by examination Treated with lotion, cream, or shampoo
Scabies *(Sarcoptes scabiei)*	First human disease with known cause; worldwide distribution; most recent outbreak in the United States began in 1971, subsided in 1981; transmitted by close skin-to-skin contact, typically occurring within families or between sexual partners Predominant manifestation is intense itching	Diagnosed from clinical manifestations, microscopic identification Treated with topical cream or lotion
Trichomoniasis *(Trichomonas vaginalis)*	Common cause of lower genital tract infection; found in both partners; urethra most common site of infection in men, primarily involves vagina in women Manifestations range from none to severe, including pain on intercourse, dysuria, and spotting; most men remain asymptomatic	Definitive diagnosis through microscopic confirmation of trichomonads in vaginal secretions Treat with antibiotics for both sexual partners

NOTE: AIDS is discussed extensively in Chapter 7.

DNA, Deoxyribonucleic acid; *VDRL,* Venereal Disease Research Laboratory test; *RPR,* rapid plasma reagin test; *STI,* sexually transmitted infection; *IV,* intravenous.

Bacterial Sources

Gonococcal infections

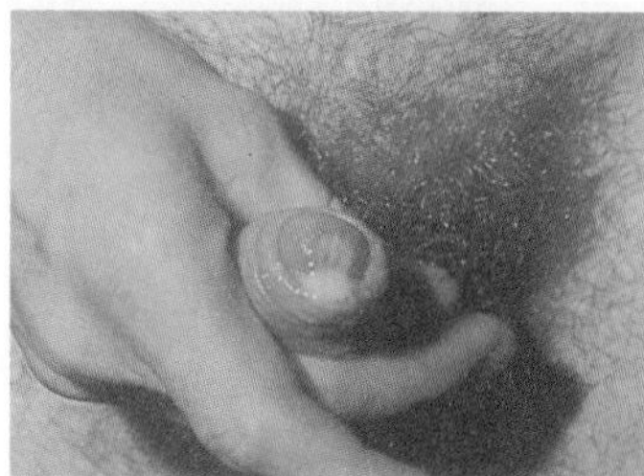

Symptomatic gonococcal urethritis.

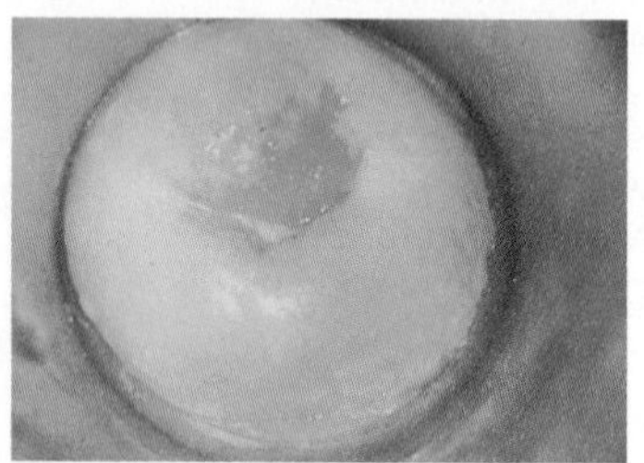

Endocervical gonorrhea.

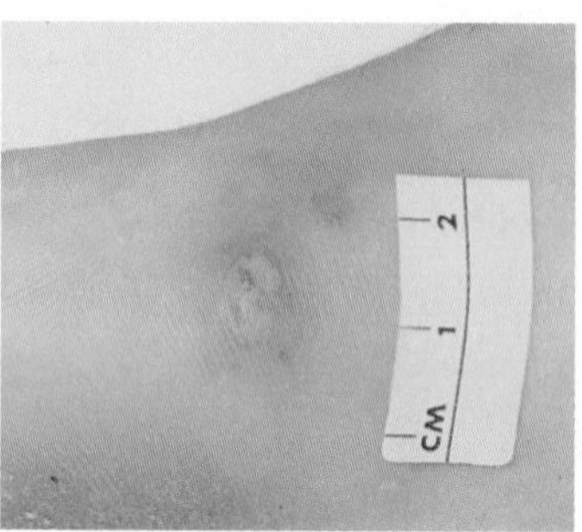

Skin lesions of disseminated gonococcal infection.

Bacterial vaginosis

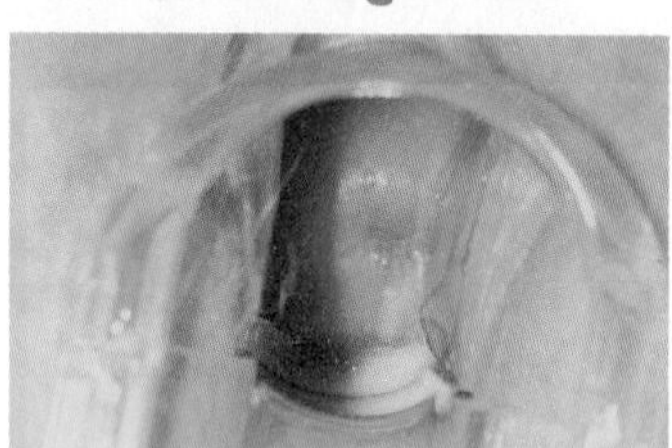

Vaginal examination showing mild bacterial vaginosis.

Syphilis

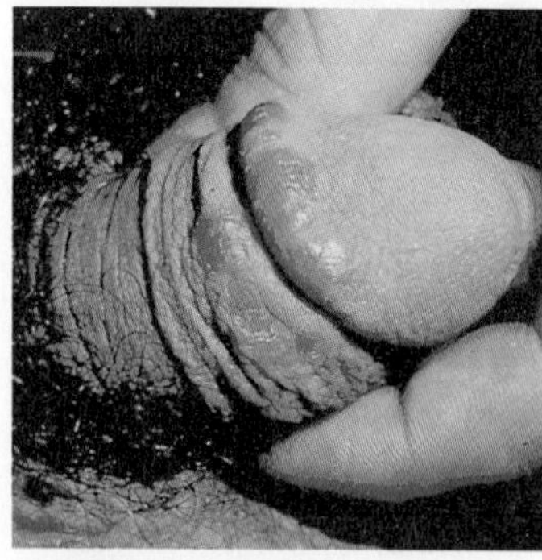

Erythematous penile plaques of secondary syphilis.

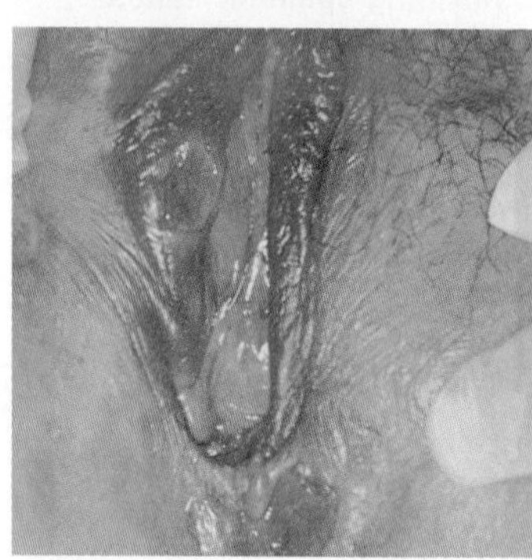

Multiple primary syphilitic chancres of labia and perineum.

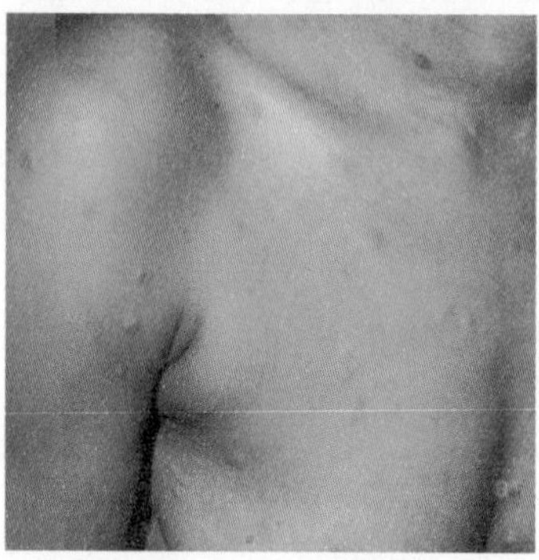

Papular secondary syphilis.

Lymphogranuloma

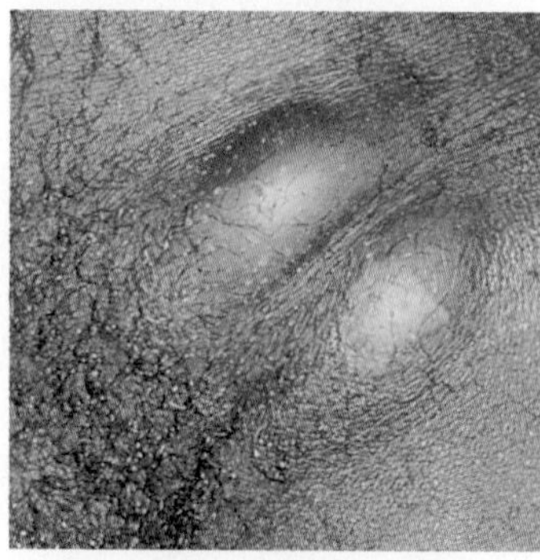

"Groove sign" in man with lymphogranuloma venereum (LV).

Chlamydial infections

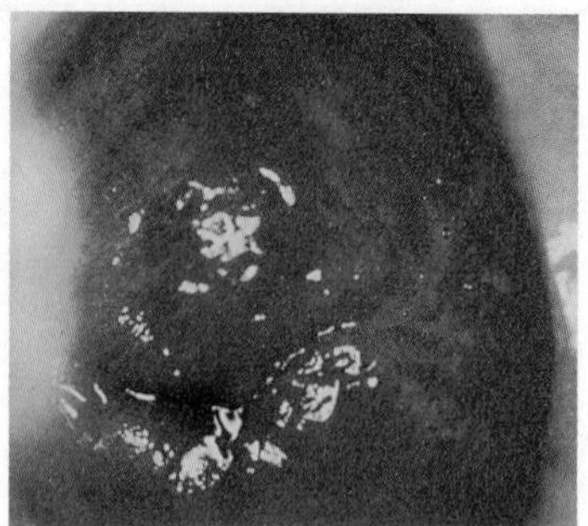

Beefy red mucosa in chlamydial infection.

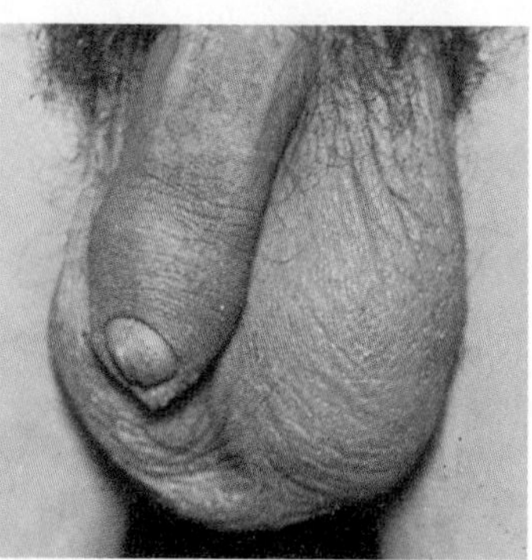

Chlamydial epididymitis

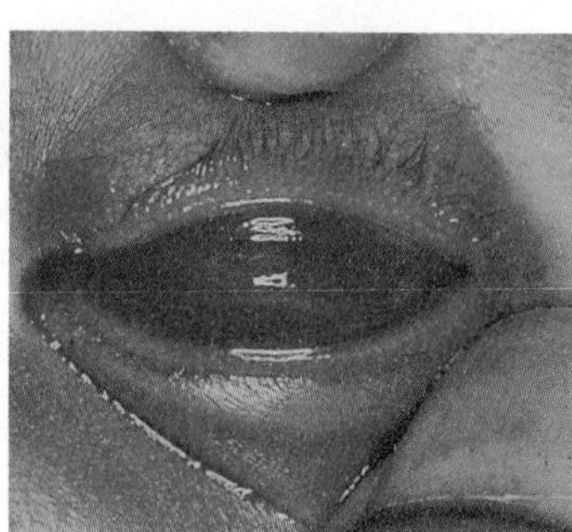

Chlamydial ophthalmia: erythematous conjunctiva in infant.

From Morse SA, Moreland AA, Holmes KK: *Atlas of sexually transmitted diseases and AIDS,* ed 2, London, 1996, Mosby.

Viral Sources

Genital herpes

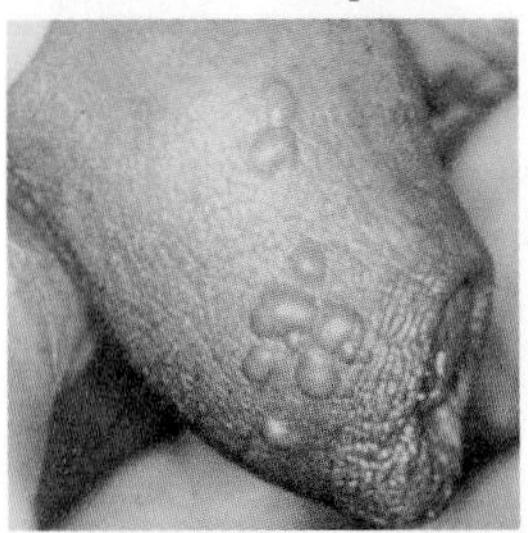

Early lesions of primary genital herpes.

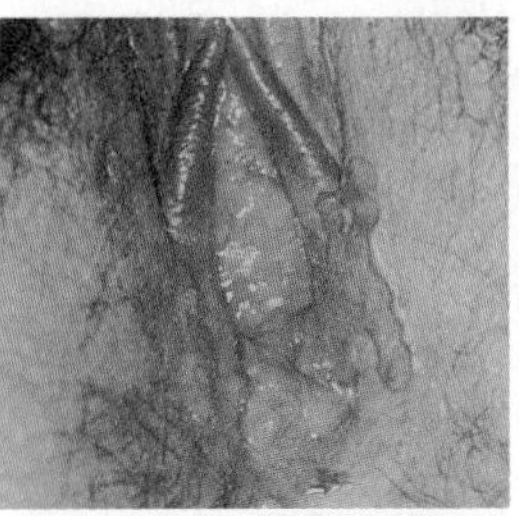

Primary vulvar herpes.

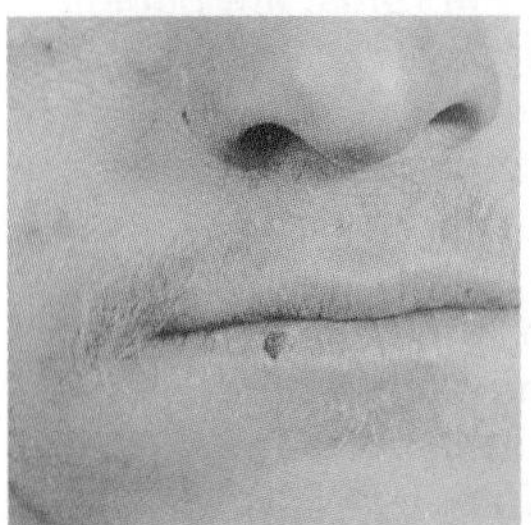

Generalized herpes simplex in patient with atopic dermatitis.

Human papillomavirus (HPV)

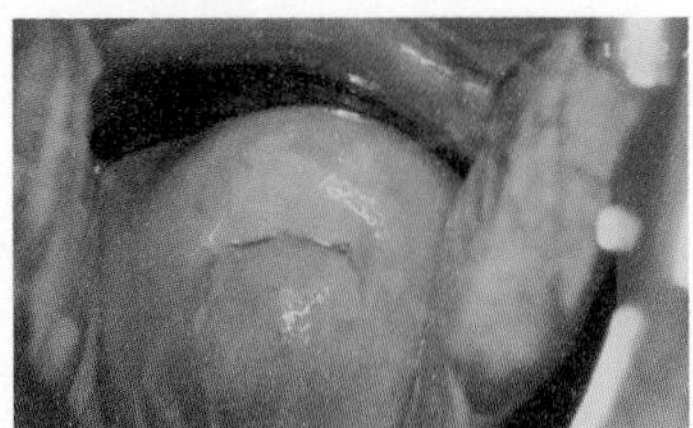

Human papillomavirus (HPV) infection of the cervix.

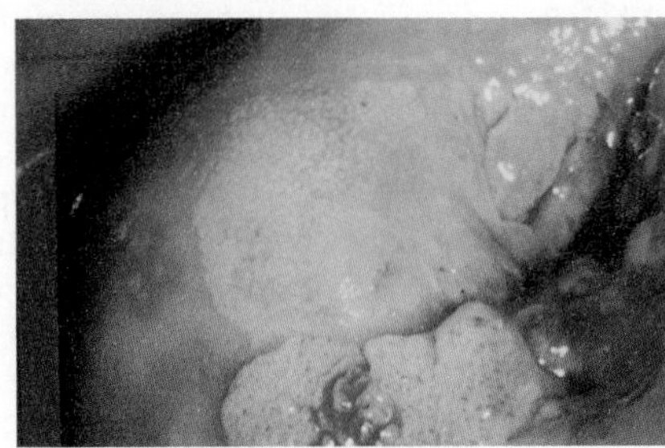

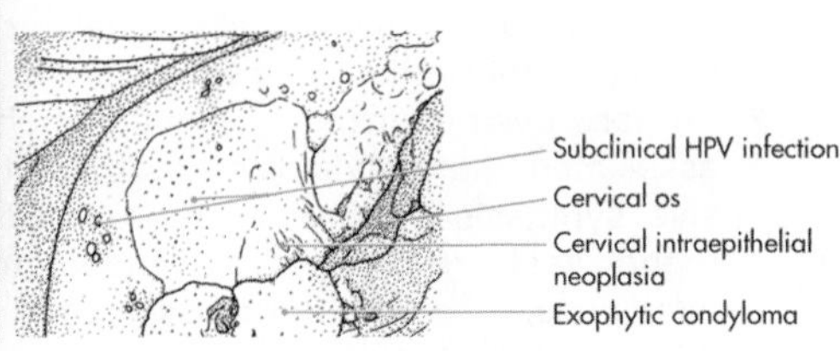

Exophytic (outward-growing) condyloma, subclinical human papillomavirus (HPV) infection, and high-grade cervical intraepithelial neoplasia (CIN).

Condylomata acuminata

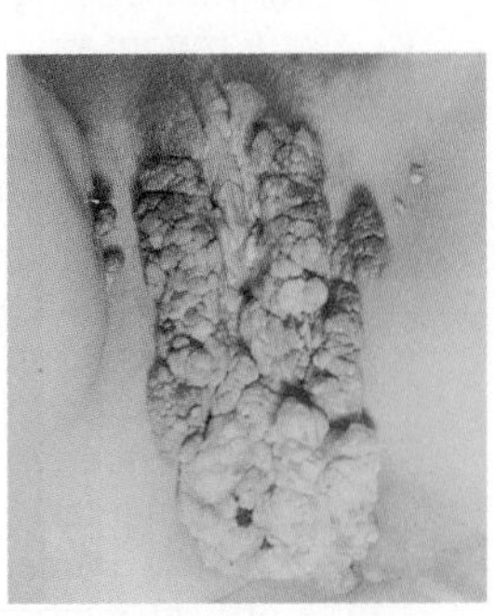

Condylomata acuminata: vulva and perineum.

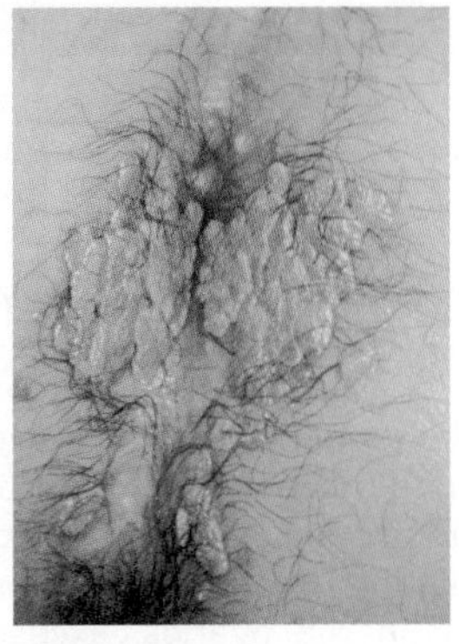

Condylomata acuminata: perianal.

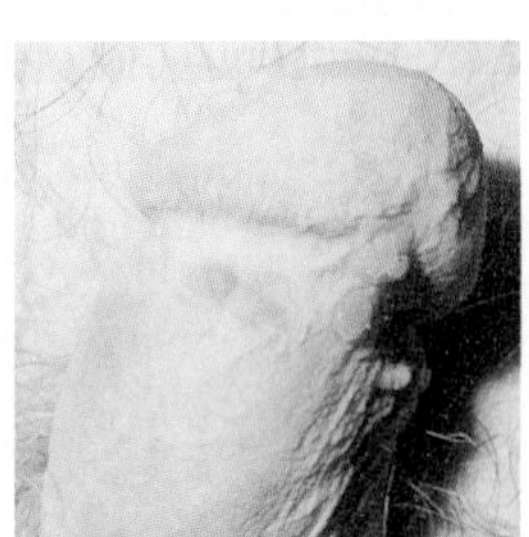

Condylomata acuminata: penile.

Parasite Sources

Trichomonisasis

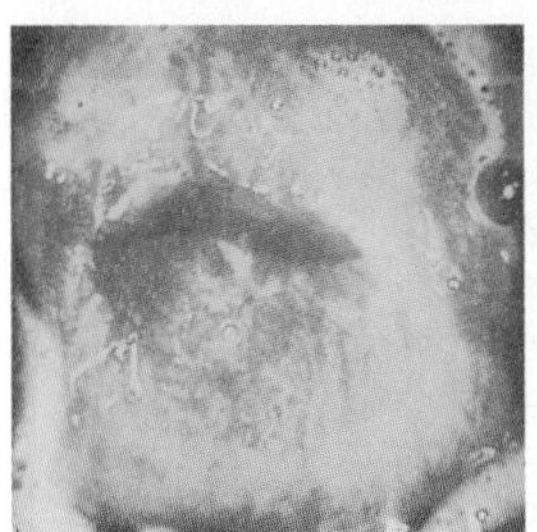

"Strawberry cervix" seen with trichomoniasis.

Scabies

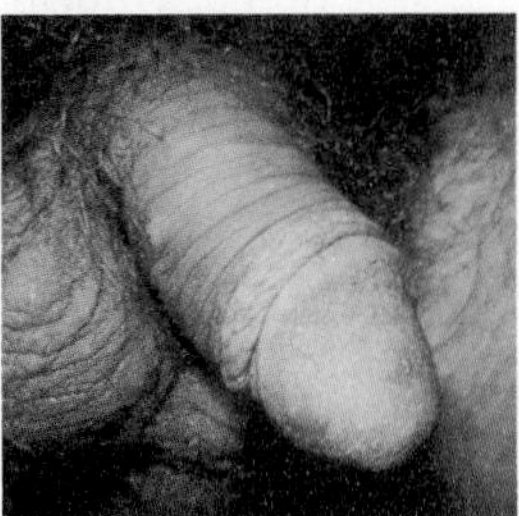

Nodular lesions of scabies on male genitalia.

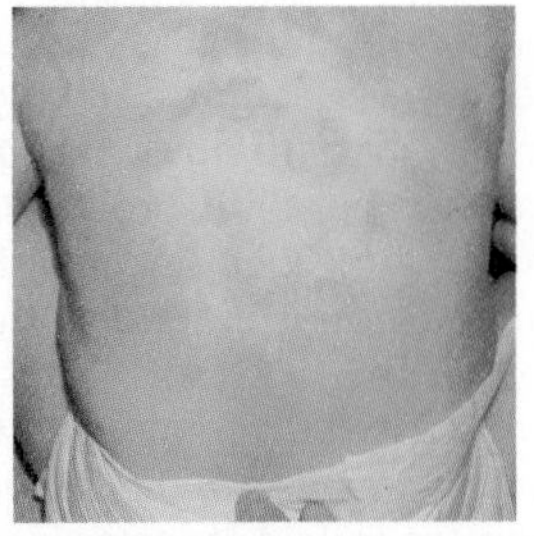

Urticaria associated with scabies.

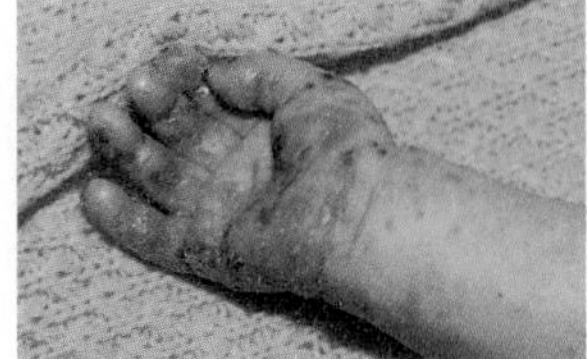

Scabies of palm with secondary pyoderma in infant.

Pediculosis pubis (*Phthirus pubis* [crablouse])

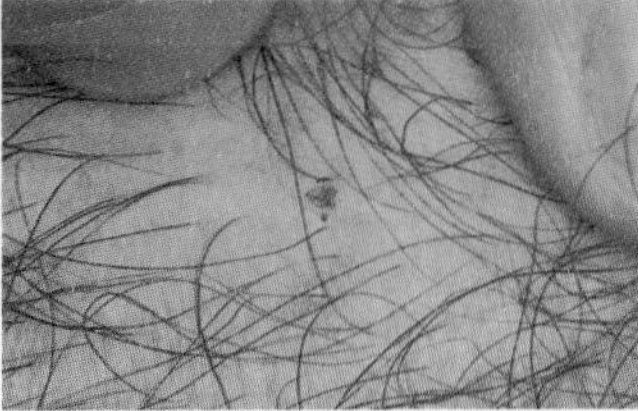

Phthirus pubis feeding on its host.

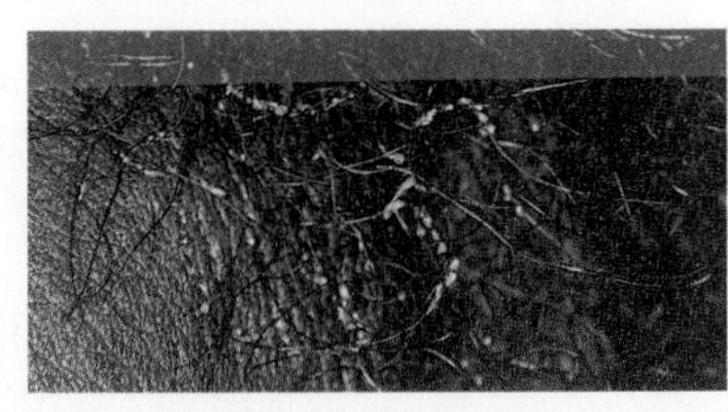

Pubic hair with multiple nits.

Did You Understand?

Alterations of Sexual Maturation

1. Sexual maturation, or puberty, should begin in girls between the ages of 8 and 13 years and in boys between the ages of 9 and 14 years.
2. Delayed puberty is the onset of sexual maturation after these ages; precocious puberty is the onset before these ages. Treatment depends on the cause.

Disorders of the Female Reproductive System

1. The female reproductive system can be altered by hormonal imbalances, infectious microorganisms, inflammation, structural abnormalities, and benign or malignant proliferative conditions.
2. Primary dysmenorrhea is painful menstruation not associated with pelvic disease. It results from excessive synthesis of prostaglandin F. Secondary dysmenorrheal results from endometriosis, pelvic adhesions, inflammatory disease, uterine fibroids, or adenomyosis.
3. Primary amenorrhea is the continued absence of menarche and menstrual function by 14 years of age without the development of secondary sex characteristics or by 16 years of age if these changes have occurred.
4. Secondary amenorrhea is the absence of menstruation for a time equivalent to more than 3 cycles or 6 months in women who have previously menstruated. Secondary amenorrhea is associated with anovulation.
5. Dysfunctional uterine bleeding (DUB) is heavy or irregular bleeding caused by a disturbance of the menstrual cycle.
6. Polycystic ovary (PCO) is a condition in which excessive androgen production is triggered by inappropriate secretion of gonadotropins. This hormonal imbalance prevents ovulation and causes enlargement and cyst formation in the ovaries, excessive endometrial proliferation, and often hirsutism. Hyperinsulinemia plays a key role in androgen excess.
7. Premenstrual syndrome (PMS) is the cyclic recurrence of physical, psychologic, or behavioral changes distressing enough to disrupt normal activities or interpersonal relationships. Emotional symptoms, particularly depression, anger, irritability, and fatigue, are reported as the most distressing symptoms; physical symptoms tend to be less problematic. Treatment is symptomatic and includes self-help techniques, lifestyle changes, counseling, and medication.
8. Infection and inflammation of the female genitalia can result from microorganisms from the environment or overproliferation of microorganisms that normally populate the genital tract.
9. Pelvic inflammatory disease (PID) is an acute ascending infection of the upper genital tract caused by a sexually transmitted pathogen. Untreated PID can lead to infertility.
10. Vaginitis, or vaginal infection, is usually caused by sexually transmitted pathogens or *Candida albicans*, which causes candidiasis.
11. Cervicitis, which is infection of the cervix, can be acute (mucopurulent cervicitis) or chronic. Its most common cause is a sexually transmitted pathogen.
12. Vulvitis is an inflammation of the skin of the vulva. It can be caused by chemical irritants, allergens, skin disorders, irritation from tight-fitting clothing, or spread of vaginal infections, such as candidiasis.
13. Bartholinitis, also called Bartholin cyst, is an infection of the ducts that lead from the Bartholin glands to the surface of the vulva. Infection blocks the glands, preventing the outflow of glandular secretions.
14. The pelvic relaxation disorders—uterine displacement, uterine prolapse, cystocele, rectocele, and urethrocele—are caused by the relaxation of muscles and fascial supports, usually with age or after childbirth or other trauma, and are more likely to occur in women with a familial or genetic predisposition.
15. Benign ovarian cysts develop from mature ovarian follicles that do not release their ova (follicular cysts) or from a corpus luteum that persists abnormally instead of degenerating (corpus luteum cyst). Cysts usually regress spontaneously.
16. Endometrial polyps consist of overgrowths of endometrial tissue and often cause abnormal bleeding in the premenopausal woman.
17. Leiomyomas, also called *uterine fibroids,* are benign tumors arising from the muscle layer of the uterus, the myometrium.
18. Adenomyosis is the presence of endometrial glands and stroma within the uterine myometrium.
19. Endometriosis is the presence of functional endometrial tissue (i.e., tissue that responds to hormonal stimulation) at sites outside the uterus. Endometriosis causes an inflammatory reaction at the site of implantation and is a cause of infertility.
20. Most cancers of the female genitalia involve the uterus (particularly the endometrium), the cervix, and the ovaries. Cancer of the vagina is rare.
21. Cervical cancer arises from the cervical epithelium and is triggered by human papillomavirus (HPV). The progressively serious neoplastic alterations are cervical intraepithelial neoplasia (cervical dysplasia), cervical carcinoma in situ, and invasive cervical carcinoma. Smoking is a cofactor.
22. Most vaginal cancers are not invasive. Like cervical cancers, they arise from the epithelium and are identified as intraepithelial neoplasia (dysplasia), carcinoma in situ, or invasive carcinoma.
23. Risk factors for endometrial cancer include exposure to unopposed estrogen, obesity, high-fat diet, infertility or no pregnancies, late menopause, diabetes, and hypertension. Hormonal contraception protects against endometrial and ovarian cancers. Incidence of endometrial cancer is greatest among women in their 50s and early 60s.
24. Risk factors for ovarian cancer include family history, residence in an industrialized country, prior breast or endometrial cancer, infertility, early menopause, obesity, a high-fat diet, and exposure to asbestos or talc. Ovarian cancer causes more deaths than any other genital cancer in women.
25. Infertility, or the inability to conceive after 1 year of unprotected intercourse, affects approximately 15% of all couples. Fertility can be impaired by factors in the male, female, or both partners.

Did You Understand?—Cont'd

26. Chronic illness, medications, infection, sexual trauma, and a variety of psychosocial concerns have been implicated as causes of female sexual dysfunction.

Disorders of the Male Reproductive System

1. Disorders of the urethra include urethritis (infection of the urethra) and urethral strictures (narrowing or obstruction of the urethral lumen caused by scarring).
2. Most cases of urethritis result from sexually transmitted pathogens. Urologic instrumentation, foreign body insertion, trauma, or an anatomic abnormality can cause urethral inflammation with or without infection.
3. Urethritis causes urinary symptoms, including a burning sensation during urination (dysuria), frequency, urgency, urethral tingling or itching, and clear or purulent discharge.
4. The scarring that causes urethral stricture can be caused by trauma or by severe untreated urethritis.
5. Manifestations of urethral stricture include those of bladder outlet obstruction: urinary frequency and hesitancy, diminished force and caliber of the urinary stream, dribbling after voiding, and nocturia.
6. Phimosis and paraphimosis are penile disorders involving the foreskin (prepuce). In phimosis, the foreskin cannot be retracted over the glans. In paraphimosis, the foreskin is retracted and cannot be reduced (returned to its normal anatomic position over the glans). Phimosis is caused by poor hygiene and chronic infection and can lead to paraphimosis. Paraphimosis can constrict the penile blood vessels, preventing circulation to the glans.
7. Peyronie disease consists of fibrosis affecting the corpora cavernosa, which causes penile curvature during erection. Fibrosis prevents engorgement on the affected side, causing a lateral curvature that can prevent intercourse.
8. Priapism is a prolonged, painful erection that is not stimulated by sexual arousal. The corpora cavernosa (but not the corpus spongiosum) fill with blood that does not drain out, probably because of venous obstruction. Priapism is associated with spinal cord trauma, sickle cell disease, leukemia, and pelvic tumors. It can also be idiopathic.
9. Balanitis is an inflammation of the glans penis. It is associated with phimosis, inadequate cleansing under the foreskin, skin disorders, and pathogens (e.g., *Candida albicans*).
10. Cancer of the penis is rare. Penile carcinoma in situ tends to involve the glans; invasive carcinoma of the penis involves the shaft as well.
11. A varicocele is an abnormal dilation of the veins within the spermatic cord caused by either congenital absence of valves in the internal spermatic vein or acquired valvular incompetence.
12. A hydrocele is a collection of fluid between the testicular and scrotal layers of the tunica vaginalis. Hydroceles can be idiopathic or caused by trauma or infection of the testes.
13. A spermatocele is a cyst located between the testis and epididymis that is filled with fluid and sperm.
14. Cryptorchidism is a congenital condition in which one or both testes fail to descend into the scrotum. Uncorrected cryptorchidism is associated with infertility and significantly increased risk of testicular cancer.
15. Testicular torsion is the rotation of a testis, which twists blood vessels in the spermatic cord. This interrupts the blood supply to the testis, resulting in edema and, if not corrected within 6 hours, necrosis and atrophy of testicular tissues.
16. Orchitis is an acute infection of the testes. Complications of orchitis include hydrocele and abscess formation.
17. Testicular cancer is the most common malignancy in males 15 to 35 years of age. Although its cause is unknown, high androgen levels, genetic predisposition, and history of cryptorchidism, trauma, or infection may contribute to tumorigenesis.
18. Spermatogenesis (sperm production by the testes) can be impaired by disruptions of the hypothalamic-pituitary-testicular axis that reduce testosterone secretion and by testicular trauma, infection, or atrophy from any cause. Sperm production is also impaired by neoplastic disease, cryptorchidism, or any factor that causes testicular temperature to rise (e.g., circulatory impairment, wearing tight clothing).
19. Epididymitis, an inflammation of the epididymis, is usually caused by a sexually transmitted pathogen that ascends through the vasa deferentia from an already infected urethra or bladder.
20. Benign prostatic hyperplasia (BPH), also called benign prostatic hypertrophy, is the enlargement of the prostate gland. This condition becomes symptomatic as the enlarging prostate compresses the urethra, causing symptoms of bladder outlet obstruction and urine retention.
21. Bacterial prostatitis is an infection of the prostate. Acute bacterial prostatitis causes an inflammatory response in which the prostate becomes enlarged, tender, and firm. Infection may spread to the bladder. Chronic bacterial prostatitis is recurrent prostatic infection that eventually causes fibrosis.
22. Prostate cancer is the second leading cause of cancer deaths in men (after lung cancer). Possible causes include genetic predisposition, environmental and dietary factors, and alterations in hormones (testosterone, dihydrotestosterone, and estradiol) and growth factor (IGF-1). Incidence is greatest among northwestern European and North American men (particularly blacks) older than 65 years.
23. Most cancers of the prostate are adenocarcinomas that develop at the periphery of the gland. Routine screening is recommended for early detection of disease.
24. Sexual dysfunction in males can be caused by any physical or psychologic factor that impairs erection, emission, or ejaculation.

Disorders of the Breast

1. Most disorders of the breast are disorders of the mammary gland—that is, the female breast.

(Continued)

Did You Understand?—Cont'd

2. Galactorrhea, or inappropriate lactation, is the persistent secretion of a milky substance by the breasts of a woman who is not in the postpartum state or nursing an infant. Its most common cause is nonpuerperal hyperprolactinemia, a rise in serum prolactin levels.
3. Benign breast conditions are numerous and involve both ducts and lobules. Benign epithelial lesions can be broadly classified according to their future risk of developing breast cancer as (1) nonproliferative breast lesions, (2) proliferative breast disease, and (3) atypical hyperplasia.
4. Nonproliferative lesions include fibrocystic changes (FCC). In addition to FCC, many women experience several other types of benign breast tumors.
5. Proliferative breast lesions without atypia are characterized by proliferation of ductal epithelium or stroma or both without cellular signs of malignancy.
6. Atypical hyperplasia is an increase in the number of cells, and the cells have some variation in structure.
7. Ductal carcinoma in situ (DCIS) refers to a heterogenous group of lesions, presumably malignant epithelial cells, within the ductal system. It is unclear whether the increase in incidence of DCIS reflects an increase in cancer or increased detection by mammography.
8. Breast cancer is the most common form of cancer in women and second to lung cancer as the most common cause of cancer death.
9. The major risk factors for breast cancer are reproductive factors, such as nulliparity; hormonal factors and growth factors, such as excessive estradiol and IGF-1; familial factors, such as a family history of breast cancer; and environmental factors, such as ionizing radiation. Physical activity and human chorionic gonadotrophin hormone may be protective factors.
10. Pathogenesis involves several steps including modification of DNA, alteration of chromosomes, suppression of apoptosis, alterations of breast stroma, and modifications of oncogenes or tumor-suppressor genes or both. Approximately one third of breast cancers are hormone dependent (progesterone-receptor positive or estrogen-receptor positive). Treatment protocols are often based on whether the tumor is receptor positive or negative.
11. Most breast cancers arise from the ductal epithelium and then may metastasize to the lymphatics, opposite breast, abdominal cavity, lungs, bones, kidneys, liver, adrenal glands, ovaries, and pituitary glands.
12. The first clinical manifestation of breast cancer is usually a small, painless lump in the breast. Other manifestations include palpable lymph nodes in the axilla, dimpling of the skin, nipple and skin retraction, nipple discharge, ulcerations, reddened skin, and bone pain associated with bony metastases.
13. Gynecomastia is the overdevelopment (hyperplasia) of breast tissue in a male. It is first seen as a firm, palpable mass at least 2 cm in diameter and is located in the subareolar area.
14. Gynecomastia affects 32% to 40% of the male population. Incidence is greatest among adolescents and men older than 50 years of age.
15. Gynecomastia is caused by hormonal or breast tissue alterations that cause estrogen to dominate. These alterations can result from systemic disorders, drugs, neoplasms, or idiopathic causes.
16. Breast cancer is relatively uncommon in males, but it has a poor prognosis because men tend to delay seeking treatment until the disease is advanced. Incidence is greatest in men in their 60s.
17. Most breast cancers in men are estrogen receptor positive.

Sexually Transmitted Infections

1. Sexually transmitted diseases are infections contracted by intimate as well as sexual contact and include systemic infections, such as tuberculosis and hepatitis, that can spread to a sexual partner.
2. The etiology of an STI may be bacterial, viral, protozoan, parasitic, or fungal.
3. Although the majority of STIs can be treated, viral-induced STIs are considered incurable.

Key Terms

Key Terms—Cont'd

Nonpuerperal hyperprolactinemia, 885
Oophoritis, 855
Orchitis, 874
Ovarian torsion, 861
Papilloma, 886
Paraphimosis, 870
Pelvic inflammatory disease (PID), 855
Pessary, 858
Peyronie disease ("bent nail syndrome"), 871
Phimosis, 870
Polycystic ovary syndrome (PCOS), 852
Precocious puberty, 849
Premenstrual dysphoric disorder (PMDD), 853
Premenstrual syndrome (PMS), 853
Priapism, 871
Primary amenorrhea, 850
Primary dysmenorrhea, 850
Prolactin-inhibiting factor (PIF), 885
Prostate-specific antigen (PSA), 878
Prostate-specific antigen density (PSAD), 878
Prostatic antibacterial factor (PAF), 879
Prostatitis, 878
Prostatodynia, 878
Radial scar, 886
Rectocele, 858
Salpingitis, 855
Sclerosing adenosis, 886
Secondary amenorrhea, 850
Secondary dysmenorrhea, 850
Sexual dysfunction, 884
Spermatocele, 873
Stress incontinence, 858
Torsion of the testis, 874
Urethral stricture, 869
Urethritis, 869
Urethrocele, 858
Uterine prolapse, 858
Vaginismus, 868
Vaginitis, 856
Varicocele, 872
Vulvitis, 857
Xenoestrogen, 894

References

1. American Cancer Society: *Cancer facts & figures 2007*, Atlanta, 2007, American Cancer Society.
2. Reid RL: Amenorrhea, In Copeland LJ, Farrell JF, editors: *Textbook of gynecology*, ed 2, Philadelphia, 2000, Saunders.
3. Herman-Giddens ME: Recent data on pubertal milestones in United States children: the secular trend toward earlier development, *Int J Androl* 29(1):241–246, 2006, discussion 286–290.
4. Emans SJ: Delayed puberty, In Emans SJ et al, editors: *Pediatric and adolescent gynecology*, ed 5, Philadelphia, 2005, Lippincott Williams & Wilkins.
5. Speroff L, Fritz MA: *Clinical gynecologic endocrinology and infertility*, ed 7, Philadelphia, 2005, Lippincott Williams & Wilkins.
6. Faucher MA, Schuiling KD: Normal and abnormal uterine bleeding, In Schuiling KD, Likis FE et al, editors: *Women's gynecologic health*, Sudbury, Mass, 2006, Jones & Bartlett.
7. Legro RS: A 27-year-old woman with a diagnosis of polycystic ovary syndrome, *JAMA* 297(5):509–519, 2007.
8. Hart R, Hickey M, Franks S: Definitions, prevalence and symptoms of polycystic ovaries and polycystic ovary syndrome, *Best Pract Res Clin Obstet Gynaecol* 18(5):671–683, 2004.
9. Leung PCK, Adashi EY: *The ovary*, ed 2, San Diego, Calif, 2004, Elsevier Academic Press.
10. Rotterdam ESHRE/ASRM-sponsored PCOS consensus workshop group: revised 2003 consensus on diagnostic criteria and long-term health risks related to polycystic ovary syndrome, *Hum Reprod* 19(1):41–47, 2004.
11. Diamanti-Kandarakis E et al: Controversies in endocrinology. A modern medical quandary: polycystic ovary syndrome, insulin resistance, and oral contraceptive pills, *J Clin Endocrinol Metab* 88(5):1927–1932, 2003.
12. Legro RS: Polycystic ovarian syndrome, In Leung PC, Adashi EY, editors: *The ovary*, ed 2, St Louis, 2004, Elsevier Academic Press.
13. Taylor D, Schuiling KD, Sharp BA: Menstrual cycle pain and discomforts, In Schuiling KD, Likis FE, editors: *Women's gynecologic health*, Sudbury Mass, 2006, Jones & Bartlett.
14. Cohen LS et al: Prevalence and predictors of premenstrual dysphoric disorder (PMDD) in older premenopausal women: the Harvard Study of Moods and Cycles, *J Affect Disord* 70(2):125–132, 2002.
15. Halbreich U: The diagnosis of premenstrual syndromes and premenstrual dysphoric disorder: clinical procedures and research perspectives, *Gynecol Endocrinol* 19(6):320–334, 2004.
16. Wyatt KM, Dimmock PW, O'Brien PM: Selective serotonin reuptake inhibitors for premenstrual syndrome, *Cochrane Database Syst Rev* (4):CD001396, 2002.
17. Wyatt KM et al: Prescribing patterns in premenstrual syndrome, *BMC Womens Health* 2(1):4, 2002.
18. Centers for Disease Control: Sexually transmitted disease treatment guidelines 2006, *MMWR Recomm Rpt* 55:R11, 2006.
19. Stenchever MA et al: *Comprehensive gynecology*, ed 4, p. 710, St Louis, 2001, Mosby.
20. Viera AJ, Larkins-Pettigrew M: Practical use of the pessary, *Am Fam Physician* 61(9):2719–2726, 2000.
21. Forrest DE: Common gynecologic pelvic disorders, In Youngkin EQ, Davis MS, editors: *Women's health: a primary care clinical guide*, ed 3, Stamford, Conn, 2004, Appleton & Lange.
22. McCartney CR et al: Hypothalamic regulation of cyclic ovulation: evidence that the increase in gonadotropin releasing hormone pulse frequency during the follicular phase reflects the gradual loss of the restraining effects of progesterone, *J Clin Endocrinol Metab* 87(5):2194–2200, 2002.
23. Adelson MD, Adelson KL: Miscellaneous benign disorders of the upper genital tract, In Copeland LJ, Farrell JF, editors: *Textbook of gynecology*, ed 2, Philadelphia, 2000, Saunders.
24. Chabbert-Buffet N et al: Selective progesterone receptor modulators and progesterone antagonists: mechanisms of action and clinical applications, *Hum Reprod Update* 11(3):293–307, 2005.
25. Karaer O, Oruc S, Koyuncu FM: Aromatase inhibitors: possible future applications, *Acta Obstet Gynecol Scand* 83(8): 699–706, 2004.
26. Gupta JK et al: Uterine artery embolization for symptomatic uterine fibroids, *Cochrane Database Syst Rev* (1):CD005073, 2006.
27. Fong K et al: Transvaginal US and hysterosonography in postmenopausal women with breast cancer receiving tamoxifen: correlation with hysteroscopy and pathologic study, *Radiographics* 23(1):137–150, discussion 151–155, 2003.
28. Kovacs P: Endometriosis conference report from the 49th annual meeting of the Society for Gynecologic Investigation, *Medscape Ob Gyn Women's Health* 7:1, 2002.
29. O'Shaughnessy JA et al: Special article: treatment and prevention of intraepithelial neoplasia: an important target for accelerated new agent development, *Clin Cancer Res* 8(2):314–346, 2002.
30. Bosch FX et al: The causal relation between human papillomavirus and cervical cancer, *J Clin Patho* 55(4):241–242, 2002.

References—Cont'd

31. Moodley M: Update on pathophysiologic mechanisms of human papillomavirus, *Curr Opin Obstet Gynecol* 17(1): 61–64, 2005.
32. Nappi L et al: Cervical squamous intraepithelial lesions of low-grade in HIV-infected women: recurrence, persistence, and progression, in treated and untreated women, *Eur J Obstet Gynecol Reprod Biol* 121(2):226–232, 2005.
33. Wallin KL et al: A population-based prospective study of *Chlamydia trachomatis* infection and cervical carcinoma, *Int J Cancer* 101(4):371–374, 2002.
34. Creasman WT: Vaginal cancers, *Curr Opin Obstet Gynecol* 17:71–76, 2005.
35. Canavan TP: Vulvar cancer, *Am Fam Physician* 66(7): 1269–1274, 2002.
36. American Cancer Society: *Overview: endometrial cancer. How is endometrial cancer treated?*, New York, 2005, American Cancer Society.
37. Brewer MA et al: Prevention of ovarian cancer: intraepithelial neoplasia, *Clin Cancer Res* 9(1):20–30, 2003.
38. American Cancer Society: *Overview: ovarian cancer. How is ovarian cancer found?*, New York, 2006, American Cancer Society.
39. Blast RC, Mills GB: Molecular pathogenesis of ovarian cancer. In Mendelsohn J et al, editors: *The molecular basis of cancer*, Philadelphia, 2001, Saunders.
40. Gershenon D: Epithelial ovarian cancer. In Copeland LJ, Farrell JF, editors: *Textbook of gynecology*, ed 2, Philadelphia, 2000, Saunders.
41. Nelson HD et al: Genetic risk assessment and BRCA mutation testing for breast and ovarian cancer susceptibility: systemic evidence review for the U.S. Preventive Services Task Force, *Ann Intern Med* 143(5):362–379, 2005.
42. Vigano P et al: Molecular mechanisms and biologic plausibility underlying the malignant transformation of endometriosis: a critical analysis, *Hum Reprod Update* 12(1):77–89, 2006.
43. Olshansky E: Infertilty, In Schuiling KD, Likis FE, editors: *Women's gynecologic health*, Sudbury, Mass, 2006, Jones & Bartlett.
44. Tanagho EA, McAninch JW, editors: *Smith's general urology*, ed 13, Norwalk, Conn, 1992, Appleton-Lange.
45. Noble J, editor: *Textbook of primary care medicine*, ed 2, St Louis, 1996, Mosby.
46. Bella AJ et al: Minimally invasive intracoporeal incision of Peyronie's plaque: initial experience with a new technique, *Urology* 68(4):852–857, 2006.
47. Burnett AL et al: Long term oral phosphodiesterase 5 inhibitor therapy alleviates recurrent priapism, *Urology* 67(5): 1043–1048, 2006.
48. American Cancer Society: *Penile cancer*, New York, 2003, American Cancer Society.
49. Trussell JC et al: High prevalence of bilateral varicoceles confirmed with ultrasonography, *Int Urol Nephrol* 35(1):15–18, 2003.
50. McAninch JW: Disorders of the testis, scrotum, and spermatic cord. In Tanagho EA, McAninch JW, editors: *Smith's general urology*, ed 14, Norwalk, Conn, 1995, Appleton & Lange.
51. Nielsen ME et al: Insight of pathogenesis of varicoceles: relationship of varicocele and body mass index, *Urology* 68(2): 392–396, 2006.
52. Galejs LE: Diagnosis and treatment of the acute scrotum, *Am Fam Physician* 59(4):817–824, 1999.
53. Rosenthal MS: *The fertility sourcebook*, Los Angeles, 1998, Lowell House.
54. Lanum DL: Carcinoma of the genitourinary system. In Nseyo UO, Weinman E, Lamm DL, editors: *Urology for primary care physicians*, Philadelphia, 1999, Saunders.
55. LaRock DR, Sant GR: Lower urinary tract infections. In Nseyo UO, Weinman E, Lamm DL, editors: *Urology for primary care physicians*, Philadelphia, 1999, Saunders.
56. Raivio T, Wikstrom AM, Dunkel L: Treatment of gonadotrophin-deficient boys with recombinant human FSH: long term observation and outcome, *Eur J Endocrinol* 156(1):105–111, 2007.
57. Ferlin A et al: The human Y chromosome's azoospermia factor b (AZFb) region: sequence, structure, and deletion analysis in infertile men, *J Med Genet* 40(1):18–24, 2003.
58. Brugh VM III, Maduro MR, Lamb DJ: Genetic disorders and infertility, *Urol Clin North Am* 30(1):143–152, 2003.
59. Lewis-Jones I et al: Sperm chromosomal abnormalities are linked to sperm morphologic deformities, *Fertil Steril* 79 (1):212–215, 2003.
60. Padrich DA: Testicular cancer and male infertility, *Curr Opin Urol* 16(6):419–427, 2006.
61. Pagani R, Brugh VM III, Lamb DJ: Y chromosome genes and male infertility, *Urol Clin North Am* 29(4):745–753, 2002, review.
62. Turek PJ, Pera RA: Current and future genetic screening for male infertility, *Urol Clin North Am* 29(4):767–792, 2002.
63. Check JH: The infertile male: diagnosis, *Clin Exp Obstet Gynecol* 33(3):133–139, 2006.
64. Foratos DL, de La Rosette JJ: Heat treatment for the prostate: where do we stand in 2000? *Curr Opin Urol* 11(1):35, 2000.
65. American Cancer Society: Prostate cancer resource center, 1999; www3.cancer.org/cancerinfo.
66. Fried NM: New laser treatment approaches for benign prostatic hyperplasia, *Curr Urol Rep* 8(1):47–52, 2007.
67. Ghafar MA et al: Does the prostatic vascular system contribute to the development of benign prostatic hyperplasia? *Curr Urol Rep* 3(4):292–296, review, 2002.
68. Brown CT, Das G: Assessment, diagnosis, and management of lower urinary tract symptoms in men, *Int J Clin Pract* 56(8): 591–603, review, 2002.
69. Reynard JM et al: The ICS-'BPH' Study: uroflometry, lower urinary tract symptoms and bladder outlet obstruction, *Br J Urol* 82(5):619–623, 1998.
70. Burke JP et al: Association of anthropometric measures with the presence and progression of benign prostatic hyperplasia, *Am J Epidemiol* 164(1):41–46, 2006.
71. Kasturi S, Russell S, McVary KT: Metabolic syndrome and lower urinary tract symptoms secondary to benign prostatic hyperplasia, *Curr Urol Rep* 7(4):288–292, 2006.
72. Garg G et al: Management of benign prostate hyperplasia: an overview of alpha-adrenergic antagonist, *Biol Pharm Bull* 29(8):1554–1558, 2006.
73. Wilt TJ, Mac Donald R, Rutks I: Tamsulosin for benign prostatic hyperplasia (Cochrane review), *Cochrane Database Syst Rev* (1):CD002081, 2003.
74. Shibata A, Ma J, Whittemore AS: Prostate cancer incidence and mortality in the United States and the United Kingdom, *J Natl Cancer Inst* 90(16):1230–1231, 1998.
75. Chu KC, Tarone RE, Freeman HP: Trends in prostate cancer mortality among black and white men in the United States, *Cancer* 97(6):1507–1516, 2003.
76. Palapattu GS et al: Prostate carcinogenesis and inflammation: emerging insights, *Carcinogenesis* 26(7):1170–1181, 2005.
77. Bosland MC: Sex steroids and prostate carcinogenesis: integrated, multifactorial working hypothesis, *Ann NY Acad Sci* 1089:168–176, 2006.
78. Hayes RB et al: Dietary factors and risks for prostate cancer among blacks and whites in the United States, *Cancer Epidemiol Biomarkers Prev* 8(1):25–34, 1999.

References—Cont'd

79. Wolk A: Diet, lifestyle and risk of prostate cancer, *Aeta Oncol* 44(3):277–281, 2006.
80. Signorello LB, Adami H: Prostate cancer. In Adami H, Hunter D, Trichopoulos D, editors: *Textbook of cancer epidemiology*, New York, 2002, Oxford Press.
81. Meinbach DS, Lokeshwar BL: Insulin-like growth factors and their binding proteins in prostate cancer: cause or consequence? *Urol Oncol* 24(4):294–306, 2006.
82. Kanagaraj P et al: Effect of lycopene on insulin-like growth factor-1, IGF binding protein 3, and IGF type-1 receptor in prostate cancer cells, *Cancer Res Clin Oncol.* (Epub Jan 12, 2007.)
83. CaP CURE Nutrition Project: *Nutrition and prostate cancer: a monograph from the CaP CURE Nutrition Project*, ed 3, p. 4, January, 1999.
84. Denis L et al: Diet and its preventive role in prostatic disease, *Eur Urol* 35(5–6):377–387, 1999.
85. Gonzalez CA: Nutrition and cancer: the current epidemiological evidence, *Br J Nutr* 96(suppl 1):S42–S45, 2006.
86. Yang M, Sytkowski AJ: Differential expression and androgen regulation of the human selenium-binding protein gene hSP56 in prostate cancer cells, *Cancer Res* 58(14):3150–3153, 1998.
87. Zhao XY et al: 1-alpha,25-dihydroxyvitamin D3 inhibits prostate cancer cell growth by androgen-dependent and androgen-independent mechanisms, *Endocrinology* 141 (7):2548–2556, 2000.
88. Arnot R: *The prostate cancer protection plan: the powerful foods, supplements, and drugs that could save your life*, Boston, 2000, Little, Brown.
89. Giovannucci E et al: Insulin-like growth factors and colon cancer: a review of the evidence, *J Nutr* 131(11 suppl): 3109S–3120S, review, 2001.
90. Singh RP, Agarwal R: Mechanisms of action of novel agents for prostate cancer chemoprevention, *Endocr Relat Cancer* 13 (3):751–778, review, 2006.
91. Ebling DW et al: Development of prostate cancer after pituitary dysfunction: a report of 8 patients, *Urology* 49(4): 564–568, 1997.
92. Oosthuzien JM et al: Melatonin and steroid-dependent carcinomas, *Andrologia* 21(5):429–431, 1989.
93. Roberts JT, Essenhigh DM: Adenocarcinoma of prostate in 40-year-old body-builder, *Lancet* 2(8509):742, 1986.
94. Bosland MC: The role of steroid hormones in prostate carcinogenesis, *J Natl Cancer Inst Mongr* (27):39–66, 2000.
95. Thompson IM et al: The influence of finasteride on the development of prostate cancer, *N Engl J Med* 349:215–224, 2003.
96. Peterson DE et al: Vasectomy and the risk of prostate cancer, *Am J Epidemiol* 135(3):324–325, 1992.
97. Honda GD et al: Vasectomy, cigarette smoking, and age at first sexual intercourse as risk factors for prostate cancer in middle-aged men, *Br J Cancer* 57(3):326–331, 1988.
98. MacLennan GT et al: The influence of chronic inflammation in prostatic carcinogenesis: a 5-year follow-up study, *J Urol* 176(3):1012–1016, 2006.
99. Klein EA: An update on prostate cancer, *Cleve Clin J Med* 62(5):325–338, 1995.
100. Narayan P: Neoplasms of the prostate gland. In Tanagho EA, McAninch JW, editors: *Smith's general urology*, ed 14, Norwalk, Conn, 1995, Appleton & Lange.
101. Giovannucci E et al: Smoking and risk of total fatal prostate cancer in United States health professionals, *Cancer Epidemiol Biomarkers Prev* 8(4 pt 1):277–282, 1999.
102. Brown SL, Resnick MI: Transrectal ultrasound and the prostate biopsy: clinical and pathologic issues. In Lepor H, editor: *Prostatic diseases*, Philadelphia, 2000, Saunders.
103. Parnes HL, Thompson IM, Ford LG: Review article: prevention of hormone-related cancers: prostate cancer, *J Clin Oncol* 23(2):368–377, 2005.
104. Chan JM et al: Insulin-like growth factor 1 (IGF-1), IGF-binding protein-3 and prostate cancer risk: epidemiological studies, *Growth Horm IGF Res* 10(suppl A):S32–S33, 2000.
105. Djavan B et al: Insulin-like growth factors and prostate cancer, *World J Urol* 19(4):225–233, 2001.
106. Moschos SJ, Mantzoros CS: The role of the IGF system in cancer: from basic to clinical studies and clinical applications, *Oncology* 63(4):317–332, 2002.
107. Chung LW et al: Molecular insights into prostate cancer progression: the missing link of tumor microenvironment, *J Urol* 173(1):10–20, 2005.
108. Stamey TA: The era of serum prostate specific antigens as a marker for biopsy of the prostate and detecting prostate cancer is now over in the USA, *BJU Int* 94(7):963–964, 2004.
109. American Cancer Society: Available at www.cancer.org/docroot/CRI/content, accessed, February, 2007.
110. Jefferson Health System, Men's Health: *Overview of impotence* 1997; www.jeffersonhealth.orgdiseases/mens_health/impotenc.htm.
111. Carson CC: Long-term use of sildenafil, *Expert Opin Pharmacother* 4(3):397–405, 2003.
112. Speroff L, Glass RH, Kase NG: *Clinical gynecologic endocrinology and infertility*, ed 6, Baltimore, 1999, Williams & Wilkins.
113. Kase N, Weingold AB, Gershenon DM, editors: *Principles and practice of clinical gynecology*, ed 2, New York, 1990, Churchill Livingstone.
114. Lester SC: The breast. In Kumar V, Abbas AK, Fausto N, editors: *Robbins & Cotran pathologic basis of disease*, ed 7, Philadelphia, 2005, Elsevier-Saunders.
115. Jacobs TW: Radial scars in benign breast-biopsy specimens and the risk of breast cancer, *N Engl J Med* 340(6):430, 1999.
116. Sharkey FE, Allred DC, Valente PT: Breast. In Damjanov I, Linder J, editors: *Anderson's pathology*, ed 10, St Louis, 1996, Mosby.
117. Berg JW: Clinical implications of risk factors for breast cancer, *Cancer* 53(3 suppl):589–591, 1984.
118. American Cancer Society: *Cancer facts & figures 2006*, New York, 2006, American Cancer Society.
119. Lindegarrds JC et al: A retrospective analysis of 82 cases of cancer of the penis, *Br J Urol* 77(6):883, 1996.
120. Swanson SM, Unterman TG: The growth hormone deficient spontaneous dwarf rat is resistant to chemically induced mammary carcinogenesis, *Carcinogenesis* 23(6):977–982, 2002.
121. Henderson B et al: Breast cancer. In Schottenfeld D, Fraumeni J Jr, editors: *Cancer epidemiology and prevention*, p 1022–1039, New York, 1996, Oxford Press.
122. MacMahon B et al: Age at menarche, urine estrogens and breast cancer risk, *Int J Cancer* 30(4):427–431, 1982.
123. Seifert M, Galid A: Oral contraceptives and breast cancer: a causal relationship? *Gynakologisch-Geburtschilfliche Rundschau* 38:101–104, 1998.
124. Cordera F, Jordan VC: Steroid receptors and their role in the biology and control of breast cancer growth, *Semin Oncol* 33(6):631–641, 2006.
125. Kaaks R et al: Postmenopausal serum androgens, oestrogens, and breast cancer risk: the European prospective investigation into cancer and nutrition, *Endocr Relat Cancer* 12(4): 1017–1082, 2005.

125a. Chebowski RT et al: Influence of estrogen plus progestin on breast cancer and mammography in healthy postmenopausal women: the Women's Health Initiative Randomized Trial, *JAMA* 289(24):3243–3243, 2003.

References—Cont'd

126. Micheli A et al: Endogenous sex hormones and subsequent breast cancer in premenopausal women, *Int J Cancer* 112:213–218, 2004.
127. Beral V et al: Breast cancer and hormone-replacement therapy in the Million Women Study, *Lancet* 362(9382):419–427, 2003.
128. Rossouw JE et al: Risks and benefits of estrogen plus progestin in healthy postmenopausal women: principle results from the Women's Health Initiative randomized controlled trial, *JAMA* 288(3):321–333, 2002.
129. Kondro W: Decline in breast cancer since HRT study, *CMAJ* 176(2):160–161, 2007.
130. Fleming RM: Do women taking hormone replacement therapy (HRT) have a higher incidence of breast cancer than women who do not? *Integr Cancer Ther* 2(3):235–237, 2003.
131. Fisher B et al: Treatment of lymph-node-negative, oestrogen-receptor-positive breast cancer: long-term findings from National Surgical Adjuvant Breast and Bowel Project randomised clinical trials, *Lancet* 364(9437):858–868, 2004.
132. Russo I, Russo J: *Molecular basis of breast cancer: prevention and treatment*, Germany, 2004, Springer.
133. Pasqualini JR, Chetrite GS: Recent insight on the control of enzymes involved in estrogen formation and transformation in human breast cancer, *J Steroid Biochem Mol Biol* 93(2–5): 221–236, 2005.
134. Cavalieri E, Rogan E: Catechol quinines of estrogen in the initiation of breast, prostate, and other cancers: keynote lecture, *Ann NY Acad Sci* 1089:286–301, 2006.
135. Pollack M: IGF-1 physiology and breast cancer, *Recent Results Cancer Res* 152:63–70, 1998.
136. Byrne C et al: Plasma insulin-like growth factor (IGF) I, IGF-binding protein 3, and mammographic density, *Cancer Res* 60(14):3744–3748, 2000.
137. Kleinberg DL, Feldman M, Ruan W: IGF-1: an essential factor in terminal end bud formation and ductal morphogenesis, *J Mammary Gland Biol Neoplasia* 5(1):7–17, review, 2000.
138. Tanaka Y et al: Gonadotropins stimulate growth of MCF-7 human breast cancer cells by promoting intercellular conversion of adrenal androgens to estrogens, *Oncol* 59(suppl 11): 19–23, 2000.
139. Lange CA, Richer JK, Horwitz KB: Hypothesis: progesterone primes breast cancer cells for cross-talk with proliferative or antiproliferative signals, *Molecular Endocrinol* 13(6):829–836, 1999.
140. Wu J, Brandt S, Hyder SM: Ligand- and cell-specific effects of signal transduction pathway inhibitors on progestin-induced vascular endothelial growth factor levels in human breast cancer cells, *Molecular Endocrinol* 19(2):312–326, 2005.
141. Kuller LH: The etiology of breast cancer: from epidemiology to prevention, *Public Health Rev* 23(2):157–213, 1995.
142. Fung TT et al: Dietary patterns and the risk of postmenopausal breast cancer, *Int J Cancer* 116(1):116–121, 2005.
143. Adebamowo CA et al: Dietary flavonols and flavonol-rich foods intake and the risk of breast cancer, *Int J Cancer* 114(4):628–633, 2005.
144. Byers T: Nutritional risk factors for breast cancer, *CA Cancer J Clin* 74(suppl 1):288, 1994.
145. Bartsch H et al: Dietary polyunsaturated fatty acids and cancer of the breast and colorectum: emerging evidence for their role as risk modifiers, *Carcinogenesis* 20(12):2209, 1999.
146. Cognault S et al: Effect of an alpha-linolenic acid–rich diet on rat mammary tumor growth depends on the dietary oxidative status, *Nutr Cancer* 36(1):33, 2000.
147. Nakagawa H et al: Effects of genistein and synergistic action in combination with eicosapentaenoic acid on the growth of breast cancer cell lines, *J Cancer Res Clin Oncol* 126(8):448, 2000.
148. Thoennes SR et al: Differential transcriptional activation of peroxisome proliferator-activated receptor gamma by omega-3 and omega-6 fatty acids in MCF-7 cells, *Mol Cell Endocrinol* 160(1–2):67, 2000.
149. Simopoulos AP: The importance of the ratio of omega-6/omega-3 essential fatty acids, *Biomed Pharmacother* 56(8): 365–379, 2002.
150. Frankenberg D et al: Enhanced neoplastic transformation by mammography X rays relative to 200 kVp X rays: indication for a strong dependence on photon energy of the RBE(M) for various end points, *Radiat Res* 157(1):99–105, 2002.
151. Petrakis NL: Nipple aspirate fluid in epidemiologic studies of breast disease, *Epidemiol Rev* 15(1):188–195, 1993.
152. Venturi S: Is there a role for iodine in breast disease? *The Breast* 10:379–382, 2001.
153. Deslypere JP: Obesity and cancer, *Metabolism* 44(suppl 9):14, 1995.
154. Holmes MD, Willett WC: Does diet affect breast cancer risk? *Breast Cancer Res* 6(4):170–178, 2004.
155. Wenten M et al: Associations of weight, weight change, and body mass with breast cancer risk in Hispanic and non-Hispanic white women, *Ann Epidemiol* 12(6):435–444, 2002.
156. Trentham-Diaz A et al: Weight change and risk of postmenopausal breast cancer (United States), *Cancer Causes Control* 11(6):533–542, 2000.
157. Le Marchand L et al: Body size at different periods of life and breast cancer risk, *Am J Epidemiol* 128(1):137–152, 1988.
158. Morimoto LM et al: Obesity, body size, and risk of postmenopausal breast cancer: the Women's Health Initiative (United States), *Cancer Causes Control* 13(8):741–751, 2002.
159. Endogenous Hormones Breast Cancer Collaborative Group: Body mass index, serum sex hormones, and breast cancer risk in postmenopausal women, *J Natl Cancer Inst* 95(6): 1218–1226, 2003.
160. Tretli S, Gaard M: Lifestyle changes during adolescence and risk of breast cancer: an ecologic study of the effect of World War II in Norway, *Cancer Causes Control* 7(5):507–512, 1996.
161. Mahabir S et al: Usefulness of body mass index as a sufficient adiposity measurement for sex hormone concentration associations in postmenopausal women, *Cancer Epidemiol Biomarkers Prev* 15(12):2502–2507, 2006.
162. Korner A et al: Total and high molecular weight adiponectin in breast cancer: in vitro and in vivo studies, *J Clin Endocrinol Metab* Dec 27, 2006. (Epub ahead of print.)
163. Surmacz E: Obesity hormone leptin: a new target in breast cancer? *Breast Cancer Res* 9(1):301, 2007.
164. Arditi JD et al: Antiproliferative effect of adiponectin on MCF7 breast cancer cells: a potential hormonal link between obesity and cancer, *Horm Metab Res* 39(1):9–13, 2007.
165. Merzenich H, Boeing H, Wahrendorf J: Dietary fat and sports activity as determinants of age at menarche, *Am J Epidemiol* 138(4):217–224, 1993.
166. Chen J, Campbell TC, Junyao L: Diet, lifestyle, and mortality in China: a study of the characteristics of 65 Chinese counties, Oxford, England, 1990, Oxford University Press.
167. Cho E et al: Premenopausal dietary carbohydrate, glycemic index, glycemic load, and fiber in relation to risk of breast cancer, Toronto, Canada, 2003, American Association for Cancer Research.
168. Terry P et al: No association among total dietary fiber, fiber-fractions, and risk of breast cancer, *Cancer Epidemiol Biomarkers Prev* 11(11):1507–1508, 2002.

References—Cont'd

169. Witte JS et al: Diet and premenopausal bilateral breast cancer: a case-control study, *Breast Cancer Res Treat* 42(3): 243–251, 1997.
170. Stampfer MJ, Bechtel SD, Hunter D: Fat, alcohol, selenium, and breast cancer risk, *Contemp Oncol* 3(7):28, 33–35, 1993.
171. Rohan TE et al: Dietary intake folate consumption and breast cancer risk, *J Natl Cancer Inst* 92(3):266–269, 2000.
172. Ginsburg ES et al: The effect of acute ethanol ingestion on estrogen levels in postmenopausal women using transdermal estradiol, *J Soc Gynecol Investig* 2(1):26–29, 1995.
173. Sellers TA et al: Dietary folate intake, alcohol, and risk of breast cancer in a prospective study of postmenopausal women, *Epidemiology* 12(4):420–428, 2001.
174. Zhang S et al: A prospective study of folate intake and the risk of breast cancer, *JAMA* 281(17):1632–1637, 1999.
175. Takada H et al: Inhibition of 7,12-dimethyl-benz(a)anthracene–induced lipid peroxidation and mammary tumor development in rats by vitamin E in conjunction with selenium, *Nutr Cancer* 17(2):115–122, 1992.
176. Willett WC et al: Relation of serum vitamins A and E and carotenoids to the risk of cancer, *N Engl J Med* 310(7): 430–434, 1983.
177. Verhoeven DT et al: Vitamins C and E, retinol, beta-carotene, and dietary fibre in relation to breast cancer risk: a prospective cohort study, *Br J Cancer* 75(1):149–155, 1997.
178. Wu K et al: A prospective study of plasma ascorbic acid concentrations and breast cancer (United States), *Cancer Causes Control* 11(3):279–283, 2000.
179. Ip C, Hayes C: Tissue selenium levels in selenium-supplemented rats and their relevance in mammary cancer protection, *Carcinogenesis* 10(5):921–925, 1989.
180. Cross HS et al: Phytoestrogens and vitamin D metabolism: a new concept for the prevention and therapy of colorectal, prostate, and mammary carcinomas, *J Nutr* 134(5): 1207S–1212S, 2004.
181. Krieger N et al: Breast cancer and serum organochlorines: a prospective study among white, black, and Asian women, *J Natl Cancer Inst* 86(8):589–599, 1994.
182. Petrakis NL et al: Stimulatory influence of soy protein isolate on breast secretion in pre- and postmenopausal women, *Cancer Epidemiol Biomarkers Prev* 5(10):785–794, 1996.
183. Ito T, Warnken SP, May WS: Protein synthesis inhibition of flavonoids: roles of eukaryotic initiation factor 2 alpha kinase, *Biochem Biophys Res Com* 265(2):3890, 1999.
184. Aceves C, Anguiano B, Delgado G: Is iodine a gatekeeper of the integrity of the mammary gland? *J Mammary Gland Biol Neoplasia* 10(2):189–196, 2005.
185. Funahashi H et al: Seaweed prevents breast cancer, *Jpn J Cance Res* 92(5):483–487, 2001.
186. Smyth PP: Role of iodine in antioxidant defense in thyroid and breast disease, *Biofactors* 19(3–4):121–130, 2003.
187. Friedenreich CM, Orenstein MR: Physical activity and cancer prevention: etiologic evidence and biological mechanisms, *J Nutr* 132(11 suppl):3464S–3465S, 2002.
188. Kaaks R, Lukanova A: Effects of weight control and physical activity in cancer prevention: role of endogenous hormone metabolism, *Ann N Y Acad Sci* 963:268–281, 2002.
189. Garber JE, Offit K: Hereditary cancer predisposition syndromes, *J Clin Oncol* 23(2):276–292, 2005.
190. Sprague BL et al: Lifetime recreational and occupational physical activity and risk of in situ and invasive breast cancer, *Cancer Epidemiol Biomarkers Prev* 16(2):236–243, 2007.
191. Sjöblom T et al: The consensus coding sequences of human breast and colorectal cancers. *Sciencexpress*; www.scienceexpress.org/7sept2006/pg1-7.
192. Newman B et al: Frequency of breast cancer attributable to BRCA1 in population-based series of American women, *JAMA* 279(12):915–921, 1998.
193. Miki Y et al: A strong candidate for the breast and ovarian cancer susceptibility gene BRCA1, *Science* 266(5182):66–71, 1994.
194. Sullivan A et al: Concomitant inactivation of p53 and ChK2 in breast cancer, *Oncogene* 21(9):1316–1324, 2002.
195. Weber F et al: Total-genome analysis of BRCA1/2-related invasive carcinomas of the breast identifies tumor stroma as potential landscaper for neoplastic initiation, *Am J Hum Genet* 78:961–972, 2006.
196. Russo IH, Calaf G, Russo J: Hormones and proliferative activity in breast tissue. In Stoll BA, editor: *Approaches to breast cancer prevention*, Dordrecht, Netherlands, 1991, Kluwer Academic.
197. Zhu BT, Conney AH: Is 2-methoxyestradiol an endogenous estrogen metabolite that inhibits mammary carcinogenesis? *Cancer Res* 58(11):2269–2277, 1998.
198. Russo J, Russo IH: The role of estrogen in the initiation of breast cancer, *J Steroid Biochem Mol Biol* 102(1–5):89–96, 2006.
199. Lester SC: The breast, In Kumar V, Abbas AK, Fausto N, editors: *Robbins & Cotran pathologic basis of disease*, ed 7, Philadelphia, 2005, Saunders.
200. Buerger H et al: Different genetic pathways in the evolution of invasive breast cancer are associated with distinct morphological subtypes, *J Pathol* 189(4):521–526, 1999.
201. Buerger H et al: Genetic characterisation of invasive breast cancer: a comparison of CGH and PCR based multiplex microsatellite analysis, *J Clin Pathol* 54(11):836–840, 2001.
202. Silverstein MJ, Baril NB: In situ carcinoma of the breast. In Donegan WL, Spratt JS, editors: *Cancer of the breast*, Philadelphia, 2002, Saunders.
203. Stratton MR, Wooster R: Hereditary predisposition to breast cancer, *Curr Opin Genet Dev* 6(1):93–97, 1996.
204. Centers for Disease Control: National surveillance data for chlamydia, gonorrhea, and syphilis, *Trends in reportable sexually transmitted diseases in the United States, 2004*; www.cdc.gov.std.stats.
205. Joura EA et al: Efficacy of a quadrivalent prophylactic human papillomavirus (types 6, 11, 16, and 18) L1 virus-like-particle vaccine against high-grade vulval and vaginal lesions: a combined analysis of three randomised clinical trials, *Lancet* 369(9574):1693–1927, 2007.
206. The FUTURE II Study Group: Quadrivalent vaccine against human papillomavirus to prevent high-grade cervical lesions, *N Engl J Med* 356(19):1915–1927, 2007.
207. Villa LL et al: Prophylactic quadrivalent human papillomavirus (types 6, 11, 16, and 18) L1 virus-like particle vaccine in young women: a randomised double-blind placebo-controlled multicentre phase II efficacy trial, *Lancet* 6(5): 271–278, 2005.

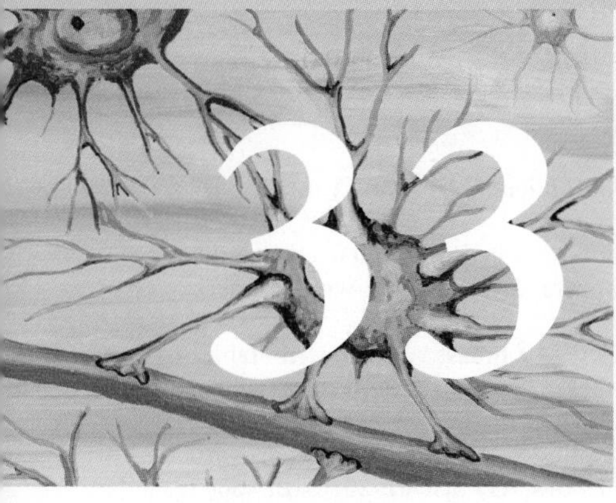

33 STRUCTURE AND FUNCTION OF THE DIGESTIVE SYSTEM

Sue E. Huether

CHAPTER OUTLINE

ELECTRONIC RESOURCES

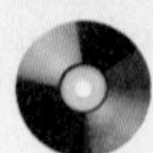

Companion CD
- Review Questions and Answers
- Animations

evolve Website
http://evolve.elsevier.com/Huether/
- Quick Check Answers
- Key Terms Exercises
- Critical Thinking Questions with Answers
- Algorithm Completion Exercises
- WebLinks

The digestive system breaks down ingested food, prepares it for uptake by the body's cells, provides body water, and eliminates wastes. This system consists of the gastrointestinal tract and accessory organs of digestion: the salivary glands, liver, gallbladder, and exocrine pancreas.

Food breakdown begins in the mouth with chewing and continues in the stomach, where food is churned and mixed with acid, mucus, enzymes, and other secretions. From the stomach, the fluid and partially digested food pass into the small intestine, where biochemical agents and enzymes secreted by the liver and exocrine pancreas break it down into absorbable components of proteins, carbohydrates, and fats. These nutrients pass through the walls of the small intestine into blood vessels and lymphatics that carry them to the liver for storage or further processing.

Ingested substances and secretions that are not absorbed in the small intestine pass into the large intestine, where fluid continues to be absorbed. Fluid wastes travel to the kidneys and are eliminated in the urine. Solid wastes pass into the rectum and are eliminated from the body through the anus.

Except for chewing, swallowing, and defecation of solid wastes, the movements of the digestive system (gastrointestinal motility) are all controlled by hormones and the autonomic nervous system. The autonomic innervation, both sympathetic and parasympathetic, is controlled by centers in the brain and by local stimuli that are mediated at plexuses (networks of nerve fibers) within the gastrointestinal walls.

THE GASTROINTESTINAL TRACT

The **alimentary canal,** or **gastrointestinal tract,** consists of the mouth, esophagus, stomach, small intestine, large intestine, rectum, and anus (Figure 33-1). It carries out the following digestive processes:

1. Ingestion of food
2. Propulsion of food and wastes from the mouth to the anus
3. Secretion of mucus, water, and enzymes
4. Mechanical digestion of food particles
5. Chemical digestion of food particles
6. Absorption of digested food
7. Elimination of waste products by defecation

Histologically, the gastrointestinal tract consists of four layers. From the inside out they are the mucosa, submucosa, muscularis, and serosa or adventitia. These concentric layers vary in thickness, and each layer has sublayers (Figure 33-2). A network of intrinsic nerves that controls mobility, secretion, sensation, and blood flow is located solely within the gastrointestinal tract and controlled by local and autonomic nervous system stimuli through the **enteric plexus** located in different layers of the gastrointestinal walls (see Figure 33-2).

Mouth and Esophagus

The **mouth** is a reservoir for the chewing and mixing of food with saliva. As food particles become smaller and move around in the mouth, the taste buds and olfactory nerves are continuously stimulated, adding to the satisfaction of eating. The tongue's surface contains thousands of

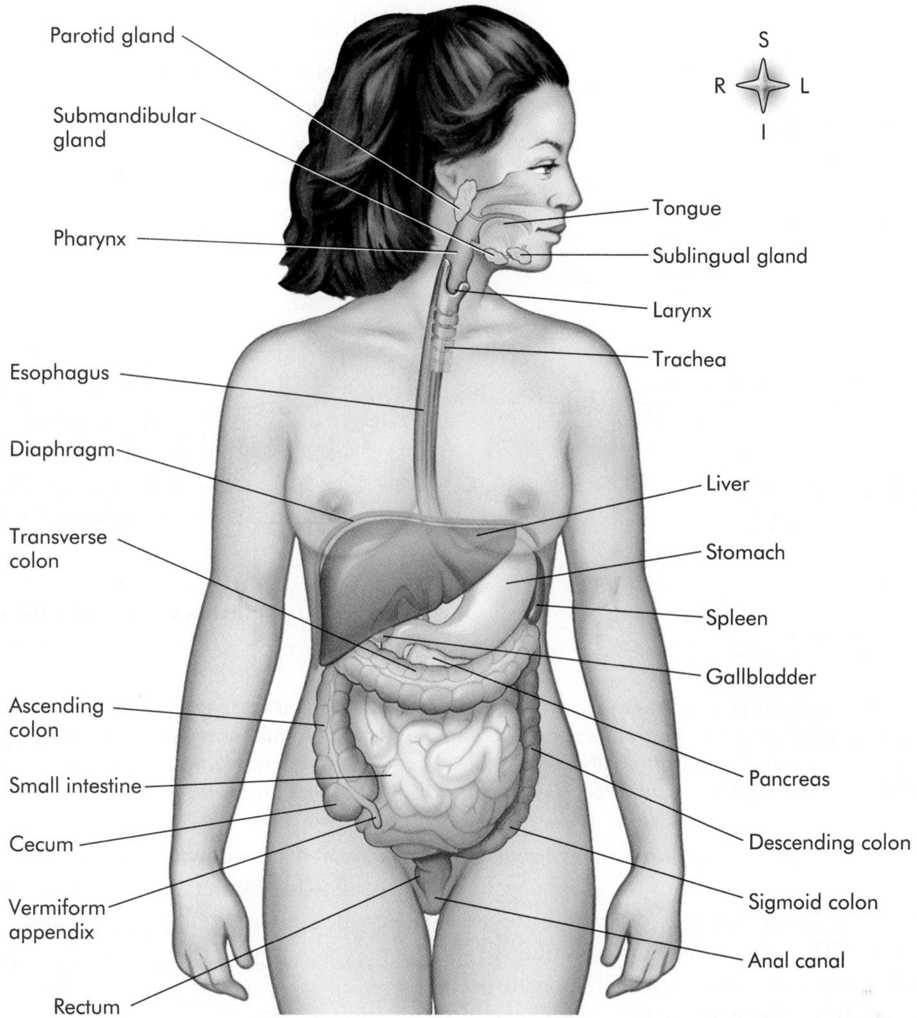

Figure 33-1 ■ **Structure and Function of the Digestive System.** Digestion begins in the mouth with chewing, which breaks down food mechanically and mixes it with saliva. Swallowing propels chewed food through the esophagus to the stomach, where acids and stomach motility liquefy it further. Next the liquefied food enters the small intestine, where secretions of the intestinal walls, liver, gallbladder, and pancreas digest it into absorbable nutrients. Nutrients are absorbed through intestinal walls, and unabsorbed wastes enter the large intestine (colon), where fluids are removed. Solid wastes then enter the rectum and leave the body through the anus. (From Thibodeau GA, Patton KT: *Anatomy & physiology,* ed 6, St Louis, 2007, Mosby.)

chemoreceptors, or taste buds, which can distinguish salty, sour, bitter, and sweet tastes. Tastes and food odors help to initiate salivation and the secretion of gastric juice in the stomach. There are 32 permanent teeth in the adult mouth, and they are important for speech and mastication.

Salivation

The three pairs of **salivary glands**—the submandibular, sublingual, and parotid glands (Figure 33-3)—secrete about 1 L of saliva per day. **Saliva** consists mostly of water with mucus, sodium, bicarbonate, chloride, potassium, and **salivary α-amylase (ptyalin),** an enzyme that initiates carbohydrate digestion in the mouth and stomach.

Both sympathetic and parasympathetic divisions of the autonomic nervous system control salivation. Cholinergic parasympathetic fibers stimulate the salivary glands, and atropine (an anticholinergic agent) inhibits salivation and makes the mouth dry. β-Adrenergic stimulation from sympathetic fibers also increases salivary secretion. The salivary glands are not regulated by hormones.

The composition of saliva depends on the rate of secretion (Figure 33-4). Aldosterone can increase an exchange of sodium for potassium, increasing sodium conservation and potassium excretion. The bicarbonate concentration of saliva sustains a pH of about 7.4, which neutralizes bacterial acids and prevents tooth decay. Saliva also contains immunoglobulin A (IgA) and other antimicrobial substances, which helps prevent infection. Exogenous fluoride (e.g., fluoride in drinking water) is also secreted in the saliva, providing additional protection against tooth decay.

Swallowing

The **esophagus** is a hollow, muscular tube approximately 25 cm long that conducts substances from the oropharynx to the stomach (see Figure 33-1). Swallowed food is moved to the stomach by **peristalsis,** the coordinated sequential

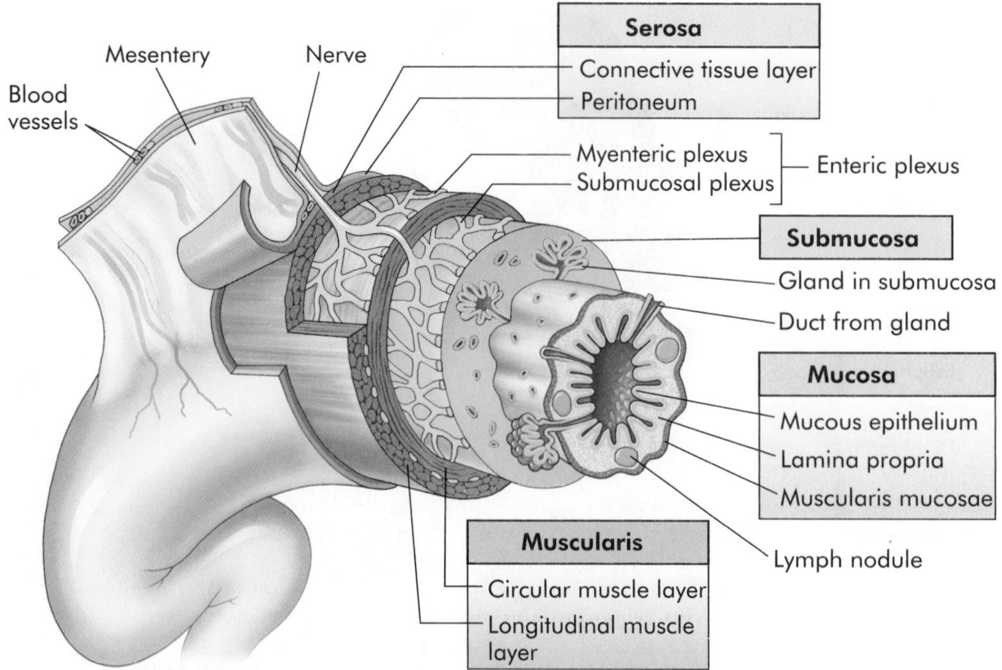

Figure 33-2 ■ **Wall of the Gastrointestinal Tract.** The wall of the gastrointestinal tract is made up of four layers with a network of nerves between the layers. This generalized diagram shows a segment of the gastrointestinal tract. Note that the serosa is continuous with a fold of serous membrane called a *mesentery.* Note also that digestive glands may empty their products into the lumen of the gastrointestinal tract by way of ducts. (From Thibodeau GA, Patton KT: *Anatomy & physiology,* ed 6, St Louis, 2007, Mosby.)

contraction and relaxation of outer longitudinal and inner circular layers of muscles. The upper third of the esophagus contains striated muscle (voluntary) that is directly innervated by motor neurons. The lower two thirds contains smooth muscle (involuntary) that is innervated by preganglionic cholinergic fibers from the vagus nerve. The fibers are activated in a downward sequence and coordinated by the swallowing center in the medulla. Peristalsis is stimulated when afferent fibers distributed along the length of

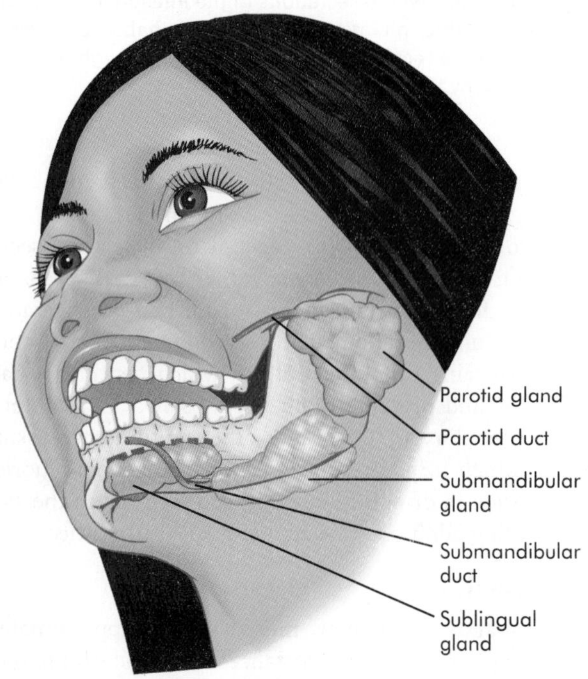

Figure 33-3 ■ **Salivary Glands.** (From Thibodeau GA, Patton KT: *Anatomy & physiology,* ed 6, St Louis, 2007, Mosby.)

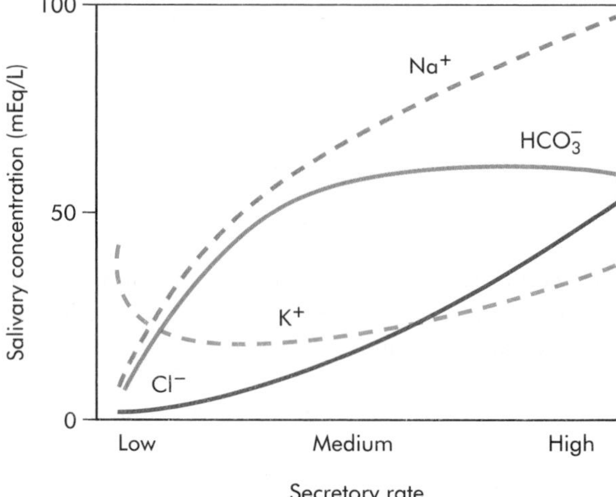

Figure 33-4 ■ **Salivary Electrolyte Concentrations and Flow Rate.** Changes in concentration of sodium (Na^+), potassium (K^+), chloride (Cl^-), and bicarbonate (HCO_3^-) increases in flow rate of saliva. *Green line,* sodium; *orange line,* bicarbonate; *red line,* chloride; *blue line,* potassium. At low rates of salivary flow (i.e., between meals), sodium, chloride, and bicarbonate are reabsorbed in the collecting ducts of the salivary glands, and the saliva contains fewer of these electrolytes (i.e., is more hypotonic). At higher flow rates (i.e., stimulated by food), reabsorption decreases and saliva is hypertonic. By this mechanism, sodium, chloride, and bicarbonate are recycled until they are released to help with digestion and absorption.

the esophagus sense changes in wall tension caused by stretching as food passes. The greater the tension, the greater the intensity of esophageal contraction. Occasionally, intense contractions cause pain similar to "heartburn" or angina.

Each end of the esophagus is opened and closed by a sphincter. The **upper esophageal sphincter** keeps air from entering the esophagus during respiration. The **lower esophageal sphincter (cardiac sphincter)** prevents regurgitation from the stomach and caustic injury to the esophagus.

Swallowing is coordinated primarily by the swallowing center in the medulla. During the **oropharyngeal (voluntary) phase,** the following steps occur:

1. Food is segmented into a bolus by the tongue and forced posteriorly toward the pharynx.
2. The superior constrictor muscle of the pharynx contracts so the food cannot move into the nasopharynx.
3. Respiration is inhibited, and the epiglottis slides down to prevent the food from entering the larynx and trachea.

This entire sequence takes place in less than 1 second.

The **esophageal phase** proceeds as follows:

1. The bolus of food enters the esophagus.
2. Waves of relaxation travel the esophagus, preparing for the movement of the bolus.
3. Peristalsis, the sequential waves of muscular contractions that travel down the esophagus, transport the food to the lower esophageal sphincter, which is relaxed at that point.
4. The bolus enters the stomach, and the sphincter muscles return to their resting tone.

This phase takes 5 to 10 seconds, with the bolus moving 2 to 6 cm/sec.

Peristalsis that immediately follows the oropharyngeal phase of swallowing is called **primary peristalsis.** If a bolus of food becomes stuck in the esophageal lumen, **secondary peristalsis**—a wave of contraction and relaxation independent of voluntary swallowing—occurs. This is in response to stretch receptors stimulated by increased wall tension, which increase impulses from the swallowing center of the brain.

The lower esophageal sphincter is normally constricted and serves as a barrier between the stomach and esophagus. The muscle tone of the lower sphincter changes with neural and hormonal stimulation and relaxes with swallowing. Cholinergic vagal input and the digestive hormone gastrin increase sphincter tone. Nonadrenergic, noncholinergic vagal impulses relax the lower esophageal sphincter, as do the hormones progesterone, secretin, and glucagon.[1]

QUICK CHECK 33-1

1. Describe the layers of the walls of the gastrointestinal tract.
2. What are the major functions of the gastrointestinal tract? How are they controlled?
3. What are the functions of the upper and lower esophageal sphincters?

Stomach

The **stomach** is a hollow, muscular organ just below the diaphragm that stores food during eating, secretes digestive juices, mixes food with these juices, and propels partially digested food, called **chyme,** into the duodenum of the small intestine. The anatomy of the stomach is presented in Figure 33-5. Its major anatomic boundaries are the lower esophageal sphincter, where food passes through the **cardiac orifice** into the stomach; the greater and lesser

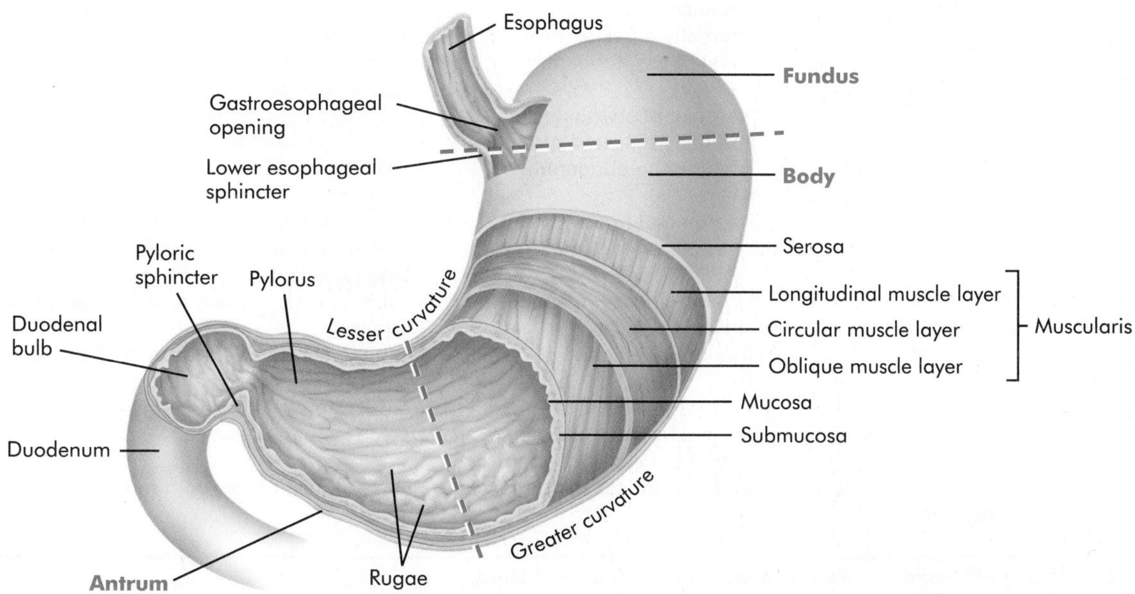

Figure 33-5 ■ **Stomach.** A portion of the anterior wall has been cut away to reveal the muscle layers of the stomach wall. Note that the mucosa lining the stomach forms folds called *rugae.* The dotted lines distinguish the fundus, body, and antrum of the stomach. (Modified from Thibodeau GA, Patton KT: *Anatomy & physiology,* ed 6, St Louis, 2007, Mosby.)

curvatures; and the **pyloric sphincter,** which relaxes as food is propelled through the **pylorus (gastroduodenal junction)** into the duodenum. Functional areas are the **fundus** (upper portion), **body** (middle portion), and **antrum** (lower portion).

The tunica muscularis has a circular muscle layer and a longitudinal layer (see Figure 33-5). The oblique muscle of the stomach wall is the most prominent and lies between the submucosa and the circular muscle layer. These layers become progressively thicker in the body and antrum. The glandular epithelium is discussed in the section about secretory functions of the stomach (see p. 917).

The stomach's blood supply is so abundant that nearly all arterial vessels must be occluded before ischemic changes occur in the stomach wall. The splenic vein drains the right side of the stomach, and the gastric vein drains the left side.

Sympathetic and parasympathetic divisions of the autonomic nervous system innervate the stomach. Some of the autonomic fibers are extrinsic—that is, they originate outside the stomach and are controlled by nerve centers in the brain. Others are intrinsic: they originate within the stomach and also respond to local stimuli. Extrinsic sympathetic fibers reach the stomach through the celiac plexus (solar plexus), whereas extrinsic parasympathetic fibers enter through the gastric branch of the vagus nerve.

Gastric motility

In its resting state, the stomach is small and contains about 50 ml fluid. There is no wall tension, and the muscle layers in the fundus contract very little. Swallowing causes the fundus to relax (receptive relaxation) to receive a bolus of food from the esophagus. Relaxation is coordinated by efferent, nonadrenergic, noncholinergic vagal fibers and is facilitated by **gastrin** and **cholecystokinin**—two polypeptide hormones secreted by the gastrointestinal mucosa. (The actions of digestive hormones are summarized in Table 33-1.) Food is stored in vertical or oblique layers as it arrives in the fundus, whereas fluids flow relatively quickly down to the antrum.

Gastric (stomach) motility increases with the initiation of peristaltic waves, which sweep over the body of the

TABLE 33-1

Selected Hormones and Neurotransmitters of the Digestive System

Source	Hormone	Stimulus for Secretion	Action
Mucosa of the stomach	Gastrin	Presence of partially digested proteins in the stomach	Stimulates gastric glands to secrete hydrochloric acid and pepsinogen; growth of gastric mucosa
	Histamine	Gastrin	Stimulates acid secretion
	Somatostatin	Acid in the stomach	Inhibits acid and pepsinogen secretion and release of gastrin
	Acetylcholine	Vagus and local nerves in stomach	Stimulates release of pepsinogen and acid secretion
	Gastrin-releasing peptide (bombesin)	Vagus and local nerves in stomach	Stimulates release of pepsinogen and acid secretion
Mucosa of the small intestine	Motilin	Presence of acid and fat in the duodenum	Increases gastrointestinal motility
	Secretin	Presence of chyme (acid, partially digested proteins, fats) in the duodenum	Stimulates pancreas to secrete alkaline pancreatic juice and liver to secrete bile; decreases gastrointestinal motility; inhibits gastrin and gastric acid secretion
	Cholecystokinin	Presence of chyme (acid, partially digested proteins, fats) in the duodenum	Stimulates gallbladder to eject bile and pancreas to secrete alkaline fluid; decreases gastric motility; constricts pyloric sphincter; inhibits gastrin
	Enteroglucagon	Intraluminal fats and carbohydrates	Weakly inhibits gastric and pancreatic secretion and enhances insulin release, lipolysis, ketogenesis, and glycogenolysis
	Gastric inhibitory peptide (GIP)	Fat and glucose in small intestine	Inhibits gastric secretion, stimulates insulin release
	Peptide YY	Intraluminal fat and bile acids	Inhibits postprandial gastric acid and pancreatic secretion and delays gastric and small bowel emptying
	Pancreatic polypeptide	Protein, fat, and glucose in small intestine	Decreases pancreatic HCO_3^- and enzyme secretion
	Vasoactive intestinal peptide	Intestinal mucosa and muscle	Relaxes intestinal smooth muscle

Modified from Johnson LR: *Gastrointestinal physiology,* ed 7, St Louis, 2007, Mosby.
Additional data from Rehfeld JF: *Horm Metab Res* 36(11–12):735–741, 2004; Small CJ, Bloom SR: *Trends Endocrinol Metab* 5(6):259–263, 2004; Druce MR, Bloom SR: *Endocrinology* 145(6):2660–2665, 2004.
NOTE: The digestive hormones are not secreted into the gastrointestinal lumen but rather into the bloodstream, in which they travel to target tissues. There are more than 30 peptide hormone genes expressed in the gastrointestinal tract and more than 100 hormonally active peptides.

stomach toward the antrum. The rate of peristaltic contractions is approximately three per minute and is influenced by neural and hormonal activity. Gastrin, **motilin** (an intestinal hormone), and the vagus nerve increase contraction by lowering the threshold potential of muscle fibers. (The neural and biochemical mechanisms of muscle contraction are described in Chapter 36. Sympathetic activity and **secretin** (another intestinal hormone) are inhibitory and raise the threshold potential. The rate of peristalsis is mediated by pacemaker cells that initiate a wave of depolarization (basic electrical rhythm), which moves from the upper part of the stomach to the pylorus.

The mixing and emptying of food (chyme) from the stomach take several hours. Mixing occurs as food is propelled toward the antrum. As food approaches the pylorus, the velocity of the peristaltic wave increases. This forces the contents back toward the body of the stomach. This **retropulsion** effectively mixes food with digestive juices, and the oscillating motion breaks down large food particles. With each peristaltic wave, a small portion of the gastric contents (chyme) passes through the pylorus and into the duodenum. The pylorus is about 1.5 cm long and is always open about 2.0 mm. It opens wider during antral contraction. Normally there is no regurgitation from the duodenum into the antrum.

The rate of **gastric emptying** (movement of gastric contents into the duodenum) depends on the volume, osmotic pressure, and chemical composition of the gastric contents. Larger volumes of food increase gastric pressure, peristalsis, and rate of emptying. Solids, fats, and nonisotonic solutions delay gastric emptying. (Osmotic pressure and tonicity are described in Chapters 1 and 4.) Products of fat digestion, which are formed in the duodenum by the action of bile from the liver and enzymes from the pancreas, stimulate the secretion of cholecystokinin. This hormone inhibits gastric motility and decreases gastric emptying so that fats are not emptied into the duodenum at a rate that exceeds the rate of bile and enzyme secretion. Osmoreceptors in the wall of the duodenum are sensitive to the osmotic pressure of duodenal contents. The arrival of hypertonic or hypotonic gastric contents activates the osmoreceptors, which delay gastric emptying to facilitate formation of an isosmotic duodenal environment. The rate at which acid enters the duodenum also influences gastric emptying. Secretions from the pancreas, liver, and duodenal mucosa neutralize gastric acid in the duodenum. The rate of emptying is adjusted to the duodenum's ability to neutralize the incoming acidity.[2]

Gastric secretion

Stimulated by eating, the stomach secretes large volumes of gastric juices or gastric secretions, including mucus, acid, enzymes, hormones, intrinsic factor, and gastroferrin. Intrinsic factor is necessary for the intestinal absorption of vitamin B_{12}, and gastroferrin facilitates small intestinal absorption of iron. The hormones are secreted into the blood and travel to target tissues in the bloodstream. The other gastric secretions are released directly into the stomach lumen.

In the fundus and body of the stomach, the **gastric glands** of the mucosa are the primary secretory units (Figure 33-6). The composition of gastric juice depends on volume and flow rate (Figure 33-7). Potassium remains relatively constant, but its concentration is greater in gastric juice than in plasma. The rate of secretion varies with the time of day. Generally, the rate and volume of secretion are lowest in the morning and highest in the afternoon and evening. Loss of gastric juices through vomiting, drainage, or suction may decrease body stores of sodium and potassium.

Gastric secretion is inhibited by unpleasant odors and tastes and by rage, fear, or pain. A discharge of sympathetic impulses inhibits parasympathetic impulses. Increased secretions are associated with aggression or hostility and may contribute to some forms of gastric pathology.

Acid

The major functions of gastric acid are to dissolve food fibers, act as a bactericide against swallowed microorganisms, and convert pepsinogen to pepsin. The production of acid by the parietal cells requires the transport of hydrogen and chloride from the parietal cells to the stomach lumen. Acid is formed in the parietal cells, primarily through the hydrolysis of water (Figure 33-8). At a high

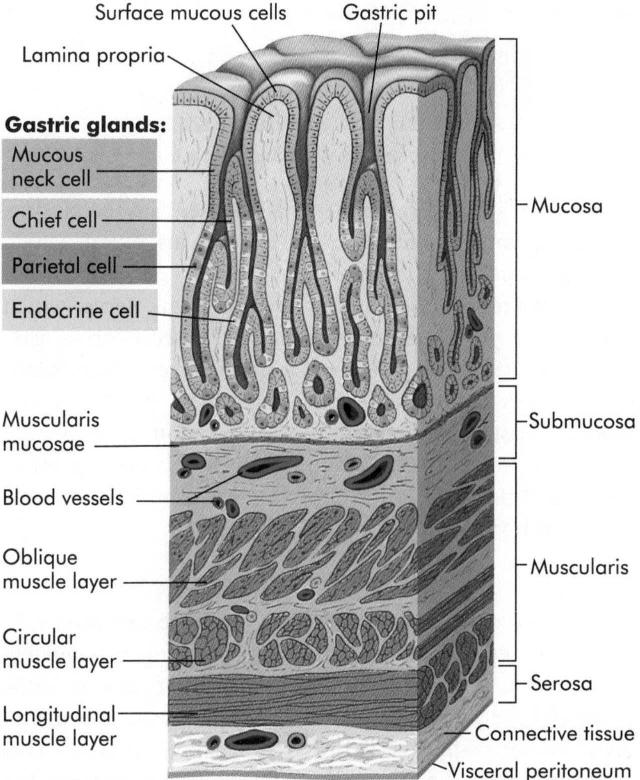

Figure 33-6 ■ **Gastric Pits and Gastric Glands.** Gastric pits are depressions in the epithelial lining of the stomach. At the bottom of each pit is one or more tubular *gastric glands.* Chief cells produce the enzymes of gastric juice (such as pepsinogen), parietal cells produce stomach acid, and G cells produce the hormone gastrin. (From Thibodeau GA, Patton KT: *Anatomy & physiology,* ed 6, St Louis, 2007, Mosby.)

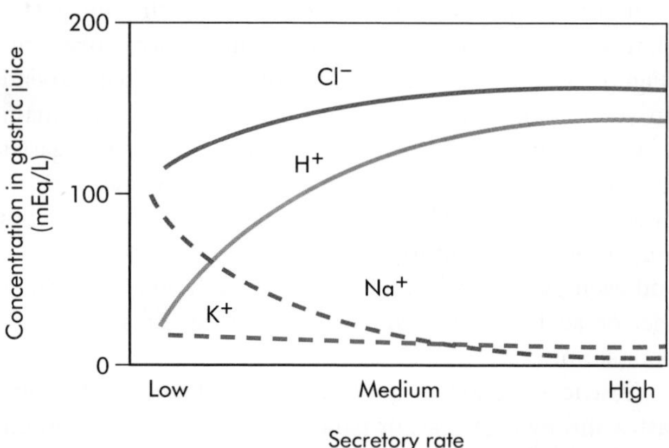

Figure 33-7 ■ Relationship Between Secretory Rate and Electrolyte Composition of the Gastric Juice. Sodium (Na^+) concentration is lower in the gastric juice than in the plasma, whereas hydrogen (H^+), potassium (K^+), and chloride (Cl^-) concentrations are higher. *Red line,* chloride; *orange line,* hydrogen; *green line,* sodium; *blue line,* potassium.

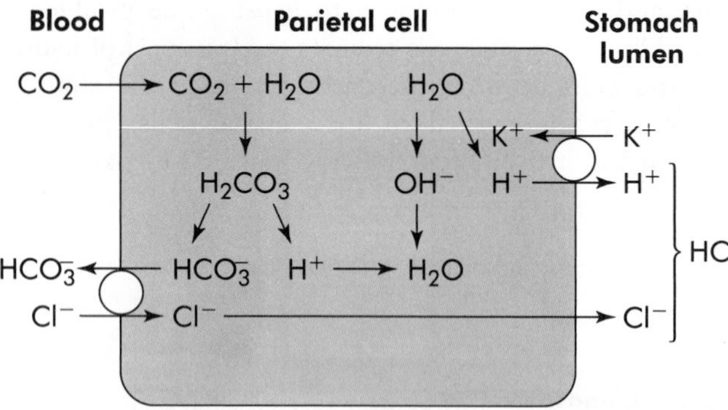

Figure 33-8 ■ Hydrochloric Acid Secretion by Parietal Cell.

rate of gastric secretion, bicarbonate moves into the plasma, producing an "alkaline tide" in the venous blood, which also may result in a more alkaline urine.[3]

Acid secretion is stimulated by the vagus nerve, which releases acetylcholine and stimulates the secretion of gastrin, which stimulates release of histamine from enterochromaffin cells (mast cells; see Chapter 5) in the gastric mucosa. Histamine stimulates acid secretion by activating histamine receptors (H_2 receptors) on acid secreting parietal cells. Acid secretion is inhibited by secretin and other intestinal hormones.[4]

Pepsin

Acetylcholine, gastrin, and secretin stimulate the **chief cells** to release pepsinogen during eating. Pepsinogen is quickly converted to **pepsin** in the acid gastric environment (optimum pH for pepsin activation = 2.0). Pepsin is a proteolytic enzyme—that is, it breaks down protein and forms polypeptides in the stomach. Once chyme has entered the duodenum, the alkaline environment of the duodenum inactivates pepsin.

Mucus

The gastric mucosa is protected from the digestive actions of acid and pepsin by a coating of mucus called the **mucosal barrier.** The quality and quantity of mucus and the tight junctions between epithelial cells make gastric mucosa relatively impermeable to acid. Prostaglandins protect the mucosal barrier by stimulating the secretion of mucus and bicarbonate and by inhibiting secretion of acid. Mucosal blood flow is important to maintaining mucosal protective functions. A break in the protective barrier may occur because of exposure to *Helicobacter pylori,* aspirin, ethanol, regurgitated bile, or ischemia. Breaks cause inflammation and ulceration.

Phases of gastric secretion

The secretion of gastric juice is influenced by numerous stimuli that together facilitate the process of digestion. The phases of gastric secretion are the *cephalic phase* (stimulated by the thought, smell, and taste of food), the *gastric phase* (stimulated by distention of the stomach), and the *intestinal phase* (stimulated by histamine and digested protein). All phases promote the secretion of acid by the stomach.

QUICK CHECK 33-2

1. Why are there three layers of stomach muscle?
2. What hormones are involved in gastric motility?
3. What are the phases of gastric secretion?

Small Intestine

The **small intestine** is about 5 to 6 meters long and is functionally divided into three segments: the **duodenum, jejunum,** and **ileum** (Figure 33-9). The duodenum begins at the pylorus and ends where it joins the jejunum at a suspensory ligament called the *Treitz ligament.* The end of the jejunum and beginning of the ileum are not distinguished by an anatomic marker. These structures are not grossly different, but the jejunum has a slightly larger lumen. The **ileocecal valve,** or **sphincter,** controls the flow of digested material from the ileum into the large intestine and prevents reflux into the small intestine.[5]

The **peritoneum** is the serous membrane surrounding the organs of the abdomen and pelvic cavity. It is analogous to the pericardium and pleura, which surround the heart and lungs, respectively. The visceral peritoneum lies over the organs, and the parietal peritoneum lines the wall of the abdominal cavity. The space between these two layers is called the **peritoneal cavity** and normally contains just enough fluid to lubricate the two layers and prevent friction during organ movement.

The duodenum lies behind the peritoneum, or retroperitoneally, and is attached to the posterior abdominal wall. The ileum and jejunum are suspended in loose folds from the posterior abdominal wall by a peritoneal membrane called the **mesentery.** The mesentery facilitates intestinal motility and supports blood vessels, nerves, and lymphatics.

The arterial supply to the duodenum arises primarily from the gastroduodenal artery. The jejunum and ileum

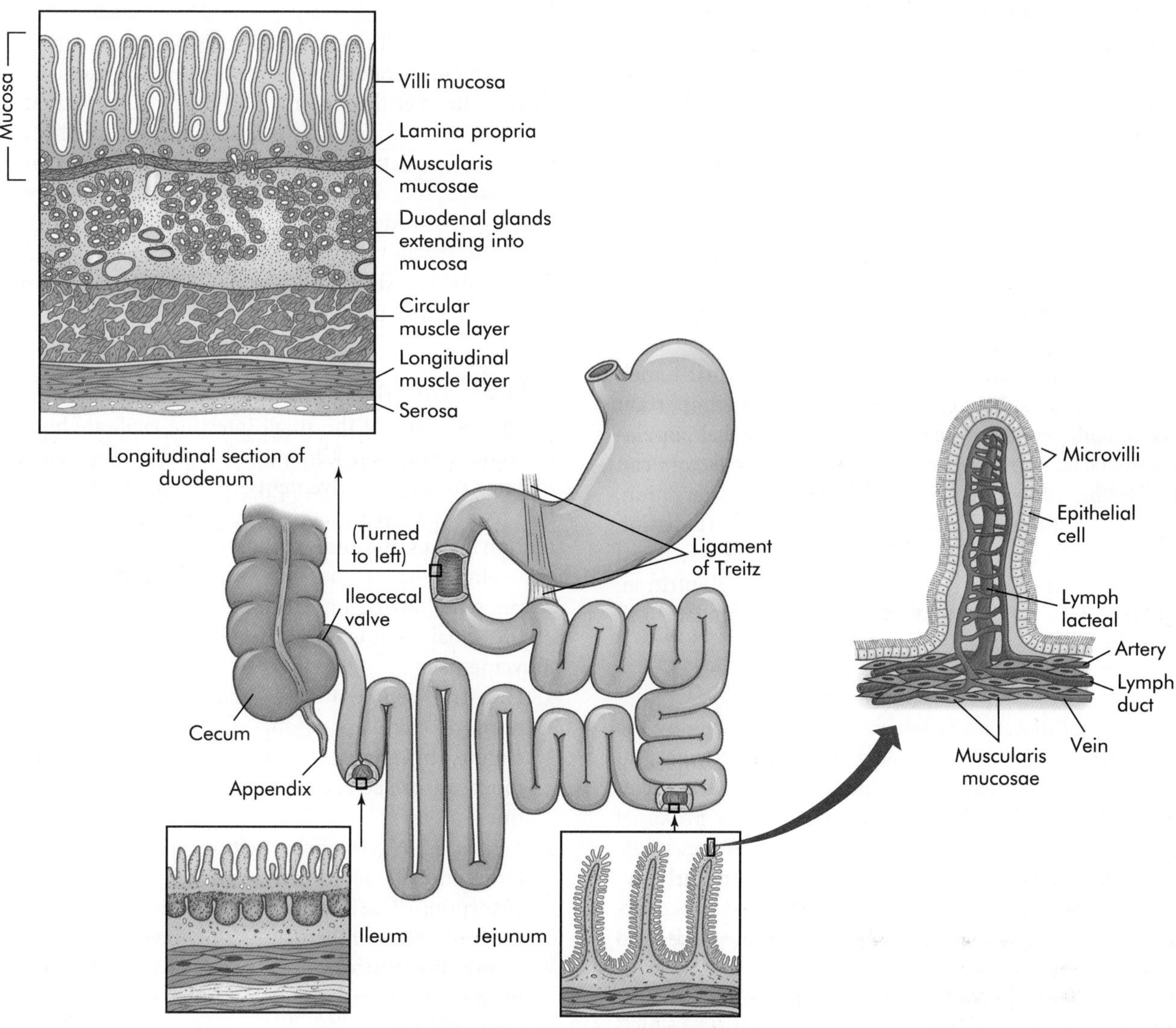

Figure 33-9 ■ **The Small Intestine.**

are supplied by branches of the superior mesenteric artery. The superior mesenteric vein joins the splenic vein and empties into the portal circulation to the liver. The regional lymph nodes and lymphatics drain into the thoracic duct. Both divisions of the autonomic nervous system innervate the small intestine. Secretion, motility, pain sensation, and intestinal reflexes (e.g., relaxation of the lower esophageal sphincter) are mediated by parasympathetic nerves. Sympathetic activity inhibits motility and produces vasoconstriction. Intrinsic motor innervation is mediated by the **myenteric plexus (Auerbach plexus)** and the **submucosal plexus (Meissner plexus).**

The smooth muscles of the small intestine are arranged in two layers: a longitudinal outer layer and a thicker inner circular layer (see Figure 33-9). Mucosal folds (plica) within the small intestine slow the passage of food, thereby providing more time for digestion and absorption. The folds are most numerous and prominent in the jejunum and upper ileum (see Figure 33-9).

Absorption occurs through **villi** (*sing.*, **villus**), which cover the mucosal folds and are the functional units of the intestine. Each villus (see Figure 33-9) secretes some of the enzymes necessary for digestion and absorbs nutrients. A villus is composed of absorptive columnar cells and mucus-secreting goblet cells of the mucosal epithelium. Near the surface, columnar cells closely adhere to each other at sites called *tight junctions.* Water and electrolytes are absorbed through these intercellular spaces. The surface of each columnar epithelial cell contains tiny projections called **microvilli** (*sing.*, **microvillus**) (see Figure 33-9). Together the microvilli create a mucosal surface known as the **brush border.** The villi and microvilli greatly increase the surface area available for absorption. Coating the brush border is an "unstirred" layer of fluid that is important for the absorption of substances other than water and electrolytes. The **lamina propria** (a connective tissue layer of the mucous membrane) lies beneath the epithelial cells of the villi and contains lymphocytes; plasma cells, which produce immunoglobulins; and macrophages.

Central arterioles ascend within each villus and branch into a capillary array that extends around the base of the columnar cells and cascades down to the venules that lead to the portal circulation (see Figure 33-9). A central **lacteal,** or lymphatic channel, is also contained within each villus and is important for the absorption and transport of fat molecules. Contents of the lacteals flow to regional nodes and channels that eventually drain into the thoracic duct.[6]

Between the bases of the villi are the crypts of Lieberkühn, which extend to the submucosal layer. Undifferentiated and secretory cells are located there. The undifferentiated cells arise from the base of the crypt and move toward the tip of the villus, maturing in shape and function as they progress. After becoming columnar cells and completing their migration to the tip of the villus, they function for a few days and then are sloughed into the intestinal lumen and digested. Sloughed epithelial cells are an important source of endogenous protein. The entire epithelial population is replaced about every 4 to 7 days. Many factors can influence this process of cellular proliferation. Starvation, vitamin B_{12} deficiency, and cytotoxic drugs or irradiation suppress cell division and shorten the villi. The decreased absorption that results can cause diarrhea and malnutrition. Nutrient intake and intestinal resection stimulate cell production.

Intestinal digestion and absorption

The process of digestion is initiated in the stomach by the actions of hydrochloric acid and pepsin. The chyme that passes into the duodenum is a liquid with small particles of undigested food. Digestion continues in the proximal portion of the small intestine by the action of pancreatic enzymes, intestinal enzymes, and bile salts. There carbohydrates are broken down to monosaccharides and disaccharides; proteins are degraded further to amino acids and peptides; and fats are emulsified and reduced to fatty acids (Box 33-1) and monoglycerides (Figure 33-10). These nutrients, along with water, vitamins, and electrolytes, are absorbed across the intestinal mucosa by active transport, diffusion, or facilitated diffusion. Products of carbohydrate and protein breakdown move into villus capillaries and then to the liver through the portal vein. Digested fats move into the lacteals and eventually reach the liver through the systemic circulation. Intestinal motility exposes nutrients to a large mucosal surface area by mixing chyme and moving it through the lumen. Different segments of the gastrointestinal tract absorb different nutrients. Sites of absorption are shown in Figure 33-11. Box 33-2 outlines the major nutrients involved in this process.

Intestinal motility

The movements of the small intestine facilitate both digestion and absorption. Chyme coming from the stomach stimulates intestinal movements that mix in secretions from the liver, pancreas, and intestinal glands. A churning motion brings the luminal contents into contact with the absorbing cells of the villi. Propulsive movements then advance the chyme toward the large intestine.

Intestinal motility is affected by the following two movements:

1. **Haustral segmentation.** Localized rhythmic contractions of circular smooth muscles divide and mix the chyme, bringing it into contact with the absorbent mucosal surface and propelling it toward the large intestine.
2. *Peristalsis.* Waves of contraction along short segments of longitudinal smooth muscle allow time for digestion and absorption. The intestinal villi move with contractions of the muscularis mucosae, a thin layer of muscle separating the mucosa and submucosa, with absorption promoted by the swaying of the villi in the luminal contents.

BOX 33-1 Dietary Fat

Saturated Fatty Acids (Palmitic Acid [$C_{16}H_{32}O_2$])

Each carbon atom in the chain is linked by single bonds to adjacent carbon and hydrogen atoms:

1. Solid at room temperatures; include animal fat and tropical oils (coconut and palm oil).
2. Increase low-density lipoprotein (LDL) cholesterol ("bad" cholesterol) blood levels.
3. Increase the risk of coronary artery disease.

Unsaturated Fatty Acids

Soft or liquid at room temperature; omega-6 fatty acids found in plants and vegetables (olive, canola, and peanut oils); omega-3 fatty acids found in fish and shellfish.

Monounsaturated Fatty Acids (Oleic Acid [$C_{18}H_{34}O_2$])

Contain one double bond in the carbon chain:

1. Found in both plants and animals.
2. May be beneficial in reducing blood cholesterol, glucose levels, and systolic blood pressure.
3. Do not lower high-density lipoprotein (HDL) cholesterol ("good" cholesterol) level.
4. Low HDL levels have been associated with coronary heart disease.

Polyunsaturated Fatty Acids (Linoleic Acid [$C_{18}H_{32}O_2$])

Contain two or more double bonds in the carbon chain:

1. Found in plants and fish oils.
2. Omega-6 fatty acids lower total and LDL cholesterol blood levels.
3. High levels of polyunsaturated fatty acids may lower LDL; omega-3 fatty acids lower blood triglyceride levels and reduce platelet aggregation and reduce blood-clotting tendency.
4. Necessary for growth and development and may prevent coronary artery disease, hypertension, inflammatory and immune disorders.

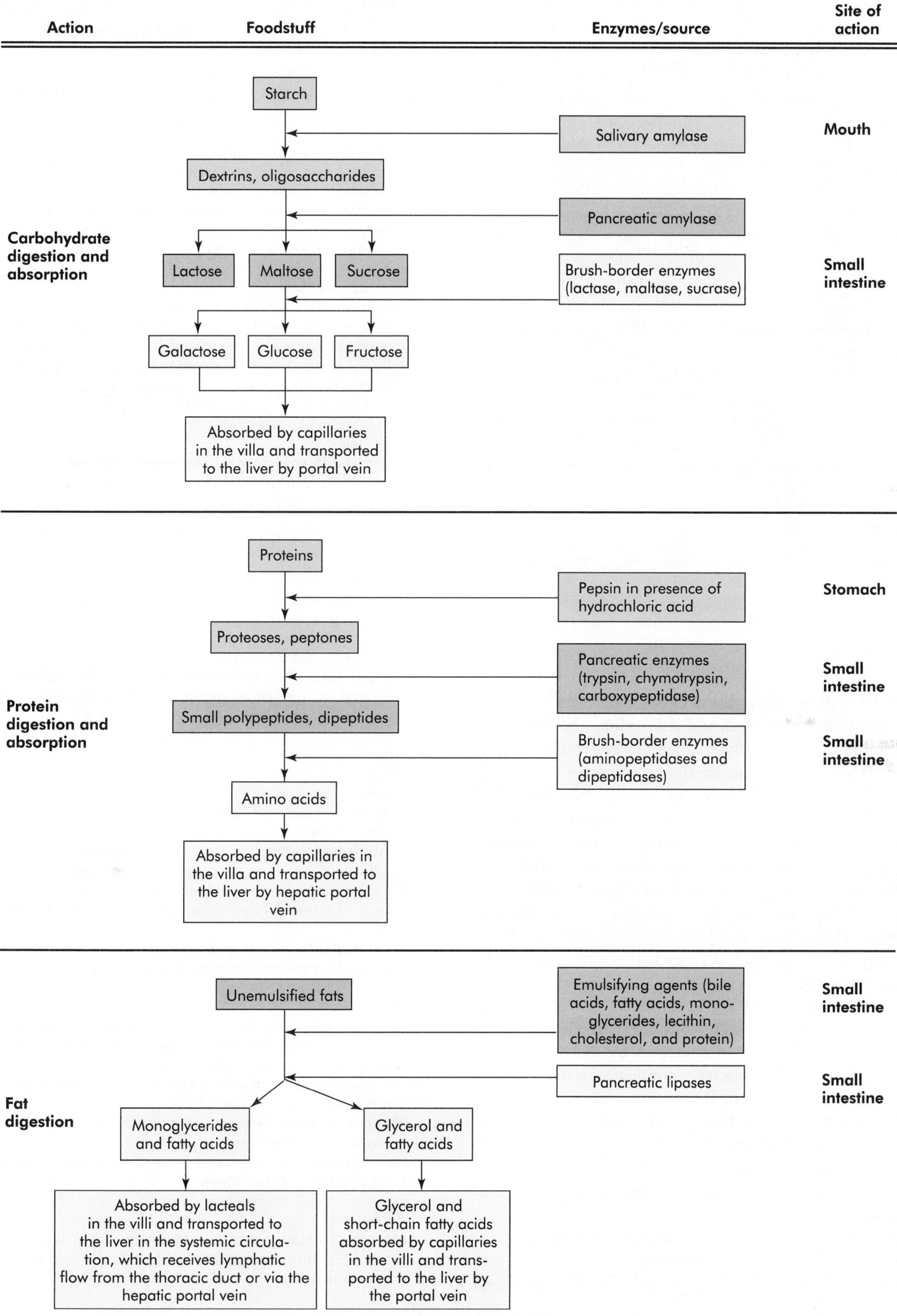

Figure 33-10 ■ **Digestion and Absorption of Foodstuffs.**

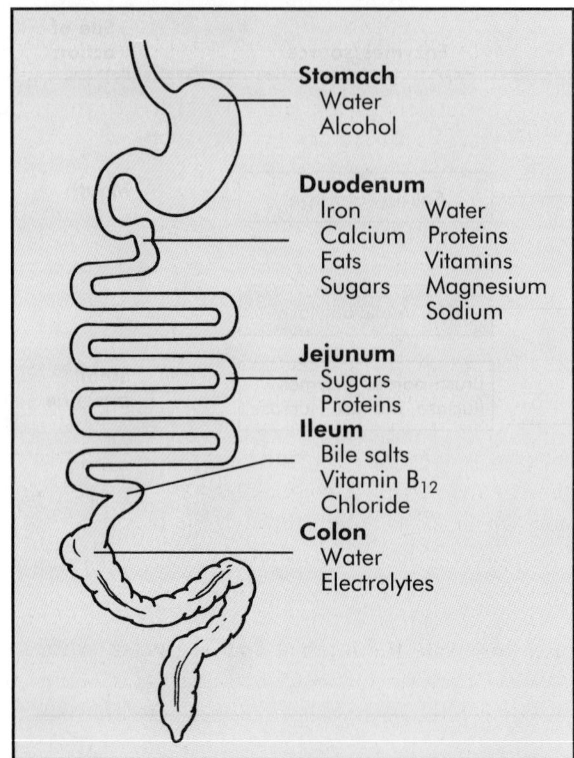

Figure 33-11 ■ **Sites of Absorption of Major Nutrients.**

Neural reflexes along the length of the small intestine facilitate motility, digestion, and absorption. The **ileogastric reflex** inhibits gastric motility when the ileum becomes distended. This prevents the continued movement of chyme into an already distended intestine. The **intestinointestinal reflex** inhibits intestinal motility when one part of the intestine is overdistended. Both of these reflexes require extrinsic innervation. The **gastroileal reflex,** which is activated by an increase in gastric motility and secretion, stimulates an increase in ileal motility and relaxation of the ileocecal sphincter. This empties the ileum and prepares it to receive more chyme. The gastroileal reflex is probably regulated by the hormone gastrin.

During prolonged fasting or between meals, particularly overnight, slow waves sweep along the entire length of the intestinal tract from the stomach to the terminal ileum. This interdigestive myoelectric complex appears to propel residual gastric and intestinal contents into the colon.

The ileocecal valve (sphincter) marks the junction between the terminal ileum and the large intestine. This valve is intrinsically regulated and is normally closed. The arrival of peristaltic waves from the last few centimeters of the ileum causes the ileocecal valve to open, allowing a small amount of chyme to pass through. Distention of the upper large intestine causes the sphincter to constrict, preventing further distention or retrograde flow of intestinal contents.

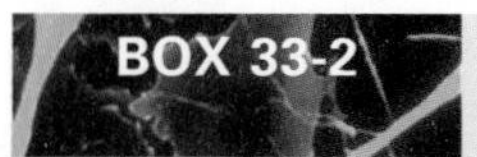

BOX 33-2 Major Nutrients Absorbed in the Small Intestine

Water and Electrolytes

Approximately 85% to 90% of the water that enters the gastrointestinal tract is absorbed in the small intestine.

Sodium passes through tight junctions and is actively transported across cell membranes; it is exchanged for bicarbonate to maintain electroneutrality in the ileum; sodium absorption is enhanced by glucose transport.

Potassium moves passively across tight junctions with changes in the electrochemical gradient.

Carbohydrates

Only monosaccharides are absorbed by intestinal mucosa, so complex carbohydrates must be hydrolyzed to simplest form.

Salivary and pancreatic amylases break down starches to oligosaccharides (sucrose, maltose, lactose) in stomach and duodenum; brush-border enzymes hydrolyze them in intestine so they can pass through unstirred layer by diffusion.

Fructose diffuses into the bloodstream; glucose and galactose diffuse or are actively transported.

Cellulose remains undigested and stimulates large intestine motility.

Proteins

From 90% to 95% of protein is absorbed; major hydrolysis is accomplished in small intestine by pancreatic enzymes trypsin, chymotrypsin, and carboxypeptidase.

Brush-border enzymes break down proteins into smaller peptides that can cross cell membranes when the cytosol breaks them down into amino acids, specifically, neutral amino acids, basic amino acids, and proline and hydroxyproline.

Fats

Digestion and absorption occur in four phases:

1. Emulsification and lipolysis—agents cover small fat particles and prevent them from reforming into fat droplets; then lipolysis breaks them into diglycerides, monoglycerides, free fatty acids, and glycerol.
2. Micelle formation—products are made water soluble.
3. Fat absorption—move from micelle to absorbing surface of intestinal epithelium and diffuse through resynthesis.
4. Triglycerides and phospholipids—become chylomicrons that eventually enter the systemic circulation.

Minerals

Calcium—absorbed by passive diffusion and transported actively across cell membranes bound to a carrier protein; absorption primarily in ileum.

Magnesium—50% absorbed by active transport or passive diffusion in jejunum and ileum.

Phosphate—absorbed by passive diffusion and active transport in small intestine.

Iron—absorbed by epithelial cells of duodenum and jejunum; vitamin C facilitates.

Vitamins

Absorbed mainly by sodium-dependent active transport, with vitamin B_{12} bound to intrinsic factor and absorbed in terminal ileum.

QUICK CHECK 33-3

1. What cells arise from the crypts of Lieberkühn?
2. How are fats absorbed from the small intestine?
3. Which reflexes inhibit intestinal motility? Which promote it?

Large Intestine

The **large intestine** is approximately 1.5 meters long and consists of the cecum, appendix, colon (ascending, transverse, descending, and sigmoid), rectum, and anal canal (Figure 33-12). The **cecum** is a pouch that receives chyme from the ileum. Attached to it is the **vermiform appendix,** an appendage having little or no physiologic function. From the cecum, chyme enters the **colon,** which loops upward, traverses the abdominal cavity, and descends to the anal canal. The four parts of the colon are the **ascending colon, transverse colon, descending colon,** and **sigmoid colon.** Two sphincters control the flow of intestinal contents through the cecum and colon: the ileocecal valve, which admits chyme from the ileum to the cecum, and the **O'Beirne sphincter,** which controls the movement of wastes from the sigmoid colon into the rectum. A thick (2.5 to 3 cm) portion of smooth muscle surrounds the anal canal, forming the **internal anal sphincter.** Overlapping it distally is the striated muscle of the **external anal sphincter**.

In the cecum and colon, the longitudinal muscle layer consists of three longitudinal bands called **teniae coli** (see Figure 33-12). They are shorter than the colon and give it a gathered appearance. The circular muscles of the colon separate the gathers into outpouchings called **haustra** (*sing.*, **haustrum**). The haustra become more or less prominent with the contractions and relaxations of the circular muscles. The mucosal surface of the colon has rugae (folds), particularly between the haustra, and **Lieberkühn crypts** but no villi. Columnar epithelial cells and mucus-secreting goblet cells form the mucosa throughout the large intestine. The columnar epithelium absorbs fluid and electrolytes, and the mucus-secreting cells lubricate the mucosa.

The myenteric plexus regulates motor and secretory activity independently of the extrinsic system. Extrinsic parasympathetic innervation occurs through the vagus and extends from the cecum up to the first part of the transverse colon. Vagal stimulation increases rhythmic contraction of the proximal colon. Extrinsic parasympathetic fibers reach the distal colon through the pelvic nerves and can increase motility throughout the colon. The internal anal sphincter is usually contracted, and its reflex response is to relax when the rectum is distended. The intrinsic nerve plexuses innervate the internal anal sphincter, which also receives sympathetic innervation to maintain contraction and parasympathetic innervation that facilitates relaxation when the rectum is full. Branches of the sacral division of the spinal cord innervate the external anal sphincter. Sympathetic activity in the entire large intestine modulates intestinal reflexes, conveys somatic sensations of fullness and pain, participates in the defecation reflex, and constricts blood vessels. The blood supply of the large intestine and rectum is derived primarily from branches of the superior and inferior mesenteric arteries (Figure 33-13).[7]

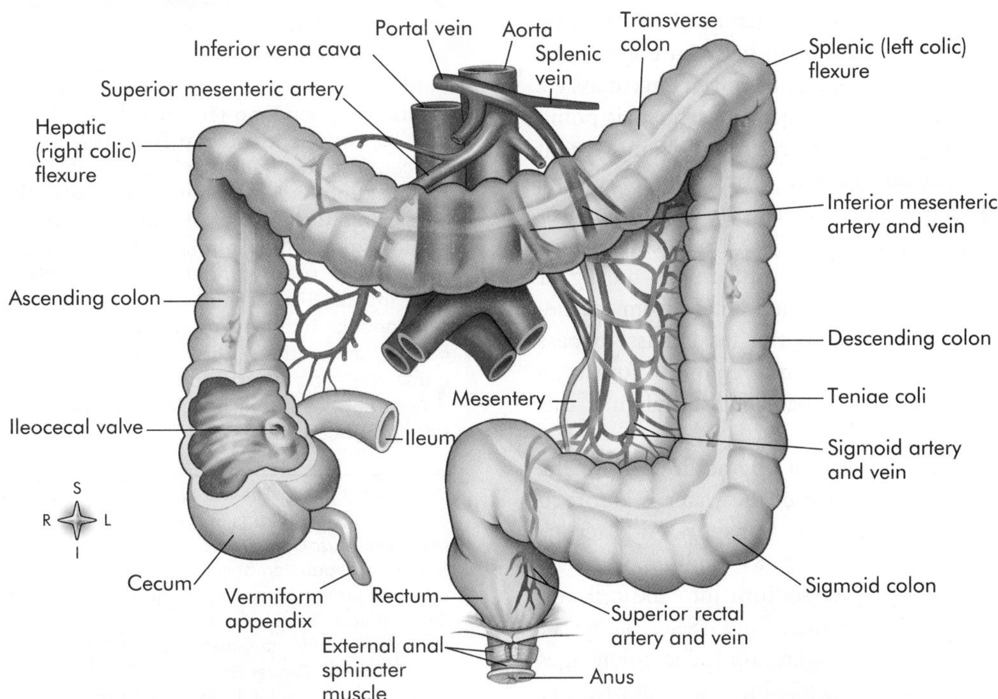

Figure 33-12 ■ **Division of the Large Intestine.** (From Thibodeau GA, Patton KT: *Anatomy & physiology,* ed 6, St Louis, 2007, Mosby.)

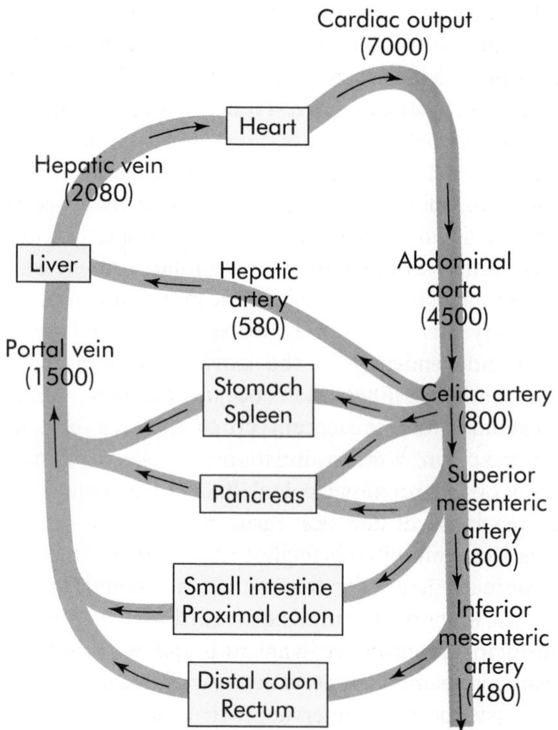

Figure 33-13 ■ The Major Blood Vessels and Organs Supplied with Blood in the Splanchnic Circulation. Numbers in parentheses reflect approximate blood flow values (ml/minute) for each major vessel in an 80-kg normal, resting, adult human subject. Arrows indicate the direction of blood flow. (Modified from Johnson LR: *Gastrointestinal pathophysiology,* St Louis, 2001, Mosby.)

The primary colonic movement is segmental. The circular muscles contract and relax at different sites, shuttling the intestinal contents back and forth between the haustra, most commonly during fasting. The movements massage the intestinal contents, called the **fecal mass** at that point, and facilitate the absorption of water. Propulsive movement occurs with the proximal-to-distal contraction of several haustral units. Peristaltic movements also occur and promote the emptying of the colon. The **gastrocolic reflex** initiates propulsion in the entire colon, usually during or immediately after eating, when chyme enters from the ileum. The gastrocolic reflex causes the fecal mass to pass rapidly into the sigmoid colon and rectum, stimulating defecation. Gastrin may participate in stimulating this reflex.

Approximately 500 to 700 ml of chyme flows from the ileum to the cecum per day. Most of the water is absorbed in the colon by diffusion and active transport. Aldosterone increases membrane permeability to sodium, thereby increasing both the diffusion of sodium into the cell and its active transport to the interstitial fluid. (See Chapter 17 for a discussion of aldosterone secretion.) The colon does not absorb sugars and amino acids, but some short-chain free fatty acids, which are produced by fermentation, are absorbed.

Absorption and epithelial transport occur in the cecum, ascending colon, transverse colon, and descending colon. By the time the fecal mass enters the sigmoid colon, the mass consists entirely of wastes and is called the *feces,* consisting of food residue, unabsorbed gastrointestinal secretions, shed epithelial cells, and bacteria.

The movement of feces into the sigmoid colon and **rectum** stimulates the **defecation reflex (rectal reflex).** The rectal wall stretches, and the tonically constricted internal anal sphincter (smooth muscle with autonomic nervous system control) relaxes, creating the urge to defecate. The defecation reflex can be overridden voluntarily by contraction of the external anal sphincter and muscles of the pelvic floor. The rectal wall gradually relaxes, reducing tension, and the urge to defecate passes. Retrograde contraction of the rectum may displace the feces out of the rectal vault until a more convenient time for evacuation. Pain or fear of pain associated with defecation (e.g., rectal fissures or hemorrhoids) can inhibit the defecation reflex.

Squatting and sitting facilitate defecation because these positions straighten the angle between the rectum and anal canal and increase the efficiency of straining (increasing intraabdominal pressure). Intra-abdominal pressure is increased by initiating the Valsalva maneuver—that is, inhaling and forcing the diaphragm and chest muscles against the closed glottis to increase both intrathoracic and intraabdominal pressure, which is transmitted to the rectum. (The Valsalva maneuver is lost in individuals who have undergone radical neck dissection. This group of individuals may need to alter dietary habits and rely on chemical agents to aid in defecation.)

HEALTH ALERT
Diet and Colon Cancer Prevention

Epidemiologic and experimental studies suggest an association between long-term use of a diet high in fiber, folic acid, calcium, and vitamin D in reducing the risk of colon cancer. The mechanism of fiber protection appears to be related to the natural tumor suppressor effect of butyrate, a fermentation product of fiber. Lack of controlled studies regarding fiber type, amount of intake, and duration of diet are needed to fully understand colorectal cancer risk and fiber intake. Similar studies are needed to understand the relationship between calcium, vitamin D, and colorectal cancer prevention. The most recent reports for nitric oxide-donating aspirin (or nonsteroidal anti-inflammatory drugs) suggests that it holds promise for safe chemoprevention of cancer.

Data from Rigas B: The use of nitric oxide-donating nonsteroidal anti-inflammatory drugs in the chemoprevention of colorectal neoplasia, *Curr Opin Gastroenterol* 23(1):55–9, 2007; Bhagavathula N et al: Upregulation of calcium-sensing receptor and mitogen-activated protein kinase signaling in the regulation of growth and differentiation in colon carcinoma, *Br J Cancer* 93(12):1364–1371, 2005; Rock CL: Primary dietary prevention: is the fiber story over? *Recent Results Cancer Res* 174:171–7, 2007; Weingarten MA, Zalmanovici A, Yaphe J: Dietary calcium supplementation for preventing colorectal cancer and adenomatous polyps, *Cochrane Database Syst Rev* (3):CD003548, 2005.

QUICK CHECK 33-4

1. What are the two veins of the liver, and what blood flows into them?
2. What are haustra?
3. What two functions does the large intestine play in relation to the fecal mass?

Intestinal Bacteria

The number of bacteria increases from the stomach to the distal colon. The stomach is relatively sterile because of the secretion of acid that kills ingested pathogens or inhibits bacterial growth. Bile acid secretion, intestinal motility, and antibody production suppress bacterial growth in the duodenum, and in the duodenum and jejunum there is a low concentration of aerobes (10^{-1} to 10^{-4}/ml), primarily streptococci, lactobacilli, staphylococci, and enterobacteria. Anaerobes are found distal to the ileocecal valve but not proximal to the ileum. They constitute about 95% of the fecal flora in the colon and contribute one third of the solid bulk of feces. *Bacteroides,* clostridia, anaerobic lactobacilli, and coliforms are the most common microorganisms from the ileum to the cecum.

The intestinal tract is sterile at birth but becomes colonized with *Escherichia coli, Clostridium welchii,* and *Streptococcus* within a few hours. Within 3 to 4 weeks after birth, the normal flora are established. The intestinal bacteria do not have major digestive or absorptive functions but do play a role in metabolism of bile salts, estrogens, androgens, lipids, carbohydrates, various nitrogenous substances and drugs, and protection against infection. The normal flora do not have the virulence factors associated with pathogenic microorganisms, thus permitting immune tolerance.[8]

Endogenous infections of the gastrointestinal tract occur by three major mechanisms: proliferation or overgrowth of bacteria, perforation of the intestine, and contamination of neighboring structures.

Splanchnic Blood Flow

The **splanchnic blood flow** provides blood to the esophagus, stomach, small and large intestine, liver, gallbladder, pancreas, and spleen (see Figure 33-13). Blood flow is regulated by cardiac output and blood volume, the autonomic nervous system, hormones, and local autoregulatory blood flow mechanisms. The splanchnic circulation serves as an important reservoir of blood volume to maintain circulation to the heart and lungs when needed.

ACCESSORY ORGANS OF DIGESTION

The liver, gallbladder, and exocrine pancreas all secrete substances necessary for the digestion of chyme. These secretions are delivered to the duodenum through ducts (Figure 33-14). The liver produces bile, which contains salts necessary for fat digestion and absorption. Between meals, bile is stored in the gallbladder. The exocrine pancreas produces (1) enzymes needed for the complete digestion of carbohydrates, proteins, and fats and (2) an alkaline fluid that neutralizes chyme, creating a duodenal pH that supports enzymatic action.

The liver also receives nutrients absorbed by the small intestine and metabolizes or synthesizes them into forms that can be absorbed by the body's cells. It then releases the nutrients into the bloodstream or stores them for later use.

Liver

The **liver** weighs 1200 to 1600 g. It is located under the right diaphragm and is divided into right and left lobes. The larger, right lobe is divided further into the caudate and quadrate lobes (Figure 33-15). The falciform ligament separates the right and left lobes and attaches the liver to the anterior abdominal wall. The round ligament (ligamentum teres) extends along the free edge of the falciform ligament, extending from the umbilicus to the inferior surface of the liver. The coronary ligament branches from the falciform ligament and extends over the superior surface of the right and left lobes, binding the liver to the inferior surface of the diaphragm. The liver is covered by the **Glisson capsule,** which contains blood vessels, lymphatics, and nerves. When the liver is diseased or swollen, distention of the capsule causes pain and the lymphatics may ooze fluid into the peritoneal space.

The metabolic functions of the liver require a large amount of blood. The liver receives blood from both arterial and venous sources. The hepatic artery branches from the abdominal aorta and provides oxygenated blood at the rate of 400 to 500 ml/min (about 25% of the cardiac

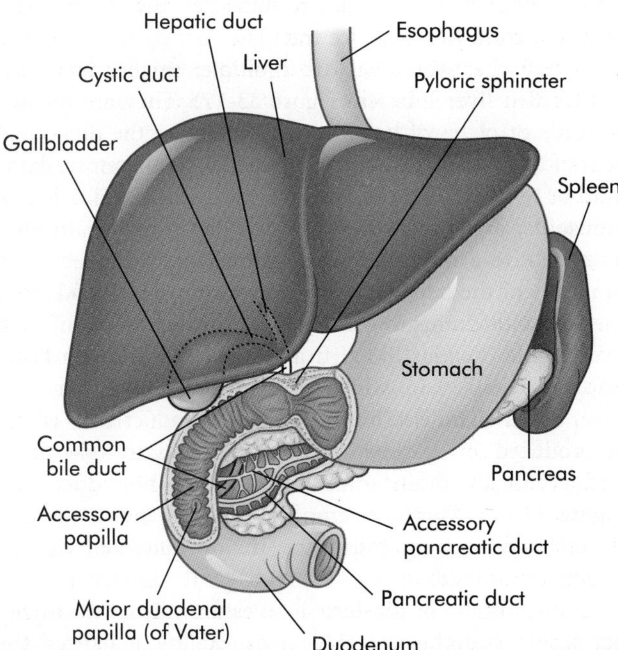

Figure 33-14 ■ **Location of the Liver, Gallbladder, and Exocrine Pancreas, Which Are the Accessory Organs of Digestion.**

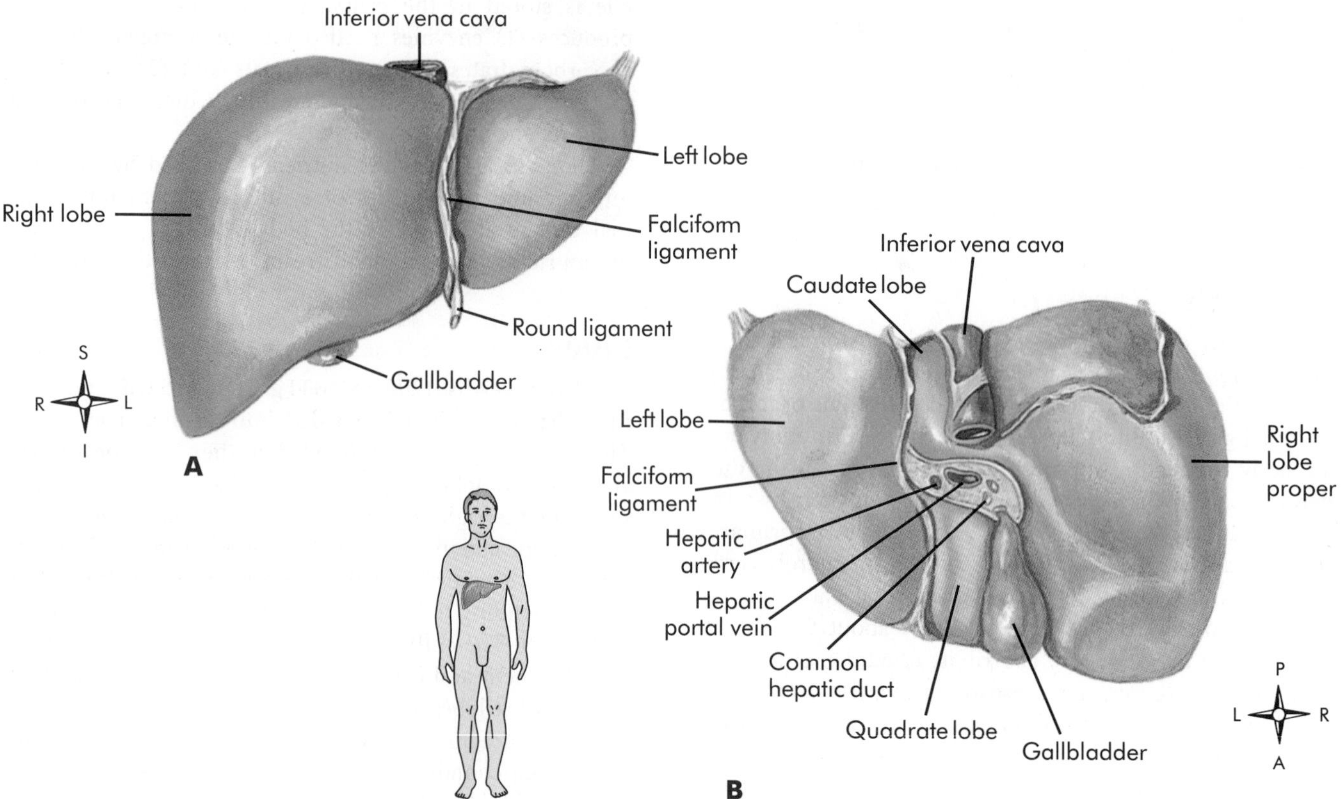

Figure 33-15 ■ **Gross Structure of the Liver. A,** Anterior view. **B,** Inferior view. (From Thibodeau GA, Patton KT: *Anatomy & physiology,* ed 6, St Louis, 2007, Mosby.)

output). The **hepatic portal vein,** which receives deoxygenated blood from the inferior and superior mesenteric veins and the splenic vein, delivers about 1000 to 1200 ml/min to the liver (Figure 33-16). Portal venous blood constitutes 70% of the blood supply to the liver. This blood carries some oxygen and is rich in nutrients that have been absorbed from the digestive tract.

Within the liver lobes are multiple, smaller anatomic units called **liver lobules** (Figure 33-17). They are formed of cords or plates of **hepatocytes,** which are the functional cells of the liver. These cells can regenerate; therefore, damaged or resected liver tissue can regrow. Small capillaries, or **sinusoids,** are located between the plates of hepatocytes. They receive a mixture of venous and arterial blood from branches of the hepatic artery and portal vein. Blood from the sinusoids drains to a central vein in the middle of each liver lobule. Venous blood from all the lobules then flows into the hepatic vein, which empties into the inferior vena cava. Small channels **(bile canaliculi)** conduct bile, which is produced by the hepatocytes, outward to bile ducts and eventually drain into the **common bile duct** (see Figure 33-17). This duct empties bile into the duodenum through an opening called the **major duodenal papilla** (sphincter of Oddi).

The sinusoids of the liver lobules are lined with highly permeable endothelium. This permeability enhances the transport of nutrients from the sinusoids into the hepatocytes, where they are metabolized. The sinusoids are also lined with phagocytic **Kupffer cells (tissue macrophages),** which are part of the mononuclear phagocyte system. They remove foreign substances from the blood and trap bacteria. Between the endothelial lining of the sinusoid and the hepatocyte is the **Disse space,** which drains interstitial fluid into the hepatic lymph system.

QUICK CHECK 33-5

1. Where does blood in the portal vein come from?
2. What is the function of hepatocytes?
3. What are sinusoids?

Secretion of bile

The liver assists intestinal digestion by secreting 700 to 1200 ml of bile per day. **Bile** is an alkaline, bitter-tasting, yellowish green fluid that contains bile salts (conjugated bile acids), cholesterol, bilirubin (a pigment), electrolytes, and water. It is formed by hepatocytes and secreted into the canaliculi. **Bile salts,** which are conjugated bile acids, are required for the intestinal emulsification and absorption of fats. Having facilitated fat emulsification and absorption, most bile salts are actively absorbed in the terminal ileum and returned to the liver through the portal circulation for resecretion. The recycling of bile salts is termed the **enterohepatic circulation** (Figure 33-18).

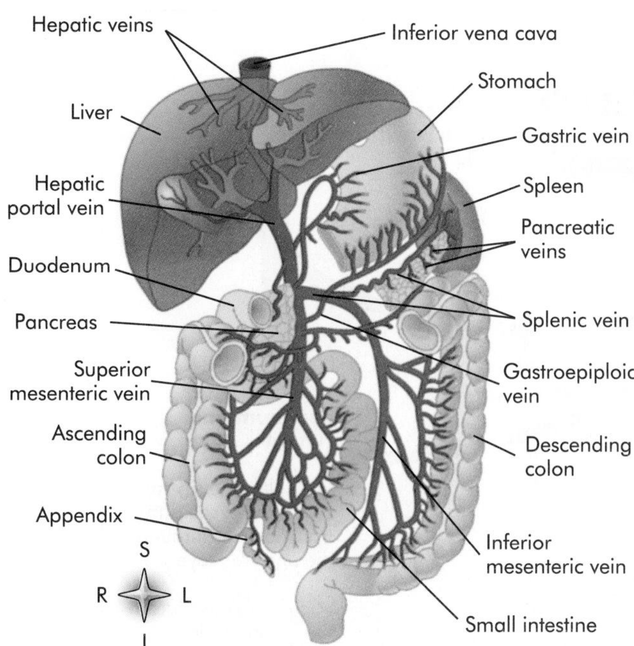

Figure 33-16 ■ Hepatic Portal Circulation. In this unusual circulatory route, a vein is located between two capillary beds. The hepatic portal vein collects blood from capillaries in visceral structures located in the abdomen and empties into the liver. Hepatic veins return blood to the inferior vena cava. (Organs are not drawn to scale.) (From Thibodeau GA, Patton KT: *Anatomy & physiology*, ed 6, St Louis, 2007, Mosby.)

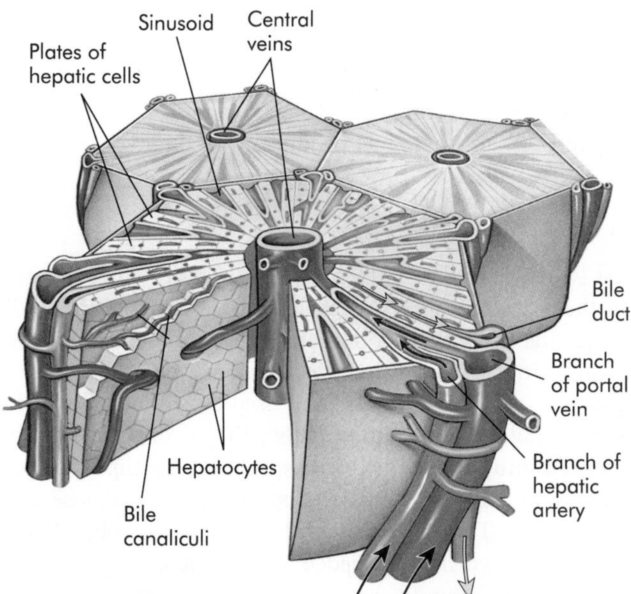

Figure 33-17 ■ Diagrammatic Representation of a Liver Lobule. A central vein is located in the center of the lobule with plates of hepatic cells disposed radially. Branches of the portal vein and hepatic artery are located on the periphery of the lobule and blood from both perfuse the sinusoids. Peripherally located bile ducts drain the bile canaliculi that run between the hepatocytes. (Modified from Thibodeau GA, Patton KT: *Anatomy & physiology*, ed 6, St Louis, 2007, Mosby.)

Bile has two fractional components: the acid-dependent fraction and the acid-independent fraction. Hepatocytes secrete the **bile acid-dependent fraction,** which consists of bile acids, cholesterol, lecithin (a phospholipid), and bilirubin (a bile pigment). The **bile acid-independent fraction,** which is secreted by the hepatocytes and epithelial cells of the bile canaliculi, is a bicarbonate-rich aqueous fluid that gives bile its alkaline pH.

Bile salts are conjugated in the liver from primary and secondary bile acids. The **primary bile acids** are cholic acid and chenodeoxycholic (chenic) acid. These acids are synthesized from cholesterol by the hepatocytes. The **secondary bile acids** are deoxycholic and lithocholic acid. These acids are formed in the small intestine by intestinal bacteria, after which they are absorbed and flow to the liver (see Figure 33-18). Both forms of bile acids are conjugated with amino acids (glycine or taurine) in the liver to form bile salts. Conjugation makes the bile acids more water soluble, thus restricting their diffusion from the duodenum and ileum. The primary and secondary bile acids together form the **bile acid pool.**

Some bile salts are deconjugated by intestinal bacteria to secondary bile acids. These acids diffuse passively into the portal blood from both small and large intestines. An increase in the plasma concentration of bile acids accelerates the uptake and resecretion of bile acids and salts by the hepatocytes. The cycle of hepatic secretion, intestinal absorption, and hepatic resecretion of bile acids completes the enterohepatic circulation.

Bile secretion is called **choleresis.** A **choleretic agent** stimulates the liver to secrete bile. One strong stimulus is a high concentration of bile salts. Other choleretics include secretin, which increases the rate of bile flow by promoting the secretion of bicarbonate from canaliculi and other intrahepatic bile ducts; cholecystokinin; and vagal stimulation.

Metabolism of bilirubin

Bilirubin is a by-product of the destruction of aged red blood cells. It gives bile a greenish black color and produces the yellow tinge of jaundice. Aged red blood cells are taken up and destroyed by macrophages of the mononuclear phagocyte system (also called the **reticuloendothelial system**), primarily in the spleen and liver. (In the liver these macrophages are Kupffer cells.) Within these cells, hemoglobin is separated into its component parts, heme and globin (Figure 33-19). The globin component is further degraded into its constituent amino acids, which are recycled to form new protein. The heme moiety is converted to biliverdin by the enzymatic cleavage of iron. The iron attaches to transferrin in the plasma and can be stored in the liver or used by the bone marrow to make new red blood cells. The biliverdin is enzymatically converted to bilirubin in the macrophage of the mononuclear phagocytic system and then is released into the plasma, where it binds to albumin and is known as **unconjugated bilirubin,** or free bilirubin, which is lipid soluble.

In the liver, unconjugated bilirubin moves from plasma in the sinusoids into the hepatocyte. Within hepatocytes,

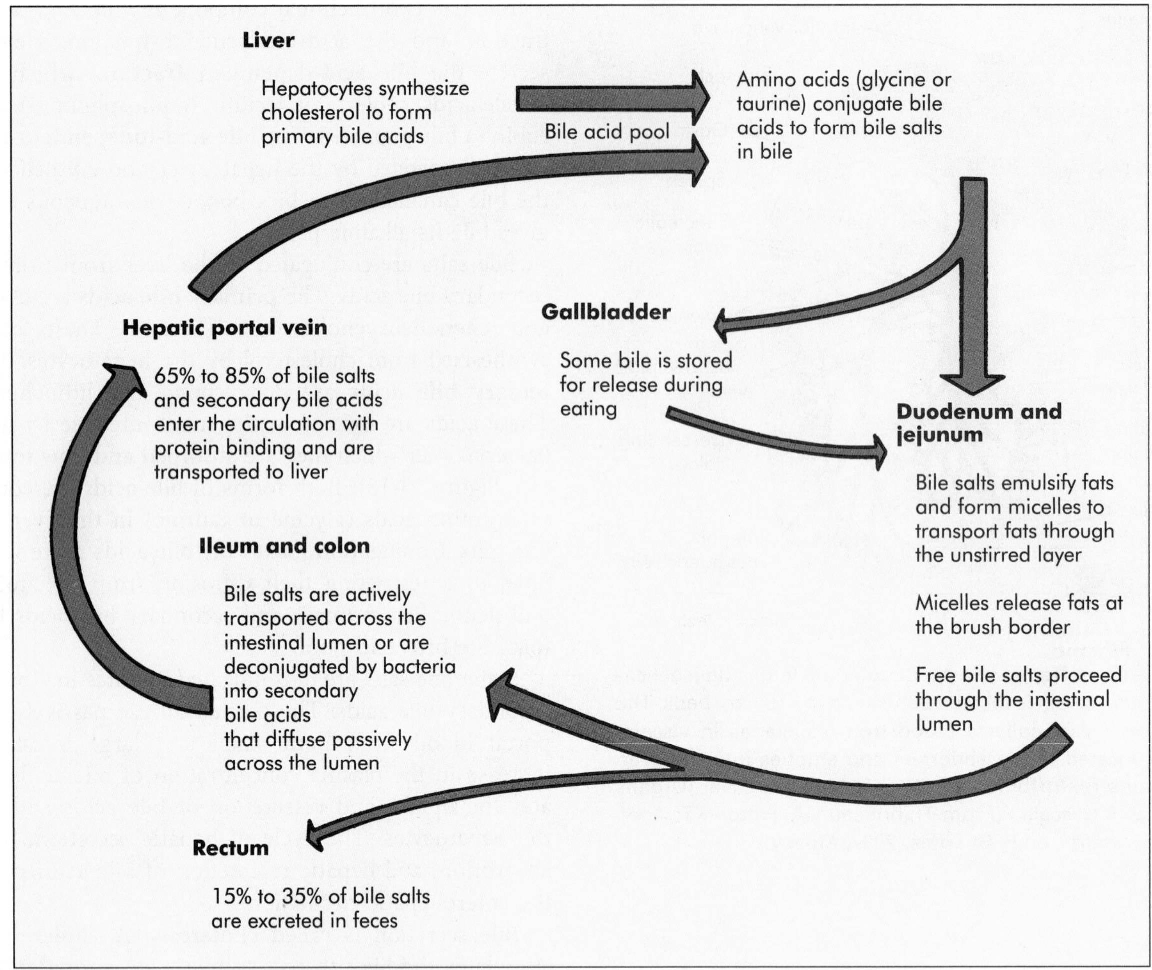
Liver
Hepatocytes synthesize cholesterol to form primary bile acids
Bile acid pool
Amino acids (glycine or taurine) conjugate bile acids to form bile salts in bile
Gallbladder
Some bile is stored for release during eating
Duodenum and jejunum
Bile salts emulsify fats and form micelles to transport fats through the unstirred layer
Micelles release fats at the brush border
Free bile salts proceed through the intestinal lumen
Hepatic portal vein
65% to 85% of bile salts and secondary bile acids enter the circulation with protein binding and are transported to liver
Ileum and colon
Bile salts are actively transported across the intestinal lumen or are deconjugated by bacteria into secondary bile acids that diffuse passively across the lumen
Rectum
15% to 35% of bile salts are excreted in feces

Figure 33-18 ■ **The Enterohepatic Circulation of Bile Salts.**

it joins with glucuronic acid to form **conjugated bilirubin,** which is water soluble. When conjugated bilirubin reaches the distal ileum and colon, it is deconjugated by bacteria and converted to **urobilinogen.** Most of the urobilinogen is then excreted in the urine, and a small amount is eliminated in feces.

Vascular and hematologic functions

Because of its extensive vascular network, the liver can store a large volume of blood. The amount stored at any one time depends on pressure relationships in the arteries and veins. The liver also can release blood to maintain systemic circulatory volume in the event of hemorrhage.

Kupffer cells in the sinusoids of the liver remove bacteria and foreign particles from the portal blood. Because the liver receives all the venous blood from the gut and pancreas, the Kupffer cells play an important role in destroying intestinal bacteria and preventing infections.

The liver also has hemostatic functions. It synthesizes prothrombin, fibrinogen, and factors I, II, VII, IX, and X, all of which are necessary for effective clotting (see Chapter 19). Vitamin K, a fat-soluble vitamin, is essential for the synthesis of other clotting factors. Because bile salts are needed for reabsorption of fats, vitamin K absorption depends on adequate bile production in the liver.

Metabolism of nutrients

Fats

Fat is synthesized from carbohydrate and protein, primarily in the liver. Fat absorbed by lacteals in the intestinal villi enters the liver through the lymphatics, primarily as triglycerides. In the liver, the triglycerides can be hydrolyzed to glycerol and free fatty acids and used to produce metabolic energy (adenosine triphosphate [ATP]), or they can be released into the bloodstream as lipoproteins (lipids bound to proteins). Blood carries the lipoproteins to adipose cells for storage. The liver also synthesizes phospholipids and cholesterol, which are needed for the hepatic production of bile salts, steroid hormones, components of plasma membranes, and other special molecules.

Proteins

Protein synthesis requires the presence of all the essential amino acids (obtained only from food), as well as nonessential amino acids. Proteins perform many important roles in the body; these are summarized in Table 33-2.

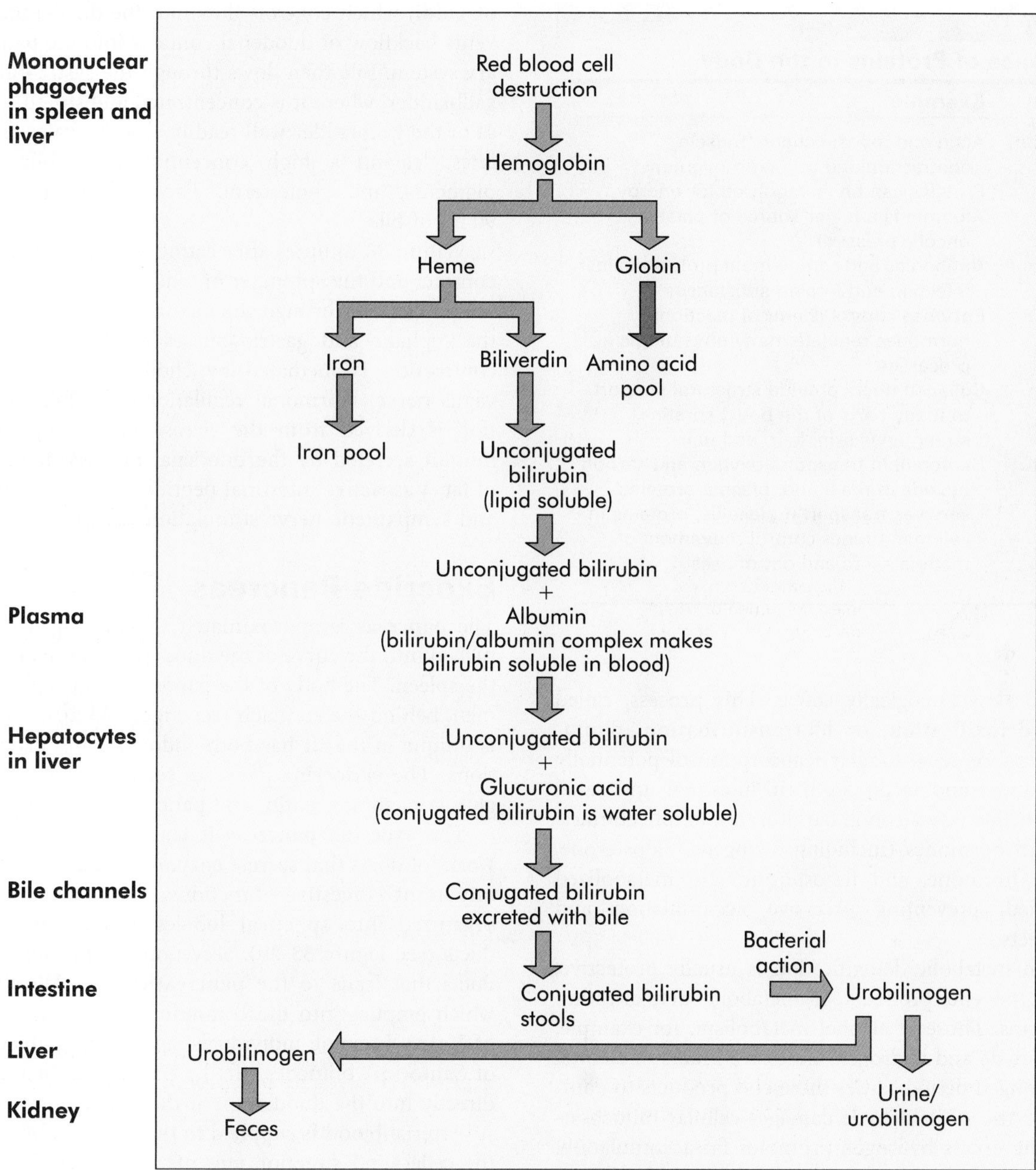

Figure 33-19 ■ **Bilirubin Metabolism.**

Within hepatocytes, amino acids are converted to carbohydrates (ketoacids) by the removal of ammonia (NH_3), a process known as **deamination.** The ammonia is converted to urea by the liver and passes into the blood to be excreted by the kidneys. Depending on need, the ketoacids are converted to fatty acids for fat synthesis and storage or are oxidized by the Krebs tricarboxylic acid cycle (see Chapter 1) to provide energy for the liver cells.

The plasma proteins, including albumins and globulins (with the exception of γ-globulin, which is formed in lymph nodes and lymphoid tissue), are synthesized by the liver. They play an important role in maintaining blood volume and pressure by maintaining plasma oncotic pressure. The liver also synthesizes several nonessential amino acids and serum enzymes, including aspartate aminotransferase (AST; previously SGOT), alanine aminotransferase (ALT; previously SGPT), lactate dehydrogenase (LDH), and alkaline phosphatase.

Carbohydrates

The liver contributes to the stability of blood glucose levels by releasing glucose during hypoglycemia (low blood sugar) and taking up glucose during hyperglycemia (high blood sugar) and storing it as glycogen (glyconeogenesis) or converting it to fat. When all glycogen stores have been used, the liver can convert amino acids and glycerol to glucose (gluconeogenesis).

Metabolic detoxification

The liver alters exogenous and endogenous chemicals (e.g., drugs), foreign molecules, and hormones to make them

TABLE 33-2

Importance of Proteins in the Body

Function	Example
Contraction	Actin and myosin enable muscle contraction and cellular movement
Energy	Proteins can be metabolized for energy
Fluid balance	Albumin is a major source of plasma oncotic pressure
Protection	Antibodies and complement protect against infection and foreign substances
Regulation	Enzymes control chemical reactions; hormones regulate many physiologic processes
Structure	Collagen fibers provide structural support to many parts of the body; keratin strengthens skin, hair, and nails
Transport	Hemoglobin transports oxygen and carbon dioxide in the blood; plasma proteins serve as transport molecules; proteins in cell membranes control movement of materials into and out of cells

less toxic or less biologically active. This process, called **metabolic detoxification,** or **biotransformation,** diminishes intestinal or renal tubular reabsorption of potentially toxic substances and facilitates their intestinal and renal excretion. In this way alcohol, barbiturates, amphetamines, steroids, and hormones (including estrogens, aldosterone, antidiuretic hormone, and testosterone) are metabolized or detoxified, preventing excessive accumulation and adverse effects.

Although metabolic detoxification is usually protective, sometimes the end products of metabolic detoxification become toxins. Those of alcohol metabolism, for example, are acetaldehyde and hydrogen. Excessive intake of alcohol over a prolonged period causes these end products to damage hepatocytes. Acetaldehyde damages cellular mitochondria, and the excess hydrogen promotes fat accumulation. This is how alcohol impairs the liver's ability to function.

Storage of minerals and vitamins

The liver stores certain vitamins and minerals, including iron and copper, in times of excessive intake and releases them in times of need. The liver can store vitamins B_{12} and D for several months and vitamin A for several years. The liver also stores vitamins E and K. Iron is stored in the liver as ferritin, an iron-protein complex, and is released as needed for red blood cell production. Common tests of liver function are listed in Table 33-3.

Gallbladder

The **gallbladder** is a saclike organ on the inferior surface of the liver (Figure 33-20). Its primary function is to store and concentrate bile between meals. Bile flows from the liver through the right or left hepatic duct into the common hepatic duct and meets resistance at the closed **sphincter of Oddi,** which controls flow into the duodenum and prevents backflow of duodenal contacts into the pancreatobiliary system. Bile then flows through the **cystic duct** into the gallbladder, where it is concentrated and stored. The mucosa of the gallbladder wall readily absorbs water and electrolytes, leaving a high concentration of bile salts, bile pigments, and cholesterol. The gallbladder holds about 90 ml of bile.

Within 30 minutes after eating, the gallbladder begins to contract and the sphincter of Oddi relaxes, forcing bile into the duodenum through the major duodenal papilla. During the cephalic and gastric phases of digestion, gallbladder contraction is mediated by cholinergic branches of the vagus nerve. Hormonal regulation of gallbladder contraction is derived from the release of cholecystokinin and motilin secreted by the duodenal mucosa in the presence of fat. Vasoactive intestinal peptide, pancreatic polypeptide, and sympathetic nerve stimulation relax the gallbladder.

Exocrine Pancreas

The **pancreas** is approximately 20 cm long, with its head tucked into the curve of the duodenum and its tail touching the spleen. The body of the pancreas lies deep in the abdomen, behind the stomach (see Figure 33-20). The pancreas is unique in that it has both endocrine and exocrine functions. The endocrine pancreas secretes hormones: insulin, glucagon, somatostatin, and pancreatic polypeptide.[9]

The **exocrine pancreas** is composed of acini and networks of ducts that secrete enzymes and alkaline fluids with important digestive functions. The acinar cells are organized into spherical lobules around small secretory ducts (see Figure 33-20). Secretions drain into a system of ducts that leads to the **pancreatic duct (Wirsung duct),** which empties into the common bile duct at the **ampulla of Vater.** In some individuals, an accessory duct (the duct of Santorini) branches off the pancreatic duct and drains directly into the duodenum at the minor duodenal papilla.

Arterial blood is supplied to the pancreas by branches of the celiac and superior mesenteric arteries. Venous blood leaves the head of the pancreas through the portal vein, with the body and tail being drained through the splenic vein. All hormonal pancreatic secretions also pass through the portal vein into the liver.

Pancreatic innervation arises from preganglionic parasympathetic fibers of the vagus nerve. These fibers activate postganglionic fibers, which stimulate enzymatic and hormonal secretion. Sympathetic postganglionic fibers from the celiac and superior mesenteric plexuses innervate the blood vessels, cause vasoconstriction, and inhibit pancreatic secretion.

The aqueous secretions of the exocrine pancreas are isotonic and contain potassium, sodium, bicarbonate, and chloride. The highly alkaline pancreatic juice neutralizes the acidic chyme that enters the duodenum from the stomach and provides the alkaline medium needed for the actions of digestive enzymes and intestinal absorption of fat.

TABLE 33-3
Selected Tests of Liver Function

Test	Normal Value	Clinical Significance
SERUM ENZYMES		
Alkaline phosphatase	20–125 U/L	Increases with biliary obstruction and cholestatic hepatitis
Aspartate aminotransferase (AST; previously SGOT)	6–21 U/L	Increases with hepatocellular injury
Alanine aminotransferase (ALT; previously SGPT)	0–48 U/L	Increases with hepatocellular injury
Lactic dehydrogenase (LDH)	0–250 U/L	Isoenzyme LD_5 is elevated with hypoxic and primary liver injury
5′-Nucleotidase	2–11 U/L	Increases with increase in alkaline phosphatase and cholestatic disorders
BILIRUBIN METABOLISM		
Serum bilirubin		
Indirect (unconjugated)	0–1.0 mg/dl	Increases with hemolysis (lysis of red blood cells)
Direct (conjugated)	0–0.3 mg/dl	Increases with hepatocellular injury or obstruction
TOTAL	0–1.0 mg/dl	Increases with biliary obstruction
Urine bilirubin	0.2–1.3 mg/dl	Increases with biliary obstruction
Urine urobilinogen	0.3–2.1 mg/2 hr (male) 0.1–1.1 mg/2 hr (female)	Increases with hemolysis or shunting of portal blood flow
SERUM PROTEINS		
Albumin	4.0–6.0 g/dl	Reduced with hepatocellular injury
Globulin	2.0–4.0 g/dl	Increases with hepatitis
TOTAL	6–8 g/dl	
A/G ratio	1.5:1 to 2.5:1	Ratio reverses with chronic hepatitis or other chronic liver disease
Transferrin	250–300 μg/dl	Liver damage with decreased values; iron deficiency with increased values
α-Fetoprotein	<10 ng/ml	Elevated values in primary hepatocellular carcinoma
BLOOD CLOTTING FUNCTIONS		
Prothrombin time (PT)	10–14 sec or 90%-100% of control	Increases with chronic liver disease (cirrhosis) or vitamin K deficiency
Partial thromboplastin time (PTT)	25–40 sec	Increases with severe liver disease or heparin therapy
Bromsulphalein (BSP) excretion	<6% retention in 45 min	Increases retention with hepatocellular injury

In the pancreas, transport of water and electrolytes through the ductal epithelium involves both active and passive mechanisms. The secretory cells of the acini actively transport hydrogen into the blood and bicarbonate into the duct lumen. Potassium and chloride are secreted by diffusion according to changes in electrochemical potential gradients. As the secretion flows down the duct, water is osmotically transported into the juice until it becomes isosmotic. At low flow rates, bicarbonate is exchanged passively for chloride, but at higher flow rates, there is less time for this exchange and bicarbonate concentration increases. Because eating stimulates the flow of pancreatic juice, the juice is most alkaline when it needs to be: during digestion.

The pancreatic enzymes can hydrolyze proteins, carbohydrates, and fats. The proteolytic (protein-digesting) enzymes include trypsin, chymotrypsin, carboxypeptidase, and elastase. These enzymes are secreted in their inactive forms—that is, as trypsinogen, chymotrypsinogen, and procarboxypeptidase—to protect the pancreas from the digestive effects of its own enzymes. For further protection, the pancreas produces **trypsin inhibitor,** which prevents the activation of proteolytic enzymes while they are in the pancreas. Once in the duodenum, the inactive forms (proenzymes) are activated by **enterokinase,** an enzyme secreted by the duodenal mucosa. Trypsinogen is the first proenzyme to be activated. Its conversion to trypsin stimulates the conversion of chymotrypsinogen to chymotrypsin and procarboxypeptidase to carboxypeptidase. Each of these enzymes cleaves specific peptide bonds to reduce polypeptides to smaller peptides.

Secretion of the aqueous and enzymatic components of pancreatic juice is controlled by hormonal and vagal stimuli. Secretin stimulates the acinar and duct cells to secrete the bicarbonate-rich fluid that neutralizes chyme and prepares it for enzymatic digestion. As chyme enters the duodenum, its acidity (pH of 4.5 or less) stimulates the **S cells** (secretin-producing cells) of the duodenum to release secretin, which is absorbed by the intestine and delivered to the pancreas in the bloodstream. In the pancreas, secretin causes ductal and acinar cells to release alkaline fluid.

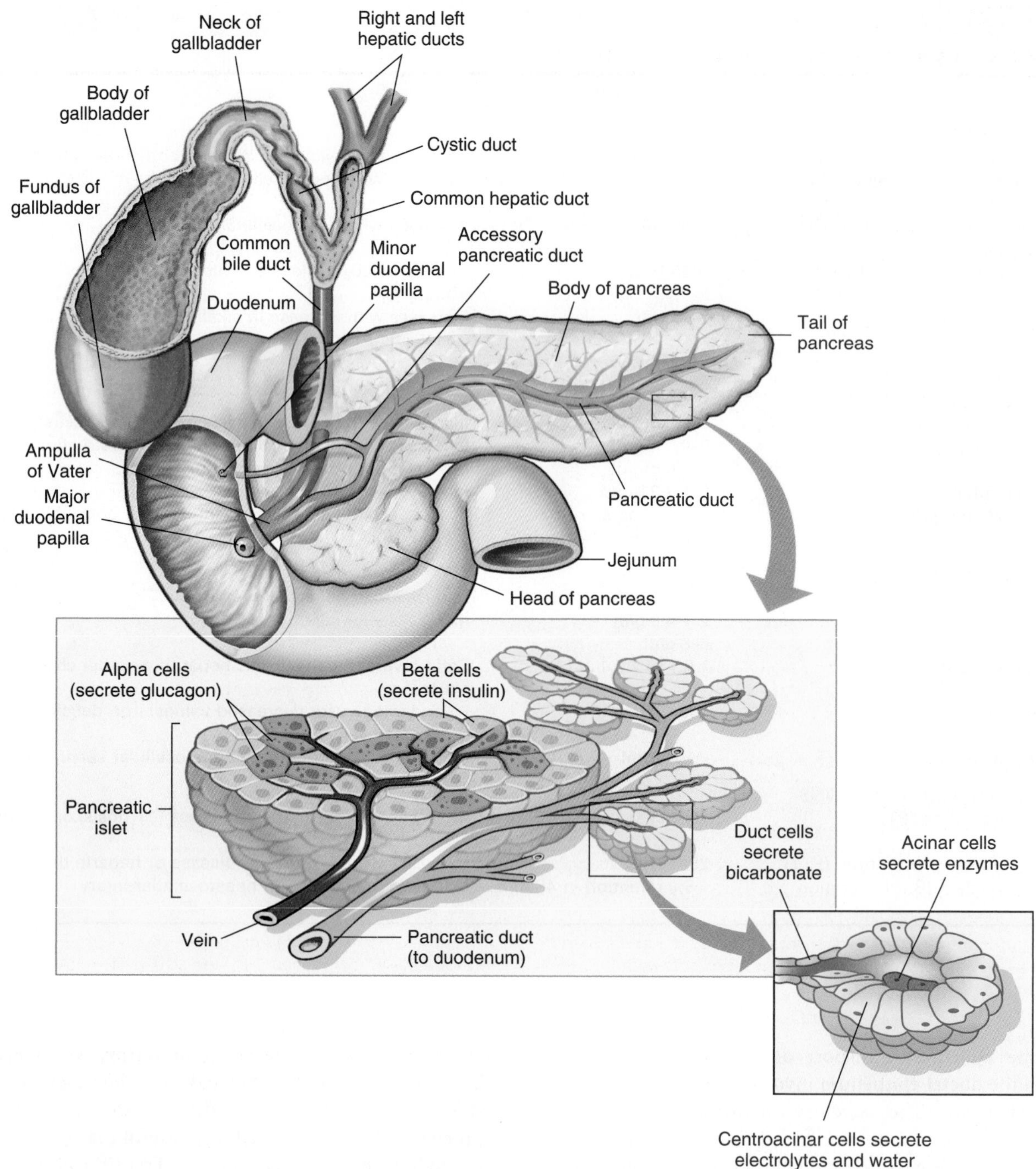

Figure 33-20 ■ **Associated Structures of the Gallbladder, Pancreas, and Pancreatic Acinar Cells and Duct.** (Main illustration from Thibodeau GA, Patton KT: *Anatomy & physiology*, ed 6, St Louis, 2007, Mosby.)

Secretin also inhibits the actions of gastrin, thereby decreasing gastric acid secretion and motility. The overall effect is to neutralize contents of the duodenum.

Enzymatic secretion follows, stimulated by cholecystokinin and acetylcholine. Cholecystokinin is released in the duodenum in response to the essential amino acids and fatty acids already present in chyme. Cholecystokinin and acetylcholine both act on the acinar cells, causing enzyme release. Once in the small intestine, activated pancreatic enzymes inhibit the release of more cholecystokinin and acetylcholine. This feedback mechanism inhibits the secretion of more pancreatic enzymes. Acetylcholine is liberated from pancreatic branches of the vagus nerve during the cephalic phase of digestion. Pancreatic polypeptide is released after eating and inhibits postprandial pancreatic exocrine secretion. (See Table 33-1 for a summary of hormonal stimulation of pancreatic secretions.) Selected tests of pancreatic function are listed in Table 33-4.

TABLE 33-4
Selected Laboratory Tests of Pancreatic Function

Test	Normal Value	Clinical Significance
Serum amylase	27–131 U/L	Elevated levels with pancreatic inflammation
Serum lipase	20–180 U/L	Elevated levels with pancreatic inflammation (may be elevated with other conditions; differentiates with amylase isoenzyme study)
Urine amylase	2–19 U/hr	Elevated levels with pancreatic inflammation
Secretin test	Volume 1.8 ml/kg/hr Bicarbonate concentration: >80 mEq/L Bicarbonate output: >10 mEq/L/30 sec	Decreased volume with pancreatic disease because a secretin stimulates pancreatic secretion
Stool fat	2–5 g/24 hr	Measures fatty acids; decreased pancreatic lipase increases stool fat

AGING & The Gastrointestinal System

Age-related changes in gastrointestinal function include the following:

Oral Cavity and Esophagus

1. Tooth enamel and dentin wear down, so cavities are more likely.
2. Teeth are lost as a result of periodontal disease and brittle roots that break easily.
3. Taste buds decline in number.
4. Sense of smell diminishes.
5. Salivary secretion decreases.
6. Dysphagia is much more common.

Result: Eating is less pleasurable, appetite is reduced, and food is not chewed or lubricated enough, so swallowing is difficult.

Stomach and Intestines

1. Gastric motility, blood flow, and volume and acid content of gastric juice may be reduced, particularly with gastric atrophy.
2. Protective mucosal barrier decreases.
3. Intestinal villi become shorter and more convoluted, with diminished reparative capacity.
4. Intestinal absorption, motility, and blood flow decrease, impairing nutrient absorption.
5. Nutritive substances are absorbed more slowly and in smaller amounts.
6. Rectal muscle mass decreases, and the anal sphincter weakens.
7. Constipation is common and is related to immobility, low-fiber diet, and changes in enteric nervous system functions.

Liver

1. Size and weight decrease.
2. Ability to detoxify drugs decreases.
3. Blood flow decreases, influencing efficiency of drug metabolism.

Pancreas and Gallbladder

1. Fibrosis, fatty acid deposits, and pancreatic atrophy occur.
2. Secretion of digestive enzymes, particularly proteolytic enzymes, decreases.
3. No changes in gallbladder and bile ducts occur, but there is an increased prevalence of gallstones and cholecystitis.

Data from Newton JL: Changes in upper gastrointestinal physiology with age, *Mech Ageing Dev* 125(12):867–870, 2004; Drozdowski L, Thomson AB: Aging and the intestine, *World J Gastroenterol* 12(47):7578–84, 2006; Wynne H: Drug metabolism and ageing, *J Br Menopause Soc* 11(2):51–56, 2005.

QUICK CHECK 33-6

1. Trace the route of bile salts and acids from formation to recycling.
2. What are the two types of bilirubin?
3. What function does the gallbladder perform?
4. How do pancreatic beta cells differ from acinar cells?

Did You Understand?

The Gastrointestinal Tract

1. The major functions of the gastrointestinal tract are the mechanical and chemical breakdown of food and the absorption of digested nutrients.
2. The gastrointestinal tract is a hollow tube that extends from the mouth to the anus.
3. The walls of the gastrointestinal tract have several layers: mucosa, muscularis mucosae, submucosa, tunica muscularis (circular muscle and longitudinal muscle), and serosa.
4. The peritoneum is a double layer of membranous tissue. The visceral layer covers the abdominal organs, and the parietal layer extends along the abdominal wall.
5. Except for swallowing and defecation, which are controlled voluntarily, the functions of the gastrointestinal tract are controlled by extrinsic and intrinsic autonomic nerves and intestinal hormones.
6. Digestion begins in the mouth, with chewing and salivation. The digestive component of saliva is α-amylase, which initiates carbohydrate digestion.
7. The esophagus is a muscular tube that transports food from the mouth to the stomach. The tunica muscularis in the upper part of the esophagus is striated muscle, and that in the lower part is smooth muscle.
8. Swallowing is controlled by the swallowing center in the reticular formation of the brain. The two phases of swallowing are the oropharyngeal phase (voluntary swallowing) and the esophageal phase (involuntary swallowing).
9. Food is propelled through the gastrointestinal tract by peristalsis: waves of sequential relaxations and contractions of the tunica muscularis.
10. The lower esophageal sphincter opens to admit swallowed food into the stomach and then closes to prevent regurgitation of food back into the esophagus.
11. The stomach is a baglike structure that secretes digestive juices, mixes and stores food, and propels partially digested food (chyme) into the duodenum.
12. The vagus nerve stimulates gastric (stomach) secretion and motility.
13. The hormones gastrin and motilin stimulate gastric emptying; the hormones secretin and cholecystokinin delay gastric emptying.
14. Mucus is secreted throughout the stomach and protects the stomach wall from acid and digestive enzymes.
15. Gastric glands in the fundus and body of the stomach secrete intrinsic factor, which is needed for vitamin B_{12} absorption, and hydrochloric acid, which dissolves food fibers, kills microorganisms, and activates the enzyme pepsin.
16. Chief cells in the stomach secrete pepsinogen, which is converted to pepsin in the acid environment created by hydrochloric acid.
17. Acid secretion is stimulated by the vagus nerve, gastrin, and histamine and is inhibited by sympathetic stimulation and cholecystokinin.
18. The three phases of acid secretion by the stomach are the cephalic phase (anticipation and swallowing), the gastric phase (food in the stomach), and the intestinal phase (chyme in the intestine).
19. The small intestine is 5 meters long and has three segments: the duodenum, jejunum, and ileum.
20. The duodenum receives chyme from the stomach through the pyloric valve. The presence of chyme stimulates the liver and gallbladder to deliver bile and the pancreas to deliver digestive enzymes. Bile and enzymes flow through an opening guarded by the sphincter of Oddi.
21. Bile is produced by the liver and is necessary for fat digestion and absorption. Bile's alkalinity helps to neutralize chyme, thereby creating a pH that enables the pancreatic enzymes to digest proteins, carbohydrates, and sugars.
22. Enzymes secreted by the small intestine (maltase, sucrase, lactase), pancreatic enzymes, and bile salts act in the small intestine to digest proteins, carbohydrates, and fats.
23. Digested substances are absorbed across the intestinal wall and then transported to the liver, where they are metabolized further.
24. The ileocecal valve connects the small and large intestines and prevents reflux into the small intestine.
25. Villi are small finger-like projections that extend from the small intestinal mucosa and increase its absorptive surface area.
26. Sugars, amino acids, and fats are absorbed primarily by the duodenum and jejunum; bile salts and vitamin B_{12} are absorbed by the ileum. Vitamin B_{12} absorption requires the presence of intrinsic factor.
27. Bile salts emulsify and hydrolyze fats and incorporate them into water-soluble micelles, which transport them through the unstirred layer to the brush border of the intestinal mucosa. The fat content of the micelles readily diffuses through the epithelium into lacteals (lymphatic ducts) in the villi. From there, fats flow into lymphatics and into the systemic circulation, which delivers them to the liver.
28. Minerals and water-soluble vitamins are absorbed by both active and passive transport throughout the small intestine.
29. Peristaltic movements created by longitudinal muscles propel the chyme along the intestinal tract, and contractions of the circular muscles (haustral segmentation) mix the chyme.
30. The ileogastric reflex inhibits gastric motility when the ileum is distended.
31. The intestinointestinal reflex inhibits intestinal motility when one intestinal segment is overdistended.
32. The gastroileal reflex increases intestinal motility when gastric motility increases.
33. The large intestine consists of the cecum, appendix, colon (ascending, transverse, descending, and sigmoid), rectum, and anal canal.
34. The teniae coli are three bands of longitudinal muscle that extend the length of the colon.
35. Haustra are pouches of colon formed with alternating contraction and relaxation of the circular muscles.
36. The mucosa of the large intestine contains mucus-secreting cells and mucosal folds, but no villi.
37. The large intestine massages the fecal mass and absorbs water and electrolytes.

Did You Understand?—Cont'd

38. Distention of the ileum with chyme causes the gastrocolic reflex, or the mass propulsion of feces to the rectum.
39. Defecation is stimulated when the rectum is distended with feces. The conically contracted internal anal sphincter relaxes, and if the voluntarily regulated external sphincter relaxes, defecation occurs.
40. The largest number of intestinal bacteria is in the colon. They are anaerobes consisting of *Bacteroides,* clostridia, coliforms, and lactobacilli.
41. The intestinal tract is sterile at birth and becomes totally colonized within 3 to 4 weeks.
42. Endogenous infections of the gastrointestinal tract occur by excessive proliferation of bacteria, perforation of the intestine, or contamination from neighboring structures.
43. The splanchnic blood flow provides blood to the esophagus, stomach, small and large intestine, gallbladder, pancreas, and spleen.

Accessory Organs of Digestion

1. The liver is the second largest organ in the body. It has digestive, metabolic, hematologic, vascular, and immunologic functions.
2. The liver is divided into the right and left lobes and is supported by the falciform, round, and coronary ligaments.
3. Liver lobules consist of plates of hepatocytes, which are the functional cells of the liver.
4. The hepatocytes synthesize 700 to 1200 ml of bile per day and secrete it into the bile canaliculi, which are small channels between the hepatocytes. The bile canaliculi drain bile into the common bile duct and then into the duodenum through an opening called the *major duodenal papilla (sphincter of Oddi).*
5. Sinusoids are capillaries located between the plates of hepatocytes. Blood from the portal vein and hepatic artery flows through the sinusoids to a central vein in each lobule and then to the hepatic vein and inferior vena cava.
6. Kupffer cells, which are part of the mononuclear phagocyte system, line the sinusoids and destroy microorganisms in sinusoidal blood.
7. The primary bile acids are synthesized from cholesterol by the hepatocytes. The primary acids are then conjugated to form bile salts. The secondary bile acids are the product of bile salt deconjugation by bacteria in the intestinal lumen.
8. Most bile salts and acids are recycled. The absorption of bile salts and acids from the terminal ileum and their return to the liver are known as the *enterohepatic circulation of bile.*
9. Bilirubin is a pigment liberated by the lysis of aged red blood cells in the liver and spleen. Unconjugated bilirubin is fat-soluble and can cross cell membranes. Unconjugated bilirubin is converted to water-soluble, conjugated bilirubin by hepatocytes and is secreted with bile.
10. The gallbladder is a saclike organ located in the inferior surface of the liver. The gallbladder stores bile between meals and ejects it when chyme enters the duodenum.
11. Stimulated by cholecystokinin, the gallbladder contracts and forces bile through the cystic duct and into the common bile duct. The sphincter of Oddi relaxes, enabling bile to flow through the major duodenal papilla into the duodenum.
12. The pancreas is a gland located behind the stomach. The endocrine pancreas produces hormones (glucagon, insulin) that facilitate the formation and cellular uptake of glucose. The exocrine pancreas secretes an alkaline solution and the enzymes (trypsin, chymotrypsin, carboxypeptidase, α-amylase, lipase) that digest proteins, carbohydrates, and fats.
13. Secretin stimulates pancreatic secretion of alkaline fluid, and cholecystokinin and acetylcholine stimulate secretion of enzymes. Pancreatic secretions originate in acini and ducts of the pancreas and empty into the duodenum through the common bile duct or an accessory duct that opens directly into the duodenum.

Key Terms

Alimentary canal (gastrointestinal tract), 912
Ampulla of Vater, 930
Antrum of stomach, 916
Ascending colon, 923
Bile, 926
Bile acid pool, 927
Bile acid-dependent fraction, 927
Bile acid-independent fraction, 927
Bile canaliculi, 926
Bile salt, 926
Bilirubin, 927
Body of stomach, 916
Brush border, 919
Cardiac orifice, 915
Cecum, 923
Chief cell, 918
Cholecystokinin, 916
Choleresis, 927
Choleretic agent, 927
Chyme, 915
Colon, 923
Common bile duct, 926
Conjugated bilirubin, 928
Cystic duct, 930
Deamination, 929
Defecation reflex (rectal reflex), 924
Descending colon, 923
Disse space, 926
Duodenum, 918
Enteric plexus, 912
Enterohepatic circulation, 926
Enterokinase, 931
Esophageal phase of swallowing, 915
Esophagus, 913
Exocrine pancreas, 930
External anal sphincter, 923
Fecal mass, 924
Fundus of stomach, 916
Gallbladder, 930
Gastric emptying, 917
Gastric gland, 917

Key Terms—Cont'd

Gastrin, 916
Gastrocolic reflex, 924
Gastroileal reflex, 922
Glisson capsule, 925
Haustral segmentation, 920
Haustrum (*pl.* haustra), 923
Hepatic portal vein, 926
Hepatocyte, 926
Ileocecal valve (sphincter), 918
Ileogastric reflex, 922
Ileum, 918
Internal anal sphincter, 923
Intestinointestinal reflex, 922
Jejunum, 918
Kupffer cell (tissue macrophage), 926
Lacteal, 920
Lamina propria, 919
Large intestine, 923
Lieberkühn crypts, 923
Liver lobule, 926
Liver, 925
Lower esophageal sphincter (cardiac sphincter), 915
Major duodenal papilla, 926
Mesentery, 918
Metabolic detoxification (biotransformation), 930
Microvillus (*pl.*, microvilli), 919
Motilin, 917
Mouth, 912
Mucosal barrier, 918
Myenteric plexus (Auerbach plexus), 919
O'Beirne sphincter, 923
Oropharyngeal (voluntary) phase of swallowing, 915
Pancreas, 930
Pancreatic duct (Wirsung duct), 930
Pepsin, 918
Peristalsis, 913
Peritoneal cavity, 918
Peritoneum, 918
Primary bile acid, 927
Primary peristalsis, 915
Pyloric sphincter, 916
Pylorus (gastroduodenal junction), 916
Rectum, 924
Reticuloendothelial system, 927
Retropulsion, 917
S cell, 931
Saliva, 913
Salivary α-amylase (ptyalin), 913
Salivary gland, 913
Secondary bile acid, 927
Secondary peristalsis, 915
Secretin, 917
Sigmoid colon, 923
Sinusoid, 926
Small intestine, 918
Sphincter of Oddi, 930
Splanchnic blood flow, 925
Stomach, 915
Submucosal plexus (Meissner plexus), 919
Swallowing, 915
Teniae coli, 923
Transverse colon, 923
Trypsin inhibitor, 931
Unconjugated bilirubin, 927
Upper esophageal sphincter, 915
Urobilinogen, 928
Vermiform appendix, 923
Villus (*pl.*, villi), 919

References

1. Boeckxstaens GE: The lower oesophageal sphincter, *Neurogastroenterol Motil* 17(suppl 1):13–21, 2005.
2. Guyton AC, Hall JE: *Textbook of medical physiology*, ed 11, pp 786 Philadelphia, 2006, Elsevier Saunders.
3. Malbert CH: The ileocolonic sphincter, *Neurogastroenterol Motil* 17(suppl 1):41–49, 2005.
4. Johnson LR: Gastrointestinal physiology, In Johnson LR, editor, *Mosby physiology monograph series*, ed 7, St Louis, 2007, Mosby.
5. Malbert CH: The ileocolonic sphincter, *Neurogastroenterol Motil* 17(suppl 1):41–49, 2005.
6. Chandi G, Harsha BS, Booshanam BV: The morphology and development of the small intestine, In Ratnaike RN, editor: *Small bowel disorders*, London, 2000, Arnold.
7. Rosenblum JD, Boyle CM, Schwartz LB: The mesenteric circulation: anatomy and physiology, *Surg Clin North Am* 77(2): 289–306, 1997.
8. Kelly D, Conway S, Aminov R: Commensal gut bacteria: mechanisms of immune modulation, *Trends Immunol* 26(6): 26–33, 2005.
9. Thibodeau GA, Patton KT: *Anatomy & physiology*, ed 6, St Louis, 2007, Mosby.

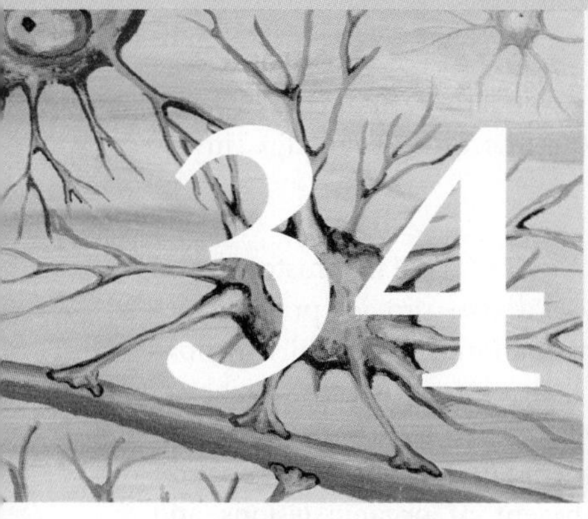

ALTERATIONS OF DIGESTIVE FUNCTION

Sue E. Huether

CHAPTER OUTLINE

ELECTRONIC RESOURCES

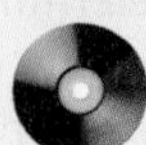

Companion CD
- Review Questions and Answers
- Animations

evolve Website
http://evolve.elsevier.com/Huether/
- Quick Check Answers
- Key Terms Exercises
- Critical Thinking Questions with Answers
- Algorithm Completion Exercises
- WebLinks

The gastrointestinal tract is a continuous, hollow organ that extends from the mouth to the anus. It includes the esophagus, stomach, small intestine, large intestine, and rectum. The accessory organs of digestion include the salivary glands, liver, gallbladder, and pancreas.

Disorders of the gastrointestinal tract disrupt one or more of its functions. Structural and neural abnormalities can slow, obstruct, or accelerate the movement of chyme at any level of the gastrointestinal tract. Inflammatory and ulcerative conditions of the gastrointestinal wall disrupt secretion, motility, and absorption. Inflammation or obstruction of the liver, pancreas, or gallbladder can alter metabolism and result in local and systemic symptoms. Many clinical manifestations of gastrointestinal tract disorders are nonspecific and can be caused by a variety of impairments.

DISORDERS OF THE GASTROINTESTINAL TRACT

Clinical Manifestations of Gastrointestinal Dysfunction

Anorexia

Anorexia is lack of a desire to eat despite physiologic stimuli that would normally produce hunger. This nonspecific symptom is often associated with nausea, abdominal pain, and diarrhea and often accompanies disorders of other organ systems, including cancer, heart disease, and renal disease. Anorexia also can be related to psychosocial distress.

Vomiting

Vomiting (emesis) is the forceful emptying of stomach and intestinal contents (chyme) through the mouth. Stimuli initiating the vomiting reflex include severe pain; distention of the stomach or duodenum; the presence of ipecac or copper salts in the duodenum; torsion or trauma affecting the ovaries, testes, uterus, bladder, or kidney; motion; and activation of the chemoreceptor trigger zone in the medulla.

Nausea and retching usually precede vomiting. **Nausea** is a subjective experience associated with various conditions, including abnormal pain and labyrinthine stimulation (i.e., spinning movement). Specific neural pathways have not been identified, but hypersalivation and tachycardia are common associated symptoms. **Retching** begins with deep inspiration. The glottis closes, intrathoracic pressure falls, and the esophagus becomes distended. Simultaneously the abdominal muscles contract, creating a pressure gradient from abdomen to thorax. The lower esophageal sphincter (LES) and body of the stomach relax, but the duodenum and antrum of the stomach go into spasm. The reverse peristalsis and pressure gradient force chyme from the stomach and duodenum up into the esophagus. Because the upper esophageal sphincter is closed, chyme does not enter the mouth. As the abdominal muscles relax, the contents of the esophagus drop back into the stomach. This process may be repeated several times before vomiting occurs. A diffuse sympathetic discharge causes the tachycardia, tachypnea, and sweating that accompany retching and vomiting. The parasympathetic system mediates copious salivation, increased gastric motility, and relaxation of the upper and lower esophageal sphincters.

Vomiting is usually associated with nausea and follows retching. The duodenum and antrum of the stomach produce reverse peristalsis, while the body of the stomach and esophagus relax. When the stomach is full of gastric contents, the diaphragm is forced high into the thoracic cavity by strong contractions of the abdominal muscles. The higher intrathoracic pressure forces the upper esophageal sphincter to open, and chyme is expelled from the mouth. Then the stomach relaxes and the upper part of the esophagus contracts, forcing the remaining chyme back into the stomach. The lower esophageal sphincter then closes. The cycle is repeated if there is a volume of chyme remaining in the stomach.

Spontaneous vomiting not preceded by nausea or retching is called **projectile vomiting.** It is caused by direct stimulation of the vomiting center by neurologic lesions (e.g., tumors or aneurysms) involving the brain stem or can be a symptom of gastrointestinal obstruction (pyloric stenosis). The metabolic consequences of vomiting are fluid, electrolyte, and acid-base disturbances (see Chapter 4).

Constipation

Constipation is difficult or infrequent defecation. It is a common complaint caused by personal habits and various disorders and drugs. It usually means a decrease in the number of bowel movements per week, hard stools, and difficult evacuation, but the definition must be individually determined. Normal bowel habits range from one to three evacuations per day to one per week.

PATHOPHYSIOLOGY Constipation can be caused by neurogenic disorders of the large intestine in which neural pathways or neurotransmitters are altered and delay transit time.[1] A low-residue diet (the habitual consumption of highly refined foods) decreases the volume and number of stools and causes constipation. A sedentary lifestyle and lack of regular exercise are common causes of constipation. Hypothyroidism decreases bowel motility. Lack of access to toilet facilities and consistent suppression of the urge to empty the bowel are other causes. Excessive use of antacids containing calcium carbonate or aluminum hydroxide often results in constipation. Opiates, particularly codeine, tend to inhibit bowel motility. Aging may result in changes in neuromuscular function causing constipation.[2]

CLINICAL MANIFESTATIONS Changes in bowel evacuation patterns, such as less frequent defecation, smaller stool volume, difficulty in evacuating the rectum, or a feeling of bowel fullness and discomfort, require investigation.

EVALUATION AND TREATMENT The history and physical examination and stool diaries provide precise clues regarding the nature of constipation. Functional constipation—that is, constipation resulting from lifestyle or bowel habits—usually has a long history. Dysfunctional constipation is more likely to be sudden. Sudden-onset constipation can accompany the development of organic lesions and requires careful evaluation.

The individual's description of frequency, stool consistency, associated pain, and presence of blood is significant. In assessing frequency, it is important to discover whether evacuation was stimulated by enemas or cathartics (laxatives). Palpation discloses colonic distention, masses, and tenderness. Digital examination of the rectum is performed to assess sphincter tone and detect anal lesions. Stool transit time is evaluated. Proctosigmoidoscopy is used to visualize the lumen directly. A barium enema may be required if no lesions are directly visualized and symptoms continue after simple treatment.

The treatment for dysfunctional constipation is to manage the underlying lesion or disease. Management of functional constipation usually consists of bowel retraining, in which the individual establishes a satisfactory bowel evacuation routine without becoming preoccupied with bowel movements. The individual also may need to engage in moderate exercise, drink more fluids, and increase fiber intake. Bulk supplements (e.g., Metamucil, Konsyl), stool softeners, and laxative agents are useful for some individuals. Enemas can be used to establish bowel routine, but they should not be used habitually.

Diarrhea

Diarrhea is an increase in the frequency of defecation and the fluidity and volume of feces. More than three stools per day is considered abnormal. Many factors determine stool volume and consistency, including water content of the colon and the presence of unabsorbed food, unabsorbable material, and intestinal secretions. Stool volume in the normal adult averages less than 200 g/day. Stool volume in children depends on age and size. An infant may pass up to 100 g/day. The adult intestine processes approximately 9 L of luminal content per day: 2 L is ingested, and the remaining 7 L consists of intestinal secretions. Of this volume, 99% of the fluid is absorbed: 90% (7 to 8 L) in the small intestine and 9% (1 to 2 L) in the colon. Normally, approximately 150 ml of water is excreted daily in the stool.

PATHOPHYSIOLOGY Diarrhea in which the volume of feces is increased is called *large-volume diarrhea.* It generally is caused by excessive amounts of water or secretions or both in the intestines. *Small-volume diarrhea,* in which the volume of feces is not increased, usually results from excessive intestinal motility.

The three major mechanisms of diarrhea are osmotic, secretory, and motile:

1. **Osmotic diarrhea.** A nonabsorbable substance in the intestine draws excess water into the intestine and increases stool weight and volume, producing large-volume diarrhea. Causes include lactase and pancreatic enzyme deficiency and excessive ingestion of synthetic, nonabsorbable sugars.
2. **Secretory diarrhea.** Excessive mucosal secretion of fluid and electrolytes produces large-volume diarrhea. Causes include bacterial enterotoxins (e.g., *Escherichia coli*), neoplasms, or exotoxins from overgrowth of *Clostridium difficile* following antibiotic therapy.[3] Small-volume diarrhea is usually caused by an inflammatory disorder of the intestine, such as ulcerative colitis or Crohn disease, but also can result from fecal impaction.
3. **Motility diarrhea.** Food is not mixed properly, digestion is impaired, and motility is increased. Causes include resection of the small intestine, surgical bypass of an area of the intestine, or fistula formation between loops of intestine and excessive motility of the intestine caused by diabetic neuropathy.

CLINICAL MANIFESTATIONS Diarrhea can be acute or chronic, depending on its cause. Systemic effects of prolonged diarrhea are dehydration, electrolyte imbalance, and weight loss. Manifestations of acute bacterial or viral infection include fever, with or without cramping pain. Fever, cramping pain, and bloody stools accompany diarrhea caused by inflammatory bowel disease. Steatorrhea (fat in the stools) and diarrhea are common signs of malabsorption syndromes.

EVALUATION AND TREATMENT A thorough history is taken to document the onset and frequency of diarrhea. Exposure to contaminated food or water is indicated if the individual has traveled in foreign countries or areas where drinking water might be contaminated. Iatrogenic diarrhea is suggested if the individual has undergone abdominal radiation therapy, intestinal resection, or treatment with selected drugs (e.g., antibiotics, diuretics, antihypertensives, laxatives) or probiotics (i.e., lactobacillus) to support normal intestinal bacteria.[4] Physical examination helps identify underlying systemic disease. Stool culture, examination of stool specimens for blood, abdominal x-ray films, and intestinal biopsies provide more specific data.

Treatment for diarrhea includes restoration of fluid and electrolyte balance, management of distressing symptoms, and treatment of causal factors. Nutritional deficiencies need to be corrected in cases of chronic diarrhea or malabsorption.

Abdominal pain

The causal mechanisms of abdominal pain are *mechanical, inflammatory,* or *ischemic.* Generally, the abdominal organs are not sensitive to mechanical stimuli, such as cutting, tearing, or crushing. These organs are, however, sensitive to stretching and distention, which activate nerve endings in both hollow and solid structures. Pain accompanies rapid distention rather than gradual distention. Traction on the peritoneum caused by adhesions, distention of the common bile duct, or forceful peristalsis resulting from intestinal obstruction causes pain because of increased tension. Capsules that surround solid organs, such as the liver and gallbladder, contain pain fibers that are stimulated by stretching if these organs swell.

Biochemical mediators of the inflammatory response, such as histamine, bradykinin, and serotonin, stimulate organic nerve endings and produce abdominal pain. The edema and vascular congestion that accompany chemical, bacterial, or viral inflammation also cause painful stretching. Obstruction of blood flow from the distention of bowel obstruction or mesenteric vessel thrombosis produces the pain of ischemia, and increased concentrations of tissue metabolites stimulate pain receptors.

Abdominal pain can be parietal (somatic), visceral, or referred. **Parietal pain,** from the parietal peritoneum, is more localized and intense than visceral pain, which arises from the organs themselves. Parietal pain lateralizes because, at any particular point, the parietal peritoneum is innervated from only one side of the nervous system.

Visceral pain arises from a stimulus acting on an abdominal organ. It is usually poorly localized with a radiating pattern. Visceral pain is diffuse and vague because nerve endings in abdominal organs are sparse and multisegmented. Pain arising from the stomach, for example, is experienced as a sensation of fullness, cramping, or gnawing in the midepigastric area.

Referred pain is visceral pain felt at some distance from a diseased or affected organ. It is usually well localized and is felt in skin or deeper tissues that share a central afferent pathway with the affected organ. Generally, referred pain develops as the intensity of a visceral pain stimulus increases.

Gastrointestinal bleeding

Upper gastrointestinal bleeding, which is defined as bleeding in the esophagus, stomach, or duodenum, is characterized by frank, bright red bleeding or "coffee ground" material that has been affected by stomach acids. Upper gastrointestinal bleeding is commonly caused by bleeding varices (varicose veins) in the esophagus, peptic ulcers, or a Mallory-Weiss tear at the esophageal gastric junction from severe retching. **Lower gastrointestinal bleeding,** or bleeding from the jejunum, ileum, colon, or rectum, can be caused by polyps, inflammatory disease, cancer, or hemorrhoids. Acute, severe gastrointestinal bleeding is life threatening, depending on the volume and rate of blood loss, associated disease, age, and effectiveness of treatment.

The signs of gastrointestinal bleeding are described in Table 34-1. Physiologic response to gastrointestinal bleeding depends on the amount and rate of the loss (Figure 34-1). Changes in blood pressure and heart rate are the best indicators of massive blood loss in the gastrointestinal tract. During the early stages of blood volume depletion, the peripheral vascular compartment constricts

TABLE 34-1

Presentations of Gastrointestinal Bleeding

Presentations	Definition
ACUTE BLEEDING	
Hematemesis	Bloody vomitus; either fresh, bright red blood or dark grainy digested blood with "coffee grounds" appearance
Melena	Black, sticky, tarry, foul-smelling stools caused by digestion of blood in the gastrointestinal tract
Hematochezia	Fresh, bright red blood passed from the rectum
OCCULT BLEEDING	Trace amounts of blood in normal-appearing stools or gastric secretions; detectable only with a guaiac test

to shunt blood to vital organs, including the brain. A sign that this is happening is postural hypotension (a drop in blood pressure that occurs with a change from the recumbent position to a sitting or upright position), lightheadedness, and loss of vision. If blood loss continues, hypovolemic shock progresses. Diminished blood flow to the kidneys causes decreased urine output and may lead to oliguria (low urine output), tubular necrosis, and renal failure. Ultimately, insufficient cerebral and coronary blood flow causes irreversible anoxia and death.

The accumulation of blood in the gastrointestinal tract is irritating and increases peristalsis, causing diarrhea. If bleeding is from the lower gastrointestinal tract, the diarrhea is frankly bloody. Bleeding from the upper gastrointestinal tract also can be rapid enough to produce **hematochezia** (bright red stools), but generally some digestion of the blood components will have occurred, producing melena—black or tarry stools that are sticky and have a characteristic foul odor. The digestion of blood proteins originating from massive upper gastrointestinal bleeding is reflected by an increase in blood urea nitrogen (BUN) levels (see Figure 34-1).

The hematocrit and hemoglobin values are not the best indicators of acute gastrointestinal bleeding because plasma volume and red cell volume are lost proportionately. As the plasma volume is replaced, the hematocrit and hemoglobin values begin to reflect the extent of blood loss. The interpretation of these values is modified to account for exogenous replacement of fluids and the hydration status of the tissues.

QUICK CHECK 34-1

1. How is visceral pain "referred"?
2. How does osmotic diarrhea differ from secretory diarrhea?
3. Why is hematocrit not a good indicator of acute GI bleeding blood loss?

Disorders of Motility

Dysphagia

PATHOPHYSIOLOGY **Dysphagia** is difficulty swallowing. It can result from *mechanical obstruction* of the esophagus or a disorder that impairs esophageal motility. Intrinsic obstructions originate in the wall of the esophageal lumen and include tumors, strictures, and diverticular herniations (outpouchings). Extrinsic mechanical obstructions originate outside the esophageal lumen and narrow the esophagus by pressing inward on the esophageal wall. The most common cause of extrinsic mechanical obstruction is tumor.

Functional dysphagia is caused by neural or muscular disorders that interfere with voluntary swallowing or peristalsis. Disorders that affect the striated muscles of the upper esophagus interfere with the oropharyngeal (voluntary) phase of swallowing. Typical causes are dermatomyositis (a muscle disease) and neurologic impairments caused by cerebrovascular accidents, Parkinson disease, or achalasia.

Achalasia is a rare form of dysphagia characterized by loss of esophageal peristalsis and failure of the lower esophageal sphincter (LES) to relax. Achalasia results from loss of neurons in the myenteric plexus and dysfunction of the vagal nerve outside the esophagus.[5] Disrupted innervation results in loss of neuromuscular coordination and decreased peristalsis of the middle esophagus. Decreased relaxation of the LES after swallowing allows food to accumulate above the obstruction, which distends the esophagus (Figure 34-2). As hydrostatic pressure increases, food is slowly forced past the obstruction into the stomach. Psychosocial achalasia has been documented and may be the result of life stressors.

CLINICAL MANIFESTATIONS Distention and spasm of the esophageal muscles during eating or drinking may cause a mild or severe stabbing pain at the level of obstruction. Discomfort occurring 2 to 4 seconds after swallowing is associated with upper esophageal obstruction. Discomfort occurring 10 to 15 seconds after swallowing is more common in obstructions of the lower esophagus. If obstruction results from a growing tumor, dysphagia begins with difficulty swallowing solids and advances to difficulty swallowing semisolids and liquids. If motor function is impaired, both solids and liquids are difficult to swallow. Regurgitation of undigested food, unpleasant taste, vomiting, aspiration, and weight loss are common manifestations of all types of dysphagia. Aspiration of esophageal contents can lead to pneumonia.

EVALUATION AND TREATMENT Knowledge of the patient's history and clinical manifestations contributes significantly to a diagnosis of dysphagia. A barium swallow is used to visualize the contours of the esophagus and identify structural defects. Manometry documents the duration and amplitude of abnormal pressure changes associated with obstruction or loss of neural regulation. Esophageal

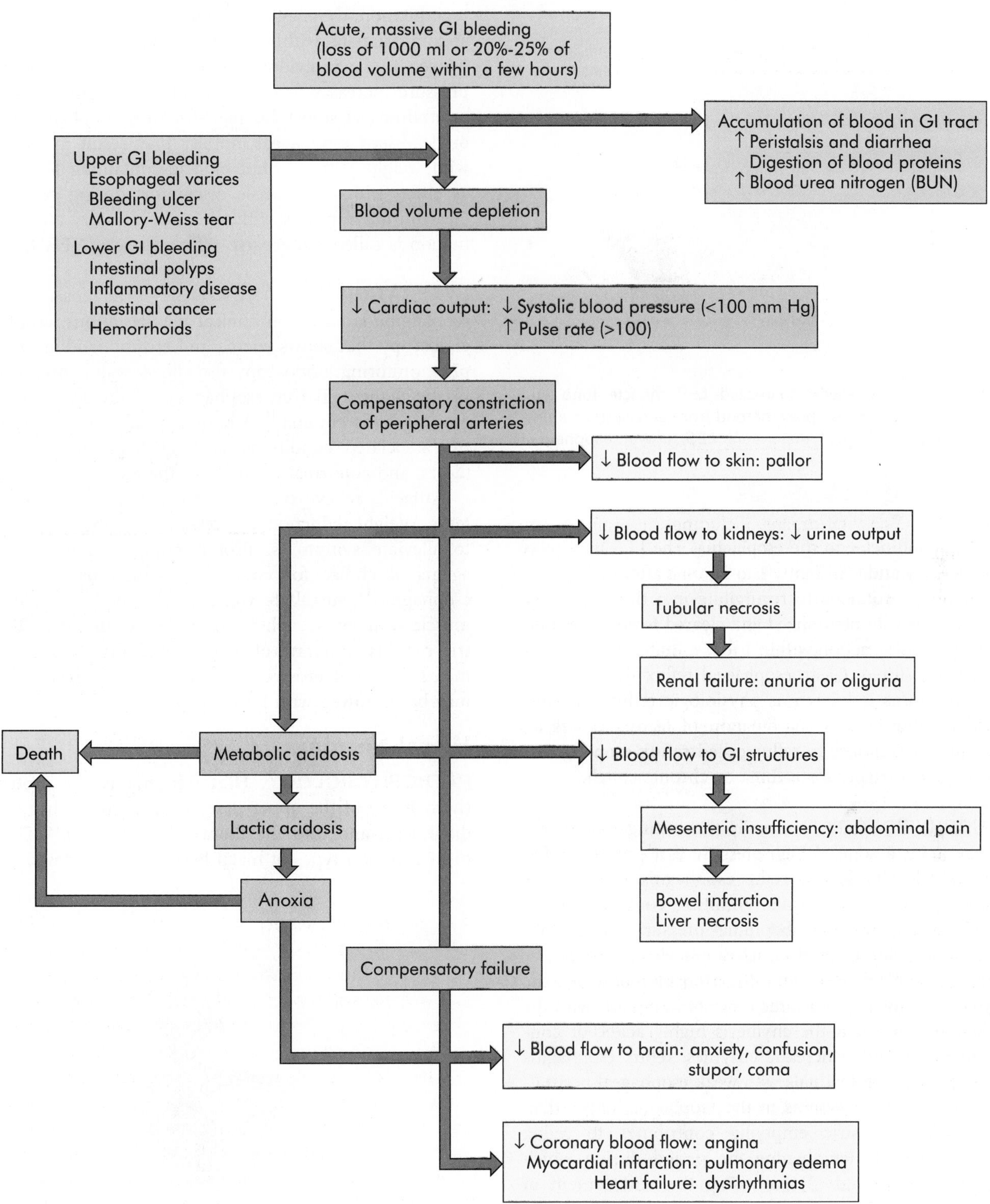

Figure 34-1 ■ **Pathophysiology of Gastrointestinal (GI) Bleeding.**

endoscopy is performed to examine the esophageal mucosa and obtain biopsy specimens.

The individual is taught to manage symptoms by eating slowly, eating small meals, taking fluid with meals, and sleeping with the head elevated to prevent regurgitation and aspiration. Anticholinergic drugs (e.g., botulism toxin) may relieve symptoms of dysphagia.[6] Mechanical dilation of the esophageal sphincter and surgical separation of the lower esophageal muscles with a longitudinal incision (myotomy) may alleviate achalasia.

Gastroesophageal reflux

Gastroesophageal reflux (GER) is the reflux of chyme (acid and pepsin) from the stomach through the lower

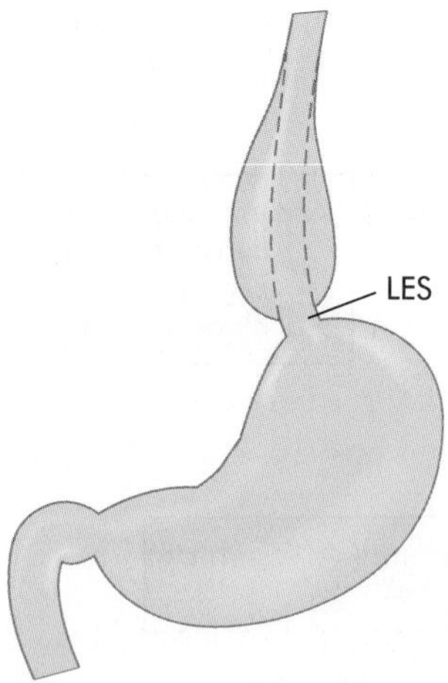

Figure 34-2 ■ **Achalasia.** Increased LES muscle tone and loss of peristaltic function prevent food from entering the stomach, causing esophageal distention. *LES,* Lower esophageal sphincter.

esophageal sphincter to the esophagus. The LES may relax spontaneously and transiently 1 to 2 hours after eating, permitting gastric contents to regurgitate into the esophagus. The acid is usually neutralized and cleared from the esophagus by peristaltic action within 1 to 3 minutes, and sphincter tone is restored. Gastroesophageal reflux that does not cause symptoms is known as physiologic reflux. In some individuals, however, a combination of factors causes an inflammatory response to reflux called **reflux esophagitis.**[7] GER may be a trigger for asthma or chronic cough.[7]

PATHOPHYSIOLOGY Normally the resting tone of the LES maintains a zone of high pressure that prevents GER. In individuals who develop reflux esophagitis, this pressure tends to be lower than normal. Vomiting, coughing, lifting, or bending that increases abdominal pressure can contribute to the development of reflux esophagitis. The severity of the esophagitis depends on the composition of the gastric contents and the length of time they are in contact with the esophageal mucosa. If the chyme is highly acidic or contains bile salts and pancreatic enzymes, reflux esophagitis can be severe. In individuals with weak esophageal peristalsis, refluxed chyme remains in the esophagus longer than usual. Delayed gastric emptying contributes to reflux esophagitis by (1) lengthening the period during which reflux is possible and (2) increasing the acid content of chyme. Disorders that delay emptying include gastric or duodenal ulcers, which can cause pyloric edema; strictures that narrow the pylorus; and hiatal hernia, which can weaken the LES.[8]

Reflux esophagitis causes inflammatory responses in the esophageal wall, such as hyperemia, increased capillary permeability, edema, tissue fragility, and erosion. Fibrosis and thickening may develop.

CLINICAL MANIFESTATIONS The clinical manifestations of erosive reflux esophagitis are heartburn, acid regurgitation, dysphagia, chronic cough, asthma, and upper abdominal pain within 1 hour of eating. The symptoms worsen if the individual lies down or if intra-abdominal pressure increases (e.g., as a result of coughing, vomiting, or straining at stool). Edema, strictures, esophageal spasm, or decreased esophageal motility may result in dysphagia with weight loss. Alcohol or acid-containing foods, such as citrus fruits, can cause discomfort during swallowing. Heartburn symptoms without mucosal injury and inflammation is called **nonerosive reflux disease (NERD).**[9]

EVALUATION AND TREATMENT Diagnosis of reflux esophagitis is based on clinical manifestations, esophageal endoscopy that shows edema and erosion, and ambulatory pH monitoring. Endoscopy also allows evaluation for metaplastic changes (Barrett esophagus) and the development of esophageal carcinoma.[10] A barium swallow is used to identify associated conditions, such as hiatal hernia, gastric ulcers, and abnormal contours of the esophageal lumen.

Antacids relieve symptoms by neutralizing gastric contents. Weight reduction and cessation of smoking also help to alleviate symptoms. Proton pump inhibitors are the agents of choice for controlling symptoms and healing esophagitis.[11] Sucralfate will coat ulcerated tissue; smooth muscle stimulants, such as cisapride, can increase LES gastric motility and rate of gastric emptying. If other treatments fail or if erosive esophagitis fails to heal, the LES may be narrowed with laparoscopic surgery.

Hiatal hernia

PATHOPHYSIOLOGY **Hiatal hernia** is the protrusion (herniation) of the upper part of the stomach through the diaphragm and into the thorax (Figure 34-3).[12] The two most common types of hiatal hernia are as follows:

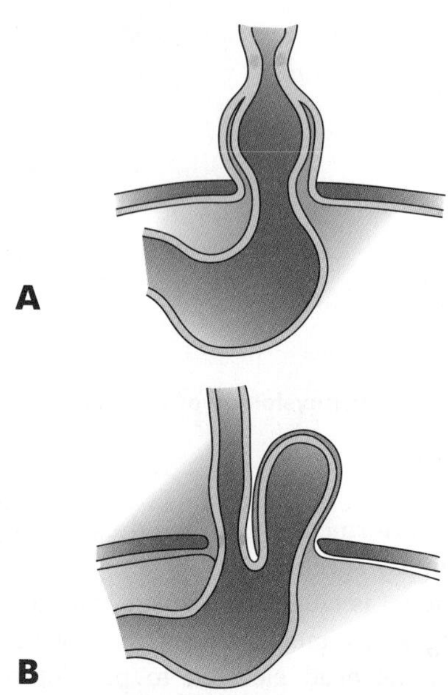

Figure 34-3 ■ **Types of Hiatal Hernia. A,** Sliding hiatal hernia. **B,** Paraesophageal hiatal hernia.

1. **Sliding hiatal hernia.** The stomach slides or moves into the thoracic cavity through the esophageal hiatus; a congenitally short esophagus, trauma, or weakening of the diaphragmatic muscles at the gastroesophageal junction is contributory. Coughing, bending, tight clothing, ascites, obesity, and pregnancy accentuate the hernia.
2. **Paraesophageal hiatal hernia.** The greater curvature of the stomach herniates through a secondary opening in the diaphragm and lies alongside the esophagus. Symptoms include congestion of mucosal blood flow leading to gastritis and ulcer formation. Strangulation of the hernia is a major complication.

Hiatal hernias of both types tend to occur in conjunction with several other diseases, including reflux esophagitis, peptic ulcer, cholecystitis (gallbladder inflammation), cholelithiasis (gallstones), chronic pancreatitis, and diverticulosis.

CLINICAL MANIFESTATIONS Hiatal hernias are often asymptomatic. Generally, a wide variety of symptoms develop later in life and are associated with other gastrointestinal disorders as well. Manifestations include gastroesophageal reflux, dysphagia, heartburn, and epigastric pain. Regurgitation and substernal discomfort after eating are common.

EVALUATION AND TREATMENT Diagnostic procedures include (1) examinations using barium as a contrast medium and (2) endoscopy. A chest x-ray film often will show the protrusion of the stomach into the thorax, indicating paraesophageal hiatal hernia.

Treatment for sliding hiatal hernia is usually conservative. The individual can diminish reflux by eating small, frequent meals and avoiding the recumbent position after eating. Abdominal supports and tight clothing should be avoided, and weight control is recommended for obese individuals. Antacids alleviate reflux esophagitis. Individuals who are uncomfortable at night benefit from sleeping in a semi-upright position. Surgery (fundoplication) may be performed if medical management fails to control symptoms.

Pyloric obstruction

PATHOPHYSIOLOGY **Pyloric obstruction** is the narrowing or blocking of the opening between the stomach and the duodenum. This condition can be congenital (see Chapter 35) or acquired. Acquired obstruction is caused by peptic ulcer disease or carcinoma near the pylorus. Duodenal ulcers are more likely than gastric ulcers to obstruct the pylorus. Ulceration causes obstruction resulting from inflammation, edema, spasm, fibrosis, or scarring. Tumors cause obstruction by growing into the pylorus.

CLINICAL MANIFESTATIONS Early in the course of pyloric obstruction, the individual experiences vague epigastric fullness, which becomes more distressing after eating and later in the day. Nausea and epigastric pain may occur as the muscles of the stomach contract in attempts to force chyme past the obstruction. These symptoms disappear when the chyme finally moves into the duodenum. As obstruction progresses, anorexia develops, sometimes accompanied by weight loss. Severe obstruction causes gastric distention and atony (lack of muscle tone and gastric motility). Gastric distention stimulates gastric secretion, which increases the feeling of fullness. Rolling or jarring of the abdomen produces a sloshing sound called the *succussion splash.* At this stage, vomiting is a cardinal sign of obstruction. It is usually copious and occurs several hours after eating. The vomitus contains undigested food but no bile. Prolonged vomiting leads to dehydration, which is accompanied by a hypokalemic and hypochloremic metabolic alkalosis caused by loss of potassium and gastric acid. Because food does not enter the intestine, stools are infrequent and small. Prolonged pyloric obstruction causes malnutrition, dehydration, and extreme debilitation.

EVALUATION AND TREATMENT Diagnosis is based on clinical manifestations, a history of ulcer disease, and examination of residual gastric contents. Endoscopy is performed if gastric carcinoma is the suggested cause of pyloric obstruction. Barium studies are contraindicated.

Obstructions resulting from ulceration often resolve with conservative management. A large-bore tube is used to aspirate stomach contents and relieve distention. Then nasogastric suction is maintained for 2 to 3 days to decompress the stomach and restore normal motility. Gastric secretions that contribute to inflammation and edema can be suppressed with proton pump inhibitors or cimetidine. Fluids and electrolytes (saline and potassium) are given intravenously to effect rehydration and correct hypokalemia and alkalosis (see Chapter 4). Severely malnourished individuals may require parenteral hyperalimentation (intravenous nutrition). Surgery or the placement of stents may be required to treat gastric carcinoma or persistent obstruction caused by fibrosis and scarring.

Intestinal obstruction

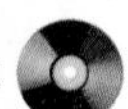

Intestinal obstruction can be caused by any condition that prevents the normal flow of chyme through the intestinal lumen (Table 34-2). Obstructions can occur in either the small or the large intestine (Table 34-3). Criteria for classifying intestinal obstruction are summarized in Table 34-4. Intestinal obstruction is classified by cause as simple or functional. *Simple obstruction* is mechanical blockage of the lumen by a lesion; *functional obstruction* is a failure of motility (paralytic ileus), often occurring after abdominal surgery. Simple obstruction of the small intestine is the most common type of intestinal obstruction. Acute obstructions usually have mechanical causes, such as adhesions or hernias (Figure 34-4). Chronic or partial obstructions are more often associated with tumors or inflammatory disorders, particularly of the large intestine.

PATHOPHYSIOLOGY The major pathophysiologic alterations are presented in Figure 34-5. Postoperative

TABLE 34-2
Common Causes of Intestinal Obstruction

Cause	Pathophysiology
Hernia	Protrusion of the intestine through a weakness in the abdominal muscles or through the inguinal ring
Intussusception	Telescoping of one part of the intestine into another; this usually causes strangulation of the blood supply; more common in infants 10–15 months of age than in adults
Torsion (volvulus)	Twisting of the intestine on its mesenteric pedicle, with occlusion of the blood supply; often associated with fibrous adhesions; occurs most often in middle-aged and elderly men
Diverticulosis	Inflamed saccular herniations (diverticuli) of the mucosa and submucosa through the tunica muscularis of the colon; diverticuli are interspersed between thick, circular, fibrous bands; most common in obese individuals older than 60 yr
Tumor	Tumor growth into the intestinal lumen; adenocarcinoma of the colon and rectum is the most common tumoral obstruction; most common in individuals older than 60 yr
Paralytic (adynamic) ileus	Loss of peristaltic motor activity in the intestine; associated with abdominal surgery, peritonitis, hypokalemia, ischemic bowel, spinal trauma, or pneumonia
Fibrous adhesions	Peritoneal irritation from surgery or trauma leads to formation of fibrin and adhesions that attach to intestine, omentum, or peritoneum and can cause obstruction; most common in small intestine

TABLE 34-3
Large and Small Bowel Obstruction

Type of Obstruction	Cause
Small bowel obstruction	Adhesions: secondary to previous abdominal surgeries—50%-70%
	Hernia: inguinal, ventral, or femoral—20%-25%
	Tumors: may be associated with intussusception—10%
	Mesenteric ischemia—3%-5%
	Crohn disease—<1%
	Hernia—<1%
Large bowel obstruction	Colon/rectal cancer—90%
	Volvulus—4%-5%
	Diverticular disease—3%
	Other causes (inflammatory bowel disease, adhesions, hernia)

Data from Turnage RH, Bergen P: Intestinal obstruction and ileus. In Feldman M et al: *Sleisenger & Fordtran's gastrointestinal and liver disease*, ed 7, Philadelphia, 2002, Saunders.

TABLE 34-4
Classifications of Intestinal Obstruction

Criteria for Classification	Definition
ONSET	
Acute	Sudden onset; often caused by torsion, intussusception, or herniation
Chronic	Protracted onset; more commonly from tumor growth or progressive formation of strictures
EXTENT OF OBSTRUCTION	
Partial	Incomplete obstruction of intestinal lumen
Complete	Complete obstruction of intestinal lumen
LOCATION OF OBSTRUCTING LESION	
Intrinsic	Obstruction develops within intestinal lumen; examples: gut wall edema or hemorrhage, foreign bodies (gallstones), tumors, or gut wall fibrosis
Extrinsic	Obstruction originates outside the intestine; examples: tumors, torsion, fibrosis, hernia, intussusception
EFFECTS ON INTESTINAL WALL	
Simple	Luminal obstruction without impairment of blood supply
Strangulated	Luminal obstruction with occlusion of blood supply
Closed loop	Obstruction at each end of a segment of the intestine
CASUAL FACTORS	
Mechanical	Blockage of the intestinal lumen by intrinsic or extrinsic lesions; usually treated surgically
Functional (paralytic ileus)	Paralysis of the intestinal musculature caused by trauma, peritonitis, electrolyte imbalances, or spasmolytic agents; usually treated by decompression with suction or surgery if death of tissue.

paralytic ileus results from inhibitory neural reflexes, inflammatory mediators, and the influence of exogenous and endogenous opioids.[13] If the obstruction is at the pylorus or high in the small intestine, metabolic alkalosis develops initially as a result of excessive loss of hydrogen ions that normally would be reabsorbed from the gastric juice. With prolonged obstruction or obstruction lower in the intestine, metabolic acidosis is more likely to occur because bicarbonate from pancreatic secretions and bile cannot be reabsorbed. Hypokalemia can be extreme, promoting acidosis and atony of the intestinal wall. Metabolic acidosis also may be accentuated by ketosis, the result of declining carbohydrate stores caused by starvation. If pressure from the distention is severe enough, it occludes the arterial circulation and causes strangulation leading to perforation. Continued intestinal secretion and decreased absorption lead to decreased blood volume; lack of circulation permits the buildup of significant amounts of lactic acid, which worsen the metabolic acidosis. Bacteria also proliferate and may cross the mucosal barrier and cause peritonitis or sepsis.

CLINICAL MANIFESTATIONS Colicky pains followed by vomiting are the cardinal symptoms. Typically the pain occurs intermittently and intensifies for seconds or minutes as a peristaltic wave of muscle contraction meets the obstruction. Sweating, nausea, and hypotension occur as an autonomic response. The passing of the wave is followed by a pain-free interval. With severe distention, the pain may diminish in intensity. If strangulation occurs, the pain looses its colicky character, becoming more constant and severe as ischemia progresses to necrosis, perforation, and peritonitis.

Vomiting and distention vary, depending on the level of the obstruction. Obstruction at the pylorus causes early, profuse vomiting of clear gastric fluid. Obstruction in the proximal small intestine causes mild distention and vomiting of bile-stained fluid. Obstruction lower in the intestine causes more pronounced distention, and vomiting may not occur or may occur later and contain fecal material. Partial obstruction can cause diarrhea or constipation, but complete obstruction usually causes constipation only. Early in the course of complete obstruction, the frequency of bowel sounds increases and they may be tinkly and accompanied by peristaltic rushes and crampy abdominal pain as the bowel contracts to overcome the obstruction. Signs of dehydration, hypovolemia, and metabolic acidosis may be observed as early as 24 hours after the occurrence of complete obstruction. Distention may be severe enough to push against the diaphragm and decrease lung volume. This can lead to atelectasis and pneumonia, particularly in debilitated individuals.

EVALUATION AND TREATMENT Evaluation is based on clinical manifestations. Successful management requires early identification of the site and type of obstruction. Postoperative ileus requires a multimodal approach, including thoracic epidural blockade with local anesthetic, nasogastric suction, early enteral feeding, mu opioid receptor blockade,

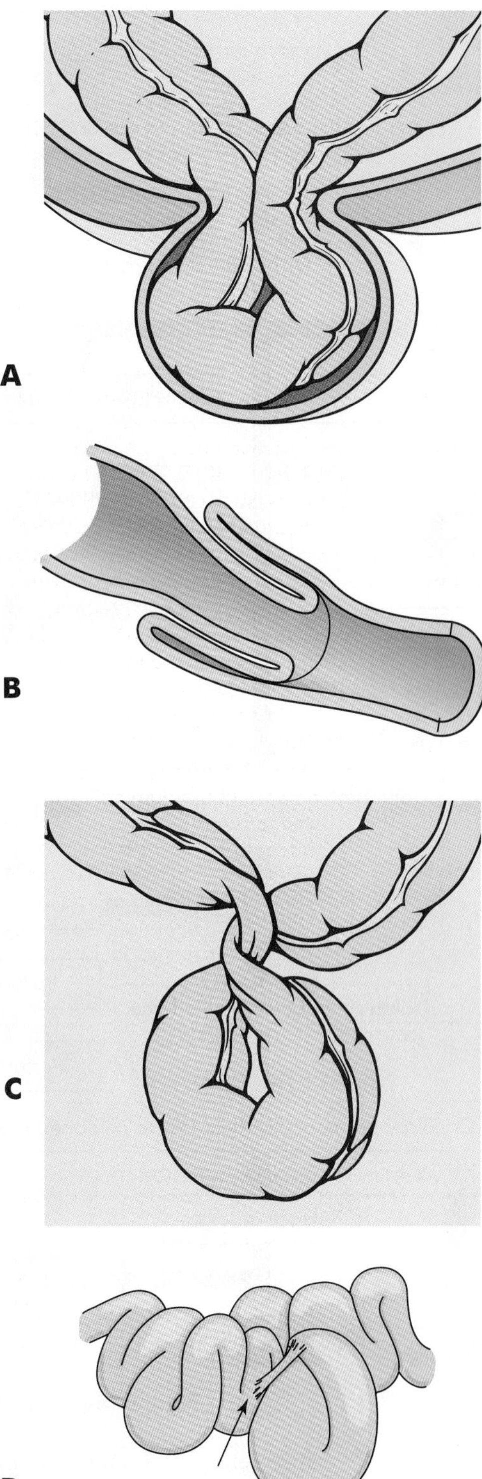

Figure 34-4 ■ **Intestinal Obstructions. A,** Hernia. **B,** Intussusception. **C,** Volvulus. **D,** Constriction adhesions. (**A, B,** and **C** from Damjanov I: *Pathology for the health professions*, ed 3, Philadelphia, 2006, Saunders. **D** from Monahan FD et al: *Phipps' medical-surgical nursing: concepts and clinical practice,* ed 8, St Louis, 2007, Mosby.)

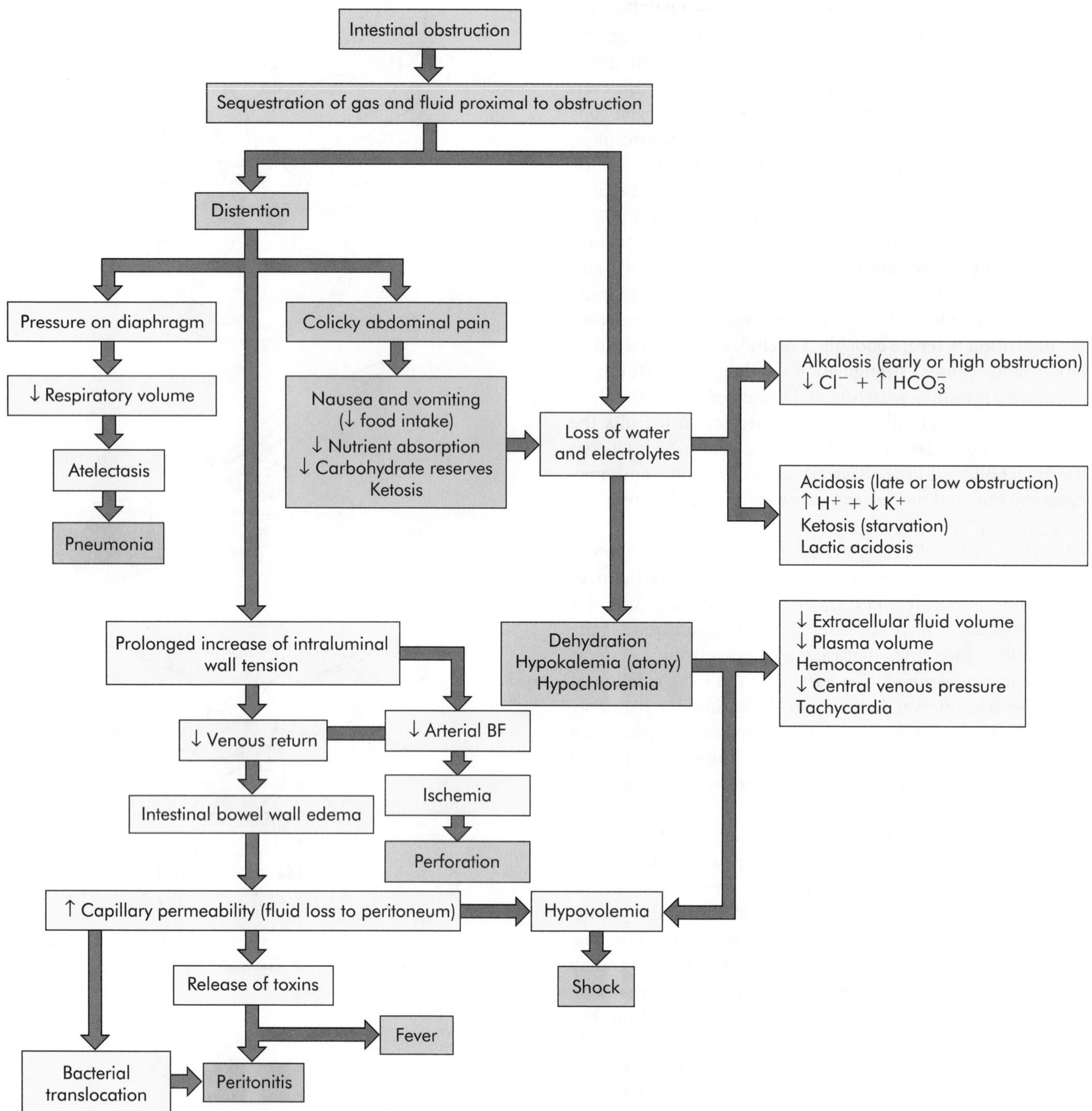

Figure 34-5 ■ **Pathophysiology of Intestinal Obstruction.**

and mobilization.[14] Antisecretory and intestinal motility agents may be helpful. Replacement of fluid and electrolytes and decompression of the lumen with gastric or intestinal suction are essential forms of therapy. Immediate surgical intervention is required for complete obstruction, strangulation, or perforation.

QUICK CHECK 34-2

1. Why is heartburn associated with gastroesophageal reflux?
2. How does peritonitis develop with bowel obstruction?

Gastritis

Gastritis is an inflammatory disorder of the gastric mucosa. It can be acute or chronic and affect the fundus or antrum or both.

Acute gastritis erodes the surface epithelium in a diffuse or localized pattern. The erosions are usually superficial. Acute gastritis is usually the result of injury of the protective mucosal barrier caused by drugs or chemicals. Anti-inflammatory drugs cause gastritis, perhaps because they inhibit prostaglandins, which normally stimulate the secretion of mucus. Alcohol, histamine, digitalis, and metabolic disorders such as uremia are contributing factors. The clinical manifestations of acute gastritis can include vague abdominal discomfort, epigastric tenderness, and bleeding. Healing usually occurs spontaneously within a few days. Discontinuing injurious drugs, using antacids, or decreasing acid secretion with cimetidine facilitates healing.

Chronic gastritis tends to occur in elderly individuals and causes thinning and degeneration of the stomach wall. Chronic gastritis is classified as type A (fundal) or type B (antral), depending on the pathogenesis and location of the lesions.

Chronic fundal gastritis, also called *atrophic gastritis,* is the most severe type. The gastric mucosa degenerates extensively in the body and fundus of the stomach, leading to gastric atrophy. Loss of chief cells and parietal cells diminishes acid secretion, so the feedback mechanism that normally inhibits gastrin secretion is impaired, causing elevated plasma levels of gastrin. Pernicious anemia develops because intrinsic factor is less available to facilitate vitamin B_{12} absorption in the ileum.

A significant number of individuals with chronic fundal gastritis have antibodies to parietal cells, intrinsic factor, and gastric cells in their sera, suggesting that an autoimmune mechanism is involved in pathogenesis of the disease. The fact that chronic fundal gastritis occurs in association with other autoimmune diseases strengthens this association. *Helicobacter pylori* infection also can promote mucosal atrophy and tissue injury.[15] Chronic fundal gastritis is a risk factor for gastric carcinoma, particularly in individuals who develop pernicious anemia.

Chronic antral gastritis generally involves the antrum only and occurs approximately four times more often than fundal gastritis. It is not associated with decreased hydrochloric acid secretion, pernicious anemia, or presence of parietal cell antibodies. *H. pylori* also is a major causative factor,[15] and mucosal atrophy is rare. In approximately 10% of cases, antibodies to gastrin-secreting cells are found in the serum. Chronic reflux of bile and pancreatic enzymes may contribute to the gastritis by persistently disrupting the mucosal barrier (Figure 34-6).

Signs and symptoms of chronic gastritis often do not correlate with the severity of the disease. Gastroscopic examination and biopsy may show a long-standing inflammatory process and gastric atrophy in an individual with no history of abdominal distress. Failure to stimulate acid secretion confirms achlorhydria (diminished secretion of hydrochloric acid). The gastric secretions also can be evaluated for the presence of intrinsic factor. Individuals may report vague symptoms, including anorexia, fullness, nausea, vomiting, and epigastric pain. Gastric bleeding may be the only clinical manifestation of gastritis.

Symptoms can usually be managed with smaller meals; a soft, bland diet; and avoidance of alcohol and aspirin. *H. pylori* infection is treated with antibiotics, and vitamin B_{12} is administered to correct pernicious anemia.

Peptic Ulcer Disease

A **peptic ulcer** is a break, or ulceration, in the protective mucosal lining of the lower esophagus, stomach, or duodenum. Such breaks expose submucosal areas to gastric secretions and autodigestion. Peptic ulcers can be acute or chronic, superficial or deep. Superficial ulcerations are called *erosions* because they erode the mucosa but do not penetrate the muscularis mucosae (see Figure 34-6). True ulcers extend through the muscularis mucosae and damage blood vessels, causing hemorrhage, or perforate the gastrointestinal wall. Risk factors for peptic ulcer disease are summarized in *Risk Factors:* Peptic Ulcer.

Psychologic stress may be a risk factor for peptic ulcer disease, although studies of life stress and ulcer disease are inconclusive. Individuals with multiple stressors, poor coping skills, and persistent anxiety and depression in the presence of recurrent peptic ulcers may require psychiatric management.[16,17]

RISK FACTORS Peptic Ulcer

- Smoking
- Advanced age
- Habitual use of nonsteroidal anti-inflammatory drugs (NSAIDs)
- Alcohol
- Chronic diseases, such as emphysema, rheumatoid arthritis, cirrhosis, and diabetes
- Infection of the gastric and duodenal mucosa with *Helicobacter pylori*

Data from Hawkey CJ et al: *Gut* 51(3):336–343, 2002; Yuan Y, Padol IT, Hunt RH: Peptic ulcer disease today, *Nat Clin Pract Gastroentrol Hepatol* 3(2):80–89.

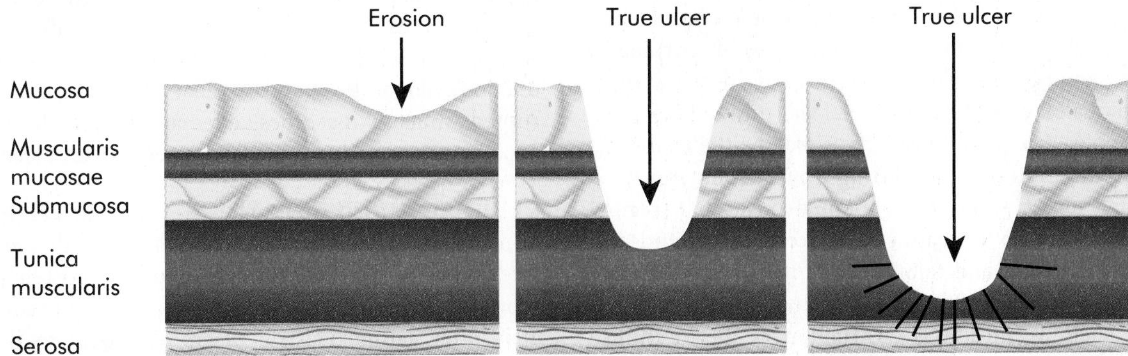

Figure 34-6 ■ Lesions Caused by Peptic Ulcer Disease.

Duodenal ulcers

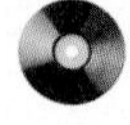

Duodenal ulcers occur with greater frequency than other types of peptic ulcers and tend to develop in younger persons and perhaps in individuals with type O blood.[18]

PATHOPHYSIOLOGY Infection with *H. pylori* and non-steroidal anti-inflammatory drugs (NSAIDs) are the major cause of duodenal ulcer.[19] Hypersecretion of acid and pepsin is the primary cause of duodenal ulcers, but inadequate secretion of bicarbonate by the duodenal mucosa also may be a factor.[20] Factors that contribute to ulcer formation include the following:

1. A greater than usual number of parietal (acid-secreting) cells in the gastric mucosa.
2. High serum gastric levels that remain high longer than normal after eating and continue to stimulate secretion of acid and pepsin (may be caused by *H. pylori*).
3. Failure of the feedback mechanism, whereby acid in the gastric antrum inhibits gastrin release.
4. Rapid gastric emptying, which overwhelms the buffering capacity of the bicarbonate-rich pancreatic secretions
5. Association of *H. pylori* with death of mucosal epithelial cells and elevated levels of gastrin and pepsinogen.
6. *H. pylori* release of toxins and enzymes that promote inflammation and ulceration.
7. Use of NSAIDs, which inhibit prostaglandins.
8. Acid production stimulated by cigarette smoking.
9. Decreased mucosal bicarbonate secretion or clearing of acid.

All these factors, singly or in combination, cause acid and pepsin concentrations in the duodenum to penetrate the mucosal barrier and cause ulceration (Figure 34-7).

CLINICAL MANIFESTATIONS The characteristic manifestation of a duodenal ulcer is chronic intermittent pain in the epigastric area. The pain begins 2 or 3 hours after eating, when the stomach is empty. It is not unusual for pain to occur in the middle of the night and disappear by morning. Pain is relieved rapidly by ingestion of food or antacids, creating a typical pain-food-relief pattern. Some individuals with duodenal ulcer may have no symptoms; the first manifestation may be hemorrhage or perforation, particularly with history of aspirin or anticoagulant use.

Complications of duodenal ulcer include bleeding, perforation, and obstruction of the duodenum or outlet of the stomach. Bleeding is the most common cause of mortality, particularly among the elderly. Perforation occurs with destruction of all layers of the duodenal wall and causes sudden severe epigastric pain. Obstruction may be the result of edema from inflammation or scarring from chronic injury.

Duodenal ulcers often heal spontaneously but recur within months without treatment. Exacerbations tend to develop in the spring and fall. Relief of pain accompanies healing. Constant, unremitting pain may be caused by complications, such as intestinal obstruction or perforation. Bleeding from duodenal ulcers causes hematemesis or melena.

EVALUATION AND TREATMENT Several diagnostic approaches are used to differentiate duodenal ulcers from gastric ulcers or gastric carcinoma. X-ray examinations using barium may show an anatomic deformity created by the ulcer crater. If the x-ray examination is inconclusive, flexible endoscopic evaluations may be performed. Radioimmune assays of gastrin levels are evaluated to identify ulcers associated with gastric carcinomas. *H. pylori* can be detected by endoscopic evaluation and biopsy, serology, or noninvasively with a urea breath test or stool antigen.[21]

Management of duodenal ulcers is aimed at (1) relieving the causes and effects of hyperacidity and (2) administering antacids and drugs that suppress acid secretion (omeprazole). *H. pylori* is treated with a combination of antibiotics and proton pump inhibitors.[22] Research is in progress for an *H. pylori* vaccine.[23] Risk of duodenal ulcer may be reduced with a high vitamin A and fiber diet.[24] Endoscopic heater probes are effective to stop bleeding. Complications are treated with either endoscopic or surgical approaches.

Gastric ulcers

Gastric ulcers are ulcers of the stomach and occur about equally in males and females, usually between the ages of 55 and 65 years. They are about one fourth as common as duodenal ulcers (Table 34-5).

PATHOPHYSIOLOGY Use of nonsteroidal anti-inflammatory drugs and *H. pylori* infection are major causes of gastric ulcer. Generally, gastric ulcers develop in the antral region, adjacent to the acid-secreting mucosa of the body. The primary defect is an abnormality that increases the mucosal barrier's permeability to hydrogen ions. Gastric secretion may be normal or less than normal.

Chronic gastritis is often associated with development of gastric ulcers and may precipitate ulcer formation by limiting the mucosa's ability to secrete a protective layer of mucus (Figure 34-8). Other factors include the following:

1. Decreased mucosal synthesis of prostaglandin
2. Duodenal reflux of bile and pancreatic enzymes
3. Use of ulcerogenic drugs

An increased concentration of bile salts disrupts the gastric mucosa and may decrease the electrical potential across the gastric mucosal membrane. The break permits hydrogen ions to diffuse into the mucosa, where they disrupt permeability and cellular structure. A vicious cycle can be established as the damaged mucosa liberates histamine, which stimulates the increase of acid and pepsinogen production, blood flow, and capillary permeability. The disrupted mucosa becomes edematous and loses plasma proteins. Destruction of small vessels causes bleeding.

CLINICAL MANIFESTATIONS The clinical manifestations of gastric ulcers are similar to those of duodenal ulcers (see Table 34-5). The pattern of pain-food-relief is common, but the pain of gastric ulcers also may occur immediately after eating. Gastric ulcers also tend to be chronic rather than alternating between periods of remission and exacerbation. Gastric ulcers cause more anorexia, vomiting,

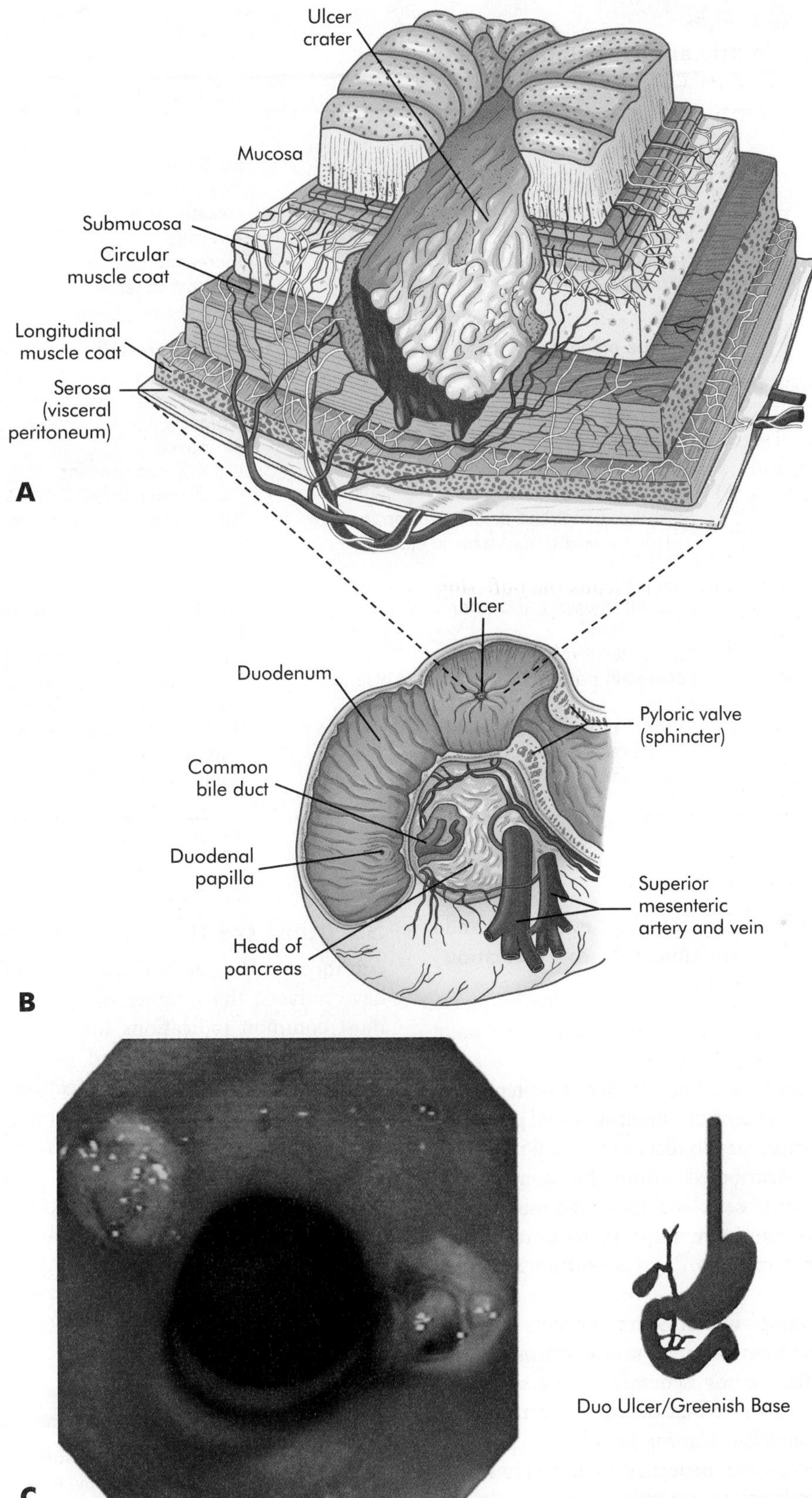

Figure 34-7 ■ **Duodenal Ulcer. A,** A deep ulceration in the duodenal wall extending as a crater through the entire mucosa and into the muscle layers. **B,** Sequence of ulcerations from normal mucosa to duodenal ulcer. **C,** Bilateral (kissing) duodenal ulcers in a person using nonsteroidal anti-inflammatory drugs (NSAIDs). (**C** courtesy David Bjorkman, MD, University of Utah School of Medicine, Department of Gastroenterology.)

TABLE 34-5

Characteristics of Gastric and Duodenal Ulcers

Characteristics	Gastric Ulcer	Duodenal Ulcer
INCIDENCE		
Age at onset	50–70 yr	20–50 yr
Family history	Usually negative	Positive
Gender (prevalence)	Equal in women and men	Greater in men
Stress factors	Increased	Average
Ulcerogenic drugs	Normal use	Increased use
Cancer risk	Increased	Not increased
PATHOPHYSIOLOGY		
Abnormal mucus	May be present	May be present
Parietal cell mass	Normal or decreased	Increased
Acid production	Normal or decreased	Increased
Serum gastrin	Increased	Normal
Serum pepsinogen	Normal	Increased
Associated gastritis	More common	Usually not present
Helicobacter pylori	May be present (60%–80%) Stimulates reduced acid secretion, gastric atrophy, and risk of gastric cancer	Often present (95%–100%) Stimulates acid hypersecretion
CLINICAL MANIFESTATIONS		
Pain	Located in upper abdomen Intermittent Pain-antacid-relief pattern Food-pain pattern (when food in stomach)	Located in upper abdomen Intermittent Pain-antacid or food-relief pattern Pain when stomach empty Nocturnal pain common
Clinical course	Chronic ulcer without pattern of remission and exacerbation Heals more slowly	Pattern of remissions and exacerbation for years Heals more quickly

and weight loss than duodenal ulcers. The evaluation and treatment of gastric ulcers are similar to the evaluation and treatment of duodenal ulcers.

Stress ulcers

A **stress ulcer** is an acute form of peptic ulcer that tends to accompany severe illness, systemic trauma, or neural injury.[25] Emotional stress may cause peptic ulcer.[17] Usually multiple sites of ulceration are distributed within the stomach or duodenum. Decreased mucosal blood flow, mucosal ischemia, and reperfusion injury are important contributing events in stress ulcer formation.[26] Stress ulcers may be classified as follows:

1. **Ischemic ulcer.** Develops within hours of events such as hemorrhage, multisystem trauma, severe burns, heart failure, or sepsis that causes ischemia of the stomach and duodenal mucosa; those that develop as a result of burn injury are often called *Curling ulcers.*
2. **Cushing ulcer.** Stress ulcer associated with severe head trauma or brain surgery that results from decreased mucosal blood flow and hypersecretion of acid caused by overstimulation of the vagal nuclei.

The primary clinical manifestation of stress ulcers is bleeding. Acid suppression with antacids and proton pump inhibitors may provide the best prophylactic treatment.[25] Stress ulcers seldom become chronic.

Surgical treatment of ulcer

Advances in the medical treatment of peptic ulcer disease have reduced the number of cases requiring surgery. The most common indications for ulcer surgery are recurrent or uncontrolled bleeding and perforation of the stomach or duodenum. The primary objectives of surgical treatment are to reduce stimuli for acid secretion, decrease the number of acid-secreting cells in the stomach, and correct complications of ulcer disease.

Acute complications of gastrectomy or anastomosis are relatively uncommon except in debilitated persons. Chronic complications, however, are likely to develop if a large portion of the stomach has been removed. These complications and their pathophysiologic mechanisms are described in the next section.

QUICK CHECK 34-3

1. What is the most common surgical emergency of the abdomen? How does it develop?
2. Compare the three types of peptic ulcers.
3. What is Cushing ulcer?

Postgastrectomy syndromes

Postgastrectomy syndromes are a group of signs and symptoms that occur after gastric resection. They are caused by

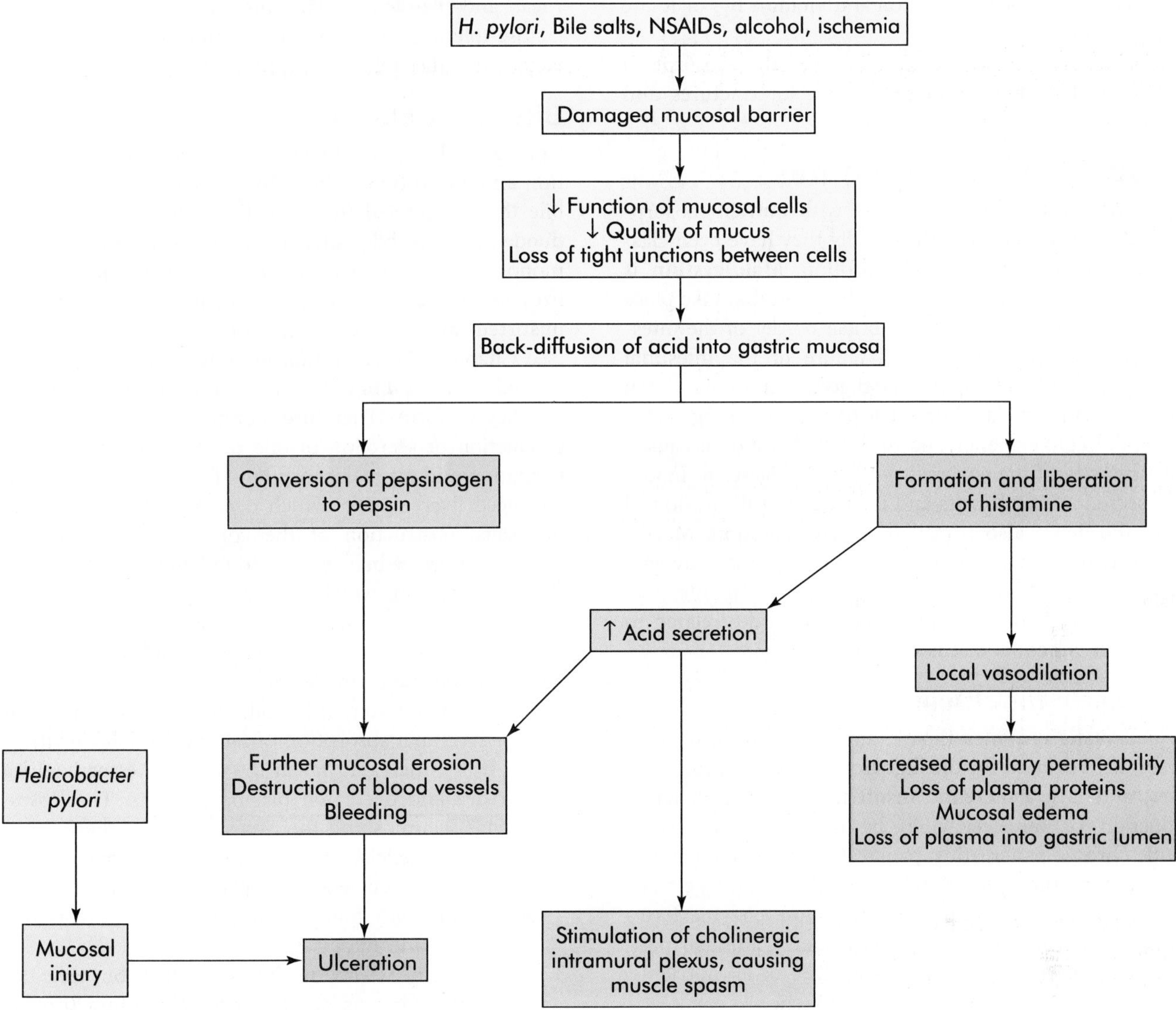

Figure 34-8 ■ **Pathophysiology of Gastric Ulcer Formation.** *NSAIDs,* nonsteroidal antiinflammatory drugs.

changes in motor and control functions of the stomach and upper small intestine[27] and include the following:

1. **Dumping syndrome.** Rapid emptying of hypertonic chyme from the surgically residual stomach (the stomach component remaining after surgical resection) into small intestine 10 to 20 minutes after eating; promoted by loss of gastric capacity, loss of emptying control when pylorus is removed, and loss of feedback control by duodenum when it is removed; responds to dietary management. Symptoms include cramping pain, nausea, vomiting, osmotic diarrhea, weakness, pallor, and hypotension.
2. **Alkaline reflux gastritis.** Stomach inflammation caused by reflux of bile and alkaline pancreatic secretions containing proteolytic enzymes that disrupt the mucosal barrier; symptoms include nausea, bilious vomiting, and sustained epigastric pain that worsens after eating and is not relieved by antacids; responds somewhat to avoidance of aspirin and alcohol, but surgical correction may be required.
3. **Afferent loop obstruction.** Intermittent severe pain and epigastric fullness after eating as a result of volvulus, hernia, adhesion, or stenosis of the duodenal stump on the proximal side of the gastrojejunostomy; vomiting relieves symptoms; management includes low-fat diet, but surgery is required for complete obstruction.
4. **Diarrhea.** Either frequent, persistent elimination of liquid stool or intermittent, precipitous, and unpredictable elimination of a large volume of stool; related to rapid gastric emptying and osmotic attraction of water into the gut, especially after large intake of high-carbohydrate liquids; small, dry meals and anticholinergic drugs are effective control measures.
5. **Weight loss.** Commonly caused by inadequate caloric intake because individual cannot tolerate carbohydrates or a normal-size meal; stomach is also less able to mix, churn, and break down food.
6. **Anemia.** Iron malabsorption may result from decreased acid secretion or lack of duodenum after Billroth II

procedure; deficiencies of iron and vitamin B_{12} or folate may result.

7. **Bone disorders.** Related to altered calcium absorption and metabolism with increased risk for fractures and deformity.

Malabsorption Syndromes

Malabsorption syndromes interfere with nutrient absorption in the small intestine. Historically they have been classified as maldigestion or malabsorption. **Maldigestion** is failure of the chemical processes of digestion that take place in the intestinal lumen or at the brush border of the intestinal mucosa. **Malabsorption** is failure of the intestinal mucosa to absorb (transport) the digested nutrients. Often these two are interrelated or occur together, making classification difficult. Generally, however, maldigestion is caused by deficiencies of the enzymes needed for digestion. Inadequate secretion of bile salts and inadequate reabsorption of bile in the ileum also contribute to maldigestion. Malabsorption is the result of mucosal disruption caused by gastric or intestinal resection, vascular disorders, or intestinal disease. Celiac disease, an autoimmune disorder related to cereal grain gluten, is discussed in Chapter 35.

Pancreatic insufficiency

The pancreatic enzymes (lipase, amylase, trypsin, chymotrypsin) are required for the digestion of proteins, carbohydrates, and fats. **Pancreatic insufficiency** is the deficient production of these enzymes by the pancreas. Causes include chronic pancreatitis, pancreatic carcinoma, pancreatic resection, and cystic fibrosis. Significant damage to or loss of pancreatic tissue must occur before enzyme levels decrease sufficiently to cause maldigestion. Although pancreatic insufficiency causes poor digestion of all nutrients, fat maldigestion is the chief problem. Absence of pancreatic bicarbonate in the duodenum and jejunum causes an acidic pH that worsens maldigestion by precipitating bile salts and preventing activation of the pancreatic enzymes that are present. A large amount of fat in the stool (steatorrhea) is the most common sign of pancreatic insufficiency.

Lactase deficiency

Deficiency of disaccharidase at the brush border of the small intestine is caused by a genetic defect in which a single enzyme, usually lactase, is lacking. **Lactase deficiency** inhibits the breakdown of lactose (milk sugar) into monosaccharides and therefore prevents lactose digestion and absorption across the intestinal wall. Lactase deficiency is most common in blacks, Latinos, and Native Americans and usually does not develop until adulthood. Secondary (acquired) lactase deficiency can be caused by several diseases of the intestine, including gluten-sensitive enteropathy, enteritis, and bacterial overgrowth.

The undigested lactose remains in the intestine, where bacterial fermentation causes gases to form. Undigested lactose also increases the osmotic gradient in the intestine, causing irritation and osmotic diarrhea. Clinical manifestations of lactase deficiency are bloating, crampy pain, diarrhea, and flatulence. The disorder is diagnosed by a lactose-tolerance test. Avoiding milk and adhering to a lactose-free diet relieve symptoms.

Bile salt deficiency

Conjugated bile acids (bile salts) are necessary for the digestion and absorption of fats. Bile salts are conjugated in the bile that is secreted from the liver. When bile enters the duodenum, the bile salts aggregate with fatty acids and monoglycerides to form micelles. Micelle formation solubilizes fat molecules and allows them to pass through the unstirred layer at the brush border of the small intestine (see Chapter 33). A minimum concentration of bile salts, termed the *critical micelle concentration,* is required to allow micelles to form. Therefore, conditions that decrease the production or secretion of bile result in decreased micelle formation and fat malabsorption. These conditions include advanced liver disease, which decreases the production of bile salts; obstruction of the common bile duct, which decreases flow of bile into the duodenum; intestinal stasis (lack of motility), which permits overgrowth of intestinal bacteria that deconjugate bile salts; and diseases of the ileum, which prevent the reabsorption and recycling of bile salts (enterohepatic circulation).

Clinical manifestations of bile salt deficiency are related to poor intestinal absorption of fat and fat-soluble vitamins (A, D, E, K). Increased fat in the stools (steatorrhea) leads to diarrhea and decreased plasma proteins. The losses of fat-soluble vitamins and their effects include the following:

1. Vitamin A deficiency results in night blindness.
2. Vitamin D deficiency results in decreased calcium absorption with bone demineralization (osteoporosis), bone pain, and fractures.
3. Vitamin K deficiency prolongs prothrombin time, leading to spontaneous development of purpura (bruising) and petechiae.
4. Vitamin E deficiency has uncertain effects but may cause testicular atrophy and neurologic defects in children.

The most effective treatment for fat-soluble vitamin deficiency is to increase medium-chain triglycerides in the diet, for example, by using coconut oil for cooking. Vitamins A, D, and K are given parenterally. Oral bile salts are an effective therapy.

Inflammatory Bowel Disease

Ulcerative colitis and Crohn disease together are known as the inflammatory bowel diseases (IBD). Although the diseases have some unique differences, genetics, immune dysregulation, epithelial barrier dysfunction, and microbial flora have some role for both in disease pathogenesis.

Ulcerative colitis

Ulcerative colitis is a chronic inflammatory disease that causes ulceration of the colonic mucosa, usually in the rectum and sigmoid colon. The lesions appear in susceptible individuals between 20 and 40 years of age. Risk factors include family history of disease and Jewish descent, and the disease is more prevalent among white populations.

Although the cause of ulcerative colitis is unknown, infectious, genetic, and immunologic factors are all suggested causes.[28] The familial tendency to develop ulcerative colitis and the occurrence of disease in identical twins support a genetic theory of causation. Perhaps most significant are humoral immunologic factors and activated macrophages associated with the disease. Anticolon antibodies have been identified in the sera of individuals with ulcerative colitis. Lymphocytes (T cells) in individuals with ulcerative colitis may have cytotoxic effects on the epithelial cells of the colon. Furthermore, autoimmune disorders, such as systemic lupus erythematosus and erythema nodosum, may accompany ulcerative colitis.

PATHOPHYSIOLOGY The primary lesion of ulcerative colitis begins with inflammation at the base of the crypt of Lieberkühn in the large intestine. The disease is most severe in the rectum and sigmoid colon. The mucosa is hyperemic and may appear dark red and velvety. Small erosions form and coalesce into ulcers. Abscess formation, necrosis, and ragged ulceration of the mucosa ensue. Edema and thickening of the muscularis mucosae may narrow the lumen of the involved colon. Mucosal destruction causes bleeding, cramping pain, and an urge to defecate. Frequent diarrhea, with passage of small amounts of blood and purulent mucus, is common. Loss of the absorptive mucosal surface and rapid colonic transit time cause large volumes of watery diarrhea.

CLINICAL MANIFESTATIONS The course of ulcerative colitis consists of intermittent periods of remission and exacerbation. Mild ulcerative colitis involves less mucosa, so that frequency of bowel movements, bleeding, and pain are minimal. Severe forms may involve the entire colon and are characterized by fever, elevated pulse rate, frequent diarrhea (10 to 20 stools/day), urgency, obviously bloody stools, and continuous, crampy pain. Dehydration, weight loss, anemia, and fever result from fluid loss, bleeding, and inflammation. Complications include anal fissures, hemorrhoids, and perirectal abscess. Severe hemorrhage is rare. Edema, strictures, or fibrosis can obstruct the colon. Perforation is an unusual but possible complication. The risk of colon cancer increases significantly after 10 years of ulcerative colitis. The systemic manifestations include polyarthritis, episcleritis, disorders of the liver, and alterations in coagulation.

EVALUATION AND TREATMENT Diagnosis of ulcerative colitis is based on the medical history and clinical manifestations. Sigmoidoscopy, barium enema, and x-ray films are used in addition to laboratory data. Infectious causes are ruled out by stool culture. The symptoms of ulcerative colitis are similar to those of Crohn disease, making differential diagnosis difficult.

Treatment is individualized and depends on the severity of symptoms and the extent of mucosal involvement. The disease is often treated with sulfasalazine (a combination of a sulfa drug and aspirin) or mesalazine. Steroids and aminosalicylates suppress the inflammatory response and help to alleviate the cramping pain. Immunomodulary agents may prevent relapse. Broad-spectrum antibiotics may be prescribed if bacterial infection is suggested. Severe, unremitting disease can require hospital admission and administration of intravenous fluids. Extreme malnutrition may require intravenous hyperalimentation. Smoking may be of some benefit.[29] Surgical resection of the colon may be performed if other forms of therapy are unsuccessful or if there are acute serious complications (sepsis, hemorrhage, perforation, or obstruction). Proctocolectomy and ileal pouch anal anastomosis (IPPA) has become the standard surgery for mucosal ulcerative colitis.[30]

Crohn disease

Crohn disease (granulomatous colitis, regional enteritis) is an inflammatory disorder that affects both the large and small intestines. In a small percentage of cases, Crohn disease is difficult to differentiate from ulcerative colitis (Table 34-6). The rectum is seldom involved. Risk factors and theories of causation are the same as those for ulcerative colitis, including genetic predisposition and an altered immune response to normal bowel flora.[31] Of affected individuals, 10% to 20% have a positive family history. Increased suppressor T cell activity, alterations in immunoglobulin A (IgA) production, macrophage activation, luminal flora, antigens, and susceptibility genes are factors associated with Crohn disease.[32] Psychologic stresses have been suggested as a cause of both Crohn disease and ulcerative colitis. Although stressful events may exacerbate illness, the role of stress in inflammatory bowel disease is not clear.[33]

PATHOPHYSIOLOGY The inflammation process of Crohn disease begins in the intestinal submucosa and spreads inward and outward to involve the mucosa and serosa. Activated neutrophils and macrophages promote inflammation and cause tissue injury. The ascending colon and the transverse colon are the most common sites of the disease, but both the large and small intestines may be involved, particularly the ileum. The inflammation can affect some segments of the intestine but not others, creating "skip lesions." One side of the intestinal wall may be affected and not the other. The ulcerations of Crohn disease produce fissures that extend inflammation into lymphoid tissue. The typical lesion is a granuloma (granulomas are described in Chapter 5) with a cobblestone appearance from projections of inflamed tissue surrounded by ulceration. Fistulae may form in the perianal area between loops of intestine or extend into the bladder. Strictures may develop promoting obstruction. Smoking increases the risk of developing severe disease.[34]

CLINICAL MANIFESTATIONS Individuals with Crohn disease may have no specific symptoms other than an "irritable bowel" for several years. Diarrhea is the most

TABLE 34-6

Features of Ulcerative Colitis and Crohn Disease

Feature	Ulcerative Colitis	Crohn Disease
INCIDENCE		
Age at onset	Any age; 10–40 yr most common	Any age; 10–30 yr most common
Family history	Less common	More common
Gender	Prevalence equal in women and men	Prevalence about equal in women and men
Cancer risk	Increased	Increased
PATHOPHYSIOLOGY		
Location of lesions	Large intestine, no "skip" lesions Left side more common	Large and small intestine, "skip" lesions common Right side more common
Inflammation and ulceration	Mucosal layer involved	Entire intestinal wall involved
Granulomas	Rare	Common
Friable mucosa	Common	Less common
Anal and perianal fistulae	Rare	Common; abscesses
Narrowed lumen and possible obstruction	Rare	Common; obstruction
CLINICAL MANIFESTATIONS		
Abdominal pain	Mild to severe	Moderate to severe
Diarrhea	Common; 4 times/day	Common; 4 times/day
Bloody stools	Common	Less common
Abdominal mass	Rare	Common
Small intestinal malabsorption	Rare	Common
Steatorrhea	Rare	Common
Clinical course	Remissions and exacerbations	Remissions and exacerbations

common sign and, occasionally, colonic bleeding. Weight loss and lower abdominal pain accompany Crohn disease. If the ileum is involved, the individual may be anemic as a result of malabsorption of vitamin B_{12}. There also may be deficiencies in folic acid and vitamin D absorption. In addition, proteins may be lost, leading to hypoalbuminemia. Extraintestinal complications are similar to those occurring in ulcerative colitis. There is increased risk for colon cancer and cancer of the small intestine with long-standing disease.[35]

EVALUATION AND TREATMENT The diagnosis and treatment of Crohn disease are similar to the diagnosis and treatment of ulcerative colitis. Surgery generally is performed to manage complications such as fistula, abscess, or obstruction. Routine endoscopy for cancer screening should be performed for long-standing disease.

Diverticular disease of the colon

Diverticula are herniations or saclike outpouchings of mucosa through the muscle layers, usually in the wall of the sigmoid colon (Figure 34-9). **Diverticulosis** is asymptomatic diverticular disease. **Diverticulitis** represents inflammation. Diverticular disease is most common in elderly persons, but the incidence is increasing in younger individuals, particularly when much of the diet consists of refined foods.

PATHOPHYSIOLOGY Although diverticula can occur anywhere in the gastrointestinal tract, the most common site is the left sigmoid colon. The diverticula form from increases in intraluminal pressure, particularly at weak points in the colon wall, usually where arteries penetrate the tunica muscularis to nourish the mucosal layer. A common associated finding is thickening of the circular and longitudinal (teniae coli) muscles surrounding the diverticula.[36] Hypertrophy and contraction of these muscles increase intraluminal pressure and degree of herniation. Habitual consumption of a low-residue diet reduces fecal bulk, thus reducing the diameter of the colon. According to the law of Laplace (see Chapter 22), wall pressure

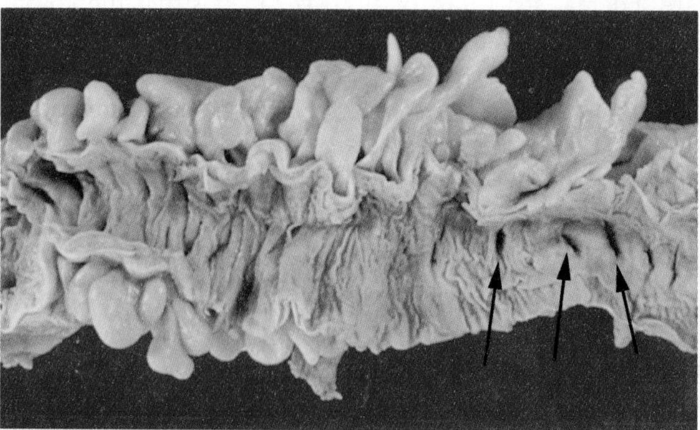

Figure 34-9 ■ **Diverticular Disease.** In diverticular disease, the outpouches *(arrows)* of mucosa seen in the sigmoid colon appear as slitlike openings from the mucosal surface of the opened bowel. (Modified from Stevens A, Lowe, J: *Pathology,* ed 2, Edinburgh, 2000, Mosby.)

increases as the diameter of a cylindrical structure decreases. Therefore, pressure within the narrow lumen can increase enough to rupture the diverticula. Diverticulitis can cause fistula, abscess formation, perforation, and peritonitis.[37]

CLINICAL MANIFESTATIONS Symptoms of diverticular disease may be vague or absent. Cramping pain of the lower abdomen can accompany constriction of the hypertrophied colonic muscles. Diarrhea, constipation, distention, or flatulence may occur. If the diverticula become inflamed or abscesses form, the individual develops fever, leukocytosis (increased white blood cell count), and tenderness of the lower left quadrant. Severe complications, such as hemorrhage, peritonitis, bowel obstruction, and fistula formation, are rare.

EVALUATION AND TREATMENT Diverticula are often discovered during diagnostic procedures performed for other problems. Sigmoidoscopy permits direct observation of the lesions. Ultrasound and barium enema reveals the muscle hypertrophy, but barium may become trapped in the diverticula and form hard masses. Abdominal computed tomography is used for complicated cases.

An increase of dietary fiber intake often relieves symptoms. Surgical resection may be required for diverticulitis or if there are severe complications.[38]

Appendicitis

Appendicitis is an inflammation of the vermiform appendix, which is a projection from the apex of the cecum. It is the most common surgical emergency of the abdomen and affects 7% to 12% of the population. It generally occurs between 20 and 30 years of age, although it may develop at any age.

PATHOPHYSIOLOGY The exact mechanism of the cause of appendicitis is controversial. Obstruction of the lumen with stool, tumors, or foreign bodies with consequent bacterial infection is the most common theory. The obstructed lumen does not allow drainage of the appendix, and as mucosal secretion continues, intraluminal pressure increases. The increased pressure decreases mucosal blood flow, and the appendix becomes hypoxic. The mucosa ulcerates, promoting bacterial or other microbial invasion with further inflammation and edema. Inflammation may involve the distal or entire appendix. Gangrene develops from thrombosis of the luminal blood vessels, followed by perforation.[39]

CLINICAL MANIFESTATIONS Gastric or periumbilical pain is the typical symptom of an inflamed appendix. The pain may be vague at first, increasing in intensity over 3 to 4 hours. It may subside and then recur in the right lower quadrant, indicating extension of the inflammation to the surrounding tissues. Nausea, vomiting, and anorexia follow the onset of pain, and a low-grade fever is common. Diarrhea occurs in some individuals, particularly children; others have a sensation of constipation. Perforation, peritonitis, and abscess formation are the most serious complications of appendicitis.

EVALUATION AND TREATMENT In addition to clinical manifestations, the clinician can usually locate the painful site with one finger. Rebound tenderness is usually referred to the right lower quadrant. The white blood cell count ranges from 10,000 to 16,000 cells/mm^3 with increased neutrophils. Ultrasonography and computed tomography (CT) scans can assist in differentiating appendicitis from perforated ulcer or cholecystitis. Laparoscopy may be necessary.

Appendectomy is the treatment for simple or perforated appendicitis. Surgery provides quick recovery for simple appendicitis. Recovery is more complicated in cases of perforation or abscess formation.

Irritable Bowel Syndrome

Irritable bowel syndrome (IBS) is a functional gastrointestinal disorder with no specific structural or biochemical alterations as a cause of disease. It is broadly characterized by abdominal pain and discomfort associated with altered bowel habits. About 20% of the world's population is estimated to have the disorder, and it is more common in women with a higher prevalence during youth and middle age. Individuals with symptoms of IBS are also more likely to have anxiety and depression. Symptoms of IBS can negatively affect quality of life and activity and present a significant economic burden.[40]

PATHOPHYSIOLOGY The pathophysiology of IBS is complex, but there is increasing evidence for organic disease, Several mechanisms are proposed to explain the causes for the symptoms listed here.

1. Visceral hypersensitivity or hyperalgesia particularly with distention of the rectum but also other areas of the gut. The mechanism may be related to a dysregulation of the "brain-gut axis," the role of serotonin in the enteric nervous system or alterations in autonomic or central nervous system processing of information.[41]
2. Abnormal gastrointestinal motility and secretion. Individuals with diarrhea type IBS have more rapid colonic transit times, whereas those with bloating and constipation have delayed transit times. The mechanism may also be related to visceral hypersensitivity as wells as dysregulation of the brain-gut axis or to the role of serotonin in the function of the enteric nervous system.
3. Intestinal infection (bacterial enteritis) has been associated with symptoms of IBS, and postinfectious IBS appears to be related to ongoing low-grade inflammation and an abnormal immune response in gut tissues.[42]
4. Overgrowth of intestinal flora (normal gut bacteria) may precipitate IBS symptoms, and it is proposed that methane gas may slow intestinal transit time resulting in constipation and bloating.[43,44]
5. Food allergy or food intolerance. Food antigens may activate the mucosal immune system mediating

hypersensitivity reactions and IBS symptoms. Food elimination approaches are helpful in some cases.[45]
6. Psychosocial factors including emotional stress influence brain-gut interations including neuroendocrine, autonomic nervous system and pain modulatory responses contributing to the symptoms of IBS.[46]

CLINICAL MANIFESTATIONS IBS is characterized by lower abdominal pain or discomfort, diarrhea-predominant, constipation-predominant, or alternating diarrhea/constipation, gas, bloating, and nausea. Symptoms are usually relieved with defecation and do not interfere with sleep.

EVALUATION AND TREATMENT The diagnosis of IBS is based on signs and symptoms and includes the exclusion of structural or biochemical causes of disease. Diagnostic procedures to rule out other causes of symptoms may include endoscopic evaluations, CT scans or abdominal ultrasound, blood tests, and tests for lactose intolerance, celiac disease, or other disorders. The patient may be evaluated for food allergies, parasites, or bacterial growth. The Rome III criteria for diagnosing IBS have been released to guide evaluation (see Box 34-1).

There is no cure for IBS, and treatment is individualized. Treatment of symptoms may include laxatives and fiber, antidiarrheals, antispasmodics, low-dose antidepressants, visceral analgesics, and serotonin agonists or antagonists. For more severe constipation, 5-hydroxytryptomine 4 agonists (e.g., tegaserod) may be used, and for more severe diarrhea, 5-hydroxytryptomine 3 antagonists (e.g., alosetron) may be used to normalize bowel habits. Alternative therapies including probiotics, hypnosis, and psychotherapy are treatment options. Research continues to advance the management of this complex syndrome.[47]

Vascular Insufficiency

Three branches of the abdominal aorta supply the stomach and intestines: the celiac axis and the superior and inferior mesenteric arteries. Because of the rich collateral circulation, at least two of the supplying vessels must be compromised to cause ischemia.[48] Atherosclerotic lesions, thrombi, and emboli can develop in these vessels, occluding blood flow and causing ischemia or necrosis in the gastrointestinal tract.

Chronic mesenteric arterial insufficiency is rare but can develop secondary to congestive heart failure, acute myocardial infarction, hemorrhage, stenosis, thrombus formation, or any condition that decreases arterial blood flow. Elderly individuals with arteriosclerosis are particularly susceptible. Chronic occlusion is often accompanied by formation of collateral circulation. The collateral vessels may be able to nourish the resting intestine, but after eating, when the intestine requires more blood, the arterial supply may be insufficient. Ischemia develops, causing a cramping abdominal pain (abdominal angina). Progressive vascular obstruction eventually causes continuous abdominal pain and necrosis of the intestinal tissue.

Acute mesenteric arterial insufficiency results from dissecting aortic aneurysms (rare) or emboli. Embolic obstruction is associated with atrial fibrillation, mitral valve disease, and heart valve prostheses. The superior mesenteric artery has a more direct line of flow from the aorta; therefore, emboli enter it more readily than the inferior branch, causing ischemia and necrosis of the small intestine. Ischemia and necrosis alter membrane permeability. Increased motility followed by absence of motility result.[49] The damaged intestinal mucosa cannot produce enough mucus to protect itself from digestive enzymes. Fluid moves from the blood vessels into the bowel wall and peritoneum, and its loss causes hypovolemia and further decreases intestinal blood flow. As intestinal infarction progresses, shock, fever, bloody diarrhea, leukocytosis, and abdominal distention develop. Abdominal pain may be severe.

Colicky abdominal pain after eating is a cardinal symptom of chronic mesenteric insufficiency. Some individuals suffer significant weight loss because they stop eating to control the pain. Acute mesenteric insufficiency causes severe continuous pain, rigid abdomen, and bloody diarrhea. Manifestations of unrelieved acute obstruction are distended abdomen, loss of bowel sounds, shock, peritonitis, fever, and tachycardia.

Diagnosis of mesenteric artery occlusion is based on clinical manifestations, mesenteric artery angiography, and abdominal imaging. Often a bruit can be heard over the occluded artery. After angiography, a vasodilating agent may be injected into the vessels to improve the circulation. Surgery is required to remove necrotic tissue or repair sclerosed vessels. Mortality is high for individuals with acute occlusion, compromised cardiac output, coexisting systemic disease, or delayed diagnosis.[50]

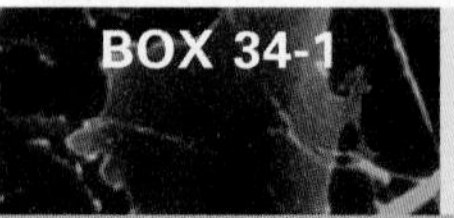

Rome III—Diagnostic Criteria for Irritable Bowel Syndrome

For a disorder to be diagnosed as irritable bowl syndrome, at least two or more of the following conditions will have existed for at least 3 months, with onset occurring at least 6 months before the beginning of the recurrent abdominal pain or discomfort (an uncomfortable sensation not described as pain):

1. Improvement with defecation
2. Onset associated with a change in frequency of stool
3. Onset associated with a change in form (appearance) of stool

Modified from Longstreth GF et al: Functional bowel disorders, *Gastroenterology* 130(5):1480–1491, 2006.

Disorders of Nutrition

Obesity

Obesity is an increase in body fat mass and a metabolic disorder that has increased in rate of incidence significantly since the 1980s. Over 60% of adults are overweight or obese in the United States, and the rate is rapidly increasing among children and adolescents.[51] Obesity generally develops when caloric intake exceeds caloric expenditure. **Obesity** is defined as a body mass index (body mass index [BMI] = kg/m^2) that exceeds 30. Obesity is a major risk for morbidity and death.

The causes and consequences of obesity are multiple and complex with rapidly advancing research regarding risk factors, causal mechanisms, and complications. Obesity is known to occur in families and genotypes,[52] and gene-environment interactions are important predisposing factors. Environmental factors include culture, socioeconomic status, food intake habits, and exercise. Metabolic abnormalities associated with obesity include Cushing syndrome, Cushing disease, polycystic ovarian syndrome, hypothyroidism, and hypothalamic injury.

PATHOPHYSIOLOGY Adipocytes (fat cells) secrete a number of hormones and cytokines known as adipocytokines[53] (Box 34-2). These adipocytokines are signaling molecules and participate in the neuroendocrine regulation of food intake, lipid storage, metabolism, insulin sensitivity, and female reproduction. Adipocytokines also influence the alternative complement system, vascular homeostasis, blood pressure regulation, angiogenesis, and the inflammatory and immune responses. Excessive increase in fat cell mass causes dysfunction in the regulation and interaction of these hormones and contributes to the complications and consequences of obesity.

Neuroendocrine regulation of appetite, eating behavior, energy metabolism, and body fat mass is controlled by a dynamic circuit of signaling molecules from the periphery acting on the hypothalamus.[54] An imbalance in this system is usually associated with excessive caloric intake in relation to exercise with the consequence of weight gain and obesity.

Many different hormones and signaling systems control appetite and body weight. The sources include insulin from the beta cells of the pancreas; ghrelin from the stomach; peptide YY from the intestines; and leptin, adiponectin, and resistin from adipose tissue. These hormones circulate in the blood at concentrations proportional to body fat mass and serve as peripheral signals to the hypothalamus where appetite and metabolism are regulated. Obesity is associated with increased circulating plasma levels of leptin, insulin, ghrelin, and peptide YY and decreased levels of adiponectin. Interaction of these hormones with neuropeptides at the level of the hypothalamus may be an important determinant of excessive fat mass.

Leptin, a product of the obesity gene (Ob gene), is a hormone that is being studied in relation to obesity. One of the functions of leptin is to act on the hypothalamus to suppress appetite and function to regulate body weight within a fairly narrow range. Leptin increases as adipocytes increase; however, for unknown reasons, high leptin levels are ineffective at decreasing appetite and energy expenditure, a condition is known as *leptin resistance.* Leptin resistance disrupts hypothalamic satiety signaling and promotes overeating and excessive weight gain and may be a factor in the development of obesity[55] (Figure 34-10). Leptin also may be associated with the cardiovascular complications of obesity.[56] Decreases in adiponectin are associated with insulin resistance, coronary artery disease, and hypertension and also may contribute to the complications of obesity.[57]

CLINICAL MANIFESTATIONS Obesity usually presents with two different forms of adipose tissue distribution. **Central obesity** (also known as intra-abdominal, visceral, or masculine obesity) occurs when the distribution of body fat is localized around the abdomen and upper body, resulting in an apple shape. Central obesity has an increased risk for hyperlipidemia, cardiovascular disease, and insulin resistance with the development of type 2 diabetes mellitus.[58] This combination of traits, also known as *metabolic syndrome,*[59] is discussed in detail in Chapters 17 and 23). **Peripheral obesity** (also known as gluteal-femoral or feminine obesity) occurs when the distribution of body fat is around the thighs and buttocks, resulting in a pear shape.

Three leading causes of death in the United States are associated with obesity: coronary artery disease, type 2 diabetes mellitus, and cancer (colon, breast in postmenopausal women, endometrial, prostate, kidney, and esophagus). Obesity is also a risk factor for hypertension, stroke, hepatobiliary disease (gallstones and nonalcoholic steatohepatitis), and osteoarthritis. Pulmonary function can be compromised by a large amount of adipose tissue overlying the chest cage, and obstructive sleep apnea syndrome can occur as a consequence (see Chapter 13).

BOX 34-2 Examples of Adipocytokines and Hormones From Adipose Tissue

Adipocytokines

Leptin: Hunger/appetite suppression at hypothalamus; promotes insulin sensitivity

Adiponectin: Insulin sensitizing for regulation of blood glucose; promotes anti-inflammatory vascular effects and reduces atherosclerosis.

Resistin: Promotes insulin resistance and increases blood glucose levels.

Vistatin: Mimics insulin and binds to insulin receptors

Other Hormones

Tumor necrosis factor alpha (TNFα): A proinflammatory hormone

Angiotensinogen: Regulates blood pressure and blood volume

Plasminogen activator inhibitor-1 (PAI-1): Promotes clot formation by inhibiting plasminogen and urokinase

Interleukins 6 and 8: Proinflammatory hormones

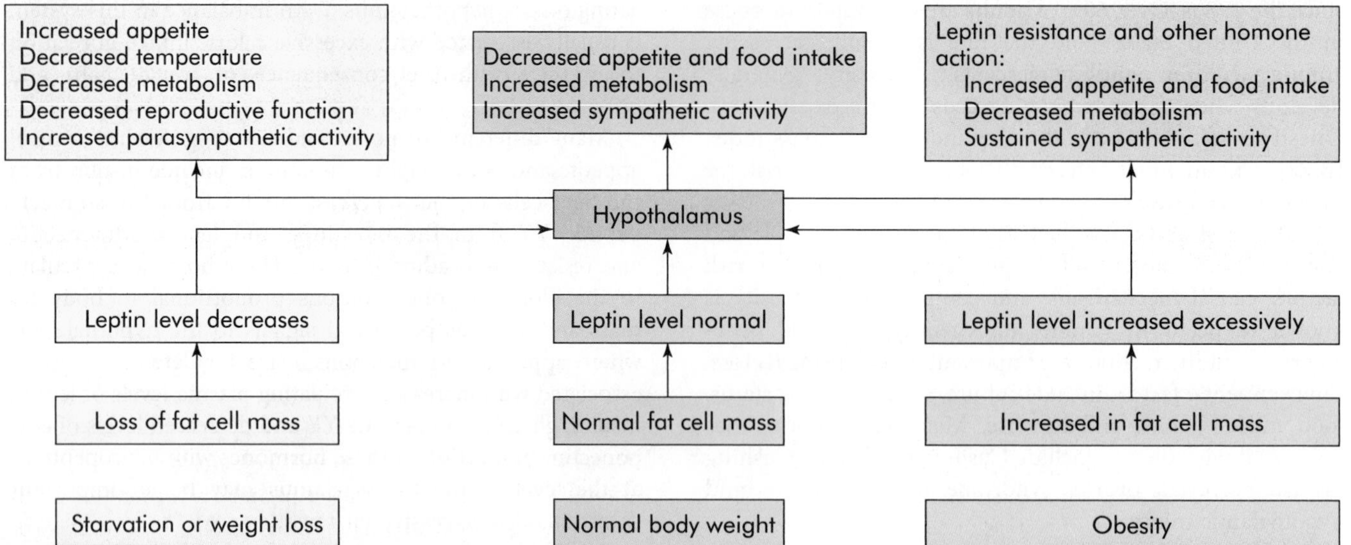

Figure 34-10 ■ **Leptin Theory of Obesity.** The hypothalamus controls appetite, fat cell mass, and energy expenditure by responding to circulating levels of leptin and other hormones. Regulation of normal body weight is presented in the green boxes. Changes occurring with obesity are presented in the orange boxes, and changes occurring with starvation or weight loss are presented in the yellow boxes.

EVALUATION AND TREATMENT There are several methods for measuring or estimating body fat mass, including computed tomography (CT) and magnetic resonance imaging (MRI) techniques; bioimpedance analysis; underwater weighing; and anthropometric measurements, such as skinfold thickness, circumferences, and various body diameters (i.e., waist-to-hip ratios and waist circumference, and body mass index [BMI—kg/m^2] tables).[60,61] The BMI and waist-to-hip ratios are most commonly used because they are the easiest to measure. Overweight is defined as a BMI greater than 25 and obesity is a BMI greater than 30. BMI charts are available for children ages 2 to 20 years; these can be used for comparison during adulthood because obese children generally become obese adults.[62,63] No specific diagnostic criteria for obesity have been established.

Obesity is a chronic disease for which various approaches to treatment have been used; these include correction of metabolic abnormalities, individually tailored weight reduction diets, and exercise programs.[64–69] A combination of weight reduction and exercise are the most effective treatments.[70] Self-motivation and support systems are critical aspects of treatment. Additional treatments, such as psychotherapy, behavioral modification, medications, and bariatric surgery (i.e., the Roux-en-Y gastric bypass or gastric banding) are also prescribed and when successful significantly reduce comorbidities and decrease insulin resistance.[71] Unraveling the causes of obesity will lead to more specific prevention and pharmacotherapeutic strategies.[72]

Anorexia nervosa and bulimia nervosa

Many young adults and adolescents—5 to 10 million young and adult women and 1 million males—are affected by two complex and related eating disorders: anorexia nervosa and bulimia nervosa. Both conditions have a familial tendency and may be associated with other disorders such as anxiety, depression, and obsessive compulsive disorder.[73]

Anorexia nervosa is a psychologic and physiologic syndrome characterized by the following:

1. Fear of becoming obese despite progressive weight loss
2. Distorted body image: the perception that the body is fat when it is actually underweight
3. Body weight 15% less than normal for age and height because of refusal to eat
4. In women and girls, absence of three consecutive menstrual periods

Persons with anorexia nervosa often deny they have an eating problem. As the disease progresses, muscle and fat depletion give the individual a skeleton-like appearance. Postural hypotension, edema, bradycardia, hypothermia, constipation, and sleep disturbances may ensue. The loss of 25% to 30% of ideal body weight can eventually lead to death caused by starvation-induced cardiac failure. Diagnosis of anorexia nervosa involves a thorough medical history, a physical and psychologic examination, and ruling out other causes of anorexia and malnutrition.

Treatment objectives for anorexia nervosa include reversing the compromised physical state, promoting insights and knowledge about the disorder, setting mutual goals, promoting interaction with family members, restoring developmental growth, modifying food habits, and restoring weight. Correction of nutritional status can require hospitalization. When the individual demonstrates the willingness to eat food for nourishment, dietary protein, carbohydrate, and fat are introduced in tolerable amounts. Psychotherapy begins as soon as the physical symptoms are stabilized and may continue for several years.[74]

HEALTH ALERT
Refeeding Syndrome

Refeeding syndrome occurs in severely malnourished individuals when parenteral or enteral nutritional therapy is initiated. During starvation, loss of body minerals causes the movement of phosphate, magnesium, and potassium out of the cells and into the plasma. When refeeding starts, an increase in insulin levels stimulates the intracellular movement of glucose and these ions and the plasma concentrations can decrease to dangerously low levels causing hypophosphatemia, hypomagnesaemia, and hypokalemia. Rapid expansion of the extracellular fluid volume can also occur with carbohydrate refeeding and may cause fluid overload. Hypophosphatemia contributes to alterations in red blood cell shape and function contributing to tissue hypoxia and increased respiratory drive. The consequence of these alterations includes life-threatening dysrhythmias, congestive heart failure, muscle weakness (including respiratory muscles), and death. Individuals at greatest risk are those with starvation from any cause including anorexia nervosa, chronic alcoholism, morbid obesity with massive weight loss, and prolonged fasting. Refeeding syndrome is prevented by slowly reinstituting feeding (about 20 kcal/kg/day for the first few days) and monitoring plasma phosphate, potassium, magnesium, and calcium.

Data from Marinella MA: Refeeding syndrome and hypophosphatemia, *J Intensive Care Med* 20(3):155–159, 2005; Azumagawa K, Kambara Y, Kawamura N, Takenaka Y, Yamasaki T, Tanaka H, Tamai H: Anorexia nervosa and refeeding syndrome: a case report, *Scientific World J* 7:400–403, 2007; Ladage E: Refeeding syndrome, *ORL Head Neck Nurs* 21(3):18–20, 2003.

Bulimia nervosa is characterized by bingeing—the consumption of normal to large amounts of food, often several thousand calories at a time—followed by self-induced vomiting or purging of the intestines with laxatives. The group at risk is the same as that for anorexia nervosa, except that bulimia nervosa tends to occur in slightly older, less affluent women. Approximately 50% of individuals with anorexia nervosa are bulimic as well.[75] Many young women stimulate vomiting inappropriately to control weight but are not classified as bulimic unless the pattern is obsessional or normal health or activity is interrupted. Diagnosis of bulimia nervosa is based on the following findings:

1. Recurrent episodes of binge eating during which the individual fears not being able to stop
2. Self-induced vomiting, use of laxatives, or fasting to oppose the effect of binge eating
3. Two binge-eating episodes per week for at least 3 months

Although individuals with bulimia nervosa are afraid of gaining weight, their weight usually remains within normal range. Because of negative connotations associated with self-stimulated vomiting and purging, individuals who have bulimia nervosa binge and purge secretly. They may binge and purge as often as 20 times each day. Continual vomiting of acidic chyme can cause pitted teeth, pharyngeal and esophageal inflammation, and tracheoesophageal fistulae. Overuse of laxatives can cause rectal bleeding. Secret bingeing isolates the bulimic individual and leads to depression and anger that is turned inward. A vicious cycle of depression, overeating to try to feel better, vomiting and purging to maintain a normal weight, and returning depression perpetuates this eating disorder.

Because persons with bulimia are usually older than individuals with anorexia nervosa and have usually separated from a family core, individual or group counseling is the treatment focus. Individuals with bulimia nervosa rarely have physical problems requiring hospital care.

Malnutrition and starvation

Malnutrition is lack of nourishment from inadequate amounts of calories, protein, vitamins, or minerals and is caused by improper diet, alterations in digestion or absorption, or a combination of these factors. **Starvation** is a state of extreme malnutrition and hunger from lack of nutrients. Short-term starvation (1 to 14 days of fasting) and long-term starvation (14 to 60 days of fasting) have different effects.[76,77] Therapeutic short-term starvation is part of many weight-reduction programs because it causes an initial rapid weight loss that reinforces the individual's motivation to diet. Therapeutic long-term starvation is used in medically controlled environments to facilitate rapid weight loss in morbidly obese individuals. Pathologic long-term starvation can be caused by poverty (particularly among those living in third world countries); chronic diseases of the cardiovascular, pulmonary, hepatic, renal, and digestive systems; malabsorption syndromes; and cancer. **Cachexia** is physical wasting with loss of weight and muscle atrophy, fatigue, and weakness. Inflammatory mediators (i.e., TNFα, interferon gamma, or interleukin 6) associated with advanced cancer (see Chapter 10), AIDS, tuberculosis, and other major chronic progressive diseases contribute to cachexia. Anorexia and cachexia often occur together. Cachexia is not the same as starvation. A healthy person's body can adjust to starvation by slowing metabolism, but in cachexia the body does not make this adjustment.

Short-term starvation, or extended fasting, consists of several days of total dietary abstinence or deprivation. Once all available energy has been absorbed from the intestine, glycogen in the liver is converted to glucose through **glycogenolysis,** the splitting of glycogen into glucose. This process peaks within 4 to 8 hours, and gluconeogenesis begins. **Gluconeogenesis** is the formation of glucose from noncarbohydrate molecules: lactate, pyruvate, amino acids, and the glycerol portion of fats. Like glycogenolysis, gluconeogenesis takes place within the liver. Both of these processes deplete stored nutrients and thus cannot meet the body's energy needs indefinitely. Proteins continue to be catabolized to a minimal degree, providing carbon for the synthesis of glucose. The kidney converts glutamine to glucose, significantly contributing to glucose production. Fatigue decreases physical activity and energy expenditure.

Long-term starvation begins after several days of dietary abstinence and eventually causes death. The major characteristic of long-term starvation is a decreased dependence on gluconeogenesis and an increased use of ketone bodies (products of lipid and pyruvate metabolism) as a cellular energy source. Depressed insulin and glucagon levels promote lipolysis in adipose tissue. Lipolysis liberates fatty acids, which supply energy to cardiac and skeletal muscle cells, as well as ketone bodies, which sustain brain tissue. Fatty acid or ketone body oxidation meets most energy needs of the cells. (Some glucose is still needed as fuel for brain tissue.) Once the supply of adipose tissue is depleted, proteolysis begins. The breakdown of muscle protein is the last process to supply energy for life. Death results from severe alterations in electrolyte balance and loss of renal, pulmonary, and cardiac function.

Adequate ingestion of appropriate nutrients is the obvious treatment for starvation. In medically induced starvation, the body is maintained in a ketotic state until the desired amount of adipose tissue has been lysed. Starvation imposed by chronic disease, long-term illness, or malabsorption is treated with enteral or parenteral nutrition.

✔ QUICK CHECK 34-4

1. Why are Crohn disease and ulcerative colitis called *inflammatory bowel diseases*?
2. List the manifestations of anorexia nervosa.
3. How do child-onset obesity and adult-onset obesity differ?

DISORDERS OF THE ACCESSORY ORGANS OF DIGESTION

The accessory organs of digestion (liver, gallbladder, pancreas) secrete substances necessary for digestion and, in the case of the liver, carry out metabolic functions needed to maintain life. Causes are inflammatory disease, obstruction of ducts, and tumors. (Cancers of the digestive tract are described at the end of this chapter.)

Clinical Manifestations of Liver Disorders

Of all the accessory organ disorders, acute or chronic liver disease leads to significant systemic, life-threatening complications. These complications include portal hypertension, ascites, hepatic encephalopathy, jaundice, and hepatorenal syndrome.

Portal hypertension

Portal hypertension is abnormally high blood pressure in the portal venous system. Pressure in this system is normally 3 mm Hg; portal hypertension is an increase to at least 10 mm Hg.

PATHOPHYSIOLOGY Portal hypertension is caused by disorders that obstruct or impede blood flow through any component of the portal venous system or vena cava. *Intrahepatic causes* result from thrombosis, inflammation, or fibrosis of the sinusoids, as occurs in cirrhosis of the liver, viral hepatitis, or schistosomiasis (a parasitic infection). *Posthepatic causes* occur from hepatic vein thrombosis or cardiac disorders that impair the pumping ability of the right heart. This causes blood to back up and increases pressure in the portal system. The most common cause of portal hypertension is obstruction caused by cirrhosis of the liver[78] (see p. 697).

Long-term portal hypertension causes several problems that are difficult to treat and can be fatal:

1. **Varices** (distended, tortuous, collateral veins). Prolonged elevation of pressure in collateral veins causes their transformation into varices, particularly in the lower esophagus and stomach, but also in the rectum (Figure 34-11). Rupture of varices can cause life-threatening hemorrhage.
2. **Splenomegaly** (enlargement of the spleen) caused by increased pressure in the splenic vein, which branches from the portal vein.
3. **Ascites** (the accumulation of fluid in the peritoneal cavity) caused by increased pressure in the mesenteric tributaries of the portal vein. Hydrostatic pressure forces water out of these vessels and into the peritoneal cavity.
4. **Hepatic encephalopathy,** also called *portal-systemic encephalopathy,* which is characterized by central nervous

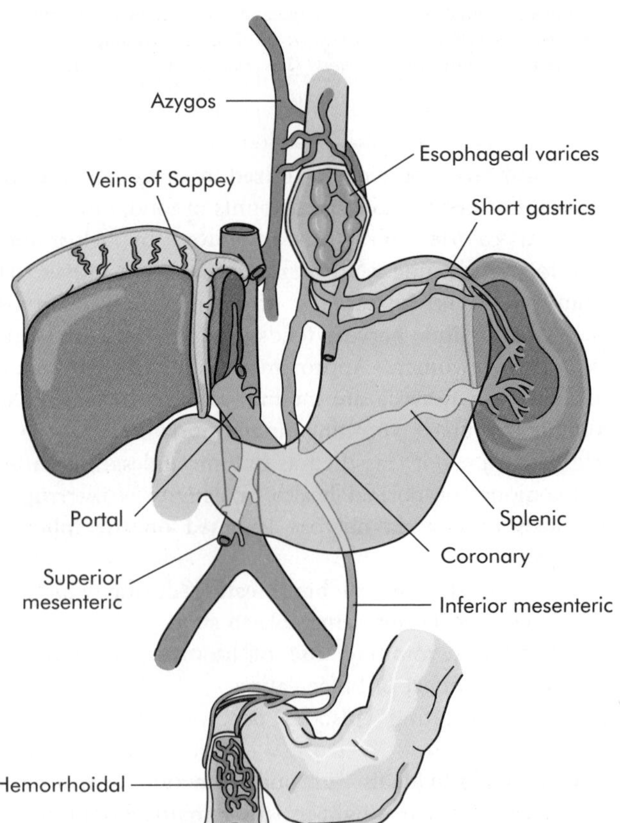

Figure 34-11 ■ Varices Related to Portal Hypertension. Portal vein, its major tributaries, and the most important shunts (collateral veins) between the portal and caval systems. (From Mohahan FD et al: *Phipps' medical-surgical nursing: concepts and clinical practice,* ed 8, St Louis, 2007, Mosby.)

system disturbances, particularly reversible alterations of consciousness. Blood that is shunted through collateral vessels to the systemic veins bypasses the liver, where toxins, hormones, and other harmful substances normally are removed. Hepatic encephalopathy results from the presence of these substances, particularly ammonia, in blood that reaches the brain.

CLINICAL MANIFESTATIONS Vomiting of blood from bleeding esophageal varices is the most common clinical manifestation of portal hypertension. Slow, chronic bleeding from varices causes anemia and the presence of digested blood in the stools. Usually the bleeding is from varices that have developed slowly over a period of years.

Rupture of esophageal varices causes hemorrhage and voluminous vomiting of dark-colored blood. The ruptured varices are usually painless. Rupture is caused by a combination of erosion by gastric acid and elevated venous pressure. Mortality from ruptured esophageal varices ranges from 30% to 60%. Recurrent bleeding of esophageal varices indicates a poor prognosis. Most individuals die within 1 year.

EVALUATION AND TREATMENT Portal hypertension is often diagnosed at the time of variceal bleeding and confirmed by endoscopy and evaluation of portal venous pressure. Distended collateral veins may radiate over the abdomen, giving rise to the description of caput medusae (Medusa head). The individual usually has a history of jaundice, hepatitis, or alcoholism.

Emergency management of bleeding varices includes use of vasopressors and compression of the varices with an inflatable Sengstaken-Blakemore tube, sclerotherapy, or variceal ligation. Surgical shunts may decompress the varices, but this treatment can precipitate encephalopathy or liver failure. Liver transplant is an alternative with end-stage liver disease.[79]

Ascites

Ascites is the accumulation of fluid in the peritoneal cavity. Ascites traps body fluid in a "third space" from which it cannot escape. The effect is to reduce the amount of fluid available for normal physiologic functions. Cirrhosis is the most common cause of ascites, but others include heart failure, constrictive pericarditis, abdominal malignancies, nephrotic syndrome, and malnutrition.[80] Of individuals who develop ascites caused by cirrhosis, 25% die within 1 year. Continued heavy drinking of alcohol is associated with this mortality.

PATHOPHYSIOLOGY Several factors contribute to the development of ascites. Impaired excretion of sodium by the kidneys promotes water retention. Portal hypertension and reduced serum albumin levels cause capillary hydrostatic pressure to exceed capillary osmotic pressure. This imbalance pushes water into the peritoneal cavity. Portal hypertension also increases the production of hepatic lymph, which "weeps" into the peritoneal cavity. Peripheral vasodilation associated with increased nitric oxide "underfills" the vascular system with hormonal stimulation that promotes renal sodium and water retention.

With cirrhosis, both portal hypertension and decreased production of albumin by hepatocytes contribute to the ascites. Besides reducing albumin synthesis, deranged liver metabolism permits the accumulation of hormones that regulate sodium and water balance. As ascites sequesters more and more body fluid, the kidneys respond by retaining sodium and water in amounts exceeding intake, particularly in response to increased aldosterone and antidiuretic hormone. This expands plasma volume, thereby accelerating portal hypertension and ascites formation.[81]

Ascites can be complicated by bacterial peritonitis, an inflammatory response that increases mesenteric capillary permeability. As plasma seeps out of the permeable mesenteric capillaries, it adds to the volume of ascitic fluid. Figure 34-12 summarizes the mechanisms by which cirrhosis of the liver causes ascites.

CLINICAL MANIFESTATIONS The accumulation of ascitic fluid causes weight gain, abdominal distention, and increased abdominal girth (Figure 34-13). Large volumes of fluid (10 to 20 L) displace the diaphragm and cause dyspnea by decreasing lung capacity. Respiratory rate increases, and the individual assumes a semi-Fowler position to relieve the dyspnea. Approximately 10% of individuals with ascites develop bacterial peritonitis, which causes fever, chills, abdominal pain, decreased bowel sounds, and cloudy ascitic fluid.

EVALUATION AND TREATMENT Diagnosis is usually based on clinical manifestations and identification of liver disease. Paracentesis is used to aspirate ascitic fluid for bacterial culture, biochemical analysis, and microscopic examination. The goal of treatment is to relieve discomfort. If the restoration of liver function is possible, the ascites diminishes spontaneously. In the meantime, dietary salt restriction and potassium-sparing diuretics can reduce ascites. Serum electrolytes are monitored carefully because the individual is at risk for hyponatremia and hypokalemia.

Palliative measures include paracentesis to remove 1 or 2 L of ascitic fluid and relieve respiratory distress. However, the removal of too much fluid relieves pressure on blood vessels and carries the risk of hypotension, shock, or death. Despite repeated paracentesis, ascitic fluid reaccumulates in individuals with irreversible disease. Paracentesis is also likely to cause peritonitis. Other procedures include peritoneovenous shunt, transjugular intrahepatic portosystemic shunt, and liver transplant.[73] Individuals with ascites and portal hypertension have a poor prognosis.

Hepatic encephalopathy

Hepatic encephalopathy (portal-systemic encephalopathy) is a complex neurologic syndrome characterized by impaired cerebral function, flapping tremor (asterixis), and electroencephalogram (EEG) changes. The syndrome may develop rapidly during acute fulminant hepatitis or

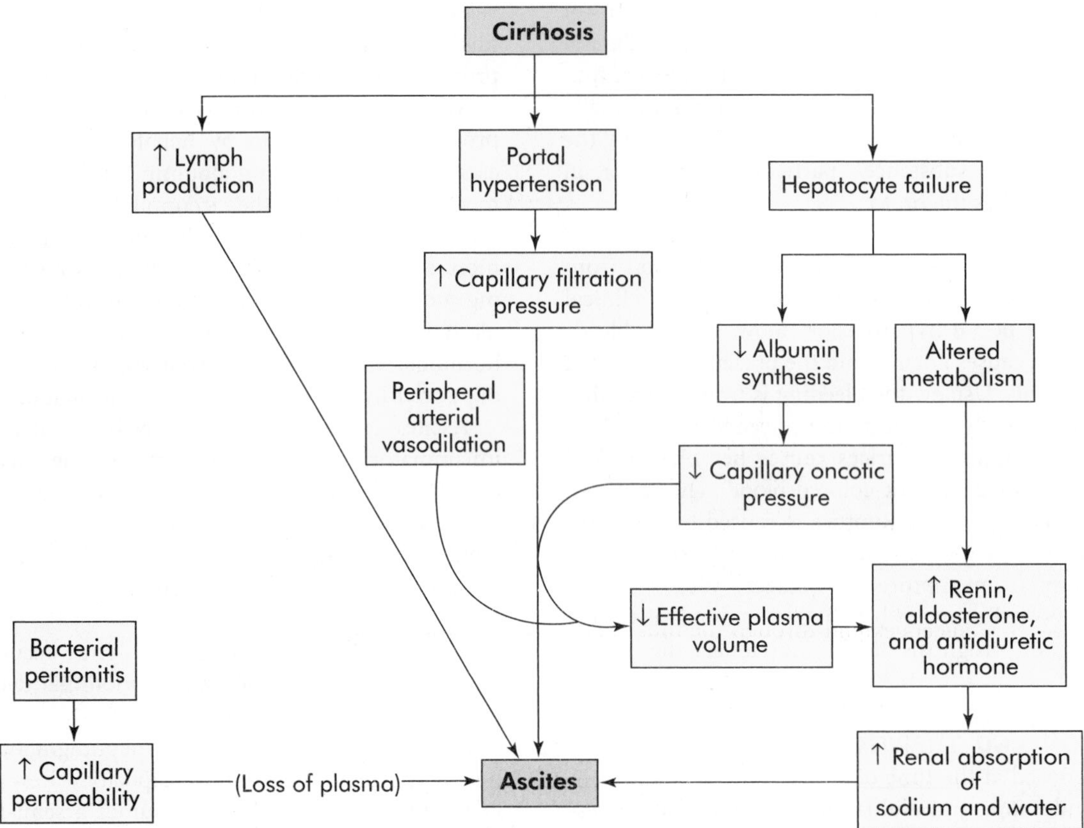

Figure 34-12 ■ **Mechanisms of Ascites Caused by Cirrhosis.**

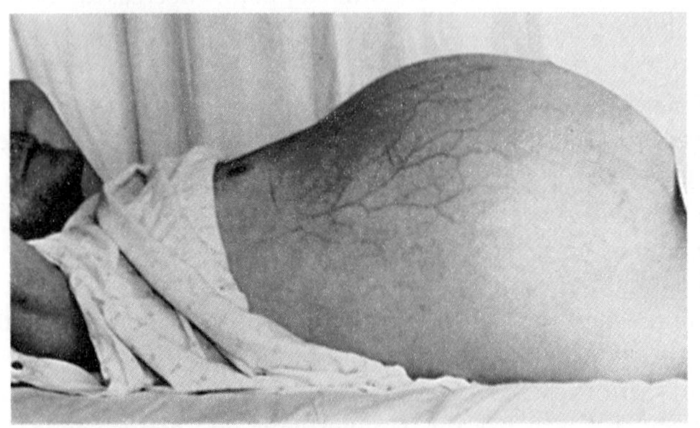

Figure 34-13 ■ Massive Ascites in an Individual With Cirrhosis. Distended abdomen, dilated upper abdominal veins, and inverted umbilicus are classic manifestations. (From Prior JA, Silberstein JS, Stang JM: *Physical diagnosis: the history and examination of the patient,* ed 6, St Louis, 1981, Mosby.)

slowly during the course of chronic liver disease and the development of portal hypertension.

PATHOPHYSIOLOGY Hepatic encephalopathy probably results from a combination of biochemical alterations that affect neurotransmission. Liver dysfunction and collateral vessels that shunt blood around the liver to the systemic circulation both permit toxins absorbed from the gastrointestinal tract to circulate freely to the brain. The most hazardous substances are end products of intestinal protein digestion, particularly ammonia. Ammonia that reaches the brain may alter cerebral energy metabolism or interfere with neurotransmitters.

Blood levels of ammonia do not account for all symptoms associated with hepatic encephalopathy. The accumulation of short-chain fatty acids, serotonin, tryptophan, and false neurotransmitters probably contributes to neural derangement.[82] Infection, hemorrhage, electrolyte imbalance including zinc deficiency, sedatives, and analgesics also can precipitate stupor and coma in the presence of liver disease.[83]

CLINICAL MANIFESTATIONS Subtle changes in personality, memory loss, irritability, lethargy, and sleep disturbances are common initial manifestations of hepatic encephalopathy. Symptoms then can progress to confusion, flapping tremor of the hands, stupor, convulsions, and coma. Coma is usually a sign of liver failure and ultimately results in death.

EVALUATION AND TREATMENT Diagnosis of hepatic encephalopathy is based on a history of liver disease and clinical manifestations. Electroencephalography and blood chemistry tests provide supportive data.

Correction of fluid and electrolyte imbalances and withdrawal of depressant drugs metabolized by the liver are first steps in the treatment of hepatic encephalopathy. Restricting dietary protein intake and eliminating intestinal bacteria reduce blood ammonia levels. Neomycin is effective in sterilizing the bowel, but it can be nephrotoxic. Lactulose may be administered to prevent ammonia absorption in the colon.[84]

Jaundice

Jaundice, or **icterus,** is a yellow or greenish pigmentation of the skin caused by **hyperbilirubinemia** (plasma bilirubin concentrations above 2.5 to 3.0 mg/dl). Hyperbilirubinemia and jaundice can result from excessive hemolysis of red blood cells or obstructive disorders of the bile ducts or liver cells (Figure 34-14). Jaundice in newborns is caused by impaired bilirubin uptake and conjugation (see Chapter 35).

PATHOPHYSIOLOGY **Obstructive jaundice** can result from extrahepatic or intrahepatic obstruction.[85] *Extrahepatic obstructive jaundice* develops if the common bile duct is occluded (e.g., by a gallstone or tumor). Bilirubin conjugated by the hepatocytes cannot flow into the duodenum. Therefore, it accumulates in the liver and enters the bloodstream, causing hyperbilirubinemia and jaundice. Because conjugated bilirubin is water soluble, it appears in the urine.

Intrahepatic obstructive jaundice involves disturbances in hepatocyte function and obstruction of bile canaliculi.[86] The uptake, conjugation, and excretion of bilirubin are affected with elevated levels of both conjugated and unconjugated bilirubin. Obstruction of bile canaliculi diminishes flow of conjugated bilirubin into the common bile duct. In mild cases, some of the bile canaliculi open. Consequently the amount of bilirubin in the intestinal tract may be only slightly decreased.

Excessive hemolysis (breakdown) of red blood cells can cause **hemolytic jaundice** *(prehepatic jaundice).* Increased unconjugated bilirubin is formed through metabolism of the heme component of destroyed red blood cells and exceeds the conjugation ability of the liver, causing blood levels of unconjugated bilirubin to rise. Unconjugated hyperbilirubinemia is the major cause of hemolytic jaundice. Because it is not water soluble, it is not excreted in the urine. The reserve conjugation ability of the liver usually prevents long-term unconjugated hyperbilirubinemia greater than 4 to 5 mg/dl. Severe hemolytic crisis, such as that which occurs with sickle cell disease (see Chapter 20) and hemolytic drugs, can cause jaundice. If unconjugated hyperbilirubinemia exceeds 5 mg/dl, both hemolytic and liver disorders are indicated. The causes of jaundice are summarized in Table 34-7.

CLINICAL MANIFESTATIONS Conjugated hyperbilirubinemia may cause the urine to darken several days before the onset of jaundice. The complete obstruction of bile flow from the liver to the duodenum causes light-colored stools. With partial obstruction, the stools are normal in color and bilirubin is present in the urine.

Fever, chills, and pain often accompany jaundice resulting from viral or bacterial inflammation of the liver (e.g., viral hepatitis). Manifestations of liver injury from any

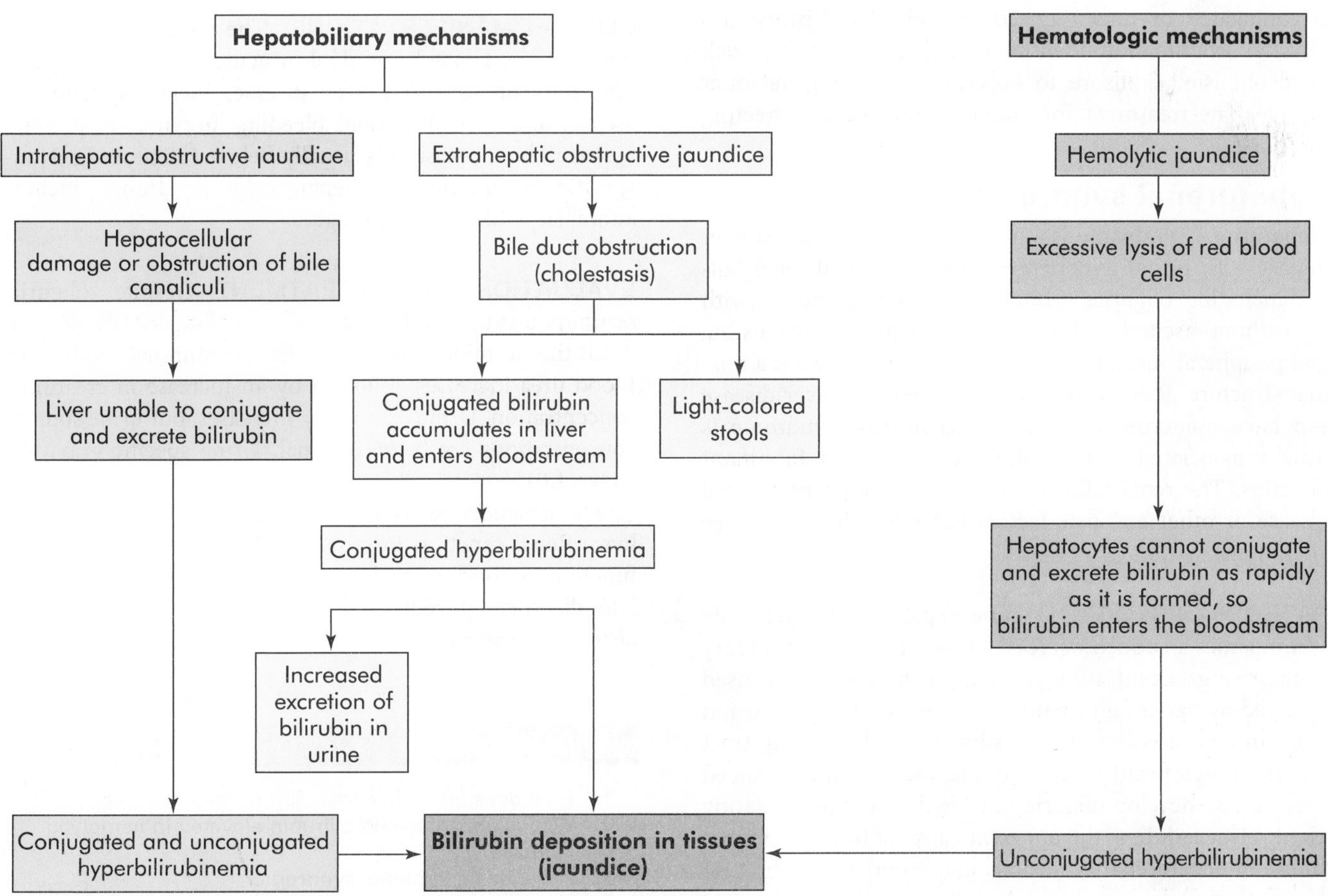

Figure 34-14 ■ **Mechanisms of Jaundice.**

TABLE 34-7
Three Common Types of Jaundice

Type	Mechanism	Causes
Hemolytic (prehepatic) jaundice (predominately unconjugated bilirubin)	Destruction of erythrocytes (increased bilirubin production)	Hemolytic anemias Severe infection Toxic substances in the circulation (e.g., snake venom) Transfusion of incompatible blood
Obstructive (posthepatic) jaundice (predominately conjugated bilirubin)	Obstruction of passage of conjugated bilirubin from liver to intestine	Obstruction of bile duct by gallstones or tumor (extrahepatic obstructive jaundice) Obstruction of bile flow through the liver (intrahepatic obstructive jaundice) Drugs
Hepatocellular (hepatic) jaundice (both conjugated and unconjugated bilirubin)	Failure of liver cells (hepatocytes) to conjugate bilirubin and of bilirubin to pass from liver to intestine	Genetic defect of hepatocyte (decreased enzymes), such as occurs in premature infants (see Chapter 35) Severe infections (i.e., hepatitis) Alcoholic liver disease or biliary cirrhosis

cause commonly include anorexia, malaise, and fatigue. Yellow discoloration may first occur in the sclera of the eye and then progress to the skin as bilirubin attaches to elastic fibers. Pruritus often accompanies jaundice because bilirubin accumulates in the skin.

EVALUATION AND TREATMENT Laboratory evaluation of serum establishes whether elevated plasma bilirubin is conjugated or unconjugated or both. The history and physical examination identify underlying disorders, such as alcoholism, exposure to hepatitis virus, or gallbladder disease. The treatment for jaundice consists of correcting the cause.

Hepatorenal syndrome

Hepatorenal syndrome is a complication of advanced liver disease with portal hypertension and functional renal failure including oliguria, sodium and water retention (with or without ascites and peripheral edema), hypotension, and peripheral vasodilation.[87] The kidney usually has a normal structure. Renal disorders associated with liver disease can have numerous causes, but hepatorenal syndrome is usually associated with alcoholic cirrhosis and fulminant hepatitis. The renal failure is not caused by primary renal disease or other extrinsic factors but rather by circulatory alterations.

PATHOPHYSIOLOGY Oliguric hepatic failure generally accompanies a sudden decrease in blood volume secondary to massive gastrointestinal bleeding or hypotension caused by bleeding varices and failing liver function. Hypotension also can be caused by the excessive use of diuretics to treat ascites. A significant number of individuals with advanced liver disease develop oliguria unrelated to any precipitating event. Liver failure is the apparent cause of functional renal failure in hepatorenal syndrome. Inappropriate constriction of renal arterioles is proposed as the causative mechanism for decreased glomerular filtration and oliguria. Intrarenal vasoconstriction may result from the selective effects of vasoactive substances that accumulate in the blood because of liver failure. Vasoconstriction also may be a compensatory response to portal hypotension and the pooling of blood in the splanchnic circulation. The exact reason for the vasoconstriction is unknown.

CLINICAL MANIFESTATIONS The onset of hepatorenal manifestations may be gradual or acute. Oliguria and complications of advanced liver disease, including jaundice, ascites, and gastrointestinal bleeding, are usually present. Systolic blood pressure is usually below 100 mm Hg. Nonspecific symptoms of hepatorenal syndrome include anorexia, weakness, and fatigue.

EVALUATION AND TREATMENT Despite oliguria, serum potassium levels do not become dangerously elevated until the terminal stages of the hepatorenal syndrome. Blood urea increases, followed by an increase in creatinine concentration. Urine osmolality increases, but urine sodium concentrations are below normal. Urine specific gravity is above 1.015.

The prognosis is usually poor and is related to a failing liver. Renal function improves with improvement in liver function. Secondary problems, including fluid and electrolyte disorders, bleeding, infections, and encephalopathy, also are vigorously treated.

QUICK CHECK 34-5

1. How does portal hypertension promote ascites?
2. Why is unconjugated bilirubin elevated in hemolytic jaundice?
3. Describe hepatorenal syndrome.

Disorders of the Liver

Viral hepatitis

Viral hepatitis is a relatively common systemic disease that affects primarily the liver. Five strains of viruses cause different types of hepatitis: hepatitis A virus (HAV), hepatitis B virus (HBV), hepatitis D virus (HDV), hepatitis C virus (HCV), and hepatitis E virus (HEV, most common in Asia and Africa). Hepatitis A formerly was known as infectious hepatitis and hepatitis B as serum hepatitis. The first five viruses can cause acute hepatitis, and types B and C also cause chronic liver disease, hepatocellular carcinoma, and liver failure.[88] Hepatitis G virus (HGV) is a flavivirus discovered in 1995 that is transmitted parenterally and sexually. The virus can be carried for years, usually without significant liver damage. Characteristics of the different types of viruses that cause hepatitis are presented in Table 34-8.

PATHOPHYSIOLOGY All five types of viral hepatitis can cause acute, icteric illness. The pathologic lesions of hepatitis are similar to those caused by other viral infection. Hepatic cell necrosis, scarring (with chronic disease), Kupffer cell hyperplasia, and infiltration by mononuclear phagocytes occur with varying severity. Regeneration of hepatic cells begins within 48 hours of injury. The inflammatory process can damage and obstruct bile canaliculi, leading to cholestasis and obstructive jaundice. In milder cases, the liver parenchyma is not damaged. Damage tends to be most severe in cases of hepatitis B and C. Hepatitis B is also associated with acute fulminating hepatitis, a rare form of the disease that is characterized by massive hepatic necrosis.

TABLE 34-8
Characteristics of Viral Hepatitis

Characteristic	Hepatitis A	Hepatitis B	Hepatitis D	Hepatitis C	Hepatitis E
Virus	27-nm RNA virus	42-nm DNA virus	36-nm RNA virus	30–60-nm RNA-virus	32-nm RNA virus
Antigens or antibodies	Anti-HAV	HBsAg HBcAg HbeAg	Anti-HDV	Anti-HCV	Anti-HEV
Incubation period	30 days	60–180 days	30–180 days	35–60 days	15–60 days
Route of transmission	Fecal-oral, parenteral, sexual	Parenteral, sexual	Parenteral (?), fecal-oral, sexual	Parenteral, sexual	Fecal-oral
Onset	Nonspecific Acute with fever	Insidious	Insidious	Insidious	Acute
Carrier state	Negative	Positive	Positive	Positive	Negative
Severity	Mild	Severe; may be prolonged or chronic	Severe	Unknown	Severe in pregnant women
Chronic hepatitis	No	Yes Increased risk of HCC	Yes	Yes Increased risk of HCC	No
Age-group affected	Children and young adults	Any	Any	Any	Children and young adults
Prophylaxis	Hygiene, immune serum globulin, HAV vaccine	Hygiene, HBV vaccine Blood screening	Hygiene, HBV vaccine	Hygiene, blood screening, interferon alpha	Hygiene, safe water
Pathophysiology	Hepatocyte injury caused by cellular immune responses (T cells, NK cells, and cytokines)	Viral replication, coinfection with viral mutation, inflammation, and cellular necrosis	Coinfection with HBV Severe cell injury, inflammation progressing to cirrhosis	Hepatocyte injury caused by immune response, inflammation, and fibrosis leading to cirrhosis	Viral replication Liver is cytotoxic Immune response causes inflammation and cholestasis
Treatment	Symptomatic support	Interferon-alpha Peginterferon-alpha Antivirals (lamivudine, adefovir, entecavir, emtricidine, telbivudine)	Interferon-alpha	Interferon alpha Peginterferon-alpha Antivirals (ribavirin)	Symptomatic support similar to HAV

RNA, Ribonucleic acid; *DNA,* deoxyribonucleic acid; *HAAg,* hepatitis A antigen; *HBsAg,* hepatitis B surface antigen; *HBcAg,* hepatitis B core antigen; *HBeAg,* hepatitis B e antigen (a fragment derived from the same propeptide for HBcAg); *HDV,* hepatitis D virus; *HCV,* hepatitis C virus; *HEV,* hepatitis E virus; *HBV,* hepatitis B virus, *HCC,* hepatocellular carcinoma.

Acute fulminating hepatitis causes severe encephalopathy, which is manifested as confusion, stupor, and coma. Liver failure can occur, leading to intestinal bleeding, cardiorespiratory insufficiency, and renal failure.

Coinfection of hepatitis B virus (HBV), hepatitis C virus (HCV), hepatitis D virus (HDV), and human immunodeficiency virus (HIV) occur as these viruses share the same route of transmission. Progression of liver disease is more rapid in these cases.[89]

CLINICAL MANIFESTATIONS The spectrum of manifestations ranges from absence of symptoms to fulminating hepatitis, with rapid onset of liver failure and coma. Acute viral hepatitis causes abnormal liver function test results. The serum aminotransferase values, aspartate transaminase (AST) and alanine transaminase (ALT), are elevated but not consistent with the extent of cellular damage. The clinical course of hepatitis usually consists of three phases:

1. **Prodromal phase.** Begins about 2 weeks after exposure and ends with the appearance of jaundice; marked by fatigue, anorexia, malaise, nausea, vomiting, headache, hyperalgia, cough, and low-grade fever; infection is highly transmissible during this phase.
2. **Icteric phase.** Begins 1 to 2 weeks after prodromal phase and lasts 2 to 6 weeks; jaundice, dark urine, and clay-colored stools are common; liver is enlarged, smooth, and tender, and percussion causes pain; this is the actual phase of illness.
3. **Recovery phase.** Begins with resolution of jaundice, about 6 to 8 weeks after exposure; symptoms diminish, but liver remains enlarged and tender; liver function returns to normal 2 to 12 weeks after the onset of jaundice.

Chronic active hepatitis is the persistence of clinical manifestations and liver inflammation after acute hepatitis B, hepatitis C, and hepatitis D. Liver function tests remain abnormal for longer than 6 months, and hepatitis B surface antigen (HBsAg) persists. Chronic, active hepatitis B is a predisposition to cirrhosis and primary hepatocellular carcinoma. Extrahepatic manifestations, including arthralgias, fatigue, neurologic, and renal symptoms, occur in some individuals.[90]

EVALUATION AND TREATMENT The most specific diagnostic test for viral hepatitis is serologic analysis for specific hepatitis virus antigens (i.e., HBsAg, which is the marker for HBV). Diagnosis of type A hepatitis is based on the presence of antigen antibodies (i.e., anti-HAV), as is the diagnosis of HCV. The assay for HDV is the total antibody to hepatitis D and antigen (anti-HDV). A test for HEV has not been developed. Liver function tests, including liver enzyme levels, are sensitive for liver cell injury and also can indicate other viral liver diseases, drug toxicity, or alcoholic hepatitis.

There is no specific treatment for acute viral hepatitis. For most individuals the disease is self-limiting with full recovery. Physical activity may be restricted. A low-fat, high-carbohydrate diet is beneficial if bile flow is obstructed. For chronic hepatitis, treatment is directed at suppressing viral replication before irreversible liver cell damage occurs. Antiviral therapies include interferon-alpha and specific antiviral agents. Cyclic and combination therapy may prevent drug resistance, and new agents are being developed.[91]

After ingestion and gastrointestinal uptake, HAV replicates in the liver and is secreted into the bile. To prevent transmission of hepatitis A, handwashing and the use of gloves for disposing of bedpans and fecal matter are imperative. HAV may be shed in the feces for up to 3 months after onset of symptoms. The administration of immune globulin before exposure or early in the incubation period can prevent hepatitis A and hepatitis B. Vaccines are available to protect against HAV and HBV infection. A vaccine for HEV is in development.[92] Prophylaxis is recommended for health care workers and others who are at risk for contact with infected body fluids, particularly children.

HEALTH ALERT
Hepatitis

Chronic hepatitis B virus (HBV) and C virus (HCV) infections affect millions of individuals in the United States and worldwide. Both diseases can progress to cirrhosis, or hepatocellular carcinoma. Immunotherapy with interferon-alpha has been the standard treatment with about 50% response rate. Combination therapy with interferon and nucleoside analogs (i.e., lamivudine, adefovir, entecavir, tenofovir, telbivudine and clevudine) for HBV and interferon with ribavirin for HCV have been more effective in controlling viral replication than monotherapy, particularly for nonresponders. Trials with pegylated interferons (peginterferon combined with ribavirin) are demonstrating superior response for HCV, and new antivirals are being evaluated for resistant viral strains (pegylation of the interferon molecule increases its size and slows absorption and lowers the rate of clearance from the plasma, thus increasing the duration of biologic activity).

Cost of treatment is expensive and drugs are sometimes poorly tolerated. Viral resistance limits drug use and advances are continuing to be made in the development of new drugs and hepatoprotective agents. With progression to end-stage liver disease, transplantation becomes the only option. Aggressive vaccination for prevention of hepatitis is needed.

Data from Farrell GC, Teoh NC: Management of chronic hepatitis B virus infection: a new era of disease control, *Intern Med J* 36(2):100–113, 2006; Forton D, Karayiannis P: Established and emerging therapies for the treatment of viral hepatitis, *Dig Dis* 24(1–2):160–173, 2006.

Fulminant hepatitis

Fulminant hepatitis is a clinical syndrome resulting in severe impairment or necrosis of liver cells and potential liver failure. The disorder rarely occurs with HAV and may occur as a complication of hepatitis C or hepatitis B, particularly HBV infection compounded by infection with the delta virus. Toxic reactions to drugs and congenital metabolic disorders also can cause fulminant hepatitis.

Edematous hepatocytes and patchy areas of necrosis and inflammatory cell infiltrates disrupt the parenchyma. The death of hepatocytes may be caused by viral or immunologic damage.

Acute liver failure usually develops within 6 to 8 weeks after the initial symptoms of viral hepatitis or a metabolic liver disorder. Anorexia, vomiting, abdominal pain, and progressive jaundice are initial signs, followed by ascites and gastrointestinal bleeding. Hepatic encephalopathy is manifested as lethargy, altered motor functions, and coma and is related to cerebral edema, ischemia, and brain stem herniation. Liver function tests show elevations of both direct and indirect serum bilirubin, serum transaminases, and blood ammonia. Prothrombin time is prolonged. Renal failure and pulmonary distress can occur.[93]

Antiviral reverse transcriptase inhibitors are available to treat chronic hepatitis B or C. Treatment of acute liver failure is supportive. The hepatic necrosis is irreversible, and 60% to 90% of affected children die. Liver transplantation may be lifesaving and should be considered early. Survivors usually do not develop cirrhosis or chronic liver disease.

Cirrhosis

Cirrhosis is an irreversible inflammatory disease that disrupts liver structure and function and is a leading cause of death in the United States. Disorganization of hepatic tissues is caused by diffuse fibrosis and nodular regeneration between fibrous bands that give the liver a cobbly appearance. The liver may be larger or smaller than normal, and usually it is firm or hard when palpated. Cirrhosis is often classified by cause (Table 34-9).

Cirrhosis develops slowly over a period of years. Its severity and rate of progression depend on the cause. If toxins, such as alcohol, are involved, the rate of cell death and the severity of inflammation depend on the amount of toxin present. Removal of the toxin slows the progression of liver damage and enhances the process of regeneration.[94]

Alcoholic liver disease

Deaths from alcohol-related liver disease have increased since the 1990s. However, high alcohol consumption among women leads to earlier and more severe cirrhosis.[95] The incidence of alcoholic cirrhosis is greatest in middle-aged men. In the United States, mortality resulting from cirrhosis is highest among nonwhites. Although alcoholic cirrhosis is the most prevalent of the different types of cirrhosis, the occurrence of cirrhosis among persons with alcoholism is relatively low (approximately 25%). The amount and duration of alcohol consumption are positively related to the extent of liver damage. Abuse of any type of alcoholic beverage can cause cirrhosis. Malnutrition may add to the risk of cirrhosis in alcohol abusers.

PATHOPHYSIOLOGY **Alcoholic cirrhosis** is caused by the toxic effects of alcohol on the liver, immunologic alterations, inflammatory cytokines, and oxidative stress from lipid peroxidation. Alcohol is transformed to acetaldehyde, and excessive amounts significantly alter hepatocyte function. Mitochondrial function is impaired, decreasing oxidation of fatty acid. Enzyme and protein synthesis may be depressed or altered, and hormone and ammonia degradation is diminished. Acetaldehyde inhibits export of proteins from the liver, alters metabolism of vitamins and minerals, and induces malnutrition.[96] Cellular damage initiates an inflammatory response that, along with necrosis, results in excessive collagen formation. Fibrosis and scarring alter the structure of the liver and obstruct biliary and vascular channels.[97]

TABLE 34-9
Cirrhosis of the Liver

Type and Disease Name	Causal Mechanisms	Pathophysiology
Alcoholic cirrhosis, Laennec cirrhosis, portal cirrhosis, fatty cirrhosis	Toxic effects of chronic, excessive alcohol intake; acetaldehyde formed by alcohol metabolism damages hepatocytes	Fatty liver, inflammation (alcoholic hepatitis), and derangement of the lobular architecture by necrosis and fibrosis (cirrhosis)
Biliary cirrhosis (intrahepatic or extra hepatic obstruction of bile flow)		
Primary biliary cirrhosis	Unknown; possibly an autoimmune mechanism	Inflammation and scarring of lobular bile ducts
Secondary biliary cirrhosis	Obstruction by neoplasms, strictures, or gallstones	Inflammation and scarring of bile ducts proximal to the obstruction
Postnecrotic cirrhosis	Viral hepatitis caused by HBV or HCV; drugs or toxins; autoimmune destruction	Replacement of necrotic tissue with cirrhosis tissue, particularly fibrous, nodular scar tissue
Metabolic cirrhosis	Metabolic defects and storage disease, such as α_1-antitrypsin deficiency, glycogen storage disease, hemochromatosis, Wilson disease, galactosemia	Inflammation and scarring with specific morphologic changes related to cause

HBV, Hepatitis B virus; *HCV,* hepatitis C virus.

Alcoholic cirrhosis progresses with fatty infiltration, fibrosis, and cirrhosis. Fat deposition (deposition of triglycerides) within the liver is caused primarily by increased lipogenesis and decreased fatty acid oxidation by hepatocytes. Lipids mobilized from adipose tissue or dietary fat intake may contribute to fat accumulation. Cessation of alcohol intake reverses the fatty accumulation, but fibrosis and liver damage are irreversible.

Fatty liver (steatosis) is the mildest form of alcoholic liver disease. It can be caused by relatively small amounts of alcohol, may be asymptomatic, and is reversible with cessation of drinking.[98]

Alcoholic hepatitis is a precursor of cirrhosis characterized by inflammation, degeneration, and necrosis of hepatocytes and infiltration of polymorphonuclear leukocytes and lymphocytes. The injured hepatocytes contain Mallory bodies (hyaline endoplasmic reticulum), indicating the onset of fibrosis. The mechanism of hepatocyte injury is not clearly understood, but immunologic factors and inflammatory mediators are involved. Serum IgA is often elevated in individuals with alcoholic hepatitis, and liver antigens and antibodies have been identified in those with progressive alcoholic liver disease. The inflammation and necrosis caused by alcoholic hepatitis stimulate the irreversible fibrosis characteristic of the cirrhotic stage of disease.

CLINICAL MANIFESTATIONS Fatty infiltration causes no specific symptoms or abnormal liver function test results. The liver is usually enlarged, however, and the individual has a history of continuous alcohol intake during the previous weeks or months. Anorexia, nausea, jaundice, and edema develop with advanced fatty infiltration or the onset of alcoholic hepatitis (Figure 34-15).

The clinical manifestations of alcoholic hepatitis can be mild or severe. Nonspecific symptoms include fatigue, weight loss, and anorexia. Toxic effects of alcohol also can cause testicular atrophy, reduced libido, azoospermia, and decreased testosterone in men. Manifestations of acute

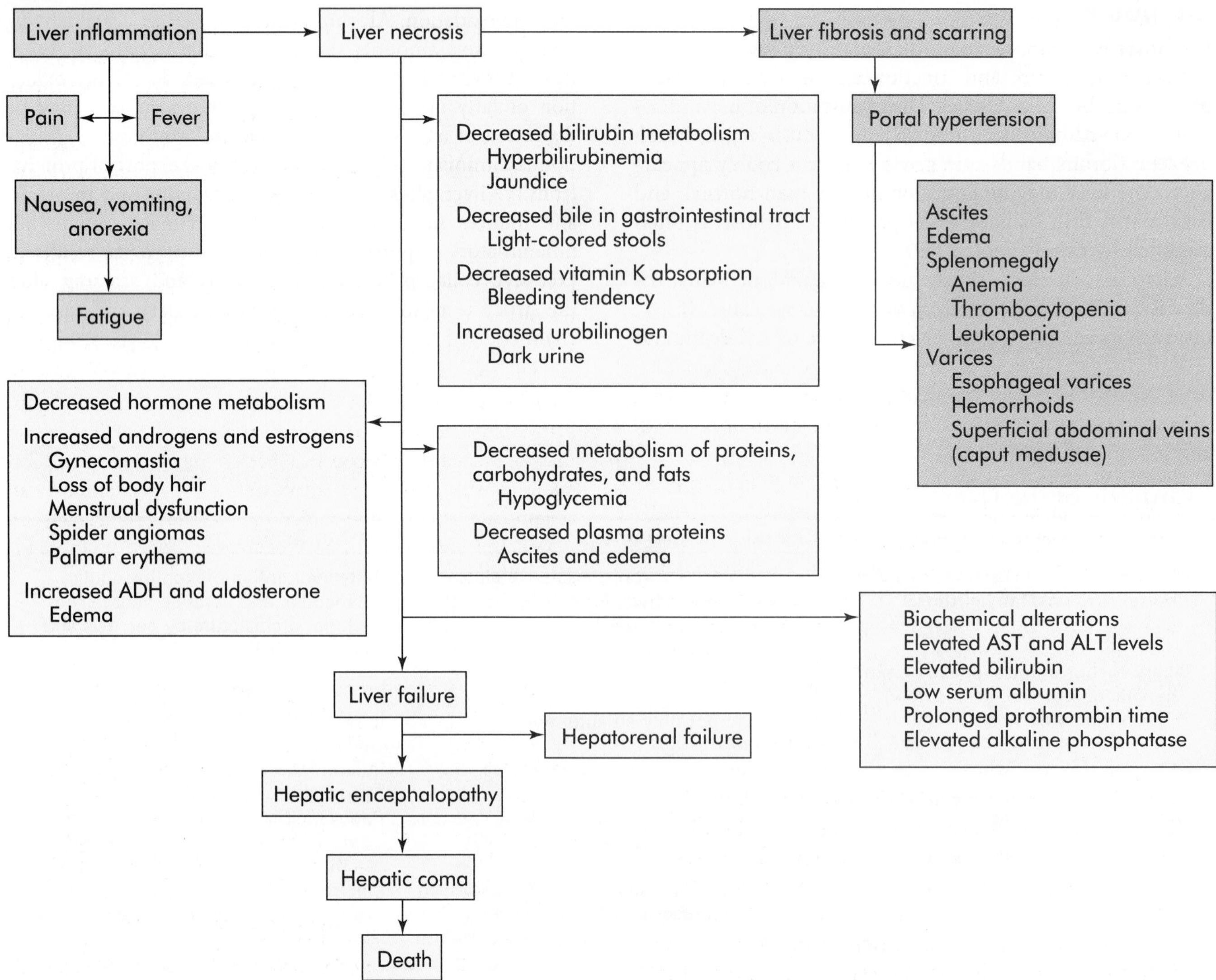

Figure 34-15 ■ **Clinical Manifestations of Cirrhosis.** *ADH,* Antidiuretic hormone; *AST,* aspartate transaminase; *ALT,* alanine transaminase.

illness include nausea, anorexia, fever, abdominal pain, and jaundice. Cirrhosis is a multiple-system disease and causes hepatomegaly, splenomegaly, ascites, gastrointestinal hemorrhage, portal hypertension, hepatic encephalopathy, and esophageal varices. Anemia results from blood loss, poor nutrition, and hypersplenism. Renal failure is often a late complication of hepatorenal failure. The presence of numerous and severe manifestations increases the risk of death.

EVALUATION AND TREATMENT The diagnosis of alcoholic hepatitis is based on the individual's history and clinical manifestations. The results of liver function tests are abnormal, and serologic studies show elevated serum enzymes and bilirubin, decreased serum albumin, and prolonged prothrombin time. Liver biopsy can confirm the diagnosis of cirrhosis, but biopsy is not necessary if clinical manifestations of cirrhosis are evident.

There is no specific treatment for alcoholic cirrhosis. Rest, vitamin supplements, a nutritious diet, and management of complications, such as ascites, gastrointestinal bleeding, and encephalopathy, are essential. Cessation of drinking is essential and slows the progression of liver damage, improves clinical symptoms, and prolongs life. Individuals with severe symptoms are treated with a regimen of corticosteroids and other drugs, including antioxidants and tumor necrosis factor alpha (TNFα) inhibition, which are being evaluated.[99] Orthotopic liver transplantation can be successful for treatment of end-stage liver disease.

Biliary cirrhosis

Biliary cirrhosis differs from alcoholic cirrhosis in that the damage and inflammation leading to cirrhosis begin in bile canaliculi and bile ducts, rather than in the hepatocytes. The two types of biliary cirrhosis are *primary* and *secondary.* Although both involve bile duct pathology, they differ with respect to cause, risk factors, and mechanisms of obstruction and inflammation as follows:

1. **Primary biliary cirrhosis.** Caused by autoimmune inflammation and destruction of the small intrahepatic bile ducts; affects women and those older than 30 years; progresses insidiously from pruritus, hyperbilirubinemia, jaundice, and light-colored stools to cirrhosis, portal hypertension, and encephalopathy; life expectancy is 5 to 10 years after onset of symptoms. Primary biliary cirrhosis can be detected by identifying the disease-specific antibodies. Treatment with ursodeoxycholic acid slows disease progression and liver transplant is highly effective.[100]
2. **Secondary biliary cirrhosis.** Caused by prolonged partial or complete obstruction of common bile duct or branches by gallstones, tumors, fibrotic strictures, or chronic pancreatitis; biliary atresia and cystic fibrosis are causative in children; necrotic areas develop and lead to proliferation and inflammation of portal ducts, producing edema and fibrosis; surgery or endoscopy relieves obstruction, prolongs survival, and diminishes or resolves symptoms.

✔ QUICK CHECK 34-6

1. What are the major pathologic differences between alcoholic and biliary cirrhosis?
2. How does hepatitis A virus (HAV) differ from hepatitis B virus (HBV)?
3. How are varices and ascites associated with portal hypertension?

Disorders of the Gallbladder

Obstruction and inflammation are the most common disorders of the gallbladder. Obstruction is caused by **gallstones,** which are aggregates of substances in the bile. The gallstones may remain in the gallbladder or be ejected, with bile, into the cystic duct. Gallstones that become lodged in the cystic duct obstruct the flow of bile into and out of the gallbladder and cause inflammation. Gallstone formation is termed **cholelithiasis.** Inflammation of the gallbladder or cystic duct is known as **cholecystitis.**

Cholelithiasis

Cholelithiasis is a prevalent disorder in developed countries, where incidence is 10% to 20%, although many individuals are asymptomatic. Gallstones are of two types: cholesterol and pigmented. Cholesterol stones are the most common. Risk factors include obesity, middle age, female gender, rapid weight loss, Native American ancestry, genetic predisposition and gallbladder, pancreatic, or ileal disease.[101,102]

PATHOPHYSIOLOGY Cholesterol gallstones form in bile that is supersaturated with cholesterol produced by the liver.[103] Supersaturation sets the stage for cholesterol crystal formation, or the formation of "microstones." More crystals then aggregate on the microstones, which grow to form "macrostones." This process usually occurs in the gallbladder, which may have decreased motility. The stones may lie dormant or become lodged in the cystic or common duct, causing pain and cholecystitis.[104] The stones can accumulate and fill the entire gallbladder (Figure 34-16). Pigmented stones form from increased levels of unconjugated bilirubin, which binds with calcium.

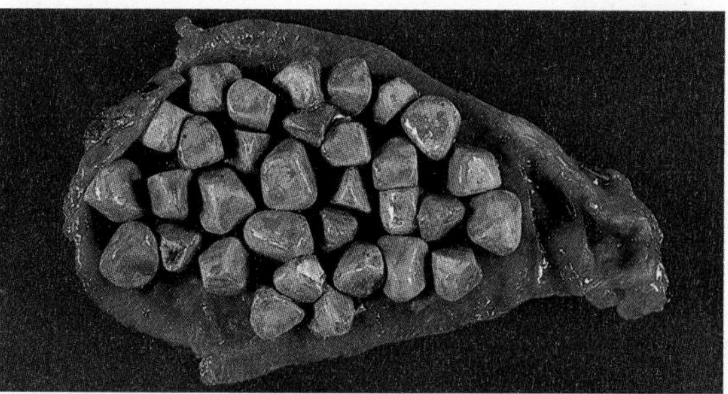

Figure 34-16 ■ Resected Gallbladder Containing Mixed Gallstones. (From Kissane JM, editor: *Anderson's pathology,* ed 9, St Louis, 1990, Mosby.)

CLINICAL MANIFESTATIONS Abdominal pain and jaundice are the cardinal manifestations of cholelithiasis. Vague symptoms include heartburn, flatulence, epigastric discomfort, and food intolerances, particularly to fats and cabbage. The pain (biliary colic) is caused by the lodging of one or more gallstones in the cystic or common duct. It can be intermittent or steady and usually occurs in the right upper quadrant, radiating to the mid-upper area of the back. Jaundice indicates that the stone is located in the common bile duct.

EVALUATION AND TREATMENT Diagnosis is based on the history, physical examination, and ultrasound or computed tomography. An oral cholecystogram usually outlines the stones. Intravenous cholangiography is used to differentiate cholelithiasis from other causes of extrahepatic biliary obstruction if the cholecystogram is negative. Endoscopic or percutaneous cholangiography is also a diagnostic option. Laparoscopic cholecystectomy is the preferred treatment for uncomplicated gallstones that cause obstruction or inflammation. Shockwave lithotripsy and laser lithotripsy may be used to fragment large bile duct stones before endoscopic removal.[105]

Cholecystitis

Cholecystitis can be acute or chronic, but both forms are almost always caused by a gallstone lodged in the cystic duct.[106] The gallbladder becomes distended and inflamed, with pain similar to that caused by gallstones. Pressure against the distended wall of the gallbladder decreases blood flow and may result in ischemia, necrosis, and perforation. Fever, leukocytosis, rebound tenderness, and abdominal muscle guarding are common findings. Serum bilirubin and alkaline phosphatase levels may be elevated. The acute abdominal pain of cholecystitis must be differentiated from that caused by pancreatitis, myocardial infarction, and acute pyelonephritis of the right kidney. Cholangiography or radioactive scan can confirm the diagnosis.

Narcotics may be required to control pain, and antibiotics (e.g., gentamicin, clindamycin) often are prescribed to manage bacterial infection in severe cases. Persistent symptoms or development of chronic cholecystitis punctuated by recurrent, acute attacks usually requires gallbladder resection (cholecystectomy). Obstruction may also lead to acute pancreatitis. If pancreatic abscesses develop, they are usually resected.[105]

Disorders of the Pancreas

Pancreatitis, or inflammation of the pancreas, is a relatively rare and potentially serious disorder that occurs equally in men and women in their 50s. Pancreatitis can be acute or chronic and is associated with conditions such as alcoholism, obstructive biliary tract disease (particularly cholelithiasis), peptic ulcers, trauma, and hyperlipidemia, as well as certain drugs.[107]

Acute pancreatitis

PATHOPHYSIOLOGY **Acute pancreatitis (acute hemorrhagic pancreatitis)** is usually a mild disease, but about 20% of those with the disease develop a severe pancreatic inflammation requiring hospital care. Although the precise pathogenic mechanism or sequence of events often is unknown, alcoholism and biliary tract obstruction because of gallstones are commonly associated.[107] The most common theory is that pancreatitis develops because of obstruction to the outflow of pancreatic enzymes by bile and pancreatic duct obstruction, which permits leakage of pancreatic enzymes into pancreatic tissue. The leaked enzymes become activated, initiating autodigestion and acute pancreatitis. Proinflammatory mediators are released into the bloodstream and cause coagulation abnormalities and injury to vessels and other organs, such as the lungs and kidneys. Myocardial depression and shock can develop secondary to the release of vasoactive peptides. Translocation of bacteria may cause sepsis. These systemic effects are major causes of multiple organ involvement, morbidity, and mortality.[108,109]

CLINICAL MANIFESTATIONS Epigastric or midabdominal pain ranging from mild abdominal discomfort to severe, incapacitating pain is caused by (1) edema, which distends the pancreatic ducts and capsule; (2) chemical irritation and inflammation of the peritoneum; and (3) irritation or obstruction of the biliary tract. Fever and leukocytosis accompany the inflammatory response. Nausea and vomiting are caused by hypermotility or paralytic ileus secondary to the pancreatitis or peritonitis.

Abdominal distention accompanies bowel hypermotility and the accumulation of fluids in the peritoneal cavity. Hypotension and shock occur often because plasma volume is lost as enzymes and kinins released into the circulation increase vascular permeability and dilate vessels. Hypovolemia, hypotension, and myocardial insufficiency result. A small percentage of individuals develop tachypnea and hypoxemia secondary to pulmonary edema, atelectasis, or pleural effusions caused by circulating pancreatic enzymes. In severe cases, hypovolemia decreases renal blood flow sufficiently to impair renal function. Tetany may develop as a result of calcium deposited in areas of fat necrosis or as a decreased response to parathormone. Transient hyperglycemia also can occur if glucagon is released from damaged alpha cells in the pancreatic islets. Multiple organ failure accounts for most deaths with severe acute pancreatitis.

EVALUATION AND TREATMENT Diagnosis is based on clinical findings, identification of associated disorders, and laboratory studies. Elevated serum amylase is a characteristic but is not diagnostic of severity or specificity of disease. Serum lipase elevations are a sensitive marker of pancreatic injury, particularly of acute alcoholic pancreatitis. Urine amylase and serum lipase are also elevated. Elevated serum lactic dehydrogenase and C-reactive protein levels are associated with severe pancreatitis.[110]

The goal of treatment for acute pancreatitis is to stop the process of autodigestion and prevent systemic complications. Narcotic medications may be needed to relieve pain. To decrease pancreatic secretions and "rest the gland," oral food and fluids are withheld and continuous gastric suction is instituted. Nasogastric suction may not be necessary with mild pancreatitis, but it helps to relieve pain and prevent paralytic ileus in individuals who are nauseated and vomiting. Parenteral fluids are essential to restore blood volume and prevent hypotension and shock. Parenteral hyperalimentation should be initiated to reverse the catabolic state associated with severe pancreatitis. Drugs that decrease gastric acid production (e.g., cimetidine) can decrease stimulation of the pancreas by secretin. Antibiotics may control infection. The risk of mortality increases significantly with the development of infection or pulmonary, cardiac, and renal complications.[111]

Chronic pancreatitis

Structural or functional impairment of the pancreas leads to **chronic pancreatitis.** Chronic alcohol abuse is the most common cause, and smoking increases risk of chronic pancreatitis.[112] Chronic pancreatitis causes continuous or intermittent abdominal pain, which usually intensifies after a meal. Occasionally manifestations of pancreatic enzyme deficiency, such as steatorrhea or a malabsorption syndrome, are present. To correct enzyme deficiencies and prevent malabsorption, oral enzyme replacements are taken before and during meals. Loss of islet cell function can cause insulin-dependent diabetes. Cessation of alcohol intake is essential for the management of chronic pancreatitis.

Fibrosis, strictures, continued inflammation, calcification, and pancreatic cysts are common lesions of chronic pancreatitis. The cysts are walled-off areas or pockets of pancreatic juice, necrotic debris, or blood within or adjacent to the pancreas. Surgical drainage or partial resection of the pancreas may be required to relieve pain and to prevent cystic rupture.[113] Chronic pancreatitis is a risk factor for pancreatic cancer.

CANCER OF THE DIGESTIVE SYSTEM

Cancer of the Gastrointestinal Tract

Cancer of the esophagus

Carcinoma of the esophagus is a rare type of cancer, but the incidence is increasing among white males.[114] The incidence is about 1% of all new cancers (Table 34-10) in the United States.[115] In the United States, it occurs more in blacks than in whites and peaks at about 60 years of age.

PATHOGENESIS Carcinoma of the esophagus is usually squamous cell carcinoma or, less commonly, adenocarcinoma. Adenocarcinomas are often secondary to infiltration by a gastric carcinoma or to the presence of Barrett epithelium (columnar rather than squamous epithelium in the lower esophagus), which is associated with chronic gastroesophageal reflux.[116] Carcinomas can occur at any level of the esophageal tract but are most common at the gastroesophageal junction.

The pathogenesis of esophageal carcinoma is facilitated by (1) alterations of esophageal structure and function that permit food and drink to remain in the esophagus for prolonged periods; (2) ulceration and metaplasia caused by esophageal reflux; (3) chronic exposure to irritants, such as alcohol and tobacco, that cause neoplastic transformation; and (4) obesity[114] (see Chapter 10). Chronic inadequate nutrition can impair esophageal structure and function (see *Risk Factors:* Esophageal Cancer).

RISK FACTORS Esophageal Cancer

- Age greater than 70 years
- Male
- African American
- Tobacco use
- Alcoholism
- Dietary factors: deficiencies of trace elements and vitamins
- Malnutrition associated with poor economic conditions or special dietary habits
- Reflux esophagitis with dysplasia
- Sliding hiatal hernia
- Obesity

With data from American Cancer Society: *What are the risk factors for cancer of the esophagus?* www.cancer.org/docroot/CRI/content/CRI_2_4_2X_What_are_the_risk_factors_for_esophagus_ cancer_12.asp?sitearea=.

CLINICAL MANIFESTATIONS The two frequent symptoms of esophageal carcinoma are chest pain and dysphagia. The most common type of pain is heartburn (pyrosis). It is initiated by eating spicy or highly seasoned foods and by lying down. Dysphagia (difficulty swallowing) is usually pressure-like and may radiate posteriorly between the scapulae. Odynophagia (pain on swallowing) may be initiated by the swallowing of cold liquids. Spontaneous chest pain is more difficult to diagnose positively. Some individuals with esophageal cancer complain of a constant retrosternal pain that radiates to the back. Dysphagia usually progresses rapidly. It is mostly painless during the early stages of esophageal carcinoma.

EVALUATION AND TREATMENT Individuals with dysphagia undergo endoscopy so that specimens can be obtained and examined for neoplastic change. Endoscopic ultrasound is also used for staging. CT studies of the thorax are also used for diagnosis. Prevention of gastroesophageal reflux is essential to the management of Barrett esophagus. Esophageal cancer metastasizes rapidly and therefore has a poor prognosis. It is impossible to remove all lymph nodes with the tumor, but removal of the primary lesion and the local lymph nodes can benefit the individual with esophageal cancer. If the malignancy has not spread beyond

TABLE 34-10

Cancer of the Gut, Liver, and Pancreas

Organ	Deaths Out of All Cancers Combined	Risks	Cell Type	Common Manifestations
Esophagus	2.4%	Malnutrition Alcohol Tobacco Chronic reflux	Squamous cell Adenocarcinoma	Chest pain Dysphagia
Stomach	2%	Salty food Nitrates-nitrosamines	Adenocarcinoma Squamous cell	Anorexia Malaise Weight loss Upper abdominal pain Vomiting Occult blood
Colorectal	9%	Polyps Ulcerative colitis Diverticulitis High-refined carbohydrates, low-fiber, high-fat diets	Adenocarcinoma (left colon grows in ring; right colon grows as mass)	Pain Mass Anemia Bloody stool Obstruction Distention
Liver	2.9%	HBV, HCV, HDV Cirrhosis Intestinal parasite Aflatoxin from moldy peanuts	Hepatomas Cholangiomas	Pain Anorexia Bloating Weight loss Portal hypertension Ascites Jaundice
Pancreas	5.9%	Chronic pancreatitis Cigarette smoking Alcohol (?) Diabetic women	Adenocarcinoma (exocrine part of gland, ductal epithelium)	Weight loss Weakness Nausea Vomiting Abdominal pain Depression ± jaundice May have insulin-secreting tumors with symptoms of hypoglycemia

From American Cancer Society: *Cancer facts & figures—2007,* Atlanta, 2007, American Cancer Society.
HBV, Hepatitis B virus; *HVC,* hepatitis C virus; *HDV,* hepatitis D virus.

these sites, cure is likely. If spread has occurred, however, an incomplete resection is of little survival benefit. Treatment is combined radiation and chemotherapy.[117]

Cancer of the stomach

Although the incidence of gastric adenocarcinoma has declined in the United States, it still represents about 1% to 2% of all new cancer cases annually.[115] In Japan, the British Isles, and Iceland, the incidence of stomach cancer has remained high consistently. Studies of Japanese immigrants to the United States show that offspring who are born and raised in the United States have an incidence rate comparable with that of other Americans. These data illustrate the importance of environmental factors, such as diet, to carcinogenesis.

The most important environmental causative factors of gastric cancer are (1) infection with *Helicobacter pylori,* (2) heavily salted and preserved foods (e.g., nitrates in pickled or salted foods such as bacon), (3) low intake of fruits and vegetables, and (4) use of tobacco and alcohol. Dietary salt enhances the conversion of nitrates to carcinogenic nitrosamines in the stomach. Salt is also caustic to the stomach and can cause chronic atrophic gastritis. Finally, hypertonic salt solutions delay gastric emptying. Delayed emptying increases the time during which carcinogenic nitrosamines can exert their effects on the stomach mucosa. Nitrates interact with amino acids in the stomach to form nitrosamines, enhanced at a low pH by iodides and thiocyanates. Nitrates are thought to be active only when converted to nitrites and to cause stomach cancer once atrophic gastritis has occurred. *H. pylori*–associated gastritis increases the risk for gastric adenocarcinoma and gastric mucosa–associated lymphoid tissue (MALT) lymphoma.[118]

The incidence of gastric cancer is greater in males than in females. Other nonenvironmental risk factors are a family history of gastric adenocarcinoma, blood type (blood group A), and pernicious anemia, which results from atrophy of the gastric mucosa in the same locations where gastric tumors arise. Loss of tumor suppressor genes and other genetic alterations may be important in gastric cancer.[119]

PATHOGENESIS Gastric adenocarcinoma usually begins in the glands of the distal stomach mucosa. Approximately 50% develop in the prepyloric antrum (Figure 34-17). Inflammation and atrophic gastritis associated with *H. pylori* infection and intestinal metaplasia are strongly linked to the development of gastric cancer. Insufficient acid secretion by the atrophic mucosa creates a relatively alkaline environment that permits bacteria to multiply and act on nitrates. The resulting increase in nitrosamines damages the deoxyribonucleic acid (DNA) of mucosal cells further, promoting metaplasia and neoplasia. Duodenal reflux also may contribute to intestinal metaplasia. The reflux contains caustic bile salts that destroy the mucosal barrier that normally protects the stomach.

CLINICAL MANIFESTATIONS The early stages of gastric cancer are generally asymptomatic or produce vague symptoms such as loss of appetite (especially for meat), malaise, and indigestion. Later manifestations of gastric cancer include unexplained weight loss, upper abdominal pain, vomiting, change in bowel habits, and anemia caused by persistent occult bleeding. The prognosis is poor because symptoms do not occur until the tumor has penetrated the muscle layers of the stomach, spread to surrounding tissues, and entered the draining lymph nodes and veins, causing distant metastases, particularly to the liver and peritoneal structures. Generally the first manifestations of carcinoma are caused by distant metastases, and the disease is already in an advanced stage.

EVALUATION AND TREATMENT Most symptoms suggest a problem in the upper gastrointestinal tract, and a barium x-ray film shows the lesion. Direct endoscopic visualization and biopsy usually establish the diagnosis. Another definitive technique is microscopic examination of exfoliated cells obtained by lavage during endoscopy.

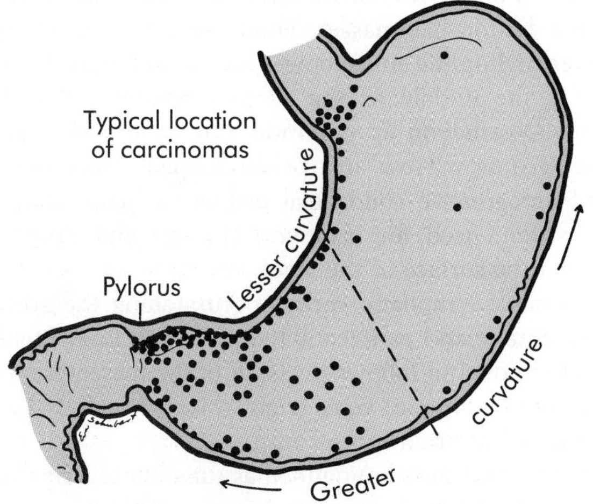

Figure 34-17 ■ **Typical Sites of Stomach Cancer.** (From del Regato JA, Spjut HJ, Cox JD: *Cancer: diagnosis, treatment, and prognosis,* ed 2, St Louis, 1985, Mosby.)

Surgery is the usual treatment for gastric cancer. Staging is determined by pathologic findings after resection. Radiation therapy is generally unsuccessful, and immunotherapy is still experimental. Chemotherapy combined with radiation reduces the tumor.[120] Individuals who respond well to chemotherapy generally live longer than those who do not.

QUICK CHECK 34-7

1. How do gallstones form?
2. Compare acute and chronic pancreatitis.
3. What factors are associated with cancer of the esophagus?

Cancer of the colon and rectum

Cancer of the lower intestinal tract (colorectal cancer) is the third most common cause of cancer and cancer death in the United States, for both men and women. Colorectal cancer accounts for 9% to 10% of all cancer deaths in the United States.[115] Cancer of the colon tends to occur in individuals older than 50 years and is rare in children. Clustering in families is common; *familial adenomatous polyposis (FAP)* has been mapped to chromosome 5 (the APC gene),[121] and *hereditary nonpolyposis colorectal cancers (HNPCC)* are mapped to chromosome 2.[122] Other colorectal cancers are caused by multiple gene interactions. **Familial adenomatous polyposis (FAP),** also known as **adenomatous polyposis coli (APC),** is a rare autosomal dominant inheritance trait that accounts for about 1% to 5% of colorectal cancer.[123] FAP is usually associated with hundreds of adenomas that distribute through the colon with a high risk for malignant transformation by 35 to 40 years of age. Worldwide, the prevalence of colorectal cancer is highest in populations with high socioeconomic standards, possibly because of dietary habits (see *Risk Factors:* Cancer of the Colon and Rectum). Cancer of the small intestine is rare and represents less than 1% of gastrointestinal cancers.[124]

PATHOGENESIS Cancer of the colon may be a sporadic event or associated with genetic and epigenetic events. Deletion of genes is linked to the transformation of normal

RISK FACTORS Cancer of the Colon and Rectum

- Advanced age
- High-fat (especially egg consumption), low-fiber diet
- High consumption of alcohol
- Cigarette smoking
- Obesity
- Familial polyposis or family history of colorectal cancer
- Low levels of physical activity
- Ulcerative colitis after 10 years
- Gastrectomy

Data from American Cancer Society: *Cancer facts & figures—2007,* Atlanta, 2007, American Cancer Society.

colon epithelial cells to benign and malignant adenomas. Mutations of oncogenes, tumor suppressor, and repair genes are associated with colon cancer.[125] Dietary factors, including high fat, low fiber, and low calcium, may promote somatic mutations. Promoting mechanisms also are related to prolonged contact of the fecal mass with colon mucosa.[126]

Colorectal polyps are closely associated with development of cancer. A polyp, or papilloma, is a finger-like projection arising from the mucosal epithelium. Most polyps are benign. **Neoplastic polyps** are premalignant lesions and are classified as tubular (the most prevalent), villous, or tubulovillous, adenomas (Figure 34-18).

Adenocarcinoma of the colon and rectum usually arise from adenomatous polyps. Once the malignant cells of an adenoma traverse the muscularis mucosae, the tumor becomes invasive and highly malignant. Adenomas can be detected early, however, and the submucosa may not be penetrated for several years (Figure 34-19). The larger the polyp, the greater the risk of colorectal cancer. Although lesions larger than 1.5 cm occur less often, they are more likely to be malignant than those smaller than 1.0 cm. For other conditions commonly confused with colorectal cancer, see Table 34-11.

Most colorectal cancers are moderately differentiated adenocarcinomas. These tumors have a long preinvasive phase, and when they invade, they tend to grow slowly. Colorectal carcinoma starts in the glands of the mucosal lining. Because the lymphatic channels are located under the muscularis mucosae, the lesions must traverse this layer before metastasis can occur (Figure 34-20).

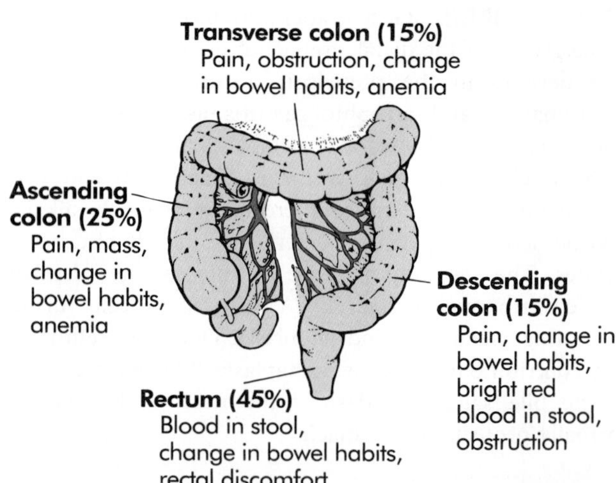

Figure 34-19 ■ **Signs and Symptoms of Colorectal Cancer by Location of Primary Lesion.** Clinical manifestations are listed in order of frequency for each region (lymphatics of colon also shown).

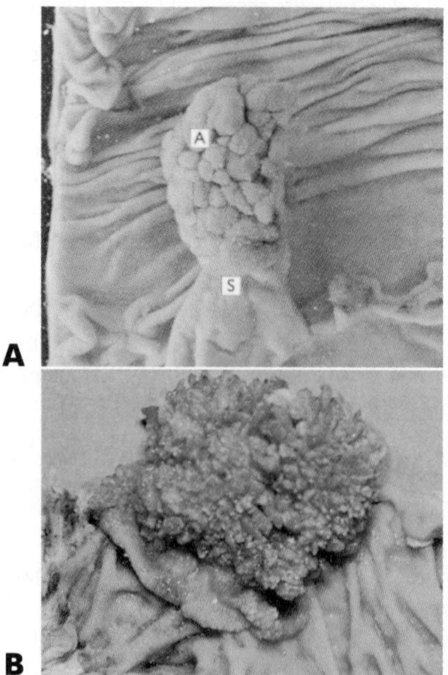

Figure 34-18 ■ **Neoplastic Polyps. A,** Tubular adenomata *(A)* are rounded lesions 0.5 to 2 cm in size that are generally red and sit on a stalk *(S)* of normal mucosa that has been dragged up by traction of the polyp in the bowel lumen. **B,** Villous adenomata are velvety lesions about 0.6 cm thick that occupy a broad area of mucosa generally 1 to 5 cm in diameter. (From Stevens A, Lowe J: *Pathology,* ed 2, Edinburgh, 2000, Mosby.)

CLINICAL MANIFESTATIONS Symptoms of colorectal cancer depend on the location, size, and shape of the lesion. Tumors of the right (ascending) colon and left (descending) colon evolve into two distinct tumor types.[127] On the right side, the lesions are polypoid and extend along one wall of the cecum and ascending colon. These tumors may be silent, evolving to pain, palpable mass in the lower right quadrant, anemia, fatigue, and dark-red or mahogany-colored blood mixed with the stool (see Figure 34-19). These tumors can become large and bulky with necrosis and ulceration, contributing to persistent blood loss and anemia. Obstruction is unusual because the growth does not readily encircle the colon.

Tumors of the left, or descending, colon start as small, elevated, button-like masses. This type grows circumferentially, encircling the entire bowel wall, and eventually ulcerating in the middle as the tumor penetrates the blood supply. Obstruction is common but occurs slowly and stools become narrow and pencil shaped. Manifestations include progressive abdominal distention, pain, vomiting, constipation, need for laxatives, cramps, and bright red blood on the surface of the stool.

Systematic lymphatic spread occurs along the aorta to the mesenteric and pancreatic lymph nodes. Liver metastasis is common and follows invasion of the mesenteric veins (left colon) or superior veins (right colon), which drain into the portal circulation.

Rectal carcinomas are defined as tumors occurring up to 15 cm from the anal opening. Tumors of the rectum can spread through the rectal wall to nearby structures: the prostate in men and the vagina in women. Penetration occurs more readily in the lower third of the rectum

TABLE 34-11

Conditions Commonly Confused With Colorectal Cancer

Condition	Significant Characteristics
Diverticulitis	Left-sided pain similar to that of appendicitis; tender lower left quadrant; associated findings: nausea, vomiting, fever, obstruction, anorexia, and leukocytosis; mucosa is intact, and perforation, peritonitis, and abscesses occur more often than in cancer; proctosigmoidoscopy or barium enema used to distinguish from cancer
Chronic ulcerative colitis	Younger people with chronic attacks of bloody diarrhea, crampy abdominal pain, fever, malnutrition, and dehydration; usually involves the left colon and rectum; endoscopy, barium enema, and biopsy performed for definitive diagnosis
Crohn disease (granulomatous colitis)	Generally involves the right colon; chronic diarrhea with abdominal cramps, fever, weight loss, and often a palpable abdominal mass; difficult at times to distinguish Crohn disease from ulcerative colitis; endoscopic examination and barium enema used to distinguish from cancer
Appendicitis	Vague abdominal symptoms, often with a tender or nontender mass in the lower right quadrant; associated symptoms: mild fever and leukocytosis; barium enema used to distinguish from cancer
Thrombosed hemorrhoids	Examination shows a tender, swollen, bluish painful mass in the anus; patient will have a history of hemorrhoids

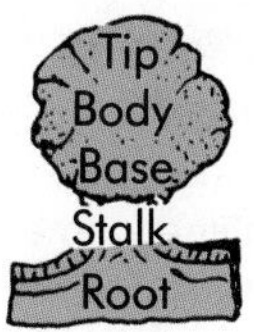

Adenomatous polyp

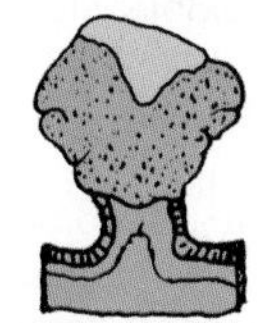

Focal atypia (cancer in situ)

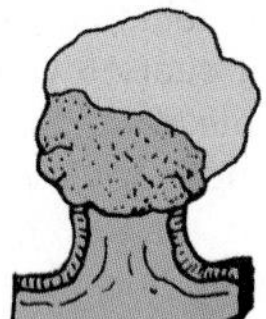

Focal cancer (malignant adenoma)

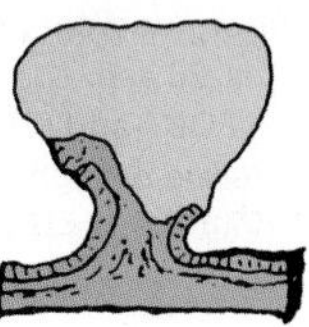

Focal cancer invading stalk with some "benign" polyp still in body

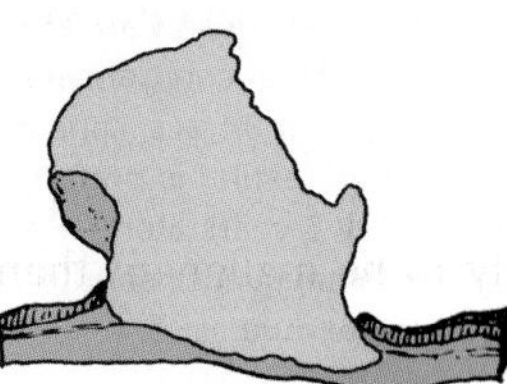

Invasive cancer containing piece of polyp

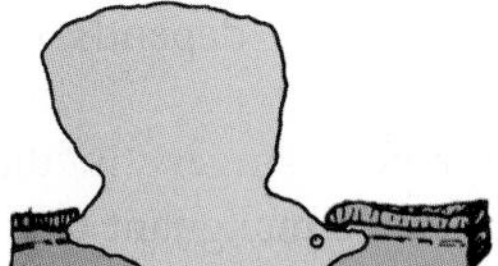

Polypoid invasive cancer without polyp remnant

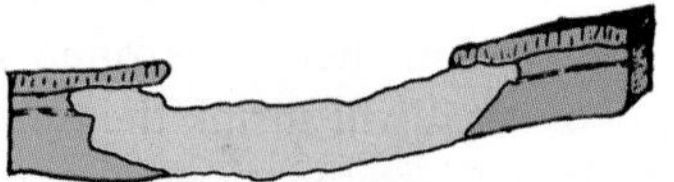

Ulcerated invasive cancer without polyp remnant

Figure 34-20 ■ Development of Cancer of the Colon From Adenomatous Polyps. The tumor becomes invasive if it penetrates the muscularis mucosae and enters the submucosal layer. (From del Regato JA, Spjut HJ, Cox JD: *Cancer: diagnosis, treatment, and prognosis,* ed 2, St Louis, 1985, Mosby.)

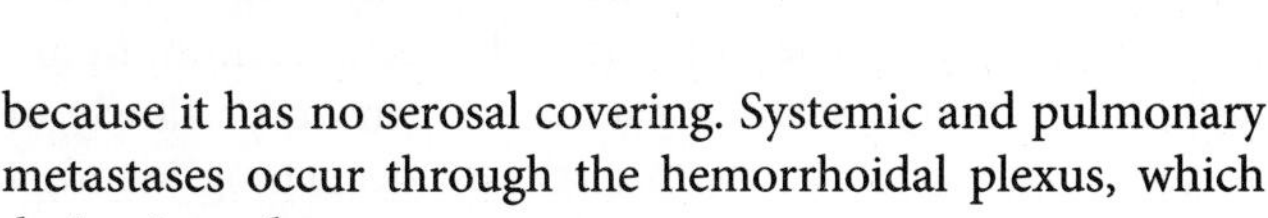

because it has no serosal covering. Systemic and pulmonary metastases occur through the hemorrhoidal plexus, which drains into the vena cava.

EVALUATION AND TREATMENT Early detection screening procedures are summarized in Box 34-3. Individuals with a family history of polyps should be screened using colonoscopy with removal of polyps when they are found.[128] A diet rich in vegetables, grains, fruit folate, calcium, and low in fat can modify cancer risk.[129]

The staging of colorectal cancer involves endoscopic ultrasonography and operative exploration. Physical examination of the abdomen detects liver enlargement and ascites; appropriate lymph nodes are palpated. Elevations of carcinoembryonic antigen (CEA) are often detected in the sera of individuals with colorectal carcinoma, but it is not a screening marker for colorectal cancer as it is elevated with other intestinal diseases. Operative staging consists of careful exploration during surgery and biopsy of possible metastases. The Dukes classification for staging of colorectal cancer is as follows:

- Stage A: Cancer limited to the bowel wall
- Stage B: Cancer extending through the bowel wall
- Stage C: Nodal metastases regardless of extension into the bowel wall
- Stage D: Distant metastases regardless of primary size

Treatment for cancer of the colon is always surgical. Resection and anastomosis can be performed for cancer of the ascending, transverse, descending, or sigmoid colon and upper rectum. These surgeries are performed through abdominal incisions, and natural defecation is preserved.

Growths in the lower portion of the rectum require removal of the entire rectum with the formation of a

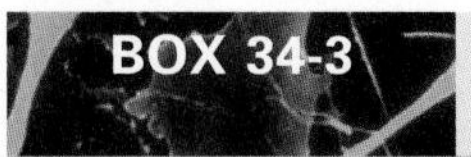

Screening for Colorectal Cancer

Beginning at age 50, men and women should follow one of the examination schedules noted here:

- A fecal occult blood test (FOBT) or fecal immunochemical test (FIT) every year
- A flexible sigmoidoscopy (FSIG) every 5 years
- Annual fecal, occult blood test and flexible sigmoidoscopy every 5 years*
- A double-contrast barium enema every 5 years
- A colonoscopy every 10 years
- Genetic testing is available for familial adenomatous polyposis and hereditary nonpolyposis colon cancer
- Stool DNA testing provides noninvasive, early detection of colorectal cancer
- All positive tests should be followed up with colonoscopy.

Data from American Cancer Society: *Guidelines for Early Detection of Cancer,* American Cancer Society; www.cancer.org/docroot/ped/content/ped_2_3x_acs_cancer_detection_guidelines_36.asp.
*Combined testing is preferred over either annual FOBT and FIT or FSIG every 5 years alone. People who are at moderate or high risk for colorectal cancer should talk with a doctor about a different testing schedule.

permanent colostomy. Resection of liver metastases can prolong survival.[130] Prognosis after surgery depends on the stage and location of the tumor.

Radiation therapy is often given before surgery in the hope that it will shrink the tumor, alter the malignant cells, or do both, so that these cells will not survive after surgery. Chemotherapy is used to treat metastatic disease and cases with a high risk of recurrence. New chemotherapeutic agents are improving first-line therapy. Immunotherapy may boost the immune response.[131] Vaccines and viral vectors for the treatment of colon cancer are under development.[132,133]

Cancer of the Accessory Organs of Digestion

Cancer of the liver

Cancer of the liver usually develops secondarily and is caused by metastatic spread from a primary site elsewhere in the body. Primary liver cancer is relatively rare in the United States but is common in densely populated parts of the Far East, Southern Africa, China, and Greece. In the United States, the incidence of primary liver cancer is higher in blacks than in whites and higher in males than in females. Primary liver cancer is rare before the age of 40 years and is most common during the sixth decade. Together, primary and secondary liver cancers account for about 2% to 3% of all cancer deaths in the United States[104] (see *Risk Factors:* Primary Liver Cancer). Chronic hepatitis (B and C), cirrhosis, and dietary exposure to the fungal toxin aflatoxin are significant risk factors.[134]

RISK FACTORS Primary Liver Cancer

- Exposure to mycotoxins. The most significant mycotoxins are the aflatoxins, particularly those produced by *Aspergillus flavus,* a mold found on spoiled corn, peanuts, and grain.
- Alcohol abuse
- Obesity
- Chronic liver disease, especially cirrhosis.
- Infection with hepatitis B virus (HBV), hepatitis C virus (HCV), and hepatitis D virus (HDV), particularly in conjunction with cirrhosis. These infections act either as carcinogens or as cocarcinogens in chronically infected hepatocytes.

PATHOGENESIS Primary carcinomas of the liver are hepatocellular or cholangiocellular. **Hepatocellular carcinoma (hepatocarcinoma)** develops in the hepatocytes, whereas **cholangiocellular carcinoma (cholangiocarcinoma)** develops in the bile ducts. Hepatocellular carcinoma can be nodular (consisting of multiple, discrete nodules), massive (consisting of a large tumor mass having satellite nodules), or diffuse (consisting of small nodules distributed throughout most of the liver). It is closely associated with chronic hepatitis cirrhosis. Because carcinoma of the liver invades the hepatic and portal veins, it often spreads to the heart and lungs. Other sites of metastases are the brain, kidney, and spleen.

Cholangiocellular carcinoma occurs less often than hepatocellular carcinoma in the United States and is most common where liver fluke infestation is prevalent, such as Southeast China. Cholangiocellular carcinoma can occur anywhere along the bile duct and extend directly into the liver, usually as a solitary lesion. It is difficult to distinguish an invasion of cholangiocellular carcinoma from a metastatic adenocarcinoma except by neoplastic changes found in nearby ducts.

CLINICAL MANIFESTATIONS The clinical presentation of liver cancer in adults is characterized by vague abdominal symptoms, such as nausea and vomiting, fullness, pressure, and dull ache in the right hypochondrium. Manifestations of hepatocellular carcinoma can occur slowly or abruptly. In individuals with cirrhosis, deepening jaundice or abrupt lack of appetite is a sign of hepatocellular carcinoma. Obstruction by the tumor can cause sudden worsening of portal hypertension and development of ascites. As the tumor enlarges, it causes pain. Cholangiocellular carcinoma more commonly presents insidiously as pain, loss of appetite, weight loss, and gradual onset of jaundice. Some carcinomas of the liver rupture spontaneously, causing hemorrhage. Others are discovered accidentally during evaluation of a bone fracture or surgical exploration.

EVALUATION AND TREATMENT There is no specific test for the diagnosis of liver cancer. The diagnosis is based on clinical manifestations, laboratory findings, radiologic examination, and exploratory laparotomy and tissue pathology. In individuals without cirrhosis, liver scans can document filling defects. CT or ultrasonography is used to detect solid tumors, but neither can distinguish benign from malignant tumors. A liver biopsy can be diagnostic unless the examiner misses scattered nodules. Primary prevention may be achieved with vaccination against hepatitis B and reduced contamination of food with aflatoxins.[135]

Surgical resection is possible only if the tumor is localized to a removable lobe of the liver. Chemotherapeutic agents are administered systemically or locally, but their use may be limited to the presence of advanced cirrhosis.

The overall median survival rate for those with symptomatic liver cancer is only 3 to 4 months. Surgery is hazardous and usually not undertaken if the individual has cirrhosis. Most individuals develop metastases after surgical resection, but long-term survival is possible. Liver transplant offers a cure if the waiting time is short.[136] Gene and immunotherapy are being explored.[137]

Cancer of the gallbladder

Cancer of the gallbladder occurs in about 6800 people each year in the United States.[115] It is more common in women than in men by a ratio of about 2 to 1. It occurs rarely before the age of 40 years and is most common between the ages of 50 and 60 years. Most gallbladder cancer is caused by metastasis. Primary carcinoma of the gallbladder is rare and usually is associated with cholelithiasis.

PATHOGENESIS Most primary carcinomas of the gallbladder are adenocarcinomas, and they are rare. A few are squamous cell carcinomas. Invasion of the liver occurs early. Spreading to the cystic and periportal lymph nodes occurs with invasion of the pancreas and retroperitoneal lymph nodes. Direct invasion of the stomach and the duodenum can cause pyloric obstruction. Infection often accompanies cancer of the gallbladder. Generalized peritonitis, gangrene, perforation, and liver abscesses are potential complications of infection.

CLINICAL MANIFESTATIONS Early stages of gallbladder carcinoma are asymptomatic. A typical presentation of carcinoma of the gallbladder is steady, upper right quadrant pain for about 2 months. Other manifestations include diarrhea, belching, weakness, loss of appetite, weight loss, and vomiting. Obstructive jaundice can occur if an enlarging tumor presses on the extrahepatic ducts.

EVALUATION AND TREATMENT Early diagnosis of cancer of the gallbladder is rare. Therefore, individuals with gallstones, especially older women, are evaluated carefully. Inflammatory disorders, such as cholangitis (bile duct inflammation) and peritonitis, often obscure an underlying malignancy. Diagnostic procedures include upper gastrointestinal barium study, ultrasonography, cholangiography, and CT scan.

Complete surgical resection of the gallbladder is the only effective treatment. Because advanced malignancies cannot be resected, gallbladders containing stones are removed as a preventive measure. The prognosis of gallbladder cancer is extremely poor; most individuals die within 1 year after surgery.[138]

Cancer of the pancreas

Pancreatic cancer now ranks fourth as a cause of cancer deaths in the United States. The incidence of pancreatic cancer rises steadily with age. Males are affected slightly more often than females, and blacks more often than whites. Pancreatic cancer accounts for about 33,300 deaths annually in the United States.[115] Mortality is nearly 100%. The cause of pancreatic cancer is not known, but there are modest risks associated with cigarette smoking, certain dietary factors, obesity, diabetes mellitus, and chronic pancreatitis.[139]

PATHOGENESIS Cancer of the pancreas can arise from exocrine or endocrine cells. Most pancreatic tumors arise from exocrine cells in the ducts and are called *ductal adenocarcinomas.* Tumors arising in small ducts invade nearby glandular tissue, penetrate the covering of the pancreas, and extend into surrounding tissues.[140]

Ductal adenocarcinomas can occur in the head, body, or tail of the pancreas. Tumors of the head quickly spread to obstruct the common bile duct and portal vein. These tumors can then infiltrate the superior mesenteric artery, the vena cava, and the aorta and form emboli. Tumors of the body and tail infiltrate the posterior abdominal wall. Lymphatic invasion occurs early and rapidly and involves local and regional lymph nodes. Venous invasion causes metastases to the liver. Tumor implants on the peritoneal surface can obstruct veins and promote development of ascites.

Ductal adenocarcinomas arising in the head of the pancreas cause biliary obstruction somewhat early in the disease. Individuals with such tumors survive slightly longer than those with cancer of the body and tail, presumably because they seek medical attention earlier.

CLINICAL MANIFESTATIONS Cancer of the body and tail of the pancreas is generally asymptomatic until there is intraductal destruction or the tumor invades adjacent tissue. Often vague back pain is an initial symptom. Jaundice develops in most cases, usually caused by obstruction of the bile duct. Because obstruction impairs enzyme secretion and flow to the duodenum, pancreatic cancer causes fat and protein malabsorption, resulting in weight loss.[141] Distant metastases are found in the neck nodes, the lungs, and the brain. Most individuals die of hepatic failure, malnutrition, or systemic diseases.

EVALUATION AND TREATMENT A laparotomy is often performed, particularly if jaundice is present. Ultrasonography and CT may be needed to confirm the need for a laparotomy, especially in individuals without jaundice. Laparotomy is used to establish a definitive diagnosis, evaluate the extent of disease, and determine whether palliative bypass surgery (i.e., cholecystojejunostomy and gastrojejunostomy) is needed. Most individuals require palliative double bypass of the blocked bile ducts, as well as gastrojejunostomy to prevent duodenal obstruction.

Many surgeons recommend a total pancreatectomy because cancer of the pancreas seldom consists of a single lesion. Chemotherapy and radiation adjuvant therapy are used as palliative measures. Because almost all pancreatic cancers are advanced at the time of diagnosis, staging has little relevance in determining treatment.[142] Five-year survival is less than 5%.

QUICK CHECK 34-8

1. What are the primary risk factors for gastric carcinoma?
2. Compare tumors of the right colon with those of the left colon.
3. What is the most common cause of liver cancer?

Did You Understand?

Disorders of the Gastrointestinal Tract

1. Anorexia (loss of appetite), vomiting, constipation, diarrhea, abdominal pain, and evidence of gastrointestinal bleeding are clinical manifestations of many disorders of the gastrointestinal tract.
2. Vomiting is the forceful emptying of the stomach effected by gastrointestinal contraction and reverse peristalsis of the esophagus. It is usually preceded by nausea and retching, with the exception of projectile vomiting, which is associated with direct stimulation of the vomiting center in the brain.
3. Constipation is often caused by unhealthy dietary and bowel habits combined with lack of exercise. Constipation also can result from a disorder that impairs intestinal motility or obstructs the intestinal lumen.
4. Diarrhea can be caused by excessive fluid drawn into the intestinal lumen by osmosis (osmotic diarrhea), excessive secretion of fluids by the intestinal mucosa (secretory diarrhea), or excessive gastrointestinal motility.
5. Abdominal pain is caused by stretching, inflammation, or ischemia (insufficient blood supply). Abdominal pain originates in the organs themselves (visceral pain) or in the peritoneum (parietal pain). Visceral pain is often referred to the back.
6. Obvious manifestations of gastrointestinal bleeding are hematemesis (vomiting of blood), melena (dark, tarry stools), and hematochezia (frank bleeding from the rectum). Occult bleeding can be detected only by testing stools or vomitus for presence of blood.
7. Dysphagia is difficulty swallowing. It can be caused by a mechanical or functional obstruction of the esophagus. Functional obstruction is an impairment of esophageal motility.
8. Achalasia is a form of functional dysphagia caused by loss of esophageal innervation.
9. Gastroesophageal reflux is the regurgitation of chyme from the stomach into the esophagus. An inflammatory response (reflux esophagitis) ensues if the esophageal mucosa is repeatedly exposed to acids and enzymes in the regurgitated chyme.
10. Hiatal hernia is the protrusion of the upper part of the stomach through the hiatus (esophageal opening in the diaphragm) at the gastroesophageal junction. Hiatal hernia can be sliding or paraesophageal.
11. Pyloric obstruction is the narrowing or blockage of the pylorus, which is the opening between the stomach and the duodenum. It can be caused by a congenital defect, inflammation and scarring secondary to a gastric ulcer, or tumor growth.
12. Intestinal obstruction prevents the normal movement of chyme through the intestinal tract. It is usually mechanical—that is, it is caused by torsion, herniation, or tumor.
13. The most severe consequences of intestinal obstruction are fluid and electrolyte losses, hypovolemia, shock, intestinal necrosis, and perforation of the intestinal wall.
14. Gastritis is an acute or chronic inflammation of the gastric mucosa.
15. Regurgitation of bile, use of anti-inflammatory drugs or alcohol, and some systemic diseases are associated with gastritis.
16. Chronic gastritis of the fundus and body is the most severe form of gastritis. It can result in gastric atrophy and decreased secretion of hydrochloric acid, pepsinogen, and intrinsic factor.
17. Chronic gastritis of the antrum, the most common type, is not usually associated with impaired secretion or gastric atrophy.
18. A peptic ulcer is a circumscribed area of mucosal inflammation and ulceration caused by excessive secretion of gastric acid, disruption of the protective mucosal barrier, or both.
19. There are three types of peptic ulcers: duodenal, gastric, and stress ulcers.
20. Duodenal ulcers, the most common peptic ulcers, are associated with increased numbers of parietal (acid-secreting) cells in the stomach, elevated gastrin levels, and rapid gastric emptying. Pain occurs when the stomach is empty, and it is relieved with food or antacids. Duodenal ulcers tend to heal spontaneously and recur frequently.
21. Gastric ulcers develop near parietal cells, generally in the antrum, and tend to become chronic. Gastric secretions may be normal or decreased, and pain may occur after eating.
22. Ischemic stress ulcers develop suddenly after severe illness, systemic trauma, or neural injury. Ulceration follows mucosal damage caused by ischemia (decreased blood flow to the gastric mucosa).
23. Cushing ulcer is a stress ulcer caused by head trauma. Ulceration follows hypersecretion of hydrochloric acid caused by overstimulation of the vagal nuclei.

Did You Understand?—Cont'd

24. Postgastrectomy syndromes are long-term complications that follow gastrectomy, the resection of all or part of the stomach. The postgastrectomy syndromes include dumping syndrome, alkaline reflux gastritis, afferent loop obstruction, diarrhea, weight loss, and anemia.
25. Dumping syndrome is the rapid emptying of chyme into the small intestine. It causes an osmotic shift of fluid from the vascular compartment to the intestinal lumen, which decreases plasma volume.
26. Alkaline reflux gastritis is stomach inflammation caused by the reflux of bile and pancreatic secretions from the duodenum into the stomach. These substances disrupt the mucosal barrier and cause inflammation.
27. Afferent loop obstruction is an obstruction of the duodenal stump on the proximal side of a gastrojejunostomy. Biliary and pancreatic secretions accumulate in the stump, causing distention, intermittent pain, and vomiting.
28. Malabsorption syndromes result in impaired digestion or absorption of nutrients.
29. Pancreatic insufficiency causes malabsorption associated with impaired digestion. The pancreas does not produce sufficient amounts of the enzymes that digest protein, carbohydrates, and fats into components that can be absorbed by the intestine.
30. Deficient lactase production in the brush border of the small intestine inhibits the breakdown of lactose. This prevents lactose absorption and causes osmotic diarrhea.
31. Bile salt deficiency causes fat malabsorption and steatorrhea (fatty stools). Bile salt deficiency can result from inadequate secretion of bile, excessive bacterial deconjugation of bile, or impaired reabsorption of bile salts caused by ileal disease.
32. Ulcerative colitis is an inflammatory disease that causes ulceration, abscess formation, and necrosis of the colonic and rectal mucosa. Cramping pain, bleeding, frequent diarrhea, dehydration, and weight loss accompany severe forms of the disease. A course of frequent remissions and exacerbations is common.
33. Crohn disease is similar to ulcerative colitis, but it affects both the large and small intestines and ulceration tends to involve all the layers of the lumen. "Skip lesion" fissures and granulomas are characteristic of Crohn disease. Abdominal tenderness, diarrhea, and weight loss are the usual symptoms.
34. Diverticula are outpouchings of colonic mucosa through the muscle layers of the colon wall. Diverticulosis is the presence of these outpouchings; diverticulitis is inflammation of the diverticula.
35. Appendicitis is the most common surgical emergency of the abdomen. Obstruction of the lumen leads to increased pressure, ischemia, and inflammation of the appendix. Without surgical resection, inflammation may progress to gangrene, perforation, and peritonitis.
36. Irritable bowel syndrome is a functional disorder with no known structural or biochemical alterations that can be diarrhea prevalent, constipation prevalent, or may alternate between diarrhea and constipation. Alterations in the brain-gut axis with intestinal hypersensitivity and alterations in motility and secretion are associated with the symptoms.
37. Vascular insufficiency in the intestine is most often associated with occlusion or obstruction of the mesenteric vessels or insufficient arterial blood flow. The resulting ischemia and necrosis produce abdominal pain, fever, bloody diarrhea, hypovolemia, and shock.
38. Obesity is a metabolic disorder with an increase in body fat mass and a BMI greater than 30.
39. The causes of obesity are complex and involve the interaction of adipokines produced by fat cells and other body weight control signals at the level of the hypothalamus. Hypothalamic resistance to leptin increases body fat mass.
40. Central obesity increases the risk of developing hypertension, coronary artery disease, type 2 diabetes mellitus, cancer, and pulmonary disorders.
41. Anorexia nervosa, or self-imposed starvation, is a psychogenic disorder of primarily adolescent and young women. It causes significant weight loss and developmental delays and can be fatal.
42. Bulimia nervosa, or binging and purging, involves eating normal or large amounts of food and then purging by inducing vomiting or abusing laxatives. Severe weight loss is rare, but frequent vomiting causes tooth decay, pharyngitis, and esophagitis.
43. Malnutrition is lack of nourishment from inadequate amounts of calories, protein, vitamins, or minerals. Starvation is an extreme state of malnutrition. Cachexia is physical wasting associated with chronic disease.
44. Short-term starvation, or lack of dietary intake for 3 or 4 days, stimulates mobilization of stored glucose by two metabolic processes: glycogenolysis (splitting of glycogen into glucose) and gluconeogenesis (formation of glucose from noncarbohydrate molecules).
45. Long-term starvation triggers the breakdown of ketone bodies and fatty acids. Eventually proteolysis (protein breakdown) begins, and death ensues if nutrition is not restored.

Disorders of the Accessory Organs of Digestion

1. Portal hypertension, ascites, hepatic encephalopathy, jaundice, and hepatorenal syndrome are complications of many liver disorders.
2. Portal hypertension is an elevation of portal venous pressure to at least 10 mm Hg. It is caused by increased resistance to venous flow in the portal vein and its tributaries, including the sinusoids and hepatic vein.
3. Portal hypertension is the most serious complication of liver disease because it can cause potentially fatal complications, such as bleeding varices, ascites, and hepatic encephalopathy.
4. Ascites is the accumulation and sequestration of fluid in the peritoneal cavity, often as a result of portal hypertension and decreased concentrations of plasma proteins.
5. Hepatic encephalopathy (portal-systemic encephalopathy) is impaired cerebral function caused by blood-borne toxins (particularly ammonia) not metabolized by the liver. Toxin-bearing blood may bypass the liver in collateral vessels opened as a result of portal hypertension, or diseased hepatocytes may be unable to carry out their metabolic functions.

(Continued)

Did You Understand?—Cont'd

6. Manifestations of hepatic encephalopathy range from confusion and asterixis (flapping tremor of the hands) to loss of consciousness, coma, and death.
7. Jaundice (icterus) is a yellow or greenish pigmentation of the skin or sclera of the eyes caused by increases in plasma bilirubin concentration (hyperbilirubinemia).
8. Obstructive jaundice is caused by obstructed bile canaliculi (intrahepatic obstructive jaundice) or obstructed bile ducts outside the liver (extrahepatic obstructive jaundice). Bilirubin accumulates proximal to sites of obstruction, enters the bloodstream, and is carried to the skin and deposited.
9. Hemolytic jaundice is caused by destruction of red blood cells at a rate that exceeds the liver's ability to metabolize unconjugated bilirubin.
10. Hepatorenal syndrome is functional kidney failure caused by advanced liver disease, particularly cirrhosis with portal hypertension. Renal failure is caused by a sudden decrease in blood flow to the kidneys, usually caused by massive gastrointestinal hemorrhage or liver failure. Its chief clinical manifestation is oliguria.
11. Viral hepatitis is an infection of the liver caused by a strain of the hepatitis virus (i.e., hepatitis A virus [HAV], hepatitis B virus [HBV], or hepatitis C virus [HCV]). Although they differ with respect to modes of transmission and severity of acute illness, all can cause hepatic cell necrosis, Kupffer cell hyperplasia, and infiltration of liver tissue by mononuclear phagocytes. These changes obstruct bile flow and impair hepatocyte function.
12. The clinical manifestations of viral hepatitis depend on the stage of infection. Fever, malaise, anorexia, and liver enlargement and tenderness characterize the prodromal phase (stage 1). Jaundice and hyperbilirubinemia mark the icteric phase (stage 2). During the recovery phase (stage 3), symptoms resolve. Recovery takes several weeks.
13. Fulminant hepatitis is a complication of hepatitis B (with or without hepatitis D infection) or hepatitis C virus. It causes widespread hepatic necrosis and is often fatal.
14. Cirrhosis is an inflammatory disease of the liver that causes disorganization of lobular structure, fibrosis, and nodular regeneration. Cirrhosis can result from hepatitis or exposure to toxins, such as acetaldehyde (a product of alcohol metabolism). The disease causes progressive irreversible liver damage, usually over a period of years.
15. Alcoholic cirrhosis impairs the hepatocytes' ability to oxidize fatty acids, synthesize enzymes and proteins, degrade hormones, and clear portal blood of ammonia and toxins. The inflammatory response includes excessive collagen formation, fibrosis, and scarring, which obstruct bile canaliculi and sinusoids. Bile obstruction causes jaundice. Vascular obstruction causes portal hypertension, shunting, and varices.
16. Primary biliary cirrhosis is the inflammatory destruction of intrahepatic bile ducts. Its cause is unknown.
17. Secondary biliary cirrhosis develops from prolonged obstruction of bile flow with increased pressure in the hepatic bile ducts that causes pooling of bile and necrosis of tissue. Relief of obstruction allays symptoms of jaundice and pruritus. Continued obstruction causes cirrhosis and liver failure.
18. Cholelithiasis (the formation of gallstones) is a common disorder of the gallbladder. Gallstones form in the bile as a result of the aggregation of cholesterol crystals (cholesterol stones) or precipitates of unconjugated bilirubin (pigmented stones). Gallstones that fill the gallbladder or obstruct the cystic or common bile duct cause abdominal pain and jaundice.
19. Cholecystitis is an inflammation of the gallbladder. It is usually associated with obstruction of the cystic duct by gallstones.
20. Acute pancreatitis (pancreatic inflammation) is a serious but relatively rare disorder. Some unknown factor injures the pancreatic ducts or acini. Injury permits leakage of digestive enzymes into pancreatic tissue where they become activated and begin the process of autodigestion, inflammation, and destruction of tissues. Release of pancreatic enzymes into the bloodstream or abdominal cavity causes damage to other organs.
21. Chronic pancreatitis results from structural or functional impairment of the pancreas. It causes recurrent abdominal pain and digestive disorders.

Cancer of the Digestive System

1. Cancer of the esophagus is rare and tends to occur in people older than 60 years of age. Alcohol and tobacco use, reflux esophagitis, and nutritional deficiencies are associated with esophageal carcinoma.
2. Dysphagia and chest pain are the primary manifestations of esophageal cancer. Early treatment of tumors that have not spread into the mediastinum or lymph nodes results in a good prognosis.
3. Gastric carcinoma is associated with high salt intake, food preservatives (nitrates, nitrites), and atrophic gastritis.
4. Approximately 50% of all gastric cancers are located in the prepyloric antrum. Clinical manifestations (weight loss, upper abdominal pain, vomiting, hematemesis, anemia) develop only after the tumor has penetrated the wall of the stomach.
5. Cancer of the colon and rectum (colorectal cancer) is the third most common cause of cancer death in the United States. Preexisting polyps are highly associated with adenocarcinoma of the colon.
6. Tumors of the right (ascending) colon are usually large and bulky; tumors of the left (descending, sigmoid) colon develop as small, button-like masses. Manifestations of colon tumors include pain, bloody stools, and a change in bowel habits.
7. Rectal carcinoma is located up to 15 cm from the opening of the anus. The tumor spreads transmurally to the vagina in women or prostate in men.
8. Metastatic invasion of the liver is more common than primary cancer of the liver.
9. Primary liver cancers are associated with chronic liver disease (cirrhosis, hepatitis B). Hepatocellular carcinomas arise from the hepatocytes, whereas cholangiocellular carcinomas arise from the bile ducts. Primary liver cancer spreads to the heart, lungs, brain, kidney, and spleen through the circulation.

Did You Understand?—Cont'd

10. Cancer of the gallbladder is relatively rare and tends to occur in women older than 50 years. Adenocarcinoma is most common. Because clinical manifestations occur late in the disease, metastases to lymph channels have usually occurred by the time of diagnosis and the prognosis is poor.
11. Cancer of the pancreas now ranks fifth as a cause of cancer deaths. The one known risk factor is heavy cigarette smoking. Most tumors are adenocarcinomas that arise in the exocrine cells of ducts in the head, body, or tail of the pancreas. Symptoms may not be evident until the tumor has spread to surrounding tissues. Treatment is palliative, and mortality is nearly 100%.

Key Terms

Achalasia, 940
Acute gastritis, 946
Acute pancreatitis (acute hemorrhagic pancreatitis), 970
Afferent loop obstruction, 951
Alcoholic cirrhosis, 967
Alcoholic hepatitis, 968
Alkaline reflux gastritis, 951
Anemia, 951
Anorexia, 937
Anorexia nervosa, 958
Appendicitis, 955
Ascites, 960, 961
Biliary cirrhosis, 969
Bone disorder, 952
Bulimia nervosa, 959
Cachexia, 959
Central obesity, 957
Cholangiocellular carcinoma (cholangiocarcinoma), 976
Cholecystitis, 969
Cholelithiasis (gallstone), 969
Chronic active hepatitis, 966
Chronic gastritis, 947
Chronic pancreatitis, 971
Cirrhosis, 967
Colorectal polyp, 974
Constipation, 938
Crohn disease, 953
Cushing ulcer, 950
Diarrhea, 938, 951
Diverticula, 954
Diverticulitis, 954
Diverticulosis, 954
Dumping syndrome, 951
Duodenal ulcer, 948
Dysphagia, 940
Familial adenomatous polyposis (FAP) (adenomatous polyposis coli [APC]), 973
Fatty liver (steatosis), 968
Fulminant hepatitis, 966
Gallstone, 969
Gastric ulcer, 948
Gastritis, 946
Gastroesophageal reflux (GER), 941
Gluconeogenesis, 959
Glycogenolysis, 959
Hematochezia, 940
Hemolytic jaundice, 963
Hepatic encephalopathy, 960, 961
Hepatocellular carcinoma (hepatocarcinoma), 976
Hepatorenal syndrome, 964
Hiatal hernia, 942
Hyperbilirubinemia, 963
Icteric phase of hepatitis, 966
Intestinal obstruction, 943
Irritable bowel syndrome, 955
Ischemic ulcer, 950
Jaundice (icterus), 963
Lactase deficiency, 952
Leptin, 957
Long-term starvation, 959
Lower gastrointestinal bleeding, 939
Malabsorption, 952
Maldigestion, 952
Malnutrition, 959
Motility diarrhea, 939
Nausea, 937
Neoplastic polyp, 974
Nonerosive reflux disease (NERD), 942
Obesity, 957
Obstructive jaundice, 963
Osmotic diarrhea, 939
Pancreatic insufficiency, 952
Pancreatitis, 970
Paraesophageal hiatal hernia, 943
Parietal pain, 939
Peptic ulcer, 947
Peripheral obesity, 957
Portal hypertension, 960
Primary biliary cirrhosis, 969
Prodromal phase of hepatitis, 966
Projectile vomiting, 938
Pyloric obstruction, 943
Recovery phase of hepatitis, 966
Referred pain, 939
Reflux esophagitis, 942
Retching, 937
Secondary biliary cirrhosis, 969
Secretory diarrhea, 939
Short-term starvation, 959
Sliding hiatal hernia, 943
Splenomegaly, 960
Starvation, 959
Stress ulcer, 950
Ulcerative colitis, 952
Upper gastrointestinal bleeding, 939
Varices, 960
Viral hepatitis, 965
Visceral pain, 939
Vomiting (emesis), 937
Weight loss, 951

References

1. Wald A: Pathophysiology, diagnosis and current management of chronic constipation, *Nat Clin Pract Gastroenterol Hepatol* 3(2):90–100, 2006.
2. Hsieh C: Treatment of constipation in older adults, *Am Fam Physician* 72(11):2277–2284, 2005.
3. Oldfield EC 3rd: Clostridium difficile-associated diarrhea: resurgence with a vengeance, *Rev Gastroenterol Disord* 6(2): 79–96, 2006.
4. Sazawal S et al: Efficacy of probiotics in prevention of acute diarrhea: a meta-analysis of masked, randomized, placebo-controlled trials, *Lancet Infect Dis* 6(6):374–382, 2006.
5. Park W, Vaezi MF: Etiology and pathogenesis of achalasia: the current understanding, *Am J Gastroenterol* 100(6):1404–1414, 2005.
6. Jost WH: Other indications of botulinum toxin therapy, *Eur J Nerol* 13(suppl 1):65–69, 2006.
7. Jones R, Galmiche JP: Review: what do we mean by GERD?—definition and diagnosis, *Aliment Pharmacol Ther* 22(suppl 1): 2–10, 2005.
8. Moayyedi P, Talley NJ: Gastro-oesophageal reflux disease, *Lancet* 367(9528):2086–2100, 2006.

References—Cont'd

9. Fass R: Erosive esophagitis and nonerosive reflux disease (NERD): comparison of epidemiologic, physiologic, and therapeutic characteristics, *J Clin Gastroenterol* 41(2):131–137, 2007.
10. Merola E, Claudio PP, Giordano A: p53 and the malignant progression of Barrett's esophagus, *J Cell Physiol* 206(3): 574–577, 2006.
11. Armstrong D: Gastroesophageal reflux disease, *Curr Opin Pharmacol* 5(6):589–595, 2005.
12. van Herwaarden MA, Samsom M, Smout AJ: The role of hiatus hernia in gastro-oesophageal reflux disease, *Eur J Gastroenterol Hepatol* 16(9):831–835, 2004.
13. Jones MP, Wessinger S: Small intestinal motility, *Curr Opin Gastroenterol* 22(2):111–116, 2006.
14. Saclarides TJ: Current choices—good or bad—for the proactive management of postoperative ileus: a surgeon's views, *J Perianesth Nurs* 21(2A suppl):S7–S15, 2006.
15. Peck RM Jr, Crabtree J: Helicobacter infection and gastric neoplasia, *J Pathol* 208(2):233–248, 2006.
16. Levenstein S: The very model of a modern etiology: a biopsychosocial view of peptic ulcer, *Psychosom Med* 62(2):176–185, 2000.
17. Jones MP: The role of psychosocial factors in peptic ulcer disease: beyond Helicobacter pylori and NSAIDs, *J Psychosom Res* 60(4):407–412, 2006.
18. Cohen H: Peptic ulcer and, *Helicobacter pylori, Gastroenterol Clin North Am* 29(4):775–789, 2000.
19. Zapata-Colindres JC et al: The association of *Helicobacter pylori,* infection and nonsteroidal anti-inflammatory drugs in peptic ulcer disease, *Can J Gastroentrol* 20(4):277–280, 2006.
20. Savoye G, Oors J, Smout A: Duodenal acid clearance in humans: observations made with intraluminal impedance recording, *Dig Dis Sci* 50(8):1553–1560, 2005.
21. Tummala S et al: Quantifying gastric *Helicobacter pylori* infection: a comparison of quantitative culture, urease breath testing, and histology, *Dig Dis Sci* 52(2):396–401, 2007.
22. Ables AZ, Simon I, Melton ER: Update on *Helicobacter pylori* treatment, *Am Fam Physician* 75(3):351–358, 2007.
23. Chmiela M, Michetti P: Inflammation, immunity, vaccines for Helicobacter infection, *Helicobacter* 11(suppl 1): 21–26, 2006.
24. Mozsik G et al: Mechanisms of action of retinoids in gastrointestinal mucosal protection in animals, human healthy subjects and patients, *Life Sci* 69(25–26):3103–3112, 2001.
25. Stollman N, Metz DC: Pathophysiology and prophylaxis of stress ulcer in intensive care unit patients, *J Crit Care* 20(1): 35–45, 2005.
26. Metz DC: Preventing the gastrointestinal consequences of stress-related mucosal disease, *Curr Med Res Opin* 21(1): 11–18, 2005.
27. Ukleja A: Dumping syndrome: pathophysiology and treatment, *Nutr Clin Pract* 20(5):517–525, 2005.
28. Sands BE: Inflammatory bowel disease: past, present, and future, *J Gastroenterol* 42(1):16–25, 2007.
29. Nayar M, Rhodes JM: Management of inflammatory bowel disease, *Postgrad Med J* 80(942):206–213, 2004.
30. Bach SP, Mortensen NJ: Revolution and evolution: 30 years of ileoanal pouch surgery, *Inflamm Bowel Dis* 12(2):131–145, 2006.
31. Chamberlin WM, Naser SA: Integrating theories of the etiology of Crohn's disease: On the etiology of Crohn's disease: questioning the hypotheses, *MedSci Monit* 12(2):RA25–RA33, 2006.
32. Chamaillard M et al: Advances and perspectives in the genetic of inflammatory bowel diseases, *Clin Gastroentrol Hepatol* 4(2): 143–151, 2005.
33. Bernstein CN, Walker JR, Graff LA: On studying the connection between stress and IBD, *Am J Gastroenterol* 101(4): 782–785, 2006.
34. Thomas GA et al: Role of smoking in inflammatory bowel disease: implications for therapy, *Postgrad Med J* 76(895): 273–279, 2000.
35. Friedman S: Cancer in Crohn's disease, *Gastroenterol Clin North Am* 35(3):621–639, 2006.
36. Parra-Blanco A: Colonic diverticular disease: pathophysiology and clinical picture, *Digestion* 73(suppl 1):47–57, 2006.
37. West A Brian: The pathology of diverticulosis: classical concepts and mucosal changes in diverticula, *J Clin Gastroenterol* 40(7 suppl 3):S126–S131, 2006.
38. Frieri G, Pimpo MT, Scarpignato C: Management of colonic diverticular disease, *Digestion* 73(suppl 1):58–66, 2006.
39. Birnbaum BA, Wilson SR: Appendicitis at the millennium, *Radiology* 215(2):337–348, 2000.
40. Talley NJ: Irritable bowel syndrome, *Intern Med J* 36(11): 724–728, 2006.
41. Chey WD, Cash BD: Irritable bowel syndrome: update on colonic neuromuscular dysfunction and treatment, *Curr Gastroenterol Rep* 8(4):273–281, 2006.
42. Rhodes DY, Wallace M: Post-infectious irritable bowel syndrome, *Curr Gastroenterol Rep* 8(4):327–332, 2006.
43. Lee HR, Pimentel M: Bacteria and irritable bowel syndrome: the evidence for small intestinal bacterial overgrowth, *Curr Gastroenterol Rep* 8(4):305–311, 2006.
44. Fanigliulo L et al: Role of gut microflora and probiotic effects in the irritable bowel syndrome, *Acta Biomed* 77(2):85–89, 2006.
45. MacDermott RP: Treatment of irritable bowel syndrome in outpatients with inflammatory bowel disease using a food and beverage intolerance, food and beverage avoidance diet, *Inflamm Bowel Dis* 13(1):91–96, 2007.
46. Bach DR et al: Emotional stress reactivity in irritable bowel syndrome, *Eur J Gastroenterol Hepatol* 18(6):629–636, 2006.
47. Podovei M, Kuo B: Irritable bowel syndrome: a practical review, *South Med J* 99(11):1235–1242, 2006.
48. Moneta GL: Screening for mesenteric vascular insufficiency and follow-up of mesenteric artery bypass procedures, *Semin Vasc Surg* 14(3):186–192, 2001.
49. Chang RW, Chang JB, Longo WE: Update in management of mesenteric ischemia, *World J Gastroenterol* 12(20):3243–3247, 2006.
50. Menon NJ et al: Acute mesenteric ischaemia, *Acta Chir Belg* 105(4):344–354, 2005.
51. Wyatt SB, Winters IP, Dubbert PM: Overweight and obesity: prevalence, consequences and causes of a growth public health program, *Am J Med Sci* 331(4):166–174, 2006.
52. Herbert A et al: A common genetic variant is associated with adult and childhood obesity, *Sci* 312(5771):279–283, 2006.
53. Rondinone CM: Adipocyte-derived hormones, cytokines, and mediators, *Endocrine* 29(1):81–90, 2006.
54. Trayhurn P, Bing C: Review: appetite and energy balance signals from the adipocytes, *Philos Trans R Soc Lond B Biol Sci* 361(1471):1237–1249, 2006.
55. Klok MD, Jakobsdottir S, Drent ML: The role of leptin and ghrelin in the regulation of food intake and body weight in humans: a review, *Obes Rev* 8(1):21–34, 2007.
56. Schulze PC, Kratzsch J: Leptin as a new diagnostic tool in chronic heart failure, *Coin Chim Acta* 362(1–2):1–11, 2005.
57. Ouchi N, Shibata R, Walsh K: Cardioprotection by adiponectin, *Trends Cardiovasc Med* 16(5):141–146, 2006.
58. Poirier P et al: Obesity and cardiovascular disease: pathophysiology, evaluation, and effect of weight loss, *Arterioscler Thromb Vasc Biol* 26(5):968–976, 2006.

References—Cont'd

59. Bray GA, Bellanger T: Epidemiology, trends, and morbidities of obesity and metabolic syndrome, *Endocrine* 29(1): 109–117, 2006.
60. Dagenais GR et al: Prognostic impact of body weight and abdominal obesity in women and men with cardiovascular disease, *Am Heart J* 149(1):54–60, 2005.
61. Hoffman DJ et al: Human body composition. In Eckel RH, Ed. *Obesity: mechanisms and clinical management*, Philadelphia, Lippincott, 2003, Williams & Wilkins.
62. National Heart, Lung, and Blood Institute, National Institutes of Health: *Clinical guidelines on the identification, evaluation, and treatment of overweight and obesity in adults: executive summary*, 1998, www.nhlbi.nih.gov/guidelines/obesity/sum_intr.htm.
63. Centers for Disease Control and Prevention: *BMI—body mass index: BMI calculator for children and teens*, 2004; www.cdc.gov/growthcharts.
64. Thompson WG et al: Treatment of obesity, *Mayo Clin Proc* 82(1):93–101, 2007.
65. Ruser CB, Federman DG, Kashaf SS: Whittling away at obesity and overweight: small lifestyle changes can have the biggest impact, *Postgrad Med* 117(1):31–34, 37–40, 2005.
66. Teixeira PJ et al: A review of psychosocial pre-treatment predictors of weight control, *Obes Rev* 6(1):43–65, 2005.
67. Tsai AG, Wadden TA: Systematic review: an evaluation of major commercial weight loss programs in the United States, *Ann Intern Med* 142(1):56–66, 2005.
68. Volek JS, Vanheest JL, Forsythe CE: Diet and exercise for weight loss: a review of current issues, *Sports Med* 35(1):1–9, 2005.
69. Fujioka K, Lee MW: Pharmacologic treatment options for obesity: current and potential medications, *Nutr Clin Pract* 22(1):50–54, 2007.
70. Orzano AJ, Scott JG: Diagnosis and treatment of obesity in adults: an applied evidence based review, *J Am Board Fam Pract* 17(5):359–369, 2004.
71. Puzziferri N, Blankenship J, Wolfe BM: Surgical treatment of obesity, *Endocrine* 29(1):11–19, 2006.
72. Aja S, Moran TH: Recent advances in obesity: adiposity signaling and fat metabolism in energy homeostasis, *Adv Psychosom Med* 27:1–23, 2006.
73. Balik CM: Exploring the gene-environment nexus in eating disorders, *J Psychiatry Neurosci* 30(5):355–359, 2005.
74. le Grange D, Lock J: The dearth of psychological treatment studies for anorexia nervosa, *Int J Eat Disord* 37(2):79–91, 2005.
75. Garrow JS, James WPT: *Human nutrition and dietetics*, Edinburgh, 1993, Churchill Livingstone.
76. Feldman M, Friedman LS, Sleisenger MH: *Sleisenger and Fordtran's gastrointestinal and liver disease*, ed 8, Philadelphia, 2002, Saunders, p. 271.
77. Emery PW: Metabolic changes in malnutrition, *Eye* 19(10): 1029–1034, 2005.
78. Laleman W et al: Portal hypertension: from pathophysiology to clinical practice, *Liver Int* 25(6):1079–1090, 2005.
79. Wright AS, Rikkers LF: Current management of portal hypertension, *J Gastrointest Surg* 9(7):992–1005, 2005.
80. Sandhu BS, Sanyal AJ: Management of ascites in cirrhosis, *Clin Liv Dis* 9(4):715–732, viii, 2005.
81. Cardenas A, Arroyo V: Refractory ascites, *Dig Dis* 23(1): 30–38, 2005.
82. Faint V: The pathophysiology of hepatic encephalopathy, *Nurs Crit Care* 11(2):69–74, 2006.
83. Mas A: Hepatic encephalopathy: from pathophysiology to treatment, *Digestion* 73(suppl 1):86–93, 2006.
84. Wright G, Jalan R: Management of hepatic encephalopathy in patients with cirrhosis, *Best Pract Res Clin Gastroenterol* 21(1): 95–110, 2007.
85. Roche SP, Kobos R: Jaundice in the adult patient, *Am Fam Physician* 69(2):299–304, 2004.
86. Scott-Conner CE, Grogan JB: The pathophysiology of biliary obstruction and its effect on phagocytic and immune function, *J Surg Res* 57(2):316–336, 1994.
87. Arroyo V, Terra C, Gines P: New treatments of hepatorenal syndrome, *Semin Liver Dis* 26(3):254–264, 2006.
88. Parikh S, Hyman D: Hepatocellular cancer: a guide for the internist, *Am J Med* 120(3):194–202, 2007.
89. Shukla NB, Poles MA: Hepatitis B virus: coinfection with hepatitis C virus, hepatitis D virus, and human immunodeficiency virus, *Clin Liver Dis* 8(2):445–460, viii, 2004.
90. Sterling RK, Bralow S: Extrahepatic manifestations of hepatitis C virus, *Curr Gastroenterol Rep* 8(1):53–59, 2006.
91. Tanikawa K: Recent advances in antiviral agents: antiviral drug discovery for hepatitis viruses, *Curr Pharm Des* 12(11): 1371–1377, 2006.
92. Shrestha MP et al: Safety and efficacy of a recombinant hepatitis E vaccine, *N Engl J Med* 356(9):895–903, 2007.
93. Khan SA et al: Acute liver failure: a review, *Clin Liver Dis* 10(2):239–258, 2006.
94. Siegmund SV, Brenner DA: Molecular pathogenesis of alcohol-induced hepatic fibrosis, *Alcohol Clin Exp Res* 29(11 suppl): 102S–109S, 2005.
95. Day CP: Who gets alcoholic liver disease: nature or nurture, *J R Coll Physicians Lond* 34(6):557–562, 2002.
96. Roongpisuthipong C et al: Nutritional assessment in various stages of liver cirrhosis, *Nutrition* 17(9):761–765, 2001.
97. Tsukada S, Parsons CJ, Rippe RA: Mechanisms of liver fibrosis, *Clin Chim Acta* 364(1–2):33–60, 2006.
98. Baraona E, Lieber CS: Alcohol and lipids, *Recent Dev Alcohol* 14:97–134, 1998.
99. Sougioultzis S et al: Alcoholic hepatitis: from pathogenesis to treatment, *Curr Med Res Opin* 21(9):1337–1346, 2005.
100. Bhatia AS, Mihas AA: Cholestatic liver disease: recognizing the clinical signs, *Postgrad Med* 119(1):67–75, 82, 2006.
101. Wittenburg H, Lammert F: Genetic predisposition to gallbladder stones, *Semin Liver Dis* 27(1):109–121, 2007.
102. Shaffer EA: Gallstone disease: epidemiology of gallbladder stone disease, *Best Pract Res Clin Gastroenterol* 20(6): 981–996, 2006.
103. Portincasa P, Moschetta A, Palasciano G: Cholesterol gallstone disease, *Lancet* 368(9531):230–239, 2006.
104. Portincasa P et al: Gallstone disease: symptoms and diagnosis of gallbladder stones, *Best Pract Res Clin Gastroenterol* 20(6): 1017–1029, 2006.
105. Bellows CF, Berger DH, Crass RA: Management of gallstones, *Am Fam Physician* 72(4):637–642, 2005.
106. Middelfart HV et al: Pain patterns after distension of the gallbladder in patients with acute cholecystitis, *Scand J Gastroenterol*, 33(9):982–987, 1998.
107. Perez-Mateo M: How we predict the etiology of acute pancreatitis, *JOP* 7(3):257–261, 2006.
108. Browne GW, Pitchumoni CS: Pathophysiology of pulmonary complications of acute pancreatitis, *World J Gastroenterol* 12(44):7087–7096, 2006.
109. Kakafika A et al: Coagulation, platelets, and acute pancreatitis, *Pancreas* 34(1):15–20, 2007.
110. Mayerle J, Hlouschek V, Lerch MM: Current management of acute pancreatitis, *Nat Clin Pract Gasteroentrol Hepatol* 2(10): 473–483, 2005.
111. Sargent S: Pathophysiology, diagnosis and management of acute pancreatitis, *Br J Nurs* 15(18):999–1005, 2006.
112. DeMagno MJ, DiMagno EP: Chronic pancreatitis, *Curr Opin Gastroenterol* 21(5):544–554, 2005.

References—Cont'd

113. Leppaniemi A, Kemppainen E: Recent advances in the surgical management of necrotizing pancreatitis, *Curr Opin Crit Care* 11(4):349–352, 2005.
114. Pera M et al: Epidemiology of esophageal adenocarcinoma, *J Surg Oncol* 92(3):151–159, 2005.
115. American Cancer Society: *Cancer facts & figures—2007*, Atlanta, 2007, American Cancer Society.
116. Holmes RS, Vaughan TL: Epidemiology and pathogenesis of esophageal cancer, *Semin Radiat Oncol* 17(1):2–9, 2007.
117. Wong R, Malthaner R: Combined chemotherapy and radiotherapy (without surgery) compared to radiotherapy alone in localized carcinoma of the esophagus, *Cochrane Database Syst Rev* (1):CD002092, 2006.
118. Matysiak-Budnik T, Megraud F: Helicobacter pylori infection, and gastric cancer, *Eur J Cancer* 42(6):708–716, 2006.
119. Sutter AP, Fechner H: Gene therapy for gastric cancer: is it promising, *World J Gastroenterol* 12(3):380–387, 2006.
120. Sastre J, Garcia-Saenz JA, Diaz-Rubio E: Chemotherapy for gastric cancer, *World J Gastroenterol* 12(2):204–213, 2006.
121. Galiatsatos P, Foulkes WD: Familial adenomatous polyposis, *Am J Gastroenterol* 101(2):385–398, 2006.
122. Wagner A et al: A 10-Mb paracentric inversion of chromosome arm 2p inactivates MSH2 and is responsible for hereditary nonpolyposis colorectal cancer in a North-American kindred, *Genes Chromosomes Cancer* 35(1):49–57, 2002.
123. Bodmer WF: Cancer genetics: colorectal cancer as a model, *J Hum Genet* 51(5):391–396, 2006.
124. Gore RM et al: Diagnosis and staging of small bowel tumours, *Cancer Imaging* 6:209–212, 2006.
125. Calvert PM, Frucht H: The genetics of colorectal cancer, *Ann Intern Med* 137(7):603–612, 2002.
126. Wakai K et al: Dietary risk factors for colon and rectal cancers: a comparative case-control study, *J Epidemiol* 16(3):125–135, 2006.
127. Distler P, Holt PR: Are right- and left-sided colon neoplasms distinct tumors, *Dig Dis* 15(4–5):302–311, 1997.
128. Kronborg O: Colon polyps and cancer, *Endoscopy* 34(1):69–72, 2002.
129. Willett WC: Diet and cancer, *Oncologist* 5(5):393–404, 2002.
130. Wei AC et al: Survival after hepatic resection for colorectal metastases: a 10-year experience, *Ann Surg Oncol* 13(5):668–676, 2006.
131. Pallis AG, Mouzas IA: Adjuvant chemotherapy for colon cancer, *Anticancer Res* 26(6C):4809–4815, 2006.
132. Hanna MG Jr et al: Active specific immunotherapy with autologous tumor cell vaccines for stage II colon cancer: logistics, efficacy, safety and immunological pharmacodynamics, *Hum Vaccin* 2(4):185–191, 2006.
133. Morse MA: Virus-based therapies for colon cancer, *Expert Opin Biol Ther* 5(12):1627–1633, 2005.
134. Motola-Kuba D et al: Hepatocellular carcinoma: a review, *Ann Hepatol* 5(1):16–24, 2006.
135. Fecht WJ Jr, Befeler AS: Hepatocellular carcinoma: updates in primary prevention, *Curr Gastroenterol Rep* 6(1):37–43, 2004.
136. Lubienski A: Hepatocellular carcinoma: interventional bridging to liver transplantation, *Transplantation* 80(1 suppl):S113–S119, 2005.
137. Blum HE: Hepatocellular carcinoma: therapy and prevention, *World J Gastroenterol* 11(47):7391–7400, 2005.
138. Sicklick JK, Choti MA: Controversies in the surgical management of cholangiocarcinoma and gallbladder cancer, *Semin Oncol* 32(6 suppl 9):S112–S117, 2005.
139. Freelove R, Walling AD: Pancreatic cancer: diagnosis and management, *Am Fam Physician* 73(3):485–492, 2006.
140. Schafer M, Mullhaupt B, Clavien PA: Evidence-based pancreatic head resection for pancreatic cancer and chronic pancreatitis, *Ann Surg* 236(2):137–148, 2002.
141. Ellison NM et al: Supportive care for patients with pancreatic adenocarcinoma: symptom control and nutrition, *Hematol Oncol Clin North Am* 16(1):105–121, 2002.
142. Boeck S et al: Importance of performance status for treatment outcome in advanced pancreatic cancer, *World J Gastroenterol* 13(2):224–227, 2007.

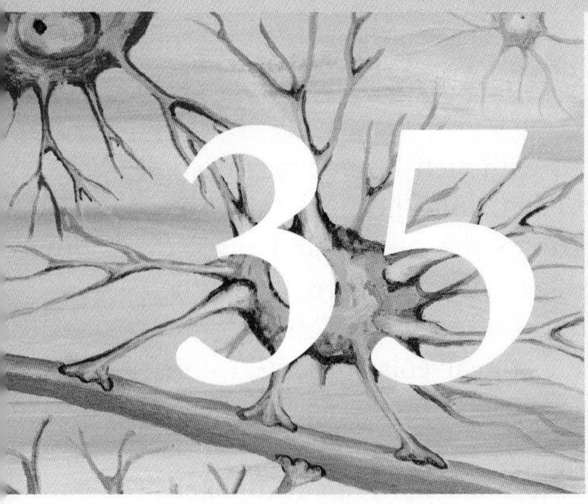

ALTERATIONS OF DIGESTIVE FUNCTION IN CHILDREN

Sue E. Huether

CHAPTER OUTLINE

ELECTRONIC RESOURCES

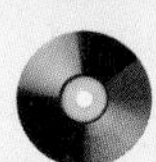

Companion CD
- Review Questions and Answers
- Animations

evolve Website
http://evolve.elsevier.com/Huether/
- Quick Check Answers
- Key Terms Exercises
- Critical Thinking Questions with Answers
- Algorithm Completion Exercises
- WebLinks

Disorders of the gastrointestinal tract in children include anomalies with structural and functional alterations, as well as enzyme deficiencies. Structural alterations can occur throughout the gastrointestinal tract and include cleft lip and palate, esophageal atresia, tracheoesophageal fistula, pyloric stenosis, aganglionic megacolon, and imperforate anus. Gastroesophageal reflux, hepatic and pancreatic enzyme deficiencies, and bacterial or viral invasions of the gastrointestinal tract also contribute to the diseases and gastrointestinal clinical manifestations in children.

Deborah B. Evers, DNS, RN, CPN, contributed to this chapter in the previous edition.

DISORDERS OF THE GASTROINTESTINAL TRACT

Congenital Impairment of Motility

Cleft lip and cleft palate

Cleft lip (harelip) and **cleft palate** are developmental anomalies of the first branchial arch (Figure 35-1). These defects, which occur during embryonic development, vary in severity. In whites, the incidence of cleft lip or cleft palate ranges from 1 in 600 to 1 in 1250 births. The incidence of cleft lip, with or without cleft palate, is 1 in 1000 births, whereas the incidence of cleft palate alone is about 1 in 2500 births. The incidence is lower in black populations and higher in Asian populations. Cleft lip, with or without cleft palate, is more common in females. Both anomalies can be unilateral or bilateral, partial or complete.

In most cases, cleft lip and cleft palate are caused by multiple factors, both genetic and nongenetic, each of which contributes only a minor developmental defect. (This phenomenon, called *multifactorial inheritance,* is discussed in Chapter 2.) Together, these factors reduce the amount of neural crest mesenchyme that migrates into the area that will develop into the face of the embryo. The cleft can be part of a syndrome determined by single mutant genes or part of a chromosomal defect, usually trisomy 13.[1] Rarely, the cleft is caused by a teratogenic agent, such as an anticonvulsant drug.[2] Maternal tobacco and alcohol use, maternal diabetes mellitus, and maternal hyperhomocysteinemia have been associated with having offspring with orofacial clefts.[3]

PATHOPHYSIOLOGY

Cleft lip

Cleft lip is caused by the incomplete fusion of the nasomedial or intermaxillary process during the second month of embryonic development. The cleft causes structures of the face and mouth to develop without the normal restraints of encircling lip muscles. The facial cleft may affect not only the lip but also the external nose, nasal cartilages, nasal septum, and alveolar processes.

The cleft is usually just beneath the center of one nostril. The defect may occur bilaterally and may be symmetric or asymmetric. The more complete the cleft lip, the greater the chance that teeth in the line of the cleft will be missing or malformed.

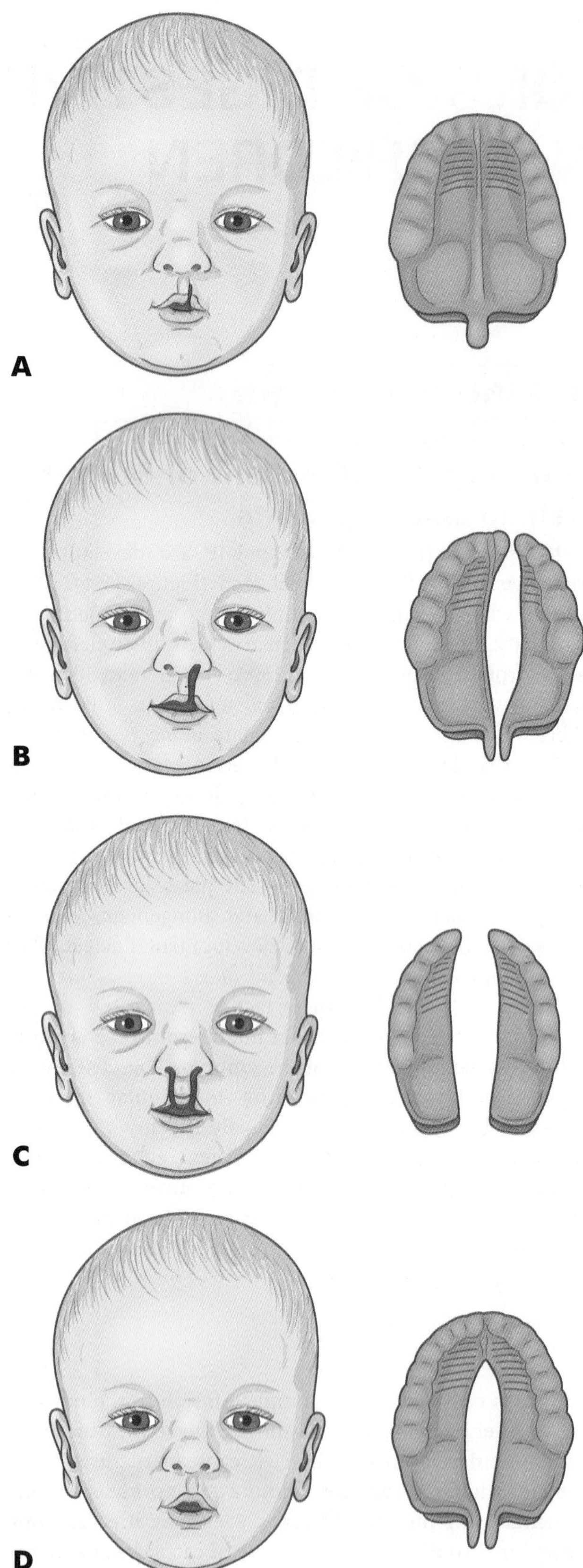

Figure 35-1 ■ **Variations in Clefts of the Lip and Palate.** **A,** Notch in vermilion border. **B,** Unilateral cleft lip and palate. **C,** Bilateral cleft lip and cleft palate. **D,** Cleft palate.

Cleft palate

Cleft palate is often associated with cleft lip but may occur without it. The fissure may affect only the uvula and soft palate or may extend forward to the nostril and involve the hard palate and the maxillary alveolar ridge. It may be unilateral or bilateral, with the cleft occupying the midline posteriorly and as far forward as the alveolar process, where it deviates to the involved side. Clefts involving the palate only are usually but not necessarily in the midline. In some cases, the vomer and nasal septum are partly or completely undeveloped. When these facial bones are involved, the nasal cavity may freely communicate with the oral cavity.

CLINICAL MANIFESTATIONS Feeding the infant with cleft lip usually presents no difficulty if the cleft lip is simple and the palate intact. A baby with cleft palate usually requires large, soft nipples with crosscut openings. Breast-feeding may be impossible for some infants. An orthodontic prosthesis for the roof of the mouth may facilitate sucking for some infants.[4]

EVALUATION AND TREATMENT Prenatal diagnosis is made by 3D ultrasound.[5] Postnatal facial x-ray films confirm the extent of bone deformity. Soft tissue alterations are evaluated by physical examination.

The nature and extent of the cleft, the infant's condition, and the method of surgical correction proposed determine the course of treatment. Surgical correction is often planned in stages.[6] Speech training and special attention by a prosthodontist and orthodontist are almost always required.[7,8]

Both before and after surgery, children with cleft palate tend to have repeated infections of the paranasal sinuses. Excessive dental decay is not unusual. Hypertrophy of tonsils and adenoids and otitis media are frequent accompaniments, and the child should be evaluated for hearing loss.[9] Periconceptual B vitamins, folate, and folic acid intake may prevent orofacial clefts.[10,11]

Esophageal malformations

Congenital malformations of the esophagus occur in 1 of 3000 to 4500 live births. In **esophageal atresia,** the esophagus ends in a blind pouch. It is usually accompanied by a fistula between the esophagus and the trachea **(tracheoesophageal fistula [TEF]).** Either defect can occur alone, however (Figure 35-2).

PATHOPHYSIOLOGY Esophageal abnormalities are thought to arise from defective differentiation as the trachea separates from the esophagus during the fourth to sixth weeks of embryonic development. Defective growth of endodermal cells leads to atresia. Incomplete fusion of the lateral walls of the foregut leads to incomplete closure of the laryngotracheal tube and fistula formation.

CLINICAL MANIFESTATIONS Polyhydramnios (excessive amniotic fluid) is reported to occur in 14% to 90% of mothers of affected infants because of alterations in fetal

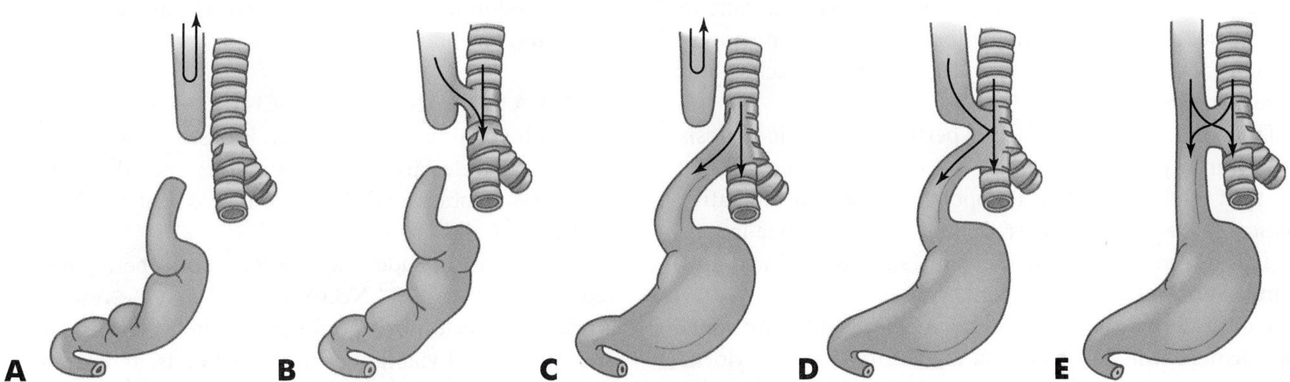

Figure 35-2 ■ **Five Types of Esophageal Atresia and Tracheoesophageal Fistulas. A,** Simple esophageal atresia. Proximal esophagus and distal esophagus end in blind pouches, and there is no tracheal communication. Nothing enters the stomach; regurgitated food and fluid may enter the lungs. **B,** Proximal and distal esophageal segments end in blind pouches, and a fistula connects the proximal esophagus to the trachea. Nothing enters the stomach; food and fluid enter the lungs. **C,** Proximal esophagus ends in a blind pouch, and a fistula connects the trachea to the distal esophagus. Air enters the stomach; regurgitated gastric secretions enter the lungs through the fistula. **D,** Fistula connects both proximal and distal esophageal segments to the trachea. Air, food, and fluid enter the stomach and the lungs. **E,** Simple tracheoesophageal fistula between otherwise normal esophagus and trachea. Air, food, and fluid enter the stomach and the lungs. Between 85% and 90% of esophageal anomalies are type C; 6% to 8% are type A; 3% to 5% are type E; and fewer than 1% are type B or D.

swallowing.[12] If a fistula connects the trachea with the distal esophagus, the abdomen fills with air and becomes distended, possibly interfering with breathing (see Figure 35-2, *C* to *E*). Intermittent cyanosis may result.

Pulmonary complications are compounded by reflux of air and gastric secretions into the tracheobronchial tree through the fistula, causing severe chemical irritation. Infants with esophageal atresia but no fistula have scaphoid (boat-shaped), gasless abdomens. In fistula without atresia (see Figure 35-2, *E*), the usual symptoms are recurrent aspiration, pneumonia, and atelectasis that remains unexpressed for days or even months.

In at least 50% of infants with esophageal defects, other congenital anomalies are present as well. Cardiovascular anomalies are the most common, but other digestive tract, urinary, vertebral, and central nervous system defects can accompany esophageal atresia and tracheoesophageal fistula.

EVALUATION AND TREATMENT Esophageal atresia is usually diagnosed at birth, when attempts to pass a catheter into the stomach fail. X-ray films will show the catheter coiled in the upper esophageal pouch.

Treatment is surgical. Esophageal continuity is restored, and the fistula is eliminated. The child may continue to have problems with aspiration, gastroesophageal reflux, esophageal strictures, and esophagitis after surgical repair.[13] The overall survival rate for infants with esophageal defects is approximately 90%.[14]

Pyloric stenosis

Pyloric stenosis is an obstruction of the pyloric sphincter caused by hypertrophy of the sphincter muscle, and the cause is unknown. One of the most common disorders of early infancy, it affects infants between the ages of 1 and 2 weeks and 3 and 4 months. The incidence of pyloric stenosis among males is approximately 2 to 5 in 1000, whereas that among females is only 1 in 1000.[15] Whites are affected more often than blacks or Asians, and full-term infants are affected more often than premature infants.

PATHOPHYSIOLOGY Individual muscle fibers thicken, so the whole pyloric sphincter becomes enlarged and inelastic. The mucosal lining of the pyloric opening is folded and narrowed by the encroaching muscle. Because of the extra peristaltic effort necessary to force the gastric contents through the narrow pylorus, the muscle layers of the stomach may become hypertrophied as well.

CLINICAL MANIFESTATIONS Between 2 and 3 weeks after birth, an infant who has fed well and gained weight begins to vomit without apparent reason. The vomiting gradually becomes more forceful (projectile). Food is often regurgitated through the nose. The vomiting usually occurs immediately after eating, and the vomitus consists of the bulk of the feeding plus some food retained from previous feedings but is almost always free of bile.

Prolonged retention of food in the stomach is characteristic. Constipation occurs because little food reaches the intestine.

In severe, untreated cases, increased gastric peristalsis and vomiting lead to severe fluid and electrolyte imbalances, malnutrition, and weight loss that can be fatal within 4 to 6 weeks. Infants with pyloric stenosis are irritable because of hunger, and they may have esophageal discomfort caused by repeated vomiting and esophagitis. The vomitus may be blood streaked because of rupture of gastric and esophageal vessels.

EVALUATION AND TREATMENT Diagnosis is based on the history, clinical manifestations, and findings on ultrasound.[16] Occasionally, gastric peristalsis is observable over the abdomen. A firm, small, movable mass, approximately the size of an olive, is felt in the right upper quadrant in 70% to 90% of infants with pyloric stenosis. Sonography clearly shows the hypertrophied pyloric muscles and narrowed pyloric channel.

The standard treatment for hypertrophic pyloric stenosis is a pyloromyotomy, in which the muscles of the pylorus are split and separated. Preoperative and postoperative medical management to correct fluid and electrolyte imbalance has been the key to the high success rate and low complication rates with this surgery.[17]

Some infants may respond to medical and nutritional management, which is based on the theory that the pylorus will open spontaneously by 6 to 8 months of age if nutrition can be maintained. Antispasmodic drugs are given to relax the pylorospasm, and the infant is re-fed after vomiting. Endoscopic balloon dilation and treatment with oral or intravenous atropine sulfate have also shown some success.[18]

Intestinal malrotation

In **intestinal malrotation of the colon,** there is incomplete rotation around the superior mesenteric artery during fetal development. Additionally, an abnormal membrane (periduodenal band) may press on and obstruct the duodenum. This **periduodenal band (Ladd bands)** is one of the most significant findings in malrotation. Associated abnormalities are seen in some children with duodenal and jejunal atresia.[19]

PATHOPHYSIOLOGY In malrotation, the small intestine lacks a normal posterior fixation because it has only a rudimentary attachment near the origin of the superior mesenteric artery. Therefore, the entire mass can twist when the mobile loops of intestine from the duodenojejunal junction to the middle of the transverse colon twist on themselves. The twisting is known as *volvulus* leading to symptoms of bowel obstruction (see Chapter 34). Intestinal twisting around the rudimentary mesentery angulates and obstructs the intestinal lumen and can partly or completely occlude the superior mesenteric artery, causing infarction and necrosis of the entire midgut.

CLINICAL MANIFESTATIONS Although most cases of malrotation-associated volvulus and infarction develop during the neonatal period (50%) or infancy (85% are younger than 1 year), some develop during childhood or even adulthood. In infants, the obstruction causes intermittent or persistent bile-stained vomiting after feedings. Abdominal distention is limited initially to the epigastrium because only the stomach and duodenum are dilated. Dehydration and electrolyte imbalance may occur rapidly because large amounts of pancreatic juice, bile, and gastric secretions are lost through vomiting (bilious vomiting). Fever usually ensues. Pain, scanty stools, diarrhea, and bloody stools are associated with progressive volvulus, vascular compression, and infarction of the intestine in infants. Intermittent or partial volvulus may be seen in older children and in adults. This condition may be asymptomatic and discovered during unrelated abdominal surgery, or it may cause minor abdominal complaints, such as nausea after meals, vomiting, or abdominal pain.

EVALUATION AND TREATMENT Diagnosis of malrotation with volvulus and infarction is based on a review of the clinical manifestations. X-ray films of the abdomen show gas bubbles and distention proximal to the site of obstruction and barium studies.

Treatment includes laparoscopic or open surgery to reduce the volvulus.[20] Necrotic bowel may be resected and a primary anastomosis performed. When there is gangrene and question of viability of the bowel ends, an enterostomy may be performed. Second-look operations may be done to avoid resection of viable bowel. In cases of malrotation without duodenal obstruction, operative survival is 80%. Operative survival is 40% to 50% in cases of malrotation complicated by obstruction caused by periduodenal bands or other intra-abdominal anomalies. Resection of large segments of the small intestine results in short bowel syndrome and its long-term sequelae.[21]

✔ QUICK CHECK 35-1

1. What structures are affected in cleft palate and cleft lip?
2. What is esophageal atresia?
3. What produces pyloric stenosis?

Meconium ileus

Meconium is a substance that fills the entire intestine before birth. It consists of intestinal gland secretions and some amniotic fluid. Normally, meconium is passed from the rectum during the first 12 to 72 hours after birth.

Meconium ileus is an intestinal obstruction caused by meconium formed in utero that is abnormally sticky and adheres firmly to the mucosa of the small intestine, resisting passage beyond the terminal ileum. The cause is usually a lack of digestive enzymes during fetal life. This meconium is also found to contain albumin, which is not normally found in meconium. This has been used as a screening test for cystic fibrosis. Most cases of meconium ileus are caused by cystic fibrosis.[22] In the cases *not* associated with cystic fibrosis, the cause usually is unknown. Partial aplasia of the pancreas is an associated factor, however, and one fifth of infants with meconium ileus are premature or have a history of maternal hydramnios (excessive amniotic fluid). After intestinal atresia and malrotation with volvulus, meconium ileus is the most common cause of small intestinal obstruction in newborns.

PATHOPHYSIOLOGY The terminal ileum is plugged with thick, viscous meconium resulting from the formation of an insoluble, calcium-glycoprotein compound in abnormal mucus. The segment of the ileum proximal to the obstruction is distended with liquid contents, and its walls may be hypertrophied. The segment distal to the obstruction is collapsed and filled with small pellets of pale-colored stool. Meconium in the obstructed segment has the consistency of thick syrup or glue. Peristalsis fails to propel this viscous material through the ileum, and it becomes impacted. Volvulus, atresia, or perforation of the bowel sometimes accompanies meconium ileus.

CLINICAL MANIFESTATIONS Abdominal distention usually develops during the first few days after birth. The infant begins to vomit within hours or days of birth. Infants with cystic fibrosis may have signs of pulmonary involvement, such as tachypnea, intercostal retractions, and grunting respirations. The distended abdomen shows patterns of dilated intestinal loops that feel doughlike when palpated. Some of the loops contain scattered, firm, movable masses. Despite hyperactive peristalsis, the rectal ampulla is empty.

EVALUATION AND TREATMENT Radiologic examination confirms the presence of meconium ileus. The sweat test, which is accurate in 90% of infants, is performed to detect or rule out cystic fibrosis. In approximately 50% of cases not complicated with volvulus or perforation, a hyperosmolar radiopaque (Gastrografin) enema done using fluoroscopy evacuates the meconium. If this is not possible, the meconium is removed surgically.[23]

Survival of infants with meconium ileus is improving, with 85% to 100% survival at 1 year.[24] Mortality increases to 70% if obstruction is complicated by peritonitis. After recovery from neonatal meconium ileus, the long-term outlook depends on the severity and progression of pulmonary disease. Research demonstrates a clear association of meconium ileus with intestinal complications and challenges to nutrition maintenance in children with cystic fibrosis related to surgical treatment for the ileus.[25]

Distal intestinal obstruction syndrome

Distal intestinal obstruction syndrome (DIOS) affects approximately 15% of older children and adults with cystic fibrosis. Intestinal contents may become abnormally thick and impact the intestinal lumen, particularly after episodes of dehydration or lack of pancreatic enzymes. The child displays signs and symptoms of intestinal obstruction. In most cases, the obstruction is relieved by hypertonic enemas. Meconium ileus and DIOS have been shown to be risk factors for the development of cirrhosis in individuals with cystic fibrosis.[26,27]

Obstructions of the duodenum, jejunum, and ileum

Congenital obstruction of the duodenum can be caused by intrinsic malformations or external pressure. An annular pancreas—a defect in which the head of the pancreas surrounds part of the duodenum—can obstruct the duodenum. Congenital obstructions of the jejunum and ileum can be attributable to atresia, stenosis, meconium ileus, megacolon (Hirschsprung disease), intussusception, Meckel diverticulum, intestinal duplication, or strangulated hernia.

In **ileal** or **jejunal atresia,** the intestine ends blindly, proximal and distal to an interruption in its continuity, with or without a gap in the mesentery. Stenosis (narrowing of the lumen) causes dilation proximal to the obstruction and luminal collapse distal to it.

Meckel diverticulum

Meckel diverticulum is an outpouching of all layers of the small intestinal wall (usually in the ileum) and is the most common congenital malformation of the gastrointestinal tract.[28]

It develops when there is failure to obliterate the omphalomesenteric duct which normally leaves a fibrous band that connects the small intestine to the umbilicus during the first months of fetal development. Ectopic gastric mucosal cells are contained in the diverticuli. It occurs in about 2 percent of the population, primarily affects males, is symptomatic in about 2 percent of those with the malformation usually by the age of two years. Although most Meckel diverticulum are asymptomatic, the most common symptom is painless rectal bleeding. Intestinal obstruction, intussusception and volvulus can occur, more commonly in adults, with severe abdominal pain. Peptic ulcer disease may develop from the presence of the gastric mucosal cells. Diagnosis is made by symptom presentation and radionucleotide scintingraphy. The scan shows the gastric mucosal cells in the diverticuli. Treatment in those with symptoms is surgical resection.[29]

Congenital aganglionic megacolon

Congenital aganglionic megacolon (Hirschsprung disease) is a functional obstruction of the colon caused by inadequate motility. The exact cause is unknown but involves a complex inheritance pattern.[30] It is the most common cause of colon obstruction, accounting for about one third of all gastrointestinal obstructions in infants. The incidence is 1 in 5000, with a preponderance in males. There is an increased incidence in children with Down syndrome.[31]

PATHOPHYSIOLOGY Congenital aganglionic megacolon is caused by a malformation of the parasympathetic nervous system and is characterized by an absence of the intramural ganglion cells in the enteric nerve plexuses (Meissner and Auerbach plexuses). In 80% of cases, the aganglionic segment is limited to the rectal end of the sigmoid colon. In 3% of cases, the entire colon lacks ganglion cells. The abnormally innervated colon obstructs fecal movements, causing the proximal colon to become distended—hence the term *megacolon* (Figure 35-3).

CLINICAL MANIFESTATIONS Mild to severe constipation is the usual manifestation of congenital aganglionic megacolon. Diarrhea may be the first sign, however, because only water can travel around the impacted feces.

The most serious complication in the neonatal period is enterocolitis related to fecal impaction. Bowel dilation stretches and partly occludes the encircling blood and lymphatic vessels, causing edema, ischemia, infarction of the mucosa, and significant outflow of fluid into the bowel

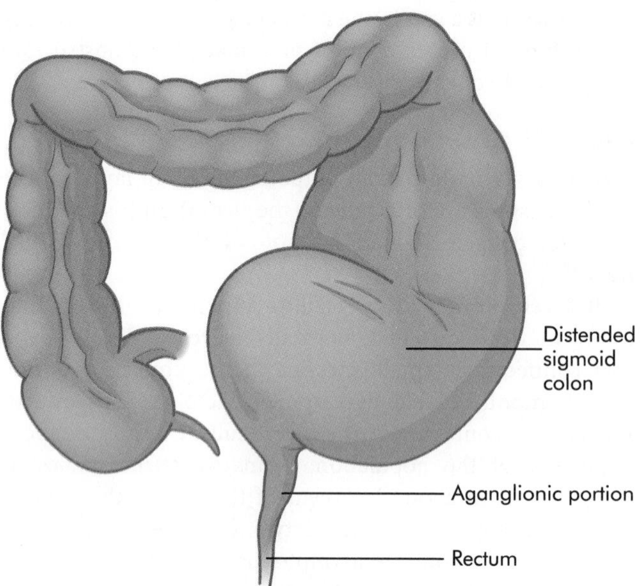

Figure 35-3 ■ Congenital Aganglionic Megacolon (Hirschsprung Disease).

lumen. Copious liquid stools result. Infarction and destruction of the mucosa enable enteric microorganisms to penetrate the bowel wall. Frequently, gram-negative sepsis occurs, accompanied by fever and vomiting. Severe and rapid electrolyte changes may take place, causing collapse and death.

EVALUATION AND TREATMENT Anorectal manometry is a reliable screening tool for the diagnosis of Hirschsprung disease. Serial manometries may be required in neonates. The definitive diagnosis is made by rectal biopsy showing an absence of ganglion cells in the submucosa of the colon. X-ray films show dilated loops of colon, and contrast films show aganglionic areas.[32]

The involved segment is resected within the first few months of life. Alternatively, enemas are given until the lumen is clear and then stool softeners are prescribed for life. The child is not treated for diarrhea.

After surgery, enterocolitis sometimes recurs, and if it is allowed to persist, pseudopolyps may appear. Because these are essentially identical to the lesions of ulcerative colitis, they have malignant potential. Therefore, a colectomy is indicated if pseudopolyps develop.[33]

In general, the prognosis of congenital megacolon is satisfactory for children who undergo surgical treatment. Bowel training may be prolonged, but most children achieve bowel continence before puberty.

Anorectal malformations

Several congenital malformations of anorectal structures can obstruct the passage of feces. The incidence of minor abnormalities is approximately 1 in 500, and that of major anomalies is approximately 1 in 5000.

Congenital anorectal malformations range from mild anal stenosis, which is corrected by simple dilation, to complex deformities, such as anal or rectal agenesis, atresia, and fistula (Figure 35-4). Deformities that cause complete obstruction are known collectively as **imperforate anus.**

Approximately 40% of infants with anorectal malformations have other developmental anomalies as well. The most commonly associated major anomalies are Down syndrome, congenital heart disease, renal abnormalities, esophageal atresia, and malformations of the spine.[34]

Imperforate anus can be detected by gentle insertion of a rectal tube. X-ray films show dilations throughout the intestinal tract. Anal stenosis can be treated by dilations, but all other anorectal malformations require surgical correction. Overall mortality is approximately 10%. Children with a low (anal) anomaly usually achieve bowel continence, but those with a high (rectal) anomaly rarely do.

Acquired Impairment of Motility

Intussusception

The most common cause of acquired intestinal obstruction in infants is **intussusception**—the telescoping or invagination of one portion of the intestine into another. Usually, the ileum invaginates the cecum and part of the ascending colon by collapsing through the ileocecal valve. Intussusception involving the ileum and colon (ileocolic intussusception) accounts for 80% to 90% of intestinal obstructions in infants and is two to three times more common in males than in females. Nearly 75% of intussusceptions occur before the age of 2 years; 70% occur before the age of 1 year.[35] Intussusception is rare in infants younger than 3 months of age and is uncommon after 36 months. Intussusception has rarely occurred in children of all ages recovering from abdominal surgery;[36] intussusception has been found in children with cystic fibrosis and symptoms of bowel obstruction who were initially misdiagnosed as having distal intestinal obstruction syndrome (see p. 989).[37]

PATHOPHYSIOLOGY The proximal portion of the intestine (the intussusceptum) collapses into the distal portion (the intussuscipiens) in the direction of peristaltic flow (Figure 35-5). The intussusceptum then drags its mesentery into the enveloping lumen causing an intussusception. Initially, the mesentery is constricted, obstructing venous return. Compression of the mesenteric vessels between the two layers of intestinal wall and at the U-shaped angle at either end of the intussusceptum leads within hours to venous stasis, engorgement, edema, exudation, and further vascular compression The tension of the mesentery on the intussusceptum tends to arch the bowel in a curve having its center at the mesenteric root. Edema and compression obstruct the flow of chyme through the intestine. Unless the intussusception is treated, gangrene ensues.

CLINICAL MANIFESTATIONS The affected infant suddenly develops abdominal pain, becomes irritable (colicky), and draws up the knees. Vomiting occurs soon afterward. A single normal stool may be passed, evacuating the colon distal to the apex of the intussusception. After that, 60% of infants pass "currant jelly" stools, which appear dark

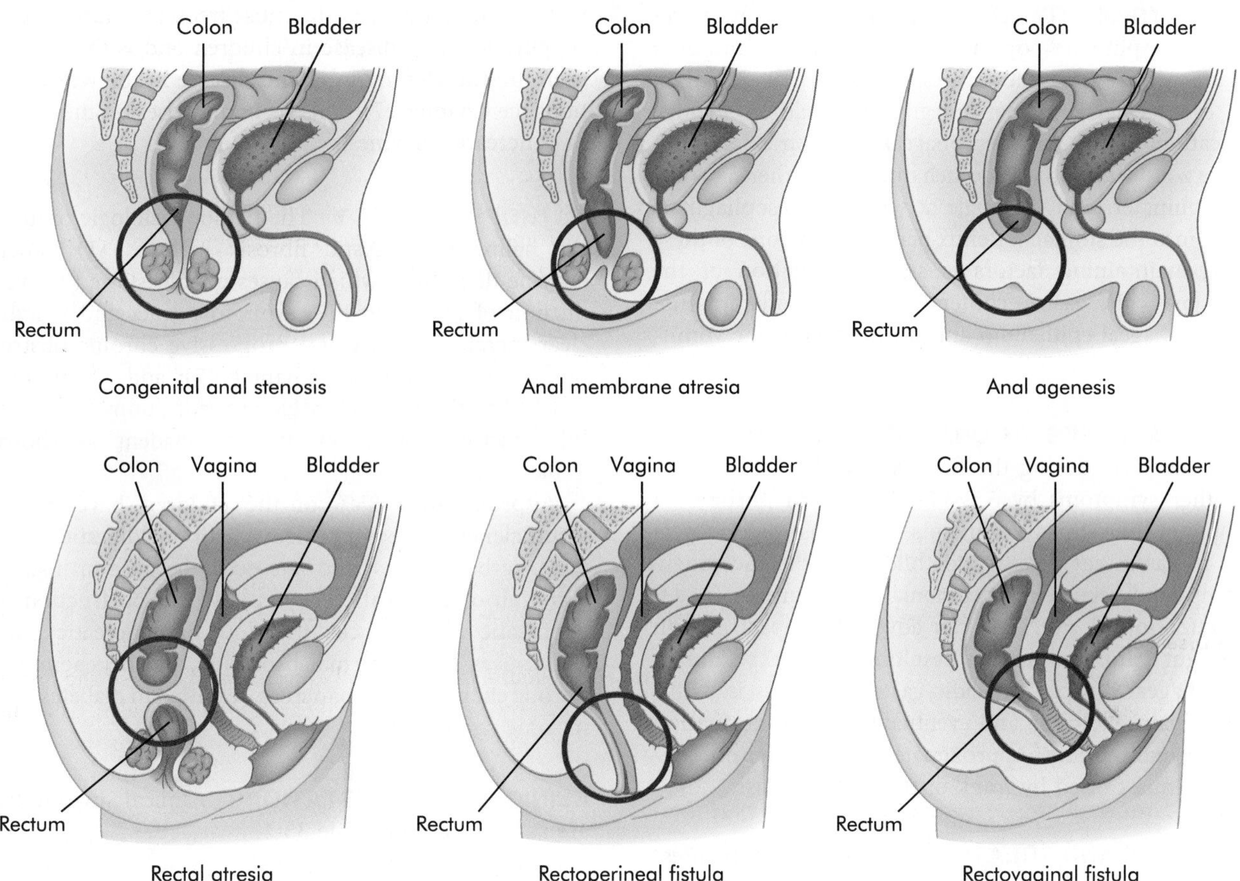

Figure 35-4 ■ **Anorectal Stenosis and Imperforate Anus.**

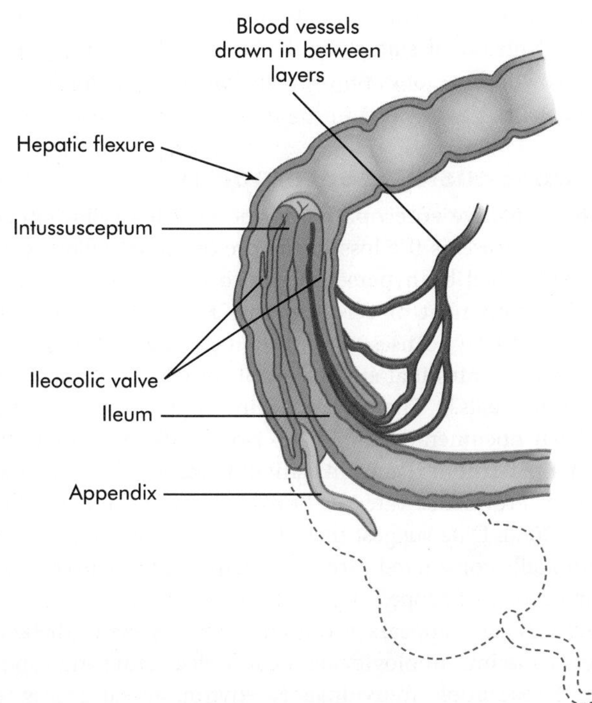

Figure 35-5 ■ **Ileocolic Intussusception.**

and gelatinous because of their blood and mucus content. Abdominal tenderness and distention develop as intestinal obstruction becomes more acute.

EVALUATION AND TREATMENT Diagnosis is based on clinical manifestations, onset of symptoms, and ultrasonography. Reduction is an emergency procedure involving hydrostatic pressure exerted by an enema given under fluoroscopic guidance and is successful 60% to 70% of the time. Surgical reduction is done on children who fail or are not candidates for hydrostatic reduction. Untreated intussusception in infants is nearly always fatal. Most infants recover if the intussusception is reduced within 24 hours.[38,39]

Gastroesophageal reflux

Gastroesophageal reflux (**GER**) is the return of stomach contents into the esophagus because of relaxation or incompetence of the lower esophageal sphincter. In newborns, reflux is normal because neuromuscular control of the gastroesophageal sphincter is not fully developed. The frequency of reflux is highest in premature infants and decreases during the first 6 to 12 months of life. Normal infants and children have been shown to have some reflux but may be asymptomatic. **Gastroesophageal reflux disease (GERD)** is different from GER and occurs when complications such as bleeding, dysphagia, or failure to thrive develop.[40]

PATHOPHYSIOLOGY Delayed maturation of the lower esophageal sphincter or impaired hormonal response mechanisms are possible causes. Factors that maintain lower esophageal sphincter integrity in children include the location of the gastroesophageal junction in a high-pressure zone within the abdomen, mucosal gathering within the sphincter, and the angle at which the esophagus is inserted into the stomach. Reflux persists if any one of these pressure-maintaining factors is altered. Irritation of the mucosa by acidic gastric contents results in inflammation of the esophageal epithelium and stimulation of the vomiting reflex.

CLINICAL MANIFESTATIONS Of affected infants, 85% vomit excessively during the first week of life and usually have other symptoms by 6 weeks. Aspiration pneumonia develops in one third of infants with gastroesophageal reflux. In cases that persist into childhood, chronic cough, wheezing, and recurrent pneumonia are common. Inadequate retention of nutrients can adversely impact growth and weight gain. Esophagitis resulting from exposure of the esophageal mucosa to acidic gastric contents is manifested by pain, bleeding, and eventually stricture formation and abnormal motility. Approximately 25% have iron deficiency anemia caused by frank or occult blood loss.[41]

EVALUATION AND TREATMENT The clinical manifestations are often adequate to confirm a diagnosis of gastroesophageal reflux. A barium swallow and esophageal pH monitoring with a probe are useful diagnostic procedures in complex cases.

Mild gastroesophageal reflux resolves without treatment. Small, frequent feedings and frequent burping are also accepted strategies for managing reflux. Medications to increase motility, to increase lower esophageal sphincter pressure, or to decrease gastric acid production have been used to treat GER. If no improvement is seen with medical management or the child has life-threatening events with reflux, an antireflux surgical procedure, including gastropexy and fundoplication, is performed.[42]

✓ QUICK CHECK 35-2

1. Describe the pathologic defect in meconium ileus.
2. Why is there poor bowel motility with Hirschsprung disease?
3. Describe the defect in intussusception.

Impairment of Digestion, Absorption, and Nutrition

Cystic fibrosis

Cystic fibrosis (CF) of the pancreas, which is also called *mucoviscidosis* or *fibrocystic disease of the pancreas,* is a genetically transmitted disease that involves many organs and systems and usually causes death in childhood or young adulthood. It is the most frequent cause of chronic suppurative lung disease in children and is the most common life-threatening inherited disease in the white population (see Chapter 27). This section focuses on the deficiency of pancreatic enzymes.

PATHOPHYSIOLOGY The pathophysiologic triad that is the hallmark of cystic fibrosis includes (1) pancreatic enzyme deficiency, which causes maldigestion; (2) overproduction of mucus in the respiratory tract and inability to clear secretions that cause progressive chronic obstructive pulmonary disease (see Chapter 27); and (3) abnormally elevated sodium and chloride concentrations in sweat. The full spectrum of involvement is evident as shown in Table 35-1.

Approximately 85% of the children have pancreatic insufficiency. Severe problems with maldigestion of proteins, carbohydrates, and fats occur because of insufficient secretion of pancreatic enzymes. Mucus obstruction of the pancreatic ducts blocks the flow of pancreatic enzymes and causes intestinal malabsorption and degenerative and fibrotic changes in the pancreas, resulting in diabetes mellitus in some children.[43]

CLINICAL MANIFESTATIONS Clinical manifestations are summarized in Table 35-1.

EVALUATION AND TREATMENT Seventy-two-hour stool fat measurements are used to determine the extent of pancreatic function. Stools also may be examined for absence of pancreatic enzymes, including lipase and elastase, trypsin, and chymotrypsin.[44] Pancreatic replacement enzymes (i.e., lipase) are administered before or with meals. High-caloric, high-protein diets with frequent snacks and vitamin supplements are used to treat the malnutrition. Nutritional status should be carefully monitored,[45] and growth hormone may be included with nutritional supplements.[46]

Gluten-sensitive enteropathy

Gluten-sensitive enteropathy, formerly called **celiac sprue** or *celiac disease,* is the loss of mature intestinal villous epithelium caused by hypersensitivity to gluten (gliadin), the protein component of cereal grains. The gluten in wheat, rye, and barley causes a T cell–mediated autoimmune injury to the intestinal epithelial cells of genetically susceptible individuals.[47] The disease occurs largely in whites and has been documented in Asians from India and Pakistan but is almost nonexistent in native Africans, Japanese, and Chinese. Prevalence rates in Europe range from 1 in 1000 to 1 in 3000. Data suggest that gluten-sensitive enteropathy, traditionally considered rare in the United States, may be as common as in Europe.[48]

Pathogenesis appears to be complex, involving dietary, genetic, and immunologic factors, as well as requiring exposure of susceptible individuals to environmental agents in addition to gluten. Gluten-sensitive enteropathy has been

TABLE 35-1

Pathophysiology, Clinical Manifestations, and Complications of Cystic Fibrosis

Organ Involved	Secretory Dysfunction	Clinical Manifestations	Complications
Sweat glands	Elevated concentration of sodium and chloride in sweat	Hyponatremia; hypochloremia	Heat prostration; shock
INTESTINE			
Newborn	Viscid meconium	Meconium ileus with intestinal obstruction	Meconium peritonitis
Older child and adult	Inspissated (dried out) mucofecal masses (intestinal sludging)	Partial intestinal obstruction with severe cramping pains	Volvulus (obstruction), intussusception (prolapse)
Pancreas (enzyme deficiency)	Inspissation and precipitation of pancreatic secretions, causing obstruction of pancreatic ducts	Absence of pancreatic enzymes, causing malabsorption of food and fatty, bulky stools	Hypoproteinemia; iron deficiency anemia; malnutrition
		Decreased vitamin A, D, E, and K absorption	Vitamins A, D, E, and K deficiency and rectal prolapse
	Insulin deficiency	Glucose intolerance	Diabetes mellitus
Liver	Inspissation and precipitation of bile and biliary system	Focal biliary cirrhosis; shrunken, "hobnail" liver	Portal hypertension with esophageal varices and hematemesis
Salivary glands	Inspissation and precipitation of secretions in small ducts of submaxillary and sublingual salivary glands	Mild patchy fibrosis of salivary glands	None
Paranasal structures	Viscid mucus	Retention of mucus; clouding seen on sinus roentgenograms	Mucopyoceles (pus accumulations) with nasal deformity or orbital cavity extension
Nose	Nasal polyps	Obstruction of nasal air flow	None
Lungs	Viscid mucus in bronchioles and bronchi	Obstruction of bronchioles causing bronchiolectasis, bronchiectasis, and chronic lung infection	Hemoptysis; pneumothorax; cor pulmonale; respiratory failure
REPRODUCTIVE TRACT			
Male	Viscid genital tract secretions during embryologic development, causing failure of formation of normal vas deferens	Sterility	None
Female	Distention of endocervical epithelial cells with cytoplasmic mucin	Decreased fertility	Polypoid cervicitis (cervical inflammation) while taking oral contraceptives

Data from Rudolph CD et al: *Rudolph's pediatrics,* ed 21, New York, 2003, McGraw-Hill.

associated with other immune disorders, including diabetes mellitus and thyroid disease.[49]

PATHOPHYSIOLOGY The major pathophysiologic characteristics of celiac disease are atrophy and flattening of villi in the upper small intestine and malabsorption of most nutrients in the presence of cereal gluten (Figure 35-6). The mucosa of the upper small intestine appears shiny, cobble-stoned, and thin in children with gluten-sensitive enteropathy.

Damage to the mucosa of the duodenum and jejunum exacerbates malabsorption. The secretion of intestinal hormones, such as secretin and cholecystokinin-pancreozymin, may be diminished, so secretion of pancreatic enzymes and expulsion of bile from the gallbladder decrease, contributing to malabsorption.

Destruction of mucosal cells causes inflammation, and water and electrolytes are secreted, leading to watery diarrhea. Potassium loss leads to muscle weakness. Magnesium and calcium malabsorption can cause seizures or tetany. Unabsorbed fatty acids combine with calcium, and secondary hyperparathyroidism increases phosphorus excretion, resulting in bone reabsorption. Calcium is no longer available to bind oxalate in the intestine and is absorbed, which causes hyperoxaluria. Gallbladder function may be abnormal, and bile salt conjugation may decrease.

Fat malabsorption in the jejunum is the major cause of steatorrhea (fatty stools). Deficiencies of fat-soluble

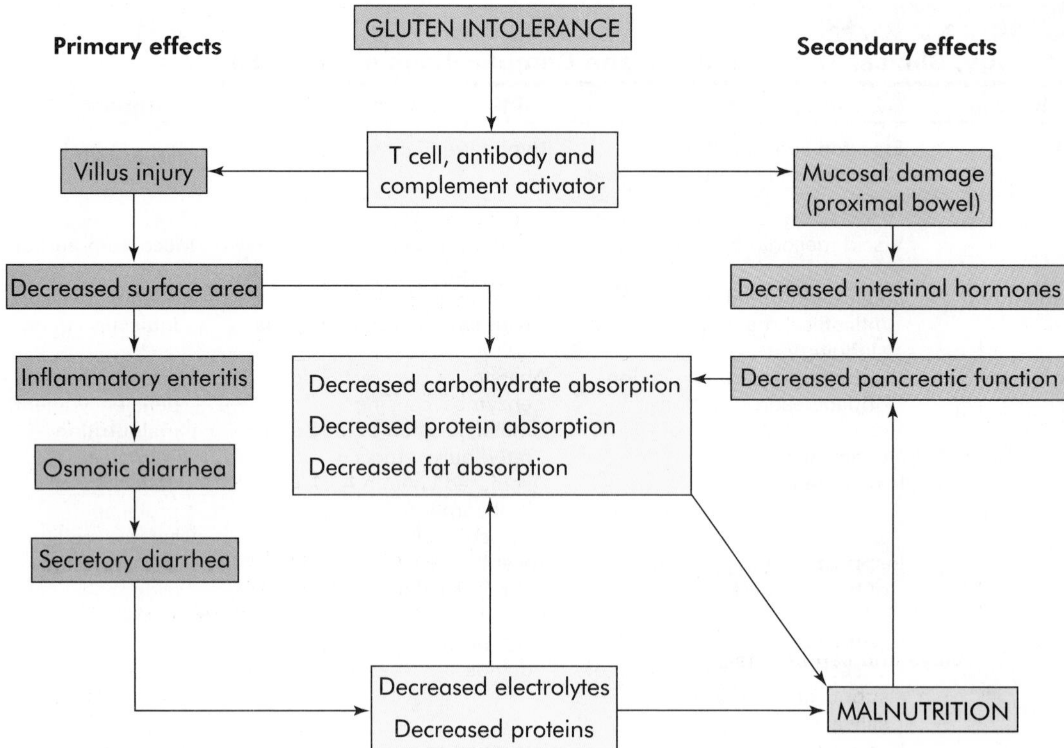

Figure 35-6 ■ **Pathophysiology of Gluten-Sensitive Enteropathy.**

vitamins are common in children with gluten-sensitive enteropathy. Vitamin K malabsorption leads to hypoprothrombinemia. In one third of cases, iron and folic acid malabsorption is manifested as cheilosis, anemia, and a smooth red tongue. Vitamin B_{12} absorption is impaired in those with extensive ileal disease, and folate and iron deficiencies are common.

CLINICAL MANIFESTATIONS The onset of clinical manifestations of gluten-sensitive enteropathy depends on the age of the infant when gluten-containing substances are added to the diet. In 50% of affected children, onset occurs by 18 months of age, with latent intervals varying from months to years.

Diarrhea is an early sign in most infants. The stools are pale, bulky, greasy, and foul smelling, and they may contain oil droplets. Three to five such movements occur daily. As early as 3 or 4 months of age, growth failure, anorexia, and constipation can begin. In older children, constipation is occasionally seen despite steatorrhea. Vomiting and abdominal pain are prominent in infants but unusual in older children. Anorexia is prevalent. The classic physical manifestations of organic failure to thrive, such as abdominal protuberance, wasted buttocks and limbs, and hypotonia, occur in fewer than 50% of infants with gluten-sensitive enteropathy. Growth is usually diminished.[50]

Manifestations of malabsorption, such as rickets, anemia, tetany, frank bleeding, or anemia, may be obvious. Some children urinate more at night. The tongue is smooth and red, and the child may bruise and bleed easily. Hypomagnesemia and hypocalcemia cause irritability, tremor, convulsions, tetany, bone pain, osteomalacia, and dental abnormalities. If vitamin D deficiency is prolonged, rickets and clubbing of the terminal phalanges are likely. Eighty-six percent of older children have fingerprint changes (ridge atrophy). In older children, delayed puberty and infertility may be manifestations of otherwise subtle gluten-sensitive enteropathy.[51]

An unusual complication of gluten-sensitive enteropathy in infancy is **celiac crisis.** Celiac crisis is characterized by severe diarrhea, dehydration, and hypoproteinemia as a result of malabsorption and protein loss.

EVALUATION AND TREATMENT Serologic assay for autoantibodies (immunoglobulins A and G [IgA, IgG] antigliadin [from gluten] antibodies and antitissue transglutaminase) and intestinal biopsy is mandatory to detect the classic mucosal changes caused by gluten-sensitive enteropathy. The initial biopsy is generally followed by a second intestinal biopsy to demonstrate regeneration of intestinal villi after treatment with a gluten-free diet. A wide variety of screening tests for malabsorption also may be useful.

Treatment consists of the immediate and permanent institution of a diet free of cereal grains (wheat, rye, barley, malt). Lactose intolerance is presumed; therefore, lactose (milk sugar) is also excluded from the diet. Infants are routinely given vitamin D, iron, and folic acid supplements to treat deficiencies.

Approximately 25% of children experience recurrent relapses that interfere with growth. For most children, however, the long-term prognosis is excellent. There is an increased incidence of malignant disease, particularly lymphoma, in individuals who fail to respond to gluten-free diets.[52,53]

Protein energy malnutrition

Kwashiorkor and marasmus are the two most common types of malnutrition in children. These disorders are known collectively as **protein energy malnutrition (PEM).** Both are states of long-term starvation. **Kwashiorkor** is a severe protein deficiency, and **marasmus** is a severe deficiency of all nutrients. Kwashiorkor is a widespread nutritional problem among children in developing countries and economically destitute populations. The disease usually occurs in infants or children from 1 to 4 years of age who have been weaned from breast milk to a high-starch, protein-deficient diet.

Marasmus can occur at any age, but it is common in children younger than 1 year. In marasmus, starvation is attributable to lack of protein and carbohydrates and, in neglected children, to a psychogenic basis. In developing countries and impoverished populations, early weaning of breast-fed infants to overdiluted commercial formulas is a risk factor for marasmus.

Protein energy malnutrition is also a complication of diseases, such as chronic fever, tuberculosis, malignancy, digestive and malabsorptive disorders, and psychogenic illness. Radiation therapy and chemotherapy can also contribute to protein energy malnutrition.

PATHOPHYSIOLOGY In kwashiorkor, the deficit of dietary amino acids reduces protein synthesis in all tissues. Physical growth and mental growth are stunted, and maintenance of minimal life processes is in jeopardy. The lack of sufficient plasma proteins results in generalized edema with a substantial loss of potassium. The liver swells with stored fat because no hepatic proteins are synthesized to form and release lipoproteins. Pancreatic atrophy and fibrosis may be present. Kwashiorkor also causes malabsorption, reduced bone density, and impaired renal function. If the condition is not reversed, the prognosis is very poor.

Because the intake of all dietary nutrients is reduced to a minimum in marasmus, metabolic processes, including liver function, are preserved, but growth is severely retarded. Caloric intake is too low to support protein synthesis for growth or the storage of fat. Muscle wasting also occurs. Fat wasting and anemia are common and can be severe. Severe vitamin A deficiency commonly results in blindness.[54]

CLINICAL MANIFESTATIONS Retarded physical, mental, and psychologic development; muscle wasting; diarrhea; dermatosis; low hemoglobin; and infection characterize marasmus. The presence of subcutaneous fat, hepatomegaly, and fatty liver distinguishes kwashiorkor from marasmus.

EVALUATION AND TREATMENT Evaluation of protein energy malnutrition is based on nutritional history and clinical manifestations. Mid–upper arm circumference and weight-for-height ratios are inexpensive assessments.[55] The provision of deficient nutrients will resolve clinical symptoms in 4 to 6 weeks. Physical and mental retardation may not be reversible, however. Nutritional rehabilitation with appropriate environmental stimulation for infants and young children has been shown to resolve or improve cerebral shrinkage, physical growth, and psychomotor development.

Failure to thrive

Failure to thrive (FTT) is the inadequate physical development of an infant or child. It is manifested as a deceleration in weight gain, a low weight/height ratio, or a low weight/height/head circumference ratio. In the United States, FTT usually affects infants and young children. It is a nutritional disorder that has organic or nonorganic causes. Nonorganic FTT is most common among psychosocially and economically deprived populations, whereas organic FTT occurs equally in all populations. The incidence of nonorganic FTT is more than that of organic FTT.[56]

PATHOPHYSIOLOGY **Organic FTT** has a pathophysiologic cause, for example, gastroesophageal reflux, pyloric stenosis, gastroenteritis, infection by intestinal parasites, or congenital anomalies or chronic diseases of major body systems. All these disorders reduce the availability of nutrients for maintenance and growth. A chronic disease or congenital anomaly that causes weakness or reduced stature also can create developmental problems, psychosocial problems, and emotional problems for the child.

Nonorganic FTT is a syndrome with many psychosocial causes and may be complicated by inadequate economic resources and lack of knowledge. The problem in nonorganic FTT is ineffective nurturing by primary caregivers. Infants and children are at risk for nonorganic FTT if their parents or primary caregivers are unable to provide nurturance. Various parental stressors may be involved, including the following:

- Lack of nurturance in the parents' own childhood
- Unwanted pregnancy
- Inability to bond with the infant because of health or other problems
- Postpartum depression
- Family crisis, such as the occurrence of a death or marital problems
- Stress caused by single parenthood or social isolation
- Mental, emotional, or physical illness

CLINICAL MANIFESTATIONS Clinical manifestations of organic FTT are retarded growth accompanied by manifestations of the underlying disease. Manifestations of nonorganic FTT are retarded growth plus reduced energy level, reduced responsiveness and interaction with the environment, social isolation, spasticity and rigidity when held or touched, inability to make eye contact or smile, refusal to eat, and rejection of foods. Weight loss and decelerated growth are accompanied by developmental retardation in many areas. Nonorganic FTT is a complex syndrome involving psychosocial, emotional, and parent-child problems that compound the pathophysiologic abnormalities.[57]

EVALUATION AND TREATMENT FTT is suggested if a child falls below the third percentile on the growth curve or is falling off a previously established growth curve. Organic FTT is manifested in infancy by weight, height, and head circumference growth that may be parallel to but below the normal ranges. If no genetic, endocrine, or other systemic disorder is identified and if the physical and laboratory examinations show no abnormalities other than delayed growth, an environmental cause is indicated.

Hospital admission is recommended if the diagnosis is unclear or the child is in nutritional or emotional jeopardy. Eating patterns, food preferences, caloric intake, and family interactions can be assessed during the hospital stay. If the cause is environmental, the hospitalized child with FTT usually begins to gain weight.

If an organic problem has been identified, management of FTT consists of treating the cause. Management of nonorganic FTT involves the immediate total care of the child and measures to address (1) the psychosocial and emotional problems of the caregivers and (2) parent-child interactions. Counseling, parental modeling, and long-term family support are sometimes required.[58]

Necrotizing enterocolitis

Necrotizing enterocolitis (NEC) is an ischemic, inflammatory condition of the bowel that causes necrosis, perforation, and death if untreated. NEC occurs primarily in premature infants; affected infants have a mean gestational age of 31 weeks and weigh less than 1500 g. The risk of necrotizing enterocolitis decreases as the gastrointestinal tract matures. The cause is unknown.[59]

PATHOPHYSIOLOGY Factors contributing to the development of NEC include maternal age older than 35 years, infections, immunologic injury, perinatal stress, and the effects of medications and feeding practices. Accumulation of gas in the mucosa and submucosa leads to reduced mucosal blood flow, ischemia, and necrosis of intestinal segments. The injury leads to release of inflammatory mediators and bacterial invasion or perforation of the bowel wall, or both.[60]

CLINICAL MANIFESTATIONS Manifestations of NEC usually appear within 2 weeks of birth. They range from mild abdominal distention to bowel perforation, sepsis, and death. Abdominal pain, unstable temperature, bradycardia, and apnea are nonspecific signs. Affected infants have occult or grossly bloody stools, gastric retention, abdominal distention, and septicemia with elevated white blood cell and falling platelet counts. Premature infants often have more severe disease and other disorders, such as respiratory distress syndrome and immune compromise.

EVALUATION AND TREATMENT Diagnosis is based on clinical manifestations, laboratory results, and plain films of the abdomen that show gas accumulation in the intestine. Prevention of NEC includes prenatal glucocorticoids and standardized feeding schedules.[61,62] Treatments include cessation of feeding, gastric suction to decompress the intestines, fluid and electrolyte maintenance, and administration of antibiotics to control sepsis. Surgical resection and peritoneal drainage are the treatment of choice for perforation[63,64]; however, for very ill infants weighing less than 1000 g, peritoneal drainage without laparotomy may improve survival.[65] Overall mortality is 20% to 40%; however, the incidence is decreasing.[66]

✔ QUICK CHECK 35-3

1. Why do individuals with cystic fibrosis have pancreatic insufficiency?
2. Why is there loss of villi with gluten-sensitive enteropathy?
3. Compare kwashiorkor and marasmus.

Diarrhea

Diarrhea is a common gastrointestinal problem during infancy and early childhood and is the leading cause of death in children younger than 5 years of age.[67] Severe diarrhea occurs one to three times during the first 3 years of life. Most episodes are self-limiting and resolve within 72 hours. The pathophysiologic mechanisms of diarrhea in children are similar to those described for adults. Prolonged diarrhea is more dangerous in children, however, because they have much smaller fluid reserves than adults. Therefore, dehydration can develop rapidly if any disturbance increases fluid secretion into the gastrointestinal lumen (secretory diarrhea), draws fluid into the lumen by osmosis (osmotic diarrhea), or prevents fluid absorption in the intestine.

Infant diarrhea is of special concern because its cause may be a congenital or metabolic anomaly. Infants have low fluid reserves and relatively rapid peristalsis and metabolism. Therefore, the danger of dehydration is great.

Common causes of acute diarrhea in infants include congenital aganglionic megacolon, infections, milk protein allergies, and necrotizing enterocolitis. Less common causes are adrenogenital syndrome, impaired chloride-bicarbonate exchange, congenital lactase deficiency, glucose-galactose malabsorption, and sucrase-isomaltase deficiency.

Infectious diarrhea in newborns is usually associated with nursery epidemics involving pathogens such as *Escherichia coli*, *Klebsiella*, staphylococci, *Salmonella*, and *Shigella*. Diarrhea caused by these agents has a rapid onset, and acidosis and shock can occur quickly. *Clostridium difficile*, often associated with previous antibiotic therapy, can cause acute, profuse, watery diarrhea and symptoms of colitis.[68] True milk protein allergy, which is uncommon, causes bloody, explosive stools after the introduction of bovine milk into the diet.[69]

Acute diarrhea

Acute diarrhea in children is almost synonymous with acute viral or bacterial gastroenteritis. **Rotavirus** is the single most significant cause of gastroenteritis in infants and young children. Severe dehydration results from vomiting and diarrhea.[70] Viral gastroenteritis tends to be self-limiting. Bacterial gastroenteritis is treated with antibiotics if the causal pathogen can be identified. Other causes of acute diarrhea in the older child include antibiotic therapy, appendicitis, chemotherapy, inflammatory bowel disease, parasitic infestation, parenteral infections, and ingestion of toxic substances.

HEALTH ALERT

Rotavirus Vaccine

Rotavirus is the leading cause of severe diarrhea and dehydration in infants and young children. Most children are infected by the age of 5 years, and it is a leading cause of death because of diarrhea in developing countries. The first vaccine (Rotashield) was released in 1998 and withdrawn 1 year later because of complications, including intussusception. Rotarix, an oral vaccine, has been approved for use in Mexico, the European Union, and 33 other countries. RotaTeq, an oral vaccine, has been approved for use in the United States. It is administered in three doses at ages 2, 4 and 6 months with all doses given by 32 weeks and can be given with other childhood vaccines (see Table 7-11).

Data from O'Ryan M: Rotarix (RIX4414): an oral human rotavirus vaccine, *Expert Rev Vaccines* 6(1):11–19, 2007; Centers for Disease Control and Prevention (CDC): Postmarketing monitoring of intussusception after RotaTeq vaccination—United States, February 1, 2006–February 15, 2007. *MMWR Morb Mortal Wkly Rep* 56(10):218–222, 2007.

Chronic diarrhea

Children with acute gastroenteritis often remain mildly symptomatic for up to 4 weeks; therefore, diarrhea that persists longer than 4 weeks is considered to be chronic. Children with chronic diarrhea can be divided into two groups: (1) otherwise well children whose growth is normal and (2) ill children whose growth is retarded. Causes of chronic diarrhea in the first group include abnormal colonic motility, lactose intolerance, encopresis, parasitic infestation, and antibiotic use. Chronic diarrhea in the second group is usually caused by a disease that impairs absorption.

Chronic nonspecific diarrhea

In **chronic nonspecific diarrhea**, uncoordinated colonic motility causes forceful expulsion of feces. In some instances, there is a family history of bowel complaints. As an infant, the child is likely to have experienced colic and diarrhea associated with teething and immunizations. In more than 90% of cases, chronic nonspecific diarrhea resolves by 3 to 4 years of age. The cure often accompanies toilet training. Many children with chronic nonspecific diarrhea develop irritable bowel syndrome (also called *mucous colitis*) as adults.[71] Children with chronic nonspecific diarrhea usually do well with normal food and fluid intake with a balance of fluid, fiber, fat, and fruit juices.

Primary lactose intolerance

Lactose intolerance, the inability to digest milk sugar, is caused by inadequate production of lactase. It is a common cause of diarrhea. The malabsorption of lactose results in osmotic diarrhea accompanied by abdominal pain, bloating, and flatulence. These symptoms begin before the age of 7 years in half of affected blacks. Hydrogen lactose breath testing provides a formal diagnosis. Treatment consists of reducing milk consumption or oral lactase supplementation. Some children can tolerate lactose in fermented forms, such as cheese and yogurt, or by adding soy food.[72]

DISORDERS OF THE LIVER

Disorders of Biliary Metabolism and Transport

Neonatal jaundice

Neonatal jaundice is usually a transient, benign icterus that occurs during the first week of life in otherwise healthy, full-term infants and is common in preterm infants.[73] It is caused by mild unconjugated (indirect-reacting) hyperbilirubinemia.

PATHOPHYSIOLOGY Physiologic jaundice results from the complex interaction of factors that (1) increase bilirubin production, (2) impair hepatic uptake and excretion of bilirubin, and (3) promote reabsorption of bilirubin in the small intestine. The most common cause is hemolytic disease of the newborn (ABO blood incompatibility) (see Chapter 21). Serum bilirubin values increase to 5 to 6 mg/dl by the second to fourth day after birth in full-term infants, and to 10 to 15 mg/dl by the fifth to seventh days in premature infants. A high level of indirect hyperbilirubinemia (15 to 20 mg/dl) is considered pathologic. There is a risk of brain damage **(kernicterus)** as the bilirubin passes across neonatal brain capillaries (the blood-brain barrier) and into brain cells of the basal ganglia.[74]

CLINICAL MANIFESTATIONS Physiologic jaundice develops during the second or third day after birth and usually subsides in 1 to 2 weeks in full-term infants and in 2 to 4 weeks in premature infants. After this, increasing bilirubin values and persistent jaundice indicate pathologic hyperbilirubinemia. Premature infants with respiratory distress, acidosis, or sepsis are at greater risk for encephalopathy and the development of athetoid cerebral palsy and speech and hearing impairment.[75]

EVALUATION AND TREATMENT Both total and direct (conjugated) bilirubin levels are measured; the direct bilirubin should not exceed 1 mg/dl.[76] Other causes of jaundice must be eliminated to confirm physiologic jaundice. Treatment depends on the degree of hyperbilirubinemia. Physiologic jaundice is usually treated by phototherapy (ultraviolet light). Pathologic jaundice requires an exchange transfusion and treatment of the underlying disorder.

Biliary atresia

Biliary atresia is a rare congenital malformation characterized by the absence or obstruction of intrahepatic or extrahepatic bile ducts. The cause of the intrauterine injury to the ducts is not clear but is thought to be related to chromosomal abnormality, an immune response, or viral injury. The disease expression is a continuum in which the principal process is one of bile duct destruction.[77]

The atresia or obstruction of the bile ducts leads to plugging, inflammation, fibrosis of the bile canaliculi, and cholestasis. Progressive obstruction may lead to biliary cirrhosis (see Chapter 34), portal hypertension, or liver failure.

Jaundice is the primary clinical manifestation of biliary atresia, along with hepatomegaly and acholic (clay-colored) stools. Fat absorption is impaired for lack of bile salts, and the infant may fail to gain weight. Cirrhosis and liver failure can lead to death.

Early diagnosis of biliary atresia is essential and is based on clinical manifestations and liver biopsy. Liver function test results are abnormal. Serum transaminase and alkaline phosphatase values are elevated, and conjugated (direct) serum bilirubin levels rise progressively.

Extrahepatic atresia can be relieved by the Kasai portoenterostomy. Even with initial restoration of bile flow, however, obliteration of intrahepatic bile ducts continues and cirrhosis results. Liver transplantation is the long-term therapy for biliary atresia. Of children with biliary atresia, 80% die before the age of 3 years if not treated.[78]

Inflammatory Disorders

Hepatitis

More detailed information about viral and fulminant hepatitis is described in Chapter 34 (see Table 34-8).

Hepatitis A (HAV)

Approximately 20% to 30% of the reported cases of hepatitis A (HAV) occur in children,[79] particularly children of nursery school age. Outbreaks tend to occur in day care centers with large numbers of children who are not toilet trained and staff members who practice poor handwashing techniques.[80] HAV in children is usually mild and asymptomatic, but it may involve nausea, vomiting, and diarrhea. Because jaundice is absent, infected children appear to have the flu. Almost all children recover from hepatitis A without residual liver damage. Vaccination programs are successfully reducing the incidence of HAV in the United States (See Table 7-11 in Chapter 7).

HEALTH ALERT

Hepatitis Vaccines for Children

Hepatitis A vaccine: Recommended for children 12–23 months of age (2 doses) and older and for high-risk populations.

Hepatitis B vaccine: Recommended for all unvaccinated children up to 18 years of age; for infants, the vaccines are administered at birth, 1 month, and 6 months of age.

Hepatitis B Vaccine Guidelines

1. Establish standing orders for administration of hepatitis B vaccination beginning at birth;
2. Institute delivery hospital policies and procedures and case management programs to improve identification of and administration of immunoprophylaxis to infants born to mothers who are hepatitis B surface antigen (HBsAg) positive and to mothers with known HBsAg status at the time of delivery; and
3. Implement vaccination record reviews for all children 11 to 12 years of age and children and adolescents younger than 19 years of age who were born in countries with intermediate and high levels of HBV epidemicity, adopting hepatitis B vaccine requirements for school entry, and integrating hepatitis B vaccination services into settings that serve adolescents (see Table 7-11).

Data from Centers for Disease Control: Recommended Immunization Schedules for Persons Aged 0–18 Years—United States, 2007. January 5, 2007, *MMWR* 55(51);Q1-Q4. http://www.cdc.gov/mmwr/preview/mmwrhtml/mm5551a7.htm?s_cid=mm5551a7_e.

Hepatitis B (HBV)

Infants of mothers who are chronic hepatitis B (HBV) surface antigen (HBsAg) carriers, children with hemophilia who receive frequent blood transfusions, children who abuse parenteral drugs, and children who live in institutions for mentally retarded persons are all at risk for HBV infection. Of newborns infected by their mothers, 90% develop chronic hepatitis and become carriers. Chronic hepatitis may develop because the infant's immune system is immature. Infected infants are at risk for cirrhosis and hepatocellular carcinoma.[81] The most serious consequence of HBV infection is fulminant hepatitis, which occurs in 1% of cases. Hepatitis D virus (HDV) infection depends on active infection with HBV. There is evidence that the risk of fulminant hepatitis is higher in individuals with combined infection of HBV and HDV than in those with HBV infection alone.[82] Aggressive vaccination programs reduce the incidence of HBV.

Hepatitis C (HCV)

Hepatitis C (HCV) in children is associated primarily with blood transfusions or perinatal transmission from infected mothers. Children who received frequent transfusions before 1992 are at highest risk. The disease is usually mild in children, and cirrhosis is rare.[83]

Chronic hepatitis

Hepatitis B (HBV) and hepatitis C (HCV) are the main causes of chronic hepatitis in children. Manifestations of chronic hepatitis include malaise, anorexia, fever, gastrointestinal bleeding, hepatomegaly, edema, and transient joint pain. Serum alanine aminotransferase and bilirubin levels are elevated. There may be evidence of impairment of synthetic functions of the liver: prolonged prothrombin time and hypoalbuminemia. Diagnosis is based on the clinical manifestations and liver biopsy. There is no curative therapy for chronic HBV or chronic HCV. Some success has been achieved with human alpha interferon and lamivudine.[81] Liver transplant may ultimately be required.

Cirrhosis

Cirrhosis is fibrotic scarring of the liver resulting in obstruction to the flow of blood and bile. Most forms of chronic liver diseases in children can progress to cirrhosis, but they seldom do so. The complications of cirrhosis in children are the same as those in adults: portal hypertension, the opening of collateral vessels between the portal and systemic veins, and varices. In addition, children with cirrhosis experience growth failure caused by nutritional deficits, as well as developmental delay, particularly in gross motor function because of ascites and weakness. The cause of cirrhosis may influence its severity and course. Some types of cirrhosis can be stabilized if the cause is identified and treated early.[84]

Portal Hypertension

There are two basic causes of portal hypertension in children: (1) increased resistance to blood flow within the portal system and (2) increased volume of portal blood flow. The second cause is rare in children and is not discussed here. Increased resistance to flow can occur anywhere in the portal circulatory system. Portal hypertension can accompany cirrhosis, intra-abdominal infections, portal vein thrombosis, congenital anomalies of the portal vein, and congenital hepatic fibrosis.

Types of portal hypertension

Extrahepatic portal hypertension

Extrahepatic (prehepatic) portal venous obstruction causes 50% to 70% of **extrahepatic portal hypertension** in children. In approximately two thirds of these children, no specific cause can be found.[85] Obstruction is almost always in the portal vein and is usually caused by thrombosis as a complication of abdominal trauma, pancreatitis, abdominal infections, and some systemic disorders; however, these causes are rare. The liver is usually normal in extrahepatic portal hypertension.

Intrahepatic portal hypertension

Cirrhosis is the primary cause of **intrahepatic portal hypertension.** The most common finding is fibrosis, which increases resistance to portal blood flow by constricting and reducing the compliance of the hepatic sinusoids.

Course of the disease

The important consequences of portal hypertension in children are the development of collateral circulation, with portal-systemic shunting; hypersplenism; esophageal varices; and ascites.

CLINICAL MANIFESTATIONS The clinical manifestations of portal hypertension are (1) splenomegaly, (2) upper gastrointestinal bleeding, (3) ascites, and (4) hepatic encephalopathy (see Chapter 34).

EVALUATION AND TREATMENT The objectives of the clinical investigation are to (1) locate the site of the venous block and (2) identify the disease responsible for the portal hypertension. Thorough physical examination, laboratory tests of liver function, imaging procedures, and biopsy may be included in the diagnostic evaluation. Sclerotherapy is the initial treatment of choice for severe esophageal varices in children. Surgical venous shunts are rarely performed on small children because of the high failure rate secondary to vessel occlusion, but they may be an alternative in older children.[86]

The outcome of portal hypertension depends almost entirely on its cause. Children with extrahepatic disease are expected to recover with little morbidity. For children with intrahepatic disease, the prognosis varies.

Metabolic Disorders

More than 5000 genetically determined metabolic pathways have been identified in liver tissue. The earliest possible identification of metabolic disorders is essential because (1) early treatment may prevent permanent damage to vital organs, such as the liver or brain; (2) precise genetic counseling may be possible with prenatal diagnosis; and (3) complications can be minimized, even if cure is not possible. **Galactosemia, fructosemia,** and **Wilson disease** are treatable metabolic disorders that have hepatic clinical manifestations. The mechanisms of disease, clinical manifestations, evaluation, and treatment of these disorders are presented in Table 35-2.

QUICK CHECK 35-4

1. Why is diarrhea such a serious disorder in infants and children?
2. What is biliary atresia?
3. What are the three most common metabolic disorders that cause liver damage in children?

TABLE 35-2

Galactosemia, Fructosemia, and Wilson Disease

	Galactosemia	Fructosemia	Wilson Disease
Mechanism of disease	Deficiency of galactose-1-phosphate uridyl transferase An autosomal recessive trait Cannot convert galactose to glucose Toxic accumulation of galactose in body tissues, liver, and brain	Deficiency of fructose-1-phosphate aldolase An autosomal recessive trait Cannot metabolize fructose, sucrose, or honey; occurs when breast milk is replaced with cow's milk Toxic accumulation of fructose in body tissues	Autosomal recessive: defect on chromosome 13 (ATP 7B) Defect in copper excretion by liver Impaired transport of copper into bile/blood caused by diminished transport protein (ceruloplasmin) Toxic accumulations of copper in liver, brain, kidney, corneas
Clinical manifestation	High levels of blood galactose Vomiting Hypoglycemia May have failure to thrive Symptoms of cirrhosis at 2–6 mo—jaundice Mental retardation if not treated Cataracts if not treated	High levels of blood fructose Vomiting Hypoglycemia May have failure to thrive Hepatomegaly Jaundice Seizures	Intention tremors Indistinct speech Dystonia Greenish yellow rings in cornea Hepatomegaly Jaundice Anorexia Renal tubular defects
Evaluation	Newborn screening Presence of reducing substances in urine when infant is receiving lactose	Detailed dietary history Liver or intestinal mucosa biopsy	Low plasma ceruloplasmin
Treatment	Galactose-free diet	Fructose-, sucrose-, honey-free diet Vitamin C supplementation	Chelation therapy to remove copper from body Decreased dietary intake of copper Liver transplant

Did You Understand?

Disorders of the Gastrointestinal Tract

1. Most alterations of digestive function in children include congenital obstructions of the intestinal tract; disorders of digestion, absorption, or nutrition; or liver disease.
2. Cleft lip (harelip) and cleft palate (failure of the bony palate to fuse in the midline) may occur separately or together. The fissure may affect the uvula, soft palate, hard palate, nostril, and maxillary alveolar ridge.
3. Esophageal atresia, a condition in which the esophagus ends in a blind pouch, may occur with or without tracheoesophageal fistula, or connection between the esophagus and the trachea. As the infant swallows oral secretions or ingests milk, the pouch fills, causing either drooling or aspiration into the lungs.
4. Pyloric stenosis, one of the most common disorders requiring surgery in early infancy, is an obstruction of the pyloric outlet caused by hypertrophy of circular muscles in the pyloric sphincter.
5. Intestinal malrotation occurs during fetal development with an obstructing band and volvulus (twisting of the bowel on itself) that may partly or completely occlude the gastrointestinal tract and its blood vessels.
6. Meconium ileus is a newborn condition in which intestinal secretions and amniotic waste products produce a thick, tarry plug that obstructs the intestine. Of children with cystic fibrosis, 10% to 15% present with meconium ileus as a neonate.
7. Duodenal, jejunal, and ileal obstructions can be caused by meconium ileus, atresia, congenital aganglionic megacolon, and acquired obstructive disorders.
8. Meckel diverticulum is a congenital malformation of the gastrointestinal tract involving all layers of the small intestinal wall usually in the ileum.
9. Congenital aganglionic megacolon (Hirschsprung disease) is caused by a malformation of the parasympathetic nervous system in a segment of the colon. It is characterized by the absence of nerves needed for peristalsis and causes colon obstruction.
10. Malformations of the anus and rectum range from mild congenital stenosis of the anus to complex deformities, all of which are classified as imperforate anus.
11. Intussusception is a condition in which one portion of the bowel telescopes, or invaginates, into another, most commonly in the area of the ileocecal junction causing obstruction.
12. Gastroesophageal reflux is the return of stomach contents into the esophagus caused by relaxation or incompetence of the lower esophageal sphincter that results from immaturity of the gastroesophageal sphincter.

Did You Understand?—Cont'd

13. Cystic fibrosis of the pancreas is an inherited fibrocystic disease of the pancreas that involves many organs and causes pancreatic enzyme deficiency with maldigestion.
14. Gluten-sensitive enteropathy is caused by hypersensitivity to gluten protein with autoimmune injury and loss of the villous epithelium. It results in malabsorption and growth failure.
15. Protein energy malnutrition is a group of disorders resulting from a severe dietary deficiency of proteins, carbohydrates, or both. Starvation causes stunted mental and physical development.
16. Kwashiorkor is a severe protein deficiency that occurs in children who have stopped breast-feeding and subsist on a high-carbohydrate diet. Marasmus is a deficiency of all dietary nutrients, including carbohydrates.
17. Failure to thrive is inadequate physical growth of a child. Organic failure to thrive is caused by genetic, anatomic, or pathophysiologic factors that retard normal growth and development. Nonorganic failure to thrive is caused by nutritional deficits associated with inadequate nurturing.
18. Necrotizing enterocolitis is an ischemic, inflammatory disorder in neonates, particularly premature infants, thought to result from stress and anoxia of the bowel wall. Bacteria invade the mucosa and submucosa, resulting in colitis, necrosis, and even perforation of the intestinal wall.
19. Diarrhea in infants and children can rapidly cause dehydration and electrolyte imbalances because fluid reserves are relatively small.
20. The most common cause of acute diarrhea in children is bacterial or viral enterocolitis (infection of the gastrointestinal tract).
21. Chronic diarrhea (diarrhea persisting longer than 4 weeks) can be caused by a wide variety of underlying conditions and often leads to growth failure and slow development.
22. Primary lactose intolerance is the inability to digest milk sugar because of a lack of lactose and results in osmotic diarrhea.

Disorders of the Liver

1. Physiologic jaundice of the newborn is caused by mild hyperbilirubinemia that subsides in 1 or 2 weeks. Pathologic jaundice is caused by severe hyperbilirubinemia and can cause brain damage (kernicterus).
2. Biliary atresia is a congenital malformation of the bile ducts that obstructs bile flow. Atresia causes jaundice, cirrhosis, and liver failure.
3. Acute hepatitis is usually caused by a virus, and hepatitis A is the most common form of childhood hepatitis. Chronic hepatitis B or C usually occurs by perinatal transmission.
4. Cirrhosis results from fibrotic scarring of the liver and is rare in children, but it can develop from most forms of chronic liver disease.
5. Portal hypertension in children usually is caused by extrahepatic obstruction. Thrombosis of the portal vein is the most common cause of portal hypertension in children, and splenomegaly is the most common sign.
6. The three most common metabolic disorders that cause liver damage in children are galactosemia, fructosemia, and Wilson disease. All three are inherited as genetic traits and allow toxins to accumulate in the liver.

Key Terms

Biliary atresia, 998
Celiac crisis, 994
Chronic nonspecific diarrhea, 997
Cirrhosis, 999
Cleft lip (harelip), 985
Cleft palate, 985
Congenital aganglionic megacolon (Hirschsprung disease), 989
Cystic fibrosis (CF), 992
Distal intestinal obstruction syndrome (DIOS), 989
Esophageal atresia, 986
Extrahepatic portal hypertension, 999
Failure to thrive (FTT), 995
Fructosemia, 999
Galactosemia, 1000
Gastroesophageal reflux (GER), 991
Gastroesophageal reflux disease (GERD), 991
Gluten-sensitive enteropathy (celiac sprue), 992
Ileal atresia, 989
Imperforate anus, 990
Infant diarrhea, 996
Intestinal malrotation of the colon, 988
Intrahepatic portal hypertension, 999
Intussusception, 990
Jejunal atresia, 989
Kernicterus, 997
Kwashiorkor, 995
Lactose intolerance, 997
Marasmus, 995
Meckel diverticulum, 989
Meconium, 988
Meconium ileus, 988
Necrotizing enterocolitis, 996
Neonatal jaundice, 997
Nonorganic FTT, 995
Organic FTT, 995
Periduodenal band (Ladd band), 988
Protein energy malnutrition (PEM), 995
Pyloric stenosis, 987
Rotavirus, 997
Tracheoesophageal fistula (TEF), 986
Wilson disease, 999

References

1. Stanier P, Moore GE: Genetics of cleft lip and palate: syndromic genes contribute to the incidence of non-syndromic clefts, *Hum Mol Genet* 13(Spec No 1):R73–R81, 2004. (Epub Jan 13, 2004.)
2. Holmes LB: The teratogenicity of anticonvulsant drugs: a progress report, *J Med Genet* 39(4):245–247, 2002.
3. Little J et al: Smoking and orofacial clefts: a United Kingdom–based case-controlled study, *Cleft Palate Craniofac J* 41(4):381–386, 2004.
4. Turner L et al: The effects of lactation education and a prosthetic obturator appliance on feeding efficiency in infants with cleft lip and palate, *Cleft Palate Craniofac J* 38(5):519–524, 2001.
5. Campbell S et al: Ultrasound antenatal diagnosis of cleft palate by a new technique: the 3D "reverse face" view, *Ultrasound Obstet Gynecol* 25(1):12–80, 2005.
6. Stein S et al: One- or two-stage palate closure in patients with unilateral cleft lip and palate: comparing cephalometric and occlusal outcomes, *Cleft Palate Craniofac J* 44(1):13–22, 2007.
7. Lisson J et al: Suggestions for orthodontic and speech improving measures in CLP patients, *J Orofac Orthoped* 62(5):367–374, 2001.
8. Rosenstein SW: Case report: surgeon and orthodontist work together from patient's birth, *World J Orthod* 7(3):293–298, 2006.
9. Sheahan P et al: Incidence and outcome of middle ear disease in cleft lip and/or cleft palate, *Int J Pediatr Otorhinolaryngol* 67(7):785–793, 2003.
10. Wilcox AJ et al: Folic acid supplements and risk of facial clefts: national population based case-control study, *BMJ* 334 (7591):464, 2007.
11. Shaw GM et al: Maternal nutrient intakes and risk of orofacial clefts, *Epidemiology* 17(3):285–291, 2006.
12. Langer JC et al: Prenatal diagnosis of esophageal atresia using sonography and magnetic resonance imaging, *J Pediatr Surg* 36(5):804–807, 2001.
13. Kovesi T, Rubin S: Long-term complications of congenital esophageal atresia and/or tracheoesophageal fistula, *Chest* 136(3):915–925, 2004.
14. Goyal A et al: Oesophageal atresia and tracheo-oesophageal fistula, *Arch Dis Child Fetal Neonatal Ed* 91(5):F381–384, 2006.
15. MacMahon B: The continuing enigma of pyloric stenosis of infancy: a review, *Epidemiology* 17(2):195–201, 2006.
16. Vasavada P: Ultrasound evaluation of acute abdominal emergencies in infants and children, *Radiol Clin North Am* 42(2):445–456, 2004.
17. Aspelund G, Langer JC: Current management of hypertrophic pyloric stenosis, *Semin Pediatr Surg* 16(1):27–33, 2007.
18. Singh UK, Kumar R, Prasad R: Oral atropine sulfate for infantile hypertrophic pyloric stenosis, *Indian Pediatr* 42(5):473–476, 2005.
19. Sweeney B, Surana R, Puri P: Jejunoileal atresia and associated malformations: correlation with the timing of in utero insult, *J Pediatr Surg* 36(5):774–776, 2001.
20. Millar AJ, Rode H, Cywes S: Malrotation and volvulus in infancy and childhood, *Semin Pediatr Surg* 12(4):229–236, 2003.
21. Murphy FL, Sparnon AL: Long-term complications following intestinal malrotation and the Ladd's procedure: a 15 year review, *Pediatr Surg Int* 22(4):326–329, 2006.
22. Blackman SM et al: Relative contribution of genetic and nongenetic modifiers to intestinal obstruction in cystic fibrosis, *Gastroenterology* 131(4):1030–1039, 2006.
23. Nagar H: Meconium ileus: is a single surgical procedure adequate? *Asian J Surg* 29(3):161–164, 2006.
24. Evans AK, Fitzgerald DA, McKay KO: The impact of meconium ileus on the clinical course of children with cystic fibrosis, *Eur Respir J* 18(5):784–789, 2001.
25. Escobar MA et al: Surgical considerations in cystic fibrosis: a 32-year evaluation of outcomes, *Surgery* 138(4):560–571, 2005.
26. Dray X et al: Distal intestinal obstruction syndrome in adults with cystic fibrosis, *Clin Gastroenterol Hepatol* 2(6):498–503, 2004.
27. Wyllie R: Gastrointestinal manifestations of cystic fibrosis, *Clin Pediatr (Phila)* 38(12):735–738, 1999.
28. Sagar J, Kumar V, Shah DK: Meckel's diverticulum: a systematic review, *J R Soc Med* 99(10):501–505, 2006.
29. Sai Prasad TR et al: Meckel's diverticular complications in children: is laparoscopy the order of the day? *Pediatr Surg Int* 23(2):141–147, 2007.
30. de Pontual L et al: Mutations of the RET gene in isolated and syndromic Hirschsprung's disease in human disclose major and modifier alleles at a single locus, *J Med Genet* 43(5):419–423, 2006.
31. Catto-Smith AG, Trajanovska M, Taylor RG: Long-term continence in patients with Hirschsprung's disease and Down syndrome, *J Gastroenterol Hepatol* 21(4):748–753, 2006.
32. Kessmann J: Hirschsprung's disease: diagnosis and management, *Am Fam Physician* 74(8):1319–1322, 2006.
33. Dasgupta R, Langer JC: Hirschsprung disease, *Curr Probl Surg* 41(12):942–988, 2004.
34. Cho S, Moore SP, Fangman T: One hundred three consecutive patients with anorectal malformations and their associated anomalies, *Arch Pediatr Adolesc Med* 155(5):587–591, 2001.
35. Wang NL et al: Prenatal and neonatal intussusception, *Pediatr Surg Int* 13(4):232–236, 1998.
36. Turkyilmaz Z et al: Postoperative intussusception in children, *Acta Chir Belg* 105(2):187–189, 2005.
37. Eggermont E, De Boeck K: Small-intestinal anomalies in cystic fibrosis patients, *Eur J Pediatr* 150(12):824–828, 1991.
38. Blanch AJ, Perel SB, Acworth JP: Paediatric intussusception: epidemiology and outcome, *Emerg Med Australas* 19(1):45–50, 2007.
39. Klein EJ, Kapoor D, Shugerman RP: The diagnosis of intussusception, *Clin Pediatr* 43(4):343–347, 2004.
40. Henry SM: Discerning differences: gastroesophageal reflux and gastroesophageal reflux disease in infants, *Adv Neonatal Care* 4(4):235–247, 2004.
41. McGovern MC, Smith MB: Causes of apparent life threatening events in infants: a systematic review, *Arch Dis Child* 89 (11):1043–1048, 2004.
42. Suwandhi E, Ton MN, Schwarz SM: Gastroesophageal reflux in infancy and childhood, *Pediatr Ann* 35(4):259–266, 2006.
43. Baker SS et al: Pancreatic enzyme therapy and clinical outcomes in patients with cystic fibrosis, *J Pediatr* 146(2):189–193, 2005.
44. Littlewood JM, Wolfe SP, Conway SP: Diagnosis and treatment of intestinal malabsorption in cystic fibrosis, *Pediatr Pulmonol* 41(1):35–49, 2006.
45. Murphy AJ et al: The nutritional status of children with cystic fibrosis, *Br J Nutr* 95(2):321–324, 2006.
46. Hardin DS et al: Growth hormone treatment enhances nutrition and growth in children with cystic fibrosis receiving enteral nutrition, *J Pediatr* 146(3):324–328, 2005.
47. Stepniak D, Koning F: Celiac disease: sandwiched between innate and adaptive immunity, *Hum Immunol* 67(6):460–468, 2006.
48. Fasano A et al: Prevalence of celiac disease in at-risk and non-at-risk groups in the United States: a large multi-center study, *Arch Int Med* 163(3):286–292, 2003.

References—Cont'd

49. Iughetti L et al: Endocrine aspects of coeliac disease, *J Pediatr Endocrinol Metab* 16(6):805–818, 2003.
50. Catassi C, Fasano A: Celiac disease as a cause of growth retardation in children, *Curr Opin Pediatr* 16(4):445–449, 2004.
51. Rossi T: Celiac disease, *Adolesc Med Clin* 15(1):91–103, 2004.
52. Cereda S et al: Celiac disease and childhood cancer, *J Pediatr Hematol Oncol* 28(6):346–349, 2006.
53. Silano M et al: Collaborating centers of the Italian registry of the complications of coeliac disease: delayed diagnosis of coeliac disease increases cancer risk, *BMC Gastroenterol* 7:8, 2007.
54. Kello AB, Gilbert C: Causes of severe visual impairment and blindness in children in schools for the blind in Ethiopia, *Br J Ophthalmol* 87(5):526–530, 2003.
55. Berkley J et al: Assessment of severe malnutrition among hospitalized children in rural Kenya: comparison of weight for height and mid upper arm circumference, *JAMA* 294(5): 591–597, 2005.
56. Bergman P, Graham J: An approach to "failure to thrive," *Aust Fam Physician* 34(9):725–729, 2005.
57. Feldman R et al: Mother-child touch patterns in infant feeding disorders: relation to maternal, child, and environmental factors, *J Am Acad Child Adolesc Psychiatry* 43(9):1089–1097, 2004.
58. Chatoor I: Feeding disorders in infants and toddlers: diagnosis and treatment, *Child Adolesc Psychiatr Clin North Am* 11(2): 163–183, 2004.
59. Lin PW, Stoll BJ: Necrotising enterocolitis, *Lancet* 368 (9543):1271–1283, 2006.
60. Gibbs K, Lin J, Holzman IR: Necrotising enterocolitis: the state of the science, *Indian J Pediatr* 74(1):67–72, 2007.
61. Kamitsuka MD, Horton MK, William MA: The incidence of necrotizing enterocolitis after introducing standardized feeding schedules for infants between 1250 and 1500 grams and less than 35 weeks of gestation, *Pediatrics* 105(2):379–384, 2000.
62. Nanthakumar NN et al: Glucocorticoid responsiveness in developing human intestine: possible role in prevention of necrotizing enterocolitis, *AmJ Physiol Gastrointest Liver Physiol* 288(1):G85–G92, 2005.
63. Blakely ML et al: Laparotomy versus peritoneal drainage for necrotizing enterocolitis or isolated intestinal perforation in extremely low birth weight infants: outcomes through 18 months adjusted age, *Pediatrics* 117(4):e680–e687, 2006.
64. Rees CM et al: Surgical strategies for necrotizing enterocolitis: a survey of practice in the United Kingdom, *Arch Dis Child Fetal Neonatal Ed* 90(2):F152–F155, 2005.
65. Ahmed T, Ein S, Moore A: The role of peritoneal drains in treatment of perforated necrotizing enterocolitis: recommendations from recent experience, *J Pediatr Surg* 33(10): 1468–1470, 1998.
66. Luig M, Lui K, NSW & ACT NICUS Group: Epidemiology of necrotizing enterocolitis—part I: changing regional trends in extremely preterm infants over 14 years, *J Paediatr Child Health* 41(4):169–173, 2005.
67. Ocha TJ, Salazar-Lindo E, Cleary TG: Management of children with infection-associated persistent diarrhea, *Semin Pediatr Infect Dis* 15(4):229–236, 2004.
68. Surawicz CM: *Clostridium difficile*, disease: diagnosis and treatment, *Gastroenterologist* 6(1):60–65, 1998.
69. Ewing WM, Allen PJ: The diagnosis and management of cow mild protein intolerance in the primary care setting, *Pediatr Nurs* 31(6):486–493, 2005.
70. Leung AK, Kellner JD, Davies HD: Rotavirus gastroenteritis, *Adv Ther* 22(5):476–487, 2005.
71. Besedovsky A, Li BU: Across the developmental continuum of irritable bowel syndrome: clinical and pathophysiologic considerations, *Curr Gastroenterol Rep* 6(3):247–253, 2004.
72. Heyman MBCommittee on Nutrition: Lactose intolerance in infants, children, and adolescents, *Pediatrics* 118(3): 1279–1286, 2006.
73. Truman P: Jaundice in the preterm infant, *Pediatr Nurs* 18(5): 20–22, 2006.
74. Wennberg RP et al: Toward understanding kernicterus: a challenge to improve the management of jaundiced newborns, *Pediatrics* 117(2):474–485, 2006.
75. Blackmon LR, Faranoff AA, Raju TNNational Institute of Child Health and Human Development: Research on prevention of bilirubin-induced brain injury and kernicterus: National Institute of Child Health and Human Development conference executive summary, *Pediatrics* 114(1):29–223, 2004.
76. Behrman RE, Kliegman R, Jenson HB: *Nelson textbook of pediatrics*, ed 16, Philadelphia, 2001, Saunders.
77. Davenport M: Biliary atresia, *Semin Pediatr Surg* 14(1):42–48, 2005.
78. Escobar MA et al: Effect of corticosteroid therapy on outcomes in biliary atresia after Kasai portoenterostomy, *J Pediatr Surg* 41(1):99–103, 2006.
79. Wasley A, Samandari T, Bell BP: Incidence of hepatitis A in the United States in the era of vaccination, *JAMA* 294(2): 194–201, 2005.
80. Muecke CJ et al: Hepatitis A seroprevalence and risk factors among day care educators, *Clin Invest Med* 27(5):259–264, 2004.
81. Slowik MK, Jhaveri R: Hepatitis B and C viruses in infants and young children, *Semin Pediatr Infect Dis* 16(4):296–305, 2005.
82. Shukla NB, Poles MA: Hepatitis B virus infection: co-infection with hepatitis C virus, hepatitis D virus, and human immunodeficiency virus, *Clin Liver Dis* 8(2):445–460, 2004.
83. Mast EE et al: Risk factors for perinatal transmission of hepatitis C virus (HCV) and the natural history of HCV infection acquired in infancy, *J Infect Dis* 192(11):1880–1889, 2005 (Epub Oct 28, 2005.)
84. Badizadegan K et al: Histopathology of the liver in children with chronic hepatitis C viral infection, *Hepatology* 28(5): 1416–1423, 1998.
85. Mack CL et al: Surgically restoring portal blood flow to the liver in children with primary extrahepatic portal vein thrombosis improves fluid neurocognitive ability, *Pediatrics* 117(3): e405–e412, 2006.
86. Ryckman FC, Alonso MH: Causes and management of portal hypertension in the pediatric population, *Clin Liver Dis* 5(3): 789–818, 2001.

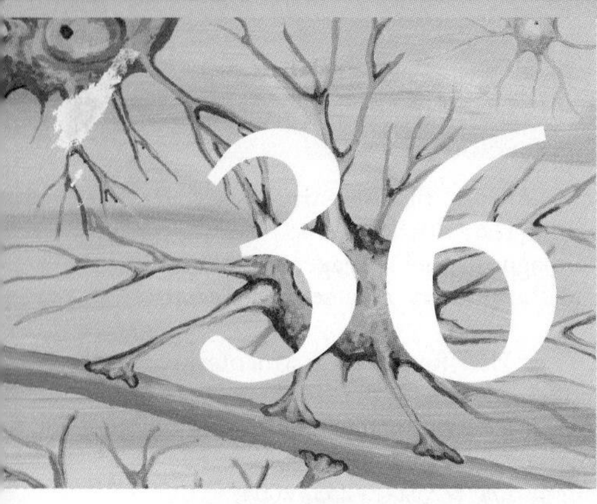

36 STRUCTURE AND FUNCTION OF THE MUSCULOSKELETAL SYSTEM

Christy L. Crowther

CHAPTER OUTLINE

ELECTRONIC RESOURCES

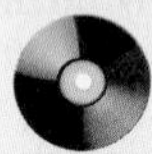

Companion CD
- Review Questions and Answers
- Animations

evolve Website
http://evolve.elsevier.com/Huether/
- Quick Check Answers
- Key Terms Exercises
- Critical Thinking Questions with Answers
- Algorithm Completion Exercises
- WebLinks

The way an individual functions in daily life, moves about, or manipulates objects physically depends on the integrity of the musculoskeletal system. The musculoskeletal system is actually two systems: (1) the skeleton composed of bones and joints and (2) skeletal muscles. Each system contributes to mobility. The skeleton supports the body and provides leverage to the skeletal muscles so that movement of various parts of the body is possible. Contraction of the skeletal muscles and bending or rotation at the joints facilitate movements of the various body parts.

STRUCTURE AND FUNCTION OF BONES

Bones give form to the body, support tissues, and permit movement by providing points of attachment for muscles. Many bones meet in movable joints that determine the type and extent of movement possible. Bones also protect many of the body's vital organs. For example, the bones of the skull, thorax, and pelvis are hard exterior shields that protect the brain, heart, lungs, and reproductive and urinary organs.

The marrow cavities within certain bones serve as sites of blood cell formation. In adults, blood cells originate exclusively in the marrow cavities of the skull, vertebrae, ribs, sternum, shoulders, and pelvis. Bones also have a crucial role in mineral homeostasis, storing minerals (i.e., calcium, phosphate, carbonate, magnesium) that are essential for the proper working of many delicate cellular mechanisms.

Elements of Bone Tissue

Mature bone is a rigid connective tissue consisting of cells, fibers, a gelatinous material termed **ground substance,** and large amounts of crystallized minerals, mainly calcium, that give bone its rigidity. Ground substance consists of proteoglycans and hyaluronic acid secreted by chondroblasts. The structural elements of bone are summarized in Table 36-1.

Bone cells enable bone to grow, repair itself, change shape, and continuously synthesize new bone tissue and **resorb** (dissolve or digest) old tissue. The fibers in bone are made of collagen, which gives bone its tensile strength (the ability to hold itself together). Ground substance acts as a medium for the diffusion of nutrients, oxygen, metabolic wastes, biochemicals, and minerals between bone tissue and blood vessels.

Bone formation begins during fetal life with the growth of cartilage—the precursor of bone tissue. In mature bone, the formation of new tissue begins with the production of an organic matrix by the bone cells. This **bone matrix** consists of ground substances, collagen, and other proteins (see Table 36-1) that take part in bone formation and maintenance.

The next step in bone formation is **calcification**, in which minerals are deposited and then crystallize. Minerals bind tightly to collagen fibers, producing tensile and

TABLE 36-1
Structural Elements of Bone

Structural Elements	Function
BONE CELLS	
Osteoblasts	Synthesize collagen and proteoglycans: stimulate osteoclast resorptive activity
Osteocytes	Maintain bone matrix
Osteoclasts	Resorb bone; assist with mineral homeostasis
BONE MATRIX	
Collagen fibers	Lend support and tensile strength
Proteoglycans	Control transport of ionized materials through matrix
Bone morphogenic proteins	Induce bone and cartilage formation
BMP-1	Plays key role in ECM formation
BMP-2A	Promotes chondrogenesis
BMP-4	Involved in cartilage repair
GLYCOPROTEINS	
Sialoprotein	Promotes calcification
Osteocalcin	Inhibits calcium-phosphate precipitation; promotes bone resorption
Laminin	Stabilizes basement membranes in bones
Osteonectin	Binds calcium in bones
Albumin	Transports essential elements to matrix; maintains osmotic pressure of bone fluid
α-glycoproteins	Promotes calcification
MINERALS (ELEMENTS)	
Calcium	Crystallizes to lend rigidity and compressive strength
Phosphate	Regulates vitamin D and thereby promotes mineralization

compressional strength in bone and allowing it to withstand pressure and weight bearing.

Bone cells

Bone contains three types of cells: osteoblasts, osteocytes, and osteoclasts (Figure 36-1). Osteoblasts are the bone-forming cells. Their primary function is to lay down new bone. Once this function is complete, osteoblasts become osteocytes. Osteocytes are osteoblasts that have become imprisoned within the mineralized bone matrix. They help maintain bone by synthesizing new bone matrix molecules. Osteoclasts function primarily to resorb (remove) bone during processes of growth and repair.

Osteoblast

An **osteoblast** is a cell derived from osteogenic mesenchymal stromal cells that produces type I collagen and is the major bone-forming cell. Osteoblasts are responsive to parathyroid hormone (PTH) and produce osteocalcin when stimulated by 1,25-dihydroxyvitamin D. Osteoblasts are active on the outer surfaces of bones, where they form a single layer of cells. Osteoblasts bring about new bone formation by their synthesis of **osteoid** (nonmineralized bone matrix). Osteoblasts also mineralize newly formed bone matrix. Stimulation of bone formation of new bone and the orderly mineralization of bone matrix occur by concentrating some of the plasma proteins (growth factors) found in the bone matrix and by facilitating the deposit and exchange of calcium and other ions at the site. Growth factors, including bone morphogenic proteins (BMPs) and other members of the transforming growth factor-beta (TGF-βa) superfamily, are critical components of bone formation, maintenance, and remodeling (Table 36-2).[1]

Coupling bone formation with bone resorption has been extensively studied.[2] Studies have shown that osteoblasts use intercellular calcium signaling to include osteoclastic activity. One of the most important discoveries linking osteoblast and osteoclast function is that of the cytokine receptor activator nuclear factor kappa-B ligand, or RANKL. RANKL is expressed on osteoblasts and is necessary for forming osteoclasts (see the Osteoclast section).[3] In contact with bone mineral, osteoclasts can be further stimulated by colony-stimulating factor and interleukins-1, -3, and -6 produced by macrophage cells in the presence of PTH.[4] Thus, the cells of the osteoblastic lineage (osteoblasts, osteocytes) form a network of cells in bone that sense the shape and structure of bone and determine where it is appropriate that bone be formed or resorbed, according to Wolff's law (bone is shaped according to its function).

Originating from mesenchymal stem cells (MSCs), osteoblasts are specialized fibroblasts that have both an active and a resting state. Osteoblasts synthesize and secrete osteoid when active and when in the resting state are termed *satellite cells.* If appropriately stimulated, however, the resting osteoblasts are capable of resuming activity.

Osteoclast

Osteoclasts are large (typically 20 to 100 microns in diameter), multinucleated cells that develop from the hematopoietic monocyte-macrophage lineage. Osteoclasts are the major resorptive cells of bone.[5] They migrate over bone surfaces to resorption areas that have been prepared and stripped of osteoid by enzymes, such as collagenases, produced by osteoblasts in the presence of PTH, which is necessary for the resorptive process. Osteoclasts travel over the prepared bone surfaces, creating irregular, scalloped cavities, known as *Howship lacunae* or *resorption bays,* as they resorb bone areas and then acidify hydroxyapatite in order to dissolve it.

A specific area of the cell membrane forms adjacent to the bone surface and forms multiple infoldings to permit intimate contact with the resorption bay. These infoldings, known as the **ruffled border,** greatly increase the cell's surfaces under their scalloped or ruffled borders. Osteoclasts resorb bone by secretion of hydrochloric acid and acid

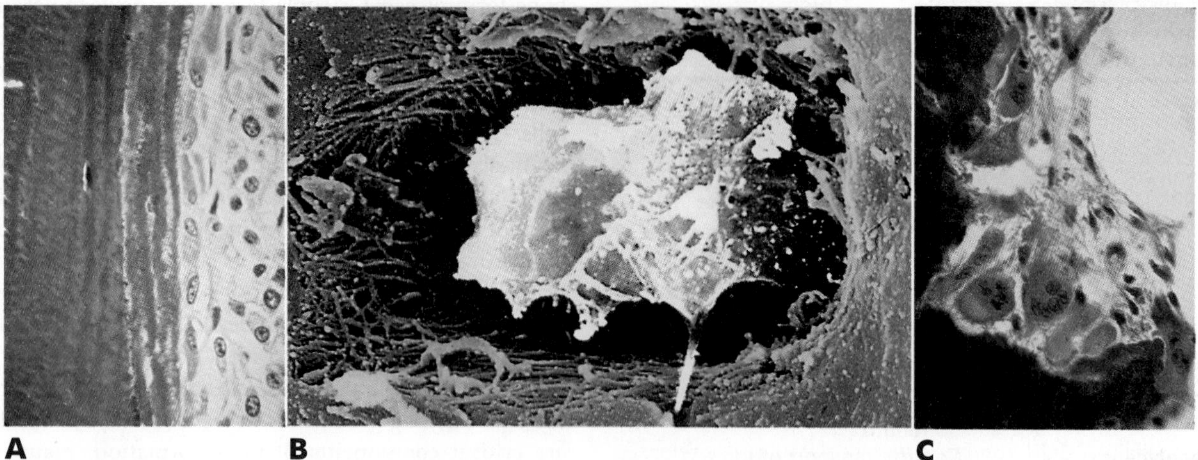

Figure 36-1 ■ **Bone Cells. A,** Osteoblasts are responsible for the production of collagenous and noncollagenous proteins that compose osteoid. Active osteoblasts are lined up on the osteoid. Note the eccentrically located nuclei. **B,** Scanning electron micrograph showing an osteocyte within a lacuna. The cell is surrounded by collagen fibers and mineralized bone. **C,** Osteoclasts actively resorb mineralized tissue. The scalloped surface in which the multinucleated osteoclasts rest is termed *Howship lacuna.* (**A** and **C** from Damjanov I, Linder J, editors: *Anderson's pathology,* ed 10, St Louis, 1996, Mosby; **B** from Erlandsen S, Magney J: *Color atlas of histology,* St Louis, 1992, Mosby.)

TABLE 36-2

Effects of Selected Cytokines (Growth Factors) on Skeletal Tissues

Cytokine (Growth Factor)	Target Tissue	Formation	Resorption
Transforming growth factor-beta	Bone	+, −	+, −
	Cartilage	+, −	−
Transforming growth factor-alpha or epidermal growth factor	Bone	+, −	+
	Cartilage	+	
Insulin-like growth factor	Bone	−	0
	Cartilage	−	?
Fibroblast growth factor	Bone	+, −	0
	Cartilage		?
Platelet-derived growth factor	Bone	+	0
Colony-stimulating factors	Bone	0	+
	Cartilage	?	?
Interferon-gamma	Bone	−	−
	Cartilage	−	?
Tumor necrosis factor	Bone	−	+
	Cartilage	−	+
Interleukin-1, -3, and -6	Bone	+, −	+
	Cartilage	−	+

+, −, Both stimulatory and inhibitory properties on the specific cell listed; 0, no effects presently known; ?, possible effects on cell listed.

proteinases, such as cathepsin K, that help digest collagen, along with the action of cytokines (see Table 36-2). Osteoclasts also resorb bone through the action of lysosomes (digestive vacuoles) filled with hydrolytic enzymes in their mitochondria.

Osteoclasts bind to the bone surfaces through attachments called **integrins.**[6] Once resorption is complete, the osteoclasts retract and loosen from the bone surface under the ruffled border through the action of calcitonin. Calcitonin binds to receptor areas of the osteoclasts' cell membranes to effectively loosen the osteoclasts from the bone surfaces. Once resorption is completed, osteoclasts disappear by the process of degeneration, either by reverting to the form of their parent cells or through cell movements away from the site, in which the osteoclast becomes an inactive or resting osteoclast.

Osteocyte

An **osteocyte** is a transformed osteoblast that is trapped or surrounded in osteoid as it hardens as a result of minerals that enter during calcification (see Figure 36-1, *B*). The osteocyte is within a space in the hardened bone matrix called a **lacuna.** Each osteocyte has a high nucleus/cytoplasm ratio with a thin layer of nonmineralized osteoid around it, like the egg white surrounding an egg yolk.

The function of osteocytes is not fully known, but it is known that they synthesize certain matrix molecules, thereby assisting bone calcification. Osteocytes are the most numerous bone cells. They also help concentrate nutrients in the matrix. Osteocytes obtain nutrients from capillaries in the canaliculi, which contain nutrient-rich fluids. Osteocytes help determine bone structure by acting as mechanosensory cells that direct functional adaptation of bone.[7] Through exchanges among these cells, hormone catalysts, and minerals, optimal levels of calcium, phosphorus, and other minerals are maintained in blood plasma. The osteocyte also aids in modifying bone matrix through the release of enzymes to dissolve the mineralized walls of the lacunae to prepare the bone for remodeling. Remodeling is described on page 1008.

Bone matrix

Bone matrix is made of the *extracellular elements* of bone tissue, specifically collagen fibers, proteins, carbohydrate-protein complexes, ground substance, and minerals.

Collagen fibers

Collagen fibers make up the bulk of bone matrix. They are formed as follows:

1. Osteoblasts synthesize and secrete type I collagen.
2. Collagen molecules assemble into three thin chains (alpha chains) to form **fibrils.**
3. Fibrils organize into the staggered pattern, with each fibril overlapping its nearest neighbor by about one fourth its length. This creates gaps into which mineral crystals are deposited.
4. After mineral deposition, fibrils link together and twist to form ropelike fibers.
5. The fibers join to form the framework that gives bone its tensile and supportive strength.

Proteoglycans

Proteoglycans are large complexes of numerous polysaccharides attached to a common protein core. They strengthen bone by forming compression-resistant networks between the collagen fibers. Proteoglycans also control the transport and distribution of electrically charged particles (ions), particularly calcium, through the bone matrix, thereby playing a role in bone calcium deposition and calcification.

Glycoproteins

Glycoproteins are carbohydrate-protein complexes that control the collagen interactions that lead to fibril formation. They also may function in calcification. Four glycoproteins are present in bone: **sialoprotein,** which binds easily with calcium; **osteocalcin,** which binds preferentially to crystallized calcium; **bone albumin,** which is identical to serum albumin and possibly transports essential nutrients to and from bone cells and maintains the osmotic pressure of **bone fluid;** and **alpha-glycoprotein (α-glycoprotein),** which probably plays a significant role in calcification and also may facilitate bone resorption by activating osteoclasts (see Table 36-1).

Bone minerals

Mineralization (crystallization) is the final step in bone formation, after collagen synthesis and fiber formation. Mineralization has two distinct phases: (1) formation of the initial mineral deposit (initiation) and (2) proliferation or accretion of additional mineral crystals on the initial mineral deposits (growth). The majority of the mineral in the body is an analog of the naturally occurring mineral, *hydroxyapatite.*

Table 36-3 lists the sequence in which calcium and phosphate form amorphous (fluid) calcium phosphate compounds that are converted, in stages, to solid hexagonal crystals of **hydroxyapatite (HAP).** As the calcium and phosphorus concentrations increase in the bone matrix, the first precipitate to form is dicalcium phosphate dihydrate (DCPD). Once DCPD precipitation begins, the remaining phases of bone crystal formation proceed until insoluble HAP is produced, with approximately 80% to 90% of the HAP incorporated into the collagen fibers. Amorphous calcium phosphate is distributed throughout the bone matrix.

Types of Bone Tissue

Bone is composed of two types of bony (osseous) tissue: **compact bone (cortical bone)** and **spongy bone (cancellous bone)** (Figure 36-2). Cortical bone comprises about 85% of the skeleton; cancellous bone makes up the remaining 15%. Both types of bone tissue contain the same structural elements, and with a few exceptions, both compact tissue and spongy tissue are present in every bone. The major difference between the two types of tissue is the organization of the elements.

Compact bone is highly organized, solid, and extremely strong. The basic structural unit in compact bone is the **haversian system** (Figure 36-3). Each haversian system is made up of the following:

TABLE 36-3

Sequence of Calcium and Phosphate Compound Formation and Crystallization

Formula	Name	Abbreviation
$Ca(HPO_4) \cdot 2\,H_2O$	Dicalcium phosphate dihydrate	DCPD
$Ca_4H(PO_4)_3$	Octacalcium phosphate	OCP
$Ca_9(PO_4)_6$ (var.)	Amorphous calcium phosphate	ACP
$Ca_3(PO_4)_2$	Tricalcium phosphate	TCP
$Ca_5(PO_4)_3OH$	Hydroxyapatite	HAP

NOTE: Compounds are listed in the order in which precipitation and crystal formation occur.

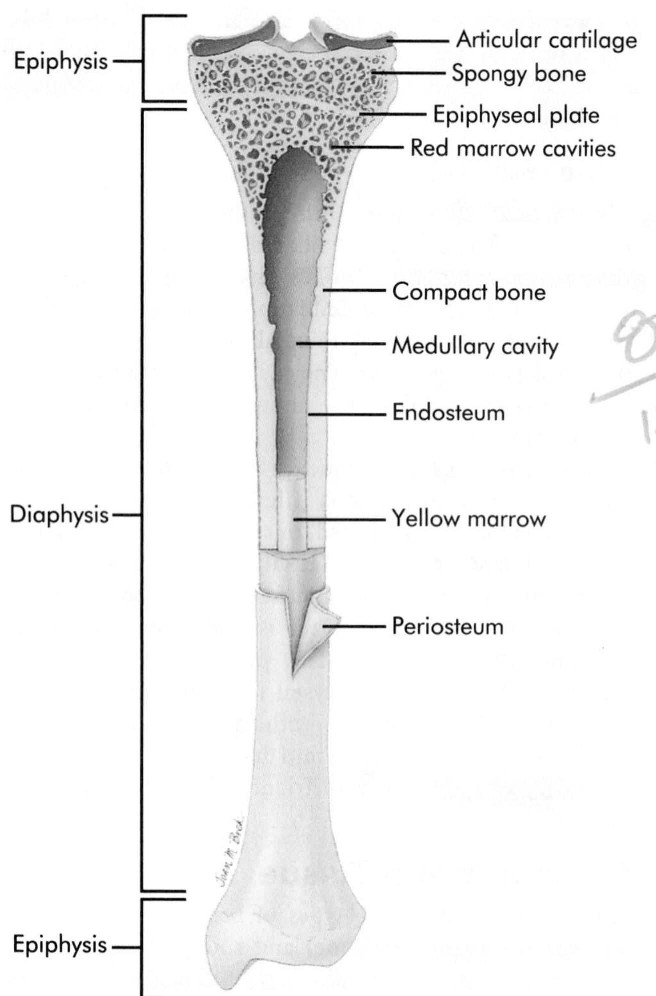

Figure 36-2 ■ **Cross Section of Bone.** Longitudinal section of long bone (tibia) showing spongy (cancellous) and compact bone. (From Thibodeau GA, Patton KT: *Anatomy & physiology*, ed 6, St Louis, 2007, Mosby.)

1. A central canal called the **haversian canal**
2. Concentric layers of bone matrix called **lamellae** (*sing.*, lamella)
3. Tiny spaces (lacunae) between the lamellae
4. Bone cells (osteocytes) within the lacunae
5. Small channels or canals called **canaliculi** (*sing.*, canaliculus)

Spongy bone is less complex and lacks haversian systems. In spongy bone, the lamellae are not arranged in concentric layers but in plates or bars termed **trabeculae** (*sing.*, trabecula) that branch and unite with one another to form an irregular meshwork. The pattern of the meshwork is determined by the direction of stress on the particular bone. The spaces between the trabeculae are filled with red bone marrow. The osteocyte-containing lacunae are distributed between the trabeculae and interconnected by canaliculi. Capillaries pass through the marrow to nourish the osteocytes.

All bones are covered with a double-layered connective tissue called the **periosteum.** The outer layer of the periosteum contains blood vessels and nerves, some of which penetrate to the inner structures of the bone through channels called *Volkmann canals* (see Figure 36-3). The inner layer of the periosteum is anchored to the bone by collagenous fibers (Sharpey fibers) that penetrate the bone. Sharpey fibers also help hold or attach tendons and ligaments to the periosteum of bones.

Characteristics of Bone

The 206 bones of the human skeleton are distributed between the axial skeleton and the appendicular skeleton. Eighty bones are in the **axial skeleton,** making up the skull, vertebral column, and thorax. The other 126 bones of the **appendicular skeleton** make up the upper and lower extremities, the shoulder girdle (pectoral girdle), and the pelvic girdle (os coxae) (Figure 36-4). The skeleton contributes approximately 14% of an adult's body weight.

Bones can be classified by shape as long, flat, short (cuboidal), or irregular. **Long bones** are longer than they are wide and consist of a narrow tubular midportion **(diaphysis)** that merges into a broader neck **(metaphysis)** and a broad end **(epiphysis)** (see Figure 36-2).

The diaphysis consists of a shaft of thick, rigid compact bone that is able to tolerate bending forces. Contained within the diaphysis is the elongated marrow (medullary) cavity. The marrow cavity of the diaphysis contains primarily fatty tissue, which is referred to as *yellow marrow.* The yellow marrow assists red bone marrow in hematopoiesis only during times of stress. The yellow marrow cavity of the diaphysis is continuous with marrow cavities in the spongy bone of the metaphysis and diaphysis. The marrow contained within the epiphysis is red because it contains primarily blood-forming tissue (see Chapter 19). A layer of connective tissue, the **endosteum,** lines the outer surfaces of both types of marrow cavity.

The broadness of the epiphysis allows weight bearing to be distributed over a wide area. The epiphysis is made up of spongy bone covered by a thin layer of compact bone. In a child, the epiphysis is separated from the metaphysis by a cartilaginous **growth plate (epiphyseal plate).** After puberty, the epiphyseal plate calcifies and the epiphysis and metaphysis merge. By adulthood, the line of demarcation between the epiphysis and metaphysis is undetectable.

In **flat bones,** such as the ribs and scapulae, two plates of compact bone are roughly parallel to each other. Between the compact bone plates is a layer of spongy bone. **Short bones,** such as the bones of the wrist or ankle, are often cuboidal in shape. They consist of spongy bone covered by a thin layer of compact bone.

Irregular bones, such as the vertebrae, mandibles, or other facial bones, have various shapes that include thin and thick segments. The thin part of an irregular bone consists of two plates of compact bone with spongy bone in between. The thick part consists of spongy bone surrounded by a layer of compact bone.

Maintenance of Bone Integrity

Remodeling

The internal structure of bone is maintained by **remodeling,** a three-phase process in which existing bone is resorbed

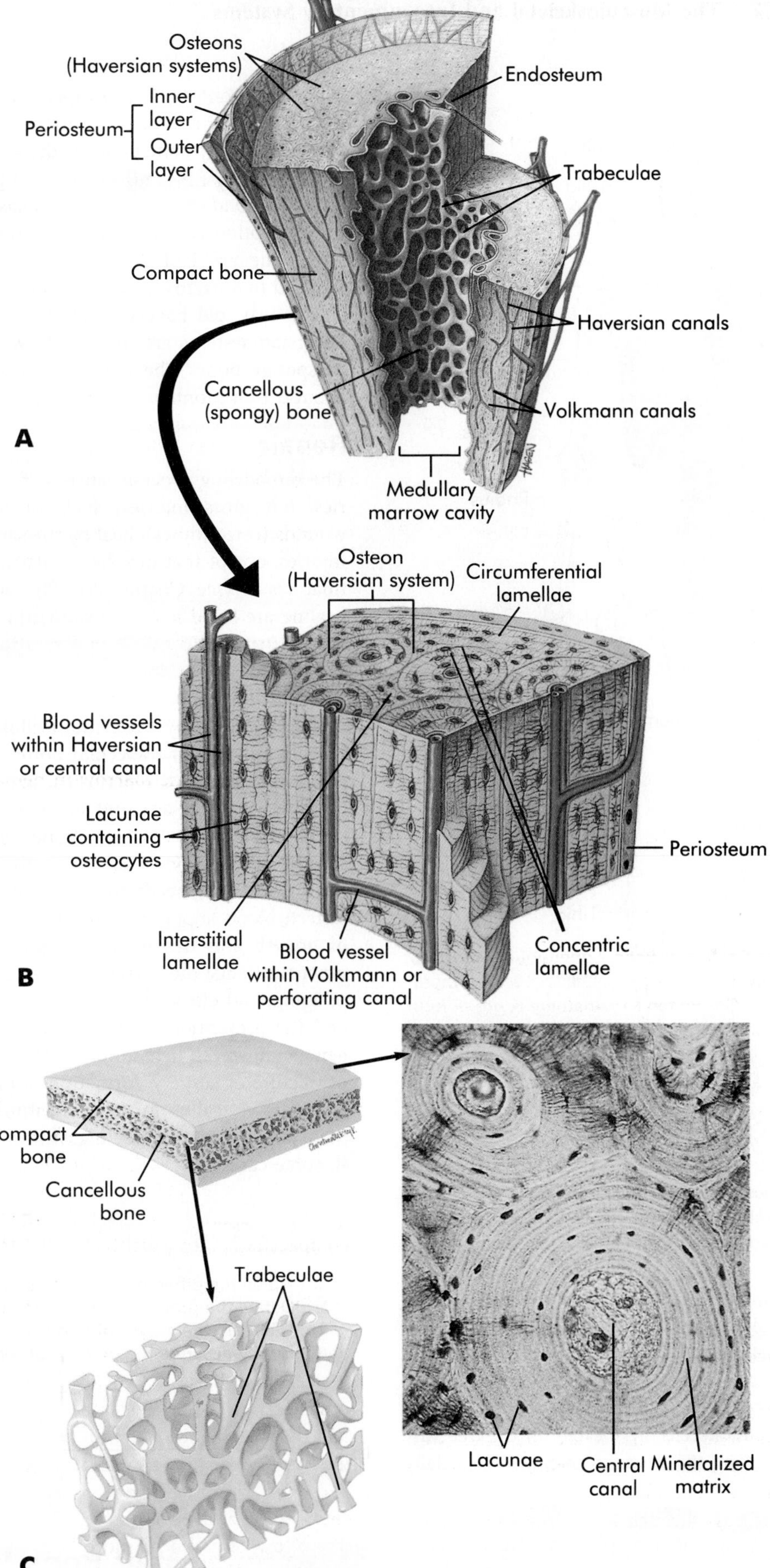

Figure 36-3 ■ **Structure of Compact and Cancellous Bone. A,** Longitudinal section of a long bone showing both cancellous and compact bone. **B,** A magnified view of compact bone. **C,** Section of a flat bone. Outer layers of compact bone surround cancellous bone. Fine structure of compact and cancellous bone is shown to the right. (From Thibodeau GA, Patton KT: *Anatomy & physiology,* ed 6, St Louis, 2007, Mosby.)

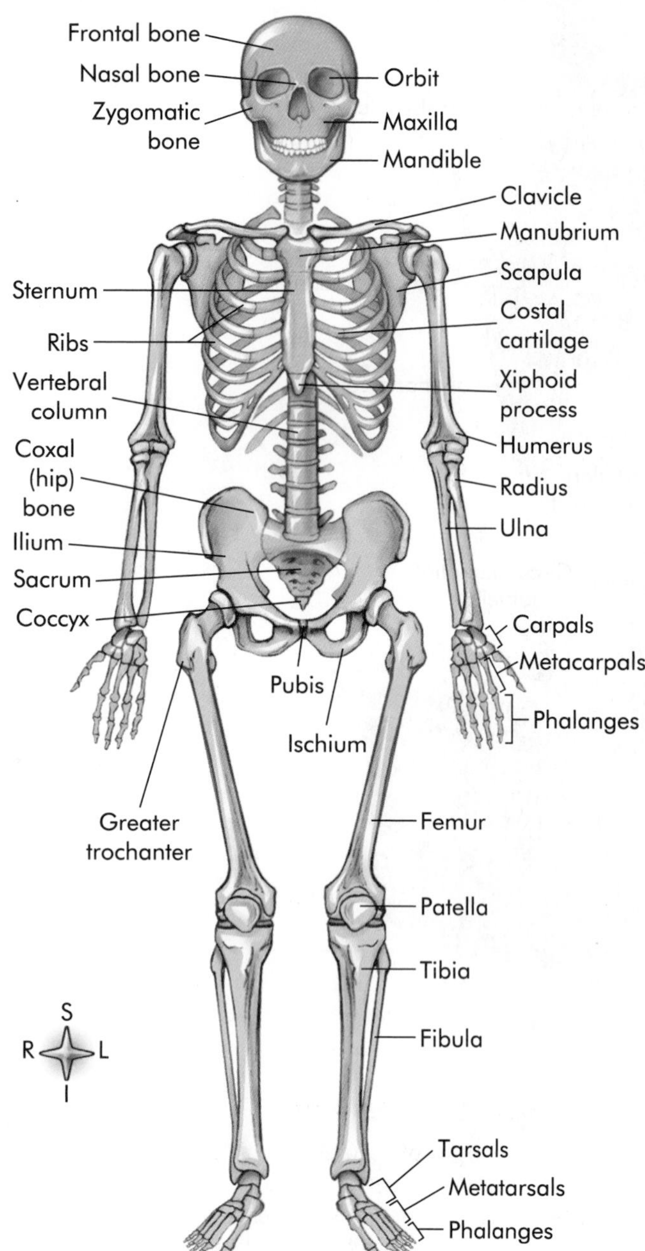

Figure 36-4 ■ **Anterior View of Skeleton.** Axial skeleton in blue; appendicular skeleton in tan. (From Thibodeau GA, Patton KT: *Anatomy & physiology,* ed 6, St Louis, 2007, Mosby.)

and new bone is laid down to replace it. Remodeling is carried out by clusters of bone cells termed **basic multicellular units.** The basic multicellular units are made up of bone precursor cells that differentiate into osteoclasts and osteoblasts. Precursor cells are located on the free surfaces of bones and along the vascular channels (especially the marrow cavities).

In phase 1 (activation) of the remodeling cycle, a stimulus (e.g., hormone, drug, vitamin, physical stressor) activates the bone cell precursors in a localized area of bone to form osteoclasts. In phase 2 (resorption), the osteoclasts form a "cutting cone," which gradually resorbs bone, leaving behind an elongated cavity termed a *resorption cavity.* The resorption cavity in compact bone follows the longitudinal axis of the haversian system, whereas the resorption cavity in spongy bone parallels the surface of the trabeculae.

Phase 3 (formation) is the laying down of new bone, termed *secondary bone,* by osteoblasts lining the walls of the resorption cavity. Successive layers (lamellae) in compact bone are laid down, until the resorption cavity is reduced to a narrow haversian canal around a blood vessel. In this way, old haversian systems are destroyed and new haversian systems are formed. New trabeculae are formed in spongy bone. The entire process of remodeling takes about 3 to 4 months.

Repair

The remodeling process can repair microscopic bone injuries, but gross injuries, such as fractures and surgical wounds (osteotomies), heal by the same stages as soft tissue injuries, except that new bone, instead of scar tissue, is the final result (see Chapter 5). The stages of bone wound healing are listed here and shown in Figure 36-5:

1. Inflammation/hematoma formation
2. Procallus formation
3. Callus formation
4. Replacement, by basic multicellular units, of the callus with lamellar or trabecular bone
5. Remodeling of the periosteal and endosteal surfaces of the bone to the size and shape of the bone before injury

The speed with which bone heals depends on the severity of the bone disruption; the type and amount of bone tissue that needs to be replaced (spongy bone heals faster); blood supply and oxygen to the site; the presence of growth and thyroid hormones, insulin, vitamins, and other nutrients; the presence of systemic disease; the effects of aging; and effective treatment, including immobilization and the prevention of complications such as infection. In general, however, hematoma formation occurs within hours of fracture or surgery, formation of procallus by osteoblasts within days, callus formation within weeks, and replacement and contour modeling within years—up to 4 years in some cases.

QUICK CHECK 36-1

1. Name the different types of bone cells.
2. Define the process of bone resorption.
3. What are the stages of bone wound healing?
4. Briefly describe the process of remodeling.

STRUCTURE AND FUNCTION OF JOINTS

The site where two or more bones are attached is called a **joint,** or **articulation** (Figure 36-6). The primary function of joints is to provide stability and mobility to the skeleton. Whether a joint provides stability or mobility depends on its location and its structure. Generally, joints that stabilize

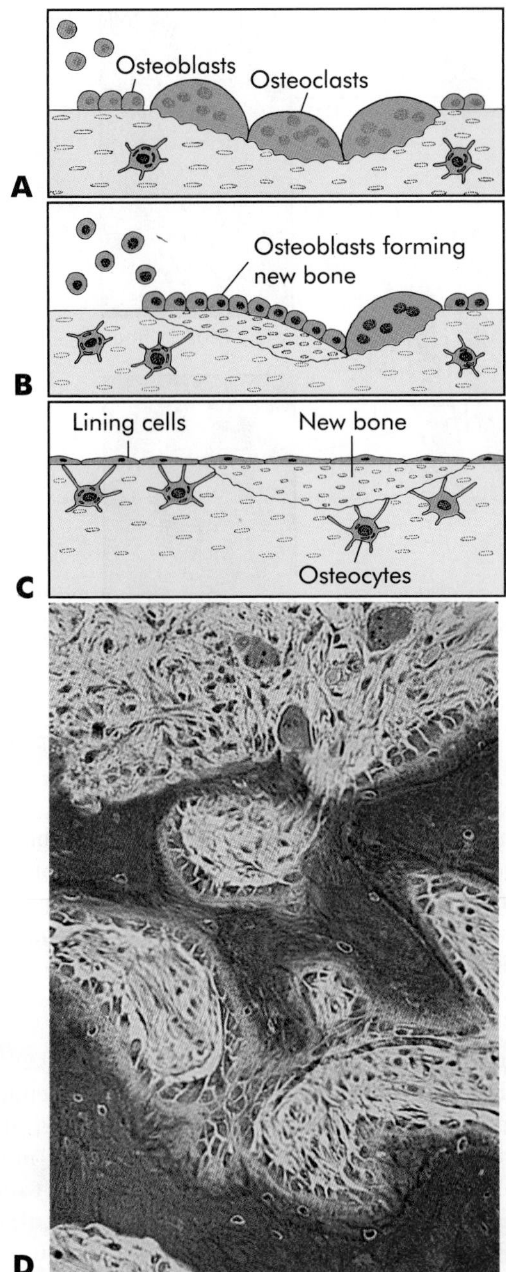

Figure 36-5 ■ Bone Remodeling. In the remodeling sequence, bone sections are removed by bone-resorbing cells (osteoclasts) and replaced with a new section laid down by bone-forming cells (osteoblasts). The cells work in response to signals generated in that environment. Only the multinucleated osteoclastic cells mediate the first phase of remodeling. They are activated, scoop out bone **(A)**, and resorb it; then the work of the osteoblasts begins **(B)**. They form new bone that replaces bone removed by the resorption process **(C)**. The sequence takes 4 to 5 months. **D,** Micrograph of active bone remodeling seen in the settings of primary or secondary hyperparathyroidism. Note the active osteoblasts surmounted on red-stained osteoid. Marrow fibrosis is present. (**D** from Damjanov I, Linder J, editors: *Anderson's pathology,* ed 10, St Louis, 1996, Mosby.)

the skeleton have a simpler structure than those that enable the skeleton to move. Most joints provide both stability and mobility to some degree (Figure 36-7).

Joints are classified based on the degree of movement they permit or on the connecting tissues that hold them together. Based on movement, a joint is classified as a **synarthrosis (immovable joint),** an **amphiarthrosis (slightly movable joint),** or a **diarthrosis (freely movable joint).** On the basis of connective structures, joints are classified broadly as fibrous, cartilaginous, or synovial. Each of these three structural classifications can be subdivided according to the shape and contour of the articulating surfaces (ends) of the bones and the type of motion the joint permits.

Fibrous Joints

A joint in which bone is united directly to bone by fibrous connective tissue is called a **fibrous joint.** These joints have no joint cavity and allow little, if any, movement.

Fibrous joints are further subdivided into three types: sutures, syndesmoses, and gomphoses. A **suture** has a thin layer of dense fibrous tissue that binds together interlocking flat bones in the skulls of young children. Sutures form an extremely tight union that permits no motion. By adulthood, the fibrous tissue has been replaced by bone. A **syndesmosis** is a joint in which the two bony surfaces are united by a ligament or membrane. The fibers of ligaments are flexible and stretch, permitting a limited amount of movement. The paired bones of the lower arm (radius and ulna) and the lower leg (tibia and fibula) and their ligaments are syndesmotic joints. A **gomphosis** is a special type of fibrous joint in which a conical projection fits into a complementary socket and is held there by a ligament. The teeth held in the maxilla or mandible are gomphosis joints.

Cartilaginous Joints

There are two types of cartilaginous joints: symphyses and synchondroses. A **symphysis** is a cartilaginous joint in which bones are united by a pad or disk of fibrocartilage. A thin layer of hyaline cartilage usually covers the articulating surfaces of these two bones, and the thick pad of fibrocartilage acts as a shock absorber and stabilizer. Examples of symphyses are the symphysis pubis, which joins the two pubic bones, and the intervertebral disks, which join the bodies of the vertebrae. A **synchondrosis** is a joint in which hyaline cartilage, rather than fibrocartilage, connects the two bones. The joints between the ribs and the sternum are synchondroses. The hyaline cartilage of these joints is called *costal cartilage.* Slight movement at the synchondroses between the ribs and the sternum allows the chest to move outward and upward during breathing.

Joint (articular) capsule

The **joint (articular) capsule** is fibrous connective tissue that covers the ends of bones where they meet in a joint; Sharpey fibers firmly attach the proximal and distal capsule to the periosteum, and ligaments and tendons also may reinforce the capsule. It is composed of parallel, interlacing

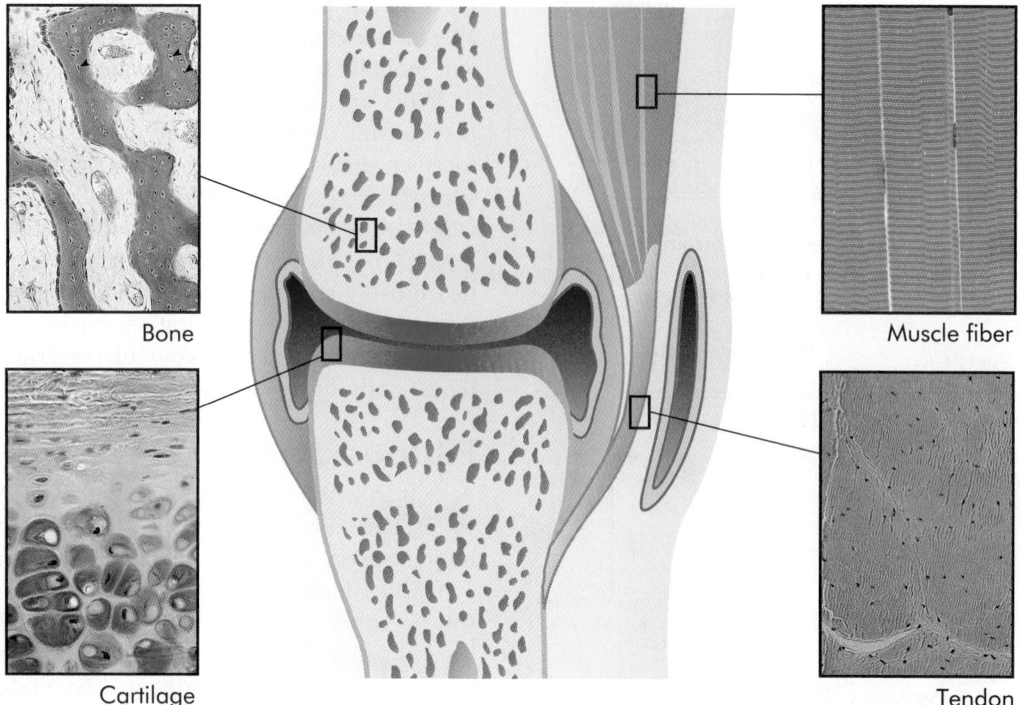

Figure 36-6 ■ **Main Tissues of a Joint.** (Micrographs from Gartner LP, Hiatt JL: *Color textbook of histology,* ed 3, Philadelphia, 2007, Saunders.)

bundles of dense, white fibrous tissue richly supplied with nerves, blood vessels, and lymphatic vessels. Nerves in and around the joint capsule are sensitive to rate and direction of motion, compression, tension, vibration, and pain.

Synovial membrane

The **synovial membrane** is a smooth, delicate inner lining of joint capsule found in the nonarticular portion of the synovial joint and any ligaments or tendons that traverse this cavity. It is composed of two layers: vascular subintima and thin cellular intima. Vascular intima merges with the fibrous joint capsule and is composed of loose fibrous connective tissue, elastin fibers, fat cells, fibroblasts, macrophages, and mast cells; intima consists of rows of synovial cells embedded in fiber-free intercellular matrix and contains two types of cells—A and B. A cells ingest and remove (phagocytose) bacteria and particles of debris in the joint cavity; B cells secrete hyaluronate, which gives synovial fluid its viscous quality. The synovial membrane is richly supplied with blood and lymphatic vessels and is capable of rapid repair and regeneration.

Joint (synovial) cavity

The **joint (synovial) cavity** is an enclosed, fluid-filled space between articulating surfaces of two bones, also called *joint space.* It enables two bones to move "against" one another and is surrounded by synovial membrane and filled with synovial fluid.

Synovial fluid

Synovial fluid is superfiltrated plasma from blood vessels that lubricates the joint surfaces, nourishes the pad of the articular cartilage, and covers the ends of the bones. Hyaluronic acid in the synovial fluid gives it important biomechanical properties. It also contains free-floating synovial cells and various leukocytes that phagocytose joint debris and microorganisms.

Articular cartilage

Articular cartilage is a layer of hyaline cartilage that covers the end of each bone; it may be thick or thin, depending on the size of the joint, the fit of the two bone ends, and the amount of weight and shearing force the joint normally withstands. The function of articular cartilage is to reduce friction in the joint and to distribute the forces of weight bearing. Articular cartilage is composed of **chondrocytes** (cartilage cells) (making up about 2% of the tissue) and an intercellular matrix made up of collagen (making up about 10% to 30% of weight), protein polysaccharides (making up 5% to 10% of weight), and water. The water content ranges from 60% to almost 80% of the net weight of the cartilage, and individual molecules rapidly enter or exit the articular cartilage to contribute to the resiliency of the tissue.

At the surface of articular cartilage, the collagen fibers run parallel to the joint surface and are closely compacted into a dense, protective mat. (Loss of this dense, compacted configuration at the surface subjects the underlying fibers to splitting and thinning, in which case the cartilage is unable to tolerate weight bearing.) In the middle layer (the proliferative zone) of the cartilage, the fibers are arranged tangential to the surface, which allows them to deform and absorb some of the weight bearing. In the bottom layer (the hypertrophic zone) of the cartilage, the fibers are perpendicular to the joint surface, allowing them to resist

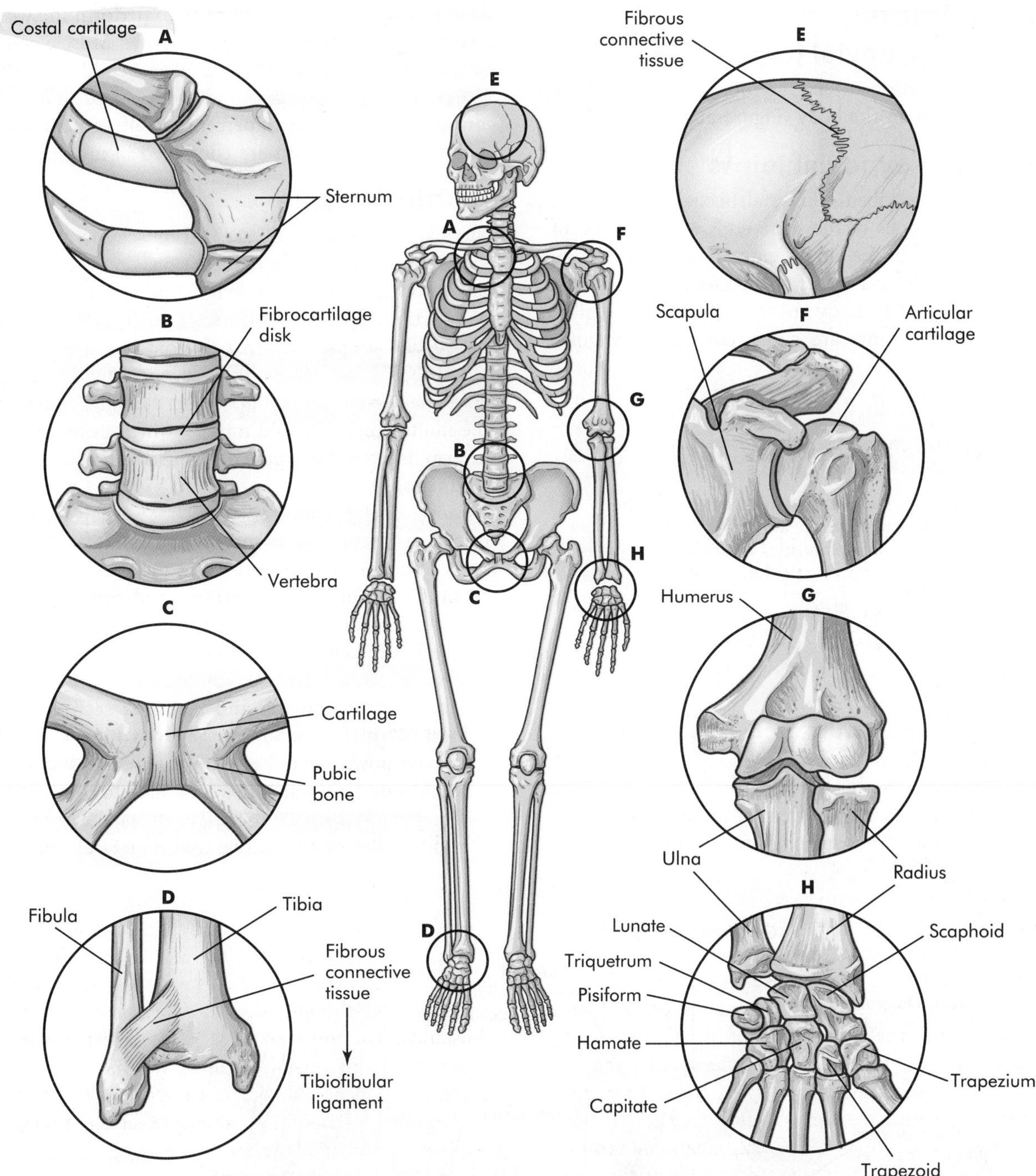

Figure 36-7 ■ **Types of Joints.** Cartilaginous (amphiarthrodial) joints, which are slightly movable, include **(A)** a synchondrosis that attaches ribs to costal cartilage, **(B)** a symphysis that connects vertebrae, and **(C)** the symphysis that connects the two pubic bones. Fibrous (synarthrodial) joints, which are immovable, include **(D)** the syndesmosis between the tibia and fibula and **(E)** sutures that connect the skull bones and the gomphosis (not shown), which holds teeth in their sockets. The synovial joints include **(F)** the spheroid type at the shoulder, **(G)** the hinge type at the elbow, and **(H)** the gliding joints of the hand.

shear forces, and are embedded in a calcified layer of cartilage called the *tidemark*. The **tidemark** anchors the collagen fibers to the underlying (subchondral) bone. Collagen fibers are important components of the cartilage matrix because they account for approximately 60% of the dry weight and because they (1) anchor the cartilage securely to underlying bone, (2) provide a taut framework for the cartilage, (3) control the loss of fluid from the cartilage, and (4) prevent the escape of protein polysaccharides (proteoglycans) from the cartilage. The proteoglycans give articular cartilage its stiff quality and regulate the movement of synovial fluid through the cartilage. The proteoglycans are macromolecules consisting of proteins, carbohydrates (glycosaminoglycans), and hyaluronic acid.

Synovial Joints

Structure of synovial joints

Synovial joints (diarthroses) are the most movable and the most complex joints in the body (Figure 36-8).

Movement of synovial joints

Synovial joints are described as uniaxial, biaxial, or multiaxial according to the shapes of the bone ends and the type of movement occurring at the joint (Figure 36-9). Usually, one of the bones is stable and serves as an axis for the motion of the other bone. The body movements made possible by various synovial joints are either circular or angular (Figure 36-10).

QUICK CHECK 36-2

1. How do each of these joints differ from each other: synarthrosis, amphiarthrosis, and diarthrosis?
2. Name at least two characteristics of each of the joints in the previous question that either facilitate or hinder movement.
3. Why is articular cartilage important?

STRUCTURE AND FUNCTION OF SKELETAL MUSCLES

Skeletal muscles arise from mesodermal precursor cells that then form myoblasts. The millions of individual fibers of skeletal muscle contract and relax to perform the work necessary to move the body (Figure 36-11). Muscle constitutes 40% of adults' body weight and 50% of children's. Muscle is 75% water, 20% protein, and 5% organic and inorganic compounds. Thirty-two percent of all protein stores for energy and metabolism are contained in muscle.

Whole Muscle

There are more than 600 skeletal muscles in the body. The body's muscles vary dramatically in size and shape. They range from 2 to 60 cm in length and are shaped according to function. **Fusiform muscles** are elongated muscles shaped like straps and can run from one joint to another. **Pennate muscles** are broad, flat, and slightly fan shaped, with fibers running obliquely to the muscle's long axis. The multipennate deltoid muscle, which flexes and extends the arm, is a good example of a muscle shaped according to its function.

Each skeletal muscle is a separate organ, encased in a three-part connective tissue framework called **fascia.** The layers of connective tissue protect the muscle fibers, attach the muscle to bony prominences, and provide a structure for a network of nerve fibers, blood vessels, and lymphatic channels. The layers are as follows:

1. The outermost layer, the **epimysium,** is located on the surface of the muscle and tapers at each end to form the **tendon** (Figure 36-12). Tendons allow short muscles to exert power on a distant joint, whereas a thick muscle would interfere with the joint's mobility.
2. The **perimysium** further subdivides the muscle fibers into bundles of connective tissue, or **fascicles.**

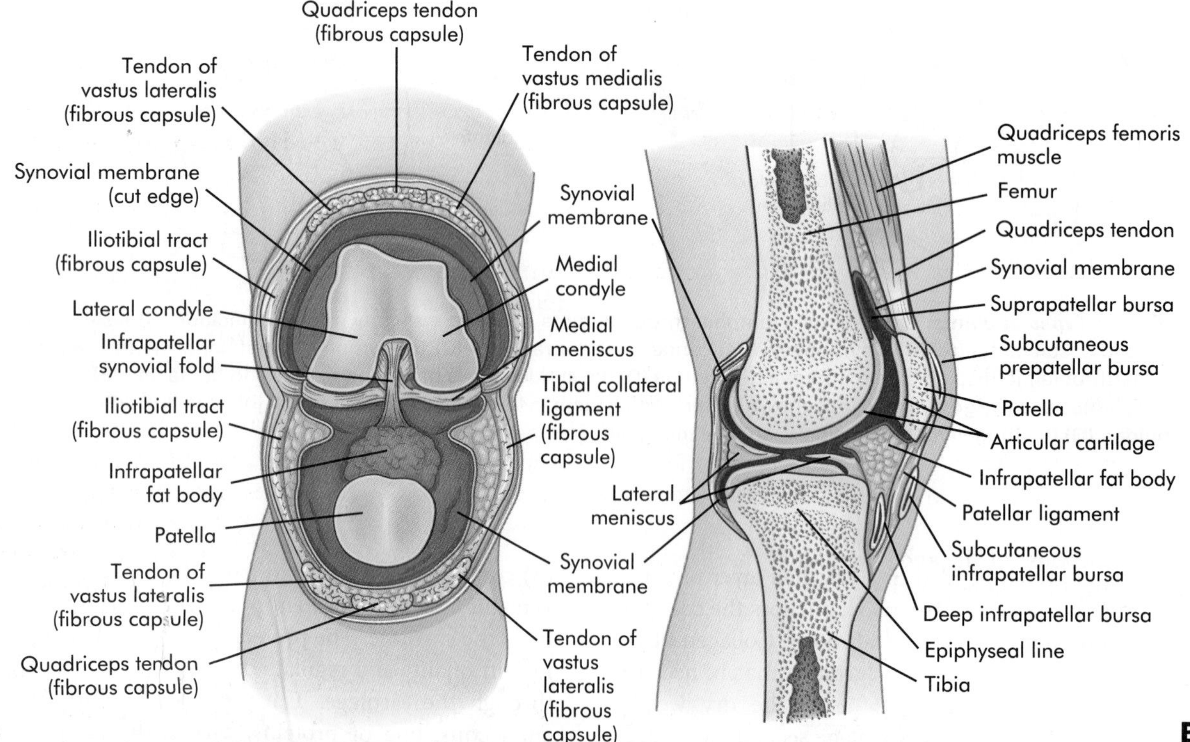

Figure 36-8 ■ **Knee Joint (Synovial Joint). A,** Frontal view. **B,** Lateral view.

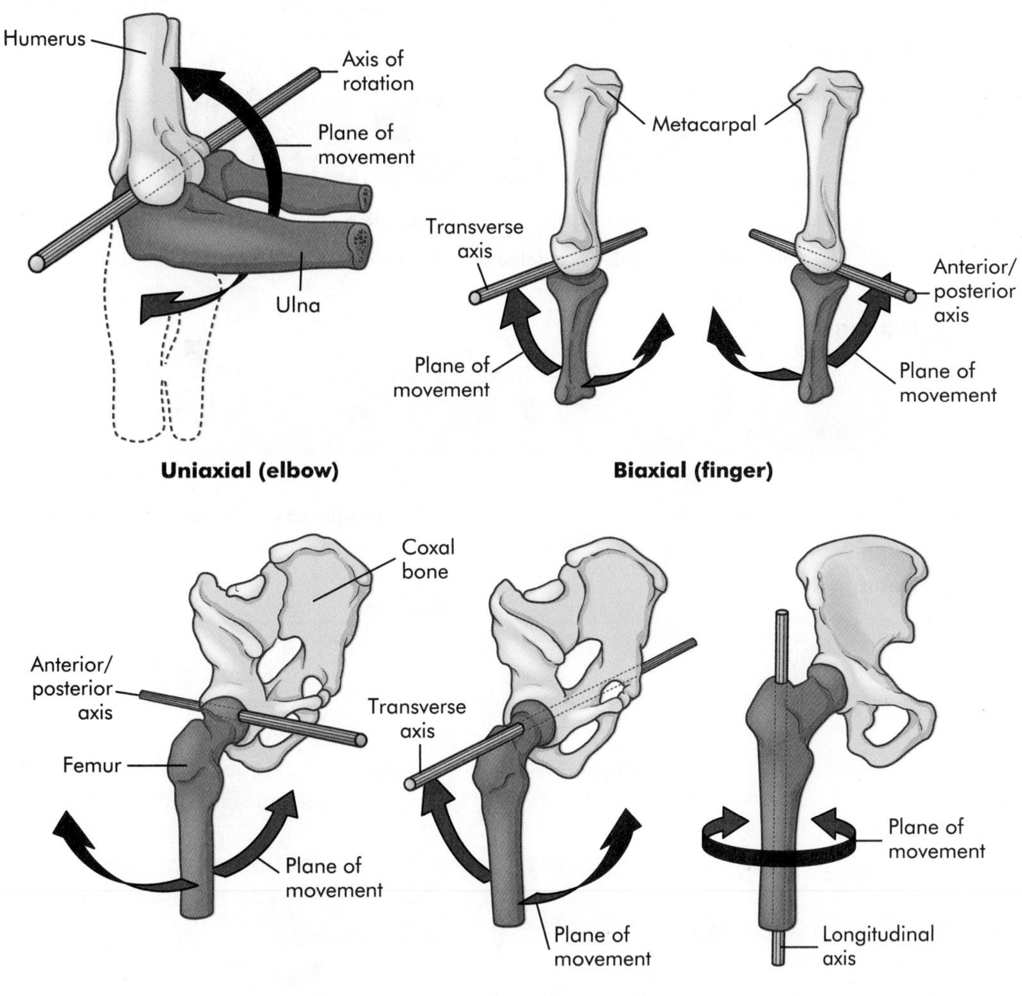

Figure 36-9 ■ **Movements of Synovial (Diarthrodial) Joints.**

3. The smallest unit of muscle visible without a microscope is the **endomysium,** which surrounds the muscle.

The ligaments, tendons, and fascia are made up of connective tissue that also buffers the limbs from the effects of sudden strains or changes in speed. The rapid recovery necessary for strenuous exercise is supported by the elastic property of muscle and its connective tissue.

Skeletal muscle has been termed **voluntary** (controlled directly by the nervous system), **striated** (has a striped pattern when viewed under a light microscope), or **extrafusal** (to distinguish from other contractile fibers in the sensory organ of the muscle). Components that are visible on gross inspection of the whole muscle include the motor and sensory nerve fibers. These function together with the muscle, innervating portions of it and providing the electrical impulses needed for motor function.

Motor unit

From the anterior horn cell of the spinal cord, the axons of motor nerves branch out to innervate a specific group of muscle fibers. Each anterior horn cell, its axon (part of the lower motor neuron; see Chapter 12), and the muscle fibers innervated by it are called a **motor unit** (Figure 36-13). The motor units are composed of lower motor neurons, which extend to skeletal muscles. Often termed the *functional unit* of the neuromuscular system, the motor unit behaves as a single entity and contracts as a whole when it receives an electrical impulse.

The whole muscle may be controlled by several motor nerve axons. These branch to innervate many motor units within the muscle. The whole muscle then may be made up of many motor units. The number of motor units per individual muscle varies greatly. In the calf, for example, one motor axon innervates approximately 2000 muscle fibers, out of a total of 1,200,000 muscle fibers. This is a high innervation ratio of muscle fibers to axons, and it contrasts markedly with the low innervation ratio in the laryngeal muscles. There, two to three muscle fibers constitute each motor unit, and the innervation ratio can be of great functional significance. The greater the innervation ratio of a particular organ, the greater its endurance. Higher innervation ratios prevent fatigue, whereas lower innervation ratios allow for precision of movement.

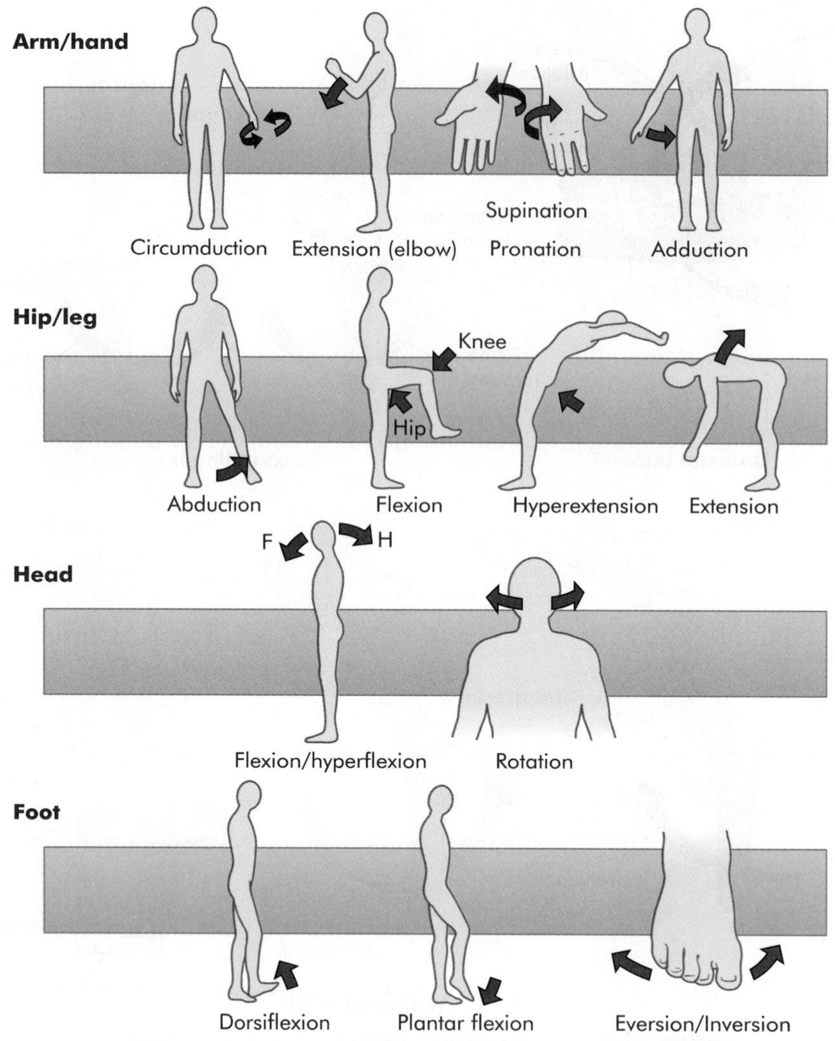

Figure 36-10 ■ **Body Movements Made Possible by Synovial (Diarthrodial) Joints.**

Sensory receptors

Although muscles function as effector organs, they also contain sensory receptors and are involved in sending different signals to the central nervous system. Among these are the muscle spindles and Golgi tendon organs. **Spindles** are mechanoreceptors that lie parallel to muscle fibers and respond to muscle stretching. **Golgi tendon organs** are dendrites that terminate and branch to tendons near the neuromuscular junction. The muscle spindles, Golgi tendon organs, and free nerve endings provide a means of reporting changes in length, tension, velocity, and tone in the muscle. This system of afferent signals is responsible for the muscle stretch response and maintenance of normal muscle tone.

Muscle fibers

Each **muscle fiber** is a single **muscle cell,** cylindrical in structure and surrounded by a membrane capable of excitation and impulse propagation. The muscle fiber contains bundles of **myofibrils,** the fiber's functional subunits, in a parallel arrangement along the longitudinal axis of the muscle (Figure 36-14). At birth, the muscle fibers have completed development from precursor cells called **myoblasts.** All **voluntary muscles** are derived from the mesodermal layer of the embryo. Genetic transcription factors, most notably myod induce skeletal muscle differentiation.[8] Myoblasts are the main cells responsible for muscle growth and regeneration. Myoblasts are termed *satellite cells* when in a dormant state.[9]

The type of peripheral nerve influences the muscle fiber and motor unit considerably. Whether motor nerves are fast or slow determines the type of muscle fibers in the motor unit. White muscle **(type II fibers [white fast-motor fibers])** is innervated by relatively large type II alpha motor neurons with fast conduction velocities. These fibers rely on a short-term anaerobic glycolytic system for rapid energy transfer; red muscle **(type I fibers [slow-twitch fibers])** depends on aerobic oxidative metabolism. Table 36-4 describes the specific characteristics of type I and type II fibers.

The overlap of muscle fibers that appears with staining gives the checkerboard appearance of muscle biopsy specimens and provides an equal distribution of fiber types throughout the muscle. This overlap also helps to compensate

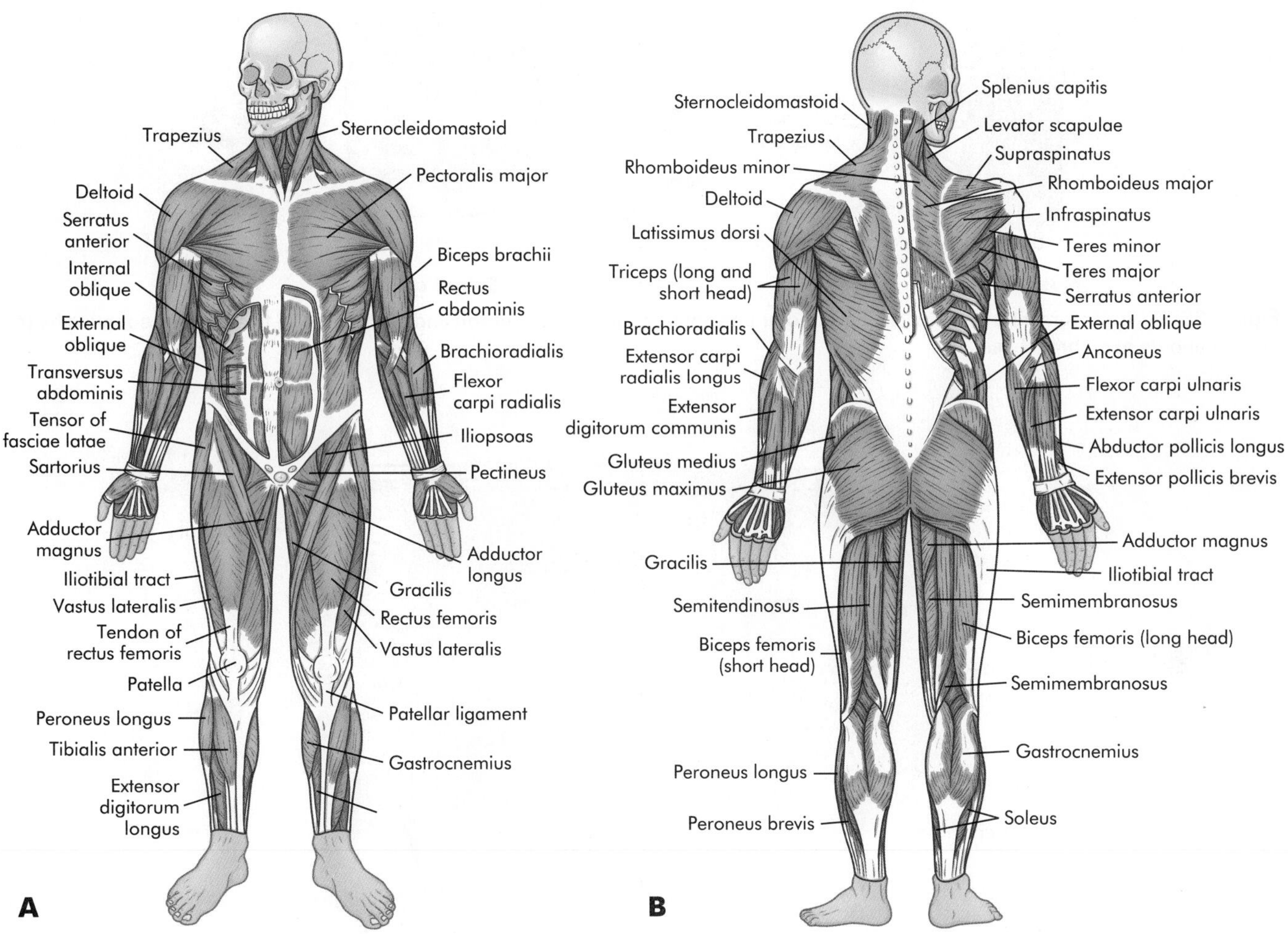

Figure 36-11 ■ **Skeletal Muscles of Body. A,** Anterior view. **B,** Posterior view.

for muscle fiber loss and fatigue of individual motor units during activity. In spite of this, some muscles contain proportionally more of one fiber type than another. The postural muscles have more type I fibers, allowing them the high resistance to fatigue that is necessary to maintain the same position for extended periods. The ocular muscles have more type II muscle fibers, allowing them to respond rapidly to visual changes.

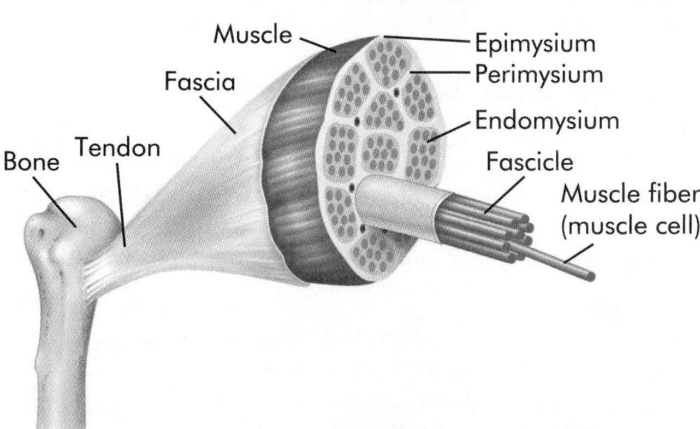

Figure 36-12 ■ **Cross Section of Skeletal Muscle Showing Muscle Fibers and Their Coverings.** (From Thibodeau GA, Patton KT: *Anatomy & physiology,* ed 6, St Louis, 2007, Mosby.)

The number of muscle fibers varies according to location. Large muscles, such as the gastrocnemius, have more fibers (1,200,000) than smaller muscles, such as the lumbrical muscles in the hand (10,000). The diameter of muscle fibers also varies. The closely packed polygons are small (10 to 20 μm) until puberty, when they attain the normal adult diameter of 40 to 80 μm. Women usually have smaller-diameter fibers than men. Small muscles, such as the ocular muscles, are 15 μm in diameter; larger, more proximal muscles are 40 μm. Fiber size can have functional significance. Studies have shown that larger fiber diameter is associated with generation of greater forces. Fiber diameter can be increased by exercise or occupational overuse, activities that cause hypertrophied muscle.

The major components of the muscle fiber include the muscle membrane, myofibrils, sarcotubular system, sarcoplasm, and mitochondria (see Figure 36-14). The **muscle membrane** is a two-part membrane. It includes the **sarcolemma,** which contains the plasma membrane of the muscle cell, and the cell's **basement membrane.** The sarcolemma is 7.5 μm thick and is capable of propagating electrical impulses to initiate contraction. At the motor

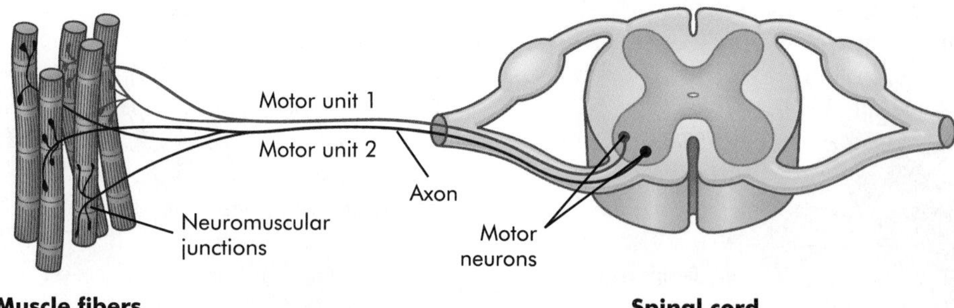

Figure 36-13 ■ **Motor Units of a Muscle.** Each motor unit consists of a motor neuron and all the muscle fibers (cells) supplied by the neuron and its axon branches.

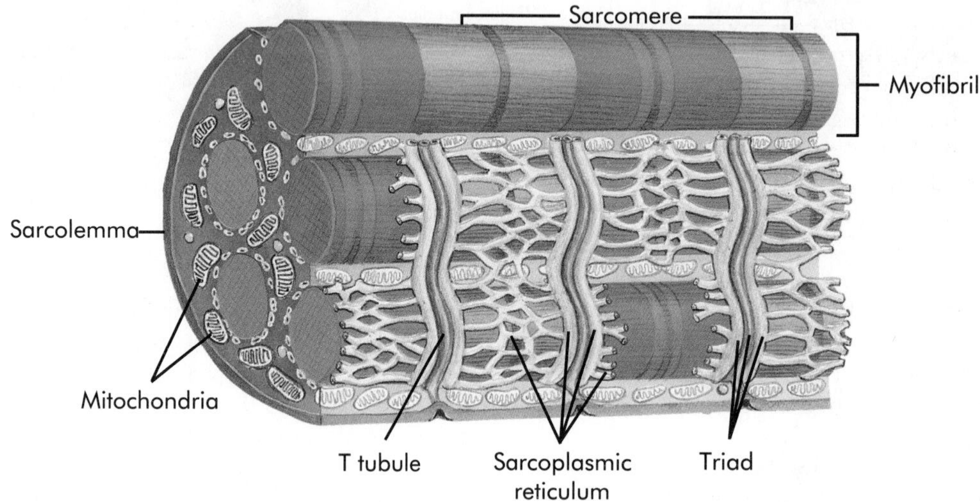

Figure 36-14 ■ **Myofibrils.** Myofibrils of a skeletal muscle fiber (cells) and overall organization of skeletal muscle. (From Thibodeau GA, Patton KT: *Anatomy & physiology,* ed 6, St Louis, 2007, Mosby.)

TABLE 36-4

Characteristics of Muscle Fibers

Characteristics	Type I (Red)	Type II (White)
Anatomic location	Deep axial portion of surface muscle	Surface portion of surface muscle
Contraction speed	Slow	Fast
Motor neuron type	Type I, α	Type II, A
Firing frequency	Low, long duration	Rapid, short duration
Resistance to fatigue	High	Low
Myoglobin	High	Low
Capillary supply	Profuse	Intermediate to sparse
Metabolism	Oxidative	Glycolysis
Mitochondria	Many	Few
Enzymes	Lactate dehydrogenase, types I-III	Lactate dehydrogenase, types IV and V
Creatine kinase	Cardiac type	Fast, skeletal
Example (most muscles are mixed)	Greater proportion of slow-contracting fibers in soleus	Greater proportion of fast-contracting fibers in laryngeal and ocular muscles
Glycogen content	Low	High
Intensity of contraction	Low	High
Aerobic metabolic capacity	High	Low
Fiber diameter	Small	Large
Myosin-ATPase activity	Low	High

From Spence AP, Mason EE: *Human anatomy and physiology,* ed 4, St Paul, Minn, 1992, West Publishing.

nerve end plate, where the nerve impulse is transmitted, the sarcolemma forms the highly convoluted synaptic cleft. The sarcolemma is made up of lipid molecules and protein systems. The protein systems perform special functions, such as transport of nutrients and protein synthesis. They also provide the sodium-potassium pump and include the cell's cholinergic receptor. The basement membrane is 50 μm thick and is composed primarily of proteins and polysaccharides. It also serves as the cell's microskeleton and maintains the shape of the muscle cell. The basement membrane also may function in some way to restrict further diffusion of electrolytes once they have crossed the sarcolemma.

The **sarcoplasm** is the cytoplasm of the muscle cell and contains the intracellular components that are common to all cells (see Chapter 1). The sarcoplasm is an aqueous substance that provides a matrix that surrounds the myofibrils. It contains numerous enzymes and proteins that are responsible for the cell's energy production, protein synthesis, and oxygen storage. The mitochondria house enzyme systems for energy production, particularly those that regulate processes such as the citric acid cycle and adenosine triphosphate (ATP) formation. Many other structures are present in the sarcoplasm. The ribosomes are composed of primarily ribonucleic acid (RNA) and participate in the process of protein synthesis. The cell nucleus, satellite cells, glycogen granules, and lipid droplets are suspended in the sarcoplasmic matrix. Blood vessels, nerve endings, muscle spindles, and Golgi tendon organs are also directly located within this structure.

Unique to the muscle is the **sarcotubular system,** a network that includes the transverse tubules and the sarcoplasmic reticulum, which crosses the interior of the cell. The **sarcoplasmic reticulum** is made like the endoplasmic reticulum in other cells. In the muscle cells, the sarcoplasmic reticulum is involved in calcium transport, which initiates muscle contraction at the **sarcomere,** a portion of the myofibril. The sarcoplasmic reticulum is composed of tubules that run parallel to the myofibrils. The longitudinal tubules are termed **sarcotubules.** The **transverse tubules,** which are closely associated with the sarcotubules, run across the sarcoplasm and communicate with the extracellular space. Together, the tubules of this membrane system allow for intracellular calcium uptake, regulation, release during muscle contraction, and storage of calcium during muscle relaxation.

Myofibrils

The myofibrils are the functional units of muscle contraction. Each myofibril contains sarcomeres, which appear at intervals (see Figure 36-14). The speed with which sarcomeres lengthen and shorten during movement directly influences the strength of skeletal muscles. Sprinters tend to have more fast-twitch (FT) fibers than slow-twitch (ST) fibers in their leg muscles, and endurance runners have more ST fibers in their leg muscles.[10] The sarcomeres are composed of two contractile proteins: **actin** and **myosin.**

The myofibrils are the most abundant subcellular muscle component, equaling 85% to 90% of the total volume. On cross section, they are seen to be irregular polygons with a mean diameter of less than 1 μm. Each myofibril is composed of serially repeating sarcomeres, separated by Z lines, which give the muscle its striped, cross-striated appearance. Each sarcomere has a dark A band and is flanked by two light I bands (Figure 36-15). The A band is 1.5 to 1.6 μm long and contains the thick myosin filaments. Included in the A band is a lighter zone called the *H band,* and in the center of the H band is the dark *M band,* or *M line.* The *I band,* which contains actin, is divided at the midpoint of each sarcomere by the *Z line.* Its length varies with the start of muscle contraction.

Myofibrils are composed of myofilaments. Each myofilament is structured in a closely packed hexagonal arrangement, with two thin filaments for every thick filament. The thick filament, along with C protein and M line protein, is made up of myosin. Myosin has two subunits, heavy and light meromyosin, which resemble twisted golf club shafts. The thin filaments are twisted double strands made up of actin, troponin, and tropomyosin (see Chapter 22 and Figures 22-14 and 22-15).

Muscle proteins

Currently, 12 proteins have been identified in the muscle fibrils. (Table 36-5 outlines their distribution, location, and possible functional significance.) The contractile and regulatory functions of actin, myosin, and the troponin-tropomyosin complex (associated with actin) are the most commonly known. They also account for most of the protein found in the myofibril.

Nonprotein constituents of muscle

Substances such as nitrogen, creatine, creatinine, phosphocreatine, purines, uric acid, and amino acids all serve in the complex process of muscle metabolism. Energy is provided by glycogen and its derivatives.

Creatine metabolism and creatinine metabolism have been used to measure muscle mass. Plasma creatine is taken up by muscle and converted into the high-energy phosphate compound phosphocreatine by the enzyme creatine kinase. Creatinine is formed in muscle from creatine at a constant rate of 2%/day. (Tests for plasma creatine are discussed in Chapter 28.) Creatine excretion is increased in muscle wasting. This change reflects the reduction in total body creatine stores and loss of muscle mass.

Inorganic compounds, anions (phosphate, chloride), and cations (calcium, magnesium, sodium, potassium) are important in the regulation of protein synthesis, muscle contraction, enzyme systems, and membrane stabilization. Total body potassium (TBK), measured by the K40 method, has been used to measure muscle mass, also called *lean body mass.* Total body potassium levels reflect changes in muscle mass seen during growth, malnutrition, and muscle wasting.

Components of Muscle Function

The ultimate function of muscle is to accomplish work. Although variously expressed in such measures as foot-pounds or kilogram-meters, work usually refers to the amount of energy liberated or force exerted over a

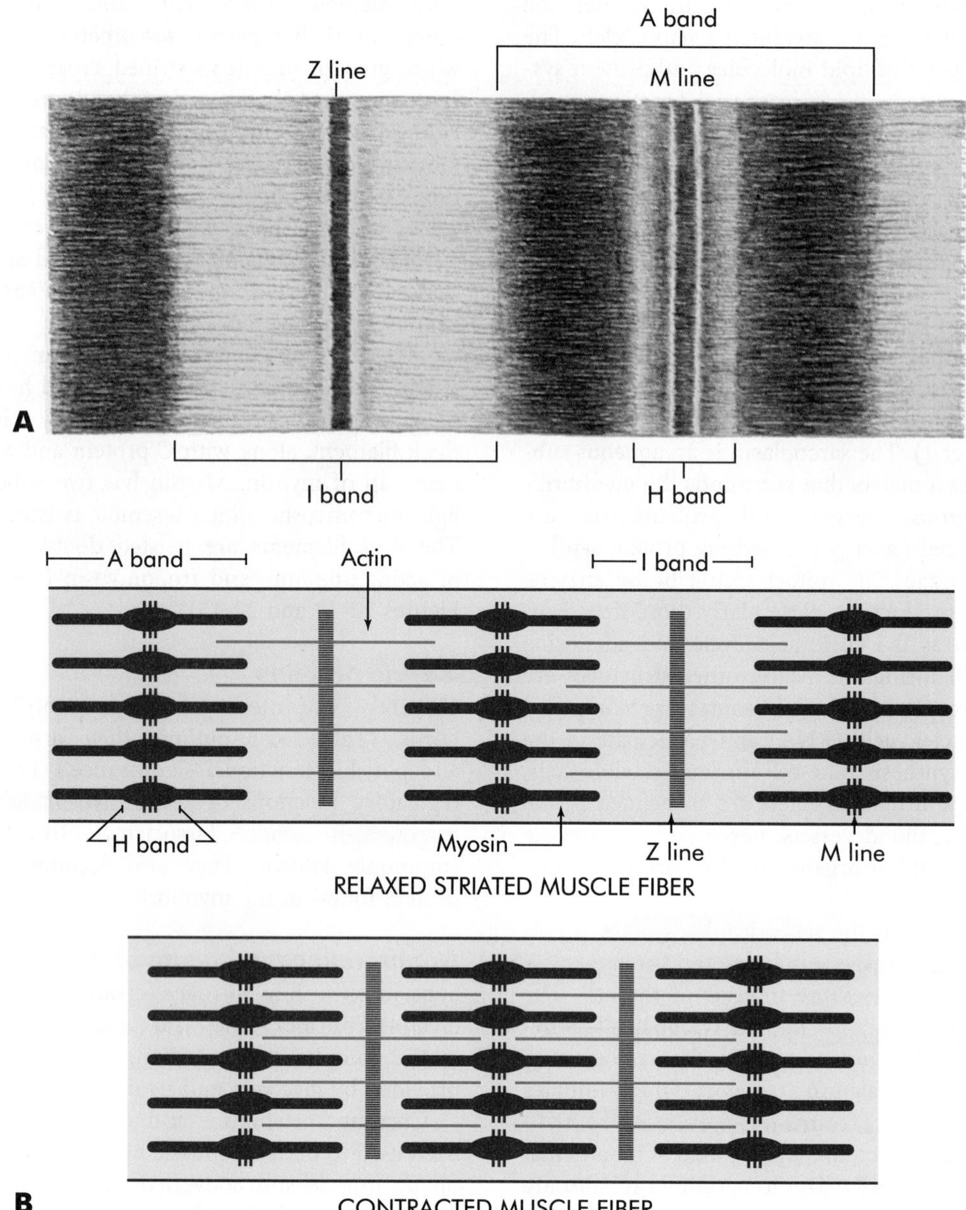

Figure 36-15 ■ **Muscle Fibers. A,** Lines and bands in striated muscle. **B,** Relationships of bands, actin, myosin, and lines in relaxed and contracted muscle fibers. (**A** modified from Thompson JM et al: *Mosby's clinical nursing,* ed 5, St Louis, 2002, Mosby.)

distance (work = force × distance). Muscles usually contract or tense while doing work. Muscle contraction occurs on the molecular level and leads to the observable phenomenon of muscle movement.

Muscle contraction at the molecular level

The four steps of muscle contraction are (1) excitation, (2) coupling, (3) contraction, and (4) relaxation. The process involves the electrical properties of all cells and the movement of ions across the plasma membrane (see Chapter 1). The muscle fiber is an excitable tissue. At rest, an electric charge of −90 mV is continually maintained across the sarcolemma. This resting potential, generated by the separation of positive and negative charges on either side of the membrane, creates an electrochemical equilibrium caused by the selective permeability of the sarcolemma to electrolytes in the intracellular and extracellular fluids, particularly potassium and sodium.

Excitation, the first step of muscle contraction, begins with the spread of an action potential from the nerve terminal to the neuromuscular junction. The rapid depolarization of the membrane initiates an electrical impulse in the muscle fiber membrane called the **muscle fiber action potential.** As the action potential advances along the sarcolemmal membrane, it spreads to the transverse tubules. (The velocity of conduction is much slower in muscle fibers

TABLE 36-5

Contractile Proteins of Skeletal Muscle Fibrils

Name	Approximate Percentage of Myofibrillar Protein	Location	Function
Myosin	50–55	A band (thick filament)	Contraction; hydrolyzes ATP and develops tension
Actin	20	I band (thin filaments)	Contraction; activates myosin-ATPase and interacts with myosin
Troponin	7	Thin filament	Regulatory protein; in presence of Ca^{++}, promotes actin-myosin activation
Tropomyosin	5-7	Thin filament	Regulatory and structural function; links filaments, controls filament length
Alpha (α) actin	10	Z band	Regulatory and structural function; links filaments, controls filament length
Beta (β) actin	2	Z band	Regulatory and structural function; links filaments, controls filament length
M protein	2	M line (center of thick filament)	Regulatory and structural function; provides enzyme creatine kinase
C protein	2	A band (thick filament)	Binds to myosin
Titin (connectin)	Unknown	Z line (thick filament)	Responsible for passive elasticity of sarcomere
Creatine kinase	Unknown	M line	Catalyzes the phosphorylation of ADP to form ATP
Desmin	Unknown	Z line	Structural role; connects multiple macromolecules, transmits mechanical load signals to muscle; possible regulation of gene expression

Data from Buckwater JA, Einhorn TA, Simon SR, editors: *Orthopaedic basic science,* ed 2, Chicago, 2000, American Academy of Orthopaedic Surgeons; Costa ML et al: Desmin: molecular interactions and punitive functions of the muscle intermediate filament protein, *Braz J Med Biol Res* 37(12):1819–1830, 2004; Liu X, Pollack GH: Stepwise sliding of single actin and myosin filaments, *Biophysical J* 86:353–358, 2004.
ATP, Adenosine triphosphate; *ATPase,* adenosine triphosphatase; *ADP,* adenosine diphosphate.

than in myelinated nerve fibers—only 3 to 5 m/sec compared with 54 to 90 m/sec in nerve fibers.)

The second stage, **coupling,** follows the depolarization of the transverse tubules. This triggers the release of calcium ions from the sarcoplasmic reticulum, exposing binding sites on the actin molecule. Calcium affects troponin and tropomyosin, muscle proteins that bind with actin when the muscle is at rest. In the presence of calcium, however, both these proteins are attracted to calcium ions, leaving the actin free to bind with myosin.

Contraction begins as the calcium ions combine with troponin, a reaction that overcomes the inhibitory function of the troponin-tropomyosin system. Myosin binds to actin forming cross-bridges. The myosin heads attach to the exposed actin-binding sites, pulling actin (the thin filament) inward.[11] The thin filament, actin, then slides toward the thick filament, myosin. The two ends of the myofibril shorten after contraction when the myosin heads attach to the actin molecules, forming a cross-bridge that constitutes an actin-myosin complex. ATP, located on the actin-myosin complex, is released when the cross-bridges attach. This is the **sliding filament theory** described by A.F. Huxley in the 1950s, but it is now called the **cross-bridge theory** because of the formation of the actin-myosin cross-bridges, the process of contraction. The process is so named because the actin actually slides onto the myosin, causing the sarcomere to shorten. The useful distance of contraction of a skeletal muscle is approximately 25% to 35% of the muscle's length.

The last step, **relaxation,** begins as calcium ions are actively transported back into the sarcoplasmic reticulum, removing ions from interaction with troponin. The cross-bridges detach, and the sarcomere lengthens. (The cross-bridge theory of muscle contraction is discussed in Chapter 22.)

Muscle metabolism

Skeletal muscle requires a constant supply of ATP and phosphocreatine. These substances are necessary to fuel the complex processes of muscle contraction, driving the cross-bridges of actin and myosin together and transporting calcium from the sarcoplasmic reticulum to the myofibril. Other internal processes of the muscular system that require ATP include protein synthesis, which replenishes muscle constituents and accommodates growth and repair. The rate of protein synthesis is related to hormone levels (particularly insulin), amino acid substrates, and overall nutritional status. At rest, the rate of ATP formation by oxidation of glucose or acetoacetate is sufficient to maintain internal processes, given normal nutritional status. During activity, the need for ATP increases 100-fold. The metabolic pathways for muscle activity in Table 36-6 show reactions to the immediate need for increased ATP caused by contraction. Activity lasting longer than 5 seconds expends the available stored ATP and phosphocreatine.

TABLE 36-6

Energy Sources for Muscular Activity

Sources	Reactions
Short-term (anerobic) sources	Adenosine triphosphate (ATP)→ Adenosine diphosphate (ADP) + Inorganic phosphate (P_i) + Energy
	Phosphocreatine + ADP ⇌ Creatine + ATP
	Glycogen/glucose + P_i + ADP → Lactate + ATP
Long-term (aerobic) sources	Glycogen/glucose + ADP + P_i + O_2 → H_2O + CO_2 + ATP
	Free fatty acids + ADP + P_i + O_2 → H_2O + CO_2 + APT
	Creatine kinase catalyzes the reversible reaction of ATP to ADP: Creatine phosphate + ATP $\xrightleftharpoons{\text{Creatine kinase}}$ Creatine + ATP

From Spence AP, Mason EE: *Human anatomy and physiology*, ed 4, St Paul, Minn, 1992, West Publishing.

HEALTH ALERT

Soft Tissue Repair

Developments in identifying musculoskeletal progenitor cells (myogenic stem cells) have opened up a new realm of tissue repair. It may soon be much easier to manage difficult problems involving severe tendon or muscle injuries. Mesenchymal progenitor cells are programmed to form fat, bone, muscle, tendon, and cartilage. Transcriptional factors, including the transforming growth factor beta superfamily and other related intracellular proteins, transmit signals from surface cells to the nucleus.

One group of intracellular proteins known as *Smads* has been shown to induce osteoblast formation and appear to promote and enhance skeletal muscle differentiation and assist in formation of tendon cells. Satellite cells found in muscle are capable of tissue regeneration and have been grown in culture. Because they are already established as muscle cells, satellite cells form muscle more precisely than even myogenic cells.

These discoveries present the real opportunity to engineer new tissues that can successfully treat conditions such as muscular dystrophy, severe traumatic injuries, burns, and anatomic defects. The regeneration and formation of new tissue holds great promise for the fields of orthopaedics, plastic surgery, trauma, and rehabilitation.

Data from: Bach AD et al: Skeletal muscle tissue engineering, *J Cell Mol Med* 8(4):413–422, 2004; Towler DA, Gelberman RH: The alchemy of tendon repair: a primer for the (S) mad scientist, *J Clin Investig* 116(4):863–866, 2006.

Stored glycogen and blood glucose are converted anaerobically to sustain brief activity without increasing the demand for oxygen. Anaerobic glycolysis is much less efficient than aerobic glycolysis, using six to eight times more glycogen to produce the same amount of ATP. With increased activity, such as intense exercise, or with ischemia, an increase in lactic acid occurs because of the breakdown of glycogen, thus causing a shift in muscle pH (see Table 36-6). This short-term mechanism buys time by allowing ATP formation in spite of inadequate energy stores or oxygen supply. When the anaerobic threshold is reached and more oxygen is required, physiologic changes occur, including an increase in lactic acid and increases in oxygen consumption, heart rate, respiratory rate, and muscle blood flow.

Strenuous exercise requires oxygen, which activates the aerobic glycogen pathway for ATP formation. During maximal exercise, free fatty-acid mobilization and the aerobic glycogen pathways provide ATP over an extended time. These pathways require oxygen both to maintain maximal activity and to return the muscle to the resting state. Maximal exercise increases oxygen uptake by 15 to 20 times over the resting state. When this system becomes exhausted or inadequate to respond to the need for ATP, fatigue and weakness finally force the muscle to reduce activity with a resultant buildup of lactic acid in muscle fibers. Creatine supplementation may provide short-term benefit in exercises lasting less than 30 seconds by making additional phosphate for rapid resynthesis of ATP during strenuous muscle activity.[12]

Sustaining maximal muscular activity accumulates an **oxygen debt,** which is the amount of oxygen needed to oxidize the residual lactic acid, convert it back to glycogen, and replenish ATP and phosphocreatine stores. For example, after running at maximal speed for 10 seconds, the average person has consumed 1 L of oxygen. At rest, oxygen consumption for the same period is approximately 40 ml. As the person recovers, the measured oxygen debt is 4 L greater than the amount used during activity.

Oxygen consumption is measured to calculate the metabolic cost of activity in normal and diseased muscle. It is an indirect measure of energy expenditure, along with timed tests of activity, heart rate, and respiratory quotient (ratio of carbon dioxide to expired oxygen consumed). Energy expenditure is measured directly by heat production because heat is released whenever work is accomplished.

Another factor that changes energy requirements is muscle fiber type. Type II fibers rely on anaerobic glycolytic metabolism and fatigue readily. Type I fibers can resist fatigue for longer periods because of their capacity for oxidative metabolism.

Muscle mechanics

Muscle contraction cannot be viewed in isolation. Several factors determine how force is transmitted from the crossbridges on individual muscle fibers to accomplish whole-muscle contraction. First, when a motor unit responds to a single nerve stimulus, it develops a phasic contraction, also called a *twitch.* Because the motor unit contracts in an all-or-nothing manner, the contraction that is generated will be a maximal contraction. The central nervous system smoothly grades the force generated by recruiting additional motor units and varying the discharge frequency of each active motor unit. This adding of motor units within the muscle is called **repetitive discharge.**

Recruitment and repetitive discharge of motor units allow the muscle to activate the number of motor units needed to generate the desired force. The total force developed is the sum of the force generated by each motor unit. As the strength, speed, and duration of stimuli increase, the summation of contractions reaches a critical frequency called **physiologic tetanus.**

Other variables, such as fiber type, innervation ratio, muscle temperature, and muscle shape, influence the efficiency of muscular contraction. The two muscle fiber types differ in their responses to electrical activity. Tetanus and duration of phasic contractions, which take microseconds to accomplish, are achieved more rapidly in type II (white fast-twitch) than in type I (red slow-twitch) muscle fibers. Low innervation ratios promote control and coordination, whereas high ratios promote strength and endurance. Muscles work best at normal body temperature, 98.6° F (37° C). Finally, muscles with a large cross-sectional area, such as the fan-shaped pennate muscles, develop greater contractile forces than smaller-diameter muscles. The initial length of a muscle and the range of shortening that occur when the muscle contracts also determine the force it can generate. The long fusiform muscles have a greater range of shortening and can contract up to 57% of their resting length. A certain amount of elongation is necessary to generate sufficient tension and muscular force. The elongation that occurs during the swing of a golf club or tennis racket is an example of how stretch improves contractile force.

Types of muscle contraction

During **isometric contraction,** the muscle maintains constant length as tension is increased (Figure 36-16). Isometric contraction occurs, for example, when the arm or leg is pushed against an immovable object. The muscle contracts, but the limb does not move. Isometric contraction is also called a **static (holding) contraction.**

During **isotonic contraction,** the muscle maintains a constant tension as it moves. Isotonic contractions can be **eccentric (lengthening)** or **concentric (shortening).** Positive work is accomplished during concentric contraction, and energy is released to exert force or lift a weight. In contrast, during an eccentric contraction the muscle lengthens and absorbs energy. Negative work is accomplished on the muscle by the load. Eccentric contraction requires less energy to accomplish and has been said to result in the development of pain and stiffness after unaccustomed exercise.

Movement of muscle groups

Muscles do not act alone but in groups, often under automatic control. When a muscle contracts and acts as a prime mover, or **agonist,** its reciprocal muscle, or **antagonist,** relaxes. This is easily tested by holding the right arm in the horizontal position in front of the body, then bending the elbow while feeling the biceps in the front and the triceps in the back with the other hand. The biceps is firm, and the triceps is soft. As the arm is flexed, the muscles change. When the elbow is completely flexed, the biceps is soft and the triceps firm. Completing this movement causes the agonist and antagonist to change automatically; only the movement is commanded, not the alternate contraction and relaxation of the specific muscle groups.

Other associated actions may be seen during walking; as the foot leaves the ground, the paravertebral and gluteal muscles on the opposite sides of the body contract to maintain balance. One notices the loss of the associated muscle's action when paralysis offsets this process and decreases balance. If a person is paralyzed, difficulty in maintaining balance is noticeable.

AGING & The Musculoskeletal System

Aging of Bones

Aging is accompanied by the loss of bone tissue. Bones become less dense, less strong, and more brittle with aging. The bone remodeling cycle takes longer to complete, and the rate of mineralization also slows. With aging, women experience loss of bone density, accelerated with the rapid bone loss that occurs during early menopause from increased osteoclastic bone resorption. By age 70 years, susceptible women have, on the average, lost 50% of their peripheral cortical bone mass (see Chapter 37). Bone mass losses to such an extent lead to deformity, pain, stiffness, and high risk for fractures. Men experience bone loss also but at later ages and much slower rates than women. Also, initial bone masses in men are approximately 30% higher than in women; therefore, bone loss in men causes less risk of disability than for women. Men's peak bone mass is related to their race, heredity, hormonal factors, physical activity, and calcium intake during childhood. Bone loss in both sexes is related to smoking, calcium deficiency, alcohol intake, and physical inactivity. Bone mass can be gained in healthy young women up to the third decade through physical activity, intake of dietary calcium and other minerals, and use of oral contraceptives. Height is also lost with aging because of intervertebral disk degeneration and, sometimes, osteoporotic spinal fractures.

Stem cells in the bone marrow perform less efficiently, predisposing older persons to acute and chronic illnesses. Such illnesses cause weakness and confusion in older persons and may increase the risk of injury or falling.

Aging of Joints

With aging, cartilage becomes more rigid, fragile, and susceptible to fibrillation because of more cross-linking of collagen and elastin, decreasing water content in the cartilage ground substance, and decreasing concentrations of glycosaminoglycans. Decreased range of motion of the joint is related to the changes in ligaments and muscles. Bones in joints develop evidence of osteoporosis with fewer trabeculae and thinner, less dense bones, making them prone to

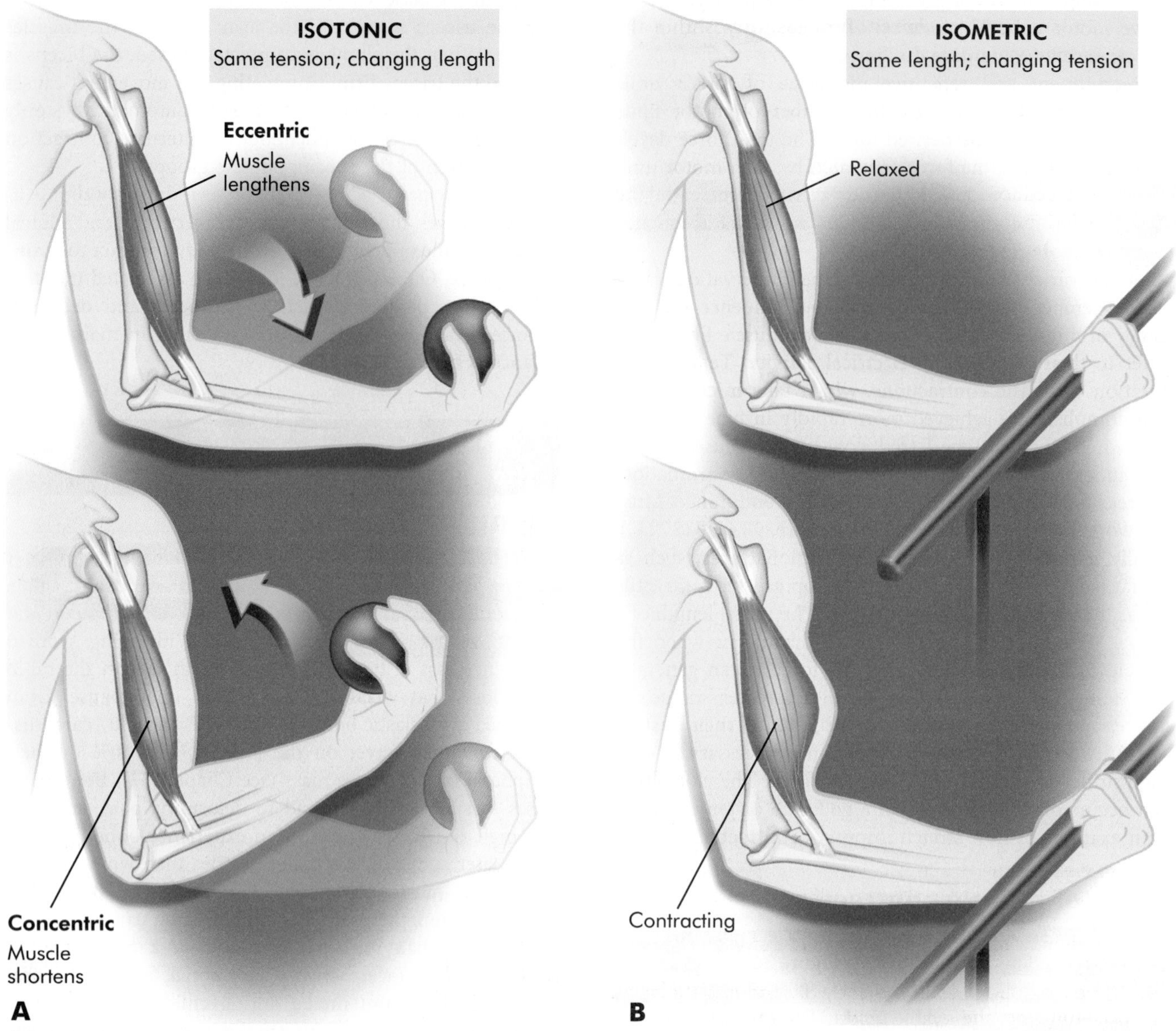

Figure 36-16 ■ **Isotonic and Isometric Contraction. A,** In isotonic contraction, the muscle shortens, producing movement. **B,** In isometric contraction, the muscle pulls forcefully against a load but does not shorten. (From Thibodeau GA, Patton KT: *Anatomy & physiology,* ed 6, St Louis, 2007, Mosby.)

fractures. Intervertebral disk spaces decrease in height. The rate of loss of height accelerates at age 70 years and beyond. Tendons shrink and harden.

Aging of Muscles

The function of skeletal muscle depends on many influences that are affected by aging, including nervous, vascular, and endocrine systems. In the young child, the development of muscle tissue depends greatly on continuing neurodevelopmental maturation. Muscle fiber composition in adults does not change until late in life, but the variation among individuals increases with age. Muscle function remains trainable even into advanced age. Maintaining musculoskeletal fitness at any age can improve overall health.[13] Muscle diseases have a definite association with specific age groups. Muscular dystrophies occur in children, and muscle disabilities related to rheumatic diseases usually occur in advancing age.

Age-related loss in skeletal muscle is referred to as **sarcopenia** and is a direct cause of the age-related decrease in muscle strength. As the body ages, muscle mass and strength decline slowly; thus, strength is maintained into the 50s, with a slow decline in dynamic and isometric strength evident after age 70 years. Type II fibers also decrease. There is reduced RNA synthesis, loss of mitochondrial function,[14] and reduction in the size of motor units. The regenerative function of muscle tissue remains normal in aging persons. As much as 30% to 40% of skeletal muscle mass and strength may be lost from the third to ninth decades. Muscle fatigue also may contribute to loss of function with aging.[15] Sarcopenia is thought to be secondary to progressive neuromuscular changes and diminishing anabolic hormones. There is an age-related decline in synthesis of mixed proteins, myosin heavy chains, and mitochondrial protein.[14] Changes in these muscle proteins are related to declines in insulin-like growth factor-1 (IGF-1), testosterone, and dehydroepiandrosterone (DHEA)-sulfate.

Maximal oxygen intake declines with age. Basal metabolic rate is reduced and lean body mass decreases in the aged population.

QUICK CHECK 36-3

1. Why is one particular type of muscle used for lifting one's legs?
2. Why is adenosine triphosphate (ATP) used for muscle contraction?
3. Describe significant changes in the musculoskeletal system with aging.

Did You Understand?

Structure and Function of Bones

1. Bones provide support and protection for the body's tissues and organs and are important sources of minerals and blood cells.
2. Bone formation begins with the production of an inorganic matrix by bone cells. Bone minerals crystallize in and around collagen fibers in the matrix, giving bone its characteristic hardness and strength.
3. Bone tissue is continuously being resorbed and synthesized by basic multicellular units of osteoclasts and osteoblasts.
4. Bones in the body are made up of compact bone tissue and spongy bone tissue. Compact bone is highly organized into haversian systems that consist of concentric layers of crystallized matrix surrounding a central canal that contains blood vessels and nerves. Dispersed throughout the concentric layers of crystallized matrix are small spaces containing osteocytes. Smaller canals, called *canaliculi,* interconnect the osteocyte-containing spaces. The crystallized matrix in spongy bone is arranged in bars or plates. Spaces containing *osteocytes* are dispersed between the bars or plates and interconnected by canaliculi.
5. There are 206 bones in the body divided into the axial skeleton and the appendicular skeleton. Bones are classified by shape as long, short, flat, or irregular. Long bones have a broad end (epiphysis), broad neck (metaphysis), and narrow midportion (diaphysis) that contains the medullary cavity.
6. Bone injuries are repaired in stages. Hematoma formation provides the fibrin framework for formation and organization of granulation tissue. The granulation tissue provides a cartilage model for the formation and crystallization of bone matrix. Remodeling restores the original shape and size to the injured bone.

Structure and Function of Joints

1. A joint is the site where two or more bones attach. Joints provide stability and mobility to the skeleton.
2. Joints are classified as synarthroses, amphiarthroses, or diarthroses, depending on the degree of movement they allow. Joints are also classified by the type of connecting tissue holding them together. Fibrous joints are connected by dense fibrous tissue, ligaments, or membranes. Cartilaginous joints are connected by fibrocartilage or hyaline cartilage. Synovial joints are connected by a fibrous joint capsule. Within the capsule is a small fluid-filled space. The fluid in the space nourishes the articular cartilage that covers the ends of the bones meeting in the synovial joint.
3. Articular cartilage is a highly organized system of collagen fibers and proteoglycans. The fibers firmly anchor the cartilage to the bone, and the proteoglycans control the loss of fluid from the cartilage.
4. Joints help move bones and muscle.

Structure and Function of Skeletal Muscles

1. Skeletal muscle is made up of millions of individual fibers.
2. Whole muscles vary in size (2 cm to 60 cm) and shape (fusiform, pennate). They are encased in a three-part connective tissue framework. The fundamental concept of muscle function is the motor unit, defined as those muscle fibers innervated by a single motor nerve, its axon, and anterior horn cell.
3. Satellite cells are dormant myoblasts; however, they can regenerate muscle when activated.
4. Muscle fibers contain bundles of myofibrils arranged in parallel along the longitudinal axis and include the muscle membrane, myofibrils, sarcotubular system, aqueous sarcoplasm, and mitochondria. There are two types of muscle fibers, type I and type II, determined by motor nerve innervation.
5. Myofibrils and myofilaments contain the major muscle proteins, actin and myosin, which interact to form cross-bridges during muscle contraction. The nonprotein muscle constituents provide an energy source for contraction and regulate protein synthesis, enzyme systems, and membrane stabilization.
6. Muscle contraction includes excitation, coupling, contraction, and relaxation.
7. Muscle strength is graded by the all-or-nothing phenomenon and recruitment. Speed of contraction is affected by several factors: muscle fiber type, temperature, stretch, and weight of the load.
8. There are two types of muscle contraction: isometric and isotonic. Muscle shortening occurs during contraction but can be seen also during pathologic and physiologic contracture.
9. Skeletal muscle requires a constant supply of adenosine triphosphate (ATP) and phosphocreatine to fuel muscle contraction and for growth and repair. ATP and phosphocreatine can be generated aerobically or anaerobically.

(Continued)

Did You Understand?—Cont'd

AGING & the Musculoskeletal System

1. Sarcopenia, or age-related loss in skeletal muscle, is a direct cause of decrease in muscle strength. A slow decline in dynamic and isometric strength is evident after age 70 years.
2. The regenerative function of muscle tissue remains normal in elderly persons.
3. On average, people lose about one third of a pound of muscle every year after age 40 years and gain at least as much body fat.
4. Reduced basal metabolic rate and decreased lean body mass are also noted in the elderly population.

Key Terms

Actin, 1019
Agonist, 1023
Alpha-glycoprotein (α-glycoprotein), 1007
Amphiarthrosis (slightly movable joint), 1011
Antagonist, 1023
Appendicular skeleton, 1008
Articular cartilage, 1012
Axial skeleton, 1008
Basement membrane, 1017
Basic multicellular unit, 1010
Bone albumin, 1007
Bone fluid, 1007
Bone matrix, 1004
Calcification, 1004
Canaliculus (*pl.*, canaliculi), 1008
Chondrocyte, 1012
Collagen fiber, 1007
Compact bone (cortical bone), 1007
Contraction, 1021
Coupling, 1021
Cross-bridge theory, 1021
Diaphysis, 1008
Diarthrosis (freely movable joint), 1011
Endomysium, 1015
Endosteum, 1008
Epimysium, 1014
Epiphysis, 1008
Excitation, 1020
Fascia, 1014
Fascicle, 1014
Fibril, 1007
Fibrous joint, 1011
Flat bone, 1008
Fusiform muscle, 1014
Glycoprotein, 1007
Golgi tendon organ, 1016
Gomphosis, 1011
Ground substance, 1004
Growth plate (epiphyseal plate), 1008
Haversian canal, 1008
Haversian system, 1007
Hydroxyapatite (HAP), 1007
Integrin, 1006
Irregular bone, 1008
Isometric contraction (static or holding contraction), 1023
Isotonic contraction (eccentric [lengthening] or concentric [shortening]), 1023
Joint (articular) capsule, 1011
Joint (articulation), 1010
Joint (synovial) cavity, 1012
Lacuna, 1007
Lamella, 1008
Long bone, 1008
Metaphysis, 1008
Mineralization (crystallization), 1007
Motor unit, 1015
Muscle fiber (muscle cell), 1016
Muscle fiber action potential, 1020
Muscle membrane, 1017
Myoblast, 1016
Myofibril, 1016
Myosin, 1019
Osteoblast, 1005
Osteocalcin, 1007
Osteoclast, 1005
Osteocyte, 1006
Osteoid, 1005
Oxygen debt, 1022
Pennate muscle, 1014
Perimysium, 1014
Periosteum, 1008
Physiologic tetanus, 1023
Proteoglycan, 1007
Relaxation, 1021
Remodeling, 1008
Repetitive discharge, 1023
Resorb, 1004
Ruffled border, 1005
Sarcolemma, 1017
Sarcomere, 1019
Sarcopenia, 1024
Sarcoplasm, 1019
Sarcoplasmic reticulum, 1019
Sarcotubular system, 1019
Sarcotubule, 1019
Short bone, 1008
Sialoprotein, 1007
Skeletal muscle (voluntary, striated, or extrafusal muscle), 1015
Sliding filament theory, 1021
Spindle, 1016
Spongy bone (cancellous bone), 1007
Suture, 1011
Symphysis, 1011
Synarthrosis (immovable joint), 1011
Synchondrosis, 1011
Syndesmosis, 1011
Synovial fluid, 1012
Synovial joint, 1014
Synovial membrane, 1012
Tendon, 1014
Tidemark, 1013
Trabecula, 1008
Transverse tubule, 1019
Type I fiber (slow-twitch fiber), 1016
Type II fiber (white fast-motor), 1016
Voluntary muscle, 1016

References

1. Kuo P-L et al: Bone morphogenic protein-2 and -4 (BMP-2 and -4) mediates fraxetin-induced maturation and differentiation in human osteoblast-like cell lines, *Biol Pharm Bull* 29 (1):119–124, 2006.
2. Jorgensen NR: Short-range intercellular calcium signaling in bone, *APMIS Suppl* 118:5–36, 2005.
3. Hofbauer LC, Schoppert M: Clinical implications of the osteoprotegerin/RANKL/RANK system for bone and vascular diseases, *JAMA* 292(4):490–495, 2004.
4. Dequeker J: Bone structure and function, In Klippel JH, Dieppe PA, editors: *Rheumatology*, St Louis, 1998, Mosby.
5. Yin T, Li L: The stem cell niches in bone, *J Clin Invest* 116(5): 1195–1201, 2006.

References—Cont'd

6. Ross FP, Christiano AM: Nothing but skin and bone, *J Clin Invest* 116(5):1140–1149, 2006.
7. Han Y et al: Mechanotransduction and strain amplification in osteocyte cell processes, *Proc Natl Acad Sci* 101(4): 16689–16694, 2004.
8. Tapscott SJ: The circuitry of a master switch: myoD and the regulation of skeletal muscle gene transcription, *Development* 132:2585–2595, 2005.
9. Chen Y, Zajac JD, MacLean HE: Androgen regulation of satellite cell function, *J Endocrinol* 186:21–31, 2005.
10. Zierath JR, Hawley JA: Skeletal muscle fiber type: influence on contractile and metabolic properties, *PLoS Biol* 2(10):e348, 2004.
11. Liu X, Pollack GH: Stepwise sliding of single actin and myosin filaments, *Biophysical J* 86:353–358, 2004.
12. Paddon-Jones D, Bϕrsheim E, Wolfe RR: Potential ergogenic effects of arginine and creatine supplementation, *J Nutr* 134 (10 suppl):2888S–2894S, 2004.
13. Rennie MJ: Body maintenance and repair: how food and exercise keep the musculoskeletal system in good shape, *Exp Physiol* 80(4):427–436, 2005.
14. Nair KS: Aging muscle, *Am J Nutr* 81:953–963, 2005.
15. Katsiaras A et al: Skeletal muscle fatigue, strength, and quality in the elderly: the Health ABC study, *J Appl Physiol* 99:210–216, 2005.

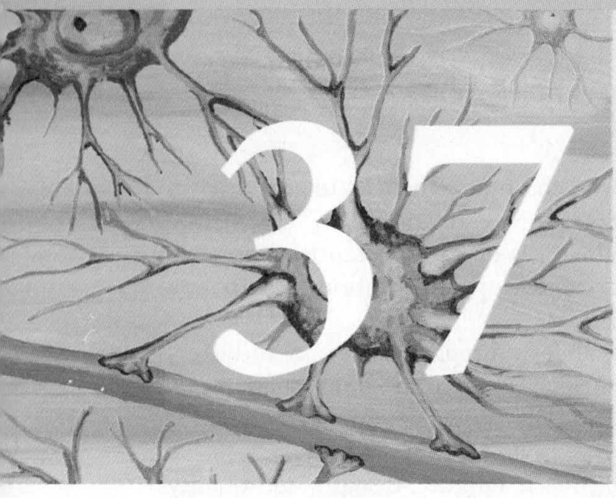

37 ALTERATIONS OF MUSCULOSKELETAL FUNCTION

Christy L. Crowther ■ Kathryn L. McCance

CHAPTER OUTLINE

ELECTRONIC RESOURCES

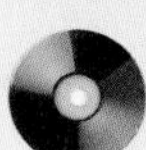

Companion CD
- Review Questions and Answers
- Animations

evolve Website
http://evolve.elsevier.com/Huether/
- Quick Check Answers
- Key Terms Exercises
- Critical Thinking Questions with Answers
- Algorithm Completion Exercises
- WebLinks

Musculoskeletal injuries include fractures, dislocations, sprains, and strains. Fractures are the most serious. Alterations in bones, joints, and muscles may be caused by metabolic disorders, infections, inflammatory or noninflammatory diseases, or tumors. The most common disease affecting bone is osteoporosis; much attention and debate has been focused on its risk factors and pathophysiology. A group of disorders, known collectively as *myositis,* that cause inflammatory changes in muscles are increasing in incidence as well.

MUSCULOSKELETAL INJURIES

Trauma is referred to as the "neglected disease." It is the leading cause of death of people ages 1 to 44 years of all races and socioeconomic levels. Each year, more than 150,000 persons in the United States die from accidents and 500,000 are permanently disabled.[1]

Musculoskeletal injuries have a major impact on patients, families, and society in general because of the physical and psychologic effects of limitation on daily activities, pain, and decreased quality of life; direct costs of diagnosis and treatments; and the indirect economic costs related to the loss of employment and decreased productivity.

Skeletal Trauma

Fractures

A **fracture** is a break in the continuity of a bone. A break occurs when force is applied that exceeds the tensile or compressive strength of the bone. The incidence of fractures varies for individual bones according to age and gender, with the highest incidence of fractures in young males (between the ages of 15 and 24 years) and older persons (65 years of age and older). Fractures of healthy bones, particularly the tibia, clavicle, and lower humerus, tend to occur in young persons and to be the result of trauma. Fractures of the hands and feet are usually caused by accidents in the workplace. The incidence of fractures of the upper femur, upper humerus, vertebrae, and pelvis is highest in older adults and is often associated with osteoporosis (see p. 1036). Hip fractures, the most serious outcome of osteoporosis are occurring much more often because the world's population is aging.[2]

Classification of fractures

Fractures can be classified as complete or incomplete and open or closed (Figure 37-1). In a **complete fracture,** the bone is broken all the way through, whereas in an **incomplete fracture,** the bone is damaged but is still in one piece. Complete and incomplete fractures also can be called **open** (formerly referred to as compound) if the skin is broken and **closed** (formerly called simple) if it is not. A fracture in which a bone breaks into two or more fragments is termed a **comminuted fracture.** Fractures are also classified according to the direction of the fracture line. A **linear fracture** runs parallel to the long axis of the bone. An **oblique fracture** occurs at an oblique angle to the shaft of the bone.

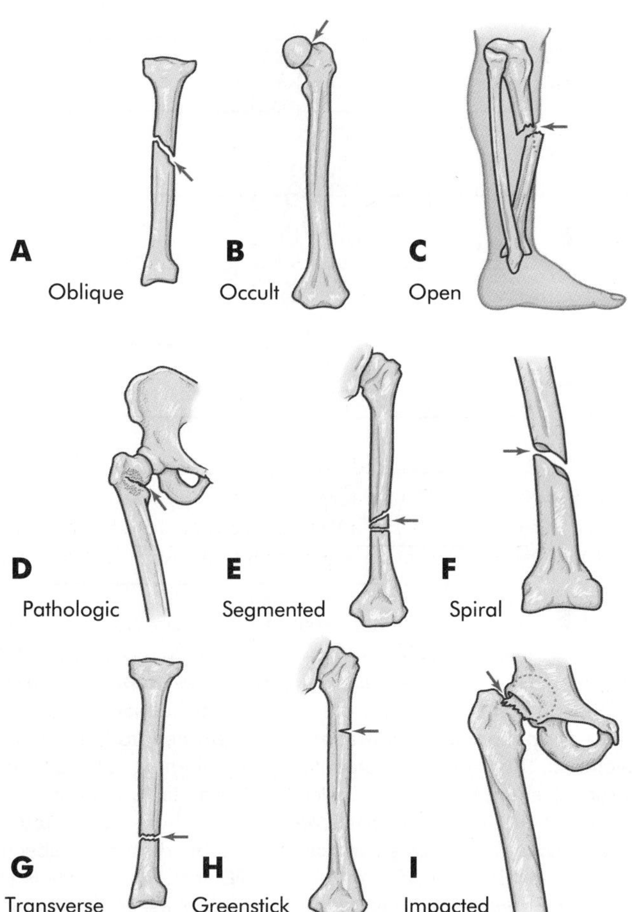

Figure 37-1 ■ Examples of Types of Bone Fractures. A, Oblique: fracture at oblique angle across both cortices. *Cause:* Direct or indirect energy, with angulation and some compression. **B,** Occult: Fracture that is hidden or not readily discernible. *Cause:* Minor force or energy. **C,** Open: Skin broken over fracture; possible soft tissue trauma. *Cause:* Moderate to severe energy that is continuous and exceeds tissue tolerances. **D,** Pathologic: transverse, oblique, or spiral fracture of bone weakened by tumor pressure or presence. *Cause:* Minor energy or force, which may be direct or indirect. **E,** Comminuted: Fracture with two or more pieces or segments. *Cause:* Direct or indirect moderate to severe force. **F,** Spiral: Fracture that curves around cortices and may become displaced by twist. *Cause:* Direct or indirect twisting energy or force with distal part held or unable to move. **G,** Transverse: horizontal break through bone. *Cause:* Direct or indirect energy toward bone. **H,** Greenstick: Break in only one cortex of bone. *Cause:* Minor direct or indirect energy. **I,** Impacted: Fracture with one end wedged into opposite end of inside fractured fragment. *Cause:* Compressive axial energy or force directly to distal fragment. (Redrawn from Mourad L: Musculoskeletal system. In Thompson JM et al, editors: *Mosby's clinical nursing,* ed 7, St Louis, 2002, Mosby.)

A **spiral fracture** encircles the bone, and a **transverse fracture** occurs straight across the bone.

Incomplete fractures tend to occur in the more flexible, growing bones of children. The three main types of incomplete fractures are greenstick, torus, and bowing fractures. A **greenstick fracture** perforates one cortex and splinters the spongy bone. The name is derived from the damage sustained by a young tree branch (a green stick) when it is bent sharply. The outer surface is disrupted, but the inner surface remains intact. Greenstick fractures typically occur in the proximal metaphysis or diaphysis of the tibia, radius, and ulna. In a **torus fracture,** the cortex buckles but does not break. **Bowing fractures** usually occur when longitudinal force is applied to bone. This type of fracture is common in children and usually involves the paired radius-ulna or the fibula-tibia. A complete diaphyseal fracture occurs in one of the bones of the pair, which disperses the stress sufficiently to prevent a complete fracture of the second bone, which bows rather than breaks. A bowing fracture resists correction (reduction) because the force necessary to reduce it must be equal to the force that bowed it. Treatment of bowing fractures is also difficult because the bowed bone interferes with reduction of the fractured bone. Types of fractures are summarized in Table 37-1.

TABLE 37-1

Types of Fractures

Type of Fracture	Definition
TYPICAL COMPLETE FRACTURES	
Closed	Noncommunicating wound between bone and skin
Open	Communicating wound between bone and skin
Comminuted	Multiple bone fragments
Linear	Fracture line parallel to long axis of bone
Oblique	Fracture line at an angle to long axis of bone
Spiral	Fracture line encircling bone (as a spiral staircase)
Transverse	Fracture line perpendicular to long axis of bone
Impacted	Fracture fragments pushed into each other
Pathologic	Fracture at a point where the bone has been weakened by disease, for example, by tumors or osteoporosis
Avulsion	A fragment of bone connected to a ligament or tendon breaks off from the main bone
Compression	Fracture wedged or squeezed together on one side of bone
Displaced	Fracture with one, both, or all fragments out of normal alignment
Extracapsular	Fragment close to the joint but remains outside the joint capsule
Intracapsular	Fragment within the joint capsule
TYPICAL INCOMPLETE FRACTURES	
Greenstick	Break in one cortex of bone with splintering of inner bone surface, commonly occurs in children and elderly persons
Torus	Buckling of cortex
Bowing	Bending of bone
Stress	Microfracture
Transchondral	Separation of cartilaginous joint surface (articular cartilage) from main shaft of bone

Fractures may be further classified by cause as pathologic, stress, or transchondral fractures. A **pathologic fracture** is a break at the site of a preexisting abnormality, usually by force that would not fracture a normal bone. Any disease process that weakens a bone (especially the cortex) predisposes the bone to pathologic fracture. Pathologic fractures are commonly associated with tumors, osteoporosis, infections, and metabolic bone disorders.

Stress fractures occur in normal or abnormal bone that is subjected to repeated stress, such as occurs during athletics. The stress is less than the stress that usually causes a fracture. Two types of stress fractures are recognized: fatigue fracture and insufficiency fracture. A **fatigue fracture** is caused by abnormal stress or torque applied to a bone with normal ability to deform and recover. Fatigue fractures usually occur in individuals who engage in a new or different activity that is both strenuous and repetitive (e.g., joggers, skaters, dancers, military recruits). Because gains in muscle strength occur more rapidly than gains in bone strength, the newly developed muscles place exaggerated stress on the bones that are not yet ready for the additional stress. The imbalance between muscle and bone development causes microfractures to develop in the cortex. If the activity is controlled and increased gradually, new bone formation catches up to the increased demands and microfractures do not occur.

Insufficiency fractures are stress fractures that occur in bones lacking the normal ability to deform and recover; a fracture can occur as a result of normal weight bearing or activity. Rheumatoid arthritis, osteoporosis, Paget disease, osteomalacia, rickets, hyperparathyroidism, and radiation therapy all cause bone to lose its normal ability to deform and recover (i.e., the stress of normal weight bearing or activity fractures the bone).

A **transchondral fracture** consists of fragmentation and separation of a portion of the articular cartilage that covers the end of a bone at a joint. (Joint structures are defined in Chapter 36.) Single or multiple sites may be fractured, and the fragments may consist of cartilage alone or cartilage and bone. Typical sites of transchondral fracture are the distal femur, the ankle, the kneecap, the elbow, and the wrist. Transchondral fractures are most prevalent in adolescents.

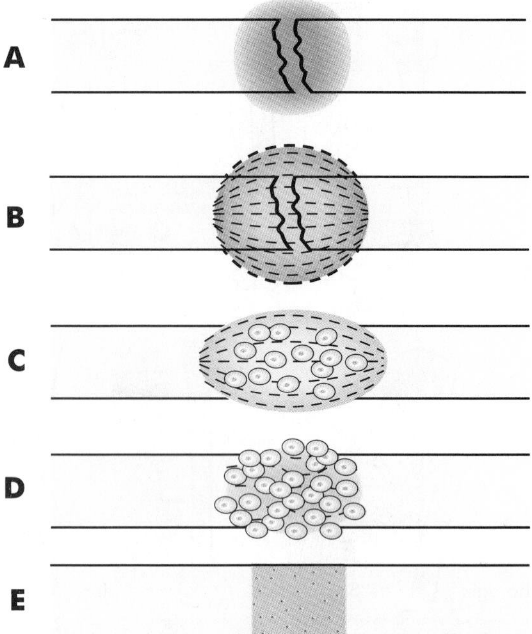

Figure 37-2 ■ **Bone Healing (Schematic Representation).** **A**, Bleeding at broken ends of the bone with subsequent hematoma formation. **B**, Organization of hematoma into fibrous network. **C**, Invasion of osteoblasts, lengthening of collagen strands, and deposition of calcium. **D**, Callus formation; new bone is built up as osteoclasts destroy dead bone. **E**, Remodeling is accomplished as excess callus is reabsorbed and trabecular bone is laid down. (From Monahan FD et al: *Phipps' Medical-surgical nursing: health and illness perspectives,* ed 8, St Louis, 2007, Mosby.)

PATHOPHYSIOLOGY When a bone is broken, the periosteum and blood vessels in the cortex, marrow, and surrounding soft tissues are disrupted. Bleeding occurs from the damaged ends of the bone and from the neighboring soft tissue. A clot (hematoma) forms within the medullary canal, between the fractured ends of the bone, and beneath the periosteum (Figure 37-2). Bone tissue immediately adjacent to the fracture dies. This dead tissue (along with any debris in the fracture area) stimulates an intense inflammatory response characterized by vasodilation, exudation of plasma and leukocytes, and infiltration by inflammatory leukocytes, growth factors, and mast cells that simultaneously decalcify the fractured bone ends. Within 48 hours after the injury, vascular tissue from surrounding soft tissue and the marrow cavity invades the fracture area, and blood flow to the entire bone increases. Bone-forming cells in the periosteum, endosteum, and marrow are activated to produce subperiosteal procallus along the outer surface of the shaft and over the broken ends of the bone (see Figure 37-2). Osteoblasts within the procallus synthesize collagen and matrix, which becomes mineralized to form callus. As the repair process continues, remodeling occurs, during which unnecessary callus is resorbed and trabeculae are formed along lines of stress as the repair tissues bring it in line with the tissue cells of the host (Figure 37-3). Except for the liver, bone is unique among all body tissues in that it will form new bone, not scar tissue, when it heals after a fracture.

CLINICAL MANIFESTATIONS The signs and symptoms of a fracture include unnatural alignment (deformity), swelling, muscle spasm, tenderness, pain, and impaired sensation and decreased mobility. The position of the bone segments is determined by the pull of attached muscles, gravity, and the direction and magnitude of the force that caused the fracture.

Immediately after a bone is fractured, usually there is numbness in the fracture site because of trauma to the nerve or nerves at the site. The numbness may last up to 20 minutes, during which time the injured person may use the fractured bone or bones to crawl or move from the area. However, once the numbness dissipates, the subsequent

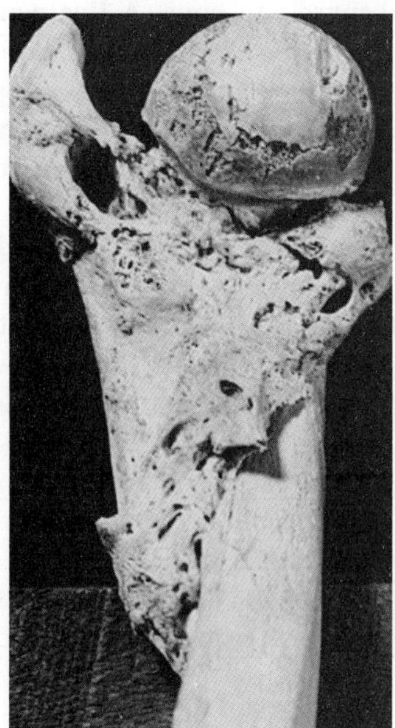

Figure 37-3 ■ Exuberant Callus Formation Following Fracture. (From Rosai J: *Ackerman's surgical pathology,* ed 8, St Louis, 1996, Mosby.)

pain is quite severe and incapacitating until relieved with medication and treatment of the fractured bones. The pain is related to muscle spasms at the fracture site, overriding of the fracture segments, or damage to adjacent soft tissues.

Pathologic fractures usually cause angular deformity, painless swelling, or generalized bone pain. Stress fractures are painful because of accelerated remodeling. The pain occurs during activity and is usually relieved by rest. Stress fractures also cause local tenderness and soft tissue swelling. Transchondral fractures may be entirely asymptomatic or may be painful during movement. Range of motion in the joint is limited, and movement may evoke audible clicking sounds (crepitus).

EVALUATION AND TREATMENT Treatment of a displaced fracture involves realigning the bone fragments **(reduction)** close to their normal or anatomic position and holding the fragments in place **(immobilization)** so that bone union can occur. Several methods are available to reduce a fracture: closed manipulation, traction, and open reduction. Adequate immobilization is often all that is required for healing of fractures that are *not* misaligned.

Most fractures can be reduced by closed manipulation and reduction. The bone is moved or manipulated into place without opening the skin. Closed reduction is used when the contour of the bone is in fair alignment and can be maintained well with immobilization.

Traction may be used to accomplish or maintain reduction. When bone fragments are displaced (not in their anatomic position), weights are used to apply firm, steady traction (pull) and countertraction to the long axis of the bone. Traction stretches and fatigues muscles that have pulled the bone fragments out of place, allowing the distal fragment to align with the proximal fragment. Traction can be applied to the skin (skin traction), directly to the involved bone, or distal to the involved bone (skeletal traction). Skin traction is used when only a few pounds of pulling force are needed to realign the fragments or when the traction will be used for brief times only, such as before surgery or, for children with femoral fractures, for 3 to 7 days before applying a cast. A traction boot is applied to the skin, closed with self-adhering straps, and then weights are attached to the foot area of the traction boot. In skeletal traction, a pin or wire is drilled through the bone below the fracture site, and a traction bow, rope, and weights are attached to the pin or wire to apply tension and to provide the pulling force to overcome the muscle spasm and help realign the fracture fragments.

Open reduction is a surgical procedure that exposes the fracture site; the fragments are brought into alignment under direct visualization. Some form of prosthesis, screw, plate, nail, or wire is used most often to maintain the reduction **(internal fixation). External fixation,** a system of surgically placed pins and stabilizing bars, is another method of maintaining fracture alignment. Bone grafts, using donor bone from the individual (autograft), cadaver (allograft), or bone substitutes (ceramic composites, bioactive cement), can fill voids in the bone.

Splints and plaster casts are used to immobilize and hold a reduction in place. Improper reduction or immobilization of a fractured bone may result in nonunion, delayed union, or malunion. **Nonunion** is failure of the bone ends to grow together. The gap between the broken ends of the bone fills with dense fibrous and fibrocartilaginous tissue instead of new bone. Occasionally, the fibrous tissue contains a fluid-filled space that resembles a joint and is termed a *false joint,* or *pseudoarthrosis.* **Delayed union** is union that does not occur until approximately 8 to 9 months after a fracture. **Malunion** is the healing of a bone in an incorrect anatomic position.

Dislocation and subluxation

Dislocation and subluxation are usually caused by trauma. **Dislocation** is the temporary displacement of one or more bones in a joint in which the opposing bone surfaces lose contact entirely. If the contact between the opposing bone surfaces is only partially lost, the injury is called a **subluxation.**

Dislocation and subluxation are most common in persons younger than 20 years of age and are generally associated with fractures. However, they may be the result of congenital or acquired disorders that cause (1) muscular imbalance, as occurs with congenital dislocation of the hip or neurologic disorders; (2) incongruities in the articulating surfaces of the bones, as occur with rheumatoid arthritis (see p. 1048); or (3) joint instability.

The joints most often dislocated or subluxated are the joints of the shoulder, elbow, wrist, finger, hip, and knee. The shoulder joint most often injured is the glenohumeral joint.

Traumatic dislocation of the elbow joint is common in the immature skeleton. In adults, an elbow dislocation is usually associated with a fracture of the ulna or head of the radius. Traumatic dislocation of the wrist usually involves the distal ulna and carpal bones. Any one of the eight carpal bones can be dislocated after an injury. Dislocation in the hand usually involves the metacarpophalangeal and interphalangeal joints.

Considerable trauma is needed to dislocate the hip. Anterior hip dislocation is rare; it is caused by forced abduction, for example, when an individual lands on his or her feet after falling from an elevated height. Posterior dislocation of the hip can occur as a result of an automobile accident in which the flexed knee strikes the dashboard, causing the head of the femur to be pushed posteriorly from the hip joint.

The knee is an unstable weight-bearing joint that depends heavily on the soft tissue structures around it for support. It is exposed to many different types of motion (flexion, extension, rotation) and is one of the most commonly injured joints. A knee dislocation can be anterior, posterior, lateral, medial, or rotary. It is usually the result of an injury that occurs during sports activities.

PATHOPHYSIOLOGY Dislocations and subluxations are often accompanied by fracture because stress is placed on areas of bone not usually subjected to stress. In addition, as the bone separates from the joint, it may bruise or tear adjacent nerves, blood vessels, ligaments, supporting structures, and soft tissue. Dislocations of the shoulder may damage the shoulder capsule and the axillary nerve. Damage to axillary nerves can causes anesthesia in the sensory distribution of the nerve and paralysis of the deltoid muscle. Dislocations also may disrupt circulation, leading to ischemia and possibly permanent disability of the affected extremity tissues.

CLINICAL MANIFESTATIONS Signs and symptoms of dislocations or subluxations include pain, swelling, limitation of motion, and joint deformity. Pain may be caused by effusion of inflammatory exudate into the joint or associated tendon and ligament injury. Joint deformity is usually caused by muscle contractions that exert pull on the dislocated or subluxated joint. Limitation of motion results from effusion into the joint or the displacement of bones.

EVALUATION AND TREATMENT Evaluation of dislocations and subluxations is based on clinical manifestations and roentgenograms. Treatment consists of reduction and immobilization for 2 to 6 weeks and exercises to maintain normal range of motion in the joint. Depending on which joint is injured, healing is usually complete within months to sometimes years.

Support Structures

Sprains and strains of tendons and ligaments

Tendon and ligament injuries can accompany fractures and dislocations. A **tendon** is a fibrous connective tissue that attaches skeletal muscle to bone. A **ligament** is a band of fibrous connective tissue that connects bones where they meet in a joint. Tendons and ligaments support the bones and joints and either facilitate or limit motion. Tendons and ligaments can be torn, ruptured, or completely separated from bone at their points of attachment.

A tear in a tendon is commonly known as a **strain.** Major trauma can tear or rupture a tendon at any site in the body. Most commonly injured are the tendons of the hands and feet, the knee (patellar), the upper arm (biceps and triceps), the thigh (quadriceps), the ankle, and the heel (Achilles).

Ligament tears are commonly known as **sprains.** Ligament tears and ruptures can occur at any joint but are most common in the wrist, ankle, elbow, and knee joints. A complete separation of a tendon or ligament from its bony attachment site is known as an **avulsion** and is commonly seen in young athletes, especially sprinters, hurdlers, and runners.

Strains and sprains are classified as first degree (least severe), second degree, and third degree (most severe).

PATHOPHYSIOLOGY When a tendon or ligament is torn, an inflammatory exudate develops between the torn ends. Later, granulation tissue containing macrophages, fibroblasts, and capillary buds grows inward from the surrounding soft tissue and cartilage to begin the repair process. Within 4 to 5 days after the injury, collagen formation begins. At first, collagen formation is random and disorganized. As the collagen fibers interweave and connect with preexisting tendon fibers, they become organized parallel to the lines of stress. Eventually vascular fibrous tissue fuses the new and surrounding tissues into a single mass. As reorganization takes place, the healing tendon or ligament separates from the surrounding soft tissue. Usually a healing tendon or ligament lacks sufficient strength to withstand strong pull for 4 to 5 weeks after the injury. If strong muscle pull does occur during this time, the tendon or ligament ends may separate again, which causes the tendon or ligament to heal in a lengthened shape with an excessive amount of scar tissue that renders the tendon or ligament functionless.

CLINICAL MANIFESTATIONS Tendon and ligament injuries are painful and are usually accompanied by soft tissue swelling, changes in tendon or ligament contour, and dislocation or subluxation of bones. The pain is generally sharp and localized, and tenderness persists over the distribution of the tendon or ligament. Depending on the tendon or ligament involved, such injuries may result in decreased mobility, instability, and weakness of the affected joints, even with prompt treatment.

EVALUATION AND TREATMENT Evaluation is based on clinical manifestations, stress radiography, arthroscopy, or arthrography. When possible, treatment consists of suturing the tendon or ligament ends in close approximation. If this is not possible because of the extent of damage, tendon or ligament grafting may be necessary. Prolonged rehabilitation exercises help ensure regaining of nearly normal functions, but recovery may be complicated by posttraumatic arthritis.

Tendonitis, epicondylitis, and bursitis

Trauma can also cause painful inflammation of tendons (**tendonitis [tendinopathy]**) and bursae (bursitis). Other causes, however, of damage to tendons include reduced tissue perfusion, mechanical irritation, crystal deposits, postural misalignment, and hypermobility in a joint. Thus, *tendinopathy* is a more accurate term than *tendonitis* in most cases. The histopathology of common conditions, such as lateral epicondylitis ("tennis elbow") or medial epicondylitis ("golfer's elbow"), is a degenerative process (Figure 37-4)[3] brought about by submaximal overload of the tendon. Achilles tendonitis is inflammation of the Achilles tendon, one that is often inflamed.

Epicondylitis is inflammation of a tendon where it *attaches* to a bone at its origin. Epicondylar areas of the humerus, radius, or ulna, and around the knee are most often inflamed. **Lateral epicondylitis,** commonly called **tennis elbow,** although most affected people are not tennis players, is likely caused by irritation of the extensor carpi radialis brevis tendon and the resulting degradation. **Medial epicondylitis,** referred to as **golfer's elbow,** is inflammation of the medial humeral epicondyle (see Figure 37-4). Epicondylitis is also related to work activities that involve cyclic flexion and extension of the elbow, or cyclic pronation, supination, extension, and flexion of the wrist that generate loads to the elbow and forearm region. A longitudinal study indicates that three sets of risk factors affect the incidence of epicondylitis. They include biochemical constraints and psychosocial and personal factors (including social support at work).

Bursae are small sacs lined with synovial membrane and filled with synovial fluid that are located between tendons, muscles, and bony prominences (Figure 37-5). Their primary function is to separate, lubricate, and cushion these structures. Acute bursitis occurs primarily in the middle years and is caused by trauma. Chronic bursitis can result from repeated trauma. Septic bursitis is caused by wound infection or bacterial infection of the skin overlying the bursae. Bursitis commonly occurs in the shoulder, hip, knee, and elbow.

PATHOPHYSIOLOGY In addition to tearing of the tendon in tendinopathy, evidence also exists of tissue degeneration and disorganized collagen formation.[4] Initial inflammatory changes cause thickening of the sheath, limiting movements and causing pain. Microtears cause bleeding, edema, and pain in the involved tendon or tendons. At times, after repeated inflammations, calcium may be deposited in the tendon origin area.

Usually bursitis is an inflammation that is reactive to overuse or excessive pressure. The inflamed bursal sac becomes engorged, and the inflammation can spread to adjacent tissues. The inflammation may decrease with rest, ice, and aspiration of the fluid. (Inflammation is discussed in Chapter 6.)

CLINICAL MANIFESTATIONS Clinical manifestations are usually localized to one side of the joint. Generally there

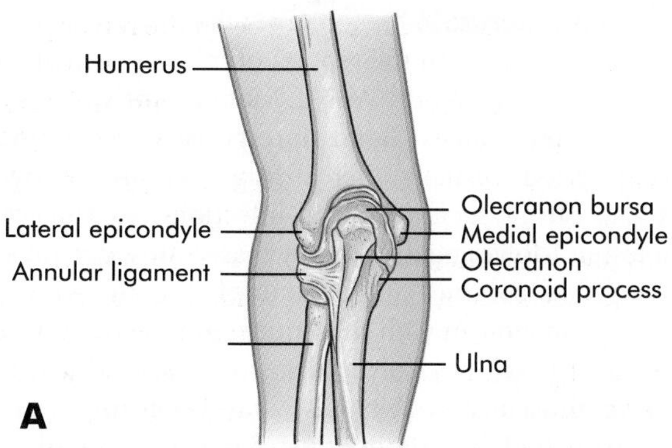

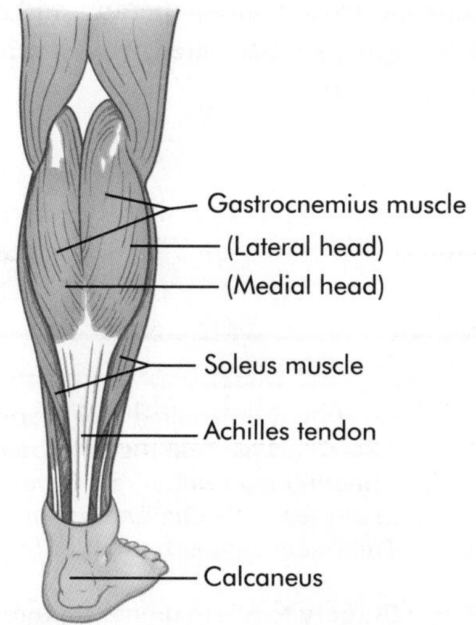

Figure 37-4 ■ **Tendionitis and Epicondylitis. A,** Medial or lateral epicondyles of humerus, site of epicondylitis. **B,** Achilles tendon, site of commonly occurring tendonitis.

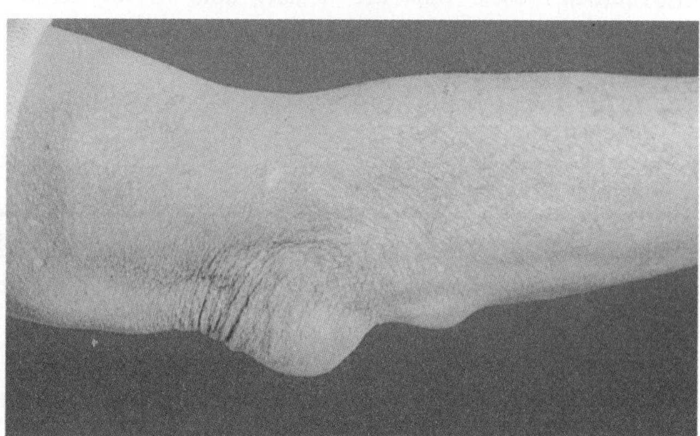

Figure 37-5 ■ **Olecranon Bursitis.** A case of olecranon bursitis in a patient with rheumatoid arthritis. A rheumatoid nodule is also shown. (From Klippel JH, Deippe PA, editors: *Rheumatology,* ed 2, London, 1998, Mosby.)

is local tenderness and more pain with active motion than with passive motion. With tendonitis, the pain is localized over the involved tendon. Pain, and sometimes weakness, limit joint movement. The onset of pain may be gradual or sudden in bursitis, and pain may limit active movement in the joint. Shoulder bursitis impairs arm abduction. Bursitis in the knee produces pain when climbing stairs, and crossing the legs is painful in bursitis of the hip. Lying on the side of the inflamed trochanteric bursa is also very painful. Signs of infectious bursitis may include the presence of a puncture site, warmth and erythema, prior corticosteroid injection, severe inflammation, or an adjacent source of infection, such as an infected total joint replacement.

EVALUATION AND TREATMENT The evaluation of tendonitis, epicondylitis, and bursitis is based on clinical manifestations, physical examination, arthroscopy, arthrography, and possibly magnetic resonance imaging (MRI). Treatment includes immobilization of the joint with a sling, splint, or cast; systemic analgesics; ice or heat applications; or local injection of an anesthetic and a corticosteroid to reduce inflammation. Physical therapy to prevent loss of function begins after acute inflammation subsides.

Muscle strains

Mild injury such as **muscle strain** is usually seen after traumatic or sports injuries. *Muscle strain* is a general term for local muscle damage. It is often the result of sudden, forced motion causing the muscle to become stretched beyond normal capacity. Knife and gunshot wounds also cause traumatic rupture. Strains often involve the tendon as well. Muscles are ruptured more often than tendons in young people; the opposite is true in the older population. Muscle strain may be chronic when the muscle is repeatedly stretched beyond its usual capacity. There is evidence of tissue disruption with subsequent signs of muscle regeneration and connective tissue repair when a biopsy is performed. Hemorrhage into the surrounding tissue and signs of inflammation also may be present. Regardless of the cause of trauma, muscle cells are usually able to regenerate. Regeneration may take up to 6 weeks, and the affected muscle should be protected during that time. (Degrees of acute muscle strain, together with their manifestations and treatment, are summarized in Table 37-2.)

A late complication of localized muscle injury is **myositis ossificans.** Also known as **heterotropic ossification,** this condition is thought to be caused by scar tissue calcification and subsequent ossification. It is often associated with trauma to the musculoskeletal system, spinal cord, or central nervous system.[5] Examples include "rider's bone," in which the adductor muscle of the thigh of equestrians becomes calcified, and "drill bone," in which the same complication is seen in the deltoid and pectoral muscles of fencers and infantry soldiers, as well as football players, after injury to thigh muscles.

Myoglobinuria

Myoglobinuria, also called **rhabdomyolysis,** can be a life-threatening complication of severe muscle trauma, or secondary to malignant hyperthermia. Myoglobinuria is named for the principal manifestation of the condition—an excess of myoglobin (an intracellular muscle protein) in the urine. Muscle damage, with disruption of the sarcolemma, releases the myoglobin. The most severe form is often called *crush syndrome.* Less severe and more localized forms are called **compartment syndromes,** which can lead to **Volkmann ischemic contracture** in the forearm or leg. Crush syndrome first gained notoriety in the reports of injuries seen after the London air raids in World War II. More recently, it has been reported in individuals found unresponsive and immobile for long periods, usually after a drug overdose. Myoglobinuria also can be seen after viral infections, administration of cholesterol-lowering drugs known as statins, certain anesthetic agents, cocaine, amphetamines, heroin, strychnine poisoning, alcoholism with subsequent muscle tremors, tetanus, heat stroke, electrolyte disturbances, and fractures. Excessive muscular activity also has been implicated in reports of myoglobinuria in athletes (such as long-distance runners, ice skaters, and skiers) and military recruits. Status epilepticus, electroconvulsive therapy, and high-voltage electrical shock are also associated with severe and sometimes fatal myoglobinuria.

TABLE 37-2
Muscle Strain

Type	Manifestations	Treatment
First degree (example: bench press in untrained athlete)	Muscle overstretched	Ice should be applied 5 or 6 times in the first 24–48 hr; gradual resumption of full weight bearing after initial rest for up to 2 weeks Exercises individualized to specific injury
Second degree (example: any muscle strain with bruising and pain)	Muscle intact with some tearing of fibers, pain	Treatment similar to that for first-degree strains
Third degree (example: traumatic injury)	Caused by tearing of fascia	Surgery to approximate ruptured edges; immobilization and nonweight bearing for 6 weeks

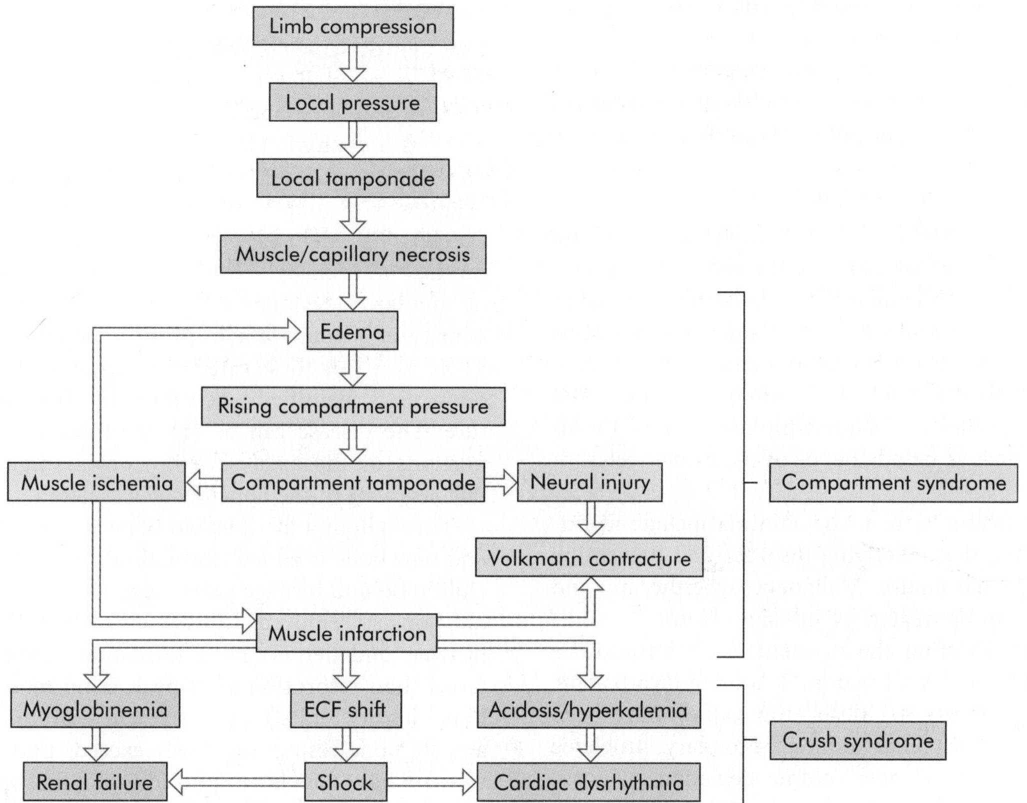

Figure 37-6 ■ Pathogenesis of Compartment Syndrome and Crush Syndrome Caused by Prolonged Muscle Compression. *ECF,* Extracellular fluid.

If the myoglobinuria is caused by fulminant malignant hyperthermia, severe muscle spasm and rhabdomyolysis can lead to renal failure. Other complications include intraoperative rigidity, tachycardia, cardiac dysrhythmias, metabolic and respiratory acidosis, and rising temperature elevations up to 43° C, which can occur at a rapid rate. Cerebral edema, cardiogenic and hypovolemic shock, pulmonary edema, and disseminated intravascular clotting can contribute to the death of an individual with **malignant hyperthermia.**

PATHOPHYSIOLOGY The weight of a limp extremity can generate enough pressure to produce muscle ischemia (Figures 37-6 and 37-7). This causes edema, rising compartment pressure, and tamponade that leads to muscle infarction and neural injury and, finally, results in cell loss. Physical interruptions in the sarcolemmal membrane, called *holes* or *delta lesions,* suggest that the sarcolemmal membrane may be the route by which muscle constituents are released. (The sarcolemmal membrane, the plasma membrane of the muscle cell, is described in Chapter 36.)

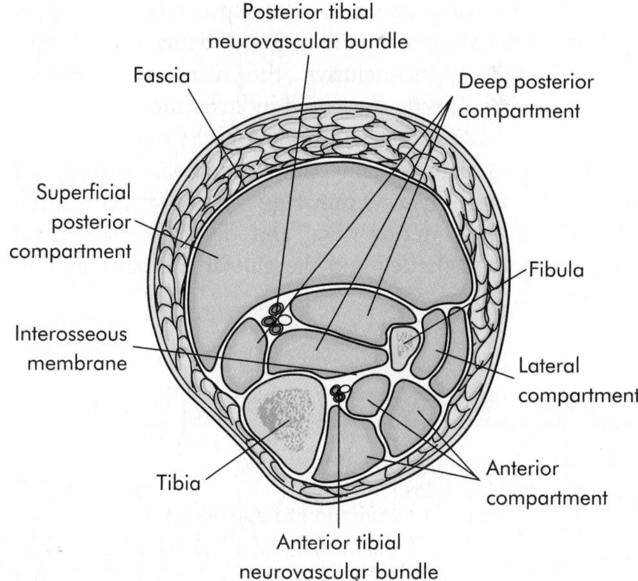

Figure 37-7 ■ The Muscle Compartments of the Lower Leg. (From Mohahan FD et al: *Phipps' Medical-surgical nursing: health and illness perspectives,* ed 8, St Louis, 2007, Mosby.)

CLINICAL MANIFESTATIONS When myoglobin is released from the muscle cells into the circulation, it can cause a visible, dark reddish brown pigmentation of the urine.[6] The renal threshold for myoglobin is low, approximately 0.5 mg/dl of urine, so only 200 g of muscle need be damaged to cause visible changes in the urine. Along with the release of myoglobin, creatine kinase (CK) and other serum enzymes are released in massive quantities. The CK level may reach 2000 times normal (5 to 25 U/ml for women and 5 to 35 U/ml for men). The efflux of proteins and enzymes also includes loss of potassium, phosphate, nucleotides, creatinine, and creatine. Serum hypocalcemia is seen early in the course of myoglobinuria and is followed by late hypercalcemia. The risk of renal failure increases directly with the height of serum CK, potassium, and phosphorus levels.

EVALUATION AND TREATMENT Careful and thorough preoperative assessment should alert the anesthesiologist to the possibility of an individual being susceptible to malignant hyperthermia. A family history of anesthetic problems and previous untoward anesthetic experiences (muscle cramping, unexplained fevers, dark urine) are criteria that require further clarification before administration of a volatile anesthetic, such as halothane, or of the muscle relaxant succinylcholine.

Priorities in treatment of myoglobinuria include identifying and treating the underlying disorder and preventing life-threatening renal failure. Malignant hyperthermia and myoglobinuria can be treated by infusing dantrolene sodium (Dantrium). Diluting the pigment using intravenous fluids and administration of mannitol, sodium bicarbonate, and furosemide (Lasix) to "flush" the kidney have been advocated to prevent renal failure. Secondary problems include electrolyte imbalance, volume depletion, acidosis, hyperuricemia, hyperkalemia, and calcium imbalance. These need specific treatment. Short-term dialysis also may be necessary.

Compartment syndromes may require emergency treatment when blood flow to the affected extremity is compromised because of increased venous pressure, leading to decreased arterial inflow, ischemia, and edema.[7] When clinical evaluation is inconclusive, the rising compartment pressure can be directly measured by inserting a wick catheter, needle, or slit catheter into the muscle. Immediate fasciotomy and débridement have been advocated for pressures of more than 30 mm Hg.[8,9] Compartments often affected are the anterior tibial and deep posterior tibial compartments in the leg and the gluteal compartments in the buttocks.

QUICK CHECK 37-1

1. What is the incidence of fractures?
2. How are fractures classified?
3. How does the inflammation of epicondylitis occur?

DISORDERS OF BONES

Metabolic Bone Diseases

Metabolic bone disease is characterized by abnormal bone structure that is caused by altered or inadequate biochemical reactions, which may be attributable to genetics, diet, or hormones.

Osteoporosis

Osteoporosis, or porous bone, is a disease in which bone tissue is normally mineralized but the mass (density) of bone is decreased and the structural integrity of trabecular bone is impaired. Cortical bone becomes more porous and thinner, making bone weaker and prone to fractures (Figures 37-8 and 37-9). The World Health Organization (WHO) has defined postmenopausal osteoporosis based on the bone density.[10] Bone density is based on the number of standard deviations away from the mean bone mineral density of a young-adult reference population (a T-score). Table 37-3 lists these categories. Severe or established osteoporosis is identified when there has been a fragility fracture. The disease can be (1) generalized, involving major portions of the axial skeleton, or (2) regional, involving one segment of the appendicular skeleton.

Throughout a lifetime, old bone is removed (resorption) and new bone is added (formation) to the skeleton. During childhood and teenage years, new bone is added faster than old bone is removed. Consequently, bones become larger, heavier, and denser. Bone formation continues at a pace faster than resorption until **peak bone mass** or maximum bone density and strength is reached, around age 30. After age 30, bone resorption slowly exceeds bone formation. In women, bone loss is most rapid in the first years after menopause but persists throughout the postmenopausal years. Based on year 2000 census data, it is estimated that 55% of people age 50 and older have either osteoporosis or low bone mass.[11] The major risks for persons with osteoporosis are fractures. Men lose bone density with aging but because they begin with a higher bone density, they reach osteoporotic levels at an older age than do women (see *Health Alert:* Osteoporosis and Men). By the age of 90, about 17% of males have had a hip fracture, compared to 32% of females. Over half of all adults hospitalized for hip fracture do not return to their former level of functioning.[12]

Vertebral fractures also occur in the later years of life, however, they are more difficult to ascertain because people are unaware of the fracture. The degree of compression

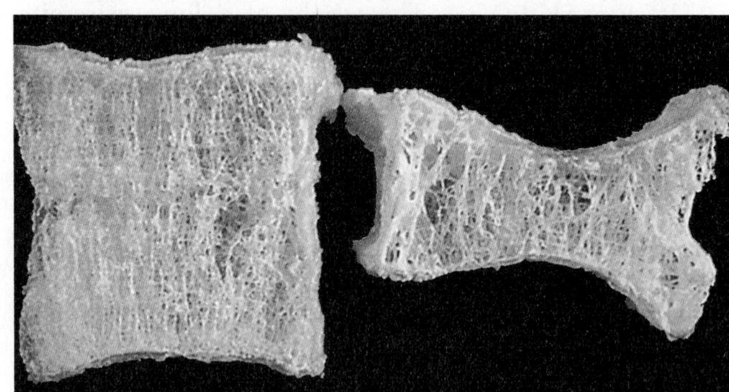

Figure 37-8 ■ Vertebral Body. Osteoporotic vertebral body (right) shortened by compression fractures compared with a normal vertebral body. Note that the osteoporotic vertebra has a characteristic loss of horizontal trabeculae and thickened vertical trabeculae. (From, Kumar V et al: *Robbins and Cotran pathologic basis of disease,* ed 7, Philadelphia, 2005, Saunders.)

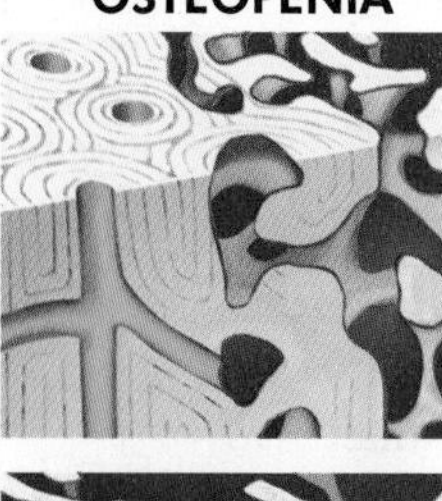
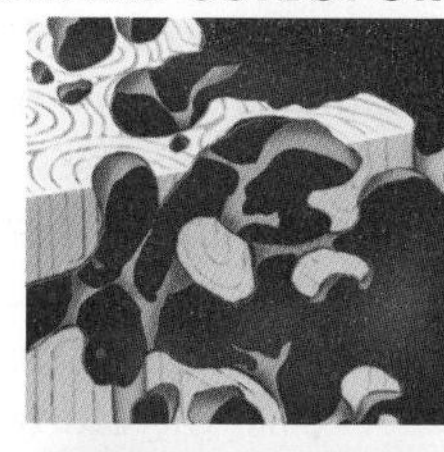
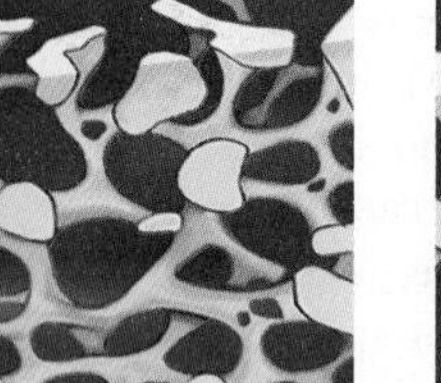
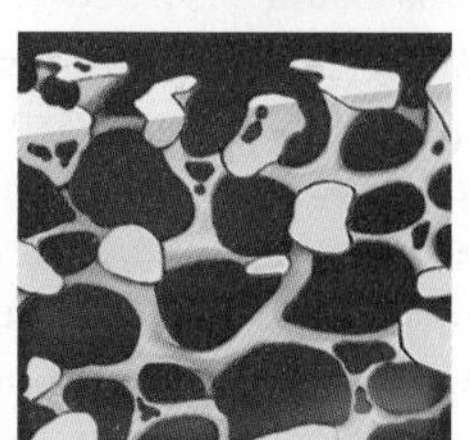
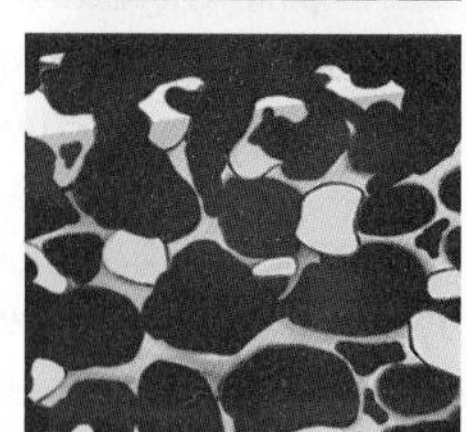

Figure 37-9 ■ **Osteoporosis in Cortical and Trabecular Bone.**

HEALTH ALERT
Osteoporosis in Men

With the emphasis on osteoporosis in women, the cellular and molecular aspects of male idiopathic osteoporosis (MIO, i.e., unknown cause) are poorly understood. The major difference in bone physiology between males and females is in the *level* of gonadal hormones. Although hypogonadism is related to bone loss in men, and androgen levels decline with age in men, it is not at all clear that reduced androgen levels are related to bone loss in older men. Testosterone is possibly anabolic at the bone level, and testosterone increases muscle mass, which indirectly results in higher bone density. In peripheral tissue, testosterone is converted to estrogen, which prevents excessive bone resorption. Estrogen is necessary to bone in men as well as in women. Men who have a deficiency of the enzyme that converts testosterone to estrogen develop osteoporosis and are excessively tall because of the failure to fuse growth plates. Thus, estrogen plays a vital role in the maintenance of bone in men as well as women. Some studies have shown that for a given bone mineral density (BMD), males and females have the same fracture risk, although other studies demonstrate a higher fracture risk in men with a higher BMD than in women.

Data from Byers RJ et al: *J Endocrinol* 168(3):353–362, 2002, review; Seeman E: Pathogenesis of bone fragility in women and men, *Lancet* 359(9320):1841–1850, 2002; Vescini F et al: Does bone mineral density predict fractures comparatively in women and men? *J Endocrin Invest* 28(10 suppl):48–51, 2005.

TABLE 37-3
T-score and World Health Organization Diagnosis of Bone Density

T-score	Diagnosis
0 to −0.99 SD	Normal BMD
−1.0 to −2.49 SD	Low bone density (osteopenia)
≤2.5 SD	Osteoporosis
≤2.5 SD with any fracture	Severe osteoporosis

Adapted from Licata AA: Diagnosing primary osteoporosis: it's more than a T-score, *Clev Clin J Med* 73(5):473–476, 2006.
SD, Standard deviation; *BMD,* bone mineral density.

HEALTH ALERT
Osteoporosis Facts and Figures at a Glance

- Osteoporosis is the foremost underlying cause of fractures in the elderly.
- Approximately 10 million Americans over age 50 have osteoporosis.
- Approximately 34 million Americans have low bone density.
- Four out of 10 white women over age 50 will experience a hip, spine, or wrist fracture sometime during their lives.
- It is estimated that 61 million Americans will have low bone mass or osteoporosis by the year 2020.
- Annual direct medical costs to treat osteoporotic fractures range from $12.2 to $17.9 billion.

Data from Office of the Surgeon General: *Bone health and osteoporosis: a report of the surgeon general,* Rockville, MD, 2004, US Department of Health and Human Services, Office of the Surgeon General.

necessary to define a vertebral fracture is not standardized.[13] Thus, the true prevalence is unknown, but fractures do increase in frequency by the sixth and seventh decades. Vertebral fracture prevalence in men is close to that in women.[14] (See *Health Alert:* Osteoporosis Facts and Figures at a Glance.)

Osteoporosis is most common in whites but affects all races. Whites are more susceptible than other races to osteoporosis caused by loss of bone density with age. Blacks have only about half the fracture rate of whites, probably related to their higher peak bone mass.[15] The cause of generalized osteoporosis remains uncertain.

Bone quality is not defined by bone mass alone (as measured by **bone mass density [BMD]**) but also by the microarchitecture of the bone. Thus, other variables include crystal size and shape, brittleness, vitality of the bone cells, structure of the bone proteins, integrity of the trabecular network, and the ability to repair tiny cracks.[16,17] Because bone density relates to *quantity* of bone, *quality* of bone is not accurately identified by bone density testing. Therefore, bone density testing may or may not accurately identify those who will go on to suffer a fracture.

Osteoporosis is a complex, multifactorial, chronic disease that often progresses silently for decades until fractures occur. It is the most common disease that affects bone. It is not necessarily a consequence of the aging process because some elderly people retain strong, relatively dense bones.[18] In osteoporosis, the old bone is being resorbed faster than new bone is being made, causing the bones to lose density, becoming thinner and more porous. A progressive loss of bone mass may continue until the skeleton is no longer strong enough to support itself. Eventually, bones can fracture spontaneously. As bone becomes more fragile, falls or bumps that would not have caused fracture previously now do cause a fracture. Osteoporosis appears to be most severe in the spine, wrists, and hip.

Postmenopausal osteoporosis is bone loss that occurs in middle-aged and older women. It can occur because of estrogen deficiency as well as estrogen-independent age-related mechanisms (e.g., secondary causes such as hyperparathyroidism and decreased mechanical stimulation). Estrogen deficiency can also increase with stress, excessive exercise, and low body weight. Postmenopausal changes include a substantial increase in bone turnover—that is, a remodeling imbalance between the activity of osteoclasts (bone destroyers) and osteoblasts (bone formers). Increased formation of osteoclasts that causes removal or resorption of bone results in a cascade of proinflammatory cytokines. Increased cytokine activation, especially tumor necrosis factor (TNF), can occur with declining estrogen levels.[19] In addition, estrogen helps osteoclast apoptosis so its decline is associated with *survival* of the bone removing osteoclasts. Biologically, these processes involve the receptor activator nuclear factor κβ ligand (RANKL), osteoprotegerin (OPG) signaling pathways (see the Pathophysiology section), and insulin-like growth factor (IGF). Other causes may include a combination of inadequate dietary calcium intake and lack of vitamin D, possibly decreased magnesium, lack of exercise, low body mass, and family history.[20] IGF is known to help in fracture healing and collagen synthesis and improves conditions for bone mineralization. IGF levels significantly decline by age 60. Excessive phosphorus intake, chiefly through the intake of sodas and junk foods, interferes with the calcium/phosphorus balance.

Estrogen replacement can slow bone loss around the time of menopause; however, osteoporosis and fractures are still common in older women who have used estrogen continuously since menopause.[21,22] In clinical studies of women, data have suggested that serum androgens may influence bone density in pre-, peri-, and postmenopausal women.[14,23] Androgens (i.e., testosterone and dihydrotestosterone) have long been recognized as stimulants of bone formation. Increasing age in both men and women is associated with declining levels of estradiol and androgen, leading to losses in BMD. In addition, progesterone deficiency may be related to osteoporosis. Decreases in weight-bearing exercise is associated with osteoporosis as well. Other risk factors are identified in *Risk Factors:* Osteoporosis.

RISK FACTORS Osteoporosis

Genetic
Family history of osteoporosis
White race
Increased age
Female sex

Anthropometric
Small stature
Fair or pale skinned
Thin build
Low bone mineral density

Hormonal and Metabolic
Early menopause (natural or surgical)
Late menarche
Nulliparity
Obesity
Hypogonadism
Gaucher disease
Cushing syndrome
Weight below healthy range
Acidosis

Dietary
Low dietary calcium and vitamin D
Low endogenous magnesium
Excessive protein*
Excessive sodium intake
High caffeine intake
Anorexia
Malabsorption

Lifestyle
Sedentary
Smoker
Alcohol consumption (excessive)
Low impact fractures as an adult
Inability to rise from a chair without using one's arms

Concurrent
Hyperparathyroidism

Illness and Trauma
Renal insufficiency, hypocalciuria
Rheumatoid arthritis
Spinal cord injury
Systemic lupus

Liver Disease
Marrow disease (myeloma, mastocytosis, thalassemia)

Drugs
Corticosteroids
Dilantin
Gonadotropin-releasing hormone agonists
Loop diuretics
Methotrexate
Thyroid
Heparin
Cyclosporin
Depo-medroxyprogesterone acetate
Retinoids

*Low levels of protein intake also have been reported.

Insufficient intake or malabsorption of dietary minerals is a factor in the development of osteoporosis.[24] Calcium absorption from the intestine decreases with age, and studies of individuals with osteoporosis show that their calcium intake is lower than that of age-matched controls. Other mineral deficiencies also may be important, including magnesium. Deficiencies of vitamins, particularly vitamins C and D, and both deficiencies and excesses of protein also contribute to bone loss. Excessive intakes of caffeine, phosphorus, alcohol, and nicotine along with low body fat (weight less than 125 pounds) also have been considered risk factors. In addition, significant differences in the trace elements (zinc, copper, manganese) were noted in the bones and hair of unaffected individuals compared to those with osteoporosis.[25]

Skeletal homeostasis depends on a narrow range of plasma calcium and phosphate concentrations, which are maintained by the endocrine system. Therefore, endocrine dysfunction ultimately can cause metabolic bone disease. In addition to declining levels of sex steroids, the hormones most commonly associated with osteoporosis are parathyroid hormone, cortisol, thyroid hormone, and growth hormone. (Endocrine function is discussed in Chapters 17 and 18.)

Iatrogenic osteoporosis sometimes develops temporarily in individuals receiving large doses of heparin, perhaps because heparin promotes bone resorption by decreasing collagen synthesis or by increasing collagen breakdown. Osteoporosis caused by heparin therapy usually resolves when therapy ceases. Other medications increasing risk of osteoporosis include glucocorticoids and lithium, methotrexate, anticonvulsants, cyclophosphamide, and cyclosporine.

Regional osteoporosis—osteoporosis confined to a region or segment of the appendicular skeleton—usually has a known cause. Classic regional osteoporosis is associated with disuse or immobilization of a limb because of fractures, motor paralysis, or bone or joint inflammation.[26] A negative calcium balance develops early and continues throughout the period of immobilization. After 8 weeks of immobilization, significant osteoporosis is present, although it may develop earlier in persons younger than 20 years or older than 50 years. A uniform distribution of osteoporosis also has been observed in astronauts and in individuals treated with air suspension therapy as a result of weightlessness.

PATHOPHYSIOLOGY Whatever the cause, osteoporosis develops when the remodeling cycle (coupling)—bone resorption (destruction) and bone formation—is disrupted leading to an imbalance in the coupling process. Osteoclasts are differentiated cells that function to resorb bone. The explosion of new information in the field of bone biology has lead to new understandings of osteoclast biology and bone pathophysiology. Of primary importance is the osteoclast differentiation pathway that is dependent on processes including proliferation, maturation, fusion, and activation. These processes, in turn, are dependent on the availability of stem cells to allow differentiation to occur and controlled by hormones, cytokines, and paracrine stromal-cell interactions.[27,28] Thus, the intracellular communication in bone is key and the molecular regulators are necessary for bone homeostasis. Numerous interleukins, tumor necrosis factor (TNF), transforming growth factor-beta (TGF-β), prostaglandin E_2, and hormones interact to control osteoclasts[29] (Figure 37-10). Staggering in its importance to understand

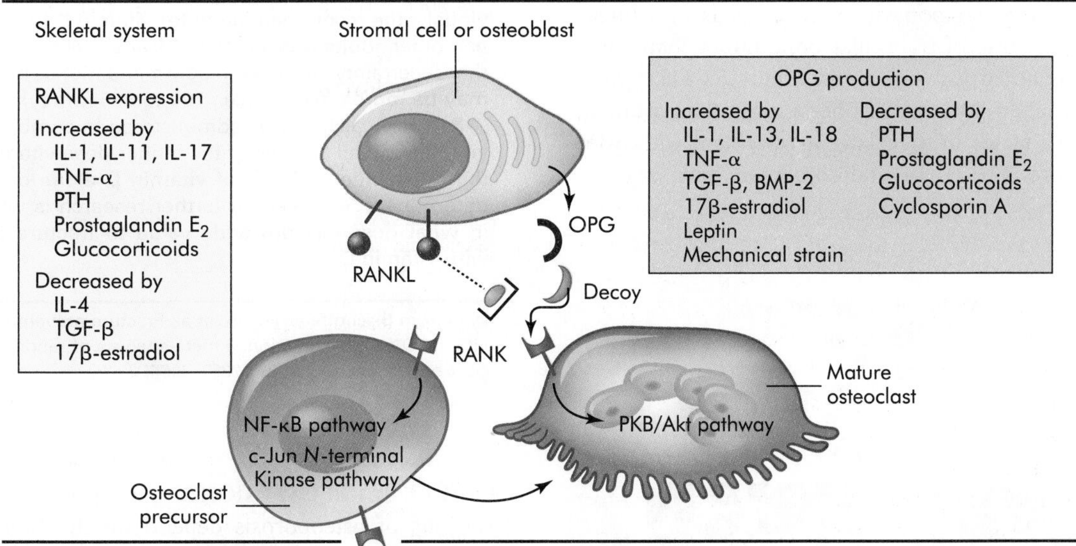

Figure 37-10 ■ **OPG/RANKL/RANK System.** RANKL, receptor activator of nuclear factor κβ ligand, a cytokine and part of the tumor necrosis factor (TNF) family, expression and OPG, a glycoprotein receptor antagonist, are modulated by various cytokines, hormones, drugs, and mechanical strains *(see inserts)*. In bone, RANKL is expressed by both stromal cells and osteoblasts. RANKL stimulates the receptor RANK on osteoclast precursor cells and mature osteoclasts and activates intracellular signaling pathways to promote osteoclast differentiation and activation, as well as cytoskeletal reorganization and survival (PKB/Akt pathway) that increases resorption and bone loss. OPG, secreted by stromal cells and osteoblasts, acts as a "decoy" receptor and blocks RANKL binding to and activating RANK. *BMP,* Bone morphogenic protein; *IL,* interleukin; *TGF-β,* transforming growth factor beta; *TNF-α,* tumor necrosis factor alpha; *PTH,* parathyroid hormone. (Adapted from Hofbauer LC, Schoppet M: *JAMA* 292(4):490–495, 2004.)

osteoclast biology is the cytokine **receptor activator of nuclear factor κβ ligand (RANKL)**; its **receptor activator nuclear factor κβ (RANK)**; and its decoy receptor **osteoprotegerin (OPG)**, a glycoprotein.

Basically, OPG is key in the interaction between osteoblasts and osteoclasts. Osteoblasts and osteoclasts cooperate to maintain normal bone homeostasis. RANKL is an essential cytokine needed for the formation and activation of osteoclasts. RANKL, like an automobile's accelerator, increases bone loss. OPG, similar to the car brakes, decreases bone loss because when it is activated it promotes bone formation. When RANKL binds to its receptor RANK on osteoclast precursor cells, it triggers their proliferation and increases bone resorption. OPG secreted by the bone matrix serves as a decoy by binding to RANK—preventing RANKL binding to RANK—thus preventing bone resorption. Therefore, the overall balance between RANKL and OPG determines the amount of bone loss (Figure 37-11). The balance between RANKL and OPG is regulated by cytokines and hormones. Alterations of the RANKL/RANK/OPG system can lead to dysregulation and pathologic conditions, including primary osteoporosis, immune mediated bone diseases, malignant bone disorders, and inherited skeletal diseases.[29,30]

Glucocorticoid- (e.g., cortisone) **induced osteoporosis** is characterized by increased bone resorption and decreased bone formation. Glucocorticoids increase RANKL expression and inhibit OPG production by osteoblasts.

Age-related bone loss begins in the fourth decade. The cause remains unclear, but it is known that decreased serum growth hormone (GH) and insulin-like growth factor (IGF) levels, along with increased binding of RANKL and decreased OPG, affect osteoblast and osteoclast function. Loss of trabecular bone in men proceeds in a linear fashion with thinning of trabecular bone rather than complete loss, as is noted in women (see Figure 37-11).[31] Men have approximately 30% greater bone mass than women, which may be a factor in their later involvement with osteoporosis (Figure 37-12). In addition, men have a more gradual decrease in testosterone and estradiol (and possibly progesterone), thereby maintaining their bone mass longer than women.[29] The reduction in physical activity in older persons also may be a factor.

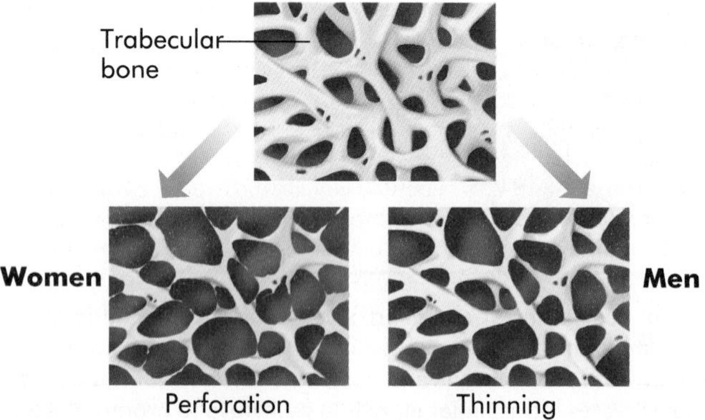

Figure 37-11 ■ **Mechanism of Loss of Trabecular Bone in Women and Trabecular Thinning in Men.** Bone thinning predominates in men because of reduced bone formation. Loss of connectivity and complete trabeculae predominates in women.

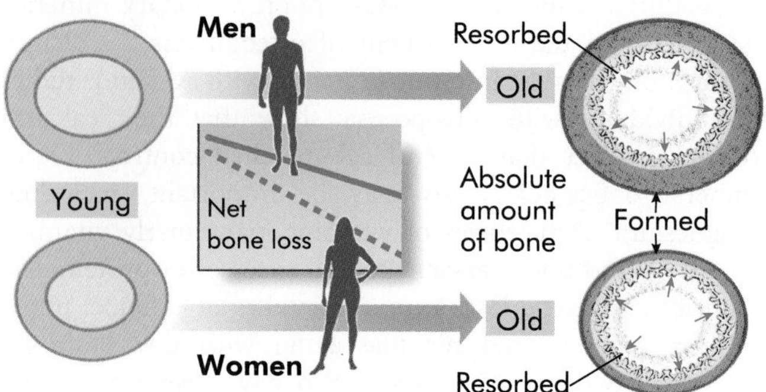

Figure 37-12 ■ **Bone Loss in Men and Women.** Absolute amount of bone resorbed on the inner bone surface and formed on the outer bone surface is more in men than women during aging.

HEALTH ALERT
Vitamin D and Fracture Risk

The beneficial effects of vitamin D on fracture risk are attributed to two explanations: (1) the decrease in bone loss in older persons and (2) the increase in muscle strength and balance mediated through vitamin D receptors in muscle tissue.

In addition, vitamin D has been correlated with a significant (22%) reduction in the risk of falling in older people. Pooled analyses reveal that higher doses (700 to 800 IU/day) are better for reducing fractures than 400 IU/day. Previously, the recommendation for vitamin D in middle-aged and older adults was 400 to 600 IU/day. With new data and the uncertainty of intake recommendations, higher doses may be more effective (i.e., 700 to 800 IU/day).

Because calcium was administered in combination with vitamin D in all but one of the higher-dose vitamin D trials, the independent effects of vitamin D alone could not be determined. Still needing further research is whether and in what dose calcium adds value to fracture prevention with vitamin D.

Data from Bischoff-Ferrari HA, et al: Fracture prevention with vitamin D supplementation: a meta-analysis of randomized controlled trials, *JAMA* 293:2257–2264, 2005.

CLINICAL MANIFESTATIONS The specific clinical manifestations of osteoporosis depend on the bones involved. The most common manifestations, however, are pain and bone deformity. Unfortunately, these manifestations occur only in an advanced disease state. Fractures are likely to occur because the trabeculae of spongy bone become thin and sparse, and compact bone becomes porous. As the bones lose volume, they become brittle and weak and may collapse or become misshapen. Vertebral collapse causes **kyphosis** (hunchback) and diminishes height (Figure 37-13). Fractures

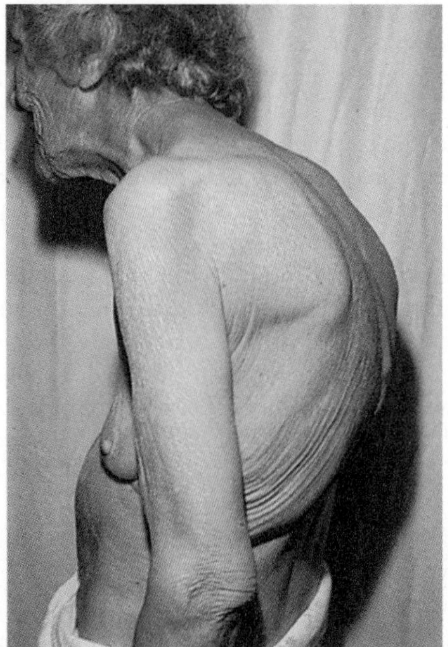

Figure 37-13 ■ **Kyphosis.** This elderly woman's condition was caused by a combination of spinal osteoporotic vertebral collapse and chronic degenerative changes in the vertebral column. (From Kamal A, Brocklehurst JC: *Color atlas of geriatric medicine,* ed 2, St Louis, 1992, Mosby.)

of the long bones (particularly the femur and humerus), distal radius, ribs, and vertebrae are most common. Fracture of the neck of the femur—the so-called broken hip—tends to occur in older or elderly women with osteoporosis. Fatal complications of fractures include fat or pulmonary embolism, pneumonia, hemorrhage, and shock. Approximately 20% of persons may die as a result of surgical complications. Male osteoporosis is usually secondary osteoporosis. Adequate dietary intake of calcium, vitamin D, magnesium, and possibly boron; a regular regimen of weight-bearing exercise; avoidance of tobacco and glucocorticoids; and no alcoholism seem to help prevent primary osteoporosis.

EVALUATION AND TREATMENT Generally, osteoporosis is detected radiographically as increased radiolucency of bone. By the time abnormalities are detected by radiologic examination, up to 25% to 30% of bone tissue may have been lost.

Dual x-ray absorptiometry (DXA) is the gold standard for detecting and monitoring osteoporosis. Quantitative computed tomography (QCT) scans also are helpful. Other evaluation procedures include tests for levels of serum calcium, phosphorus, and alkaline phosphatase, and protein electrophoresis. Serum and urinary biochemical markers are useful in monitoring bone turnover (Box 37-1).[32]

The goals of osteoporosis treatment are to slow down the rate of calcium and bone loss and to stop the disease before it progresses too far. New medications formulated to prevent or treat osteoporosis are currently being prescribed and evaluated. There are new treatments that may rebuild the skeleton (see *Health Alert:* Newer Treatments for Osteoporosis: Strontium and Teriparatide). Treatment includes increasing the dietary intake of calcium to 1500 mg/day along with vitamin D supplements to increase the intestinal absorption of calcium. High intake of phosphorus may neutralize calcium interfering with its benefits. Magnesium supplementation may increase bone growth by stimulating cytokine activity in bone.[33,34] Postmenopausal women may be given estrogen and progestins to prevent bone loss. However, combined estrogen-progestin therapy increases the risk for invasive breast cancer, heart disease, stroke, and pulmonary embolism and is not warranted for routine osteoporosis prevention Other steroid agents—for example, raloxifene—may also be prescribed (see Chapter 32). Regular, moderate weight-bearing exercise can slow down the bone loss and, in some cases, reverse demineralization because the mechanical stress of exercise stimulates bone formation. It is important to reduce the risk of falls and enhance bone quality. An exercise program to enhance strength has the added benefits of reducing the risk of falls and promoting bone quality.

BOX 37-1 Biochemical Markers of Bone Turnover

Biochemical markers of bone turnover are useful in monitoring osteoporosis treatment. Markers of resorption include urinary N-telopeptide (NTx), C-telopeptide (CTx), and deoxypyridinoline. Markers of bone formation include bone-specific alkaline phosphatase (BSAP) and osteocalcin. However, these tests have diurnal variability within the same individual, so there must be significant changes in levels to indicate a difference in bone turnover.

HEALTH ALERT
Newer Treatments for Osteoporosis: Strontium and Teriparatide

A Cochran Database review showed a 37% reduction in vertebral fractures and a 14% reduction in nonvertebral fractures with 2 grams of strontium ranelate daily in a treatment population (O'Donnell et al, 2006). An increase in bone mineral density (BMD) was shown at all BMD sites after 2 to 3 years in studied populations. Lower doses were also superior to placebo and the highest doses revealed the greatest reduction in vertebral fractures. Strontium ranelate did not increase the risk of gastritis or death but slightly increased vascular and nervous system side effects.

Teriparatide is a recombinant form of parathyroid hormone used as a bone formation drug and increases both bone mass and strength (Delmas et al, 2006). Teriparatide significantly reduced the risk of fracture. Much research is still needed on both therapies to understand benefits versus risks.

Data from O'Donnell S et al: Strontium ranelate for preventing and treating postmenopausal osteoporosis, *Cochrane Database Syst Rev* Oct 18(4):CD005326, 2006; Delmas PD et al: Fracture risk reduction during treatment with teriparatide is independent of pretreatment bone turnover, *Bone* 39(2):237–243, 2006.

The anabolic or bone-building drug parathyroid hormone (PTH) has been widely studied, and the results are encouraging. PTH directly stimulates bone formation, particularly in trabecular bone[35] (see *Health Alert:* Newer Treatments for Osteoporosis: Strontium and Teriparatide).

Osteomalacia

Osteomalacia is a metabolic disease characterized by inadequate and delayed mineralization of osteoid in mature compact and spongy bone. In osteomalacia, the remodeling cycle proceeds normally through osteoid formation, but mineral calcification and deposition do not occur. Bone volume remains unchanged, but the replaced bone consists of soft osteoid instead of rigid bone. Rickets is similar to osteomalacia in pathogenesis, but it occurs in the growing bones of children, whereas osteomalacia occurs in adult bone. (Rickets is described in Chapter 38.)

Both osteomalacia and rickets are rare in the United States and western Europe but are significant health problems in Great Britain, Ethiopia, Pakistan, Iran, and India. In the United States, these diseases are prevalent in elderly persons, in premature infants of very low birth weight, and in individuals adhering to rigid macrobiotic vegetarian diets. Breast-fed African-American infants who do not receive vitamin D supplementation have been shown to be at risk for developing nutritional rickets.[36]

Many factors contribute to the development of osteomalacia, but the most important is a deficiency of vitamin D. The major risk factors in vitamin D deficiency are diets deficient in vitamin D, decreased endogenous production of vitamin D, intestinal malabsorption of vitamin D, renal tubular diseases, and anticonvulsant therapy. Classic vitamin D deficiency is rare in the United States because of the addition of synthetic vitamin D to dairy products and bread.

Disorders of the small bowel, hepatobiliary system, and pancreas are causes of vitamin D deficiency in the United States. In malabsorptive disease of the small bowel, vitamin D and calcium absorption are decreased, so vitamin D is lost in feces. Liver disease interferes with the metabolism of vitamin D to its more active form, and diseases of the pancreas and biliary system cause a deficiency of bile salts, which are necessary for normal intestinal absorption of vitamin D.

The mechanism by which anticonvulsant drug therapy results in vitamin D deficiency is not completely understood, but researchers think that the anticonvulsants phenobarbital and phenytoin interfere with calcium absorption and increase degradation of vitamin D metabolism in the liver. Renal osteodystrophy is another cause of osteomalacia.

PATHOPHYSIOLOGY Crystallization of minerals in osteoid requires adequate concentrations of calcium and phosphate. When the concentrations are too low, crystallization (and hence ossification) does not proceed normally.

Vitamin D deficiency disrupts mineralization because vitamin D normally regulates and enhances the absorption of calcium ions from the intestine. A lack of vitamin D causes the plasma calcium concentrations to fall. Low plasma calcium levels stimulate increased synthesis and secretion of PTH. Although the increase in circulating PTH raises the plasma calcium concentration, it also stimulates increased renal clearance of phosphate. When the concentration of phosphate in the bone decreases below a critical level, mineralization cannot proceed normally. Newer research has identified a complex interplay of matrix proteins, hormones, metallopeptidases, and certain proteins as also being involved in the development of osteomalacia.

Abnormalities occur in both spongy and compact bone. Trabeculae in spongy bone become thinner and fewer, whereas haversian systems in compact bone develop large channels and become irregular. Because osteoid continues to be produced but not mineralized, abnormal quantities of osteoid build up, coating the trabeculae and the linings of the haversian canals. Excessive osteoid also can accumulate in areas beneath the periosteum. The excess of osteoid leads to gross deformities of the long bones, spine, pelvis, and skull.

CLINICAL MANIFESTATIONS Osteomalacia causes varying degrees of diffuse skeletal pain and tenderness. Pain is noted particularly in the hips, and the individual may be hesitant to walk. Muscular weakness is common and may contribute to a waddling gait. Bone fractures and vertebral collapse occur with minimal trauma. Low back pain may be an early complaint, but pain may also involve ribs, feet, other areas of the vertebral column, and other sites. Uremia may be present in renal osteodystrophy.

EVALUATION AND TREATMENT Laboratory data may include elevated blood urea nitrogen (BUN) and creatinine levels, normal or low serum calcium levels, and a serum inorganic phosphate level that is usually over 5.5 mg. Alkaline phosphatase and PTH levels are usually elevated. Radiographic findings show pseudofractures and radiolucent bands perpendicular to the surface of involved bones. A bone biopsy is used to evaluate the presence of renal osteodystrophy to determine bone aluminum deposits.

Treatment of osteomalacia includes the following:

1. Adjusting serum calcium and phosphorus levels to normal
2. Suppressing secondary hyperthyroidism
3. Chelating bone aluminum if needed
4. Administration of calcium carbonate to decrease hyperphosphatemia
5. Dietary supplements of vitamin D
6. Renal dialysis
7. Renal transplant for renal osteodystrophy

Paget disease

Paget disease (osteitis deformans) is a state of increased metabolic activity in bone characterized by abnormal and excessive bone remodeling, both resorption and formation. Chronic accelerated remodeling eventually enlarges and softens the affected bones.

Paget disease can occur in any bone but most often affects the vertebrae, skull, sacrum, sternum, pelvis, and femur. The disease process may occur in one or more bones without causing significant clinical manifestations.

Paget disease occurs with equal frequency in men more than 55 years of age and women older than 40 years of age. It is often symptomless, and diagnosis is made by x-ray and radioisotope bone scan. Autopsy data from England and Germany indicate that approximately 3% to 4% of the population older than 40 years of age have Paget disease. It is most prevalent in Australia, Great Britain, New Zealand, and the United States. Paget disease affects several members of the same family in 5% to 25% of individuals.

The cause of Paget disease is unknown, but there appears to be a strong genetic component.[37] A viral connection to Paget disease has also been proposed.[38] The disease arises as a consequence of disorderly bone resorption and formation.

PATHOPHYSIOLOGY Paget disease begins with excessive resorption of spongy bone. The trabeculae diminish, and bone marrow is replaced by extremely vascular fibrous tissue.

The resorption phase of Paget disease is followed by the formation of abnormal new bone at an accelerated rate. The collagen fibers are disorganized, and glycoprotein levels in the matrix decrease. Mineralization may extend into the bone marrow. Bone formation is excessive around partially resorbed trabeculae, causing them to thicken and enlarge. Eventually, Paget disease progresses to an inactive phase, in which abnormal remodeling is minimal or absent.

CLINICAL MANIFESTATIONS In the skull, abnormal remodeling is first evident in the frontal or occipital regions; then it encroaches on the outer and inner surfaces of the entire skull. The skull thickens and assumes an asymmetric shape. Thickened segments of the skull may compress areas of the brain, producing altered mentality and dementia. Impingement of new bone on cranial nerves causes sensory abnormalities, impaired motor function, deafness (because of involvement of the middle ear ossicles or compression of the auditory nerve), atrophy of the optic nerve, and obstruction of the lacrimal duct. Headache is commonly noted.

Extensive alterations of the facial bones are rare except in the jaw, where sclerosis and thickening of the maxilla and mandible displace teeth and produce malocclusion. In long bones, resorption begins in the subchondral regions of the epiphysis and extends into the metaphysis and diaphysis. Occasionally, Paget disease affects both ends of a tubular bone. In the femur, Paget disease produces an exaggerated lateral curvature. In the tibia, anterior curvature is also exaggerated. Stress fractures are common in the lower extremities.

Clinical manifestations of Paget disease in the vertebral column depend on the level of involvement and are caused by compression of adjacent structures. In the cervical spine, cord compression can lead to spastic quadriplegia. Approximately 1% of persons with Paget disease develop osteogenic sarcoma.

EVALUATION AND TREATMENT Evaluation of Paget disease is made on the basis of radiographic findings of irregular bone trabeculae with a thickened and disorganized pattern. Early disease is detected by bone scanning that shows increased uptake of bone radionuclides. Alkaline phosphatase and urinary hydroxyproline are elevated.

Many individuals require no treatment if the disease is localized and does not cause symptoms. Treatment during active disease is for pain relief, prevention of deformity, or fracture. Bisphosphonates are the treatment of choice. Cytotoxic drugs are sometimes used to slow excessive resorption.

Infectious Bone Disease: Osteomyelitis

Infectious bone disease is expensive, difficult to treat, and often culminates in extensive physical disability. Several factors contribute to the difficulty in treating bone infection:

1. Bone contains multiple microscopic channels that are impermeable to the cells and biochemicals of the body's natural defenses. Once bacteria gain access to these channels, they are able to proliferate unimpeded.
2. The microcirculation of bone is highly vulnerable to damage and destruction by bacterial toxins. Vessel damage causes local thrombosis (blockage) of the small vessels, which leads to ischemic necrosis (death) of bone.
3. Bone cells have a limited capacity to replace bone destroyed by infections. Initially, osteoclasts are stimulated by infection to resorb bone, which opens up isolated bone channels so that cells of the inflammatory and immune systems can gain access to the infected bone. At the same time, however, resorption weakens the structural integrity of the bone. New bone formation usually lags behind resorption, and the haversian systems in the new bone are incomplete.

Osteomyelitis is a bone infection most often caused by bacteria; however, fungi, parasites, and viruses also can cause bone infection (Figure 37-14). It is further categorized according to the pathogen's mode of entry into bone tissue. **Exogenous osteomyelitis** is an infection that enters from outside the body, for example, through open fractures, penetrating wounds, or surgical procedures. In exogenous osteomyelitis, the infection spreads from soft tissues into adjacent bone. **Endogenous (hematogenous) osteomyelitis** is caused by pathogens carried in the blood from sites of infection elsewhere in the body. In hematogenous osteomyelitis, the infection spreads from bone to adjacent soft tissues. Hematogenous osteomyelitis is commonly found in infants, children, and elderly persons. (Osteomyelitis in children is discussed in Chapter 38.) In infants, incidence rates among males and females are approximately equal. In children and older adults, however, males are most commonly affected. Osteomyelitis is a common complication of sickle cell anemia and low oxygen tension.

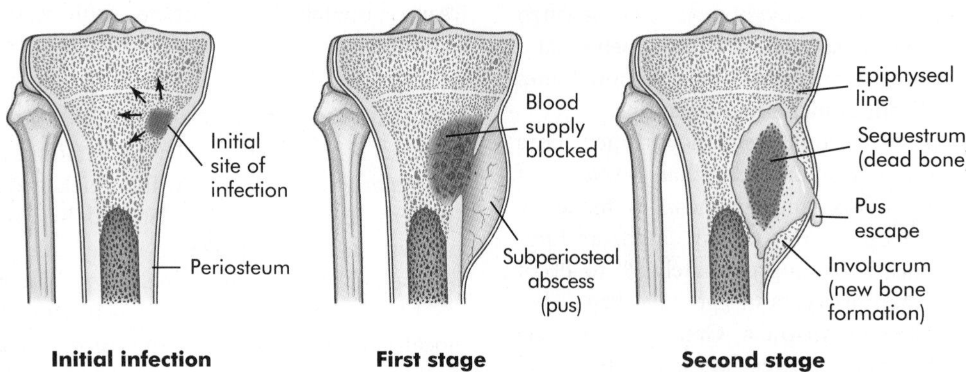

Figure 37-14 ■ **Osteomyelitis Showing Sequestration and Involucrum.**

Staphylococcus aureus is the usual cause of hematogenous osteomyelitis.[39,40] Other microorganisms include group B streptococcus, *Haemophilus influenzae, Salmonella,* and gram-negative bacteria. Group B streptococcus and *H. influenzae* tend to infect young children; *Salmonella* infection is associated with sickle cell anemia; and gram-negative infections are most common in older adults and immunocompromised individuals with impaired immunity. Mycobacterial, viral, and fungal infections occur in immunocompromised individuals.

Cutaneous, sinus, ear, and dental infections are the primary sources of bacteria in hematogenous bone infections. Soft-tissue infections, disorders of the gastrointestinal tract, infections of the genitourinary system, and respiratory infections are also sources of bacterial contamination. In addition, infections that occur after total joint replacements are sometimes the cause. The vulnerability of specific bone depends on the anatomy of its vascular supply.

In adults, hematogenous osteomyelitis is more common in the spine, pelvis, and small bones. Microorganisms reach the vertebrae through arteries, veins, or lymphatic vessels. The spread of infection from pelvic organs to the vertebrae is well documented. Vaginal, uterine, ovarian, bladder, and intestinal infections can lead to iliac or sacral osteomyelitis.

Exogenous osteomyelitis can be caused by human bites or fist blows to the mouth. Superficial animal or human bites inoculate local soft tissue with bacteria that later spread to underlying bone. Deep bites can introduce microorganisms directly onto bone. The most common infecting organism in human bites is *S. aureus.* In animal bites, the most common infecting organism is *Pasteurella multocida,* which is part of the normal mouth flora of cats and dogs.

Direct contamination of bones with bacteria can also occur in open fractures or dislocations with an overlying skin wound. Intervertebral disk surgery and operative procedures involving implantation of large foreign objects, such as metallic plates or artificial joints, are associated with exogenous osteomyelitis. Local injections and venous punctures are significant causes of exogenous osteomyelitis. Exogenous osteomyelitis of the arm and hand bones tends to occur in persons who abuse drugs. *S. aureus* is the most common pathogen. In general, persons who are chronically ill, have diabetes or alcoholism, or are receiving large doses of steroids or immunosuppressive drugs are particularly susceptible to exogenous osteomyelitis or recurring episodes of this disease.

PATHOPHYSIOLOGY Regardless of the source of the pathogen, the pathologic features of bone infection are similar to those in any other body tissue (see Chapters 5 and 6). First, the invading pathogen provokes an intense inflammatory response. Inflammation in bone is characterized by vascular engorgement, edema, leukocyte activity, and abscess formation. Once inflammation is initiated, the small terminal vessels thrombose and exudate seals the bone's canaliculi. Inflammatory exudate extends into the metaphysis and the marrow cavity and through small metaphyseal openings into the cortex. In children, exudate that reaches the outer surface of the cortex forms abscesses that lift the periosteum off underlying bone. Lifting of the periosteum disrupts blood vessels that enter bone through the periosteum, which deprives underlying bone of its blood supply; this leads to necrosis and death of the area of bone infected, producing **sequestrum,** an area of devitalized bone (Figure 37-15). Lifting of the periosteum also stimulates an intense osteoblastic response. Osteoblasts lay down new bone that can partially or completely surround the infected bone. This layer of new bone surrounding the infected bone is called an **involucrum.** Openings in the involucrum allow the exudate to escape into surrounding soft tissue and ultimately through the skin by way of sinus tracts.

In adults, this complication is rare because the periosteum is firmly attached to the cortex and resists displacement. Instead, infection disrupts and weakens the cortex, which predisposes the bone to pathologic fracture.

CLINICAL MANIFESTATIONS Clinical manifestations of osteomyelitis vary with the age of the individual, the site of involvement, the initiating event, the infecting organism, and whether the infection is acute, subacute, or chronic. Acute osteomyelitis causes abrupt onset of inflammation (see Figure 37-15). If an acute infection is not completely eliminated, the disease may become subacute or chronic. In subacute osteomyelitis, signs and symptoms are usually vague. In the chronic stage, infection is indolent or silent between exacerbations. The microorganisms persist in small

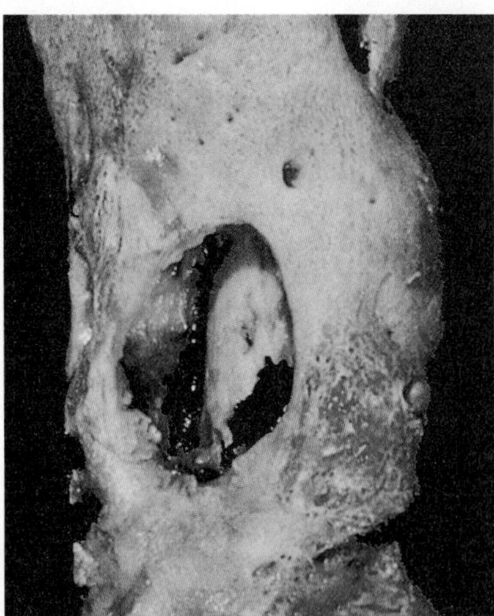

Figure 37-15 ■ **Resected Femur in a Patient With Draining Osteomyelitis.** The drainage tract in the subperiosteal shell of viable new bone (involucrum) reveals the inner native necrotic cortex (sequestrum). (From Kumar V et al: *Robbins and Cotran pathologic basis of disease,* ed 7, Philadelphia, 2005, Saunders.)

abscesses or fragments of necrotic bone and produce occasional flareups of acute osteomyelitis. The progression from acute to subacute osteomyelitis may be the result of inadequate or inappropriate therapy or the development of drug-resistant microorganisms.

In the adult, hematogenous osteomyelitis has an insidious onset. The symptoms are usually vague and include fever, malaise, anorexia, weight loss, and pain in and around the infected areas. Edema may or may not be evident. Recent infection (urinary, respiratory, skin) or instrumentation (catheterization, cystoscopy, myelography, diskography) usually precedes onset of symptoms.

Single or multiple abscesses (Brodie abscesses) characterize subacute or chronic osteomyelitis. Brodie abscesses are circumscribed lesions 1 to 4 cm in diameter, usually in the ends of long bones and surrounded by dense ossified bone matrix. The abscesses are thought to develop when the infectious microorganism has become less virulent or the individual's immune system is resisting the infection somewhat successfully.

In exogenous osteomyelitis, signs and symptoms of soft-tissue infection predominate. Inflammatory exudate in the soft tissues disrupts muscles and supporting structures and forms abscesses. Low-grade fever, lymphadenopathy, local pain, and swelling usually occur within days of contamination by a puncture wound.

EVALUATION AND TREATMENT Laboratory data show an elevated white cell count. Radiographic studies include radionuclide bone scanning, computed tomography, and MRI. MRI scanning with gadolinium contrast shows both bone and soft tissue, providing more accurate assessment of infection.[41] Treatment of osteomyelitis includes antibiotics and débridement with bone biopsy. Biodegradable antibiotic-impregnated bioabsorbable beads has also benefited many individuals.[42,43] Chronic conditions may require surgical removal of the inflammatory exudate followed by continuous wound irrigation with antibiotic solutions in addition to systemic treatment with antibiotics. The ideal antibiotic regimen for treating osteomyelitis has not yet been developed. **Hyperbaric oxygen therapy** of 100% oxygen may stimulate healing by suppressing proinflammatory cytokines and prostaglandins.[44] Implants for total joint replacements may be removed to treat the infected joint more thoroughly.

✔ QUICK CHECK 37-2

1. What are the causes associated with osteoporosis in women and men?
2. What are the risk factors for osteoporosis?
3. How does osteoporosis differ from osteomalacia? Name three differences.

DISORDERS OF JOINTS

The American Rheumatism Association recognizes 13 groups of joint disease (arthropathies). Most of these disorders can be placed into two major categories: noninflammatory joint disease and inflammatory joint disease. With the improvement in detection methods, however, inflammatory pathways are now identified in previously classified conditions as noninflammatory, such as osteoarthritis.

Osteoarthritis

Traditionally, **noninflammatory joint disease** was differentiated from inflammatory joint disease by (1) the absence of synovial membrane inflammation, (2) the lack of systemic signs and symptoms, and (3) normal synovial fluid. **Degenerative joint disease (osteoarthritis)** was the most prevalent noninflammatory joint disease. Because of the use of MRI and arthroscopy, inflammation has been identified and is emerging as an important feature of osteoarthritis (Figure 37-16).

Osteoarthritis tends to occur in men and women older than 40 years and becomes more common with increasing age. Although incidence rates are quite similar in men and women, women are more severely affected. It usually occurs in those persons who put exceptional stress on joints, as do gymnasts; long-distance runners or marathoners; basketball, soccer, or football players; and others; many develop osteoarthritis at earlier ages than usual. A previously torn anterior cruciate ligament or meniscectomy increases the risk for accelerated osteoarthritis of the knee.[45]

Types of osteoarthritis

Osteoarthritis (OA) is a common, age-related disorder of synovial joints. It is characterized by local areas of loss and damage of articular cartilage, new bone formation of joint margins (osteophytosis), subchondral bone changes, variable degrees of mild synovitis, and thickening of the

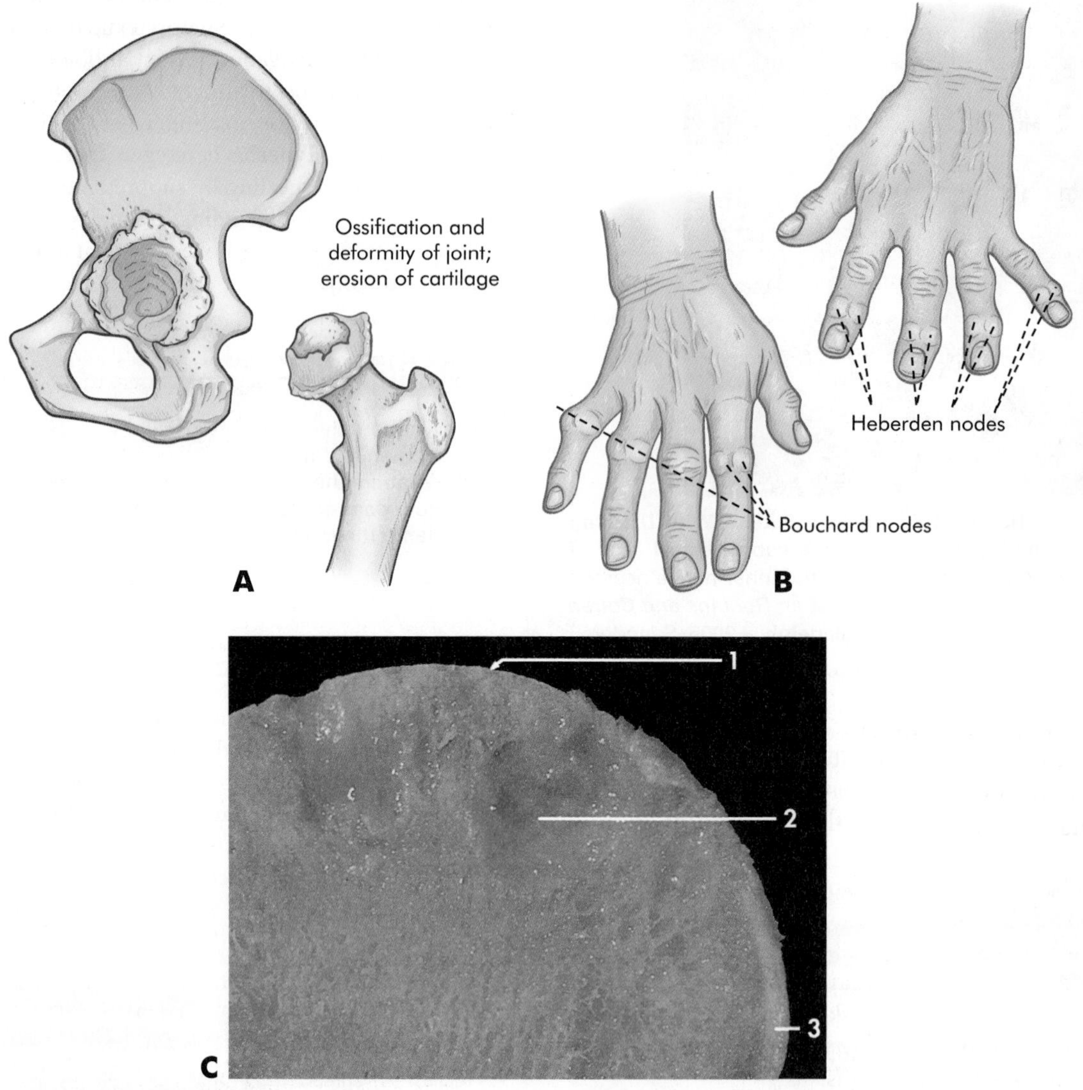

Figure 37-16 ■ **Osteoarthritis (OA). A,** Cartilage and degeneration of the hip joint from osteoarthritis. **B,** Heberden nodes and Bouchard nodes. **C,** Severe osteoarthritis with small islands of residual articular cartilage next to exposed subchondral bone. *1,* Eburnated articular surface. *2,* Subchondral cyst. *3,* Residual articular cartilage. (**C** from Kumar V, et al: *Robbins and Cotran pathologic basis of disease,* ed 7, Philadelphia, 2005, Saunders.)

joint capsule (see Figure 37-16). Pathology centers on load-bearing areas. Advancing disease reveals narrowing of the joint space because cartilage loss, bone spurs (**osteophytes**), and sometimes changes in the subchondral bone. OA can arise in any synovial joint but is commonly found in the hands, hips, and spine. It is less common in people younger than 40 years of age but rises with age. With improved understanding of OA, the designation into primary and secondary no longer seems viable.[46] Although the exact causes of OA are unclear, they involve low-grade inflammation, calcification of articular cartilage, genetic alterations, and metabolic disorders.[47] OA involves a complex interaction of cytokines, growth factors, matrix molecules, and enzymes (see the Pathophysiology section).

PATHOPHYSIOLOGY The primary defect in OA is loss of articular cartilage.[48] Early in the disease, the articular cartilage loses its glistening appearance, becoming yellow-gray or brownish gray. As the disease progresses, surface areas of the articular cartilage flake off and deeper layers develop longitudinal fissures (fibrillation). The cartilage becomes thin and may be absent over some areas, leaving the underlying bone (subchondral bone) unprotected. Consequently, the unprotected subchondral bone becomes sclerotic (dense and hard). Cysts sometimes develop within the subchondral bone and communicate with the longitudinal fissures in the cartilage. Pressure builds in the cysts until the cystic contents are forced into the synovial cavity, breaking through the articular cartilage on the way. As the articular cartilage erodes, cartilage-coated osteophytes may grow outward from the underlying bone and alter the bone contours and joint anatomy. These spurlike bony projections enlarge until small pieces, called *joint mice,* break off into the synovial cavity. If osteophyte fragments irritate the synovial membrane, synovitis and joint effusion result. The joint capsule also becomes thickened and at times adheres to the deformed underlying bone, which may figure in the limitation of movement (see Figure 37-16).

Articular cartilage is lost through a cascade of cytokine and anabolic growth factor pathways.[49] Enzymatic processes (including matrix metalloproteinases) assist in breaking down the macromolecules of proteoglycans, glycosaminoglycans, and collagen into large, diffusible fragments. Then the fragments are taken up by the cartilage cells (chondrocytes) and digested by the cell's own lysosomal enzymes. (Processes of cellular uptake and lysosomal digestion are described in Chapter 1.) The loss of proteoglycans from articular cartilage is a hallmark of the osteoarthritic process.[49]

Enzymatic destruction of articular cartilage begins in the matrix, with destruction of proteoglycans and collagen fibers. Enzymes, particularly stromelysin and acid metalloproteinase, affect proteoglycans by interfering with assembly of the proteoglycan subunit or the proteoglycan aggregate (see Chapter 36); these enzymes are markedly elevated in OA. Changes in the conformation of proteoglycans disrupt the pumping action that regulates movement of water and synovial fluid into and out of the cartilage. Without the regulatory action of the proteoglycan pump, cartilage imbibes too much fluid and becomes less able to withstand the stresses of weight bearing. With aging, the proteoglycan content is decreased, and water content in cartilage can be increased by as much as 8%, affecting the strength of the cartilage. Persons with OA, even those with fairly extensive cartilage destruction, have elevated levels of proteoglycans/fragments in their synovial fluid, perhaps indicative of the degree of disease activity. Other studies indicate that cytokines, such as interleukin-1 (see Chapter 6 for discussion of cytokines) may play a major role in cartilage degradation as a result of release and activation of proteolytic and collagenolytic enzymes associated with an imbalance of cell responses to growth factor activity.

Enzymes that degrade collagen (i.e., collagenases) probably originate in the chondrocytes or in leukocytes. Collagen breakdown destroys the fibrils that give articular cartilage its tensile strength and exposes the chondrocytes to mechanical stress and enzyme attack. Thus, a cycle of destruction begins that involves all the components of articular cartilage: proteoglycans, collagen fibers, and chondrocytes.

CLINICAL MANIFESTATIONS Clinical manifestations of idiopathic or secondary OA typically appear during the fifth or sixth decade of life, although asymptomatic, articular surface changes are common after the age of 40 years. Pain in one or more joints, usually weight bearing or load bearing, is the first and most predominant symptom of the disease. It is usually aggravated by weight bearing or use of the joint and relieved by resting the joint. Nocturnal pain is usually not relieved by rest and may be accompanied by paresthesias (numbness, tingling, or prickling). Sometimes pain is referred to another part of the body. For example, osteoarthritis of the lumbosacral spine may mimic sciatica, causing severe pain in the back of the thigh along the course of the sciatic nerve. OA in the lower cervical spine may cause brachial neuralgia (pain in the arm) aggravated by movement of the neck. Osteoarthritic conditions in the hip cause pain that may be referred to the lower thigh and knee area. Sleep deprivation adds to the stress of the chronic pain of OA. Physical examination of the person with OA usually shows general involvement of both peripheral and central joints. Peripheral joints most often involved are in the hands, wrists, knees, and feet. Central joints most often afflicted are in the lower cervical spine, lumbosacral spine, shoulders, and hips.

Joint structures are capable of generating a limited number of signs and symptoms. The primary signs and symptoms of joint disease are pain, stiffness, enlargement or swelling, tenderness, limited range of motion, muscle wasting, partial dislocation, and deformity (see *Risk Factors: Osteoarthritis*).

RISK FACTORS Osteoarthritis

- Trauma, sprains, strains, joint dislocations, and fractures
- Long-term mechanical stress—athletics, ballet dancing, or repetitive physical tasks
- Inflammation in joint structures
- Joint instability from damage to supporting structures
- Neurologic disorders (e.g., diabetic neuropathy, Charcot neuropathic joint) in which pain and proprioceptive reflexes are diminished or lost
- Congenital or acquired skeletal deformities
- Hematologic or endocrine disorders, such as hemophilia, which causes chronic bleeding into the joints, or hyperparathyroidism, which causes bone to lose calcium
- Drugs (e.g., colchicine, indomethacin, steroids) that stimulate the collagen-digesting enzymes in the synovial membrane

The origin of joint stiffness is unknown. **Joint stiffness** is generally defined as difficulty in initiating joint movement, immobility, or a loss of range of motion. The stiffness usually occurs as joint movement begins, and it dissipates rapidly after a few minutes. Enlargement and bulging of joint contour, commonly described as swelling, may be caused by bone enlargement or the proliferation of osteophytes around the margins of the joint. Swelling also occurs if inflammatory exudate or blood enters the joint cavity, thereby increasing the volume of synovial fluid. This condition, termed **joint effusion,** is caused by (1) the presence of osteophyte fragments in the synovial cavity, (2) drainage of cysts from diseased subchondral bone, or (3) acute trauma to joint structures, resulting in hemorrhage and inflammatory exudation into the synovial cavity (see Figure 37-16, *C*).

Range of motion is limited to some degree, depending on the extent of cartilage degeneration. Frequently, joint motion is accompanied by sounds of crepitus, creaking, or grating. Hypermobility and subluxation of joints occur in OA secondary to a neurologic disorder. Knee alignment (either varus or valgus of more than 5 degrees) has been shown to increase progression of the disease.[50]

As OA of the lower extremity progresses, the person may begin to limp noticeably (Figure 37-17). Having a limp is distressing because it affects the person's independence and ability to do usual activities of daily living. The affected joint is also more symptomatic after use, such as at the end of a period of strenuous activity.

EVALUATION AND TREATMENT Evaluation consists of clinical assessment and radiologic studies, CT scan, arthroscopy, and MRI. Treatment is either conservative or surgical. Conservative treatment includes rest of the involved joint until inflammation, if present, subsides; range of motion to prevent joint capsule contraction; use of a cane, crutches, or walker to decrease weight bearing; weight loss if obesity is present (obese persons are five times more likely to have OA of the knees and twice as likely to have OA of the hips as normal-weight persons); and analgesic and anti-inflammatory drug therapy to reduce swelling and pain. Glucosamine and possibly chondroitin (see *Health Alert:* Body Weight and Osteoarthritis), so-called nutraceuticals, have shown some success in reducing the pain and progression of OA.[51] Intra-articular injection of high-molecular-weight viscose supplements, particularly hyaluronic acid, also has been successful in decreasing knee pain with OA.[52] Surgery is used to improve joint movement, correct deformity or malalignment, or create a new joint with artificial implants. More than 250,000 total hip replacements are performed yearly in the United States, most of which are related to OA. It is estimated that by 2030, primary knee joint replacements will increase to 3.48 million and hip replacements will rise to 572,000 annually.[53]

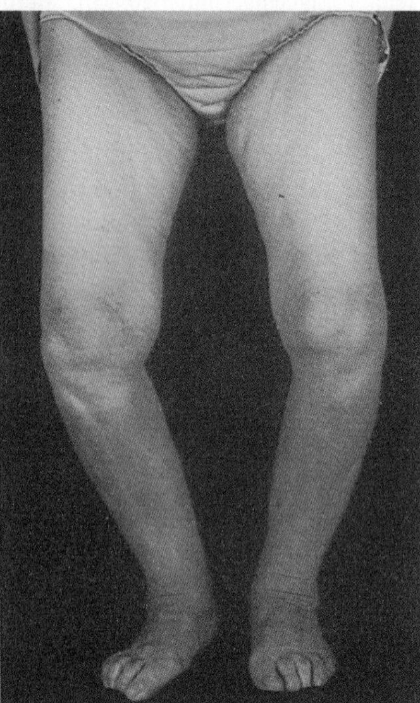

Figure 37-17 ■ Typical Varus Deformity of Knee Osteoarthritis. (From Doherty M: *Color atlas and text of osteoarthritis,* London, 1994, Wolfe.)

HEALTH ALERT

Body Weight and Osteoarthritis

Longitudinal studies have shown obesity to be a major risk factor in developing osteoarthritis of the knee. In addition to altered biomechanics, increased weight may make subchondral bone stiffer and thus less capable of handling joint impact loading.

Data from Powell A et al: Obesity: a preventable risk factor for large joint osteoarthritis which may act through biomechanical factors, *Br J Sports Med* 39:4–5, 2005.

Classic Inflammatory Joint Disease

Inflammatory joint disease is commonly called **arthritis.** Inflammatory joint disease is characterized by inflammatory damage or destruction in the synovial membrane or articular cartilage and by systemic signs of inflammation (fever, leukocytosis, malaise, anorexia, hyperfibrinogenemia).

Inflammatory joint disease can be infectious or noninfectious. In infectious inflammatory joint disease, inflammation is caused by invasion of the joint by bacteria, mycoplasmas, viruses, fungi, or protozoa. These agents can invade the joint through a traumatic wound, surgical incision, or contaminated needle, or they can be delivered by the bloodstream from sites of infection elsewhere in the body, typically bones, heart valves, or blood vessels. In noninfectious inflammatory joint disease, which is the most common form, inflammation is caused by immune reactions or the deposition of crystals of monosodium urate in and around the joint. Rheumatoid arthritis and ankylosing spondylitis are noninfectious inflammatory diseases caused by immune reactions and possibly hypersensitivity reactions[54,55]; gouty arthritis is a noninfectious inflammatory disease caused by crystal deposition.

Rheumatoid arthritis

Rheumatoid arthritis (RA) is a systemic, inflammatory autoimmune disease associated with swelling and pain in multiple joints. (Autoimmune disease is described in Chapter 7.) The first joint tissue to be affected is the synovial membrane, which lines the joint cavity (see Chapter 36, Figure 36-8). Eventually, inflammation may spread to the articular cartilage, fibrous joint capsule, and surrounding ligaments and tendons, causing pain, joint deformity, and loss of function (Figure 37-18). The joints most commonly affected are in the fingers, feet, wrists, elbows, ankles, and knees, but the shoulders, hips, and cervical spine also may be involved, as well as the tissues of the lungs, heart, kidneys, and skin.

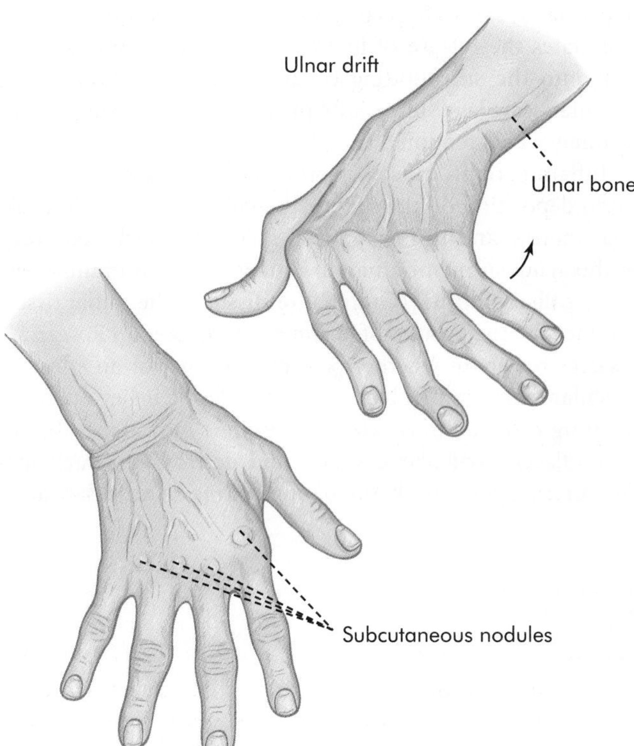

Figure 37-18 ■ **Rheumatoid Arthritis of the Hand.** Note swelling from chronic synovitis of metacarpophalangeal joints, marked ulnar drift, subcutaneous nodules, and subluxation of metacarpophalangeal joints with extension of proximal interphalangeal joints and flexion of distal joints. Note also deformed position of thumb. Hand has wasted appearance. (Redrawn from Mourad LA: *Orthopedic disorders,* St Louis, 1991, Mosby.)

RA affects 1% to 2% of adults and, like most autoimmune diseases, develops most often in women, with a female/male ratio of 3:1. The frequency of RA increases from the third decade on, affecting 5% or more of the population aged 70 years and older. Besides inflammation of the joints, RA can cause fever, malaise, rash, lymph node or spleen enlargement, and Raynaud phenomenon (transient lack of circulation to the fingertips and toes).

Despite intensive research, the cause of RA remains obscure. It is likely a combination of genetic factors interacting with inflammatory mediators. The chronic inflammation characteristics of RA result from an intricate interplay of chemokines that are powerful mediators of inflammation. Ligand/receptor chemokines attract T cells and produce inflammatory changes.[56] A key genetic element has been localized to the HLA-DR4, HLA-DQ, and HLA-DP areas of the major histocompatibility complex. Infectious microorganisms that may play a role in the cause of RA include bacteria, mycoplasmas, and viruses (especially Epstein-Barr virus). With long-term or intensive exposure to the antigen, normal antibodies (immunoglobulins [Ig]) become autoantibodies—antibodies that attack host tissues (self-antigens). Because they are usually present in individuals with RA, the transformed antibodies are termed **rheumatoid factors (RFs).** The RFs usually consist of two classes of immunoglobulin antibodies (antibodies for IgM and IgG) but occasionally involve antibodies for IgA. Their main antigenic targets are portions of the immunoglobulin molecules. RFs bind with their target self-antigens in blood and synovial membrane, forming immune complexes (antigen-antibody complexes). (See Chapter 5 for a discussion about antigen-antibody binding in the immune response.)

RA has a higher incidence in women, with evidence of hormonal involvement because disease symptoms lessen during pregnancy and exacerbate in the postpartal period. Long-term smoking, silicate exposure, and positive family history are associated with development of RA.[57,58] RA also has seasonal variations and is worse in winter months.

PATHOPHYSIOLOGY Basically, cartilage damage in RA is the result of at least three processes: (1) neutrophils and other cells in the synovial fluid become activated, degrading the surface layer of articular cartilage; (2) cytokines, particularly tumor necrosis factor alpha (TNF-α), stimulate synthesis of proinflammatory compounds, including interleukin-1 (IL-1), interleukin-6 (IL-6), and interleukin-8 (IL-8), and cause the chondrocytes to attack cartilage; and (3) the synovium digests nearby cartilage, releasing inflammatory molecules containing TNF-α and IL-1.

Several types of leukocytes are attracted out of the circulation and to the synovial membrane. The phagocytes of inflammation (neutrophils, macrophages) ingest the immune complexes and, in the process of doing so, release powerful enzymes that degrade synovial tissue and articular cartilage (Figure 37-19). The immune system's B and T lymphocytes are also activated. The B lymphocytes are stimu-

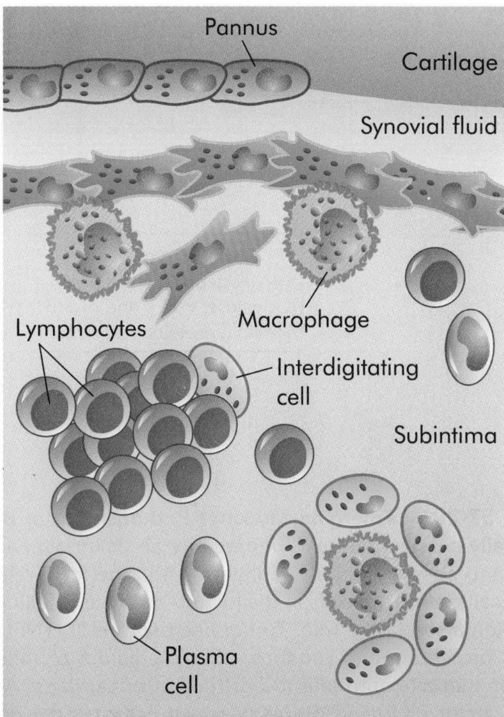

Figure 37-19 ■ **Synovitis.** Inflamed synovium showing typical arrangements of macrophages *(red)* and fibroblastic cells.

lated to produce more RFs, and the T lymphocytes produce enzymes that amplify and perpetuate the inflammatory response. The newly targeted self-antigens (immunoglobulins) are in relatively constant supply and can thus perpetuate inflammation and the formation of immune complexes indefinitely (Figure 37-20).

Inflammatory and immune processes have several damaging effects on the synovial membrane. Along with the swelling caused by leukocyte infiltration, the synovial membrane undergoes hyperplastic thickening as its cells proliferate and enlarge abnormally. As synovial inflammation progresses to involve its blood vessels, small venules become occluded by hypertrophied endothelial cells, fibrin, platelets, and inflammatory cells, which decrease vascular flow to the synovial tissue. Compromised circulation, coupled with increased metabolic needs as a result of hypertrophy and hyperplasia, causes hypoxia and metabolic acidosis. Acidosis stimulates the release of hydrolytic enzymes from synovial cells into the surrounding tissue, initiating erosion of the articular cartilage and inflammation in the supporting ligaments and tendons.

Inflammation causes hemorrhage, coagulation, and fibrin deposition on the synovial membrane, in the intracellular matrix, and in the synovial fluid. Over denuded areas of the synovial membrane, fibrin develops into granulation tissue called **pannus.** (Granulation tissue is the initial tissue produced in the process of healing; see Chapter 6.) Researchers disagree about whether pannus is a cause or an effect of articular cartilage involvement in RA. Some believe that, as RA progresses, pannus extends from the synovial membrane into adjacent articular cartilage and destroys the cartilage. Other researchers think that pannus forms on articular carti-

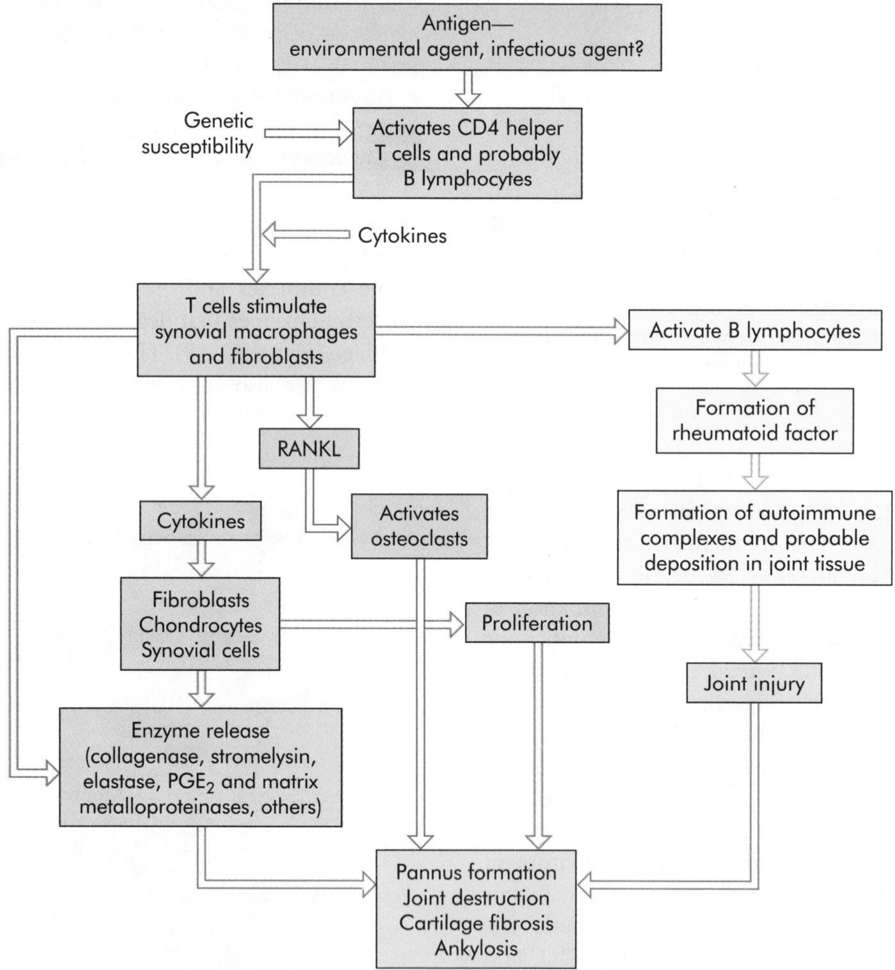

Figure 37-20 ■ **Emerging Model of Pathogenesis of Rheumatoid Arthritis.** Rheumatoid arthritis is an autoimmune disease of a genetically susceptible host triggered by an unknown antigenic agent. Chronic autoimmune reaction with activation of $CD4^+$ helper T cells and possibly other lymphocytes and the local release of inflammatory cytokines and mediators that eventually destroys the joint. T cells stimulate cells in the joint to produce cytokines that are key mediators of synovial damage. Apparently, immune complex deposition also plays a role. Tumor necrosis factor (TNF) and interleukin-1 (IL-1), as well as some other cytokines, stimulate synovial cells to proliferate and produce other mediators of inflammation, such as prostaglandins (PGE_2) matrix metalloproteinases, and enzymes that all contribute to destruction of cartilage. Activated T cells and synovial fibroblasts also produce receptor activator of nuclear factor κβ ligand (RANKL), which activates the osteoclasts and promotes bone destruction. Pannus is a mass of synovium and synovial stroma with inflammatory cells, granulation tissue, and fibroblasts that grows over the articular surface and causes its destruction.

lage after the cartilage has been destroyed by inflammation. In any case, pannus formation does not lead to synovial or articular regeneration but rather to formation of scar tissue that immobilizes the joint.

CLINICAL MANIFESTATIONS The onset of RA is usually insidious, although as many as 15% of cases have an acute onset. RA begins with general systemic manifestations of inflammation, including fever, fatigue, weakness, anorexia, weight loss, and generalized aching and stiffness. Local manifestations also appear gradually over a period of weeks or months. Typically, the joints become painful, tender, and stiff. Pain early in the disease is caused by pressure from swelling. Later in the disease, pain is caused by sclerosis of subchondral bone and new bone formation. Stiffness usually lasts for about 1 hour after arising in the morning and is thought to be related to synovitis. Initially the joints most commonly involved are the metacarpophalangeal (MCP) joints, proximal interphalangeal (PIP) joints, and wrists, with later involvement of larger weight-bearing joints.

Joint swelling, which is widespread and symmetric, is caused by increasing amounts of inflammatory exudate (leukocytes, plasma, plasma proteins) in the synovial membrane, hyperplasia of inflamed tissues, and formation of new bone. On palpation, the swollen joint feels warm and the synovial membrane feels boggy. The skin over the joint may have a ruddy, cyanotic hue and may look thin and shiny.

An inflamed joint may lose some of its mobility. Even mild synovitis can lead to loss of range of motion, which becomes evident after inflammation subsides. Extension becomes limited and is eventually lost if flexion contractures form. Loss of range of motion can progress to permanent deformities of the fingers, toes, and limbs, including ulnar deviation of the hands, boutonniere and swan-neck deformities of the finger joints, plantar subluxation of the metatarsal heads of the foot, and hallux valgus (angulation of the great toe toward the other toes). Flexion contractures of the knees and hips are also common.

Joint deformities cause the physical limitations experienced by persons with RA (see Figure 37-18). Loss of joint motion is quickly followed by secondary atrophy of the surrounding muscles. With secondary muscle atrophy, the joint becomes unstable, which further aggravates joint pathology.

Two complications of chronic RA are caused by excessive amounts of inflammatory exudate in the synovial cavity. One complication is the formation of cysts in the articular cartilage or subchondral bone. Occasionally, these cysts communicate with the skin surface (usually the sole of the foot) and can drain through passages called *fistulae*. The second complication is rupture of a cyst or of the synovial joint itself, usually caused by strenuous physical activity that places excessive pressure on the joint. Rupture releases inflammatory exudate into adjacent tissues, thereby spreading inflammation.

Extrasynovial **rheumatoid nodules,** or swellings, are observed in areas of pressure or trauma in 20% of individuals with RA. Each nodule is an aggregate of inflammatory cells surrounding a central core of fibrinoid and cellular debris. T lymphocytes are the predominant leukocytes in the nodule. B lymphocytes, plasma cells, and phagocytes are found around the periphery. Nodules are most often found in subcutaneous tissue over the extensor surfaces of elbows and fingers. Less common sites are the scalp, back, feet, hands, buttocks, and knees.

Rheumatoid nodules also may invade the skin, cardiac valves, pericardium, pleura, lung parenchyma, and spleen. These nodules are identical to those encountered in some individuals with rheumatic fever and are characterized by central tissue necrosis surrounded by proliferating connective tissue. Also noted are large numbers of lymphocytes and occasional plasma cells. Acute glaucoma may result with nodules forming on the sclera. Pulmonary involvement may result in diffuse pleuritis or multiple intraparenchymal nodules. Together, the occurrence of pulmonary nodules and pneumoconiosis (chronic inflammation of the lungs from inhalation of dust) creates the syndrome called **Caplan syndrome.** Diffuse pulmonary fibrosis may occur because of immunologically mediated immune complex deposition.

Rheumatoid nodules within the heart may cause valvular deformities, particularly of the aortic valve leaflets, and pericarditis. Lymphadenopathy of the nodes close to the affected joints may develop. Rheumatoid nodules within the spleen result in splenomegaly. Involvement of blood vessels results in an acute necrotizing vasculitis, characteristic of that noted in other immunologic/inflammatory states. Thromboses of such involved vessels may give rise to myocardial infarctions, cerebrovascular occlusions, mesenteric infarction, kidney damage, and vascular insufficiency in the hands and fingers (Raynaud phenomenon). The vascular changes are primarily noted in individuals receiving steroid therapy; thus, there is some concern that the therapy may play a role in initiating these lesions. Changes in skeletal muscle are often noted in the form of nonspecific atrophy secondary to joint dysfunction.

EVALUATION AND TREATMENT Evaluation of RA is done by physical examination, roentgenography of the joint, and serologic tests for rheumatoid factor and circulating immune complexes. The American College of Rheumatology lists the following diagnostic criteria for RA[59]:

1. Morning stiffness lasting more than 1 hour
2. Arthritis of three or more joint areas
3. Arthritis of hand joints
4. Symmetric arthritis
5. Rheumatoid nodules over extensor surfaces or bony prominences
6. Serum rheumatoid factor
7. Radiographic changes

The presence of four or more criteria is diagnostic of RA. Criteria 1 through 4 with joint signs or symptoms must be present for 6 weeks.

Treatment is nonsurgical or surgical. Nonsurgical treatment includes rest of the inflamed joint and whole-body rest for several hours daily; use of hot and cold packs; physical therapy; patient education; aggressive, early intervention using disease-modifying antirheumatic drugs (DMARDs) and biologic response modifiers (BRMs); a diet high in calories and vitamins; corticosteroids; and anti-inflammatory drugs taken orally or injected into the joint. Intra-articular injection of a radionuclide can be used to treat synovitis. Surgical synovectomy may be done early in the disease to decrease inflammatory effusion and remove pannus. Surgery is used to correct deformity or mechanical deficiency in intermediate or late stages of the disease and includes arthrodesis, arthroplasty, or total joint replacement. There is evidence that total fasting induces a substantial reduction in joint pain, swelling, morning stiffness, and other symptoms in individuals with RA.

HEALTH ALERT
New Rheumatoid Arthritis Treatments

Innovative new therapies for rheumatoid arthritis (RA) treatment continue to emerge. In addition to pharmaceutic agents, biologic and genetic agents are gaining increasing attention. New treatments are targeted at specific cytokines, inhibition of chemokines, and complement activation and investigational therapies include T cell or T cell receptor vaccination. High-dose intravenous immunoglobulins and plasmapheresis also are also being used. Experimental intra-articular gene transfer may one day prove successful as a "gene scalpel" for removing inflammatory synovial tissue.

Data from Breeveld FC, Kalden JR: Appropriate and effective management of rheumatoid arthritis, *Ann Rheum Dis* 63:627–633, 2004; Zhang H et al: Elimination of rheumatoid synovium in situ using a Fas ligand "gene scalpel," *Arthritis Res Ther* 7(6):R1235-R1243, 2005.

Ankylosing spondylitis

Ankylosing spondylitis (AS) is the most common of a group of inflammatory arthropathies known as *spondyloarthropathies.* It is a chronic, inflammatory joint disease characterized by stiffening and fusion (ankylosis) of the spine and sacroiliac joints. Like RA, ankylosing spondylitis is a systemic, immune inflammatory disease. Although inflammation is the primary pathologic process in both RA and ankylosing spondylitis, the two diseases differ in the primary site of inflammation and the end result. In RA, the primary site of inflammation is the synovial membrane, resulting in the destruction and instability of synovial joints. In ankylosing spondylitis, the primary pathologic site is the **enthesis** (the point at which ligaments, tendons, and the joint capsule are inserted into bone), and the end result is fibrosis, ossification, and fusion of the joint, primarily the sacroiliac joints and the vertebral column.

AS primarily affects white men between the ages of 15 and 40. In women, AS may affect the peripheral joints of the appendicular skeleton rather than the axial skeleton, progress less rapidly, and cause less dramatic spinal changes.

The prevalence of AS in the United States is approximately 0.5% to 1% among whites, 3% to 4% among blacks, and 18% to 50% in various tribes of Native Americans. Worldwide, the disease appears to be most prevalent in whites. The prevalence of AS in males is at least 10 times more than previously considered, and the disease is more prevalent even in females. Many individuals with AS remain undiagnosed.

Primary AS usually develops in late adolescence and young adulthood, with peak incidence at about 20 years of age. Secondary AS affects older age groups and is often associated with other inflammatory diseases (e.g., psoriatic arthropathy, inflammatory bowel disease, Reiter syndrome).

The cause of ankylosing spondylitis is unknown, but the disease is strongly associated with the presence of histocompatibility antigen HLA-B27 on the chromosome of affected individuals, suggesting a genetic predisposition to the disease.[60]

PATHOPHYSIOLOGY Ankylosing spondylitis begins with inflammation of fibrocartilage in cartilaginous joints, primarily in the vertebrae. Inflammatory cells infiltrate the fibrous tissue of the joint capsule, the cartilage that surrounds intervertebral disks, the entheses, and periosteum. As inflammatory cells (chiefly macrophages) and lymphocytes infiltrate and erode bone and fibrocartilage in joint structures, repair begins. Repair of cartilaginous structures begins with the proliferation of fibroblasts. Fibroblasts synthesize and secrete collagen. The collagen becomes organized into fibrous scar tissue that eventually undergoes calcification and ossification. With time, all the cartilaginous structures of the joint are replaced by ossified scar tissue, causing the joint to fuse, or lose flexibility.

Repair of eroded bone begins with osteoblast activation and proliferation. Osteoblasts lay down new bone (callus), which is remodeled and replaced by compact, lamellar bone. Bone repair changes the contour of the bone's surface because the new bone grows outward to form a new enthesis with the end of the eroded ligament. The new enthesis, which forms on top of the old one, is called **syndesmophyte.** As calcification of the spinal ligaments progresses, the vertebral bodies lose their concave anterior contour and appear square. The spine assumes the classic bamboo spine appearance of ankylosing spondylitis.

CLINICAL MANIFESTATIONS The most common signs and symptoms of early AS are low back pain and stiffness. Typically, the individual with primary disease develops low back pain during the early 20s. The pain is at first insidious but progressively becomes persistent. It is often worse after prolonged rest and is alleviated by physical activity. Early morning stiffness usually accompanies the low back pain, and the individual typically has difficulty sitting up or twisting the spine. Forward flexion, rotation, and lateral flexion of the spine are restricted and painful. Early pain and resultant loss of motion are caused by the underlying inflammation and reflex muscle spasm rather than by soft tissue or bony fusion.

As the disease progresses, the normal convex curve of the lower spine (lumbar lordosis) diminishes and concavity of the upper spine (kyphosis) increases. The individual becomes increasingly stooped. The thoracic spine becomes rounded, the head and neck are held forward on the shoulders, and the hips are flexed (Figure 37-21).

Inflammation in the tendon insertions of the many costosternal and costovertebral muscles can cause pleuritic chest pain and restricted chest movement. The pain is usually worse on inspiration. Movement in the diaphragm is normal and full. Pressure on the anterior chest wall over the sternum, ribs, and costal cartilages may cause tenderness. Tenderness over the pelvic brim may cause discomfort at night and interfere with sleep because turning onto the iliac crests causes pain. Tenderness over the ischial tuberosities may make sitting on hard seats unbearable. Tenderness in the heels may contribute to a limp or cautious placement of the feet during walking.

Along with low back pain, many individuals have peripheral joint involvement, uveitis, fibrotic changes in the lungs, and cardiomegaly, aortic incompetence, amyloidosis, and Achilles tendonitis. Symptoms may include fatigue, weight loss, low-grade fever, hypochromic anemia, and an increased erythrocyte sedimentation rate.

EVALUATION AND TREATMENT Diagnosis of AS is made from the history and physical examination, roentgenograms, and serum analysis for the presence of the histocompatibility antigen HLA-B27. Erythrocyte sedimentation rate and C-reactive protein are elevated throughout the disease. Alkaline phosphatase levels are often elevated.

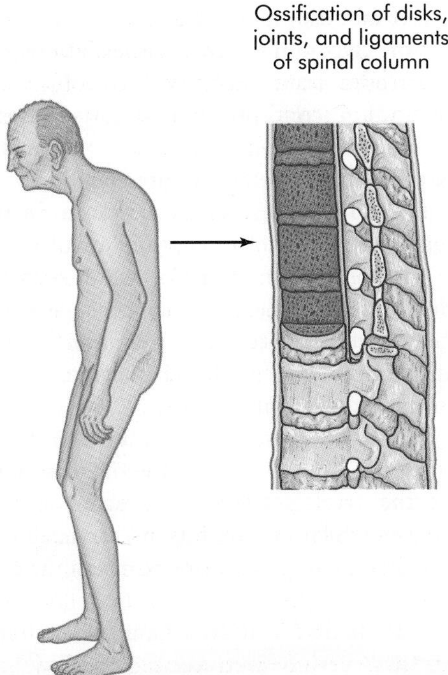

Figure 37-21 ■ **Ankylosing Spondylitis.** Characteristic posture and primary pathologic sites of inflammation and resulting damage. (Redrawn from Mourad LA: *Orthopedic disorders,* St Louis, 1991, Mosby.)

Treatment of individuals with AS consists of patient education, as well as physical therapy to maintain skeletal mobility and prevent the natural progression of contractures. Prevention of deformity and maintenance of mobility require a continuous program of physical therapy. Exercises are performed several times each day to maintain chest expansion, full extension of the spine, and complete range of motion in the proximal joints.

Nonsteroidal anti-inflammatory drugs (NSAIDs) will often provide temporary symptom relief within 48 hours. Analgesic medications are prescribed to suppress some of the pain and stiffness and to facilitate exercise. The medications do not prevent disease progression, but they do provide relief from symptoms. Biologic response modifying agents, such as infliximab, which inhibits tumor necrosis factor-alpha, may be useful in treating ankylosing spondylitis.[61,62] Surgical procedures, such as osteotomy, total hip replacement, and cervical spinal fusion, and radiation therapy are sometimes used to provide relief for individuals with end-stage disease or intolerable deformity. Individuals should stop smoking to lessen pulmonary problems.

Gout

Gout is a syndrome caused by defects in uric acid metabolism and characterized by inflammation and pain of the joints. Either excessive uric acid production or underexcretion of uric acid by the kidneys will cause hyperuricemia. When the uric acid reaches a certain concentration in fluids, it crystallizes, forming insoluble precipitates that are deposited in connective tissues throughout the body. Crystallization in synovial fluid causes acute, painful inflammation of the joint, a condition known as **gouty arthritis.** With time, crystal deposition in subcutaneous tissues causes the formation of small, white nodules, or **tophi,** that are visible through the skin. Crystal aggregates deposited in the kidneys can form urate renal stones and lead to renal failure.

In classic gouty arthritis, monosodium urate crystals form and cause joint inflammation. Pseudogout is caused by the formation of calcium *pyrophosphate*-dihydrate crystals. The effect of either crystal is the same—the onset of an acute inflammatory response (see Chapter 6).

Gout is rare in children and premenopausal women and is uncommon in males younger than 30 years. The peak age of onset in males is between 40 and 50 years, whereas it is somewhat later in females. The risk of developing gouty arthritis is similar in males and females for a particular urate concentration. The plasma urate concentration is the single most important determinant of the risk of developing gout (Table 37-4).

Uric acid is a weak acid that is ionized at normal body pH and thus occurs in the blood or tissues in the form of urate ion. When ionized, uric acid can form salts with various cations, but 98% of extracellular uric acid is in the form of monosodium urate (uric acid salt). At any time the

TABLE 37-4

Mean Urate Concentrations by Age and Gender

Characteristic	Mean Urate Levels
Prepuberty	3.5 mg/dl
Males (at puberty)	Steep rise to 5.2 mg/dl
Females (puberty to after premenopause)	Slow rise to ≈ 4.0 mg/dl
Females (after menopause)	4.7 mg/dl
Hyperuricemia	
Males	7.0 mg/dl
Females	6.0 mg/dl

proportion of uric acid or urate is pH dependent, so the ratio of these two forms varies considerably in urine.

The solubility of urate and uric acid is critical to the development of crystals. Urate is more soluble in plasma, synovial fluid, and urine than in aqueous solutions. The solubility of uric acid in urine rises dramatically as the pH increases above 4. There is little change, however, in the solubility of urate within the normal pH range that exists in the plasma, synovial fluid, and other tissues. Decreasing temperatures cause both urate and uric acid solubility to fall. The pathways of production of uric acid are shown in Figure 37-22.

PATHOPHYSIOLOGY The pathophysiology of gout is closely linked to purine metabolism (or cellular metabolism of purines) and kidney function. Most mammals, except humans, have the enzyme uricase, which catalyzes uric acid to allantoin, thus preventing overproduction of uric acid. At the cellular level, purines are synthesized to purine nucleotides, which are used in the synthesis of nucleic acids, adenosine triphosphate, cyclic adenosine monophosphate (AMP), and cyclic guanosine monophosphate (GMP). Uric acid is a breakdown product of purine nucleotides (urate synthesis and elimination are illustrated in Figure 37-23). Some individuals with gout have an accelerated rate of purine synthesis accompanied by an overproduction of uric acid. Even with restricted purine consumption, these individuals continue to overproduce uric acid. Other individuals break down purine nucleotides at an accelerated rate that also results in an overproduction of uric acid. In addition, production of uric acid can be caused by an increased turnover of nucleic acids, which is associated with an increased turnover of cells at other body sites. The increased turnover of nucleic acids leads to increased levels of uric acid with a compensatory increase in purine synthesis.

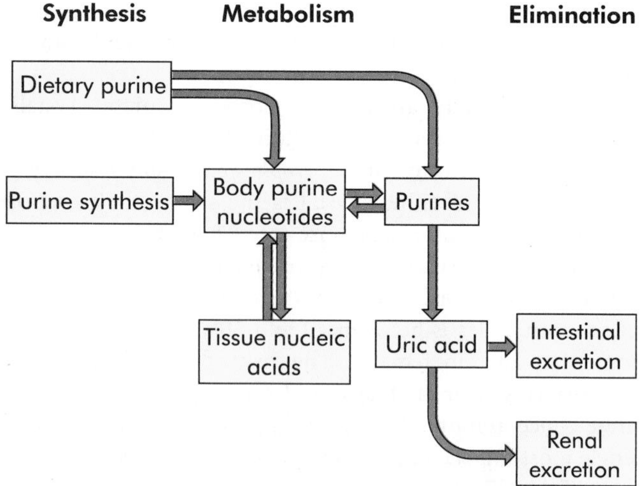

Figure 37-22 ■ **Uric Acid Synthesis and Elimination.** Uric acid is derived from purines ingested or synthesized from ingested foods, as well as being recycled after cell breakdown. Uric acid is then eliminated through the kidneys and gastrointestinal tract. (Redrawn from Klippel JH, Dieppe PA, editors: *Rheumatology,* ed 2, St Louis, 1998, Mosby.)

Most uric acid is eliminated from the body through the kidneys. Urate is filtered at the glomerulus and undergoes both reabsorption and excretion within the renal tubules. In primary gout, urate excretion by the kidneys is sluggish. The sluggish excretion may be the result of a decrease in glomerular filtration of urate or acceleration in urate reabsorption. In addition, monosodium urate crystals are deposited in renal interstitial tissues, causing impaired urine flow. (Kidney function is described in Chapter 28.)

The exact process by which crystals of monosodium urate are deposited in joints and induce gouty arthritis is unknown, but several mechanisms may be involved, including the following:

1. Monosodium urate precipitates at the periphery of the body, where lower body temperatures may reduce the solubility of monosodium urate.
2. Albumin or glycosaminoglycan levels decrease, which causes decreased urate solubility.
3. Changes in ion concentration and decreases of pH enhance urate deposition.
4. Trauma promotes urate crystal precipitation.

The monosodium urate crystals may form in the synovial fluid or in the synovial membrane, cartilage, or other connective tissues in joints and elsewhere, such as in the heart, earlobes, and kidneys. Evidence suggests that an acute attack of gout is the result of the *formation* of crystals rather than the releasing of the crystals from connective tissues into the synovial fluid.

Monosodium urate crystals can stimulate and perpetuate the inflammatory response (see Figure 37-24, *A* and *B*). The presence of the crystals triggers the acute inflammatory response, during which neutrophils are attracted out of the circulation and begin to phagocytose (ingest) the crystals.

CLINICAL MANIFESTATIONS Gout is manifested by (1) an increase in serum urate concentration (hyperuricemia); (2) recurrent attacks of monarticular arthritis (inflammation of a single joint); (3) deposits of monosodium urate monohydrate (tophi) in and around the joints; (4) renal disease involving glomerular, tubular, and interstitial tissues

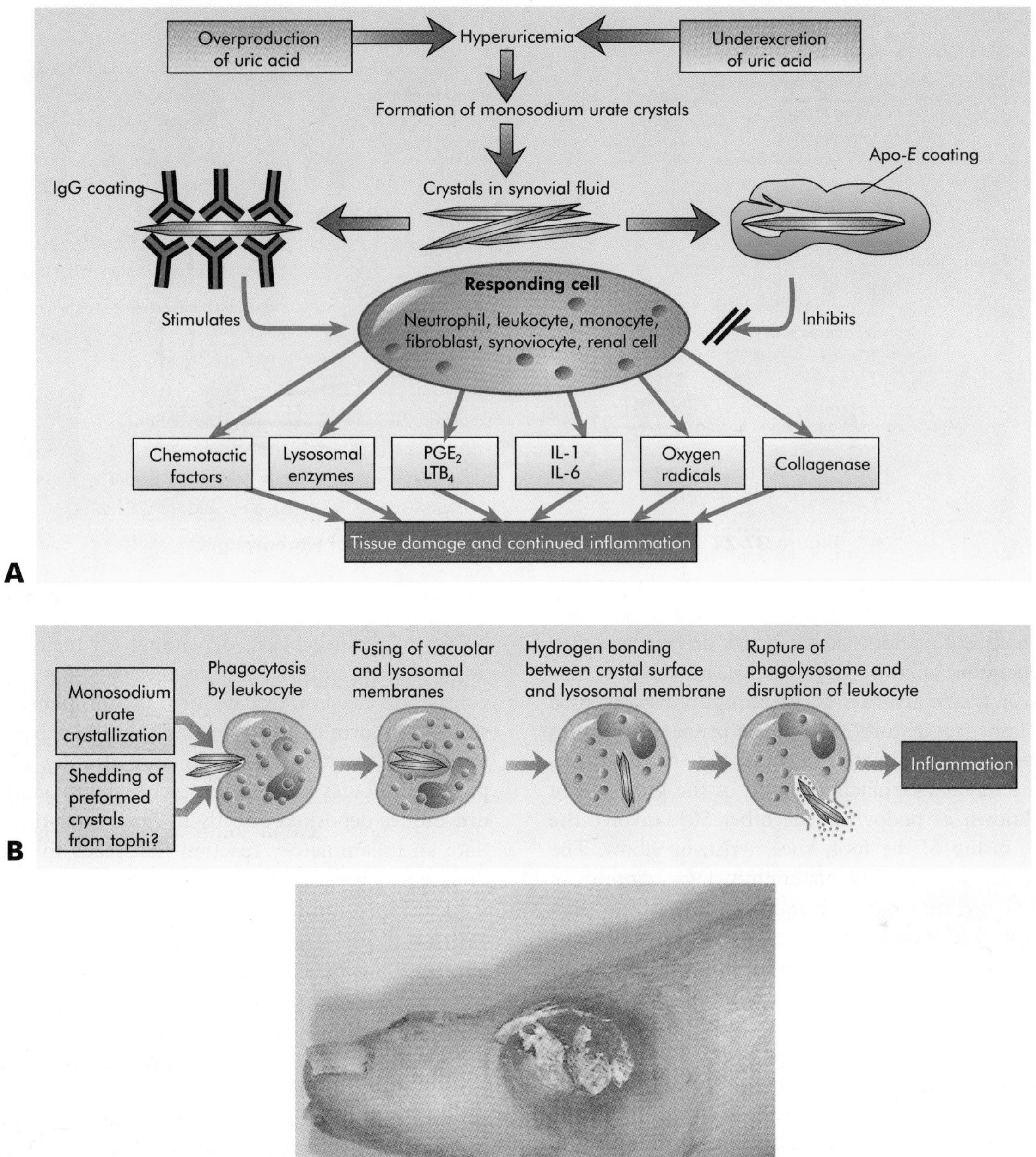

Figure 37-23 ■ **Pathogenesis of Acute Gouty Arthritis. A,** Depending on the urate crystal coating, a variety of cells may be stimulated to produce a wide range of inflammatory mediators. *IgG,* Immunoglobulin G; *Apo E,* apolipoprotein E; *PGE_2,* prostaglandin E2; *LTB_4,* leukotriene B4; *IL,* interleukin. **B,** Sequence of events in the production of inflammatory response to urate crystals. **C,** Gouty tophus on right foot. (**C** from Dieppe PA et al: *Arthritis and rheumatism in practice,* London, 1991, Gower.)

and blood vessels; and (5) the formation of renal stones. These manifestations appear in three clinical stages:

1. **Asymptomatic hyperuricemia.** The serum urate level is elevated but arthritic symptoms, tophi, and renal stones are not present; may persist throughout life.
2. **Acute gouty arthritis.** Attacks develop with increased serum urate concentrations; tends to occur with sudden or sustained increases of hyperuricemia but also can be triggered by trauma, drugs, and alcohol.
3. **Tophaceous gout.** The third and chronic stage of disease; can begin as early as 3 years or as late as 40 years after the initial attack of gouty arthritis. Progressive inability to excrete uric acid expands the urate pool until urate crystal deposits (tophi) appear in cartilage, synovial membranes, tendons, and soft tissue.

Trauma is the most common aggravating factor. The great toe is subject to chronic strain in walking, and subsequently an acute gout attack may follow long walks. Trauma

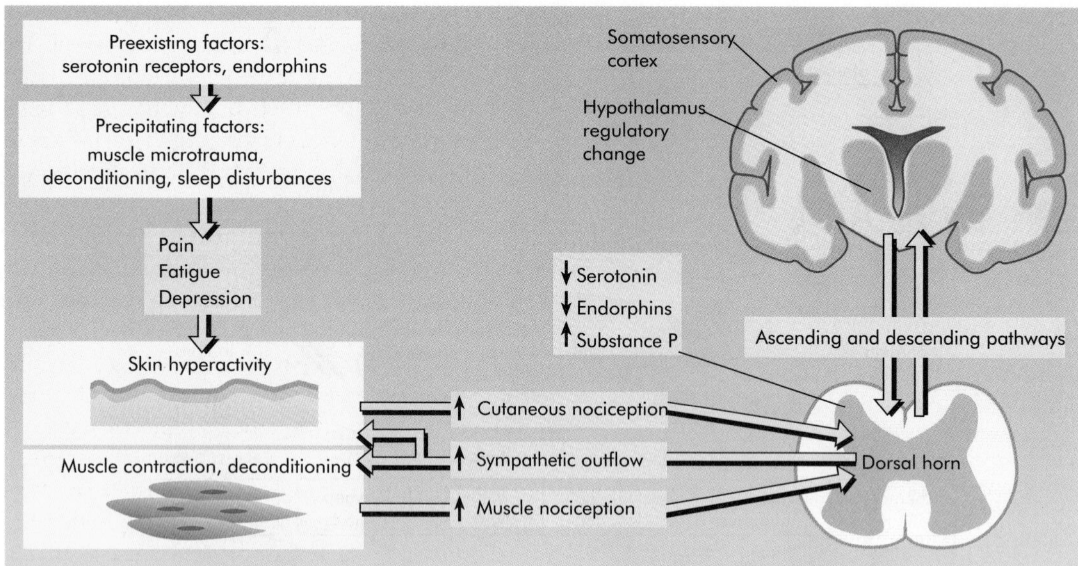

Figure 37-24 ■ Theoretic Pathophysiologic Model of Fibromyalgia.

associated with occupations such as truck driving also may precipitate an attack.

Attacks of gouty arthritis occur abruptly, usually in a peripheral joint (see Figure 37-23). The primary symptom is severe pain. Approximately 50% of the initial attacks occur in the metatarsophalangeal joint of the great toe (a condition known as podogra). The other 50% involve the heel, ankle, instep of the foot, knee, wrist, or elbow. The pain is usually noted at night. Within a few hours the affected joint becomes hot, red, and extremely tender and may be slightly swollen. Lymphangitis and systemic signs of inflammation (leukocytosis, fever, elevated sedimentation rate) are occasionally present. Untreated, mild attacks usually subside in several hours but may persist for 1 or 2 days. Severe attacks may persist for several days or weeks. When the individual recovers, the symptoms resolve completely. The helix of the ear is the most common site of tophi, which are the characteristic diagnostic lesions of chronic gout.

Tophaceous deposits produce irregular swellings of the fingers, hands, knees, and feet. Tophi commonly form lumps along the ulnar surface of the forearm, the tibial surface of the leg, the Achilles tendon, and olecranon bursae. Tophi may produce marked limitation of joint movement and eventually cause grotesque deformities of the hands and feet. Although the tophi themselves are painless, they often cause progressive stiffness and persistent aching of the affected joint. Tophi in the upper extremities may cause nerve compressions, such as carpal tunnel syndrome. Tophi in the lower extremities may cause tarsal tunnel syndrome. They also may erode and drain through the skin.

Renal stones are 1000 times more prevalent in individuals with primary gout than in the general population. The stones can be the size of a grain of sand or a piece of gravel, or they can accumulate in massive deposits called *staghorn calculi.* They range in color from pale yellow to brown to reddish black, depending on their composition. Some stones consist of pure monosodium urate; others consist of calcium oxalate or calcium phosphate. Renal stones can form in the collecting tubules, pelvis, or ureters, causing obstruction, dilation, and atrophy of the more proximal tubules and leading eventually to acute renal failure. Stones deposited directly in renal interstitial tissue initiate an inflammatory reaction that leads to chronic renal disease and progressive renal failure.

TREATMENT The aims of gout treatment are to terminate the acute gouty attack as promptly as possible, prevent recurring attacks, prevent or reverse complications associated with urate deposits in the joints and kidneys, and prevent formation of kidney stones. Acute gouty arthritis is treated with anti-inflammatory drugs. The drugs of choice are colchicine, nonsteroidal anti-inflammatory agents (NSAIDs, especially indomethacin), and allopurinol. Colchicine is useful in persons unable to take NSAIDs. Once infection has been ruled out, hydrocortisone may be injected into the joint to relieve pain. Ice also may relieve some of the inflammation of the joint. Weight bearing on the involved joint is avoided until the acute attack subsides. The individual is put on a low-purine diet, with high fluid intake to increase urinary output. Antihyperuricemic drugs are given to reduce serum urate concentrations.

✔ QUICK CHECK 37-3

1. How does noninflammatory joint disease differ from inflammatory joint disease? Describe two principal features of each.
2. How does rheumatoid arthritis affect the skin, heart, lungs, and kidneys?
3. How does uric acid (or urates) cause gout to develop?

DISORDERS OF SKELETAL MUSCLE

Muscle weakness and fatigue are common symptoms. In many cases, neural, traumatic, and psychogenic causes provide an adequate explanation for the failure to generate force (weakness) or sustain force (fatigue) seen in myopathies. The pathophysiologic mechanisms in some of the metabolic and inflammatory muscle diseases have been explored, but the cause of many of the myopathies remains obscure. The complex interaction between muscles and nerves affects muscular function as well. Only inherited and acquired disorders of skeletal muscles are discussed here.

Secondary Muscular Dysfunction

Muscular symptoms arise from a variety of causes unrelated to the muscle itself. Secondary muscular phenomena (contracture, stress-related muscle tension, immobility) are common disorders that influence muscular function.

Contractures

Contractures can be pathologic or physiologic. A physiologic muscle contracture occurs in the absence of a muscle action potential in the sarcolemma. Muscle shortening is explained on the basis of failure of the calcium pump in the presence of plentiful adenosine triphosphate (ATP). A physiologic contracture is seen in McArdle disease (muscle myophosphorylase deficiency) and malignant hyperthermia. The contracture is usually temporary if the underlying pathology is reversed.

A pathologic contracture is a permanent muscle shortening caused by muscle spasm or weakness. Heel cord (Achilles tendon) contractures are examples of pathologic contractures. They are associated with plentiful ATP and occur in spite of a normal action potential. The most common form of contracture is seen in conditions such as muscular dystrophy (see p. 1079) and central nervous system (CNS) injury. Contractures also may develop secondary to scar tissue contraction in the flexor tissues of a joint, for example, contracture of burned tissues in the antecubital area of the forearm leading to a flexion contracture.

Stress-induced muscle tension

Abnormally increased muscle tension has been associated with chronic anxiety as well as a variety of stress-related muscular symptoms, including neck stiffness, back pain, and headache. Abnormalities in the CNS, reticular activating system, and autonomic nervous system (ANS) have been implicated. For example, as an individual progressively relaxes, the amplitude of the knee jerk reflex diminishes. Conversely, individuals with absent reflexes increase tension by such maneuvers as clenching the teeth or handgrip. The underlying pathophysiology may be related to the fact that as a muscle contracts, the muscle spindle is activated. This gamma-feedback system produces a series of impulses that are transmitted to the brain by the sensitive 1A afferent fibers. Unconscious tension is thought to increase the activity of the reticular activating system as well. This influences increasing firing of the efferent loop of the gamma fibers, produces further muscle contraction, and increases muscle tension. ANS function that regulates increased blood flow to the muscle during sympathetic activity may be related to increased muscle contraction tension.

Various forms of treatment have been used to reduce the muscle tension associated with stress. Progressive relaxation training, yoga, meditation, and biofeedback are examples of stress reduction therapies. **Biofeedback** uses an integrated electromyogram (EMG) to make recordings from the skin surface. The goal is to teach the individual to control tension that has been functioning maladaptively. It is particularly useful in individuals who have a connection between skeletal muscle tension and pain. **Progressive relaxation training** emphasizes the individual's ability to perceive the difference between tension and relaxation. This technique involves sequential tensing and a relaxing environment. The individual is taught to practice this routine daily, often with the use of audiotaped instructions. By teaching the individual to recognize excessive contraction of skeletal muscle, one hopes to enhance the person's ability to relax specific muscle groups to relieve tension and thus reduce CNS arousal as well as ANS arousal.

Disuse atrophy

The term **disuse atrophy** describes the pathologic reduction in normal size of muscle fibers after prolonged inactivity from bed rest, trauma (casting), or local nerve damage. Decreased muscle activity reduces muscle mass through reduced protein synthesis and increased proteolysis, probably by reactive oxygen radical regulation.[63] The effects of muscular deconditioning associated with lack of physical activity may be apparent in a matter of days. The normal individual on bed rest loses muscle strength from baseline levels at a rate of 3% per day. Bed rest also is associated with cardiovascular, skeletal, and other organ system changes. Also, as people age, their muscles atrophy and become weaker (sarcopenia).

Measures to prevent atrophy include frequent forceful isometric muscle contractions and passive lengthening exercises. If reuse is not restored within 1 year, regeneration of muscle fibers becomes impaired.

Fibromyalgia

Fibromyalgia is a chronic musculoskeletal syndrome characterized by diffuse pain, fatigue, and tender points. Increased sensitivity to touch (i.e., tender points), the absence of systemic or localized inflammation, and the presence of fatigue and nonrestorative sleep are common. Because the symptoms are vague (see the following list), fibromyalgia has often been misdiagnosed or completely dismissed by clinicians. A common misdiagnosis has been chronic fatigue syndrome. Eighty to ninety percent of individuals affected are women, and the peak age is 30 to 50 years. Although the incidence is unknown, the prevalence is reported to be

2% and increases with age.[64] It is more common than rheumatoid arthritis, yet its cause is still unknown.

The etiology of fibromyalgia has been debated for over a century. It is unlikely that it is caused by a single factor. The most common precipitating factors include the following:

- Flulike viral illness
- Chronic fatigue syndrome
- Human immunodeficiency virus (HIV) infection
- Lyme disease
- Physical trauma
- Persistent stress
- Chronic sleep disturbance

Certain rheumatic diseases, such as RA or systemic lupus erythematosus (SLE), may coexist if not initially present with fibromyalgia (Table 37-5).[65]

TABLE 37-5

Comparison of Fibromyalgia and Myofascial Pain Syndromes

Variable	Fibromyalgia	Myofascial Pain
Location	Generalized	Regional
Examination	Tender points	Trigger points
Response to local therapy	Not sustained	Curative
Gender	Female/male ratio: 10:1	Equal or unknown
Systemic features	Characteristic	Unknown

PATHOPHYSIOLOGY It is unproven but long suspected that muscle is the end organ responsible for the pain and fatigue. Some studies have documented metabolic alterations—lower ATP, lower adenosine diphosphate (ADP), and higher concentrations of AMP—and more alterations in the number of capillaries and fiber area in individuals with fibromyalgia than in study control subjects. Most studies have demonstrated that increased muscle tenderness in fibromyalgia is a result of generalized pain intolerance, possibly related to functional abnormalities within the CNS (Figure 37-24).[66]

A chronic stress response may be involved in producing lower peripheral (e.g., at the muscle site) and central levels of serotonin. There is increasing evidence that fibromyalgia involves the sympathetic nervous system. Individuals with fibromyalgia may have an adrenal hyporesponsiveness.

CLINICAL MANIFESTATIONS The prominent symptom of fibromyalgia is diffuse, chronic pain. The locations of 9 pairs (18) of tender points for diagnostic classification of fibromyalgia are shown in Figure 37-25. Tenderness in 11 of these 18 points is necessary for diagnosis along with a history of diffuse pain. The only reliable finding on examination is the presence of multiple tender points. The pain often begins in one location, especially the neck and shoulders, but then becomes more generalized. People describe the pain as *burning* or *gnawing*. Fatigue is profound. The effect on everyday life is considerable. Fatigue is most notable when arising from sleep and in midafternoon. Headaches and memory loss are common complaints. There is a strong

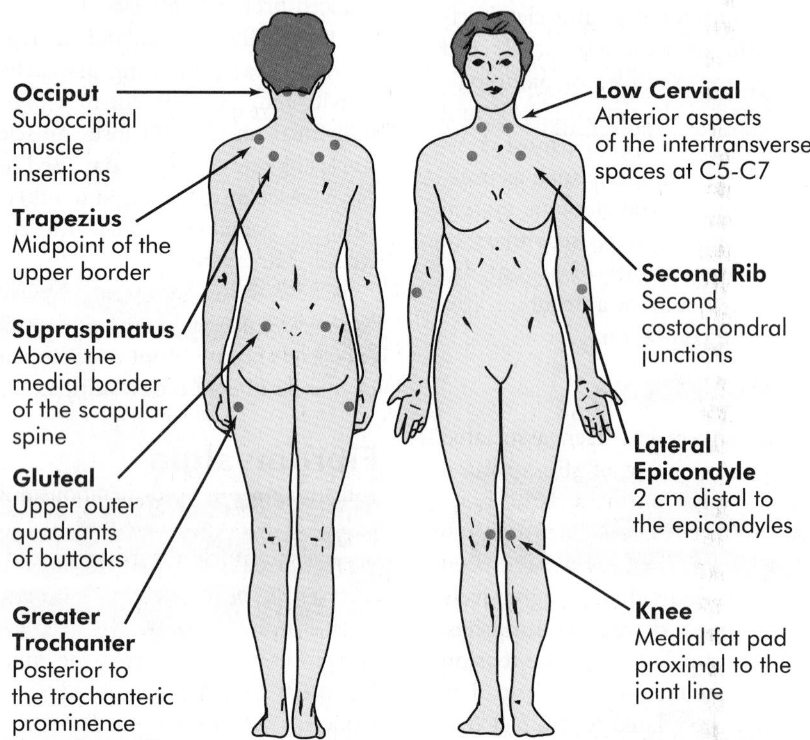

Figure 37-25 ■ **Location of Specific Tender Points for Diagnostic Classification of Fibromyalgia.** (Redrawn from Freundlich B, Leventhal L: The fibromyalgia syndrome. In Schumacher HR Jr, Klippel JH, Koopman WJ, editors: *Primer on the rheumatic diseases,* ed 11, Atlanta, 1997, Arthritis Foundation.)

association between fibromyalgia, Raynaud phenomenon, and irritable bowel syndrome. Individuals with fibromyalgia are light sleepers and awake frequently.

Almost 25% of individuals seek psychologic support for depression. Anxiety, particularly in regard to their diagnosis and future, is almost universal.

EVALUATION AND TREATMENT Because the manifestations of chronic, generalized pain and fatigue are present in many musculoskeletal (e.g., rheumatic) disorders, these disorders should be considered in the diagnosis of fibromyalgia. Treatment should be highly individualized.[64]

No one regimen of medication has proved successful for fibromyalgia. Anti-inflammatory medications have been used despite the fact there is no evidence of tissue inflammation. These medications have not been effective. Certain CNS-active medications, most notable the tricyclic antidepressants, amitriptyline, and cyclobenzaprine, were significantly better than placebos in controlled trials.[64] Amitriptyline significantly improved pain, morning stiffness, and sleep but not tender points. One of the most important aspects of treatment is education and reassurance (Box 37-2).

Muscle Membrane Abnormalities

Two defects of the muscle membrane (plasma membrane of the muscle fiber) have been linked to clinical syndromes: the hyperexcitable membrane seen in the myotonic disorders and the intermittently unresponsive membrane seen in the periodic paralyses. Although these are infrequent disorders, research into the pathologic processes has led to an improved understanding of the cell membrane.

Myotonia

Myotonia is a delayed relaxation after voluntary muscle contraction, such as grip, eye closure, or muscle percussion. The distinctive "dive bomber" noise, audible on needle EMG, is caused by the prolonged depolarization of the muscle membrane. Because the depolarization is not terminated by neuromuscular blocking agents, such as curare, the abnormality has been localized at the muscle membrane; the basic defect is the result of ion channel dysfunction. (These structures are described in Chapter 12.)

Myotonia is seen in several disorders: myotonia congenita, paramyotonia congenita, myotonic muscular dystrophy, and some forms of periodic paralysis. Most are inherited disorders and are mild in symptomatology, with the exception of myotonic muscular dystrophy (see p. 1059). Myotonia is treated by drugs that reduce muscle fiber excitability, such as procaine, procainamide, phenytoin, and quinine preparations. Treatments include acetazolamide, a carbonic anhydrase inhibitor, and verapamil, a calcium channel blocker.

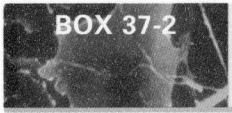

BOX 37-2 Educating and Providing Reassurance for Individuals With Fibromyalgia

- Stress that the illness is real, not imagined.
- Explain that fibromyalgia is presumably not caused by infection.
- Explain that fibromyalgia is not a deforming or deteriorating condition.
- Explain that fibromyalgia is neither life-threatening nor markedly debilitating, although it is an irritating presence.
- Discuss the role of sleep disturbances and the relationship of neurohormones to pain, fatigue, abnormal sleep, and mood.
- Reassure that although the cause is unknown, some information is known about the physiologic changes responsible for the symptoms.
- Use muscle "spasms" and, perhaps, low muscle blood flow to lay the groundwork for exercise recommendations.
- Assist the individual to use aerobic exercise to reduce stress and increase rapid eye movement (REM) sleep.

Periodic paralysis

Periodic paralysis encompasses a group of muscle diseases characterized by episodes of flaccid weakness. Most are hereditary and are caused by potassium, chloride, or sodium channel abnormalities. Exercise or thyrotoxicosis can cause symptoms. The disorder is often inherited in an autosomal dominant pattern, although it can be seen in hyperthyroidism. During an attack of periodic paralysis, the muscle membrane is unresponsive to neural stimuli, and the resting membrane potential is reduced from −90 to −45 mV.

The paralysis, which leaves the individual flaccid and weak, does not affect the respiratory muscles. Many individuals have myotonia present on examination. In most cases, the weakness is accompanied by a change in serum potassium, although in some individuals the change may be negligible. Cardiac dysrhythmias have been present during attacks. Genetic mutations are responsible for most periodic paralyses.

Hypokalemic periodic paralysis is usually caused by hyperthyroidism that causes a sudden shift of potassium into cells resulting in serum hypokalemia. (The effect of potassium on the resting membrane potential is discussed in Chapter 17.) Glucose and insulin infusions and oral potassium loading are used as provocative tests; oral and intravenous potassium can relieve acute attacks. Treatment includes thiazide diuretics and a high-salt diet. Acetazolamide and a low-salt diet are useful for long-term therapy.

Metabolic Muscle Diseases

Disorders in muscle metabolism can be caused by endocrine abnormalities or diseases of energy metabolism, such as glycogen storage disease, enzyme deficiencies, and abnormalities in lipid metabolism and mitochondrial function. The term *metabolic myopathies* refers to a group of hereditary muscle disorders caused by defective genes.

Endocrine disorders

Often the systemic effects of hormonal imbalance overshadow the individual's muscular symptoms. For example, individuals with thyrotoxicosis may have signs of proximal weakness, paresis of the extraocular muscles (exophthalmic ophthalmoplegia), and, rarely, hypokalemic periodic paralysis. Hypothyroidism is often associated with a decrease in muscle mass and strength, with weak, flabby skeletal muscles and sluggish movements.

Thyroid hormone is believed to regulate muscle protein synthesis and electrolyte balance. Changes in muscle protein synthesis and electrolyte balance may therefore explain the changes in muscle mass and contractility seen in endocrine disorders. The muscular symptoms subside with appropriate treatment of the primary hormonal disorder.

Diseases of energy metabolism

Muscle relies on carbohydrates, such as glycogen and lipids (free fatty acids), for energy. When stored glycogen or lipids cannot be used because of a lack of the enzyme necessary to convert energy for contraction, the individual experiences cramps, fatigue, and exercise intolerance. Disorders of muscle metabolism can be self-limiting, such as in McArdle disease and some lipid disorders, or they can cause widespread irreparable muscle destruction, as in acid maltase deficiency.

McArdle disease

McArdle disease, or myophosphorylase deficiency, was the first myopathy in which a single enzyme defect was identified. It is now one of nine diseases identified to date that have in common an underlying defect in glycogen synthesis, glycogenolysis, or glycolysis. These diseases are often referred to as the **glycogen storage diseases (GSDs)** because each defect results in the abnormal deposition and accumulation of glycogen in skeletal muscle. Individuals with McArdle disease lack muscle phosphorylase, which is responsible for the breakdown of glycogen in muscle. Normally, after the body uses the short-term ATP and phosphocreatine stores, intramuscular lactic acid accumulates as glycogen is used (see Chapter 17). The individual with McArdle disease is not able to break down glycogen or produce lactic acid.

The altered energy production manifests itself in exercise intolerance, fatigue, and painful muscle cramps. When exercise is carried to an extreme, painful muscle contracture and myoglobinuria develop. Some individuals describe a "second wind" phenomenon, in which exercise tolerance increases if they slow their pace once the initial sensation of fatigue commences. This may be caused by the use of free fatty acids as a secondary source of energy. As the disease progresses, some individuals have pronounced muscle weakness and wasting. Other organs are not involved, because the absence of phosphorylase is limited to muscle. Generally, individuals with McArdle disease learn to adapt their daily routine to avoid muscle symptoms.

Acid maltase deficiency

Acid maltase deficiency is an uncommon glycogen storage disease associated with an accumulation of glycogen in the lysosomes of muscle cells and the cells of other tissues. The usual pathways of glycogen degradation are preserved. The absence of the enzyme acid maltase is responsible for the abnormality in glycogen metabolism, although the exact mechanism is unknown. It is an autosomal recessive disorder, with the gene located on the long arm of chromosome 17.

The infantile form is called **Pompe disease** and is recognized shortly after birth by hypotonia, dysreflexia, and an enlarged heart, tongue, and liver. Hypertrophy of these tissues is thought to be the result of glycogen deposition. Children die of cardiac or respiratory failure within 1 year of diagnosis. The adult variety becomes evident subacutely. The muscular symptoms resemble those of muscular dystrophy or polymyositis (see p. 1079). A distinguishing feature in adults may be the presence of severe respiratory muscle weakness.

Myoadenylate deaminase deficiency

An enzyme deficiency that produces changes in skeletal muscle and is associated with exercise intolerance is **myoadenylate deaminase deficiency (MDD)**. Because these individuals lack myoadenylate deaminase, they have a poor capacity for sustained energy production. Myoadenylate deaminase is the catalytic enzyme that forms phosphocreatine and ATP during exercise through a metabolic pathway that binds the purine and phosphate molecules that constitute ATP. Persons with MDD differ from those with McArdle disease in that, during the ischemic exercise test, lactate production is normal when ATP and phosphocreatine are synthesized. The enzyme defect has been reported to be quite common, but in practice it may be rarely recognized as a cause of exercise intolerance.

Lipid deficiencies

Disorders of lipid metabolism are uncommon but account for severe changes in muscle metabolism. These disorders are caused by abnormalities in the transport and processing of fatty acids for energy. The lipid content of muscle cells consists of the free fatty acids, which are oxidized in the mitochondria. These acids require carnitine and the enzyme carnitine palmitoyltransferase (CPT) to transport long-chain fatty acids to the mitochondria. There are two types of CPT: CPT1 is found in liver, muscle, and brain tissue; and CPT2 is considered a ubiquitous protein.[67] CPT2 deficiency is an autosomal recessive disorder that invariably causes attacks of severe myalgia and myoglobinuria.[67] Carnitine deficiency causes abnormal lipid deposition in skeletal muscles.

Measuring the CPT and carnitine content in muscle aids in the diagnosis. Cells in the muscle biopsy show vacuoles and lipid deposits. Treatments with riboflavin, medium-chain triglyceride, oral carnitine, prednisone, and propranolol have been beneficial to some individuals.[67]

Inflammatory Muscle Diseases: Myositis

Viral, bacterial, and parasitic myositis

Viral, bacterial, and parasitic infections of varying severity are known to produce inflammatory changes in skeletal muscle, a group of conditions collectively described by the term **myositis.** In tuberculosis and sarcoidosis, chronic inflammatory changes and granulomas are found in muscle as well as in other affected tissues. In trichinosis, *Trichinella* larvae reside in infected pork and, after ingestion, migrate to the intestinal mucosa and from there to the lymphatics. Symptoms include severe pain, rash, and muscle stiffness. Treatment includes the administration of corticosteroids, immunotherapy, and the antiparasitic agent thiabendazole. Toxoplasmosis, a common parasitic infection, is also associated with a generalized polymyositis that responds rapidly to therapy.

In the tropics, more prevalent disorders include bacterial infections with *Staphylococcus aureus* and parasites such as cysticercus, the larva of the tapeworm *Taenia solium*. Viral infections can be associated with an acute myositis. Muscle pain, tenderness, signs of inflammation, and creatine kinase (CK) elevation are common manifestations of viral myositis. The self-limiting symptoms of muscle aches and pains during a bout of influenza may actually be a subacute form of viral myopathy.

Polymyositis, dermatomyositis, and inclusion-body myositis

Idiopathic inflammatory myopathies are characterized by symmetrical proximal muscle weakness, decreased physical endurance, and changes in muscle. There are three principal types: polymyositis (PM), dermatomyositis (DM), and inclusion-body myositis (IBM).

Polymyositis (PM) (generalized muscle inflammation) and **dermatomyositis (DM)** (polymyositis accompanied by skin lesions) are the most common inflammatory muscle diseases requiring long-term care. Prevalence rates may be about 8.4 per 1 million persons. The incidence appears to be increasing, although this may simply reflect a more accurate diagnosis. **Inclusion-body myositis (IBM)** is an inflammatory muscle disease with the abnormal finding of inclusion bodies or granular material in muscle fibers.

PATHOPHYSIOLOGY PM and inclusion-body myositis (IBM) have a distinct autoimmune component with symptoms resulting from invasion of intact muscle fibers by cytotoxic T cells causing muscle death. DM is primarily a vascular problem that affects skin and muscles through the accumulation of complement in tissues leading to muscle ischemia.[68] This family of diseases is now designated as autoimmune because of the presence of autoantibodies in the serum of many individuals.[68] Studies of DM have shown that the inflammatory cells that surround the perimysial and perivascular sites are selectively enriched in B cells and helper T cells. There is less vascular involvement in PM and IBM where the inflammatory cells, including B cells, T cells, and macrophages, surround the muscle fibers and fascicles. Genetic markers have been located that are associated with IBM, PM, and DM. These markers include human leukocyte antigens (HLAs) in both children and adults.

CLINICAL MANIFESTATIONS The acute symptoms include many of those seen in any inflammatory process: malaise, fever, muscle swelling, pain and tenderness, lethargy, listlessness, morning stiffness, anorexia, and weight loss. These illnesses are usually associated with a symmetric proximal muscle weakness and can be initially confused with other myopathies. A thorough evaluation is required to exclude other disorders. Clinical features common in both PM and DM are dysphagia, reduced esophageal motility, vasculitis, Raynaud phenomenon, cardiomyopathy, and interstitial pulmonary fibrosis. Reduced mobility with frequent falls is a common symptom in IBM because both proximal and distal muscles are affected.[69] Some individuals have other coexisting collagen vascular disorders, such as rheumatoid arthritis, systemic lupus erythematosus, and progressive systemic sclerosis (formerly called *scleroderma*).

The presence of skin rash, calcinosis, and eyelid edema most often suggests DM (Figure 37-26). The rash is often the presenting complaint and may antedate the onset of myopathic symptoms by more than 1 year. The skin rash is a purple (heliotrope) color and involves the eyelids, face, chest, and extensor surfaces of the extremities. DM is slightly more common in children and older adults, with an onset before the age of 15 years or after the age of 50 years. The adult with DM occasionally has underlying malignancies. Calcinosis, with calcium deposition in the subcutaneous tissue, can be a severe long-term complication of DM.

EVALUATION AND TREATMENT The muscle biopsy is striking in DM, with most individuals showing inflammatory cells grouped around blood vessels and atrophy of cells in muscle fascicle. This change, perifascicular atrophy, is absent in PM. Creatinine kinase (CK) is often extremely elevated in both disorders and is a helpful indicator of disease activity. Other muscle enzymes, including aldolase, aspartate aminotransferase (AST), alanine aminotransferase (AST), and lactic dehydrogenase (LDH), are also found to be elevated in most individuals. Serum antinuclear antibodies (ANA) also may be helpful. Muscle biopsy is indispensable for a diagnosis of PM or DM as opposed to

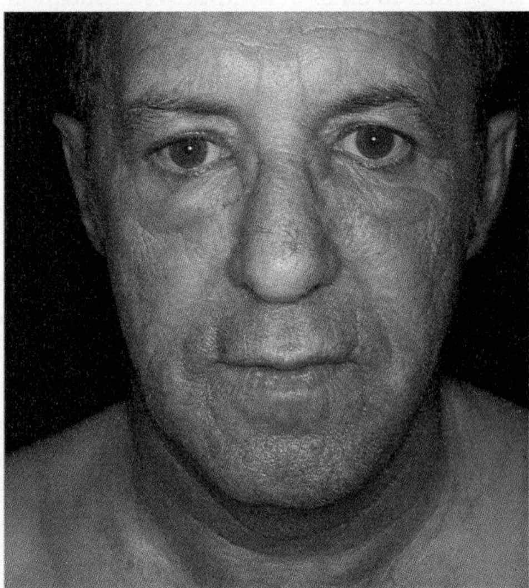

Figure 37-26 ■ **Dermatomyositis.** Heliotrope (violaceous) discoloration around the eyes and periorbital edema. (From Habif TP: *Clinical dermatology,* ed 3, St Louis, 1996, Mosby.)

other myotonic disease. MRI reveals inflammation and edema of the muscles. Electromyography (EMG) is useful in guiding the site for muscle biopsy.[68]

Treatment primarily includes immunosuppressive drugs, although they are not always successful if uniformly applied. Most clinicians choose corticosteroids initially, usually prednisone on a daily or alternating day schedule, tapering the dosage as the symptoms subside. Successful treatment with azathioprine, methotrexate, and cyclophosphamide also has been reported. High-dose intravenous immunoglobulin administration is sometimes used during active disease. Individuals with muscle weakness require careful physiotherapy to design a regular exercise program that prevents contractures and maximizes functional ability.

Toxic Myopathies

Muscle damage caused by drugs or toxins is also called **toxic myopathy**. Alcohol, lipid-lowering agents (fibrates and statins), antimalarial drugs, steroids, thiol derivatives, and narcotics (particularly heroin) can all cause symptoms. Alcohol remains the most common cause of toxic myopathy. Two clinical syndromes are prevalent: (1) an acute attack of muscle weakness, pain, and swelling after a binge or (2) a more chronic, progressive proximal weakness in a drinker of long duration. The incidence of acute alcoholic myopathy has been estimated as being up to 20% of individuals admitted with acute alcoholic withdrawal.

The pathologic abnormalities include necrosis of individual muscle fibers; whole segments can be found in the same stage of degeneration. The mechanism by which alcohol affects the muscle fiber is uncertain, but a direct toxic effect and nutritional deficiency have both received experimental support.

Acute alcoholic myopathy can range from benign cramps and pain resolving in a matter of hours to severe weakness and markedly increased CK associated with myoglobinuria and renal failure. Individuals are prone to repeated attacks following recovery. The only treatment is abstinence from alcohol and improved nutrition.[70] The individual with chronic alcoholic myopathy often has coexisting peripheral neuropathy that complicates the diagnosis.

Chemical agents also have been implicated in the development of myopathy. The drug chloroquine, an antimalarial and amebicidal agent, in high doses has been associated with the development of generalized muscle weakness, particularly of the proximal muscles. Myopathy also has been caused by emetine (the major constituent of ipecac), vincristine, corticosteroids, and the toxic denatured rapeseed oil.

The most severe complication of toxic myopathy is rhabdomyolysis (acute muscle fiber necrosis with leakage of muscle protein into the bloodstream) that leads to myoglobinuria and acute renal failure. Rhabdomyolysis and myoglobinuria can be caused by a crush injury, overexertion, sedatives and narcotics (particularly street heroin), clofibrate (a hypolipidemic agent), and the antifibrinolytic ε-aminocaproate. Drugs that induce hypokalemia, such as amphotericin B, licorice, and azathioprine, also have been reported. In addition, any drug or hormone that can raise or lower serum concentrations of sodium, potassium, calcium, phosphorus, or magnesium can induce myopathic symptoms.

Repeated intramuscular injections have been associated also with changes in muscle fibers. Local necrosis of muscle fiber and elevated CK have been reported after intramuscular injections of cephalothin, lidocaine, diazepam, and digoxin; these effects were not produced with injections of saline. When drugs are injected over long periods, a chronic focal myopathy develops. Proliferation of connective tissue in both the muscle fiber and overlying skin and subcutaneous tissue has been reported. Over time, segments of the muscles, particularly the deltoid and quadriceps, are converted into fibrotic bands. Pathophysiologic mechanisms for these changes include repeated needle trauma and infection, along with the nonphysiologic acidity or alkalinity of the injected material.

✓ QUICK CHECK 37-4

1. How does stress affect muscle tension?
2. How do metabolic muscle diseases develop? What causes them?
3. Name one toxic myopathy, and explain why it develops.

MUSCULOSKELETAL TUMORS

Bone Tumors

Many different types of tumors involve the skeleton. **Bone tumors** may originate from bone cells, cartilage, fibrous tissue, marrow, or vascular tissue. Based on the tissue of origin, bone tumors are classified as osteogenic, chondrogenic, collagenic, or myelogenic. Each of the four types arises from one of the four stem cells that are ultimately derived from the primitive mesoderm (Figure 37-27). In addition, bone tumors may be classified as being of histiocytic, notochordal, lipogenic, or neurogenic origin.

The mesoderm contributes the primitive fibroblast and reticulum cells. The fibroblast is the progenitor of the osteoblast and the chondroblast cell. Each cell synthesizes a specific type of intercellular ground substance, and the tumor derived from the cell is generally characterized by the type of ground substance produced by the cell. For example, osteogenic tumors usually contain cells that have the appearance of osteoblasts and produce an intercellular substance that can be recognized as osteoid. Chondrogenic tumors contain chondroblasts and produce an intercellular substance similar to chondroid (cartilage). Collagenic tumors contain fibrous tissue cells and produce an intercellular substance similar to the type of collagen found in fibrous connective tissue.

Tumors are also classified as benign or malignant (see Chapter 9). The criteria used to identify tumor cells as malignant are (1) an increased nuclear/cytoplasmic ratio, (2) an irregular nuclear border, (3) excess chromatin, (4) a prominent nucleolus, and (5) an increase in the number of cells undergoing mitosis. However, many young, rapidly

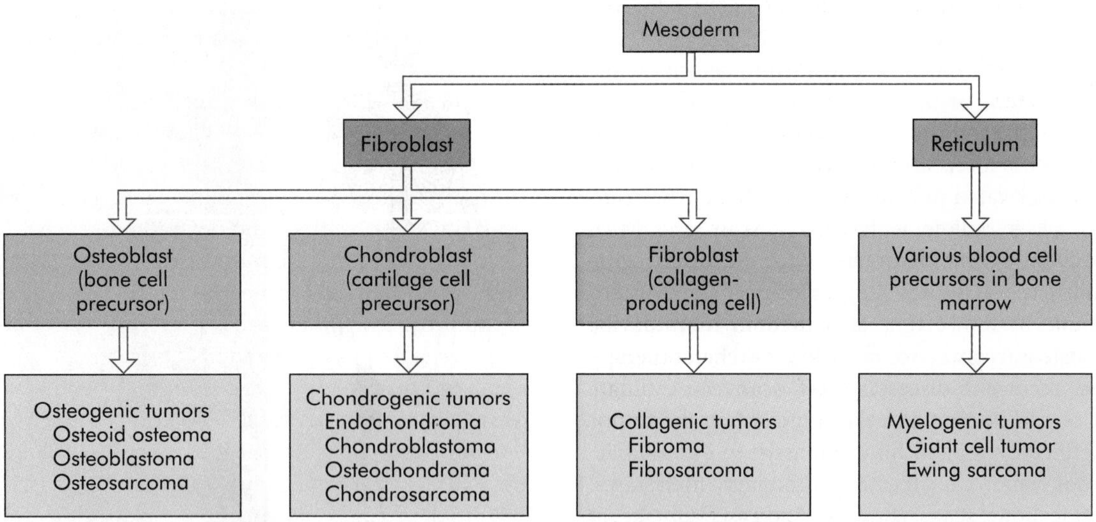

Figure 37-27 ■ **Derivation of Bone Tumors.**

growing, normal cells and cells subjected to inflammation and change in their blood supply also exhibit many of these same characteristics. (Tumor characteristics in general are described in Chapter 9.)

Epidemiology

The incidence rate of bone tumors varies with age. In children younger than 15 years, the rate of bone tumors is relatively low, constituting approximately 5% of all malignancies. Adolescents have the highest incidence of bone tumors, and adults between the ages of 30 and 35 have the lowest incidence. After age 35 years, the incidence rate slowly increases until, at age 60 years, it equals the incidence rate in adolescents, primarily related to secondary metastatic tumors.

Patterns of bone destruction

The general pathologic features of bone tumors include bone destruction, erosion or expansion of the cortex, and periosteal response to changes in underlying bone. The least amount of pathologic damage occurs with benign bone tumors, which push against neighboring tissue. Because they usually have a symmetric, controlled growth pattern, benign bone tumors tend to compress and displace neighboring normal bone tissue, which weakens the bone's structure until it is incapable of withstanding the stress of ordinary use, leading to pathologic fracture. Other tumors invade and destroy adjacent normal bone tissue by producing substances that promote resorption by increasing osteoclast activity or by interfering with a bone's blood supply. Three patterns of bone destruction by bone tumors have been identified: (1) the geographic pattern, (2) the moth-eaten pattern, and (3) the permeative pattern (Table 37-6).

Tumors that erode the cortex of the bone usually stimulate a periosteal response—that is, new bone formation at the interface between the surface of the bone and the periosteum. Slow erosion of the cortex usually stimulates a uniform periosteal response. Additional layers of bone are added to the exterior surface of the bone to buttress the cortex. Eventually, the additional layers expand the bone's contour. Aggressive penetration of the cortex usually elevates the periosteum and stimulates erratic patterns of new bone formation. Examples of erratic patterns include concentric layers of new bone; a sunburst pattern, in which delicate rays of new bone radiate toward the periosteum from a single focus on the underlying surface; and rays of new bone that grow perpendicularly, creating a brush or bristle pattern.

Evaluation

A malignant bone tumor must be identified early to allow the survival of the individual and the preservation of the affected limb. However, individuals often have only vague symptoms that may be attributed to minor trauma, degen-

TABLE 37-6

Patterns of Bone Destruction Caused by Bone Tumors

Type	Features
Geographic pattern	Least aggressive type Generally indicative of slow-growing or benign tumor Well-defined margins on tumor, easily separated from surrounding normal bone Uniform and well-defined lytic area in bone Margin smooth or irregular, demarcated by short zone of transition between normal and abnormal bone tissue
Moth-eaten pattern	Characteristic of rapidly growing, malignant bone tumors More aggressive pattern Tumor margin less defined or demarcated; cannot easily be separated from normal bone Areas of partially destroyed bone adjacent to completely lytic areas
Permeative pattern	Caused by aggressive malignant tumor with rapid growth potential Margins of tumor poorly demarcated Abnormal bone merges imperceptibly with normal bone

erative changes, or inflammatory conditions. In addition, other conditions may obscure the diagnosis.

Thorough diagnostic studies are needed to determine the exact type and extent of bone tumor present, which also helps determine the optimal treatment regimen. Serum alkaline phosphatase levels are elevated in bone lytic tumors and significantly elevated in osteosarcoma. Radiologic studies, including plain radiologic films, CT scan, and MRI, have become the examination of choice for the local staging of bone tumors, especially the staging of peripheral osteosarcomas (Table 37-7). MRI is also used to monitor the response of osteosarcomas to radiation or chemotherapy and to detect recurrent disease. A CT scan can evaluate involvement of osteosarcoma in flat bones when the tumor is not well defined on a plain film, can assist in differentiating the tumor, and can locate pulmonary metastases. Radionucleotide bone scans show an increased uptake at the tumor site. (Tumor staging is discussed in Chapter 9.)

Additional diagnostic studies done for specific bone tumors include a complete blood count and erythrocyte sedimentation rate (to rule out infection or myeloma) and serum levels of calcium and phosphorus to detect hypercalcemia. Serum glucose levels may be elevated in chondrosarcoma. Acid phosphatase may show moderate elevations in bone metastases, multiple myeloma, and advanced Paget disease. Serum protein electrophoresis and immunoelectrophoresis are done to rule out other diseases. Fine needle biopsy is done, usually at the time of surgery, to determine the exact tumor type.

Types

A large number of lesions are classified as bone tumors. The bone tumors most representative of the four derivative types—osteogenic, chondrogenic, collagenic, and myelogenic tumors—are described here (Figure 37-28).

Osteogenic tumors: osteosarcoma

Osteogenic (bone-forming) tumors are characterized by the formation of bone or osteoid tissue with a sarcomatous tissue. The tissue can have the appearance of callus or compact or spongy bone. The most common malignant bone-forming tumor is the **osteosarcoma.**

Osteosarcomas account for 38% of bone tumors. The male/female ratio is 2:1, and osteosarcoma occurs predominantly in adolescents and young adults. Sixty percent of osteosarcomas occur in persons younger than 20 years. A secondary peak incidence for osteosarcoma occurs in the 50- to 60-year age group, primarily in individuals with a history of radiation therapy several years previously for pelvic or other malignancies (see Figure 37-28).

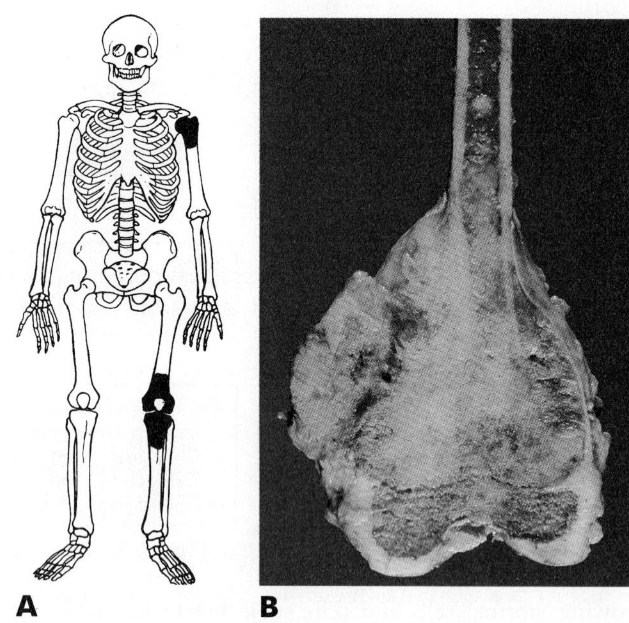

Figure 37-28 ■ **Osteosarcoma. A,** Common locations of osteosarcoma. **B,** Femur has a large mass involving the metaphysis of the bone; the tumor has destroyed the cortex, forming a soft tissue component. (From Damjanov I, Linder J, editors: *Anderson's pathology,* ed 10, St Louis, 1996, Mosby.)

An osteosarcoma is a malignant bone-forming tumor. It is large, destructive, and most often found in bone marrow; it has a moth-eaten pattern of bone destruction. The borders of the tumor are indistinct and merge into adjacent normal bone. Osteosarcomas contain osteoid, produced by anaplastic stromal cells, which are atypical, abnormal cells not seen in normal developing bone; they are neither normal nor embryonal. Many tumors are heterogenous; for example, the osteosarcoma also may contain chondroid (cartilage) and fibrinoid tissue that may form the bulk of the tumor. The osteoid is deposited as thick masses or "streamers," which infiltrate the normal compact bone, destroy it, and replace it with masses of osteoid. Demonstrating the presence of osteoid aids in the diagnosis of osteosarcoma. Bone tissue produced by osteosarcomas never matures to compact bone.

TABLE 37-7

Surgical Staging System for Bone Tumors

Stage	Grade	Site (T)	Metastasis (M)
IA	Low (G_1)	Intracompartmental (T_1)	None (M_0)
IB	Low (G_1)	Extracompartmental (T_2)	None (M_0)
IIA	High (G_2)	Intracompartmental (T_1)	None (M_0)
IIB	High (G_2)	Extracompartmental (T_2)	None (M_0)
IIIA	Low (G_1)	Intracompartmental or extracompartmental (T_1 or T_2)	Regional or distant (M_1)
IIIB	High(G_2)	Intracompartmental or extracompartmental (T_1 or T_2)	Regional or distant (M_1)

Data from Simon SR, editor: *Orthopaedic basic science,* Chicago, 1994, American Academy of Orthopaedic Surgeons.

Ninety percent of osteosarcomas are located in the metaphyses of long bones, especially the distal femoral metaphysis, with 50% around the knee area. The tumor typically breaks through the cortex, lifts the periosteum, and forms a soft tissue mass that is not covered by a smooth shell of new bone. Lifting of the periosteum stimulates bizarre patterns of new bone formation called a *periosteal reaction.* Distinct osteosarcomas occur on the surface of long bones, called parosteal, periosteal, and high-grade surface osteosarcomas; dedifferentiated parosteal and central osteosarcomas also occur.

The most common initial symptoms are pain and swelling. Initially, the pain is slight and intermittent, but within a short time the pain increases in severity and duration. Pain is usually worse at night and gradually requires medication. Systemic symptoms are uncommon. Usually, a coincidental history of trauma is noted. Occasionally, the individual may present with a pathologic fracture.

Surgery is a major treatment of choice, with the location of the tumor, its size, malignancy grade, and evidence of metastasis dictating the type and extent of surgery (see Table 37-7). Preoperative chemotherapy has greatly increased the number of individuals qualifying for limb salvage surgery. Limb-salvaging procedures have been made possible by advances in reconstructive techniques and endoprosthetics. Limb salvage ultimately may be successful in as many as 80% of persons. Individuals must have achieved most of their bone growth to be a candidate for limb salvage procedures.

If an amputation is done, individuals are monitored closely with chest roentgenograms and CT. Pulmonary metastases are surgically resected, and chemotherapy is now a common therapy given both before and after operation, using combinations of chemotherapeutic agents.

Chondrogenic tumors: chondrosarcoma

Chondrogenic (cartilage-forming) tumors produce cartilage or chondroid, a primitive cartilage or cartilage-like substance. The most common chondrogenic tumor is chondrosarcoma.

Chondrosarcoma is a tumor of middle-aged and older adults. Most cases of primary chondrosarcoma are found in persons between 50 and 70 years of age. Secondary chondrosarcoma (a chondrosarcoma derived from an **endochondroma**) occurs most often in young adults between 20 and 30 years of age. The tumor is found more often in men than in women.

A chondrosarcoma is a large, ill-defined malignant tumor that infiltrates trabeculae in spongy bone. It occurs most often in the metaphysis or diaphysis of long bones, especially the femur, and in the bones of the pelvis. If located near the end of the bone, the tumor will infiltrate into the joint space. The tumor expands and enlarges the contour of the bone, causes extensive erosion of the cortex, and expands into the soft tissues.

Symptoms associated with the chondrosarcoma have an insidious onset. Local swelling and pain are the usual presenting symptoms. At first the pain is dull and intermittent; then it gradually intensifies and becomes constant. It may waken the person at night.

Diagnostic studies include radiographs, which must be reviewed carefully for an accurate diagnosis. Biopsy is done at the time of surgery. (If biopsy is done before scheduled surgical incision, seeding of tumor cells could occur.) Sufficient tumor material must be obtained to facilitate an accurate diagnosis.

Surgical excision is generally regarded as the treatment of choice. Many surgically treated individuals demonstrate recurrences, however, so amputation is becoming one treatment of choice. Therefore individuals with tumors located in the limbs have a better prognosis than those with pelvic lesions.

Collagenic tumors: fibrosarcoma

Collagenic (collagen-forming) tumors produce fibrous connective tissue. The most typical collagenic tumor is the fibrosarcoma.

Fibrosarcomas represent 4% of the primary malignant bone tumors, with a broad age distribution. They may occur at any age but are most common in adults between 30 and 50 years of age. The incidence is slightly greater in females. Fibrosarcoma also may be a secondary complication of radiation therapy, Paget disease, and long-standing osteomyelitis.

Fibrosarcoma is a solitary tumor that most often affects the metaphyseal region of the femur or tibia. The tumor is composed of a firm fibrous mass of tissue that contains collagen, malignant fibroblasts, and occasional osteoclast-like giant cells.[71]

The tumor begins in the marrow cavity of the bone and infiltrates the trabeculae. It demonstrates a permeative growth pattern, destroys the cortex, and extends into the soft tissue. Metastasis to the lung is common.

Symptoms associated with the tumor have an insidious onset, which delays diagnosis. Pain and swelling are the usual presenting symptoms and usually indicate that the tumor has broken through the cortex. Local tenderness, a palpable mass, and limitation of motion also may be present. A pathologic fracture in the affected bone is often the reason for seeking medical help. Diagnostic studies include radiographs and MRI.

Radical surgery and amputation are the treatments of choice for fibrosarcoma. There is a high probability of metastases. Radiation therapy is generally considered ineffective treatment for this tumor.

Myelogenic tumors

Myelogenic tumors originate from various bone marrow cells. Two types of myelogenic tumors are giant cell tumor and myeloma.

Giant cell tumor

Giant cell tumor is the sixth most common of the primary bone tumors, accounting for 4% to 5% of bone tumors. It is generally benign but can become malignant after radiation treatment. Giant cell tumors have a wide age distribution;

however, they are rare in persons younger than 10 years or older than 70 years. Most giant cell tumors are found in persons between 20 and 40 years of age. Unlike most other bone tumors, giant cell tumors affect females more often than males.

The giant cell tumor is a solitary, circumscribed tumor that causes extensive bone resorption because of its osteoclastic origin. The giant cell tumor is located in the center of the epiphysis in the femur, tibia, radius, or humerus. The tumor has a slow, relentless growth rate and is usually contained within the original contour of the affected bone. It may, however, extend into the articular cartilage. When the tumor extends, it is usually covered by periosteum or periosteal bone growth. The tumor also may extend into local soft tissue, but it has a low rate of metastasis to other organs or tissues, although it has a high recurrence rate.

The most common symptoms associated with the giant cell tumor are pain, local swelling, and limitation of movement. Diagnostic studies include radiographs, CT, and MRI. Cryosurgery and resection of the tumor with the use of adjuvant polymethylmethacrylate (PMMA) for bone grafts decrease recurrence and are more successful treatments than curettage and radiation. Depending on the extent of the tumor and its recurrence, amputation may be necessary.

Muscle Tumors

Rhabdomyoma

Rhabdomyoma is an extremely rare benign tumor of muscle that generally occurs in the tongue, neck muscles, larynx, uvula, nasal cavity, axilla, vulva, and heart. These tumors are usually treated by surgical excision and do not recur.

Rhabdomyosarcoma

The malignant tumor of striated muscle is called **rhabdomyosarcoma.** Infants, children, and teenagers account for over 85% of cases. This tumor is highly malignant with rapid metastasis. Rhabdomyosarcomas are located in the muscle tissue of the head, neck, and genitourinary tract in 75% of cases. The remainder are in the trunk and extremities.

Three types of rhabdomyosarcoma are differentiated on pathologic section: pleomorphic, embryonal, and alveolar. The pleomorphic, or spindle cell, type is considered to be one of the most highly malignant tumors of the extremities seen in adulthood. Fortunately, it is very rare. Embryonal tumors are most often seen in infancy and childhood and appear to be shaped like a tadpole or tennis racquet. Alveolar-type tumors appear lattice-like and look like lung tissue alveoli.

The diagnosis of rhabdomyosarcoma is made by incisional biopsy and examination of the specimen by a pathologist. CT scan also helps define the tissue borders. Staging is based on pathologic grade of the tumor and is helpful in determining prognosis and treatment.

Treatment consists of a combination of surgical excision, radiation therapy, and systemic chemotherapy. Cure with distant metastasis is unlikely.

Other tumors

Metastatic deposits of tumors in muscles are rare in spite of the extensive vascular supply of skeletal muscles. It is suggested that local pH or metabolic changes prevent metastatic involvement from other tumors. When adjacent carcinomas do cause muscle damage, it is usually related to the compression of tissue and resultant muscle atrophy.

QUICK CHECK 37-5

1. From what cells do bone tumors originate?
2. Compare five major characteristics of benign bone tumors with those of malignant bone tumors.
3. How does the presence of metastatic tumors affect treatment options and prognosis of persons with osteosarcoma?

Did You Understand?

Musculoskeletal Injuries

1. The most serious musculoskeletal injury is a fracture. A bone can be completely or incompletely fractured. A closed fracture leaves the skin intact. An open fracture has an overlying skin wound. The direction of the fracture line can be linear, oblique, spiral, or transverse. Greenstick, torus, and bowing fractures are examples of incomplete fractures that occur in children. Stress fractures occur in normal or abnormal bone that is subjected to repeated stress. Fatigue fractures occur in normal bone subjected to abnormal stress. Normal weight bearing can cause an insufficiency fracture in abnormal bone.
2. Dislocation is complete loss of contact between the surfaces of two bones. Subluxation is partial loss of contact between two bones. As a bone separates from a joint, it may damage adjacent nerves, blood vessels, ligaments, tendons, and muscle.
3. Tendon tears are called strains, and ligament tears are called sprains. A complete separation of a tendon or ligament from its attachment is called an avulsion.
4. Myoglobinuria (rhabomyolysis) can be a serious life-threatening complication of severe muscle trauma.

Did You Understand?—Cont'd

Disorders of Bones

1. Metabolic bone diseases are characterized by abnormal bone structure. In osteoporosis the density or mass of bone is reduced because the bone-remodeling cycle is disrupted. Osteomalacia is a metabolic bone disease characterized by inadequate bone mineralization. Excessive and abnormal bone remodeling occurs in Paget disease.
2. Osteomyelitis is a bone infection caused *most often* by bacteria. Bacteria can enter bone from outside the body (exogenous osteomyelitis) or from infection sites within the body (hematogenous osteomyelitis).

Disorders of Joints

1. Because of improved imaging technology, inflammation has been identified as an important feature of osteoarthritis.
2. Osteoarthritis (OA) is a common, age-related disorder of synovial joints. The primary defect in OA is loss of articular cartilage.
3. Rheumatoid arthritis is an inflammatory joint disease characterized by inflammatory destruction of the synovial membrane, articular cartilage, joint capsule, and surrounding ligaments and tendons. Rheumatoid nodules also may invade the skin, lung, and spleen and involve small and large arteries. Rheumatoid arthritis is a systemic disease that affects the heart, lungs, kidneys, and skin, as well as the joints.
4. Ankylosing spondylitis is a chronic, inflammatory joint disease characterized by stiffening and fusion of the spine and sacroiliac joints. It is a systemic, immune inflammatory disease.
5. Gout is a syndrome caused by defects in uric acid metabolism with high levels of uric acid in the blood and body fluids. Uric acid crystallizes in the connective tissue of a joint where it initiates inflammatory destruction of the joint.

Disorders of Skeletal Muscle

1. A pathologic contracture is permanent muscle shortening caused by muscle spasticity, as seen in central nervous system (CNS) injury or severe muscle weakness.
2. Stress-induced muscle tension is presumably caused by increased activity in the reticular activating system and gamma loop in the muscle fiber. The use of progressive relaxation training and biofeedback has been advocated to reduce muscle tension.
3. Fibromyalgia is a chronic musculoskeletal syndrome characterized by diffuse pain and tender points. Unknown but suspected is that muscle is the end organ responsible for the pain and fatigue. Most cases are women, and the peak age is 30 to 50 years.
4. Atrophy of muscle fibers and overall diminished size of the muscle are seen after prolonged inactivity. Isometric contractions and passive lengthening exercises decrease atrophy to some degree in immobilized patients.
5. Hyperexcitable membranes cause the physical and electrical phenomenon of myotonia. The disorder is treated with drugs that reduce muscle fiber excitability. Periodic paralysis is caused by an unresponsive muscle membrane and is accompanied by changes in serum potassium. The biochemical defect is possibly related to changes in the muscle membrane and sarcoplasmic reticulum.
6. Metabolic muscle diseases are caused by endocrine disorders, glycogen storage diseases, enzyme deficiencies, and abnormal lipid function. The muscle depends on a complex system of carbohydrates and fats converted by enzymes to produce energy for the muscle cell. Abnormalities in these pathways can inhibit function or cause damage to the muscle fiber. These illnesses are rare, yet they account for significant functional abnormalities.
7. Viral, bacterial, and parasitic infections of muscles produce the characteristic clinical and pathologic changes associated with inflammation. These are usually treatable and self-limiting disorders.
8. Polymyositis (generalized muscle inflammation) and dermatomyositis (polymyositis accompanied by skin rash) are characterized by inflammation of connective tissue and muscle fibers and muscle fiber necrosis. Cell-mediated and humoral immune factors have been implicated. Treatment with immunosuppressive agents is effective in many cases.
9. The most common toxic myopathy is caused by alcohol abuse. Direct toxic effects of alcohol-producing necrosis of muscle fibers and nutritional deficiency have been suggested. The only treatment is abstinence and improved nutrition. The toxic effects of many drugs on muscle fibers cause local trauma to the muscle fibers caused by direct effects of the needle, secondary infection, and changes caused by nonphysiologic acidity and alkalinity in the fibers.

Musculoskeletal Tumors

1. Sarcomas of muscle tissue are rare. Rhabdomyosarcoma has a uniformly poor prognosis because of an aggressive invasion and early, widespread dissemination. The usual treatment includes surgical excision, radiation therapy, and systemic chemotherapy.
2. Bone tumors originate from bone cells, cartilage cells, fibrous tissue cells, or vascular marrow cells. Each cell produces a specific type of ground substance that is used to classify the tumor as osteogenic (bone cell), chondrogenic (cartilage cell), collagenic (fibrous tissue cell), or myelogenic (vascular marrow cell). Malignant bone tumors are usually large, aggressively destroy surrounding bone, invade surrounding tissue, and initiate independent growth outside the site of origin. Benign bone tumors are less destructive, limit their growth to the anatomic confines of the bone, and have a well-demarcated border.

Key Terms

Acid maltase deficiency, 1060
Acute gouty arthritis, 1055
Age-related bone loss, 1040
Ankylosing spondylitis (AS), 1052
Asymptomatic hyperuricemia, 1055
Avulsion, 1032
Biofeedback, 1057
Bone mass density (BMD), 1037
Bone tumor, 1062
Bowing fracture, 1029
Bursa (*pl.*, bursae), 1033
Caplan syndrome, 1051
Chondrogenic (cartilage-forming) tumor, 1065
Chondrosarcoma, 1065
Closed (simple) fracture, 1028
Collagenic (collagen-forming) tumor, 1065
Comminuted fracture, 1028
Compartment syndrome, 1034
Complete fracture, 1028
Contracture, 1057
Degenerative joint disease (osteoarthritis), 1045
Delayed union, 1031
Dermatomyositis (DM), 1061
Dislocation, 1031
Disuse atrophy, 1057
Dual x-ray absorptiometry (DXA), 1041
Endochondroma, 1065
Endogenous (hematogenous) osteomyelitis, 1043
Enthesis, 1052
Epicondylitis, 1033
Exogenous osteomyelitis, 1043
External fixation, 1031
Fatigue fracture, 1030
Fibromyalgia, 1057
Fibrosarcoma, 1065
Fracture, 1028
Giant cell tumor, 1065
Glucocorticoid-induced osteoporosis, 1040
Glycogen storage disease (GSD), 1060
Gout, 1053
Gouty arthritis, 1053
Greenstick fracture, 1029
Hyperbaric oxygen therapy, 1045
Iatrogenic osteoporosis, 1039
Immobilization (of a fracture), 1031
Inclusion-body myositis (IBM), 1061
Incomplete fracture, 1028
Inflammatory joint disease (arthritis), 1048
Insufficiency fracture, 1030
Internal fixation, 1031
Involucrum, 1044
Joint effusion, 1047
Joint stiffness, 1047
Kyphosis, 1040
Lateral epicondylitis (tennis elbow), 1033
Ligament, 1032
Linear fracture, 1028
Malignant hyperthermia, 1035
Malunion, 1031
McArdle disease, 1060
Medial epicondylitis (golfer's elbow), 1033
Muscle strain, 1034
Myelogenic tumor, 1065
Myoadenylate deaminase deficiency (MDD), 1060
Myoglobinuria (rhabdomyolysis), 1034
Myositis ossificans (heterotropic ossification), 1034
Myositis, 1060
Myotonia, 1059
Noninflammatory joint disease, 1045
Nonunion, 1031
Oblique fracture, 1028
Open (compound) fracture, 1028
Osteoarthritis (OA), 1045
Osteogenic (bone-forming) tumor, 1064
Osteomalacia, 1042
Osteomyelitis, 1043
Osteophyte, 1046
Osteoporosis, 1036
Osteoprotegerin (OPG), 1040
Osteosarcoma, 1064
Paget disease (osteitis deformans), 1042
Pannus, 1050
Pathologic fracture, 1030
Peak bone mass, 1036
Periodic paralysis, 1059
Polymyositis (PM), 1061
Pompe disease, 1060
Postmenopausal osteoporosis, 1038
Progressive relaxation training, 1057
Receptor activator nuclear factor κβ (RANK), 1040
Receptor activator of nuclear factor κβ ligand (RANKL), 1040
Reduction (of a fracture), 1031
Regional osteoporosis, 1039
Rhabdomyoma, 1066
Rhabdomyosarcoma, 1066
Rheumatoid arthritis (RA), 1048
Rheumatoid factor (RF), 1049
Rheumatoid nodule, 1051
Sequestrum, 1044
Spiral fracture, 1029
Sprain, 1032
Strain, 1032
Stress fracture, 1030
Subluxation, 1031
Syndesmophyte, 1052
Tendon, 1032
Tendonitis (tendinopathy), 1033
Tophaceous gout, 1055
Tophus (*pl.*, tophi), 1053
Torus fracture, 1029
Toxic myopathy, 1062
Transchondral fracture, 1030
Transverse fracture, 1029
Volkmann ischemic contracture, 1034

References

1. Vyrostek SB et al: Surveillance for fatal and nonfatal injuries—United States 2001, *MMWR Morb Mortal Wkly Rep* 53:SS-7, 1–57, 2004.
2. Shumway-Cook A et al: Incidence of and risk factors for falls following hip fractures in community-dwelling older adults, *Phys Ther* 85(7):648–655, 2005.
3. Wilson JJ, Best TM: Common overuse tendon problems: a review and recommendations for treatment, *Am Fam Physician* 72(5):811–818, 2005.
4. Whaley AL, Baker CL: Lateral epicondylitis, *Clin Sports Med* 23:677–691, 2004.
5. Shehab D, Elgazzar AH, Collier BD: Heterotopic ossification, *J Nucl Med* 43(3):346–353, 2002.
6. Sauret JM, Marinides G, Wang GK: Rhabdomyolysis, *Am Fam Physician* 65(5):907–912, 2002.
7. Allan D, Jones B: Compartment syndrome: a forgotten diagnosis, *Lancet* 359(9325):2248, 2002.
8. Yamaguchi S, Viegas SF: Causes of upper extremity compartment syndrome, *Hand Clin* 14(3):365–370, 1998.
9. Trice M, Colwell CW: A historical review of compartment syndrome and Volkmann's ischemic contracture, *Hand Clin* 14(3):335–341, 1998.
10. Kanis JA: Assessment of fracture risk and its application to screening for postmenopausal osteoporosis: synopsis of a WHO report, WHO Study Group, *Osteoporos Int* 4:368–381, 1994.
11. National Osteoporosis Foundation: *America's bone health: the state of osteoporosis and low bone mass in our nation*, Washington, DC, 2002, National Osteoporosis Foundation.
12. Binder EF, Brown M, Sinecore DR: Effects of extended outpatient rehabilitation after hip fracture, *JAMA* 292:837–846, 2004.
13. Old JL, Calvert M: Vertebral compression fractures in the elderly, *Am Fam Physician* 69(1):111–116, 2004.
14. Rochira Z et al: Osteoporosis and male age-related hypogonadism: role of sex steroids on bone (patho)physiology, *Eur J Endocrinol* 154:175–185, 2006.

References—Cont'd

15. US Department of Health and Human Services: *Bone health and osteoporosis: a report of the surgeon general*, Rockville, MD, 2004.
16. Licata AA: Diagnosing primary osteoporosis: it's more than a T-score, *Clev Clin J Med* 73(5):473–476, 2006.
17. Nelson DA, Megyesi MS: Sex and ethnic differences in bone architecture, *Curr Osteoporosis Rep* 2(2):65–69, 2004.
18. Nguyen TV, Sambrook PN, Eisman JA: Bone loss, physical activity, and weight change in elderly women: the Dubbo Osteoporosis Epidemiology Study, *J Bone Miner Res* 13(9): 1458–1467, 1998.
19. Weitzmann MN, Pacifici R: Estrogen regulation of immune cell bone interactions, *Ann NY Acad Sci* 1068:256–274, 2006.
20. Ueland, T et al: Age-related changes in cortical bone contents of insulin-like growth factor binding protein (IGCBP)-3, osteoprotegerin, and calcium in postmenopausal osteoporosis: a cross-sectional study. *J Clin Indocrinol Metab*, 85(3):1014–2003.
21. Sammartino A et al: Osteoporosis and cardiovascular disease: benefit-risk of hormone replacement therapy, *J Endocrinol Invest* 28(10 suppl):80–84, 2005.
22. Tormy SM et al: Current status of combined hormone replacement therapy in clinical practice, *Clin Breast Can* 6(suppl 2):S51–S57, 2006.
23. Amin S et al: Estradiol, testosterone, and the risk for hip fractures in elderly men from the Framingham Study, *Am J Med* 119(5):426–433, 2006.
24. Nieves J: Osteoporosis: the role of micronutrients, *Am J Clin Nutr* 81(suppl):1232S–1239S, 2005.
25. Cashman K, Flynn A: Trace elements and bone metabolism, *Bibliotheca Nutritio et Dieta* 54:150–164, 1998.
26. Bauman WA et al: Effect of pamidronate administration on bone in patients with acute spinal cord injury, *J Rehab Res Develop* 42:305–314, 2005.
27. Blair HC, Carrington JL: Bone cell precursors and the pathophysiology of bone loss, *Ann NY Acad Sci* 1068:244–249, 2006.
28. Sambrook P, Cooper C: Osteoporosis, *Lancet* 367(9527): 2010–2018, 2006.
29. Hofbauer LC, Schoppet M: Clinical implications of the osteoprotegerin/RANKL/RANK system for bone and vascular diseases, *JAMA* 292(4):490–495, 2004.
30. Riggs BL, Khosla S, Melton LJ III: Sex steroids and the construction and conservation of the adult skeleton, *Endocr Rev* 23(3):279–302, 2002.
31. Stevens JA, Olson S: Reducing falls and resulting hip fractures among older women, *MMWR Recomm Rep* 49(RR-2):3–12, 2000.
32. Greenspan SL, Resnick NM, Parker RA: Early changes in biochemical markers of bone turnover are associated with long-term changes in bone mineral density in elderly women on alendronate, hormone replacement therapy, or combination therapy: a three-year, double-blind, placebo-controlled randomized clinical trial, *J Clin Endocrinol Metab* 90(5):2762–2767, 2005.
33. Cohen L: The role of magnesium, *Isr Med Assoc J* 4(3):232–233, 2002.
34. Rude RK et al: Magnesium deficiency: effect on bone and mineral metabolism in the mouse, *Calcif Tissue Int* 72(1):32, 41, 2003.
35. Potts JT: Parathyroid hormone: past and present, *J Endocrinol* 187:311–325, 2005.
36. Weisberg P et al: Nutritional rickets among children in the United States: review of cases reported between 1986 and 2003, *Am J Clin Nutr* 8(6 suppl):1697S–1705S, 2004.
37. Walsh JP: Paget's disease of bone, *Med J Austral* 181(5): 262–265, 2004.
38. Reddy SV, et al: Paget's disease of the bone: a disease of the osteoclast, *Rev Endocr Metab Disord* 2(2):195–201, 2001.
39. De Boeck H: Osteomyelitis and septic arthritis in children, *Acta Orthop Belg* 71:505–515, 2005.
40. Kaplan SL: Osteomyelitis in children, *Infect Dis Clin North Am* 19:787–797, 2005.
41. Restrepo CS et al: Imaging findings in musculoskeletal complications of AIDS, *Radio Graphics* 24(4):1029–1049, 2004.
42. Garvin K, Feschuk C: Polylactide-polyglycolide antibiotic implants, *Clin Orthop Relat Res* 437:105–110, 2005.
43. Witso E et al: Cortical allograft as a vehicle for antibiotic delivery, *Acta Orthop* 76(4):481–486, 2005.
44. Al-Waili NS, Butler GJ: Effects of hyperbaric oxygen on inflammatory response to wound and trauma: possible mechanism of action, *Scientific World J* 6:425–441, 2006.
45. Rijk PC: Meniscal allograft transplantation—part II: background, results, graft selection and preservation, and surgical considerations, *Arthroscopy* 20(7):728–743, 2004.
46. Dieppe PA, Lohmander LS: Pathogenesis and management of pain in osteoarthritis, *Lancet* 365(9463):965–973, 2005.
47. Rutsch F, Terkeltaub R: Deficiencies of physiologic calcification inhibitors and low grade inflammation in arterial calcification: lessons for cartilage calcification, *Joint Bone Spine* 72(2):110–118, 2005.
48. Aigner T, McKenna L: Molecular pathology and pathobiology of osteoarthritic cartilage, *Cell Molec Life Sci* 59(1):5–18, 2002.
49. Pufe T et al: The influence of biomechanical parameters on the expression of VEGF and endostatin in the bone and joint system, *Annal Anat* 187(5–6):461–472, 2005.
50. Krohn K: Footwear alterations and bracing as treatments for knee osteoarthritis, *Curr Opin Rheumatol* 17(5):653–656, 2005.
51. Towheed TE et al: Glucosamine therapy for treating osteoarthritis, *Cochran Database Syst Rev* 2, CD002946, 2005.
52. Bellamy N et al: Viscosupplementation for the treatment of osteoarthritis of the knee, *Cochrane Database Syst Rev* 2: CD005321, 2005.
53. Kurtz S et al: Prevalence of primary and revision total hip and knee arthroplasty in the United States from 1990 through 2002, *J Bone Joint Surg Am* 87(7):1487–1497, 2005.
54. Klareskog L et al: What precedes development of rheumatoid arthritis? *Ann Rheum Dis* 63(suppl 2):ii28–ii31, 2004.
55. Mimori T: Clinical significance of anti-CCP antibodies in rheumatoid arthritis, *Intern Med* 44(11):1122–1126, 2005.
56. Haringman JJ, Ludikhuize J, Tak PP: Chemokines in joint disease: the key to inflammation? *Ann Rheum Dis* 63:1186–1194, 2004.
57. Firestein GS: Etiology and pathogenesis of rheumatoid arthritis. In Ruddy S et al, editors: *Kelley's textbook of rheumatology*, ed 7, Philadelphia, 2005, Saunders.
58. Harris ED: Clinical features of rheumatoid arthritis. In Ruddy S et al, editors: *Kelley's textbook of rheumatology*, ed 7, Philadelphia, 2005, Saunders.
59. American College of Rheumatology Subcommittee on Rheumatoid Arthritis Guidelines: guidelines for the management of rheumatoid arthritis, *Arthritis Rheum* 46(2):328–346, 2002.
60. Kim TH, Uhm WS, Inman RD: Pathogenesis of ankylosing spondylitis and reactive arthritis, *Curr Opin Rheumatol* 17(4): 400–405, 2005.
61. Braun J et al: International ASAS consensus statement for the use of anti-tumor necrosis factor agents in patients with ankylosing spondylitis, *Ann Rheum Dis* 62:817–824, 2003.
62. Zochling J et al: ASAS/EULAR recommendations for the management of ankylosing spondylitis, *Ann Rheum Dis* 65(4): 442–452, 2006.

References—Cont'd

63. Powers SK, KaVASI SK, DeRuisseau KC: Mechanisms of disuse muscle atrophy: role of oxidative stress, *Ann J Physiol Regul Integ Comp* 288(2):R377, 2005.
64. Goldenberg DL, Burckhardt C, Crofford L: Management of fibromyalgia syndrome, *JAMA* 292(19):2388–2395, 2004.
65. Nampiaparampil DE, Shmerling RH: A review of fibromyalgia, *Am J Manag Care* 10(11 pt 1):794–800, 2004.
66. McBeth J et al: Hypothalamic-pituitary-adrenal stress axis function and the relationship with chronic widespread pain and its antecedents, *Arthritis Res Ther* 7(5):R992–R1000, 2005.
67. Bonnefont JP et al: Carnitine palmitoyltransferases 1 and 2: biochemical, molecular, and medical aspects, *Mol Aspects Med* 25(5–6):495–520, 2004.
68. Dalakas MC: Inflammatory disorders of muscle: progress in polymyositis, dermatomyositis and inclusion-body myositis, *Curr Opin Neurol* 17(5):561–567, 2004.
69. Gupta SJ: The idiopathic inflammatory myopathies: current perspectives and management, *J Indian Rheumatol Assoc* 12:58–69, 2004.
70. Urbano-Marquez A, Fernandez-Sola J: Effects of alcohol on skeletal and cardiac muscle, *Muscle Nerve* 30(6):689–707, 2004.
71. Papagelopoulos PJ et al: Clinicopathologic features, diagnosis, and treatment of fibrosarcoma of bone, *Am J Orthop* 31(5): 253–257, 2002.

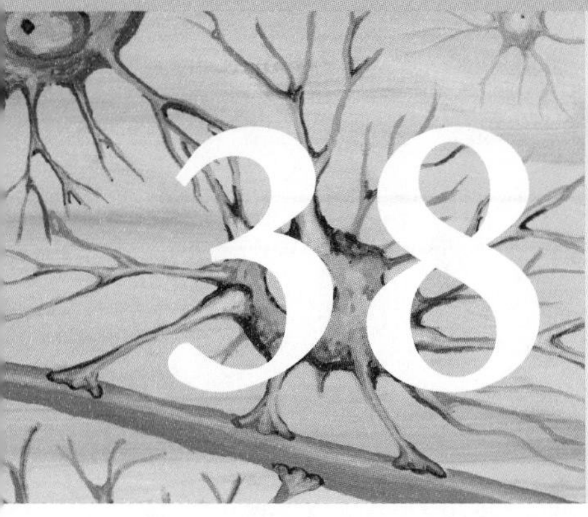

ALTERATIONS OF MUSCULOSKELETAL FUNCTION IN CHILDREN

Kristen Lee Carroll

CHAPTER OUTLINE

ELECTRONIC RESOURCES

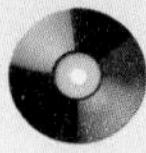

Companion CD
- Review Questions and Answers
- Animations

evolve Website
http://evolve.elsevier.com/Huether/
- Quick Check Answers
- Key Terms Exercises
- Critical Thinking Questions with Answers
- Algorithm Completion Exercises
- WebLinks

Musculoskeletal problems in children can be either congenital or acquired. Both pathology and treatment can cause long-term sequelae because of the growing nature of the immature skeleton. In addition, the emotional trauma of an injured or malformed child is substantial and requires that careful attention be paid to the emotional health of both the child and his or her family.

CONGENITAL DEFECTS

Clubfoot

Clubfoot, or congenital equinovarus, describes a deformity in which the forefoot is adducted and supinated (Table 38-1) and the heel is in varus (inwardly deviated) and equines (pointing down) (Figures 38-1 and 38-2). The clubfoot deformity can be positional (correctable passively), idiopathic, or teratologic (as a result of another syndrome, such as spina bifida). The idiopathic clubfoot occurs in 1:1000 live births, with males twice as likely as females to be affected.

In the idiopathic clubfoot, manipulation and casting above the knee, as described by Ponseti,[1] begun soon after birth can correct the forefoot deformity in 70% to 90% of feet.[2] The hindfoot equinus often requires lengthening of the Achilles tendon, which can be performed in a clinic under local anesthetic. Achilles tenotomy (complete transaction of the tendon) can be safely performed with local anesthetic until 8 of 9 months. After this age, a formal lengthening and repair under general anesthesia is required. Bracing is required until age 3. Idiopathic feet recalcitrant to these procedures require a surgical posteromedial release (PMR). The posterior medial release includes lengthening of the Achilles, posterior tibialis, and flexor tendons, and surgical release of the capsules of the ankle, subtalar, and midfoot joints. Teratologic feet are usually stiffer, and up to 90% require PMR. From 25% to 50% of children requiring PMR may need a second operative procedure with growth; a large number of those with teratologic feet also may need a second procedure.

Developmental Dysplasia of the Hip

Developmental dysplasia of the hip (DDH) describes imperfect development of the hip joint and can affect the femoral head, the acetabulum, or both. Although most often present congenitally, dysplasia may develop later in the newborn or infant period. Like clubfoot, DDH can be idiopathic or teratologic. Teratologic hips (because of another cause such as cerebral palsy, spina bifida, or arthrogryposis) are more difficult to treat and often need operative intervention. In idiopathic DDH, 70% of cases involve the left side only, 10% to 15% are bilateral, and girls are four times as likely to be affected. Positive family history,

TABLE 38-1

Terms Used to Describe Foot Abnormalities

Term	Definition
POSITION	
Abduction	Lateral deviation away from the midline of the body
Adduction	Lateral deviation toward the midline of the body
Eversion	Twisting of the foot outward along its long axis
Inversion	Twisting of the foot inward on its long axis
Dorsiflexion	Bending of the foot upward and backward
Plantar flexion	Bending of the foot downward and forward
ABNORMALITY	
Talipes	Congenital abnormality of the foot (clubfoot)
Pes	Acquired deformity of the foot
Varus	Inversion and adduction of the heel and forefoot
Valgus	Eversion and abduction of the heel and forefoot
Equinus	Plantar flexion of the foot in which the heel is lower than the toes
Calcaneus	Dorsiflexion of the foot in which the heel is lower than the toes
Planus	Flattening of the medial longitudinal arch of the foot (flatfoot)
Cavus	Elevation of the medial longitudinal arch of the foot (high arch)
Equinovarus	Coexistent equinus and varus deformities
Calcaneovarus	Coexistent calcaneus and varus deformities
Equinovalgus	Coexistent equinus and valgus deformities
Calcaneovalgus	Coexistent calcaneus and valgus deformities

NOTE: The positions listed can all be achieved by voluntary movement of the normal foot; an abnormality exists if the foot is fixed in one or more of the positions while at rest.

breech presentation, and oligohydramnios (low intrauterine fluid) all predispose children to DDH. Children in these groups are considered high risk and must be carefully evaluated with physical examination and, possibly, ultrasound.[3] Variants of idiopathic DDH are **dislocated hip** (no contact between femoral head and acetabulum), **subluxated hip** (partial contact only), and **acetabular dysplasia** (the femoral head is located properly but the acetabulum is shallow). Idiopathic instability of the hip ranges from 3 to 7:1000, but a true dislocation is only 1:1000.

Clinical examination is the mainstay of diagnosis. The examination must be performed on a relaxed infant for

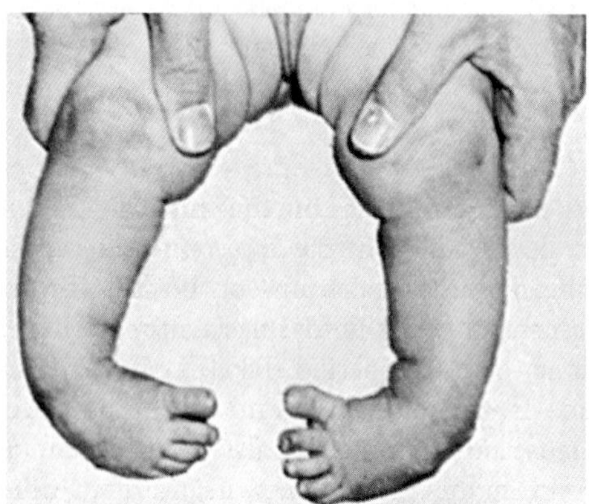

Figure 38-1 ■ Infant with Bilateral Congenital Talipes Equinovarus. (From Brashear HR, Raney RB: *Shand's handbook of orthopedic surgery,* ed 9, St Louis, 1978, Mosby.)

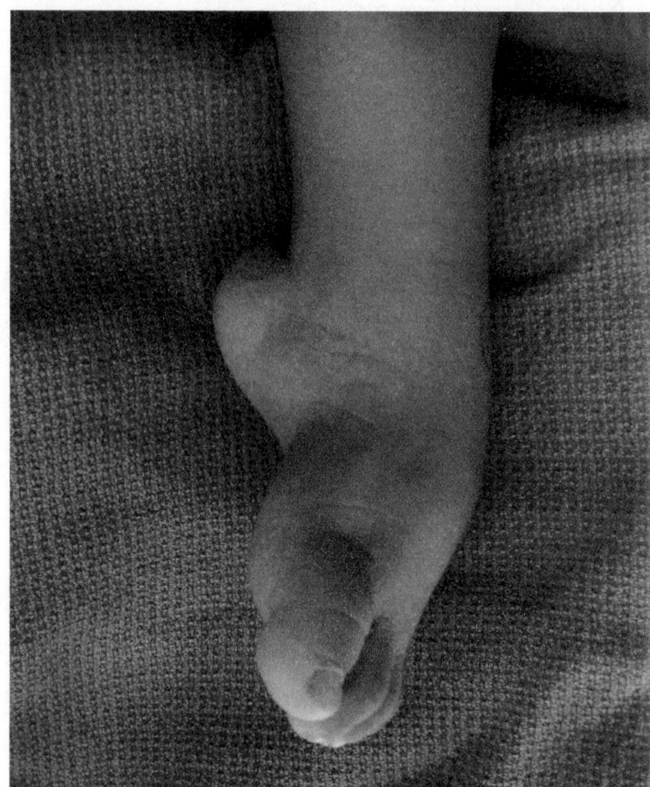

Figure 38-2 ■ Idiopathic Clubfoot. Idiopathic clubfoot displaying forefoot adduction (toward midline of body), supination (upturning), and hindfoot equinus (pointed downward). Note skin creases along arch and back of heel.

accuracy. A positive Ortolani sign (hip dislocated, but reducible) or Barlow sign (hip reduced but, dislocatable) are absolute indications for treatment. Other indicators for further evaluation are limitation of abduction,[4] or apparent shortening of the femur (Galeazzi sign). Asymmetric skin folds at the groin crease also may be observed.

In children younger than 4 months old, bracing with a Pavlik harness is successful in 90% of DDH cases. A Barlow positive hip (hip reduced, but dislocatable) is easier to treat with a Pavlik harness, and success reaches 95% to 98%. An Ortolani positive hip (hip dislocated, but reducible) must be followed closely with ultrasound and exam; the success rate with Pavlik is 70% in this situation. If a stable reduction is not attained within 2 to 3 weeks of treatment, the Pavlik harness should be abandoned. A partially reduced hip puts pressure on the rim of the acetabulum by the femoral head and can worsen dysplasia and make treatment more difficult. In older children, or failed Pavlik, closed reduction of the hip and spica (body) casting under general anesthesia is required. The spica cast is worn for 3 months. Children older than 12 months of age require surgery either on the joint, the femur, the acetabulum, or all three (Figure 38-3). The incidence of excellent outcome falls steadily with age, underscoring the need for early diagnosis and treatment.

Osteogenesis Imperfecta

Osteogenesis imperfecta (OI) (brittle bone disease) is a spectrum of disease caused by genetic mutation in the gene that encodes for type I collagen, the main component of bone and blood vessels. The Sillence classification defines four types. Types I and IV are milder forms and are inherited in an autosomal dominant pattern. Types II and III are more severe and are inherited in a recessive pattern. Children with type II often die during infancy.

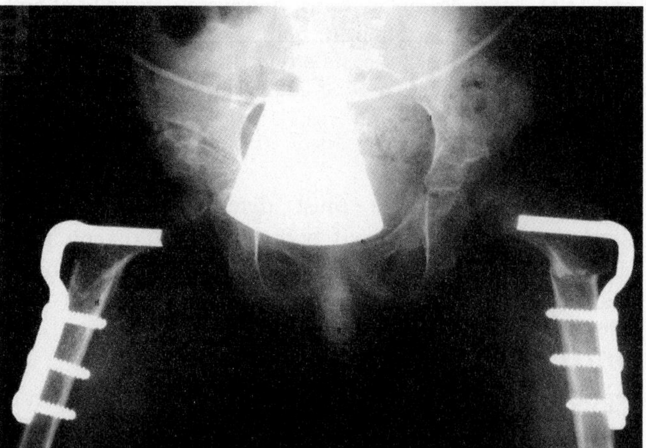

Figure 38-3 ■ Surgically Treated Bilateral Hip Dislocation. Postoperative x-ray of 5-year-old child after femoral, acetabular, and joint surgery bilaterally. The plates will be removed once the child heals. The extent of surgery necessitated staged (i.e., one side at a time) intervention.

The classic clinical manifestations of osteogenesis imperfecta (OI) are osteopenia (decreased bone mass) and an increased rate of fractures. With recurrent fractures, bone deformity (bowing) often occurs. In type III OI, the most severe form compatible with life, children are of short stature and have triangular faces, possibly blue sclera, and poor dentition. Because type I collagen also is the main component of blood vessels, vascular deformity, such as aortic aneurysm, can occur. Type IV OI can be subtle with more normal stature and fractures often not occurring until children are older; it can be misdiagnosed as child abuse. Analysis of skin fibroblast is diagnostic in 85% of children with OI.

Treatment is a combination of medical and surgical approaches (Figure 38-4). For fractures and deformity, intramedullary rodding of the long bones improves position and also splints new fractures. Telescoping rods, which grow with the child, are improving in efficacy. Unfortunately, these children may have to undergo multiple surgeries and reroddings with growth. The medical treatment, classically involving increased calcium and vitamin D, is under intense study. Pamidronate and other biphosphates, such as Alendronate (Fosamax) are now being used with encouraging results. In a multicenter trial,[5] Pamidronate was given at 2- to 4-month intervals to children with severe (type III) and mild (type IV) OI. Pamidronate inhibits bone resorption by decreasing osteoclastic activity. In the 30 children in the study, bone mineral density increased by 41.9% and fractures decreased by 1.7% per year and mobility increased in 51% of the children. All children claimed their fatigue and chronic bone pain improved. Fracture healing remained unchanged. A large multicenter study is now trying to refine these treatments for all children with OI.

BONE INFECTION

Osteomyelitis

Osteomyelitis, or bone infection, is caused by either bacterial or granulomatous (i.e., tuberculosis) infective processes (Box 38-1). Antibiotic drugs and often surgical interventions are used to fight these infections. Morbidity and mortality resulting from osteomyelitis has fallen drastically. With present management, serious long-term sequelae are under 15%.

Acute hematogenous osteomyelitis is the most common form in children. The infection usually begins as an abscess in the metaphysis of a long bone where blood flow is sluggish and bacteria can collect. With increasing pressure, the infection will rupture out of the periosteum and spread along the diaphysis. A new shell of bone can develop under the elevated periosteum and can become an **involucrum.** The portion of bone that is separated from adequate blood supply by the infection can die, thereby leading to an involucrum. All three of these changes are apparent on radiograph and signify the need for surgical débridement as well as antibiotic treatment.

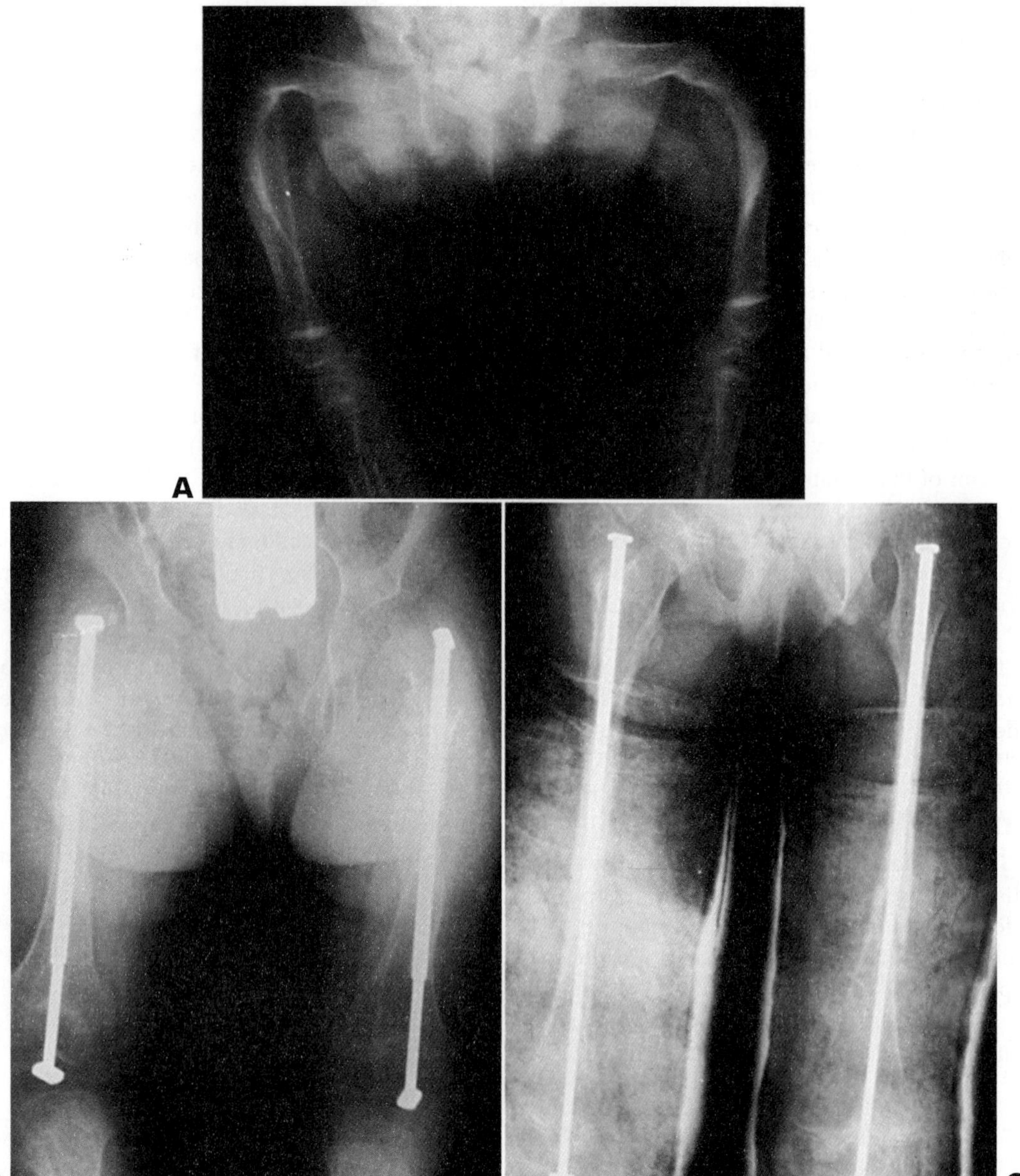

Figure 38-4 ■ **Osteogenesis Imperfecta Treated With Osteotomies and Telescoping Medullary Rods. A,** Severe deformity of both femurs. **B,** Same individual after multiple osteotomies with telescoping medullary rod fixation. C, Same individual 4 years later demonstrating growth of femurs, no recurrence of deformity, and elongation of rods. (Plaster casts are in place for immobilization of tibial osteotomies.) (From Crenshaw AH, editor: *Campbell's operative orthopaedics,* ed 8, vol 3, St Louis, 1992, Mosby.)

These radiographic bone changes take 2 to 3 weeks to develop. Initially, osteomyelitis presents as pain, swelling, and warmth. Children often will present with fever, elevated white blood cell count (50% to 70%), elevated C-reactive protein (98%), and elevated erythrocyte sedimentation rate (ESR) (90%). Blood culture is positive in only 40% of cases. Without changes on plain radiograph, bone scan can help define the location of infection. In infants, where osteomyelitis can be multifocal in up to 40%, bone scan identifies other locations of infection that may need surgical intervention (Figures 38-5 and 38-6).

Treatment of osteomyelitis consists of appropriate antibiotic management for 6 weeks. If blood cultures are negative, bone aspirate must determine the bacterial etiology of the infection. If bony changes exist on plain radiographs, surgical debridement accompanies antibiotic treatment.

Septic Arthritis

Septic arthritis is a bacterial or granulomatous infection of the joint space. This is always a surgical emergency. The bacteria, and the lysosomes created by white cells fighting the bacteria, can quickly destroy the articular cartilage of the joint and affect the blood supply to the epiphyseal bone nearby. Both of these complications have no good solution and can lead to a lifetime of disability.

BOX 38-1 Causative Microorganisms of Osteomyelitis According to Age

Newborns
Staphylococcus aureus
Group B streptococcus
Gram-negative enteric rods

Infants
Staphylococcus aureus
Haemophilus influenzae (decreasingly less common secondary to immunization)

Older Children
Staphylococcus aureus
Pseudomonas
Salmonella
Neisseria gonorrhoeae

Adolescents and Adults
Pseudomonas
Mycobacterium tuberculosis

Septic arthritis can occur primarily or secondary to osteomyelitis that breaks out of the metaphysis of the bone into the joint space. The metaphysis of the pediatric hip, shoulder, proximal radius, and distal lateral tibia are all located within the joint capsule, and therefore osteomyelitis in these regions must be carefully monitored for secondary septic arthritis. The most common sites for septic arthritis are knees, hips, ankles, and elbows.

Children with septic arthritis present with severe joint pain, "pseudoparalysis" or marked guarding to motion of the joint, inability to bear weight, and malaise, often with anorexia. Children appear quite ill with this diagnosis. Nonpyogenic arthritis, such as juvenile rheumatoid arthritis, can be difficult to distinguish clinically from septic arthritis because both can lead to malaise and elevated ESR. An elevation in CRP, fever, and complete inability to bear weight is more common with septic arthritis. Blood cultures are positive in 30% to 40%. Joint aspirate positive for pus defines the diagnosis and determines bacterial etiology. As in osteomyelitis. *Staphylococcus aureus* is the most common bacteria.

After surgical debridement of the joint, antibiotics are required for 2 to 3 weeks. Long-term follow-up to assess articular or physeal damage is required.

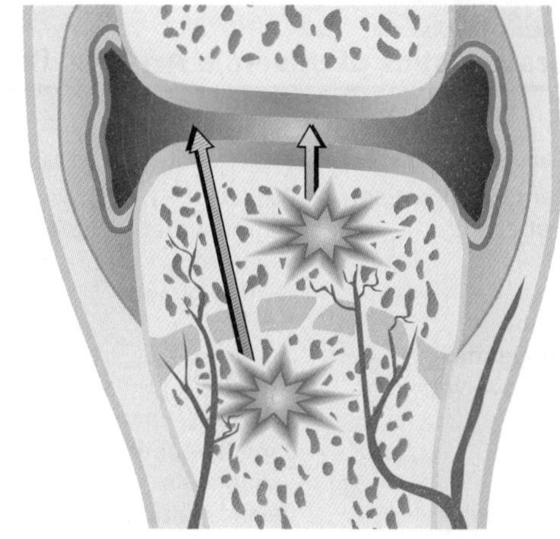

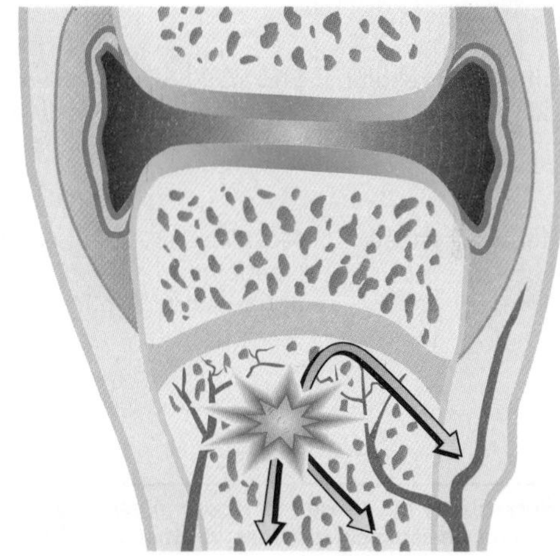

Figure 38-5 ■ **Pathogenesis of Acute Osteomyelitis Differs With Age. A,** In infants younger than 1 year the epiphysis is nourished by arteries penetrating through the physis, allowing development of the condition within the epiphysis. **B,** In children up to 15 years of age, the infection is restricted to below the physis because of interruption of the vessels.

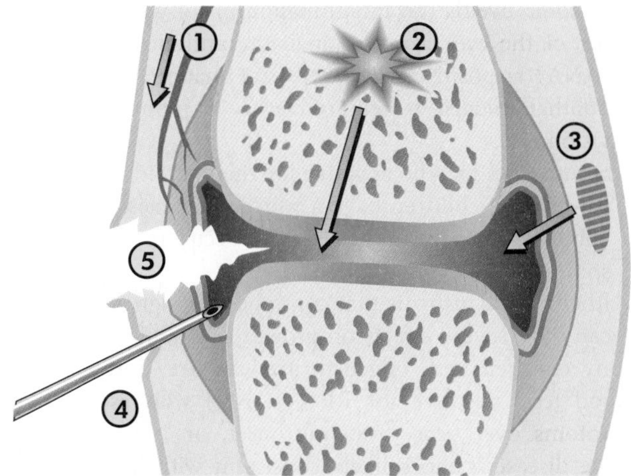

Figure 38-6 ■ **The Routes of Infection to the Joint.** *1,* The hematogenous route. *2,* Dissemination from osteomyelitis. *3,* Spread from an adjacent soft tissue infection. *4,* Diagnostic or therapeutic measures. *5,* Penetrating damage by puncture or cutting.

JUVENILE RHEUMATOID ARTHRITIS

Juvenile rheumatoid arthritis (JRA) is the childhood form of rheumatoid arthritis (see Chapter 37) and accounts for 5% of all cases of rheumatoid arthritis. Juvenile rheumatoid arthritis has three distinct modes of onset: **oligoarthritis** (fewer than three joints), **polyarthritis** (more than three joints), and **Stills disease** (severe systemic onset)

TABLE 38-2
Characteristics of Juvenile Arthritis Related to Mode of Onset

	Systemic Onset	Pauciarticular (Two or Three Subtypes)	Polyarticular (Two Subtypes)
Percentage of patients	30%	45%	25%
Age at onset	Bimodal distribution 1–3 yr of age 8–10 yr of age	Type I: younger than 10 yr Type II: older than 10 yr	Throughout childhood and adolescence
Sex ratio (female/male)	1.5:1	Type I: Almost all female Type II: 1:9	Mostly female
Joints involved	Any Only 20% have joint involvement at time of diagnosis	Usually confined to lower extremities—knee, ankle, and eventually sacroiliac; sometimes elbow	Any joints; usually symmetric involvement of small joints Hip involvement in 50% Spine involvement in 50%
Extra-articular manifestations	Fever, malaise, myalgia, rash, pleuritis or pericarditis, adenomegaly, splenomegaly, hepatomegaly	Type I: chronic iridocyclitis; mucocutaneous lesions Type II: acute iridocyclitis; sacroiliitis common; eventual ankylosing spondylitis in many	Systemic signs minimal Possible low-grade fever, malaise, weight loss, rheumatoid nodules, or vasculitis
Laboratory test results	Elevated ESR, CRP levels; RF negative; ANA rarely positive; anemia; leukocytosis	Elevated ESR, CRP levels; ANA positive Type I: HLA-DRW5 positive Type II: HLA-B27 positive Type III: HLA-TMo positive	Elevated ESR, CRP levels Type I: RF positive Type II: RF negative
Long-term prognosis	Mortality: 1%-2% of all JRA patients Joint destruction in 40%	Continuous disease; eventual remission in 60% Type I: ocular damage; functional blindness in 10% Type II: ankylosing spondylitis Type III: best outlook for recovery	Longer duration; more crippling; remission in 25% Type I: high incidence of crippling arthritis Type II: outlook good

From Hockenberry MJ, Wilson D: *Wong's nursing care of infants and children*, ed 8, St Louis, 2007, Mosby.
ESR, Erythrocyte sedimentation rate; *RF*, rheumatoid factor; *ANA*, antinuclear antibody; *HLA*, human leukocyte antigen; *JRA*, juvenile rheumatoid arthritis; *CRP*, C-reactive protein.

(Table 38-2). JRA differs from rheumatoid arthritis in several ways:

1. Large joints are most commonly affected.
2. Chronic uveitis (an inflammation of the anterior chamber of the eye) is common if the antinuclear antibody (ANA) is positive; slit lamp examination by a trained ophthalmologist is required every 6 months to avoid vision loss.
3. Serum tests may be negative for rheumatoid factor (RF); RF-positive children have a worse prognosis.
4. Subluxation and ankylosis may occur in the cervical spine if disease progresses.
5. Rheumatoid arthritis that continues through adolescence can have severe effects on growth and adult morbidity.

Many children with oligoarthritis who are "seronegative" (blood tests negative for RF or ANA) will resolve their symptoms over time. Systemic onset, or "seropositivity," of the disease is more likely consistent with lifelong arthritis. Treatment is, therefore, supportive, not curative. Nonsteroidal anti-inflammatories are a mainstay, and methotrexate is also being used with success. The aims are to minimize inflammation and deformity.

QUICK CHECK 38-1

1. Why is an early diagnosis of developmental dysplasia of the hip imperative?
2. How does osteomyelitis develop?
3. How does juvenile rheumatoid arthritis differ from the adult form?

OSTEOCHONDROSES

The **osteochondroses** are a series of childhood diseases involving areas of significant tensile or compressive stress (i.e., tibial tubercle, Achilles insertion, hip). The pathophysiology is partial loss of blood supply, death of bone (osseous necrosis), progressive bony weakness, and then microfracture. The cause of the decreased blood supply is controversial; trauma, a change in clotting sensitivity, vascular injury, or a combination of these is presently considered most likely.

Treatment with reparative processes by neovascularization is the rule, although years may be required for full healing, and deformity from compression during the period of osseous necrosis can persist.

Legg-Calvé-Perthes Disease

Legg-Calvé-Perthes (LCP) disease is a common osteochondrosis usually occurring in children between the ages of 3 and 10 years, with a peak incidence at 6 years. The disorder is bilateral in 10% to 20% of children, and boys are affected five times more often than girls. Boys have a more poorly developed blood supply to the femoral head than do girls of the same age, and this is felt to be the reason for male predilection. The role of genetics is unclear, but LCP is more common in northern European and Japanese children and rare in black children; family history is positive in 20%. This self-limited disease of the hip, which runs its natural course in 2 to 5 years, is presumably produced by recurrent interruption of the blood supply to the femoral head. The ossification center first becomes necrotic (osteonecrosis) and then is gradually replaced by live bone.

PATHOPHYSIOLOGY Several causative theories have been proposed, including a generalized disorder of epiphyseal cartilage growth, thyroid deficiency, trauma, infection, and blood clotting disorders. However, a Harvard study did not show increases in thrombotic disorders in consecutive children with LCP.[6] Children are often delayed in skeletal age by 2 years, making some believe LCP disease is actually a systemic skeletal dysplasia. Another study has shown the risk of LCP is five times greater in children exposed to passive smoke than those who are not.[7]

In the first stage of LCP, the soft tissues of the hip (synovial membrane and joint capsule) are swollen, edematous, and hyperemic, often with fluid present in the joint (Figure 38-7). In the second necrotic stage, the anterior 50% or greater of the epiphysis of the femoral head dies due to a lack of blood supply, and the metaphyseal bone at the junction of the femoral neck and capital epiphyseal plate is softened because of increased blood supply and decalcification. Granulation tissue (procallus) and blood vessels then invade the dead bone. The third, or regenerative healing stage, ordinarily lasts 2 to 4 years. The dead bone in the femoral head is replaced by procallus, and new bone is laid down (see Figure 38-7). In the fourth, or residual, stage, remodeling takes place and the newly formed bone is organized into a live spongy bone.

CLINICAL MANIFESTATIONS Injury or trauma precedes the onset of LCP in approximately 30% to 50% of children with Legg-Calvé-Perthes disease. For several months the child complains of a limp and pain that can be referred to the knee, inner thigh, and the groin, following the path of the obturator nerve. The pain is usually aggravated by activity and relieved by rest and anti-inflammatories.

The typical physical findings include spasm on rotation of the hip, limitation of internal rotation and abduction, and hip flexion–adduction deformity. If the child is walking, an abnormal gait termed an **antalgic abductor lurch,** or "Trendelenburg" gait, is apparent. If the hip pain or limp has been present for a prolonged period, muscles of the hip and thigh atrophy.

EVALUATION AND TREATMENT The goals of treatment are to preserve normal congruity of the femoral head and acetabulum and maintain spasm-free and pain-free range of motion in the hip joint. Currently, most children can be managed with anti-inflammatory medications and activity modification during periods of synovitis. Serial radiographs are obtained to monitor the progress of the disease and to ensure that the femoral head remains congruent in the acetabulum. Surgery may be necessary if the femoral head becomes subluxated or incongruent with the acetabulum (Figures 38-8 and 38-9).[8–10] Children older than age 6 (by bone age) have a worse prognosis due to poorer remodeling potential. Older children require surgery more often to avoid poor congruence of the hip. Poor congruence predisposes to early osteoarthritis, with nearly 50% requiring hip replacement by age 40.

Osgood-Schlatter Disease

Osgood-Schlatter disease consists of osteochondrosis of the tubercle of the tibia and associated patella tendonitis. Osgood-Schlatter disease occurs most often in preadolescents and adolescents who participate in sports and is more prevalent in boys than in girls. Osgood-Schlatter disease is one of the most common ailments reported in the 30 million children who are involved in sports.[11]

The severity of the lesion varies from mild tendonitis to a complete separation of the anterior tibial apophysis, a part of the tibial tubercle. The mildest form of Osgood-Schlatter disease causes ischemic (avascular) necrosis in the region of

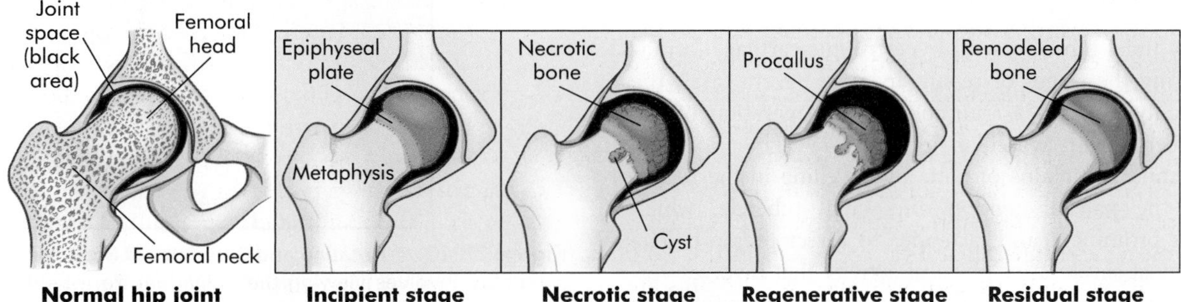

Figure 38-7 ■ Stages of Legg-Calvé-Perthes Disease, a Form of Osteochondrosis.

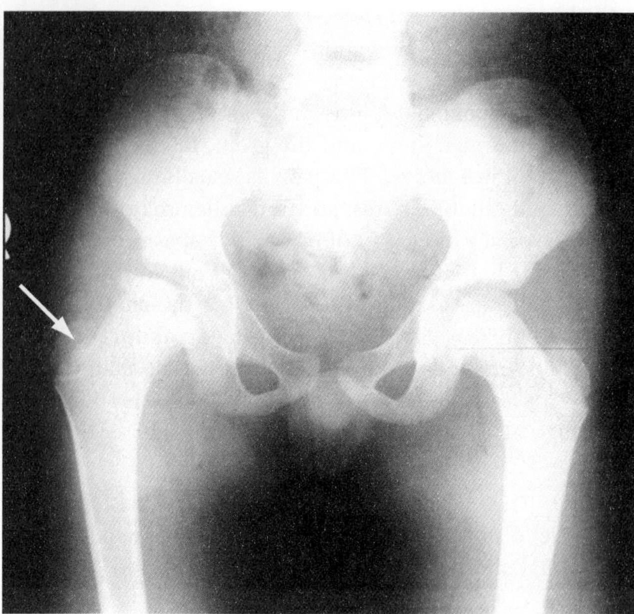

Figure 38-8 ■ Pelvis of a 7-Year-Old Boy With Legg-Calvé-Perthes Disease. The femoral head is flat and extruded from the edge of the joint. This hip is at risk for early arthritis if left to revascularize and heal in this position.

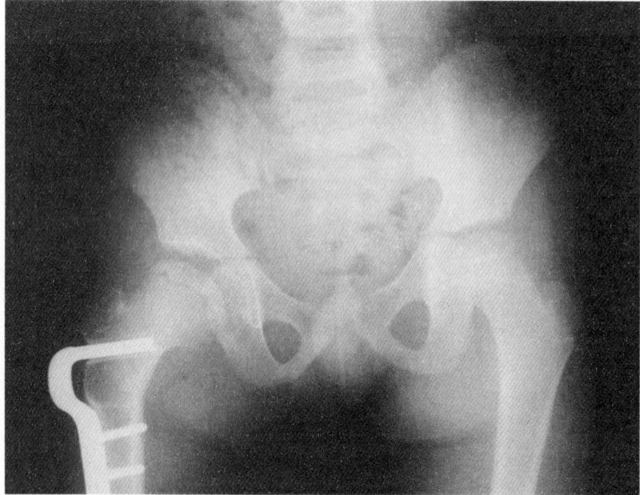

Figure 38-9 ■ Surgical Replacement of Femoral Head of a 7-Year-Old Boy With Legg-Calvé-Perthes Disease. As the Perthes heals, the ball has taken on a round shape that matches the socket well.

the bony tibial tubercle, with hypertrophic cartilage formation during the stages of repair. In more severe cases, the abnormality involves a true apophyseal separation of the tibial tubercle with avascular necrosis.

The child complains of pain and swelling in the region around the patellar tendon and tibial tubercle, which becomes prominent and is tender to direct pressure. The pain is most severe after physical activity that involves vigorous quadriceps contraction (jumping or running) or direct local trauma to the tibial tubercle area.

The goal of treatment for Osgood-Schlatter disease is to decrease the stress at the tubercle. Often a period of 4 to 8 weeks of restriction from strenuous physical activity is sufficient. Bracing with a tubercle band can be very helpful. If the pain is not relieved, a cast or knee immobilizer is required, a situation that is particularly difficult if the condition is bilateral.

Gradual resumption of activity is permitted after 8 weeks, but return to unrestricted athletic participation requires an additional 8 weeks to allow for revascularization, healing, and ossification of the tibial tubercle.[8,12] With skeletal maturity and closure of the apophysis, Osgood-Schlatter disease resolves.

SCOLIOSIS

There are three main types of **scoliosis:** idiopathic; congenital (due to bony deformity such as hemivertebrae); and teratologic (because of another systemic syndrome such as cerebral palsy). Eighty percent of all scoliosis is idiopathic, which may have a genetic component. True structural scoliotic deformity involves not only a side-to-side curve but also rotation; curves without rotation may result from another cause such as limb length inequity or splinting from pain (Figure 38-10). Although girls and boys are equally affected, once the curve becomes more than 20 degrees, girls are five times more likely to be affected. Ninety-eight percent of curves are apex right thoracic. If a left thoracic curve appears in the adolescent with idiopathic scoliosis, MRI is done to rule out a neurologic etiology. MRI also should be performed with kypho- (round back) scoliosis, loss of abdominal reflexes, children who also have exertional headaches, or a congenital curve.[13]

Idiopathic curves progress while a child is growing, and progression can be very rapid during growth spurts. When

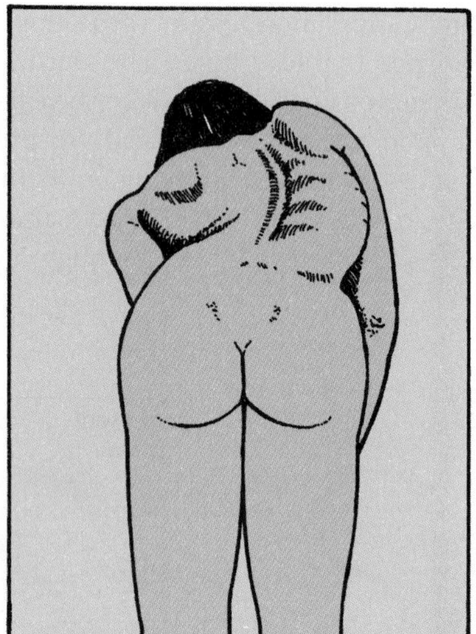

Figure 38-10 ■ Rotation and Curvature of Scoliosis. Scoliosis screening involves viewing the individual from behind, which discloses scapular asymmetry caused by not only curvature but also true rotation of the spine.

idiopathic curves progress to 25 degrees or greater, and the child is skeletally immature, bracing is required. Curves of more than 50 degrees will progress after skeletal maturity, so spinal fusion is required to stop progression. Early diagnosis is therefore necessary so that bracing can be attempted in the hopes of halting progression before surgical indicators are reached. Children are required to wear the brace 16 hours per day, and full compliance can be difficult to attain. Nevertheless, bracing is the only nonoperative measure known to slow scoliotic progression. Chiropractic manipulation, physical therapy, exercise, and diet regimens have not been shown to alter natural history. Bracing is less successful in teratologic or congenital curves; therefore, these conditions may require surgical intervention more often.

MUSCULAR DYSTROPHY

The **muscular dystrophies** are a group of familial disorders that cause degeneration of skeletal muscle fibers. Ongoing genetic research has helped define not only the inheritance pattern and carrier detection but also the biochemical aberration of the various types. The major muscular dystrophy syndromes are contained in Table 38-3. The most common singular type, Duchenne muscular dystrophy (DMD), is discussed here.

Duchenne Muscular Dystrophy

PATHOPHYSIOLOGY **Duchenne muscular dystrophy (DMD)** is a myopathy caused by mutations in the dystrophin gene located on the short arm of the X chromosome. A protein called **dystrophin** is present in normal muscle cells; it is abnormal in structure, reduced, or absent in those with Duchenne muscular dystrophy (Figure 38-11). Dystrophin is thought to be involved in maintaining the structural integrity of the cell's cytoskeleton. Dystrophin also occurs in the brain, and about one third of people with DMD show mental retardation. As an X-linked inherited disorder, DMD affects only boys, with any male child of a known female carrier having a 50% risk. The overall incidence is 1:3500 male births.

CLINICAL MANIFESTATIONS Duchenne muscular dystrophy causes muscle bulk to diminish and interstitial fibrous connective tissue and fat to eventually replace muscle fibers. Although fibers regenerate in the younger child, they are abnormal in many ways and become nonfunctional with time.

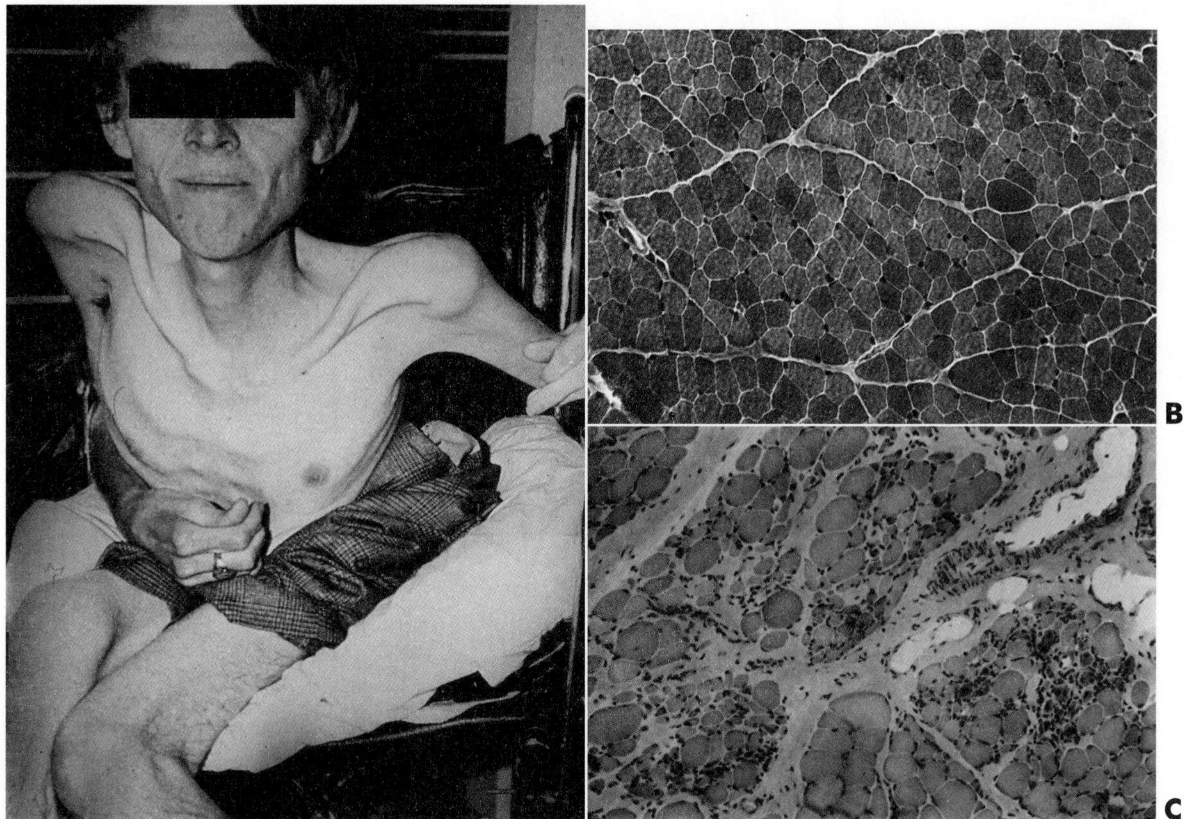

Figure 38-11 ■ **Duchenne Muscular Dystrophy. A,** Patient with late-stage Duchenne muscular dystrophy showing severe muscle loss. **B,** Transverse section of gastrocnemius muscle from a normal boy. **C,** Transverse section of gastrocnemius muscle from a boy with Duchenne muscular dystrophy. Normal muscle fiber is replaced with fat and connective tissue. (From Jorde LB et al: *Medical genetics,* ed 3, updated, St Louis, 2006, Mosby.)

TABLE 38-3

Major Muscular Dystrophy Syndromes

Disease	Mode of Inheritance	Age at Clinical Onset	Usual Distribution	Rate of Progression	Mental Retardation	Distinguishing Findings
Duchenne muscular dystrophy	X-linked recessive, sporadic	1–3 yr	Hips and shoulders, quadriceps femoris, gastrocnemius (pseudohypertrophy)	Rapid	Frequent	Elevated serum enzymes A (CK, LDH, AST [formerly SGOT], aldolase)
Facioscapulo-humeral (FSH)	Autosomal dominant	Early adolescence; older than 8 yr	Shoulder girdle, neck, face, pelvic girdle (late)	Moderate	Occasional	Several distinct muscle pathologic conditions
Limb girdle (LG) dystrophy	Poorly defined or recessive	Late childhood or during adolescence; older than 8 yr	Pelvic and shoulder girdles	Variable	Variable	Collection of several diseases
Myotonic dystrophy (MyD)	Autosomal dominant	Variable—birth to fifth decade	Distal extensor muscle, eyelids, face, neck, hands, pharynx	Slow; related to age at clinical onset; faster with younger patients	Frequent	Percussion myotonia, cataracts, diabetic GTT despite increased insulin, testicular atrophy, decreased IgG

CK, Creatine kinase; *LDH,* lactic dehydrogenase; *AST,* aspartate transaminase; *SGOT,* serum glutamic oxaloacetic transaminase; *GTT,* glucose tolerance test; *IgC,* immunoglobulin C.

Duchenne muscular dystrophy is usually identified at about 3 years of age, with parents noting slow motor development or regression of motor tasks. Sitting, standing, and walking become labored, and the child is clumsy, falls frequently, and has difficulty climbing stairs.

Muscular weakness always begins in the pelvic girdle, causing a waddling gait. Hypertrophy of the calf muscles is apparent in 80% of cases. The method of rising from the floor by "climbing up the legs" (Gowers sign) is characteristic and is caused by weakness of the lumbar and gluteal muscles. The foot assumes a talipes equinovarus position, and the child tends to walk on the toes because of weakness of the anterior tibial and peroneal muscles. The deep tendon reflexes are usually depressed or absent. Contractures and wasting of the muscles contribute to muscular atrophy and deformity of the skeleton. Scoliosis can occur and is relentlessly progressive; curves of more than 20 degrees are treated surgically to maintain pulmonary function and slow the progression to a wheelchair. Children usually lose their ability to walk by age 8 to 10 years. Progressive osteopenia, due to inactivity, leads to pathologic fractures. Studies cite that bisphosphonates, such as those used in OI or orthoporosis, slow bone loss.[14] Death, usually from progressive pulmonary or cardiac weakness, ensues by the 20s. Only 25% of individuals with Duchenne reach the age of 21 years.

EVALUATION AND TREATMENT Diagnosis is confirmed by measurement of the serum enzyme, creatinine kinase. Creatine kinase (CK), is increased to more than 20 times normal because CK leaks into the bloodstream with muscle death.

Although there is no effective cure for Duchenne muscular dystrophy, maintaining function for as long as possible is the primary goal. Activity fosters maintenance of muscle function, but strenuous exercise may hasten the breakdown of muscle fibers. A consensus statement by the American Academy of Neurology recommends treatment with steroids to maintain muscle strength and function. This significantly lengthens the period of time a child can still walk. Range-of-motion exercises, bracing, and surgical release of contracture deformities are used to maintain normal function. Genetic counseling is recommended. With X-linked inheritance, male siblings of an affected child have a 50% chance of being affected, and female siblings have a 50% chance of being carriers.

Because of its tragic course, prenatal screening for Duchenne muscular dystrophy can be done. Possible female carriers are encouraged to have serum CK levels determined, which can be elevated in 60% to 80% of those affected.

✔ QUICK CHECK 38-2

1. What is the most common osteochondrosis?
2. What is the cause of Duchenne muscular dystrophy?
3. Why are only boys affected with Duchenne muscular dystrophy?

MUSCULOSKELETAL TUMORS

Benign Bone Tumors

The two most common forms of benign bone tumors are osteochondroma and nonossifying fibroma.

Osteochondroma

Osteochondroma (or exostosis) can occur as a solitary lesion or as an inherited syndrome of **hereditary multiple exostoses (HME).** HME is an autosomal dominant condition with exostoses occurring throughout the skeleton. Osteochondromas appear as bony protuberances, either sessile or pedunculated lesions appearing in the periphyseal area. They are most common near active growth plates of the proximal humerus, distal femur, or proximal tibia. The most common presentation is a palpable mass that is painful when traumatized. Rarely, the lesion can cause neurologic or vascular problems, or tendon rupture from local compression. The lesions can lead to growth disturbance and mildly short stature. Knee valgus (knock knee), ankle valgus, and hip problems are common. Upper extremity lesions can lead to a pronounced deformity in the forearm with a very short ulna bone. Three genetic loci have been identified on chromosomes 8, 11, and 19. Two of these loci (8 and 11) have been associated with the very rare (1%) but serious complication of malignant degeneration to chondrosarcoma after skeletal maturity. These lesions grow until skeletal maturity; growth or pain after skeletal maturity is a sign of possible malignant transformation, especially in the pelvis or scapular region.

Treatment involves minimizing growth disturbance, local tissue compression, and pain by resection of symptomatic lesions. The regrowth rate is 30% when lesions are removed in early childhood; therefore, only symptomatic lesions should be surgically addressed in the growing child.[15]

Nonossifying fibroma

Of all benign bone tumors, 50% are nonossifying fibromas or fibrous cortical defects. **Nonossifying fibromas** are sharply demarcated, cortically based lesions of fibrocytes that have replaced normal bone. The lesion can occur in any bone, at any age. Nearly 30% of all children have at least one.

Microscopically, these benign nonmetastasizing lesions appear as whorled bundles of fibroblasts and osteoclast-like giant cells. As the tumor grows, lipids make the fibroblasts foamy in appearance, and they are known as *foam cells.*

Treatment is observational only. If these lesions grow too large, however, they will compromise the biomechanical strength of the bone and lead to pathologic fractures. Curettage and bone grafting is suggested after pathologic fracture or if impending fracture (nonossifying fibroma greater than 50% of the diameter of the bone or greater than 3 or 4 cm) is noted radiographically.

Malignant Bone Tumors

Malignant bone tumors are uncommon tumors in childhood, accounting for fewer than 5% of childhood malignancies and occurring mostly during adolescence. The two main tumors are osteosarcoma and Ewing sarcoma.

Osteosarcoma

Osteosarcoma is the most common malignant bone tumor found during childhood and originates in bone-producing mesenchymal cells. Tumors can be broadly classified as those arising within the bone and those arising on the surface of bone. Three fourths occur in children between the ages of 10 and 25 years, with most being diagnosed between 15 and 19 years of age during the adolescent growth spurt. Incidence is the same for males and females.

Osteosarcoma may develop as a result of rapid local growth, which increases the likelihood of mutation. It can be induced by ionizing radiation, even with relatively low doses, and can be a tragic consequence of therapeutic radiation for other forms of cancer. The latent period after radiation exposure is 5 to 40 years. There also has been a link to individuals with retinoblastoma (a hereditary eye tumor).

Osteosarcoma has not been linked to chemical carcinogens or viruses. No deoxyribonucleic acid (DNA) or ribonucleic acid (RNA) virus has been isolated.

Molecular analysis has demonstrated deletion of genetic material on the long arm of chromosome 13, which led to the identification of a tumor suppressor gene as being part of the mechanism for tumor development. The oncogene *src* also has been associated with osteosarcoma.

PATHOPHYSIOLOGY Osteosarcoma occurs mainly in the metaphyses of long bones near sites of active physeal growth. The tumor most commonly occurs at the distal femur, proximal tibia, or proximal humerus. As a tumor of mesenchymal cells, osteosarcoma demonstrates production of osteoid cells.

Osteosarcoma is a bulky tumor that extends beyond the bone into a soft tissue mass. It may encircle the bone and destroy the trabeculae of the diseased area. Osteosarcoma disseminates through the bloodstream, usually to the lung. As many as 25% of children diagnosed with osteosarcoma exhibit lung metastases at diagnosis. Other sites of metastatic spread include other bones and visceral organs.

CLINICAL MANIFESTATIONS The most common presenting complaint is pain. Night pain, awakening a child from sleep, is a particularly foreboding sign. There may be swelling, warmth, and redness caused by the vascularity of the tumor. Symptoms also may include cough, dyspnea, and chest pain if lung metastasis is present. If a lower extremity is involved, a child may limp or suffer a pathologic fracture. Although osteosarcoma is not the result of trauma, trauma may call attention to a preexisting tumor.

EVALUATION AND TREATMENT The five histologic types of osteosarcoma are determined by the predominant cell type. The tumor is graded according to degree of malignancy; the higher the grade, the worse the prognosis.

Surgery and chemotherapy are the primary treatments for osteosarcoma. The tumor is resistant to radiation. Traditionally, surgery includes amputation at the joint above the involved bone; however, more recent limb salvage procedures have gained acceptance, and amputation may be avoided in many children.

Chemotherapy is an important component of treatment. Children routinely receive chemotherapy preoperatively; then the disease is restaged with MRI and surgical biopsy to determine rate of "tumor kill." If over 90% of tumor cells are killed by chemotherapy, prognosis is markedly improved. Chemotherapy is then used after surgery for any additional cell spill during surgery. The use of chemotherapy with surgery has increased the 5-year survival rate to 60% or more.[16]

A number of approaches have been used to treat pulmonary metastases. Because pulmonary metastases are generally solitary, thoracotomy with wedge resection has proven to be the most effective treatment.

Ewing sarcoma

Ewing sarcoma is the second most common and most lethal malignant bone tumor that occurs during childhood. This tumor is named after James Ewing, who first identified it as a separate clinical diagnosis in 1921. The most common period of diagnosis is between 5 and 15 years of age; it is rare after age 30 years. Ewing sarcoma is slightly more common in males than females. Cytogenic studies have shown a translocation of chromosome 11 and 22 resulting in a fusion protein (EWS-FLI 1) forming at the chromosomal junction.

PATHOPHYSIOLOGY Ewing sarcoma is most commonly located in the midshaft of long bones or in flat bones. The most common sites include the femur, pelvis, and humerus (Figure 38-12).

Arising from bone marrow, Ewing sarcoma can break through the cortex of the bone to form a soft tissue mass. Unlike osteosarcoma, Ewing sarcoma does not make bone and radiographically appears as a permeative, destructive lesion (Figure 38-13). Ewing sarcoma metastasizes to nearly every organ. Metastasis occurs early and is usually apparent at diagnosis or within 1 year. The most common sites are the lung, other bones, lymph nodes, bone marrow, liver, spleen, and central nervous system.

CLINICAL MANIFESTATIONS As with osteosarcoma, the most common complaint is pain that increases in severity. A soft tissue mass is often present. Additional symptoms may include fever, malaise, and anorexia. The radiographic appearance is similar to osteomyelitis, and diagnosis is only confirmed with biopsy.

EVALUATION AND TREATMENT No specific laboratory test is diagnostic; however, the sedimentation rate will be elevated and lactic dehydrogenase (LDH) often is elevated,

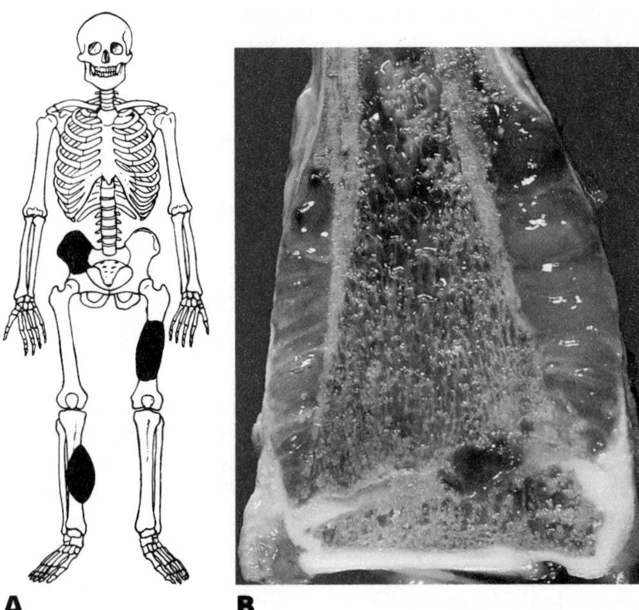

Figure 38-12 ■ **Ewing Sarcoma. A,** Most common anatomic sites. **B,** Closeup view of Ewing sarcoma of the distal end of the tibia. Tumor extends into the soft tissue. (From Damjanov I, Linder J, editors: *Anderson's pathology,* ed 10, St Louis, 1996, Mosby.)

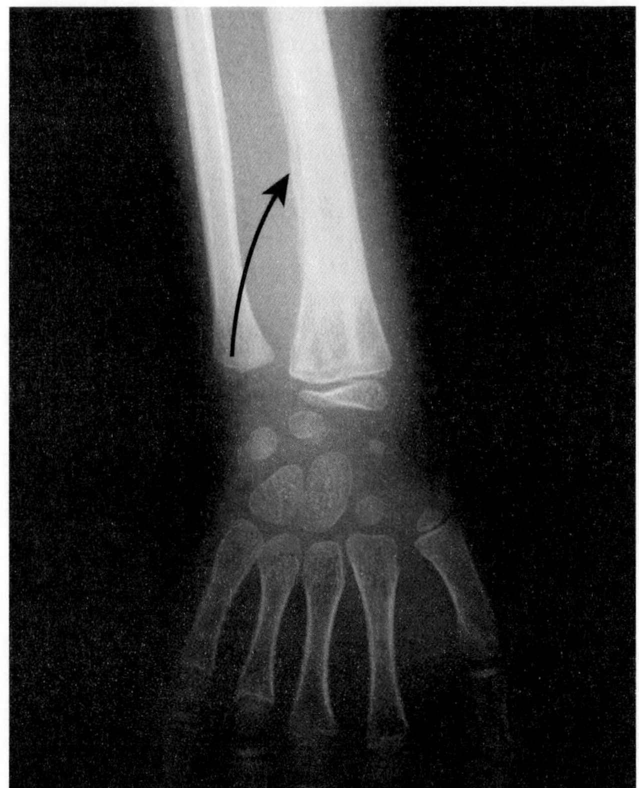

Figure 38-13 ■ **Ewing Sarcoma of the Distal Radius.** Radiograph of an 8-year-old boy showing a permeative lesion of the distal radius. Note the loss of bone cortex on the ulnar border suggesting an aggressive process. Bone biopsy revealed Ewing sarcoma.

which is a poor prognostic sign. Biopsy is used to conclusively establish the diagnosis of a small round cell tumor.

Present treatment includes radiation, chemotherapy, and, if possible, surgical débridement. Chemotherapy is continued for 12 to 18 months after resection. Present 5-year survival with this tri-therapeutic approach is 60%; however, tumors of the pelvis have a markedly worse prognosis. Metastasis at diagnosis is another poor prognostic indicator, with 5-year survival rate dropping to under 40%.

QUICK CHECK 38-3

1. What are the most common benign bone tumors of children?
2. What are the two malignant bone tumors found in children?
3. Why is rapid growth associated with osteosarcoma?

NONACCIDENTAL TRAUMA

It is estimated that more than 1.5 million children are abused per year in the United States. Maltreatment may be psychologic, sexual, or physical. Thirty percent of children who have been physically abused are seen by an orthopedist. Accurate and appropriate referrals to child protection agencies are not only legally mandated but also essential for the well-being of the child. An abused child who is returned to the same situation without intervention has a 10% to 15% chance of subsequent mortality.

Fractures in Nonaccidental Trauma

Children who are not yet ambulatory and present with a long bone fracture have more than a 75% chance of that fracture being caused by nonaccidental trauma.[17] "Corner" metaphyseal fractures are nearly always pathognomonic of abuse but occur only 25% of the time. Fractures at multiple stages of healing also suggest abuse; however, osteogenesis imperfecta or other causes of systemic osteomalacia must be ruled out. The most common presentation is a transverse tibia fracture. After walking age, only 2% of long bone fractures are the result of nonaccidental trauma.[18]

Evaluation

Nonaccidental trauma necessitates early consultation with child protective services. The child should undergo skeletal survey (especially if less than 2 years of age) and have a complete physical examination to evaluate for pattern bruising, burns, or multiple soft tissue injuries. A thorough history must be obtained for all identified injuries. It is important to remember that social isolation can lead to an increased likelihood of abuse, but no social status is immune. One study reported that nonwhite children were three times more likely than whites to be reported for nonaccidental trauma; however, it is important to remember that all races are at risk.[19]

When the cause of injury is unclear, bone scan can be helpful in diagnosing subtle injuries, especially rib fractures.

Posterior rib fractures are especially likely to be the result of abuse. MRI/CT of the brain to check for subdural hematoma and retinal examination to look for hemorrhages is essential.

TREATMENT The treating health care provider must have a nonjudgmental attitude. The child and family involved in nonaccidental trauma are emotionally delicate and require not only physical but also emotional care. Social workers need to be involved early to ensure that the child receives appropriate medical care. Fortunately, fractures tend to heal quickly for those in this age group. Neurologic injury and social disease, however, are much more difficult to cure.

Did You Understand?

Congenital Defects

1. Clubfoot is a common deformity in which the foot is twisted out of its normal shape or position. Clubfoot can be positional, idiopathic, or teratologic.
2. Developmental dysplasia of the hip (DDH) is an abnormality in the development of the femoral head, acetabulum, or both. Like clubfoot, DDH can be idiopathic or teratologic. It is a serious and disabling condition in children if not diagnosed and treated.
3. Osteogenesis imperfecta (brittle bone disease) is an inherited disorder of collagen that affects primarily bones and results in serious fractures of many bones.

Bone Infection

1. Osteomyelitis is a local or generalized bacterial or granulomatous (i.e., tuberculosis) infection of bone and bone marrow. Bacteria are usually introduced by direct extension from a nearby infection, through the bloodstream, or by trauma.
2. Septic arthritis can occur de novo or secondary to osteomyelitis in very young children where the metaphysis is still located within the joint capsule of certain joints.

Juvenile Rheumatoid Arthritis

1. Juvenile rheumatoid arthritis is an inflammatory joint disorder characterized by pain and swelling. Large joints are most commonly affected.

Osteochondroses

1. Avascular diseases of the bone are collectively referred to as osteochondroses and are caused by an insufficient blood supply to growing bones.
2. Legg-Calvé-Perthes disease is one of the most common osteochondroses. This disorder is characterized by epiphyseal necrosis or degeneration of the head of the femur followed by regeneration or recalcification.
3. Osgood-Schlatter disease is characterized by tendonitis of the anterior patellar tendon and inflammation or partial separation of the tibial tubercle caused by chronic irritation, usually as a result of overuse of the quadriceps muscles. The condition is seen primarily in muscular, athletic adolescent males.

Scoliosis

1. Scoliosis is a lateral curvature of the spinal column that can be caused by congenital malformations of the spine, poliomyelitis, skeletal dysplasias, spastic paralysis, and unequal leg length, but it is most often idiopathic.

Muscular Dystrophy

1. The muscular dystrophies are a group of genetically transmitted diseases characterized by progressive atrophy of skeletal muscles. There is an insidious loss of strength in all forms of the disorder with increasing disability and deformity. The most common type is Duchenne muscular dystrophy.

Musculoskeletal Tumors

1. The two most common forms of benign bone tumors are osteochondroma and nonossifying fibroma.
2. The two main types of malignant childhood bone tumors are osteosarcoma and Ewing sarcoma.
3. Osteosarcoma, the most common malignant childhood bone tumor, originates in bone-producing mesenchymal cells and is most often located near active growth plates, such as distal femur, proximal tibia, or proximal humerus.
4. Most children with osteosarcoma are diagnosed between 15 and 19 years of age, and osteosarcoma occurs equally in males and females.
5. Ewing sarcoma originates from cells within the bone marrow space and is most often located in the midshaft of long bones or in flat bones. The most common sites include the femur, pelvis, and humerus.
6. Ewing sarcoma is more common in males and is diagnosed most often between the ages of 5 and 15 years.
7. Pain is the usual presenting symptom for either osteosarcoma or Ewing sarcoma.
8. The primary treatments for osteosarcoma are surgery and chemotherapy. The primary treatment for Ewing sarcoma is a combination of chemotherapy, radiation, and surgery.

Nonaccidental Trauma

1. Nonaccidental trauma must be considered with any long bone injury in the preambulatory child.
2. The presence of soft tissue injury, corner fractures, and multiple fractures at different stages of healing is extremely helpful for making a diagnosis of nonaccidental trauma.
3. When nonaccidental trauma is suspected, a child must be evaluated radiographically for other fractures, heat trauma, and retinal hemorrhage.
4. All social strata are at risk.
5. The health care provider is legally responsible to report suspected nonaccidental trauma.

Key Terms

Acetabular dysplasia, 1072
Acute hematogenous osteomyelitis, 1073
Antalgic abductor lurch, 1077
Clubfoot, 1071
Developmental dysplasia of the hip (DDH), 1071
Dislocated hip, 1072
Duchenne muscular dystrophy (DMD), 1079
Dystrophin, 1079
Ewing sarcoma, 1082
Hereditary multiple exostoses (HME), 1081
Involucrum, 1073
Juvenile rheumatoid arthritis (JRA), 1075
Legg-Calvé-Perthes (LCP) disease, 1077
Malignant bone tumor, 1082
Muscular dystrophy, 1079
Nonossifying fibroma, 1081
Oligoarthritis, 1075
Osgood-Schlatter disease, 1077
Osteochondroma, 1081
Osteochondrosis, 1076
Osteogenesis imperfecta (OI) (brittle bone disease), 1073
Osteomyelitis, 1073
Osteosarcoma, 1082
Polyarthritis, 1075
Scoliosis, 1078
Septic arthritis, 1074
Stills disease, 1075
Subluxated hip, 1072

References

1. Morcuende JA et al: Plaster cast treatment of clubfoot: the Ponseti method of manipulation and casting, *J Pediatr Orthop* 3(2):161–167, 1994.
2. Noonan, KJ, Richards, BS: Nonsurgical management of idiopathic clubfoot, *J Am Acad Orthop Surg* 11(6):392–402, 2003.
3. Woolacott NF et al: Ultrasonography in screening for developmental dysplasia of the hip in newborns: systematic review, *Br Med J* 330(7505):1413, 2005.
4. Jari, S, Paton, RW, Srinivasan, MS: Unilateral limitation of abduction of the hip: a valuable clinical sign for DDH? *J Bone Joint Surg Br* 84(1):104–107, 2002.
5. Glorieux FH et al: Cyclic administration of Pamidronate in children with severe osteogenesis imperfecta, *N Engl J Med* 339(14):947–952, 1998.
6. Hresko MT et al: Prospective reevaluation of the association between thrombotic diathesis and Legg-Perthes disease, *J Bone Joint Surg Am* 84(9):1613–1618, 2002.
7. Mata SG et al: Legg-Calvé-Perthes disease and passive smoking, *J Pediatr Orthop* 20(3):326–330, 2000.
8. McCullough L, Lyman KS: Musculoskeletal considerations across the life span, In Gates SJ, Mooar PA, editors: *Musculoskeletal primary care*, Philadelphia, 1998, Lippincott.
9. Morrissy R, Weinstein S, editors: *Lovell and Winter's pediatric orthopaedics*, ed 4, Philadelphia, 1996, Lippincott-Raven.
10. Jorde LB et al: *Medical genetics*, ed 3, updated, St Louis, 2006, Mosby.
11. Cassas, KJ, Cassettari-Wayhs A: Childhood and adolescent sports-related overuse injuries, *Am Fam Physician* 73(6): 1014–1022, 2006.
12. Kaeding CC, Whitehead R: Musculoskeletal injuries in adolescents, *Prim Care* 25(1):211–223, 1998.
13. Davis JR, Chamberlin E, Blackhurst DW: Indications for magnetic resonance imaging in presumed adolescent idiopathic scoliosis, *J Bone Joint Surg Am* 86:2187–2195, 2004.
14. McDonald DG et al: Fracture prevalence in Duchenne muscular dystrophy, *Dev Med Child Neurol* 44(10):695–698, 2002.
15. Cummings RJ et al: Congenital clubfoot, *Instr Course Lect* 51:385–400, 2002.
16. Heyden, JB, Hoang, BH: Osteosarcoma: basic science and clinical implications, *Orthop Clin North Am* 37(1):1–7, 2006.
17. Rex, C, Kay, PR: Features of femoral fractures in nonaccidental injury, *J Pediatr Orthop* 20(3):411–413, 2000.
18. Thomas SA et al: Long-bone fractures in young children: distinguishing accident injuries from child abuse, *Pediatrics* 88(3):471–476, 1991.
19. Lane WG et al: Racial differences in the evaluation of pediatric fractures for physical abuse, *JAMA* 288(13):1603–1609, 2002.

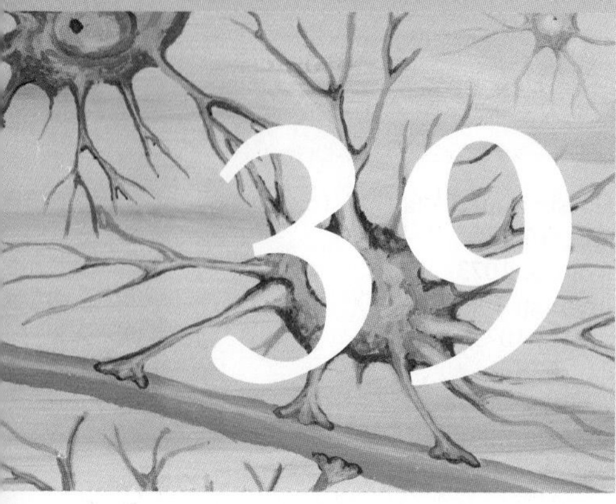

39 STRUCTURE, FUNCTION, AND DISORDERS OF THE INTEGUMENT

Sue E. Huether

CHAPTER OUTLINE

ELECTRONIC RESOURCES

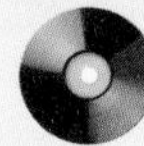

Companion CD
- Review Questions and Answers
- Animations

evolve Website
http://evolve.elsevier.com/Huether/
- Quick Check Answers
- Key Terms Exercises
- Critical Thinking Questions with Answers
- Algorithm Completion Exercises
- WebLinks

The skin is the largest organ of the body. Combined with the accessory structures of hair, nails, and glands, it forms the integumentary system. The skin covers the entire body and accounts for approximately 20% of the body's weight. The primary function of the skin is to protect the body from the environment by serving as a barrier against microorganisms, ultraviolet radiation, loss of body fluids, and the stress of mechanical forces. The skin also regulates body temperature and is involved in immune regulation and the activation of vitamin D. Touch and pressure receptors provide important protective functions and pleasurable sensations. The commensal organisms of the skin protect against pathologic bacteria.

STRUCTURE AND FUNCTION OF THE SKIN

Layers of the Skin

The skin is formed of two major layers: (1) a superficial or outer layer of **epidermis** and (2) a deeper layer of **dermis** (the true skin) (Figure 39-1). The **hypodermis** is an underlying layer of connective tissue that contains macrophages, fibroblasts, and fat cells. Each skin layer contains cells that represent progressive stages of skin cell differentiation as the skin grows. These are summarized in Table 39-1.

HEALTH ALERT
Tissue Adhesives for Closure of Skin Lacerations

A liquid adhesive bandage or glue (octyl-2-cyanoacrylate) is a pliable, waterproof adhesive film that can be applied to a laceration and left in place until it disintegrates in 7 to 14 days. It is appropriate for use in simple lacerations in areas where there is not excessive mobility or tension. The adhesives are particularly useful in children because they are painless and easy to apply and have good health and cosmetic results when compared with monofilament sutures. Fibrin-based glues have also gained a major role as a suture substitute for attaching biologic tissues and as surface sealants including use in ophthalmology. Many other adhesives are being developed and show promise as surface sealants and protective membranes.

Data from Dowson CC et al: A prospective, randomized controlled trial comparing n-butyl cyanoacrylate tissue adhesive (LiquiBand) with sutures for skin closure after laparoscopic general surgical procedures, *Surg Laparosc Endosc Percutan Tech* 16(3):146–150, 2006; Kuo F, Lee D, Rogers GS: Prospective, randomized, blinded study of a new wound closure film versus cutaneous suture for surgical wound closure, *Dermatol Surg* 32(5):676–681, 2006; Zeikus P, Dufresne R: Novel technique for use of cyanoacrylate in Mohs surgery, *Dermatol Surg* 32(7):943–944, 2006.

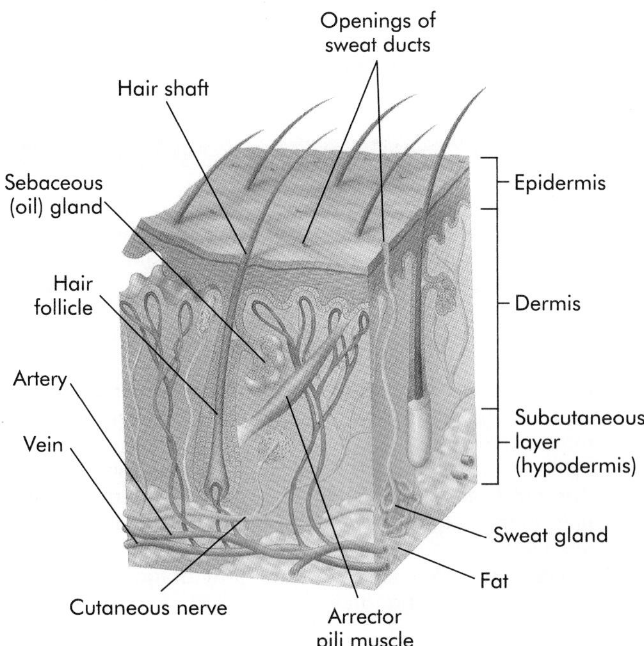

Figure 39-1 ■ **Structure of the Skin.** (From Thibodeau GA, Patton KT: *Anatomy & physiology,* ed 5, St Louis, 2003, Mosby.)

Dermal appendages

The **dermal appendages** include the nails, hair, sebaceous glands, and the eccrine and apocrine sweat glands. The nails are protective keratinized plates that appear at the ends of fingers and toes. They have four structural units: (1) the proximal nail fold, (2) the matrix from which the nail grows, (3) the hyponychium (the nail bed), and (4) the nail plate (Figure 39-2). Nail growth continues throughout life at 1 mm or less per day.

Hair color, density, grain, and pattern of distribution vary considerably among people and depend on age, gender, and race. Hair follicles arise from the matrix (or bulb) located deep in the dermis. They extend from the dermis at an angle and have an erector pili muscle attached near the middermis that straightens the follicle when contracted,

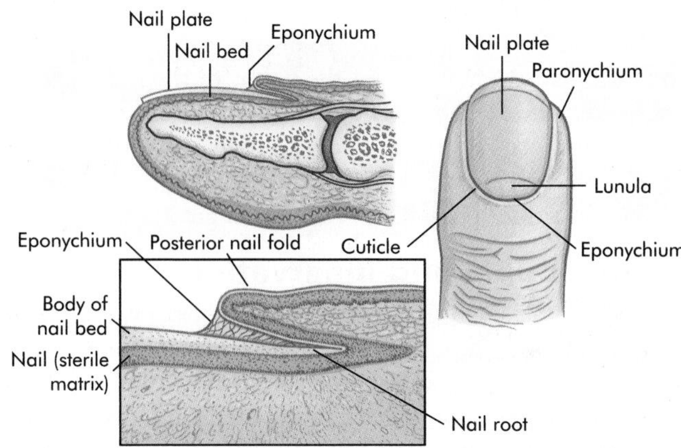

Figure 39-2 ■ **Structures of the Nail.** (Redrawn from Thompson JM et al: *Mosby's clinical nursing,* ed 5, St Louis, 2002, Mosby.)

TABLE 39-1
Layers of the Skin

Structure	Cell Types	Characteristics
EPIDERMIS	Keratinocytes	Most important layer of skin; normally very thin (0.12 mm) but can thicken and form corns or calluses with constant pressure or friction
	Langerhans cells	Cells with dendrite process and immune functions
Stratum corneum	Keratinocytes	Tough superficial layer covering the body
Stratum lucidum	Keratinocytes	Clear layers of cells containing eleidin, which becomes keratin as cells move up to the corneum layer
Stratum granulosum	Keratinocytes Melanocytes	Keratohyalin gives a granular appearance to this layer
Stratum spinosum	New keratinocytes	Polygonal-shaped with spinous processes projecting between adjacent keratinocytes
Stratum basale (germinativum)	Keratinocytes	Basal layer where keratinocytes divide and move upward to replace cells shed from the surface
	Melanocytes	Melanocytes synthesize the pigment melanin
	Merkel cells	The function of Merkel cells is not clearly known; they are associated with sensory nerve endings
DERMIS Papillary layer (thin) Reticular layer (thick)	Macrophages Mast cells Histiocytes	Irregular connective tissue layer with rich blood, lymphatic, and nerve supply; contains sensory receptors and special glands Histiocytes are wandering macrophages that collect pigments and inflammatory debris
SUBCUTANEOUS TISSUE		Subcutaneous tissue or superficial fascia of varying thickness that connects the overlying dermis to underlying muscle

causing the hair to stand up. Hair growth begins in the bulb, with cellular differentiation occurring as the hair progresses up the follicle. Hair is fully hardened, or cornified, by the time it emerges at the skin surface. Hair growth is cyclic, with periods of growth and rest that vary over different body surfaces.

The **sebaceous glands** open onto the surface of the skin through a canal. They are found in greatest numbers on the face, chest, and back, with modified glands on the eyelids, lips, nipples, glans penis, and prepuce. Sebaceous glands secrete sebum, composed primarily of lipids, which oils the skin and hair and prevents drying. Androgens stimulate the growth of sebaceous glands, and their enlargement is an early sign of puberty.

The **eccrine sweat glands** are distributed over the body, with the greatest numbers in the palms of the hands, soles of the feet, and forehead. They are important in thermoregulation and cooling of the body through evaporation. The **apocrine sweat glands** are fewer in number and are located in the axillae, scalp, face, abdomen, and genital area.

Blood supply and innervation

The blood supply to the skin is limited to the **papillary capillaries,** or plexus, of the dermis. These capillary loops are supplied by a deeper arterial plexus. Branches from the deep plexus also supply hair follicles and sweat glands. A subpapillary network of veins drains the capillary loops. Arteriovenous anastomoses in the dermis facilitate the regulation of body temperature. Heat loss can be regulated by varying blood flow through the skin by opening and closing the arteriovenous anastomoses in conjunction with evaporative heat loss of sweat. The sympathetic nervous system regulates both vasoconstriction and vasodilation through α-adrenergic receptors in the skin. The lymphatic vessels of the skin arise in the papillary dermis and drain into larger subcutaneous trunks, removing cells, proteins, and immunologic mediators.

QUICK CHECK 39-1

1. Describe the two layers of the skin.
2. How do the skin blood vessels regulate body temperature?
3. What cells of the skin regulate immune function?

Clinical Manifestations of Skin Dysfunction

Lesions

Identification of the morphologic structure and appearance of the skin in combination with a health history is necessary to identify underlying pathophysiology. Table 39-2 describes and illustrates the basic lesions of the skin. Clinical manifestations of select skin lesions are described in Table 39-3.

Pressure ulcers

Pressure ulcers are ischemic ulcers resulting from unrelieved pressure, shearing forces, friction, and moisture. The term *decubitus ulcer* refers to ulcers or pressure sores that develop when an individual lies in the recumbent position for a long time. The risks for pressure ulcers are summarized in *Risk Factors:* Pressure Ulcer.[1]

RISK FACTORS Pressure Ulcer

- Immobilization
- Elderly persons in hospitals and nursing homes
- Neurologic disorders (coma, spinal cord injuries, dementia, or cerebrovascular disease)
- Incontinence
- Fractured femur
- Debilitation
- Lying in bed or sitting in chair or wheel chair without changing position or relieving pressure over an extended period
- Lying for hours on hard x-ray and operating tables
- Chronic diseases accompanied by anemia, edema, renal failure, malnutrition, sepsis, and urinary or fecal incontinence
- Coarse bed sheets used for turning by dragging, which produces a shearing force

Pressure sores usually develop over bony prominences, such as the sacrum, heels, ischia, and greater trochanters. Continuous pressure on tissue between the bony prominence and a resistant outside surface distorts capillaries and occludes the blood supply. If the pressure is relieved within a few hours, a brief period of reactive hyperemia (redness) occurs with no lasting tissue damage. If the pressure continues unrelieved, the endothelial cells lining the capillaries become disrupted with platelet aggregation, forming microthrombi that block blood flow and cause anoxic necrosis of surrounding tissues (Figure 39-3). One classification of pressure ulcer grades or stages is as follows[2]:

1. Nonblanchable erythema of intact skin
2. Partial-thickness skin loss involving epidermis or dermis

Text continued on p. 1094

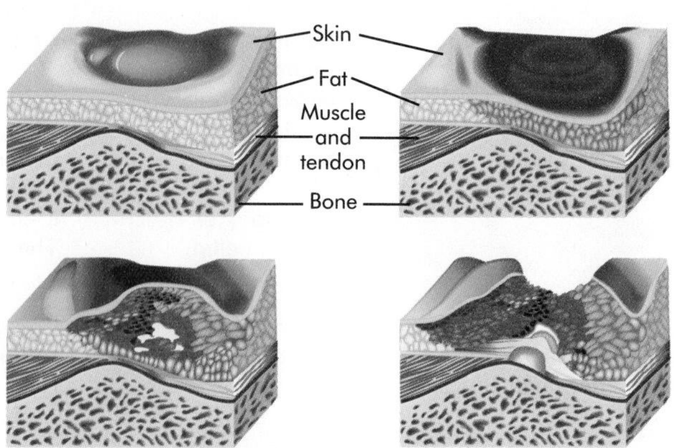

Figure 39-3 ■ Progression of Decubitus Ulcer. Sustained pressure over a bony prominence compresses the tissue and reduces blood flow resulting in progressive ischemia and necrosis of tissue.

TABLE 39-2

Primary and Secondary Skin Lesions

Primary Skin Lesions	Examples
MACULE A flat, circumscribed area that is a change in the color of the skin; less than 1 cm in diameter	Freckles, flat moles (nevi), petechiae, measles, scarlet fever

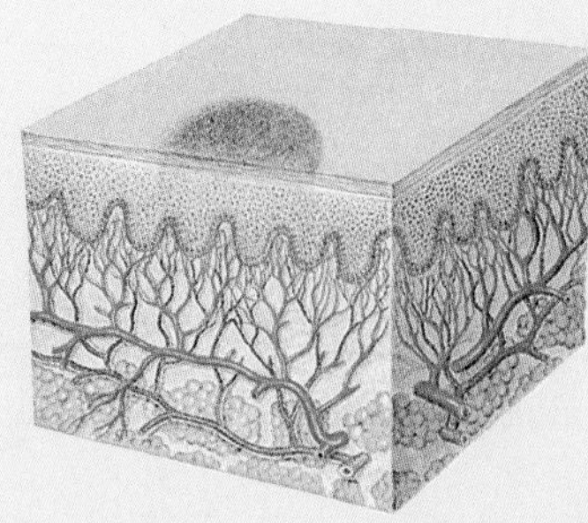

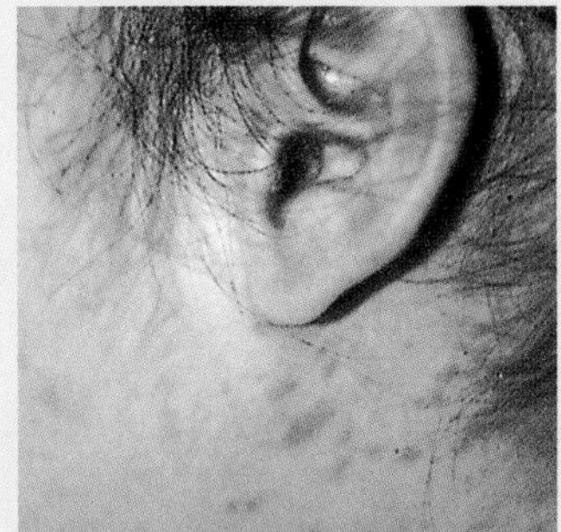

Macules[c]

Primary Skin Lesions	Examples
PAPULE An elevated, firm, circumscribed area less than 1 cm in diameter	Wart (verruca), elevated moles, lichen planus

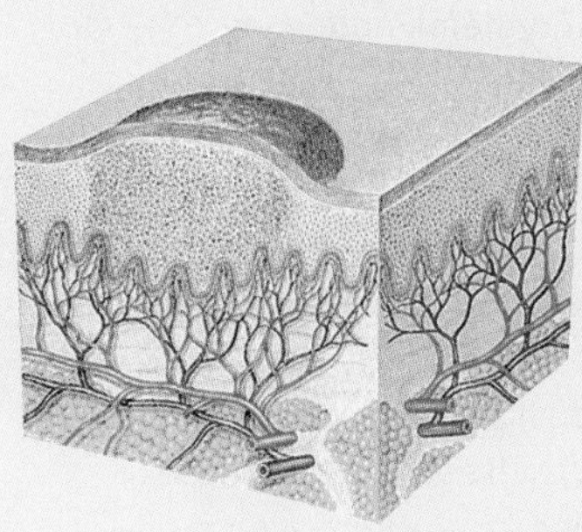

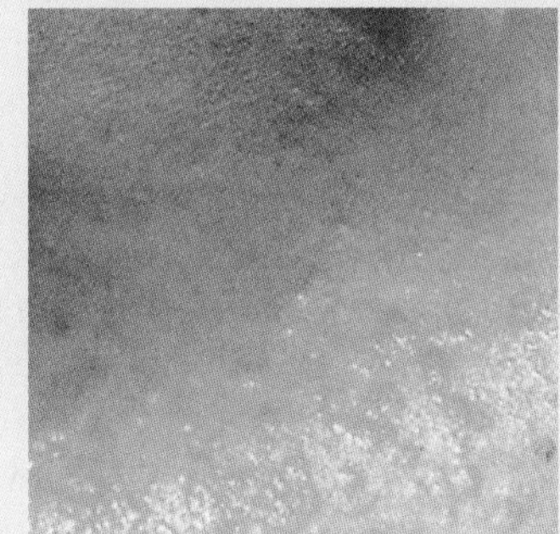

Flat warts[c]
(Courtesy Dr. E Sahn.)

Primary Skin Lesions	Examples
PATCH A flat, nonpalpable, irregular-shaped macule more than 1 cm in diameter	Vitiligo, port-wine stains, Mongolian spots, café au lait spots

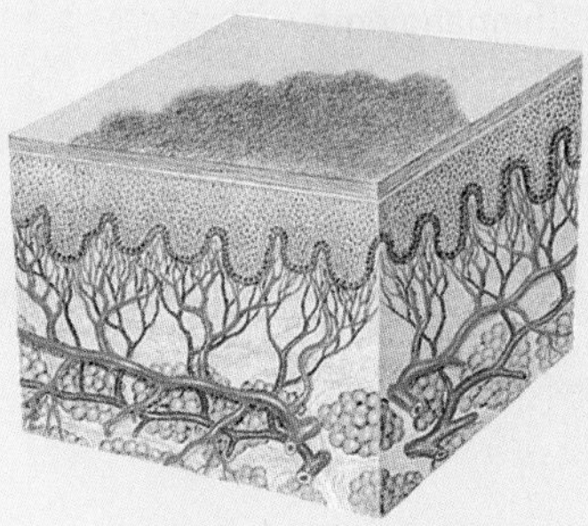

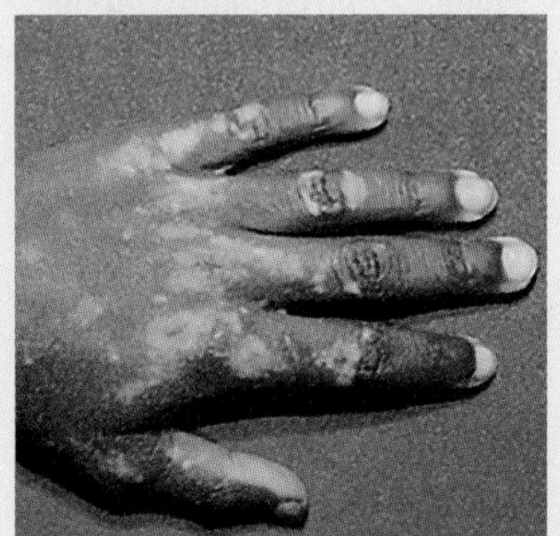

Vitiligo[h]

Primary Skin Lesions	Examples
PLAQUE Elevated, firm, and rough lesion with flat top surface more than 1 cm in diameter	Psoriasis, seborrheic and actinic keratoses

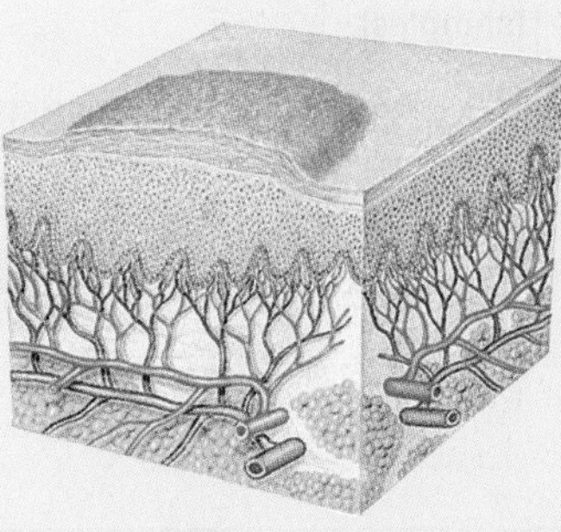

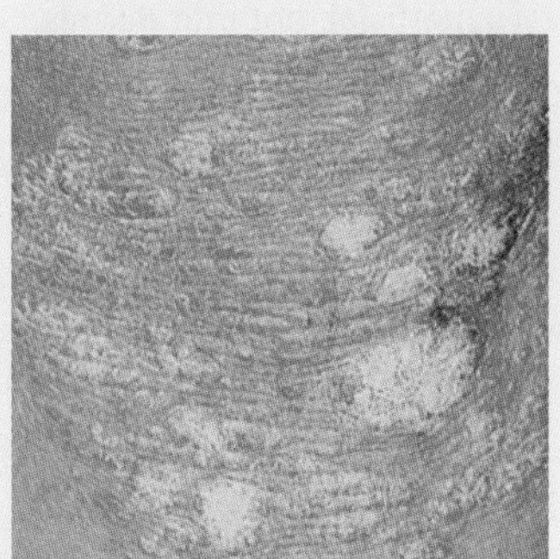

Plaque[e]

(Continued)

TABLE 39-2

Primary and Secondary Skin Lesions—Cont'd

Primary Skin Lesions	Examples		
WHEAL Elevated irregular-shaped area of cutaneous edema; solid, transient; variable diameter	Insect bites, urticaria, allergic reaction	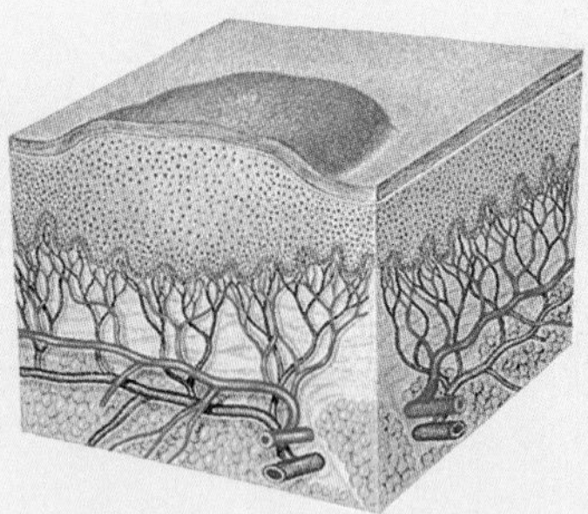	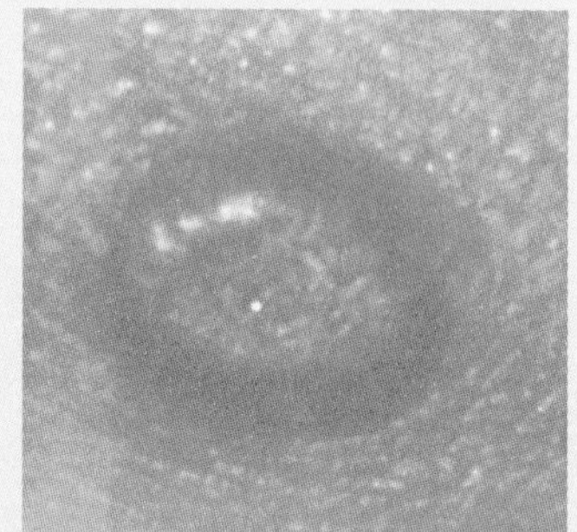 Wheal[c]
NODULE Elevated, firm, circumscribed lesion; deeper in dermis than a papule; 1–2 cm in diameter	Erythema nodosum, lipomas	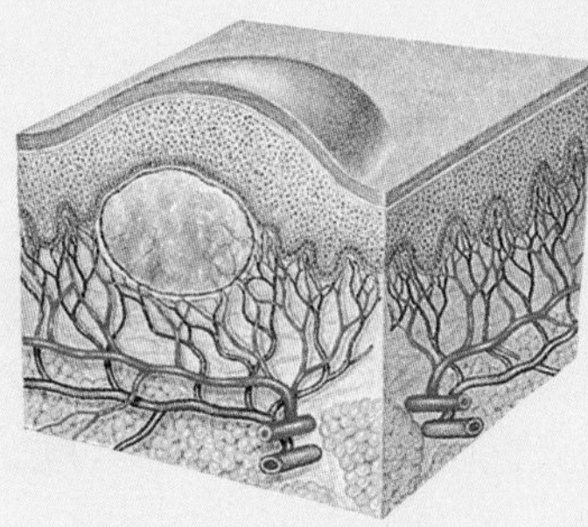	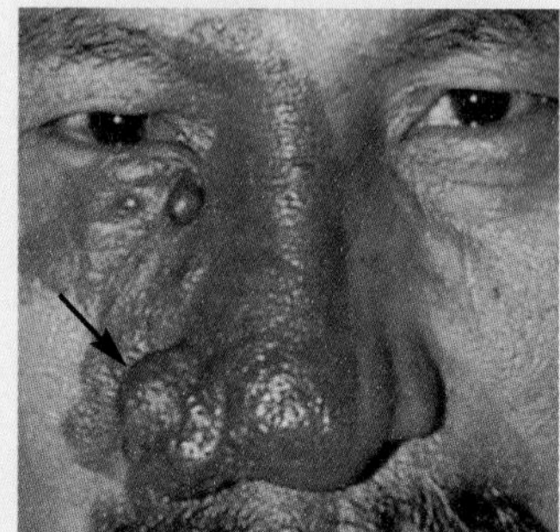 Hypertrophic nodule[d]
TUMOR Elevated, solid lesion; may be clearly demarcated; deeper in dermis; more than 2 cm in diameter	Neoplasms, benign tumor, lipoma, hemangioma	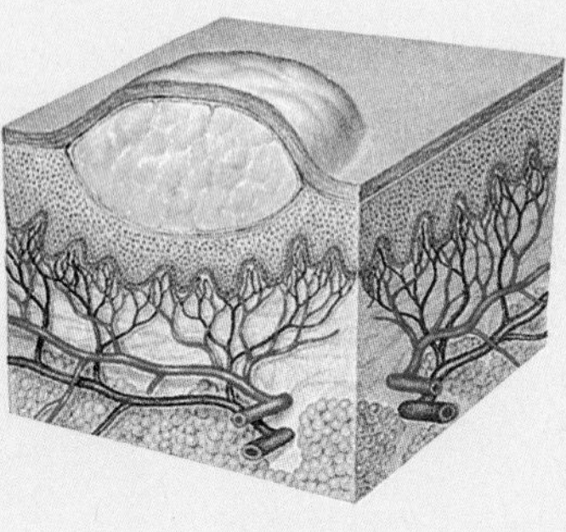	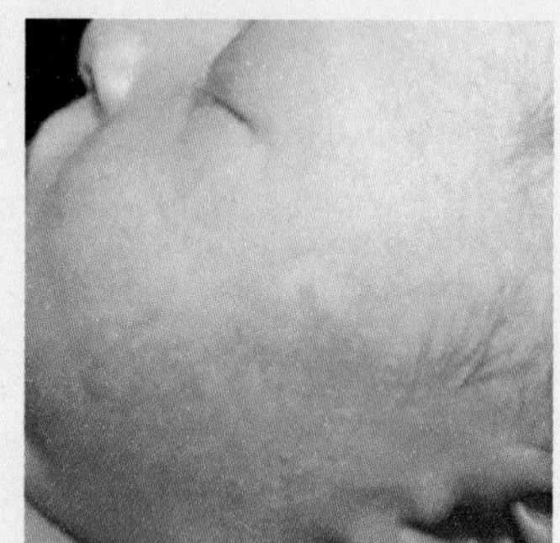 Hemangioma[h]
VESICLE Elevated, circumscribed, superficial, not into dermis; filled with serous fluid; less than 1 cm in diameter	Varicella (chickenpox), herpes zoster (shingles)	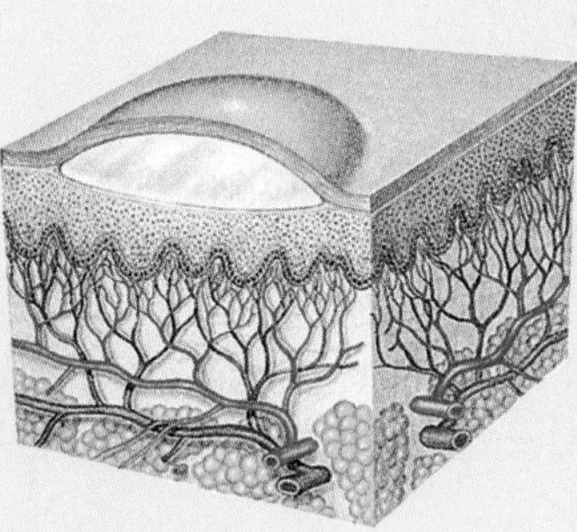	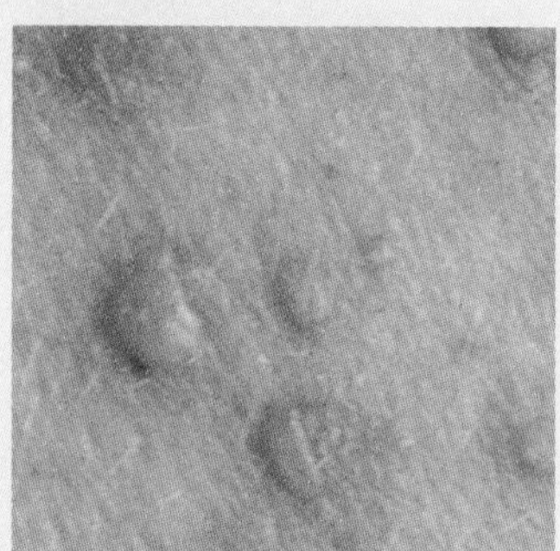 Vesicles[c]

TABLE 39-2

Primary and Secondary Skin Lesions—Cont'd

Primary Skin Lesions	Examples		
BULLA Vesicle more than 1 cm in diameter	Blister, pemphigus vulgaris	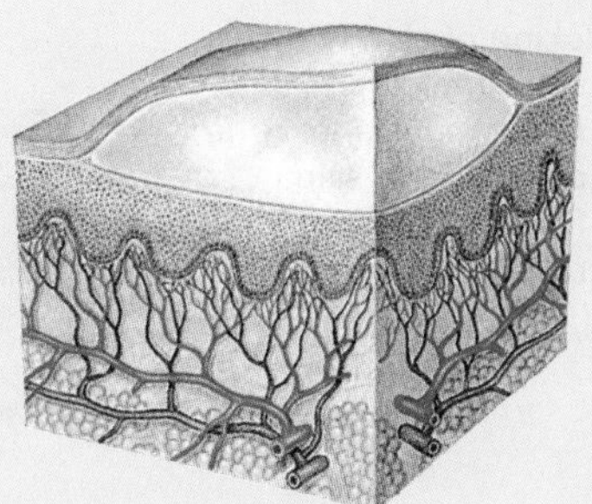	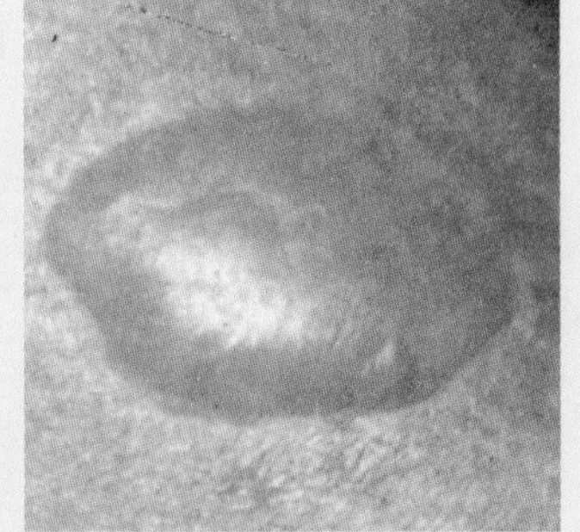 Bulla[c] (Courtesy Dr. KA Riley.)
PUSTULE Elevated, superficial lesion; similar to a vesicle but filled with purulent fluid	Impetigo, acne	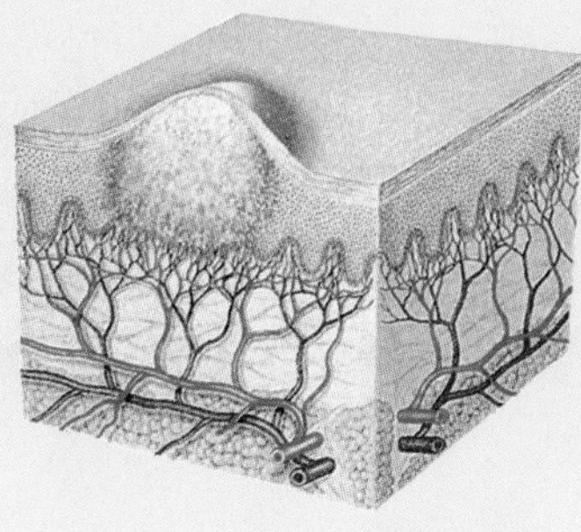	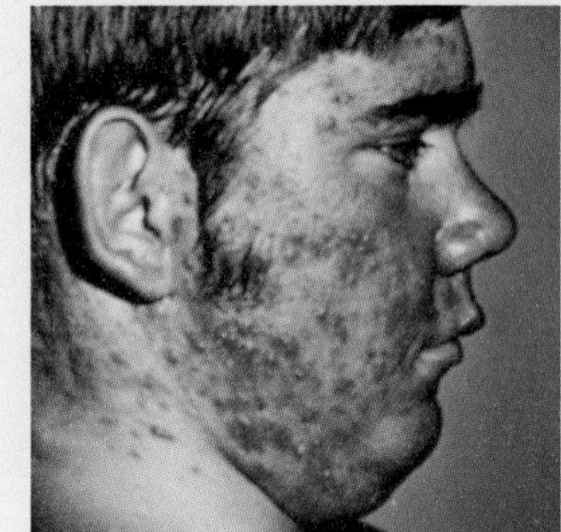 Acne[h]
CYST Elevated, circumscribed, encapsulated lesion; in dermis or subcutaneous layer; filled with liquid or semisolid material	Sebaceous cyst, cystic acne	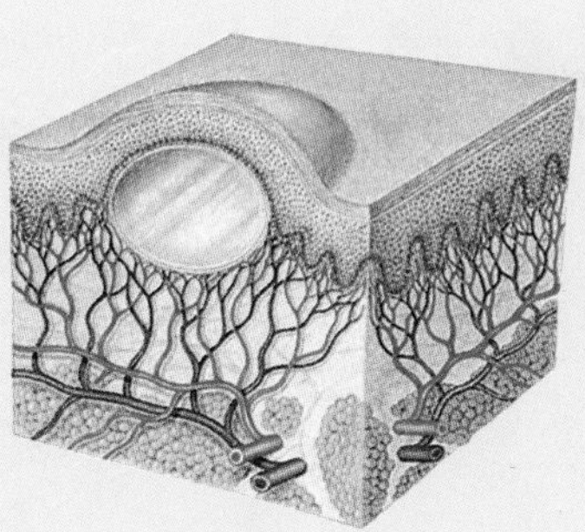	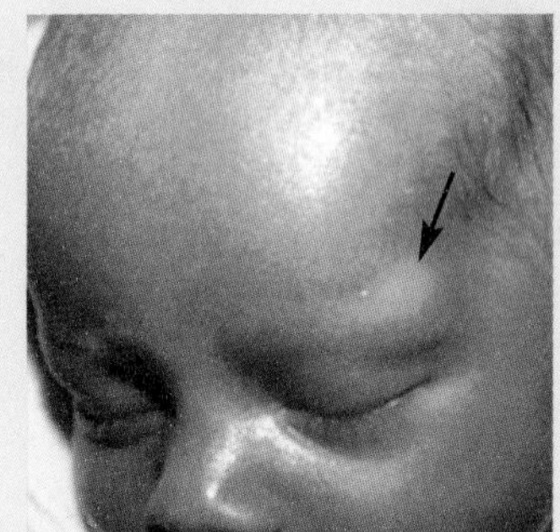 Sebaceous cyst[h]
TELANGIECTASIA Fine, irregular red lines produced by capillary dilation	Telangiectasia in rosacea	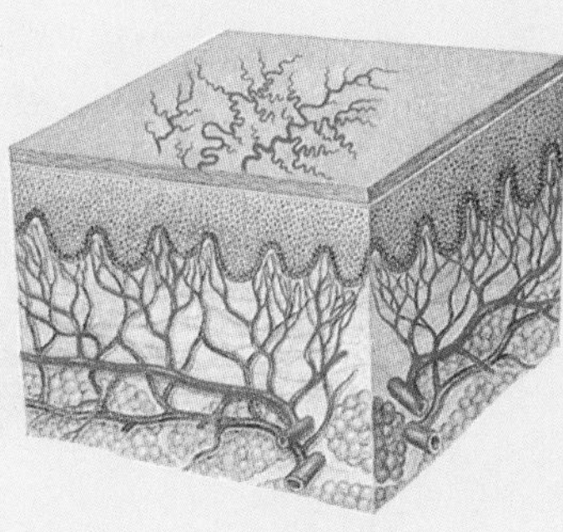	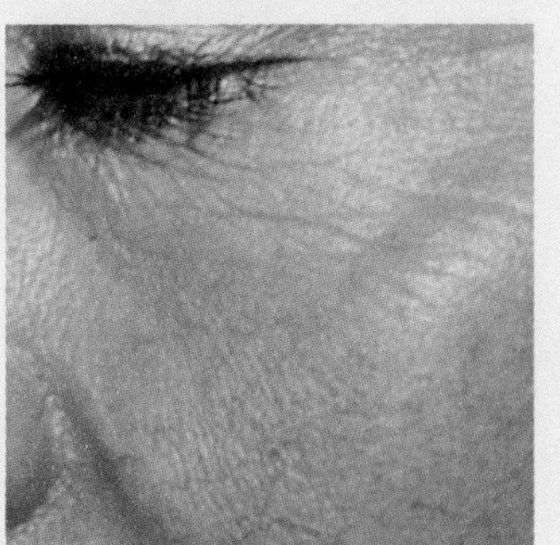 Telangiectasia[d]

(Continued)

TABLE 39-2

Primary and Secondary Skin Lesions—Cont'd

Secondary Skin Lesions	Examples		
SCALE Heaped-up, keratinized cells; flaky skin; irregular; thick or thin; dry or oily; variation in size	Flaking of skin with seborrheic dermatitis following scarlet fever, or flaking of skin following a drug reaction; dry skin	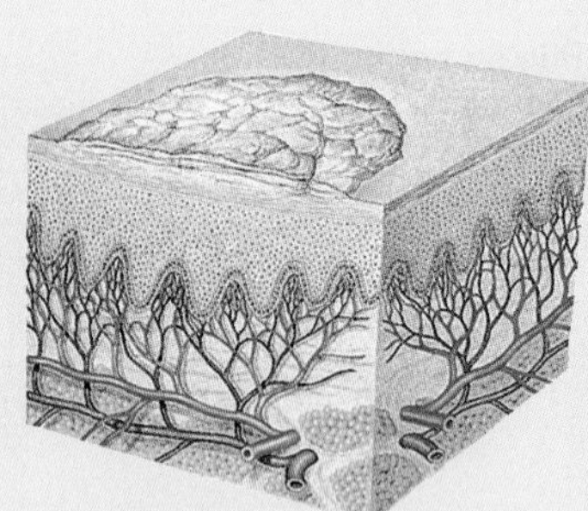	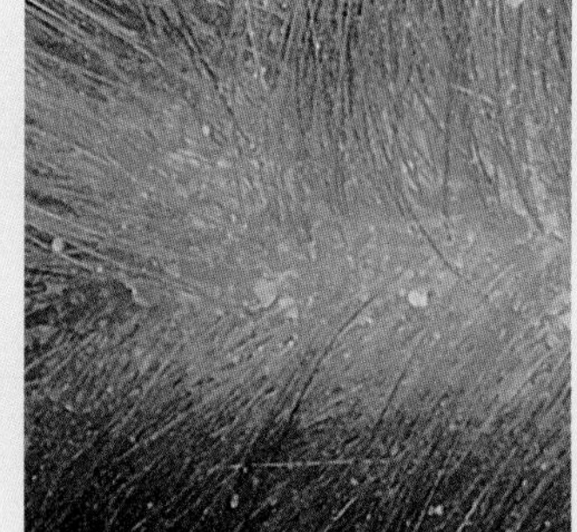 Fine scaling[a]
LICHENIFICATION Rough, thickened epidermis secondary to persistent rubbing, itching, or skin irritation; often involves flexor surface of extremity	Chronic dermatitis	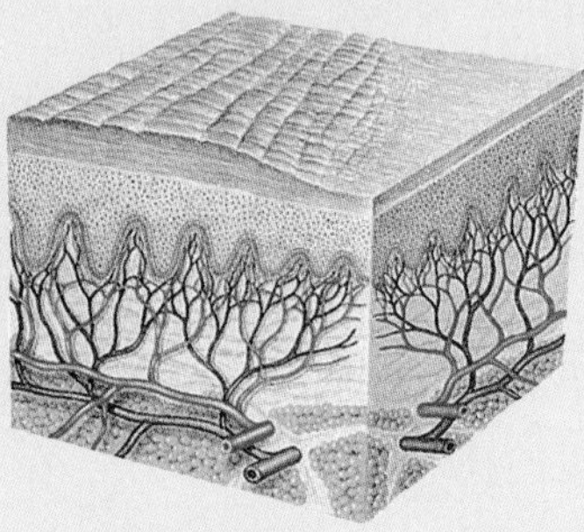	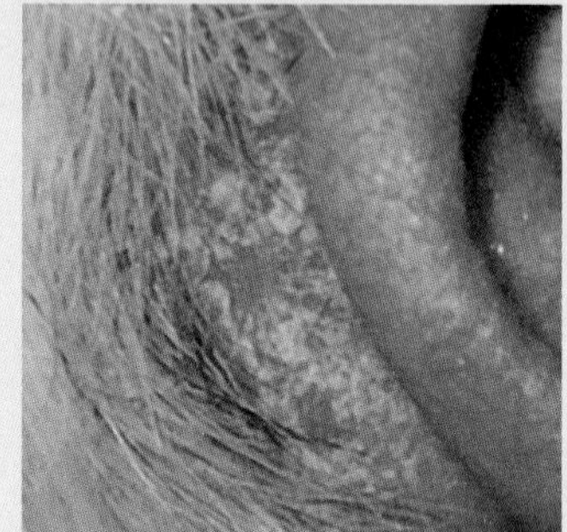 Stasis dermatitis in early stage[f]
KELOID Irregular-shaped, elevated, progressively enlarging scar; grows beyond the boundaries of the wound; caused by excessive collagen formation during healing	Keloid formation following surgery	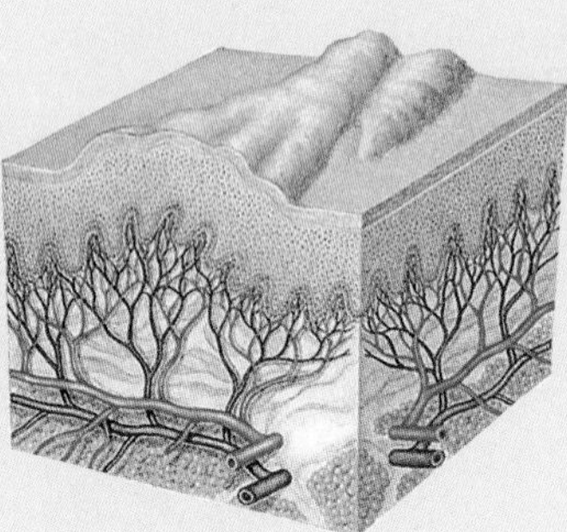	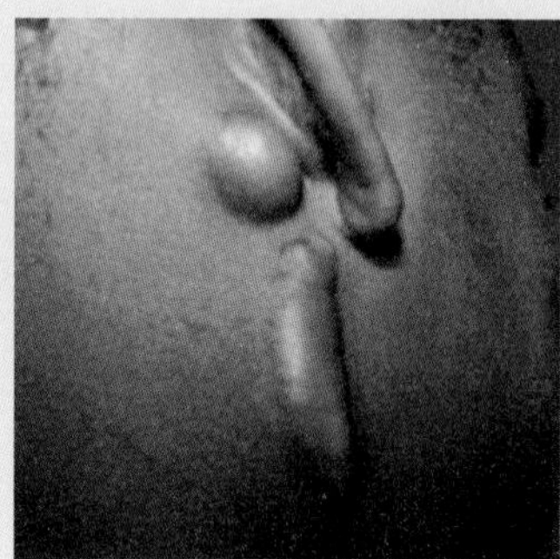 Keloid[h]
SCAR Thin to thick fibrous tissue that replaces normal skin following injury or laceration to the dermis	Healed wound or surgical incision	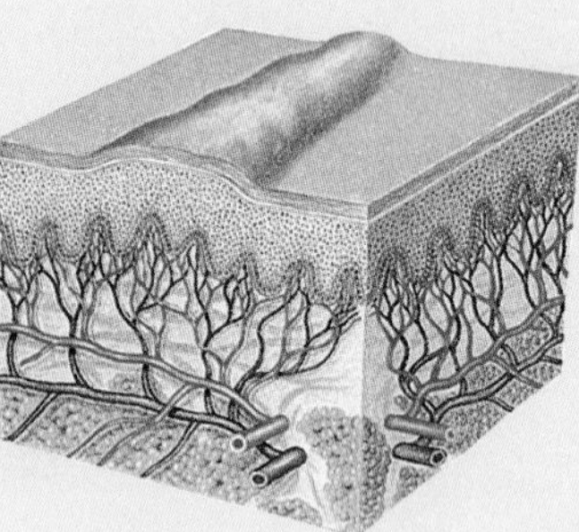	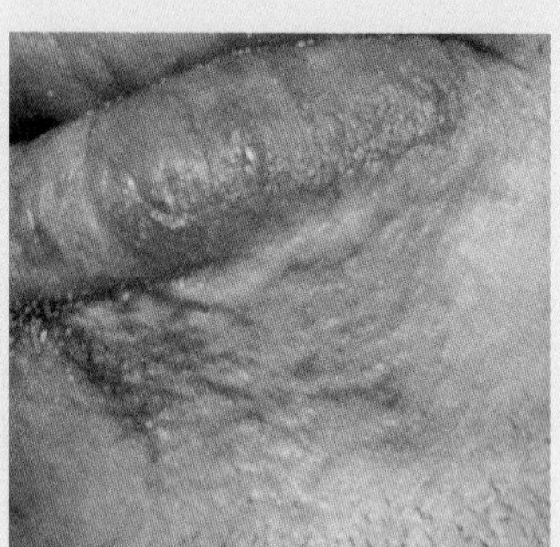 Hypertrophic scar[d]

TABLE 39-2

Primary and Secondary Skin Lesions—Cont'd

Secondary Skin Lesions	Examples
EXCORIATION Loss of the epidermis; linear, hollowed-out, crusted area	Abrasion or scratch, scabies

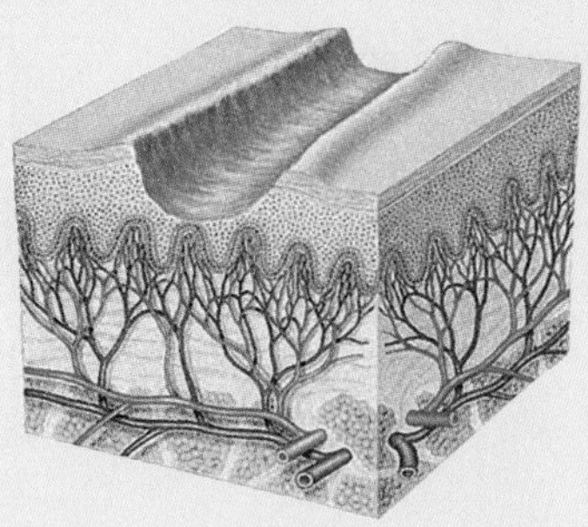

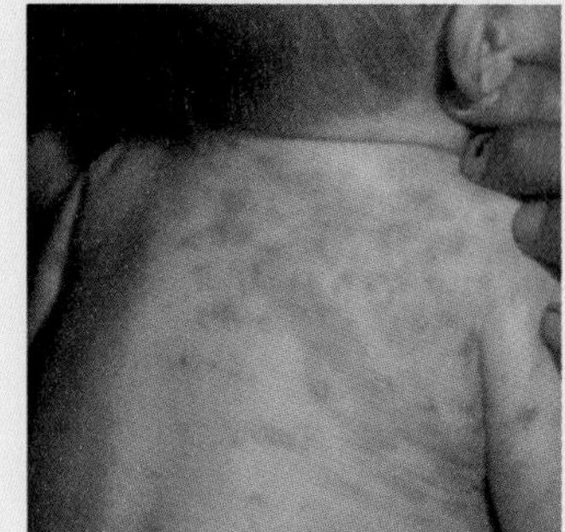

Scabies[h]

Secondary Skin Lesions	Examples
FISSURE Linear crack or break from the epidermis to the dermis; may be moist or dry	Athlete's foot, cracks at the corner of the mouth

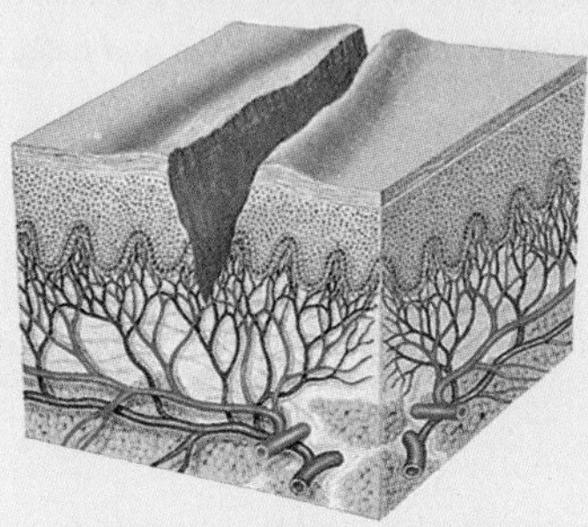

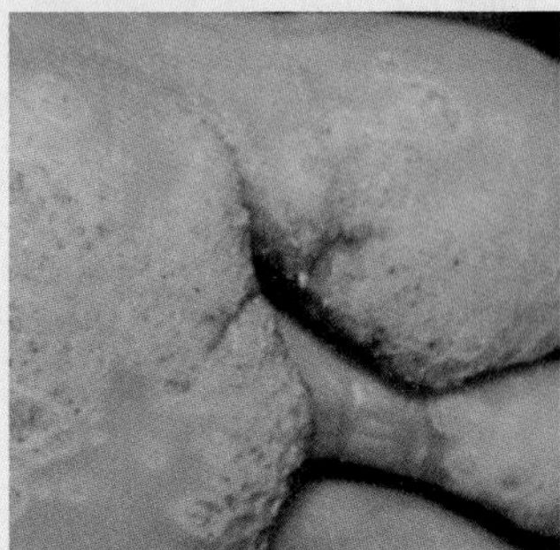

Fissures[d]

Secondary Skin Lesions	Examples
EROSION Loss of part of the epidermis; depressed, moist, glistening; follows rupture of a vesicle or bulla	Varicella, variola after rupture

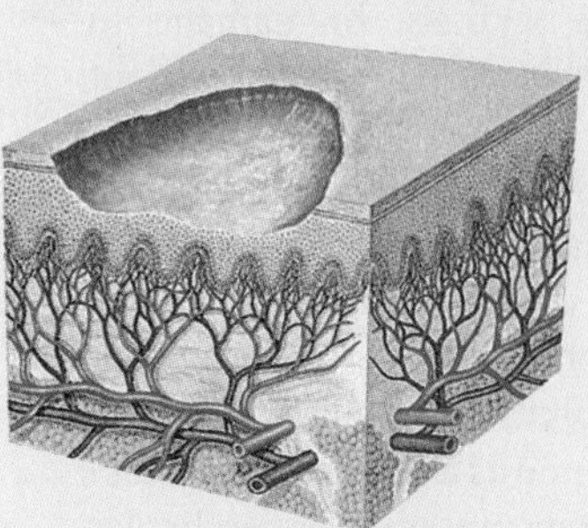

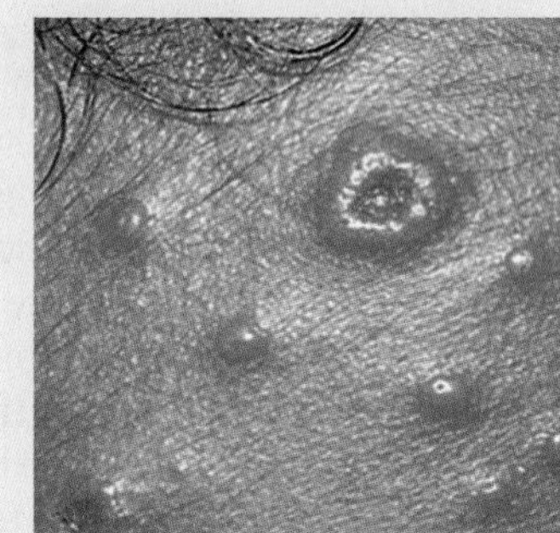

Erosion[b]

Secondary Skin Lesions	Examples
ULCER Loss of epidermis and dermis; concave; varies in size	Decubiti, stasis ulcers

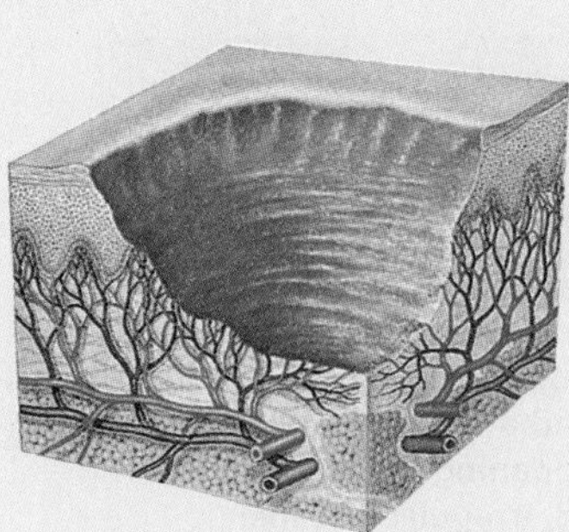

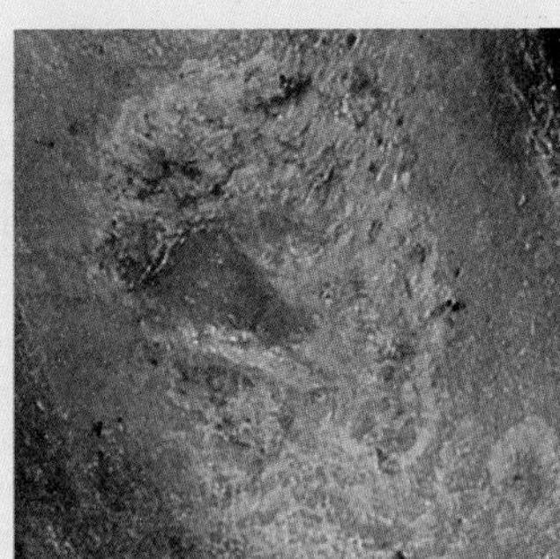

Stasis ulcer[e]

(Continued)

TABLE 39-2
Primary and Secondary Skin Lesions—Cont'd

Secondary Skin Lesions	Examples
ATROPHY	
Thinning of the skin surface and loss of skin markings; skin appears translucent and paper-like	Aged skin, striae

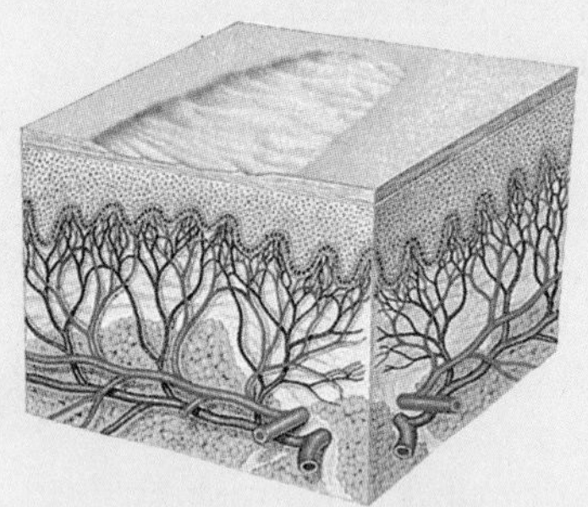

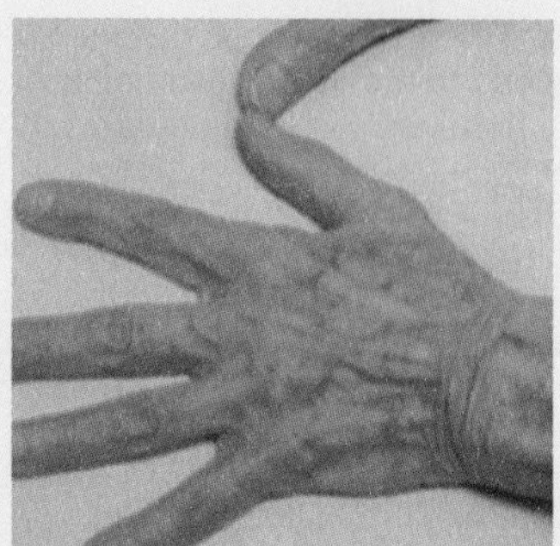

Aged skin[g]

From Thompson JM, Wilson SF: *Health assessment for nursing practice,* ed 2, St Louis, 2002, Mosby.
[a]Baran R, Dawber RR, Levene GM: *Color atlas of the hair, scalp, and nails,* St Louis, 1991, Mosby.
[b]Cohen BA: *Pediatric dermatology,* London, 1993, Wolfe.
[c]Farrar WE et al: *Infectious diseases,* ed 2, London, 1992, Gower.
[d]Goldman MP, Fitzpatrick RE: *Cutaneous laser surgery: the art and science of selective photo thermolysis,* ed 2, St Louis, 1998, Mosby.
[e]Habif TP: *Clinical dermatology,* ed 4, St Louis, 2004, Mosby.
[f]Marks JG Jr, DeLeo VA: *Contact and occupational dermatitis,* St Louis, 1991, Mosby.
[g]Seidel HM et al: *Mosby's guide to physical examination,* ed 6, St Louis, 2007, Mosby.
[h]Weston WL, Lane AT: *Color textbook of pediatric dermatology,* ed 3, St Louis, 2002, Mosby.

3. Full-thickness skin loss involving damage or necrosis of subcutaneous tissue that may extend to, but not through, underlying fascia
4. Extensive destruction, tissue necrosis, or damage to muscle, bone, or supporting structures with or without full-thickness skin loss.

A layer of dead tissue forms as what appears as an abrasion or blister when there is superficial damage or as a reddish blue discoloration when there is deeper tissue damage. Superficial sores are more common on the sacrum as a result of shearing or friction forces (forces parallel to the skin). Deep sores develop closer to the bone as a result of tissue distortion and vascular occlusion from pressure perpendicular to the tissue (over the heels, trochanter, and ischia).

TABLE 39-3
Clinical Manifestations of Select Skin Lesions

Type	Clinical Manifestation
Comedone	A plug of sebaceous and keratin material lodged in the opening of a hair follicle; an open comedone has a dilated orifice (blackhead), and a closed comedone has a narrow opening (whitehead)
Burrow	A narrow, raised, irregular channel caused by a parasite
Petechiae	A circumscribed area of blood less than 0.5 cm in diameter
Purpura	A circumscribed area of blood greater than 0.5 cm in diameter
Telangiectasia	Dilated, superficial blood vessels

The necrotic tissue initiates an inflammatory response, with pain, fever, and leukocytosis. Although bacteria colonize the dead tissue, the infection is usually localized and self-limiting. Proteolytic enzymes from bacteria and macrophages dissolve necrotic tissues and cause a foul-smelling discharge that resembles, but is not, pus.

Pressure sores are painful and cause an inflammatory response with hyperemia, fever, and increased white blood cell count. If the ulceration is large, toxicity and pain lead to loss of appetite, debility, and renal insufficiency. Individuals who are immunosuppressed or have diabetes mellitus may develop infection and inflammation of adjacent tissues (cellulitis) or septicemia.

The primary goal for those at risk for pressure ulcers is prevention. Turning every 2 hours, use of flotation devices and alternating pressure mattresses, and elimination of excessive moisture and drainage are effective preventive techniques. Adequate nutrition, oxygenation, and fluid balance must be maintained.[3,4]

Superficial ulcers should be covered with flat, nonbulky dressings (e.g., hydrogel dressings) that cannot wrinkle and cause increased pressure or friction. Spontaneous healing occurs more quickly using moist dressings.[5] Successful healing requires continued adequate relief of pressure. Large, deep pressure ulcers may require surgical débridement of necrotic tissue and opening of deep pockets for drainage.

Keloids

Keloids are sharply elevated, irregular or claw shaped, progressively enlarging scars caused by excessive amounts of collagen in the corneum during connective tissue repair. Seemingly inconsequential trauma may result in a keloidal reaction, particularly in darkly pigmented skin and in burn scars.

Excessive or poorly aligned tension on a wound, introduction of foreign material into the skin, and certain types of trauma (e.g., burns) are all provocative factors. Those parts of the body at risk include shoulders, back, chin, ears, and lower legs. Most keloids appear within 1 year of trauma. Individuals 10 to 30 years of age develop lesions much more commonly than do children before puberty or older adults. A familial tendency for keloid formation has been found.[6]

Keloids start as pink or red, firm, well-defined, rubbery plaques that persist for several months after trauma. Later, uncontrolled overgrowth causes extension beyond the site of the original wound, and the tumor becomes smoother, irregularly shaped, hyperpigmented, harder, and more symptomatic. The fibrous tissue that accumulates in keloids is associated with increased cellularity and metabolic activity of fibroblasts. The tendency to send out **clawlike prolongations** is typical (Figure 39-4).

Preventive measures, such as avoiding unnecessary, elective surgeries, are of paramount importance. When surgery is necessary for cosmetic reasons, having it done in early childhood is best. Many keloids are unresponsive to silicone gel sheeting or steroids. Radiation therapy has been successful, as have local chemotrophic agents, such as Bleomycin, 5-fluorouracil, and immiquamod.[7]

Pruritus

Pruritus, or itching, is a symptom associated with many primary skin disorders, such as eczema or lice infestations, or it can be a manifestation of systemic disease (e.g., chronic renal failure, cholestatic liver disease, thyroid disorders, iron deficiency) or the use of opiate drugs. It may be localized or generalized and may move from one location to another.

Multiple stimuli can produce itching, and there is interaction between itch and pain sensations. Peripheral itch mediators include histamine, serotonin, prostaglandins, bradykinins, neuropeptides, and acetylcholine. Small unmyelinated nerve fibers transmit itch sensations and specific spinal pathways may carry itch sensations to the brain.[8,9]

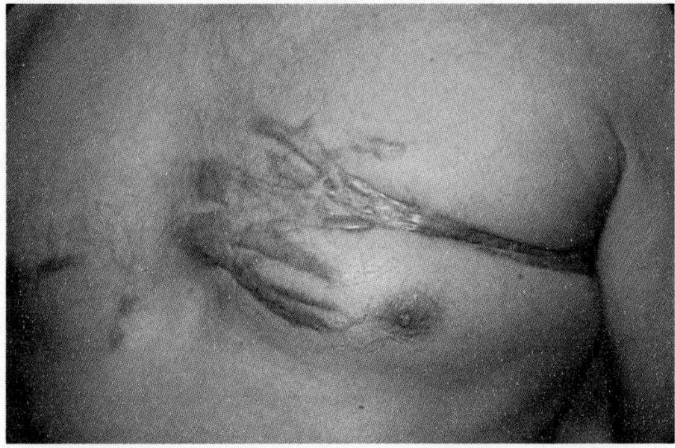

Figure 39-4 ■ **Keloid Formation.** (Courtesy Department of Dermatology, School of Medicine, University of Utah.)

Management of localized itching depends on the cause, and the primary condition must be treated. Symptomatic relief may be obtained from antihistamines, which also have a sedative effect. Minor tranquilizers, such as promethazine, may be effective for some causes of pruritus. Itching related to dry, rough skin (xerosis) can be managed with applications of emollients and increased environmental humidity. Topical steroids are immediately effective with some occurrences of pruritus, and opioid antagonists may relieve some cases of severe chronic itch. Phototherapy may provide some relief, and some pruritus is resistant to any type of therapy.[10,11]

✔ QUICK CHECK 39-2

1. What areas are at greatest risk of pressure ulcers?
2. How does a keloid differ from a normal scar?
3. What stimulates pruritus?

AGING & Changes in Skin Integrity

Skin becomes thinner, dryer, and more wrinkled.
Epidermal cells contain less moisture and change shape.
The dermoepidermal border flattens, shortening and decreasing number of capillary loops.
DNA repair of damaged skin decreases.
There are fewer melanocytes, giving decreased protection from ultraviolet radiation and leading to graying of hair.
Pigmentation becomes irregular.
There is a loss of the rete pegs, giving skin a smooth, shiny appearance.
There is a loss of elastin, producing wrinkling.
The dermis thins, producing translucent, paper-thin quality.
There is a loss of flexibility of collagen fibers, so skin cannot stretch and regain shape as readily.
The barrier function of the stratum corneum reduces.
Dermis becomes more permeable and less able to clear substances, so they accumulate and cause irritation.
Atrophy of eccrine, apocrine, and sebaceous glands causes dry skin.
Significantly decreased Langerhans cells reduce the skin's immune response.
Pressure and touch receptors and free nerve endings decrease, causing reduced sensory perception.
Wound healing decreases as a result of decreased blood flow and slower rate of basal cell turnover.
With compromised temperature regulation, loss of cutaneous vasomotion, and decreased eccrine sweat production, there is an increased risk of heat stroke and hypothermia.
The nail plate thin, and nails are more brittle.

Data from Fore J: A review of skin and the effects of aging on skin structure and function, *Ostomy Wound Manage* 52(9):24–35, quiz 36–37, 2006; McCullough JK, Kelly KM: Prevention and treatment of skin aging, *Ann N Y Acad Sci* 1067:323–331, 2006; Verdier-Sevrain S, Bonte F, Gilchrest B: Biology of estrogens in skin: implications for skin aging, *Exp Dermatol* 15(2):83–94, 2006; Wickremaratchi MM, Llewelyn JG: Effects of ageing on touch, *Postgrad Med J* 82(967):301–304, 2006.

DISORDERS OF THE SKIN

Disruptions in skin integrity may be precipitated by trauma, abnormal cellular function, infection and inflammation, and systemic diseases.

Inflammatory Disorders

The most common inflammatory disorders of the skin are eczema or dermatitis. **Eczema** and **dermatitis** are general terms that describe a particular type of inflammatory response in the skin and can be used interchangeably. Eczematous disorders are generally characterized by pruritus, lesions with indistinct borders, and epidermal changes. These lesions can appear as erythema, papules, or scales; they can present in an acute, subacute, or chronic phase. Edema, serous discharge, and crusting occur with continued irritation and scratching. In chronic eczema, the skin becomes thickened, leathery, and hyperpigmented from recurrent irritation and scratching. The location of eczema is related to the underlying cause. Eczematous inflammations need to be differentiated from other rashes and dermatoses, particularly psoriasis.

Allergic contact dermatitis

Allergic contact dermatitis is a common form of cell-mediated or delayed hypersensitivity. (See Chapter 7 for different types of allergic responses.) The response is an interaction of skin barrier function, reaction to irritants, and neuronal responses, such as itching. Various allergens (e.g., microorganisms, chemicals, foreign proteins, latex, drugs, metals) can form the sensitizing antigen. Contact with poison ivy is a common example (Figure 39-5). As the allergen comes in contact with the skin, the allergen is bound to a carrier protein, forming a sensitizing antigen. The Langerhans cells process the antigen and carry it to T cells. T cells then become sensitized to the antigen inducing the release of cytokines and symptoms of dermatitis.[12] In latex allergy, there is an increase in immunoglobulin E (IgE) antibodies.[13]

Delayed hypersensitivity is characterized by the passing of several hours before an immunologic response is apparent. The T cells play an important role because they differentiate and secrete lymphokines that affect macrophage movement and aggregation, coagulation, and other inflammatory responses (see Chapter 6). Sensitization usually develops with first exposure to the antigen, and symptoms of dermatitis occur with reexposure.

The manifestations of allergic contact dermatitis include erythema and swelling with pruritic (itching) vesicular lesions in the areas of allergen contact. The pattern of distribution provides clues to the source of the antigen (i.e., hands exposed to chemical solutions or boundaries from rings and bracelets). The antigen must be removed for the inflammatory response to resolve and tissue repair to begin. Treatment may require topical or systemic steroids.

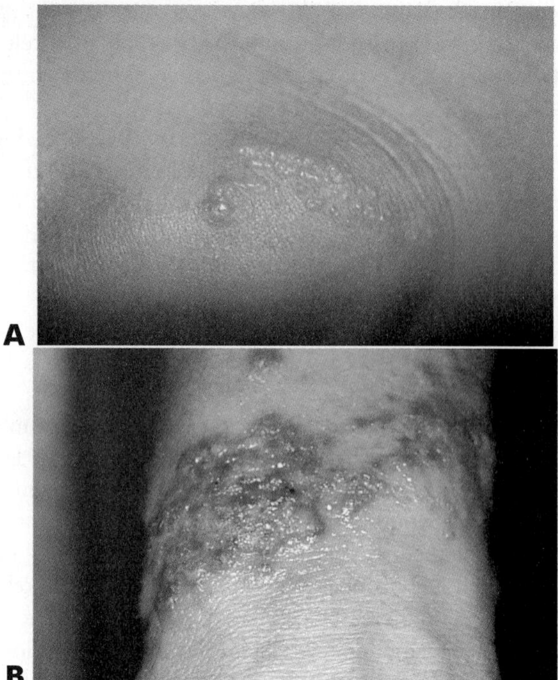

Figure 39-5 ■ **Poison Ivy. A,** Poison ivy on knee. **B,** Poison ivy dermatitis. (Courtesy Department of Dermatology, School of Medicine, University of Utah.)

Irritant contact dermatitis

Irritant contact dermatitis is a commonly occurring nonimmunologically mediated inflammation of the skin that may promote systemic involvement.[14] The severity of the inflammation is related to concentration of the irritant and exposure time. Chemical irritation from acids and prolonged exposure to soaps, detergents, and various agents used in industry can cause inflammatory lesions. The skin lesions resemble allergic contact dermatitis. Removing the source of irritation and using topical agents provide effective treatment.

Atopic dermatitis

Atopic dermatitis is more common in infancy and childhood; however, some individuals are affected throughout life. Specific details of this disorder are presented in Chapter 40 (p. 1121).

Stasis dermatitis

Stasis dermatitis usually occurs on the legs as a result of venous stasis and edema and is associated with varicosities, phlebitis, and vascular trauma. First, erythema and pruritus develop and then scaling, petechiae, and hyperpigmentation. Progressive lesions become ulcerated, particularly around the ankles and tibia (Figure 39-6).

Treatment includes elevating the legs as often as possible, not wearing tight clothes around the legs, and not standing for long periods. Acute inflammations are treated with antibiotics. Chronic lesions with ulceration are treated with wet dressings of Burow solution or silver nitrate. Edema is controlled with external compression.

Seborrheic dermatitis

Seborrheic dermatitis is a common chronic inflammation of the skin involving the scalp, eyebrows, eyelids, ear canals,

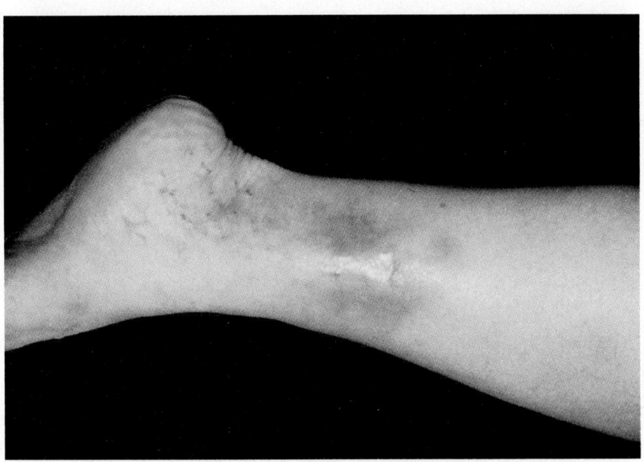

Figure 39-6 ■ **Stasis Ulcer.** (Courtesy Department of Dermatology, School of Medicine, University of Utah.)

nasolabial folds, axillae, chest, and back (Figure 39-7). In infants it is known as *cradle cap.* The cause is unknown, but Malassezia yeasts have been implicated. The lesions appear from infancy to old age with periods of remission and exacerbation. The lesions appear as scaly, white or yellowish inflammatory plaques with mild pruritus. Mild cases are treated with shampoos containing sulfur, salicylic acid, or tar. Topical therapy includes antifungals and low-dose steroids.[15] Corticosteroid applications suppress severe symptoms but should not be used for maintenance therapy.

Papulosquamous Disorders

Psoriasis, pityriasis rosea, and lichen planus are characterized by papules, scales, plaques, and erythema. Collectively they are described as **papulosquamous disorders.**

Psoriasis

Psoriasis is a chronic, relapsing, proliferative skin disorder that occurs at any age and affects 1% to 4% of the population. The onset is generally established by 20 years of age. A family history of psoriasis is often established. Inflammatory cytokines (i.e., tumor necrosis factor alpha) from activated T-cells cause the lesions of psoriasis.[16] The types of psoriasis include plaque (psoriasis vulgaris), inverse, guttate, pustular, and erythrodermic.

Both the dermis and epidermis are thickened with cellular proliferation and inflammation. The turnover time for shedding the epidermis is decreased to 3 to 4 days, with many more germinative cells and increased transit time through the dermis. Cell maturation and keratinization are bypassed, and the epidermis thickens and plaques form. The loosely cohesive keratin gives the lesion a silvery appearance. Capillary dilation and increased vascularization accommodate the increased cell metabolism but also cause erythema. The disease can be mild, moderate, or severe, depending on the size, distribution, and inflammation of the lesions. Psoriasis is marked by remissions and exacerbations. Arthritis develops in approximately 5% of individuals with psoriasis.

The typical plaque psoriatic lesion is a well-demarcated, thick, silvery, scaly, erythematous plaque surrounded by normal skin (Figure 39-8). Small erythematous papules enlarge and coalesce into larger inflammatory lesions on the face, scalp, elbows, and knees and at sites of trauma. Lesions that develop in the axilla and groin are smooth and have a deep red color. The scales are usually loosely adherent and may cause small bleeding points when removed.

In guttate psoriasis, small papules appear suddenly on the trunk and extremities (Figure 39-9) a few weeks after a streptococcal respiratory infection. Guttate psoriasis may resolve spontaneously in weeks or months.

Treatment is related to reducing epidermal cell turnover and immunomodulation. Mild lesions are usually treated with emollients, keratolytic agents, and corticosteroids. Moderate to severe lesions may respond to ultraviolet light, methotrexate, acitretin, vitamin D analogs, cyclosporin, interleukin-2 inhibitors, or one of the new biologics.[17] Severe disease may require hospitalization. Lesions of the scalp, nails, and genitalia are treated with different lotions and shampoos.

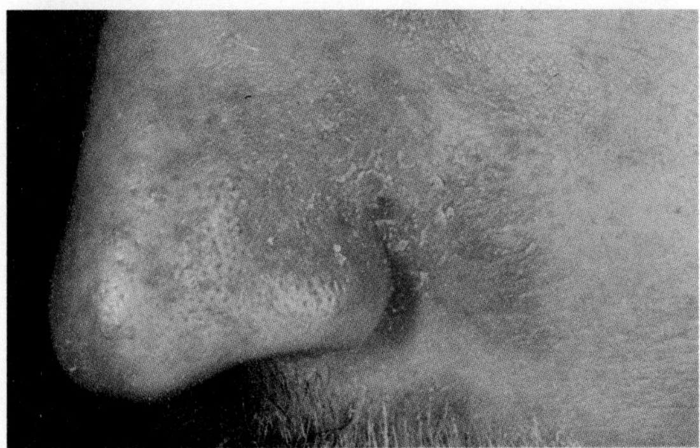

Figure 39-7 ■ **Seborrheic Dermatitis.** (Courtesy Department of Dermatology, School of Medicine, University of Utah.)

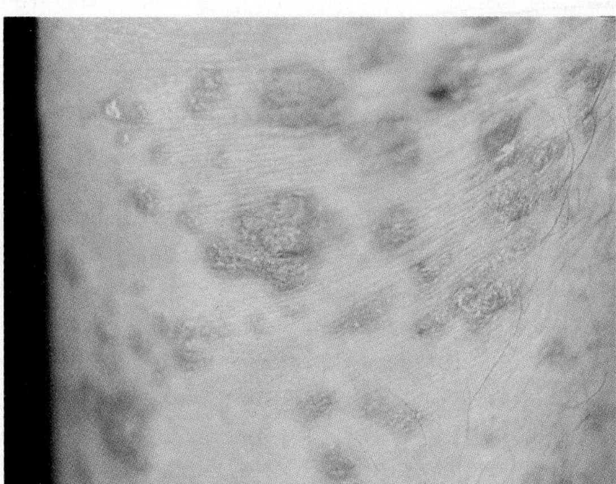

Figure 39-8 ■ **Psoriasis.** Typical oval plaque with well-defined borders and silvery scale. (Courtesy Department of Dermatology, School of Medicine, University of Utah.)

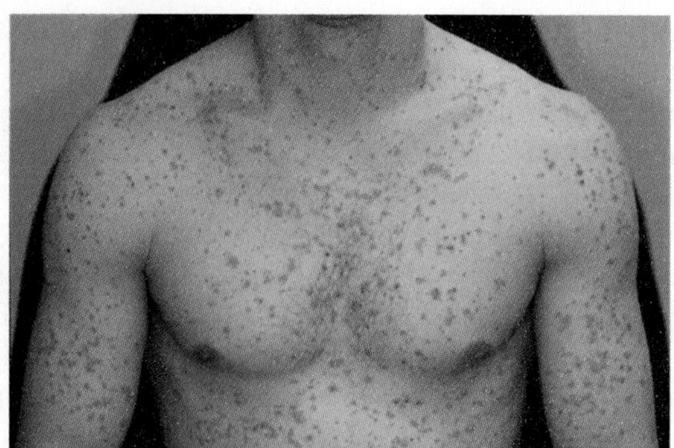

Figure 39-9 ■ Guttate Psoriasis Following Streptococcal Infection. Numerous uniformly small lesions may abruptly occur following streptococcal pharyngitis. (Courtesy Department of Dermatology, School of Medicine, University of Utah.)

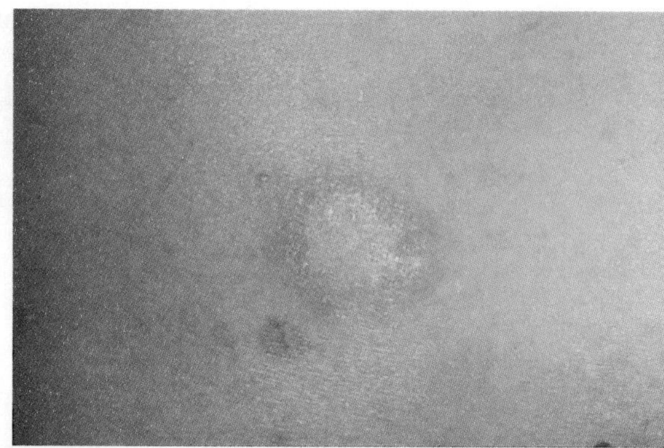

Figure 39-10 ■ Pityriasis Rosea Herald Patch. A collarette pattern has formed around the margins. (Courtesy Department of Dermatology, School of Medicine, University of Utah.)

HEALTH ALERT
Biologic Treatment for Psoriasis

Psoriasis is a chronic inflammatory disease of the skin. The disease develops when an unknown antigen activates T cells trafficked into the skin where they release cytokines such as tumor necrosis factor-alpha (TNFα) that maintain the plaque of psoriasis. New immunomodulation therapies are providing beneficial outcomes and new insights for treatment of this disease. *Alefacept* works primarily by decreasing the life span of T lymphocytes through increased activity of natural killer cells, causing depletion of T cells. Efalizumab modifies T cell receptor sites so the antigen is unable to activate naïve T cells in lymph nodes and suppresses trafficking to and activation in the skin. This results in decreased plaque formation. *Etanercept, adalimumab,* and *infliximab* block tumor necrosis factor-alpha released from the T lymphocytes that have trafficked to the skin. The consequence is decreased inflammation and a decrease in the hyperproliferation of skin cells. Etanercept also has been used for the treatment of psoriatic arthritis. Continuing advances in new biologic therapies will continue to improve the safety and effectiveness of treatment for psoriasis.

Data from Boehncke WH, Prinz J, Gottlieb AB: Biologic therapies for psoriasis: a systematic review, *J Rheumatol* 33(7):1447–1451, 2006; Lowes MA, Bowcock AM, Krueger JG: Pathogenesis and therapy of psoriasis, *Nature* 445(7130):866–873, 2007.

Pityriasis rosea

Pityriasis rosea is a self-limiting inflammatory disorder that occurs more often in young adults, usually during the winter months. The cause is thought to be a herpes-like virus.[18] Pityriasis rosea begins as a single lesion **(herald patch)** that is circular, demarcated, and salmon-pink, approximately 3 to 4 cm in diameter, and usually located on the trunk. Early lesions are macular and papular. Secondary lesions develop within 14 to 21 days and extend over the trunk and upper part of the extremities (Figure 39-10), although rarely on the face. The small erythematous papules expand into characteristic oval lesions. The pattern of distribution follows the skin lines around the trunk and resembles a drooping pine tree. The scales flake off from the margin of the lesions, forming a collarette pattern. Itching is the most common symptom. Occasionally headache, fatigue, or sore throat precedes the development of the lesions.[19]

The diagnosis of pityriasis rosea follows the clinical appearance of the lesion. It can be confused with secondary syphilis, psoriasis, or seborrheic dermatitis. The disorder is usually self-limiting and resolves in a few months with symptomatic treatment for pruritus. Ultraviolet light or systemic corticosteroids may be used to control itching. Sun exposure facilitates resolution of the lesions.

Lichen planus

Lichen planus is a benign autoimmune inflammatory disorder of the skin and mucous membranes. Some individuals develop lichenoid lesions after exposure to drugs or film processing chemicals. The age of onset is usually between 30 and 70 years. The disorder begins with nonscaling, violet-colored pruritic papules, 2 to 4 mm in size, usually located on the wrists, ankles, lower legs, and genitalia (Figure 39-11). The papules are flat-topped and have a polygonal shape. New lesions are pale pink and evolve into a dark violet color. Persistent lesions may be thickened and

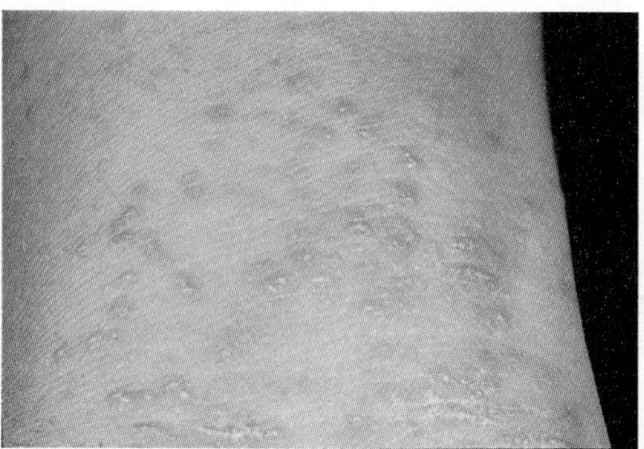

Figure 39-11 ■ Hypertrophic Lichen Planus on Arms. (Courtesy Department of Dermatology, School of Medicine, University of Utah.)

red, forming hypertrophic lichen planus. The lesions often involve the oral mucous membranes, appearing as lacy white rings that must be differentiated from leukoplakia or oral candidiasis.[20,21] The cause may be an abnormal T cell–mediated immune response where epithelial cells are recognized as foreign. Mucous membrane lesions also can develop on the penis and vulvovaginal area. Usually, oral lesions do not ulcerate, but localized or extensive painful ulcerations can occur, and there may be increased risk for oral cancer. Chronic ulcerated lesions become malignant in 1% of individuals with the disease. Thinning and splitting of nails are common, and part or all of the nail may be shed.[22]

Pruritus is the most distressing symptom. The lesions are self-limiting and may last for months or years, with an average duration of 6 to 18 months. Postinflammatory hyperpigmentation is a common consequence of the lesion. Approximately 20% of individuals have a recurrence. Diagnosis is made by the clinical appearance of the lesion. Antihistamines may be given for itching, and topical or systemic corticosteroids may be used to control inflammation. Acitretin is a first-line therapy with cutaneous lesions. Low-molecular-weight heparin and sulfasalazine also have been effective.

QUICK CHECK 39-3

1. Why is there inflammation with contact dermatitis?
2. What factors are associated with atopic dermatitis?
3. What lesions are associated with papulosquamous disorders?
4. Give three examples of papulosquamous disorders.

Acne vulgaris

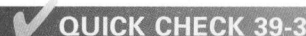

Acne vulgaris is an inflammatory disorder of the pilosebaceous follicle (the sebaceous gland contiguous with a hair follicle) that usually occurs during adolescence. It is discussed in Chapter 40 (p. 1122).

Acne rosacea

Acne rosacea is a chronic inflammation of the skin that develops in middle-aged adults.[23] The cause is unknown. The most common lesions are erythema, papules, pustules, and telangiectasia. They occur in the middle third of the face, including the forehead, nose, cheeks, and chin (Figure 39-12). The lesions are associated with chronic, inappropriate vasodilation resulting in flushing and sun sensitivity. Hypertrophy of the sebaceous glands may be severe enough to produce an irreversible bulbous appearance of the nose (rhinophyma). Disorders of the eye often accompany rosacea, particularly conjunctivitis and keratitis, which can result in visual impairment. Facial application of fluorinated topical steroids may precipitate rosacea-like lesions that are difficult to treat.

Hot drinks or alcohol should be taken cautiously because the heat and vasodilation accentuate erythema. Photoprotection, using sunscreens, is essential. Therapeutic options for rosacea include topical agents, oral therapies, and laser and light treatments. Surgical excision of excessive tissue may be required for rhinophyma.[24]

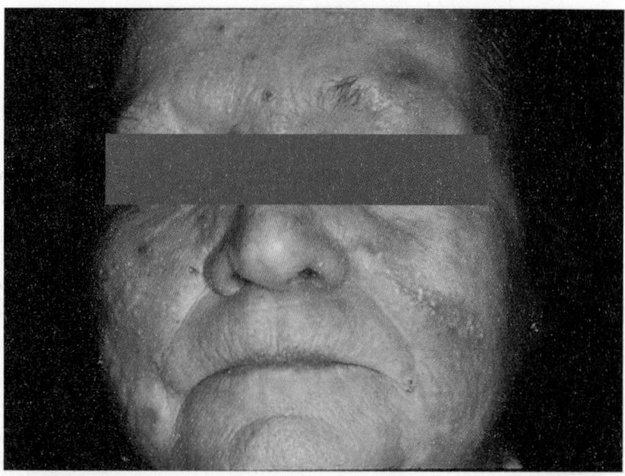

Figure 39-12 ■ **Granulomatous Rosacea.** Pustules and erythema occur on the forehead, cheeks, and nose. (Courtesy Department of Dermatology, School of Medicine, University of Utah.)

Lupus erythematosus

Lupus erythematosus is an autoimmune, systemic, inflammatory disease that expresses cutaneous manifestations. Discoid, or cutaneous, lupus erythematosus (DLE) is limited to the skin and can lead to systemic lupus erythematosus in about 5% of cases. (Systemic lupus erythematosus [SLE], a diffuse, multisystem disease, is discussed in Chapter 7.)

Discoid lupus erythematosus

Discoid lupus erythematosus (DLE) usually occurs in adults, particularly women in their late 30s or early 40s, but people of any age can be affected. The lesions may be single or multiple and of various sizes. Often the lesions are located on light-exposed areas of the skin, and photosensitivity is common. The face is the most common site of lesion involvement.

The cause is related to both genetic and environmental factors and is thought to be an altered immune response. DLE may be described as a subset of SLE, with cutaneous manifestations as the only symptom[25] (Figure 39-13). On skin biopsy with immunofluorescent observation, there are lumpy deposits of immunoglobulins, especially IgM.

The early lesion is asymmetric, with a 1- to 2-cm raised red plaque with a brownish scale. The scale penetrates the hair follicle and leaves a carpet-tack appearance when removed. The lesions persist for months and then resolve spontaneously or atrophy. Healing progresses from the center of the lesion, with a residual telangiectasia and hypopigmented scarring. Atrophy of the dermis and epidermis can cause a depressed scar. Scalp lesions may lead to hair loss. Other symptoms of cutaneous lupus erythematosus include alopecia (hair loss), telangiectasias, urticaria, and Raynaud phenomenon. Raynaud phenomenon is characterized by an initial stage of vasospasm that leads to white, numb,

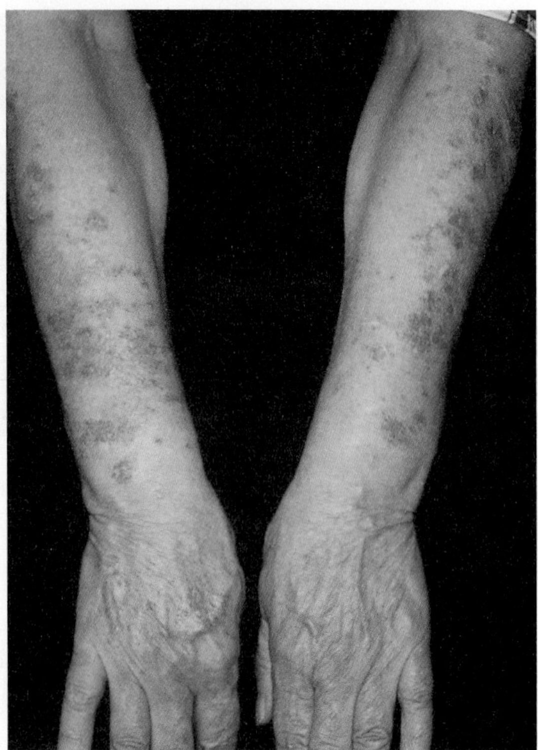

Figure 39-13 ■ Subacute Cutaneous Lupus (Discoid Lupus Erythematosus). (Courtesy Department of Dermatology, School of Medicine, University of Utah.)

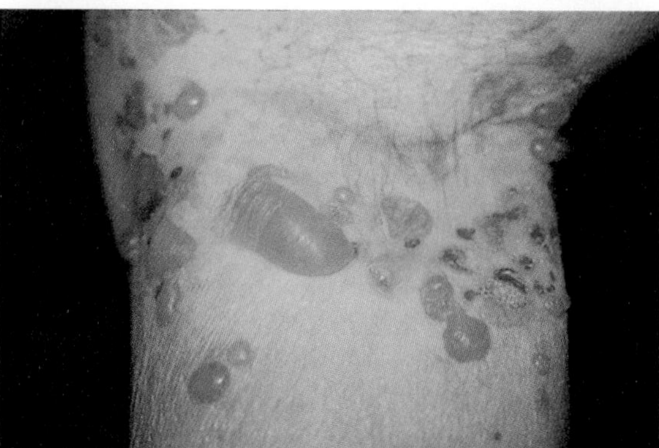

Figure 39-14 ■ Bullous Pemphigoid. Generalized eruption with blisters arising from an edematous, erythematous annular base. (Courtesy Department of Dermatology, School of Medicine, University of Utah.)

and cold digits followed by cyanosis and then a reactive hyperemia as the vasospasm relaxes.

Presenting symptoms and biopsy of skin lesions with direct immunofluorescence lead to a diagnosis of DLE. Individuals with DLE should use sunscreen or limit direct exposure to the sun. Initial treatment with topical steroids relieves symptoms. Pimecrolimus 1% cream has shown some success.[26] Systemic therapy with antimalarial drugs (i.e., hydroxychloroquine sulfate, sulfasalazine) usually leads to clinical improvement within 1 to 3 months. Thalidomide is effective in severe refractory cases but must not be used in women who may become pregnant because it causes birth defects.[27]

Vesiculobullous Disorders

Vesiculobullous skin disorders share a common characteristic of vesicle, or blister, formation. Two such diseases are pemphigus and erythema multiforme.

Pemphigus

Pemphigus (meaning to blister or bubble) is a rare autoimmune blistering disease of the skin and oral mucous membranes caused by circulating autoantibodies directed against the cell surface adhesion molecule desmoglein at the desmosomal cell junction in the suprabasal layer in the epidermis. Immunoglobulin G (IgG) autoantibodies and C3 complement bind to the desmoglein adhesion molecules, resulting in the destruction of cell-to-cell adhesion (acantholysis) in the epidermis with fluid accumulation and the resulting symptom of blister formation[28] (Figure 39-14). IgA and IgM autoantibodies have been found in some individuals.[29] Pemphigus can occur in all age groups but is more prevalent in persons between 40 and 50 years of age. Pemphigus presents in varying forms:

- **Pemphigus vulgaris** is the most common form with acantholysis at the deeper suprabasal level. Oral lesions precede the onset of skin blistering, which is more prominent on the face, scalp, and axilla. The blisters rupture easily because of the thin, fragile overlying portion of the epidermis.
- **Pemphigus vegetans** is a variant of pemphigus vulgaris in which large blisters occurring in tissue folds of the axilla and groin.
- **Pemphigus foliaceus** is a milder form of the disease and involves acantholysis at the more superficial, subcorneal level with blistering, erosions, scaling, crusting, and erythema usually of the face and chest. Oral mucous membranes are rarely involved.
- **Pemphigus erythematosus** is a subset of pemphigus foliaceus often associated with system lupus erythematosus with positive antinuclear antibodies. The lesions are generally less widely distributed.

The diagnosis of pemphigus results from the clinical manifestations and histologic examination of the skin. Immunofluorescence demonstrates the presence of antibodies at the site of blister formation. The clinical course of the disease may range from rapidly fatal to relatively benign. The primary treatment for pemphigus is systemic corticosteroids, usually in high doses during acute episodes or when there is widespread involvement. Azathioprine or mycophenolate also may be used and decreases the steroid dosage requirement. Newer methods of treatment and a clearer understanding of the pathogenesis have improved the prognosis.[30] Individuals are frequently managed in a burn unit.

Erythema multiforme

Erythema multiforme is a syndrome characterized by inflammation of the skin and mucous membranes, often associated with immunologic or toxic reactions to a drug or herpesvirus. It is relatively rare and can occur at any age but occurs more often in individuals between 20 and 40 years of age. Immune complex formation and deposition of C3, IgM, and fibrinogen around the superficial dermal blood vessels, basement membrane, and keratinocytes are found in most individuals with erythema multiforme. Edema develops in the superficial dermis, so vesicles and bullae form. The lesions vary in clinical presentation and may involve the skin or mucous membranes or both. The characteristic "bull's-eye," or "target," lesions occur on the skin surface with a central erythematous region surrounded by concentric rings or alternating edema and inflammation. The lesions usually occur suddenly in groups over a period of 2 to 3 weeks. Urticarial plaques, 1 to 2 cm in diameter, can develop without the target lesion. A vesiculobullous form is characterized by mucous membrane lesions and erythematous plaques on the extensor surfaces of the extremities. Single or multiple vesicles or bullae may arise on a part of the plaque accompanied by pruritus and burning. The lesions heal within 3 to 4 weeks.

The most common forms of erythema multiforme in children and young adults are **Stevens-Johnson syndrome** (severe bullous form) and **toxic epidermal necrolysis (TEN),** in which numerous erythematous bullous lesions occur on the skin and mucous membranes. An immune mechanism is probably related to drug reactions.[31,32] Prodromal symptoms of fever, headache, malaise, sore throat, and cough develop in approximately one third of the cases. The bullous lesions form erosions and crusts when they rupture. There is necrosis of the epidermis in TEN. The mouth, air passages, esophagus, urethra, and conjunctiva may be involved. Blindness can result from corneal ulcerations. Difficulty eating, breathing, and urinating may develop with severe manifestations. The disease can involve the kidneys and extend from the upper respiratory passages into the lungs. Severe forms of the disease can be fatal.

Diagnosis follows (1) recognition of the target lesion or by skin biopsy if the target lesion is absent and (2) medication history. Mild acute forms of the disease last 10 to 14 days and require no treatment. Ongoing drug therapy should be reevaluated and underlying infections treated. Fluid and electrolyte balance should be monitored in severe forms of the disease, and mucous membranes should be carefully managed with a bland diet, warm saline eyewashes, topical anesthetics, or corticosteroids to maintain comfort and prevent infection. Cutaneous blisters can be treated with wet compresses of Burow solution. Ophthalmic, kidney, and lung involvement require special care. Resolution occurs in 8 to 10 days, usually without scarring. Mucosal lesions may take 6 weeks to heal.

QUICK CHECK 39-4

1. Describe the inflammatory lesion associated with lupus erythematosus.
2. Compare the three forms of pemphigus.
3. What is Stevens-Johnson syndrome?

Infections

Cutaneous infections are common forms of skin disease. They generally remain localized, although serious complications can develop with systemic involvement. The types of skin infection include bacterial, viral, and fungal. Most infections occur superficially; however, systemic signs and symptoms occasionally develop and can be life threatening. The normal flora of the skin consists of aerobes, yeast, and anaerobes. These flora often provide protection against pathogens that cause skin infections, including *Staphylococcus* and *Streptococcus.*

Community-acquired methicillin-resistant *Staphylococcus aureus* (ca-MRSA) is increasing with the most common presentation being an abscess or folliculitis. Cultures of the lesions guide treatment, which includes incision and drainage, systemic antimicrobial therapy, and adjuvant topical antibacterial treatment.[32a]

Bacterial infections

Most bacterial infections of the skin are caused by local invasion of pathogens. Coagulase-positive *S. aureus* and, less often, β-hemolytic streptococci are the common causative microorganisms.[33]

Folliculitis

Folliculitis is a bacterial infection of the hair follicle. *S. aureus* commonly causes the infection, which develops from proliferation of the microorganism around the opening of the follicle with spread into the follicle. Inflammation is caused by the release of chemotactic factors and enzymes from the bacteria. The lesions appear as pustules with a surrounding area of erythema. They are most prominent on the scalp and extremities and rarely cause systemic symptoms. Prolonged skin moisture, skin trauma, and poor hygiene are associated contributing factors. Cleaning with soap and water and topical application of antibiotics are effective treatments.

Furuncles and carbuncles

Furuncles, or "boils," are inflammations of hair follicles (Figure 39-15). They may develop after folliculitis that

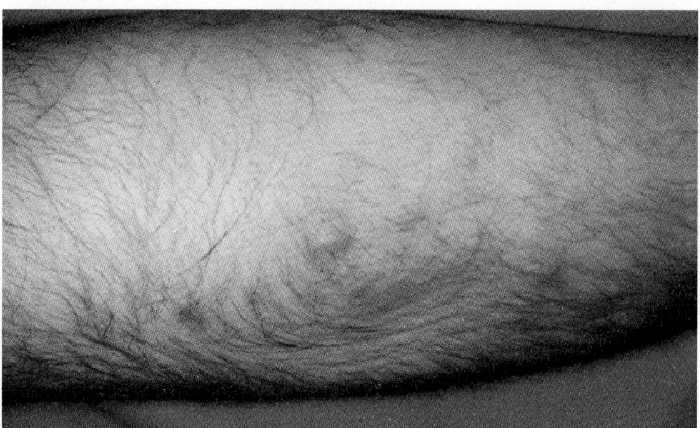

Figure 39-15 ■ **Furuncle of the Forearm.** (Courtesy Department of Dermatology, School of Medicine, University of Utah.)

spreads through the follicular wall into the surrounding dermis. The invading microorganism is usually *S. aureus.* The infecting strain may spread to the skin from the anterior nares. Any skin area with hair can be infected, and one or several lesions may be present. The initial lesion is a deep, firm, red, painful nodule 1 to 5 cm in diameter. Within a few days, the erythematous nodules change to a large fluctuant and tender cystic nodule accompanied by cellulitis. No systemic symptoms are present, and the lesion may drain large amounts of pus and necrotic tissue.

Carbuncles are a collection of infected hair follicles and usually occur on the back of the neck, the upper back, and the lateral thighs. The lesion begins in the subcutaneous tissue and lower dermis as a firm mass that evolves into an erythematous, painful, swollen mass that drains through many openings. Abscesses may develop. Chills, fever, and malaise can occur during the early stages of lesion development.

Furuncles and carbuncles are treated with warm compresses to provide comfort and promote localization and spontaneous drainage. Abscess formation requires incision and drainage, and recurrent infections are treated with systemic antibiotics.

Cellulitis

Cellulitis is an infection of the dermis and subcutaneous tissue usually caused by *Staphylococcus.* Cellulitis can occur as an extension of a skin wound, as an ulcer, or from furuncles or carbuncles. The infected area is warm, erythematous, swollen, and painful. The infection is usually in the lower extremities and responds to systemic antibiotics, as well as Burow soaks to relieve pain.

Erysipelas

Erysipelas is an acute superficial infection of the upper dermis most often caused by group A beta hemolytic streptococci. The face, ears, and lower legs are involved. Chills, fever, and malaise precede the onset of lesions by 4 hours to 20 days. The initial lesions appear as firm, red spots that enlarge and coalesce to form a clearly circumscribed, advancing, bright red, hot lesion with a raised border. Vesicles may appear over the lesion and at the border. Itching, burning, and tenderness are present. Cold compresses provide symptomatic relief, and systemic antibiotics are required to arrest the infection.

Impetigo

Impetigo is a superficial lesion of the skin that is caused by coagulase-positive *Staphylococcus* or β-hemolytic streptococci. The disease occurs in adults but is more common in children (see Chapter 40, p. 1123).

Viral infections

Herpes simplex virus

Infections with herpes simplex virus (HSV) are commonly caused by two types of viruses: HSV-1 and HSV-2. Their differences can be distinguished by laboratory tests. HSV-1 is generally associated with oral infections (cold sore or fever blister), and HSV-2 is associated with genital infections, although infections can occur anywhere on the skin. HSV-1 is transmitted by contact with infected saliva. With initial infection or primary infection, the virus is imbedded in sensory nerve endings and is moves by retrograde axonal transport to the dorsal root ganglion, where the virus develops lifelong latency. During the secondary phase, the lesions occur at the same site from reactivation of the virus. The virus travels down the peripheral nerve to the site of the original infection where it is shed.[34] Exposure to ultraviolet light, skin irritation, fever, fatigue, or stress may cause reactivation.

The lesions for HSV-1 appear as a rash or clusters of inflamed and painful vesicles within the mouth, over the tongue, or on the lips and around the nose (Figure 39-16). Increased sensitivity, paresthesias, and mild burning may occur before onset of the lesions. The vesicles rupture, forming a crust. Lesions may last from 2 to 6 weeks. Treatment is symptomatic and lesions usually resolve within 2 weeks.

HSV-2 genital infection is spread by skin-to-skin mucous membrane contact during viral shedding. Risk of infection is high after sexual contact with infected individuals. The initial infection is asymptomatic. With recurrent exposure, the lesions begin as small vesicles that progress to ulceration within 3 to 4 days with pain, itching, and weeping.[35]

Treatment is symptomatic and includes topical or oral antiviral agents. A vaccine has been effective in controlling recurrent infection, and progress is being made with prophylactic vaccines.[36]

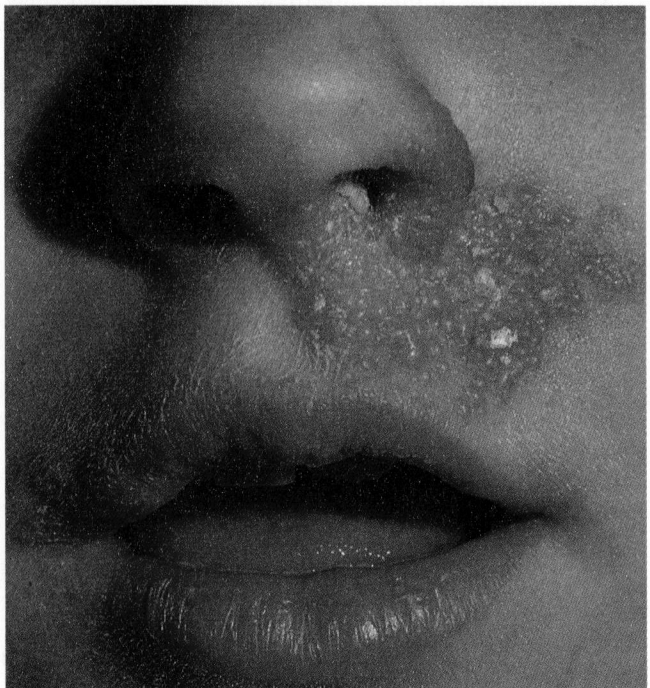

Figure 39-16 ■ Herpes Simplex Labialis. Typical presentation with tense vesicles appearing on the lips and extending onto the skin. (From Habif TP: *Clinical dermatology: a color guide to diagnosis and therapy,* ed 4, St Louis, 2004, Mosby.)

Herpes zoster and varicella

Herpes zoster (shingles) and **varicella (chickenpox)** are caused by the same herpesvirus, varicella-zoster virus (VZV). Varicella occurs as a primary infection followed years later by activation of the virus to cause herpes zoster (shingles). During this time, the virus remains latent in trigeminal and dorsal root ganglia.

Herpes zoster has initial symptoms of pain and paresthesia localized to the affected dermatome (the cutaneous area innervated by a single spinal nerve; see Chapter 12), followed by vesicular eruptions that follow along a facial, cervical, or thoracic lumbar dermatome (Figure 39-17). Infections are more common with advancing age and in immunocompromised individuals. Local symptoms are alleviated with compresses, calamine lotion, or baking soda. Antiviral drugs (vidarabine, acyclovir, brivudin) are useful and should be used within 72 hours to prevent postherpetic neuralgia. Approximately 20% of individuals experience postherpetic neuralgia (pain) and are treated with tricyclic antidepressants.[37] A new vaccine (Zostavax) is available to reduce risk of shingles in individuals 60 years and older.[37a]

Warts

Warts (verrucae) are benign lesions of the skin caused by the many different types of human papillomavirus (HPV). The lesions are round and elevated with a rough, grayish surface, and they can occur anywhere on the skin. Warts are transmitted by touch. Common warts (verruca vulgaris) occur most often in children and are usually on the fingers, although they may be located on any skin surface or mucous membrane. Warts vary in shape, size (flat, round, or fusiform), and location and are commonly treated with topical salicylic acid or cryotherapy.[38] Plantar warts are usually located at pressure points on the bottom of the feet (Figure 39-18).

Condylomata acuminata (venereal warts) are cauliflower-like lesions that occur in moist areas, along the glans of the penis, vulva, and anus (see Chapter 32). It is one of the most common sexually transmitted infections. Exposure

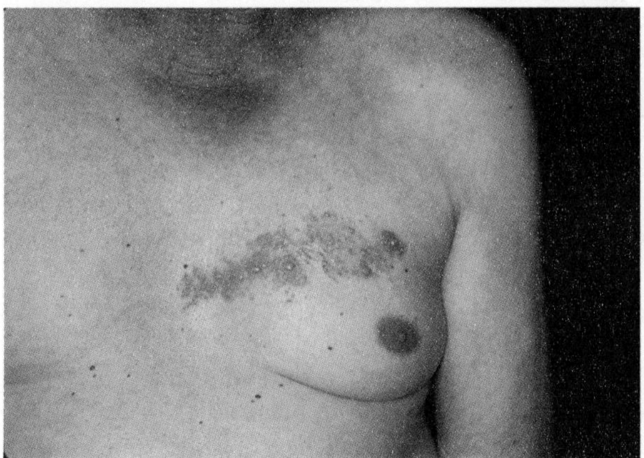

Figure 39-17 ■ **Herpes Zoster.** Diffuse involvement of a dermatome. (Courtesy Department of Dermatology, School of Medicine, University of Utah.)

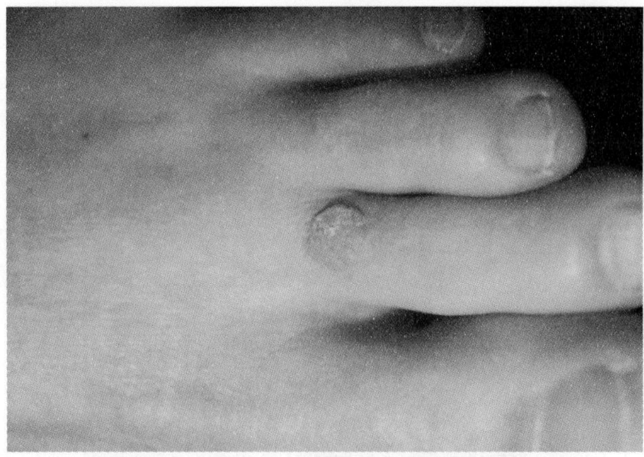

Figure 39-18 ■ **Verruca Vulgaris.** (Courtesy Department of Dermatology, School of Medicine, University of Utah.)

to this virus in women increases the risk of cervical cancer.[39] Epidermodysplasia verruciformis is a rare condition and is associated with warts all over the body.

Genital HPV is usually symptomless and diagnosed through visualization. Treatment involves consideration of the age of the individual and the size and location of the lesion. Warts can be removed by freezing with liquid nitrogen, electrocautery, vaporization with lasers, application of keratolytics, or application of irritants and corrosives, such as salicylic acid, formaldehyde, interferons, or saturated solution of potassium iodide. Imiquimod cream 5% has been approved for use in anogenital warts. Recurrence is not unusual, and many warts resolve spontaneously. A vaccine for the prevention of HPV is available and will contribute to the prevention of cervical cancer.[40]

Fungal infections

The fungi causing superficial skin infections are called *dermatophytes,* and they thrive on keratin (stratum corneum, hair, nails). Fungal disorders are known as *mycoses;* when caused by dermatophytes, the mycoses are termed *tinea* (dermatophytosis or ringworm). **Tinea pedis** is a chronic, superficial fungal infection of the skin of the foot common in adults (Figure 39-19). In prepubertal children most scaling disorders of the toes and feet are eczema. **Tinea corporis (ringworm)** and **tinea capitis** (a fungal infection of the scalp) are much more common in children than adults (see Chapter 40).

Tinea infections

Tinea infections are classified according to their location on the body. The most common sites are summarized in Table 39-4. Tinea is diagnosed by culture, microscopic examination of skin scrapings prepared with potassium hydroxide wet mount, or observation of the skin with an ultraviolet light (Wood lamp). Cultures establish the particular type of fungus; these are necessary for diagnosis of hair and nail infections. Fungi have characteristic spores and filaments known as *hyphae* that are more prominent when prepared in potassium hydroxide. The spores fluoresce

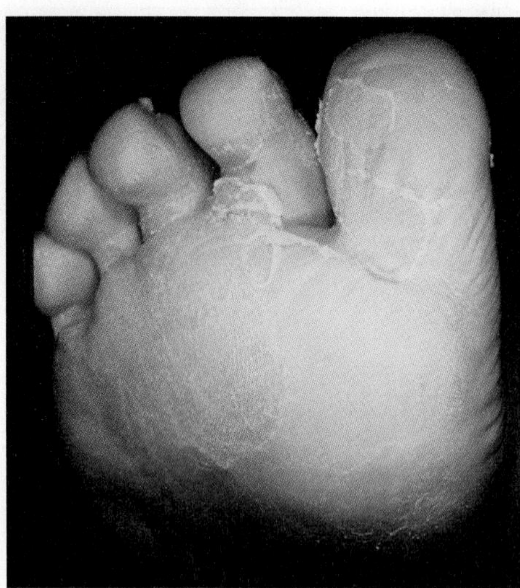

Figure 39-19 ■ **Tinea Pedis.** Inflammation has extended from the web area onto the dorsum of the foot. (Courtesy Department of Dermatology, School of Medicine, University of Utah.)

blue-green when exposed to ultraviolet light. Treatment is related to the type of fungi and includes both topical and systemic antifungal medication.[41]

Candidiasis

Candidiasis is caused by the yeastlike fungus *Candida albicans* and normally can be found on mucous membranes, on the skin, in the gastrointestinal tract, and in the vagina. *C. albicans* can, under certain circumstances, change from a commensal microorganism to a pathogen, particularly when the immune system is depressed. Among those factors that predispose to infection are (1) local environment of moisture, warmth, maceration, or occlusion; (2) the systemic administration of antibiotics; (3) pregnancy; (4) diabetes mellitus; (5) Cushing disease; (6) debilitated states; (7) infants younger than 6 months of age, as a result of decreased immune reactivity; (8) immunosuppressed persons; and (9) certain neoplastic diseases of the blood and monocyte/macrophage system. The resident bacteria on the skin, mainly cocci, inhibit proliferation of *C. albicans*. *C. albicans* can activate the complement system by the alternative pathway and produce small abscesses. Candidiasis affects only the outer layers of mucous membranes and skin and occurs in the mouth, vagina, uncircumcised penis, and large skin folds. Table 39-5 lists the points of differentiation of various sites of candidiasis habitation.

The initial lesion is a thin-walled pustule that extends under the stratum corneum with an inflammatory base that may burn or itch. The accumulation of inflammatory cells and scale produces a whitish yellow curdlike substance over the infected area. The lesion ceases to spread when it reaches dry skin.[42] Treatments are use of topical or systemic antifungal agents.

TABLE 39-4

Common Sites of Tinea Infections

Site	Clinical Manifestations
Tinea capitis (scalp)	Scaly, pruritic scalp with bald areas; hair breaks easily
Tinea corporis (skin areas, excluding scalp, face, hands, feet, groin)	Circular, clearly circumscribed, mildly erythematous scaly patches with a slightly elevated ringlike border; some forms are dry and macular, and other forms are moist and vesicular
Tinea cruris (groin, also known as "jock itch")	Small, erythematous and scaling vesicular patches with well-defined borders that spread over the inner and upper surfaces of the thighs; occurs with heat and high humidity
Tinea pedis (foot; also known as "athlete's foot)	Occurs between the toes and may spread to the soles of feet, nails, and skin or toes; slight scaling; macerated, painful skin, occasionally with fissures and vesiculation
Tinea manus (hand)	Dry, scaly, erythematous lesions, or moist, vesicular lesions that begin with clusters of intensely itching, clear vesicles; often associated with fungal infection of the feet
Tinea unguium or onychomycosis (nails)	A superficial or deep inflammation of the nail that develops yellow-brown accumulations of brittle keratin over all or portions of the nail

Vascular Disorders

Vascular abnormalities are commonly associated with skin diseases, may be congenital, or may involve vascular responses to local or systemic vasoactive substances. Blood vessels may increase in number, dilate, constrict, or become obliterated by disease processes.

Cutaneous vasculitis

Vasculitis (angiitis) is an inflammation of the blood vessel wall that can result in bleeding aneurysm formation, or occlusion with ischemia or infection. The extensive vascular bed in the skin results in the involvement of vasculitic syndromes that may be localized and self-limiting or generalized with multiorgan involvement.[43] The initiating site may be the blood, the vessel wall, or the adjacent tissue. Small vessels are usually affected.

Cutaneous vasculitis develops from the deposit of immune complexes in small blood vessels as a toxic response to drugs (phenothiazines, barbiturates, sulfonamides) or allergens or as a response to streptococcal or viral infection. The deposits activate complement, which is chemotactic for polymorphonuclear leukocytes.

The disorder is also known as *cutaneous leukocytoclastic angiitis* (from the presence of leukocytes in and around vessel walls). A systemic form (cutaneous systemic vasculitis) can involve other organs, including the kidneys, lungs, and gastrointestinal tract. The pattern of skin involvement includes palpable purpura in the lower legs and feet (from the leakage of blood from damaged vessels) that may progress to hemorrhagic bullae with necrosis and ulceration from occlusion of the vessel. Lesions appear in clusters

TABLE 39-5

Sites of Candidiasis Infection

Site	Risk Factors	Clinical Manifestations	Treatment
Vagina (vulvovaginitis)	Heat, moisture, occlusive clothing Pregnancy Systemic antibiotic therapy Diabetes mellitus Sexual intercourse with infected male	Vaginal itching; white, watery, or creamy discharge Red, swollen vaginal and labial membranes with erosions Lesions may spread to anus and groin	Miconazole cream Clotrimazole tablets or cream Nystatin tablets Ketoconazole cream Loose cotton clothing
Penis (balanitis)	Uncircumcised Sexual intercourse with infected female	Pinpoint, red, tender papules and pustules on glans and shaft of penis	Any of creams listed above Topical steroids for severe inflammation
Mouth	Diabetes mellitus Immunosuppressive therapy Inhaled steroid therapy	Red, swollen, painful tongue and oral mucous membranes Localized erosions and plaques appear with chronic infection	Nystatin oral suspension Clotrimazole troches Ketoconazole

and remain from 1 to 4 weeks. The disease may be self-limiting and occur as a single episode. Biopsy confirms the diagnosis.

Identifying and removing the antigen (chemical, drug, or source of infection) are the first steps of treatment. Corticosteroids and immunosuppressants may be used when symptoms are severe.[44]

Urticaria

Urticarial lesions are most commonly associated with type 1 hypersensitivity reactions to drugs (penicillin, aspirin), certain foods (strawberries, shellfish), systemic diseases (intestinal parasites, lupus erythematosus), or physical agents (heat or cold)[45] (see Chapter 7). The lesions are mediated by histamine release from sensitized mast cells, which causes the endothelial cells of skin blood vessels to contract. The leak of fluid from the vessel appears as wheals, welts, or hives, and there may be few or many and may be distributed over the entire body. Most lesions resolve spontaneously within 24 hours, but new lesions may appear. All possible causes of the reaction should be removed. Antihistamines usually reduce hives and provide relief of itching. Corticosteroids and β-adrenergic agonists may be required for severe attacks. Chronic urticaria is either idiopathic or autoimmune. Angioedema (welts or swelling of the skin) is associated with both groups. The autoimmune group has histamine-releasing autoantibodies and may have antithyroid antibodies.[46]

Scleroderma

Scleroderma (systemic sclerosis) means sclerosis of the skin and is an autoimmune disease. The disease is associated with vascular, immunologic, and fibrotic processes[47] and is more prominent in women. It may affect the visceral organs or remain localized to the skin. *Systemic sclerosis* involves the connective tissues of many organs, including the kidneys, gastrointestinal tract, and lungs. The cutaneous lesions are most often on the face and hands, the neck, and the upper chest, although the entire skin can be involved.

There are massive deposits of collagen with fibrosis, accompanied by inflammatory reactions, vascular changes in the capillary network with a decrease in the number of capillary loops, and dilation of the remaining capillaries.[48] Autoimmunity and an immune reaction to a toxic substance are both possible initiating mechanisms of the disease, and autoantibodies are often recovered from the skin and serum of individuals with scleroderma. Impaired regulation of collagen gene expression by fibroblasts probably underlies the persistent fibrosis.[49]

The skin is hard, hypopigmented, taut, shiny, and tightly connected to the underlying tissue. The tightness of the facial skin projects an immobile masklike appearance, and the mouth may not open completely. The nose may assume a beaklike appearance. The hands are shiny and sometimes red and edematous. The fingers become tapered and flexed, often with depressed scars and loss of fingertips from atrophy. Raynaud phenomenon with episodic arteriolar vasoconstriction of the fingers contributes to ulcer formation. The nails may be shed (Figure 39-20). Calcium deposits

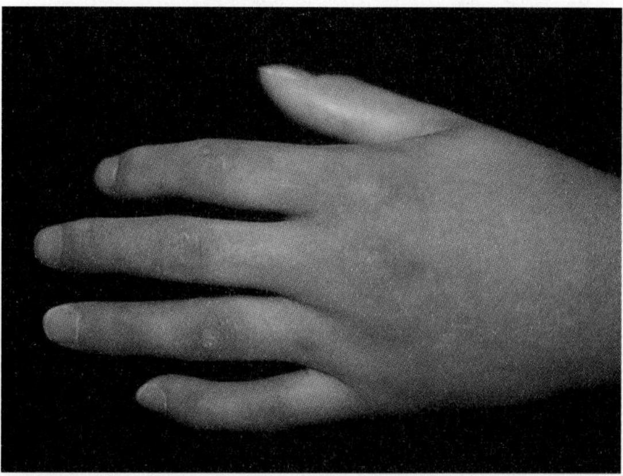

Figure 39-20 ■ **Scleroderma (Acrosclerosis).** Note inflammation and shiny skin. (Courtesy Department of Dermatology, School of Medicine, University of Utah.)

develop in the subcutaneous tissue and erupt through the skin. Progression to body organs may occur, and death is caused by subsequent respiratory failure, renal failure, cardiac dysrhythmias, or esophageal or intestinal obstruction or perforation.[50] There is no specific treatment, and 50% of individuals die within 5 years from onset.

Suitable clothing and a warm environment are essential for protecting the hands. Trauma and smoking should be avoided. Vasodilator drugs or sympathectomy rarely has lasting effects. Advances are being made in immunosuppressive therapy and autologous stem-cell transplantation.[51]

QUICK CHECK 39-5

1. Name two bacterial skin infections, and describe the typical lesions.
2. Compare herpes zoster and varicella.
3. What features distinguish urticarial lesions?

Insect Bites

Insect bites and stings are the cause of local and systemic toxic and allergic reactions. Local reactions include immediate pain, itching, and swelling. Systemic responses include generalized itching, hives, or anaphylaxis. Bites from scabies, lice, fleas, ticks, and bedbugs are discussed in Chapter 40. Other bites and stings are discussed next.

Mosquitoes, flies, and bees

There are thousands of species of **mosquitoes** throughout the world. Species from the Culicidae family are responsible for malaria, yellow fever, dengue fever, filariasis, and St. Louis encephalitis. Mosquitoes can bite through thin, loose clothing and are attracted to warmth and sweat. The edema, pruritus, and papular lesions of the mosquito bite are caused by the disruption of the skin that results from the insertion of a blood tube by a female mosquito. Irritating salivary secretions also contain anticoagulants. Reactions vary depending on the sensitivity of the victim.

Several species of **flies** are bloodsuckers. The blackfly (Simuliidae family) is usually found in swarms, near moving bodies of water in the late spring and early summer, and is a vicious biter. The initial bite is painless because the fly injects an anesthetic with it. Subsequent lesions are painful and accompanied by significant swelling of surrounding tissues. Systemic reactions, such as fever, headache, and nausea, are common.

Very small flies of the Ceratopogonidae family, also known as *no-see-ums, midges, punkies,* or *sand fleas,* are also bloodsuckers. The bite of the female is particularly miserable and produces immediate pain, erythema, and vesicles. Itching and vesicular reactions may persist for weeks.

The fiercest blood-sucking flies are the Tabanidae, or horseflies, deerflies, gadflies, greenheads, and clegs. These flies vary in size from 1 to 5 cm and produce painful, bleeding bites because of their large mouthparts. The bites produce urticaria that may be accompanied by weakness, dizziness, and wheezing.

Bees, wasps, hornets, and yellow jackets are stinging insects. The stinger is implanted in the skin with the release of venom. The stinger should be flicked away and not pinched and pulled to prevent the release of more venom. Reactions to venom can be localized or generalized depending on individual sensitivity.[42] Wounds produced by biting insects should be cleansed with soap and water and a local antiseptic applied. Local applications of steroid creams or antihistamine will reduce symptoms. Systemic reactions may require emergency care.

Benign Tumors

Most benign tumors of the skin are associated with aging. Benign tumors include seborrheic keratosis, keratoacanthoma, actinic keratosis, and moles.

Seborrheic keratosis

Seborrheic keratosis is a benign proliferation of basal cells that produces elevated lesions that may be smooth or warty in appearance. They are usually seen in older people and occur as multiple lesions on the chest, back, and face. The color varies from tan to waxy yellow, flesh-colored, or dark brown-black. Lesion size varies from a few millimeters to several centimeters, and they are often oval and greasy appearing with a hyperkeratotic scale (Figure 39-21). Cryotherapy with liquid nitrogen is an effective treatment, and the lesions usually slough 2 to 3 weeks after treatment.

Keratoacanthoma

A **keratoacanthoma** is a benign, self-limiting tumor of squamous cell differentiation arising from hair follicles. It usually occurs on sun-damaged skin of elderly individuals. Incidence is highest among smokers and males. The most commonly affected sites are the face, back of the hands, forearms, neck, and legs. The lesion develops over a period of 1 to 2 months with a histologic pattern resembling squamous cell carcinoma:[52]

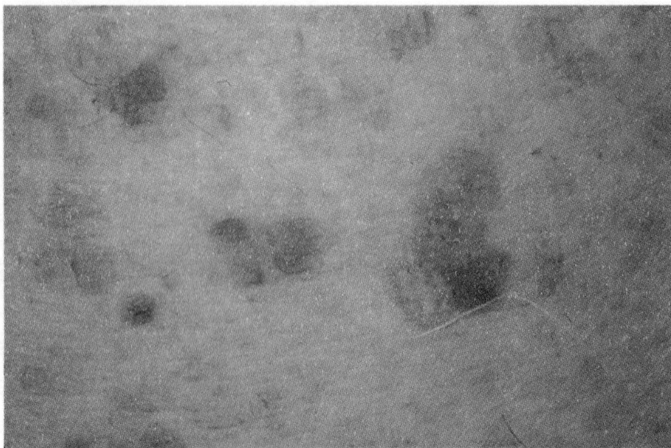

Figure 39-21 ■ **Seborrheic Keratosis.** Typical lesion that is broad, flat, and comparatively smooth surfaced. (Courtesy Department of Dermatology, School of Medicine, University of Utah.)

1. *Proliferative stage.* Rapid-growing, dome-shaped nodule with central crust
2. *Mature stage.* Lesion fills with whitish-colored keratin and requires differentiation from squamous cell carcinoma
3. *Involution stage.* Occurs over a 3- to 4-month period with regression of lesion

Although the lesions will resolve spontaneously, they can be removed by curettage or excision to improve cosmetic appearance.

Actinic keratosis

Actinic keratosis is a premalignant lesion found on skin surfaces exposed to the ultraviolet radiation of the sun. The prevalence is highest in individuals with unprotected, light-colored skin and rare in those with black skin. The lesions appear as rough, poorly defined papules, which may be felt more than seen. Surrounding areas may have telangiectasias. Freezing with liquid nitrogen provides quick, effective treatment. Topical modulators, such as 5-fluorouracil, diclofenac sodium gel, or imiquimod cream, are used.[53] Excisions also may be performed, providing tissue for cellular analysis. The lesions should continue to be evaluated for progression to squamous cell carcinoma. Protection from the sun with clothing or a sun-blocking agent to prevent lesions from developing elsewhere is advised.

Nevi (moles)

Nevi (*sing.*, **nevus**) are pigmented or nonpigmented lesions that form from melanocytes beginning at ages 3 to 5 years. During the early stages of development, the cells accumulate at the junction of the dermis and epidermis and are macular lesions. Over time, the cells move down into the dermis and the nevi become nodular and palpable. Nevi may appear on any part of the skin and vary in size. They occur singly or in groups and are not disfiguring. Nevi may undergo transition to malignant melanoma (see p. 1108). Nevi irritated by clothing should be excised.

QUICK CHECK 39-6

1. List two diseases caused by insect bites.
2. Compare keratoacanthoma and actinic keratosis.

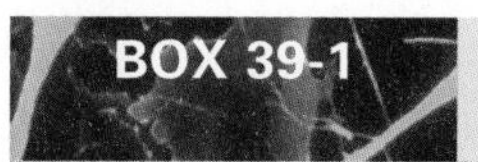

BOX 39-1 Important Trends for Skin Cancer

Incidence

More than 1 million new cases per year with the majority being the highly curable *basal* (90%) or *squamous cell cancers*

Not as common is the most serious malignant melanoma with an estimated 59,940 new cases per year

Mortality

Total estimated deaths in 2007 were 10,850: 8110 from malignant melanoma, 2740 from other skin cancers

Risk Factors

Excessive exposure to ultraviolet radiation from the sun or tanning salons

Fair complexion

Occupational exposure to coal tar, pitch, creosote, arsenic compounds, and radium

Skin cancer is negligible in blacks because of heavy skin pigmentation

Warning Signals

Any unusual skin condition, especially a change in the size or color of a mole or other darkly pigmented growth or spot

Prevention and Early Detection

Avoid the sun when ultraviolet light is strongest (e.g., 10 a.m. to 3 p.m.), seek shade, use sunscreen preparations, especially those containing ingredients such as PABA (para-aminobenzoic acid), wear protective clothing.

Basal and squamous cell skin cancers often form a pale, waxlike pearly nodule or a red, scaly, sharply outlined patch.

Melanomas usually have dark brown or black pigmentation; they start as small molelike growths that increase in size, change color, become ulcerated, and bleed easily from slight injury.

Treatment

Options for treatment include surgery, electrodessication (tissue destruction by heat), radiation therapy, or cryosurgery (tissue destruction by freezing).

Malignant melanomas require wide and often deep excisions and removal of nearby lymph nodes or selective lymphadenectomy, or immunotherapy; vaccines and gene therapy are in development.

Survival

For basal cell and squamous cell cancers, cure is virtually ensured with early detection and treatment; malignant melanoma, however, metastasizes quickly and accounts for a lower 5-year survival rate for white persons with the disease.

Cancer

Skin cancers are the most prevalent form of cancer, and nearly all persons living beyond age 65 years will have had at least one skin cancer. The most common types are basal cell carcinoma and squamous cell carcinoma with 1 million cases occurring annually.[54] These carcinomas are 50% more common in men than in women, and incidence increases steadily with age. Malignant melanoma is the most serious skin cancer with 59,940 new cases per year and increasing at a rate of about 3% per year.[54] An estimated 10,850 people die of skin cancer each year, 8110 from malignant melanoma.[54] Important trends related to skin cancer are described in Box 39-1.

Solar radiation causes most skin cancers.[55] Protection from the sun during the first 10 to 20 years of life significantly reduces the risk of skin cancer.[56] Areas widely exposed to the sun's rays—the face, neck, and hands—are highly vulnerable for such lesions. Outdoor workers (farmers, sailors, fishermen) are high-risk skin cancer populations. Box 39-1 summarizes the risk factors for skin cancer.

Basal cell carcinoma

Basal cell carcinoma of the skin is the most common human cancer. The originating cells are in interfollicular basal cells, hair follicles, or sebaceous glands, and deeper than squamous cell carcinoma. The tumors grow upward and laterally or downward to the dermal/epidermal junction (Figure 39-22). They usually have depressed centers and rolled borders. Early tumors are so small they are not clinically apparent. Generally, these tumors do not invade blood or lymph vessels; thus, they usually do not metastasize beyond the skin but grow by direct extension to adjacent structures.

The risk for basal cell carcinoma is sunlight exposure in fair-skinned individuals. Lesions are seen most often in regions with intense sunlight (ultraviolet radiation) and on those areas most exposed, the face and neck. In dark-skinned persons, basal cells contain the pigment *melanin,* a protective factor against sun exposure. Although ultraviolet radiation seems to be the primary causative agent, arsenic and genetic factors, with alterations in tumor suppressor genes, are also implicated.[57]

The growth rate for these tumors is slow. The lesion starts as a nodule (more than 5 mm across) that is pearly or ivory in appearance and slightly elevated above the skin surface with small blood vessels on the surface. As the lesion grows, it often ulcerates, develops crusting, and is firm to the touch. If left untreated, basal cell lesions invade surrounding tissues and, over months or years, can destroy a nose, eyelid, or ear (for treatment, see Box 39-1).

Squamous cell carcinoma

Squamous cell carcinoma of the skin is a tumor of the epidermis generally characterized by two types: in situ and invasive. Because of the invasive nature of some tumors, squamous cell carcinoma is significantly more malignant if left untreated.

Sunlight exposure causes squamous cell carcinoma. Areas affected are the head and neck (75%) and the hands (15%), with 10% of cases elsewhere on the body.[58] In countries where arsenic is at a higher level in drinking water, these tumors are more predominant. X-rays and gamma rays are also associated with squamous cell carcinoma. In addition, individuals who are immunosuppressed experience a greater occurrence.

The exact mechanism for producing squamous cell carcinoma is unknown. It is unclear whether ultraviolet light produces its harmful effects because of problems in deoxyribonucleic acid (DNA) synthesis, repair, or replication; activation of proto-oncogenes; or inactivation of tumor-suppressor genes.[59]

Premalignant lesions include sun-damaged skin or dysplasias (actinic dermatitis); leukoplakia, or whitish discolored areas; scars; radiation-induced keratosis; tar and oil keratosis; chronic ulcers and sinuses; and Bowen disease. Bowen disease is a dysplastic epidermal lesion often found on unexposed areas of the body such as the penis and demonstrated by flat, reddish, scaly patches. These lesions may enlarge to more than 1 cm in diameter, rarely invading surrounding tissue and almost never metastasizing. Other cellular components in the skin (e.g., sweat glands, hair follicles) can give rise to skin cancer, but these are relatively uncommon. The invasive type grows more rapidly than basal cell carcinomas and can spread to regional lymph nodes. These tumors are firm and increase in both elevation and diameter. The surface may be granular and bleed easily (Figure 39-23).

Invasive squamous cell carcinoma can arise from premalignant lesions of the skin and rarely develops from normal-appearing skin. Squamous cell carcinoma is usually confined to the epidermis (intraepidermal) but may extend into the reticular dermis.

Malignant melanoma

Cutaneous melanoma is a malignant tumor of the skin originating from melanocytes, or cells that synthesize the pigment melanin. Early recognition of cutaneous melanomas can have a major impact on surgical cure of this disease. The ABCDE rule is used as a guide (*A*symmetry, *B*order irregularity, *C*olor variation, *D*iameter larger than 6 mm, *E*volving or rapid enlargement).[60]

Causative factors implicated in melanoma induction include genetic predisposition, solar radiation, and steroid

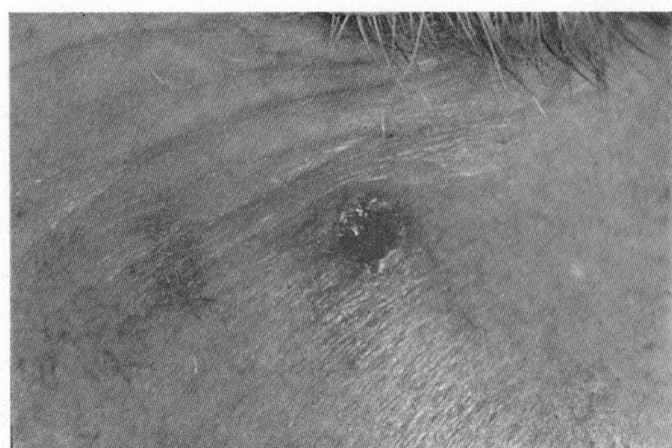

Figure 39-22 ■ **Basal Cell Carcinoma.** Center has ulcerated. (Courtesy Department of Dermatology, School of Medicine, University of Utah.)

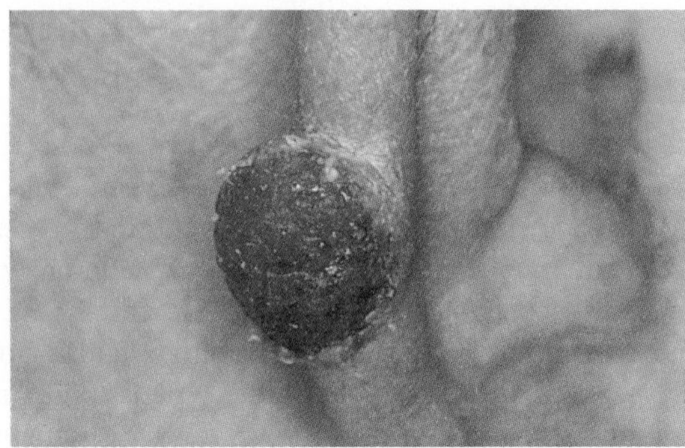

Figure 39-23 ■ **Squamous Cell Carcinoma.** The sun-exposed ear is a common site for squamous cell carcinoma. (Courtesy Department of Dermatology, School of Medicine, University of Utah.)

hormone activity. Sunlight is an important promotional factor. Melanomas arise as a result of malignant degeneration of melanocytes located either along the basal layer of the epidermis or in a benign melanocytic nevus. The relationship between nevi and melanoma makes it important for the clinician to understand the various neval forms (Table 39-6). Most nevi never become suspicious; however, suspicious pigmented nevi need to be removed.[61] Indications for biopsy include color change, size change, irregular notched margin, itching, bleeding or oozing, nodularity, scab formation, and ulceration. The clinical varieties of cutaneous melanoma include lentigo malignant melanoma (LMM) (Figure 39-24), superficial spreading melanoma (SSM), primary nodular melanoma (PNM), and acral lentiginous melanoma (ALM). Staging is determined by lesion thickness.

Treatment of melanoma is guided by size and depth of the lesion. No evidence of metastatic disease involves surgical excision of the primary lesion site, and there also may be selective regional lymph node dissection. Radiation therapy, chemotherapy, and biologic response modifiers may be prescribed. Lesions of the extremities have the best surgical prognosis, next best are head and neck lesions, and trunk lesions have the poorest prognosis. Depth of invasion is also associated with prognosis. Immunotherapy, antibody-based vaccines and gene therapy are under investigation.[62,63] Less than 10% with regional metastasis are alive after 5 years.

TABLE 39-6

Classification of Nevi

Type	Common Characteristics
Junctional nevus	Flat, well-circumscribed, vary in size up to 2 cm, dark color hairs may be present; originate in basal layer of epidermis and can eventually reach the cutaneous surface; most likely to develop into a melanoma
Compound nevus	Most common in adolescents; the majority of pigmented lesions in children; rarely does this lesion develop into melanoma; usually 1 cm in size; hairs may be present; surface is elevated and smooth
Intradermal nevus	Small, less than 1 cm, with regular edges and bristle-like hairs; color ranges from fair skin tone to light brown; has a slight likelihood of developing into a melanoma

Kaposi sarcoma

Kaposi sarcoma (KS) is a vascular malignancy associated with immunodeficiency states and occurs among transplant recipients taking immunosuppressive drugs. A rapidly progressive form of KS appears with acquired immunodeficiency syndrome (AIDS) and is associated with human herpesvirus-8 (HHV-8) (see Chapter 32). KS is also common among middle-aged black males in equatorial Africa and persons of Mediterranean or Jewish descent. Four forms of the disease have been described: classic, epidemic, posttransplant, and acquired immunodeficient associated virus.[64]

The endothelial cell is thought to be the progenitor of KS. The lesions emerge as purplish brown macules and develop into plaques and nodules with angioproliferation. They tend to be multifocal rather than spreading by metastasis. The lesions initially appear over the lower extremities in the classic form (Figure 39-25). The rapidly progressive form associated with AIDS tends to spread symmetrically over the upper body, particularly the face and oral mucosa. The lesions are often pruritic and painful. About 75% of individuals with epidemic KS have involvement of lymph nodes, particularly in the gastrointestinal tract and lungs. Organ involvement is much less common in the classic form. The rapidly progressive form has a poor prognosis and shorter survival rates than the classic form. (See Chapter 7 for a further discussion of AIDS.)

Diagnosis is by skin biopsy, with a high index of suspicion for those with immunodeficiency. Local lesions can be excised. Multiple disseminated lesions may be treated with a combination of α-interferon, radiotherapy, and cytotoxic drugs. Antiangiogenic agents are being tested. Indivi-

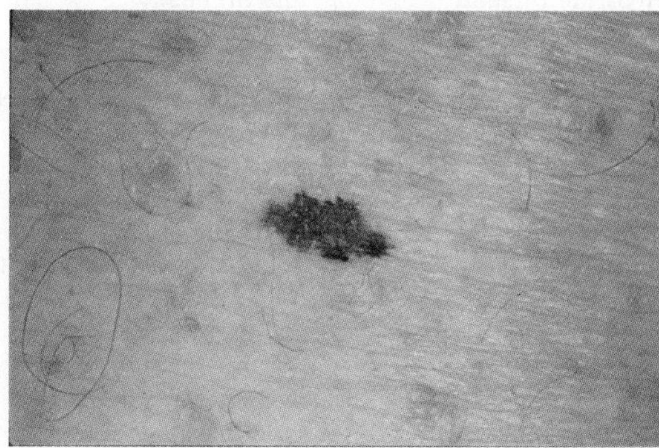

Figure 39-24 ■ **Lentigo Malignant Melanoma.** (Courtesy Department of Dermatology, School of Medicine, University of Utah.)

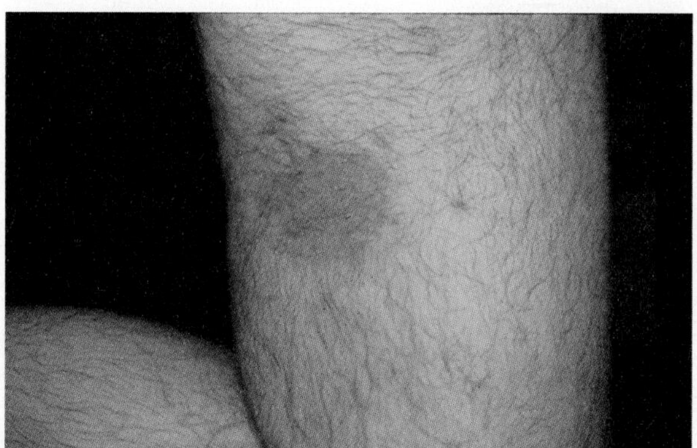

Figure 39-25 ■ **Kaposi Sarcoma.** The purple lesion commonly seen on the skin. (Courtesy Department of Dermatology, School of Medicine, University of Utah.)

duals receiving highly active antiretroviral therapy (HAART) have a markedly reduced incidence of KS.[65]

QUICK CHECK 39-7

1. What is the most common skin cancer?
2. What malignancy can arise from melanocytes?
3. How is Kaposi sarcoma related to AIDS?

Burns

The incidence of burn injuries has declined in the past several years. About 1 million people are burned in the United States each year, with 45,000 people hospitalized and 4500 burn-related deaths.[66] Most significant burns occur in the home, and the highest percentage of deaths (70%) are from home fires.[67]

Burns may be caused by thermal or nonthermal sources including chemical, electrical, or radioactive sources. Thermal injuries result from exposure to direct flames, hot liquids, or radiation. Direct contact, inhalation, and ingestion of acids, alkalis, or blistering agents cause chemical burns. Electrical burns occur with the passage of electrical current through the body to the ground. Associated electrical flames or flashes also can burn the skin.

Burn wound depth

The depth of injury identifies the level of tissue destruction; the extent of injury determines clinical management and mortality. The depth of the burn is divided into four categories (Table 39-7).

First-degree burns are a **partial-thickness injury** involving only the epidermis, without injury to the underlying dermal or subcutaneous tissue. The skin maintains water vapor and bacterial barrier functions. Many instances of sunburn are first-degree injuries caused by the exposure of skin to the ultraviolet radiation from the sun. Initially, there is local pain and erythema, but no blisters appear for about 24 hours. An extensive first-degree burn may cause systemic responses, such as chills, headache, localized edema, and nausea or vomiting. No treatment of extensive first-degree burns is required unless the person is elderly or an infant, in which case severe nausea and vomiting may lead to inadequate fluid intake and dehydration. Therapy consists of intravenous hydration until the nausea and vomiting subside at 24 to 72 hours after burn injury. Comfort measures for previously healthy children or adults with extensive first-degree burns consist of aspirin for adults or acetaminophen for children every 4 hours in age-appropriate dosages and frequent application of a water-soluble lotion. First-degree burns heal in 3 to 5 days without scarring.

TABLE 39-7
Depth of Burn Injury

		SECOND DEGREE		THIRD DEGREE
Characteristic	**First Degree**	**Superficial Partial-Thickness**	**Deep Partial-Thickness**	**Full-Thickness**
Morphology	Destruction of epidermis only	Destruction of epidermis and some dermis	Destruction of epidermis and dermis, leaving only skin appendages	Destruction of epidermis, dermis, and underlying subcutaneous tissue
Skin function	Intact	Absent	Absent	Absent
Tactile and pain sensors	Intact	Intact	Intact but diminished	Absent
Blisters	Present only after first 24 hr	Present within minutes; thin-walled and fluid filled	May or may not appear as fluid-filled blisters; often is layer of flat, dehydrated tissue paper–like skin that lifts off in sheets	Blisters rare; usually is a layer of flat, dehydrated tissue paper–like skin that lifts off easily
Appearance of wound after initial débridement	Skin peels at 24–48 hr; normal or slightly red underneath	Red to pale ivory, moist surface	Mottled with areas of waxy, white, dry surface	White, cherry red, or black; may contain visible thrombosed veins; dry, hard, leathery surface
Healing time	3–5 days	21–28 days	30 days to many months	Will not heal; may close from edges as secondary healing if wound is small
Scarring	None	May be present; low incidence influenced by genetic predisposition	Highest incidence because of slow healing rate promoting scar tissue development; also influenced by genetic predisposition	Skin graft; scarring minimized by early excision and grafting; influenced by genetic predisposition

Second-degree burns describe two categories of burn depth—superficial and deep partial thickness—with markedly different characteristics. **Superficial partial-thickness injuries** involve thin-walled, fluid-filled blisters that develop within just a few minutes after injury. As blisters break or are removed, nerve endings are exposed to air (Figure 39-26). Tactile and pain sensors remain intact throughout the healing process, with each wound care procedure causing extreme pain. Wounds heal in 3 to 4 weeks, provided the individual is adequately nourished and no complications develop (Figure 39-27). Scar formation is unusual with this injury and is genetically determined.

Deep partial-thickness burns involve the entire dermis, sparing skin appendages such as hair follicles and sweat glands (see Table 39-7 and Figure 39-28). These wounds look waxy white and take weeks to heal. Current therapy consists of surgical removal of the burn wound (excision) followed by application of the person's own unburned skin from another body area (autograft). The ultimate healing of deep partial-thickness burns commonly results in hypertrophic scarring with poor functional and cosmetic results.

Third-degree burns, or **full-thickness burns,** involve destruction of the entire epidermis, dermis, and often underlying subcutaneous tissue (see Table 39-7). On occasion, all underlying subcutaneous tissue is destroyed and muscle or bone may be destroyed as well. Elasticity of the dermis is destroyed, giving the wound a dry, leathery appearance (Figure 39-29). Distal circulation may be compromised in areas of circumferential burns from pressure caused by edema. **Escharotomies** (tissue decompression by cutting through burned skin) are performed to release pressure and prevent compartment syndrome (the compression of blood vessels, veins, muscle or abdominal organs resulting in irreversible injury). Full-thickness burns are painless because all nerve endings have been destroyed by the injury.

The extent of the **total body surface area (TBSA)** burn is estimated using either the "rule of nines" (Figure 39-30) or the Lund and Browder chart.[68] The severity of a burn injury is determined by a combination of many factors, including age, medical history, extent and depth of injury,

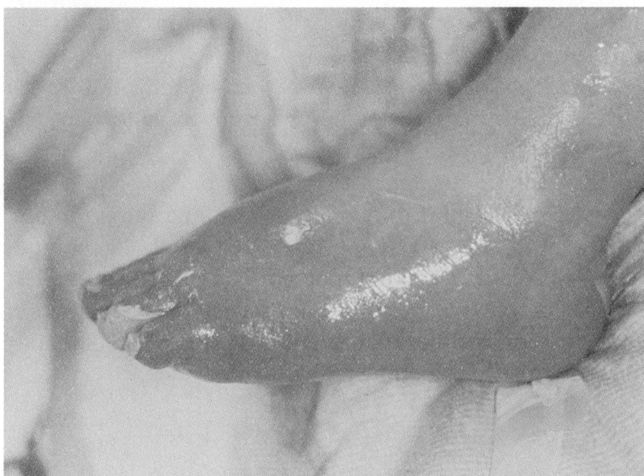

Figure 39-26 ■ **Superficial Partial-Thickness Injury.** Scald injury following débridement of overlying blister and nonadherent epithelium. (Courtesy Intermountain Burn Center, University of Utah.)

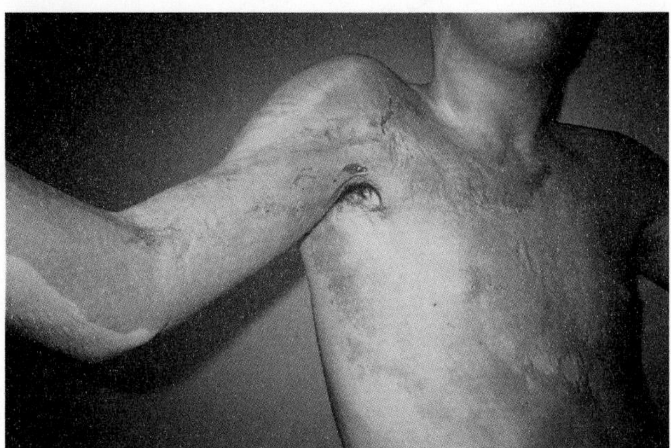

Figure 39-27 ■ **Axillary Burn Scar Contracture.** Note the blanching of the anterior axillary fold and small ulceration from a deep partial thickness burn, both indicating the diminished range of motion. (Courtesy Intermountain Burn Center, University of Utah.)

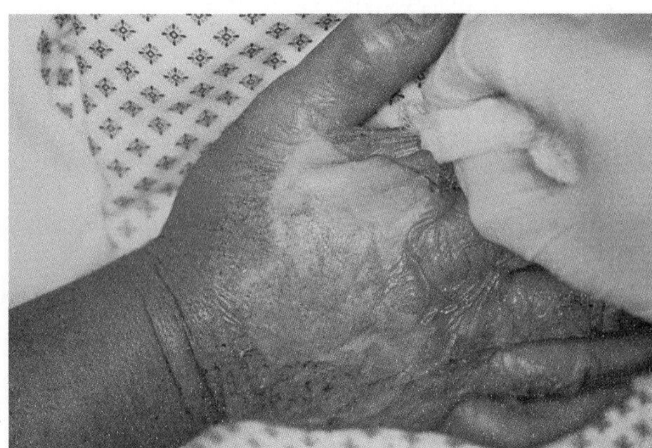

Figure 39-28 ■ **Deep Partial-Thickness Wound.** Note pale appearance and minimal exudate. (Courtesy Intermountain Burn Center, University of Utah.)

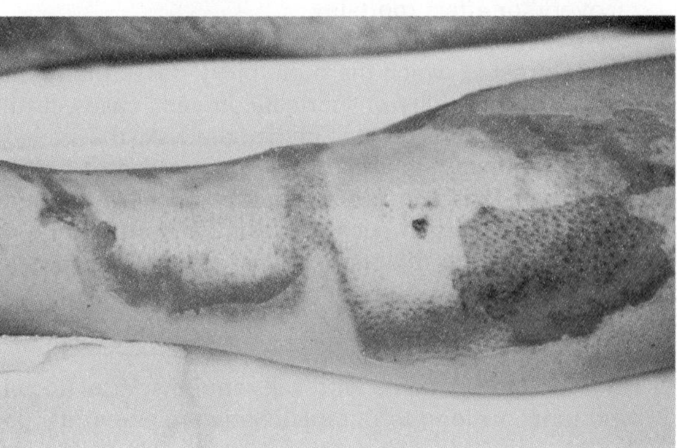

Figure 39-29 ■ **Full-Thickness Thermal Injury.** The wound is dry and insensate. (Courtesy Intermountain Burn Center, University of Utah.)

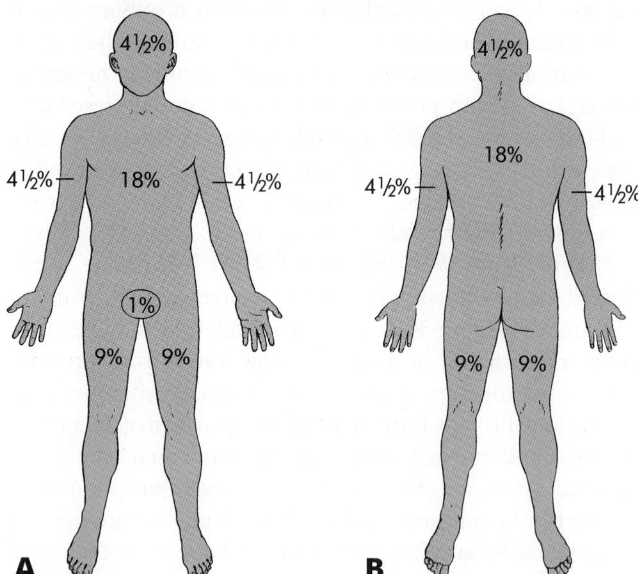

Figure 39-30 ■ Estimation of Burn Injury: Rule of Nines. A commonly used assessment tool with estimates of the percentages (in multiples of 9) of the total body surface area burned. **A,** Adults (anterior view). **B,** Adults (posterior view).

and body area involved. The American College of Surgeons has defined criteria to assist health care professionals in identifying who should be cared for at a specialized burn center (Box 39-2).

BOX 39-2 Burn Unit Referral Criteria

A burn unit may treat adults or children or both. Burn injuries that should be referred to a burn unit include the following:

1. Partial-thickness burns greater than 10% total body surface area (TBSA)
2. Burns that involve the face, hands, feet, genitalia, perineum, or major joints
3. Third-degree burns in any age group
4. Electrical burns, including lightning injury
5. Chemical burns
6. Inhalation injury
7. Burn injury in patients with preexisting medical disorders that could complicate management, prolong recovery, or affect mortality
8. Any patient with burns and concomitant trauma (such as fractures) in which the burn injury poses the greatest risk of morbidity or mortality; in such cases, if the trauma poses the greater immediate risk, the patient may be initially stabilized in a trauma center before being transferred to a burn unit; physician judgment will be necessary in such situations and should be in concert with the regional medical control plan triage protocols
9. Burned children in hospitals without qualified personnel or equipment for the care of children
10. Burn injury in patients who will require special social, emotional, or long-term rehabilitative intervention

From Committee on Trauma: *Resources for optimal care of the injured patient,* Chicago, 1999, American College of Surgeons.

PATHOPHYSIOLOGY AND CLINICAL MANIFESTATIONS Burn injury results in dramatic changes in most physiologic functions of the body within the first few minutes after the event. The effect of burn depends on two parameters: the extent of body surface affected and the depth of cutaneous injury. Burns exceeding 20% TBSA in most adults are considered to be major burn injuries and are associated with massive evaporative water losses and flux of large amounts of fluid and electrolytes in the body tissues, manifested as generalized edema, circulatory hypovolemia, and hypotension.

With a major burn injury, both local and systemic alterations ensue that require therapeutic intervention to sustain life. The local zones of burn injury and surrounding tissue are described as the[68a]:

Zone of coagulation—a zone of maximum, irreversible tissue injury and loss due to protein coagulation

Zone of ischemia or stasis—the zone immediately surrounding the zone of coagulation with microvascular injury. The tissue can survive with adequate fluid resuscitation and prevention of infection.

Zone of hyperemia—a zone of vasodilation with increased perfusion due to release of inflammatory mediators from adjacent injured tissue.

The immediate (acute) systemic physiologic consequences of major burn injury center around the profound, life-threatening hypovolemic shock that occurs in conjunction with cellular and immunologic disruption within a few minutes of injury (Figure 39-31). **Burn shock** is a condition consisting of both a hypovolemic cardiovascular component and a cellular component.

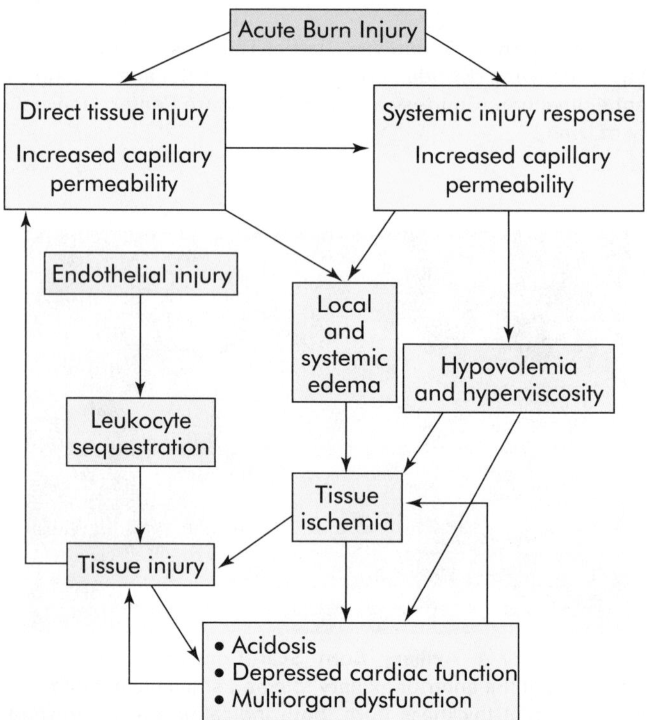

Figure 39-31 ■ Immediate Cellular and Immunologic Alterations of Burn Shock.

Hypovolemia associated with burn shock is the result of massive fluid losses and shifts to the interstitial space from the circulating blood volume. The losses are caused by an increase in capillary endothelial permeability that persists for approximately 24 hours after burn injury. **Fluid resuscitation** (Box 39-3) is the administration of intravenous fluids, often lactated Ringer solution, in an effort to restore the circulating blood volume during the period of increasing capillary permeability. In addition to hypovolemia, most other organ systems are affected. Cardiac contractility diminishes during the initial 24-hour resuscitation period with shunting of blood away from the liver, kidney, and gut, and other viscera with attendant decreased function of these organs. Decreased perfusion of the viscera can decrease gut barrier function and result in translocation of bacteria and endotoxemia with sepsis.[69]

There is also evidence that cellular metabolism is disrupted with onset of the burn wound, resulting in altered cell membrane permeability and loss of normal electrolyte homeostasis, which contributes to burn shock. Many cytokines and inflammatory mediators play a role in the cellular, cardiovascular, and systemic responses to burn injury. Evaporative water loss must also be considered.

Evaporative water loss

One of the major purposes of intact skin is to serve as a barrier to evaporative water loss (EWL) from the body. With major burn injury, this ability of the skin to regulate evaporative water loss is totally disrupted. Calculation of the amount of fluid lost by evaporative water loss includes losses from all sources. Normally, the skin is the major source of insensible loss (75%), and the lungs are minor sources (25%), with a total loss of only approximately 600 to 800 ml/day. This changes dramatically with burns because not only does skin loss increase, but also lung loss increases because of hypermetabolism and hyperventilation, especially in an intubated individual. Total evaporative losses exceed many liters per day in an adult with large burn wounds. Replacement of the loss is mandatory to prevent volume deficit.

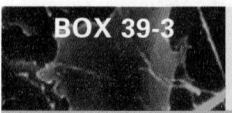

Maintenance Fluid Replacements After Major Burn Injury*

1. *Basal fluid* replacements per day
   1500 ml/day/m^2 body surface area = 24-hour requirements
2. *Evaporative water loss* from burn wound
   a. Adults: (25 + % total body surface area burn) (m^2 body surface area) = ml/hr
   b. Children: (35 + % total body surface area burn) (m^2 body surface area) = ml/hr
3. *Total hourly maintenance fluids*
   Basal fluid requirements per day ÷ 24 hours + evaporative water loss per hour = ml/hr maintenance fluids

Example: A 70-kg adult with a 50% total body surface area burn and a body surface area of 2 m requires the following:

Basal = (1500 ml/day) (2 m^2 body surface area)
= 3000 ml/24 hr, or **125 ml/hr**

Evaporative = (25 + 50% total body surface burn) (2 m^2 total body surface area)
= (75) (2) = **150 ml/hr**

Total maintenance fluids = **125 ml** + **150 ml** = **275 ml/hr**

*From end of burn shock until wound closes.

Cardiovascular response to burn

The clinical manifestations of burn shock are the result of alterations in cellular function throughout the body. The hallmark of burn shock is decreased cardiac output with inadequate capillary perfusion in most tissues. Decreased cardiac output is related to myocardial depressant factors, as well as decreased intravascular volume. The fluid and protein movement out of the vascular compartment results in an elevated hematocrit and white blood cell count, and hypoproteinemia. If not treated immediately, profound hypovolemic shock and inadequate perfusion leads to irreversible shock and death within a few hours. Restoration of capillary integrity and a functional lymphatic system are required for resolution of the edema. Usually this occurs within 24 hours, but in extensive burns, it may take days or weeks. After the individual has reached the end point of burn shock, the term used to describe the person's condition is **capillary seal.**

Cellular response to burn injury

In addition to capillary endothelial permeability changes resulting in vascular fluid losses, there are transmembrane potential changes in cells not directly damaged by heat. Such membrane potential changes may be caused by a circulating shock factor.[70] Other changes can be categorized as (1) metabolic responses and (2) immunologic responses to the burn injury.

The cellular dysfunction of burn injury results from impairment of the sodium-potassium pump, which results in increased intracellular sodium and water and decreased potassium and disruption of the transmembrane potential. Intracellular calcium also may be elevated, thereby influencing myocardial function.[71] Loss of intracellular magnesium and phosphate[72] and elevated serum lactic dehydrogenase (LDH) occurs.[73] Thus, impairments of basic cellular function may be the underlying cause of the diminished membrane potentials and contribute to burn shock.

Metabolic response to burn injury

Metabolic reactions to the stress of a major burn injury involve the response of the sympathetic nervous system and other homeostatic regulators. Catecholamines are found in elevated amounts in both the serum and urine of burned individuals. Cortisol, glucagon, and insulin levels are elevated with a corresponding increase in gluconeogenesis, lipolysis, and proteolysis. Changes in lipid metabolism are reflected as an elevation in plasma free fatty acids (FFAs) and a decrease in plasma cholesterol and phospholipids.[74] Glucose and lactate kinetics are altered after burn injury. Although tissue hypoxia produces lactic acidosis, its persistence in the presence of adequate tissue perfusion suggests an increased rate of glycogenolysis.[75]

Burn injury and release of inflammatory cytokines induces a *hypermetabolic state* that persists until wound closure. The metabolic rate increases with burn size in a curvilinear relationship, with oxygen consumption rarely exceeding two times basal levels. Evaporative water loss and surface cooling are not the primary stimulus for the hypermetabolic state; rather, the hypermetabolism is related to an increase and resetting of the thermal regulatory set point. A core body temperature of 38.5° C is typical, and there is persistent tachycardia, hypercapnia, and body wasting. Wound healing may be impaired contributing to increased risk for infection.[76]

The inflammatory response and release of cytokines at the wound level is magnified into a generalized systemic inflammatory response that is often deleterious.[77–79] Vasodilation, increased capillary permeability, and edema occur to facilitate healing of the local area but at high metabolic cost that continues during sleep and rest. The hepatic response alters clotting factors and leads to a hypercoagulable state.[80]

Immunologic response to burn injury

The immunologic/inflammatory response to burn injury is immediate, prolonged, and severe. The end result in individuals surviving burn shock is *immunosuppression* with increased susceptibility to potentially fatal systemic burn wound sepsis. White blood cells are altered at a time when their need to inhibit sepsis is vital.[81] Phagocytosis is impaired, and cellular and humoral immunity is abnormal. Macrophages, neutrophils, and platelets also release large amounts of inflammatory cytokines and, when combined with bacterial products, produce peripheral vasodilation, distant organ dysfunction, and multiple organ failure.[82] Inflammatory mediators circulating to the lung result in pulmonary edema that can be life threatening.[83] Normally, opsonin renders bacteria susceptible to phagocytosis, but the burn injury triggers a consumptive decrease in opsonins with a greater risk for infection. Individuals with altered immunocompetence or chronic disease before burn injury are at additional risk for complications.[84]

EVALUATION AND TREATMENT Burn recovery is long and stormy, with complications the rule rather than the exception. Severity of inhalation injury is also a significant morbidity and mortality factor. The goal of burn management is wound closure in a manner that promotes survival. Scar formation with contractures is often a consequence of healing in deep partial-thickness and third-degree burns (Figure 39-32).

The three essential elements of survival of major burn injury are (1) adequate fluids and nutrition, (2) meticulous wound management, and (3) early surgical excision and grafting (Figure 39-33).[85] Burn pain is almost always acute, and treatment strategies usually differ from strategies for chronic pain. In addition to opioid-based agents, strategies for treatment may include antianxiety agents, hypnosis, and relaxation techniques.[86] Nutritional therapy focuses on early enteral therapy to reduce gut-mediated sepsis.[69] Advancements in skin replacement technology are effective and promising.[87]

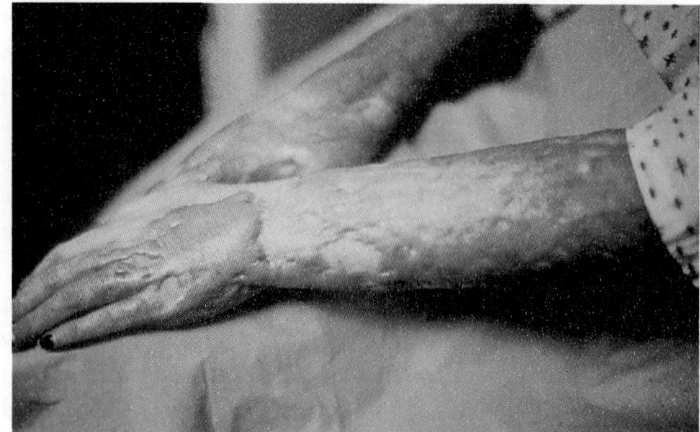

Figure 39-32 ■ **Hypertrophic Scarring.** Deep partial-thickness thermal injury can result in extensive hypertrophic scarring. (Courtesy Intermountain Burn Center, University of Utah.)

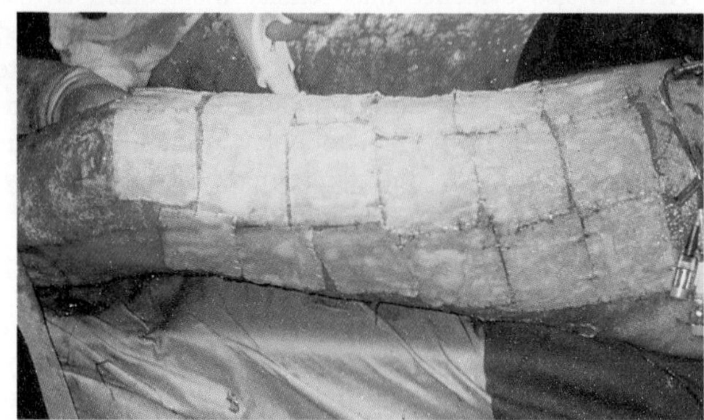

Figure 39-33 ■ **Application of Cultured Epithelial Autografts.** The thin sheets of keratinocytes are attached to gauze backing to allow application onto the clean, excised thigh. (Courtesy Intermountain Burn Center, University of Utah.)

Frostbite

Frostbite is injury to the skin caused by exposure to extreme cold. The most common areas affected are fingers, toes, ears, nose, and cheeks. The mechanism of injury appears to be related to direct cold injury to cells, indirect injury from ice crystal formation, and impaired circulation with anoxia to the exposed area and the release of inflammatory mediators, including thromboxanes and prostaglandins.[88] Frozen skin becomes white or yellowish and has a waxy texture. There is numbness and no sensation of pain.

Mild frostbite causes redness and discomfort during rewarming, followed by a return to normal in a few hours. Cyanosis and mottling develop followed by redness, swelling, and burning pain on rewarming in more severe cases. Within 24 to 48 hours, vesicles and bullae appear that resolve into crusts that eventually slough off, leaving thin, newly formed skin. The most severe cases result in gangrene with loss of the affected part. Frostbite may be classified by depth of injury: superficial includes partial skin freezing (first degree) and full-thickness skin freezing (second degree); deep includes full-thickness skin and subcutaneous freezing (third degree) and deep tissue freezing (fourth degree).

Immediate treatment of frostbite is to cover affected areas with other body surfaces and warm clothing. The area should not be rubbed or massaged. Immersion in a warm water bath (40° C to 44° C) until frozen tissue is thawed is the best treatment. Pain is severe and should be treated with potent analgesics, including epidural narcotics. Gentle cleansing and no pressure on the skin should be maintained during healing. Vasodilators, thrombolytics, hyperbaric oxygen, and sympathectomy may improve healing responses.[89] Amputation of necrotic tissue is delayed for 1 to 3 months after a clear line of demarcation is established.

DISORDERS OF THE HAIR

Alopecia

Male-pattern alopecia (androgenic alopecia)

Alopecia means loss of hair. Localized hair loss in men is not a disease but a genetically predisposed response to androgens. Within the distribution of hair over the scalp, androgen-sensitive hair follicles are on top and androgen-insensitive follicles are on the sides and back. In genetically predisposed men, the androgen-sensitive follicles are transformed into vellus follicles. The normal hair is shed and replaced by fine, light, short hair. Male-pattern baldness begins with frontotemporal recession and progresses to loss of hair over the top of the scalp. Minoxidil and finasteride (a 5-alpha reductase inhibitor) decrease the effect of androgens on hair follicles and are used to stimulate hair growth.[90] Affected men may choose to wear wigs or have hair transplants.

Female-pattern alopecia

Some women in their 20s and 30s experience progressive thinning and loss of hair over the central part of the scalp, and prevalence increases with advancing age. Contrary to male-pattern baldness, there is no loss of hair along the frontal hairline. Many of these women have elevated levels of serum adrenal androgen dehydroepiandrosterone sulfate (DHEAS), but the role of androgens is not fully known. Genetic mechanisms are also suspected.[91] Treatment may include minoxidil or oral antiandrogens.

Alopecia areata

Alopecia areata is an autoimmune T cell–mediated chronic inflammatory disease directed against hair follicles and results in hair loss. There is rapid onset of hair loss in multiple areas of the scalp, usually in round patches. The eyebrows, eyelashes, beard, and other areas of body hair are rarely involved. Stressful events, cell-mediated immune factors, genetic susceptibility, and metabolic disorders, such as Addison disease, thyroid disease, and lupus erythematosus, are associated with alopecia areata.[92]

The affected areas of skin are smooth or may have short shafts of hair. The hair shaft is poorly developed and breaks at the surface. Regrowth occurs within 1 to 3 months, but there may be recurrent hair loss at the same site. Permanent regrowth usually occurs. Some young people experience total loss of hair (alopecia totalis), and the long-term prognosis for regrowth is poor.

Diagnosis is made by observation of the pattern of hair loss. Biopsy may show a lymphocytic infiltrate around the follicle. Intralesional steroids may be used to stimulate hair growth when there are a few small areas of hair loss. Systemic steroids are used for larger areas of alopecia. Topical applications of anthralin are also used to stimulate hair growth. Minoxidil and topical immunotherapy are used in resistant cases.[93]

Hirsutism

Hirsutism occurs in women and is the abnormal growth and distribution of hair on the face, body, and pubic area in a male pattern. There is also frontotemporal hair recession. These areas of hair growth are androgen sensitive. Variations of hair growth in women are great, and a male pattern may be normal. Women who develop hirsutism may be secreting hormones associated with ovarian or adrenal disease, and such women should be evaluated for polycystic ovaries, adrenal hyperplasia, or adrenal tumors. If no hormonal pathologic conditions exist, treatment may include cosmetic removal of hair, oral contraceptives, glucocorticoids, cimetidine, or finasteride.[94]

DISORDERS OF THE NAIL

Paronychia

Paronychia is an acute or chronic infection of the cuticle. Acute paronychia is manifest by the rapid onset of painful inflammation of the cuticle, usually after minor trauma. An abscess may develop requiring incision and drainage for relief of pain. The most common causative microorganisms are staphylococci and streptococci. Occasionally *Candida* is present.[95]

Chronic paronychia develops slowly, with tenderness and swelling around the proximal or lateral nail folds. One or more fingers or toes may be involved. Individuals whose hands are frequently exposed to moisture are at greatest risk. Manipulation of the cuticle opens the space between the proximal nail fold and nail plate, leaving a moist, warm medium for the incubation of pathogenic microorganisms. The skin around the nail becomes more edematous and painful with progressive infection. Pus may be expressed from the proximal nail fold. The nail plate is usually not affected, although it can become discolored with ridges.

Treatment includes keeping the hands dry. Oral antibiotics are not effective because they do not penetrate the affected tissues. Topical application of thymol is usually effective.

Onychomycosis

Onychomycosis is a fungal or dermatophyte infection of the nail plate. The most common pattern is a nail plate that turns yellow or white and becomes elevated with the accumulation of hyperkeratotic debris within the plate. Fungal infections of the nail are differentiated from psoriasis, lichen planus, and trauma by culture and microscopy and the absence of pitting on the nail surface, which is characteristic of psoriasis. Treatment is difficult because topical or systemic antifungal agents do not penetrate the nail plate readily. New antifungal drugs are more effective.[96] Surgical excision of the nail may be required. Education is essential to preventing recurrence.

QUICK CHECK 39-8

1. Describe the three degrees of burn injury.
2. What dangers accompany frostbite?
3. What is alopecia? Compare the different types.
4. What disorders of the nail are seen?

Did You Understand?

Structure and Function of the Skin

1. Skin is the largest organ of the body and equals 20% of body weight.
2. The skin has two layers—the dermis and epidermis. The hypodermis contains underlying connective tissue, fat cells, fibroblasts, and macrophages.
3. The underlying epidermis contains a basal and spinous layer with melanocytes, Langerhans cells, and Merkel cells.
4. The dermis is composed of connective tissue elements, hair follicles, sweat glands, sebaceous glands, blood vessels, nerves, and lymphatic vessels.
5. The papillary capillaries provide the major blood supply to the skin, arising from deeper arterial plexuses.
6. The dermal appendages include nails, hair, and eccrine and apocrine sweat glands.
7. Heat loss and heat conservation are regulated by arteriovenous anastomoses that lead to the papillary capillaries.
8. Pressure ulcers develop from pressure and shearing forces that occlude capillary blood flow with resulting ischemia and necrosis. Areas at greatest risk are pressure points over bony prominences, such as the greater trochanters, sacrum, ischia, and heels.
9. Keloids are sharply elevated scars that extend beyond the border of traumatized skin.
10. Pruritus is itching and is associated with many skin disorders. Small unmyelinated nerve fibers transmit itch sensation.

Disorders of the Skin

1. Contact dermatitis is a form of delayed hypersensitivity that develops with sensitization to allergens, such as metal, chemicals, or poison ivy.
2. Irritant contact dermatitis develops from prolonged exposure to chemicals, such as acids or soaps.
3. Atopic or allergic dermatitis is associated with a family history of allergies, hay fever, elevated IgE levels, and increased histamine sensitivity. Pruritus and scratching predispose the skin to infection, scaling, and thickening.
4. Stasis dermatitis occurs on the legs and results from venous stasis and edema.
5. Seborrheic dermatitis involves scaly, yellowish, inflammatory plaques of the scalp, eyebrows, eyelids, ear canals, chest, axillae, and back. The cause is unknown but Malassezia yeasts have been implicated.
6. Papulosquamous disorders are characterized by papules, scales, plaques, and erythema.
7. Psoriasis is a chronic inflammatory skin disease associated with T cell activation and thickening of both the epidermis and dermis, characterized by scaly, erythematous, pruritic plaques.
8. Pityriasis rosea is a self-limiting disease characterized by oval lesions with scales around the edges located along skin lines of the trunk and may be caused by a herpes-like virus.
9. Lichen planus is an autoimmune papular, violet-colored inflammatory lesion of unknown origin manifested by severe pruritus.
10. Acne vulgaris is an inflammation of the pilosebaceous follicle.
11. Acne rosacea develops on the middle third of the face with hypertrophy and inflammation of the sebaceous glands.
12. Lupus erythematosus is an autoimmune disease that can affect only the skin (discoid) or have a systemic presentation. The cutaneous inflammatory lesions usually occur in sun-exposed areas with a butterfly distribution over the nose and cheeks.
13. Pemphigus is a chronic, autoimmune, blistering disease that begins in the mouth or on the scalp and spreads to other parts of the body, often with a fatal outcome.
14. Erythema multiforme is an acute inflammation of the skin and mucous membranes with lesions that appear target-like with alternating rings of edema and inflammation, often associated with allergic reactions to drugs.
15. Folliculitis is a bacterial infection of the hair follicle.
16. A furuncle is an infection of the hair follicle that extends to the surrounding tissue.
17. A carbuncle is a collection of infected hair follicles that forms a draining abscess.
18. Cellulitis is a diffuse infection of the dermis and subcutaneous tissue.
19. Erysipelas is a superficial streptococcal infection of the skin commonly affecting the face, ears, and lower legs.
20. Impetigo may have a bullous or an ulcerative form and is caused by *Staphylococcus* or *Streptococcus*.

Did You Understand?—Cont'd

21. Herpes simplex virus type 1 (HSV-1) causes cold sores but can infect the cornea, mouth, and labia. HSV-2 causes genital lesions and is usually spread by sexual contact.
22. Herpes zoster (shingles) and varicella (chickenpox) are both caused by the same herpesvirus.
23. Warts are benign, rough, elevated lesions caused by papillomavirus. Condylomata acuminata, or venereal warts, are spread by sexual contact.
24. Tinea infections (fungal infections) can occur anywhere on the body and are classified by location (i.e., tinea pedis, tinea corporis, tinea capitis).
25. Candidiasis is a yeastlike fungal infection occurring on skin, mucous membranes, and the gastrointestinal tract.
26. Cutaneous vasculitis is an inflammation of skin blood vessels related to immune complex deposition with purpura, ischemia, and necrosis resulting from vessel necrosis.
27. Urticarial lesions are commonly associated with type 1 hypersensitivity responses and appear as wheals, welts, or hives.
28. Scleroderma is an autoimmune mediated sclerosis of the skin that may also affect systemic organs and cause renal failure, bowel obstruction, or cardiac dysrhythmias.
29. Mosquitoes can transmit infectious diseases, and the saliva from their bite produces the characteristic itching and wheal formation.
30. Blood-sucking flies are represented by many species and their bites are usually painful and produce bleeding, and the itching and local reactions may last for days with systemic symptoms of fever and malaise.
31. Bee sting venom may produce a local or systemic reaction that can be anaphylactic.
32. Seborrheic keratosis is a proliferation of basal cells that produce elevated, smooth, or warty lesions of varying size. They are most common among the elderly population.
33. Keratoacanthoma arises from hair follicles on sun-exposed areas. Three stages of development characterize the lesion, which results in a dome-shaped, crusty lesion filled with keratin that resolves in 3 to 4 months.
34. Actinic keratosis is a pigmented scaly lesion that develops in sun-exposed individuals with fair skin. The lesion may become malignant in the form of a squamous cell carcinoma.
35. Nevi arise from melanocytes and may be pigmented or fleshy pink. They occur singly or in groups and may undergo transition to malignant melanoma.
36. Basal cell carcinoma is the most common skin cancer and occurs most often on sun-exposed areas of the skin.
37. Squamous cell carcinoma is a tumor of the epidermis and can be localized (in situ) or invasive.
38. Malignant melanoma arises from melanocytes, and if not excised early, metastasis occurs through the lymph nodes.
39. Kaposi sarcoma is a vascular malignancy associated with immunodeficiency states and herpes virus-8.
40. Burns are classified according to depth and extent of injury as first, second, or third degree burns.
41. Severe burns cause profound edema and burn shock related to an inflammatory response throughout the cardiovascular system with loss of capillary seal. Fluid resuscitation is critical to prevent shock and death.
42. Burns cause a hypermetabolic response with increased cortisol, glucagon, and insulin levels.
43. Immune suppression associated with inflammatory cytokine release from burned tissue increases risk for infection and can delay wound healing.
45. Frostbite usually occurs on cheeks and digits, with direct injury to cells and impaired circulation.

Disorders of the Hair

1. Male-pattern alopecia is an inherited form of irreversible baldness with hair loss in the central scalp and recession of the temporofrontal hairline.
2. Female-pattern alopecia is a thinning of the central hair of the scalp beginning in women at 20 to 30 years of age.
3. Alopecia areata is an autoimmune mediated loss of hair and may be associated with stress or metabolic diseases; it is usually reversible.
4. Hirsutism is a male pattern of hair growth in women that may be normal or the result of excessive secretion of androgenic hormones.

Disorders of the Nail

1. Paronychia is an inflammation of the cuticle that can be acute or chronic and is usually caused by staphylococci or streptococci.
2. Onychomycosis is a fungal infection of the nail plate.

Key Terms

Acne rosacea, 1099
Acne vulgaris, 1099
Actinic keratosis, 1107
Allergic contact dermatitis, 1096
Alopecia, 1115
Alopecia areata, 1115
Apocrine sweat gland, 1088
Atopic dermatitis, 1096
Basal cell carcinoma, 1108
Burn shock, 1112
Candidiasis, 1104
Capillary seal, 1113
Carbuncle, 1102
Cellulitis, 1102
Clawlike prolongation, 1095
Condylomata acuminata (venereal warts), 1103
Cutaneous melanoma, 1108
Cutaneous vasculitis, 1104
Deep partial-thickness burn, 1111
Dermal appendage, 1087
Dermatitis, 1096
Dermis, 1086

Key Terms—Cont'd

Discoid lupus erythematosus (DLE), 1099
Eccrine sweat gland, 1088
Eczema, 1096
Epidermis, 1086
Erysipelas, 1102
Erythema multiforme, 1100
Escharotomy, 1111
First-degree burn, 1110
Fluid resuscitation, 1113
Fly, 1106
Folliculitis, 1101
Frostbite, 1114
Furuncle, 1101
Herald patch, 1098
Herpes zoster (shingles), 1103
Hirsutism, 1115
Hypodermis, 1086
Impetigo, 1102
Irritant contact dermatitis, 1096
Kaposi sarcoma (KS), 1109
Keloid, 1094
Keratoacanthoma, 1106
Lichen planus, 1098
Lupus erythematosus, 1099
Mosquito, 1106
Nevus (*pl.* nevi), 1107
Onychomycosis, 1116
Papillary capillary, 1088
Papulosquamous disorder, 1097
Paronychia, 1115
Partial-thickness injury, 1110
Pemphigus, 1100
Pemphigus erythematosus, 1100
Pemphigus foliaceus, 1100
Pemphigus vegetans, 1100
Pemphigus vulgaris, 1100
Pityriasis rosea, 1098
Psoriasis, 1097
Scleroderma (systemic sclerosis), 1105
Sebaceous gland, 1088
Seborrheic dermatitis, 1096
Seborrheic keratosis, 1106
Second-degree burn, 1111
Squamous cell carcinoma, 1108
Stasis dermatitis, 1096
Stevens-Johnson syndrome, 1101
Superficial partial-thickness injury, 1111
Third-degree burn (full-thickness burn), 1111
Tinea capitis, 1103
Tinea corporis (ringworm), 1103
Tinea infection, 1103
Tinea pedis, 1103
Total body surface area (TBSA), 1111
Toxic epidermal necrolysis (TEN), 1101
Urticarial lesion, 1105
Varicella (chicken pox), 1103
Wart, 1103

References

1. de Laat EH et al: Epidemiology, risk and prevention of pressure ulcers in critically ill patients: a literature review, *J Wound Care* 15(6):269–275, 2006.
2. Stott NA: Assessing a patient with pressure ulcer, In Morison MJ, editor: *The prevention and treatment of pressure ulcers*, St Louis, 2001, Mosby.
3. Brem H, Lyder C: Protocol for the successful treatment of pressure ulcers, *Am J Surg* 188(1A suppl):9–17, 2004.
4. Reddy M, Gill SS, Rochon PA: Preventing pressure ulcers: a systematic review, *JAMA* 296(8):974–984, 2006.
5. Bergstrom N et al: The National Pressure Ulcer Long-Term Care Study: outcomes of pressure ulcer treatments in long-term care, *J Am Geriatr Soc* 53(10):1721–1729, 2005.
6. Bayat A et al: Genetic susceptibility to keloid disease: mutation screening of the TGFbeta3 gene, *Br J Plast Surg* 58(7):914–921, 2005.
7. Al-Attar A et al: Keloid pathogenesis and treatment, *Plast Reconstr Surg* 117(1):286–300, 2006.
8. Steinhoff M et al: Neurophysiological, neuroimmunological, and neuroendocrine basis of pruritus, *J Invest Dermatol* 126 (8):1705–1718, 2006.
9. Paus R et al: Frontiers in pruritus research: scratching the brain for more effective itch therapy, *J Clin Invest* 116(5): 1174–1186, 2006.
10. Dawn AG, Yosipovitch G: Butorphanol for treatment of intractable pruritus, *J Am Acad Dermatol* 54(3):527–531, 2006.
11. Lovell P, Vender RB: Management and treatment of pruritus, *Skin Therapy Lett* 12(1):1–6, 2007.
12. Saint-Mezard P et al: Allergic contact dermatitis, *Eur J Dermatol* 14(5):284–295, 2004.
13. Weissman DN, Lewis DM: Allergic and latex-specific sensitization: route, frequency and amount of exposure that are required to initiate IgE production, *J Allergy Clin Immunol* 110(2 suppl):S57–S63, 2002.
14. Li LY, Cruz PD Jr: Allergic contact dermatitis: pathophysiology applied to future therapy, *Dermatol Ther* 17(3):219–223, 2004.
15. Schwartz RA, Janusz CA, Janniger CK: Seborrheic dermatitis: an overview, *Am Fam Physician* 74(1):125–130, 2006.
16. Lowes MA, Bowcock AM, Krueger JG: Pathogenesis and therapy of psoriasis, *Nature* 45(7130):866–873, 2007.
17. Myers WA, Gottlieb AB, Mease P: Psoriasis and psoriatic arthritis: clinical features and disease mechanisms, *Clin Dermatol* 24(5):438–447, 2006.
18. Malnati MS: Additional evidence that pityriasis rosea is associated with reactivation or human herpesvirus-6 and -7, *J Invest Dermatol* 124(6):1234–1240, 2005.
19. Allen RA, Janniger CK, Schwartz RA: Pityriasis rosea, *Cutis* 56(4):198–202, 1995.
20. DeRossi SS, Ciarrocca KN: Lichen planus, lichenoid drug reactions, and lichenoid mucositis, *Dent Clin North Am* 49(1): 77–89, 2005.
21. Mignogna MD, Lo Russo L, Fedele S: Gingival involvement of oral lichen planus in a series of 700 patients, *J Clin Periodontaol* 32(10):1029–1033, 2005.
22. Tosti A et al: Lichen planus of the nails and fingertips, *Eur J Dermatol* 8(6):447–448, 1998.
23. Diamantis S, Waldorf HA: Rosacea: clinical presentation and pathophysiology, *J Drugs Dermatol* 5(1):8–12, 2006.
24. Nally JB, Berson DS: Topical therapies for rosacea, *J Drugs Dermatol* 5(1):23–26, 2006.
25. Pramatarov KD: Chronic cutaneous lupus erythematosus: clinical spectrum, *Clin Dermatol* 22(2):113–120, 2004.
26. Kreuter A et al: Pimecrolimus 1% cream for cutaneous lupus erythematosus, *J Am Acad Dermatol* 51(3):407–410, 2004.
27. Coelho A et al: Long-term thalidomide use in refractory cutaneous lesions of lupus erythematosus: a 65 series of Brazilian patients, *Lupus* 14(6):434–439, 2005.
28. Lanza A et al: How does acantholysis occur in pemphigus vulgaris: a critical review, *J Cutan Pathol* 33(6):401–412, 2006.
29. Hashimoto T: Recent advances in the study of the pathophysiology of pemphigus, *Arch Dermatol Res* 295(suppl 1):S2–S11, 2003.
30. Beissert S et al: A comparison of oral methylprednisolone plus azathioprine or mycophenolate mofetil for the treatment of pemphigus, *Arch Dermatol* 142(11):1447–1454, 2006.
31. Lamoreux MR, Sternbach MR, Hsu WT: Erythema multiforme, *Am Fam Physician* 74(11):1883–1888, 2006.
32. Williams PM, Conklin RJ: Erythema multiforme: a review and contrast from Stevens-Johnson syndrome/toxic epidermal necrolysis, *Dent Clin North Am* 49(1):67–76, 2005.

References—Cont'd

32a. Elston DM: Community-acquired methicillin-resistant *Staphylococcus aureus, J Am Acad Dermatol* 56(1):1–16, 2007.
33. Rogers RL, Perkins J: Skin and soft tissue infections, *Prim Care* 33(3):697–710, 2006.
34. Cunningham AL et al: The cycle of human herpes simplex virus infection: virus transport and immune control, *J Infect Dis* 194(suppl 1):S11–S18, 2006.
35. Sacks SL et al: HSV-2 transmission, *Antiviral Res* 63(suppl 1): S27–S35, 2004.
36. Koelle DM: Vaccines for herpes simplex virus infections, *Curr Opin Investig Drugs* 7(2):136–141, 2006.
37. Johnson RW: Pain following herpes zoster: implications for management, *Herpes* 11(3):63–65, 2004.
37a. Vaccine approved for shingles in older people, *FDA Consum* 40(5):38–39, 2006.
38. Bacelieri R, Johnson: Cutaneous warts: an evidence-based approach to therapy, *Am Fam Physician* 72(4):647–652, 2005.
39. Cox JT: Epidemiology and natural history of HPV, *J Fam Pract* (suppl):3–9, 2006.
40. Schiller JT, Lowy DR: Prospects for cervical cancer prevention by human papillomavirus vaccination, *Cancer Res* 66(21): 10229–10232, 2006.
41. Weinstein A, Berman B: Topical treatment of common superficial tinea infections, *Am Fam Physician* 65(10):2095–2102, 2002.
42. Habif TP: *Clinical dermatology*, ed 4, p. 440. St Louis, 2004, Mosby.
43. Hayat S, Berney SM: Cutaneous vasculitis, *Curr Rhematol Rep* 7(4):276–278, 2005.
44. Carlson JA et al: Cutaneous vasculitis: diagnosis and management, *Clin Dermatol* 24(5):414–429, 2006.
45. Dibbern DA Jr: Urticaria: selected highlights and recent advances, *Med Clin North Am* 17(1):56–61, 2005.
46. Kaplan AP: Chronic urticaria: pathogenesis and treatment, *J Allergy Clin Immunol* 114(3):465–474, 2004.
47. Denton CP, Black CM, Abraham DJ: Mechanisms and consequences of fibrosis in systemic sclerosis, *Nat Clin Pract Rheumatol* 2(3):134–144, 2006.
48. Chizzolini C: Update on pathophysiology of scleroderma with special reference to immunoinflammatory events, *Ann Med* 39 (1):42–53, 2007.
49. Trojanowska M: What did we learn by studying scleroderma fibroblasts? *Clin Exp Rheumatol* 22(3 suppl 33):S59–S63, 2004.
50. Mayes MD: Scleroderma epidemiology, *Rheum Dis Clin North Am* 29(2):239–254, 2003.
51. Charles C, Clements P, Furst DE: Systemic sclerosis: hypothesis-driven treatment strategies, *Lancet* 367(9523): 1683–1691, 2006.
52. Clausen OP et al: Are keratoacanthomas variants of squamous cell carcinomas? A comparison of chromosomal aberrations by comparative genomic hybridization, *J Invest Dermatol* 126 (10):2308–2315, 2006.
53. Gold MH, Nestor MS: Current treatments of actinic keratosis, *J Drugs Dermatol* 5(2 suppl):17–25, 2006.
54. American Cancer Society: *Cancer facts & figures—2007,* Atlanta, American Cancer Society, 2007.
55. Cleaver JE, Crowley E: UV damage, DNA repair and skin carcinogenesis, *Front Biosci* 7:d1024–d1043, 2002.
56. Green A et al: Sun exposure, skin cancers and related skin conditions, *J Epidemiol* 9(6 suppl):S7–S13, 1999.
57. Pons M, Quintanilla M: Molecular biology of malignant melanoma and other cutaneous tumors, *Clin Transl Oncol* 8(7): 466–474, 2006.
58. Franceschi S et al: Site distribution of different types of skin cancer: new aetiologic clues, *Int J Cancer* 67(1):24–28, 1996.
59. Backvall H et al: The density of epidermal p53 clones is higher adjacent to squamous cell carcinoma in comparison with basal cell carcinoma, *Br J Dermatol* 150(2):259–266, 2004.
60. Abbasi NR et al: Early diagnosis of cutaneous melanoma, revisiting the ABCD criteria, *JAMA* 292(22):2771–2776, 2004.
61. Cummins DL et al: Cutaneous malignant melanoma, *Mayo Clin Proc* 81(4):500–507, 2006.
62. Queirolo P, Acquati M: Targeted therapies in melanoma, *Cancer Treat Rev.* 32(7):524–531, 2006.
63. Pilla L et al: Vaccination: role in metastatic melanoma, *Expert Rev Anticancer Ther* 6(8):1305–1318, 2006.
64. Gessain A, Duprez R: Spindle cells and their role in Kaposi's sarcoma, *Int J Biochem Cell Biol* 37(12):2457–2465, 2005.
65. Martinez V et al: Remission from Kaposi's sarcoma on HAART is associated with suppression of HIV replication and is independent of protease inhibitor therapy, *Br J Cancer* 94(7):1000–1006, 2006.
66. American Burn Association: Burn incidence and treatment in the US: 2000 fact sheet [online], 2000; www.ameriburn.org/resources_factsheet.php?PHPSESSID=3377a1bd04a77df-d0a6a5601066c092e.
67. Centers for Disease Control and Prevention: Fire Deaths and Injuries: Fact Sheet, March, 2007 http://www.cdc.gov/ncipc/factsheets/fire.htm.
68. Wachtel TL et al: The inter-rater reliability of estimating the size of burns from various burn area chart drawings, *Burns* 26(2):156–170, 2000.
68a. Jackson DM: The diagnosis of the depth of burning, *Br J Surg* 40:588–596, 1953.
69. Magnotti LJ, Deitch EA: Burns, bacterial translocation, gut barrier function, and failure, *J Burn Care Rehabil* 26(5): 383–391, 2005.
70. Button B et al: Quantitative assessment of a circulating depolarizing factor in shock, *Shock* 15(3):239–244, 2001.
71. White DJ et al: Cardiomyocyte intracellular calcium and cardiac dysfunction after burn trauma, *Crit Care Med* 30(1): 14–22, 2002.
72. Klein GL, Herndon DN: Magnesium deficit in major burns: role in hypoparathyroidism and end-organ parathyroid hormone resistance, *Magnes Res* 11(2):103–109, 1998.
73. Liu ZJ, Wang W, He CS: Comparison of serum and plasma lactate dehydrogenase in postburn patients, *Burns* 26(1): 46–48, 2000.
74. Pratt VC et al: Fatty acid content of plasma lipids and erythrocyte phospholipids are altered following burn injury, *Lipids* 36(7):675–682, 2001.
75. Sayeed MM: Signaling mechanisms of altered cellular responses in trauma, burn, and sepsis: role of Ca^2, *Arch Surg* 135(12):1432–1442, 2000.
76. Pereira CT, Murphy KD, Herndon DN: Altering metabolism, *J Burn Care Rehabil* 26(3):194–199, 2005.
77. Gump FE, Price JB Jr, Kinney JM: Blood flow and oxygen consumption in patients with severe burns, *Surg Gynecol Obstet* 130(1):23–28, 1970.
78. Finnerty CC et al: Cytokine expression profile over time in severely burned pediatric patients, *Shock* 26(1):13–19, 2006.
79. Murphy KD, Lee JO, Herndon DN: Current pharmacotherapy for the treatment of severe burns, *Expert Opin Pharmacother* 4(3):369–384, 2003.
80. Nishiura T et al: Gene expression and cytokine and enzyme activation in the liver after a burn injury, *J Burn Care Rehabil* 21(2):135–141, 2000.
81. Goebel A et al: Injury induces deficient interleukin-12 production, but interleukin-12 therapy after injury restores resistance to infection, *Ann Surg* 231(2):253, 2000.

References—Cont'd

82. Wright K et al: Burn-activated neutrophils and tumor necrosis factor-alpha alter endothelial cell actin cytoskeleton and enhance monolayer permeability, *Surgery* 128(2):259–265, 2000.
83. Turnage RH et al: Mechanisms of pulmonary microvascular dysfunction during severe burn injury, *World J Surg* 26(7): 848–853, 2002.
84. Kelley D, Lynch JB: Burns in alcohol and drug users result in longer treatment times with more complications, *J Burn Care Rehabil* 13(2 pt 1):218–220, 1992.
85. Sheridan RL: Burns, *Crit Care Med* 30(11 suppl):S500–S514, 2002.
86. Young A: Rehabilitation of burn injuries, *Phys Med Rehabil Clin N Am* 13(1):vi, 85–108, 2002.
87. Atiyeh BS, Hayek SN, Gunn SW: New technologies for burn would closure and healing: review of the literature, *Burns* 31 (8):944–956, 2005.
88. Murphy JV et al: Frostbite: pathogenesis and treatment, *J Trauma* 48(1):171–178, 2000.
89. Jurkovich GJ: Environmental cold-induced injury, *Surg Clin North Am* 87(1):247–256, 2007.
90. Stough D et al: Psychological effect, pathophysiology, and management of androgenic alopecia in men, *Mayo Clin Proc* 80(10):1316–1322, 2005.
91. Birch MP, Lalla SC, Messenger AG: Female pattern hair loss, *Clin Exp Dermatol* 27(5):383–388, 2002.
92. Bertolino AP: Alopecia areata: a clinical overview, *Postgrad Med* 107(7):81–85, 89–90, 2000.
93. Dombrowski NC, Bergfeld WF: Alopecia areata: what to expect from current treatments, *Cleve Clin J Med* 72(9):760–761, 765–767 passim, 758, 2005.
94. Sahin Y, Kelestimur F: Medical treatment regimens of hirsutism, *Reprod Biomed Online* 8(5):538–546, 2004.
95. Shaw J, Body R: Best evidence topic report: incision and drainage preferable to oral antibiotics in acute paronychial nail infection? *Emerg Med J* 22(11):813–814, 2005.
96. Gupta AK, Tu LQ: Therapies for onychomycosis: a review, *Dermatol Clin* 24(3):375–379, 2006.

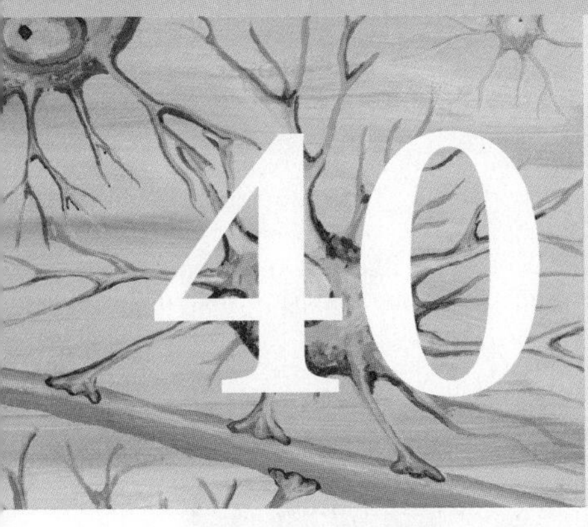

ALTERATIONS OF THE INTEGUMENT IN CHILDREN

Sue E. Huether

CHAPTER OUTLINE

ELECTRONIC RESOURCES

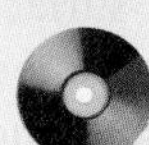

Companion CD
- Review Questions and Answers
- Animations

evolve Website
http://evolve.elsevier.com/Huether/
- Quick Check Answers
- Key Terms Exercises
- Critical Thinking Questions with Answers
- Algorithm Completion Exercises
- WebLinks

Children frequently develop alterations of the skin. The lesions may be minor or severe and localized or generalized. There are often no prodromal symptoms. Skin diseases in children may have different mechanisms of expression than those found in adults, although the causative mechanisms may be similar. Some skin diseases resolve spontaneously and require no treatment. Diagnosis is commonly made from the history, appearance, and distribution of the lesion or lesions. This chapter presents common skin diseases of childhood.

DERMATITIS

Atopic Dermatitis

Atopic dermatitis (AD) is the most common cause of eczema in children, with a prevalence of about 25% to 35% and the incidence is increasing.[1] The etiology is unknown and complex. From 75% to 80% of individuals with atopic dermatitis have a personal or family history of asthma or allergic rhinitis (hay fever). Onset is usually from 2 to 6 months of age, and 85% of cases occur within the first 5 years of life. There are no specific laboratory features of AD that can be used for diagnostic purposes. Most affected individuals show an increased serum immunoglobulin E (IgE) level, elevated interleukin-4, elevated eosinophils, and positive skin tests to a variety of common food and inhalant allergens.[2] Similarly, blood eosinophilia is a common finding in AD.

AD has a constellation of clinical features that include severe pruritus, chronic course with frequent exacerbations, and characteristic eczematoid appearance and age-dependent distribution of skin lesions. The skin becomes increasingly dry, sensitive, itchy, and easily irritated because the barrier function of the skin is impaired. Microscopic epidermal cracks that let water out and irritants and allergens in lead to further drying and cracking, which results in rubbing and scratching. Rubbing and scratching to relieve the itch are actually responsible for many of the clinical changes. In young children, the rash appears primarily on the face, scalp, trunk, and extensor surfaces of the arms and legs (Figure 40-1). In older children and adults, the rash tends to be found on the neck, antecubital and popliteal fossae, and hands and feet. Individuals with AD also tend to develop viral, bacterial, and fungal skin infections in the eczematous areas.

Management of patients with AD includes accurate diagnosis, identification and elimination of exacerbating factors, such as irritants and allergens, and reduction of emotional stresses. Hydration of the skin is the key to good therapy. Anti-inflammatory agents, such as topical corticosteroids or tar preparations, are necessary during active flares of eczema. Immunomodulator therapy is used for severe eczema. Systemic therapy includes the use of sedating antihistamines and antibiotics.

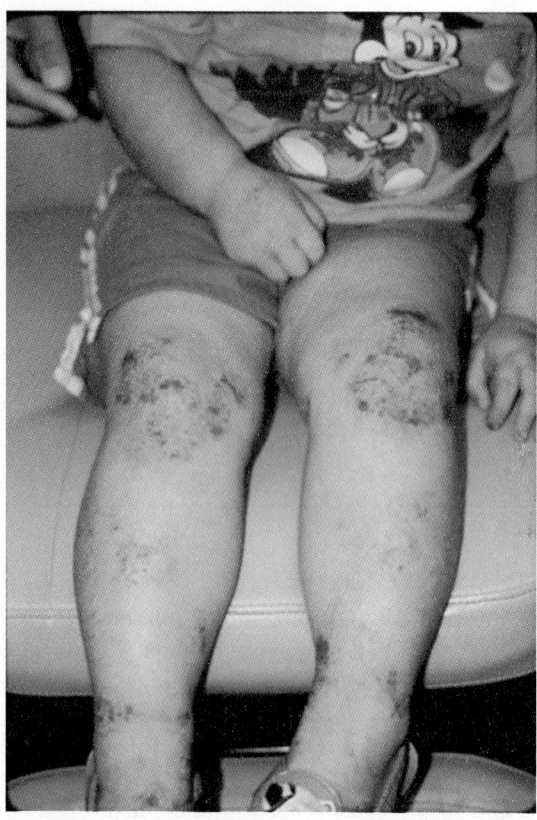

Figure 40-1 ■ **Atopic Dermatitis.** Characteristic lesions with crusting from irritation and scratching over knees and around ankles. (Courtesy Department of Dermatology, School of Medicine, University of Utah.)

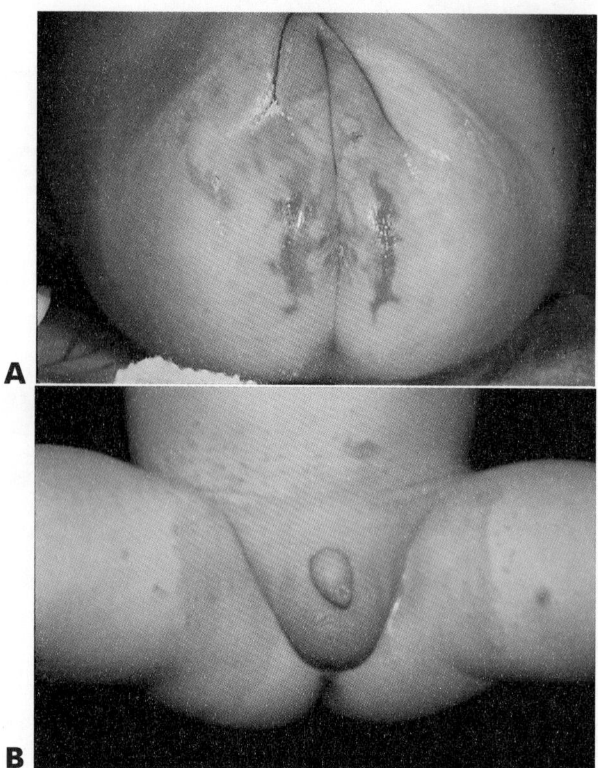

Figure 40-2 ■ **Diaper Dermatitis. A,** Diaper dermatitis with erosions. **B,** Diaper dermatitis with *Candida albicans* secondary infection. (Courtesy Department of Dermatology, School of Medicine, University of Utah.)

Diaper Dermatitis

Diaper dermatitis is a form of irritant contact dermatitis initiated by a combination of factors including prolonged exposure to and irritation by urine and feces, maceration by wet diapers, and airtight plastic diaper covers. Often, diaper dermatitis is secondarily infected with *Candida albicans.* The resulting inflammation affects the lower aspect of the abdomen, genitalia, buttock, and upper portion of the thigh.

The lesions vary from mild erythema to erythematous papular lesions. Candidal (monilial) diaper dermatitis is usually very erythematous, with sharp margination and pustulovesicular satellite lesions (Figure 40-2).

Treatment involves frequent diaper changes to keep the affected area clean and dry or frequently exposing the perineal area to air. Topical antifungal medication is used to treat *C. albicans.* Short-term use of low-potency topical steroids alternately with antifungals at each diaper change helps to reduce the inflammation. Use of various topical medications to provide a barrier between the irritating agents and the skin promotes healing.

ACNE VULGARIS

Acne vulgaris is the most common skin disease; it affects 85% of the population between the ages of 12 and 25 years. Genetic influences may determine an individual's susceptibility and the severity of the disease. The incidence of acne is the same in both genders, although severe disease affects males more often.

Acne develops at distinctive pilosebaceous units known as *sebaceous follicles.* Located primarily on the face and upper parts of the chest and back, these follicles have many large sebaceous glands, a small vellus hair, and a dilated follicular canal that is visible as a pore on the skin surface. Acne lesions may be inflammatory or noninflammatory (Figure 40-3). In **noninflammatory acne,** the comedones are open (blackheads) and closed (whiteheads), with the accumulated material causing distention of the follicle and thinning of follicular canal walls. **Inflammatory acne** develops in closed comedones when the follicular wall ruptures, expelling sebum into the surrounding dermis and initiating inflammation. Pustules form when the inflammation is close to the surface; papules and cystic nodules can develop when the inflammation is deeper, causing mild to severe scarring. Both types of lesions may exist in the same individual.

The principal causative factors are hyperkeratinization of the follicular epithelium, excessive sebum production, and follicular proliferation of *Propionibacterium acnes* with release of inflammatory mediators. Androgens (dihydrotestosterone and testosterone) increase the size and productivity of the sebaceous glands and promote *P. acnes.*[3] Acne begins with sebum accumulation that obstructs the pilosebaceous unit. The accumulated material and bacteria within

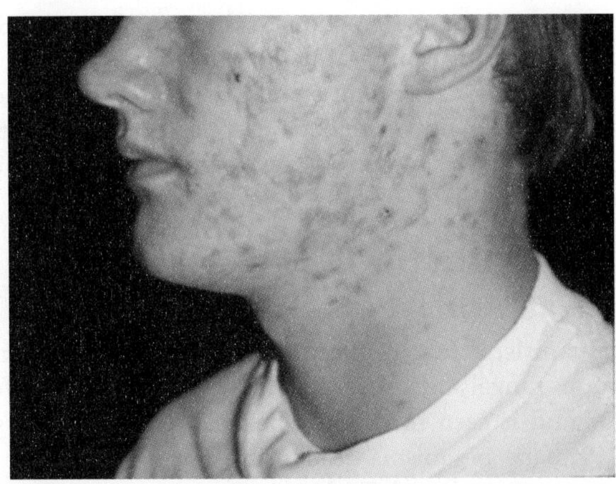

Figure 40-3 ■ **Cystic Acne.** Multiple pustules (erythematous papules and pustules) are present, and several have become confluent. Note areas of scarring. (Courtesy Department of Dermatology, School of Medicine, University of Utah.)

the follicle (see Figure 40-3) produce inflammation with rupture of a follicle.

Acne conglobata is a highly inflammatory form of acne with communicating cysts and abscesses beneath the skin that can cause scarring. Remissions tend to occur during the summer, perhaps from more exposure to sunlight.

Topical treatment, including benzoyl peroxide, salicylic acid, and retinoids, should be the first line of therapy because it is the least invasive. Use of systemic therapies, including oral antibiotics, sex hormones, corticosteroids, and isotretinoin, may be limited by side effects.[4] Acne surgery, including comedo extraction, intralesional steroids, and cryosurgery, is useful in selected patients. Severe scarring may be treated with dermabrasion, lasers, and resurfacing techniques.

QUICK CHECK 40-1

1. What causes the inflammation of acne vulgaris?
2. What lesions are typical of atopic dermatitis in children?
3. What causes diaper dermatitis?

INFECTIONS OF THE SKIN

Infectious diseases caused by bacteria, viruses, and fungi constitute the major forms of skin disease. Skin infections are caused by breaks in the skin or alterations in the protective barrier functions of the skin with resulting introduction of pathogens. Most infections tend to occur superficially; however, systemic signs and symptoms do develop occasionally and can be life threatening.

Bacterial Infections

Impetigo contagiosum

Impetigo is a common bacterial skin infection in infants and children, usually caused by staphylococcus and streptococcus. The disease is more common in midsummer to late summer, with a higher incidence in hot, humid climates. Impetigo is particularly infectious among people living in crowded conditions with poor sanitary facilities. It affects children in good health, but conditions such as anemia and malnutrition are predisposing factors. There are two types of impetigo: vesicular and, more rarely, bullous[5] (Box 40-1). Both start as vesicles with a thin vesicular roof composed of stratum corneum (Figure 40-4).

BOX 40-1 Impetigo

Vesicular Impetigo

Contagious, acute, superficial, vesiculopustular and most common form

Caused by group A *Streptococcus pyogenes* (alone or with *S. aureus*)

Spread by direct physical contact with other infected individuals or through insect bites

Presents as small vesicles with a honey-colored serum; yellow to white-brown crusts form as vesicles rupture and extend radially

Untreated lesions last for weeks and cover large area

Regional lymphadenitis common

Most significant complication is acute glomerulonephritis

Treatment is aggressive in light of this complication

Bullous Impetigo

Caused by *Staphylococcus aureus*

Bacterial toxin produced (exfoliative toxin [ET]) causes disruption in cellular adhesion with blister formation

Occurs in neonates

Highly contagious

Source is family member with pustule or asymptomatic carrier with pathogen in anterior nares, perineal region, or fingernails

Transmitted by contact with individual or contaminated equipment

Presents with vesicles that enlarge or coalesce to form superficial bullae, few localized lesions or many scattered over the skin surface; as bullae rupture, thin, flat, honey-colored crust appears (hallmark of impetigo)

Lesions found on face around the nose and mouth; hands and other exposed areas also susceptible

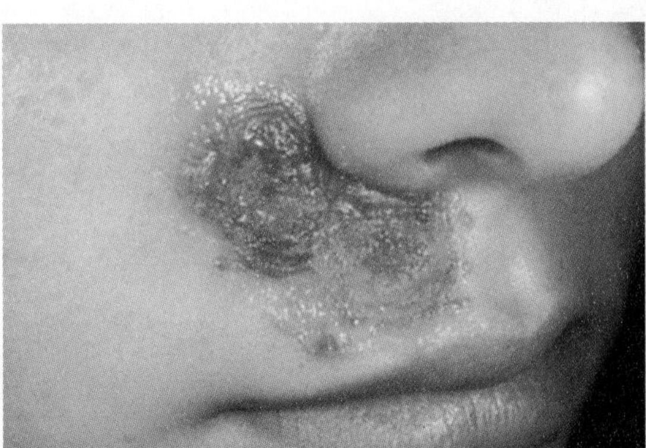

Figure 40-4 ■ **Impetigo and Herpes Simplex Virus (HSV) of Upper Lip.** Note weeping and crusting lesions. (Courtesy Department of Dermatology, School of Medicine, University of Utah.)

The treatment of choice for both types of impetigo is topical mupirocin for uncomplicated lesions or systemic antibiotics. Prompt treatment avoids complications, such as glomerulonephritis. Removal of crusts and scrubbing the lesions with antibacterial soaps has not been effective.[6] Good handwashing techniques and isolation of the infected child's washcloth, towels, drinking glass, and linen are important.

Staphylococcal scalded-skin syndrome

Staphylococcal scalded-skin syndrome (SSSS) is the most serious staphylococcal infection that affects the skin. It is caused by infection with group II staphylococci, which produce a toxin—an epidermolysin that causes a separation of the skin just below the granular layer of the epidermis. The syndrome is more common in children younger than 10 years than it is in adults. Adults have circulating antistaphylococcal antibodies and are better able to metabolize and excrete the toxin. Neonates are at the highest risk because of their lack of immunity, not having prior exposure to the toxin.

The clinical symptoms begin with fever, malaise, rhinorrhea, and irritability followed by generalized erythema with exquisite tenderness of the skin. There may be an associated impetigo, but the infection often begins in the throat or chest. The erythema spreads from the face and trunk to cover the entire body except for the palms, soles, and mucous membranes. Within 48 hours, blisters and bullae may form, and the pain is severe (Figure 40-5). Fluid loss from ruptured blisters and water evaporation from denuded areas may cause dehydration. Perioral and nasolabial crusting and fissures develop. In severe cases, the skin of the entire body may slough. When secondary infection can be prevented, healing of the involved skin occurs in 10 to 14 days, usually without scarring. Before medical intervention is initiated, culture, histology, or exfoliative cytology must be done to differentiate SSSS from *erythema multiforme* and *toxic epidermal necrolysis* (TEN), which are usually caused by an immune reaction to drugs.[7] When the SSSS infection is confirmed, treatment with oral or intravenous antibiotics begins. The skin should be treated the same as a severe burn, with meticulous aseptic technique. Special care is required when there is involvement of the lips and eyelids.

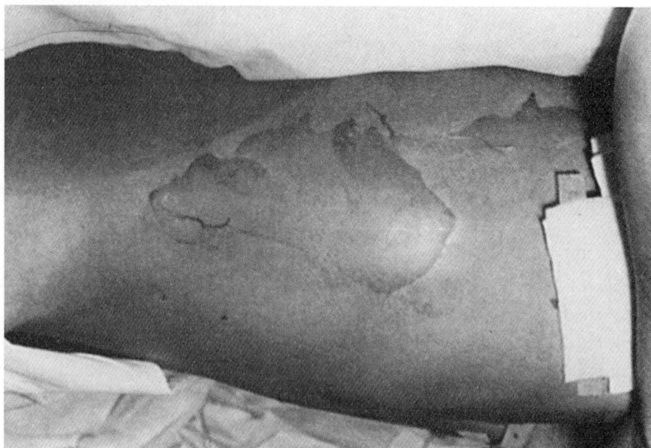

Figure 40-5 ■ Staphylococcal Scalded-Skin Syndrome (SSSS). The skin lesions, showing desquamation and wrinkling of the skin margins, appeared 1 day after drainage of a staphylococcal abscess. (From Levine G, Norden C: *N Engl J Med* 287:1339, 1972.)

Fungal Infections

Tinea capitis

Tinea capitis, a fungal infection of the scalp, is the most common fungal infection of childhood. It rarely affects infants and is seen in children between 2 and 10 years of age. Primary organisms responsible for this disease are *Microsporum canis* and *Trichophyton tonsurans. M. canis* is found on cats, dogs, and certain rodents. Humans appear to be a terminal host for *M. canis,* and children who handle such animals are possible hosts. Human-to-human transmission does not occur. *T. tonsurans* conversely is transmitted human to human, with areas of crowding the most prevalent environments of the fungus. Often, the lesions are circular and manifested by broken hairs 1 to 3 mm above the scalp, leaving a partial area of alopecia from 1 to 5 cm in diameter (Figure 40-6). A slight erythema and scaling with raised borders can be observed.

Diagnosis is best confirmed by performing Wood light examination, potassium hydroxide (KOH) examination, and fungal culture, in that order. Several oral antifungal agents, particularly griseofulvin, are available for treatment.[8]

Tinea corporis

Tinea corporis is a common superficial dermatophyte infection in children. The organisms most commonly responsible for this disease are *M. canis* and *Trichophyton mentagrophytes.* As in tinea capitis, contact with young kittens and puppies is a common source of the disorder. Tinea corporis preferentially affects the nonhairy parts of the face, trunk, and limbs. Lesions are often erythematous, round or oval scaling patches that spread peripherally with clearing in the center, creating the ring appearance, which is why this disease is commonly referred to as *ringworm.*

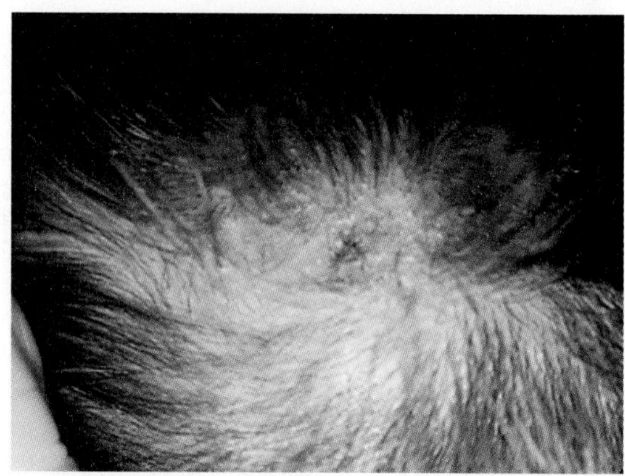

Figure 40-6 ■ Tinea Capitis. (Courtesy Department of Dermatology, School of Medicine, University of Utah.)

The lesions are distributed asymmetrically, and multiple lesions, when present, overlap. Potassium hydroxide examination of the scale from the border of the lesions confirms the diagnosis. Most lesions respond well to applications of appropriate topical antifungal medications.[9]

Thrush

Thrush is the term used to describe the presence of *Candida* in the mucous membranes of the mouth of infants and, less commonly, adults. Thrush is characterized by the formation of white plaques or spots in the mouth that lead to shallow ulcers caused by keratolytic proteases from the microorganism. The tongue may have a dense, white covering. The underlying mucous membrane is red and tender and may bleed when the plaques are removed. The disease is often accompanied by fever and gastrointestinal irritation. The infection commonly spreads to the groin, buttocks, and other parts of the body. Treatment may be difficult and may include oral antifungal washes, such as nystatin oral suspension. Simultaneous treatment of a *Candida* nipple infection or vaginitis in the mother is helpful in reducing the *C. albicans* surface colonization of the infant. Feeding bottles and nipples should be sterilized to prevent reinfection. The diaper area should be kept clean and dry.

Viral Infections

Viral infections of the skin in children are caused by poxvirus, papovavirus, and herpesvirus.

Molluscum contagiosum

Molluscum contagiosum is a common, highly contagious viral infection of the skin and, occasionally, conjunctiva that affects primarily children. The poxvirus proliferates within the follicular epithelium and induces epidermal cell proliferation. The epidermis grows down into the dermis to form saccules containing clusters of virus. The characteristic molluscum body is composed of mature, immature, and incomplete viruses and cellular debris.[10] The disease is transmitted by skin-to-skin contact or from contact with contaminated clothing, washcloths, or towels. The incidence is higher among children who swim in public pools.[11]

The lesions of molluscum are discrete, slightly umbilicated, dome-shaped papules 1 to 5 mm in diameter that appear anywhere on the skin or conjunctiva. The lesions are mainly on the trunk, face, and extremities in children (Figure 40-7). There is usually no inflammation surrounding molluscum lesions unless they are traumatized or secondary infection occurs. Scarring occurs with healing.

The best three diagnostic procedures are (1) staining smears of the expressed molluscum body, (2) examining a biopsy specimen, or (3) inoculating a molluscum suspension into cell cultures to demonstrate the cytotoxic reactions. Most lesions are self-limiting and clear in 6 to 9 months if not manipulated. The papules can be removed by curette or destroyed with liquid nitrogen. If multiple lesions are present, however, these procedures are painful to small children and then are not justified. Imiquimod 5% cream has been used to treat these lesions, but no specific treatment has been developed.[12,13] Measures to prevent spread of infection must be taken. Recurrences are common.

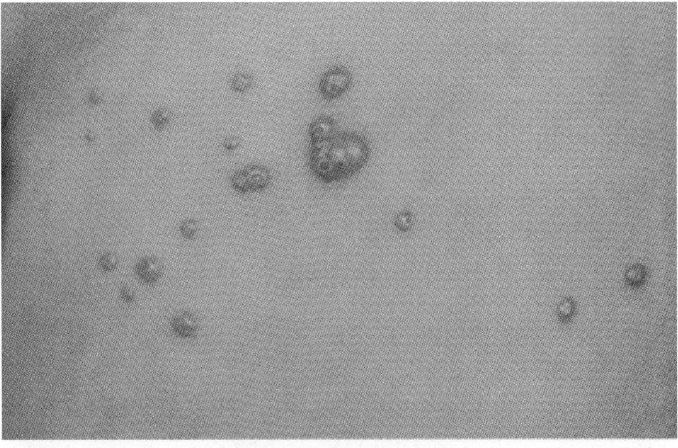

Figure 40-7 ■ **Molluscum Contagiosum.** Waxy pink globules with umbilicated centers. (From Habif TP: *Clinical dermatology: a color guide to diagnosis and therapy,* ed 4, St Louis, 2004, Mosby.)

Rubella (German or 3-day measles)

Rubella is a common communicable disease of children and young adults caused by a ribonucleic acid (RNA) virus that enters the bloodstream through the respiratory route. This disease is mild in most children. The incubation period ranges from 14 to 21 days. Prodromal symptoms include enlarged cervical and postauricular lymph nodes, low-grade fever, headache, sore throat, runny nose, and cough. A faint-pink to red coalescing maculopapular rash develops on the face with spread to the trunk and extremities 1 to 4 days after the onset of initial symptoms (Figure 40-8). The rash is thought to be the result of virus dissemination to the skin. The rash subsides after 2 to 3 days, usually without complication. Children are usually not contagious after development of the rash (Table 40-1).

Vaccination for rubella is usually combined with vaccines for mumps and measles (rubeola) (MMR) (see *Health Alert:* MMR and Varicella Vaccines). Measles is known to occur in previously immunized children.[14]

HEALTH ALERT
MMR and Varicella Vaccines

Vaccinations for measles, mumps, and rubella (MMR) are given by 12 to 15 months of age. The second vaccination is routinely administered at 4 to 6 years (if the child does not receive the second vaccine at 4 to 6 years, it should be given no later than 11 to 12 years of age as a "catchup"). The second vaccination can be given earlier but not sooner than 1 month after the first vaccine. Varicella vaccine is recommended at 12 to 18 months of age or at any time up to 13 years of age.

Data from Centers for Disease Control and Prevention: Recommended childhood and adolescent immunization schedule—United States 2006; www.cdc.gov/nip/acip.

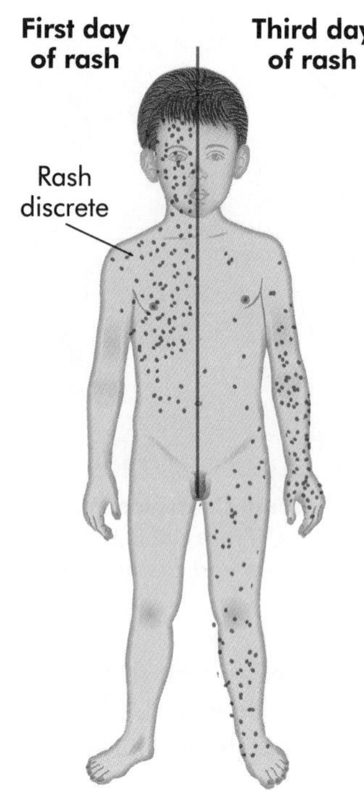

Figure 40-8 ■ **Rubella (3-Day Measles).** Typical distribution of full-blown maculopapular rash with tendency to coalesce.

There is no specific treatment for rubella. Recovery is spontaneous, although lymph nodes may remain enlarged for weeks. Supportive therapy includes rest, fluids, and use of a vaporizer. In rare cases, a mild encephalitis or peripheral neuritis may follow rubella.

Women of childbearing age are immunized if their rubella hemagglutination-inhibition titer is low. Pregnancy should be avoided for 3 months after vaccination because the attenuated virus in the vaccine may remain for this period. Pregnant women who have rubella early in the first trimester may have a fetus that develops congenital defects.

Rubeola (red measles)

Rubeola is a highly contagious, acute viral disease of children. Transmitted by direct contact with droplets from infected persons, rubeola is caused by an RNA-containing paramyxovirus with an incubation period of 7 to 12 days, during which there are no symptoms. Prodromal symptoms include high fever (up to 40.5° C), malaise, enlarged lymph nodes, runny nose, conjunctivitis, and barking cough. Within 3 to 4 days, an erythematous maculopapular rash develops over the head and spreads distally over the trunk, extremities, hands, and feet. Early lesions blanch with pressure, followed by a brownish hue that does not blanch as the rash fades. Characteristic pinpoint white spots surrounded by an erythematous ring develop over the buccal mucosa and are known as *Koplik spots.* These spots precede the rash by 1 to 2 days. The rash then subsides within 3 to 5 days.

Complications associated with measles may be caused by the primary infection or by a secondary bacterial infection. Measles encephalitis occurs in about 1 of 800 cases, and most children recover completely. Only a small minority develop permanent brain damage or die. Bacterial complications include otitis media and pneumonia, usually caused by group A hemolytic streptococcus, *Haemophilus influenzae*, or *S. aureus* infection.

Measles is prevented by vaccination. There is no specific treatment for measles, and supportive therapy is the same as for rubella. Antibiotic therapy is initiated if secondary bacterial infections develop.

Roseola (exanthema subitum)

Roseola is a presumed viral infection of infants between 6 months and 2 years of age and can be seen in children up

TABLE 40-1

Differential Presentation of Viral Diseases Producing Rashes

Viral Disease	Incubation Period	Prodromal Symptoms	Duration/ Characteristics	Clinical Symptoms
Rubella (German measles)	14–21 days	1–2 days Mild fever Malaise Respiratory symptoms	1–3 days Pink-red maculopapular Face and trunk	Enlarged and tender occipital and periauricular nodes
Rubeola (measles)	7–12 days	2–5 days Fever Cough Respiratory symptoms	3–5 days Purple-red to brown maculopapular Face, trunk, extremities	Koplik spots 1–3 days before rash
Roseola (exanthema subitum)	5–15 days	2–5 days High fever	1–3 days Red macular Neck and trunk	Rash develops when fever subsides
Varicella (chickenpox)	11–20 days	1–2 days Low-grade fever Cough May be asymptomatic	7–14 days Red papules, vesicles, pustules in clusters	Eruption of new lesions for 4–5 days Occasional ulcerative lesion in the mouth

to 4 years of age. The incubation period is 5 to 15 days, followed by the sudden onset of fever (38.9° to 40.5° C) that lasts for 3 to 5 days. After the fever, an erythematous macular rash that lasts about 24 hours develops primarily over the trunk and neck. Children usually feel well, eat normally, and have few other symptoms. There is usually no treatment.

Chickenpox, herpes zoster, and smallpox

Chickenpox

Chickenpox is a disease of early childhood, with 90% of children contracting the disease during the first decade of life. Being a highly contagious virus, chickenpox is spread by close person-to-person contact and by airborne droplets. Introduction of an infected person into a household results in 90% possibility of susceptible persons developing the disease within the incubation period, usually 14 days. Children are contagious for at least 1 day before development of the rash. Transmission of the virus may occur until approximately 5 to 6 days after the onset of the first skin lesions in normal children. In immunocompromised children, the virus is recoverable for a longer period, but infected children must be considered contagious for at least 7 to 10 days. Chickenpox occurs most commonly in the late winter and early spring. Transmission occurs more readily in temperate climates than in tropical climates.

Normally, children who develop chickenpox have no prodromal symptoms. The first sign of illness may be itching or the appearance of vesicles, usually on the trunk, scalp, or face. The rash later spreads to the extremities. Characteristically, lesions can be seen in various stages of maturation with macules, papules, and vesicles present in a particular area at the same time (Figure 40-9). The vesicular lesions are superficial and rupture easily. New lesions will erupt for 4 to 5 days, until there are approximately 100 to 300 in different stages of development. The vesicles become crusted, and over time only the crust remains, although there may be an occasional vesicle on the palm later in the disease. Although uncommon, ulcerative lesions are sometimes seen in the mouth and, less commonly, on the conjunctiva and pharynx. Fever usually lasts 2 to 3 days and ranges from 38.5° to 40° C.

Complications are rare in children but more common in adults. They can include transient hematuria (from rupture of vesicles in the bladder), epistaxis, laryngeal edema, and varicella pneumonia. One case of chickenpox produces almost complete immunity against a second attack. The fetus may be malformed if chickenpox develops in the first half of pregnancy.[15] Infants whose mothers have chickenpox at any stage of pregnancy have a higher risk of developing herpes zoster during the first few years of life.

Uncomplicated chickenpox requires no specific therapy. Baths, wet dressings, and oral antihistamines occasionally help to relieve itching and to prevent secondary infection from developing as a result of scratching. Oral antistaphylococcal drugs should be given if secondary bacterial infection

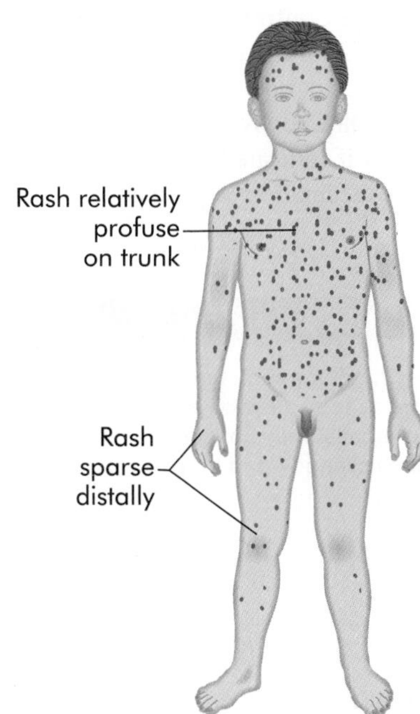

Figure 40-9 ■ **Chickenpox.** Pattern of generalized, polymorphous eruption.

is present. Zoster immune globulin may be administered to immunodeficient individuals if given within 72 hours after exposure to chickenpox. Oral acyclovir may be valuable in immunosuppressed or other select groups of children. The varicella vaccine protects against both varicella and herpes zoster. However, wild (vaccine resistant) type viruses are a continuing threat.[16]

Herpes zoster

Although **herpes zoster (shingles)** occurs mainly in adults, approximately 5% of cases are in children younger than 15 years. The course of the disease in children with an immune defect is more complicated and requires intravenous treatment with antiviral agents.[17] The chickenpox virus persists for life in sensory nerve ganglia and can reactivate to cause herpes zoster. The eruption of zoster consists of groups of vesicles situated on an inflammatory base and follows the course of a sensory nerve. Common dermatomal distribution in childhood is thoracic. The base of the lesions often appears hemorrhagic, and some of the lesions may become necrotic and ulcerative. Therapy is similar to that for chickenpox unless it is ophthalmic or disseminated zoster, for which systemic antiviral medication is indicated.

Smallpox

Smallpox (variola) was a highly contagious and deadly, but also preventable, disease caused by poxvirus variolae. Smallpox was eradicated worldwide in 1977. Routine vaccination in the United States was discontinued in 1972, and vaccine production ceased in 1983. Some samples of the virus were reported to have been stored in laboratory settings, and there has been concern that smallpox virus may be in the hands of bioterrorists. In response to this concern, the

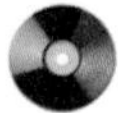

Centers for Disease Control and Prevention have proposed criteria for isolation of infected individuals (if that should occur) and for vaccination of those at risk within 4 days after exposure, followed by more widespread vaccination of the population if indicated.[18] The most serious possible complication of vaccination is postvaccinal encephalitis.

QUICK CHECK 40-2

1. Compare impetigo and staphylococcal scalded-skin syndrome as to cause and presentation.
2. Describe rubella and rubeola.
3. How are chickenpox and herpes zoster related?

INSECT BITES AND PARASITES

Insect bites and infestations are common causes of skin disorders in children and adults. Skin damage occurs by various mechanisms, including trauma of bites and stings, allergic reactions, transmission of disease, injection of substances that cause local or systemic reactions, and inflammatory reactions, resulting from embedded and retained insect mouth parts.

Scabies

Scabies is a contagious disease caused by the itch mite, Sarcoptes scabiei (Figure 40-10, *A*), that can colonize the human epidermis. It is transmitted by close personal contact and by infected clothing and bedding. Scabies is often epidemic in areas of overcrowded housing and poor sanitation. Immunocompromised individuals are at greater risk. Infestation is initiated by a female mite that tunnels into the stratum corneum, depositing eggs and creating a burrow several millimeters to 1 centimeter long. Over a 3-week period, the eggs mature into adult mites, which sometimes are recognized as tiny dots at the ends of intact burrows.

Symptoms appear 3 to 5 weeks after infestation. The primary lesions are burrows, papules, and vesicular lesions, with severe itching that worsens at night. Itching is thought to be related to sensitization to the larval stages of the parasite. In older children and adults, the lesions occur in the webs of fingers; axillae; creases of the arms and wrists; along the belt line; and around the nipples, genitalia, and lower buttocks. Infants and young children have a different pattern of distribution, with involvement of the palms, soles, head, neck, and face (Figure 40-10, *B*). Secondary infections and crusting develop as a result of scratching and eczematous changes.

Diagnosis of scabies is made by observation of the tunnels and burrows and microscopic examination of scrapings of the skin to identify the mite or its eggs or feces. Treatment involves the application of a scabicide, which is curative. All clothing and linens should be washed and dried in hot cycles or dry-cleaned.

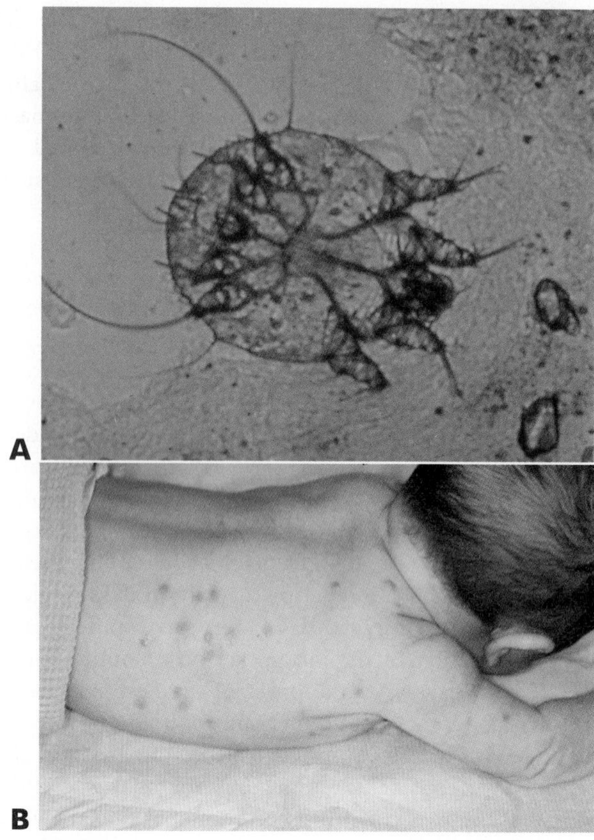

Figure 40-10 ■ **Scabies. A,** Scabies mite, as seen clinically when removed from its burrow. **B,** Characteristic scabies bites. (Courtesy Department of Dermatology, School of Medicine, University of Utah.)

Pediculosis (Lice Infestation)

The three known types of human lice are (1) the head louse *(Pediculus capitis)*, (2) the body louse *(Pediculus corporis)*, and (3) the crab or pubic louse *(Phthirus pubis)*. They are parasites and survive by sucking blood. The female louse reproduces every 2 weeks, producing hundreds of nits as newly hatched lice mate with older lice. The mouthparts are shaped for piercing and sucking and are attached to the skin of the host while the louse is feeding. When piercing the skin, the louse secretes a toxic saliva, and the mechanical trauma and toxin produce a pruritic dermatitis. Head and body lice are acquired by personal contact and sharing of combs or brushes. Crab lice are spread by close body contact, usually with an infected adult. Sharing clothing or headphones are also common sources of transmission.

Itching is the major symptom of lice infestation. With head lice, the ova attach to hairs above the ears and in the occipital region. The primary lesion caused by the body louse is a pinpoint red macule, papule, or wheal with a hemorrhagic puncture site. The primary lesion often is not seen, because it is masked by excoriations, wheals, and crusts. The crab louse is found on pubic hairs but also may be found in other body hair, such as eyelashes, mustache, beard, and underarm axillae hair. Young children in particular may become infected with crab lice on their eyebrows or eyelashes.

The live louse, 2 to 3 mm long, is rarely observed, although the ova, or nits, can be observed as oval, yellowish, pinpoint specks fastened to a hair shaft. The ova fluoresce under an ultraviolet light (Wood lamp) and are observed best with a microscope. Pediculicides, such as lindane shampoo or lotion, are the most effective treatment. All clothes, towels, bedding, combs, and brushes should be washed and dried in hot air or instead washed in boiling water, or clothes can be ironed to rid them of lice. Individuals who have close personal contact with the infected person also should be treated.

Fleas

Young children are very susceptible to **fleabites;** bites from cat, dog, and human fleas are most common.[19] Bites occur in clusters along the arms and legs or where clothing is tight fitting, such as near elastic bands that circle the thigh or waist. The bite produces an urticarial wheal with a central hemorrhagic puncture (Figure 40-11). Treatment includes spraying carpets, crevices, and furniture with Malathion or lindane powder. Infected animals should be treated, and clothes and bedding should be washed in hot water.

Ticks

Lyme disease is a multisystem (skin, joints, nervous system, heart) inflammatory disease caused by the spirochete *Borrelia burgdorferi,* which is transmitted by tick bites. The highest incidence of this disease is among children, and 50% of infected individuals are symptom free. The incidence is increasing.[20] The disease occurs in stages, and the mechanisms of injury are not well understood:

1. Soon after bite, localized infection (rash—erythema migrans, myalgia, and fatigue)
2. Nine months later, disseminated infection (secondary erythema migrans, arthralgias, meningitis, neuritis, carditis)
3. Late persistent infection continuing for years (arthritis, encephalopathy, polyneuropathy)

The microorganism is difficult to culture.

The diagnosis of Lyme disease is based on the clinical presentation; history of tick bite, if known; and serology. Culture and serologic tests confirm the diagnosis.[21] Antibiotics (such as, doxycycline or amoxicillin) are used for treatment, although the response may be slow. Prevention of tick bites is essential.

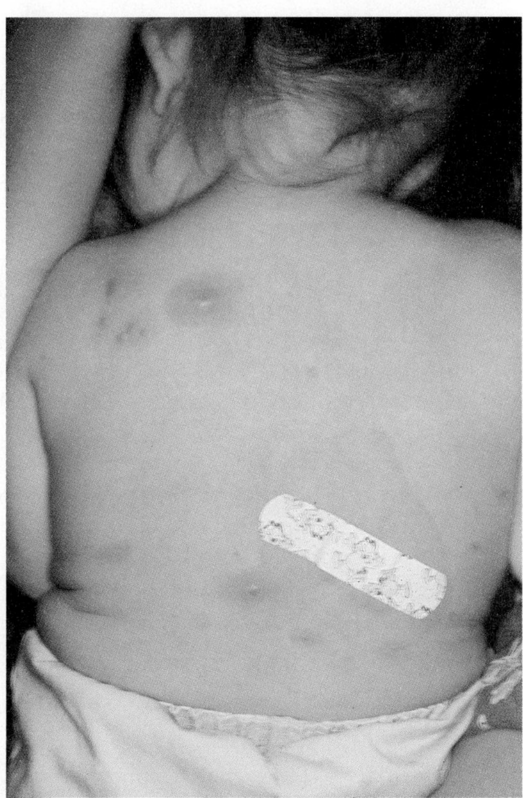

Figure 40-11 ■ **Flea Bites.** Fleabite producing an urticarial wheal with central puncture.

Bedbugs

Bedbugs *(Cimex lectularius)* are blood-sucking parasites that live in the crevices and cracks of floors, walls, and furniture and in bedding or furniture stuffing. They are 3 to 5 mm long and reddish brown. Bedbugs emerge to feed in darkness and attach to the skin to suck blood. Feeding occurs for 5 to 15 minutes, and the bedbug then leaves. It will move long distances to search for food and can travel from house to house.

If the host has not been previously sensitized, the only symptom is a red macule that develops into a nodule, lasting up to 14 days. In sensitized children and adults, pruritic wheals, papules, and vesicles may form. Secondary infections require treatment. Bedbugs are eliminated by spraying with chlordane or lindane and by cleaning or disposing of infested bedding, mattresses, and furniture.

HEMANGIOMAS AND VASCULAR MALFORMATIONS

Vascular anomalies occur in about 10% of infants and are categorized as either hemangiomas or vascular malformations.[22]

Hemangiomas

Hemangiomas are benign tumors that form from the rapid growth of vascular endothelial cells, which results in formation of extra blood vessels. Infiltration of fat cells, fibrosis, and the rich vascular network give the lesions a firm, rubbery feel. Females are affected more often than males. About 30% of hemangiomas are apparent at birth, with most emerging during the first few weeks of life. They grow rapidly during the first few years of life, then shrink or involute during childhood years. With involution the lesions become darker in color and then gradually turn to a flesh color. There may be some residual telangiectasia. Most require no treatment depending on location.

Hemangiomas located over the eye, ear, nose, mouth, urethra, or anus may require treatment because they interfere with function and have a higher risk for infection or injury. Systemic or intralesional steroids are the treatment of choice. Interferons, vincristine, and radiotherapy can suppress angiogenesis. Cryosurgery, laser surgery, and sclerotherapy are also alterative treatment options.[23] Hemangiomas can be superficial or deep. Superficial hemangiomas are known as capillary or strawberry hemangiomas, and deep lesions are known as cavernous hemangiomas.

Strawberry (capillary) hemangiomas are distinct, raised vascular lesion that may be present at birth but usually emerge 3 to 5 weeks after birth. They proliferate and become bright red and elevated with minute capillary projections that give them a strawberry appearance. Usually there is only one lesion, and it is located on the head and neck area or trunk (Figure 40-12). After the initial growth, the lesion grows at the same rate as the child and then starts to involute at 12 to 16 months of age. Approximately 90% of strawberry hemangiomas involute by 5 to 6 years of age, usually without scarring.

Cavernous hemangiomas are present at birth and have larger and more mature vessels within the lesion than strawberry hemangiomas. Some lesions, however, are composed of a mixture of strawberry and cavernous hemangiomas. They appear primarily on the head and neck area and have a bluish red color with less distinct borders (Figure 40-13). Cavernous hemangiomas grow rapidly up to 6 months of age and mature by 1 year of age. A period of involution begins and proceeds for 6 to 12 months, with complete involution by 2 to 3 years in 30% of children and by 9 years of age in 90% of children.

Vascular Malformations

Vascular malformations are congenital anomalies of blood vessels that are present at birth but may not be apparent for several years.[24] They grow proportionately with the child and never regress. The malformations occur equally among males and females. Occasionally they expand rapidly, particularly during the hormonal changes of puberty or pregnancy and in association with trauma. Vascular malformations are classified as low flow or high flow. *Low-flow malformations* involve capillaries, veins, and lymphatics. *High-flow malformations* involve arteries. In addition to locations within the skin, they may involve the gastrointestinal tract, bone (Maffucci syndrome), or nerves and meninges (Surge-Weber syndrome).[25,26] *Overgrowth syndromes* can occur with either high- or low-flow malformations, with overgrowth of the underlying structures (i.e., legs, arms, facial bones). The most common vascular malformations are nevus flammeus (port-wine stains) and salmon patches (stork bite, angel kiss).

Port-wine (nevus flammeus) stains are congenital malformations of the dermal capillaries. The lesions are flat, and their color ranges from pink to dark reddish purple. They are present at birth or within a few days after birth and do not fade with age. Involvement of the face and other body surfaces is common, and the lesions may be large (Figure 40-14). Treatments using cryosurgery or tattooing are not satisfactory. The pulsed dye laser is the treatment of choice to successfully lighten the color and flatten the more nodular and cavernous lesions.[27] Waterproof cosmetics may be used to cover the lesions.

Salmon patches are macular, pink lesions present at birth and located on the nape of the neck, forehead, upper eyelids, or nasolabial fold region. They are a variant of nevus flammeus, more superficial, and one of the most common congenital malformations in the skin. The pink color results from distended dermal capillaries, and 95% fade by 1 year of age. Those located at the nape of the neck may persist for a lifetime. They generally do not present a cosmetic problem.

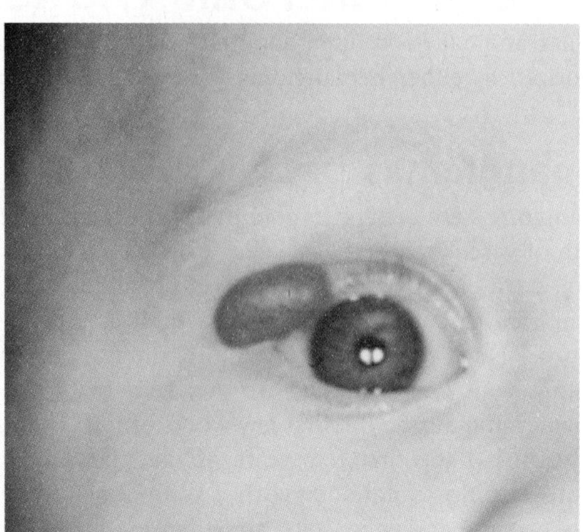

Figure 40-12 ■ **Capillary Hemangioma.** (Courtesy Department of Dermatology, School of Medicine, University of Utah.)

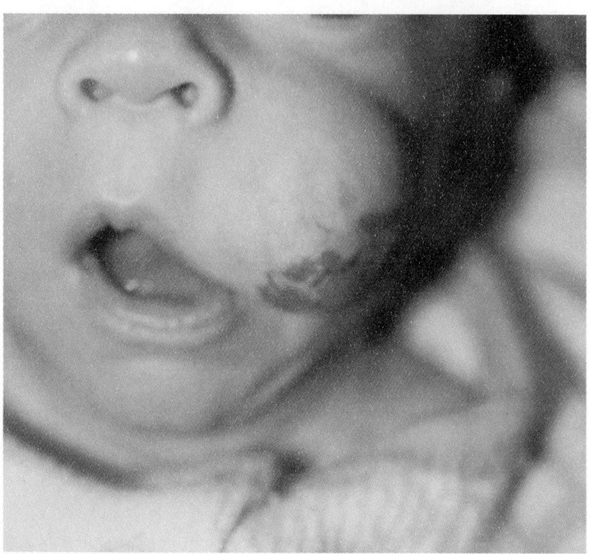

Figure 40-13 ■ **Cavernous Hemangioma.** (Courtesy Department of Dermatology, School of Medicine, University of Utah.)

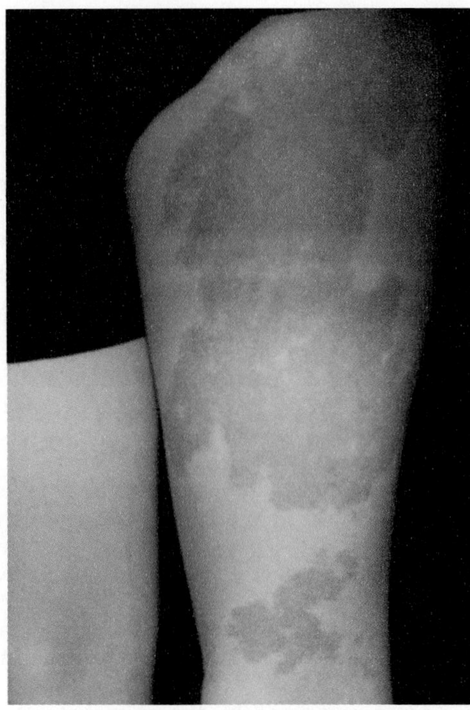

Figure 40-14 ■ **Port-Wine Hemangioma.** Port-wine hemangioma in a child. (Courtesy Department of Dermatology, School of Medicine, University of Utah.)

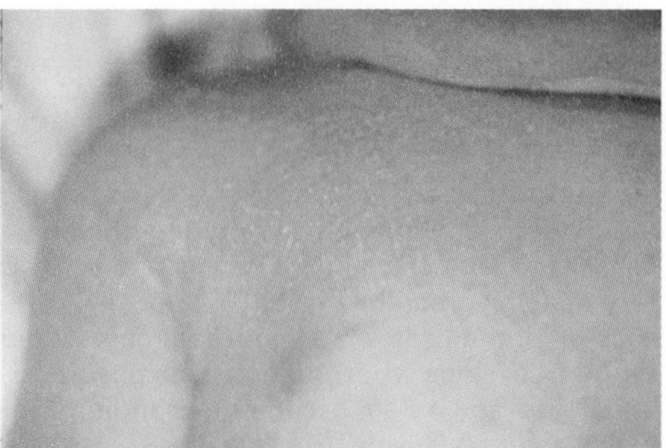

Figure 40-15 ■ **Miliaria Rubra.** Note discrete erythematous papules or papulovesicles. (Courtesy Department of Dermatology, School of Medicine, University of Utah.)

OTHER SKIN DISORDERS

Miliaria

Miliaria is a dermatosis commonly seen in infants that is characterized by a vesicular eruption after prolonged exposure to perspiration with subsequent obstruction of the eccrine ducts. There are two forms of miliaria: **miliaria crystallina** and **miliaria rubra.** In miliaria crystallina, ductal rupture occurs within the stratum corneum and appears as 1- to 2-mm clear vesicles without erythema. They rupture within 24 to 48 hours and leave a white scale. In miliaria rubra, the ductal rupture occurs in the lower epidermis with inflammatory cells attracted to the site of the rupture. Miliaria rubra (prickly heat) is characterized by 2- to 4-mm discrete erythematous papules or papulovesicles (Figure 40-15). Both forms may become secondarily infected, requiring systemic antibiotics. The key to management is avoidance of excessive heat and humidity, which cause sweating. Light clothing, cool baths, and air conditioning assist in keeping the skin surface dry and cool.

Erythema Toxicum Neonatorum

Erythema toxicum neonatorum (toxic erythema of the newborn) is a benign, erythematous accumulation of macules, papules, or pustules that appear at birth or 3 to 4 days after birth. The lesions first appear as a blotchy, macular erythematous rash. The macules vary from 1 mm to 1 cm. When papules or pustules develop, they are light yellow or white and 1 to 3 mm in diameter. There may be a few or several hundred lesions, and any body surface can be affected, with the exception of the palms and soles, where there are no pilosebaceous follicles. The cause of the lesion is unknown, and it is self-limiting. No treatment is required.

✔ QUICK CHECK 40-3

1. Give two examples of insect bites or parasites that affect children. What features are observed in each?
2. Compare a strawberry hemangioma and a cavernous hemangioma.

Did You Understand?

Dermatitis

1. Atopic dermatitis commonly occurs as red, scaly lesions on the face, cheeks, and flexor surfaces of the extremities in infants and young children and is associated with elevated IgE levels and a family history of asthma and hay fever.
2. Diaper dermatitis is a type of irritant contact dermatitis that develops from prolonged exposure to urine and feces and often becomes secondarily infected with *Candida albicans.*

Acne Vulgaris

1. Acne vulgaris is a common disorder related to obstruction of pilosebaceous follicles and proliferation of *Propionibacterium acnes*, primarily of the face, neck, and upper trunk. It is characterized by both noninflammatory and inflammatory lesions.

Infections of the Skin

1. Impetigo is a contagious bacterial disease occurring in two forms: bullous and vesicular. The toxins from the bacteria produce a weeping lesion with a honey-colored crust.
2. Staphylococcal scalded-skin syndrome (SSSS) is a staphylococcal skin infection that occurs more commonly in young children with low titers of antistaphylococcal antibody. Painful blisters and bullae form over large areas of the skin, requiring systemic antibiotics for treatment.
3. Tinea capitis and tinea corporis are fungal infections of the scalp and body caused by dermatophytes.
4. Thrush is a fungal infection of the mouth caused by *Candida albicans.*
5. Molluscum contagiosum is a poxvirus of the skin that produces pale papular lesions filled with viral and cellular debris.
6. Rubella (3-day measles) is a communicable viral disease characterized by fever, sore throat, enlarged cervical and postauricular nodes, and a generalized maculopapular rash that lasts 1 to 4 days.
7. Rubeola is a viral contagious disease with symptoms of high fever, enlarged lymph nodes, conjunctivitis, and a red rash that begins on the head, spreads to the trunk and extremities, and lasts 3 to 5 days. Both bacterial and viral complications may accompany rubeola.
8. Roseola is a benign disease of infants with a sudden onset of fever that lasts 3 to 5 days, followed by a rash that lasts 24 hours.
9. Chickenpox (varicella) is a highly contagious disease caused by the varicella-zoster virus. Vesicular lesions occur on the skin and mucous membranes. Individuals are contagious from 1 day before the development of the rash until about 5 to 6 days after the rash develops.
10. Herpes zoster (shingles) is a viral eruption of vesicles on the skin along the distribution of a sensory nerve caused by chickenpox virus that persists in sensory nerve ganglia.
11. Smallpox (variola) was a highly contagious, deadly viral disease that has been eradicated worldwide by vaccination but may be a bioterrorist threat.

Insect Bites and Parasites

1. Scabies is an itching lesion caused by the itch mite, which burrows into the skin forming papules and vesicles. The mite is very contagious and is transmitted by direct contact.
2. Pediculosis (lice infestation) is caused by blood-sucking parasites that secrete a toxic saliva and damage the skin to produce a pruritic dermatitis. Lice are spread by direct contact and are recognized by the ova or nits that attach to the shafts of body hairs.
3. Fleabites produce a pruritic wheal with a central puncture site and occur as clusters in areas of tight-fitting clothing.
4. Lyme disease is caused by the spirochete *Borrelia burgdorferi* transmitted by tick bites with cutaneous and systemic inflammatory symptoms.
5. Bedbugs are blood-sucking parasites that live in cracks of floors, furniture, or bedding and feed at night. They produce pruritic wheals and nodules.

Vascular Disorders

1. Hemangiomas are benign tumors that form from the rapid growth of vascular endothelial cells and result in formation of extra blood vessels.
2. A strawberry hemangioma is a vascular lesion present at birth that proliferates in size and then grows at the same rate as the child. Most lesions resolve spontaneously by 5 years of age.
3. A cavernous hemangioma is present at birth, with larger vessels than a strawberry hemangioma, and is bluish red. Cavernous hemangiomas usually involute by 9 years of age and may require surgical removal if located near the eyes, nares, or genitalia.
4. Salmon patches are macular pink lesions with dilated capillaries that usually resolve by 1 year of age.
5. Port-wine stains are congenital malformations of dermal capillaries that do not fade with age.

Other Skin Disorders

1. Miliaria is small pruritic papules or vesicles that result from closure of the sweat duct opening in infants.
2. Erythema toxicum neonatorum is a benign accumulation of macules, papules, and pustules that spontaneously resolves within a few weeks after birth.

Key Terms

Acne conglobata, 1123
Acne vulgaris, 1122
Atopic dermatitis (AD), 1121
Bedbug, 1129
Cavernous hemangioma, 1130
Chickenpox, 1127
Diaper dermatitis, 1122
Erythema toxicum neonatorum, 1131
Fleabite, 1129
Herpes zoster (shingles), 1127
Impetigo, 1123
Inflammatory acne, 1122
Lyme disease, 1129
Miliaria, 1131
Miliaria crystallina, 1131
Miliaria rubra, 1131
Molluscum contagiosum, 1125
Noninflammatory acne, 1122
Port-wine (nevus flammeus) stain, 1130
Roseola, 1126
Rubella, 1125
Rubeola, 1126
Salmon patch, 1130
Scabies, 1128
Smallpox (variola), 1127
Staphylococcal scalded-skin syndrome (SSSS), 1124
Strawberry (capillary) hemangioma, 1130
Thrush, 1125
Tinea capitis, 1124
Tinea corporis, 1124

References

1. Stone KD: Atopic diseases of childhood, *Curr Opin Pediatr* 14(5):634–646, 2002.
2. Abramovits W: Atopic dermatitis, *J Am Acad Dermatol* 52(1 suppl 1):S86–S94, 2005.
3. Essah PA et al: Dermatology of androgen-related disorders, *Clin Dermatol* 24(4):289–298, 2006.
4. Goodman G: Managing acne vulgaris effectively, *Aust Fam Physician* 35(9):705–709, 2006.
5. Ladhani S, Garbash M: Staphylococcal skin infections in children: rational drug therapy recommendations, *Paediatr Drugs* 7(2):77–102, 2005.
6. Hacker SM: Common infections of the skin: characteristics, causes, and cures, *Postgrad Med* 96(2):43–46, 49–52, 1994.
7. Patel GK, Finlay AY: Staphylococcal scalded skin syndrome: diagnosis and management, *Am J Clin Dermatol* 4(3): 165–175, 2003.
8. Alvarez MS, Silverberg NB: Tinea capitis, *Cutis* 78(3):189–196, 2006.
9. Weinstein A, Berman B: Topical treatment of common superficial tinea infections, *Am Fam Physician* 65(10):2095–2102, 2002.
10. Smith KJ, Skelton H: Molluscum contagiosum: recent advances in pathogenic mechanisms, and new therapies, *Am J Clin Dermatol* 3(8):535–545, 2002.
11. Braue A et al: Epidemiology and impact of childhood *molluscum contagiosum*: a case series and critical review of the literature, *Pediatr Dermatol* 22(4):287–294, 2005.
12. Smolinski KN, Yan AC: How and when to treat *molluscum contagiosum* and warts in children, *Pediatr Ann* 34(3): 211–221, 2005.
13. van der Wouden JC et al: Interventions for cutaneous molluscum contagiosum, *Cochrane Database Syst Rev* (2):CD004767, 2006.
14. Ki M et al: Rubella antibody loss rates in Korean children, *Epidemiol Infect* 129(3):557–564, 2002.
15. Chickenpox, pregnancy, and the newborn: a follow-up, *Drug Ther Bull* 43(12):94–95, 2005.
16. Leung AK, Robson WL, Leong AG: Herpes zoster in childhood, *J Pediatr Health Care* 20(5):300–303, 2006.
17. Kakourou T et al: Herpes zoster in children, *J Am Acad Dermatol* 39(2 pt 1):207–210, 1998.
18. Tom WL, Kenner JR, Friedlander SF: Smallpox: vaccine reactions and contraindications, *Dermatol Clin* 22(3):275–289, vi, 2004.
19. Demain JG: Papular urticaria and things that bite in the night, *Curr Allergy Asthma Rep* 3(4):291–303, 2003.
20. Kudish K, Sleavin W, Hathcock L: Lyme disease trends: Delaware, 2000–2004, *Del Med J* 79(2):51–58, 2007.
21. DePietropaolo DL et al: Diagnosis of Lyme disease, *Am Fam Physician* 72(2):297–304, 2005.
22. Buckmiller LM: Update on hemangiomas and vascular malformations, *Curr Opin Otolaryngol Head Neck Surg* 12(6): 476–487, 2004.
23. Marler JJ, Mulliken JB: Current management of hemangiomas and vascular malformations, *Clin Plast Surg* 32(1):99–116, ix, 2005.
24. Buckmiller LM: Update on hemangiomas and vascular malformations, *Curr Opin Otolaryngol Head Neck Surg* 12(6): 476–487, 2004.
25. Baselga E: Sturge-Weber syndrome, *Semin Cutan Med Surg* 23(2):87–98, 2004.
26. Thomas-Sohl KA, Vaslow DF, Maria BL: Sturge-Weber syndrome: a review, *Pediatr Neurol* 30(5):303–310, 2004.
27. Kelly KM et al: Description and analysis of treatments for port-wine stain birthmarks, *Arch Facial Plast Surg* 7(5): 287–294, 2005.

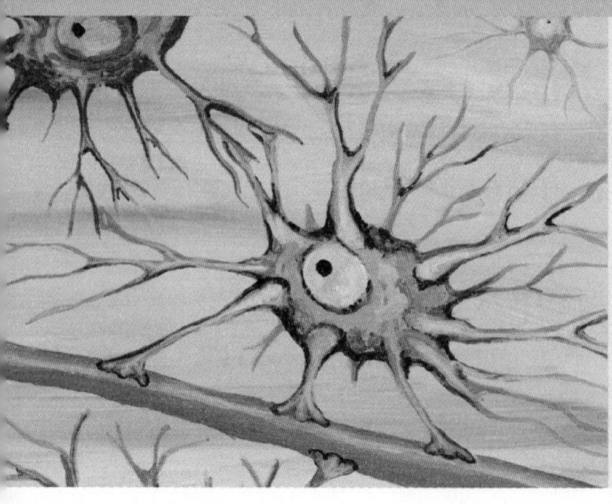

APPENDIX: MOST COMMON LABORATORY VALUES

Constituent	Normal Mean Value and Some Ranges	Normal Range in SI Units
ELECTROLYTES	Total, 1% of plasma weight	
Na^+	142 mEq/L (136-145)	136-145 mmol/L
K^+	3.5-5.0 mEq/L	3.5-5.0 mmol/L
Ca^{++} (total)	8.8-10.5 mg/dl	2.25-2.75 mmol/L
Mg^{++}	1.8-3.0 mEq/L	1.65-1.75 mmol/L
Cl^-	95-105 mEq/L	95-105 mmol/L
HCO_3^-	24-28 mEq/L	24-28 mmol/L
Phosphate (mostly $HPO_4^=$)	2.5-5.0 mg/L	0.5-1.25 mmol/L
$SO_4^=$	1 mEq/L	0.25-0.75 mmol/L
PROTEINS		
Albumins	4-6 g/dl	40.0-60.0 g/L
Gamma globulin	0.5-1.6 g/dl	5-16 g/L
Globulins	2-4 g/dl	20.0-40.0 g/L
Fibrinogen	200-400 mg/dl	2.0-4.0 g/L
BLOOD GASES		
pH	7.35-7.45	
CO_2 content (arterial)	35-45 mm Hg	4.65-5.32 kPa
O_2 content (arterial)	75-100 mm Hg	9.97-13.30 kPa
Bicarbonate	24-28 mEq/L	24-28 mmol/L
NUTRIENTS		
Glucose (fasting)	75-110 mg/dl	3.85-6.05 mmol/L
Total proteins	6-8 g/dl	60-80 gm/L
Total lipids	400-800 mg/dl	4.0-8.0 g/L
Cholesterol (total)	<200 mg/dl	< 5.20 mmol/L
Triglycerides	<160 mg/dl	< 0.45-1.81 mmol/L (males) < 0.40-1.52 mmol/L (females)
Phospholipids	150-380 mg/dl	1.50-3.80 mol/L
Free fatty acids	8.0-25.0 mg/dl	0.28-0.89 mmol
WASTE PRODUCTS		
Urea (BUN)	7-18 mg/dl	2.9-8.2 mmol/L
Uric acid	2-6 mg/dl	0.110-0.360 mmol/L
Creatinine	0.6-1.2 mg/dl	53-106 μmol/L
Creatinine clearance	107-139 ml/min	1.78-2.32 mL/s
Uric acid (from nucleic acids)	2-7 mg/dl	0.120-0.360 mmol/L
Bilirubin (direct)	Up to 0.3 mg/dl	Up to 5.1 μmol/L
Bilirubin (indirect)	0-1.0 mg/dl	1.7-5.1 μmol/L

Constituent	Normal Mean Value and Some Ranges	Normal Range in SI Units
INDIVIDUAL HORMONES		
Prolactin	<20 ng/ml	<20 μg/L
Thyroid tests		
Thyroxine (T_4) (total)	4-11 ng/dl	51-142 nmol/L
T_4 expressed as iodine	3.2-7.2 ng/dl	253-569 nmol/L
Free thyroxine (T_4)	0.8-2.4 ng/dl	10.4-30.9 nmol/L
T_3 (total)	75-220 ng/dl	1.15-3.39 nmol/L
T_3 resin uptake	25%-38% relative uptake	0.25%-0.38% relative uptake
TSH*	0.3-3.04 mIUL	0.3-3.04 mIUL
HEMATOLOGY VALUES		
Erythrocyte (red blood cell count)	4.2-6.2 million/mm^3	
Leukocyte (white blood cell count)	5000-10,000/mm^3	
Lymphocyte	25%-33% of leukocyte count (leukocyte differential)	
Monocyte and macrophage	3%-7% of leukocyte differential	
Eosinophil	1%-4% of leukocyte differential	
Neutrophil	57%-67% of leukocyte differential	
Basophil	0-0.75% of leukocyte differential	
Platelet	140,000-340,000/mm^3	
Hematocrit	40%-50%	
Hemoglobin	13.5-18.0 g/dl	
Mean corpuscular volume	80-100 fL	
OTHER		
Bile acids	0.3-3.0 mg/dl	3.00-30 mg/L
Bilirubin (total)	0.3-1.2 mg/dl	5.3-20.5 μmol/L
Bilirubin, direct (conjugated)	Up to 5.1 μmol/L	Up to 5.1 mmol/L
Bilirubin, indirect (unconjugated)	1.7-5.1 μmol/L	1.7-17.1 mmol/L
Creatine (s)	0.1-0.4 mg/dl	7.6-30.5 mmol/L
Iron, total (s)	60-150 μg/dl	11-27 μmol/L
Iron-binding capacity (s)	300-360 μg/dl	38-67 mmol/L
Lactic dehydrogenase	80-120 units at 30° C	38-62 units/L at 30° C
Acid phosphatase	Cherry-Crandall (units/dl)	0-5.5 u/L
	King-Armstrong (units/dl)	0-5.5 u/L
	Bodansky (units/dl)	0-5.5 u/L
Alkaline (units/dl)	King-Armstrong (units/dl)	30-120 u/L
	Bodansky (units/dl)	30-120 u/L
	Bessey-Lowry-Brock (units/dl)	30-120 u/L
Phosphorus, inorganic (s)	3.0-4.5 mg/dl	0.97-1.45 mmol/L
Prostate specific antigen (PSA)	<0-4 ng/mL	<0.4 μg/L

s, Serum.
*Recently changed.

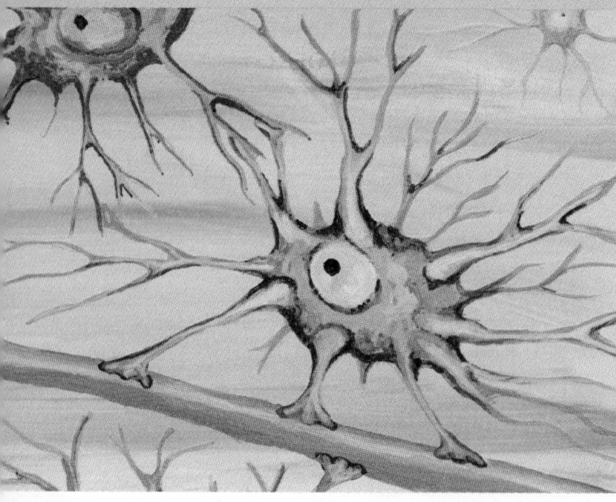

GLOSSARY

Beth A. Forshee

Absolute polycythemia A condition in which red blood cell mass increases because of a defect in the erythroid progenitor cells or an increase in circulating serum factors like erythropoietin.

Absolute refractory period A time interval during an action potential when membrane sodium channels are inactivated and cannot respond to additional stimuli.

Achalasia The failure of a sphincter, usually an esophageal sphincter, to relax completely, often because of a neuromuscular disorder of the esophagus that reduces the ability to move food down the esophagus.

Acid maltase deficiency A genetic disease in which a deficiency in lysosomal metabolism prevents the breakdown of glycogen and causes it to accumulate in the lysosomes, leading to severe muscle degradation primarily in the heart, skeletal, and respiratory muscles.

Acidosis An acid-base imbalance characterized by a reduction in arterial blood pH.

Acne conglobata A condition of severe cystic acne that is characterized by cystic lesions, abscesses, communicating sinuses, and thickened, nodular scars.

Acne rosacea A chronic form of dermatitis of the face in which the middle of the face appears red with small red lines that result from dilated capillaries.

Acne vulgaris An inflammatory eruption usually occurring on the face, upper back, and chest that consists of blackheads, cysts, papules, and pustules.

Acromegaly A condition of excessive growth hormone that originates from the anterior pituitary; it is manifest by progressive enlargement of the head, face, hands, feet, and chest.

Actinic keratosis A condition in which a premalignant small, reddish, rough spot appears on skin that has been chronically exposed to the sun.

Action potential The propagation of electrical changes in the membrane that is continued as long as the stimuli reach the electrical threshold of the membrane.

Active acquired immunity (active immunity) A form of acquired immunity in which antibody or immune lymphoid cells are formed in response to an antigen.

Active transport Movement of a substance across a membrane, which is made possible by the expenditure of energy that activates integral membrane carrier proteins; this movement is the polar opposite of the chemical or electrical gradient of the substance being transported.

Activin A protein hormone that opposes inhibin by enhancing follicle-stimulating hormone synthesis and secretion; participates in the regulation of the menstrual cycle, enhances luteinizing hormone action in the ovary and testis, and mediates spermatogenesis.

Acute bacterial prostatitis Inflammation of the prostate gland caused by a urinary tract infection; results in chills, fever, pain in the lower back and genital area, body aches, burning or painful urination, and the frequent and urgent need to urinate.

Acute epiglottitis A bacterial infection that causes inflammation of the epiglottis and surrounding tissues that may lead to upper airway blockage, which increases the work of breathing, the retention of carbon dioxide, and the reduction in oxygen intake; may cause death if left untreated.

Acute rejection Rejection of a graft within days to months after transplantation or termination of immunosuppressive drugs; caused by a cell-mediated immune response against incompatible antigens.

Acute renal failure (ARF) A condition characterized by the rapid loss of renal function resulting in retention of nitrogenous and non-nitrogenous waste products that may lead to metabolic disturbances, altered body fluid balance, or oliguria.

Acute respiratory distress syndrome (ARDS) A condition in which capillaries or alveoli of the lungs are damaged from infection, injury, blood loss, or inhalation injury causing fluid to leak from the capillaries into the alveoli and some alveoli to collapse.

Acute tubular necrosis (ATN) A condition in which the kidney undergoes ischemic or nephrotoxic injury because of severe hypotension, aminoglycosides, or radiocontrast agents; produces granular and epithelial cell casts in urine.

Adaptive immunity Immunity acquired from vaccines or prior infection.

Adenomyosis A condition characterized by benign masses of the endometrial glands in the uterine smooth muscle that typically occurs between the ages of 35 and 50 and causes painful menses.

Adhesion molecule *See* Cell adhesion molecule.

Adrenal gland Either of two small endocrine glands located above the kidney that secrete several steroid hormones, epinephrine and norepinephrine.

Adrenergic transmission Transmission of a nerve impulse using epinephrine, or norepinephrine as a neurotransmitter.

Adrenomedullin (ADM) A protein hormone discovered in human pheochromocytoma to function as a vasodilator as well as a regulator of growth cytokines and neurotransmission.

Afterload The tension or pressure that must be generated by a ventricle of the heart in order to eject blood.

Agnosia Loss of comprehension of sensory stimuli, such as sounds or images.

Aldosterone A mineralocorticoid that is synthesized and secreted by the adrenal cortex and regulates sodium and potassium balance by altering reabsorption in the kidney.

Alkalosis An acid-base imbalance characterized by elevated pH.

Allergy Hypersensitivity and immunologic protective reaction caused by exposure to an antigen.

Alloimmune disease An immune reaction in which individuals of the same species have incompatible antigens, preventing them from receiving an organ transplant from each other.

Alopecia A condition in which hair is lost because of heredity, a hormonal imbalance, certain diseases, or drugs and treatments.

Alveolar ventilation The volume of gas that reaches the alveoli per minute, or the difference between tidal volume and dead space multiplied by ventilation rate.

Amino acid Carboxylic acid with attached amino and R groups that combine with other amino acids to form a protein.

Amylin A peptide hormone secreted by the pancreatic beta cells that may function in the regulation of glucose homeostasis, gastric motor and secretory function, and gastroprotection.

Anabolism A cellular process that uses energy to synthesize complex molecules from simpler molecules.

Anaerobic glycolysis The process of adenosine triphosphate (ATP) formation in the absence of oxygen, during which carbohydrate-derived pyruvate is reduced to form lactic acid.

Anaphase Third phase of mitosis, during which centromeres are separated and sister chromatids are moved to opposite poles.

Anaphylatoxin Fragments of C3a, C4a, and C5a that degranulate mast cells, resulting in the release of histamine that vasodilates and increases capillary permeability.

Anaphylaxis A potentially life-threatening immediate hypersensitivity response caused by exposure of a sensitized individual to a specific antigen.

Anaplasia Inability of tumor cells to differentiate and orient to one another and to blood vessels.

Anemia A condition in which hemoglobin concentration is below normal because of a deficiency in red blood cells, a low level of hemoglobin in cells, or both; manifests as pallor of the skin and mucous membranes, weakness, dizziness, easy fatigability, and drowsiness resulting from oxygen deficiency.

Anencephaly Congenital abnormality in which part of the brain and skull is absent.

Aneurysm A localized dilation or ballooning of a blood vessel, usually in the arteries at the base of the brain and in the aorta.

Angina pectoris A condition in which myocardial ischemia, resulting from reduced blood flow around the heart's blood vessels, causes chest pain.

Angiogenesis The process of forming new blood vessels that occurs in the development of the embryo and fetus and in tumor formation.

Angiotensin I Inactive product of the cleavage of angiotensinogen by renin.

Angiotensin II Active hormone that is formed from the cleavage of angiotensin I by angiotensin-converting enzyme; stimulates aldosterone secretion and vasoconstriction.

Ankylosing spondylitis (AS; spondylarthritis) A condition in which the spine and sacroiliac joints are chronically inflamed, causing pain and stiffness in and around the spine and a gradual fusion of the vertebrae that immobilizes the spine.

Anomalous viscosity The alteration in viscosity of suspensions, such as blood, in which the viscosity increases as blood flow decreases.

Anorexia nervosa A mixed psychologic and physiologic disorder that begins with dieting to lose weight but over time becomes a sign of control and continued restrictive eating; may lead to starvation and eventual death.

Anoxia A lack of oxygen caused by vascular obstruction.

Antibody A protein of the adaptive immune response that interacts with the antigen that induced its synthesis.

Anticipatory response The secretion of stress hormones in anticipation of a psychologic stressor.

Anticodon Three-nucleotide sequence located on tRNA that recognizes specific codons on mRNA molecules by way of complementary base pairing.

Antidiuretic hormone (ADH) Protein hormone that is produced in the hypothalamus, is stored in and released from the posterior pituitary, and increases water reabsorption in the kidney.

Antigen A molecule that binds to an antibody and initiates an immune response because of the body's recognition of that molecule as foreign.

Antimicrobial peptide Protein released by epithelial cells that is toxic to some bacteria, fungi, and viruses and is capable of activating cells involved in innate and acquired immunity.

Antitoxin Antibody formed against a specific toxin.

Aortic stenosis A condition in which the aortic valves do not open completely, thereby increasing afterload so that more pressure must be generated in the left ventricle to eject blood; a condition that results in ventricular hypertrophy.

Aphasia The inability to articulate ideas or comprehend spoken or written language.

Aplastic crisis A condition that occurs when bone marrow temporarily ceases erythropoiesis, resulting in an acute fall in hemoglobin levels and subsequent anemia.

Apocrine sweat gland One of several sweat glands in the skin of the armpit, pubic region, and areolae of the breasts that produce a slightly viscous secretion in response to emotional stress or sexual excitement.

Apoptosis An active process in which cells self-destruct in normal and pathologic tissues.

Appendicitis A condition in which the appendix becomes inflamed because of a blockage of the opening from the appendix into the cecum; the appendix wall becomes infected and ruptures so that the infection spreads throughout the abdomen and causes pain, anorexia, fever, nausea, vomiting and diarrhea.

Arteriosclerosis A condition in which the blood vessel walls thicken, harden, lose elasticity, and typically accumulate lipids, resulting in elevated blood pressure and a decrease in the diameter of the coronary arteries as well as pain when walking from decreased perfusion to leg vessels.

Ascites A condition in which fluid accumulates in the peritoneal cavity because of liver disease, portal hypertension, tuberculosis or nephritic syndrome, resulting in abdominal distention and paraumbilical herniations of the abdominal wall.

Asphyxial injury A suffocation, strangulation, or chemical or drowning injury that results from oxygen deprivation in cells.

Aspiration The removal of a gas or fluid by suction or the sucking of fluid or a foreign body into the airway when breathing.

Aspiration pneumonitis A condition caused by the abnormal entry of fluids, particulate matter, or secretions into the lower airways; can lead to chemical pneumonitis by materials toxic to lungs such as gastric acid, bacterial infection, or mechanical obstruction of the lower airways.

Asthma A chronic inflammatory respiratory disease marked by periodic attacks of wheezing, shortness of breath, a tight feeling in the chest, and a cough that produces mucus caused by an allergic reaction, certain drugs or irritants, exercise, or emotional stress.

Astrocyte A neuroglial cell of the central nervous system that branches into many processes and fills spaces between neurons and surrounding blood vessels.

Atelectasis A condition in which part of a lung or a whole lung collapses and the alveoli deflate as a result of surgery, smoking, or blockage of a bronchiole.

Atherosclerosis A type of arteriosclerosis in which cholesterol and lipid deposits accumulate on the innermost layer of the walls of large and medium-sized arteries.

Atopic dermatitis (AD) A chronic hereditary skin disease characterized by intense itching and inflamed skin that causes redness, swelling, cracking, crusting, and scaling.

Atrial natriuretic peptide (ANP) or factor A protein hormone that is synthesized and released from the atria in response to high sodium concentration, high extracellular fluid volume, or high blood volume; it promotes sodium excretion and causes vasodilation in the circulatory system.

Atrial septal defect (ASD) Any of a group of congenital heart diseases involving the interatrial septum of the heart separating the right and left atria; results in travel of blood between the two sides of the heart.

Atrioventricular canal (AVC) defect A condition in which a large hole is present in the center of the heart where the wall between the upper chambers joins the wall between the lower chambers; the tricuspid and mitral valves are formed into a single large valve that crosses the defect.

Atrioventricular node (AV node) The tissue between the atria and the ventricles that contains pacemaker cells; capable of setting the heart rate but mainly functions to slowly conduct the normal electrical impulse from the atria to the ventricles.

Autocrine stimulation The ability of a cell to secrete a substance that can feed back and provide continued stimulation or inhibition of that cell.

Autoimmunity A condition in which the immune system considers an individual's own body tissues to be foreign antigens and initiates an immune response against the tissues.

Autonomic hyperreflexia (dysreflexia) A syndrome resulting from a lesion above the splanchnic nerves that is characterized by hypertension, bradycardia, sweating of the forehead, severe headache, and gooseflesh upon distention of the bladder and rectum.

Autoregulation Changes in blood vessel diameter to maintain a constant blood flow despite changes in arterial pressure.

Axon hillock The portion of the neuron where the cell body and axon join, and the point where an action potential begins if stimulus magnitude reaches a critical threshold.

Bacterial pneumonia An acute or chronic disease marked by inflammation of the lungs caused by bacterial infection.

Bainbridge reflex A homeostatic mechanism that increases heart rate in response to stimulation of local muscle spindles when blood pressure in the venae cavae and right atrium increase.

Balanitis Inflammation of the glans penis resulting from irritation by environmental substances, physical trauma, or infection.

Baroreceptor reflex A homeostatic mechanism consisting of baroreceptors that regulate the amount of blood being received by the tissues by altering cardiac output and resistance to maintain mean arterial blood pressure.

Baroreceptors Nerve endings located in the heart, aortic arch, and carotid sinuses that sense changes in blood pressure and volume.

Basopenia A condition in which the number of basophils decrease because of thyrotoxicosis, acute hypersensitivity reactions, or infection.

Basophilia A condition in which the number of basophils in the blood elevates because of hypothyroidism.

Bedbugs Any of a group of small, blood-sucking bugs that are flat-bodied, oval, reddish brown, and about one-quarter inch in size and that produce irritation in individuals when bit.

Benign prostatic hyperplasia (BPH) A condition in which the prostate gland becomes enlarged and may press against the urethra and bladder, interfering with urine flow.

Benign tumor Noncancerous but abnormal overgrowth or mass of cells; nonrecurrence and complete recovery after excision is common.

Biliary atresia A condition found in newborn children in which the biliary tract is blocked or absent, resulting in liver failure because of bile accumulation.

Blood group antigens Antigens present on the surface of erythrocytes that determine blood groups.

Blunt force injuries Tearing, shearing, or crushing of tissues caused by blows, impacts, or a combination of both.

B-lymphocyte (B-cell) Cell of the adaptive immune response that originates in the bone marrow and differentiates into plasma cells and memory cells in the presence of an antigen.

Bohr effect The ability to reduce the affinity of hemoglobin for oxygen in response to an increase in blood carbon dioxide levels and a decrease in pH, thereby allowing the hemoglobin to bind and remove more carbon dioxide.

Bone matrix The intercellular substance of bone tissue containing collagen fibers, ground substance, and inorganic bone salts that form the major constituent of bone.

Bowman capsule A cup-shaped region of the nephron that surrounds the glomerulus and functions as a filter to remove organic wastes, excess inorganic salts, and water from the blood.

Bradykinin A protein produced during the plasma kinin cascade that acts to stimulate vasodilation and pain receptor activation and to increase capillary permeability.

Brain death (brain stem death) Irreversible brain damage that renders an individual unresponsive to all stimuli and lacking in muscle activity, such as that required for respiration and heart activity.

Brain stem gliomas A group of tumors located in the brain stem usually classified as high-grade that results in the sudden onset of symptoms including headaches, vomiting, and visual disturbances.

Bronchiectasis A condition in which the bronchi of the lungs become dilated in response to obstruction.

Bronchiolitis Inflammation of the bronchioles usually as a result of viral infection.

Bronchiolitis obliterans A condition in which the bronchioles and possibly some of the bronchi are partly or completely obliterated by granulation and fibrotic tissue masses.

Bronchopulmonary dysplasia (BPD) A condition in which chronic pulmonary insufficiency occurs because of long-term artificial pulmonary ventilation; usually present in premature infants but may also occur in mature infants.

Brush border The luminal side of the small intestine that contains villi and microvilli; increases the surface area for absorption.

Buffer A substance that can absorb excess acids or bases without causing a significant change in pH.

Buffering The action of buffers minimizing the change in pH of a solution in response to the addition of acids or bases.

Bulimia nervosa A psychologic disorder in which recurrent binge eating—followed by intentional vomiting; using laxatives, enemas, diuretics, or other medication inappropriately; excessive exercising; and fasting in order to compensate for eating—becomes uncontrollable.

Bundle of His (atrioventricular bundle, common bundle) A bundle of specialized heart muscle cells located between the AV node and the ventricles that conducts electrical impulses from the atria to the ventricles.

Burkitt lymphoma An undifferentiated malignant lymphoma characterized by a large osteolytic lesion in the facial bones that is associated with the Epstein-Barr virus.

Cachexia Illness and malnutrition seen in individuals with cancer that results in wasting and eventual death.

Calcification Hardening of tissue by the insertion of calcium or calcium salts.

Calcitonin A protein hormone produced by the parafollicular cells of the thyroid gland that decreases plasma calcium and phosphate levels by inhibiting osteoclastic activity in bone.

Calculi An abnormal formation in the body, usually formed of mineral salts and most commonly found in the gallbladder, kidney, or urinary bladder.

Candidiasis A fungal infection caused by an overgrowth of normal bacteria that usually occurs in the skin and mucous membranes of the mouth, respiratory tract, or vagina but may invade the bloodstream in the immunocompromised.

Caplan syndrome A condition in which exposure to coal dust causes inflammation and scarring of the lungs.

Carbuncles A condition in which a bacterial infection of the hair follicle or sebaceous gland ducts becomes painful and discharges pus through various openings.

Carcinoma Epithelial cell tumor that typically invades surrounding tissue and metastasizes.

Cardiac cycle The cycle of events in the heart from the beginning of one heart beat to the beginning of the next, during which an electrical impulse is conducted through the heart muscle.

Cardiomyopathy A condition in which the cardiac muscle of the heart wall becomes dysfunctional because of ischemic or nonischemic mechanisms.

Carrier An individual that possesses genes for a disease but does not show phenotypical characteristics of the disease.

Carrier detection test A test used to determine whether an individual is a carrier of a genetic disease; evidence of a reduced amount of a critical enzyme indicates a carrier and allows for prediction of the probability that a child will inherit the disease.

Caseous necrosis A combination of coagulative and liquefactive necrosis in which dead cells disintegrate but are not completely digested, resulting in soft granular clumped cellular debris.

Catabolism Cellular process that provides energy by breaking down complex molecules into simpler molecules.

Cavernous hemangioma A birthmark that is similar to the strawberry hemangioma but is more deeply rooted and may appear as a red-blue spongy mass of tissue filled with blood.

Cell adhesion molecule (CAM) Protein that aids in maintaining cell shape by allowing cells to join and attach to the cytoskeleton.

Cell cycle Series of events during which nuclear material of a parent cell is duplicated and divided to form two daughter cells.

Cellular accumulation (infiltration) Accumulation of normal cellular substances in the cytoplasm or nucleus as a result of cellular injury or inefficient cell function.

Cellular immunity Immune protection afforded by the ability of cytotoxic T cells to lyse target cells that contain antigens that bind specific receptors.

Cellular receptor Protein molecule that can be embedded in the membrane or located within the cell in the cytoplasm or on the nucleus; this protein contains binding sites for a specific chemical (ligand) that when bound initiates a particular response.

Cellulitis A condition in which subcutaneous or connective tissue becomes infected and inflamed, causing tenderness, swelling, and redness that spreads to other regions of the body.

Centromere The site on the chromosome where chromatids are attached and held together before anaphase.

Cerebellar astrocytoma Brain tumor in which cancer (malignant) cells begin to grow in the tissues of the brain, resulting in head tilt, limb ataxia, and nystagmus when the eyes are turned toward the tumor.

Cerebral death Irreversible brain damage that renders an individual unresponsive to all stimuli but able to maintain the necessary respiratory and cardiovascular functions of life.

Cerebral palsy A developmental brain injury that occurs before or shortly after birth that causes muscular impairment that affects motor function and also may alter speech and learning abilities.

Cerebrovascular accident (CVA, stroke) A localized brain infarction that may result in facial, arm, or leg numbness and weakness, confusion, difficulty speaking or understanding, visual disturbances, dizziness, loss of balance, difficulty walking, and headache.

Cervicitis Inflammation of the mucous membrane of the uterine cervix because of infection, typically resulting from chlamydia, genital herpes, or gonorrhea.

Chemical asphyxiant Chemical or gas that prevents the delivery of oxygen to tissues or blocks its use.

Chemical synapse Region between two nerve cells where a neurotransmitter is released from one cell and stimulates or inhibits cellular activity by binding to its receptor on a target cell.

Chemotactic factor A biochemical substance that facilitates chemotaxis.

Chemotaxis Directional movement and attraction of microorganisms or phagocytes to substances released in the environment or tissues.

Cheyne-Stokes respiration An abnormality of the pattern of breathing in which tidal volume gradually increases followed by a gradual decrease and a period of apnea before returning to a normal respiratory pattern.

Chickenpox An infectious viral disease spread by direct contact or through the air by coughing or sneezing, which results in a blister-like rash that appears first on the face and trunk and can spread over the entire body, resulting in 250 to 500 itchy blisters, fatigue, & fever.

Choking asphyxiation Injury resulting from failure of cells to receive oxygen because of obstruction of internal airways.

Cholecystitis Inflammation of the gallbladder commonly resulting from impaction of a gallstone that causes right upper quadrant pain and possibly a rupture and abscess in the gallbladder.

Cholecystokinin A protein hormone produced by the duodenum in response to fat- or protein-rich chyme that stimulates the release of digestive enzymes from the pancreas and bile from the gallbladder to aid in fat and protein digestion.

Cholelithiasis The presence or formation of gallstones in the gallbladder or bile ducts. Cholinergic transmission of a nerve impulse using acetylcholine as a neurotransmitter.

Chondrocyte Cells that produce and maintain the cartilaginous matrix.

Chondrosarcoma A cancer of the cartilage usually occurring in the pelvic bones, shoulder bones, and the upper part of the arms and legs.

Chordae tendineae cordis Bands of fibrous tissue that attach on one end to the edges of the tricuspid and mitral valves of the heart and on the other end to the papillary muscles that anchor the valves.

Chromatid One of two daughter chromatids produced by chromosomal replication that are joined at the centromere.

Chromatin Chains of DNA containing proteins spaced along the chain, which gives chromosomes a granular appearance during interphase.

Chromosome Genetic material in the nucleus of a eukaryotic cell that contains the DNA of the organism.

Chromosome band A pattern on a chromosome that is visualized by preferential binding of stain to specific regions, allowing chromosomes to be distinguished from one another.

Chronic bacterial prostatitis A condition in which long-standing prostatitis and an underlying defect in the prostate makes the prostate more susceptible to bacterial urinary tract infection.

Chronic obstructive pulmonary disease (COPD) Any of a group of irreversible respiratory diseases that are characterized by airflow obstruction or limitation, usually caused by smoking.

Chronic rejection Rejection of a graft months to years after transplantation because of a gradual loss of organ function.

Chronic renal failure A slowly developing condition that can result as a complication of a large number of kidney diseases, such as IgA nephritis, glomerulonephritis, chronic pyelonephritis, and urinary retention; leads to end-stage renal failure for which dialysis is generally required while a donor kidney is found.

Chyme Partially digested food found in the stomach that has been exposed to the salivary enzyme amylase, the gastric enzyme pepsin, and hydrochloric acid.

Cirrhosis A condition in which organ tissues degenerate, resulting in fibrosis with nodule and scar formation and organ dysfunction.

Citric acid cycle (Krebs cycle, tricarboxylic acid cycle) A component of aerobic metabolism that includes a series of reactions in which acetyl CoA is oxidized into carbon dioxide, nicotinamide adenine dinucleotide (NADH), and flavin adenine dinucleotide (FADH).

Cleft lip (harelip) A deformity of the lip caused by abnormal facial development during pregnancy.

Clotting factor Any of several plasma components involved in the clotting of blood, including fibrinogen, prothrombin, thromboplastin, and calcium ion.

Coagulative necrosis Changes in albumin caused by protein denaturation, primarily in kidneys, heart, and adrenal glands that have experienced hypoxia.

Coarctation of the aorta (COA) A condition in which the aorta narrows in the area where the ductus arteriosus inserts. Narrowing usually occurs preductal in children and postductal in adults.

Cochlea A cavity of the temporal bone of the inner ear that contains the nerve endings essential for hearing.

Codominance Occurs when a heterozygote expresses two dominant alleles rather than one that dominates over the other.

Codon A triplet of nucleotides located in the mRNA that determines which amino acids will be formed during translation.

Collagen Strong fibers that form connective tissues in areas such as tendons, bone, and dermis.

Collecting duct The final section of the nephron before reaching the ureter where salts and water are reabsorbed or secreted and urine concentration is maximal.

Communicating (extraventricular) hydrocephalus A disorder in which the cerebrospinal fluid pathways are intact but cerebrospinal fluid absorption is impaired.

Compact bone (cortical bone) The bone type that makes up a large portion of skeletal mass but has a low surface area.

Compensation Adjustment of acid or base content by removal or addition in response to changes in pH; for example, a decrease in pH is accompanied by an increase in carbon dioxide removal by the lungs, causing pH to increase.

Compensatory hyperplasia An increased rate of cell division that compensates for absent or dysfunctional cells of the same tissue.

Competitive inhibitor A molecule that reversibly or irreversibly binds to a site specific for a given solute, thereby inhibiting the binding and action of the solute.

Complement receptor A receptor present on cells of the innate and acquired immune responses that removes antibody-antigen complexes when bound to complement system products.

Compliance A measure of the ease with which a structure, such as the lungs or chest wall, may be deformed or stretched.

Concentration gradient The difference in concentration of a substance found in a solution that is contained in separate areas or compartments—such as the intracellular and extracellular spaces found on either side of a cell membrane—that causes movement by way of diffusion.

Conduction system The electrical system of the heart that allows the impulse generated by the sinoatrial (SA) node to be propagated to the remaining muscle of the heart, resulting in a wave of contraction that propels the blood forward to be pumped to the body.

Congenital aganglionic megacolon (Hirschsprung disease) A congenital defect in which the nerves that innervate the anus through the wall of the bowel are absent, resulting in enlargement of the bowel above the point where the nerves are missing and a subsequent decrease in peristalsis that results in chronic constipation.

Connexon A channel composed of six protein subunits that form a hollow center through the plasma membrane at a gap junction; when two connexons in adjacent cells are aligned, chemical and electrical communication can occur between the cells.

Contact dermatitis An allergic response to an environmental antigen binding to specific carrier proteins contained in an individual's skin.

Contracture A permanent shortening of muscle or scar tissue that distorts or deforms affected joints.

Contusion A bruise produced by bleeding into the skin or underlying tissues from an insult that did not break the skin but did rupture blood vessels.

Cor pulmonale Right-sided heart failure resulting from prolonged hypertension secondary to pulmonary hypertension.

Cornea The transparent layer of the front of the eye that helps to focus light on the retina by bending the light waves.

Corpora cavernosa Erectile tissue that contains most of the blood in the male penis during erection and in the female clitoris during sexual arousal.

Corpus luteum A temporary endocrine structure that develops from an ovarian follicle after it has released an ovum; functions to secrete progesterone that thickens the uterine lining in preparation for the fertilized egg.

Corpus luteum cyst A condition in which excessive bleeding leads to the development of a cyst in the corpus luteum that may be tender and painful.

Countercurrent exchange system A mechanism by which a substance in one flowing current of fluid moves across a semipermeable membrane, down its concentration gradient, into another parallel current of fluid moving in the opposite direction, allowing the maintenance of a constant concentration gradient.

Craniopharyngioma A brain tumor that develops in the pituitary gland and most often affects children, causing headache, seizure, diabetes insipidus, early onset of puberty, and delayed growth.

Craniosynostosis Premature ossification of the skull and closure of the sutures, resulting in abnormal skull expansion and asymmetric skull growth.

Crohn disease An autoimmune condition in which the intestines, and possibly any other component of the digestive system, are chronically inflamed and ulcerated, causing chronic diarrhea, disrupted digestion, and subsequent difficulty eating and digesting food.

Cross-bridge theory of muscle contraction A proposal that during muscle contraction, sarcomeres shorten because thin filaments slide between thick filaments and form cross-bridges that provide a force that slides the two filaments past one another.

Crossing over An exchange of genetic information between two homologous chromosomes.

Cryoglobulin An immunoglobulin that precipitates at low body temperatures.

Cryptorchidism A condition in which the scrotum of one or both testes is absent because of failure of the testis to descend from the abdominal position during fetal development.

Cushing syndrome A condition caused by increased synthesis and secretion of adrenocorticotropic hormone (ACTH) from a tumor of the adrenal cortex or of the anterior lobe of the pituitary gland, resulting in weight gain, glucose intolerance, and muscle wasting.

Cutaneous vasculitis A type of vasculitis affecting the skin and other organs that is characterized by a polymorphonuclear infiltrate of the small vessels.

Cyanosis A condition in which the skin, mucous membranes, and nail beds appear blue because of a lack of oxygenated hemoglobin in the blood secondary to congenital heart defects, slowed circulation, or possibly poison.

Cyclooxygenase (COX) An enzyme responsible for formation of prostaglandins, prostacyclin, and thromboxane and subsequent inflammatory response.

Cyclopia A congenital defect in which the two eye orbits merge to form a single cavity containing one eye with a noselike appendage above the orbit.

Cystic fibrosis (CF) A genetic disorder of the exocrine glands caused by a mutation in the CF transmembrane regulator gene causing impairment in chloride transfer across cell membranes and subsequent chloride and water accumulation in organs; thickened secretions block ducts and form cysts.

Cystic fibrosis transmembrane regulator (CFTR) A chloride transporter found in the lung, liver, pancreas, digestive tract, reproductive tract, and skin.

Cystitis A condition characterized by acute or chronic inflammation of the urinary bladder, usually resulting from bacterial infection of the urethra; cause frequent burning urination, blood in the urine, pain in the pubic area, chills and fever, back pain, and nausea.

Cystocele A condition in which the muscle between a woman's bladder and vagina weaken and the bladder descends into the vagina causing discomfort, urine leakage, and incomplete emptying of the bladder.

Cytokine Molecule produced by cells of the acquired immune system that mediates interactions between cells to kill bacteria; active during the inflammatory response.

Cytokinesis The process by which the cytoplasm of a parent cell divides into two identical cells after mitosis.

Cytoplasm Liquid material of a cell enclosed within the plasma membrane.

Cytotoxic (metabolic) edema Cerebral edema resulting from tissue hypoxia and impairment of the Na^+-K^+ ATP pump, causing a loss of intracellular potassium and a gain of intracellular sodium and water.

Cytotoxic T lymphocyte (Tc cell) Killer lymphocyte that binds to and lyses specific cells containing particular antigen receptors.

Deep venous thrombosis (DVT) The formation of one or more thrombi in the deep veins, usually of the lower extremity. DVT is often asymptomatic but carries a high risk of pulmonary embolism; symptoms (principally unilateral) include pain, tenderness, swelling, warmth, and skin discoloration.

Defecation reflex (rectal reflex) A process by which the accumulation of feces in the rectum stimulates defecation.

Degenerative disk disease A condition in which intervertebral disk tissue is replaced by fibrocartilage during aging; functional capacity is rarely altered.

Deoxyribonucleic acid (DNA) Genetic information of an organism that is contained in chromatin.

Depolarization The movement of sodium across the membrane, resulting in a change in membrane charge from a negative to positive potential.

Dermatome An area of skin that is innervated by a specific spinal nerve.

Dermoid cyst A benign tumor resulting from congenital malformation of the skin or ovary.

Desmosome A region of tight adhesion between neighboring cells that provides structural strength to the tissue and allows the cells of the tissue to function as a unit.

Developmental dysplasia of the hip (DDH) A condition in which the hip joint of babies or young children is malformed with the ball being completely out of the socket or the socket being too shallow to support the ball.

Diabetes insipidus A disease caused by antidiuretic hormone deficiency or resistance characterized by excretion of large amounts of diluted urine resulting from the inability of the kidneys to concentrate urine.

Diabetic ketoacidosis (DKA) A complication of diabetes mellitus caused by the buildup of by-products of fat metabolism that occurs when glucose is not available as a fuel source for the body because of insulin deficiency.

Diabetic neuropathy Combined sensory and motor disorder often seen in older diabetic patients as a result of microvascular injury involving small blood vessels that supply nerves.

Diabetic retinopathy Damage to the retina caused by an overaccumulation of glucose or fructose that damages the blood vessels in the retina; in advanced stages, lack of oxygen in the retina causes fragile blood vessels to grow along the retina and in the vitreous fluid of the eye that may bleed and cause blurred vision.

Diaper dermatitis A type of dermatitis characterized by inflammation of the skin in the diaper area in infants and caused by exposure of the skin to feces and urine.

Diarrhea An increase in the frequency of watery bowel movements or a greater looseness of stools as a result of disease, excessive consumption of alcohol or other liquids or foods that irritate the stomach or intestine, allergy to certain food products, poisoning, hyperactivity of the nervous system, or viral or bacterial infection.

Diastole The period of time when the heart relaxes after contraction, resulting in a pressure drop in the relaxed region.

Diastolic heart failure A condition in which heart contractions are normal but the ventricle does not relax completely; therefore less blood enters the heart.

Differentiation The process by which cells mature and become specialized to perform specific functions.

Diffuse brain injury (diffuse axonal injury) Injury to neuronal axons in many areas of the brain caused by stretching and shearing forces received during brain injury.

Diploid cell A cell that contains two sets of chromosomes, giving each diploid cell 46 chromosomes.

Disseminated intravascular coagulation (DIC) A condition in which the blood coagulates throughout the entire body following the uncontrolled activation of clotting factors and fibrinolytic enzymes throughout small blood vessels, resulting in platelet and coagulation factor depletion and increased bleeding.

Distal tubule A section of the nephron between the loop of Henle and the collecting duct system that helps regulate potassium, sodium, calcium, and pH by reabsorbing bicarbonate, sodium, and calcium and secreting protons and potassium into the filtrate.

Diverticulitis Inflammation of the diverticula in the colon, usually occurring in elderly patients.

Diverticulosis A condition in which multiple bulging sacs push outward from the wall of the large intestine and may become infected and rupture, causing abdominal pain and tenderness, and fever.

Dominant An allele that can mask the effects of another allele.

Dosage compensation The phenomenon in which males are able to produce proteins expressed by sex chromosomes in an amount equal to that produced by females even though the males only have one X chromosome.

Down-regulation The process by which a cell decreases its sensitivity to a hormone or neurotransmitter by decreasing the number of receptors in response to a high concentration of that particular hormone or neurotransmitter.

Drowning Breathing in fluid that causes airway obstruction, thereby decreasing oxygen delivery to tissues.

Duchenne muscular dystrophy A genetic disorder in which fat and fibrous tissue infiltrate and weaken muscle tissues in the legs, pelvis, lungs, and heart; usually results in death before adulthood.

Dumping syndrome A condition in which the lower end of the small intestine fills too quickly with undigested food from the stomach following stomach surgery, resulting in nausea, vomiting, bloating, diarrhea, and shortness of breath during or immediately following a meal.

Dyspareunia A reversible condition in which sexual intercourse is painful.

Dysphasia Impairment of speech that manifests as the inability to arrange words in logical order.

Dyspnea Shortness of breath and difficulty in breathing usually the result of lung or heart disease.

Eccrine sweat gland One of several sweat glands at the body's surface that produce a clear, watery secretion important in regulating body temperature.

Effective osmolality Osmotic activity sustained by the presence of varying solute concentrations in two regions separated by a permeable membrane.

Eisenmenger syndrome A congenital defect in which the abnormal development of circulation causes a reversed right-to-left shunt secondary to increased pressures on the right side of the heart resulting from pulmonary hypertension.

Elastic recoil The ability of the lungs to resist stretching and return to their original shape after having been stretched.

Elastin Long, stretchable fiber that forms connective tissues in areas where elasticity is necessary, such as skin and lungs.

Electrolyte Electrically charged substance that is capable of ionizing, dissociating into ions, and conducting electricity.

Electron-transport chain A series of transfer reactions that includes transferring electrons from a donor to an acceptor, thereby releasing energy during each transfer.

Embolic stroke A stroke caused by blockage of cerebral vessels.

Embolus An air bubble, a detached blood clot, or a foreign body that travels in the bloodstream and gets stuck in a blood vessel, resulting in obstruction in vessels supplying the lungs, brain, or heart, and possibly gangrene and the need for amputation in extremities.

Empyema (infected pleural effusion) A condition in which purulent is persistently discharged into the pleural space because of complications of bacterial infections.

Encephalitis Inflammation of the brain usually caused by a virus.

Encephalocele A congenital abnormality in which a gap in the skull results in a protrusion of brain material.

Encephalopathy Any of the various diseases or syndromes of the brain.

End-diastolic volume Used as a measure of diastolic function, this volume is the amount of blood in the ventricle before a cardiac contraction.

Endocytosis A process by which extracellular substances are trapped in a section of the membrane that folds inward and separates from the membrane to form an intracellular vesicle.

Endometrial polyp A typically benign mass protruding from the mucous membrane of the endometrium.

Endometriosis A condition common in women of reproductive age in which the tissue lining the uterus is found outside of the uterus, resulting in pain and infertility.

Endomitosis A chromosomal replication in the absence of division of the cell nucleus, resulting in a polyploid nucleus.

Endothelial cell A cell of the endothelial layer that lines heart, blood, lymph vessels, and the lung cavity.

Endotoxin Lipopolysaccharide released during cell lysis from the bacterial outer membrane that causes fever, leukopenia, and possibly diarrhea and hemorrhagic shock.

Enuresis A condition in which urination is uncontrolled or involuntary.

Eosinopenia A reduction in the number of eosinophils present in the blood.

Eosinophil A phagocyte that destroys antigen-antibody complexes, allergens, and inflammatory chemicals and aids in fighting parasitic infections.

Eosinophilia A condition in which the number of eosinophils in the blood elevates because of diseases such as parasitic infections, allergies, cholesterol emboli, chronic myeloid leukemia, and some drug reactions.

Ependymoma An intracranial tumor most commonly found in children that typically arises from the inner lining of the fourth ventricle and the spinal canal.

Epicritic Extreme sensitivity, such as that required to accurately determine fine variations of touch or temperature.

Epididymis A narrow, convoluted tube that lies behind each testicle and functions as a site of spermatozoa maturation and storage before entering the vas deferens during emission.

Epididymitis A painful condition where the epididymis becomes inflamed, usually caused by a secondary bacterial infection brought about by a variety of underlying conditions, such as urinary tract or sexually transmitted infections.

Epidural hematoma A collection of blood between the inner surface of the skull and the dura caused by torn arteries secondary to skull fracture.

Epigenetic A mechanism by which changes in gene function can be inherited without alteration of gene sequence.

Epilepsy Any of a group of syndromes characterized by recurring seizures of an unknown cause.

Epiphyseal plate A plate of hyaline cartilage at the end of long bones that provides a site for lengthening of the bone.

Epispadias A birth defect in which the urethra opens on the upper penile surface.

Erysipelas A highly contagious bacterial infection that produces shiny, red, swollen areas and fever and can lead to blood poisoning and pneumonia.

Erythema multiforme A skin disease caused by allergies, seasonal changes, or drug sensitivities, resulting in the formation of red macules, papules, or subdermal vesicles on the skin and mucous membranes.

Erythema toxicum neonatorum A temporary eruption of redness of the skin, small papules, and occasionally pustules in newborns accompanied by contact dermatitis or hypersensitivity to milk or other allergens.

Erythrocyte (red blood cell) A disk-shaped cell in the blood that contains hemoglobin, lacks a nucleus, and transports oxygen and carbon dioxide to and from the tissues.

Esophageal phase The phase of swallowing during which food enters the esophagus, esophageal peristalsis moves food toward the lower esophageal sphincter, the lower esophageal sphincter relaxes, and food moves into the stomach.

Essential (primary) thrombocythemia (ET) A chronic disorder associated with sustained megakaryocyte proliferation, which increases the number of circulating platelets and results in megakaryocytic hyperplasia, splenomegaly, and complications by hemorrhagic and thrombotic episodes.

Estradiol (E2) The most potent of the estrogens, estradiol has many functions; it increases the growth and development of female sex organs and characteristics, increases secretions from the cervix and growth of the endometrium, reduces low-density lipoprotein (LDL)-cholesterol, and increases high-density lipoprotein (HDL)-cholesterol concentrations in the blood.

Eukaryotes Organisms such as plants, animals, fungi, protozoa, and most algae that are composed of cells with a nucleus and other membrane-bound organelles.

Excitation-contraction coupling The process by which an action potential depolarizes a myocyte causing calcium to be transported into the cell and released from the sarcoplasmic reticulum resulting in muscle contraction.

Excitatory postsynaptic potential (EPSP) A graded subthreshold depolarization of the postsynaptic membrane in response to neurotransmitter release from a presynaptic neuron.

Exocytosis A mechanism for cellular secretion in which vesicles containing substances such as neurotransmitters fuse with the cell membrane and discharge their contents into the extracellular space.

Exon A nucleotide sequence in an RNA molecule that codes for proteins.

Exotoxin A protein synthesized by a specific species of bacteria found outside the bacterial wall.

Exstrophy of the bladder A congenital defect in which the lower abdominal wall is malformed and ruptures, allowing communication between the bladder and the amniotic fluid; results in anomalies of the lower abdominal wall, bladder, anterior bony pelvis, and external genitalia.

Extracellular matrix (basement membrane) Fibrous proteins embedded in a carbohydrate-rich liquid secreted by the cell that functions as a pathway for diffusion of nutrients, wastes, and other substances between the blood and tissues.

Extrinsic allergic alveolitis (hypersensitivity pneumonitis) An inflammation of the lung caused by an immune reaction to small airborne particles such as bacteria, mold, and fungi; causes fever, chills, coughing, shortness of breath, and body aches.

Exudate Fluids or cells that have leaked from blood vessels.

Failure to thrive (FTT) A condition that is characterized by poor weight gain and physical growth over an extended period of time in infancy.

Fat necrosis A lipase-induced cellular dissolution of triglycerides in breast, pancreas, and other abdominal structures.

Fibrils Chains of collagen fibers that organize in a staggered pattern to create gaps where mineralization takes place and form ropelike fibers.

Fibroblast A connective tissue cell that proliferates at inflammatory sites and produces collagen fibers and ground substance to aid in wound healing.

Fibromyalgia A condition in which muscles, tendons, and joints are painful, stiff, and tender; frequently accompanied by restless sleep, fatigue, anxiety, depression, and disturbances in bowel function.

Fibrosarcoma A malignant tumor of the fibrous connective tissue usually derived from immature proliferating fibroblasts.

Focal segmental glomerulosclerosis (FSGS) A condition in which glomerular capillaries with thickened basement membranes and increased mesangial matrix collapse in segments.

Follicle stimulating hormone (FSH) Anterior pituitary hormone released in response to gonadotropin releasing hormone that increases spermatozoa production in males and follicle maturation in females.

Follicular cyst A cyst caused by the retention of secretions in a follicular space caused by the blockage of a duct, resulting in the failure of the dominant follicle to rupture or failure of the nondominant follicles to regress.

Follicular/proliferative phase These phases represent the period during which the follicle matures because of granulosa cell proliferation and increased estrogen production; the endometrium thickens because of estrogen stimulation.

Folliculitis Inflammation of a follicle damaged by friction from clothing, blockage of the follicle, or shaving that becomes infected with a bacteria.

Follistatin A protein hormone produced by the pituitary and found in the follicles that binds to and inhibits the actions of activin, resulting in a decrease in follicle stimulating hormone secretion and subsequent follicular growth.

Fovea centralis A small region of the retina filled with cones that receive the most direct light stimulation; becomes the area of greatest visual acuity.

Frailty Physiologic and immune changes that waste the body during aging and leave the affected person susceptible to falls, functional decline, disease, and death.

Frank-Starling law of the heart The idea that fluctuations in the volume of blood filling the heart will change the volume ejected by the same amount because the force of the contraction will increase as the heart is filled with more blood.

Free radical Highly reactive and destructive particle with an unpaired electron and is produced from an atom or molecule.

Fulminant hepatitis A type of viral hepatitis that has a high mortality rate and causes fatigue, nausea, jaundice, dark urine, flulike symptoms, hepatomegaly, and eventually encephalopathy.

Furuncles A condition in which staphylococcal infection produces painful, pus-filled, inflamed sites on the skin and subcutaneous tissue.

Fusiform aneurysm (giant aneurysm) A large aneurysm that stretches to affect the entire circumference of the arterial wall.

Galactorrhea (inappropriate lactation) A condition in which milklike fluid is secreted from the breast because of hormonal alterations, but it is not associated with childbirth or nursing.

Gamete A haploid reproductive cell including sperm and eggs.

Gangrenous necrosis Tissue death typically found in the lower leg as a result of severe hypoxic injury secondary to arteriosclerosis or blockage of major arteries.

Gap junction Tunnel or connexon that joins two adjacent cells and allows for the passage of molecules and electrical signals between the cells.

Gas gangrene The formation of gas bubbles and subsequent destruction of connective tissue and cell membranes resulting from the hydrolytic enzymes produced by bacterium of the *Clostridium* species.

Gastrin A protein hormone produced primarily in the antrum of the stomach by the G cells in response to stomach distension, vagal stimulation, the presence of partially digested proteins, and hypercalcemia that acts to stimulate parietal cells of the stomach to secrete hydrochloric acid and the chief cells to secrete pepsinogen.

Gastritis A condition in which the lining of the stomach is inflamed because of bacterial infection, bile reflux or excessive consumption of alcohol or certain foods.

Gastrocolic reflex A process by which food entering an empty stomach increases intestinal and colonic peristalsis.

Gastroesophageal reflux (GER) A type of injury to the esophagus caused by chronic exposure of the esophagus to stomach liquid reflux made up of acid and pepsin; creates heartburn, inflammation of the esophageal lining, strictures, dysphagia, and chronic chest pain.

Gastroileal reflex A process by which food entering an empty stomach increases ileal motility and causes the ileocecal valve to open.

Gate control theory A proposal that a pain gate is present in the spinal cord that allows or blocks pain signals to the brain depending on whether the impulse is traveling on a large or small afferent fiber.

Gating A calcium-induced decrease in permeability of a junctional complex that may aid in protecting uninjured cells from the increased calcium levels released by injured cells.

Genomic imprinting Genes that are inherited from only one parent and have variable degrees of activation.

Genotype The genetic composition of an individual.

Germline mosaicism A mechanism by which a child can inherit a genetic disease even though the parents do not express the disease; the mechanism is believed to involve a mutation during the embryonic development of the parent germ cells.

Giant cell tumor A benign tumor usually near the end of the bone near a joint in arms, legs, knee, and flat bones.

Giantism Severely increased long bone growth caused by excessive growth hormone secretion before and during puberty.

Glans A structure composed of corpus spongiosum in males (glans penis) and corpus cavernosa and vestibular tissue in females (glans clitoris) located at the tip of the genital structures involved in sexual arousal, contains the highest density of sensory receptors.

Glomerular filtration rate (GFR) the volume of plasma filtered at the glomerulus per unit time.

Glomerulonephritis An autoimmune or infectious disease characterized by inflammation of the glomeruli that may not produce symptoms or may present with hematuria and proteinuria.

Glomerulus A capillary bed surrounded by the Bowman capsule of the nephron in the kidney where filtration occurs.

Glucagon A protein hormone secreted by the alpha cells of the islets of Langerhans that increases blood sugar by promoting glycogenolysis and gluconeogenesis in the liver.

Glucocorticoid A steroid hormone produced by the adrenal cortex that facilitates carbohydrate, protein, and fat metabolism and is commonly used as an anti-inflammatory and anti-immunity agent.

Glucose-6-phosphate dehydrogenase (G6PD) deficiency An inherited condition that is asymptomatic in the absence of exposure to particular substances, such as certain medicines, mothballs, or severe infections; with exposure, the red blood cells undergo destruction that produces excessive bilirubin, which overloads the liver and causes jaundice.

Gluten-sensitive enteropathy Also known as celiac sprue, this condition is characterized by mucosal lesions in the gastrointestinal tract formed in response to a genetic predisposition for an immune response to gluten and similar proteins.

Glycolysis Catabolism of glucose or other monosaccharides to pyruvate and two molecules of ATP in the absence of oxygen.

Goiter A noncancerous enlargement of the thyroid gland that is visible as a swelling at the front of the neck.

Golgi tendon organ A specialized structure in the tendon fibers that stretches when the corresponding muscle contracts and sends information to the brain about the actual tension the muscle is achieving in contraction.

Gomphosis An immovable articulation, such as a tooth inserted into its bony socket.

Gonadostat A theory proposing that near the time of puberty the hypothalamus and pituitary loses sensitivity to sex steroid feedback, resulting in an increase in gonadotropins that initiates puberty.

Gonadotropin-releasing hormone (GnRH) A hormone produced by the hypothalamus that stimulates the anterior pituitary gland to secrete luteinizing hormone and follicle-stimulating hormone.

Gout A disorder of uric-acid metabolism that causes painful inflammation of the joints, commonly the big toe, and arthritic attacks caused by elevated levels of uric acid in the blood and the deposition of urate crystals around the joints.

Granulation tissue Vascularized tissue that replaces the fibrin clot during the reconstructive phase of wound healing.

Granulocyte A type of white blood cell, such as neutrophils, that contain enzymes capable of killing microorganisms and catabolizing debris ingested during phagocytosis.

Granulocytopenia A condition in which the number of granular white blood cells in the blood is decreased.

Granulocytosis A condition in which the number of granulocytes, usually neutrophils, in blood is increased secondary to bacterial infection, leukemia, or autoimmune disease.

Granuloma A tumor-like mass containing macrophages and fibroblasts that forms as a result of chronic inflammation and isolation of the infected area.

Granulosa cell A cell in the ovarian follicle that converts androgens into estrogens and becomes a luteal cell after ovulation.

Graves disease A condition usually caused by excessive thyroid hormone characterized by an enlarged thyroid gland, protrusion of eyeballs, a rapid heartbeat, and nervous excitability.

Growth factor A chemical messenger that mediates tissue growth and development by stimulating mitosis and cell differentiation.

Gynecomastia A condition in which abnormal breast tissue develops on adolescent boys or men usually because of an imbalance in hormones.

Haploid cell A cell that contains one copy of each chromosome, giving each cell 23 chromosomes.

Hematoma A collection of blood in soft tissue or an enclosed space.

Hematopoietic growth factor One of several glycoproteins with regulatory functions in the processes of proliferation, differentiation, and functional activation of hematopoietic progenitors and mature blood cells.

Hemizygous A male that has one X chromosome containing genes for a specific disease but has no alleles on the Y chromosome to counteract the effects of the diseased gene.

Hemolytic disease of the newborn (HDN) A condition that affects a fetus or newborn in which red blood cells break down because of antibodies made by the mother that are directed against the baby's red blood cells, potentially resulting in anemia, heart failure, jaundice, and brain damage if left untreated.

Hemolytic-uremic syndrome A condition in which platelets aggregate within the kidney's small blood vessels resulting in reduced blood flow to the kidney and subsequent kidney failure and destruction of the red blood cells.

Hemoproteins Endogenous pigments such as hemoglobin and cytochromes that accumulate in cells because of excessive iron storage.

Hemoptysis A period during which blood or blood-stained sputum is spit or coughed from bronchi, larynx, trachea, or lungs.

Hemorrhagic stroke (intracranial hemorrhage) Stroke usually caused by hypertension that results in bleeding in the brain; typically increases intracranial pressure and may lead to death.

Henoch-Schönlein purpura nephritis A condition in which the blood vessels are inflamed causing bleeding into the skin, mucous membranes, internal organs, and other tissues; pain and inflammation in the joints; abdominal pain; gastrointestinal bleeding; inflammation of the kidneys; subcutaneous edema; encephalopathy; and inflammation of the testis.

Hepatic encephalopathy A condition usually caused by liver cirrhosis and portal hypertension in which toxins produced by the gut pass into the systemic circulation and damage brain cells resulting in impaired cognition, tremor, and a decreased level of consciousness.

Hepatorenal syndrome A condition in which acute renal failure occurs because of a decrease in renal blood flow or liver and kidney damage.

Heterogeneous nuclear RNA (hnRNA) RNA recently transcribed that has not yet been converted into mature mRNA.

Heterozygote An individual that has different alleles for a specific gene.

Hiatal hernia An anatomic abnormality in which the esophageal hiatus is larger than normal, causing part of the stomach to protrude through the diaphragm and up into the chest.

Hodgkin lymphoma (HL) A chronic condition in which the lymph nodes, spleen, and liver become enlarged; is often accompanied by anemia, fever, and eventually death if not treated at an early stage.

Homozygote An individual that has identical alleles for a specific gene.

Hormonal signaling Communication between cells that originates when a hormone is released from an endocrine cell, travels through the bloodstream, and binds to a target cell to elicit a response.

Humoral immunity Immune protection afforded by the presence of antibodies in blood.

Huntington disease (HD) An autosomal dominant disease causing a progressive increase in involuntary, jerky, dyskinetic movements; mental deterioration; and premature death.

Hydrocele A condition in which serous fluid accumulates in a bodily cavity such as the testis.

Hydrostatic pressure Any pressure that is exerted by a liquid within a closed system, such as blood as it presses against vessel membranes in response to pumping of the heart.

Hydroxyapatite (HAP) The primary bone salt that provides compressional strength to bone.

Hyperaldosteronism A disorder marked by excessive secretion of aldosterone and subsequent weakness, cardiac irregularities, and abnormally high blood pressure.

Hyperhemolytic crisis A condition in which the rate of destruction of red blood cells is increased, resulting in decreased hemoglobin levels, increased reticulocyte count, elevated bilirubin, and elevated lactate dehydrogenase; caused by infections, hemolytic transfusion reactions, sickle cell crisis, or a combination of glucose 6-phosphodisterase deficiency with oxidant stress.

Hyperhomocysteinemia A condition in which plasma homocysteine concentration is elevated because of diet, vitamin B_6 or B_{12} deficiency, congenital enzyme deficiency, or renal failure, increasing the risk of developing atherosclerosis and venous thromboembolism.

Hyperpolarized The state of a membrane when the membrane potential is more negative than the resting membrane potential, thereby increasing the stimulus required to elicit an action potential.

Hypersensitivity A state in which the body undergoes an exaggerated immune response to an antigen.

Hypertonic hyponatremia Decreased sodium concentration caused by increases in plasma lipids and proteins that results in an osmotic shift.

Hyperventilation A condition in which overventilation reduces carbon dioxide concentration because of breathing faster or deeper than necessary, resulting in numbness or tingling in the hands, feet, and lips; lightheadedness; dizziness; headache; chest pain; and sometimes fainting.

Hypocortisolism A condition characterized by a decrease in cortisol synthesis and release that may be related to deficiency at the adrenal, pituitary, or hypothalamic level.

Hypoglycemia A state of low blood glucose that stimulates epinephrine and glucagon secretion, mobilizing stored glycogen and fat and their conversion into glucose.

Hypoparathyroidism A condition marked by decreased function of the parathyroid glands, resulting in hypocalcemia and associated tremor, tetany, and convulsions.

Hypoplastic anemia A condition in which anemia results from greatly depressed, inadequately functioning bone marrow and smaller-than-normal erythrocytes.

Hypoplastic left heart syndrome (HLHS) A condition in which the left side of the heart including the aorta, aortic valve, left ventricle, and mitral valve; is underdeveloped so that blood returning from the lungs must flow through an opening in the atrial septum; the right ventricle pumps the blood into the pulmonary artery then into the aorta.

Hypopolarized The state of a membrane when the membrane potential is more positive than the resting membrane potential but does not reach the threshold potential required to elicit an action potential.

Hypospadias A birth defect in which the urethral opening is abnormally placed, opening anywhere from the tip of the glans of the penis to the shaft or the junction of the penis and scrotum or perineum in males and usually opening in the vagina in females.

Hypothyroidism A condition caused by insufficient thyroid hormone synthesis and secretion, resulting in impaired memory, increased sensitivity to heat and cold, slow heart rate, depression, weight gain, slowed metabolism, and several other systemic alterations.

Hypoventilation A condition in which ventilation is inadequate for proper gas exchange, causing an increase in carbon dioxide concentration and subsequent respiratory acidosis.

Hypovolemia Decreased blood volume capable of causing hypotension, tachycardia, and decreased urine output.

Hypoxemia Insufficient oxygenation of arterial blood.

Hypoxia State in which the oxygen level reaching cells is insufficient, resulting in tissue injury; may be caused by a reduction in oxygen content of inspired air, a decrease in hemoglobin available for oxygen binding, or cardiovascular or respiratory disease.

Icterus neonatorum (neonatal jaundice) Temporary jaundice in newborn infants caused by functional immaturity of the liver.

Imperforate anus A congenital defect in which the anal opening is absent because of the presence of a membranous septum or complete absence of the anal canal.

Impetigo A contagious skin infection caused by hemolytic streptococci or staphylococci that results in small red spots or blisters that rupture, discharge, and become encrusted; can spread over the skin.

Infectious mononucleosis (IM) A disease caused by the Epstein-Barr virus or the cytomegalovirus that is transmitted by exchanging saliva or blood or by coughing and sneezing; acts by infecting the B cells and atypical T cells resulting in fever, sore throat, and fatigue.

Inflammatory acne A condition characterized by comedones that appear as red, swollen, and inflamed blemishes and larger, deeper, swollen, tender lesions that become inflamed and rupture under the skin.

Inflammatory joint disease A disease in which inflammation affects joint structures and often leads to structural derangement of the joint, structural joint problems, and pain at rest and with motion.

Inhibin A protein hormone that inhibits follicle stimulating hormone synthesis and secretion, impairs prolactin and growth hormone secretion, interferes with gonadotropin-releasing hormone receptors, and increases gonadotropin breakdown.

Inhibitory postsynaptic potential (IPSP) A graded hyperpolarization of the postsynaptic membrane in response to neurotransmitter release from a presynaptic neuron.

Innate resistance (immunity) Protection from or resistance to infection by nonimmune mechanisms such as natural, physical, mechanical, and biochemical barriers.

Insulin Protein hormone secreted by the beta cells of the islets of Langerhans that functions in carbohydrate and fat metabolism by increasing glucose uptake into muscle and by activating adipose cells to form glycogen and fat.

Integrin An integral membrane protein that facilitates the attachment of a cell to the extracellular matrix and signal transduction from the extracellular matrix to the cell.

Interphase The interval between cell divisions during which the chromosomes facilitate RNA synthesis.

Interstitial edema Cerebral edema in which interstitial fluid accumulates in conjunction with hydrocephalus.

Interstitial fluid Fluid present in the extracellular spaces of a tissue.

Intestinointestinal reflex A process by which intestinal motility is inhibited when the intestine becomes overdistended or its mucosa becomes excessively irritated.

Intracerebral hematoma (intraparenchymal hemorrhages) Blood accumulation that partially clots inside the brain, usually in the frontal and temporal lobes.

Intrarenal acute renal failure A type of acute renal failure characterized by renal parenchymal damage that disrupts glomerular filtration and eventually destructs the glomeruli.

Intravascular fluid Plasma present in the blood.

Intrinsic factor A small protein secreted by the parietal cells of gastric glands required for adequate absorption of vitamin B_{12}.

Intron Nucleotide sequence in an RNA molecule that has no known function and is spliced from the hnRNA to form mRNA.

Intussusception An infolding or prolapse of a segment of the small intestine into the adjacent but more distal segment of the intestine.

Involucrum An area of bone that has died from lack of blood supply.

Ion Positively or negatively charged molecule.

Iron deficiency anemia (IDA) A condition caused by insufficient dietary intake or absorption of iron, resulting in decreased incorporation of hemoglobin into red blood cells and subsequent feelings of fatigue, weakness, and shortness of breath, as well as pale earlobes, palms, and conjunctivae.

Ischemia Insufficient blood flow to tissues that may result in hypoxia and subsequent cell injury or death.

Ischemic/menstrual phase These phases represent the time period when the blood supply to the endometrium diminishes, causing it to disintegrate and menstruation to occur.

Islets of Langerhans The endocrine region of the pancreas that contains four cell types: alpha cells that secrete glucagon, beta cells that secrete insulin, delta cells that secrete somatostatin, and PP cells that secrete pancreatic polypeptide.

Isolated systolic hypertension A condition caused by loss of elasticity of the arteries, resulting in an increase in cardiac output or stroke volume, a systolic blood pressure consistently above 160 mm Hg, and a diastolic pressure below 90 mm Hg.

Isometric contraction (static or holding contraction) A type of muscle contraction in which the muscle is stimulated but is not allowed to lengthen or shorten and is held at a constant length.

Isotonic contraction A type of muscle contraction in which the muscle is stimulated and shortens while lifting a constant load.

Isthmus A narrow passage connecting two larger parts of an anatomic structure.

Jaundice (icterus) A yellowish brown staining of the skin and the whites of the eyes caused by high bilirubin levels in blood secondary to excessive erythrocyte breakdown, obstruction in or around the liver, or liver disease.

Junctional complex The region of the cell membrane containing desmosomes, tight junctions, and gap junctions that holds cells together and provides a passage for cell-to-cell communication.

Juvenile rheumatoid arthritis (JRA) A condition in which children under the age of 16 develop rheumatoid arthritis and experience swelling, tenderness, and pain in one or more joints and lymph node and splenic enlargement.

Kaposi sarcoma (KS) A type of fatal cancer caused by the herpes virus in which many bluish red nodules appear on the skin, especially skin of the lower extremities; occurs in a particularly virulent form in individuals with AIDS.

Kawasaki disease A vascular disease characterized by inflamed heart and vessels, coronary artery aneurysm, thickening and stenosis, a fever that lasts at least 5 days, and at least four of the following: inflammation with reddening of the whites of the eyes; red, swollen hands or feet; peeling skin; rash; swollen lymph gland in the neck; inflamed lips, throat, or red "strawberry" tongue.

Keloid A red, raised, overgrown, fibrous scar formed by excessive cell growth during tissue repair following trauma or surgical incision.

Kernicterus A form of jaundice in the newborn caused by elevated levels of unconjugated bilirubin in the blood secondary to an increase in red blood cell number and breakdown, and by jaundice-induced lesions in the cerebral gray matter that cause neurologic disorders.

Kussmaul respiration (hyperpnea) Deep, rapid respiration commonly seen in conditions causing acidosis.

Kwashiorkor A condition in which children do not receive enough protein in their diet, resulting in a swollen and severely bloated abdomen secondary to decreased albumin in the blood, skin changes resulting in a reddish discoloration of the hair and skin in black children, severe diarrhea, fatty liver, muscle atrophy, and retarded development.

Lactase deficiency A condition in which not enough lactase is present in the small intestine to digest lactose, resulting in lactose intolerance characterized by diarrhea, bloating, and gas in response to exposure to lactose.

Lactose intolerance A condition caused by lactase deficiency in which lactose is not broken down, making it impossible for the small intestine to absorb it causing excessive gas production and diarrhea when exposed to lactose-containing foods.

Laminar flow A flow pattern for liquids that is characterized by high-speed diffusion and low turbulence.

Legg-Calvé-Perthes disease A condition in which the blood supply to the head of the femur near the hip joint is interrupted, resulting in osteonecrosis of the corresponding epiphysis.

Leiomyoma A benign smooth muscle mass that can occur in any organ but most commonly occurs in the myometrium of the uterus or in the esophagus.

Leptin A protein hormone produced by adipose tissue that provides the brain with an assessment of adipose mass and regulates appetite and metabolism by altering the actions of neuropeptide Y.

Leukemia An acute or chronic disease of the bone marrow in which excessive proliferation of white blood cells occurs and is usually accompanied by anemia, impaired blood clotting, and enlargement of the lymph nodes, liver, and spleen.

Leukocyte (white blood cell) Colorless or white cell in the blood, lymphatic system, spleen, and other body tissues that helps defend the body against infection and disease through specialized neutrophils, lymphocytes, and monocytes.

Leukocytosis An increase in the number of leukocytes in the blood as a result of fever, inflammation, hemorrhage, infection, etc.

Leukopenia A condition in which the number of white blood cells in the blood decreases, increasing the risk for infection.

Leukotriene A mediator of the prolonged inflammatory response that acts to contract smooth muscle, increase vascular permeability, and attract neutrophils.

Leydig cell A cell that is located adjacent to the seminiferous tubules in the testes and produces testosterone in response to luteinizing hormone stimulation.

Lichen planus A condition in which a recurrent rash of small, flat-topped bumps and rough scaly patches appear on the skin, in the lining of the mouth, and in the vagina in response to inflammation or an allergy to a specific medication.

Lieberkühn crypt Any of the tubular glands on the mucous surface of the small and large intestines.

Life expectancy The range of years representing the average length of life for humans.

Ligand Substance that binds to a specific cellular receptor, initiating cellular events specific to that receptor.

Linkage Genes that are transmitted, inherited, and assorted together.

Lipofuscin A yellow-brown pigment produced by the breakdown of damaged blood cells in heart and smooth muscle.

Liquefactive necrosis Liquefaction of neurons and glial cells in the brain as a result of ischemic injury or bacterial infection.

Loop of Henle A section of the nephron that extends from the proximal convoluted tubule to the distal convoluted tubule; reabsorbs water from its descending limb and salts from its ascending limb.

Loss of heterozygosity Loss of a region on one chromosome that corresponds to a mutated region on the other chromosome; loss of the same loci on both chromosomes inactivates the affected gene.

Lupus erythematosus Any of a group of autoimmune connective tissue disorders that commonly produce red, scaly lesions and are accompanied by fever, malaise, myalgias, fatigue, and weight loss.

Luteal/secretory phase These phases represent the period following ovulation during which the follicular cells are forming the corpus luteum that secretes progesterone, and the endometrium is becoming more vascularized and begins secreting a clear fluid in preparation for implantation.

Luteinizing hormone (LH) Anterior pituitary hormone released in response to gonadotropin releasing hormone that increases testosterone production in males and estrogen production in females.

Lymphocyte A nonphagocytic leukocyte of the adaptive immune response that is immunologically competent and serves as the precursor for B and T lymphocytes.

Lymphocytopenia A condition in which the number of lymphocytes in the blood decreases because of diseases and conditions, such as human immunodeficiency virus, severe stress, or the administration of corticosteroids, chemotherapy, or radiation therapy.

Lymphocytosis A condition in which the number of lymphocytes in the blood increases because of infection, inflammation, or leukemia.

Lymphoma Cancer arising from cell proliferation in lymphoid tissue.

Lysosomal storage diseases A group of more than 30 disorders that results from impaired lysosomal function, leading to mucopolysaccharidoses, lipid storage disorders, mucolipidoses, leukodystrophies, and glycoprotein storage disorders.

Macrocytic anemia (megaloblastic anemia) A condition characterized by a deficiency of vitamin B_{12} or folic acid caused by inadequate intake or insufficient absorption secondary to alcoholism or drugs that inhibit DNA replication.

Macromolecule A very large molecule, such as a protein, that consists of several smaller units.

Macrophage A phagocyte produced from a monocyte that is important in cellular initiation of the inflammatory response.

Macula densa An area of the nephron composed of closely packed cells that line the distal convoluted tubule and lie next to the glomerulus where they monitor blood salt concentration and pressure and release renin when either decreases.

Major histocompatibility complex (MHC) A set of recognition molecules used to identify whether donor and recipient tissues possess antigens that make them compatible.

Malignant hypertension A complication of hypertension in which blood pressure is severely elevated and organ damage occurs in the eyes, brain, lung, or kidneys.

Malignant tumor Cancerous mass of cells that grows, invades, and metastasizes, usually causing death.

Marasmus A childhood disorder characterized by protein and energy malnutrition, resulting in dry skin, loss of adipose tissue from normal areas of fat deposits like buttocks and thighs, and fretful, irritable behavior.

Margination (pavementing) A process by which leukocytes adhere better to endothelial cells of the capillary walls and venules by the reciprocal change in adhesion molecules on leukocytes.

Mast cell A cell of the connective tissue that produces substances that cause activation of the inflammatory response, vasoconstriction, and muscle contraction.

Maximal life span A range of years representing the average age of death for humans.

McArdle disease A metabolic disorder in which a deficiency in the enzyme, muscle phosphorylase, that helps break down glycogen causes an energy deficit in the muscles, resulting in muscle pain and cramping.

Mean arterial pressure (MAP) An average blood pressure in an individual equal to diastolic pressure plus one third of the pulse pressure that is considered the perfusion pressure of organs in the body.

Meconium A dark green fecal material that accumulates in the fetal intestines and is discharged at or near the time of birth.

Meconium ileus A condition in which the intestine of a newborn is obstructed with thickened meconium resulting from a lack of trypsin; associated with cystic fibrosis of the pancreas.

Mediated transport The transport of inorganic ions and some organic compounds across the cell membrane by way of integral membrane or transmembrane proteins that contain specific receptors.

Medulloblastoma A malignant cerebellar tumor near the fourth ventricle most often found in children that consists of neoplastic cells that resemble the undifferentiated cells of the neural tube.

Melanin A brown-black pigment synthesized by melanocytes in skin that accumulates in the skin and retina.

Memory cell A T or B lymphocyte that "remembers" a specific antigen after the initial exposure and initiates a more efficient immunologic response in subsequent exposures to the same antigen.

Meningioma A slow-growing mass of the meninges that is usually benign but increases intracranial pressure.

Meningocele A neural tube defect in the skull or spinal column that forms a cyst filled with cerebrospinal fluid through which the meninges of the brain protrude.

Menstruation The flow of blood and cells from the endometrium that occurs about every 28 days in the nonpregnant woman beginning between ages 9 to 17 and ending around age 50.

Mesodermal germ layer A tissue located between the ectoderm and endoderm that gives rise to an epithelial component of genital and urinary structures, striated muscle, connective tissue, cartilage, bone, smooth muscle, and blood cells.

Messenger RNA (mRNA) An RNA molecule produced during transcription that provides the amino acid sequence for protein synthesis.

Metabolic acidosis A decrease in pH caused by an increase in noncarbonic acids or a decrease in bicarbonate.

Metabolic alkalosis An increase in pH caused by an increase in bicarbonate ions secondary to an increase in metabolic acid loss.

Metabolic syndrome A condition of unknown cause that presents with symptoms of insulin resistance, obesity, hypertension, dyslipidemia, and systemic inflammation.

Metaphase The second phase of mitosis, during which chromosomes are condensed and aligned along the equatorial plate for nuclear and cellular division.

Microcephaly A defect in which failure of normal brain growth causes delayed skull growth and production of a small head.

Microcytic-hypochromic anemia A condition in which red blood cells are smaller than normal.

Microglia A neuroglial cell that migrates and functions as a phagocyte for nerve tissue waste products.

Miliaria A skin disease caused by partially obstructed sweat glands that results in small and itchy rashes usually located in skin folds and on areas of the body that may rub against clothing, such as the back, chest, and stomach.

Mineralocorticoid A steroid hormone secreted by the adrenal cortex that regulates the balance of water and electrolytes in the body.

Minimal change nephropathy (MCN) A condition in which the foot processes of the renal capillary basement membrane are fused and deformed because of a T cell disorder that reduces the anion component of the basement membrane and allows proteins to leak into the renal tubule.

Mitosis The process of nuclear division during which two identical nuclei are produced from one parent cell after chromosomal replication.

Mitral valve A valve in the heart that lies between the left atrium and left ventricle; allows blood to flow into the left ventricle during ventricular diastole and prevents regurgitation from the ventricle to the left atrium during systole.

Mitral valve prolapse syndrome A condition in which the mitral valve cannot close properly because of one or both flaps being too large; may result in mitral valve regurgitation.

Monocyte A phagocyte produced in bone marrow that migrates into tissues and is transformed into a macrophage.

Monocytopenia A condition in which the number of monocytes in the blood decreases because of the release of toxins into the blood by bacteria or by administration of chemotherapy or corticosteroids.

Monocytosis A condition in which the number of monocytes in the blood increases because of a chronic infection, autoimmune disorder, blood disorder, or cancer.

Mononuclear phagocyte system (MPS) A collection of free and fixed macrophages derived from bone marrow cells whose phagocytic activity is primarily mediated by immunoglobulin and by the serum complement system.

Motilin A protein hormone believed to aid in control of regular gastrointestinal muscular activity.

Motility diarrhea Increased motility, impaired food mixing, and impaired digestion secondary to resection or surgical bypass of small bowel or fistula formation.

Mucopurulent cervicitis (MPC) Inflammation of the cervix with purulent endocervical exudate that may be asymptomatic or cause abnormal vaginal discharge and vaginal bleeding.

Multiple sclerosis A chronic demyelinating disease of the central nervous system that causes inflammation and scarring of myelin sheaths.

Myasthenia gravis A neuromuscular disorder caused by an autoimmune response in which antibodies to acetylcholine receptors impair neuromuscular transmission.

Myelodysplasia An abnormal formation of the spinal cord.

Myelodysplastic syndrome A group of hematologic conditions characterized by an ineffective production of blood cells, resulting in anemia that requires chronic blood transfusion.

Myoadenylate deaminase deficiency (MDD) A genetic disorder in which an enzyme deficiency prevents the conversion of adenosine monophosphate (AMP) to inosine monophosphate, resulting in increased AMP loss and the inability to synthesize adenosine triphosphate for energy.

Myocardial infarction A heart condition of sudden onset in which muscle tissue dies because of a lack of blood flow, resulting in varying degrees of chest pain or discomfort, weakness, sweating, nausea, vomiting, and possibly loss of consciousness.

Myocardial oxygen consumption ($M\dot{V}O_2$) The amount of oxygen consumed by cardiac muscle cells during work, as determined by myocyte contraction and factors that enhance or impair this contraction, such as the rate of tension development or the number of tension generating cycles per unit time.

Myosin A protein in muscle cells arranged in long filaments called thick filaments that attaches to actin filaments in a sliding motion during muscle contraction.

Myositis A condition in which a muscle, usually a voluntary muscle, is inflamed, resulting in pain, tenderness, and sometimes spasm in the affected area.

Myositis ossificans A condition in which bone is deposited in muscle tissue, causing pain and swelling.

Myotonia A neuromuscular disorder in which muscle relaxation following voluntary contraction is delayed.

Myxedema A disease caused by impaired thyroid gland activity in adults characterized by dry skin, swelling around the lips and nose, mental deterioration, and a decrease in basal metabolic rate.

Natural killer (NK) cell A lymphocyte capable of killing target cells by binding specific receptors with or without the aid of antibodies and by releasing chemicals toxic to the targeted cells.

Necrotizing enterocolitis A condition of extensive ulceration and necrosis of the ileum and colon in premature infants during the neonatal period.

Nephroblastoma Also known as Wilms tumor, this condition is characterized by a malignant renal tumor that compresses the normal kidney parenchyma, causing abdominal mass, blood in the urine, and fever; may be associated with anorexia, vomiting, and malaise.

Nephrotic syndrome A condition in which the glomerular membrane is attacked by complement, resulting in symptoms of nephritis, hematuria, hypertension, and renal failure.

Neuroblastoma A malignant tumor containing neuroblast cells that originate in the autonomic nervous system or the adrenal medulla; is most common in infants and young children.

Neurogenic bladder The underactivity or overactivity of the bladder caused by nervous system damage that prevents the bladder muscles from contracting to empty completely or that causes rapid bladder contraction that causes too rapid or frequent emptying.

Neuroglial cell A supporting cell that forms myelin, transports material and nutrients to neurons, maintains the ionic balance of neurons, and phagocytoses nerve waste products.

Neurohormonal signaling Communication between cells that originates when a hormone is released from a neurosecretory neuron and travels through the bloodstream to bind to a target cell and elicit a response.

Neuron A nerve cell of the central nervous system that contains a nucleus within the cell body, dendrites that receive messages from other cells, and axons that transmit messages to other cells.

Neuropathic pain Pain perceived as burning, pins and needles, or electric shock that is produced by the stimulation of pain, touch, and temperature receptors of the same area.

Neurotransmitter A chemical stored in vesicles in the axon terminal that is released into the synapse in response to an action potential.

Neutropenia A decrease in the number of neutrophils in the blood.

Neutrophil (polymorphonuclear neutrophil [PMN]) A phagocyte that destroys bacteria by phagocytosis, digestion, and secretion of bacteria-killing chemicals.

Neutrophilia A condition in which the number of neutrophils—especially the younger, less mature cells in the blood—increases.

Nevi (mole) A benign growth or mark on the skin that is colored by hyperpigmentation or increased vascularity; appears early in life.

Nissl substances Structures, also known as *Nissl bodies,* located in the cell bodies of neurons that are involved in protein synthesis.

Nonbacterial prostatitis A condition in which prostatitis causes chronic pain that goes away and comes back without warning, but the prostatic fluid does not show signs of bacterial infection even though the semen and other fluids from the prostate contain immune cells that the body produces in response to infection.

Nonbacterial thrombotic endocarditis A condition in which fibrin is deposited on the valve leaflets of the heart, especially on the left side, because of cancer, rheumatic fever, or arteriosclerosis.

Noncommunicating hydrocephalus Cerebrospinal fluid accumulation within the skull caused by obstruction of the cerebrospinal fluid pathways.

Non-Hodgkin lymphoma (NHL) A condition of the lymphoid tissue that mimics Hodgkin disease but does not produce the cells characteristic of Hodgkin disease; does not have a definitive cause other than association with latent Epstein-Barr virus, AIDS, or Agent Orange exposure.

Noninflammatory acne A condition characterized by open comedones resulting from the enlargement and dilation of a plug because of accumulation of oil and skin inside the hair follicle and closed comedones that form if the hair follicle pore remains closed and appears as a tiny, sometimes pink bump in the skin.

Noninflammatory joint disease A disease in which alterations in the structure or mechanics of the joint results in pain during motion.

Nonossifying fibroma (fibrous cortical deficit) A condition found in children and adolescents in which a benign fibrous tissue tumor forms in the metaphysis of any of the long bones; but usually occurs in the thigh and shin bones.

Non-REM (slow wave) sleep A period of sleep during which dreams do not occur and brain waves are slow and high voltage.

Nonvolatile A substance that does not have a vapor form.

Normocytic-normochromic anemia (NNA) A condition in which erythrocytes are of normal size and hemoglobin content but of insufficient number; usually caused by hereditary spherocytosis, drug-induced anemia, and anemia secondary to other malignancies.

Nucleolus A small structure in the nucleus that contains the DNA of the cell and the associated binding proteins and where RNA subunits of ribosomes are assembled.

Nucleotide A DNA subunit containing one deoxyribose molecule, one phosphate group, and one nitrogenous base.

Nucleus A large membrane-bound organelle that contains the cellular DNA and is located in the center of the cell.

Nystagmus Involuntary, rapid, rhythmic movements of the eyeball in the horizontal, vertical, or rotational direction.

Obstructive sleep apnea syndrome (OSAS) Airway obstruction resulting in disruption of sleep or arousal that is accompanied by snoring.

Obstructive uropathy A condition in which the flow of urine is blocked, frequently by ureteral or kidney stones, resulting in the reflux of urine and subsequent injury to kidneys.

Oligodendroglia (oligodendrocyte) A neuroglial cell of the central nervous system that coils around the axon of the neuron to form a myelin sheath.

Oligodendroglioma A slow-growing mass of the oligodendrocytes that is usually benign.

Oncogene A tumor-causing gene that increases the rate of cell proliferation if mutated.

Oncosis Formation of a tumor or tumors or the degeneration of cells because of injury-induced inflammation.

Oncotic pressure (colloid osmotic pressure) Pressure created by large molecules, such as plasma proteins, that cannot penetrate the membrane and pulls water toward the proteins.

Onychomycosis A fungal infection of the fingernails or toenails that causes thickening, roughness, and splitting of the nails.

Opsonin A C3b fragment that attaches antigens to phagocytes, thereby tagging the antigens for destruction.

Orchitis Swelling of the testicles that can result in ejaculation of blood, blood in the urine, and pain and visible swelling of a testicle or testicles.

Oropharyngeal (voluntary) phase The phase of swallowing during which the tongue segments food and forces it toward the esophagus, the pharynx muscles constrict to prevent food from entering into the nasopharynx, respirations are inhibited, and the epiglottis slides downward to prevent food from entering the larynx and trachea.

Orthostatic (postural) hypotension A condition in which blood pressure suddenly falls when assuming a standing position, resulting in dizziness, lightheadedness, blurred vision, and temporary loss of consciousness.

Osgood-Schlatter disease A disease mainly in preadolescents and adolescents that consists of osteochondrosis of the tibia and patella tendonitis.

Osmotic diarrhea Large-volume diarrhea produced by pulling of water from cells and interstitial spaces into the intestine secondary to enzyme deficiency or excessive consumption of nonabsorbable sugars.

Osmotic pressure Pressure exerted by the membrane and solutes in a solution that must be overcome for osmosis to occur.

Osteoarthritis (OA) A type of noninflammatory joint disease in which synthesis and degradation of the articular cartilage in the movable joints is imbalanced, resulting in the wearing and destruction of cartilage.

Osteoblast The primary bone-forming cell that secretes enzymes that facilitate mineral deposition on osteoids and provides some regulation of osteoclasts.

Osteocalcin A protein found in bone tissue that has an unknown function but has high affinity for bone mineral constituents; may be involved in bone formation.

Osteochondroses Also known as Osgood-Schlatter disease, this condition in children results from the tendons pulling on the epiphysis of long bones, causing pain just below the knee, irritation and swelling, and possibly abnormal bone growth.

Osteoclast A cell found in the growing bone that degrades and reabsorbs bone.

Osteocyte An osteoblast that becomes embedded in the matrix and functions in maintaining bone tissue.

Osteogenesis imperfecta (brittle bone disease) A genetic disease in which collagen production is deficient, making the bones abnormally fragile and causing recurring fractures with minimal trauma, deformity of long bones, a bluish coloration of the sclerae, and often the development of otosclerosis.

Osteoid A protein mixture composed mainly of collagen secreted by osteoblasts and becomes mineralized to form bone.

Osteomalacia A disease in which vitamin D or calcium deficiency or excessive renal phosphate loss causes a softening of the bones with accompanying pain and weakness.

Osteomyelitis A bacterial infection of the bone and bone marrow that occurs through open fractures, penetrating wounds, surgical operations, or by entering via the bloodstream; causes pain, high fever, and formation of an abscess at the site of infection.

Osteoporosis A disease in which bone becomes porous and weakened making it easily fractured and slow to heal.

Ovarian torsion A condition in which an ovary twists or turns on its supporting ligament to the point that its blood supply is compromised.

Ovulation The release of an ovum from the ovaries around midcycle or approximately 2 weeks into the menstrual cycle.

Oxidation A chemical reaction in which electrons are lost.

Oxidative phosphorylation A process by which adenosine diphosphate (ADP) is converted into adenosine triphosphate (ATP) and inorganic phosphate through reoxidation and phosphorylation of ADP.

Oxidative stress A tissue injury induced by free radicals that are produced during metabolic reactions and with exposure to some environmental agents.

Oxyhemoglobin dissociation curve A sigmoid plot of the percentage of hemoglobin bonding sites occupied by oxygen versus the partial pressure of oxygen, which illustrates the affinity of hemoglobin for oxygen.

Oxytocin A protein hormone that is produced in the hypothalamus, stored in and released from the posterior pituitary, and acts to increase milk let-down and uterine contractions.

Paget disease (osteitis deformans) A bone disorder in which excessive bone remodeling causes enlarged, weakened, and deformed bones that can result in bone pain, arthritis, deformities, or fractures.

Pancreas An endocrine/exocrine gland that regulates blood sugar by secreting insulin and glucagon and aids in food digestion by secreting enzymes into the small intestine.

Pancreatic insufficiency A condition in which the pancreas does not secrete enough hormones and digestive enzymes for normal digestion to occur, resulting in malabsorption, malnutrition, vitamin deficiencies, and weight loss.

Pancreatitis Inflammation of the pancreas, usually resulting in abdominal pain.

Papillary muscle Any of the myocardial bundles that terminate in the chordae tendineae and attach to the cusps of the atrioventricular valves to limit the movements of the mitral and tricuspid valves and prevent them from being everted.

Papilloma A benign nodular breast lesion consisting of hyperplastic distorted ductal cells.

Paraphimosis A condition in which the foreskin becomes trapped behind the glans penis and cannot return to its normal flaccid position covering the glans penis.

Parathyroid hormone (PTH) A protein hormone, secreted by the parathyroid glands, that regulates calcium and phosphate levels in the body by promoting the absorption of calcium by the intestine, encouraging mobilization of calcium and phosphate from bones and increasing the tendency of the kidney to reabsorb calcium and excrete phosphate.

Parkinson disease Degeneration of the basal ganglia dopaminergic nigrostriatal pathway that causes hypokinesia, tremor, and muscular rigidity.

Paronychia A condition in which the tissue surrounding a fingernail or toenail is inflamed.

Partial pressure The pressure of a specific gas contained in a mixture in the atmosphere if all other components of the mixture or solution were removed without changing temperature. The partial pressure of a gas is proportional to the temperature and the concentration of the gas in a mixture.

Passive acquired immunity (passive immunity) A form of acquired immunity in which the antibody or lymphocyte is provided by a donor.

Passive mediated transport (facilitated diffusion) The carrier-mediated transport of solutes across the membrane down a concentration gradient in the absence of energy expenditure.

Passive transport Movement of water and small, uncharged particles through a membrane using osmosis, diffusion, or hydrostatic pressure as a driving force requiring no energy expenditure.

Pathogen-associated molecular pattern (PAMP) Molecular patterns on infectious agents or their products that allow recognition by specific receptors.

Pattern recognition receptor (PRR) A receptor involved in innate resistance that recognizes cellular damage or specific patterns on infectious agents.

Pedigree A chart that summarizes family relationships and shows which members are affected by a genetic disease.

Pelvic inflammatory disease (PID) Inflammation of the female genital tract because of microorganisms, typically those that are sexually transmitted, such as chlamydia and gonococci; characterized by severe abdominal pain, high fever, vaginal discharge, and possibly infertility.

Pemphigus Any of a group of autoimmune skin diseases marked by groups of itching blisters and raw sores on the skin and mucous membranes.

Pepsin One of three protein-degrading enzymes in the digestive system that becomes active in an acidic environment and breaks down proteins into their components to ease absorption by the intestinal lining.

Peptic ulcer A nonmalignant stomach or duodenal wall ulceration, commonly caused by the bacterium *Helicobacter pylori* that thrives in the acidic environment of the stomach.

Perceptual dominance The inability to feel weak painful stimulation because of the presence of a stronger painful stimulus.

Periodic paralysis One of a group of diseases in which muscular weakness or flaccid paralysis occurs without loss of consciousness, speech, or sensation.

Peripheral artery disease Any of a group of diseases that may reduce blood flow and cause ischemia by obstruction of large peripheral arteries secondary to atherosclerosis, inflammatory processes, embolism, or thrombus formation.

Peristalsis The involuntary wavelike muscular contractions of the intestine or other tubular structure that moves the contents onward by alternating contraction and relaxation.

Pernicious anemia An autoimmune disorder that causes a deficiency in intrinsic factor resulting in the inability to absorb vitamin B_{12} and a subsequent increase in the production of abnormal erythrocytes.

Peroxynitrite An oxidant and nitrating agent produced by the reaction of superoxide and nitric oxide that damages DNA, proteins, and other cellular structures.

Peyronie disease (bent nail syndrome) A condition in which fibrous plaques grow in the soft tissue of the penis because of injury of the internal cavity of the penis; accompanied by bleeding and scar tissue formation at the tunica albuginea of the corpora cavernosa.

Phagocytosis A type of endocytosis sometimes referred to as "cell eating" in which substances such as bacteria and cell particulate are incorporated into large vesicles or vacuoles and digested.

Phenotype The physical characteristics of an individual as determined by genotype and environmental influences.

Phenylketonuria (PKU) A genetic disorder in which the body lacks the enzyme necessary to metabolize the amino acid phenylalanine to tyrosine, resulting in accumulation of phenylalanine and subsequent brain damage and progressive mental retardation.

Pheochromocytoma A tumor of the adrenal medulla that causes the chromaffin cells to secrete increased amounts of epinephrine or norepinephrine.

Phimosis A condition in which the foreskin of the penis of an uncircumcised male cannot be fully retracted.

Pinocytosis A type of endocytosis sometimes referred to as "cell drinking" in which extracellular substances are incorporated into small intracellular vesicles for digestion.

Pityriasis rosea A skin disorder in which patches of ovular pink rash appear primarily on the trunk and extremities; thought to be caused by a virus.

Plasma cell A B lymphocyte that secretes antibodies in response to local cytokines released during the primary immune response.

Plasma membrane receptor A protein attached to the extracellular region of an integral membrane protein that binds to a specific ligand, such as hormones, neurotransmitters, antigens, complement components, lipoproteins, infectious agents, drugs, and metabolites.

Plasma protein systems The complement, clotting, and kinin systems that provide protection from pathogens by initiating an inflammatory response.

Plasmin A degrading enzyme associated with fibrinolysis of many proteins of blood but primarily of fibrin clots.

Platelet A cellular fragment formed from megakaryocytes that circulates in the blood and is important in anticoagulation, stimulation of inflammation and tissue growth, and destroying bacteria.

Platelet-activating factor A mast cell–derived substance that increases vascular permeability, leukocyte adhesion to endothelial cells, and platelet activation.

Pneumoconiosis A chronic disease of the lungs typically seen in miners, sandblasters, and metal grinders caused by repeated inhalation of dusts, including iron oxides, silicates, and carbonates that collect in the lungs and become sites for the formation of fibrous nodules that eventually replace lung tissue.

Pneumonia An infection of one or both lungs caused by a bacterium, virus, fungus, or other organism that enters the body through respiratory passages and causes high fever, chills, pain in the chest, difficulty in breathing, cough with sputum, and possibly bluish skin from insufficiently oxygenated blood.

Pneumothorax The collapse of a lung and escape of air into the pleural cavity between the lung and the chest wall that is caused by trauma, environmental factors, or spontaneous occurrence; results in a sudden pain in the chest.

Polarity A condition in which a molecule has a region on one side that is positively charged and another on the opposite side that is negatively charged.

Polycystic kidney disease A condition in which several fluid-filled cysts grow in the kidneys that may reduce kidney function and result in kidney failure as well as damage the liver, pancreas, and possibly the heart and brain.

Polycystic ovary syndrome (PCOS) A hormonal condition in which multiple ovarian cysts form because of elevated androgens, resulting in hirsutism, obesity, menstrual abnormalities, infertility, and enlarged ovaries.

Polycythemia A condition characterized by an increase in the production of red blood cells in the blood.

Polycythemia vera A chronic, progressive disease that is characterized by overgrowth of the bone marrow, excessive red blood cell production, and an enlarged spleen; causes headache, inability to concentrate, and pain in the fingers and toes.

Polypeptide Chain of amino acids that are linked by phosphodiester bonds.

Port-wine (nevus flammeus) stain A birthmark caused by superficial and deep dilated capillaries in the skin that produce a reddish to purplish discoloration of the skin, usually on the eyelids.

Postmortem change Diffuse physiologic changes that occur within minutes after death.

Postobstructive diuresis Elevated urine output following surgery to remove an obstruction that causes the renal tubules to be unable to reabsorb water and electrolytes normally.

Postrenal acute renal failure A condition characterized by an obstruction that affects the normal flow of urine out of both kidneys and causes pressure to build in the nephrons that eventually shuts them down.

Precocious puberty Occurs when a boy or girl undergoes the changes associated with puberty at an unexpectedly early age, often caused by a pathologic process that increases the secretion of estrogens or androgens.

Preload The volume of blood in the ventricle after atrial contraction and ventricular filling.

Premenstrual syndrome (PMS) A group of symptoms that occur in many women from 2 to 14 days before menstruation begins, such as abdominal bloating, breast tenderness, headache, fatigue, irritability, depression, and emotional distress.

Prerenal acute renal failure A condition characterized by azotemia that results from a reduction in effective arterial blood volume, which causes the kidney to behave as though renal perfusion is impaired.

Presbyopia A form of farsightedness usually accompanying advanced age in which the lens loses elasticity and becomes unable to accommodate and focus light for near vision.

Priapism A painful condition in which the erect penis maintains an erection in the absence of physical or psychologic stimulation.

Primary (neoadjuvant) chemotherapy The presurgical use of chemotherapy to decrease tumor size in cancer patients.

Primary dysmenorrhea A condition in which menstruation is painful because of a functional disturbance rather than as a result of inflammation, growths, or anatomic factors.

Primary hyperparathyroidism Usually the result of a benign parathyroid tumor that loses its sensitivity to circulating calcium levels; this condition is accompanied by hypercalcemia, nausea, vomiting, lethargy, depression, muscular weakness, and an altered mental state.

Primary hypertension A condition of elevated blood pressure of unknown etiology that is accompanied by increased total peripheral vascular resistance produced by vasoconstriction, increased cardiac output, or both.

Primary immune response The time interval between the first and second exposures to an antigen, during which antibodies against the antigen are produced.

Progesterone A steroid hormone secreted by the corpus luteum and placenta that prepares the uterus for implantation of the fertilized ovum, maintains pregnancy, and promotes development of the mammary glands in preparation for breastfeeding.

Prokaryote Organisms such as bacteria and cyanobacteria that do not have a true nucleus or membrane-bound organelles.

Prolactinoma The most common type of anterior pituitary tumor; produces visual disturbances and prolactin excess, which results in infertility and changes in menstruation in females and impotence, loss of libido, and infertility in males.

Promotor site A region of DNA where RNA polymerase begins transcription.

Prophase The initial phase of mitosis during which chromosomes are condensed and visible.

Prostacyclin A lipid produced in endothelial cells from prostaglandin H_2 by the enzyme prostacyclin synthase that functions as a vasodilator to prevent platelet formation and aggregation involved in blood clotting.

Prostaglandin A mast cell–derived substance that increases vascular permeability, muscle contraction, neutrophil chemotaxis, induces pain, and potentially inhibits some aspects of inflammation.

Protopathic The sensation of pain, heat, cold, or pressure without the ability to localize the stimulus.

Proximal tubule The initial segment of the renal tubule that drains the Bowman capsule and is the location where most salt and water is reabsorbed.

Psammoma bodies Calcium salt layers present in calcified tissues.

Psoriasis A noncontagious inflammatory skin disorder in which the skin becomes scaly and inflamed when cells in the outer layer of skin reproduce faster than normal and accumulate on the skin surface.

Pulmonary circulation A circuit in the cardiovascular system that exclusively serves the lungs in which deoxygenated blood is pumped out of the right ventricle of the heart, into the pulmonary arteries, and into the lungs; oxygenated blood is drained into the left atrium by the pulmonary veins.

Pulmonary embolism A condition in which a blood clot dislodges from its site of origin and embolizes to the arterial blood supply of one of the lungs, resulting in shortness of breath and difficulty breathing, rapid breathing that is painful, cough, and in severe cases hypotension, shock, loss of consciousness, and death.

Pulmonary fibrosis Scarring of the lungs caused by any of several conditions such as sarcoidosis, hypersensitivity pneumonitis, rheumatoid arthritis, lupus, asbestosis, and certain medications; causes shortness of breath, coughing, and diminished exercise tolerance.

Pulmonary thromboembolism A condition in which the pulmonary artery or one of its branches is obstructed by a blood clot that originated in the deep venous system.

Pulmonic stenosis A condition in which the opening into the pulmonary artery from the right ventricle narrows.

Purkinje fibers Specialized muscle fibers located in the ventricular walls of the heart that function to initiate an electrical impulse that creates coordinated contraction of the heart.

Pyelonephritis A condition in which a bacterial infection of the urinary system has extended through the urethra, bladder, and ureters, causing abdominal or back pain, fever, malaise, nausea, and vomiting.

Pyloric stenosis A congenital abnormality in which the pylorus is narrow, resulting in poor feeding, weight loss, and progressively worsening vomiting.

Rapid eye movement (REM) sleep A period of sleep during which dreams occur, autonomic activities are irregular, and brain waves are fast and of low voltage.

Raynaud disease A condition in which the blood vessels spasm, which results in inadequate blood supply and discoloration of the fingers or the toes, after exposure to changes in temperature or emotional events.

Reactive response The secretion of stress hormones in response to a psychologic stressor.

Recessive An allele that has its effects masked by the effects of a dominant allele.

Recombination A physical exchange of genetic information between homologous chromosomes that results in the creation of new genotypes.

Rectocele A condition caused by childbirth or hysterectomy in which the region between the rectum and vagina bulges toward the vagina, resulting in a sense of pressure or protrusion within the vagina, the feeling of incomplete emptying of the rectum, difficulty passing stool, discomfort or pain during evacuation or intercourse, constipation, vaginal bleeding, fecal incontinence, the prolapse of the bulge through the opening of the vagina, or rectal prolapse through the anus.

Reflex arc A neural pathway that contains a receptor, an afferent nerve fiber, an efferent nerve fiber, an effector, and possibly one or more interneurons; involved in stereotyped, automatic, involuntary response to a stimulus.

Reflux esophagitis The most common form of gastroesophageal reflux disease, it is characterized by reflux damage to the esophagus that presents as recurrent heartburn.

Relative polycythemia A relative increase in the number of red blood cells resulting from a loss of the fluid portion of the blood.

Relative refractory period The time interval during an action potential when potassium permeability increases and repolarization, occurs but stronger-than-normal stimuli can produce an additional action potential.

Remodeling A process in which bone is resorbed then replaced without changing shape in order to release calcium and repair mildly damaged bones.

Renal adenoma A benign tumor originating in the renal tubules of the cortex that is similar in appearance to a renal cell carcinoma.

Renal agenesis A condition in which only one functional kidney is present at birth.

Renal cell carcinoma (RCC) A malignancy arising from the renal tubule that produces hematuria, flank pain, and an abdominal mass.

Renal colic A condition in which a tiny stone passing through the ureter produces intermittent but severe abdominal pain that begins in the side or upper abdomen and travels down to the lower abdomen and possibly radiating into the pubic region or into the penis or testis in men.

Renal dysplasia A condition in which tissue development in one or both kidneys is abnormal.

Renin An enzyme secreted by the juxtaglomerular cells of the kidney that is released in response to decreased blood pressure in the kidney and sympathetic nerve stimulation.

Renin-angiotensin system A mechanism by which sodium and water levels are regulated in the body, including the release of renin, conversion of angiotensinogen into angiotensin I, conversion of angiotensin I into angiotensin II, and the release of aldosterone and its actions on the kidney that increase water and sodium reabsorption.

Reperfusion (reoxygenation) injury Tissue injury resulting from the restoration of oxygen after an interval of hypoxia or anoxia.

Repolarization The reestablishment of the resting membrane potential by the closing of sodium channels, the opening of potassium channels, and the subsequent efflux of potassium.

Respiratory acidosis A decrease in pH caused by elevated carbon dioxide (hypercapnia) secondary to depressed ventilation.

Respiratory alkalosis An increase in pH caused by alveolar hyperventilation and reduced carbon dioxide (hypocapnia).

Respiratory distress syndrome (RDS) of the newborn Also known as hyaline membrane disease (HMD), this condition is a type of respiratory distress in newborns, most often in prematurely born infants, those born by cesarean section, or those who have a diabetic mother; the immature lungs do not produce enough surfactant to retain air so the air spaces empty completely and collapse after exhalation.

Resting membrane potential The difference in electrical charge across the membrane of an unstimulated cell that is accomplished by the unequal distribution of charged ions.

Retching Deep inspiration followed by esophageal distention, abdominal muscle contraction, duodenum and antrum spasm, and reverse peristalsis that propels chyme into the esophagus.

Retina A layer of the wall of the eye that contains the photoreceptors (rods and cones).

Retinoblastoma An autosomal dominant disorder in which a malignant tumor forms in the retina of one or both eyes; typically found in infants.

Retropulsion An involuntary backward movement of a substance or an organ.

Reye syndrome A type of encephalopathy that occurs primarily in children after a viral infection, such as chickenpox or influenza, and is characterized by fever, vomiting, fatty liver, disorientation, and coma.

Rhabdomyolysis A potentially fatal condition in which skeletal muscle breaks down because of injury such as physical damage to the muscle, high fever, metabolic disorders, excessive exertion, convulsions, or anoxia of the muscle for several hours; large amounts of myoglobin are usually excreted.

Rheumatic fever An inflammatory disease associated with a recent streptococcal infection that causes inflammation of the joints, fever, chorea (jerky movements), nodules under the skin, and skin rash. It is frequently followed by rheumatic heart disease and serious heart damage.

Rheumatoid arthritis An autoimmune disease that causes chronic inflammation of the joints and the tissue around the joints and other organs.

Ribonucleic acid (RNA) Nucleic acid composed of sugar, phosphate, and nitrogenous bases that is important in gene expression.

Ribosomal RNA (rRNA) RNA that complexes with proteins to form ribosomes.

Ribosome RNA-protein complex that is synthesized in the nucleolus, transported into the cytoplasm, and then floats in the cytoplasm or attaches to the endoplasmic reticulum to provide sites for cellular protein synthesis.

Right heart failure A condition in which the right side of the heart loses its ability to pump blood efficiently because of left-sided heart failure, lung disease, congenital heart disease, clots in pulmonary arteries, pulmonary hypertension, or heart valve disease.

RNA polymerase An enzyme that adds nucleotides to a growing RNA strand.

Roseola A viral disease in infants and young children that causes fever and a spotty rash that appears shortly after the fever has subsided.

Rotavirus A viral infection seen in young children that causes diarrhea by attacking the lining of the small intestine, resulting in the inability to absorb fluid and electrolytes and their subsequent loss.

Rubella An infectious viral disease of children and young adults spread by a droplet spray from the respiratory tract of an infected individual that causes a rash (which lasts about 3 days) and tender and swollen lymph nodes behind the ears.

Rubeola Also known as measles, this is an infectious viral disease of young children spread by a droplet spray from the nose, mouth, and throat of individuals in the infective stage; causes white spots in the mouth, a rash on the face that spreads to the rest of the body, and fever.

Saccular aneurysm (berry aneurysm) A localized, progressively growing sac that affects only a portion of the circumference of the arterial wall and may be the result of congenital anomalies or degeneration.

Salmon patches Also known as stork bites, these small, pink, flat spots are small blood vessels that are visible through the skin; usually found on the forehead, eyelids, upper lip, between the eyebrows, and the back of the neck.

Salpingitis Inflammation of one of the two fallopian tubes because of infection spreading from the vagina or uterus.

Saltatory conduction The rapid propagation of an impulse from one node of Ranvier to another in myelinated axons.

Sarcoma A tumor of the connective tissue cells.

Sarcopenia A condition in which muscle mass and strength is lost because of advanced age and decreased activity, resulting in impaired sense of balance.

Sclerosing adenosis A condition in which the number of acini per terminal duct is more than twice the number of normal terminal ducts; associated with a significantly increased risk of subsequent breast carcinoma.

Scoliosis A condition in which the spine is curved laterally to varying degrees.

Sebaceous gland A gland in the skin that secretes the oily substance called sebum; primarily located within the hair follicle but may also occur in hairless areas of the skin, except for the palms of the hand and soles of the feet.

Seborrheic dermatitis A condition in which the skin of the scalp, face, and trunk become scaly, flaky, itchy, and red, possibly because of a yeast infection.

Secondary (anamnestic) immune response The production of great amounts of antibodies in response to the second exposure to an antigen.

Secondary amenorrhea A condition in which menstruation begins at puberty but then is subsequently suppressed for three or more cycles or 6 months in women who previously menstruated.

Secondary dysmenorrhea A condition in which menstruation is altered as result of inflammation, infection, tumor, or anatomic factors.

Secondary hyperparathyroidism A condition of elevated parathyroid hormone resulting from disease, such as renal failure, in which parathyroid hormone is elevated in response to vitamin D deficiency.

Secondary hypertension A condition of elevated blood pressure that is associated primarily with renal disease by a renin-dependent mechanism or a fluid volume-dependent mechanism.

Secretin A protein hormone produced in the S cells of the duodenum in response to low pH and fatty acids that stimulates the secretion of bicarbonate and inhibits stomach acid secretion, which helps neutralize the gastric acid entering the duodenum from the stomach.

Secretory diarrhea Large-volume diarrhea caused by bacteria-induced excessive mucosal secretions of fluid and electrolytes.

Seizure A transient event of excessive, disorderly neurologic activity that results in disturbances of motor, sensory, and autonomic function and alters behavior and the state of consciousness.

Semicircular canals Three tubular structures of the inner ear that together maintain the body's sense of balance.

Semilunar valve One of three crescent-shaped cusps of a valve that prevents regurgitation of blood into the ventricles.

Seminiferous tubules One of multiple curved tubules in the testis where spermatozoa develop.

Sentinel nodes Lymph nodes that are the first to receive drainage and are the first targets during cancer metastasis.

Sequestration crisis A condition in which the cardiovascular system collapses causing blood to pool in the spleen and liver.

Sertoli cell (nondividing cell) Elongated, striated cells in the seminiferous tubules that join to form the blood-testis barrier, which controls the entry and exit of nutrients, hormones, and other chemicals into and out of the seminiferous tubules and provides a site for spermatid attachment during spermatogenesis.

Serum sickness A form of hypersensitivity caused by injection of soluble antigen, such as antiserum, that results in complement activation.

Shift-to-the-left (Leukemoid reaction) A form of leukocytosis that is similar to or mimics leukocytosis occurring in leukemia but results from some other cause.

Sialoprotein (osteopontin) A glycoprotein that may play a role in maintaining or reconfiguring tissues during the inflammatory process; required for stress-induced bone remodeling and cell-mediated immunity.

Sickle cell anemia An inherited disorder of the blood caused by abnormal hemoglobin that distorts red blood cells and makes them fragile and prone to rupture. When an excessive number of red blood cells rupture, anemia occurs, as well as pain in the joints, fever, leg ulcers, and jaundice.

Sickle cell trait An inherited condition in which an individual carries only one gene for sickle cell disease and is without symptoms.

Sideroblastic anemia (SA) A refractory anemia of varying severity caused by altered mitochondrial metabolism that is marked by sideroblasts in the bone marrow.

Signal transduction The transmission of signals from an extracellular chemical to the intracellular region where cellular activity is affected. Signal transduction occurs when environmental stimuli are translated into electrical signals in the body, as well as when a signal is transmitted between extracellular and intracellular domains.

Silencing A gene mutation that does not change the gene product.

Sinoatrial node (SA node, sinus node) A group of specialized cells located on the wall of the right atrium near the entrance of the superior vena cava; these cells set the heart rate by spontaneously depolarizing and exciting surrounding tissues.

Sliding filament theory A model of muscle contraction in which the myofibrils shorten when the myosin and actin attach and form cross-bridges.

Smallpox (variola) An infectious viral disease caused by a poxvirus that results in high fever and aches, as well as the widespread eruption of large sores that leave scars.

Somatic cell All cells other than sperm and eggs (gamete cells).

Specificity theory A proposal that pain activates specific receptors and fibers that project to the brain and that the intensity of pain is proportional to the area of tissue damage and number of receptors and fibers stimulated.

Spermatocele A cyst of the rete testis or the head of the epididymis distended with a milky fluid that contains spermatozoa.

Spina bifida A congenital defect in which the spinal column is not closed correctly causing protrusion of that part of the meninges or spinal cord.

Spinal stenosis The narrowing of the spinal canal as a result of congenital anomaly or spinal degeneration, resulting in pain, paresthesias, and neurogenic claudication.

Spindle A specialized structure in the muscle innervated by both sensory and motor neurons and sends information about muscle stretch to the central nervous system.

Spongy bone (cancellous bone) A trabecular bone that makes up a small portion of the skeleton but has a high surface area.

Stable angina A condition in which ischemic attacks occur at predictable frequencies and duration following activities that increase myocardial oxygen demands, such as exercise and stress.

Staphylococcal scalded-skin syndrome (SSSS) A disease in infants caused by an upper respiratory staphylococcal infection that results in large regions of skin to peel.

Stasis dermatitis A condition in which the skin appears brown and ulcerates because of blood pooling in the leg secondary to insufficient venous return.

Stevens-Johnson syndrome An inflammatory eruption of circular lesions that can cover the majority of the skin and mucous membranes; usually occurs following a respiratory infection or as an allergic reaction to drugs or other substances.

Strangulation Cerebral hypoxia or anoxia caused by compression and closure of the blood vessels and air passages by applying external pressure on the neck.

Strawberry hemangioma A birthmark caused by densely packed blood vessels that is red in color, and usually appears on the face, scalp, back, and chest.

Stress ulcer An acute peptic ulcer occurring in association with various other pathologic conditions, including burns, cor pulmonale, intracranial lesions, and surgical operations.

Stressor Stimuli that when exposed to the human body cause a physiologic response characterized by sympathetic nervous system activity and the release of hypothalamic, pituitary, and adrenal hormones.

Struvite stone Also called an infection stone, this urinary stone develops when a urinary tract infection neutralizes the urine, enabling the bacteria to grow more rapidly and a jagged ammoniomagnesium phosphate stone to develop.

Subdural hematoma A collection of blood between the inner surface of the dura mater and the surface of the brain caused by rupture of bridging veins of the subdural region.

Sudden infant death syndrome (SIDS) Also known as crib death, this syndrome is characterized by the sudden, unexpected, and unexplained death of an apparently healthy infant under 1 year of age.

Suffocation The failure of oxygen to reach the blood because of a lack of oxygen in the environment or the blockage of external airways.

Surface tension The force exerted along the surface of a fluid that maintains its structural integrity and causes it to form into drops when placed on a surface with which it does not mix.

Symphysis A cartilaginous joint in which two bones are joined by fibrocartilage without a synovial membrane.

Synaptic bouton A button-like swelling on the axon terminal where neurotransmitter vesicles are stored.

Synchondrosis A rigid union between two bones formed by hyaline cartilage or fibrocartilage that creates an articulation in which the bones are rigidly fused by cartilage.

Syndesmosis A fibrous joint in which opposing surfaces are united by ligaments.

Syndrome of inappropriate secretion of ADH (SIADH) A condition in which the release of ADH is elevated relative to sodium levels, resulting in increased water reabsorption in the kidneys.

Synovial joint (diarthroses) A joint in which the opposing bone surfaces are covered with hyaline cartilage or fibrocartilage and there is some degree of free movement.

Systemic circulation A circuit in the cardiovascular system in which blood circulates from the left ventricle to the organs and tissues then travels through the systemic veins to the right atrium.

Systole The period of time when the chambers of the heart contract and force blood out of the chambers.

Systolic heart failure A condition in which the heart muscle contracts weakly so that there is not enough oxygenated blood being pumped throughout the body.

Tamponade The blockage or compression of a body part, such as heart compression because of a collection of blood or fluid.

Tay-Sachs disease An autosomal recessive disorder in which an enzyme deficiency leads to the accumulation of gangliosides in the brain and nerve tissue, resulting in mental retardation, convulsions, blindness, and premature death.

Telomere The ends of a chromosome that are shortened during each cycle of DNA replication; this shortening of the telomere is believed to be a component of cellular aging because it deletes vital genetic information over time.

Telophase The final phase of mitosis during which a new nuclear membrane is formed around each group of 46 chromosomes, spindle fibers disappear, and the chromosomes begin to uncoil; the process results in two identical daughter cells.

Tetralogy of Fallot A congenital condition that is characterized by four malformations including ventricular septal defect, misplacement of the origin of the aorta, narrowing of the pulmonary artery, and enlargement of the right ventricle.

Thalassemia A potentially fatal genetic disorder in which hemoglobin molecules are abnormal, resulting in severe anemia; enlarged heart, liver, and spleen; and skeletal deformation.

Theca cell A cell in the ovarian follicle that converts cholesterol into androgens, which enter the granulosa cells where they are converted to estrogen.

Therapeutic index A ratio of the median lethal dose to the median effective dose for a drug.

Threshold potential The membrane potential that must be reached in order for an action potential to be generated and the impulse to be propagated to another cell.

Thromboangiitis obliterans (Buerger disease) A condition in which the medium-sized arteries and veins are inflamed because of thrombotic occlusion, resulting in ischemia and gangrene.

Thrombocythemia A condition in which the number of platelets in the blood increases, resulting in clot formation.

Thrombocytopenia A condition in which the number of platelets in the blood is severely decreased.

Thrombotic stroke (cerebral thrombosis) Stroke symptoms caused by thrombosis; typically secondary to atherosclerosis.

Thrombotic thrombocytopenic purpura (TTP) A disorder of blood coagulation caused by an enzymatic deficiency that is characterized by a reduced number of platelets in the blood, the formation of blood clots in tissue arterioles and capillaries, and neurologic damage.

Thromboxane (TXA_2) A lipid that is produced in platelets by thromboxane synthetase, acts as a vasoconstrictor, and facilitates the aggregation of platelets.

Thrombus A fibrinous blood clot formed in a vessel or in a chamber of the heart that remains attached at its site of origin.

Thrush A yeast infection of the mouth and throat that presents as creamy white, curdlike patches on the tongue, inside the mouth, and on the back of the throat; commonly associated with yeast infection of the esophagus.

Thyroid gland A two-lobed endocrine gland located in front of and on either side of the trachea that produces various hormones (such as triiodothyronine, thyroxine, and calcitonin) responsible for metabolism and calcium levels.

Thyroid hormones (THs) Tyrosine-derived protein hormones thyroxine and triiodothyronine that are produced by the thyroid gland, increase the basal metabolic rate, and affect protein synthesis.

Thyrotoxicosis A condition resulting from excessive concentrations of thyroid hormones in the body that is marked by increased metabolic rate, heat intolerance, goiter, reproductive disorders, excessive sweating, and other alterations in systemic function.

Tight junction An impermeable junction between neighboring cells that prevents leakage of small molecules between the cells and requires that molecules pass through the cell to get from one cell to another.

Tinea capitis A fungal infection of the scalp that causes patches of baldness, scaling, black dots, and possibly erythema and pyoderma.

Tinea corporis Also known as ringworm, this condition is a fungal infection caused by Trichophyton or Microsporum that results in a pink to red rash and itching of the areas of the skin not covered by hair.

Tinea infection One of a group of fungal skin infections that include athlete's foot, folliculitis, jock itch, ringworm, and pityriasis versicolor.

T lymphocyte (T cell) A cell of the adaptive immune response that originates in the bone marrow, matures in the thymus, and provides cell-mediated immunity.

Toll-like receptor (TLR) A receptor expressed on the surface of many cells that interacts with many pathogens to increase resistance and bridges innate resistance and acquired immune response through cytokine production.

Toxic epidermal necrolysis A condition in which a large portion of the skin becomes intensely red, peels off, and blisters.

Trabeculae Strands of connective tissue that project into an organ and provide part of the framework of that organ and mechanical strength and stiffness.

Tracheoesophageal fistula (TEF) A condition in which a connection is formed between the esophagus and the trachea because of esophageal atresia or laryngostomy.

Transfer RNA (tRNA) An RNA molecule that directs a specific amino acid to a codon on an mRNA strand during polypeptide synthesis.

Transferrin A protein loaded with iron that transports iron into the cell by binding a transferrin surface receptor and entering the cell where it releases iron ions.

Translation A process by which genetic information in an mRNA molecule is used to determine specific amino acids for a newly synthesized polypeptide.

Transport maximum (T_m) The maximal rate of secretion or reabsorption of a substance by the renal tubules as determined by the level of transporter saturation.

Transposition of the great arteries (TGA) A condition in which the aorta arises from the right ventricle and the pulmonary artery arises from the left ventricle.

Tricuspid valve A three-segmented valve of the heart that prevents regurgitation of blood from the right ventricle into the right atrium.

Troponin C A protein complex that provides calcium-binding sites to muscle cells.

Truncus arteriosus A congenital defect in which a large great vessel arises from a ventricular septal defect and does not divide into the aorta and pulmonary artery, resulting in one vessel carrying blood both to the body and to the lungs.

Tuberculosis (TB) An infectious disease of humans caused by tubercle bacillus that results in the formation of tubercles on the lungs and other tissues of the body.

Tubular secretion The movement of a substance into the renal tubule from the peritubular capillaries, mainly by active transport.

Tumor A growth of tissue caused by the uncontrolled replication of cells.

Tumor marker A biochemical marker sensitive to specific types of tumors that is used to screen, diagnose, assess prognosis and treatment, and monitor recurrence.

Tumor-suppressor gene A gene whose protein product terminates cell proliferation, thereby inhibiting tumor formation.

Turbulent flow A flow pattern for liquids that is characterized by low-speed diffusion and high turbulence as a result of obstruction.

Type 1 diabetes mellitus A disorder of carbohydrate metabolism characterized by a decrease in insulin production, resulting in hyperglycemia and eventually renal failure and coronary artery disease.

Type 2 diabetes mellitus A condition of glucose intolerance that normally appears first in adulthood and is exacerbated by obesity and an inactive lifestyle.

Type I fibers Slow twitch fibers that are used primarily during aerobic metabolism and function during activities that require high endurance.

Type II fibers Fast twitch fibers that are used primarily during anaerobic metabolism and function during activities that require low endurance when short bursts of strength are required.

Ulcerative colitis A condition in which the mucosal and submucosal lining of the large intestine is chronically inflamed and ulcerated, resulting in abdominal pain, diarrhea, and rectal bleeding.

Ultrafiltration The process of filtering blood across a barrier between the capillary of the glomerulus and the Bowman capsule of the nephron at a rate that is determined by hydrostatic and oncotic pressures.

Unstable angina A condition in which unprovoked ischemic attacks occur at unpredictable frequencies and may increase in severity, causing chest pain that is not relieved by rest.

Up-regulation The process by which a cell increases the number of receptors for a given hormone or neurotransmitter to improve sensitivity in response to low hormone concentration.

Urethritis Inflammation of the urethra usually caused by a sexually transmitted microorganism that results in painful urination.

Uric acid stone A condition in which uric acid levels in urine are elevated, preventing the uric acid from dissolving and causing uric acid stones to form.

Urinary tract infection An infection of the urinary tract that may occur anywhere from the kidneys to the urethra; much more common in females because of a decreased distance between the urethra and the anus.

Urobilinogen A product of bilirubin breakdown that is oxidized into urobilin and excreted in feces or reabsorbed.

Urticaria (hives) An allergic reaction in which capillaries become dilated and permeability increases, causing localized edema.

Uterine prolapse The descent or herniation of the uterus into or beyond the vagina because of weakness of the pelvic musculature, ligaments, and fascia or obstetrical trauma and lacerations sustained during labor and delivery.

Vaccine A suspension of attenuated or dead microorganisms or antigenic proteins from microorganisms that are injected into a person to provide immunity.

Vacuolar myelopathy HIV-induced loss of myelin and spongy degeneration of the spinal cord that may cause spastic paraparesis, sensory ataxia in lower limbs, and unsteady gait.

Vaginismus A form of sexual dysfunction caused by a psychologic disorder or vaginal inflammation in which the muscles at the entrance to the vagina contract and prevent sexual intercourse.

Vaginitis An infection of the vagina usually caused by a fungus that may cause itching or burning and a discharge.

Valvular regurgitation A condition in which one or more of the heart's valves does not close properly, producing a backflow of blood.

Valvular stenosis A condition in which one of more of the heart valves becomes narrow, stiff, thickened, fused, or blocked, and blood does not flow through it smoothly.

Varicocele A painful condition in which the veins in the scrotum that develop in the spermatic cord enlarge; if the valves that regulate blood flow from these veins become dysfunctional, blood does not leave the testis, causing swelling in the veins above and behind the testis.

Vasogenic edema An accumulation of fluid in the cerebrum that is typically caused by an increase in capillary endothelial cell permeability and usually occurs near a tumor.

Vasomotor flush A sudden, brief sensation of heat, typically occurring over the entire body, that is caused by a transient dilation of the blood vessels of the skin and possibly alterations in the temperature-regulating center of the hypothalamus secondary to decreased estrogen levels.

Vaso-occlusive crisis (thrombotic crisis) A condition that occurs when the microcirculation is obstructed by sickled red blood cells, resulting in ischemic injury to the organ supplied pain, and possibly irreversible organ damage.

Venous stasis ulcer A condition affecting the lower leg in which leaky valves, obstructions, or regurgitation in veins impairs blood flow back to heart, resulting in pooling of blood in the lower leg and subsequent tissue damage.

Ventilation-perfusion ratio ($\dot{V}/\dot{Q}$) The relationship between ventilation and blood flow in the lung that is measured by calculating the difference between the alveolar and arterial partial pressures of oxygen.

Ventricular septal defect (VSD) A congenital malformation in which the wall between the left and right ventricles has a hole that allows blood to travel between the left and right ventricles, potentially leading to congestive heart failure.

Vesicoureteral reflux (VUR) The reflux of urine from the bladder into the ureter.

Viral hepatitis A liver disease caused by one of several viral strains that may be acute or chronic, transmitted by blood, feces, and, for some strains, sexual contact; when chronic, may cause cirrhosis or liver cancer.

Volatile A substance such as carbonic acid that can evaporate rapidly.

Volkmann ischemic contracture A condition in which the distal humerus is fractured and disrupts the radial artery and median nerve, resulting in necrosis of the extensor muscles, contracture of elbow flexion, and a claw hand.

Wart An outgrowth of the skin caused by a virus easily transmitted by close contact that may persist for years.

Wheal and flare reaction A condition caused by an allergic reaction in which the area of skin around the site of antigen contact becomes flattened and red with fluid-filled blisters.

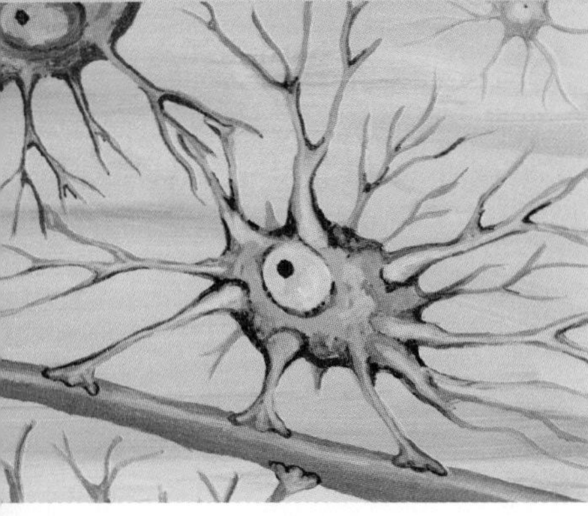

INDEX

A

Page numbers followed by f, t, or b indicate figures, tables, or boxes, respectively. Syndromes and disorders appear in **boldface**.

B

C

D

F

G

H

J

M

N

O

Q

R

T

U

V

W

X

Y

Z